THE BIOMEDICAL ENGINEERING HANDBOOK

FOURTH EDITION

Biomedical Signals, Imaging, and Informatics

THE BIOMEDICAL ENGINEERING HANDBOOK
FOURTH EDITION

Biomedical Signals, Imaging, and Informatics

Edited by

Joseph D. Bronzino
Founder and President
Biomedical Engineering Alliance and Consortium (BEACON)
Hartford, Connecticut, U.S.A.

Donald R. Peterson
Professor of Engineering
Dean of the College of Science, Technology, Engineering, Mathematics, and Nursing
Texas A&M University – Texarkana
Texarkana, Texas, U.S.A.

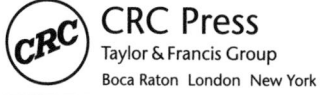

CRC Press
Taylor & Francis Group
Boca Raton London New York

CRC Press is an imprint of the
Taylor & Francis Group, an **informa** business

MATLAB® is a trademark of The MathWorks, Inc. and is used with permission. The MathWorks does not warrant the accuracy of the text or exercises in this book. This book's use or discussion of MATLAB® software or related products does not constitute endorsement or sponsorship by The MathWorks of a particular pedagogical approach or particular use of the MATLAB® software.

CRC Press
Taylor & Francis Group
6000 Broken Sound Parkway NW, Suite 300
Boca Raton, FL 33487-2742

© 2015 by Taylor & Francis Group, LLC
CRC Press is an imprint of Taylor & Francis Group, an Informa business

No claim to original U.S. Government works

Printed on acid-free paper
Version Date: 20141017

International Standard Book Number-13: 978-1-4398-2527-3 (Hardback)

Library of Congress Cataloging-in-Publication Data

Biomedical signals, imaging, and informatics / edited by Joseph D. Bronzino and Donald R. Peterson.
   p. ; cm.
   Preceded by The biomedical engineering handbook / edited by Joseph D. Bronzino. 3rd. 2006.
   Includes bibliographical references and index.
   ISBN 978-1-4398-2527-3 (hardcover : alk. paper)
   I. Bronzino, Joseph D., 1937- , editor. II. Peterson, Donald R., editor.
   [DNLM: 1. Diagnostic Imaging. 2. Signal Processing, Computer-Assisted. 3. Medical Informatics. WN 180]

   R856
   610.28--dc23
   2014035625

Visit the Taylor & Francis Web site at
http://www.taylorandfrancis.com

and the CRC Press Web site at
http://www.crcpress.com

Contents

SECTION III   Infrared Imaging

Mary Diakides

SECTION IV   Medical Informatics

Luis G. Kun

Preface

During the past eight years since the publication of the third edition—a three-volume set—of *The Biomedical Engineering Handbook*, the field of biomedical engineering has continued to evolve and expand. As a result, the fourth edition has been significantly modified to reflect state-of-the-field knowledge and applications in this important discipline and has been enlarged to a four-volume set:

- Volume I: *Biomedical Engineering Fundamentals*
- Volume II: *Medical Devices and Human Engineering*
- Volume III: *Biomedical Signals, Imaging, and Informatics*
- Volume IV: *Molecular, Cellular, and Tissue Engineering*

More specifically, this fourth edition has been considerably updated and contains completely new sections, including

- Stem Cell Engineering
- Drug Design, Delivery Systems, and Devices
- Personalized Medicine

as well as a number of substantially updated sections, including

- Tissue Engineering (which has been completely restructured)
- Transport Phenomena and Biomimetic Systems
- Artificial Organs
- Medical Imaging
- Infrared Imaging
- Medical Informatics

In addition, Volume IV contains a chapter on Ethics because of its ever-increasing role in the Biomedical Engineering arts.

Nearly all the sections that have appeared in the first three editions have been significantly revised. Therefore, this fourth edition presents an excellent summary of the status of knowledge and activities of biomedical engineers in the first decades of the twenty-first century. As such, it can serve as an excellent reference for individuals interested not only in a review of fundamental physiology but also in quickly being brought up to speed in certain areas of biomedical engineering research. It can serve as an excellent textbook for students in areas where traditional textbooks have not yet been developed and as an excellent review of the major areas of activity in each biomedical engineering sub-discipline, such as biomechanics, biomaterials, bioinstrumentation, medical imaging, and so on. Finally, it can serve as the "bible" for practicing biomedical engineering professionals by covering such topics as historical perspective of medical technology, the role of professional societies, the ethical issues associated with medical technology, and the FDA process.

Biomedical engineering is now an important and vital interdisciplinary field. Biomedical engineers are involved in virtually all aspects of developing new medical technology. They are involved in the design, development, and utilization of materials, devices (such as pacemakers, lithotripsy, etc.), and techniques (such as signal processing, artificial intelligence, etc.) for clinical research and use, and they serve as members of the healthcare delivery team (clinical engineering, medical informatics, rehabilitation engineering, etc.) seeking new solutions for the difficult healthcare problems confronting our society. To meet the needs of this diverse body of biomedical engineers, this handbook provides a central core of knowledge in those fields encompassed by the discipline. However, before presenting this detailed information, it is important to provide a sense of the evolution of the modern healthcare system and identify the diverse activities biomedical engineers perform to assist in the diagnosis and treatment of patients.

Evolution of the Modern Healthcare System

Before 1900, medicine had little to offer average citizens, since its resources consisted mainly of physicians, their education, and their "little black bag." In general, physicians seemed to be in short supply, but the shortage had rather different causes than the current crisis in the availability of healthcare professionals. Although the costs of obtaining medical training were relatively low, the demand for doctors' services also was very small, since many of the services provided by physicians also could be obtained from experienced amateurs in the community. The home was typically the site for treatment and recuperation, and relatives and neighbors constituted an able and willing nursing staff. Babies were delivered by midwives, and those illnesses not cured by home remedies were left to run their natural, albeit frequently fatal, course. The contrast with contemporary healthcare practices in which specialized physicians and nurses located within hospitals provide critical diagnostic and treatment services is dramatic.

The changes that have occurred within medical science originated in the rapid developments that took place in the applied sciences (i.e., chemistry, physics, engineering, microbiology, physiology, pharmacology, etc.) at the turn of the twentieth century. This process of development was characterized by intense interdisciplinary cross-fertilization, which provided an environment in which medical research was able to take giant strides in developing techniques for the diagnosis and treatment of diseases. For example, in 1903, Willem Einthoven, a Dutch physiologist, devised the first electrocardiograph to measure the electrical activity of the heart. In applying discoveries in the physical sciences to the analysis of the biological process, he initiated a new age in both cardiovascular medicine and electrical measurement techniques.

New discoveries in medical sciences followed one another like intermediates in a chain reaction. However, the most significant innovation for clinical medicine was the development of x-rays. These "new kinds of rays," as W. K. Roentgen described them in 1895, opened the "inner man" to medical inspection. Initially, x-rays were used to diagnose bone fractures and dislocations, and in the process, x-ray machines became commonplace in most urban hospitals. Separate departments of radiology were established, and their influence spread to other departments throughout the hospital. By the 1930s, x-ray visualization of practically all organ systems of the body had been made possible through the use of barium salts and a wide variety of radiopaque materials.

X-ray technology gave physicians a powerful tool that, for the first time, permitted accurate diagnosis of a wide variety of diseases and injuries. Moreover, since x-ray machines were too cumbersome and expensive for local doctors and clinics, they had to be placed in healthcare centers or hospitals. Once there, x-ray technology essentially triggered the transformation of the hospital from a passive receptacle for the sick to an active curative institution for all members of society.

For economic reasons, the centralization of healthcare services became essential because of many other important technological innovations appearing on the medical scene. However, hospitals remained institutions to dread, and it was not until the introduction of sulfanilamide in the mid-1930s and penicillin in the early 1940s that the main danger of hospitalization, that is, cross-infection among patients, was significantly reduced. With these new drugs in their arsenals, surgeons were able to perform their operations without prohibitive morbidity and mortality due to infection. Furthermore, even though the different blood groups and their incompatibility were discovered in 1900 and sodium citrate was used in 1913 to prevent clotting, full development of blood banks was not practical until the 1930s, when technology provided adequate refrigeration. Until that time, "fresh" donors were bled and the blood transfused while it was still warm.

Once these surgical suites were established, the employment of specifically designed pieces of medical technology assisted in further advancing the development of complex surgical procedures. For example, the Drinker respirator was introduced in 1927 and the first heart–lung bypass in 1939. By the 1940s, medical procedures heavily dependent on medical technology, such as cardiac catheterization and angiography (the use of a cannula threaded through an arm vein and into the heart with the injection of radiopaque dye) for the x-ray visualization of congenital and acquired heart disease (mainly valve disorders due to rheumatic fever) became possible, and a new era of cardiac and vascular surgery was established.

In the decades following World War II, technological advances were spurred on by efforts to develop superior weapon systems and to establish habitats in space and on the ocean floor. As a by-product of these efforts, the development of medical devices accelerated and the medical profession benefited greatly from this rapid surge of technological finds. Consider the following examples:

1. Advances in solid-state electronics made it possible to map the subtle behavior of the fundamental unit of the central nervous system—the neuron—as well as to monitor the various physiological parameters, such as the electrocardiogram, of patients in intensive care units.
2. New prosthetic devices became a goal of engineers involved in providing the disabled with tools to improve their quality of life.
3. Nuclear medicine—an outgrowth of the atomic age—emerged as a powerful and effective approach in detecting and treating specific physiological abnormalities.
4. Diagnostic ultrasound based on sonar technology became so widely accepted that ultrasonic studies are now part of the routine diagnostic workup in many medical specialties.
5. "Spare parts" surgery also became commonplace. Technologists were encouraged to provide cardiac assist devices, such as artificial heart valves and artificial blood vessels, and the artificial heart program was launched to develop a replacement for a defective or diseased human heart.
6. Advances in materials have made the development of disposable medical devices, such as needles and thermometers, a reality.
7. Advancements in molecular engineering have allowed for the discovery of countless pharmacological agents and to the design of their delivery, including implantable delivery systems.
8. Computers similar to those developed to control the flight plans of the Apollo capsule were used to store, process, and cross-check medical records, to monitor patient status in intensive care units, and to provide sophisticated statistical diagnoses of potential diseases correlated with specific sets of patient symptoms.
9. Development of the first computer-based medical instrument, the computerized axial tomography scanner, revolutionized clinical approaches to noninvasive diagnostic imaging procedures, which now include magnetic resonance imaging and positron emission tomography as well.
10. A wide variety of new cardiovascular technologies including implantable defibrillators and chemically treated stents were developed.
11. Neuronal pacing systems were used to detect and prevent epileptic seizures.
12. Artificial organs and tissue have been created.
13. The completion of the genome project has stimulated the search for new biological markers and personalized medicine.
14. The further understanding of cellular and biomolecular processes has led to the engineering of stem cells into therapeutically valuable lineages and to the regeneration of organs and tissue structures.

15. Developments in nanotechnology have yielded nanomaterials for use in tissue engineering and facilitated the creation and study of nanoparticles and molecular machine systems that will assist in the detection and treatment of disease and injury.

The impact of these discoveries and many others has been profound. The healthcare system of today consists of technologically sophisticated clinical staff operating primarily in modern hospitals designed to accommodate the new medical technology. This evolutionary process continues, with advances in the physical sciences such as materials and nanotechnology and in the life sciences such as molecular biology, genomics, stem cell biology, and artificial and regenerated tissue and organs. These advances have altered and will continue to alter the very nature of the healthcare delivery system itself.

Biomedical Engineering: A Definition

Bioengineering is usually defined as a basic research-oriented activity closely related to biotechnology and genetic engineering, that is, the modification of animal or plant cells or parts of cells to improve plants or animals or to develop new microorganisms for beneficial ends. In the food industry, for example, this has meant the improvement of strains of yeast for fermentation. In agriculture, bioengineers may be concerned with the improvement of crop yields by treatment of plants with organisms to reduce frost damage. It is clear that future bioengineers will have a tremendous impact on the quality of human life. The potential of this specialty is difficult to imagine. Consider the following activities of bioengineers:

- Development of improved species of plants and animals for food production
- Invention of new medical diagnostic tests for diseases
- Production of synthetic vaccines from clone cells
- Bioenvironmental engineering to protect human, animal, and plant life from toxicants and pollutants
- Study of protein–surface interactions
- Modeling of the growth kinetics of yeast and hybridoma cells
- Research in immobilized enzyme technology
- Development of therapeutic proteins and monoclonal antibodies

Biomedical engineers, on the other hand, apply electrical, mechanical, chemical, optical, and other engineering principles to understand, modify, or control biological (i.e., human and animal) systems as well as design and manufacture products that can monitor physiological functions and assist in the diagnosis and treatment of patients. When biomedical engineers work in a hospital or clinic, they are more aptly called clinical engineers.

Activities of Biomedical Engineers

The breadth of activity of biomedical engineers is now significant. The field has moved from being concerned primarily with the development of medical instruments in the 1950s and 1960s to include a more wide-ranging set of activities. As illustrated below, the field of biomedical engineering now includes many new career areas (see Figure P.1), each of which is presented in this handbook. These areas include

- Application of engineering system analysis (physiological modeling, simulation, and control) to biological problems
- Detection, measurement, and monitoring of physiological signals (i.e., biosensors and biomedical instrumentation)
- Diagnostic interpretation via signal-processing techniques of bioelectric data
- Therapeutic and rehabilitation procedures and devices (rehabilitation engineering)
- Devices for replacement or augmentation of bodily functions (artificial organs)

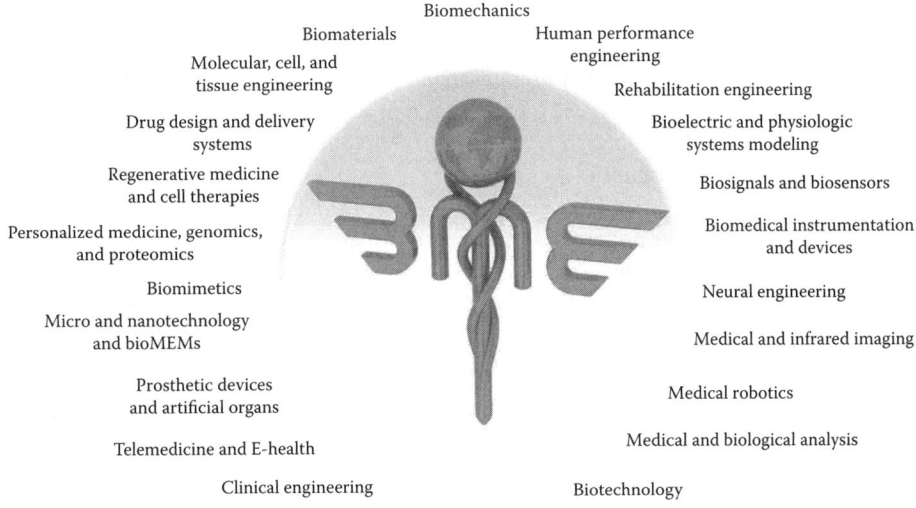

FIGURE P.1 The world of biomedical engineering.

- Computer analysis of patient-related data and clinical decision making (i.e., medical informatics and artificial intelligence)
- Medical imaging, that is, the graphic display of anatomic detail or physiologic function
- The creation of new biological products (e.g., biotechnology and tissue engineering)
- The development of new materials to be used within the body (biomaterials)

Typical pursuits of biomedical engineers, therefore, include

- Research in new materials for implanted artificial organs
- Development of new diagnostic instruments for blood analysis
- Computer modeling of the function of the human heart
- Writing software for analysis of medical research data
- Analysis of medical device hazards for safety and efficacy
- Development of new diagnostic imaging systems
- Design of telemetry systems for patient monitoring
- Design of biomedical sensors for measurement of human physiological systems variables
- Development of expert systems for diagnosis of disease
- Design of closed-loop control systems for drug administration
- Modeling of the physiological systems of the human body
- Design of instrumentation for sports medicine
- Development of new dental materials
- Design of communication aids for the handicapped
- Study of pulmonary fluid dynamics
- Study of the biomechanics of the human body
- Development of material to be used as a replacement for human skin

Biomedical engineering, then, is an interdisciplinary branch of engineering that ranges from theoretical, nonexperimental undertakings to state-of-the-art applications. It can encompass research, development, implementation, and operation. Accordingly, like medical practice itself, it is unlikely that any single person can acquire expertise that encompasses the entire field. Yet, because of the interdisciplinary nature of this activity, there is considerable interplay and overlapping of interest and effort between them. For example, biomedical engineers engaged in the development of biosensors may interact with those interested in prosthetic devices to develop a means to detect and use the same bio-electric signal to power a prosthetic device. Those engaged in automating clinical chemistry laboratories may collaborate with those developing expert systems to assist clinicians in making decisions based on specific laboratory data. The possibilities are endless.

Perhaps, a greater potential benefit occurring from the use of biomedical engineering is identification of the problems and needs of our present healthcare system that can be solved using existing engineering technology and systems methodology. Consequently, the field of biomedical engineering offers hope in the continuing battle to provide high-quality care at a reasonable cost. If properly directed toward solving problems related to preventive medical approaches, ambulatory care services, and the like, biomedical engineers can provide the tools and techniques to make our healthcare system more effective and efficient and, in the process, improve the quality of life for all.

Joseph D. Bronzino
Donald R. Peterson
Editors-in-Chief

Editors

Joseph D. Bronzino is currently the president of the Biomedical Engineering Alliance and Consortium (BEACON; www.beaconalliance.org), which is a nonprofit organization dedicated to the promotion of collaborative research, translation, and partnership among academic, medical, and industry people in the field of biomedical engineering to develop new medical technologies and devices. To accomplish this goal, Dr. Bronzino and BEACON facilitate collaborative research, industrial partnering, and the development of emerging companies. Dr. Bronzino earned a BSEE from Worcester Polytechnic Institute, Worcester, Massachusetts, in 1959, an MSEE from the Naval Postgraduate School, Monterey, California, in 1961, and a PhD in electrical engineering from Worcester Polytechnic Institute in 1968. He was recently the Vernon Roosa Professor of Applied Science and endowed chair at Trinity College, Hartford, Connecticut.

Dr. Bronzino is the author of over 200 journal articles and 15 books, including *Technology for Patient Care* (C.V. Mosby, 1977), *Computer Applications for Patient Care* (Addison-Wesley, 1982), *Biomedical Engineering: Basic Concepts and Instrumentation* (PWS Publishing Co., 1986), *Expert Systems: Basic Concepts* (Research Foundation of State University of New York, 1989), *Medical Technology and Society: An Interdisciplinary Perspective* (MIT Press and McGraw-Hill, 1990), *Management of Medical Technology* (Butterworth/Heinemann, 1992), *The Biomedical Engineering Handbook* (CRC Press, 1st Edition, 1995; 2nd Edition, 2000; 3rd Edition, 2006), *Introduction to Biomedical Engineering* (Academic Press, 1st Edition, 1999; 2nd Edition, 2005; 3rd Edition, 2011), *Biomechanics: Principles and Applications* (CRC Press, 2002), *Biomaterials: Principles and Applications* (CRC Press, 2002), *Tissue Engineering* (CRC Press, 2002), and *Biomedical Imaging* (CRC Press, 2002).

Dr. Bronzino is a fellow of IEEE and the American Institute of Medical and Biological Engineering (AIMBE), an honorary member of the Italian Society of Experimental Biology, past chairman of the Biomedical Engineering Division of the American Society for Engineering Education (ASEE), a charter member of the Connecticut Academy of Science and Engineering (CASE), a charter member of the American College of Clinical Engineering (ACCE), a member of the Association for the Advancement of Medical Instrumentation (AAMI), past president of the IEEE-Engineering in Medicine and Biology Society (EMBS), past chairman of the IEEE Healthcare Engineering Policy Committee (HCEPC), and past chairman of the IEEE Technical Policy Council in Washington, DC. He is a member of Eta Kappa Nu, Sigma Xi, and Tau Beta Pi. He is also a recipient of the IEEE Millennium Medal for "his contributions to biomedical engineering research and education" and the Goddard Award from WPI for Outstanding Professional Achievement in 2005. He is presently editor-in-chief of the Academic Press/Elsevier BME Book Series.

Donald R. Peterson is a professor of engineering and the dean of the College of Science, Technology, Engineering, Mathematics, and Nursing at Texas A&M University in Texarkana, Texas, and holds a joint appointment in the Department of Biomedical Engineering (BME) at Texas A&M University in College Station, Texas. He was recently an associate professor of medicine and the director of the

Biodynamics Laboratory in the School of Medicine at the University of Connecticut (UConn) and served as chair of the BME Program in the School of Engineering at UConn as well as the director of the BME Graduate and Undergraduate Programs. Dr. Peterson earned a BS in aerospace engineering and a BS in biomechanical engineering from Worcester Polytechnic Institute, in Worcester, Massachusetts, in 1992, an MS in mechanical engineering from the UConn, in Storrs, Connecticut, in 1995, and a PhD in biomedical engineering from UConn in 1999. He has 17 years of experience in BME education and has offered graduate-level and undergraduate-level courses in the areas of biomechanics, biodynamics, biofluid mechanics, BME communication, BME senior design, and ergonomics, and has taught subjects such as gross anatomy, occupational biomechanics, and occupational exposure and response in the School of Medicine. Dr. Peterson was also recently the co-executive director of the Biomedical Engineering Alliance and Consortium (BEACON), which is a nonprofit organization dedicated to the promotion of collaborative research, translation, and partnership among academic, medical, and industry people in the field of biomedical engineering to develop new medical technologies and devices.

Dr. Peterson has over 21 years of experience in devices and systems and in engineering and medical research, and his work on human–device interaction has led to applications on the design and development of several medical devices and tools. Other recent translations of his research include the development of devices such as robotic assist devices and prosthetics, long-duration biosensor monitoring systems, surgical and dental instruments, patient care medical devices, spacesuits and space tools for NASA, powered and non-powered hand tools, musical instruments, sports equipment, computer input devices, and so on. Other overlapping research initiatives focus on the development of computational models and simulations of biofluid dynamics and biomechanical performance, cell mechanics and cellular responses to fluid shear stress, human exposure and response to vibration, and the acoustics of hearing protection and communication. He has also been involved clinically with the Occupational and Environmental Medicine group at the UConn Health Center, where his work has been directed toward the objective engineering analysis of the anatomic and physiological processes involved in the onset of musculoskeletal and neuromuscular diseases, including strategies of disease mitigation.

Dr. Peterson's scholarly activities include over 50 published journal articles, 2 textbook chapters, 2 textbook sections, and 12 textbooks, including his new appointment as co-editor-in-chief for *The Biomedical Engineering Handbook* by CRC Press.

Contributors

Kim Abramson
Institute for BioTechnology Futures
New York, New York

P.D. Ahlgren
Ville Marie Medical and Women's Health Center
Montreal, Quebec, Canada

William C. Amalu
Pacific Chiropractic and Research Center
Redwood City, California

Amir A. Amini
Department of Electrical and Computer
    Engineering
University of Louisville
Louisville, Kentucky

Kurt Ammer
Ludwig Boltzmann Research Institute for
    Physical Diagnostics
Vienna, Austria

and

University of Glamorgan
Wales, United Kingdom

Michael Anbar
University at Buffalo, State University of
    New York
Buffalo, New York

Edward Ashton
VirtualScopics, Inc.
Rochester, New York

Raymond Balcerak
(deceased)
RSB Consulting LLC

Niranjan Balu
Department of Radiology
University of Washington
Seattle, Washington

D.C. Barber
Department of Cardiovascular Science
Sheffield University
Yorkshire, United Kingdom

Normand Belliveau
Ville Marie Medical and Women's Health Center
Montreal, Quebec, Canada

Reinhold Berz
German Society of Thermography and
    Regulation Medicine (DGTR)
Waldbronn, Germany

Anna M. Bianchi
Department of Biomedical Engineering
Politecnico di Milano
Milan, Italy

Carol J. Bickford
Department of Nursing Practice and Policy
American Nurses Association
Silver Spring, Maryland

Jeffrey S. Blair
IBM Healthcare Solutions
Atlanta, Georgia

R. Boellaard
Department of Nuclear Medicine and PET
    Research
VU University Medical Center
Amsterdam, The Netherlands

G. Faye Boudreaux-Bartels
Department of Electrical Computer and
    Biomedical Engineering
University of Rhode Island
Kingston, Rhode Island

Pradeep Buddharaju
Department of Computer Science
University of Houston
Houston, Texas

Thomas F. Budinger
Department of Electrical Engineering and
    Computer Sciences
University of California, Berkeley
Berkeley, California

Paul Campbell
Ninewells Hospital
Dundee, Scotland, United Kingdom

Gador Canton
Department of Radiology
University of Washington
Seattle, Washington

Ewart R. Carson
City University
London, United Kingdom

Sergio Cerutti
Department of Biomedical Engineering
Politecnico di Milano
Milan, Italy

Huijun Chen
Department of Radiology
University of Washington
Seattle, Washington

Wei Chen
Center for Magnetic Resonance Research
University of Minnesota Medical School
Minneapolis, Minnesota

Victor Chernomordik
National Institutes of Health
Bethesda, Maryland

David A. Chesler
Department of Radiology
Massachusetts General Hospital
Boston, Massachusetts

Steven Conolly
Department of Biomedical Engineering
Stanford University
Stanford, California

P. Constantinides
Department of Computer Science and
    Engineering
University of Warwick
Limassol, Cyprus

Timothy D. Conwell
Colorado Infrared Imaging Center
Denver, Colorado

Derek G. Cramp
City University
London, United Kingdom

Barbara Y. Croft
National Institutes of Health
Bethesda, Maryland

Ian A. Cunningham
The John P. Robarts Research Institute
University of Western Ontario
London, Ontario, Canada

Connie White Delaney
Biomedical Informatics
University of Minnesota
Minneapolis, Minnesota

Siyi Deng
Department of Cognitive Science
and
Department of Biomedical Engineering
University of California, Irvine
Irvine, California

Thomas Deserno
Department of Medical Informatics
Aachen University
Aachen, Germany

Louis de Weerd
University Hospital of North Norway
Tromsø, Norway

Mary Diakides
Advanced Concepts Analysis, Inc.
Falls Church, Virginia

Nicholas A. Diakides
(deceased)
Advanced Concepts Analysis, Inc.
Falls Church, Virginia

C. Drews-Peszynski
Laser Diagnostics and Therapy Center
Technical University of Lodz
Lodz, Poland

Ronald G. Driggers
U.S. Army CERDEC Night Vision and
   Electronic Sensors Directorate
Fort Belvoir, Virginia

Robert L. Elliot
Elliot-Elliot-Head Breast Cancer Research and
   Treatment Center
Baton Rouge, Louisiana

M. Etehadtavakol
Medical Image and Signal Processing
   Research Center
Isfahan University of Medical Science
Isfahan, Iran

Konstantinos P. Exarchos
Unit of Medical Technology and Intelligent
   Information Systems
Department of Materials Science and
   Engineering
and
Department of Medical Physics, Medical School
University of Ioannina
Ioannina, Greece

Themis P. Exarchos
Unit of Medical Technology and Intelligent
   Information Systems
Department of Materials Science and
   Engineering
and
Department of Biological Applications and
   Technology
and
Biomedical Research Institute-Forth
University of Ioannina
Ioannina, Greece

K. Whittaker Ferrara
Riverside Research Institute
Riverside, California

J. Michael Fitzmaurice
Agency for Healthcare Research and Quality
Rockville, Maryland

Dimitrios I. Fotiadis
Unit of Medical Technology and Intelligent
   Information Systems
Department of Materials Science and
   Engineering
and
Biomedical Research Institute-Forth
University of Ioannina
Ioannina, Greece

Amir H. Gandjbakhche
National Institutes of Health
Bethesda, Maryland

Israel Gannot
Department of Biomedical Engineering
Tel Aviv University
Tel Aviv, Israel

James Geiling
Geisel School of Medicine at Dartmouth
Hanover, New Hampshire

and

Veterans Affairs Medical Center
White River Junction, Vermont

N. Gheissari
Electrical and Computer Engineering Department
Isfahan University of Technology
and
Medical Image and Signal Processing Research
    Center
Isfahan University of Medical Science
Isfahan, Iran

James Giordano
Center for Neurotechnology Studies
Potomac Institute for Policy Studies
Arlington, Virginia

and

Krasnow Institute for Advanced Studies
George Mason University
Fairfax, Virginia

and

Wellcome Centre for Neuroethics
University of Oxford
Oxford, United Kingdom

Richard L. Goldberg
Department of Biomedical Engineering
University of North Carolina
Chapel Hill, North Carolina

Barton M. Gratt
School of Dentistry
University of Washington
Seattle, Washington

Michael W. Grenn
U.S. Army CERDEC Night Vision and
    Electronic Sensors Directorate
Fort Belvoir, Virginia

Moinuddin Hassan
Center for Devices and Radiological Health
U.S. Food and Drug Administration (FDA)
Silver Spring, Maryland

Jonathan F. Head
Elliot-Elliot-Head Breast Cancer Research and
    Treatment Center
Baton Rouge, Louisiana

William B. Hobbins
Women's Breast Health Center
Madison, Wisconsin

Stuart B. Horn
U.S. Army CERDEC Night Vision and
    Electronic Sensors Directorate
Fort Belvoir, Virginia

Xiaoping Hu
Center for Magnetic Resonance Research
University of Minnesota Medical School
Minneapolis, Minnesota

N. Huber
Biomedical Engineering Group
University of Sussex
Brighton, United Kingdom

Meltem Izzetoglu
School of Biomedical Engineering, Science and
    Health Systems
Drexel University
Philadelphia, Pennsylvania

T. Jakubowska
Laser Diagnostics and Therapy Center
Technical University of Lodz
Lodz, Poland

Hongjun Jia
Department of Radiology and BRIC
University of North Carolina
Chapel Hill, North Carolina

G. Allan Johnson
Departments of Biomedical Engineering and
    Physics
Duke University Medical Center
Durham, North Carolina

Bryan F. Jones
School of Computing
University of Glamorgan
Pontypridd, Wales, United Kingdom

Philip F. Judy
Department of Radiology
Brigham and Women's Hospital
Harvard Medical School
Boston, Massachusetts

A. Jung
Department of Pediatrics
Military Institute of Medicine
Warsaw, Poland

Mariusz Kaczmarek
Department of Biomedical Engineering
Gdansk University of Technology
Gdansk, Poland

Jana Kainerstorfer
National Institutes of Health
Bethesda, Maryland

B. Kalicki
Department of Pediatrics
Military Institute of Medicine
Szaserow, Warsaw, Poland

Maciej Kamiński
Department of Biomedical Physics
University of Warsaw
Warsaw, Poland

Lindsay Katona
University of New England College of
    Osteopathic Medicine
Biddeford, Maine

William S. Kerwin
Department of Radiology
University of Washington
Seattle, Washington

John R. Keyserlingk
Ville Marie Medical and Women's Health Center
Montreal, Quebec, Canada

Andrey Kondyurin
Institute for Laser and Information Technologies
    of Russian Academy of Sciences
Troitsk, Russia

Luis G. Kun
William Perry-Center for Hemispheric Defense
    Studies
National Defense University
Washington, DC

Phani Teja Kuruganti
Oak Ridge National Laboratory
Oak Ridge, Tennessee

Kenneth K. Kwong
Department of Radiology
Massachusetts General Hospital
Boston, Massachusetts

E. Kyriacou
Department of Computer Science and
    Engineering
Frederick University
Limassol, Cyprus

Joshua E. Lane
Departments of Surgery and Internal Medicine
Mercer University School of Medicine
Macon, Georgia

and

Department of Dermatology
Emory University School of Medicine
Atlanta, Georgia

Michael Lauria
Flight/Critical Care Paramedic
Dartmouth-Hitchcock Medical Center
Lebanon, New Hampshire

Richard M. Leahy
Signal and Image Processing Institute
University of Southern California
Los Angeles, California

Hualou Liang
School of Biomedical Engineering Science and
    Health Systems
Drexel University
Philadelphia, Pennsylvania

Richard F. Little
National Institutes of Health
Bethesda, Maryland

H. Helen Liu
Flow-Of-Light Natural Health
Institute of Holistic Health and Science
Houston, Texas

Zhong Qi Liu
Academy of TTM Technologies and Bioyear
    Medical Instrument
Beijing, China

M. Lubberink
Department of Biomedical Engineering and PET
   Center
Uppsala University
Uppsala, Sweden

Caro Lucas
Electrical and Computer Engineering
   Department
University of Tehran
Tehran, Iran

Jasper Lupo
Applied Research Associates, Inc.
Falls Church, Virginia

Albert Macovski
Departments of Electrical Engineering and
   Radiology
Stanford University
Stanford, California

R.P. Maguire
Novartis Institutes for Biomedical Research
Basel, Switzerland

Luca T. Mainardi
Department of Biomedical Engineering
Politecnico di Milano
Milan, Italy

Alessandro Mariotti
Department of Neurosciences and Imaging
G. d'Annunzio University
Chieti-Pescara, Italy

Kathleen A. McCormick
SAIC-F
Rockville, Maryland

James B. Mercer
University of Tromsø
Tromsø, Norway

Arcangelo Merla
University of Chieti-Pescara
Pescara, Italy

Robyn E. Mosher
Thayer School of Engineering
Dartmouth College
Hanover, New Hampshire

Jack G. Mottley
Department of Electrical and Computer
   Engineering
University of Rochester
Rochester, New York

Robin Murray
Department of Electrical Computer and
   Biomedical Engineering
University of Rhode Island
Kingston, Rhode Island

and

Environmental and Target Physics
Naval Undersea Warfare Center
Newport, Rhode Island

E.Y.K. Ng
School of Mechanical and Aerospace
   Engineering
and
College of Engineering
Nanyang Technological University
Singapore

Paul R. Norton
U.S. Army CERDEC Night Vision and
   Electronic Sensors Directorate
Fort Belvoir, Virginia

Antoni Nowakowski
Department of Biomedical Engineering
Gdansk University of Technology
Gdansk, Poland

A. Panayides
Department of Computer Science
Imperial College
Nicosia, Cyprus

Dimitrios Pantazis
Signal and Image Processing Institute
University of Southern California
Los Angeles, California

David D. Pascoe
Auburn University
Auburn, Alabama

Maqbool Patel
Center for Magnetic Resonance Research
University of Minnesota Medical School
Minneapolis, Minnesota

C.S. Pattichis
Department of Computer Science
University of Cyprus
Nicosia, Cyprus

M.S. Pattichis
Department of Electrical and Computer
    Engineering
University of New Mexico
Albuquerque, New Mexico

Jeffrey Paul
Applied Research Associates, Inc.
Alexandria, Virginia

John Pauly
Department of Electrical Engineering
Stanford University
Stanford, California

Ioannis Pavlidis
Department of Computer Science
University of Houston
Houston, Texas

Joseph G. Pellegrino
U.S. Army CERDEC Night Vision and
    Electronic Sensors Directorate
Fort Belvoir, Virginia

Philip Perconti
U.S. Army CERDEC Night Vision and
    Electronic Sensors Directorate
Fort Belvoir, Virginia

Carmen C.Y. Poon
Joint Research Centre for Biomedical
    Engineering
Department of Electronic Engineering
The Chinese University of Hong Kong
Hong Kong, China

Ron Poropatich
Center for Military Medicine Research, Health
    Sciences
University of Pittsburgh
Pittsburgh, Pennsylvania

T. Allan Pryor
University of Utah
Salt Lake City, Utah

Ram C. Purohit
Auburn University
Auburn, Alabama

Hairong Qi
Department of Electrical Engineering and
    Computer Science
University of Tennessee
Knoxville, Tennessee

Francis J. Ring
Medical Imaging Research Unit
University of Glamorgan
Pontypridd, Wales, United Kingdom

Jan Rogowski
Department of Cardiosurgery
Gdansk University of Medicine
Gdansk, Poland

Gian Luca Romani
University of Chieti-Pescara
Pescara, Italy

Joseph M. Rosen
Geisel School of Medicine at Dartmouth
and
Thayer School of Engineering
Dartmouth College
Hanover, New Hampshire

and

Veterans Affairs Medical Center
White River Junction, Vermont

A. Rustecka
Department of Pediatrics
Military Institute of Medicine
Szaserow, Warsaw, Poland

S. Sadri
Electrical and Computer Engineering Department
Isfahan University of Technology
and
Medical Image and Signal Processing Research
    Center
Isfahan University of Medical Science
Isfahan, Iran

Gerald Schaefer
Department of Computer Science
Loughborough University
Loughborough, United Kingdom

John Schenck
General Electric Corporate Research and
    Development Center
Schenectady, New York

Claus Schulte-Uebbing
German Society of Thermography and
    Regulation Medicine (DGTR)
Munich, Germany

Joyce Sensmeier
Healthcare Information and Management
    Systems Society
Chicago, Illinois

Vijay Shah
VirtualScopics, Inc.
Rochester, New York

Dinggang Shen
Department of Radiology and BRIC
University of North Carolina
Chapel Hill, North Carolina

Feng Shi
Department of Radiology and BRIC
University of North Carolina
Chapel Hill, North Carolina

Stephen W. Smith
Department of Biomedical Engineering
Duke University
Durham, North Carolina

Wesley E. Snyder
Department of Electrical and Computer
    Engineering
North Carolina State University
Raleigh, North Carolina

Juan Luis Poletti Soto
Signal and Image Processing Institute
University of Southern California
Los Angeles, California

Ramesh Srinivasan
Department of Cognitive Science
and
Department of Biomedical Engineering
University of California, Irvine
Irvine, California

Robert Strakowski
Institute of Electronics
Technical University of Lodz
Lodz, Poland

M. Strzelecki
Institute of Electronics
Technical University of Lodz
Lodz, Poland

Ron Summers
Loughborough University
Leicestershire, United Kingdom

Alexander Sviridov
Institute for Laser and Information Technologies
    of Russian Academy of Sciences
Troitsk, Russia

José G. Tamez-Peña
Tec de Monterrey
Nuevo León, México

Roderick Thomas
Swansea Institute of Technology
Swansea, Wales, United Kingdom

Saara Totterman
Qmetrics Technologies, LLC
Rochester, New York

Benjamin M.W. Tsui
Department of Radiology and Radiological
    Sciences
Johns Hopkins University
Baltimore, Maryland

Tracy A. Turner
Private Practice
Minneapolis, Minnesota

Kamil Ugurbil
Center for Magnetic Resonance
    Research
University of Minnesota Medical
    School
Minneapolis, Minnesota

Henry F. VanBrocklin
Department of Radiology
University of California, Berkeley
Berkeley, California

R. Vardasca
School of Technology and Management
Polytechnic Institute of Leiria
Leiria, Portugal

Jay Vizgaitis
U.S. Army CERDEC Night Vision and
    Electronic Sensors Directorate
Fort Belvoir, Virginia

Abby Vogel
Georgia Institute of Technology
Atlanta, Georgia

Hui Wang
Department of Electrical Engineering
University of Louisville
Louisville, Kentucky

Jinnan Wang
Philips Research North America
Briarcliff Manor, New York

Qian Wang
Department of Radiology and BRIC
and
Department of Computer Science
University of North Carolina
Chapel Hill, North Carolina

W. Wang
Biomedical Engineering Group
University of Sussex
Brighton, United Kingdom

Sven Weum
Auburn University
Auburn, Alabama

Boguslaw Wiecek
Institute of Electronics
Technical University of Lodz
Lodz, Poland

Maria Wiecek
Institute of Electronics
Technical University of Lodz
Lodz, Poland

Guorong Wu
Department of Radiology and BRIC
University of North Carolina
Chapel Hill, North Carolina

M. Wysocki
Laser Diagnostics and Therapy Center
Technical University of Lodz
Lodz, Poland

Martin J. Yaffe
Imaging/Bioengineering Research
Sunnybrook Health Sciences Centre
and
Departments of Medical Biophysics and
    Radiology
University of Toronto
Toronto, Ontario, Canada

Pew-Thian Yap
Department of Radiology and BRIC
University of North Carolina
Chapel Hill, North Carolina

Robert Yarchoan
National Institutes of Health
Bethesda, Maryland

Mariam Yassa
Ville Marie Medical and Women's
    Health Center
Montreal, Quebec, Canada

E. Yu
Ville Marie Medical and Women's
    Health Center
Montreal, Quebec, Canada

Chun Yuan
Department of Radiology
University of Washington
Seattle, Washington

Jason Zeibel
U.S. Army CERDEC Night Vision and
    Electronic Sensors Directorate
Fort Belvoir, Virginia

Yuan-ting Zhang
Joint Research Centre for Biomedical
    Engineering
Department of Electronic Engineering
The Chinese University of Hong Kong
and
Key Laboratory for Health Informatics of
    Chinese Academy of Science
Hong Kong, China

Xiaohong Zhou
Duke University Medical Center
Durham, North Carolina

J. Zuber
Department of Pediatrics
Military Institute of Medicine
Warsaw, Poland

MATLAB Statement

MATLAB® and Simulink® are registered trademarks of The MathWorks, Inc. For product information, please contact:

The MathWorks, Inc.
3 Apple Hill Drive
Natick, MA 01760-2098 USA
Tel: 508 647 7000
Fax: 508-647-7001
E-mail: info@mathworks.com
Web: www.mathworks.com

I

Biosignal Processing

Hualou Liang
Drexel University

Preface

Biosignal processing has been around for decades, but it still seems to be growing in popularity. With the rise of advanced computerized data collection systems, monitoring devices, and instrumentation technologies, large and complex datasets simply accrue as an inevitable part of biomedical enterprise. The availability of large quantities of biomedical data not only offers unprecedented opportunities to advance our understanding of the underlying biological and physiologic functions, structures, and dynamics but also drives tremendous progress toward innovative methods in biosignal processing. As such, this field has advanced to a conspicuous stage that biosignal processing has become an integral part in all phases of biomedical research and development.

The purpose of this section is to provide state-of-the-art coverage of contemporary methods in biosignal processing with an emphasis on brain signal analysis. The first two chapters in this section present fundamental aspects of biomedical signal processing, which should be accessible to the general audience. Chapter 1 provides a general overview of basic concepts in biomedical signal acquisition and processing, whereas Chapter 2 deals with the nonstationary and transient nature of signals by introducing time–frequency analysis and discusses its applications to signal analysis and detection problems in bioengineering.

The next four chapters address emerging methods for brain signal processing, each focusing on specific noninvasive imaging techniques such as electroencephalography (EEG), magnetoencephalography (MEG), magnetic resonance imaging (MRI), and functional near-infrared spectroscopy (fNIR). Chapter 3 covers a multivariate spectral analysis of EEG data using power, coherence, and second-order blind identification. Chapter 4 introduces a general linear modeling approach for the analysis of induced and evoked responses in MEG. Chapter 5 presents the progress in groupwise registration algorithms for effective MRI medical image analysis. Chapter 6 describes the basis of optical imaging, fNIR instrumentation, and signal analysis in various cognitive studies.

Chapter 7 reviews recent advances of causal influence measures such as the Granger causality for analyzing multivariate neural data. For basic applications, the emphasis is on the typical analysis of spike trains, EEG, and fMRI BOLD data, each representing a major recording modality used in neuroscience research. For clinical applications, epileptogenic seizure localization is selected as a direct demonstration.

The topics covered in this section reflect an ongoing evolution in biosignal processing. As biomedical datasets grow larger and more complicated, emerging signal processing methods that analyze and interpret these data have gained in importance. We hope that this section will aid the process for biosignal analysis and stimulate new ideas and opportunities for developing cutting-edge computational methods for biosignal processing, which will in turn accelerate laboratory discoveries into treatments for patients. All the contributors of this section share this vision and herein are gratefully recognized for donating their talent and time so that the promise of biosignal processing will be fulfilled.

1

Digital Biomedical Signal Acquisition and Processing

Luca T. Mainardi
Politecnico di Milano

Anna M. Bianchi
Politecnico di Milano

Sergio Cerutti
Politecnico di Milano

Biologic signals carry information that is useful for the comprehension of the complex pathophysiologic mechanisms underlying the behavior of living systems. Nevertheless, such information cannot be available directly from the raw recorded signals; it can be masked by other biologic signals contemporaneously detected (endogenous effects) or buried in some additive noise (exogenous effects). For such reasons, some additional processing is usually required to enhance the relevant information and to extract from it parameters that quantify the behavior of the system under study, mainly for physiologic studies, or that define the degree of pathology for routine clinical procedures (diagnosis, therapy, or rehabilitation).

Several processing techniques can be used for such purposes (they are also called preprocessing techniques): time- or frequency-domain methods, including filtering, *averaging*, spectral estimation, and others. Even if it is possible to deal with continuous time waveforms, it is usually convenient to convert them into a numerical form before processing. The recent progress of digital technology, in terms of both hardware and software, makes digital rather than analog processing more efficient and flexible. Digital techniques have several advantages: their performance is generally powerful, being able to easily implement even complex algorithms, and accuracy depends only on the truncation and round-off errors, whose effects can be predicted and controlled by the designer and are largely unaffected by other unpredictable variables such as component aging and temperature, which can degrade the performances of analog devices. Moreover, design parameters can be more easily changed because they involve software rather than hardware modifications.

A few basic elements of signal acquisition and processing will be presented in the following; our aim is to stress mainly the aspects connected with acquisition and analysis of biologic signals, leaving to the cited literature a deeper insight into the various subjects for both the fundamentals of digital signal processing and the applications.

1.1 Acquisition

A schematic representation of a general acquisition system is shown in Figure 1.1. Several physical magnitudes are usually measured from biologic systems. They include electromagnetic quantities (currents, potential differences, field strengths, etc.), as well as mechanical, chemical, or generally

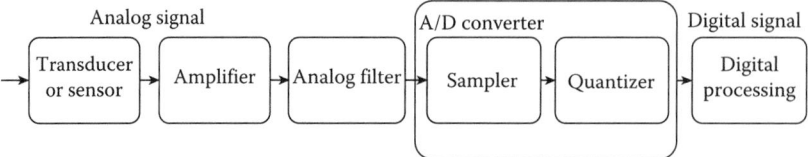

FIGURE 1.1   General block diagram of the acquisition procedure of a digital signal.

nonelectrical variables (pressure, temperature, movements, etc.). Electric signals are detected by sensors (mainly electrodes), while nonelectric magnitudes are first converted by transducers into electric signals that can be easily treated, transmitted, and stored. Several books of biomedical instrumentation give detailed descriptions of the various transducers and the hardware requirements associated with the acquisition of the different biologic signals (Tompkins and Webster, 1981; Cobbold, 1988; Webster, 2009).

An analog preprocessing block is usually required to amplify and filter the signal (in order to make it satisfy the requirements of the hardware such as the dynamic of the analog-to-digital converter), to compensate for some unwanted sensor characteristics, or to reduce the portion of undesired noise. Moreover, the continuous-time signal should be bandlimited before analog-to-digital (A/D) conversion. Such operation is needed to reduce the effect of *aliasing* induced by sampling, as will be described in the next section. Here it is important to remember that the acquisition procedure should preserve the information contained in the original signal waveform. This is a crucial point when recording biologic signals, whose characteristics may often be considered by physicians as indices of some underlying pathologies (i.e., the ST-segment displacement on an ECG signal can be considered a marker of ischemia, the peak-and-wave pattern on an EEG tracing can be a sign of epilepsy, and so on). Thus, the acquisition system should not introduce any form of distortion that can be misleading or can destroy real pathologic alterations. For this reason, the analog prefiltering block should be designed with constant modulus and linear phase (or zero-phase) *frequency response*, at least in the passband, over the frequencies of interest. Such requirements make the signal arrive undistorted up to the A/D converter.

The analog waveform is then A/D converted into a digital signal, that is, it is transformed into a series of numbers, discretized both in time and in amplitude, that can be easily managed by digital processors. The A/D conversion ideally can be divided into two steps, as shown in Figure 1.1: the sampling process, which converts the continuous signal in a discrete-time series and whose elements are named samples, and a quantization procedure, which assigns the amplitude value of each sample within a set of determined discrete values. Both processes modify the characteristics of the signal, and their effects will be discussed in the following sections.

1.1.1 Sampling Theorem

The advantages of processing a digital series instead of an analog signal have been reported previously. Furthermore, the basic property when using a sampled series instead of its continuous waveform lies in the fact that the former, under certain hypotheses, is completely representative of the latter. When this happens, the continuous waveform can be perfectly reconstructed just from the series of sampled values. This is known as the sampling theorem (or Shannon theorem) (Shannon, 1949). It states that a continuous-time signal can be completely recovered from its samples if, and only if, the sampling rate is greater than twice the signal bandwidth.

In order to understand the assumptions of the theorem, let us consider a continuous bandlimited signal $x(t)$ (up to f_b) whose Fourier transform $X(f)$ is shown in Figure 1.2a and let us suppose to uniformly sample it. The sampling procedure can be modeled by the multiplication of $x(t)$ with an impulse train:

$$i(t) = \sum_{k=-\infty,\infty} \delta(t - kT_s) \tag{1.1}$$

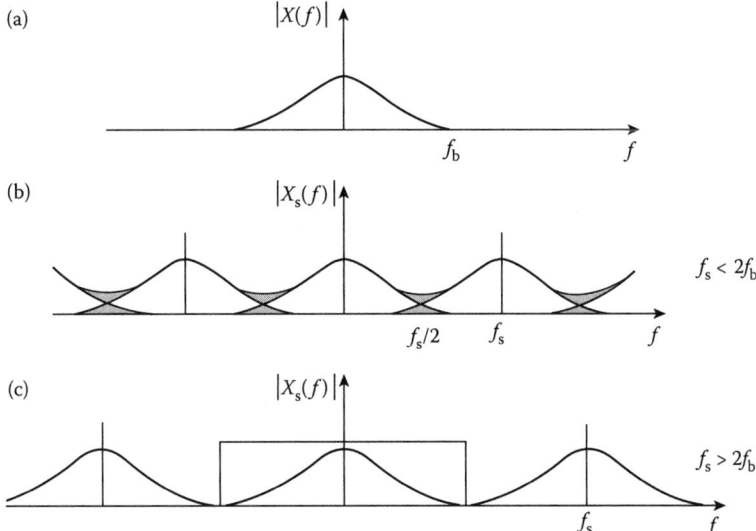

FIGURE 1.2 Effect of sampling frequency (f_s) on a bandlimited signal (up to frequency f_b). Fourier transform of the original time signal (a), of the sampled signal when $f_s < 2f_b$ (b), and when $f_s > 2f_b$ (c). The dark areas in part (b) indicate the frequency range affected by aliasing.

where $\delta(t)$ is the delta (Dirac) function, k is an integer, and T_s is the sampling interval. The sampled signal becomes

$$x_s(t) = x(t) \cdot i(t) = \sum_{k=-\infty,\infty} x(t) \cdot \delta(t - kT_s) \tag{1.2}$$

Taking into account that convolution in time domain implies multiplication in frequency domain, we obtain

$$X_s(f) = X(f) \cdot I(f) = X(f) \cdot \frac{1}{T_s} \sum_{k=-\infty,\infty} \delta(f - kf_s) = \frac{1}{T_s} \sum_{k=-\infty,\infty} X(f - kf_s) \tag{1.3}$$

where $f_s = 1/T_s$ is the sampling frequency.

Thus, $X_s(f)$, that is, the Fourier transform of the sampled signal, is periodic and consists of a series of identical repeats of $X(f)$ centered around multiples of the sampling frequency, as depicted in Figure 1.2b and c. It is worth noting in Figure 1.2b that the frequency components of $X(f)$ placed above $f_s/2$ appears, when $f_s < 2f_b$, as folded back, summing up to the lower-frequency components. This phenomenon is known as aliasing (higher component look "alias" lower components). When aliasing occurs, the original information (Figure 1.2a) cannot be recovered because the frequency components of the original signal are irreversibly corrupted by the overlaps of the shifted versions of $X(f)$.

A visual inspection of Figure 1.2 allows one to observe that such frequency contamination can be avoided when the original signal is bandlimited ($X(f) = 0$, for $f > f_b$) and sampled at a frequency $f_s > 2f_b$. In this case, as shown in Figure 1.2c, no overlaps exist between adjacent reply of $X(f)$, and the original waveform can be retrieved by low-pass filtering the sampled signal (Oppenheim and Schafer, 1975). Such observations are the basis of the sampling theorem previously reported.

The hypothesis of a bandlimited signal is hardly verified in biomedical signals due to the signal characteristics or due to the effect of superimposed wideband noise. It is worth noting that filtering

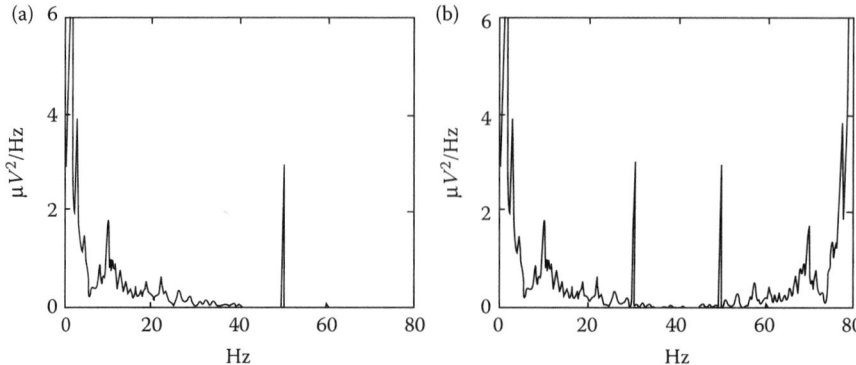

FIGURE 1.3 Power spectrum of an EEG signal (originally bandlimited up to 40 Hz). The presence of 50 Hz mains noise (a) causes aliasing error in the 30 Hz component (i.e., in the b diagnostic band) in the sampled signal (b) if $f_s = 80$ Hz.

before sampling is always needed even if we assume the incoming signal to be bandlimited. Let us consider the following example of an EEG signal whose frequency content of interest ranges between 0.5 and 40 Hz (the usual diagnostic bands are δ, 0.5–4 Hz; ϑ, 4–7 Hz; α, 8–13 Hz; β, 13–40 Hz). We may decide to sample it at 80 Hz, thus, literally respecting the Shannon theorem. If we do it without prefiltering, we could find some unpleasant results. Typically, the 50-Hz mains noise will replicate itself in the signal band (30 Hz, i.e., the β band), thus, corrupting irreversibly the information, which is of great interest from a physiologic and clinical point of view. The effect is shown in Figure 1.3a (before sampling) and Figure 1.3b (after sampling). Generally, it is advisable to sample at a frequency $>2f_b$ (Gardenhire, 1964) in order to take into account the nonideal behavior of the filter or the other preprocessing devices. Therefore, the prefiltering block of Figure 1.1 is always required to bandlimit the signal before sampling and to avoid aliasing errors.

1.1.2 Quantization Effects

The quantization produces a discrete signal (we indicate by n the discrete-time variable) whose samples can assume only certain values according to the way they are coded. Typical step functions for a uniform quantizer are reported in Figure 1.4a and b, where the quantization interval Δ between two quantization levels is evidenced in two cases, rounding and truncation, respectively.

Quantization is a heavily nonlinear procedure, but fortunately its effects can be statistically modeled. Figure 1.4c and d shows it; the nonlinear quantization block is substituted by a statistical model in which the error induced by quantization is treated as an additive noise $e(n)$ (*quantization error*) to the signal $x(n)$.

The following hypotheses are considered in order to deal with a simple mathematical problem:

1. $e(n)$ is supposed to be a white noise with uniform distribution
2. $e(n)$ and $x(n)$ are uncorrelated

First of all, it should be noted that the probability density of $e(n)$ changes according to the adopted coding procedure. If we decide to round the real sample to the nearest quantization level, we have $-\Delta/2 < \Psi e(n) < \Delta/2$, while if we decide to truncate the sample amplitude, we have $-\Delta\Psi e(n) < 0$. The two probability densities are plotted in Figure 1.4e and f.

The two ways of coding yield processes with different statistical properties. In the first case, the mean and variance value of $e(n)$ are

$$m_e = 0 \quad \sigma_e^2 = \Delta^2/12$$

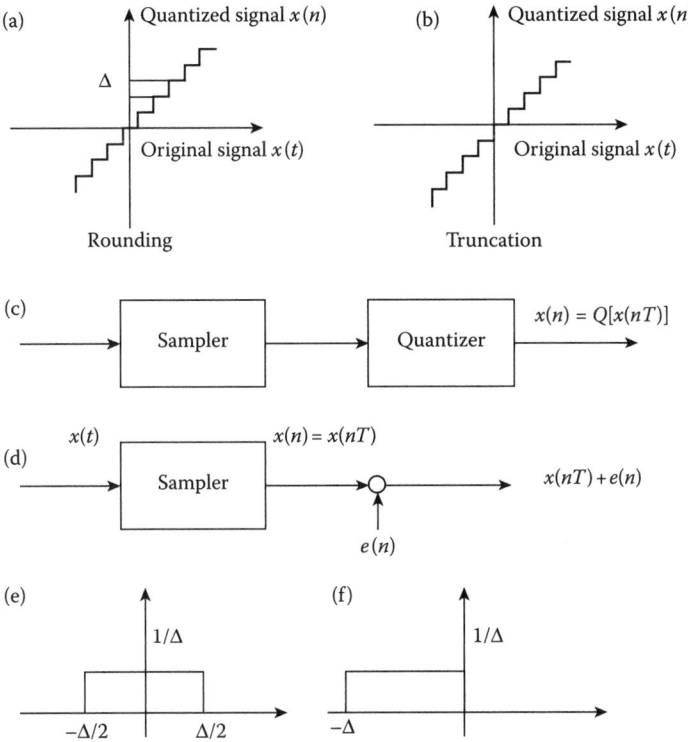

FIGURE 1.4 Nonlinear relationships for rounding (a) and truncation (b) quantization procedures. Description of quantization block (c) by a statistical model (d) and probability densities for the quantization noise $e(n)$ for rounding (e) and truncation (f). Δ is the quantization interval.

while in the second case, $m_e = -\Delta/2$, and the variance is still the same. Variance reduces in the presence of a reduced quantization interval as expected.

Finally, it is possible to evaluate the signal-to-noise ratio (SNR) for the quantization process:

$$\text{SNR} = 10\log_{10}\left(\frac{\sigma_x^2}{\sigma_e^2}\right) = 10\log_{10}\left(\frac{\sigma_x^2}{2^{-2b}/12}\right) = 6.02b + 10.79 + 10\log_{10}(\sigma_x^2) \tag{1.4}$$

having set $\Delta = 2^{-2b}$ and where σ_x^2 is the variance of the signal and b is the number of bits used for coding. It should be noted that the SNR increases by almost 6 dB for each added bit of coding. Several forms of quantization are usually employed: uniform, nonuniform (preceding the uniform sampler with a non-linear block), or roughly (small number of quantization levels and high quantization step). Details can be found in Carassa (1983), Jaeger (1982), and Widrow (1956).

1.2 Signal Processing

A brief review of different signal-processing techniques will be given in this section. They include traditional filtering, averaging techniques, and spectral estimators.

Only the main concepts of analysis and design of digital filters are presented, and a few examples are illustrated in the processing of the ECG signal. Averaging techniques will then be described briefly and their usefulness evidenced when noise and signal have similar frequency contents but different statistical properties; an example for evoked potentials enhancement from EEG background noise is illustrated.

Finally, different spectral estimators will be considered and some applications shown in the analysis of RR fluctuations (i.e., the heart rate variability (HRV) signal).

1.2.1 Digital Filters

A digital filter is a discrete-time system that operates some transformation on a digital input signal $x(n)$ generating an output sequence $y(n)$, as schematically shown by the block diagram in Figure 1.5. The characteristics of transformation $T[\cdot]$ identify the filter. The filter will be time-variant if $T[\cdot]$ is a function of time or time-invariant otherwise, while it is said to be *linear* if, and only if, having $x_1(n)$ and $x_2(n)$ as inputs producing $y_1(n)$ and $y_2(n)$, respectively, we have

$$T[ax_1 + bx_2] = aT[x_1] + bT[x_2] = ay_1 + by_2 \tag{1.5}$$

In the following, only linear, time-invariant filters will be considered, even if several interesting applications of nonlinear (Glaser and Ruchkin, 1976; Tompkins, 1993) or time-variant (Huta and Webster, 1973, 1987; Widrow et al., 1975; Cohen, 1983; Thakor, 1987; Sayed, 2003) filters have been proposed in the literature for the analysis of biologic signals.

The behavior of a filter is usually described in terms of input–output relationships. They are usually assessed by exciting the filter with different inputs and evaluating which is the response (output) of the system. In particular, if the input is the impulse sequence $\delta(n)$, the resulting output, the impulse response, has a relevant role in describing the characteristic of the filter. Such a response can be used to determine the response to more complicated input sequences. In fact, let us consider a generic input sequence $x(n)$ as a sum of weighted and delayed impulses

$$x(n) = \sum_{k=-\infty,\infty} x(k) \cdot \delta(n - k) \tag{1.6}$$

and let us identify the response to $\delta(n-k)$ as $h(n-k)$. If the filter is time-invariant, each delayed impulse will produce the same response, but time-shifted; due to the linearity property, such responses will be summed at the output:

$$y(n) = \sum_{k=-\infty,\infty} x(k) \cdot h(n - k) \tag{1.7}$$

This convolution product links input and output and defines the property of the filter. Two of them should be recalled: *stability* and *causality*. The former ensures that bounded (finite) inputs will produce bounded outputs (also called BIBO stability). Such a property can be deduced by the impulse response; it can be proved that the filter is stable if and only if

$$\sum_{k=-\infty,\infty} | h(k) | < \infty \tag{1.8}$$

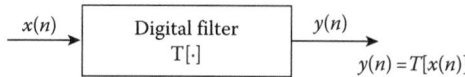

FIGURE 1.5 General block diagram of a digital filter. The output digital signal $y(n)$ is obtained from the input $x(n)$ by means of a transformation $T[\cdot]$ which identifies the filter.

Causality means that the filter will not respond to an input before the input is applied. This is in agreement with our physical concept of a system, but it is not strictly required for a digital filter that can be implemented in a noncausal form. A filter is causal if and only if

$$h(k) = 0 \quad \text{for } k < 0 \tag{1.8a}$$

Even if Equation 1.7 completely describes the properties of the filter, most often it is necessary to express the input–output relationships of linear discrete-time systems under the form of the *z*-transform operator, which allows one to express Equation 1.7 in a more useful, operative, and simpler form.

1.2.1.1 *z*-Transform

The *z*-transform of a sequence $x(n)$ is defined by (Rainer et al., 1972)

$$X(z) = \sum_{k=-\infty,\infty} x(k) \cdot z^{-k} \tag{1.9}$$

where *z* is a complex variable. This series will converge or diverge for different *z* values. The set of *z* values which makes Equation 1.9 converge is the *region of convergence*, and it depends on the series $x(n)$ considered.

Among the properties of the *z*-transform, we recall

- The delay (shift) property:

$$\text{If } w(n) = x(n - T), \quad \text{then } W(z) = X(z) \cdot z^{-T} \tag{1.9a}$$

- The product of convolution:

$$\text{If } w(n) = \sum_{k=-\infty,\infty} x(k) \cdot y(n - k), \quad \text{then } W(z) = X(z) \cdot Y(z) \tag{1.9b}$$

1.2.1.2 Transfer Function in z Domain

Thanks to the previous properties, we can express Equation 1.7 in the *z* domain as a simple multiplication:

$$Y(z) = H(z) \cdot X(z) \tag{1.10}$$

where $H(z)$, known as the *transfer function* of the filter, is the *z*-transform of the impulse response. $H(z)$ plays a relevant role in the analysis and design of digital filters. The response to input sinusoids can be evaluated as follows: assume a complex sinusoid $x(n) = e^{j\omega n T_s}$ as input; the corresponding filter output will be

$$y(n) = \sum_{k=0,\infty} h(k)e^{j\omega T_2 (n-k)} = e^{-j\omega n T_s} \sum_{k=0,\infty} h(k)e^{-j\omega k T_s} = x(n) \cdot H(z)\,|_{z=e^{j\omega T_s}} \tag{1.11}$$

Then a sinusoid in input is still the same sinusoid at the output, but multiplied by a complex quantity $H(\omega)$. Such a complex function defines the response of the filter for each sinusoid of ω pulse in input, and it is known as the frequency response of the filter. It is evaluated in the complex *z* plane by computing $H(z)$ for $z = e^{j\omega n T_s}$, namely, on the point locus that describes the unitary circle on the *z* plane ($|e^{j\omega n T_s}| = 1$).

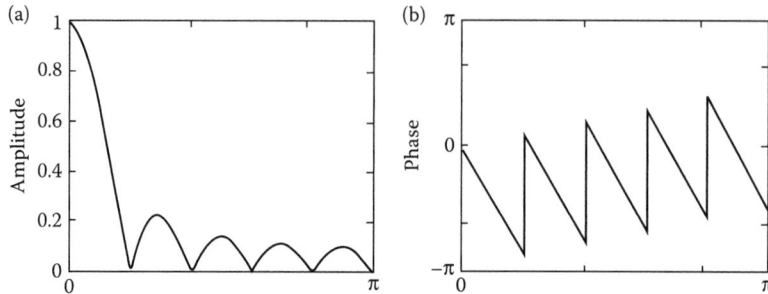

FIGURE 1.6 Modulus (a) and phase (b) diagrams of the frequency response of a moving average filter of order 5. Note that the frequency plots are depicted up to π. In fact, taking into account that we are dealing with a sampled signal whose frequency information is up to $f_s/2$, we have $\omega_{max} = 2\pi f_s/2 = \pi f_s$ or $\hat{\omega}_{max} = \pi$ if normalized with respect to the sampling rate, f_s.

As a complex function, $H(\omega)$ will be defined by its module $|H(\omega)|$ and by its phase $\angle H(\omega)$ functions, as shown in Figure 1.6 for a moving average filter of order 5. The figure indicates that the lower-frequency components will come through the filter almost unaffected, while the higher-frequency components will be drastically reduced. It is usual to express the horizontal axis of frequency response from 0 to π. This is obtained because only pulse frequencies up to $\omega_s/2$ are reconstructable (due to the Shannon theorem), and therefore, in the horizontal axis, the value of ωT_s is reported which goes from 0 to π. Furthermore, Figure 1.6b demonstrates that the phase is piecewise linear, and in correspondence with the zeroes of $|H(\omega)|$, there is a change in phase of π value. According to their frequency response, the filters are usually classified as (1) low-pass, (2) high-pass, (3) bandpass, or (4) bandstop filters. Figure 1.7 shows the ideal frequency response for such filters with the proper low- and high-frequency cutoffs.

For a large class of linear, time-invariant systems, $H(z)$ can be expressed in the following general form:

$$H(z) = \frac{\sum_{m=0,M} b_m z^{-m}}{1 + \sum_{k=1,N} a_k z^{-k}} \tag{1.12}$$

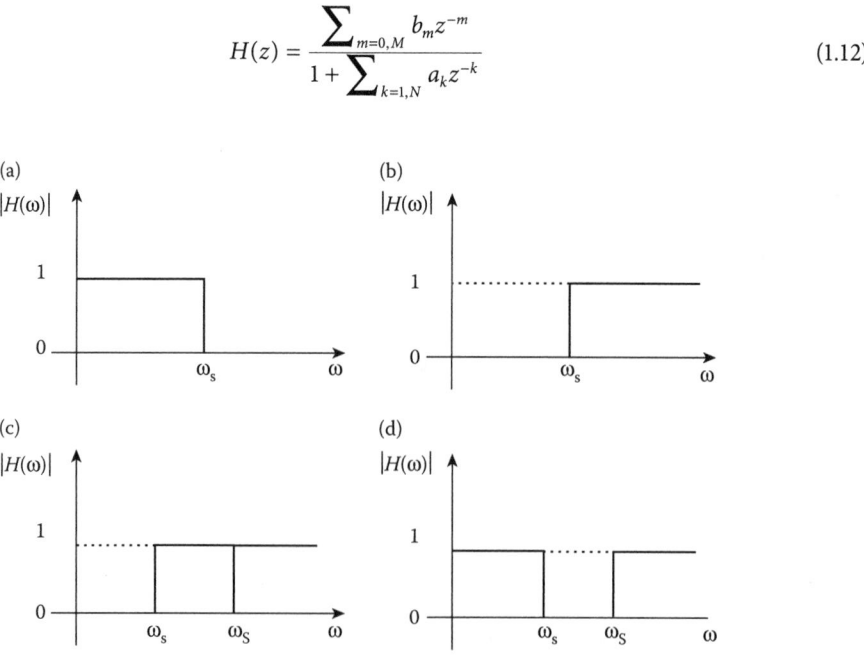

FIGURE 1.7 Ideal frequency–response moduli for low-pass (a), high-pass (b), bandpass (c), and bandstop filters (d).

which describes in the *z* domain the following *difference equation* in this discrete-time domain:

$$y(n) = - \sum_{k=1,N} a_k y(n-k) + \sum_{m=0,M} b_m x(n-m) \tag{1.13}$$

When at least one of the a_k coefficients is different from zero, some output values contribute to the current output. The filter contains some feedback, and it is said to be implemented in a recursive form. On the other hand, when the a_k values are all zero, the filter output is obtained only from the current or previous inputs, and the filter is said to be implemented in a *nonrecursive* form.

The transfer function can be expressed in a more useful form by finding the roots of both numerator and denominator:

$$H(z) = \frac{b_0 z^{N-M} \prod_{m=1,M} (z - z_m)}{\prod_{k=1,N} (z - p_k)} \tag{1.14}$$

where z_m are the zeroes and p_k are the poles. It is worth noting that $H(z)$ presents $N - M$ zeroes in correspondence with the origin of the *z* plane and *M* zeroes elsewhere (*N* zeroes totally) and *N* poles. The pole-zero form of $H(z)$ is of great interest because several properties of the filter are immediately available from the geometry of poles and zeroes in the complex *z* plane. In fact, it is possible to easily assess stability and by visual inspection to roughly estimate the frequency response without making any calculations.

Stability is verified when all poles lie inside the unitary circle, as can be proved by considering the relationships between the *z*-transform and the Laplace *s*-transform and by observing that the left side of the *s* plane is mapped inside the unitary circle (Oppenheim and Schafer, 1975; Jackson, 1986).

The frequency response can be estimated by noting that $(z - z_m)|_{z=e^{j\omega n T_s}}$ is a vector joining the *m*th zero with the point on the unitary circle identified by the angle ωT_s. Defining

$$\begin{aligned} \vec{B}_m &= (z - z_m)\,|_{z=e^{j\omega T_s}} \\ \vec{A}_k &= (z - p_k)\,|_{z=e^{j\omega T_s}} \end{aligned} \tag{1.15}$$

we obtain

$$\begin{aligned} |H(\omega)| &= \frac{b_0 \Pi_{m=1,M} |\vec{B}_m|}{\Pi_{k=1,N} |\vec{A}_k|} \\ \angle H(\omega) &= \sum_{m=1,M} \angle \vec{B}_m - \sum_{k=1,N} \angle \vec{A}_k + (N-M)\omega T_s \end{aligned} \tag{1.16}$$

Thus, the modulus of $H(\omega)$ can be evaluated at any frequency $\omega°$ by computing the distances between poles and zeroes and the point on the unitary circle corresponding to $\omega = \omega°$, as evidenced in Figure 1.8, where a filter with two pairs of complex poles and three zeroes is considered.

To obtain the estimate of $H(\omega)$, we move around the unitary circle and roughly evaluate the effect of poles and zeroes by keeping in mind a few rules (Challis and Kitney, 1982) (1) when we are close to a zero, $|H(\omega)|$ will approach zero, and a positive phase shift will appear in $\angle H(\omega)$ as the vector from the zero reverses its angle; (2) when we are close to a pole, $|H(\omega)|$ will tend to peak, and a negative phase change is found in $\angle H(\omega)$ (the closer the pole to unitary circle, the sharper is the peak until it reaches infinite and the filter becomes unstable); and (3) near a closer pole-zero pair, the response modulus will

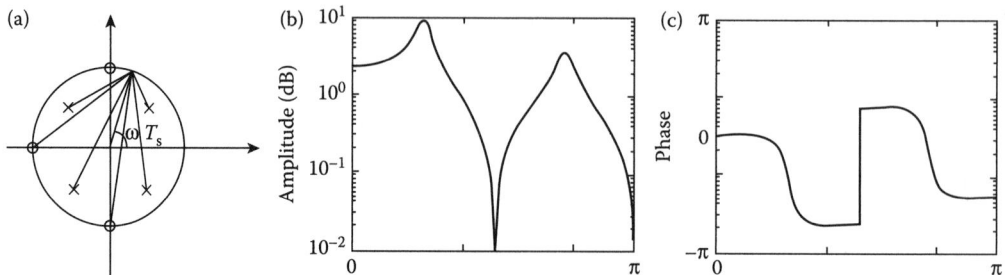

FIGURE 1.8 Poles and zeroes geometry (a); relative frequency response modulus (b); and phase (c) characteristics. Moving around the unitary circle a rough estimation of $|H(\omega)|$ and $\angle H(\omega)$ can be obtained. Note the zeroes' effects at π and $\pi/2$ and modulus rising in proximity of the poles. Phase shifts are clearly evident in part (c) closer to zeroes and poles.

tend to zero or infinity if the zero or the pole is closer, while far from this pair, the modulus can be considered unitary. As an example, it is possible to compare the modulus and phase diagram of Figure 1.8b and c with the relative geometry of the poles and zeroes of Figure 1.8a.

1.2.1.3 FIR and IIR Filters

A common way of classifying digital filters is based on the characteristics of their impulse response. For finite impulse response (FIR) filters, $h(n)$ is composed of a finite number of nonzero values, while for infinite impulse response (IIR) filters, $h(n)$ oscillates up to infinity with nonzero values. It is clearly evident that in order to obtain an infinite response to an impulse in input, the IIR filter must contain some feedback that sustains the output as the input vanishes. The presence of feedback paths requires putting particular attention to the filter stability.

Even if FIR filters are usually implemented in a nonrecursive form and IIR filters in a recursive form, the two ways of classification are not coincident. In fact, as shown by the following example, an FIR filter can be expressed in a recursive form:

$$H(z) = \sum_{k=0,N-1} z^{-k} = \sum_{k=0,N-1} z^{-k} \frac{(1-z^{-1})}{(1-z^{-1})} = \frac{1-z^{-N}}{1-z^{-1}} \tag{1.17}$$

for a more convenient computational implementation.

As shown previously, two important requirements for filters are stability and linear phase response. FIR filters can be easily designed to fulfill such requirements; they are always stable (having no poles outside the origin), and the linear phase response is obtained by constraining the impulse response coefficients to have symmetry around their midpoint. Such constrain implies

$$b_m = \pm b_{M-m}^{\bullet} \tag{1.18}$$

where the b_m are the M coefficients of an FIR filter. The sign + or − stays in accordance with the symmetry (even or odd) and M value (even or odd). This is a necessary and sufficient condition for FIR filters to have linear phase response. Two cases of impulse response that yield a linear phase filter are shown in Figure 1.9.

It should be noted that Equation 1.18 imposes geometric constrains to the zero locus of $H(z)$. Taking into account Equation 1.12, we have

$$z^M H(z) = H\left(\frac{1}{z^*}\right)z \tag{1.19}$$

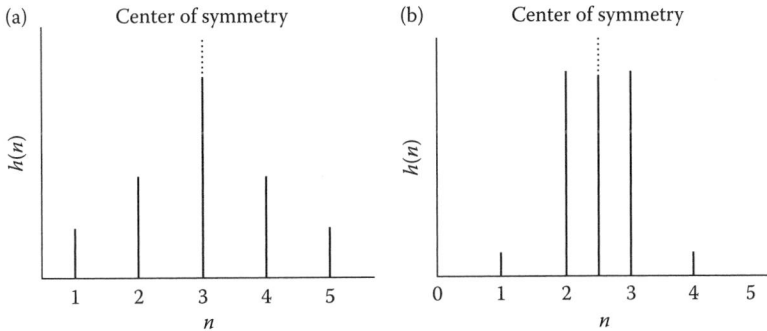

FIGURE 1.9 Examples of impulse response for linear phase FIR filters: odd (a) and even (b) number of coefficients.

Thus, both z_m and $1/z_m^*$ must be zeroes of $H(z)$. Then the zeroes of linear phase FIR filters must lie on the unitary circle, or they must appear in pairs and with inverse moduli.

1.2.1.4 Design Criteria

In many cases, the filter is designed in order to satisfy some requirements, usually on the frequency response, which depend on the characteristic of the particular application the filter is intended for. It is known that ideal filters, like those reported in Figure 1.7, are not physically realizable (they would require an infinite number of coefficients of impulse response); thus, we can design FIR or IIR filters that can only mimic, with an acceptable error, the ideal response. Figure 1.10 shows a frequency response of a nonideal low-pass filter. Here, there are ripples in passband and in stopband, and there is a transition band from passband to stopband, defined by the interval $\omega_s–\omega_p$.

Several design techniques are available, and some of them require heavy computational tasks, which are capable of developing filters with defined specific requirements. They include window technique, frequency-sampling method, or equiripple design for FIR filters. Butterworth, Chebychev, elliptical design, and impulse-invariant or bilinear transformation are instead employed for IIR filters. For detailed analysis of digital filter techniques, see Antoniou (1979), Cerutti (1983), and Oppenheim and Schafer (1975).

1.2.1.5 Examples

A few examples of different kinds of filters will be presented in the following, showing some applications on ECG signal processing. It is shown that the ECG contains relevant information over a wide range of

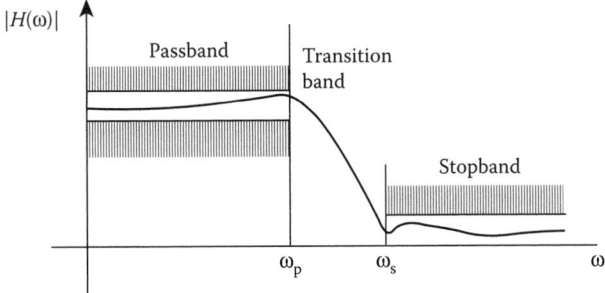

FIGURE 1.10 Amplitude response for a real low-pass filter. Ripples are admitted in both passband and stopband, but they are constrained into restricted areas. Limitations are also imposed to the width of the transition band.

frequencies; the lower-frequency contents should be preserved for correct measurement of the slow ST displacements, while higher-frequency contents are needed to correctly estimate amplitude and duration of the faster contributions, mainly at the level of the QRS complex. Unfortunately, several sources of noise are present in the same frequency band, such as higher-frequency noise due to muscle contraction (EMG noise), the lower-frequency noise due to motion artifacts (baseline wandering), the effect of respiration or the low-frequency noise in the skin–electrode interface, and others.

In the first example, the effect of two different low-pass filters will be considered. An ECG signal corrupted by an EMG noise (Figure 1.11a) is low-pass filtered by two different low-pass filters whose frequency responses are shown in Figure 1.11b and c. The two FIR filters have cutoff frequencies at 40 and 20 Hz, respectively, and were designed through window techniques (Weber–Cappellini window, filter length = 256 points) (Cappellini et al., 1978), and result more aggressive in respect to the recommended diagnostic bandwidth (0.5–200 Hz).

The output signals are shown in Figure 1.11d and e. The two drastic filterings here indicated reduce the superimposed noise but at the same time alter the original ECG waveform. In particular, the *R* wave amplitude is progressively reduced by decreasing the cutoff frequency, and the QRS width is progressively increased as well. On the other hand, *P* waves appear almost unaffected, having frequency components generally lower than 20 Hz. At this point, it is worth noting that an increase in QRS duration is generally associated with various pathologies, such as ventricular hypertrophy or bundle-branch block. It is, therefore, necessary to check that an excessive band limitation does not introduce a false-positive indication in the diagnosis of the ECG signal.

An example of an application for stopband filters (*notch filters*) is presented in Figure 1.12. It is used to reduce the 50-Hz mains noise on the ECG signal, and it was designated by placing a zero in corresponding to the frequency we want to suppress.

Finally, an example of a high-pass filter is shown for the detection of the QRS complex. Detecting the time occurrence of a fiducial point in the QRS complex is indeed the first task usually performed in ECG signal analysis. The QRS complex usually contains the higher-frequency components with respect to the other ECG waves, and thus, such components will be enhanced by a high-pass filter. Figure 1.13 shows

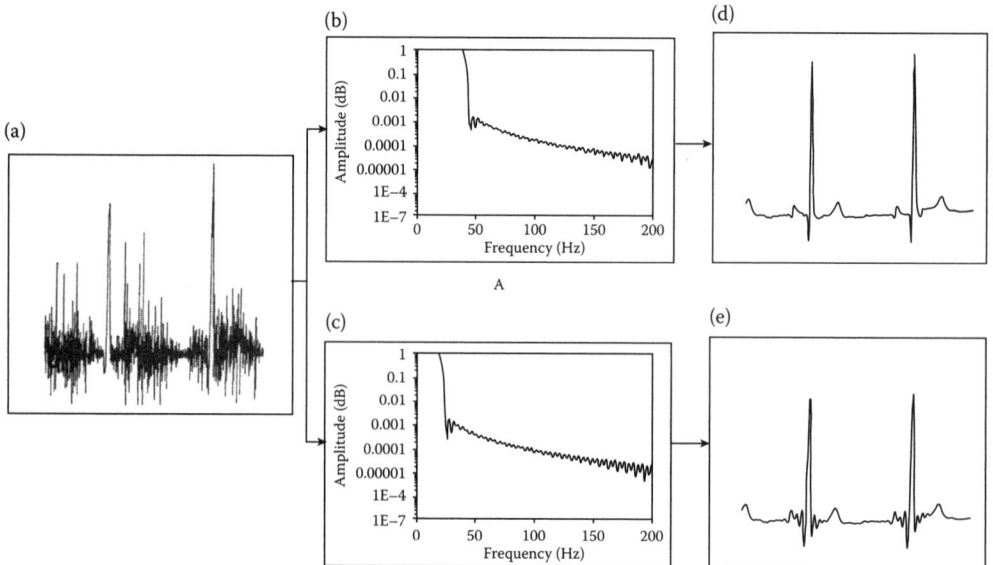

FIGURE 1.11 Effects of two different low-pass filters (b) and (c) on an ECG trace (a) corrupted by EMG noise. The resulting filtered signal is shown in panel (d) and (e). Both amplitude reduction and variation in the QRS induced by too drastic low-pass filtering are evidenced.

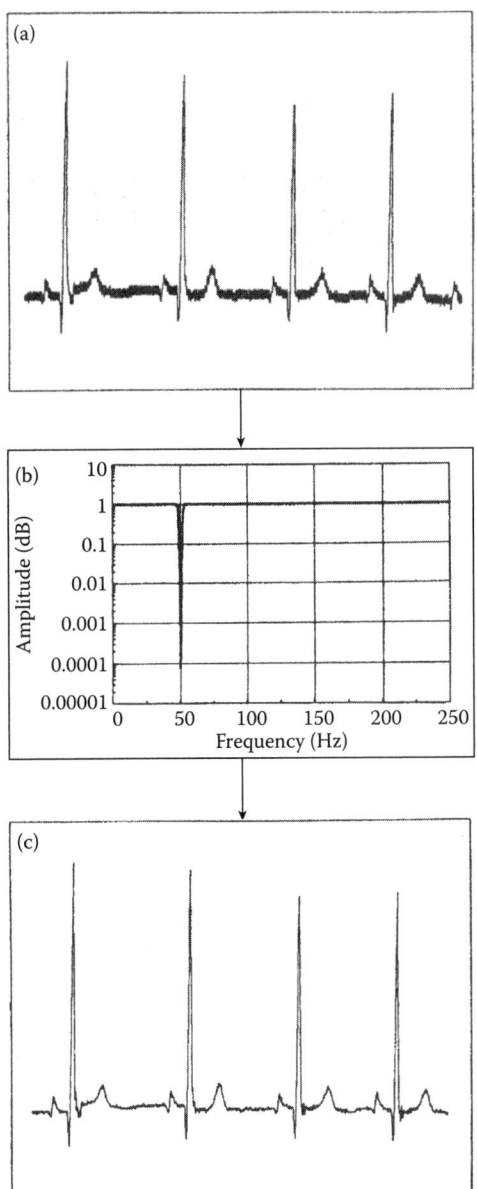

FIGURE 1.12 A 50-Hz noisy ECG signal (a); a 50-Hz rejection filter (b); and a filtered signal (c).

how QRS complexes (Figure 1.13a) can be identified by a derivative high-pass filter with a cutoff frequency to decrease the effect of the noise contributions at high frequencies (Figure 1.13b). The filtered signal (Figure 1.13c) presents sharp and well-defined peaks that are easily recognized as QRS occurrences by a threshold value.

1.2.2 Signal Averaging

Traditional filtering performs very well when the frequency content of signal and noise do not overlap. When the noise bandwidth is completely separated from the signal bandwidth, the noise can be

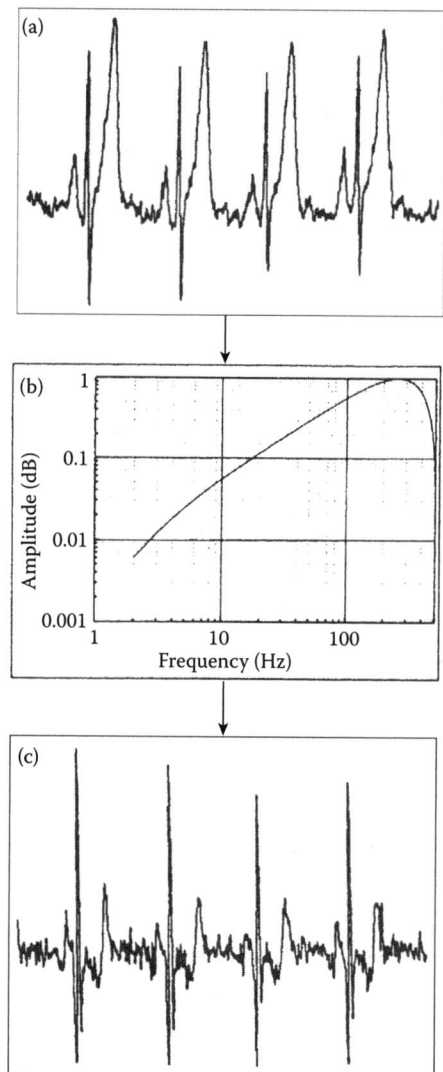

FIGURE 1.13   Effect of a derivative high-pass filter (b) on an ECG lead (a). The output of the filter (c).

decreased easily by means of a linear filter according to the procedures described earlier. On the other hand, when the signal and noise bandwidth overlap and the noise amplitude is enough to seriously corrupt the signal, a traditional filter, designed to cancel the noise, also will introduce signal cancellation or, at least, distortion. As an example, let us consider the brain potentials evoked by a sensory stimulation (visual, acoustic, or somatosensory) generally called evoked potentials (EP). Such a response is very difficult to be determined because its amplitude is generally much lower than the background EEG activity. Both EP and EEG signals contain information in the same frequency range; thus, the problem of separating the desired response cannot be approached via traditional digital filtering (Aunon et al., 1981). Another typical example is in the detection of ventricular late potentials (VLP) in the ECG signal. These potentials are very small in amplitude and are comparable with the noise superimposed on the signal and also for what concerns the frequency content (Simson, 1981). In such cases, an increase in the SNR may be achieved on the basis of different statistical properties of signal and noise.

When the desired signal repeats identically at each iteration (i.e., the EP at each sensory stimulus, the VLP at each cardiac cycle), the averaging technique can satisfactorily solve the problem of separating signal from noise. This technique sums a set of temporal epochs of the signal together with the superimposed noise. If the time epochs are properly aligned, through efficient trigger-point recognition, the signal waveforms directly sum together. If the signal and the noise are characterized by the following statistical properties:

1. All the signal epochs contain a deterministic signal component $x(n)$ that does not vary for all the epochs.
2. The superimposed noise $w(n)$ is a broadband stationary process with zero mean and variance σ^2 so that

$$E[w(n)] = 0$$
$$E[w^2(n)] = \sigma^2 \tag{1.20}$$

3. Signal $x(n)$ and noise $w_i(n)$ are uncorrelated so that the recorded signal $y(n)$ at the ith iteration can be expressed as

$$y(n)_i = x(n) + w_i(n) \tag{1.21}$$

then the averaging process yields y_t:

$$y_t(n) = \frac{1}{N}\sum_{i=1}^{N} y_i = x(n) + \sum_{i=1}^{N} w_i(n) \tag{1.22}$$

The noise term is an estimate of the mean by taking the average of N realizations. Such an average is a new random variable that has the same mean of the sum terms (zero in this case) and which has a variance of σ^2/N. The effect of the coherent averaging procedure is then to maintain the amplitude of the signal and reduce the variance of the noise by a factor of N. In order to evaluate the improvement in the SNR (in rms value) in respect to the SNR (at the generic ith sweep):

$$SNR = SNR_i \cdot \sqrt{N} \tag{1.23}$$

Thus, signal averaging improves the SNR by a factor of $\sqrt{N}$ in rms value.

A coherent averaging procedure can be viewed as a digital filtering process, and its frequency characteristics can be investigated. From Equation 1.17 through the z-transform, the transfer function of the filtering operation results in

$$H(z) = \frac{1 + z^{-h} + z^{-2h} + L + z^{-(N-1)h}}{N} \tag{1.24}$$

where N is the number of elements in the average and h is the number of samples in each response. An alternative expression for $H(z)$ is

$$H(z) = \frac{1}{N}\frac{1 - z^{Nh}}{1 - z^h} \tag{1.25}$$

This is a moving average low-pass filter as discussed earlier, where the output is a function of the preceding value with a lag of h samples; in practice, the filter operates not on the time sequence but in the sweep sequence on corresponding samples.

The frequency response of the filter is shown in Figure 1.14 for different values of the parameter N. In this case, the sampling frequency f_s is the repetition frequency of the sweeps, and we may assume it to be 1 without loss of generality. The frequency response is characterized by a main lobe with the first zero

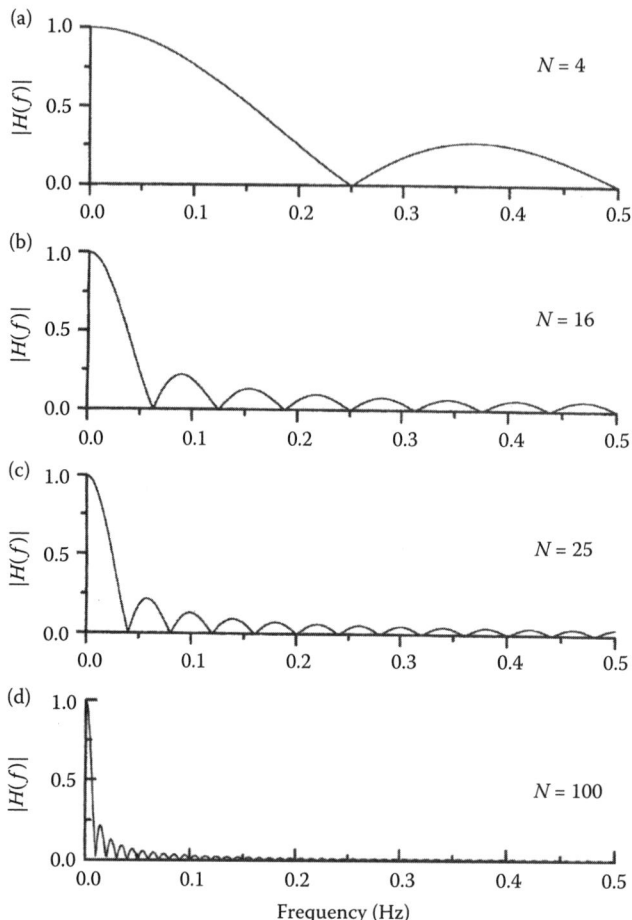

FIGURE 1.14 Equivalent frequency response for the signal-averaging procedure for different values of N. From (a) to (d) N increases.

corresponding to $f = 1/N$ and by successive secondary lobes separated by zeroes at intervals $1/N$. The width of each tooth decreases as well as the amplitude of the secondary lobes when increasing the number N of sweeps.

The desired signal is sweep-invariant, and it will be unaffected by the filter, while the broadband noise will be decreased. Some leakage of noise energy takes place in the center of the sidelobes and, of course, at zero frequency. Under the hypothesis of zero mean noise, the dc component has no effect, and the diminishing sidelobe amplitude implies the leakage to be not relevant for high frequencies. It is important to recall that the average filtering is based on the hypothesis of broadband distribution of the noise and lack of correlation between signal and noise. Unfortunately, these assumptions are not always verified in biologic signals. For example, the assumptions of independence of the background EEG and the evoked potential may be not completely realistic (Gevins and Remond, 1987). In addition, much attention must be paid to the alignment of the sweeps; in fact, slight misalignments (fiducial point jitter) will lead to a low-pass filtering effect of the final result.

1.2.2.1 Example

As mentioned previously, one of the fields in which signal-averaging technique is employed extensively is in the evaluation of cerebral evoked response after a sensory stimulation. Figure 1.15 shows the EEG recorded from the scalp of a normal subject after a somatosensory stimulation released at time $t = 0$. The

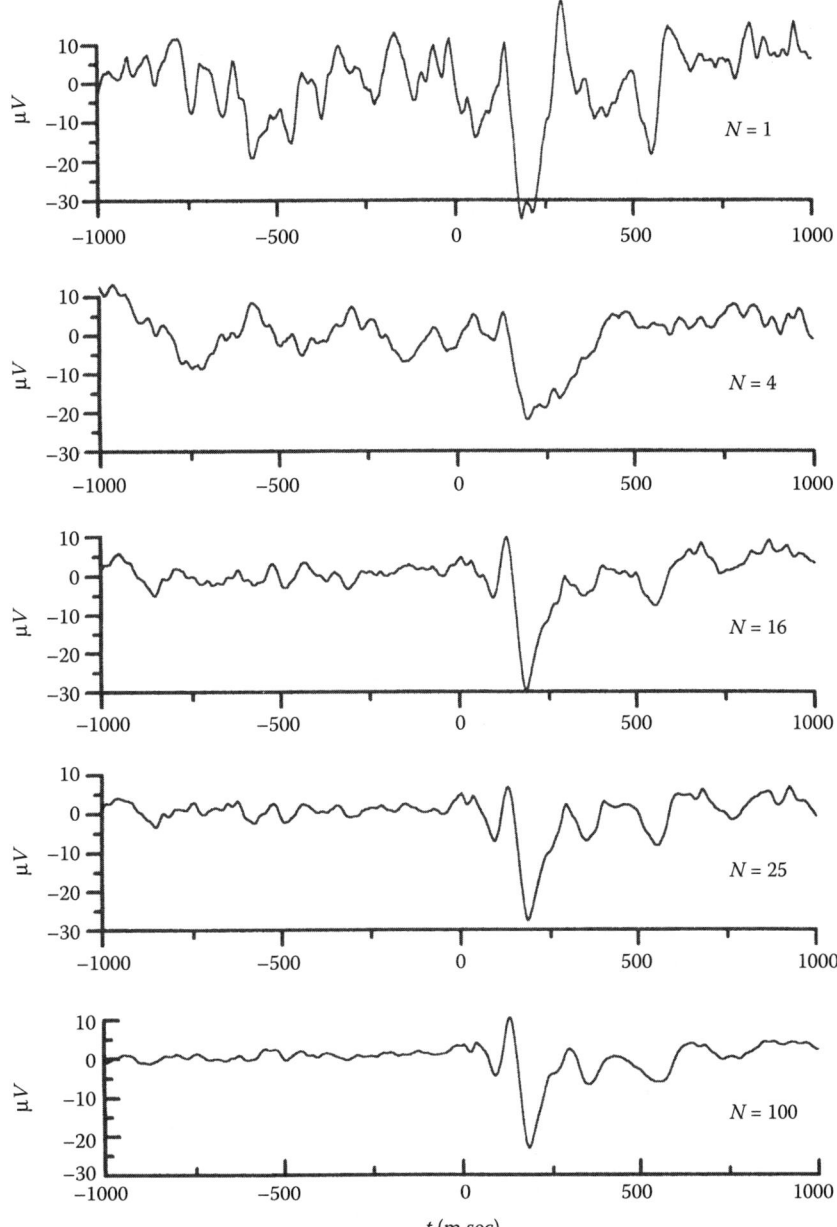

FIGURE 1.15 Enhancement of evoked potential (EP) by means of averaging technique. The EEG noise is progressively reduced, and the EP morphology becomes more recognizable as the number of averaged sweeps (N) is increased.

evoked potential ($N = 1$) is not visible because it is buried in the background EEG (upper panel). In the successive panels, there is the same evoked potential after averaging different numbers of sweeps corresponding to the frequency responses shown in Figure 1.14. As N increases, the SNR is improved by a factor $\sqrt{N}$ (in rms value), and the morphology of the evoked potential becomes more recognizable while the EEG contribution is markedly diminished. In this way, it is easy to evaluate the quantitative indices of clinical interest, such as the amplitude and the latency of the relevant waves.

1.2.3 Spectral Analysis

The various methods to estimate the power spectrum density (PSD) of a signal may be classified as *nonparametric* and *parametric*.

1.2.3.1 Nonparametric Estimators of PSD

This is a traditional method of frequency analysis based on the Fourier transform that can be evaluated easily through the fast Fourier transform (FFT) algorithm (Marple, 1987). The expression of the PSD as a function of the frequency $P(f)$ can be obtained directly from the time series $y(n)$ by using the periodogram expression

$$P(f) = \frac{1}{T_s} \left| T_s \sum_{k=0}^{N-1} y(k) e^{-j2\pi f k T_s} \right|^2 = \frac{1}{NT_s} |Y(f)|^2 \tag{1.26}$$

where T_s is the sampling period, N is the number of samples, and $Y(f)$ is the discrete-time Fourier transform of $y(n)$.

On the basis of the Wiener–Khintchin theorem, PSD is also obtainable in two steps from the FFT of the autocorrelation function $\hat{R}_{yy}(k)$ of the signal, which is estimated by means of the following expression:

$$\hat{R}_{yy}(k) = \frac{1}{N} \sum_{i=0}^{N-k-1} y(i) y^*(i+k) \tag{1.27}$$

where * denotes the complex conjugate. Thus, the PSD is expressed as

$$P(f) = T_s \cdot \sum_{k=-N}^{N} \hat{R}_{yy}(k) e^{-j2\pi f k T_s} \tag{1.28}$$

based on the available lag estimates $\hat{R}_{yy}(k)$, where $-(1/2T_s) \leq f \leq (1/2T_s)$.

FFT-based methods are widely diffused, for their easy applicability, computational speed, and direct interpretation of the results. Quantitative parameters are obtained by evaluating the power contribution at different frequency bands. This is achieved by dividing the frequency axis in ranges of interest and by integrating the PSD on such intervals. The area under this portion of the spectrum is the fraction of the total signal variance due to the specific frequencies. However, autocorrelation function and Fourier transform are theoretically defined on infinite data sequences. Thus, errors are introduced by the need to operate on finite data records in order to obtain estimators of the true functions. In addition, for the finite data set, it is necessary to make assumptions, sometimes not realistic, about the data outside the recording window; commonly, they are considered to be zero. This implicit rectangular windowing of the data results in a special leakage in the PSD. Different windows that smoothly connect the side samples to zero are most often used in order to solve this problem, even if they may introduce a reduction in the frequency resolution (Harris, 1978). Furthermore, the estimators of the signal PSD are not statistically consistent, and various techniques are needed to improve their statistical performances. Various methods are mentioned in the literature; the methods of Dariell (1946), Bartlett (1948), and Welch (1970) are the most diffused ones. Of course, all these procedures cause a further reduction in frequency resolution.

1.2.3.2 Parametric Estimators

Parametric approaches assume the time series under analysis to be the output of a given mathematical model, and no drastic assumptions are made about the data outside the recording window. The

PSD is calculated as a function of the model parameters according to appropriate expressions. A critical point in this approach is the choice of an adequate model to represent the data sequence. The model is completely independent of the physiologic, anatomic, and physical characteristics of the biologic system but simply provides the input–output relationships of the process in the so-called black-box approach.

Among the numerous possibilities of modeling, linear models, characterized by a rational transfer function, are able to describe a wide number of different processes. In the most general case, they are represented by the following linear equation that relates the input-driving signal $w(k)$ and the output of an autoregressive moving average (ARMA) process:

$$y(k) = -\sum_{i=1}^{p} a_i y(k-i) + \sum_{j=1}^{q} b_j w(k-j) + w(k) \tag{1.29}$$

where $w(k)$ is the input white noise with zero mean value and variance λ^2, p and q are the orders of AR and MA parts, respectively, and a_i and b_j are the proper coefficients.

The ARMA model may be reformulated as an AR or an MA if the coefficients b_j or a_i are, respectively, set to zero. Since the estimation of the AR parameters results in linear equations, AR models are usually employed in place of ARMA or MA models, also on the basis of the Wold decomposition theorem (Marple, 1987) that establishes that any stationary ARMA or MA process of finite variance can be represented as a unique AR model of appropriate order, even infinite; likewise, any ARMA or AR process can be represented by an MA model of sufficiently high order.

The AR PSD is then obtained from the following expression:

$$P(f) = \frac{\lambda T^2}{\left|1 + \sum_{1}^{p} a_k z^{-k}\right|^2_{\exp(j2\pi fT_s)}} = \frac{\lambda T^2}{\left|\prod_{1}^{p} (z - z_l)\right|^2_{\exp(j2\pi fT_s)}} \tag{1.30}$$

The right side of the relation puts into evidence the poles of the transfer function that can be plotted in the z-transform plane. Figure 1.16b shows the PSD function of the HRV signal depicted in Figure 1.16a, while Figure 1.16c displays the corresponding pole diagram obtained according to the procedure described in the preceding section.

Parametric methods are methodologically and computationally more complex than the nonparametric ones since they require an *a priori* choice of the structure and of the order of the model of the signal-generation mechanism. Some tests are required *a posteriori* to verify the whiteness of the prediction error, such as the Anderson test (autocorrelation test) (Box and Jenkins, 1976) in order to test the reliability of the estimation.

Postprocessing of the spectra can be performed as well for nonparametric approaches by integrating the $P(f)$ function in predefined frequency ranges; however, the AR modeling has the advantage of allowing a spectral decomposition for a direct and automatic calculation of the power and frequency of each spectral component. In the z-transform domain, the autocorrelation function (ACF) $R(k)$ and the $P(z)$ of the signal are related by the following expression:

$$R(k) = \frac{1}{2\pi j} \int_{|z|=1} P(z) z^{k-1} \, dz \tag{1.31}$$

If the integral is calculated by means of the residual method, the ACF is decomposed into a sum of dumped sinusoids, each one related to a pair of complex conjugate poles, and of dumped exponential functions, related to the real poles (Zetterberg, 1969). The Fourier transform of each one of these terms

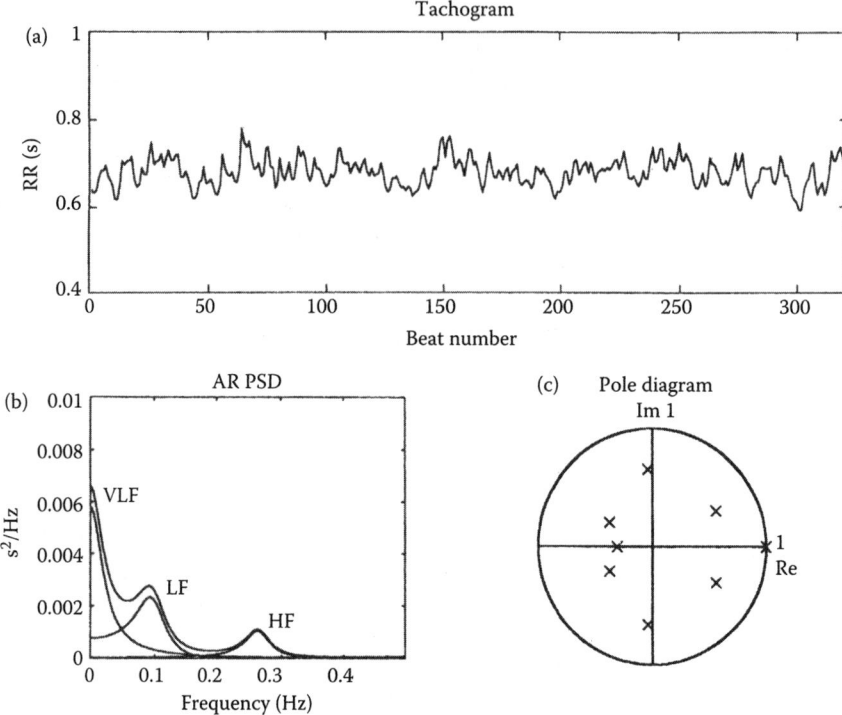

FIGURE 1.16 (a) Interval tachogram obtained from an ECG recording as the sequence of the RR time intervals expressed in seconds as a function of the beat number. (b) PSD of the signal (a) evaluated by means of an AR model (see text). (c) Pole diagram of the PSD shown in (b).

gives the expression of each spectral component that fits the component related to the relevant pole or pole pair. The argument of the pole gives the central frequency of the component, while the ith spectral component power is the residual γ_i in the case of real poles and $2\text{Re}(\gamma_i)$ in case of conjugate pole pairs. γ_i is computed from the following expression:

$$\gamma_i = z^{-1}(z - z_i)P(z)\,\big|_{z=z_i}$$

It is advisable to point out the basic characteristics of the two approaches that have been described above: the nonparametric and the parametric. The latter (parametric) has evident advantages with respect to the former, which can be summarized in the following:

- It has a more statistical consistency even on short segments of data, that is, under certain assumptions, a spectrum estimated through autoregressive modeling is a maximum entropy spectrum (MES).
- The spectrum is more easily interpretable with an "implicit" filtering of what is considered random noise.
- An easy and more reliable calculation of the spectral parameters (postprocessing of the spectrum), through the spectral decomposition procedure, is possible. Such parameters are directly interpretable from a physiologic point of view.
- There is no need to window the data in order to decrease the spectral leakage.
- The frequency resolution does not depend on the number of data.

On the other hand, the parametric approach

- Is more complex from a methodologic and computational point of view
- Requires an *a priori* definition of the kind of model (AR, MA, ARMA, or other) to be fitted and mainly its complexity defined (i.e., the number of parameters)

Some figures of merit introduced in the literature may be of help in determining their value (Akaike, 1974). Still, this procedure may be difficult in some cases.

1.2.3.3 Example

As an example, let us consider the frequency analysis of the HRV signal. In Figure 1.16a, the time sequence of the RR intervals obtained from an ECG recording is shown. The RR intervals are expressed in seconds as a function of the beat number in the so-called interval tachogram. It is worth noting that the RR series is not constant but is characterized by oscillations of up to 10% of its mean value. These oscillations are not causal but are the effect of the action of the autonomic nervous system in controlling heart rate. In particular, the frequency analysis of such a signal (Figure 1.16b shows the PSD obtained by means of an AR model) has evidenced three principal contributions in the overall variability of the HRV signal. A very low frequency (VLF) component is due to the long-term regulation mechanisms that cannot be resolved by analyzing a few minutes of signal (3–5 min are generally studied in the traditional spectral analysis of the HRV signal). Other techniques are needed for a complete understanding of such mechanisms. The low-frequency (LF) component is centered around 0.1 Hz, in a range between 0.03 and 0.15 Hz. An increase in its power has always been observed in relation to sympathetic activations. Finally, the high-frequency (HF) component, in synchrony with the respiration rate, is due to the respiration activity mediated by the vagus nerve; thus, it can be a marker of vagal activity. In particular, LF and HF power, both in absolute and in normalized units (i.e., as percentage value on the total power without the VLF contribution), and their ratio LF/HF are quantitative indices widely employed for the quantification of the sympathovagal balance in controlling heart rate (Malliani et al., 1991; Task Force, 1996).

1.3 Conclusion

The basic aspects of signal acquisition and processing have been illustrated, intended as fundamental tools for the treatment of biologic signals. A few examples also were reported relative to the ECG signal, as well as EEG signals and EPs. Particular processing algorithms have been described that use digital filtering techniques, coherent averaging, and power spectrum analysis as reference examples on how traditional or innovative techniques of digital signal processing may impact the phase of informative parameter extraction from biologic signals. They may improve the knowledge of many physiologic systems as well as help clinicians in dealing with new quantitative parameters that could better discriminate between normal and pathologic cases.

Defining Terms

Aliasing: Phenomenon that takes place when, in A/D conversion, the sampling frequency f_s is lower than twice the frequency content f_b of the signal; frequency components above $f_s/2$ are folded back and are summed to the lower-frequency components, distorting the signal.

Averaging: Filtering technique based on the summation of N stationary waveforms buried in casual broadband noise with a synchronization trigger. The SNR is improved by a factor of $\sqrt{N}$.

Frequency response: A complex quantity that, multiplied by a sinusoid input of a linear filter, gives the output sinusoid. It completely characterizes the filter and is the Fourier transform of the impulse response.

Impulse reaction: Output of a digital filter when the input is the impulse sequence $d(n)$. It completely characterizes linear filters and is used for evaluating the output corresponding to different kinds of inputs.

Notch filter: A stopband filter whose stopped band is very sharp and narrow.

Parametric methods: Spectral estimation methods based on the identification of a signal-generating model. The power spectral density is a function of the model parameters.

Quantization error: Error added to the signal, during the A/D procedure, due to the fact that the analog signal is represented by a digital signal that can assume only a limited and predefined set of values.

Region of convergence: In the z-transform plane, the ensemble containing the z complex points that makes a series converge to a finite value.

References

Akaike H. 1974. A new look at the statistical model identification. *IEEE Trans. Autom. Contr.* (AC-19): 716.

Antoniou A. 1979. *Digital Filters: Analysis and Design*. New York, McGraw-Hill.

Aunon J.L., McGillim C.D., and Childers D.G. 1981. Signal processing in evoked potential research: Averaging and modeling. *CRC Crit. Rev. Bioeng.* 5: 323.

Bartlett M.S. 1948. Smoothing periodograms from time series with continuous spectra. *Nature* 61: 686.

Box G.E.P. and Jenkins G.M. 1976. *Time Series Analysis: Forecasting and Control*. San Francisco, Holden-Day.

Cappellini V., Constantinides A.G., and Emiliani P. 1978. *Digital Filters and Their Applications*. London, Academic Press.

Carassa F. 1983. *Comunicazioni Elettriche*. Torino, Boringhieri.

Cerutti S. 1983. *Filtri numerici per l'eleborazione di segnali biologici*. Milano, CLUP.

Challis R.E. and Kitney R.I. 1982. The design of digital filters for biomedical signal processing: 1. Basic concepts. *J. Biomed. Eng.* 5: 267.

Cobbold R.S.C. 1988. *Transducers for Biomedical Measurements*. New York, John Wiley & Sons.

Cohen A. 1983. *Biomedical Signal Processing: Time and Frequency Domains Analysis*. Boca Raton, FL, CRC Press.

Dariell P.J. 1946. On the theoretical specification and sampling properties of autocorrelated time-series (discussion). *J. R. Stat. Soc.* 8: 88.

Gardenhire L.W. 1964. Selecting sample rate. *ISA J.* 4:59.

Gevins A.S. and Remond A. (eds). 1987. *Handbook of Electrophysiology and Clinical Neurophysiology*. Amsterdam, Elsevier.

Glaser E.M. and Ruchkin D.S. 1976. *Principles of Neurophysiological Signal Processing*. New York, Academic Press.

Harris F.J. 1978. On the use of windows for harmonic analysis with the discrete Fourier transform. *Proc. IEEE* 64: 51.

Huta K. and Webster J.G. 1973. 60-Hz interference in electrocardiography. *IEEE Trans. Biomed. Eng.* 20: 91.

Jackson L.B. 1986. *Digital Signal Processing*. Hingham, MA, Kluwer Academic.

Jaeger R.C. 1982. Tutorial: Analog data acquisition technology: II. Analog to digital conversion. *IEEE Micro.* 8: 46.

Malliani A., Pagani M., Lombardi F., and Cerutti S. 1991. Cardiovascular neural regulation explored in the frequency domain. *Circulation* 84: 482.

Marple S.L. 1987. *Digital Spectral Analysis with Applications*. Englewood Cliffs, NJ, Prentice-Hall.

Oppenheim A.V. and Schafer R.W. 1975. *Digital Signal Processing*. Englewood Cliffs, NJ, Prentice-Hall.

Rabiner L., Cooley J., Helms H., Jackson L., Kaiser J., Rader C., Schafer R., Steiglitz K., and Weinstein C. 1972. Terminology in digital signal processing. *IEEE Trans. Audio Electroac.* AU-20: 322.

Sayed A.H. 2003. *Fundamentals of Adaptive Filtering*, Hoboken, NJ, Wiley & Sons.

Shannon C.E. 1949. Communication in presence of noise. *Proc. IRE* 37: 10.

Simson M.B. 1981. Use of signals in the terminal QRS complex to identify patients with ventricular tachycardia after myocardial infarction. *Circulation* 64: 235.

Task Force of the European Society of Cardiology the North American Society of Pacing Electrophysiology. 1996. *Heart Rate Variability: Standards of Measurement, Physiological Interpretation, and Clinical Use*. 93: 1043.

Thakor N.V. 1987. Adaptive filtering of evoked potential. *IEEE Trans. Biomed. Eng.* 34: 1706.

Tompkins W.J. (ed). 1993. *Biomedical Digital Signal Processing*. Englewood Cliffs, NJ, Prentice-Hall.

Tompkins W.J. and Webster J.G. (eds). 1981. *Design of Microcomputer-Based Medical Instrumentation*. Englewood Cliffs, NJ, Prentice-Hall.

Webster J.G. (ed). 2009. *Medical Instrumentation Application and Design*, 4th ed. Somerset, NJ, John Wiley & Sons.

Welch D.P. 1970. The use of fast Fourier transform for the estimation of power spectra: A method based on time averaging over short modified periodograms. *IEEE Trans. Acoust.* AU-15: 70.

Widrow B. 1956. A study of rough amplitude quantization by means of Nyquist sampling theory. *IRE Trans. Cric. Theory* 3: 266.

Widrow B., Glover J.R., Jr., McCool J.M., Kaunitz J., Williams C.S., Hearn R.H., Zeidler J.R., Eugene Dong, Jr., and Goodlin R.C. 1975. Adaptive noise cancelling: Principles and applications. *Proc. IEEE* 63: 1692.

Zetterberg L.H. 1969. Estimation of parameters for a linear difference equation with application to EEG analysis. *Math. Biosci.* 5: 227.

Further Information

A book that provides a general overview of basic concepts in biomedical signal processing is *Digital Biosignal Processing*, by Rolf Weitkunat (ed) (Elsevier Science Publishers, Amsterdam, 1991). Contributions by different authors provide descriptions of several processing techniques and many applicative examples on biologic signal analysis.

A fair introduction to biomedical signal processing topics is provided by the book *Introduction to Applied Statistical Signal Analysis: Guide to Biomedical and Electrical Engineering Applications*, by R. Shiavi (CRC Press, 3rd edition, 2007).

Readers who are interested in advanced applications of biomedical signal processing methodologies can refer to the book *Bioelectrical Signal Processing in Cardiac and Neurological Applications* by L. Sornmo and P. Laguna (Academic Press, 2005) and to the book *Advanced Methods of Biomedical Signal Processing* (Wiley IEEE Press Series on Biomedical Engineering, 2009) by S. Cerutti and C. Marchesi.

Advances in signal processing are published monthly in the journal *IEEE Transactions on Signal Processing*, while the *IEEE Transaction on Biomedical Engineering* provides examples of applications in biomedical engineering fields.

2

Time–Frequency Signal Representations for Biomedical Signals

G. Faye Boudreaux-
Bartels
University of Rhode Island

Robin Murray
University of Rhode Island
Naval Undersea Warfare
Center

The Fourier transform of a signal $x(t)$

$$X(f) = \int x(t)\mathrm{e}^{-j2\pi ft}\,\mathrm{d}t \qquad (2.1)$$

is a useful tool for analyzing the spectral content of a stationary signal and for transforming difficult operations such as convolution, differentiation, and integration into very simple algebraic operations in the Fourier dual domain. The inverse Fourier transform equation

$$x(t) = \int X(f)\mathrm{e}^{j2\pi ft}\,\mathrm{d}f \qquad (2.2)$$

is a linear combination of complex sinusoids of infinite duration which implicitly assumes that each sinusoidal component is present at all times and, hence, the spectral content of the signal does not change with time. However, many signals in bioengineering are produced by biological systems whose spectral characteristics can change rapidly with time. To analyze these rapid spectral changes, one needs a two-dimensional, mixed time–frequency signal representation (TFR) that is analogous to a musical score with time represented along one axis and frequency along the other, indicating which frequency components (notes) are present at each time instant.

The first purpose of this chapter is to review several TFRs defined in Table 2.1 and to describe many of the desirable properties listed in Table 2.2 that an ideal TFR should satisfy. TFRs will be grouped into classes satisfying similar properties to provide a more intuitive understanding of their similarities, advantages, and disadvantages. Further, each TFR within a given class is completely characterized by a unique set of kernels that provide valuable insight into whether or not a given TFR (1) satisfies other ideal TFR properties, (2) is easy to compute, and (3) reduces nonlinear cross-terms. The

TABLE 2.1   List of Time–Frequency Representations of a Signal $x(t)$ Whose Fourier Transform Is $X(f)$

Ackroyd distribution	$\mathrm{ACK}_x(t,f) = \mathrm{Re}\left\{ x^*(t)X(f)e^{j2\pi ft} \right\}$
Affine Wigner distribution	$\mathrm{AWD}_X(t,f;G,F) = \int G\!\left(\dfrac{v}{f}\right) X\!\left(fF\!\left(\dfrac{v}{f}\right) + \dfrac{v}{2}\right) X^*\!\left(fF\!\left(\dfrac{v}{f}\right) - \dfrac{v}{2}\right) e^{j2\pi tv}dv$
Altes–Marinovic distribution	$\mathrm{AM}_X(t,f) = \lvert f \rvert \displaystyle\int X(fe^{u/2})X^*(fe^{-u/2})e^{j2\pi tfu}du = \lvert f \rvert \displaystyle\iint \mathrm{WAF}_X(\tau,e^{\beta})e^{j2\pi(tf\beta - f\tau)}d\tau d\beta$
(Narrowband) ambiguity function	$\mathrm{AF}_x(\tau,v) = \displaystyle\int x\!\left(t + \dfrac{\tau}{2}\right) x^*\!\left(t - \dfrac{\tau}{2}\right) e^{-j2\pi vt}dt = \displaystyle\int X\!\left(f + \dfrac{v}{2}\right) X^*\!\left(f - \dfrac{v}{2}\right) e^{j2\pi \tau f}df$
Andrieux et al. distribution	$\mathrm{AND}_x(t,f) = \displaystyle\iint \dfrac{1}{\sigma_{(t-t')}\sigma_{(f-f')}} \exp\!\left[-\left(\dfrac{(t-t')^2}{2\sigma^2_{(t-t')}} + \dfrac{(f - b_{(t-t')}(t-t'))^2}{2\sigma^2_{(f-f')}}\right)\right]$ $\times \mathrm{WD}_x(t',f')dt'df'$
	where for $x(t) = e^{j2\pi\varphi(t)}$, then $b_t = \dfrac{d^2}{dt^2}\varphi(t), \sigma_t = \left\lvert \dfrac{d^3}{dt^3}\varphi(t)\right\rvert^{-1/3}$, and $2\pi\sigma_t\sigma_f = \dfrac{1}{2}$
Autocorrelation function	
Temporal	$\mathrm{act}_x(\tau) = \displaystyle\int x^*(t)x(t+\tau)dt = \int \lvert X(f)\rvert^2 \, e^{j2\pi f\tau}df$
Spectral	$\mathrm{ACF}_X(v) = \displaystyle\int X^*(f)X(f+v)df = \int \lvert x(t)\rvert^2 \, e^{-j2\pi tv}dt$
Bertrand P_k distribution	$BkD_x(t,f;\mu_k) = \lvert f \rvert \displaystyle\int X(f\lambda_k(u))X^*(f\lambda_k(-u))\mu_k(u)e^{j2\pi tf(\lambda_k(u)-\lambda_k(-u))}du$
with $\lambda_0(u) = \dfrac{u/2e^{u/2}}{\sinh(u/2)}$,	$\lambda_1(u) = \exp\!\left[1 + \left(\dfrac{ue^{-u}}{e^{-u}-1}\right)\right], \lambda_k(u) = \left[k\dfrac{e^u-1}{e^{-ku}-1}\right]^{1/(k-1)} \quad k \neq 0,1, \mu_k(u) = \mu_k(-u) > 0$
Born–Jordan distribution	$\mathrm{BJD}_x(t,f) = \displaystyle\int \dfrac{1}{\tau}\left[\int_{t-\lvert\tau\rvert/2}^{t+\lvert\tau\rvert/2} x\!\left(t' + \dfrac{\tau}{2}\right) x^*\!\left(t' - \dfrac{\tau}{2}\right) dt'\right] e^{-j2\pi f\tau}d\tau$
Butterworth distribution	$\mathrm{BUD}_x(t,f) = \displaystyle\iint \left(1 + \left(\dfrac{\tau}{\tau_0}\right)^{2M}\left(\dfrac{v}{v_0}\right)^{2N}\right)^{-1} \mathrm{AF}_x(\tau,v)e^{j2\pi(tv - f\tau)}d\tau dv$
Choi–Williams exponential distribution	$\mathrm{CWD}_x(t,f) = \displaystyle\iint \sqrt{\dfrac{\sigma}{4\pi}}\dfrac{1}{\lvert\tau\rvert}\exp\!\left[-\dfrac{\sigma}{4}\left(\dfrac{t-t'}{\tau}\right)^2\right] x\!\left(t' + \dfrac{\tau}{2}\right) x^*\!\left(t' - \dfrac{\tau}{2}\right) e^{-j2\pi f\tau}dt'd\tau$

TABLE 2.1 (continued)   List of Time–Frequency Representations of a Signal $x(t)$ Whose Fourier Transform Is $X(f)$

Cohen's nonnegative distribution	$\mathrm{CND}_x(t,f) = \dfrac{|x(t)|^2 |X(f)|^2}{E_x}\left[1 + \varphi(\xi_x(t), \eta_x(f))\right]$
	with $\xi_x(t) = \dfrac{1}{E_x}\displaystyle\int_{-\infty}^{t} |x(\tau)|^2\,d\tau,\ \eta_x(f) = \dfrac{1}{E_x}\displaystyle\int_{-\infty}^{f} |X(f')|^2\,df',\ E_x = \displaystyle\int |x(t)|^2\,dt$
Cone–Kernel distribution	$\mathrm{CKD}_x(t,f) = \displaystyle\int g(\tau)\left[\displaystyle\int_{t-|\tau|/2}^{t+|\tau|/2} x\left(t' + \dfrac{\tau}{2}\right)x^*\left(t' - \dfrac{\tau}{2}\right)dt'\right]e^{-j2\pi f\tau}\,d\tau$
Cumulative attack spectrum	$\mathrm{CAS}_x(t,f) = \left\|\displaystyle\int_{-\infty}^{t} x(\tau)e^{-j2\pi f\tau}\,d\tau\right\|^2$
Cumulative decay spectrum	$\mathrm{CDS}_x(t,f) = \left\|\displaystyle\int_{t}^{\infty} x(\tau)e^{-j2\pi f\tau}\,d\tau\right\|^2$
Flandrin D-distribution	$\mathrm{FD}_X(t,f) = |f|\displaystyle\int X\left(f\left[1 + \dfrac{u}{4}\right]\right)^2 X^*\left(f\left[1 - \dfrac{u}{4}\right]\right)^2\left[1 - \left(\dfrac{u}{4}\right)^2\right]e^{j2\pi tfu}\,du$
Gabor expansion, $\mathrm{GE}_x(n,k;g)$	$x(t) = \Sigma_n\Sigma_k \mathrm{GE}_x(n,k;g)g(t - n\Delta T)e^{j2\pi(k\Delta F)t}$
Generalized Altes distribution	$\mathrm{GAM}_X(t,f;\alpha) = |f|\displaystyle\int e^{-\alpha u}X\left(fe^{((1/2)-\alpha)u}\right)X^*\left(fe^{-((1/2)+\alpha)u}\right)e^{j2\pi tfu}\,du$
Generalized exponential distribution	$\mathrm{GED}_x(t,f) = \displaystyle\iint \exp\left[-\left(\dfrac{\tau}{\tau_0}\right)^{2M}\left(\dfrac{v}{v_0}\right)^{2N}\right]\mathrm{AF}_x(\tau,v)e^{j2\pi(tv - ft)}\,d\tau\,dv$
Generalized rectangular distribution	$\mathrm{GRD}_x(t,f) = \displaystyle\iint rect_1\left(\dfrac{|\tau|^{\frac{M}{N}}|v|}{\sigma}\right)\mathrm{AF}_x(\tau,v)e^{j2\pi(tv - ft)}\,d\tau\,dv,$ where $rect_b(t) = \begin{cases} 1, |t| < |b| \\ 0, |t| > |b| \end{cases}$
Generalized Wigner distribution	$\mathrm{GWD}_x(t,f;\tilde\alpha) = \displaystyle\int x\left(t + \left(\dfrac{1}{2} + \tilde\alpha\right)\tau\right)x^*\left(t - \left(\dfrac{1}{2} - \tilde\alpha\right)\tau\right)e^{-j2\pi f\tau}\,d\tau$
Hyperbolic ambiguity function	$\mathrm{HAF}_X(\zeta,\beta) = \displaystyle\int_0^{\infty} X(fe^{\beta/2})X^*(fe^{-\beta/2})e^{j2\pi\zeta\ln(f/f_r)}\,df$
Hyperbolic wavelet transform	$\mathrm{HWT}_X(t,f;\Gamma) = \sqrt{\dfrac{f_r}{f}}\displaystyle\int_0^{\infty} X(\xi)\Gamma^*\left(\dfrac{f_r}{f}\xi\right)e^{j2\pi tf\ln(\xi/f_r)}\,d\xi$
Hyperbologram	$\mathrm{HYP}_X(t,f;\Gamma) = \left\|\sqrt{\dfrac{f_r}{f}}\displaystyle\int_0^{\infty} X(\xi)\Gamma^*\left(\dfrac{f_r}{f}\xi\right)e^{j2\pi tf\ln(\xi/f_r)}\,d\xi\right\|^2 = |\mathrm{HWT}_X(t,f;\Gamma)|^2$
Levin distribution	$\mathrm{LD}_x(t,f) = -\dfrac{d}{dt}\left\|\displaystyle\int_t^{\infty} x(\tau)e^{-j2\pi f\tau}\,d\tau\right\|^2$
Margineau–Hill distribution	$\mathrm{MH}_x(t,f) = \mathrm{Re}\left\{x(t)X^*(f)e^{-j2\pi ft}\right\}$
Multiform, tiltable distributions	Let $\tilde\mu(\tilde\tau,\tilde v;\alpha,r,\beta,\gamma) = \left((\tilde\tau)^2\left((\tilde v)^2\right)^\alpha + \left((\tilde\tau)^2\right)^\alpha(\tilde v)^2 + 2r\left((\tilde\tau\tilde v)^\beta\right)^\gamma\right)$

continued

TABLE 2.1 (continued) List of Time–Frequency Representations of a Signal $x(t)$ Whose Fourier Transform Is $X(f)$

Butterworth	$\displaystyle \text{MTBD}_x(t,f) = \iint \left[1 + \tilde{\mu}^{2\lambda}\left(\frac{\tau}{\tau_0}, \frac{\nu}{\nu_0}; \alpha, r, \beta, \gamma\right)\right]^{-1} \text{AF}_x(\tau,\nu)e^{j2\pi(t\nu - f\tau)} d\tau d\nu$
Exponential	$\displaystyle \text{MTED}_x(t,f) = \iint \exp\left\{-\pi\tilde{\mu}^{2\lambda}\left(\frac{\tau}{\tau_0}, \frac{\nu}{\nu_0}; \alpha, r, \beta, \gamma\right)\right\} \text{AF}_x(\tau,\nu)e^{j2\pi(t\nu - f\tau)} d\tau d\nu$
(Inverse) Chebyshev	$\displaystyle \text{MT}(I)C_x(t,f) = \iint \left[1 + \varepsilon^2 C_\lambda^{\pm 2}\left(\tilde{\mu}\left(\frac{\tau}{\tau_0}, \frac{\nu}{\nu_0}; \alpha, r, \beta, \gamma\right)^{\pm 1}\right)\right]^{-1} \text{AF}_x(\tau,\nu)e^{j2\pi(t\nu - f\tau)} d\tau d\nu$
	where $C_\lambda(a)$ is a Chebyshev polynomial of order λ
Nutall–Griffin distribution	$\displaystyle \text{ND}_x(t,f) = \iint \exp\left\{-\pi\left[\left(\frac{\tau}{\tau_0}\right)^2 + \left(\frac{\nu}{\nu_0}\right)^2 + 2r\left(\frac{\tau\nu}{\tau_0\nu_0}\right)\right]\right\} \text{AF}_x(\tau,\nu)e^{j2\pi(t\nu - f\tau)} d\tau d\nu$
Page distribution	$\displaystyle 2\,\text{Re}\left\{x^*(t)\,e^{j2\pi tf}\int_{-\infty}^{t} x(\tau)e^{-j2\pi f\tau} d\tau\right\}$
*k*th Power	
Ambiguity function	$\displaystyle B_X^{(\kappa)}(\zeta,\beta) = \text{AF}_{\mathcal{W}_\kappa X}\left(\frac{\zeta}{f_r}, f_r\beta\right), \quad (\mathcal{W}_\kappa X)(f) = \frac{1}{\sqrt{f_r \mid \tau_\kappa(f_r\xi_\kappa^{-1}(f/f_r))\mid}} X\left(f_r\xi_\kappa^{-1}\left(\frac{f}{f_r}\right)\right)$
Central member	$\displaystyle \text{AM}_X^{(\kappa)}(t,f) = \text{WD}_{\mathcal{W}_\kappa X}\left(\frac{t}{f_r\tau_\kappa(f)}, f_r\xi_\kappa\left(\frac{f}{f_r}\right)\right), \quad \tau_\kappa(f) = \frac{d}{df}\xi_\kappa\left(\frac{f}{f_r}\right)$
	where $\xi_\kappa(b) = \begin{cases} \text{sgn}(b)\mid b\mid^\kappa, & b\in\mathcal{R} \text{ for } \kappa\neq 0 \\ \ln(b), & b>0 \text{ for } \kappa=0 \end{cases}$
	and $\xi_\kappa^{-1}(b) = \begin{cases} \text{sgn}(b)\mid b\mid^{1/\kappa}, & b\in\mathcal{R}, \kappa\neq 0 \\ e^b, & b>0, \kappa=0 \end{cases}$
Power spectral density	$\displaystyle \text{PSD}_x(f) = \mid X(f)\mid^2 = \int \text{act}_x(\tau)e^{-j2\pi f\tau} d\tau$
Pseudo-Altes distribution	$\displaystyle \text{PAD}_X(t,f;\Gamma) = f_r\int_0^\infty \text{AM}_\Gamma\left(0, \frac{f_r f}{f'}\right) \text{AM}_X\left(\frac{tf}{f'}, f'\right)\frac{df'}{f'}$
Pseudo-Wigner distribution	$\displaystyle \text{PWD}_x(t,f;\eta) = \int x\left(t+\frac{\tau}{2}\right) x^*\left(t-\frac{\tau}{2}\right)\eta\left(\frac{\tau}{2}\right)\eta^*\left(-\frac{\tau}{2}\right)e^{-j2\pi f\tau} d\tau$
Radially adaptive Gaussian distribution	$\displaystyle \text{RAGD}_x(t,f) = \iint \exp\left[\frac{-(\tau/\tau_0)^2 + (\nu/\nu_0)^2}{2\sigma_x^2(\theta)}\right] \text{AF}_x(\tau,\nu)e^{j2\pi(t\nu - f\tau)} d\tau d\nu$
	where $\theta = \arctan\left[\dfrac{\nu/\nu_0}{\tau/\tau_0}\right]$
Real generalized Wigner distribution	$\displaystyle \text{RGWD}_x(t,f;\tilde{\alpha}) = \text{Re}\left\{\int x\left(t+\left(\frac{1}{2}+\tilde{\alpha}\right)\tau\right) x^*\left(t-\left(\frac{1}{2}-\tilde{\alpha}\right)\tau\right)e^{-j2\pi f\tau} d\tau\right\}$

TABLE 2.1 (continued) List of Time–Frequency Representations of a Signal $x(t)$ Whose Fourier Transform Is $X(f)$

Reduced interference distribution	$\mathrm{RID}_x(t,f;S_{\mathrm{RID}}) = \iint \dfrac{1}{|\tau|} S_{\mathrm{RID}}\left(\dfrac{t-t'}{\tau}\right) x\left(t'+\dfrac{\tau}{2}\right) x^*\left(t'-\dfrac{\tau}{2}\right) e^{-j2\pi f\tau} dt' d\tau$
	with $S_{\mathrm{RID}}(\beta) \in \mathcal{R}, S_{\mathrm{RID}}(0)=1, \left\{\dfrac{d}{d\beta} S_{\mathrm{RID}}(\beta)\Big|_{\beta=0}=0\right\}, \left\{S_{\mathrm{RID}}(\alpha)=0 \text{ for } |\alpha|>\dfrac{1}{2}\right\}$
Rihaczek distribution	$\mathrm{RD}_x(t,f) = x(t)X^*(f)e^{-j2\pi tf}$
Running spectrum, past	$\mathrm{RSP}_x(t,f) = \displaystyle\int_{-\infty}^{t} x(u)e^{-j2\pi fu} du,$
Running spectrum, future	$\mathrm{RSF}_x(t,f) = \displaystyle\int_{t}^{\infty} x(u)e^{-j2\pi fu} du$
Scalogram	$\mathrm{SCAL}_x(t,f;\gamma) = \left\| \displaystyle\int x(\tau)\sqrt{\left\|\dfrac{f}{f_r}\right\|}\gamma^*\left(\dfrac{f}{f_r}(\tau-t)\right)d\tau \right\|^2 = \|\mathrm{WT}_x(t,f;\gamma)\|^2$
Short-time Fourier transform	$\mathrm{STFT}_x(t,f;\gamma) = \displaystyle\int x(\tau)\gamma^*(\tau-t)e^{-j2\pi f\tau}d\tau = e^{-j2\pi tf}\int X(f')\Gamma^*(f'-f)e^{j2\pi tf'}df'$
Smoothed Pseudo-Altes distribution	$\mathrm{SPAD}_X(t,f;\Gamma,g) = \displaystyle\int g(tf-c)\mathrm{PAD}_X\left(\dfrac{c}{f},f;\Gamma\right)dc$
Smoothed Pseudo-Wigner distribution	$\mathrm{SPWD}_x(t,f;\gamma,\eta) = \iint \gamma(t-t')\eta\left(\dfrac{\tau}{2}\right)\eta^*\left(-\dfrac{\tau}{2}\right) x\left(t'+\dfrac{\tau}{2}\right) x^*\left(t'-\dfrac{\tau}{2}\right) e^{-j2\pi f\tau} dt' d\tau$
Spectrogram	$\mathrm{SPEC}_x(t,f;\gamma) = \left\| \displaystyle\int x(\tau)\gamma^*(\tau-t)e^{-j2\pi f\tau}d\tau \right\|^2 = \|\mathrm{STFT}_x(t,f;\gamma)\|^2$
Unterberger active distribution	$\mathrm{UAD}_X(t,f) = f\displaystyle\int_0^{\infty} X(fu)X^*(f/u)[1+u^{-2}]e^{j2\pi tf(u-1/u)}du$
Unterberger passive distribution	$\mathrm{UPD}_X(t,f) = 2f\displaystyle\int_0^{\infty} X(fu)X^*(f/u)[u^{-1}]e^{j2\pi tf(u-1/u)}du$
Wavelet transform	$\mathrm{WT}_x(t,f;\gamma) = \displaystyle\int x(\tau)\sqrt{\left\|\dfrac{f}{f_r}\right\|}\gamma^*\left(\dfrac{f}{f_r}(\tau-t)\right)d\tau = \int X(f')\sqrt{\left\|\dfrac{f_r}{f}\right\|}\Gamma^*\left(\dfrac{f_r}{f}f'\right)e^{j2\pi tf'}df'$
Wideband ambiguity function	$\mathrm{WAF}_X(\tau,\alpha) = \displaystyle\int_0^{\infty} X(f\sqrt{\alpha})X^*(f/\sqrt{\alpha})e^{j2\pi\tau f}df$
Wigner distribution	$\mathrm{WD}_x(t,f) = \displaystyle\int x\left(t+\dfrac{\tau}{2}\right)x^*\left(t-\dfrac{\tau}{2}\right)e^{-j2\pi f\tau}d\tau = \int X\left(f+\dfrac{\nu}{2}\right)X^*\left(f-\dfrac{\nu}{2}\right)e^{j2\pi t\nu}d\nu$

second goal of this chapter is to discuss applications of TFRs to signal analysis and detection problems in bioengineering. Unfortunately, none of the current TFRs is ideal; some give erroneous information when the signal's spectrum is rapidly time-varying. Researchers often analyze several TFRs side by side, keeping in mind the relative strengths and weaknesses of each TFR before drawing any conclusions.

TABLE 2.2 List of Desirable Properties for Time–Frequency Representations and Their Corresponding Kernel Constraints for Cohen's Class and the Hyperbolic Class

Property Name	TFR Property	Kernel Constraints for Cohen's Class	Kernel Constraints for Hyperbolic Class
P_1: Frequency-shift covariant	$T_y(t,f) = T_x(t, f-f_0)$ for $y(t) = x(t)e^{j2\pi f_0 t}$	Always satisfied	
P_2: Time-shift covariant	$T_y(t,f) = T_x(t-t_0, f)$ for $y(t) = x(t-t_0)$	Always satisfied	$\Psi_H(\zeta,\beta) = B_H(\beta)e^{-j2\pi\zeta \ln G(\beta)}$ with $G(\beta) = \dfrac{\beta/2}{\sinh(\beta/2)}$
P_3: Scale covariant	$T_y(t,f) = T_x(at, f/a)$ for $y(t) = \sqrt{a}\,|x(at)|$	$\Psi_C(\tau,v) = S_C(\tau v)$	Always satisfied
P_4: Hyperbolic time shift	$T_y(t,f) = T_x(t-c/f, f)$ if $Y(f) = \exp\left(-j2\pi c \ln \dfrac{f}{f_r}\right) X(f)$		Always satisfied
P_5: Convolution covariant	$T_y(t,f) = \int T_h(t-\tau, f)T_x(\tau,f)\,d\tau$ for $y(t) = \int h(t-\tau)x(\tau)\,d\tau$	$\Psi_C(\tau_1+\tau_2, v) = \Psi_C(\tau_1, v)\cdot \Psi_C(\tau_2, v)$	$\Phi_H(b_1,\beta)\Phi_H(b_2,\beta) = e^b \Phi_H(b_1,\beta)\delta(b_1-b_2)$
P_6: Modulation covariant	$T_y(t,f) = \int T_h(t, f-f')T_x(t,f')\,df'$ for $y(t) = h(t)x(t)$	$\Psi_C(\tau, v_1+v_2) = \Psi_C(\tau, v_1)\cdot \Psi_C(\tau, v_2)$	
P_7: Real-valued	$T_x^*(t,f) = T_x(t,f)$	$\Psi_C^*(-\tau,-v) = \Psi_C(\tau,v)$	$\Psi_H^*(-\zeta,-\beta) = \Psi_H(\zeta,\beta)$
P_8: Positivity	$T_x(t,f) \geq 0$	$\Psi_C(\tau,v) = AF_y(-\tau,-v)$	$\Psi_H(\zeta,\beta) = HAF_r(-\zeta,-\beta)$
P_9: Time marginal	$\int T_x(t,f)\,df = |x(t)|^2$	$\Psi_C(0,v)=1$	
P_{10}: Frequency marginal	$\int T_x(t,f)\,dt = |X(f)|^2$	$\Psi_C(\tau,0)=1$	$\Psi_H(\zeta,0)=1$
P_{11}: Energy distribution	$\iint T_x(t,f)\,dt\,df = \int |X(f)|^2\,df$	$\Psi_C(0,0)=1$	$\Psi_H(0,0)=1$
P_{12}: Time moments	$\iint t^n T_x(t,f)\,dt\,df = \int t^n |x(t)|^2\,dt$	$\Psi_C(0,v)=1$	
P_{13}: Frequency moments	$\iint f^n T_x(t,f)\,dt\,df = \int f^n |X(f)|^2\,df$	$\Psi_C(\tau,0)=1$	

P_{14}: Finite time support	$T_x(t,f) = 0$ for $t \notin (t_1,t_2)$ if $x(t) = 0$ for $t \notin (t_1,t_2)$		$\varphi_C(t,\tau) = 0, \left\lvert\frac{t}{\tau}\right\rvert > \frac{1}{2}$
P_{15}: Finite frequency support	$T_x(t,f) = 0$ for $f \notin (f_1,f_2)$ if $X(f) = 0$ for $f \notin (f_1,f_2)$	$\Phi_C(f,\nu) = 0$ if $\left\lvert\frac{f}{\nu}\right\rvert > \frac{1}{2}$	$\Phi_H(c,\zeta) = 0, \left\lvert\frac{c}{\zeta}\right\rvert > \frac{1}{2}$
P_{16}: Instantaneous frequency	$\dfrac{\int f\, T_x(t,f)\,df}{\int T_x(t,f)\,df} = \dfrac{1}{2\pi}\dfrac{d}{dt}\arg\{x(t)\}$	$\Psi_C(0,\nu) = 1$ and $\dfrac{\partial}{\partial \tau}\Psi_C(\tau,\nu)\big\vert_{\tau=0} = 0$	
P_{17}: Group delay	$\dfrac{\int t\, T_x(t,f)\,dt}{\int T_x(t,f)\,dt} = -\dfrac{1}{2\pi}\dfrac{d}{df}\arg\{X(f)\}$	$\Psi_C(\tau,0) = 1$ and $\dfrac{\partial}{\partial \nu}\Psi_C(\tau,\nu)\big\vert_{\nu=0} = 0$	$\Psi_H(\zeta,0) = 1$ and $\dfrac{\partial}{\partial \beta}\Psi_H(\zeta,\beta)\big\vert_{\beta=0} = 0$
P_{18}: Fourier transform	$T_y(t,f) = T_x(-f,t)$ for $y(t) = X(t)$	$\Psi_C(-\nu,\tau) = \Psi_C(\tau,\nu)$	
P_{19}: Frequency localization	$T_x(t,f) = \delta(f - f_0)$ for $X(f) = \delta(f - f_0)$	$\Psi_C(\tau,0) = 1$	$\Psi_H(\zeta,0) = 1$
P_{20}: Time localization	$T_x(t,f) = \delta(t - t_0)$ for $x(t) = \delta(t - t_0)$	$\Psi_C(0,\nu) = 1$	
P_{21}: Linear chirp localization	$T_x(t,f) = \delta(t - cf)$ for $X(f) = e^{-j\pi cf^2}$	$\Psi_C(\tau,\nu) = 1$	
P_{22}: Hyperbolic localization	$T_{X_C}(t,f) = \dfrac{1}{f}\delta\!\left(t - \dfrac{c}{f}\right), f > 0$ if $X_c(f) = \dfrac{1}{\sqrt{f}}e^{-j2\pi c\ln(f/f_r)}, f > 0$		$\Psi_H(0,\beta) = 1$
P_{23}: Chirp convolution	$T_y(t,f) = T_x(t - f/c, f)$ for $y(t) = \int x(t-\tau)\sqrt{\lvert c\rvert}\, e^{j\pi c\tau^2}\, d\tau$	$\Psi_C\!\left(\tau - \dfrac{\nu}{c}, \nu\right) = \Psi_C(\tau,\nu)$	
P_{24}: Chirp multiplication	$T_y(t,f) = T_x(t, f - ct)$ for $y(t) = x(t)e^{j\pi ct^2}$	$\Psi_C(\tau, \nu - c\tau) = \Psi_C(\tau,\nu)$	
P_{25}: Moyal's formula	$\displaystyle\iint T_x(t,f)T_y^*(t,f)\,dt\,df = \left\lvert \int x(t)y^*(t)\,dt \right\rvert^2$	$\lvert\Psi_C(\tau,\nu)\rvert = 1$	$\lvert\Psi_H(\zeta,\beta)\rvert = 1$

2.1 One-Dimensional Signal Representations

The instantaneous frequency and the group delay of a signal are one-dimensional representations that attempt to represent temporal and spectral signal characteristics simultaneously. The instantaneous frequency of the signal

$$f_x(t) = \frac{1}{2\pi} \frac{d}{dt} \arg\{x(t)\} \tag{2.3}$$

has been used in communication theory to characterize the time-varying frequency content of narrow-band and frequency-modulated signals. It is a generalization of the fact that the frequency f_0 of a complex sinusoidal signal $x(t) = \exp(j2\pi f_0 t)$ is proportional to the derivative of the signal's phase. A dual concept used in filter analysis is the group delay

$$\tau_H(f) = -\frac{1}{2\pi} \frac{d}{df} \arg\{H(f)\} \tag{2.4}$$

which can be interpreted as the time delay or distortion introduced by the filter's frequency response $H(f)$ at each frequency. Group delay is a generalization of the fact that time translations are coded in the derivative of the phase of the Fourier transform. Unfortunately, if the signal contains several signal components that overlap in time or frequency, then $f_x(t)$ or $\tau_H(f)$ only provides average spectral characteristics, which are not very useful.

2.2 Desirable Properties of Time–Frequency Representations

Mixed TFRs map a one-dimensional signal into a two-dimensional function of time and frequency in order to analyze the time-varying spectral content of the signal. Before discussing any particular TFR in Table 2.1, it is helpful to first investigate what types of properties an "ideal" time–frequency representation should satisfy. The list of desirable TFR properties in Table 2.2 can be broken up conceptually into the following categories: covariance, statistics, signal analysis, localization, and inner products (Claasen and Mecklenbräuker, 1980; Cohen, 1989; Boashash, 1991; Hlawatsch and Boudreaux-Bartels, 1992; Flandrin, 1993). The covariance properties P_1 to P_6 basically state that certain operations on the signal, such as translations, dilations, or convolution, should be preserved, that is, produce exactly the same operation on the signal's TFR. The second category of properties originates from the desire to generalize the concepts of the one-dimensional instantaneous signal energy $|x(t)|^2$ and power spectral density $|X(f)|^2$ into a two-dimensional statistical energy distribution $T_x(t_0, f_0)$ that provides a measure of the local signal energy or the probability that a signal contains a sinusoidal component of frequency f_0 at time t_0. Properties P_7 to P_{13} state that such an energy-distribution TFR should be real and nonnegative, have its marginal distributions equal to the signal's temporal and spectral energy densities $|x(t)|^2$ and $|X(f)|^2$, respectively, and preserve the signal energy, mean, variance, and other higher-order moments of the instantaneous signal energy and power spectral density. The next category of properties, P_{14} to P_{18}, arises from signal-processing considerations. A TFR should have the same duration and bandwidth as the signal under analysis. At any given time t, the average frequency should equal the instantaneous frequency of the signal, while the average or center of gravity in the time direction should equal the group delay of the signal. These two properties have been used to analyze the distortion of audio systems and the complex FM sonar signals used by bats and whales for echolocation. Property P_{18} is the TFR equivalent of the duality property of Fourier transforms. The group of properties P_{19} to P_{24} constitutes ideal TFR localization properties that are desirable for high-resolution capabilities. Here, $d(a)$ is the Dirac function. These properties state that if a signal is perfectly concentrated in time or frequency, that is, an impulse or a sinusoid, then its TFR also should be perfectly concentrated at the same time or

TABLE 2.3 List of Desirable Properties Satisfied by Time–Frequency Representations

Property	TFR	BAD	BJD	BUD	CWD	CAD	CKD	GAD	GED	GMD	GWD	GHD	HYD	LMD	MED	MTED	MMAD	PMD	PWD	RID	SCAD	SPAD	SPAWD	SPECD	SPUAD	SPUAPD	WD
Class(es)	c a h	a h	c a	c a	c a c	c a h	c a	c a h	c a h	c a h	c a h	a h	c	c a c	c a c	c a c	c a c p h	c a	c a	c a a h	c a	a h c	a c	c	c c	a a	c a
1. Frequency shift	✓	✓	✓	✓	✓	✓	✓	✓	✓	✓	✓	✓	✓	✓	✓	✓	✓	✓	✓	✓	✓	✓	✓	✓	✓	✓	✓
2. Time shift	✓	✓	✓	✓	✓	✓	✓	✓	✓	✓	✓	✓	✓	✓	✓	✓	✓	✓	✓	✓	✓	✓	✓	✓	✓	✓	✓
3. Scale covariance	✓	✓	✓1	✓	✓1 ✓1	✓			✓		✓	✓	✓	✓	✓9		✓	✓			✓	✓				✓	✓
4. Hyperbolic time shift	✓ ✓				✓																						
5. Convolution				✓6		✓				✓	✓10			✓	✓	✓										✓	✓
6. Modulation				✓7						✓	✓10			✓	✓		✓									✓	✓
7. Real-valued	✓	✓	✓	✓4	✓	✓	✓	✓	✓	✓	✓	✓	✓	✓	✓	✓	✓17	✓18	✓	✓	✓	✓	✓			✓	✓
8. Positivity	✓						✓				✓							✓									
9. Time marginal	✓	✓	✓	✓	✓	✓	✓	✓	✓	✓11	✓	✓	✓13	✓	✓			✓	✓							✓	✓
10. Frequency marginal	✓	✓	✓	✓	✓	✓	✓	✓	✓	✓11	✓	✓	✓	✓	✓			✓	✓							✓	✓
11. Energy distribution	✓	✓	✓	✓	✓	✓	✓8	✓	✓	✓	✓12	✓	✓	✓16	✓12	✓19	✓20	✓	✓	✓						✓	✓
12. Time moments	✓	✓	✓	✓	✓	✓	✓	✓	✓11	✓	✓13	✓	✓	✓	✓			✓	✓							✓	✓
13. Frequency moments	✓	✓	✓	✓	✓	✓	✓	✓	✓11	✓	✓	✓	✓	✓	✓			✓	✓							✓	✓
14. Finite time support	✓	✓	✓		✓5	✓		✓5			✓			✓												✓	✓
15. Finite frequency support	✓ ✓	✓	✓	✓5	✓5	✓5	✓				✓			✓												✓	✓
16. Instantaneous frequency	✓	✓2	✓		✓2	✓			✓11		✓13				✓14											✓	✓
17. Group delay	✓	✓3	✓	✓3	✓	✓			✓11		✓				✓											✓	✓
18. Fourier transform	✓	✓1	✓	✓1 ✓	✓1 ✓1	✓			✓9		✓				✓15											✓	✓

continued

TABLE 2.3 (continued)   List of Desirable Properties Satisfied by Time–Frequency Representations

Class(es)	TFCRK c a	BBAMD h	BB0JDM c a	BJDM	CUWDS c	CWKDD c	CCADSS c	CCADMD c	GGDFDS a	GGFDMD	GGEARD h	HWYLD c	M T A E c	A P M D	P P P D	P P M D	S C P W D a	S S A W A h	S S W E C c	U A P D a	U P P A a	W D D D
Property																						
19. Frequency localization	✓	✓	✓	✓	✓	✓	✓	✓	✓	✓	✓		✓11	✓	✓				✓	✓	✓	✓
20. Time localization	✓			✓		✓	✓	✓	✓	✓			✓11	✓	✓				✓	✓	✓	✓
21. Linear chirp localization										✓13			✓11	✓								✓
22. Hyperbolic localization								✓							✓							
23. Chirp convolution																				✓	✓	✓
24. Chirp multiplication																				✓	✓	✓
25. Moyal's formula	✓			✓		✓	✓		✓					✓	✓					✓	✓	✓

Note: A ✓ indicates that the TFR can be shown to satisfy the given property. A number following the ✓ indicates that the TFR defined in Table 2.1 requires additional constraints to satisfy the property. The constraints are as follows: (1): $M = N$; (2): $M > 1/2$; (3): $N > 1/2$; (4): $g(\tau)$ even; (5): $|\alpha| < 1/2$; (6): $M = 1/2$; (7): $N = 1/2$; (8): $\int_0^\infty |\Gamma(f)|^2\,df = 1$; (9): $\alpha = 1$; (10): $r = 0$, $\alpha = 1$, $\gamma = 1/4$; (11): $\alpha \neq 1$; (12): $|\rho_\Gamma(0)|^2 = (1/f_c)$; (13): $|\eta(0)| = 1$; (14): $\eta(0) = 1$; (15): $|\rho_\Gamma(0)|^2 = 1$; (16): $s_{\mathrm{RID}}(\beta)$ even; (17): $g(c) \in \Re$; (18): $\gamma(t) \in \Re$; (19): $\Gamma(0)|\eta(0)|^2 = 1$; (20): $\int|\Gamma(b)|^2 db/|b| = 1$; In the second row, the letters c, a, h, and p indicate that the corresponding TFR is a member of the Cohen, Affine, Hyperbolic, and κth Power class, respectively. The meanings of the TFR acronyms listed in the column head are given in Table 2.1.

frequency. Properties P_{21} and P_{22} state that the TFRs of linear or hyperbolic spectral FM chirp signals should be perfectly concentrated along the chirp signal's group delay. Property P_{24} states that a signal modulated by a linear FM chirp should have a TFR whose instantaneous frequency has been sheared by an amount equal to the linear instantaneous frequency of the chirp. The last property, known as *Moyal's formula* or the *unitarity property*, states that TFRs should preserve the signal projections, inner products, and orthonormal signal basis functions that are used frequently in signal detection, synthesis, and approximation theory. Table 2.3 indicates which properties are satisfied by the TFRs listed in Table 2.1.

A TFR should be relatively easy to compute and interpret. Interpretation is greatly simplified if the TFR is linear, that is

$$T_y(t, f) = \sum_{n=1}^{N} T_{x_n}(t, f) \quad \text{for } y(t) = \sum_{n=1}^{N} x_n(t). \tag{2.5}$$

However, energy is a quadratic function of the signal, and hence, so too are many of the TFRs in Table 2.1. The nonlinear nature of TFRs gives rise to troublesome cross-terms. If $y(t)$ contains N signal components or auto-terms $x_n(t)$ in Equation 2.5, then a quadratic TFR of $y(t)$ can have as many nonzero cross-terms as there are unique pairs of auto-terms, that is, $N(N-1)/2$. For many TFRs, these cross-terms are oscillatory and overlap with auto-terms, obscuring visual analysis of TFRs.

Two common methods used to reduce the number of cross-terms are to reduce any redundancy in the signal representation and to use local smoothing or averaging to reduce oscillating cross-terms. TFR analysis of real, bandpass signals should be carried out using the analytic signal representation, that is, the signal added to $\sqrt{-1}$ times its Hilbert transform, in order to remove cross-terms between the positive- and negative-frequency axis components of the signal's Fourier transform. As we will see in upcoming sections, cross-term reduction by smoothing is often achieved at the expense of significant auto-term distortion and loss of desirable TFR properties.

2.3 TFR Classes

This section will briefly review Cohen's class of shift covariant TFRs, the Affine class of affine covariant TFRs, the Hyperbolic class (developed for signals with hyperbolic group delay), and the Power class (which is useful for signals with polynomial group delay). Each class is formed by grouping TFRs that satisfy two properties. They provide very helpful insight as to which types of TFRs will work best in different situations. Within a class, each TFR is completely characterized by a unique set of TFR-dependent kernels which can be compared against a class-dependent list of kernel constraints in Tables 2.2 and 2.6 to quickly determine which properties the TFR satisfies.

2.3.1 Cohen's Class of TFRs

Cohen's class consists of all quadratic TFRs that satisfy the frequency-shift and time-shift covariance properties, that is, those TFRs with a check in the first two property rows in Table 2.3 (Claasen and Mecklenbräuker, 1980; Cohen, 1989; Hlawatsch and Boudreaux-Bartels, 1992; Flandrin, 1993). Time- and frequency-shift covariances are very useful properties in the analysis of speech, narrowband Doppler systems, and multipath environments. Any TFR in Cohen's class can be written in one of the four equivalent "normal forms":

$$C_x(t, f; \Psi_C) = \iint \varphi_C(t - t', \tau) x\left(t' + \frac{\tau}{2}\right) x^*\left(t' - \frac{\tau}{2}\right) e^{-j2\pi f \tau} dt' d\tau \tag{2.6}$$

$$= \iint \Phi_C(f - f', \nu) X\left(f' + \frac{\nu}{2}\right) X^*\left(f' - \frac{\nu}{2}\right) e^{j2\pi t\nu} df' d\nu \tag{2.7}$$

$$= \iint \psi_C(t - t', f - f')\mathrm{WD}_x(t', f')\mathrm{d}t'\mathrm{d}f' \tag{2.8}$$

$$= \iint \Psi_C(\tau, \nu)\mathrm{AF}_x(\tau, \nu)e^{j2\pi(t\nu - f\tau)}\mathrm{d}\tau\mathrm{d}\nu. \tag{2.9}$$

Each normal form is characterized by one of the four kernels $\varphi_C(t, \tau)$, $\varphi_C(f, \nu)$, $\psi_C(t, f)$, and $\Psi_C(\tau, \nu)$ which are interrelated by the following Fourier transforms:

$$\varphi_C(t, \tau) = \iint \Phi_C(f, \nu)e^{j2\pi(f\tau + \nu t)}\mathrm{d}f\,\mathrm{d}\nu = \int \Psi_C(\tau, \nu)e^{j2\pi\nu t}\mathrm{d}\nu \tag{2.10}$$

$$\psi_C(t, f) = \iint \Psi_C(\tau, \nu)e^{j2\pi(\nu t - f\tau)}\mathrm{d}\tau\mathrm{d}\nu = \int \Phi_C(f, \nu)e^{j2\pi\nu t}\mathrm{d}\nu \tag{2.11}$$

The kernels for the TFRs in Cohen's class are given in Table 2.4.

The four normal forms offer various computational and analysis advantages. For example, the first two normal forms can be computed directly from the signal $x(t)$ or its Fourier transform $X(f)$ via a one-dimensional convolution with $\varphi_C(t, \tau)$ or $\Phi_C(f, \nu)$. If $\varphi_C(t, \tau)$ is of fairly short duration, then it may be possible to implement Equation 2.6 on a digital computer in real time using only a small number of signal samples. The third normal form indicates that any TFR in Cohen's shift covariant class can be computed by convolving the TFR-dependent kernel $\psi_C(t, f)$ with the Wigner distribution (WD) of the signal, defined in Table 2.1. Hence the WD is one of the key members of Cohen's class, and many TFRs correspond to smoothed WDs, as seen in the top of Table 2.5. Equation 2.11 and the fourth normal form in Equation 2.9 indicates that the two-dimensional convolution in Equation 2.8 transforms to multiplication of the Fourier transform of the kernel $\psi_C(t, f)$ with the ambiguity function (AF) in Table 2.1; the AF is the Fourier transform of the WD. This last normal form provides an intuitive interpretation that the "AF domain" kernel $\Psi_C(\tau, \nu)$ can be thought of as the frequency response of a two-dimensional filter.

The kernels in Equations 2.6 through 2.11 are signal-independent and provide valuable insight into the performance of each Cohen class TFR, regardless of the input signal. For good cross-term reduction and little auto-term distortion, each TFR kernel $\Psi_C(\tau, \nu)$ given in Table 2.4 should be as close as possible to an ideal low-pass filter. If these kernels satisfy the constraints in the third column of Table 2.2, then the TFR properties in the first column are guaranteed to always hold (Claasen and Mecklenbräuker, 1980; Hlawatsch and Boudreaux-Bartels, 1992). For example, the last row of Table 2.2 indicates that Moyal's formula is satisfied by any TFR whose AF domain kernel, listed in the third column of Table 2.4, has unit modulus, for example, the Rihaczek distribution. Since the AF domain kernel of the WD is equal to one, that is, $\Psi_{WD}(\tau, \nu) = 1$, then the WD automatically satisfies the kernel constraints in Table 2.2 for properties P_9 to P_{13} and P_{16} to P_{21} as well as 12pt Moyal's formula. However, it also acts as an all-pass filter, passing all cross-terms. The Choi–Williams Gaussian kernel in Table 2.4 was formulated to satisfy the marginal property constraints of having an AF domain kernel equal to one along the axes and to be a low-pass filter that reduces cross-terms.

2.3.2 Affine Class of TFRs

TFRs that are covariant to scale changes and time translations, that is, properties P_2 and P_3 in Tables 2.2 and 2.3, are members of the *Affine class* (Bertrand chapter in Boashash, 1991; Flandrin, 1993). The scale covariance property P_3 is useful when analyzing wideband Doppler systems, signals with fractal structure, octave-band systems such as the cochlea of the inner ear, and detecting short-duration "transients." Any Affine class TFR can be written in four "normal form" equations similar to those of Cohen's class:

$$A_x(t, f; \Psi_A) = |f| \iint \varphi_A(f(t' - t), f\tau)x(t' + \tau/2)x^*(t' - \tau/2)\mathrm{d}t'\mathrm{d}\tau \tag{2.12}$$

TABLE 2.4 Kernels of Cohen's Shift-Invariant Class of Time–Frequency Representations

TFR	$\psi_C(t,f)$	$\Psi_C(\tau,\nu)$	$\varphi_C(t,\tau)$	$\Phi_C(f,\nu)$
ACK	$2\cos(4\pi t f)$	$\cos(\pi\tau\nu)$	$\dfrac{\delta(t+\tau/2)+\delta(t-\tau/2)}{2}$	$\dfrac{\delta(f-\nu/2)+\delta(f+\nu/2)}{2}$
BJD		$\dfrac{\sin(\pi\tau\nu)}{\pi\tau\nu}$	$\begin{cases}\dfrac{1}{\lvert\tau\rvert}, & \lvert t/\tau\rvert<1/2 \\ 0, & \lvert t/\tau\rvert>1/2\end{cases}$	$\begin{cases}\dfrac{1}{\lvert\nu\rvert}, & \lvert f/\nu\rvert<1/2 \\ 0, & \lvert f/\nu\rvert>1/2\end{cases}$
BUD		$\left(1+\left(\dfrac{\tau}{\tau_0}\right)^{2M}\left(\dfrac{\nu}{\nu_0}\right)^{2N}\right)^{-1}$		
CWD		$e^{-(2\pi\tau\nu)^2/\sigma}$	$\sqrt{\dfrac{\sigma}{4\pi}}\,\dfrac{1}{\lvert\tau\rvert}\exp\left[-\dfrac{\sigma}{4}\left(\dfrac{t}{\tau}\right)^2\right]$	$\sqrt{\dfrac{\sigma}{4\pi}}\,\dfrac{1}{\lvert\nu\rvert}\exp\left[-\dfrac{\sigma}{4}\left(\dfrac{f}{\nu}\right)^2\right]$
CKD		$g(\tau)\lvert\tau\rvert\,\dfrac{\sin(\pi\tau\nu)}{\pi\tau\nu}$	$\begin{cases}g(\tau), & \lvert t/\tau\rvert<1/2 \\ 0, & \lvert t/\tau\rvert>1/2\end{cases}$	
CAS		$\left[\dfrac{1}{2}\delta(\nu)+\dfrac{1}{j\nu}\right]e^{-j\pi\lvert\tau\rvert\nu}$		
CDS		$\left[\dfrac{1}{2}\delta(-\nu)-\dfrac{1}{j\nu}\right]e^{j\pi\lvert\tau\rvert\nu}$		
GED		$\exp\left[-\left(\dfrac{\tau}{\tau_0}\right)^{2M}\left(\dfrac{\nu}{\nu_0}\right)^{2N}\right]$	$\dfrac{\nu_0}{2\sqrt{\pi}}\left\lvert\dfrac{\tau_0}{\tau}\right\rvert^{M}\exp\left[\dfrac{-\nu_0^2\tau_0^{2M}t^2}{4\tau^{2M}}\right]$ $N=1$ only	$\dfrac{\tau_0}{2\sqrt{\pi}}\left\lvert\dfrac{\nu_0}{\nu}\right\rvert^{N}\exp\left[\dfrac{-\tau_0^2\nu_0^{2N}f^2}{4\nu^{2N}}\right]$ $M=1$ only
GRD		$\begin{cases}1, & \lVert\tau\rVert^{M/N}\lvert\nu\rvert/r\rvert<1 \\ 0, & \lVert\tau\rVert^{M/N}\lvert\nu\rvert/r\rvert>1\end{cases}$	$\dfrac{\sin(2\pi\lvert\sigma\rvert\lvert t\rvert/\lvert\tau\rvert^{M/N})}{\pi t}$ $N=1$ only	
GWD	$\dfrac{1}{\lvert\tilde\alpha\rvert}e^{j2\pi tf/\tilde\alpha}$	$e^{j2\pi\tilde\alpha\tau\nu}$	$\delta(t+\tilde\alpha\tau)$	$\delta(f-\tilde\alpha\nu)$
LD		$e^{j\pi\lvert\tau\rvert\nu}$	$\delta(t+\lvert\tau\rvert/2)$	
MH		$\cos(\pi\tau\nu)$	$\dfrac{\delta(t+\tau/2)+\delta(t-\tau/2)}{2}$	$\dfrac{\delta(f-\nu/2)+\delta(f+\nu/2)}{2}$

continued

TABLE 2.4 (continued) Kernels of Cohen's Shift-Invariant Class of Time–Frequency Representations

TFR	$\psi_C(t,f)$	$\Psi_C(\tau,\nu)$	$\varphi_C(t,\tau)$	$\Phi_C(f,\nu)$
MTBD		$\left[1+\tilde{\mu}^{2\lambda}\left(\dfrac{\tau}{\tau_0},\dfrac{\nu}{\nu_0};\alpha,r,\beta,\gamma\right)\right]^{-1}$		
MTC		$\left[1+\epsilon_p^2 C_\lambda^2\left(\tilde{\mu}\left(\dfrac{\tau}{\tau_0},\dfrac{\nu}{\nu_0};\alpha,r,\beta,\gamma\right)\right)\right]^{-1}$		
MTED		$\exp\left[-\pi\tilde{\mu}^{2\lambda}\left(\dfrac{\tau}{\tau_0},\dfrac{\nu}{\nu_0};\alpha,r,\beta,\gamma\right)\right]$		
MTIC		$\left[1+\epsilon_s^2 C_\lambda^{-2}\left(\tilde{\mu}^{-1}\left(\dfrac{\tau}{\tau_0},\dfrac{\nu}{\nu_0};\alpha,r,\beta,\gamma\right)\right)\right]^{-1}$		
ND		$\exp\left[-\pi\tilde{\mu}\left(\dfrac{\tau}{\tau_0},\dfrac{\nu}{\nu_0};0,r,1,1\right)\right]$		
PD		$e^{-j\pi|\tau||\nu|}$	$\delta(t-|\tau|/2)$	$WD_\eta(0,f)$
PWD	$\delta(t)WD_\eta(0,f)$	$\eta(\tau/2)\eta^*(-\tau/2)$	$\delta(t)\eta(\tau/2)\eta^*(-\tau/2)$	
RGWD	$\dfrac{1}{|\tilde{\alpha}|}\cos(2\pi tf/\tilde{\alpha})$	$\cos(2\pi\tilde{\alpha}\tau\nu)$	$\dfrac{\delta(t+\tilde{\alpha}\tau)+\delta(t-\tilde{\alpha}\tau)}{2}$	$\dfrac{\delta(f-\tilde{\alpha}\nu)+\delta(f+\tilde{\alpha}\nu)}{2}$
RID	$\displaystyle\int\frac{1}{\tau}s_{RID}\left(\frac{t}{\tau}\right)e^{-j2\pi tf}d\tau$	$S_{RID}(\tau\nu),$	$\dfrac{1}{|\tau|}s_{RID}\left(\dfrac{t}{\tau}\right),$	$\dfrac{1}{|\nu|}s_{RID}\left(-\dfrac{f}{\nu}\right),$
		$S_{RID}(\beta)\epsilon\text{Real},S_{RID}(0)=1$	$s_{RID}(\alpha)=0,|\alpha|>\dfrac{1}{2}$	$s_{RID}(\alpha)=0,|\alpha|>\dfrac{1}{2}$
RD	$2e^{-j4\pi tf}$	$e^{-j\pi\tau\nu}$	$\delta(t-\tau/2)$	$\delta(f+\nu/2)$
SPWD	$\gamma(t)WD_\eta(0,f)$	$\eta\left(\dfrac{\tau}{2}\right)\eta^*\left(-\dfrac{\tau}{2}\right)\Gamma(\nu)$	$\gamma(t)\eta\left(\dfrac{\tau}{2}\right)\eta^*\left(-\dfrac{\tau}{2}\right)$	$\Gamma(\nu)WD_\eta(0,f)$
SPEC	$WD_\gamma(-t,-f)$	$AF_\gamma(-\tau,-\nu)$	$\gamma\left(-t-\dfrac{\tau}{2}\right)\gamma^*\left(-t+\dfrac{\tau}{2}\right)$	$\Gamma\left(f-\dfrac{\nu}{2}\right)\Gamma^*\left(-f+\dfrac{\nu}{2}\right)$
WD	$\delta(t)\delta(f)$	1	$\delta(t)$	$\delta(f)$

Note: Here, $\tilde{\mu}(\tilde{\tau},\tilde{\nu};\alpha,r,\beta,\gamma)=((\tilde{\tau})^2((\tilde{\nu})^2)^\alpha+((\tilde{\tau})^2)^\alpha(\tilde{\nu})^2+2r((\tilde{\tau})^2)^\beta(\tilde{\nu})^2)^\gamma)$ and $C_\lambda(a)$ is a Chebyshev polynomial of order λ. Functions with lowercase and uppercase letters, for example, $\gamma(t)$ and $\Gamma(f)$, indicate Fourier transform pairs.

TABLE 2.5 Many TFRs Are Equivalent to Smoothed or Warped Wigner Distributions

TFR Name	TFR Formulation
Examples of TFRs Equivalent to Smoothed Wigner Distributions	
Cohen's class TFR	$C_x(t,f;\psi_C) = \iint \psi_C(t-t',f-f') \mathrm{WD}_x(t',f') dt' df'$
Pseudo-Wigner distribution	$\mathrm{PWD}_x(t,f;\eta) = \int \mathrm{WD}_\eta(0,f-f') \mathrm{WD}_x(t,f') df'$
Scalogram	$\mathrm{SCAL}_x(t,f;\gamma) = \iint \mathrm{WD}_\gamma\left(\dfrac{f}{f_r}(t'-t), f_r\dfrac{f'}{f}\right) \mathrm{WD}_x(t',f') dt' df'$
Smoothed Pseudo-Wigner distribution	$\mathrm{SPWD}_x(t,f;\gamma,\eta) = \iint \gamma(t-t') \mathrm{WD}_\eta(0,f-f') \mathrm{WD}_x(t',f') dt' df'$
Spectrogram	$\mathrm{SPEC}_x(t,f;\gamma) = \iint \mathrm{WD}_\gamma(t'-t,f'-f) \mathrm{WD}_x(t',f') dt' df'$
Examples of TFRs Equivalent to Warped Wigner Distributions	
Altes distribution	$\mathrm{AM}_X(t,f) = \mathrm{WD}_{\mathcal{W}X}\left(\dfrac{tf}{f}, f_r \ln\dfrac{f}{f_r}\right)$
κth Power Altes distribution	$\mathrm{AM}_X^{(\kappa)}(t,f) = \mathrm{WD}_{\mathcal{W}_\kappa X}\left(\dfrac{t}{\kappa\,\lvert f/f_r\rvert^{\kappa-1}}, f_r \mathrm{sgn}(f)\,\lvert f/f_r\rvert^\kappa\right), \kappa \neq 0$
Hyperbologram	$\mathrm{HYP}_X(t,f;\Gamma) = \displaystyle\int_{-\infty}^{\infty}\int_0^{\infty} \mathrm{WD}_{\mathcal{W}\Gamma}\left(t'-\dfrac{tf}{f_r}, f'-f_r\ln\dfrac{f}{f_r}\right) \mathrm{WD}_{\mathcal{W}X}(t',f') dt' df'$
Pseudo-Altes distribution	$\mathrm{PAD}_X(t,f;\Gamma) = f_r \displaystyle\int_0^{\infty} \mathrm{WD}_{\mathcal{W}\Gamma}\left(0, f_r \ln\dfrac{f}{f'}\right) \mathrm{WD}_{\mathcal{W}X}\left(\dfrac{tf}{f_r}, f_r \ln\dfrac{f'}{f_r}\right)\dfrac{df'}{f'}$
Smoothed Pseudo-Altes distribution	$\mathrm{SPAD}_X(t,f;\Gamma,g) = f_r \displaystyle\int_{-\infty}^{\infty}\int_0^{\infty} g(tf-c) \mathrm{WD}_{\mathcal{W}\Gamma}\left(0, f_r \ln\dfrac{f}{f'}\right) \mathrm{WD}_{\mathcal{W}X}\left(\dfrac{c}{f_r}, f_r \ln\dfrac{f'}{f_r}\right)\dfrac{df'}{f'} dc$

Note: Where $f_r > 0$ is a positive reference frequency, $(\mathcal{W}H)(f) = \sqrt{e^{f/f_r}} H(f_r e^{f/f_r})$, $(\mathcal{W}_\kappa H)(f)\,\lvert\kappa\rvert\,\lvert(f_r/f)\rvert^{\lvert(\kappa-1)/\kappa\rvert^{-1/2}}$
$H(f_r \mathrm{sgn}(f)\,\lvert f/f_r\rvert^{1/\kappa})$, $\kappa \neq 0$, and $\mathrm{sgn}(f) = \begin{cases} 1, & f > 0 \\ -1, & f < 0 \end{cases}$.

$$= \frac{1}{\lvert f\rvert}\iint \Phi_A\left(\frac{f'}{f},\frac{v}{f}\right) X(f'+v/2) X^*(f'-v/2) e^{j2\pi tv} df' dv \tag{2.13}$$

$$= \iint \psi_A\left(f(t-t'),\frac{f'}{f}\right) \mathrm{WD}_x(t',f') dt' df' \tag{2.14}$$

$$= \iint \Psi_A\left(f\tau,\frac{v}{f}\right) \mathrm{AF}_x(\tau,v) e^{j2\pi tv} d\tau dv \tag{2.15}$$

The Affine class kernels are interrelated by the same Fourier transforms given in Equations 2.10 and 2.11. Note that the third normal form of the Affine class involves an Affine smoothing of the WD. Well-known members of the Affine class are the Bertrands' P_0 distribution, the scalogram, and the Unterberger distributions. All are defined in Table 2.1, and their kernel forms and TFR property constraints are listed in Table 2.6. Because of the scale covariance property, many TFRs in the Affine class exhibit constant-Q behavior, permitting multiresolution analysis.

TABLE 2.6 Affine Class Kernels and Constraints

TFR	$\Psi_A(\zeta,\beta)$	$\Phi_A(b,\beta)$
B0D	$\dfrac{\beta/2}{\sinh\beta/2}e^{-j2\pi\zeta\left[\frac{\beta}{2}\coth\frac{\beta}{2}\right]}$	$\dfrac{\beta/2}{\sinh\beta/2}\delta\left(b-\left[\dfrac{\beta}{2}\coth\dfrac{\beta}{2}\right]\right)$
FD	$\left[1-\left(\dfrac{\beta}{4}\right)^2\right]e^{j2\pi\zeta\left[1+(\beta/4)^2\right]}$	$\left[1-\left(\dfrac{\beta}{4}\right)^2\right]\delta\left(b-\left[1+(\beta/4)^2\right]\right)$
GWD	$e^{-j2\pi\zeta[1-\tilde{\alpha}\beta]}$	$\delta(b-[1-\tilde{\alpha}\beta])$
SCAL	$AF_\gamma(-\zeta/f_r,-f_r\beta)$	$f_r\Gamma(f_r(b-\beta/2))\Gamma^*(f_r(b+\beta/2))$
UAD	$e^{-j2\pi\zeta\sqrt{1+\beta^2/4}}$	$\delta\left(b-\sqrt{1+\beta^2/4}\right)$
UPD	$\left[1+\beta^2/4\right]^{-1/2}e^{-j2\pi\zeta\sqrt{1+\beta^2/4}}$	$\left[1+\beta^2/4\right]^{-1/2}\delta\left(b-\sqrt{1+\beta^2/4}\right)$
WD	$e^{-j2\pi\zeta}$	$\delta(b-1)$

Property	Constraint on Kernel
P_1: Frequency shift	$\Psi_A(\zeta,\beta)=S_{A\cap C}(\zeta\cdot\beta)\,e^{-j2\pi\zeta}$
P_2: Time shift	Always satisfied
P_3: Scale covariance	Always satisfied
P_4: Hyperbolic time shift	$\Phi_A(b,\beta)=G_A(\beta)\delta\left(b-\dfrac{\beta}{2}\coth\dfrac{\beta}{2}\right)$
P_5: Convolution	$\Psi_A(\zeta_1+\zeta_2,\beta)=\Psi_A(\zeta_1,\beta)\cdot\Psi_A(\zeta_2,\beta)$
P_7: Real-valued	$\Psi_A(\zeta,\beta)=\Psi_A^*(-\zeta,-\beta)$
P_9: Time marginal	$\displaystyle\int\Phi_A(b,-2b)\dfrac{db}{|b|}=1$
P_{10}: Frequency marginal	$\Phi_A(b,0)=\delta(b-1)$
P_{11}: Energy distribution	$\displaystyle\int\Phi_A(b,0)\dfrac{db}{|b|}=1$
P_{14}: Finite time support	$\varphi_A(a,\zeta)=0,\quad\left|\dfrac{a}{\zeta}\right|>\dfrac{1}{2}$
P_{15}: Finite frequency support	$\Phi_A(b,\beta)=0,\quad\left|\dfrac{b-1}{\beta}\right|>\dfrac{1}{2}$
P_{17}: Group delay	$\Phi_A(b,0)=\delta(b-1)\quad\text{and}\quad\left.\dfrac{\partial}{\partial\beta}\Phi_A(b,\beta)\right|_{\beta=0}=0$
P_{19}: Frequency localization	$\Phi_A(b,0)=\delta(b-1)$
P_{25}: Moyal's formula	$\displaystyle\int\Phi_A^*(b\beta,\tilde{\eta}\beta)\Phi_A(\beta,\tilde{\eta}\beta)d\beta=\delta(b-1),\forall\tilde{\eta}$

Note: Here, $S_{A\cap C}(\cdot)$ is a one-dimensional product kernel characterizing the frequency shift members of the affine class.

2.3.3 Hyperbolic Class of TFRs

The Hyperbolic class of TFRs consists of all TFRs that are covariant to scale changes and hyperbolic time shifts, that is, properties P_3 and P_4 in Table 2.2 (Papandreou et al., 1993). They can be analyzed using the following four normal forms:

$$H_X(t,f;\Psi_H) = \iint \varphi_H(tf - c,\zeta)\upsilon_X(c,\zeta)e^{-j2\pi[\ln(f/f_r)]\zeta}\,dc\,d\zeta \tag{2.16}$$

$$= \iint \Phi_H\left(\ln\frac{f}{f_r} - b,\beta\right)f_r e^b X(f_r e^{b+\beta/2})X^*(f_r e^{b-\beta/2})e^{j2\pi tf\beta}\,db\,d\beta \tag{2.17}$$

$$= \int_{-\infty}^{\infty}\int_{0}^{\infty} \psi_H\left(tf - t'f',\ln\frac{f}{f'}\right)AM_X(t',f')\,dt'\,df' \tag{2.18}$$

$$= \iint \Psi_H(\zeta,\beta)HAF_X(\zeta,\beta)e^{j2\pi(tf\beta - [\ln(f/f_r)]\zeta)}\,d\zeta\,d\beta \tag{2.19}$$

where $AM_X(t,f)$ is the Altes distribution and $HAF_X(\zeta,\beta)$ is the hyperbolic AF defined in Table 2.1, $\upsilon_X(c,\zeta)$ is defined in Table 2.7, $(\mathcal{W}X)(f) = \sqrt{e^{f/f_r}}\,X(f_r e^{f/f_r})$ is a unitary warping on the frequency axis of the signal, and the kernels are interrelated via the Fourier transforms in Equations 2.10 and 2.11.

Table 2.3 reveals that the Altes–Marinovic, the Bertrands' P_0, and the hyperbologram distributions are members of the Hyperbolic class. Their kernels are given in Table 2.7, and kernel property constraints are given in Table 2.2. The hyperbolic TFRs give highly concentrated TFR representations for signals with hyperbolic group delay. Each Hyperbolic class TFR, kernel, and property corresponds to a warped version of a Cohen's class TFR, kernel, and property, respectively. For example, Table 2.5 shows that the Altes distribution is equal to the WD after both the signal and the time–frequency axes are

TABLE 2.7 Kernels of the Hyperbolic Class of Time–Frequency Representations

TFR	$\psi_H(c,b)$	$\Psi_H(\zeta,\beta)$	$\varphi_H(c,\zeta)$	$\Phi_H(b,\beta)$
AM	$\delta(c)\delta(b)$	1	$\delta(c)$	$\delta(b)$
B0D	$\int \delta(b + \ln\lambda(\beta))e^{j2\pi c\beta}\,d\beta$	$e^{-j2\pi\zeta\ln\lambda(\beta)}$	$\int e^{j2\pi(c\beta - \zeta\ln\lambda(\beta))}\,d\beta$	$\delta(b + \ln\lambda(\beta))$
GAM	$\dfrac{1}{\|\tilde{\alpha}\|}e^{-j2\pi cb/\tilde{\alpha}}$	$e^{j2\pi\tilde{\alpha}\zeta\beta}$	$\delta(c + \tilde{\alpha}\zeta)$	$\delta(b - \tilde{\alpha}\beta)$
HYP	$AM_\Gamma\left(\dfrac{-c}{f_r e^{-b}}, f_r e^{-b}\right)$	$HAF_\Gamma(-\zeta,-\beta)$	$\upsilon_\Gamma(-c,-\zeta)$	$V_\Gamma(-b,-\beta)$
PAD	$f_r\delta(c)AM_\Gamma(0,f_r e^b)$	$f_r\upsilon_\Gamma(0,\zeta)$	$f_r\delta(c)\upsilon_\Gamma(0,\zeta)$	$f_r AM_\Gamma(0,f_r e^b)$
SPAD	$f_r g(c)AM_\Gamma(0,f_r e^b)$	$f_r G(\beta)\upsilon_\Gamma(0,\zeta)$	$f_r g(c)\upsilon_\Gamma(0,\zeta)$	$f_r G(\beta)AM_\Gamma(0,f_r e^b)$

Note: Here, $\lambda(\beta) = (\beta/2)/(\sinh\beta/2)$, $V_\Gamma(b,\beta) = f_r e^b\Gamma(f_r e^{b+\beta/2})\Gamma^*(f_r e^{b-\beta/2})$, $\upsilon_\Gamma(c,\zeta) = \rho_\Gamma(c + \zeta/2)\rho_\Gamma^*(c - \zeta/2)$, and
$\rho_\Gamma(c) = \displaystyle\int_0^\infty \Gamma(f)(f/f_r)^{j2\pi c}\frac{df}{\sqrt{f}}$.

warped appropriately. The WD's perfect localization of linear FM chirps (P_{21}) corresponds to the Altes distribution's perfect localization for hyperbolic FM chirps (P_{22}). This one-to-one correspondence between the Cohen and Hyperbolic classes greatly facilitates their analysis and gives alternative methods for calculating various TFRs.

2.3.4 κth Power Class

The Power class of TFRs consists of all TFRs that are scale covariant and power time-shift covariant, that is

$$PC_Y^{(\kappa)}(t,f) = PC_X^{(\kappa)}\left(t - c\frac{d}{df}\xi(f/f_r), f\right) \quad \text{for } Y(f) = e^{-j2\pi c\xi_\kappa(f/f_r)}X(f) \tag{2.20}$$

where $\xi_\kappa(f) = \text{sgn}(f)\,|f|^\kappa$, for $\kappa \neq 0$ (Hlawatsch et al., 1999). Consequently, the κth Power class represents well group delay changes in the signal that are powers of frequency. When $\kappa = 1$, the Power class is equivalent to the Affine class. The central member, $AM^{(\kappa)}$ in Table 2.1, is the Power class equivalent to the Altes–Marinovic distribution.

2.4 Common TFRs and Their Use in Biomedical Applications

This section will briefly review some of the TFRs commonly used in biomedical analysis and summarize their relative advantages and disadvantages.

2.4.1 Wigner Distribution

One of the oldest TFRs in Table 2.1 is the WD, which Wigner proposed in quantum mechanics as a two-dimensional statistical distribution relating the Fourier transform pairs of position and momentum of a particle. Table 2.3 reveals that the WD satisfies a large number of desirable TFR properties, P_1 to P_3, P_5 to P_7, P_9 to P_{21}, and P_{23} and P_{25}. It is a member of both the Cohen and the Affine classes. The WD is a high-resolution TFR for linear FM chirps, sinusoids, and impulses. Since the WD satisfies Moyal's formula, it has been used to design optimal signal-detection and synthesis algorithms. The drawbacks of the WD are that it can be negative, it requires the signal to be known for all time, and it is a quadratic TFR with no implicit smoothing to remove cross-terms.

2.4.2 Smoothed Wigner Distributions

Many TFRs are related to the WD by either smoothing or warping, for example, see Equations 2.8 and 2.18 and Table 2.5. An intuitive understanding of the effects of cross-terms on quadratic TFRs can be obtained by analyzing the WD of a multicomponent signal $y(t)$ in Equation 2.5 under the assumption that each signal component is a shifted version of a basic envelope, that is, $x_n(t) = x(t - t_n)\,e^{j2\pi f_n t}$:

$$WD_y(t,f) = \sum_{n=1}^{N} WD_x(t - t_n, f - f_n) + 2\sum_{k=1}^{N-1}\sum_{q=k+1}^{N} WD_x(t - \bar{t}_{k,q}, f - \bar{f}_{k,q})$$

$$\cos(2\pi[\Delta f_{k,q}(t - \Delta t_{k,q}) - \Delta t_{k,q}(f - \Delta f_{k,q}) + \Delta f_{k,q}\Delta t_{k,q}]) \tag{2.21}$$

where $\Delta f_{k,q} = f_k - f_q$ is the difference or "beat" frequency and $\bar{f}_{k,q} = (f_k + f_q)/2$ is the average frequency between the kth and qth signal components. Similarly, $\Delta t_{k,q}$ is the difference time and $\bar{t}_{k,q}$ is the average time. The auto-WD terms in the first summation properly reflect the fact that the WD is a member of Cohen's shift covariant class. Unfortunately, the cross-WD terms in the second summation occur midway in the time–frequency plane between each pair of signal components and oscillate with a spatial frequency proportional to the distance between them. The Pseudo-WD (PWD) and the smoothed PWD (SPWD) defined in Table 2.1 use low-pass smoothing windows $\eta(\tau)$ and $\gamma(t)$ to reduce oscillatory cross-components. However, Table 2.5 reveals that the PWD performs smoothing only in the frequency direction. Short smoothing windows greatly reduce the limits of integration in the PWD and SPWD formulations and hence reduce computation time. However, Table 2.3 reveals that smoothing the WD reduces the number of desirable properties it satisfies from 18 to 7 for the PWD and to only 3 for the SPWD.

2.4.3 Spectrogram

One of the most commonly used TFRs for slowly time-varying or quasi-stationary signals is the spectrogram, defined in Tables 2.1 and 2.5 (Rabiner and Schafer, 1978). It is equal to the squared magnitude of the short-time Fourier transform, performing a local or "short-time" Fourier analysis by using a sliding analysis window $\gamma(t)$ to segment the signal into short sections centered near the output time t before computing a Fourier transformation. The spectrogram is easy to compute, using either FFTs or a parallel bank of filters, and it is often easy to interpret. The quadratic spectrogram smooths away all cross-terms except those which occur when two signal components overlap. This smoothing also distorts autoterms. The spectrogram does a poor job representing rapidly changing spectral characteristics or resolving two closely spaced components because there is an inherent trade-off between good time resolution, which requires a short analysis window, and good frequency resolution, which requires a long analysis window. The spectrogram satisfies only three TFR properties listed in Tables 2.2 and 2.3, that is, it is a nonnegative member of Cohen's shift invariant class.

2.4.4 Choi–Williams Exponential and Reduced Interference Distributions

The Choi–Williams exponential distribution (CWD) and the reduced interference distribution (RID) in Table 2.1 are often used as a compromise between the high-resolution but cluttered WD versus the smeared but easy to interpret spectrogram (Williams and Jeong, 1992). Since they are members of both the Cohen class and the Affine class, their AF domain kernels in Table 2.4 have a very special form, that is, $\Psi_C(\tau, \nu) = S_c(\tau\nu)$, called a product kernel, which is a one-dimensional kernel evaluated at the product of its time–frequency variables (Hlawatsch and Boudreaux-Bartels, 1992). The CWD uses a Gaussian product kernel in the AF plane to reduce cross-terms, while the RID typically uses a classic window function that is time-limited and normalized to automatically satisfy many desirable TFR properties (see Table 2.3). The CWD has one scaling factor σ that allows the user to select either good cross-term reduction or good auto-term preservation but, unfortunately, not always both. The generalized exponential distribution in Table 2.1 is an extension of the CWD that permits both (Hlawatsch and Boudreaux-Bartels, 1992). Because the CWD and RID product kernels have hyperbolic isocontours in the AF plane, they always pass cross-terms between signal components that occur at either the same time or frequency, and they can distort auto-terms of linear FM chirp signals whose instantaneous frequency has a slope close to 1. The multiform tiltable exponential distribution (MTED) (Costa and Boudreaux-Bartels, 1995), another extension of the CWD, works well for any linear FM chirp.

2.4.5 Scalogram or Wavelet Transform Squared Magnitude

The scalogram (Flandrin, 1993), defined in Tables 2.1 and 2.5, is the squared magnitude of the wavelet transform (WT) (Rioul and Vetterli, 1991; Daubechies, 1992; Meyer, 1993) and is a member of the Affine class. It uses a special sliding analysis window $\gamma(t)$, called the mother wavelet, to analyze local spectral information of the signal $x(t)$. The mother wavelet is either compressed or dilated to give a multiresolution signal representation. The scalogram can be thought of as the multiresolution output of a parallel bank of octave band-filters. High-frequency regions of the WT domain have very good time resolution, whereas low-frequency regions of the WT domain have very good spectral resolution. The WT has been used to model the middle- to high-frequency range operation of the cochlea, to track transients such as speech pitch and the onset of the QRS complex in electrocardiogram (ECG) signals, and to analyze fractal and chaotic signals. One drawback of the scalogram is its poor temporal resolution at low-frequency regions of the time–frequency plane and poor spectral resolution at high frequencies. Moreover, many "classical" windows do not satisfy the conditions needed for a mother wavelet. The scalogram cannot remove cross-terms when signal components overlap. Further, many discrete WT implementations do not preserve the important time-shift covariance property.

2.4.6 Biomedical Applications

The ECG signal is a recording of the time-varying electrical rhythm of the heart. The short-duration QRS complex is the most predominant feature of the normal ECG signal. Abnormal heart rhythms can be identified on the ECG by detecting the QRS complex from one cycle to the next. The transient detection capability of the WT has been exploited for detection of the QRS complex (Li and Zheng, 1995; Kadambe et al., 1999). The WT exhibits local maxima that align across successive (dyadic) scales at the location of transient components, such as QRS complexes. The advantage of using the WT is that it is robust both to noise and to nonstationarities in the QRS complex.

Other pathological features in the heart's electrical rhythm that appear only in high-resolution signal-averaged ECG signals are ventricular late potentials (VLPs). VLPs are small-amplitude, short-duration micropotentials that occur after the QRS complex and are precursors to dangerous, life-threatening cardiac arrhythmias. Tuteur (1989) used the peak of the WT at a fixed scale to identify simulated VLPs. Jones et al. (1992) and Khadra et al. (2003) compared different time–frequency techniques, such as the spectrogram, the smoothed WD, and the WT, in their ability to discriminate between normal patients and patients susceptible to dangerous arrhythmias. Morlet et al. (1993) used the transient detection capability of the WT to identify VLPs.

The WT has also been applied to the ECG signal in the context of ECG analysis and compression by Crowe et al. (1992). Furthermore, Crowe et al. (1992) exploited the capability of the WT to analyze fractal-like signals to study heart rate variability (HRV) data, which have been described as having fractal-like properties.

The recording of heart sounds, or phonocardiogram (PCG) signal, has been analyzed using many time–frequency techniques. Bulgrin et al. (1993) compared the short-time Fourier transform and the WT for the analysis of abnormal PCGs. Picard et al. (1991) analyzed the sounds produced by different prosthetic valves using the spectrogram. The binomial RID, which is a fast approximation to the CWD, was used to analyze the short-time, narrow-bandwidth features of first heart sound in mongrel dogs by Wood et al. (1992).

TFRs have also been applied to nonstationary brain wave signals, including the electroencephalogram (EEG), the electrocorticogram (ECoG), and evoked potentials (EPs). Zaveri et al. (1992) characterized the nonstationary behavior of the ECoG of epileptic patients using the spectrogram, the WD, and the CWD, with the CWD exhibiting superior results. The WT was used to identify the onset of epileptic seizures in the EEG by Schiff and Milton (1993), to extract a single EP by Bartnik et al. (1992), and to characterize changes in somatosensory EPs due to brain injury caused by oxygen deprivation by Thakor et al. (1993). A principal component analysis data reduction method to extract representative features from TFRs of ERPs was examined by Bernat et al. (2005).

Crackles are lung sounds indicative of pathological conditions. Verreault (1989) used AR models of slices of the WD to discriminate crackles from normal lung sounds.

The electrogastrogram (EGG) is a noninvasive measure of the time-varying electrical activity of the stomach. Promising results regarding abnormal EGG rhythms and the frequency of the EGG slow wave were obtained using the CWD by Lin and Chen (1994).

Widmalm et al. (1991) analyzed temporo mandibular joint (TMJ) clicking using the spectrogram, the WD, and the RID. The RID allowed for better time–frequency resolution of the TMJ sounds than the spectrogram while reducing the cross-terms associated with the WD. TMJ signals were also modeled using nonorthogonal Gabor logons by Brown et al. (1994). The primary advantage of this technique, which optimizes the location and support of each Gabor logon, is that only a few such logons were needed to represent the TMJ clicks.

Auditory applications of TFRs are intuitively appealing because the cochlea exhibits constant-bandwidth behavior at low frequencies and constant-Q behavior at middle to high frequencies. Applications include a wavelet-based model of the early stages of acoustic signal processing in the auditory system (Yang et al., 1992), a comparison of the WD and Rihaczek distribution on the response of auditory neurons to wideband noise stimulation (Eggermont and Smith, 1990), and spectrotemporal analysis of dorsal cochlear neurons in the guinea pig (Backoff and Clopton, 1991).

The importance of mammography, x-ray examination of the breast, lies in the early identification of tumors. Kaewlium and Longbotham (1993) used the spectrogram with a Gabor window as a texture discriminator to identify breast masses. Laine et al. (1994) applied multiresolution techniques, including the dyadic and hexagonal WT, for adaptive feature enhancement of mammograms blended with synthetic clinical features of interest. This technique shows promise for enhancing the visualization of mammographic features of interest without additional cost or radiation.

Magnetic resonance imaging (MRI) allows for the imaging of the soft tissues in the body. Weaver et al. (1992) reduced the long processing time of traditional phase encoding of MRI images by WT encoding. Moreover, unlike phase-encoded images, Gibb's ringing phenomena and motion artifacts are localized in WT-encoded images.

The Doppler ultrasound signal is the reflection of an ultrasonic beam due to moving red blood cells and provides information regarding blood vessels and heart chambers. Doppler ultrasound signals in patients with narrowing of the aortic valve were analyzed using the spectrogram by Cloutier et al. (1991). Guo and colleagues (1994) examined and compared the application of five different time–frequency representations (the spectrogram, short-time AR model, CWD, RID, and Bessel distributions) with simulated Doppler ultrasound signals of the femoral artery. Promising results were obtained from the Bessel distribution, the CWD, and the short-time AR model.

Another focus of bioengineering applications of TFRs has concerned the analysis of biological signals of interest, including the sounds generated by marine mammals, such as dolphins and whales, and the sonar echolocation systems used by bats to locate and identify their prey. The RID was applied to sperm whale acoustic signals by Williams and Jeong (1992) and revealed an intricate time–frequency structure that was not apparent in the original time-series data. Buck et al. (2000) developed a synthetic dolphin whistle algorithm to investigate acoustic features dolphins may use to discriminate signature whistle vocalizations. The complicated time–frequency characteristics of dolphin whistles were analyzed by Tyack et al. (1992) using the spectrogram, the WD, and the RID, with the RID giving the best results. Flandrin (1988) analyzed the time–frequency structure of the different signals emitted by bats during hunting, navigation, and identifying prey using the smoothed PWD. In addition, the instantaneous frequency of the various signals was estimated using time–frequency representations. To model the bat's ability to track amidst clutter, Saillant et al. (1993) proposed the spectrogram correlation and transformation (SCAT) receiver model of the bat's echolocation system which decomposes the bat's return echoes into a monaural temporal representation. Limitations of the SCAT model in the laboratory environment were examined in Peremans and Halam (1998). The most common application of the spectrogram is the analysis and modification of quasi-stationary speech signals (Rabiner and Schafer, 1978).

Acknowledgments

The authors would like to acknowledge the use of the personal notes of Franz Hlawatsch and Antonia Papandreou-Suppappola on TFR kernel constraints as well as the help given by Antonia Papandreou-Suppappola in critiquing the chapter and its tables.

References

Backoff P.M. and Clopton B.M. 1991. A spectrotemporal analysis of DCN single unit responses to wideband noise in guinea pig. *Hear. Res.* 53: 28.

Bartnik E.A., Blinowska K.J., and Durka P.J. 1992. Single evoked potential reconstruction by means of a wavelet transform. *Biol. Cybern.* 67: 175.

Bernat E.M., Williams W.J., and Gehring W.J. 2005. Decomposing ERP time-frequency using PCA. *Clinical Neurophysiology* 116: 1314.

Boashash B. (ed). 1991. *Time–Frequency Signal Analysis—Methods and Applications.* Melbourne, Australia, Longman-Chesire.

Brown M.L., Williams W.J., and Hero A.O. 1994. Non-orthogonal Gabor representation for biological signals. In *Proceedings of the IEEE 1994 International Conference on Acoustics, Speech and Signal Processing*, Australia, pp. 305–308.

Buck J.R., Morgenbesser, H.B., and Tyack, P.L. 2000. Synthesis and modification of the whistles of the bottlenose dolphin, *Tursiops truncates. JASA* 108: 407.

Bulgrin J.R., Rubal B.J., Thompson C.R., and Moody J.M. 1993. Comparison of short-time Fourier transform, wavelet and time-domain analyses of intracardiac sounds. *Biol. Sci. Instrum.* 29: 465.

Claasen T.A.C.M. and Mecklenbräuker W.F.G. 1980. The Wigner distribution: A tool for time-frequency signal analysis, parts I–III. *Philips J. Res.* 35: 217, 276, 372.

Cloutier G., Lemire F., Durand L., Latour Y., Jarry M., Solignac A., and Langlois Y.E. 1991. Change in amplitude distributions of Doppler spectrograms recorded below the aortic valve in patients with a valvular aortic stenosis. *IEEE Trans. Biomed. Eng.* 39: 502.

Cohen L. 1989. Time–frequency distributions—A review. *Proc. IEEE* 77: 941.

Costa A. and Boudreaux-Bartels G.F. 1995. Design of time-frequency representations using multiform, tiltable kernels. *IEEE Trans. SP* 43: 2283.

Crowe J.A., Gibson N.M., Woolfson M.S., and Somekh M.G. 1992. Wavelet transform as a potential tool for ECG analysis and compression. *J. Biomed. Eng.* 14: 268.

Daubechies I. 1992. *Ten Lectures on Wavelets.* Montpelier, VT, Capital City Press.

Eggermont J.J. and Smith G.M. 1990. Characterizing auditory neurons using the Wigner and Rihaczek distributions: A comparison. *JASA* 87: 246.

Flandrin P. 1993. *Temps-Fréquence.* Hermes, Paris, France.

Flandrin P. 1988. Time-frequency processing of bat sonar signals. In Nachtigall P.E. and Moore P.W.B., (eds.), *Animal Sonar: Processes and Performance*, pp. 797–802. New York, Plenum Press.

Guo Z., Durand L.G., and Lee H.C. 1994. Comparison of time-frequency distribution techniques for analysis of simulated Doppler ultrasound signals of the femoral artery. *IEEE Trans. Biomed. Eng.* 41: 332.

Hlawatsch F. and Boudreaux-Bartels G.F. 1992. Linear and quadratic time–frequency signal representations. *IEEE Sig. Proc. Mag.* March: 21.

Hlawatsch F., Papandreou-Suppappola A., and Boudreaux-Bartels G.F. 1999. The power classes—quadratic time-frequency representations with scale covariance and dispersive time-shift covariance. *IEEE Trans. SP* 47: 3067.

Jones D.L., Tovannas J.S., Lander P., and Albert D.E. 1992. Advanced time–frequency methods for signal averaged ECG analysis. *J. Electrocardiol.* 25: 188.

Kadambe S., Murray R., and Boudreaux-Bartels G.F. 1999. Wavelet transform based QRS complex detector. *IEEE Trans. Biomed. Eng.* 46: 838.

Kaewlium A. and Longbotham H. 1993. Application of Gabor transform as texture discriminator of masses in digital mammograms. *Biol. Sci. Instrum.* 29: 183.

Khadra, L., Dickhaus, H., and Lipp, A. 2003. Representations of ECG—late potentials in the time frequency plane. *Med. Eng. Technol.* 17: 228.

Laine A., Schuler S., and Fan J. 1994. Mammographic feature enhancement by multiscale analysis. *IEEE Trans. Med. Imag.* 13: 725

Li C. and Zheng C. 1995. Detection of ECG characteristic points using wavelet transforms. *IEEE Trans. Biomed. Eng.* 42: 21.

Lin Z.Y. and Chen J.D.Z. 1994. Time–frequency representation of the electrogastrogram: Application of the exponential distribution. *IEEE Trans. Biomed. Eng.* 41: 267.

Meyer Y. 1993. *Wavelets–Algorithms and Applications.* SIAM, Philadelphia.

Morlet D., Peyrin F., Desseigne P., Touboul P., and Rubel P. 1993. Wavelet analysis of high resolution signal averaged ECGs in postinfarction patients. *J. Electrocardiol.* 26: 311.

Murray R. 1995. Summary of biomedical applications of time-frequency representations. Technical report no. 0195-0001, University of Rhode Island, Department of Electrical Engineering, Kingston, RI, 02881.

Papandreou A., Hlawatsch F., and Boudreaux-Bartels G.F. 1993. The Hyperbolic class of quadratic time–frequency representations: I. Constant-Q warping, the hyperbolic paradigm, properties, and members. *IEEE Trans. SP* 41: 3425.

Papandreou-Suppappola A. (ed.) 2003. *Applications in Time-Frequency Signal Processing.* Boca Raton, FL, Taylor & Francis.

Peremans H. and Halam, J 1998. The spectrogram and transformation receiver, revisited. *JASA* 104: 1101.

Picard D., Charara J., Guidoin F., Haggag Y., Poussart D., Walker D., and How T. 1991. Phonocardiogram spectral analysis simulator of mitral valve prostheses. *J. Med. Eng. Technol.* 15: 222.

Rabiner L.R. and Schafer R.W. 1978. *Digital Processing of Speech Signals.* Englewood Cliffs, NJ, Prentice-Hall.

Rioul O. and Vetterli M. 1991. Wavelets and signal processing. *IEEE Sig. Proc. Mag.* October: 14.

Saillant P.A., Simmons J.A., Dear S.P., and McMullen T.A. 1993. A computational model of echo processing and acoustic imaging in frequency-modulated echo-locating bats: The spectrogram correlation and transformation receiver. *JASA* 94: 2691.

Schiff S.J. and Milton J.G. 1993. Wavelet transforms for electroencephalographic spike and seizure detection. In *Proc. SPIE—Intl. Soc. Opt. Eng.* San Diego '93, SPIE Proceedings, Vol. 2036, pp. 50–56.

Thakor N.V., Xin Rong G., Yi Chun S., and Hanley D.F. 1993. Multiresolution wavelet analysis of evoked potentials. *IEEE Trans. BME* 40: 1085.

Tuteur F.B. 1989. Wavelet transformations in signal detection. In *Proc. Intl. Conf. ASSP,* ICASSP-88, New York, NY, pp. 1435–1438.

Tyack P.L., Williams W.J., and Cunningham G. 1992. Time-frequency fine structure of dolphin whistles. In *Proc. IEEE—SP Intl. Symp. T-F and T-S Anal.* Victoria, BC, Canada, pp. 17–20.

Verreault E. 1989. Détection et Caractérisation des Rales Crépitants (French). PhD thesis, l'Université Laval, Faculté des Sciences et de Genie.

Weaver J.B., Xu Y., Healy D.M., and Driscoll J.R. 1992. Wavelet encoded MR imaging. *Magnet Reson. Med.* 24: 275.

Widmalm W.E., Williams W.J., and Zheng C. 1991. Time frequency distributions of TMJ sounds. *J. Oral. Rehabil.* 18: 403.

Williams W.J. and Jeong J. 1992. Reduced interference time–frequency distributions. In Boashash B. (ed.), *Time–Frequency Signal Analysis—Methods and Applications,* pp. 74–97. Melbourne/NY, Longman—Chesire/Wiley.

Wood J.C., Buda A.J., and Barry D.T. 1992. Tme-frequency transforms: A new approach to first heart sound dynamics. *IEEE Trans. Biomed. Eng.* 39: 730.

Yang Z., Wang K., and Shamma S. 1992. Auditory representations of acoustic signals. *IEEE Trans. Info. Theory* 38: 824.

Zaveri H.P., Williams W.J., Iasemidis L.D., and Sackellares J.C. 1992. Time–frequency representations of electrocorticograms in temporal lobe epilepsy. *IEEE Trans. Biomed. Eng.* 39: 502.

Further Information

Several TFR tutorials exist on the Cohen class (Cohen, 1989; Hlawatsch and Boudreaux-Bartels, 1992; Boashash, 1991; Flandrin, 1993), Affine class (Bertrand chapter in Boashash, 1991; Flandrin, 1993), Hyperbolic class (Papandreou et al., 1993), and Power class (Hlawatsch et al., 1999). Several special conferences or issues of IEEE journals devoted to TFRs and the WT include *Proceedings of the IEEE-SP Time Frequency and Time-Scale Workshop*, 1992, *IEEE Sig. Proc. Soc.*; Special issue on wavelet transforms and multiresolution signal analysis, *IEEE Trans. Info. Theory*, 1992; and Special issue on wavelets and signal processing, *IEEE Trans. SP*, 1993. A wide variety of TFR applications, including tutorials and pseudo-code, can be found in (Papandreou-Suppappola, 2010). An extended list of references on the application of TFRs to problems in biomedical or bioengineering can be found in Murray (1995).

3

Multivariate Spectral Analysis of Electroencephalogram: Power, Coherence, and Second-Order Blind Identification

Ramesh Srinivasan
University of California,
Irvine

Siyi Deng
University of California,
Irvine

3.1 Introduction

Clinical or research electroencephalogram (EEG) records typically consist of time series of potentials recorded with 64–256 electrodes placed on the scalp locations. This large volume of data contains information that is both redundant and difficult to interpret. A natural question is—how can we compress this information into a more concise format and extract features that can be meaningfully related to cognitive processes or clinical disease states? Because the spatial and temporal properties of EEG can vary widely, no universal answer to this question is expected. However, cognitive neuroscience research and clinical neuroscience applications of EEG including brain–computer interfaces (BCIs) almost always benefit from some form of spectral analysis in which temporal waveforms are decomposed into their discrete frequency components. Indeed, this simple approach has revealed many robust connections between different EEG frequency bands and cognitive functions or clinical diseases (Petsche and Etlinger, 1998; Pfurtsheller and Lopes da Silva, 1999; Murias et al., 2007). Spectral analysis is the obvious entry point for studying EEG dynamics, and most EEG scientists use the *power spectrum* as an essential first step in processing EEG signals.

Neuronal dynamics can be considered a stochastic (random) process having statistical properties in time and space. This general framework has important advantages over viewpoints that may prejudge the nature of EEG dynamics, for instance that one location in the brain generates the EEG observed in one frequency band. A more general (and realistic) conceptual model considers that the spatiotemporal statistics of EEG signals contain information that reflect something about the spatiotemporal statistics of current source activity in the brain. While spectral analysis is widely used to analyze the times series at each EEG channel, analyses of spatial properties of EEG are equally important to characterize statistical properties of the underlying source distribution. Across a broad range of cognitive and clinical studies, measures of phase synchronization between electrodes located over different brain regions appear especially promising approaches to identify brain networks. Brain networks are cell assemblies that coordinate neuronal action across brain regions supporting complex cognition, behavior, and consciousness. This coordination is at least partly reflected in the synchronization of EEG signals in one frequency band. *Coherence* measures the consistency of the phase difference between two channels in one frequency band. Many brain diseases, including schizophrenias, attention deficit disorders, and autism are associated with inadequate or inappropriate cell assembly formation, reflected in the strength and spatial pattern of the coherence of EEG signals.

How can we relate power and coherence measured with EEG electrodes on the scalp to statistical properties of the source activity in the brain? Mathematical models of volume conduction in the head are used to *investigate theoretical limitations on EEG dynamic properties as estimates of brain dynamics.* The resulting mathematical models provide a conceptual framework for understanding the EEG data. In this chapter, we provide a theoretical framework with which we can interpret EEG power and coherence. The effect of current flow through tissues of the head is to spatially low pass filter the signal generated in the brain. As a consequence, power at one EEG electrode depends on both the strength and spatial properties of the source activity in the brain. Coherence between electrodes also reflects this spatial filtering; as a consequence only coherence between widely spaced electrodes can be easily interpreted.

The spatial filtering due to volume conduction can be understood as a linear mixing process. Each electrode sums the activity over many sources in the brain and each electrode represented a different mixture of sources. This has led to a great deal of interest in using blind source separation (BSS) techniques to process EEG data, separating source processes according to various statistical criteria. Perhaps the most well known of these techniques, Independent Component Analysis (ICA) has been implemented using a variety of statistical criteria to separate sources from the mixtures at each electrode without any other prior information (Makeig et al., 2004). Spectral analysis can then be performed on these components. However, the source separation achieved by ICA is not optimal for spectral analysis. While ICA usually makes use of features of the joint probability density of the EEG records, the analysis is insensitive to the temporal order in which the multichannel EEG was observed. That is, if the order in which the potentials (at all electrodes) is recorded was randomized there would no effect on ICA. Second-order blind identification (SOBI) is a BSS method developed for time-series analysis (Belouchrani et al., 1997) in array processing which explicitly incorporates the temporal structure of the second-order statistics (covariance) of the signals in developing a BSS from the EEG electrode. When applied to EEG signals, they can be used to obtain a multivariate spectral analysis that can identify brain networks operating in different (or even the same) frequency bands.

3.2 Synaptic Action Generates EEG

Scalp potentials are believed to be generated by *millisecond-scale modulations* of synaptic current sources at the surfaces of neurons (Lopes da Silva and Storm van Leeuwen, 1978; Nunez, 1981, 1995, 2000a,b; Lopes da Silva, 1999).

While cortical and scalp potentials are generated by these microsources associated with synaptic action, potentials are more conveniently modeled in terms of *dipole moment per unit volume* $\mathbf{P}(\mathbf{r}, t)$ where $\mathbf{r}$ spans the volume of the brain. For convenience of this discussion, the brain volume may be parceled into N tissue masses or voxels of volume ΔV, each producing its vector dipole moment. The potential anywhere in the brain or scalp surface is then expressed as a weighted sum (or integral) of contributions from all these sources

$$\Phi_S(\mathbf{r},t) = \int_{B'} G_H(\mathbf{r},\mathbf{r}')\mathbf{P}(\mathbf{r}',t)\,dV(\mathbf{r}') \qquad (3.1)$$

If the volume element $dV(\mathbf{r}')$ is defined in terms of cortical columns, the volume integral may be reduced to an integral over the folded cortical surface. The weighting coefficients G_H is the *Green's function* which depends on the properties of the volume conductor and the locations of source $\mathbf{r}'$ and measurement location $\mathbf{r}$. The Green's function is essentially the *impulse response function* between sources and surface measurement locations. For some locations, for example, deep tissues like the thalamus or other subcortical structures, G_H is expected to be very small, while for superficial sources in the gyral crowns of the cortex, G_H is large. G_H contains all geometric and conductive information about the head volume conductor. The most common head models consist of three or four concentric spherical shells, representing brain, cerebrospinal fluid (four sphere), skull and scalp tissue with different electrical conductivities as shown in Figure 3.1 for which analytic solutions have been obtained (Nunez and Srinivasan, 2006). Numerical methods such as the boundary element method (BEM) may also be used to estimate G_H, by employing MRI to determine tissue boundaries, resulting in a more accurate geometrical model. However, the accuracy of these models may be severely limited by incomplete knowledge of tissue conductivities—they may be less accurate conductivity models (Nunez and Srinivasan, 2006; Srinivasan et al., 2007). For the purposes of the article, we make use of the analytic spherical model to estimate GH. The results have been confirmed using ellipsoidal models fit to MRI images (Srinivasan et al., 2007).

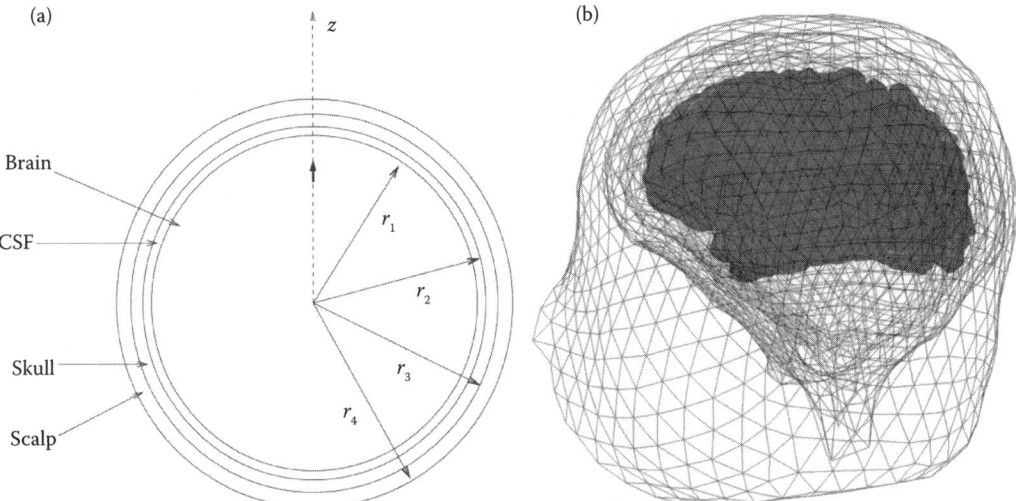

FIGURE 3.1 Volume conduction models for EEG. (a) A dipole is shown in the inner sphere of a *4-concentric spheres head model* consisting of the inner sphere (brain) and three spherical shells representing CSF (cerebrospinal fluid), skull and scalp. The parameters of model are the radii (r_1, r_2, r_3, r_4) of each shell and the conductivity ratios (σ_1/σ_2, σ_1/σ_3, σ_1/σ_4). Typical values are: radii (8, 8.1, 8.6, 9.2 cm) and conductivity ratios (0.2, 40, 1). (b) A realistic shaped BEM of the head. The brain and scalp boundaries were found by segmenting the images with a threshold, and opening and closing operation, respectively, while the outer skull boundary was obtained by dilation of the brain boundary (ASA, Netherlands). Although geometrically more accurate that the spherical model, the (geometrically) realistic BEM is potentially a less accurate model than concentric spheres because tissue resistivity is poorly known.

3.3 Time Domain Spectral Analysis

In EEG applications, spectral analysis provides a means to assess *statistical properties* of oscillations in different frequency bands. It is customary to view any experimental data record as one *realization of a random process* (or *stochastic process*) (Bendat and Piersol, 2001). In this context, the word "random" does not imply that lack of statistical structure or deterministic origins of the signals, only that its statistical properties are yet to be discovered. The spectrum obtained by applying the fast Fourier transform (FFT) to a single EEG epoch provides information about the frequency content of that particular epoch. A number of important issues in practical FFT analysis are detailed in several texts (e.g., Bendat and Piersol, 2001). For our purposes, the estimation of the Fourier coefficients for each epoch is the starting point for the development of various statistical tools based on *spectral analysis*. A number of new approaches to Fourier analysis including wavelet analysis (Lachaux et al., 2002), multitaper analysis (Percival and Walden, 1993), autoregressive models (Ding et al., 2006) and Hilbert transforms (Bendat and Piersol, 2001; Le Van Quyen et al., 2001; Deng and Srinivasan, 2010) have potential applications in EEG, particularly in the analysis of short data epochs or characterizing the variation of the spectrum during a time period following a sensory stimulus or preceding movement. All such methods yield estimates of "Fourier coefficients" that reflect the amplitude and phase of the oscillations within one frequency band (and perhaps localized to one window in time). Any of these Fourier coefficients can be used to carry out spectral analysis of time series. However, interpretations using different techniques depend on the assumptions and parameter choices built in to the specific methods chosen to estimate Fourier coefficients. These limitations are probably not as widely appreciated as those associated with conventional FFT methods, suggesting advantages of comparing multiple methods applied to the same data.

Any observed time series is just one physical realization (sample) of the underlying stochastic process, but is not sufficient to *represent* the stochastic process. Thus, the amplitude spectrum of one epoch of EEG is an exact representation of the frequency content of that particular signal epoch, but only provides one observation about the random process. An ensemble of K observations $\{V_k(t)\}$ can be used to estimate statistical properties of the random process. An important question is whether the stochastic process is stationary, that is, the statistical properties of the random process are invariant to shifts in the time where the sample records are obtained. Many studies have contrasted the EEG in different brain states such as eyes closed resting, eyes open resting, during mental calculations, and different sleep stages under the assumption that within these states the EEG can be reasonably assumed to be stationary. By contrast, EEG data collected following a sensory stimulus clearly violate the stationarity assumption—the time at which each sample record $V_k(t)$ is obtained relative to the stimulus can be expected to influence the observed EEG statistics. In this case, the ensemble mean of observations

$$\mu(t) = \frac{1}{K} \sum_{k=1}^{K} V_k(t) \tag{3.2}$$

is the evoked potential (EP) or event-related potential which varies as a function of time over the epoch. We can still use spectral analysis in this case but the interpretations of the results may be more difficult if conventional methods like the FFT are used to analyze the interval. Spectral analysis methods that capture the temporal evolution of the signal in different frequency bands, such as wavelet analysis (Lachaux et al., 2002) are then preferred.

A random process is weakly stationary if the mean (Equation 3.2) and the *power spectrum* are invariant to shifts in the time at which the sample records are obtained. The *power spectrum* (*autospectral density function*) of an EEG signal provides a decomposition of the *variance* of the signal as a function of frequency. As in the case of any other statistical measure, we can never know the *actual* power spectrum of a stochastic process. Rather, we find *estimates* of the power spectrum. The *power spectrum* may be estimated from an ensemble of observations by applying a Fourier transform and summing over K epochs, that is

$$P\left(f_n\right) = \frac{2}{K} \sum_{k=1}^{K} F_k\left(f_n\right) F_k\left(f_n\right)^* = \frac{2}{K} \sum_{k=1}^{K} \left|F_k\left(f_n\right)\right|^2 \quad n = 0,1,2,\ldots(N-1)/2 \qquad (3.3)$$

For each sample epoch $V_k(t_n)$, Fourier coefficients $F_k(f_n)$ can be obtained using the FFT. In Equation 3.3, the frequencies f_n are discrete, and depend on the length of each observation (T) as $f_n = n/T$. The factor of two occurs because we use only positive frequencies. The form of the power spectrum estimate in Equation 3.3 does not depend on the specific algorithm used to estimate the Fourier coefficients (although the discretization of frequencies does depend on the method). If the mean value of the signal is zero, the power spectrum summed over all frequencies is equal to the variance in the signal, a relationship known as *Parseval's theorem* (Bendat and Piersol, 2001). If the EEG time series is recorded in units of μV, Equation 3.3 provides a definition of the EEG power spectrum in units that depend on the bandwidth Δf. The power spectrum is sometimes normalized with respect to the bandwidth to express power in units of μV²/Hz. The *amplitude spectrum*, the square root of the power spectrum, places more emphasis on nondominant spectral peaks and is often our measure of choice for visualization.

Prior to the widespread availability of the FFT and fast computers, the autospectral density function or in the more common parlance, "power spectrum" of a time series was obtained by first estimating the autocorrelation function:

$$R_{VV}(\tau) = E\left[V(t)^* V(t - \tau)\right] \qquad (3.4)$$

Here the expectation operator indicates averaging over observations, and the lag variable τ can take positive or negative values. The autocorrelation function is the covariance of the signal with a delayed copy of the same signal. If τ spans $[-T/2, T/2]$, R_{VV} contains exactly the same information as the power spectrum defined by Equation 3.3. The Fourier transform of the autocorrelation function is the power spectrum of the signal. Modern spectral analysis methods rarely involve direct computation of the autocorrelation function. However, note that later in this chapter we will make use of this formulation of the signal statistics as the basis of a multivariate decomposition of the spectra in multichannel EEG recordings.

Implementation of Equation 3.3 forces tradeoffs involving frequency resolution, statistical power, and putative stationarity. For example, consider the choices involved in analyzing a 60 s EEG record. Figure 3.2 demonstrates power spectra of two EEG channels, one occipital and one frontal, recorded with the subject's eyes closed and at rest. The power spectral estimates were obtained using an epoch length $T = 60$ s ($\Delta f = 0.017$ Hz) and no epoch averaging ($K = 1$ epochs). With this choice, the FFT of the entire record is obtained (exact spectra of the two EEG signals), but no information about the statistical properties of the underlying random process is gained. Note that the power spectrum of the occipital channel (Figure 3.2a) contains two peaks, one below 10 Hz and a larger peak above 10 Hz. The frontal channel (Figure 3.2b) shows a larger peak below 10 Hz. By examining the other channels it was found that the two peaks have distinct spatial distributions over the scalp, suggesting they have different source distributions. Each peak is surrounded by power in sidebands (adjacent frequency bins) of the two peak frequencies. *The signals are stochastic processes occupying relatively narrow bands in the frequency spectrum.*

To analyze the 60 s signal properly, we must decide how to divide the record into epochs to implement Equation 3.3. The choice is a compromise between the advantage of good frequency resolution yielded by long epochs (large T and small K) and the statistical power of our estimate gained by using a larger number of epochs (small T small and large K). If a frequency resolution of $\Delta f = 0.5$ Hz is chosen, the

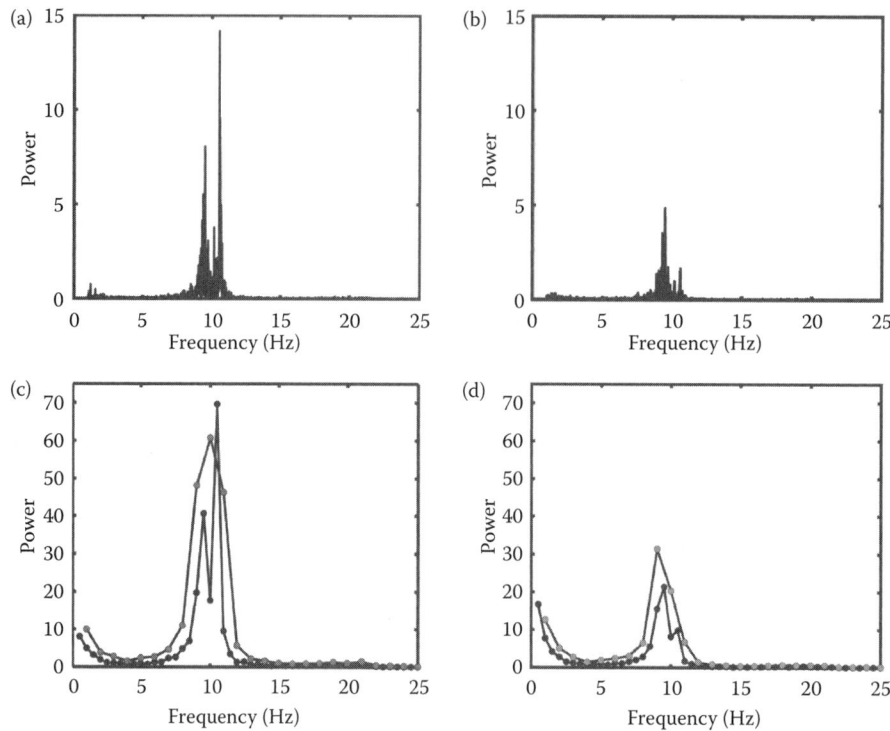

FIGURE 3.2 Example power spectra from a single subject (female, 22 years). The subject is at rest with eyes closed. (a) Power spectrum of a midline occipital channel with epoch length $T = 60$ s and $K = 1$ epochs. The power spectrum appears to have two distinct peaks one below 10 Hz and one above 10 Hz. (b) Power spectrum at a midline frontal channel with epoch length $T = 60$ s and $K = 1$ epochs. Here only the peak below 10 Hz is visible. (c) Power spectra of a midline occipital channel calculated with two different choices of epoch length T and number of epochs K. The gray circles indicate the power spectrum with $T = 1$ s and $K = 60$ epochs. The black circles indicate the power spectrum with $T = 2$ s and $K = 30$ epochs. (d) Power spectra of a midline frontal channel calculated as in Part (c).

record is segmented into $K = 30$ epochs of length $T = 2$ s. If frequency resolution is reduced to $\Delta f = 1$ Hz, we divide the record into $K = 60$ epochs of length $T = 1$ s. Figure 3.2c and d shows the power spectra of the frontal and occipital channels with $\Delta f = 1$ Hz (gray circles) and $\Delta f = 0.5$ Hz (black circles). The power spectra at the occipital and frontal channels are both dominated by alpha rhythm oscillations. At the occipital electrode (Figure 3.2c) two separate peak frequencies are at 9.5 and 10.5 Hz are evident with $\Delta f = 0.5$ Hz, but this is not revealed with $\Delta f = 1$ Hz, where only a single peak frequency at 10 Hz is evident. Lowering frequency resolution has a similar effect at the frontal channel (Figure 3.2d), but since there is very little power at 10.5 Hz, the only clear peak appears at 9 Hz. Thus, by choosing lower frequency resolution we see a signal representation having different (single) peak frequencies at the two sites, while choosing higher frequency resolution results in pairs of frequency peaks at both sites but with different relative magnitudes.

By examining the power spectra for the occipital (Figure 3.3a) and frontal sites (Figure 3.3b) for individual epochs with $\Delta f = 0.5$ Hz, support for two different oscillations within the alpha band is obtained. At the occipital channel individual epochs display two distinct peaks at 9.5 and 10.5 Hz. The first 15 epochs show a strong response at 10.5 Hz but the later epochs show a stronger response at 9.5 Hz. The dominant frequency in each epoch is summarized in the peak power histograms in Figure 3.3c showing that individual epochs displayed peak frequencies at both 9.5 and 10.5 Hz. By contrast, very few epochs have a peak frequency of 10.5 Hz at the frontal site (Figure 3.3d); most epochs have peak

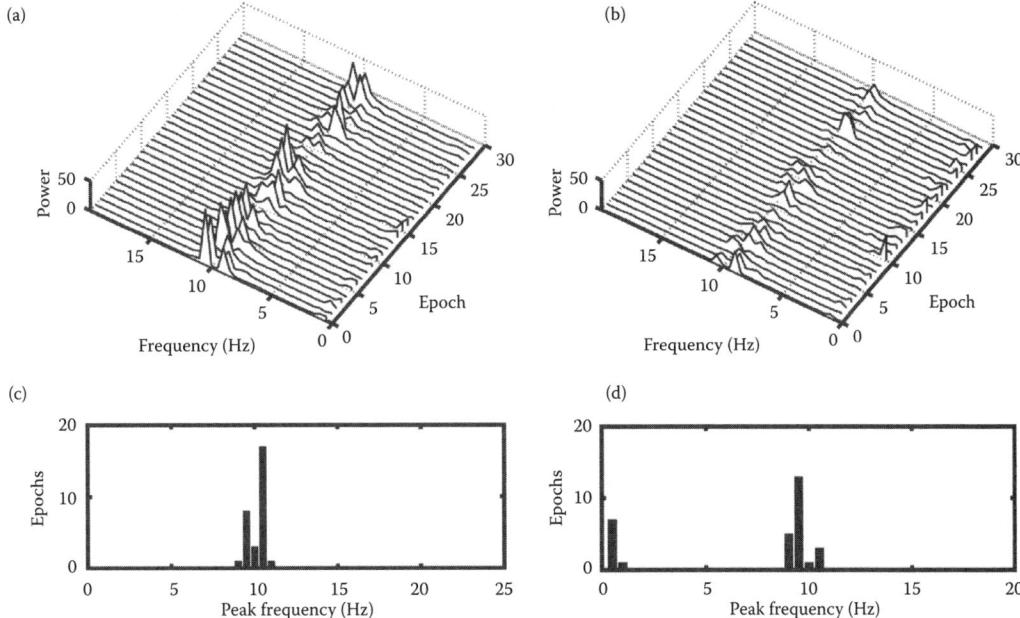

FIGURE 3.3   (a) Plots of 30 (individual epoch) power spectra for the occipital channel shown in Figure 3.2a and c. (b) Plots of the same 30 individual epoch spectra for the frontal channel. (c) Peak power histograms show the distribution of peak frequencies for the 30 epochs shown in Part (a). (d) Peak power histograms for the 30 epochs shown in Part (b).

frequencies either at 9.5 Hz or in the delta band (<2 Hz). Note that during most epochs with strong delta activity in Figure 3.3d the alpha peaks are attenuated.

In summary, estimating the *power spectrum* from an ensemble of epochs provides a decomposition of the variance of the signal as a function of frequency. This is a particularly useful approach because EEG contains oscillatory activity in distinct frequency bands that are associated with different brain states. In the simple example, we presented here of the alpha rhythm in Figures 3.2 and 3.3, electrodes at different locations show different magnitudes of two distinct oscillations with center frequencies at 9.5 and 10.5 Hz. In the next section, factors that determine the magnitude of peaks in the EEG power spectrum are considered. In later sections, methods to quantify spatial properties of EEG rhythms, which are evidently different for the two peak frequencies in this example, are investigated.

3.4 Impact of Spatial Filtering on EEG Power Spectra

Scalp potential amplitude at any frequency can change for several reasons related to "synchronization" of neurons. The large changes in scalp amplitude that occur when brain state changes are believed to be due mostly to such changes in the correlation of the synaptic activity. EEG scientists and clinicians have adopted the label *desynchronization* to indicate large amplitude reductions, particularly in the alpha band (Pfurtscheller and Lopes da Silva, 1999). However, synchronization among neurons may occur in different directions and at different spatial scales, and may occur with zero phase lag or with finite phase differences. In this section, we consider how synchronization of the underlying sources determines EEG power.

There are several (possibly overlapping) means by which synchronization can influence the EEG power spectrum. For convenience of this, we can divide the brain into several thousand volume elements (e.g., macrocolumns, 3 mm in each dimension) located along the folded gray-matter surface of the brain each having a (vector) dipole moment per unit volume $\mathbf{P}(\mathbf{r}, t)$. Volume elements in the white matter, ventricles, and other tissues of the head have very little current source activity. The strength of the dipoles (magnitude of the moment) depends strongly on the synchronization of the synapses within the volume element (Nunez and Srinivasan, 2006). As the source strength increases, we expect scalp potential to increase proportionately if there are no other changes.

A small region of the cortex, for example a gyral crown of surface area 2 cm^2, is composed of around 25 volume elements. Thus, it is more realistic to consider the EEG signals to be generated by dipole layer, consisting of many adjacent dipole sources. Figure 3.4 shows examples of dipole layers of diameter ranging from 3 to 5 cm composed only of radially oriented dipole sources in a concentric spheres model of the head. Each dipole layer is composed of dipole sources with time series that are constructed by adding

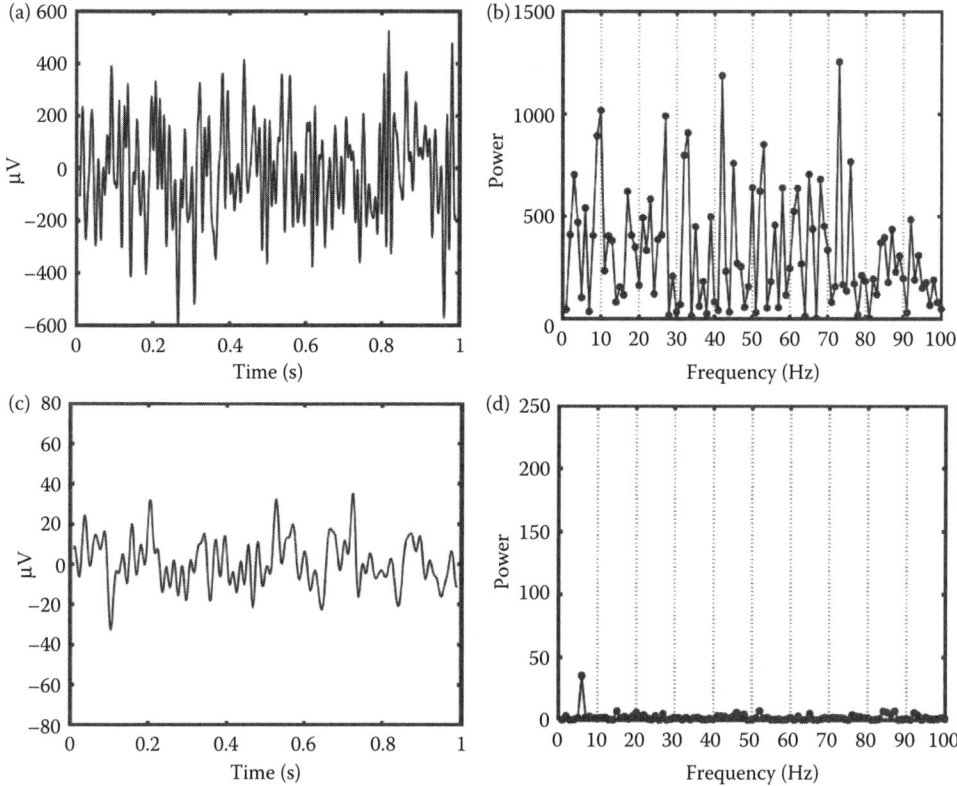

FIGURE 3.4 (a) Time series of a dipole meso-source $\mathbf{P}(\mathbf{r}, t)$ composed of a 15 µV sine wave added to Gaussian random noise with standard deviation $\sigma = 150$ µV. The Gaussian random noise was low pass filtered at 100 Hz. The sine wave has variance (power) equal 1% of the noise. (b) Power spectrum of the time series shown in Part (a). The power spectrum has substantial power at frequencies other than 6 Hz. (c) Time series recorded by an electrode on the outer sphere (scalp) of a four concentric spheres model above the center of a dipole layer of diameter 3 cm. The dipole layer is composed of 32 dipole sources $\mathbf{P}(\mathbf{r}, t)$ with time series constructed similar to Part (a) with independent Gaussian noise (uncorrelated) at each dipole source. Scalp potential was calculated for a dipole layer at a radius $r_z = 7.8$ cm in a four concentric spheres model. The model parameters were radii $(r_1, r_2, r_3, r_4) = (8, 8.1, 8.6, 9.2)$ and conductivity ratios $(\sigma_1/\sigma_2, \sigma_1/\sigma_3, \sigma_1/\sigma_4) = (0.2, 40, 1)$. Notice the time series is smoother than in the case of the individual dipole source. (d) Power spectrum of the time series shown in Part (c). Note the peak at 6 Hz. (e) Time series similar to Part (c), but due to a dipole layer of diameter of 4 cm composed of 68 dipole sources. (f) Power spectrum of the time series shown in Part (e). (g) Similar time series to Part (c), but with a dipole layer of diameter 5 cm composed of 112 dipole sources. The presence of the 6 Hz sinusoid is obvious from the time series. (h) Power spectrum of the time series shown in Part (g). Large spectral peak at 6 Hz is evident.

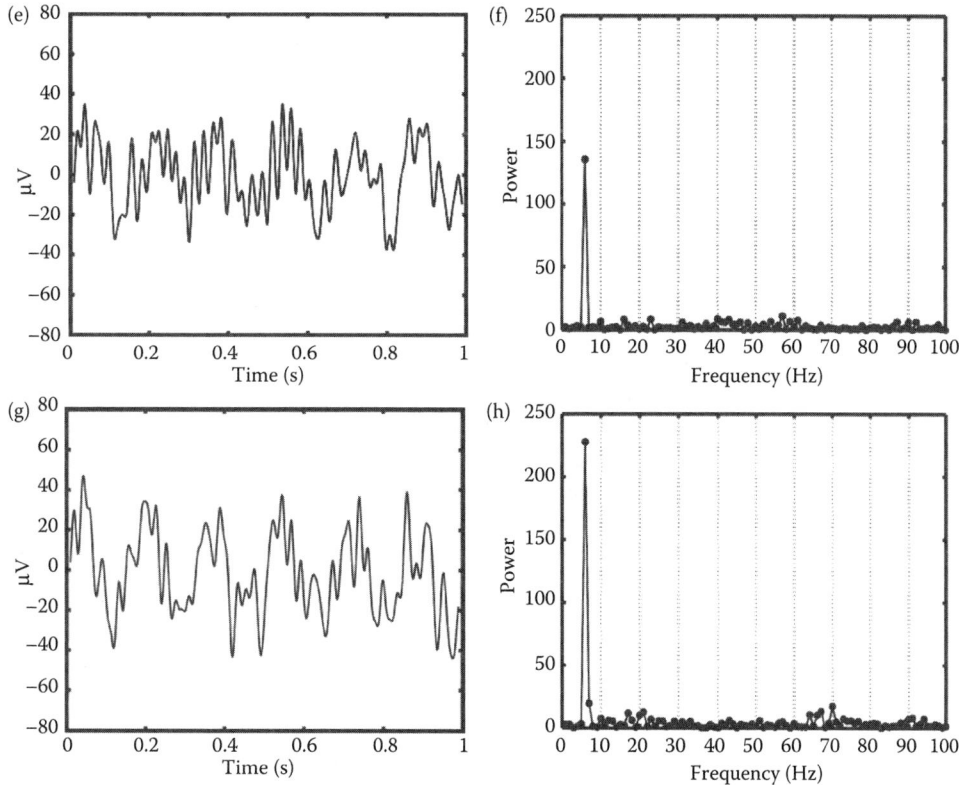

FIGURE 3.4 (Continued.)

a 6 Hz sinusoid of fixed amplitude $A = 15$ μV to a Gaussian random processes with mean $\mu = 0$ and standard deviation $\sigma = 150$ μV. *The 6 Hz components are phase locked across the dipoles, whereas all other components have random phases.* Each source signal is an independent random time series representing transcortical potential across the dipole layer. The source time series of a single dipole source (dipole layer of very small size) is plotted in Figure 3.4a and the corresponding power spectrum is plotted in Figure 3.4b. The power spectrum shows that the source signal is broadband, with some power at 6 Hz but even higher power at other frequencies. The power of the 6 Hz sinusoid is only 1% of the total power of each dipole source, and does not stand out in either the time series or the power spectrum. Figure 3.4c and d shows the estimated potential on the scalp directly above the center of a superficial dipole layer of diameter 3 cm, based on four concentric spheres model of the head. The time series shows considerably less power at higher frequencies because of cancellation of potential from asynchronous sources and exhibits a smooth appearance compared to the source time series. The corresponding power spectrum (Figure 3.4d) shows a clear peak at 6 Hz and no other peak frequencies. As the diameter of the dipole layer is increased from 3 to 4 to 5 cm, the calculated surface potential becomes more obviously sinusoidal (Figure 3.4e–h). The power substantially increases at 6 Hz, but the power distributed across the rest of the spectrum is essentially unchanged. Another factor that potentially influences the power spectrum is the relative phases of the 6 Hz sources within the dipole layer. In this example, the 6 Hz oscillation is at the same phase in every source. Variability in the phases of the sources would reduce the power.

Clearly, source synchrony is as important as source strength and source size in the generation of scalp potentials. Most (99%) of the source activity in this examples is uncorrelated; as a result, sources contribute minimally to scalp potential even as the size of the source region increases. By contrast, relatively small magnitude (1%) source activity that is synchronous across all sources in the dipole layer generates a large scalp potential that increases dramatically as dipole layer diameter increases. We have quantified this effect of the size of a dipole layer on scalp potential as a spatial filter (Srinivasan et al., 1996; 1998). *One important implication of Figure 3.4 is that spatial filtering by volume conduction can lead to temporal filtering of source activity in the scalp EEG.* If synchronous source activity in different frequency bands takes place in dipole layers of different sizes, frequency bands that are synchronized broadly over the cortical surface can easily generate higher power in the scalp potentials than a stronger but smaller dipole layer. The power at any frequency in the spectrum of scalp EEG is determined not only by the source strength but also by spatial properties of the source such as its size and synchrony. Thus, we anticipate that EEG recorded within the brain can have quite different spectra than EEG recorded on the scalp, a prediction well-supported by experimental studies. Moreover, strong correlations between EEG data recorded on the scalp and cognitive processes or clinical disease states may have no obvious correlation in EEG recorded within the brain.

In summary, these simulations demonstrate that relative EEG power in different frequency bands and power changes between brain states can easily result from changes in source synchrony, source region size, and meso-source strength. Furthermore, source strength $\mathbf{P}(\mathbf{r},t)$, measured as dipole moment per unit volume, is itself a measure of source synchrony at smaller scales because synaptic (microsource) synchrony influences effective pole separation as shown in Chapter 4. Thus, the relative power level measured by an EEG electrode at any one frequency is closely related to the degree of synchronization of synaptic currents at that frequency (with no phase lag) over tangential cortical distances roughly in the range of 5–10 cm.

3.5 Spatial Statistics of EEG

In this section, we introduce *spatial analysis* of the EEG by means of the analysis of a joint observation of time series $\{V_{mk}(t)\}$ consisting of $k = 1, K$ observations in $m = 1, M$ data channels. These joint observations of time series are the realization of a stochastic process distributed in space and time over the cortical surface and recorded on the scalp with EEG electrodes. The *coherence* between pairs of EEG channels provides an entry point to examine the spatial properties of the stochastic source activity. As in the case of other statistical measures, we can never know the coherence of a stochastic process, we can only obtain estimates. In this section, we define *coherence as a linear correlation coefficient* that primarily estimates the amount of phase synchronization between any two data channels. Coherence of a random process is a statistical measure of the relationship between two time series (or data channels) *across observations*. As we shall see, coherence is a measure very similar to a squared correlation coefficient, which measures the proportion of variance in one data channel that can be explained by a linear transformation of another data channel.

To calculate coherence we first define a *cross spectrum* (Bendat and Piersol, 2001), which is a measure of the joint spectral properties of two channels. The cross spectrum $C_{uv}(f_n)$ of two channels u and v at frequency f_n can be estimated from pairs of Fourier coefficients as an average over K epochs, that is

$$C_{uv}(f_n) = A_{uv}e^{j\phi_{uv}} = \frac{2}{K}\sum_{k=1}^{K} F_{uk}(f_n)F_{vk}^*(f_n) \quad n = 0,1,2,...(N-1)/2 \tag{3.5}$$

When $u = v$ the cross spectrum reduces to the power spectrum (2.3), and the factor of two again reflects the fact that our spectra are restricted to positive frequencies.

Unlike the power spectrum, which is real valued, the cross spectrum is complex valued, and can be expressed as magnitude (or cross-power) A_{uv} and phase φ_{uv}. The phase of the cross spectrum is the average phase difference between the two channels which we also label the *relative phase*. The cross spectrum is a measure of the covariance between two signals at one frequency across observations analogous to the ordinary *covariance* between two time series. In fact, similar to the relationship between the power spectrum and the autocorrelation function, the cross spectrum is the Fourier transform of the crosscorrelation function R_{uv}:

$$R_{uv}(\tau) = E\left[V_u(t)V_v(t+\tau)\right] \tag{3.6}$$

If t spans the interval $[-T/2, T/2]$ the crosscorrelation function contains the same information as the crossspectrum. The crosscorrelation function is at the heart of the multivariate spectral analysis methods discussed at the end of the chapter.

If we normalize the squared magnitude of the cross spectrum by the power spectrum of each channel, we obtain the coherence $\gamma_{uv}^2\left(f_n\right)$ between the two channels

$$\gamma_{uv}^2\left(f_n\right) = \frac{\left|C_{uv}\left(f_n\right)\right|^2}{P_u\left(f_n\right)P_v\left(f_n\right)} \quad n = 0,1,2,\ldots(N-1)/2 \tag{3.7}$$

The form of Equation 3.7 follows closely from the equation for a Pearson correlation coefficient (squared). The numerator is the squared magnitude of the cross spectrum (or squared cross power), analogous to squared covariance. The power spectrum is analogous to the variance of the signal. Thus, Equation 3.7 is analogous to dividing squared covariance by the variance of each channel, which is a squared correlation coefficient. Like the usual r^2 statistic, coherence $\gamma_{uv}^2\left(f_n\right)$ measures the fraction of variance of channel u at frequency f_n that can be explained by a constant linear transformation of the Fourier coefficients at frequency f_n obtained at channel v. *In the frequency domain, a constant linear transformation means both constant gain (relative amplitude) and constant relative phase.*

The form of Equation 3.7 indicates that the coherence measure is quite sensitive to the relative phases between two channels. If the relative phase is constant over epochs, the average of the product on the right-hand side of Equation 3.5 is equal to the average product of the magnitude of the Fourier coefficients and coherence is equal to one. If the relative phase varies across the K epochs, then some cancellation will take place and coherence (Equation 3.7) will be less than one. If the phase difference is purely random from epoch to epoch, the coherence estimate will approach zero as the number of epochs (K) is increased. A coherence of 0.5 in one frequency band indicates that at that frequency 50% of the variance at one channel can be explained by a linear transformation of the other channel. *This interpretation does not imply that there is a linear relationship between possible dynamic processes linking the data channels.* A coherence of 0.5 only indicates that we can only partly account for the data by a linear model. If the relationship was purely linear, the coherence estimate would be close to one if enough epochs were averaged to remove noise effects. Coherence can be less than one because the linear relationship between channels is *stochastic* as there is some randomness in the phase differences between channels but restricted to a narrow range. Another possibility is that the relationship between the channels is deterministic but nonlinear, in which case coherence provides a measure of the degree of linearity.

In describing coherence effects in EEG, we emphasize that coherence is a measure of phase synchronization. But, coherence depends both on relative amplitude and on relative phase between the two channels. If the phases at two channels are identical (phase difference = 0), coherence is still less than one if the amplitudes fluctuate independently at each channel. If our main goal is to estimate phase synchronization independent of amplitude fluctuations, we can measure coherence by normalizing each Fourier coefficient by its amplitude (phase-only coherence) or use entropy measures on the relative phase distribution across epochs to measure synchronization (Tass et al., 1998). One reason to use coherence measures rather than directly measuring phase correlation is that coherence measures are weighted in favor of epochs with large amplitudes. This makes good practical sense because phase estimates are likely to be more reliable when amplitudes are large if large amplitudes indicate large signal to noise ratio as is usually the case in EEG after obvious artifact has been removed. If only epoch phase information is used (independent of epoch amplitudes), equal emphasis is placed on low- and high-amplitude epochs in estimates of phase synchronization potentially reducing signal-to-noise ratio.

To summarize, coherence estimates provide a measure of phase synchronization between EEG channel pairs. Fluctuations in EEG amplitude are expected to produce relatively small changes in coherence, when used with epochs containing minimal artifact (Nunez, 1995). Coherence can be greater than zero or less than one for several reasons: (i) the presence of additive noise at each channel; the effects of additive noise can be minimized by averaging over a larger number of epochs; (ii) the system that gives rise to the amplitude and phase relationship between the two channels is stochastic and fluctuates across the observations; (iii) the system that gives rise to the relationship between the two channels is nonlinear; and (iv) a mutual influence between the two channels is present in the same frequency band.

3.6 Effects of Volume Conduction on EEG Coherence

Our goal in obtaining EEG coherence estimates is to estimate statistical properties of random source processes distributed in space and time over the cortical surface. In order to develop a theoretical model relating scalp potential statistics to source statistics, it is useful to think of source statistics in terms of continuous variables of time and space rather than discrete sets of sources. EEG sources are most likely dipole layers of varying size and shape which are described in terms of continuous functions of cortical location; discrete sources are simply special cases of this picture. Thus, the so-called "EEG generators" can be expressed generally in terms of the field $\mathbf{P}(\mathbf{r}, t)$ defined over the three dimensional volume of the brain, which generates a scalp potential field $V(\mathbf{r}, t)$. If the field $\mathbf{P}(\mathbf{r}, t)$ represents a random process, we can characterize it by its mean $\mu_B(\mathbf{r}, t)$ and cross-spectral density function $C_B(\mathbf{r}_1, \mathbf{r}_2, f)$. The cross-spectral density function is a spatial correlation function that depends on temporal frequency. The mean depends on brain location $\mathbf{r}$, and the cross-spectral density function depends on pairs of locations $(\mathbf{r}_1, \mathbf{r}_2)$. The mean $\mu_V(\mathbf{r}, t)$ and cross-spectral density function $C_V(\mathbf{r}_1, \mathbf{r}_2, f)$ of the scalp potential field $V(\mathbf{r}, t)$ are similarly defined, but are now continuous functions of position rather than being defined only at discrete EEG electrode locations.

For the purpose of this discussion, we assume the random process is weakly stationary, so that we can assume zero mean without loss of generality. The cross-spectral density function of the scalp potential is related to the cross-spectral density function of the source distribution by

$$C_V\left(\mathbf{r}_1, \mathbf{r}_2, f\right) = \int_{B_1'} \int_{B_2'} G_H^*\left(\mathbf{r}_1, \mathbf{r}_1'\right) C_B\left(\mathbf{r}_1', \mathbf{r}_2'\right) G_H\left(\mathbf{r}_2, \mathbf{r}_2'\right) \mathrm{d}V(\mathbf{r}_1') \mathrm{d}V(\mathbf{r}_2') \qquad (3.8)$$

where $G_H\left(\mathbf{r}, \mathbf{r}'\right)$ is the Green's function that gives the potential at location $\mathbf{r}$ due to a dipole source of unit strength located at $\mathbf{r}'$ and the integration is over the entire source distribution. In general, Equation 3.8 is an integral over the volume of the brain, but practically this volume is constrained to conform to the geometry of the cortical surface. The Green's function depends on the volume conduction properties of the head, source locations, and measurement locations.

Equation 3.8 defines a spatial filtering of the brain cross-spectral density function to obtain the scalp cross-spectral density function. Although, the exact details depend on the volume conduction model, the Green's function for scalp potentials in both spherical and realistic (BEM) volume conduction models appears to be a low pass filter (Srinivasan et al., 1998, 2007). To examine the effects of spatial filtering on the cross spectrum or coherence estimates, we consider a simple case where the source activity is a spatially uncorrelated stationary random process defined on a sphere of radius r_z in a spherical model of the head:

$$C_B\left(\theta_1, \varphi_1, \theta_2, \varphi_2, f\right) = p^2\left(f\right) \delta\left(\cos\theta_1 - \cos\theta_2\right) \delta\left(\varphi_1 - \varphi_2\right) \qquad (3.9)$$

Here φ and θ are the azimuth and elevation coordinates on a spherical surface, $p(f)$ is the source variance as a function of frequency, in other words the power spectrum of the sources. If we place the source in a concentric spheres models of the head, the cross-spectral density function of the scalp potentials can be calculated substituting the Green's function using the Green's function for a concentric sphere model to obtain (Srinivasan et al., 1998)

$$C_V\left(\theta_1,\varphi_1,\theta_2,\varphi_2,f\right) = p^2\left(f\right)\sum_{n=1}^{\infty} \frac{4\pi H_n(r_z)}{2n+1} P_n\left(\cos\chi_{12}\right) \qquad (3.10)$$

where χ_{12} is the angle between two electrodes positioned at (θ_1, φ_1) and (θ_2, φ_2), the $P_n(x)$ are the Legendre polynomials (Morse and Feshbach, 1953), and the H_n are the coefficients of the Legendre Polynomial expansion of the Green's function G_H for a concentric sphere model. The power spectral density function can be obtained from Equation 3.10 for the case of identical electrode positions, that is, $\chi_{12} = 0$. The coherence function γ_V^2 for the scalp potential can then be derived by substituting cross-spectral density function given in Equation 3.10 and the corresponding power spectral density function into Equation 3.7 to obtain:

$$\gamma_V^2(\chi_{12}) = \left[\frac{\sum_{n=1}^{\infty}(H_n(r_z)/2n+1)P_n\left(\cos\chi_{12}\right)}{\sum_{n=1}^{\infty}(H_n(r_z)/2n+1)} \right]^2 \qquad (3.11)$$

The coherence function given by Equation 3.11 is the scalp potential coherence predicted by the concentric spheres model if the source distribution is a spatially uncorrelated Gaussian random process. Thus, when coherence in the brain sphere is zero between all possible source locations, we can predict the scalp potential coherence that is due only to volume conduction.

We note immediately that the coherence function given by Equation 3.11 is independent of frequency, which does not appear as a parameter on the right-hand side of the equation. Second, we note that this theoretical coherence does not depend on the position of the electrodes but only on the angular distance between electrodes χ_{12}. Figure 3.5 shows the coherence function plotted as a function of the separation distance between electrodes measured in centimeters along the spherical scalp surface. The sources consist of a superficial spherical dipole layer placed in concentric spheres models with different assumed ratios of brain to skull conductivity. Coherence introduced by volume conduction falls off with distance, reaching a minimum at a surface distance of about 10 cm. At very large distances, there is a small rise in

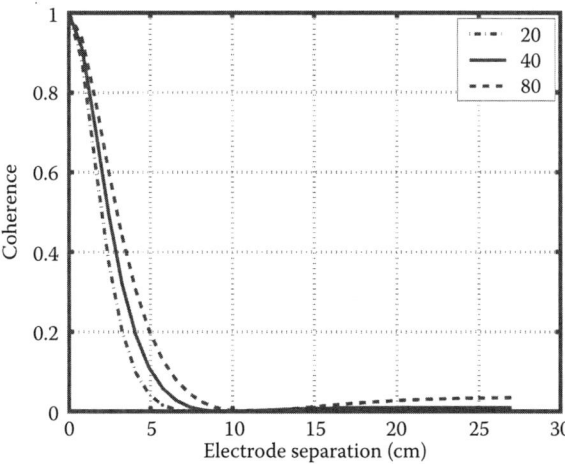

FIGURE 3.5 Theoretical predictions of coherence between scalp potentials due to volume conduction alone with an assumed spatial white-noise source distribution in the concentric spheres model of the head given by Equation 3.11. The source is a spherical dipole layer at a radial location $r_z = 7.8$ cm. The model parameters are radii $(r_1, r_2, r_3, r_4) = (8, 8.1, 8.6, 9.2)$ and conductivity ratios $(\sigma_1/\sigma_2, \sigma_1/\sigma_3, \sigma_1/\sigma_4) = (0.2, 40, 1)$. Source coherence is zero and scalp potential coherence depends only on distance.

the coherence. The implication is that over short to moderate inter-electrode distances (<10 cm in the spherical model) we may expect a significant contribution of volume conduction to coherence. This effect is similar at the three values of brain to skull conductivity ratio that spans the range of most estimates of the conductivity ratio. The same picture emerges from numerical simulations using concentric spheres and realistic models derived from MRI (Srinivasan et al., 2007).

This theoretical prediction of coherence due to volume conduction suggests that *the main effect of volume conduction is to artificially inflate coherences at short to moderate distances, and that this effect is independent of frequency.* This prediction may be evaluated with genuine EEG data. Figure 3.6 shows the coherences between an electrode labeled x and a ring of electrodes at progressively greater distances from x labeled 1–9. The subject is at rest with eyes closed, a state in which coherence is usually high in the alpha band (Nunez, 1995). The estimated coherence between electrode X and electrode n is labeled x:n. The electrode positions are indicated and the typical distance between adjacent electrodes is 2.7 cm. At the closest electrode pair x:1, coherence is very high (above 0.75) at all frequencies; coherence is

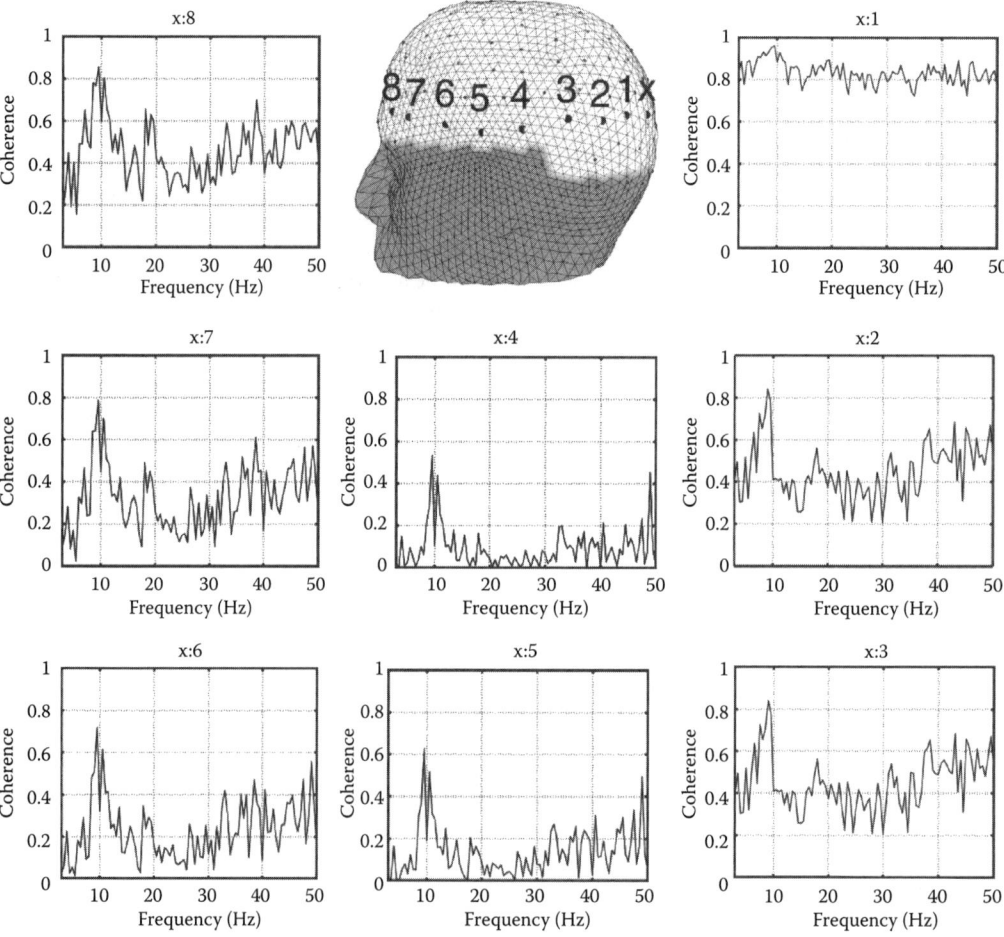

FIGURE 3.6 Scalp potential coherence spectra from a 22-year-old female subject at rest with eyes closed (to maximize alpha coherence). Coherence was estimated with $T = 2$ s ($\Delta f = 0.5$ Hz) in a 60 s record. The head plot shows the location of 9 electrodes, labeled x and 1 through 8. Coherence spectra between electrode x and each of the other electrodes 1–8 are shown, with increasing separations along the scalp. Note that very close electrodes have higher coherence independent of frequency as predicted by the theoretical model. Alpha band coherence is high for large electrode separations, apparently reflecting the large cortical source coherence. Power spectra for this subject are shown in Figure 3.2.

generally independent of temporal frequency. As the electrode separation is increased, the pair x:2 shows lower coherences, but at most frequencies coherence is still above 0.4 suggesting a strong component of coherence that is independent of frequency. A peak is visible in the alpha band at 9.5 Hz, but it is difficult to evaluate this peak, since there is also a broad elevation of coherence. As the sensor separation is further increased (x:3), the floor of the coherences reduces further to about 0.2, and a peak becomes more evident in the 18 Hz range. For pairs of electrodes involving temporal electrodes (x:4 and x:5) the floor of the coherences approaches zero at most frequencies except for the alpha band where a second peak at 10.5 Hz is visible. At very long distance, a pair with a prefrontal electrode (x:8) the coherences are again elevated across all frequencies, suggesting a very small volume conduction effect at long distances as also observed with the model shown in Figure 3.5.

The coherence spectra shown in Figure 3.6 have strong qualitative similarity to the coherence effects predicted by volume conduction of uncorrelated source activity. At short distances coherence is high across all frequencies. The level of coherence independent of frequency systematically decreases as distance increases. This suggests that it is difficult to interpret coherence between closely spaced electrodes. The electrode pair x:3 shows a clear coherence peak of about 0.4 at 18 Hz, while the pair x:2 shows many peaks of about the same size. Clearly we cannot easily determine if the source coherence of the pair x:3 is genuinely higher than x:2, since we observe a strong contribution by volume conduction that is independent of frequency. In addition, there is even a small rise in coherence at very large distances as predicted by the theoretical model (due to the head's closed surface). Many experimental papers on EEG coherence have ignored this volume conduction effect by reasoning (incorrectly) that volume conduction effects are *additive* and can be ignored in the comparison of two or more conditions in the same subject or between groups of subjects. It is important to appreciate the underlying process in filtering as expressed by Equation 3.10. *The implication of the curves shown in Figure 3.5 is that the EEG electrodes separated by less than 10 cm are averaging over many of the same sources.* Thus, if two closely spaced electrodes record from the same source region and the power of the source region increases, coherence between these electrodes will also increase. If there are two source regions, one close to each electrode, changes in source power and changes in source coherence will both cause increases in coherence when the distance between electrode pairs is small to moderate.

The implication of these results is that coherence (or any measure of correlation) between EEG electrodes can only be easily interpreted as increased coherence (or correlation) between two distinct source regions, if the electrodes are at least 10 cm apart in surface tangential directions along the scalp, but are also partly compromised at longer distances (>20 cm). This provided only a limited view of the spatial statistics of the underlying sources. Figure 3.7 shows coherence between all pairs of electrodes for the same data as Figure 3.6, but at six selected frequencies. Coherence is plotted as a function of electrode separation distance, where each point represents one pair of electrodes. Not surprisingly, at frequencies in the alpha band (9.5–12.5 Hz), coherences are very high at both short and long distances, and theta coherence (7.5 Hz) is lower than alpha coherence at long distances, but still higher than the coherence expected due to volume conduction (see Figure 3.5). At 14.5 Hz coherences are reduced and more closely resemble the characteristics of coherence due only to volume conduction. A similar pattern is observed at most higher frequencies.

High-resolution EEG methods such as the surface Laplacian (Srinivasan et al., 1996) can reduce the impact of volume conduction on coherence or correlation estimates but will also remove a substation amount of source coherence that is broadly distributed, or involves deeper sources, for instance in the sulcal walls (Srinivasan et al., 1998), also providing a limited view of the source dynamics. Despite these limitations, both conventional and high-resolution EEG coherence estimates have been used in cognitive and clinical studies to extract correlates of cognitive functions or brain disease. However, the interpretation of these coherences in terms of brain networks remains problematic and there are practical statistical problems with coherence estimates. For instance, using 128 electrodes, there are more than 8000 unique pairs of electrodes to evaluate coherence at each frequency. This is a daunting visualization problem and poses an even greater multiple comparisons problem for statistical contrasts. In the next section, we introduce a multivariate signal

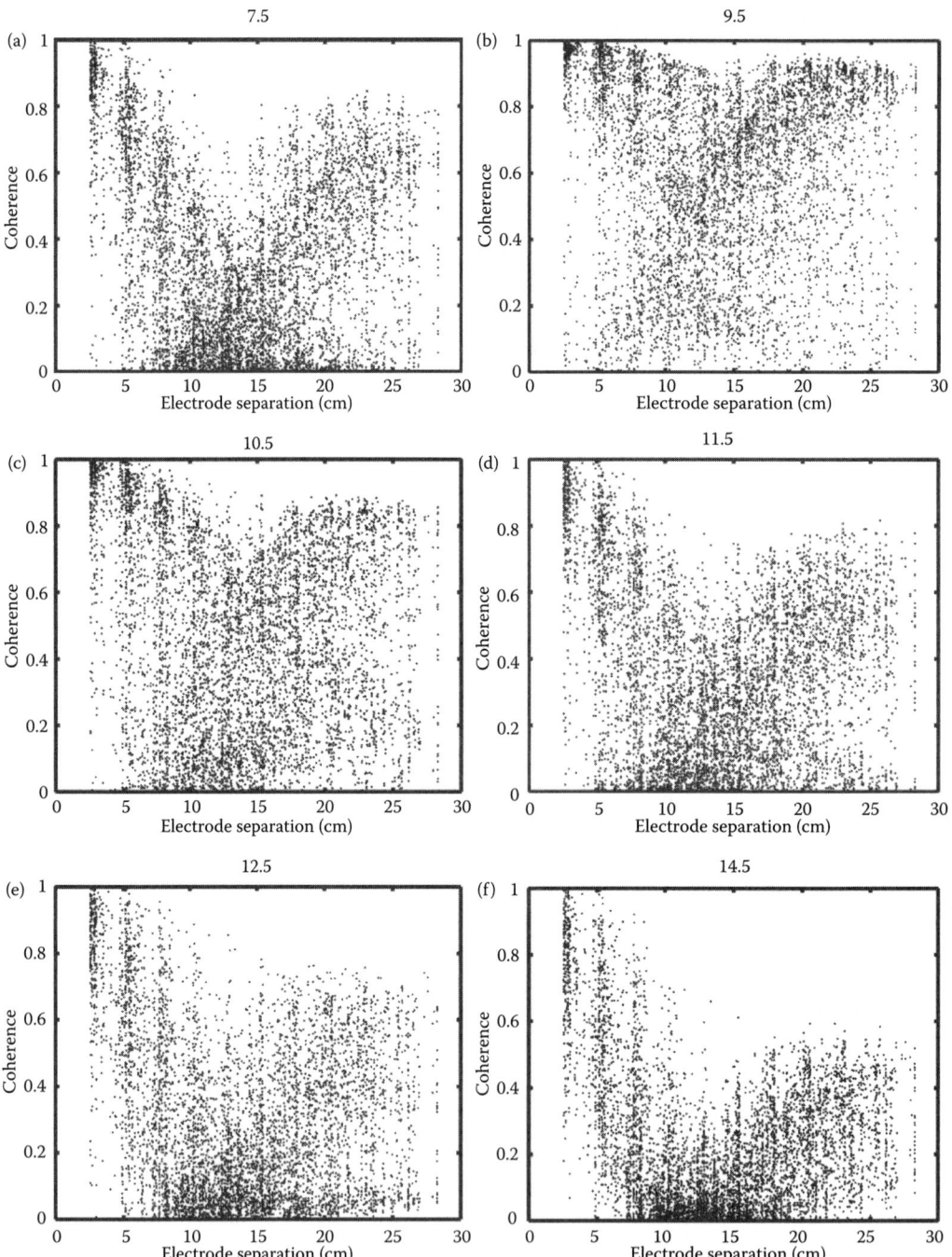

FIGURE 3.7 Scalp potential coherence at different frequencies as a function of electrode separation for the female subject at rest with eyes closed. Detailed coherence spectra for this subject are shown in Figure 3.6. (a) 7.5 Hz coherence versus electrode separation distance, (b) 9.5 Hz coherence, (c) 10.5 Hz coherence, (d) 11.5 Hz coherence, (e) 12.5 Hz, and (f) 14.5 Hz coherence. In Part (f) power is low and coherence follows electrode separation consistent with the effects of volume conduction. At the other frequencies, coherence is elevated at long distances.

processing method that has been developed for BSS using second-order statistics (correlation). In the following section, we adapt this method for multivariate spectral analysis to identify the coherent sources of EEG oscillations.

3.7 Second-Order Blind Identification

EEG signals are mixtures of potentials generated by sources distributed throughout the brain. Although we have some knowledge of the nature of the mixing process for volume conduction models (which is the Green's function G_H), the problem is more complicated because the time series of the dipole sources are not statistically independent, and have structure that reflects the dynamic functional connectivity of brain networks. Thus, EEG signals are mixtures of signals generated by multiple source distributions, each likely composed of synchronous sources distributed over the brain. Thus, there has been considerable interest in using BSS techniques to separate the source on the basis of statistical criterion. In the section we will detail the SOBI algorithm, and in the next section make use of it to obtain multivariate spectral analysis of EEG records.

The SOBI algorithm (Belchourani et al., 1997) can be described as follows. Consider an multichannel–channel time series $\{V_m, m = 1:M\}$, with mean zero. Each sample is assumed to be an instantaneous linear mixture of up to m unknown sources s, where the mixing occurs through some unknown linear mixing matrix $\mathbf{A}$:

$$\mathbf{V} = \mathbf{AS} \tag{3.12}$$

The goal of BSS analysis is to determine a separation matrix, $\mathbf{B}$ such that

$$\mathbf{S} = \mathbf{BV} \tag{3.13}$$

Each source is described by a distribution of loadings across the electrodes (the component) and the source time series. The SOBI algorithm is closely related to spectral analysis because of the criteria used to estimate $\mathbf{B}$. We will present the method in a manner to highlight the relationship between SOBI and spectral analysis, which is less compact and elegant than other discussions (Belchourani et al., 1997; Tang et al., 2004).

From the multichannel time series V, we can construct the crosscorrelation function $R_{mn}(\tau)$ for any pair of electrodes m and n following Equation 3.6. When $m = n$, the crosscorrelation function reduces to the autocorrelation function given by Equation 3.4. For each value of τ, we define the matrix $\mathbf{R}_{V,\tau}$ whose elements are $R_{mn}(\tau)$. We note that $R_{mn}(-\tau) = R_{nm}(\tau)$, so the upper and lower triangles of this matrix correspond to channel m leading n by τ and channel n leading m by τ, respectively. For a range of values of positive τ up to the period the Nyquist frequency, an ensemble of correlation matrices can be constructed $\{\mathbf{R}_{V,\tau}\}$. This ensemble of matrices contains the auto- and crosscorrelations between channels for a range of lags including both the positive and negative lags in the upper and lower triangles of each matrix.

In the SOBI algorithm, the first step is to find the eigenvalues and eigenvectors of the correlation matrix at lag $\tau = 0$ (the ordinary correlation matrix):

$$\mathbf{R}_{V,0} = \mathbf{PDP}^{\mathrm{T}} \tag{3.14}$$

Here, $\mathbf{P}$ is a matrix whose columns are the eigenvectors of the correlation matrix and $\mathbf{D}$ is a diagonal matrix whose diagonal entries are the eigenvalues. The eigenvalues and eigenvectors of the correlation can be used to "prewhiten" the data, that is, to remove all correlation between channels at lag $\tau = 0$. A whitening matrix $\mathbf{W}$ is defined as

$$\mathbf{W} = \mathbf{D}^{-1/2}\mathbf{P}^{\mathrm{T}} \tag{3.15}$$

The whitening step can be recognized as a principal components analysis (PCA), with the projection onto each component normalized by the eigenvalues to define new variables $\mathbf{Z}$:

$$\mathbf{Z} = \mathbf{WV} \tag{3.16}$$

that have a correlation matrix that is the identity matrix:

$$\mathbf{R}_{Z,0} = \mathbf{W}\mathbf{R}_{V,0}\mathbf{W}^{T} = \mathbf{I} \tag{3.17}$$

Thus the effect of the PCA is to diagonalize the correlation matrix at lag $\tau = 0$.
The entire set of correlation matrices (for all lags) can each be similarly transformed:

$$\mathbf{R}_{Z,\tau} = \mathbf{W}\mathbf{R}_{V,\tau}\mathbf{W}^{T} \tag{3.18}$$

The key procedure of SOBI is to find a unitary transformation $\mathbf{U}$ that jointly diagonalizes the set of correlation matrices $\{\mathbf{R}_{Z,\tau}\}$ by minimizing a diagonality measure M:

$$\mathbf{U} = \arg\min \sum_{\tau} M(\mathbf{U}^{T}\mathbf{R}_{Z,\tau}\mathbf{U}) \tag{3.19}$$

For example, Cardoso (1998) uses the following measure:

$$M(A) = \sum_{i \neq j} A^{2} \tag{3.20}$$

that is, minimizing the sum of squares of the off-diagonal terms. These off-diagonal terms are the correlations between the PCA components with nonzero lag τ. U can be obtained via various matrix diagonalization techniques, including classical eigenanalysis methods such as the Jacobi method (Cardoso, 1998) or the Levenberg–Marquardt algorithm (Ziehe et al., 2003). In a typical implementation the algorithm proceeds until a very small amount of correlation remains with the tolerance determined by the user (Cardoso, 1998).

After the joint-diagonalization of crosscorrelations, the estimate of the separation matrix $\mathbf{B}$ is thus obtained as

$$\mathbf{B} = \mathbf{UW} \tag{3.21}$$

After estimating the separation matrix, the source time series can be reconstructed and the statistical properties (e.g., power and coherence) of the source time series can be estimated.

3.8 Multivariate Spectral Analysis Using SOBI

The definition of the SOBI algorithm provided above was developed in the context of a single time series observed with multiple channels. We can easily generalize the above approach to account for multiple observations by extending the expectations across multiple observations (Deng et al., 2010), which is entirely consistent with the definitions of the autocorrelation and crosscorrelations.

Previous studies using SOBI (Tang et al., 2004) have typically made use of time delays that span a wide range on a logarithmic scale. The motivation for this choice is to capture the correlation structure over a wide range of time scales while minimizing the number of correlation matrices that must be diagonalized. We will consider an entirely different basis of selection of τ, which will closely tie the results of SOBI analysis to spectral analysis. Consider the analysis of 1 s of data sampled at 1000 Hz. With the second of data we can easily calculate correlations matrices with lags (in ms) from the domain {0,1,…,999}. However for very long lags, we do not have as many observations to obtain a robust estimate of the crosscorrelations. Moreover, the correlation matrices for lag τ and $\tau + 1$ ms are also not expected to vary greatly, except for the contributions of very small oscillations that are close to the Nyquist frequency. We can reasonably expect that the EEG has been sampled at a frequency at least 2.5 the highest frequency with any power present in the recording (the Engineer's Nyquist), and that analog filters in the EEG amplifier have been used to remove any power at frequencies above the Nyquist.

Consider instead the crosscorrelation matrices {$\mathbf{R}_{v,\tau}$} obtained for a set of lags τ = {0, 10, 20,…,500 ms} using a 1 s record sampled at 1000 Hz. Here we have defined a uniform step in the lags of 10 ms. These crosscorrelation matrices can accurately represent the spectral content of the signal up to 50 Hz (Nyquist criterion) or more practically 40 Hz (Engineer's Nyquist). The maximum lag chosen here is 500 ms, which can be used to capture the correlation at frequencies down to 1 Hz. Thus, between 1 Hz and 50 Hz all of the spectral information in the record has been preserved by the set of crosscorrelation matrices, and this information can always be recovered by applying a Fourier transform. Thus, applying the SOBI algorithm to this set of matrices has the goal of minimizing the crosscorrelation function between these channels over a bandwidth of 1–50 Hz.

We have applied the SOBI algorithm to the data whose power and coherence are shown in Figures 3.2, 3.3, 3.6, and 3.7 using the set of lags τ = {0, 10, 20,…, 500 ms}. In these data we have 30 epochs of duration 2 s, sampled at 1000 Hz. Figure 3.8 shows the power spectra of all the EEG channels (upper left), and the power spectra of all the SOBI components (upper right). The SOBI components have been sorted by the total variance explained by the component. The EEG channels all show highest power in the alpha band, which is also shown in the peak frequency histogram (lower left) where almost every channel is shown to peak in the alpha band, with most channels showing the peak at 9.5 Hz. The SOBI components show the largest components having power in the alpha band, with a total of 16 components showing the highest

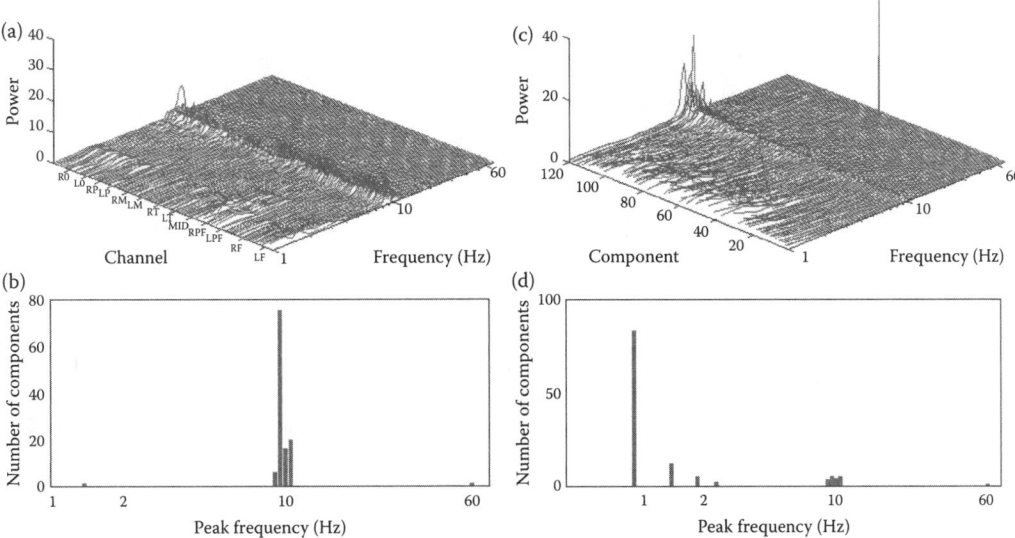

FIGURE 3.8 Average power spectra and peak histogram of the raw EEG and SOBI components. (a) The raw EEG power spectra of all 120 channels, averaged across all 30 2-s epochs. The frequency axis is in log-scale. (b) Average peak power histogram of raw EEG spectra, which shows the frequency distribution of peak power for each channel. (c) Average SOBI component spectra, ordered by power in alpha band (8–12 Hz). (d) Average peak power histogram of the 120 SOBI components.

power in the alpha band. Of these 16 components, 6 had negligible power and were discarded leaving 10 components. All of the other components had much less power and peaked at very low frequencies except for one component which contains all the 60 Hz line noise picked up by the EEG electrodes.

Figure 3.9 shows the spatial distribution of the component loading and the corresponding source power spectrum for each of the 10 components that contribute all the power in the alpha band. Each of these "alpha" components has a distinct spatial distribution. The components have been labeled C1–C10 by the total power contributed to the alpha band. Component C1 captures the main features of the broadly distributed signal which peaks at 9.5 Hz. Components C2 and C3 capture the main features of the signal that peaks at 10.5 Hz prominently at occipital and temporal channels which is less prominent at dorsal frontal channels (see Figures 3.2 and 3.3). Component C4 also peaks at 9.5 Hz and is focused on parietal channels. The other components shown correspond to independent sources of alpha rhythm power with distinct spatial distribution.

Since the SOBI analysis performed a multivariate analysis of the crosscorrelation between channels over a range of lags, we might reasonably have expected that different SOBI components would correspond to oscillations of different frequencies. However, our analysis of this simple eyes closed resting EEG record, reveals multiple components with identical peak frequency. For example, components C1, C4, C7, and C10 all have time series with peak power at 9.5 Hz. To understand why these time series are indicative of separate sources, we calculated the coherence between the source time series corresponding to the components C1–C10. We found that at all frequencies, including the alpha band, coherence between the source time series is negligible. Figure 3.10 shows the coherences between components at four frequencies in the alpha band including the dominant frequencies of 9.5 and 10.5 Hz. In all cases the highest coherences observed are <0.3. In comparison, Figure 3.7 shows that even at long electrode separations (>10 cm) very high coherences (>0.8) are observed between many electrode pairs at 9.5 Hz, but at other pairs coherence is much lower. When the SOBI decompositions separate components that oscillate centered on the same frequency, they indicate the oscillations in this frequency

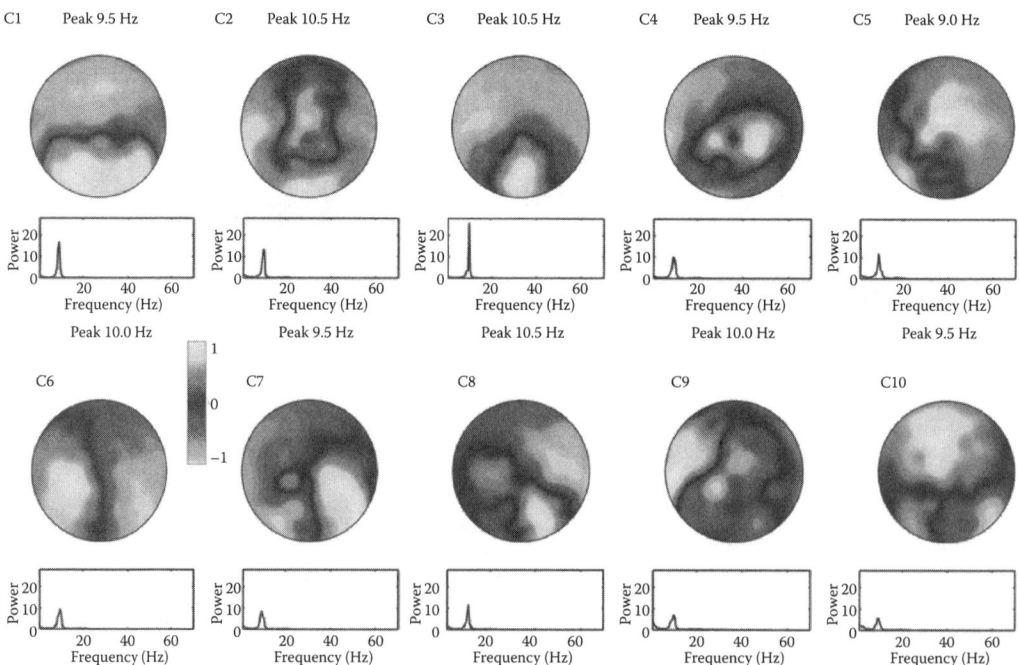

FIGURE 3.9 Spatial loading topography of first 10 SOBI components and average spectra. The SOBI components are ordered by the total power within alpha band (8–12 Hz).

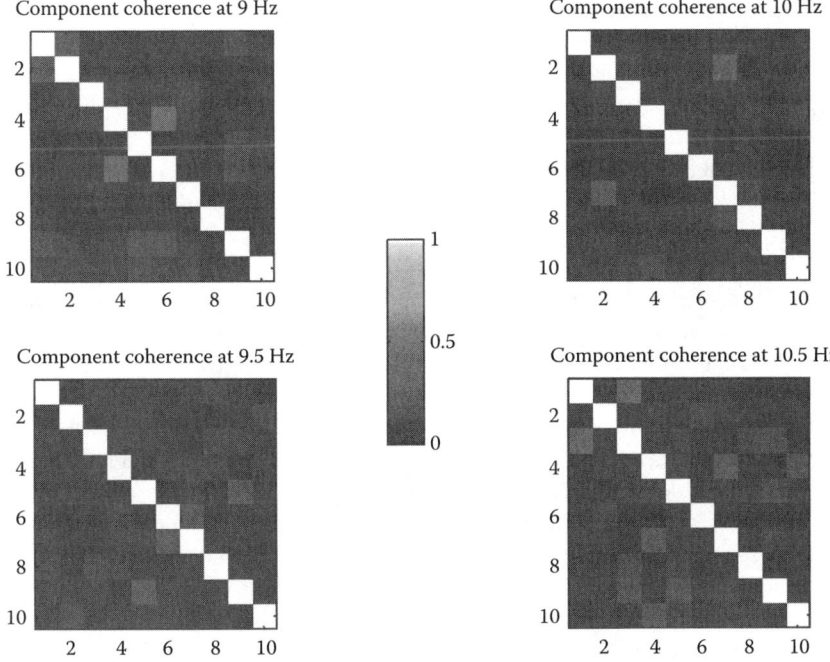

FIGURE 3.10 Coherence of the first 10 SOBI components in the alpha band. These are the same group of components as shown in Figure 3.2. Coherence was calculated between the source time series for each component. Coherence at 9, 9.5, 10, and 10.5 Hz are shown. Coherence between components is negligible, even when they peak at the same frequency.

band generated by distinct source distributions that are relatively incoherent. This picture is consistent with our understanding of alpha rhythms; there are multiple independent alpha rhythms generated by networks spanning different regions of cortex, which are selectively manipulated by different tasks. This picture is also consistent with the observation the coherence between channels in the alpha band reveals a complex pattern of high and low coherence between pairs of electrode all of whom show significant power in the alpha band (see Figure 3.8). Thus, the SOBI components identified here are a multivariate decomposition of the EEG spectra to identify the underlying coherent sources whose time series are incoherent in the sense of second-order statistics.

3.9 Summary

We view source dynamics as a stochastic (random) process having statistical properties that change with changes in behavior and cognition. This general framework has an important advantage over viewpoints that may prejudge the nature of EEG dynamics, thereby biasing experimental design. Spectral analysis is the obvious entry point for studying EEG dynamics, but the physics of volume conduction places constraints on the interpretation of the EEG spectrum. The EEG power spectrum is straightforward to estimate using Fourier methods and should be interpreted in terms of synchronization of the underlying sources, including spatial synchronization. The effects of volume conduction on EEG coherence are severe for closely spaced electrode, and limit the use of coherence to estimate spatial properties of brain networks. SOBI algorithm is a BSS method that operates on the crosscorrelation between channels over a range of lags. We show that in effect the SOBI algorithm isolates "sources" (brain networks) that oscillate at different frequencies, or within the same frequency oscillate incoherently. This provides a direct method for multivariate spectral analysis to decompose the spatio-temporal statistics of EEG signals into independent source signals.

Acknowledgment

This work was supported by a grant from NIH 2R01-MH68004.

References

Belouchrani A, Abed-Meriam K, Cardoso JF, and Moulines E, A blind source separation technique using second-order statistics. *IEEE Transactions on Signal Processing*, 45:434–444, 1997.

Bendat JS and Piersol AG, *Random Data. Analysis and Measurement Procedures*, Third Edition. New York: Wiley, 2001.

Cardoso JF, Blind signal separation: Statistical principles. *Proceedings of the IEEE*, 9:2009–2025, 1998.

Deng S, Srinivasan R, Lappas T, and D'Zmura M, EEG classification of imagined speech using Hilbert Spectrum methods. *Journal of Neural Engineering*, 7, 046006, 2010.

Deng S and Srinivasan R, Semantic and acoustic analysis of speech by functional networks with distinct time scales. *Brain Research*, 1346:132–144, 2010.

Ding JD, Sperling G, and Srinivasan R, Attentional modulation of SSVEP power depends on network tagged by flicker frequency. *Cerebral Cortex*, 16:1016–1029, 2006.

Lachaux JP, Lutz A, Rudrauf D, Cosmelli D, Le Van Quyen M, Martinerie J, Varela F, Estimating the time-course of coherence between single-trial brain signals: An introduction to wavelet coherence. *Electroencephalography and Clinical Neurophysiology*, 32(3):157–174, 2002.

Le Van Quyen M, Foucher J, Lachaux J, Rodriguez E, Lutz A, Martinerie J, and Varela FJ, Comparison of Hilbert transform and wavelet methods for the analysis of neuronal synchrony. *Journal of Neuroscience Methods*, 111(2):83–98, 2001.

Lopes da Silva FH, and Storm van Leeuwen W, The cortical alpha rhythm in dog: The depth and surface profile of phase. In: MAB Brazier MAB and H Petsche (eds) *Architectonics of the Cerebral Cortex*. New York: Raven Press, pp. 319–333, 1978.

Lopes da Silva FH, Dynamics of EEGs as signals of neuronal populations: Models and theoretical considerations. In: E Niedermeyer and FH Lopes da Silva (eds) *Electroencephalography. Basic Principals, Clinical Applications, and Related Fields. Forth Edition*. London: Williams & Wilkins, pp. 76–92, 1999.

Makeig S, Debener S, Onton J, and Delorme A, Mining event-related brain dynamics. *Trends in Cognitive Science*, 8(5):204–210, 2004.

Morse PM and Feshbach M, *Methods of Theoretical Physics*. McGraw-Hill Interamericana, 1953.

Murias M, Swanson JM, and Srinivasan R, Functional connectivity of frontal cortex in healthy and ADHD children reflected in EEG coherence. *Cerebral Cortex*, 17:1788–1799, 2007.

Nunez PL and Srinivasan R, *Electric Fields of the Brain: The Neurophysics of EEG*, 2nd Edition. New York: Oxford University Press, 2006.

Nunez PL, *Neocortical Dynamics and Human EEG Rhythms*. New York: Oxford University Press, 1995.

Nunez PL, *Electric Fields of the Brain: The Neurophysics of EEG*. Oxford University, New York, 1981.

Nunez PL, Toward a quantitative description of large scale neocortical dynamic function and EEG. *Behavioral and Brain Sciences*, 23:371–398 (target article), 2000a.

Nunez PL, Neocortical dynamic theory should be as simple as possible, but not simpler. *Behavioral and Brain Sciences*, 23:415–437 (response to commentary by 18 neuroscientists), 2000b.

Percival DB and Walden AT, *Spectral Analysis for Physical Applications: Multitaper and Conventional Univariate Techniques*. Cambridge, UK: Cambridge University Press, 1993.

Petsche H and Etlinger SC, *EEG and Thinking. Power and Coherence Analysis of Cognitive Processes*. Vienna: Austrian Academy of Sciences, 1998.

Pfurtscheller G and Lopes da Silva FH, Event-related EEG/MEG synchronization and desynchronization: Basic principles. *Electroencephalography and Clinical Neurophysiology*, 110:1842–1857, 1999.

Srinivasan R, Nunez PL., Tucker DM, Silberstein RB, and Cadusch PJ, Spatial sampling and filtering of EEG with spline Laplacians to estimate cortical potentials. *Brain Topography*, 8:355–366, 1996.

Srinivasan R, Nunez PL, and Silberstein RB, Spatial filtering and neocortical dynamics: Estimates of EEG coherence. *IEEE Transactions on Biomedical Engineering*, 45:814–826, 1998.

Srinivasan R, Anatomical constraints on source models for high-resolution EEG and MEG derived from MRI. *TCRT*, 5:389–399, 2006.

Srinivasan R, Winter WR, Ding J, and Nunez PL, EEG and MEG coherence: Measures of functional connectivity at distinct spatial scales of neocortical dynamics. *Journal of Neuroscience Methods*, 166:41–52, 2007.

Tang AC, Sutherland MT, and McKinney CJ, Validation of SOBI components from high-density EEG. *NeuroImage*, 25:539–553, 2004.

Tass P, Rosenblum MG, Weule J, Kurths J, Pikovsky A, Volkmann J, Schnitzler A, and Freund HJ, Detection of n:m phase locking from noisy data: Application to magnetoencephalography. *Physical Review Letters* 81:3291–3294, 1998.

Ziehe A, Laskov P, Muller KR, and Nolte G, A linear least-squares algorithm for joint diagonalization. *Proc. 4th Intern. Symp. on ICA and BSS 2003 (ICA2003)*, 469–474, 2003.

4

General Linear Modeling of Magnetoencephalography Data

Dimitrios Pantazis
University of Southern California

Juan Luis Poletti Soto
University of Southern California

Richard M. Leahy
University of Southern California

4.1 Introduction

Magnetoencephalography (MEG) has become increasingly popular in clinical and cognitive neuroscience as an imaging tool for studying human brain function. As more whole head systems and novel experimental paradigms become available, researchers are using MEG to explore many aspects of the workings of the human brain. To assure an objective scientific interpretation of these studies, it is important that experimental findings be accompanied by appropriate statistical analysis that effectively controls for false-positives.

This chapter reviews the statistical tools available for the analysis of distributed activation maps defined either on the 2D cortical surface or throughout the 3D brain volume. Statistical analysis of MEG data bears a great resemblance to the analysis of functional magnetic resonance imaging (fMRI) or positron emission tomography (PET) activation maps, therefore much of the methodology can be borrowed or adapted from the functional neuroimaging literature. In particular, we describe the general linear modeling (GLM) approach, where the MEG data are first mapped into brain space, and then fit to a univariate or multivariate model at each surface or volume element. A desired contrast of the estimated parameters produces a statistical map, which is then thresholded for evidence of an experimental effect.

We review several methods for generating statistical maps of brain activation based on the distributed source imaging. They all consist of these steps: process the MEG measurements to create a collection of observations, use a GLM to fit the observations at each location, and finally generate a contrast of the estimated parameters and normalize with its variance to create a map of pivotal statistics (*t*-maps, *F*-maps, etc.). This methodology is a standard approach in fMRI and PET data analysis, and together with subsequent statistical inference, is generally referred to as statistical parametric mapping (SPM) (Friston et al., 1995b).

We describe GLM formulations for the analysis of induced and evoked response in MEG. These methods include both univariate and multivariate analysis. We also extend these models to the problem of investigating large-scale cortical interactions. Finally, we describe different approaches to thresholding statistical maps to control for false-positives when testing multiple hypotheses, a problem that arises when analyzing spatial maps of cortical activity.

4.2 Special Considerations in MEG General Linear Modeling

Statistical inference in MEG distributed activation maps typically uses the GLM framework (Kiebel, 2003), which has been widely successful and is considered a standard in fMRI and PET neuroimaging studies. However, there are important differences from the other neuroimaging modalities related to how observations are created and fitted in GLM models, as well as how subsequent statistical inference is performed.

The temporal resolution of MEG is on the order of milliseconds, much higher than fMRI and PET. Standard analysis of MEG data involves the use of stimulus locked averaging over epochs to produce the evoked response. Recently there has also been a great deal of interest in analysis of the induced response, which corresponds to stimulus-related variations in power in different oscillatory bands as a function of time. This allows us to detect experimental oscillatory effects corresponding to modulations in power in specific frequency bands, even though the oscillations themselves are not phase-locked to the stimulus or response. Induced effects are typically investigated using time–frequency decomposition such as the Morlet wavelet transform (Teolis, 1998). Averaging over epochs of the power in the time–frequency maps gives us an estimate of induced components which can then be tested for experimental effects. These two forms of processing, stimulus-locked averaging and averaging of time–frequency powermaps, are the two basic approaches that are used for analyzing, respectively, evoked and induced components in the MEG data (Figure 4.1).

The fact that we often want to identify and localize experimental effects not only over space, as traditionally done in fMRI with the notion of voxels, but also in time and possibly frequency, introduces challenges that differentiate MEG analysis from that of PET and fMRI. The high dimensionality of the data (space × time × frequency × experimental design) presents challenges, in terms of the high computational costs, but also possibilities, in terms of the greater flexibility that this affords us in the design of the linear models.

Another important difference relative to fMRI is that MEG offers only limited spatial resolution. Distributed cortical imaging involves the reconstruction of thousands of elemental current sources from a few hundred measurements. The problem is highly underdetermined and requires regularization to produce a stable solution. The resulting images are typically of low resolution so that reconstructions of focal sources are blurred with extended point spread functions (PSFs). The shape of the PSF will depend on the reconstruction space, cortical or volumetric, and whether the orientations of the sources are constrained to be normal to the cortical surface. Unlike in fMRI, the PSFs for MEG are highly asymmetric and can extend over mutiple gyri or sulci. As a result, even after thresholding to control for false-positives, one can still observe false-positives at locations within the point spread of truly active regions and, therefore, care must be taken in interpreting these results. Figure 4.11, shown later in this chapter,

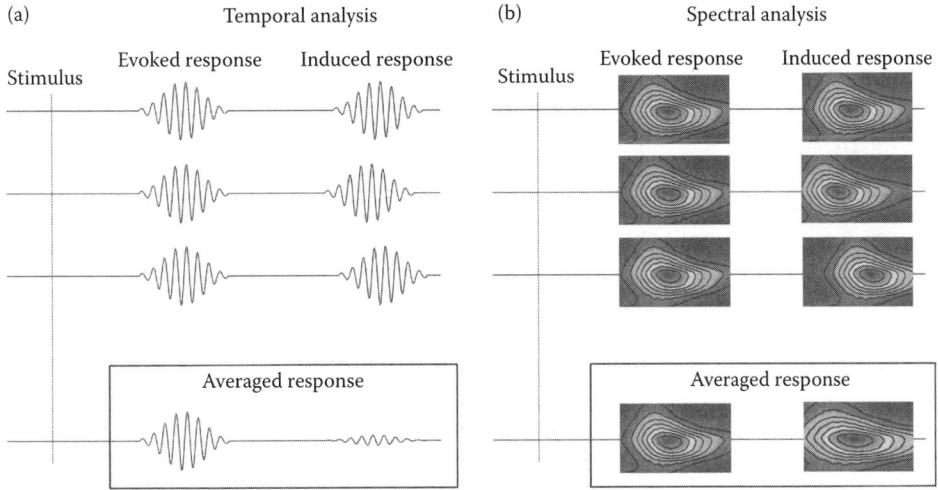

FIGURE 4.1 MEG brain activity in response to a task consists of two components: evoked responses that are phase-locked to the stimuli, and induced responses that are not. (a) Averaging the MEG time-series over epochs preserves the evoked components, but suppresses the induced (nonphase-locked) components. (b) Averaging the power time–frequency decompositions of the time-series preserves both evoked and induced components.

illustrates this issue; the reconstructed statistical map has much greater spatial extent than the single simulated cortical patch, and subsequent thresholding procedures identify significant activity in broad cortical areas.

fMRI analysis is typically performed in the 3D volumetric space while in MEG the 2D cortical surface is often chosen as the source space. Cortically constrained maps can complicate the analysis in several ways. For example, isotropic smoothing on the cortical surface when applying random field methods requires the use of the Laplace–Beltrami operator (Chung, 2001). In group analysis, the data should be brought into a common coordinate system, which requires cortical surface alignment rather than volumetric registration (Fischl et al., 1999; Joshi et al., 2007b), and the resulting areas of activation should be reported with respect to cortical anatomy rather than the standard Talairach coordinates. Orientation-free MEG reconstructions produce vector rather than scalar fields (three elemental dipoles at each location), which can also complicate analysis.

In addition to producing a nonuniform PSF, the MEG inverse operator also introduces a highly nonstationary spatial covariance structure in reconstructed images. Contributions to the covariance can include trial-to-trial variations in induced and evoked responses as well as physiological and environmental noise. Furthermore, the covariance can also vary substantially over the course of an experiment so that we can often not assume temporal stationarity. In comparison, variations in fMRI data can often reasonably be approximated as spatially and temporally stationary. As a result, statistical inference for MEG with random field theory requires the use of special formulas that correct for nonstationarity (Worsley et al., 1999).

4.3 Observations

Using source imaging methods, MEG channel measurements are converted into 2D cortical or 3D volumetric maps of brain activation. Examples of these methods include the regularized minimum-norm (Hamalainen and Ilmoniemi, 1984) and its variants depth-weighted (Fuchs et al., 1999), Tikhonov-regularized (Tikhonov and Arsenin, 1977) and noise-normalized (Dale et al., 2000), beamformers (van Veen et al., 1997), MUSIC maps (Mosher and Leahy, 1998), and sLORETA (Pascual-Marqui, 2002).

Different source assumptions underlie each of these methods, for example, the dipole model in MUSIC and beamforming versus the distributed source model in the minimum norm methods. However, in each case a statistic can be computed at each voxel in the 2D or 3D space.

To explore the spectral components of induced brain activation, it is also common to perform time–frequency decompositions of the image maps, using, for example, short-time Fourier transform (Bruns, 2004) or complex Morlet wavelet transform (Figure 4.2a). As described before, the resulting inverse solutions are of high dimension: (2D or 3D) space, time, frequency, and experimental condition for each subject. There is, therefore, tremendous flexibility in processing the MEG data; we can create observations using any of these dimensions, treat them as univariate or multivariate observations, and fit them to different GLMs.

Some form of data reduction is desirable. For example, we can summarize information by forming discrete regions or "bands" with respect to the time, frequency, and/or spatial dimensions and integrating brain activity over these bands (Figure 4.2b). Even though this reduces resolution, as we have no discrimination power within each band, it can benefit the analysis in multiple ways: reduce data storage requirements, improve the signal-to-noise ratio, and ameliorate the multiple comparison problem by reducing the number of concurrent hypothesis tests. Data reduction in the spatial, temporal, and frequency dimension is a common practice in MEG studies and we provide a few examples here: Pantazis et al. (2007) defined 10 temporal bands (100 ms each), a single α-frequency band (8–14 Hz), and 6 spatial bands (or equivalently, cortical regions of interest) and integrated power over these bands in each trial. Brooks et al. (2004) analyzed the data only in a couple of frequency bands. Kilner et al. (2005) completely collapsed the spatial information by performing time–frequency analysis on a single channel, or equivalently, a single source. Finally, Singh et al. (2003) filtered the data into four frequency bands and averaged out the temporal dimension using a spatial power map computed from an LCMV beamformer output.

If oscillatory analysis is not required, a time–frequency decomposition is not necessary and the frequency dimension is ignored (Barnes and Hillbrand, 2003; Carbonell et al., 2004b; Pantazis et al., 2005b; Sekihara et al., 2005). An alternative form of data reduction is the application of principal

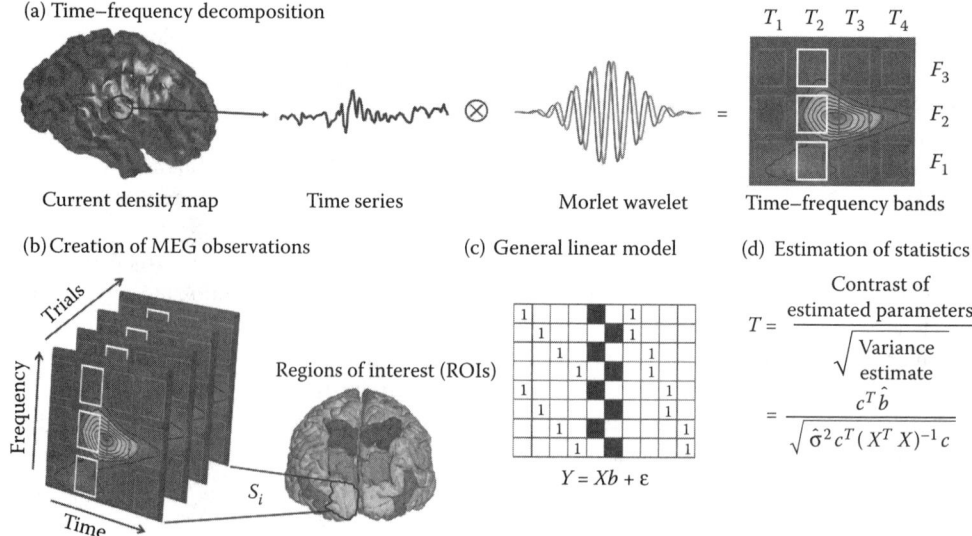

FIGURE 4.2 Creation of statistical maps of brain activation: (a) inverse methods produce distributed cortical activation maps which are expanded to time–frequency components using, for example, Morlet wavelets; (b) MEG data observations are created over several spatial-temporal-spectral bands. Alternative data reduction techniques can be used, such as singular value decomposition; (c) observations are fitted into GLMs following a mass-univariate approach or a multivariate approach; (d) a contrast of interest is defined and the statistic is normalized by its standard deviation.

components analysis (PCA) or independent component analysis (ICA) to the MEG data. For example, Friston et al. (1996) used singular value decomposition (SVD) in the spatiotemporal dimension to reduce the set of components for each multivariate observation.

4.4 Simple General Linear Modeling Example

After the construction of observations, a GLM approach is used to model the data at each location (Figure 4.2d). The MEG observations, as described before, can be current density estimates, time–frequency power maps, or others. GLM theory assumes normal distributions, which is reasonable for averaged evoked responses due to the central limit theorem. However, power time–frequency decompositions of single trial data have a χ^2-distribution. Fortunately, Kiebel et al. (2005b) has shown that, under most circumstances, one can appeal to the central limit theorem or transform the MEG power estimates with a log or square-root transform to make the error terms normal, and thus GLM theory is still appropriate.

Under the GLM framework, the MEG observations Y are predicted from the parameters b:

$$Y = Xb + \varepsilon \tag{4.1}$$

where ε is the modeling error. X is the design matrix whose elements model an experimental paradigm and consist of qualitative (0s or 1s) and/or quantitative variables.

To provide intuition on using the GLM theory for MEG data modeling, consider the following example. In an MEG visual attention study, we acquire multitrial data for two conditions: subject attends to the right (condition 1), or to the left (condition 2). By combining an inverse method with time–frequency analysis of individual trials, we produce dynamic images of brain activity in the α-frequency band. The α-power observations for a single voxel, $y_{11}, \ldots, y_{1N}$ for N trials under condition 1 and $y_{21}, \ldots, y_{2M}$ for M trials under condition 2, are fitted into a one-way analysis of variance (ANOVA) GLM model with two predictor variables, b_1 and b_2, for the two conditions:

$$y_{ij} = b_i + \varepsilon_{ij} \tag{4.2}$$

where $i = \{0,1\}$ denotes the condition, j the trial index for each condition, and ε_{ij} is the model error.

The same ANOVA model can be written in matrix notation. If the observations y_{ij} are arranged as a single observation vector Y, and the rows of the design matrix X have 0s and 1s to indicate the condition for each MEG observation, the ANOVA model becomes $Y = Xb + \varepsilon$, explicitly written as

$$\begin{bmatrix} y_{11} \\ y_{12} \\ \vdots \\ y_{1N} \\ y_{21} \\ y_{22} \\ \vdots \\ y_{2M} \end{bmatrix} = \begin{bmatrix} 1 & 0 \\ 1 & 0 \\ \vdots \\ 1 & 0 \\ 0 & 1 \\ 0 & 1 \\ \vdots \\ 0 & 1 \end{bmatrix} \begin{bmatrix} b_1 \\ b_2 \end{bmatrix} + \begin{bmatrix} \varepsilon_{11} \\ \varepsilon_{12} \\ \vdots \\ \varepsilon_{1N} \\ \varepsilon_{21} \\ \varepsilon_{22} \\ \vdots \\ \varepsilon_{2M} \end{bmatrix} \tag{4.3}$$

By assuming independent error distributions with equal variance for both conditions, $N(0, \sigma^2)$, we can solve the GLM using ordinary least squares:

$$\hat{b} = (X^T X)^{-1} X^T Y = \begin{bmatrix} \bar{y}_{1\cdot} \\ \bar{y}_{2\cdot} \end{bmatrix} \tag{4.4}$$

where the bar denotes the mean over the dotted subscript. The estimated error variance $\hat{\sigma}^2$ has $N + M - 2$ degrees of freedom, because two of them were used to estimate the model predictors. The error and error variance are estimated as

$$\hat{\varepsilon} = Y - X\hat{b} = (I - X(X^TX)^{-1}X^T)Y = PY \tag{4.5}$$

$$\hat{\sigma}^2 = \frac{\hat{\varepsilon}^T\hat{\varepsilon}}{\text{trace}\{P\}} = \frac{\sum_i (y_{1i} - \bar{y}_{1\cdot})^2 + \sum_i (y_{2i} - \bar{y}_{2\cdot})^2}{N + M - 2} \tag{4.6}$$

where P is a projection operator onto the left null space of X. Suppose we want to test whether there is a difference between the two conditions, or equivalently whether the difference $b_1 - b_2$ is significantly different from zero. The statistic of interest is, therefore, the contrast of the two parameters, $c^T\hat{b} = \begin{bmatrix} 1 \\ -1 \end{bmatrix}^T \hat{b} = b_1 - b_2$, which is then normalized with an estimate of its standard deviation. The resulting statistic T is a two-sample t-test between the two conditions.

$$T = \frac{c^T\hat{b}}{\sqrt{\hat{\sigma}^2 c^T(X^TX)^{-1}c}} = \frac{\bar{y}_{1\cdot} - \bar{y}_{2\cdot}}{\sqrt{\hat{\sigma}^2(1/N + 1/M)}} \tag{4.7}$$

Even though we could have derived the T statistic directly, it is useful to see how it is estimated in the GLM framework and gain intuition for more complex designs where the theory becomes important. The design matrix X can have multiple columns with indicator variables, as above, but also quantitative variables that correspond to covariates. The observations can be arranged in multiple ways and several contrasts can capture the experimental effect of interest.

4.5 Contrast Statistic and Normalization

After selection of a GLM approach, the MEG observations are fitted to the models and a contrast (or linear combination) of the parameters is computed (Figure 4.2d). This contrast statistic captures the effect of interest, for example, the difference between two experimental conditions or the correlation of a response variable with brain activation. It is then preferable to normalize the statistics into known parametric distributions (pivotal statistics). This allows the application of random field theory, which as we will see, requires a Gaussian distribution or one derived from Gaussian data (e.g., a t or F statistic). The normalization also helps when using nonparametric permutation methods, because it makes the variance at all voxels homogeneous under the null hypothesis, which should produce approximately uniform specificity, that is, false-positives are equally likely at all locations.

We conclude by showing that the GLM framework is parsimonious in MEG analysis. Consider, for example, the simple case where the MEG data are used to create dSPM maps (Dale et al., 2000), that is, minimum-norm inverse maps normalized with an estimate of the noise standard deviation at each location. As we will show, this corresponds to the simplest case of GLM analysis following a mass-univariate approach: the one-way ANOVA model $y_j^{it} = b^{it} + \varepsilon_j^{it}$ is fitted to the current density data y_j^{it} data separately at each spatial location i and temporal location t, where j is the trial repetition index and b^{it} is the main effect (brain response) (Pantazis et al., 2005b). We use superscripts for i and t to denote that the same model is fit separately in each spatial-temporal location. The contrast of interest is the parameter itself, which is equal to the trial average according to the minimum-norm solution: $c^T\hat{b}^{it} = [1]\hat{b}^{it} = \hat{b}^{it} = \bar{y}_{\cdot}^{it}$, where the bar indicates an average over the dotted subscript. Since the error terms ε_j^{it} are assumed to be

Gaussian, the estimated contrast is also a Gaussian statistic. Finally, to create a map of *t*-distribution statistics, we normalize with the standard deviation at each location $T^{it} = \hat{b}^{it} / \hat{\sigma}^{it} / \sqrt{J}$, where $\hat{\sigma}^{it}$ is the estimated standard deviation and J is the total number of trials. This is equivalent to the noise normalization performed in dSPM for orientation-constrained linear inverses. For the unconstrained case, the dSPM output is an *F*-map computed as the ratio of the magnitude squared of the vector current density to the noise variance at each spatial location. The sLORETA solution (Pascual-Marqui, 2002) is similar to dSPM, but with a different normalization coefficient. In this case, we normalize by the standard deviation computed from the data covariance rather than the noise only covariance. Under the null hypothesis of noise only (or equivalently a zero experimental effect), sLORETA and dSPM are identical. Similarly, the beamformer neural activity index (van Veen et al., 1997) corresponds to a *t*-map for the orientation-constrained case or an *F*-map for the orientation-free case, which can be again cast in a GLM framework (Kucukaltun-Yildirim et al., 2006).

4.6 Multisubject Studies

In multisubject studies, the measurement variance has two sources: the within-subject variance and the between-subject variance. Depending on how we model the error variance, two types of statistical analysis can be used: fixed-effect and mixed (or random) effect. Fixed-effect analysis considers only the within-subject variance and; therefore, all measurements are fitted to the same GLM in the same manner as for a single subject. Statistical inferences apply only to the particular subjects participating in the experiment. To generalize to the whole population, mixed-effect analysis is required, where both within- and between-subject variances are considered in making statistical inferences.

Mixed-effect analysis typically involves fitting hierarchical models (Friston et al., 2002; Mumford and Nichols, 2006), where we specify the complete model in stages: a first or lower level model fits the data for each subject separately, and a second level combines the different subjects. Estimation of the parameters in the two-stage analysis is a challenge since it involves iterative optimization and is generally not practical, unless we follow the summary statistics approach. This approach is computationally efficient because it dissociates estimation of the parameters of the two-stage models, and can be implemented with algorithms such as Markov chain Monte Carlo (Beckmann et al., 2003), or restricted maximum likelihood (Verbeke and Molenberghs, 2000).

Under specific assumptions, the summary statistic approach simplifies and the parameters can be estimated without the need for an iterative procedure (Holmes and Friston, 1998; Mumford and Nicholas, 2006). We describe this method here because it has become the most popular approach for multisubject analysis in MEG. The first stage model fits the data from each subject $k = 1,...,K$ separately*:

$$Y_k = X_k b_k + \varepsilon_k \tag{4.8}$$

where Y_k is the MEG observations and b_k is the model parameters for subject k. While each design matrix X_k can have a different number of rows (e.g., different number of MEG trials per subject), all the design matrices must have the same number of columns, each column expressing the same effect among subjects. The subject parameters are estimated using a generalized least squares solution, which normally requires the estimation of the error covariance matrix C_k:

$$\hat{b}_k = (X_k^T C_k^{-1} X_k)^{-1} X_k^T C_k^{-1} \tag{4.9}$$

---

* To ease notation, we now use subscripts rather than superscripts, for indices where we follow a mass-univariate approach.

The second stage model takes only one contrast $c^T \hat{b}_k$ from each subject and fits it to the group GLM:

$$
\begin{bmatrix}
c^T \hat{b}_1 \\
c^T \hat{b}_2 \\
\vdots \\
c^T \hat{b}_K
\end{bmatrix}
= X_g b_g + \varepsilon_g
\tag{4.10}
$$

where X_g and b_g are the group design matrix and group level parameters, respectively. The summary statistic model error ε_g has two variance components, the intrasubject and intersubject variance. Under the assumption of homogeneous intrasubject variance (i.e., $c^T \hat{b}_k$ has the same variance for all subjects), the intrasubject variance is a scaled identity matrix. Similarly, under the assumption of independent subjects, the intersubject variance is a scaled identity matrix. Therefore, the covariance of ε_g is also a scaled identity matrix and the generalized least squares solution of the second stage model (which normally requires estimation of the error covariance matrix) becomes equivalent to an ordinary least squares solution that does not require the covariance matrix:

$$
\hat{b}_g = (X_g^T X_g)^{-1} X_g \hat{b}
\tag{4.11}
$$

The key assumption here is the homogeneity of the intrasubject variances; without it the ordinary least squares solution could not have been used and iterations would be necessary to estimate both the intrasubject and the intersubject components of the variance.

With multisubject studies, we first coregister all subjects to a common coordinate system using either volumetric brain coregistration (Christensen and Johnson, 2001; Hellier et al., 2002; Shen and Davatzikos, 2002) or cortical surface alignment methods (Fischl et al., 1999; Thompson et al., 2001; Joshi et al., 2007a). Then the first stage model, which can be a mass-univariate approach, a multivariate approach, or a general univariate framework, estimates subject specific parameters. These parameters are then fitted to a second stage model and finally a statistic map is computed on the common coordinate system using a contrast of the group parameters b_g at each voxel. This statistic map can then be thresholded for significant activity at the group level using any of the methods described later in this chapter.

Consider the following example. In Pantazis et al. (2007), the first stage model consisted of fitting a univariate model for each subject in the α band for each of several cortically defined regions of interest and time bands. A contrast statistic was then estimated that captured an attention effect: ipsilateral minus contralateral alpha power in each spatiotemporal band. The contrast for all subjects was then fitted to a second stage GLM (Equation 4.10), whose design matrix X_g is a column of 1s. This simply leads to averaging the responses from all subjects (Equation 4.11), since the assumption of homogeneous intrasubject variance allows application of the simple summary statistic approach described above. Finally, the false discovery rate (FDR) approach, as described below, was used to threshold the resulting statistic map. Other examples of multisubject MEG studies can be found in Singh et al. (2003).

Besides the summary statistic approach, other methods for multisubject analysis have been proposed in functional neuroimaging. They consist of two steps: first, the statistic map from each subject is converted into a p-value map; then, the p-value maps from all subjects are combined into a single statistic map, which can finally be thresholded for significance with any of the error control methods described below. One important factor in determining how the individual p-value maps will be combined is the null hypothesis to be tested: one may consider, for instance, that there is a group effect if at least one subject has an effect (global null) (Friston et al., 1999), or that all subjects must have an effect for a group effect to be considered (conjunction null) (Friston et al., 2005; Nichols et al., 2005), or even that, for a group effect to be present, a predefined number of subjects having the effect is sufficient (partial conjunction null) (Benjamini and Heller, 2007; Heller et al., 2007). Once the null hypothesis is defined, we can choose between a variety of expressions for pooling individual *p*-values; some of these are due to Fisher (1950); Stouffer et al. (1949) and Worsley and Friston (2000), among others. The properties of each of these expressions are discussed elsewhere (Lazar et al., 2002; McNamee and Lazar, 2004).

4.7 Univariate versus Multivariate GLMs

We can analyze MEG data using either mass-univariate or multivariate approaches (Kiebel and Friston, 2004). The mass-univariate approach considers the data at each location in isolation. Therefore, a separate but identical GLM is fitted at each spatial-temporal-spectral location and analyzed using an ANOVA or ANCOVA approach. The data correlations in the respective dimensions are ignored at this stage, and accommodated at the inference stage through adjusting the *p*-values associated with the statistical maps. For example, even though the activation of nearby voxels is correlated, the mass-univariate approach ignores the spatial correlation, but corrects for it when random field theory or permutation tests define a threshold for significant activation. The mass-univariate approach can identify regionally specific effects, since it can test for rejection of the null hypothesis independently at each location. This property, together with its ease of implementation, has made it the most popular approach in functional neuroimaging.

In fMRI, univariate GLMs are typically fit in each cortical location to produce statistical maps that are then thresholded for significance (Friston et al., 1995a). Even though MEG does not have comparable spatial resolution, it affords high temporal resolution on the order of milliseconds (Barnes and Hillbrand, 2003; Brookes et al., 2004). This allows time–frequency decompositions of the recorded time series, which are then used as observations in mass-univariate GLMs in the spatial, temporal, and spectral dimensions (Durka et al., 2004; Kiebel et al., 2005a; Pantazis et al., 2009).

We have recently seen an increased interest in multivariate fMRI studies (Carlson et al., 2003; Cox and Savoy, 2003; Haynes and Rees, 2006; Norman et al., 2006; Pereira et al., 2009). Multivariate observations are formed across neighboring voxel locations, for example, following the searchlight approach (Kriegeskorte et al., 2006). These are then analyzed using pattern recognition techniques. Multivariate approaches offer increased sensitivity in detecting spatially distributed effects and can reveal the spatial encoding of mental states as well as assess the amount of information encoded in a particular brain region (Norman et al., 2006). Multivariate approaches should offer similar benefits for MEG data analysis. While fMRI has better spatial resolution, and multivariate observations are formed across neighboring voxels, MEG has excellent temporal resolution, allowing us to form multivariate observations across multiple frequencies. These observations are formed by first creating dynamic maps of cortical activity (regularized minimum-norm maps) through inverse mapping of MEG data (Baillet et al., 2001), and then applying time–frequency decompositions, such as the complex Morlet wavelet transform (Teolis, 1998).

In the multivariate approach we use the multivariate analysis of variance (MANOVA) or multivariate analysis of covariance (MANCOVA) framework. In this case, the MEG observations are organized into vectors and stacked as rows in an observation matrix *Y* (Figure 4.3). Classical analysis of this model proceeds by computing sample covariance matrices of the data and the residuals, and then estimating test statistics such as Roy's maximum root, Wilk's lambda, Pillai's trace, or Hotelling's trace (Seber, 2004).

An example of multivariate analysis in MEG is given in Soto et al. (2009). In this chapter, vectors of observations were formed by concatenating the power in six frequency bands and fit into separate multivariate linear models for each time band and cortical location with experimental conditions as predictor variables. The resulting Roy's maximum root statistic maps were thresholded for significance using permutation tests and the maximum statistic approach (described later in this chapter). Their results indicated that the multivariate method is more powerful than the univariate approach in detecting experimental effects when correlations exist between power across frequency bands.

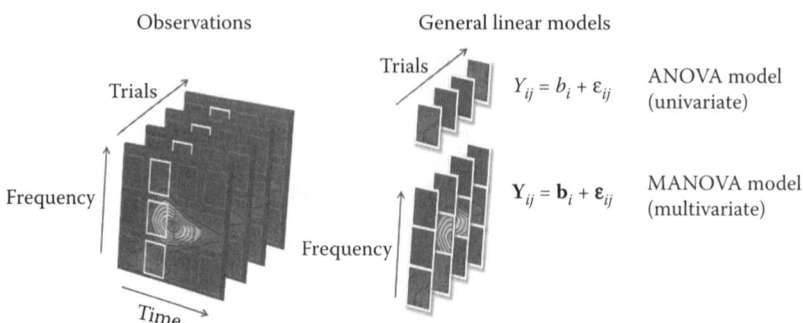

FIGURE 4.3 Power observations are fitted into GLMs using either a univariate or a multivariate approach. In the latter case, observations at multiple frequency bands are grouped together into vectors and fitted into MANOVA models.

4.8 Canonical Correlation Analysis

Until now, we have focused on investigating experimental effects by contrasting conditions between locations in space, time, and frequency. However, one may also be interested in exploring how the brain forms cortical functional networks. Given the excellent temporal resolution of MEG, we can explore functional interactions between cortical sites and even resolve these interactions at individual frequency bands.

Cortical interactions often involve several frequency bands, indicating that a multivariate (multifrequency) approach would have better sensitivity in detecting neural effects than univariate ones. Recent findings include theta–gamma coupling in visual memory (Schack et al., 2002; Bruns and Eckhorn, 2004; Schack and Weiss, 2005; Penny et al., 2008), word recognition (Mormann et al., 2005), and behavioral tasks (Canolty et al., 2006; Jensen and Colgin, 2007); delta–gamma in visual attention (Lakatos et al., 2008); alpha–gamma in mental arithmetic tasks (Palva et al., 2005) and rest (Osipova et al., 2008); beta–gamma in hand movement simulation (De Lange et al., 2008; Jerbi and Bertrand, 2009); and coupling of ultraslow rhythms with frequencies between 1 and 40 Hz during somatosensory tasks (Monto et al., 2008). Within-frequency interactions have also been reported recently (Lachaux et al., 1999; Fries, 2005; Hummel and Gerloff, 2006; Jerbi et al., 2007a; Pantazis et al., 2009).

Despite the importance of interactions across frequencies, most popular connectivity measures in MEG, such as coherence (Nunez et al., 1997; Gross et al., 2001; Le Van Quyen et al., 2001), phase synchrony (Tass et al., 1998; Lachaux et al., 1999; Lin et al., 2004), and Granger's causality (Kaminski et al., 2001; Brovelli et al., 2004; Kus et al., 2004), typically consider only interactions in amplitude or phase at the same frequency. Given the wealth of information in MEG data, analysis using a single-frequency approach requires either prior knowledge of the frequencies at which interactions will occur or, conversely, a large number of tests, one for each possible type of interaction.

Interpretation of interaction measures is further confounded by the ill-posed nature of the inverse problem in MEG, producing images of low resolution with blurred cortical sources resulting in linear mixing or crosstalk between regions, which may be mistaken as neural interactions between these regions. Approaches to reduce linear mixing when computing interactions include eliminating zero-lag correlations (Nolte et al., 2004; Gomez-Herrero et al., 2008; Marzetti et al., 2008), reconstructing current density maps that cancel interfering signals (Dalal et al., 2006; Hui and Leahy, 2006; Hui et al., 2010), and simply excluding *a priori* a number of spatial locations from the analysis (Carbonell et al., 2004a). However, all these approaches suffer from limitations and are not ideal solutions to the linear mixing problem. Because most interaction measures are sensitive to the linear mixing of sources, even small crosstalk can produce spurious interactions (Nunez et al., 1997). Here we describe a new alternative approach dealing with linear mixing: we accept as true interactions only those whose spectral profile cannot be explained by crosstalk between regions (which is equivalent to requiring canonical correlation vectors *a* and *b* to be nonparallel, as described below).

Our multivariate analysis of cortical interactions is based on canonical correlation analysis (Seber, 2004). Canonical correlation (or subspace correlation) extends the idea of simple correlation to multivariate signals; given two sets of signals, it finds the best way to linearly combine the two sets to achieve the maximum correlation. Multivariate observations are formed using the power or phase at multiple frequency bands, thus allowing us to automatically find the optimal set of frequencies contributing to neural interactions.

Time–frequency representations of brain activity are computed from MEG as described earlier in this chapter. Observations can then be formed by integrating the power of the wavelet coefficients over the frequency bands of interest, for example theta (4–7 Hz), alpha (8–14 Hz), beta (15–30 Hz), and gamma (31–50 Hz). The resulting observation matrices at each spatial location have dimension $n_{\text{trials}} \times n_{\text{bands}}$ and are normalized to have a zero mean and unit variance at each band.

Given two observation matrices $\mathbf{X}$ and $\mathbf{Y}$ from distinct voxel locations, the maximum canonical correlation seeks linear combinations of the columns of these matrices that maximize the correlation between them (Figure 4.4). In other words, we want to find vectors $\mathbf{a}$ and $\mathbf{b}$ such that ρ is maximized:

$$\rho = \frac{(\mathbf{Xa})^T (\mathbf{Yb})}{\| \mathbf{Xa} \| \| \mathbf{Yb} \|} \tag{4.12}$$

The maximum value of ρ, called the maximum canonical correlation, is given by the largest singular value of the matrix $\mathbf{M} = (\mathbf{X}^T\mathbf{X})^{1/2} (\mathbf{X}^T\mathbf{Y})(\mathbf{Y}^T\mathbf{Y})^{1/2}$ and the vectors $\mathbf{a}$ and $\mathbf{b}$ associated with the maximum ρ are $\mathbf{a} = (\mathbf{X}^T\mathbf{X})^{1/2}\mathbf{u}$ and $\mathbf{b} = (\mathbf{Y}^T\mathbf{Y})^{1/2}\mathbf{v}$, $\mathbf{u}$ and $\mathbf{v}$ being the left and right singular vectors of the largest singular value of $\mathbf{M}$, respectively. We can use the canonical vectors $\mathbf{a}$ and $\mathbf{b}$ to find the relative contribution of each frequency to the correlation between $\mathbf{X}$ and $\mathbf{Y}$ (Rencher, 1992).

To create canonical correlation statistical maps, we can either choose a seed voxel and compute the maximum canonical correlations between the seed and all other voxels on the cortical surface, or compute the canonical correlations between all possible pairs of cortical locations.

Apart from amplitude/amplitude coupling, we can also detect other forms of coupling by extending each observation vector to also include the phase of the wavelet coefficients in each band of interest. This will allow automatic detection of all possible relations: amplitude–amplitude (Bruns and Eckhorn, 2004), amplitude–phase (Canolty et al., 2006), and phase–phase (Lachaux et al., 1999).

We can use canonical vectors $\mathbf{a}$ and $\mathbf{b}$ to find the relative contribution of each frequency to the correlation between two cortical regions. However, low-resolution inverse solutions in EEG cause linear

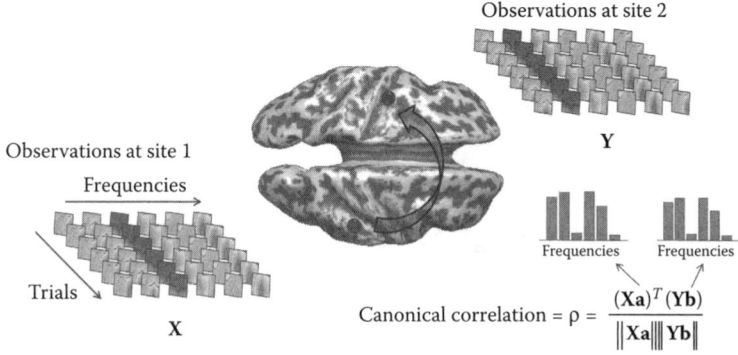

FIGURE 4.4 Observation matrices ($n_{\text{trials}} \times n_{\text{frequencies}}$) are estimated in each cortical site for a specific time band. Canonical correlation then produces the optimal combination of frequencies in one cortical site that best explains the frequencies in another site.

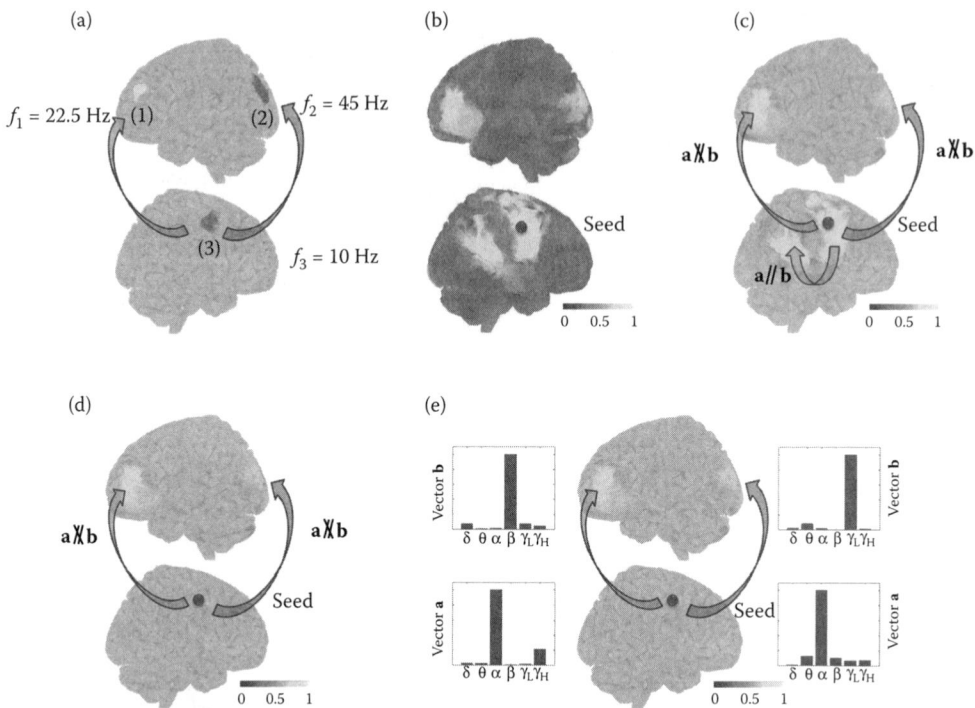

FIGURE 4.5 Identifying cortical networks with canonical correlation. (a) Simulated interactions between sources 1–3 and 2–3. Even though sources have different frequency content, their power is correlated with each other; (b) a canonical correlation map is estimated between the seed and all other cortical locations; (c) test for symmetry in cross correlation matrix to detect linear mixing; (d) interactions after controlling for linear mixing; (e) individual frequencies contributing to canonical correlation.

mixing of activation sources, causing large values in canonical correlation, even when true interaction does not exist (the same is true for simple correlations and phase synchrony). We can separate such spurious results from true cortical interactions by testing whether the cross correlation matrix between each pair of locations is symmetric. Specifically, we can show that in case of pure linear mixing, the cross correlation is symmetric. Therefore asymmetry implies true cortical interaction. Consequently the canonical correlation maps should be subjected to a statistical test, with correction for multiple comparisons, against symmetry of the cross correlation.

This procedure is illustrated in Figure 4.5. We simulate two cortical interactions and then estimate a map of canonical correlation between the seed and all other cortical locations. We successively threshold for significant canonical correlation and for asymmetry of cross correlation, to identify significant interactions that are not caused by linear mixing. Finally, vectors **a** and **b** reveal which frequencies contribute to the interaction.

4.9 Thresholding Statistical Maps

In the first half of this chapter, we reviewed several approaches to creating statistical maps of brain activation in MEG distributed cortical imaging using the GLM methodology. Arbitrary thresholding of these maps can lead to different interpretations of brain activation (Figure 4.6) and undermine the validity of a functional neuroimaging study. Objective assessment of the statistic maps requires a principled approach to identifying regions of activation. This involves testing thousands of hypotheses

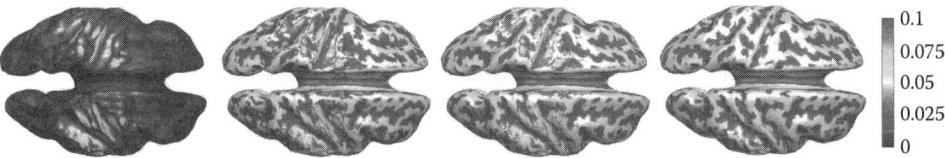

0.1
0.075
0.05
0.025
0

FIGURE 4.6 A statistic map thresholded at several arbitrary levels. Do both hemispheres show experimental effects, or just the right one? Interpretation of these activation results clearly depends on principled selection of the threshold for significance.

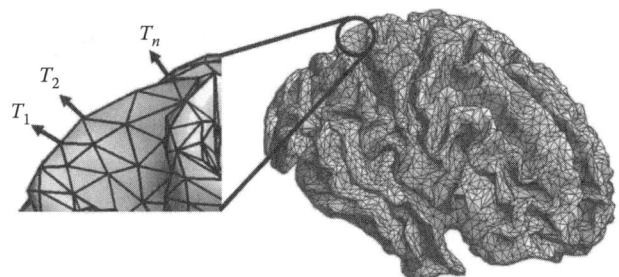

FIGURE 4.7 A statistical map typically consists of activation measures at thousands of voxels T_i on the brain surface. In the case of multidimensional statistical maps, we acquire activation measures for multiple time points and frequencies at each voxel.

(one for each spatial/temporal/frequency band or region of interest) for statistically significant experimental effects (Figure 4.7), and raises the possibility of large numbers of false-positives simply as a result of multiple hypothesis testing.

In the following, we first define measures of false-positives and show the important role that the maximum statistic plays in statistical inference. We then describe the Bonferroni correction, random field theory (RFT), permutation methods, and false discovery error rate (FDR), which provide corrected thresholds for statistical maps.

4.9.1 False-Positive Measures

Thresholding statistical maps should control some measure of the false-positive rate that takes into account the multiple hypothesis tests. Several measures of false-positives have been proposed, the most popular of which is the familywise error rate (FWER), that is, the probability of making at least one false-positive under the null hypothesis that there is no experimental effect. The Bonferroni method and two approaches based on the maximum statistic distribution, RFT and permutation tests, control the FWER. Another measure that is becoming increasingly popular is FDR, which controls the expected proportion of errors among the rejected hypotheses. Other measures of false-positives exist, such as positive false discovery rate, false discovery rate confidence, and per-family error rate confidence (Nichols and Hayasaka, 2003), but they are not as common and not covered in this chapter.

There are two types of FWER control: weak and strong. In *weak FWER control*, false-positives are controlled only when the complete null hypothesis holds, that is, when there is no experimental effect at any location in the brain. If a cortical site (or a temporal/spectral band) is truly active, control of false-positives is not guaranteed anywhere in the brain. Effectively, this implies that with weak FWER control we cannot achieve any localization of an experimental effect, but rather only reject the complete null hypothesis. Conversely, in *strong FWER control*, the false-positives are controlled for any subset where the null hypothesis holds. So, even if there is true brain activation at some locations, false-positives are still controlled at the other locations, and therefore we can localize experimental effects. Fortunately, the Bonferroni, RFT, and permutation methods achieve strong control of FWER, and therefore have localization power. On the other hand, the FDR method only has weak control of FWER.

FWER methods control the false-positives at an α level, typically 5%. This means that with 100 repetitions of the entire experiment only 5 of them will have one or more false-positives, or type I errors, at any location in the brain. We now investigate how the FWER is related to the maximum statistic.

4.9.2 Maximum Statistic

The FWER is directly related to the maximum value in the statistical image; one or more voxels T_i will exceed the threshold u_α under the null hypothesis H_0 only if the maximum exceeds that threshold:

$$
\begin{aligned}
P(\text{FWER}) &= P(\cup_i \{T_i \geq u_\alpha\} \mid H_0) \quad \text{(Probability that any voxel exceeds the threshold)} \\
&= P(\max_i T_i \geq u_\alpha \mid H_0) \quad \text{(Probability that max voxel exceeds the threshold)} \\
&= 1 - F_{\max T \mid H_0}(u_\alpha) \quad \text{(1 - cumulative density function of max voxel)} \\
&= 1 - (1 - \alpha) = \alpha
\end{aligned}
\tag{4.13}
$$

where $F_{\max}T|H_0$ is the cumulative density function of the maximum statistic under the null. Therefore, we can control the FWER if we choose the threshold u_α to be in the $(1 - \alpha)100$th percentile of the maximum distribution (Figure 4.8).

To control FWER, random field theory estimates the right tail of the maximum statistic distribution using a topological measure called the Euler Characteristic. Permutation tests, on the other hand, resample the data to estimate the empirical distribution of the maximum statistic. The Bonferroni method relies on the Bonferroni inequality and makes no use of the maximum distribution described here.

Rather than use the statistic value directly, these can first be converted to p-values by either assuming a parametric distribution or estimating an empirical distribution at each location (Pantazis et al., 2005b). In cases where the distribution of the statistic is spatially variant, p-values can improve control of FWER. We then use the distribution of the minimum p-value for control of FWER. As we see below, p-values are also used when controlling the FDR.

4.9.3 Bonferroni Correction

The simplest approach to controlling the FWER is the Bonferroni correction method (Hochberg and Tamhane, 1987; Nichols and Hayasaka, 2003). It is based on the Bonferroni inequality and assumes independence of each of the multiple hypothesis tests; under dependency Bonferroni is still valid but can be very conservative. To control false-positives at an α level, we threshold each voxel separately at the $\alpha_b = \alpha/V$ level, where V is the total number of voxels.

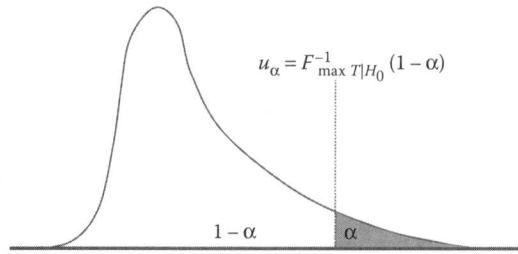

FIGURE 4.8 Probability density function of the maximum statistic. By choosing a threshold u_α which leaves only α (typically 5%) of the distribution to the right of u_α, we control the FWER at level α.

$$P(\text{FWER}) = P(\cup_i \{T_i \geq u_{\alpha_b}\} \mid H_0)$$

$$\leq \sum_i P(T_i \geq u_{\alpha_b}\} \mid H_0) \quad \text{(Bonferroni in equality)}$$

$$= \sum_i \alpha_b$$

$$= \sum_i \alpha/V = \alpha \tag{4.14}$$

The Bonferroni method requires the estimation of the marginal distribution at each location in the statistical map, or equivalently, its conversion into a *p*-value map. We can do this either parametrically, by assuming, for example, a Gaussian *t*, or *F* distribution at each voxel, or nonparametrically, by resampling the data using a permutation scheme and estimating the empirical distribution separately at each voxel. In Figure 4.11, we estimated the distributions using the later approach. Since the cortical surface was defined using 7501 nodes, the Bonferroni adjusted 5% level threshold was $\alpha_b = 0.05/7501 = 6.66 \cdot 10^{-6}$ and no voxel exceeded this very small threshold.

This is not surprising as the Bonferroni method produces very conservative thresholds unless the tests are independent or has weak dependency (Nichols and Hayasaka, 2003). This is rarely if ever the case in MEG since the number of MEG sensors rarely exceeds a few hundred, while the number of voxels in a statistical map may number several thousand. The inverse procedure that maps from sensors into brain space will inevitably introduce correlation among voxels. Many Bonferroni variants have been proposed, such as the Kounias inequality and step-up or step-down procedures (Hochberg and Tamhane, 1987). However, they offer little improvement over the original Bonferroni method.

4.9.4 Random Field Methods

As shown in Equation 4.13, the FWER can be determined directly from the probability distribution of the maximum statistic. Adler (1981) demonstrated that the expected value of the Euler Characteristic (EC), a topological measure of the suprathreshold region of a statistical map, is a good approximation of this probability when the threshold is large. Therefore, random field theory (RFT) approximates the upper tail of the maximum distribution $F_{\max}T$ using the expected value of the EC of the thresholded image (Worsley et al., 1996). Computational procedures for calculating this value are implemented in several software packages for analysis of functional imaging data (SPM—http://www.fil.ion.ucl.ac.uk, VoxBo—http://www.voxbo.org, and FSL—http://www.fmrib.ox.ac.uk/fsl among others), and are widely used in fMRI and PET functional neuroimaging studies.

Worsley et al. (1996) provides a formula for the expected value of the EC that unifies the results for all types of random fields:

$$P(\text{FWER}) = P(\cup_i \{T_i \geq u\} \mid H_0)$$

$$\approx \sum_{d=0}^{D} R_d(S)\rho_d(u) \tag{4.15}$$

This equation gives the probability of an FWER for threshold *u* in a *D*-dimensional random field T_i in a search region *S*, which can be the cortical surface ($D = 2$) or the brain volume ($D = 3$). The term $R_d(S)$ is the *d*-dimensional RESEL (RESolution Element) count, a unitless quantity that depends on the smoothness of the statistical map in the search region *S* under the null hypothesis (Figure 4.9). The term $\rho_d(u)$ is the EC density that depends only on the threshold *u* and the type of statistical field (such as *z*, *t*, χ^2, and Hotelling's T^2). In Equation 4.15, the lower dimensional terms ($d < D$) compensate for the case when the excursion set, that is, the regions of voxels in a field above a threshold *u*, touches the boundary. They can usually be omitted because they have only a small impact on the RESEL count.

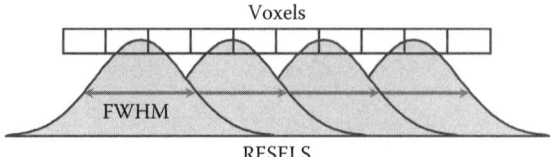

FIGURE 4.9   Random field theory uses the topological features of a statistical map to convert the voxels into RESELS, a dimensionless quantity that represents the image with interpretable units of smoothness. Under the null hypothesis of no experimental effects, it is the degree of spatial correlation in the noise in the statistical maps that determines the RESEL count.

While in fMRI and PET the random fields can be assumed to be statistically stationary, in MEG we need to compensate for nonstationarity in the spatial, temporal, and spectral dimensions (Worsley et al., 1999), both for maximum statistic inference and cluster size tests (Hayasaka et al., 2004). Such corrections in the spatial dimension were applied by Pantazis et al. (2005b) and Barnes and Hillbrand (2003) to threshold 2D cortical maps and 3D volumetric maps, respectively. Singh et al. (2003) and Park et al. (2002) used RFT as implemented in the SPM software to threshold beamformer and LORETA (Pascual-Marqui et al., 1994) volumetric maps from a multisubject MEG/EEG study. Kilner et al. (2005) used single channel EEG data to create time–frequency maps that were thresholded with SPM under the assumption of stationarity. Finally, Carbonell et al. (2004b) applied RFT on a 1D Hotelling T^2 statistical map created from multichannel EEG data in the temporal dimension.

To derive corrected thresholds for statistical maps, RFT relies on several assumptions including the following: the image has the same parametric distribution at each spatial location, the point spread function has two derivatives at the origin, the field has sufficient smoothness to justify application of continuous RFT, and the threshold is sufficiently high for the asymptotic results to be accurate. When these assumptions hold, RFT is a very powerful method; when this is not possible, for example with statistical maps of nonstandard distributions, nonparametric alternatives should be considered.

To apply RFT in Figure 4.11, the statistical map was first smoothed with the Laplace–Beltrami operator (Chung, 2001), a generalization of Gaussian smoothing on an arbitrary Riemannian manifold. The spatial filtering corresponded to a 16.7 mm full-width half-maximum (FWHM). Since the mean distance between the vertices in the tessellated cortical surface was 5.7 mm, the spatial filtering was equivalent to 2.93 vertices FWHM, which is considered sufficient when smoothing 3D Gaussian images (Hayasaka and Nichols, 2003). On the smoothed statistical map, RFT produced 334.91 RESELS from 7501 cortical vertices or voxels. Using Equation 4.15, the adjusted 5% level threshold was 4.12.

RFT results are available not only for the maximum statistic (peak statistic height), but also for the size of a cluster, the number of clusters, and joint inference on peak height and cluster size (Poline et al., 1997; Hayasaka and Nichols, 2004; Hayasaka et al., 2004). Furthermore, the theory is applicable to the multivariate analog of the *F*-statistic, Roy's maximum root, and therefore multivariate GLM modeling can also be used in conjunction with RFT (Worsley et al., 2004).

4.9.5 Permutation Methods

The standard approach to permutation tests is to find units exchangeable under the null hypothesis. Units are exchangeable if by randomly rearranging these units we can create permutation samples that are statistically equivalent under the null hypothesis to the original data. The simplest example involves a study in which we want to detect differences between two experimental conditions. Under the null hypothesis that there is no difference, epochs from the two conditions can be exchanged, provided that equal numbers of samples (in time, space, and frequency) are collected under each condition.

A test statistic is computed from each permutation sample that, including the statistic representing the original data, constitute the reference set for determining significance. The proportion of data permutations in the reference set that have test statistic values greater than or equal to the value for the experimentally obtained results are the *p*-value (significance or probability value). An excellent treatment of permutation tests can be found in Edgington (1995) and Nichols and Holmes (2001).

For FWER control, the test statistic is the maximum in the statistical map. Therefore, unlike the RFT approach, which estimates the upper tail of the maximum distribution based on geometrical features of a parametric statistical map, permutation methods resample the data and create an empirical maximum distribution. By setting a threshold at the α100th percentile of the upper tail of the empirical distribution, we have exact control of the FWER.

Since the permutation samples must be statistically equivalent to the original data, permutations that destroy the inherent correlation structure of the MEG data are not allowed. For example, we cannot exchange channel labels or randomize time-series because the spatial or temporal structure would be altered. Therefore, it is important to apply valid permutation schemes for both single-subject and multisubject studies.

In single-subject studies, permutations are feasible between experimental conditions (Maris and Oostenveld, 2007). The MEG data are assigned to conditions either beforehand, with respect to the baseline and types of stimuli provided, or on-the-fly based on the subject's responses, such as fast/slow button presses. In between-trials design, every trial is assigned to one experimental condition; in within-trials design every trial is assigned to multiple experimental conditions in different time segments. The latter is far more common, as a baseline is typically included before the presentation of a stimulus, and therefore a single trial has two conditions. Most researchers are willing to assume statistical independence between MEG trials or between nonoverlapping time segments within trials, especially if they are separated by some minimum time interval, and thus satisfy the exchangeability requirement. Figure 4.10 shows an example permutation scheme used in Pantazis et al. (2005b) to threshold minimum-norm cortical maps while controlling for false-positives.

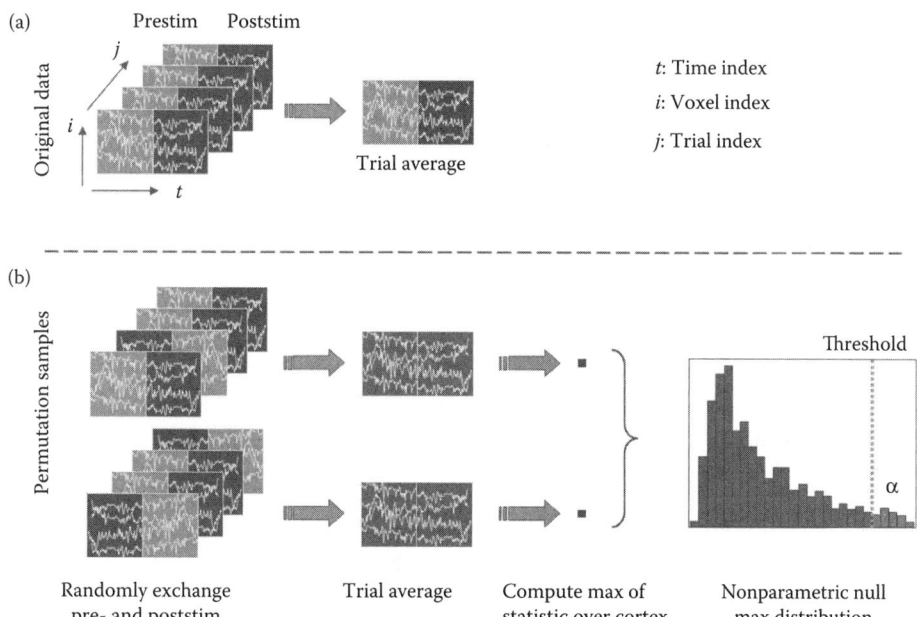

FIGURE 4.10 Permutation scheme on a single-subject multitrial MEG study. (a) Averaging of original statistical maps. (b) Generation of permutation samples by randomly exchanging pre- and poststimulus conditions within each trial. An empirical distribution of the maximum statistic is generated by averaging the permuted trials and computing the max over the cortex. The α level threshold at the upper tail of the empirical distribution is applied to the original averaged data to control the FWER.

In multisubject studies, permutations are only performed on the second-level GLM for random effect statistical inference (see Section 4.6). In the simple summary statistic approach in Equation 4.10, each subject's estimated contrast $c^T \hat{b}_k$ is assumed to have a symmetric distribution around zero under the null hypothesis. Therefore, randomly multiplying it by 1 or −1 does not change its distribution under the null hypothesis. With K subjects (and thus K contrasts), a total of 2^K permutation samples can be created, which can then each be fitted to the second-level GLM to estimate permuted group parameters that are used in turn to estimate the empirical distribution of the group-averaged map. Such an approach was followed for example by Singh et al. (2003); Pantazis et al. (2007). Unfortunately, with small K the empirical distribution may be coarsely quantized and more subjects may be necessary to achieve a desired FWER control.

Permutation tests have many advantages. They are exact, that is, give precise control of FWER, they do not assume parametric distributions, they adapt to underlying correlation patterns in the data, and they are very flexible as any test statistic can be used. The only assumptions required are those to justify permuting the labels of the conditions, such as that the distributions under the null hypothesis have the same shape or are symmetric. Even though we are free to consider any statistic summarizing evidence for the effect of interest at each location, it is usually best to use the same statistics for a nonparametric approach as we would for a comparable parametric approach. The reason is that parametric statistics often have optimal power; for example, a *t*-statistic is the most powerful in detecting differences between populations in many circumstances. Furthermore, to achieve uniform specificity, that is, equal chances of false-positives at any location in the statistical map, we should use statistics that have approximately homogeneous null permutation distributions.

On account of their flexibility, permutation tests are more commonly used in MEG than the parametric RFT. Permutation tests have been proposed to control false-positives in the channel domain: (Blair and Karnisky, 1993, 1994; Karnisky et al., 1994; Galan et al., 1997; Achim, 2001; Maris, 2004) and in the source domain: (Park et al., 2002; Pantazis et al., 2003, 2005b; Singh et al., 2003; Chau et al., 2004; Sekihara et al., 2005). These methods have been applied in multiple MEG studies: (Kaiser et al., 2000; Lutzenberger et al., 2002; Pantazis et al., 2005a, 2007; Bayless et al., 2006; Cheyne et al., 2006; Itier et al., 2006). Reviews on the application of permutation tests in MEG are available in Maris and Oostenveld (2007), Maris et al. (2007).

Various thresholding methods are illustrated in Figure 4.11. The permutation method was based on that described in Pantazis et al. (2005b) and produced a threshold of 3.99, which controls FWER over the whole cortex at a 5% level.

4.9.6 Control of False Discovery Rate

In contrast to the above methods that control the FWER, FDR controls the expected proportion of errors among the rejected hypotheses Pantazis et al. (2005b). For example, if we set $\alpha = 5\%$ FDR threshold, then on average we should expect 5% of our suprathreshold voxels to be false-positives.

The standard FDR method proposed by (Benjamini and Hochberg, 1995; Genovese et al., 2002) is conservative, as it controls the FDR at a $\frac{V_0}{V}\alpha$ level, where V is the total number of voxels and V_0 is the number of voxels where the null hypothesis is true:

$$E(\text{FDR}) = E\left(\frac{\text{False positives}}{\text{Suprathreshold voxels}} \right) \leq \frac{V_0}{V}\alpha \qquad (4.16)$$

When the true brain activation extends over broad areas, V_0 may become small and the FDR procedure too conservative. Thus, a number of adaptive procedures improve on the original FDR approach by first estimating V_0, and then using this estimate to tighten the threshold (Benjamini et al., 2006).

The FDR methods adapt to the properties of the data; when a large number of voxels are truly active, the threshold will adjust to allow for more false-positives; when no truly activated voxels exist, FDR controls the FWER, but in a weak sense (see Section 4.9.1). They are more powerful than Bonferroni,

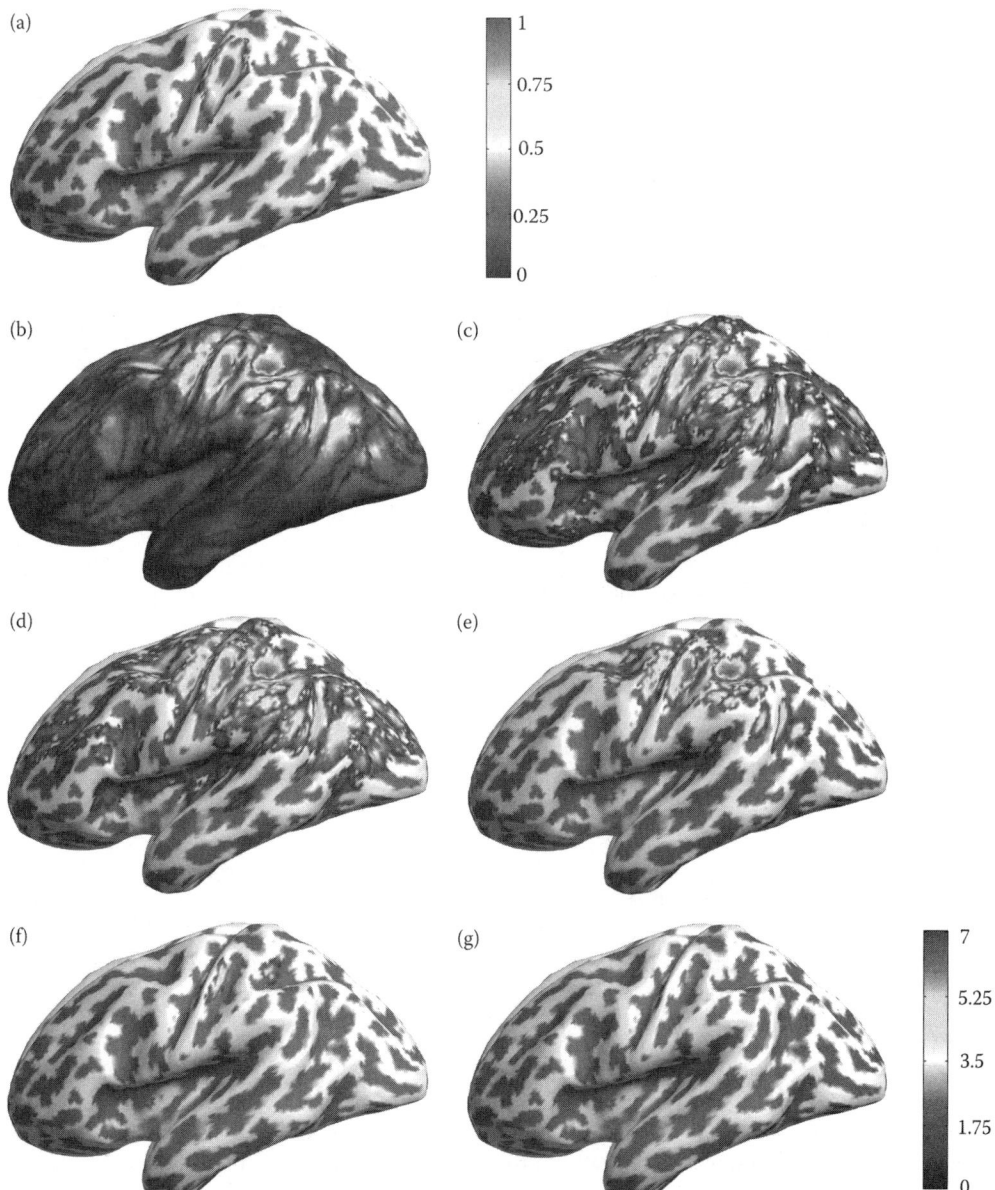

FIGURE 4.11 Simulated MEG source on the left hemisphere and reconstructed dSPM statistical map, thresholded using several methods to control false-positives. (a) Simulated sources, (b) statistical map, (c) uncorrected, (d) FDR, (e) permutations, (f) random field, and (g) Bonferroni. Uncorrected thresholding (p-value = 0.05) and FDR (p-value = 0.0065) produced many false-positives. Permutations and random field theory gave 5% FWER thresholds $t = 3.99$ and $t = 4.12$, respectively. The Bonferroni approach was very conservative (p-value 0.05/7501 = 6.6610^{-6}) and did not identify the source.

random field, and permutation control of FWER, and for this reason may become popular for thresholding MEG maps.

The FDR approach requires the estimation of the marginal distribution at each location in the statistical map, or equivalently, conversion of the statistic value at each location into an equivalent p-value. We can do this parametrically or nonparametrically, as described for the Bonferroni approach.

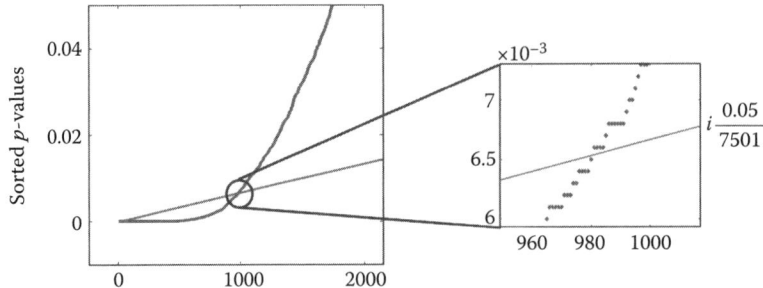

FIGURE 4.12 Graphical representation of the FDR procedure. The blue line represents the sorted p-values of the statistical map in Figure 4.11, and the red line is $i\,\alpha/V = i\,0.05/7501$. The largest p-value below the line is 0.0065 and corresponds to a 5% level FDR threshold.

Once the maps are converted to p-values, implementation of the standard FDR method is relatively straightforward (Genovese et al., 2002). If V is the total number of voxels being tested, the procedure is as follows:

1. Order the voxel p-values from smallest to largest:

$$P_{(1)} \leq P_{(2)} \leq \cdots \leq P_{(V)} \tag{4.17}$$

2. Let r be the largest i for which

$$P_{(i)} \leq \frac{i}{V}\frac{\alpha}{c(V)} \tag{4.18}$$

3. Declare all voxels corresponding to the p-values $P_{(1)}, \ldots P_{(r)}$ active.

where $c(V) = \sum_{i=1}^{V} 1/i$ if no assumptions on the joint distribution of the p-values across voxels is made, and $c(V) = 1$ if the p-values in different voxels are independent or they have positive dependence (Benjamini and Yekutieli, 2001).

The procedure is demonstrated graphically in Figure 4.12 for the FDR procedure applied to the statistical map in Figure 4.11. The estimated threshold for 7501 cortical voxels at the 5% level was 0.065, and produced an extended region of suprathreshold voxels. Unfortunately, the large extent of the significantly active region determined using FDR is a result of the limited spatial resolution of MEG; many voxels surrounding the true simulated source exhibit significant activity in the statistical map, and FDR is sensitive enough to identify them. Conversely, the more conservative thresholds from FWER control tend to reduce the size of activated regions as also shown in Figure 4.11. Other examples of the application of FDR in MEG maps include Edwards et al. (2005); Jacobs et al. (2006); Pantazis et al. (2007); Jacques and Rossion (2007).

4.10 Discussion

We have presented a GLM framework to produce statistical maps from MEG distributed cortical imaging, and subsequently threshold them while controlling for false-positives. Choosing a thresholding method depends on the data available: Bonferroni is simple and efficient for a small number of tests with minimal dependence; random fields are robust when their parametric assumptions are satisfied and strong correlation exists in the data; permutation tests are very general, adapt to the underlying data correlations, can use any statistic, and are more powerful than random fields for data with low degrees of freedom (e.g., studies with a few subjects); FDR is more powerful, works well with sparse signals, and recommended when we can afford a few false-positives. However as we have shown in our simulations, FDR can produce large regions of significant activation as a result of the limited resolution of MEG inverses.

A number of important statistical issues are beyond the scope of this chapter such as conjunction analysis (Nichols et al., 2005), that is, the identification of brain areas that are simultaneously active in multiple tasks, extraction of confidence intervals for distributed solutions using the bootstrap (DiNocera and Ferlazzo, 2000; Gross et al., 2003; Darvas et al., 2005), and thresholding using cluster size tests (Hayasaka et al., 2004). Also, the theory was developed for distributed inverse methods in MEG. However, discrete solutions are also popular in MEG, especially with well-localized activation when a few equivalent current dipoles can represent most cortical activity. In this case alternative approaches can be used to establish significance, for example the bootstrap resampling approach or Monte Carlo simulations to find localization accuracy and confidence intervals for current dipoles (Braun et al., 1997; Darvas et al., 2005).

A related problem in MEG data analysis is testing for the statistical significance of cortical interactions (Gross et al., 2001; Varela et al., 2001; Hui and Leahy, 2006; Jerbi et al., 2007b; Maris et al., 2007). In some cases, a few cortical locations are investigated and corrections for multiple comparisons are generally not employed. In the case where tests are made for interactions between multiple pairs of locations, the theory described in this chapter can be applied. The DICS algorithm, for example, can be used to investigate cortical coherence at all locations in the cortex relative to a reference, which may be a single cortical location or an electromyograph reference signal (Gross et al., 2001). The resulting maps are a measure of coherence at each cortical location for a single frequency band but can be easily extended to multiple frequency bands. The methods described in this chapter for analysis of time–frequency representations of brain activity can be adapted to testing for significant activation in these coherence maps.

References

Achim, A., 2001. Statistical detection of between-group differences in event-related potentials. *Clinical Neurophysiology* 112, 1023–1034.

Adler, R. J. (ed.), 1981. *The Geometry of Random Fields*. New York: Wiley.

Baillet, S., Mosher, J. C., Leahy, R. M., 2001. Electromagnetic brain mapping. *IEEE Signal Processing Magazine* 18, 14–30.

Barnes, G. R., Hillbrand, A., 2003. Statistical flattening of MEG beamformer images. *Human Brain Mapping* 18, 1–12.

Bayless, S. J., Gaetz, W. C., Cheyne, D. O., Taylor, M. J., 2006. Spatiotemporal analysis of feedback processing during a card sorting task using spatially filtered MEG. *Neuroscience Letters* 410, 31–36.

Beckmann, C. F., Jenkinson, M., Smith, S. M., 2003. General multilevel linear modeling for group analysis in fMRI. *NeuroImage* 20(2), 1052–1063.

Benjamini, Y., Heller, R., 2007. Screening for partial conjunction hypotheses. Technical Report RP-SOR-06-06, http://www.math.tau.ac.il/departments/st/.

Benjamini, Y., Hochberg, Y., 1995. Controlling the false discovery rate: A practical and powerful approach to multiple testing. *Journal of the Royal Statistical Society* 57, 289–300.

Benjamini, Y., Krieger, A. M., Yekutieli, D., 2006. Adaptive linear step-up procedures that control the false discovery rate. *Biometrica* 93(3), 491–507.

Benjamini, Y., Yekutieli, D., 2001. The control of the false discovery rate in multiple testing under dependency. *The Annals of Statistics* 29(4), 1165–1188.

Blair, R. C., Karnisky, W., 1993. An alternative method for significance testing of waveform difference potentials. *Psychophysiology* 30, 518–524.

Blair, R. C., Karnisky, W., 1994. Distribution-free statistical analyses of surface and volumetric maps. *Functional Neuroimaging: Technical Foundations* (R. W. Thatcher, M. Hallett, T. Zeffiro, E. R. Jony, M. Huerta, eds.), San Diego, California: Academic Press, pp. 19–28.

Braun, C., Kaiser, S., Kinces, W., Elbert, T., 1997. Confidence interval of single dipole locations based on EEG data. *Brain Topography* 10(1), 31–39.

Brookes, M., Gibson, A., Hall, S., Furlong, P., Barnes, G., Hillebrand, A., Singh, K., Holliday, I., Francis, S., Morris, P., 2004. A general linear model for MEG beamformer imaging. *NeuroImage* 23(3), 936–946.

Brooks, M. J., Gibson, A. M., Hall, S. D., Furlong, P. L., Barnes, G. R., Hillebrand, A., Singh, K. D., Holliday, I. E., Francis, S. T., Morris, P. G., 2004. A general linear model for MEG beamformer imaging. *NeuroImage* 23, 936–946.

Brovelli, A., Ding, M., Ledberg, A., Chen, Y., Nakamura, R., Bressler, S., 2004. Beta oscillations in a large-scale sensorimotor cortical network: Directional influences revealed by Granger causality. *Proceedings of the National Academy of Sciences of the United States of America* 101(26), 9849.

Bruns, A., 2004. Fourier-, Hilbert- and wavelet-based signal analysis: Are they really different approaches? *Journal of Neuroscience Methods* 137, 321–332.

Bruns, A., Eckhorn, R., 2004. Task-related coupling from high-to low-frequency signals among visual cortical areas in human subdural recordings. *International Journal of Psychophysiology* 51(2), 97–116.

Canolty, R., Edwards, E., Dalal, S., Soltani, M., Nagarajan, S., Kirsch, H., Berger, M., Barbaro, N., Knight, R., 2006. High gamma power is phase-locked to theta oscillations in human neocortex. *Science* 313(5793), 1626.

Carbonell, F., Galan, L., Valdes, P., Worsley, K., Biscay, R., Diaz-Comas, L., Bobes, M., Parra, M., 2004a. Random field-union intersection tests for EEG/MEG imaging. *NeuroImage* 22(1), 268–276.

Carbonell, F., Galan, L., Valdes, P., Worsley, K., Biscay, R. J., Diaz-Comas, L., Bobes, M. A., Parra, M., 2004b. Random field—Union intersection tests for EEG/MEG imaging. *NeuroImage* 22, 268–276.

Carlson, T., Schrater, P., He, S., 2003. Patterns of activity in the categorical representations of objects. *Journal of Cognitive Neuroscience* 15(5), 704–717.

Chau, W., McIntosh, A. R., Robinson, S. E., Schulz, M., Pantev, C., 2004. Improving permutation test power for group analysis of spatially filtered MEG data. *NeuroImage* 23, 983–996.

Cheyne, D., Bakhtazad, L., Gaetz, W., 2006. Spatiotemporal mapping of cortical activity accompanying voluntary movements using an event-related beamforming approach. *Human Brain Mapping* 27, 213–229.

Christensen, G. E., Johnson, H. J., 2001. Consistent image registration. *IEEE Transactions on Medical Imaging* 20(7), 568–582.

Chung, M. K., 2001. Statistical morphometry in neuroanatomy. Ph.D. thesis, McGill University, Montreal.

Cox, D., Savoy, R., 2003. Functional magnetic resonance imaging (fMRI). *NeuroImage* 19(2), 261–270.

Dalal, S., Sekihara, K., Nagarajan, S., 2006. Modified beamformers for coherent source region suppression. *IEEE Transactions on Biomedical Engineering* 53(7), 1357–1363.

Dale, A. M., Liu, A. K., Fischi, R. B., Buckner, R. L., Belliveau, J. W., Lewine, J. D., Halgren, E., 2000. Dynamic statistical parametric mapping: Combining fMRI and MEG for high-resolution imaging of cortical activity. *Neuron* 26, 55–67.

Darvas, F., Rautiainen, M., Pantazis, D., Baillet, S., Benali, H., Mosher, J. C., Garnero, L., Leahy, R. M., 2005. Investigations of dipole localization accuracy in MEG using the bootstrap. *NeuroImage* 25, 355–368.

De Lange, F., Jensen, O., Bauer, M., Toni, I., 2008. Interactions between posterior gamma and frontal alpha/beta oscillations during imagined actions. *Frontiers in Human Neuroscience* 2, 1–12.

DiNocera, F., Ferlazzo, F., 2000. Resampling approach to statistical inference: Bootstrapping from event-related potentials data. *Behavioral Research Methods, Instruments and Computers* 32(1), 111–119.

Durka, P., Zygierewicz, J., Klekowicz, H., Ginter, J., Blinowska, K., 2004. On the statistical significance of event-related EEG desynchronization and synchronization in the time-frequency plane. *IEEE Transactions on Biomedical Engineering* 51(7), 1167–1175.

Edgington, E. S. (ed.)., 1995. *Randomization Tests*. London, UK: Academic Press.

Edwards, E., Soltani, M., Deouell, L. Y., Berger, M. S., Knight, R. T., 2005. High gamma activity in response to deviant auditory stimuli recorded directly from human cortex. *Journal of Neurophysiology* 94, 4269–4280.

Fischl, B., Serano, M., Tootell, R., Dale, A. M., 1999. High-resolution intersubject averaging and a coordinate system for the cortical surface. *Human Brain Mapping* 8(4), 272–284.

Fisher, R., 1950. *Statistical Methods for Research Workers*, 11th edition. Edinburgh, UK: McGraw-Hill/Appleton and Lange.

Fries, P., 2005. A mechanism for cognitive dynamics: Neuronal communication through neuronal coherence. *Trends in Cognitive Sciences* 9(10), 474–480.

Friston, K., Holmes, A., Price, C., Bqchel, C., Worsley, K., 1999. Multisubject fMRI studies and conjunction analyses. *NeuroImage* 10, 385–396.

Friston, K., Holmes, A., Worsley, K., Poline, J., Frith, C., Frackowiak, R., 1995a. Statistical parametric maps in functional imaging: A general linear approach. *Human Brain Mapping* 2(4), 189–210.

Friston, K. J., Holmes, A. P., Worsley, K. J., Poline, J. B., Frith, C., Frackowiak, R. S. J., 1995b. Statistical parametric maps in functional imaging: A general linear approach. *Human Brain Mapping* 2, 189–210.

Friston, K., Penny, W., Glaser, D., 2005. Conjunction revisited. *NeuroImage* 25, 661–667.

Friston, K. J., Penny, W., Phillips, C., Kiebel, S., Hinton, G., Ashburner, J., 2002. Classical and Bayesian inference in neuroimaging: Theory. *NeuroImage* 16, 465–483.

Friston, K. J., Stephan, K. M., Heather, J. D., Frith, C. D., Ioannides, A. A., Liu, L. C., Rugg, M. D. et al., 1996. A multivariate analysis of evoked responses in EEG and MEG data. *NeuroImage* 3, 167–174.

Fuchs, M., Wagner, M., Kohler, T., Wischmann, H., 1999. Linear and nonlinear current density reconstructions. *Journal of Clinical Neurophysiology* 16, 267–295.

Galan, L., Biscay, R., Rodriguez, J. L., Abalo, M. C. P., Rodriguez, R., 1997. Testing topographic differences between event related brain potentials by using non-parametric combinations of permutation tests. *Electroencephalography and clinical Neurophysiology* 102, 240–247.

Genovese, C., Lazar, N., Nichols, T., 2002. Thresholding of statistical maps in functional neuroimaging using the false discovery rate. *NeuroImage* 15, 870–878.

Gomez-Herrero, G., Atienza, M., Egiazarian, K., Cantero, J., 2008. Measuring directional coupling between EEG sources. *NeuroImage* 43(3), 497–508.

Gross, J., Kujala, J., Hamalainen, M., Timmermann, L., Schnitzler, A., Salmelin, R., 2001. Dynamic imaging of coherent sources: Studying neural interactions in the human brain. *Proceedings of National Academy of Sciences* 98(2), 694–699.

Gross, J., Timmermann, L., Kujala, J., Salmelin, R., Schnitzler, A., 2003. Properties of MEG tomographic maps obtained with spatial filtering. *NeuroImage* 19, 1329–1336.

Hamalainen, M. S., Ilmoniemi, R. J., 1984. Interpreting magnetic fields of the brain: Minimum norm estimates. *Medical and Biological Engineering and Computing* 32(1), 35–42.

Hayasaka, S., Nichols, T. E., 2003. Validating cluster size inference: Random field and permutation methods. *NeuroImage* 20(4), 2343–2356.

Hayasaka, S., Nichols, T. E., 2004. Combining voxel intensity and cluster extent with permutation test framework. *NeuroImage* 23(1), 54–63.

Hayasaka, S., Phan, K. L., Libarzon, I., Worsley, K. J., Nichols, T. E., 2004. Nonstationary cluster-size inference with random field and permutation methods. *NeuroImage* 22, 676–687.

Haynes, J., Rees, G., 2006. Decoding mental states from brain activity in humans. *Nature Reviews Neuroscience* 7(7), 523–534.

Heller, R., Golland, Y., Malach, R., Benjamini, Y., 2007. Conjunction group analysis: An alternative to mixed/random. *NeuroImage* 37, 1178–1185.

Hellier, P., Ashburner, J., Corouge, I., Barillot, C., Friston, K. J., 2002. Inter-subject registration of functional and anatomical data using textSPM. In: *Medical Image Computing and Computer-Assisted Intervention—MICCAI 2002.* Lecture Notes in Computer Science, Vol. 2489, Dohi, T. and Kikinis, R. (Eds). pp. 590–597, Berlin/Heidelberg: Springer.

Hochberg, Y., Tamhane, A. C. (eds.), 1987. *Multiple Comparison Procedures.* Newbury Park, California: Wiley.

Holmes, A., Friston, K. J., 1998. Generalisability, random effects and population inference. *NeuroImage* 7, S754.

Hui, H., Leahy, R., 2006. Linearly constrained MEG beamformers for MVAR modeling of cortical interactions. In: *3rd IEEE International Symposium on Biomedical Imaging: Nano to Macro, 2006.* pp. 237–240, Arlington, Virginia: Institute of Electrical and Electronics Engineers (IEEE).

Hui, H., Pantazis, D., Bressler, S., Leahy, R., 2010. Identifying true cortical interactions in MEG using the nulling beamformer. *NeuroImage* 49(4), 3161–3174.

Hummel, F., Gerloff, C., 2006. Interregional long-range and short-range synchrony: A basis for complex sensorimotor processing. *Event-related Dynamics of Brain Oscillations*, 159(2006), 223–236.

Itier, R. J., Herdman, A. T., George, N., Cheyne, D., Taylor, M. J., 2006. Inversion and contrast-reversal effects on face processing. *Brain Research* 1115, 108–120.

Jacobs, J., Hwang, G., Curran, T., Kahana, M. J., 2006. EEG oscillations and recognition memory: Theta correlates of memory retrieval and decision making. *NeuroImage* 32, 978–987.

Jacques, C., Rossion, B., 2007. Early electrophysiological responses to multiple face orientations correlate with individual discrimination performance in humans. *NeuroImage* 36, 863–876.

Jensen, O., Colgin, L., 2007. Cross-frequency coupling between neuronal oscillations. Trends in cognitive sciences 11(7), 267–269.

Jerbi, K., Bertrand, O., 2009. Cross-frequency coupling in parieto-frontal oscillatory networks during motor imagery revealed by magnetoencephalography. *Frontiers in Neuroscience* 3, 00011.

Jerbi, K., Lachaux, J., N'Diaye, K., Pantazis, D., Leahy, R. M., Garnero, L., and Baillet, S., 2007a. Coherent neural representation of hand speed in humans revealed by MEG imaging. *Proceedings of the National Academy of Sciences* 104(18), 7676.

Jerbi, K., Lachaux, J. P., N'Diaye, K., Pantazis, D., Leahy, R. M., Garnero, L., 2007b. Coherent neural representation of hand speed in humans revealed by MEG imaging. *PNAS* 104(18), 7676–7681.

Joshi, A. A., Shattuck, D. W., Thompson, P. M., Leahy, R. M., April 12–15 2007a. A finite element method for elastic parameterization and alignment of cortical surfaces using sulcal constraints. In: *Biomedical Imaging: From Macro to Nano, 2007. 4th IEEE International Symposium.* pp. 640–643, Arlington, Virginia: Institute of Electrical and Electronics Engineers (IEEE).

Joshi, A. A., Shattuck, D.W., Thompson, P. M., Leahy, R. M., 2007b. Surface constrained volumetric brain registration using harmonic mappings. *IEEE Transactions on Medical Imaging* 26(12), 1657–1669.

Kaiser, J., Lutzenberger, W., Preissl, H., Mosshammer, D., Birbaumer, N., 2000. Statistical probability mapping reveals high-frequency magnetoencephalographic activity in supplementary motor area during self-paced finger movements. *Neuroscience Letters* 283(1), 81–84.

Kaminski, M., Ding, M., Truccolo, W., Bressler, S., 2001. Evaluating causal relations in neural systems: Granger causality, directed transfer function and statistical assessment of significance. *Biological Cybernetics* 85(2), 145–157.

Karnisky, W., Blair, R. C., Snider, A. D., 1994. An exact statistical method for comparing topographic maps with any number of subjects and electrodes. *Brain Topography* 6, 203–210.

Kiebel, S., 2003. The general linear model. In: Frackowiak, R., Friston, K., Frith, C., Dolan, R., Friston, K., Price, C., Zeki, S., Ashburner, J., Penny, W. (eds.), *Human Brain Function*, 2nd Edition. San Diego, California: Academic Press.

Kiebel, S., Tallon-Baudry, C., Friston, K., 2005a. Parametric analysis of oscillatory activity as measured with EEG/MEG. *Human Brain Mapping* 26(3), 170–177.

Kiebel, S. J., Friston, K. J., 2004. Statistical parametric mapping for event-related potentials: I. generic considerations. *NeuroImage* 22, 492–502.

Kiebel, S. J., Tallon-Baudry, C., Friston, K. J., 2005b. Parametric analysis of oscillatory activity as measured with EEG/MEG. *Human Brain Mapping* 26, 170–177.

Kilner, J. M., Kiebel, S. J., Friston, K. J., 2005. Applications of random field theory to electrophysiology. *Neuroscience Letters* 374, 174–178.

Kriegeskorte, N., Goebel, R., Bandettini, P., 2006. Information-based functional brain mapping. *Proceedings of the National Academy of Sciences* 103(10), 3863.

Kucukaltun-Yildirim, E., Pantazis, D., Leahy, R., 2006. Task-based comparison of inverse methods in magnetoencephalography. *IEEE Transactions on Biomedical Engineering* 53(9), 1783–1793.

Kus, R., Kamniski, M., Blinowska, K., 2004. Determination of EEG activity propagation: Pair-wise versus multichannel estimate. *IEEE Transactions on Biomedical Engineering* 51(9), 1501–1510.

Lachaux, J., Rodriguez, E., Martinerie, J., Varela, F., 1999. Measuring phase synchrony in brain signals. *Human Brain Mapping* 8(4), 194–208.

Lakatos, P., Karmos, G., Mehta, A., Ulbert, I., Schroeder, C., 2008. Entrainment of neuronal oscillations as a mechanism of attentional selection. *Science* 320(5872), 110.

Lazar, N., Luna, B., Sweeney, J., Eddy, W., 2002. Combining brains: A survey of methods for statistical pooling of information. *NeuroImage* 16(2), 538–550.

Le Van Quyen, M., Foucher, J., Lachaux, J., Rodriguez, E., Lutz, A., Martinerie, J., Varela, F., 2001. Comparison of Hilbert transform and wavelet methods for the analysis of neuronal synchrony. *Journal of Neuroscience Methods* 111(2), 83–98.

Lin, F., Witzel, T., Hamalainen, M., Dale, A., Belliveau, J., Stufflebeam, S., 2004. Spectral spatiotemporal imaging of cortical oscillations and interactions in the human brain. *NeuroImage* 23(2), 582–595.

Lutzenberger, W., Ripper, B., Busse, L., Birbaumer, N., Kaiser, J., 2002. Dynamics of gamma-band activity during an audiospatial working memory task in humans. *Journal of Neuroscience* 22(13), 5630–5638.

Maris, E., 2004. Randomization tests for ERP topographies and whole spatiotemporal data matrices. *Psychophysiology* 41, 142–151.

Maris, E., Oostenveld, R., 2007. Nonparametric statistical testing of EEG- and MEG-data. *Journal of Neuroscience Methods* 164, 177–190.

Maris, E., Schoffelen, J.-M., Fries, P., 2007. Nonparametric statistical testing of coherence differences. *Journal of Neuroscience Methods* 163, 161–175.

Marzetti, L., Del Gratta, C., Nolte, G., 2008. Understanding brain connectivity from EEG data by identifying systems composed of interacting sources. *NeuroImage* 42(1), 87–98.

McNamee, R., Lazar, N., 2004. Assessing the sensitivity of FMRI group maps. *NeuroImage* 22(2), 920–931.

Monto, S., Palva, S., Voipio, J., Palva, J., 2008. Very slow EEG fluctuations predict the dynamics of stimulus detection and oscillation amplitudes in humans. *Journal of Neuroscience* 28(33), 8268.

Mormann, F., Fell, J., Axmacher, N., Weber, B., Lehnertz, K., Elger, C., Ferńandez, G., 2005. Phase/amplitude reset and theta-gamma interaction in the human medial temporal lobe during a continuous word recognition memory task. *Hippocampus* 15(7), 890–900.

Mosher, J. C., Leahy, R. M., 1998. Recursive MUSIC: A framework for EEG and MEG source localization. *IEEE Transactions of Biomedical Engineering* 45(11), 1342–1354.

Mumford, J. A., Nichols, T., 2006. Modeling and inference of multisubject fMRI data. *IEEE Engineering in Medicine and Biology Magazine* 25(2), 42–51.

Nichols, T., Brett, M., Andersson, J., Wager, T., Poline, J.-B., 2005. Valid conjunction inference with the minimum statistic. *NeuroImage* 25, 653–660.

Nichols, T. E., Hayasaka, S., 2003. Controlling the familywise error rate in functional neuroimaging: A comparative review. *Statistical Methods in Medical Research* 12(5), 419–446.

Nichols, T. E., Holmes, A. P., 2001. Nonparametric permutation tests for functional neuroimaging: A primer with examples. *Human Brain Mapping* 15, 1–25.

Nolte, G., Bai, O., Wheaton, L., Mari, Z., Vorbach, S., Hallett, M., 2004. Identifying true brain interaction from EEG data using the imaginary part of coherency. *Clinical Neurophysiology* 115(10), 2292–2307.

Norman, K., Polyn, S., Detre, G., Haxby, J., 2006. Beyond mind-reading: Multivoxel pattern analysis of fMRI data. *Trends in Cognitive Sciences* 10(9), 424–430.

Nunez, P., Srinivasan, R., Westdorp, A., Wijesinghe, R., Tucker, D., Silberstein, R., Cadusch, P., 1997. EEG coherency. I: Statistics, reference electrode, volume conduction, Laplacians, cortical imaging, and inter-pretation at multiple scales. *Electroencephalography and Clinical Neurophysiology* 103(5), 499–515.

Osipova, D., Hermes, D., Jensen, O., 2008. Gamma power is phase-locked to posterior alpha activity. *PLoS One* 3(12), 1–7.

Palva, J., Palva, S., Kaila, K., 2005. Phase synchrony among neuronal oscillations in the human cortex. *Journal of Neuroscience* 25(15), 3962.

Pantazis, D., Merrifield, W., Darvas, F., Sutherling, W., Leahy, R. M., 2005a. Hemispheric language domi-nance using MEG cortical imaging and non-parametric statistical analysis. *WSEAS Transactions on Biology and Biomedicine* 2(3), 318325.

Pantazis, D., Nichols, T. E., Baillet, S., Leahy, R. M., 2005b. A comparison of random field theory and per-mutation methods for the statistical analysis of MEG data. *NeuroImage* 25(2), 383–394.

Pantazis, D., Nichols, T. E., Baillet, S., Leahy, R. M., July 2003. Spatiotemporal localization of significant activation in MEG using permutation tests. In: Taylor, C., Noble, J. A. (eds.), *Proceedings of the 18th Conference on Information Processing in Medical Imaging*. pp. 512–523.

Pantazis, D., Simpson, G., Weber, D., Dale, C., Nichols, T., Leahy, R., April 12–15 2007. Exploring human visual attention in an MEG study of a spatial cueing paradigm using a novel ANCOVA design. In: *2007 IEEE International Symposium on Biomedical Imaging: From Nano to Macro*.

Pantazis, D., Simpson, G., Weber, D., Dale, C., Nichols, T., Leahy, R., 2009. A novel ANCOVA design for analysis of MEG data with application to a visual attention study. *NeuroImage* 44(1), 164–174.

Pantazis, D., Weber, D., Dale, C., Nichols, T., G.V. Simpson, Leahy, R., 2005c. Imaging of oscillatory behav-ior in event-related MEG studies. In: Bouman, C., Miller, E. (eds.), *Proceedings of SPIE, Computational Imaging III*. Vol. 5674. pp. 55–63.

Park, H., Kwon, J., Youn, T., Pae, J., Kim, J., Kim, M., Ha, K., 2002. Statistical parametric mapping of LORETA using high density EEG and individual MRI: Application to mismatch negativities in schizophrenia. *Human Brain Mapping* 17, 168–178.

Pascual-Marqui, R. D., 2002. Standardized low resolution brain electromagnetic tomography (sLORETA): Technical details. *Methods and Findings in Experimental Clinical Pharmacology* 24D, 5–12.

Pascual-Marqui, R. D., Michel, C. M., Lehmann, D., 1994. Low resolution electromagnetic tomography: A new method for localizing electrical activity in the brain. *International Journal of Psychophysiology* 18, 49–65.

Penny, W., Duzel, E., Miller, K., Ojemann, J., 2008. Testing for nested oscillation. *Journal of Neuroscience Methods* 174(1), 50–61.

Pereira, F., Mitchell, T., Botvinick, M., 2009. Machine learning classifiers and fMRI: A tutorial overview. *NeuroImage* 45(1), S199–S209.

Poline, J.-B., Holmes, A. P.,Worsley, K. J., Friston, K. J., 1997. Statistical inference and the theory of ran-dom fields. In: Friston, K., Frith, C. D., Dolan, R. J., Mazziotta, J. C., Frackowiak, R. (eds.), *Human Brain Function*, 1st Edition. San Diego, California: Academic Press.

Rencher, A., 1992. Interpretation of canonical discriminant functions, canonical variates, and principal components. *American Statistician* 46(3), 217–225.

Schack, B., Vath, N., Petsche, H., Geissler, H., Moller, E., 2002. Phase-coupling of theta-gamma EEG rhythms during short-term memory processing. *International Journal of Psychophysiology* 44(2), 143–163.

Schack, B., Weiss, S., 2005. Quantification of phase synchronization phenomena and their importance for verbal memory processes. *Biological Cybernetics* 92(4), 275–287.

Seber, G. A. F., 2004. *Multivariate Observations*. Hoboken, New Jersey: John Wiley & Sons, Inc.

Sekihara, K., Sahani, M., Nagarajan, S. S., 2005. A simple nonparametric statistical thresholding for MEG spatial-filter source reconstruction images. *NeuroImage* 27, 368–376.

Shen, D., Davatzikos, C., 2002. HAMMER: Hierarchical attribute matching mechanism for elastic registration. *IEEE Transactions on Medical Imaging* 21(11), 1421–1439.

Singh, K., Barnes, G. R., Hillebrand, A., 2003. Group imaging of task-related changes in cortical synchronization using nonparametric permutation testing. *NeuroImage* 19, 1589–1601.

Soto, J., Pantazis, D., Jerbi, K., Lachaux, J.-P., Garnero, L., Leahy, R., 2009. Detection of event-related modulations of oscillatory brain activity with multivariate statistical analysis of MEG data. *NeuroImage* 30(6), 1922–1934.

Stouffer, S., Suchman, E., DeVinney, L., Star, S., Williams Jr, R., 1949. *The American Soldier: Adjustment during Army Life. (Studies in Social Psychology in World War II, Vol. 1.).* Princeton, NJ: Princeton University Press.

Tass, P., Rosenblum, M., Weule, J., Kurths, J., Pikovsky, A., Volkmann, J., Schnitzler, A., Freund, H., 1998. Detection of n: m phase locking from noisy data: Application to magnetoencephalography. *Physical Review Letters* 81(15), 3291–3294.

Teolis, A. (ed.), March 1998. *Computational Signal Processing with Wavelets (Applied and Numerical Harmonic Analysis).* Boston: Birkhauser.

Thompson, P., Mega, M., Woods, R. P., Zoumalan, C. I., Lindshield, C. J., Blanton, R. E., Moussai, J., Holmes, C., Cummings, J. L., Toga, A. W., 2001. Cortical change in Alzheimer's disease detected with a disease-specific population-based brain atlas. *Cerebral Cortex* 11(1), 1–16.

Tikhonov, A., Arsenin, V., 1977. *Solutions of Ill-Posed Problems.* Great Falls, Montana: Winston and Sons.

van Veen, B., Drongelen, W. V., Yuchtman, M., Suzuki, A., 1997. Localization of brain electrical activity via linearly constrained minimum variance spatial filtering. *IEEE Transactions of Biomedical Engineering* 44(9), 867–880.

Varela, F., Lachaux, J.-P., Rodriguez, E., Martinerie, J., 2001. The brainweb: Phase synchronization and large-scale integration. *Nature Reviews* 2, 229–239.

Verbeke, G., Molenberghs, G., 2000. *Linear Mixed Models for Longitudinal Data.* New York: Springer-Verlag.

Worsley, K., Friston, K., 2000. A test for a conjunction. *Statistics and Probability Letters* 47(2), 135–140.

Worsley, K. J., Andermann, M., Koulis, T., MacDonald, D., Evans, A. C., 1999. Detecting changes in non-isotropic images. *Human Brain Mapping* 8, 98–101.

Worsley, K. J., Marrett, S., Neelin, P., Vandal, A. C., Friston, K. J., Evans, A. C., 1996. A unified statistical approach for determining significant signals in images of cerebral activation. *Human Brain Mapping* 4, 58–73.

Worsley, K. J., Taylor, J. E., Tomaiuolo, F., Lerch, J., 2004. Unified univariate and multivariate random field theory. *NeuroImage* 23, s189–195.

5

Emergence of Groupwise Registration in MR Brain Study

Guorong Wu*
University of North Carolina

Hongjun Jia
University of North Carolina

Qian Wang
University of North Carolina

Feng Shi
University of North Carolina

Pew-Thian Yap
University of North Carolina

Dinggang Shen
University of North Carolina

5.1 Background

Modern medical imaging technologies such as magnetic resonance imaging (MRI) [1] offer a safe and noninvasive means of performing clinical diagnosis and research, involving human brain development, aging, and disease-induced anomalies. For reliable estimation of disease-related microstructural difference, accurate deformable image registration plays a key fundamental role in dealing with confounding intrasubject variability in longitudinal studies and intersubject variability in cross-sectional studies.

5.1.1 Pairwise Registration

A plethora of pairwise deformable registration algorithms have flourished in the past two decades, comprehensive surveys of which can be found in [2–6]. In general, the goal of image registration is to estimate the deformation field for warping the subject image (or moving image) to the template image (or fixed image) by maximizing a certain similarity measure between the warped subject and the template. Upon successful registration, intra- or intersubject differences are minimized, while at the same time disease-related changes and morphological variations are preserved.

The majority of image registration algorithms fall into three categories: landmark-based [7–9], intensity-based [10–15], and feature-based [16–19]. Landmark-based algorithms take advantage of

---

* Guorong Wu, Hongjun Jia, and Qian Wang contributed equally to this chapter.

anatomical prior knowledge and are thus computationally fast, since only a few landmarks out of all voxels in an image volume need to be matched. It is, however, a challenging task even for the trained experts to accurately place a sufficient number of anatomical landmarks for achieving accurate registration. Moreover, interrater landmark-placement variability could be large, thus seriously undermining the performance of landmark-based registration algorithms. Intensity-based algorithms take a different approach by aiming to maximize the intensity similarity between a pair of images, which can be fully automated by employing state-of-the-art optimization methods for deformation field estimation. However, intensity similarity does not necessarily imply anatomical correspondence. In light of this, feature-based algorithms formulate image registration as a problem of feature matching for deformation estimation. Anatomical correspondences identified by feature-based registration have been found to be more reliable than those based on intensity alone.

Hierarchical attribute matching mechanism for elastic registration (HAMMER) [17,18]—one of the most popular brain MRI registration algorithms—integrates the advantages of the methods from all three categories, and alleviates their limitations. HAMMER designates an attribute vector to each image point as its morphological signature for efficient determination of anatomical correspondences between an image pair. The attribute vector consists of a variety of image-derived features, including image intensity, edge type, and geometric moment invariants (GMIs) [20] computed for three types of tissues, that is, white matter (WM), gray matter (GM), and cerebrospinal fluid (CSF). The degree of similarity between the GMI-based features of a particular point at the anterior horn of the left ventricle (as indicated by a red cross) and the attribute vector of every other point in the image is color-coded and shown in Figure 5.1, where blue denotes high similarity and red otherwise. To achieve robust registration and to avoid local minima, only a small number of the voxels with the most distinctive attribute vectors—the driving voxels—in both template and subject are selected for guiding the initial registration. As registration progresses, an increasing number of voxels are selected as driving voxels to refine the deformation field. Figure 5.2 illustrates the hierarchical deformation mechanism in HAMMER with points in red, green, and yellow denoting the driving voxels identified in the initial, middle, and final registration stages, respectively. The gradually refined deformation field is shown in the bottom of Figure 5.2.

HAMMER has been evaluated in a number of brain studies and is found to achieve relatively high accuracy, even in the presence of significant morphological differences in cortical regions. In Figure 5.3, some representative registration results of elderly subjects from the Baltimore Longitudinal Study of Aging (BLSA [21]) are shown to demonstrate the performance of HAMMER. The abundance of anatomical details retained in the average image gives a good indication of HAMMER's capability in registering images with significant structural variations.

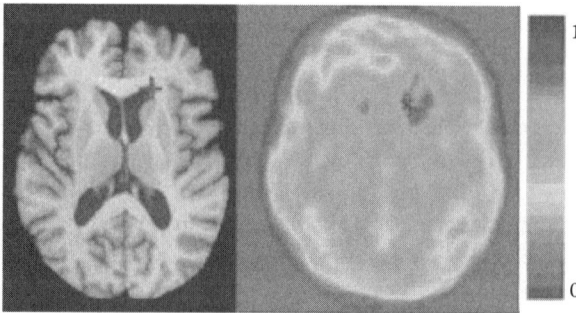

FIGURE 5.1   Color-coded map (right) of the degree of similarity between the attribute vectors of the marked point (the red cross in the left image) and every other point in the brain. Blue denotes for high similarity and red for low similarity. (Adapted from D. Shen and C. Davatzikos, *Medical Imaging, IEEE Transactions on*, 21, 1421–1439, © 2002 IEEE.)

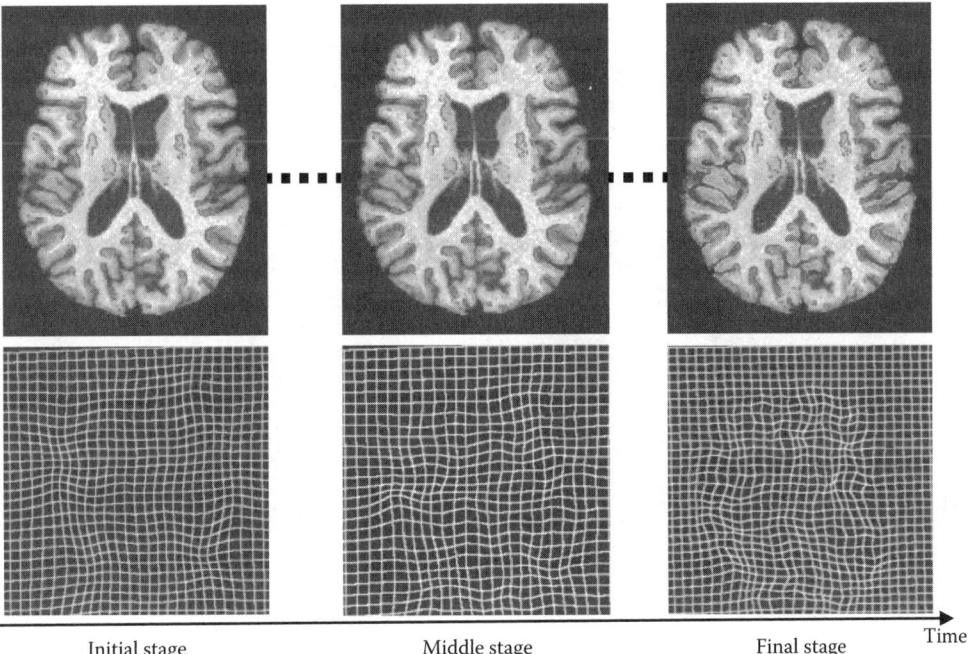

Initial stage   Middle stage   Final stage   Time

FIGURE 5.2 Hierarchical selection of the driving voxels, and evolution of deformation fields in different registration stages. In the initial stage, only a small number (around approximately 2% of total voxels) of voxels with distinctive attribute vectors (displayed in red), located at sulcal roots, gyral crowns, and ventricular boundaries, are selected to steer the registration of other less distinctive voxels. As registration progresses, more and more voxels are selected as the driving voxels, as shown in green and yellow, respectively. The bottom row shows the corresponding deformation fields estimated at three different stages. It can be observed that, as the number of the driving voxels increases, the deformation field is gradually refined. (Adapted from G. Wu et al., *NeuroImage*, 49, 2225–2233, 2010.)

5.1.2 Limitations of Pairwise Registration

Due to the high anatomic variability among individual human brains, any atlas or clinical diagnostic system based on a single subject's anatomy cannot achieve full success [23]. Although it is applicable to register each subject to the template by pairwise registration for the intra- or interpopulation analysis, registration schemes based on a single reference will introduce systematic bias toward the shape of the selected template. To increase the signal-to-noise ratio (SNR) in subsequent statistical analysis, the registration of a large number of images from different individuals needs to be considered within a unified registration framework, so that the overall registration accuracy for all images in a population can be maximized. Eventually, the anatomical shape differences within and across populations can be better delineated. Thus, groupwise registration algorithms which avoid bias in template selection are recently gaining increasing research interest.

5.1.3 Emergence of Groupwise Registration

To alleviate limitations of pairwise registration, groupwise registration aims to warp all images toward the common space by simultaneously estimating their deformations [24–43]. In other words, given an image population $I = \{I_i \mid i = 1,\ldots,N\}$, the ultimate goal of groupwise registration is to find a set of deformations $T = \{T_i \mid i = 1,\ldots,N\}$ to minimize the variation within the registered subject set $\tilde{I} = \{T_i(I_i) \mid i = 1,\ldots,N\}$. The scheme of groupwise registration is illustrated in the left panel of Figure 5.4.

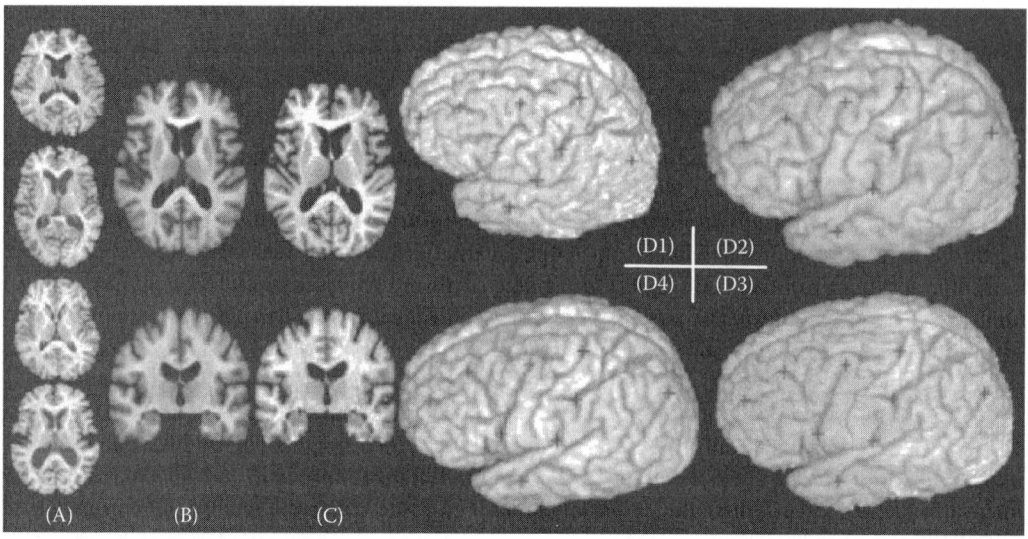

FIGURE 5.3 Results from HAMMER algorithm. (A) Four representative cross sections from BLSA dataset; (B) Representative views from the average of the 18 images after normalization onto the template in (C) by HAMMER; (D1–D4) the 3D rendering of a representative case, its warped configuration using HAMMER, the template and the average of 18 warped brains, respectively. The anatomical details seen in (B) and (D4) are the evidences of the registration accuracy. The red crosses in (D1–D4) are identically placed to allow for visual inspection of point correspondences. (Adapted from Z. Lao et al., *NeuroImage*, 21, 46–57, 2004.)

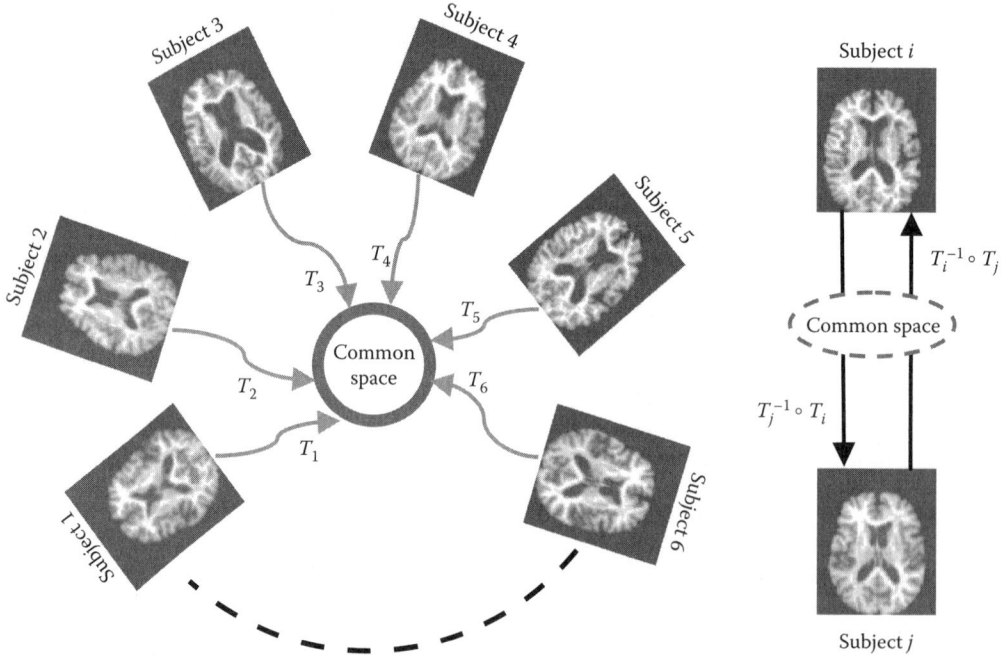

FIGURE 5.4 In groupwise registration, all subjects are warped onto a common space by following their individual deformations (as indicated by red arrows). Also, any subject I_i is connected to another subject I_j via the common space by a composed transformation, that is, $T_j^{-1} \circ T_i$, as shown in the right panel.

Specifically, subject I_i is warped to the common space, following the corresponding deformation T_i. The estimated deformation usually complies with the constraint of invertibility. Then, any two subjects can be connected via the common space. For example, in the right panel of Figure 5.4, subject i can be warped onto the space of subject j by a composed transformation and, that is, $T_j^{-1} \circ T_i$. After all images have been aligned in the common space, any quantitative analysis can be performed.

The majority of the current groupwise registration algorithms can be classified into three classes: (1) pairwise registration derived groupwise registration [24,25]; (2) population center-guided groupwise registration [26,27,32,33,38,40,42]; and (3) hidden common space-based groupwise registration [28–30,36,37,44]. The first class of methods directly applies pairwise registration to achieve the goal of groupwise registration. They attempt to determine an unbiased or least biased atlas by exhaustive pairwise registration of image pairs in a group. We will describe two typical methods of this class in Section 5.2. Recent groupwise registration algorithms take a different approach by simultaneously estimating the deformations in relation to a common space. Specifically, the second class of methods estimates the population center by explicit registration of each subject image to a group mean image. The third class of methods formulates the groupwise registration as an optimization problem with an objective function that drives all subjects toward the hidden common space. We will describe with more details these two classes of groupwise registration algorithms in Sections 5.3, 5.4, respectively. The major difference between the last two classes of methods is that, in the second class, the image in the common space is determined explicitly and is evolved with further registration, while in the third class, the image in the common space is implicit or hidden throughout the optimization. We will provide several typical applications of groupwise registration in Section 5.5, including image parcellation [22], multiple modal image population exploration [31], and infant atlas building [45].

5.2 Pairwise Registration-Derived Groupwise Registration

One of the most straightforward ways of achieving groupwise registration is to apply the pairwise registration directly on the images in the population. In this section, we briefly introduce two such groupwise registration algorithms. Seghers et al. [25] proposed to construct the brain atlas based on the exhaustive pairwise registration, with possible number of registration totaling up to $N(N-1)$. By taking in turn every image I_i in the group as the template, they estimate the deformation fields to all other $N-1$ images with respect to the template, and then warp the template with the average deformation field. Then the final atlas is obtained by the voxelwise averaging of all warped images. However, this method suffers from very heavy computation cost. For example, it takes about 170 days on one 2.6 GHz processor to perform 4032 pairwise registrations for a group of 64 subjects [25].

An alternative method can be found in the work of Park et al. [24]. They perform pairwise registrations among N subjects by taking each subject as a template in turn and registering the rest of the subjects onto this template. Next, instead of averaging all deformed images in [25], they build an $N \times N$ distance matrix with each element denoting a measure of the bending energy of a particular deformation field. Multidimensional scaling (MDS) [46] is performed on the distance matrix to choose the image that is the closest to the population center as the template. Since the distance matrix is assumed to be symmetric, this method is faster since only $N(N-1)/2$ times of pairwise registration need to be performed. Once the least biased template is determined (which is only an approximation to the real population center), all other images can be mapped onto the template space directly using a pairwise registration method. However, the potential bias introduced in the selection of the template, as well as the difficulty in registering images with large deformations to the selected template, limit its application in practice.

In brief, the goal of this kind of method is to construct an unbiased or least-biased atlas. However, the large number of required rounds of pairwise registration limits their application. Possible solution to this is discussed next.

5.3 Population Center-Guided Groupwise Registration

Groupwise registration can be implemented by aligning all images to a population center. In the literature, several groupwise registration methods have been proposed to better estimate and utilize the population center. For example, the group mean method and its extensions [26,40,41] repeatedly estimate the group mean image from the tentatively aligned images and update the deformation of each subject to the newly estimated group mean image. In the tree-based algorithms [27,42], all subjects in the population are connected by a tree structure with the root subject considered as the population center. Thus, all other subjects can be registered to the root by following the path from each individual node to the root node. To better utilize the local and global information of the manifold spanned by all subjects, a method called Atlas Building by Self-Organized Registration and Bundling (ABSORB) [32,33] has been proposed recently. In general, ABSORB warps each subject toward its selected neighbors and assures that all subjects can reach the population center. All these algorithms are detailed next.

To avoid the potential bias in groupwise registration, Joshi et al. [26] proposed to solve the groupwise registration in an iterative manner by estimating the population center via the Fréchet mean of all images. An interim population center is first built by averaging all linearly aligned images. And then all images are warped to this interim population center by a diffeomorphism registration framework. The interim population center is further updated based on all the tentatively warped images, and then the deformations for all images can be refined as well. The two steps of (1) estimating population center and (2) registering images to the population center are interleaved and iteratively performed. As illustrated in Figure 5.5, this method can provide an unbiased population center, and converge fast by a few iterations. However, the registration process of this method could be misled when trying to register individual images (with sharp anatomical structures) to a blurry group mean image (with ambiguous anatomical structures), due to the difficulty in establishing the reliable correspondences between them, especially in the beginning of the registration.

It is worth noting that other registration methods are also applicable to the group mean framework. For example, Marsland et al. [38] introduced a minimum description length (MDL)-based method, which plays as a role similar to the diffeomorphism registration method in [26], for groupwise registration. In MDL, the image population is described by not only a single mean image, but also a set of deformations and a set of residuals, which are encoded according to any given model (e.g., the histogram of the mean image). Based on the information theory, groupwise registration is accomplished when the description length of the population coding is minimized.

Fletcher et al. [40] extended the definition of the geometric median (or the L^1 estimator) to the Riemannian manifold, by adopting geodesic distances between subjects on the manifold and minimizing the distance via gradient-based optimization. The geometric median serves as the population center to guide the subsequent registration. They further proved that the geometric median exists and is unique for any nonpositively curved manifold or under certain conditions for positively curved manifolds.

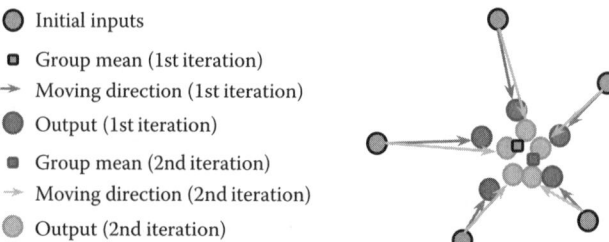

FIGURE 5.5 Illustration of the framework of the group mean method. In each iteration, the subjects are warped toward the tentatively estimated group mean. And the group mean is refined based on newly warped subjects.

In their experiments, this extension was demonstrated to be more robust to outliers than the Fréchet mean used by Joshi et al. [26].

Recently, Wu et al. [41] extended the pairwise HAMMER algorithm [17] to work in a groupwise manner. Instead of simply averaging over the intensities of the cohort of images, they proposed to average images region-by-region according to local anatomical shapes. Starting from an exemplar image which has the minimal distance to all other images, more and more anatomical details are gradually augmented to the mean image as registration progresses. In this way, the mean image can be kept sharp throughout the whole registration process, which is very important to obtain accurate registration results. In their method, each subject is treated differently (according to the alignment of local anatomical structures) in constructing the group mean based on the alignment of local anatomical shape. Two major advantages are demonstrated: (1) the group mean image has minimal anatomical difference to all subjects, and (2) the group mean retains the population information as well as sharp anatomical structures.

It is generally difficult to achieve good registration by directly registering each image to a fixed population center, especially when cross-subject anatomical variation is large. Some algorithms have been proposed to warp the individual images with the help of intermediate template [47–50]. These intermediate templates are produced to pave the path for connecting an individual image to the population center. The final registration result can be obtained by deforming each individual image along its respective path to the population center. This idea is applied to the groupwise registration by building a minimum spanning tree (MST) [51] where each node corresponds to one image and each edge indicates the distance between two connected nodes. The root node of the MST, namely the population center, can be determined by selecting a node that has the minimal edge length to all other nodes or that has the maximal number of children. In Hamm et al. [27], after learning the intrinsic manifold of the whole dataset, the population center is determined as the pseudo-geodesic median image since it minimizes the total path length from each image to the template. The corresponding geodesic paths between individual images and the population center are computed to construct a tree based on the learned manifold. The large deformation between the subject and the population center is thus decomposed into several small ones, and the accuracy of registration is improved. Nevertheless, since the population center is approximated by a fixed image (i.e., the root image) from the dataset, the bias is unavoidable in this scenario.

More recently, a new framework for groupwise registration termed as ABSORB was proposed [32,33]. The basic idea of ABSORB is illustrated in Figure 5.6. This method explores the intrinsic distributions of subjects to guide the registration. The groupwise registration problem is resolved in an iterative manner by warping each image in the population step-by-step on the learned manifold, and, at the same time, maintaining the global distribution of the population. To achieve this goal, two new strategies,

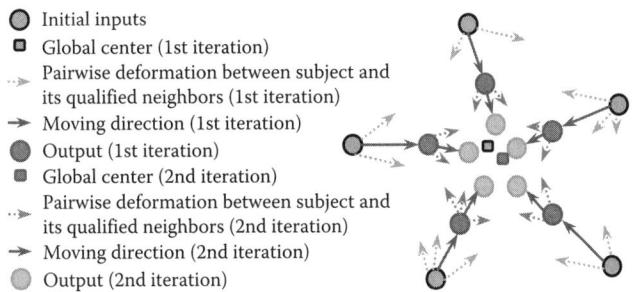

FIGURE 5.6 Illustration of the ABSORB framework. In each iteration, each subject is deformed toward its selected neighbors, which are closer to the population center. The estimated population center is updated iteratively based on the tentatively warped images. (Adapted from H. Jia et al., *NeuroImage*, 51(3), 1057–1070, 2010.)

namely self-organized registration and image bundling are employed. Specifically in the self-organized registration, each image is warped toward a subset of its neighbors that are closer to the population center, in order to condense the global distribution of the population on the manifold. The tentative population center is updated iteratively and used only to guide the selection of qualified neighbors, thereby not directly involved into registration. After several iterations, some nearby subjects become close enough to each other and are, thus, bundled together spontaneously into a subgroup. Then ABSORB jumps to the higher level, where the registration is performed on a much smaller dataset which consists of only the representative images of all subgroups. As the result of this hierarchical registration process, a pyramid of images is built automatically and the population center can be eventually generated once the registration arrives at the upmost level. With ABSORB, the possible registration error can be greatly reduced by only warping each individual subject to its neighbors with similar structures. Also, it can produce a smoother registration path, which traverses each subject image to the final population center, than other groupwise registration methods.

Similar to other approaches that solve the groupwise registration in a "relay" fashion [26,27,42], the complete path from each individual image to the final population center built by ABSORB is composed of a series of small segments. But ABSORB is inherently different from those methods in three ways. First, in ABSORB, no fixed intermediate templates are used for any image in any iteration. Instead, the movement of each individual image on the manifold is driven only by a selected set of its qualified neighboring images, not by a common explicit or implicit template. Second, the number of qualified neighboring images is adaptively determined according to the intrinsic data structure learned online, and the complete path generated from each image to the population center on the manifold is generally smoother and more conservative as ABSORB always warps one image to its nearby location, instead of moving to the population center directly. One example is demonstrated in Figure 5.7. In contrast, in [26,27,42], the direction and the amount of deformation for each image in each iteration are determined by only the selected tentative template, which can often result in a zigzag path if the selected template does not represent the data distribution very well. Finally, the registration path for each image provided by ABSORB is not predetermined before the actual registration starts. In other words, it is a fully

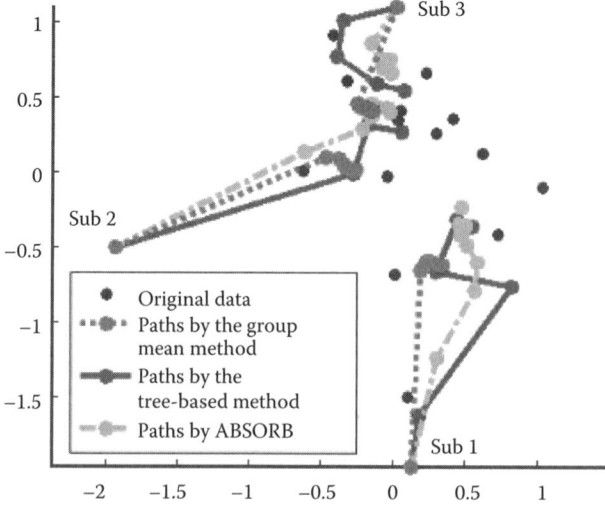

FIGURE 5.7 The registration paths produced by three different methods. The paths generated by ABSORB (with green dashed curves) are much smoother than the tree-based method (with blue solid curves), and the paths given by the group mean method (with red dotted curves) show that there is not much progress after the first iteration of registration. (Adapted from H. Jia et al., *NeuroImage*, 51(3), 1057–1070, 2010.)

data-driven groupwise registration method. On the contrary, a tree in [27,42] is built in the preprocessing step and fixed during the whole registration process.

The information provided by the population center has been demonstrated to be very useful in groupwise registration. But due to the huge gap between the limited number of available subjects and the extremely high dimensions of the data space, it is usually very difficult to estimate the population center robustly, and thus an inaccurate population center might lead the whole registration off the track and degrade the statistical analysis that follows.

5.4 Hidden Common Space-Based Groupwise Registration

For the algorithms illustrated in Section 5.3, groupwise registration is achieved under the guidance by either the selected individual image (such as the root image in the tree-based method) or the group mean image (such as the average of all aligned subjects in [26]). However, both have their limitations. For the former, the difference between the selected individual subject and the real population center cannot be simply ignored even though it might be very close to the real population center. For the latter, since the subjects are far from the good alignment in the initial stage of registration, the tentative mean image by simply averaging all the warped subjects is inevitably fuzzy. Though the mean image guarantees the generation of an unbiased atlas, registration performance might be undermined by the fuzzy mean image due to the lack of structural details for proper correspondence detection.

One common characteristic of the groupwise registration methods described in Section 5.3 is that they all need explicit approximations of the population center. However, explicit estimation of the population center is not a necessity when the goal of groupwise registration is to estimate the deformation fields for warping each subject to a common space. Given a set of images, a unified objective function is developed to help warp all images to a hidden common space in which the variation within the subject images with respect to the deformation fields is minimized. As a result, the estimated deformations for all subjects, which are usually defined in the common space, convey the anatomical diversity across population. The advantage of this kind of groupwise registration algorithm is that it bypasses the estimation of population center by introducing a hidden common space, making the group mean only a by-product of the groupwise registration. In the following, we will summarize several groupwise registration algorithms belonging to this category.

In hidden common space-based groupwise registration, pairwise registration cannot be directly applied since there is no paired relationship between any given image and the specific template. In fact, all images need to be warped to an undetermined destination simultaneously, until they are close enough to each other and converge to a hidden common space. In general, a global objective function is defined to minimize the variation between all to-be-registered images. When the objective function is gradually minimized, the images are progressively pushed to converge to the hidden common space. Therefore, groupwise registration can be regarded as a typical optimization problem, with the optimal solution to the deformations for all images estimated by minimizing the objective function.

The "congealing" method proposed by Miller et al. [28,44] is among the first methods introduced for groupwise registration. In congealing, all images are piled together from top to bottom. Then intensities of the same locations from different images are sampled to form a sequence or a stack, as in the left panel of Figure 5.8. If all input images were identical, the intensity values inside the stack would be the same. The aim of the registration algorithm is then to reduce voxel variation within a stack by minimizing the stack entropy. The local variation measurement, namely stack entropy, is further integrated over the whole image domain to obtain a unified objective function. Given the image set I and the corresponding (tentative) deformations T, the objective function f can be defined as

$$f = \int \mathcal{H}(I(T(x))) \, dx, \tag{5.1}$$

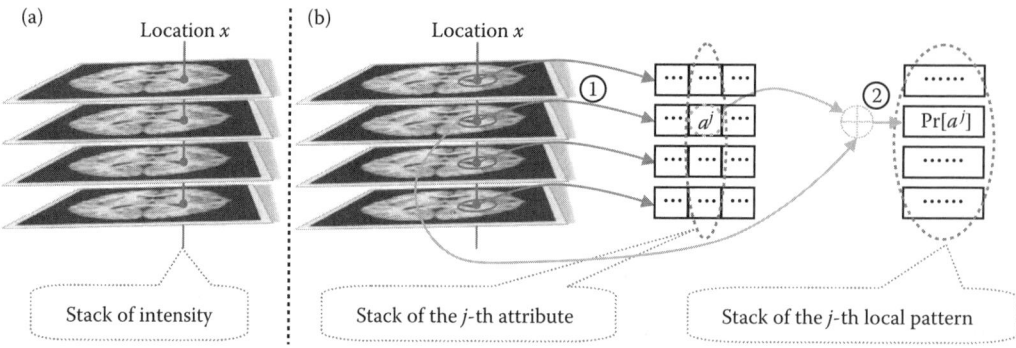

FIGURE 5.8 In (a), a stack of intensities is sampled from the identical locations of different images. (Adapted from Q. Wang et al., *NeuroImage*, 50, 1485–1496, 2010.) In (b), not only the single intensity but also more attributes are sampled to form an attribute vector as a morphological signature of each voxel. Moreover, the neighborhood of each voxel is considered as a local pattern, described by the local probability density function, to construct a robust objective function.

where $\mathcal{H}$ calculates the entropy over the sequence of intensity values sampled from location x of all images. By minimizing f, the optimal estimation of the deformations T can be obtained. Without loss of generality, the notation T will be omitted in the following for convenience, by assuming that the image set I is the tentatively warped results based on the currently estimated deformations T.

An easy way to calculate the entropy of a finite intensity sequence is to adopt the widely used Shannon entropy, although some other measurements, such as the variance in the stack, can also be used. In the case of groupwise registration, the stack sampled at location x consists of the sequence $\{I_1(x), I_2(x), \cdots I_N(x)\}$. However, the number of samples in a stack is very limited, posing great challenge to the accurate estimation of entropy. To alleviate this problem, Parzen window is often used to transfer the discrete sequence into a continuous Gaussian mixture model (GMM). The Gaussians of each GMM, corresponding to individual location x in the image space, center at the sampled pixel values, respectively. Then the cost function can be represented by

$$f = -\int \frac{1}{N}\sum_{i=1}^{N}\log\frac{1}{N}\sum_{j=1}^{N}G_\sigma(I_i(x)-I_j(x))\,\mathrm{d}x, \tag{5.2}$$

where G_σ is the Gaussian kernel with variance σ.

The deformation can be parameterized in various ways, the choice of which is often closely related to the optimization. The linear part of the deformation is usually the rigid or affine transformation, while the nonlinear part can be described by a dense deformation field. The congealing method implemented in [29] was based on affine transformations, and was then further extended nonlinearly in [30] by modeling the deformation with B-Splines [52]. For optimization, the common approach is to determine the gradient of the objective function with respect to the deformation parameters, and then search for the optimal solution along the steepest descent direction.

For example, in Wang et al. [34], where a group of point-sets are to be registered, each point-set is modeled as a continuous probability density function using GMM. The Jensen–Shannon (JS) divergence [53] is then used to measure the variation within the group of probability density functions. An objective function is built and further minimized using any gradient-based optimization for estimation of the deformation for each image.

We further note that intensity alone is insufficient for conveying all information needed by registration. It has been proven that attribute vector, consisting of additional information on the top of intensities, can better represent each voxel in an MR image. In HAMMER [17], for example, GMIs are used to determine a set of driving voxels for steering the registration. In fact, many types of features which have been shown to be effective descriptors can be incorporated as attributes for medical image registration.

Wang et al. [36,37] developed a method which integrates the attribute vector into the groupwise registration cost function. Ideally, different attributes in the attribute vector can contribute independent piece of information which is conducive for registration. In Wang et al.'s work [36,37], both intensity and intensity gradient are used as attributes for guiding groupwise registration. Intensity gradient is more sensitive than intensity alone to the subtle mismatch of anatomical boundaries. In the very beginning of registration, the variation within the population of images is high. Therefore, the contribution from intensity gradient is weighted less than that of intensity. As registration progresses, the mismatch between any two images becomes lesser. Then, to increase the accuracy in registration, the weighting for contribution of intensity gradient is increased, with simultaneous decrease in contribution from intensity. It is worth noting that, although only intensity and intensity gradient are used as attributes in Wang et al. [36,37], the framework is flexible enough to accommodate other features for guiding registration.

To further improve the robustness and accuracy of groupwise registration, local pattern is introduced in Wang et al. [36,37]. In particular, given a center voxel in the specific image, its neighborhood is viewed as a local pattern, as in the right panel of Figure 5.8. GMM is estimated to characterize the local pattern. Suppose a^j is the j-th attribute under consideration, then the local pattern centered at location x in image I_i, denoted as $Pr(a^j|i,x)$, is defined as

$$Pr(a^j|i,x) = \frac{1}{K}\sum_{\Delta x}G_\sigma\left(a^j - a^j_{i,x+\Delta x}\right),$$ (5.3)

where K is the total number of voxels in the neighborhood and Δx is the allowable offset in the neighborhood.

A single stack now actually connects a set of local patterns. These local patterns are from different images, but centering at the same locations. The variation within the stack of local patterns can be measured with the JS divergence:

$$JS(x,j) = \mathcal{H}\left(\sum_{i=1}^{N}\pi_i \cdot Pr(a^j|i,x)\right) - \sum_{i=1}^{N}\pi_i \cdot \mathcal{H}(Pr(a^j|i,x)).$$ (5.4)

By integrating the JS divergence across the image domain and combining together contributions of different attributes, the final cost function can be formulated. Similarly, gradient-based optimization methods can be used to minimize the cost function.

In general, hidden common space-based groupwise registration can be formulated as an optimization problem with the goal of minimizing variations within the image population. The way of constructing the objective function varies with applications, and should be further explored in the future. By avoiding introducing an explicit image in the common space, results yielded by groupwise registration toward the hidden common space can potentially get rid of bias introduced by inappropriate selection of template.

5.5 Applications

Image registration plays a key role in medical image analysis [23,54]. It can be used to concurrently normalize all subjects in a population, and to propagate labels from template to individual subjects. The deformation field generated from registration records the displacement of corresponding voxels between subject and template, which characterizes the global and local morphological differences. In 4D studies

[55,56], the longitudinal changes measured by the registration algorithm can be used to reveal the patterns related to brain development, aging, and neurologic or neuropsychiatric disorders. The use of groupwise registration for morphological measurement has multiple advantages. First, it needs no selection of template, thus avoiding possible bias in data analysis. Second, it is able to generate more representative group mean. Groupwise registration can be easily incorporated into most applications by using it to replace the pairwise registration, for achieving more powerful and unbiased analysis of data. We will present three typical applications of groupwise registration in this section, besides pointing out other possible applications.

5.5.1 Typical Applications

Deformable image registration serves multiple roles in many clinical studies. One of the most popular applications is the evaluation of anatomical variability in human population. By registering each individual subject to a template, a dense deformation field can be obtained, encoding dilation and contraction information of regions of each subject with respect to the template. Therefore, these deformation fields offer ways for pathology detection, identification of gender-specific anatomic patterns, and mapping of dynamic patterns of structural changes in disease-related neuro-developmental and degenerative processes. Taking HAMMER as an example, Figure 5.9 demonstrates several typical clinical

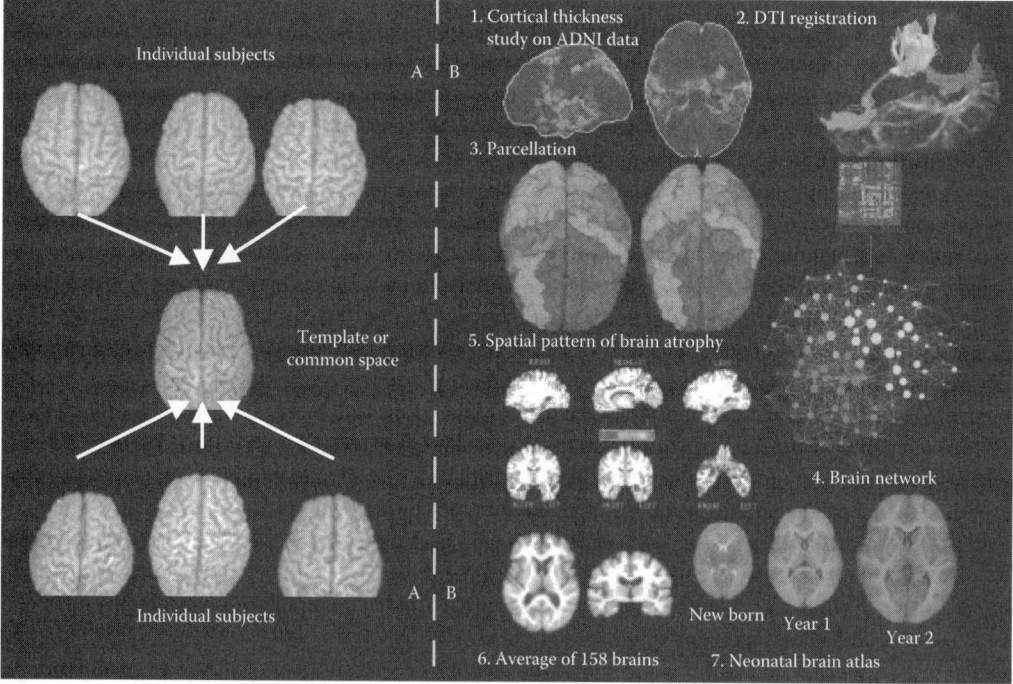

FIGURE 5.9 Illustration of various applications of image registration. Panel (A) shows the procedure of warping individuals subjects (top and bottom rows) to the template (in a pairwise scenario) or common space (in a groupwise scenario). After spatial normalization, numerous clinical applications can be performed, with some typical ones shown in the right panel (B). From (B1) to (B7), we show the illustrative results of (B1) cortical thickness study on ADNI data, (B2) DTI registration, (B3) image parcellation, (B4) brain network discovery on structural images, (B5) spatial pattern of brain atrophy with respect to MCI, (B6) normalization of elderly brains, and (B7) study on infant brain development, respectively.

applications requiring registration of the subject images to the template image (in Figure 5.9 (A)). These applications are further illustrated in Figure 5.9 (B1–B7).

1. After registering all subjects to the template space, subtle changes of cortical thickness [57,58] during pathological or physiological development can be captured, providing a powerful tool for diagnosis and study of a variety of neuro-degenerative and psychiatric disorders [59]. (B1) shows the left and interior views of statistical significance (p-value) of the correlations detected between the thickness and the CDR–SOB scores.

2. Diffusion tensor imaging (DTI) provides unprecedented insight into brain WM structures and is commonly used to delineate subtle abnormalities caused by diseases, including stroke, multiple sclerosis, dyslexia, and schizophrenia. HAMMER has also been extended to DTI image registration [60,61]. (B2) demonstrates the aligned fiber bundles in the genu, splenium, and body of the corpus callosum in green, red, and yellow, respectively.

3. Registration can be used to automatically parcellate and label the brain structures for individual brain images after estimating the deformation field between the subject and the template [22]. (B3) shows 3D renderings of the label map and a representative labeling of an individual's brain after registration to the template. It is worth noting that features extracted from the volumetric measurements of labels can also be used to classify the normal controls and diseased patients.

4. The human brain is considered as a collection of interacting networks with specialized functions to support various cognitive tasks [62]. The connectivity also changes as a consequence of the neuron degeneration, either from natural aging or from diseases such as Alzheimer's disease. After the registration and parcellation on DTI images, the connectivity of two region-of-interests (ROIs) can be identified by the common traversing fibers. This connectivity information is encoded in a connectivity matrix (in the top of (B4)). After properly thresholding the connectivity matrix, a brain network can be obtained, where the spring-embedding visualization is displayed in the bottom of (B4).

5. Computer-based pattern classification of MRI is able to detect patterns of brain structure characterizing subtle anatomical difference between normal and patient subjects after image registration. (B5) shows the representative cross-sections highlighting the brain regions that collectively form a spatial pattern of brain atrophy that is highly indicative of mild cognitive impairment (MCI) [63]. The color coding shows the relative importance of a brain region for classification.

6. HAMMER has been used as the key registration method in one of the most comprehensive longitudinal studies of aging in the world to date (Baltimore Longitudinal Study of Aging—BLSA [21]), in which HAMMER has successfully processed approximately 2100 images. Because of the high accuracy of HAMMER (as the sharp average image of all normalized subjects shown in (B6)), we can now localize longitudinal atrophy and detect abnormal anatomical changes with better spatial specificity and sensitivity.

7. Study of early brain is very challenging because of the insufficient image resolution, low SNR, dynamic myelination of WM, and lack of prior knowledge. (B7) shows the atlases of new born, year 1, and year 2 infants built from the well aligned subjects, which facilitate the infant brain analysis, such as atlas-based tissue segmentation, and brain network construction [42,45,64–66].

5.5.2 Advantages of Groupwise Registration

We demonstrate here the performance gain of groupwise registration over pairwise registration, that is, HAMMER (source code available at http://www.nitrc.org/projects/hammerwml/). Groupwise registration algorithms used in the comparison are the group mean algorithm [26], ABSORB [32,33], and the congealing algorithm [30]. Additionally, we provide the comparison results for the hierarchical groupwise registration algorithm presented in [43], which utilizes the congealing method [30] in the implementation of each level.

We first evaluate these five algorithms on 18 elderly brains from the BLSA dataset [21] by comparing the overlap ratio on WM, GM, and ventricle (VN). Here we use the Jaccard coefficient metric [67] to measure the alignment of two regions with the same tissue. For the two registered regions A and B, the Jaccard coefficient is defined as

$$J(A,B) = \frac{|A \cap B|}{|A \cup B|}, \tag{5.5}$$

where $|\cdot|$ denotes the number of voxels in the underlying region. To evaluate registration accuracy, we employ a majority vote approach by assigning each voxel with a tissue label that is the majority returned by all tissue labels at the same location of all the aligned subjects. Then the Jaccard coefficient between each of the registered label images and the voted label will be calculated. It is worth noting that this is a very strict definition for measurement of ROI overlap, and it emphasizes the importance of groupwise registration in measuring the group performance. In the following experiments, we use the average score of Jaccard coefficients as the overlap ratio for each tissue label.

Figure 5.10 shows a group of 18 elderly brain images. Each image size is of $256 \times 256 \times 124$ and resolution $0.9375 \times 0.9375 \times 1.5$ mm^3. It can be observed that the anatomical structures vary a lot across different subjects, especially for the ventricle and the cortex. To better evaluate the performance of pairwise registration (by HAMMER), we randomly select five individual subjects (shown by red boxes in Figure 5.10) as templates in reporting both the mean and the standard deviation of the overlap ratios over three different tissues (the first row of Table 5.1).

The overlap ratios on WM, GM, and VN, as well as the overall overlap ratio on the whole brain by different groupwise methods are displayed from the second to fifth row in Table 5.1. It can be observed that

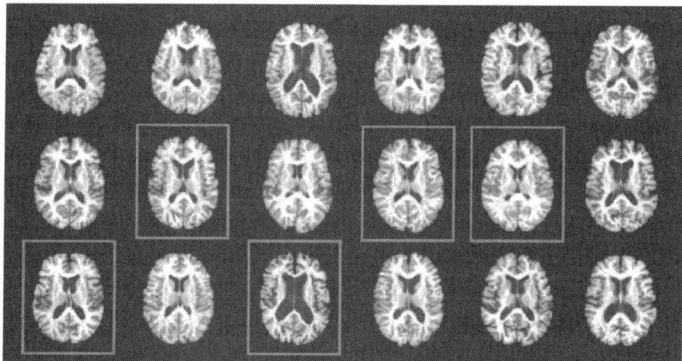

FIGURE 5.10 Eighteen elderly brain images used in evaluation of three registration methods. The five subjects with red rectangles are selected as template images in the pairwise registration algorithm for a fair performance evaluation of the pairwise registration algorithms.

TABLE 5.1 Overall Overlap Ratios of WM, GM, and VN by Five Different Registration Algorithms

	White Matter (%)	Gray Matter (%)	Ventricle (%)	Overall (%)
Pairwise HAMMER	63.86 (±3.87)	57.25 (±2.18)	76.51 (±3.70)	65.64 (±3.15)
Group mean method	73.88	60.51	78.14	70.84
ABSORB	79.01	66.82	82.33	76.05
Congealing method	59.68	51.09	70.61	59.43
Hierarchical congealing	65.64	58.36	78.60	67.54

the second class (i.e., the population center-guided groupwise registration) can achieve much higher overlap ratio than the pairwise algorithm (HAMMER). For example, the overlap ratios of the ABSORB method can reach 79.01% in WM, 66.82% in GM, and 82.33% in VN, which achieves more than 10% improvement in the overall overlap ratio. The congealing method (a hidden common space-based groupwise registration method), however, is not as good as the pairwise counterpart (HAMMER) in terms of overlap ratios at the current stage. One possible reason for this is that much more parameters, compared with those of the pairwise registration method, are involved into the optimization of the objective function (e.g., the stack entropy in the congealing method) in this class of registration methods. In pairwise registration, only the deformation of a single image needs to be estimated, while in groupwise registration the deformations have to be simultaneously refined for all images. Thus, the optimization involved in groupwise registration is more vulnerable to local minima with the same gradient-based optimization method. However, by integrating the congealing method into a hierarchical groupwise registration framework [35,43] which only performs congealing on a set of subjects with similar appearances, the registration performance in terms of the overlap ratio can be improved drastically, as shown in the last row of Table 5.1.

5.5.3 Multiple Modes in Groupwise Registration

The intersubject variation can be so large that a single common space can barely handle the groupwise registration [68]. As discussed previously, an individual subject can be connected to the final population center by a path consisting of segments linking neighboring subjects. In ABSORB, nearby images are automatically bundled together in the self-organized registration progress. A single representative image is selected from each bundle to participate into the further registration in the higher level. In general, images in a population can be better represented by multiple modes. By taking advantage of the multiple mode phenomena, groupwise registration could become more accurate and efficient.

In Wang et al. [35,43], all subjects are hierarchically clustered according to the specific pairwise similarity or distance definition. The top–down hierarchical clustering yields a pyramid, where each leaf node corresponds to an image in the population. In each class, subjects are close to each other. Then registration is always intraclass, as only the images in the identical class are warped to the center of the class in groupwise registration manner. Similar to ABSORB, only a single subject will be produced to represent the whole class when intraclass registration has finished, and contribute to registration in the higher level. From the perspective of the pyramid, the task of intraclass registration happens from the bottom of the pyramid, then climbs up, and finally ends at the top. Meanwhile, all images in the population are warped to the common space, following the path from its corresponding leaf node to the root of the pyramid. In each intraclass registration, subjects involved are much less diverse than the whole population. Therefore, to perform groupwise registration on a class of images is much easier and more accurate than to perform groupwise registration of all images directly. Moreover, the whole computation load is dispatched into several classes where only a small number of subjects are handled, leading to a faster registration algorithm.

An example with only three levels is shown in Figure 5.11, where groupwise registration has been performed on 150 brain MR images. For clarity, only a few subjects are displayed here. In the first level, each class contains a very limited number of subjects, which are quite close to each other. Then intraclass registration yields the representative image for the respective class. And in the second level, intraclass registrations perform again, resulting in fewer modes of the population. The whole process ends in the third level, where a single representative for the whole population is produced. For each image at the leaf node, it can be warped to the common space, following its individual path from the leaf node to the root node of the pyramid.

Groupwise registration can be employed to explore the existence of multiple modes in an image population. Sabuncu et al. [31] incorporated the groupwise registration into a generalized EM framework. Each subject is assigned a label. The assignments are refined, as images of the same label are warped together in a groupwise registration manner. And after the EM process converges, the intrinsic multiple

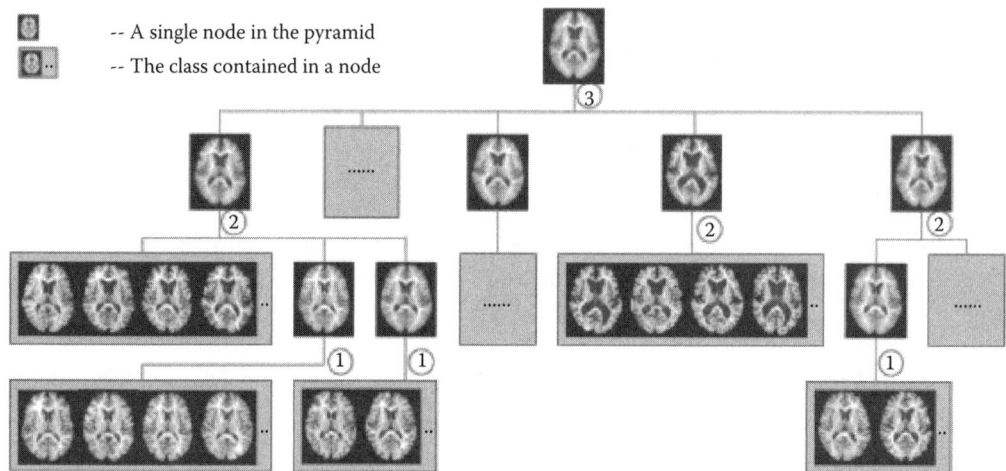

-- A single node in the pyramid

-- The class contained in a node

FIGURE 5.11   An image population of 150 brain MR images is hierarchically clustered into a pyramid, based on the similarity definition between any two images. Groupwise registration is performed in each class, producing the representative image for the class (label φ). The representative images participate into intraclass registrations in the higher level (label κ). Finally, a single representative is estimated (label λ), as the whole registration process reaches the top of the pyramid. Each input image then can be warped to the common space by following its respective deformation path. (Adapted from Q. Wang et al., *Human Brain Mapping*, 31(8), 1128–1140, 2010.)

modes of the image population are naturally manifested. For example, they can discriminate the subjects from different age groups.

5.5.4 Atlas Building for Infants

Atlas, which refers to a map or spatial record of what we know about a region, is widely used in many disciplines and applications. Brain atlases usually refer to the images incorporated with prior knowledge and take the forms of, for example, an averaged intensity model of the population, as well as the tissue probability maps of WM, GM, and CSF. In many applications, researchers use these atlases as registration templates in spatial normalization, and also as prior knowledge for guiding tissue segmentation. Atlas building is more important and challenging in infant image analysis than in adult because of the poor spatial resolution, low-tissue contrast, and high within-tissue intensity variability of the MR images [55,56,66,73]. An atlas with average-shape can normalize an infant population into the same space, and the prior probability maps can guide the tissue segmentation of infant population, which can be eventually used to disclose the brain development in the infant stage.

To build the infant atlas, we use a longitudinal dataset, in which MR scans were acquired longitudinally in neonates, 1 year old, and 2 years old [45]. We then employ the state-of-the-art longitudinal segmentation and groupwise registration methods to build infant atlases.

This dataset was collected as one of our longitudinal studies, involving 56 infants (27 males and 29 females). Each subject has a set of MR brain images scanned at 3 time points, as neonates (0.9 ± 0.3 months), 1 year old (13.2 ± 0.7 months), and 2 years old (24.9 ± 1.9 months). These healthy subjects were recruited from University of North Carolina at Chapel Hill (UNC–CH) and are free of congenital anomalies, metabolic disease, and focal lesions. Informed consent was obtained from the parents and the experimental protocols were approved by the institutional review board. All subjects were unsedated during MR imaging.

For each subject, T1 and T2 MR brain images were collected using a 3T Siemens scanner. For T1 images, 160 sagittal slices were obtained with parameters: TR = 1900 ms, TE = 4.38 ms, Flip Angle = 7, and resolution = $1 \times 1 \times 1$ mm^3. For T2 images, 70 transverse slices were acquired with parameters: TR = 7380 ms, TE = 119 ms, Flip Angle = 150, and resolution = $1.25 \times 1.25 \times 1.95$ mm^3.

All images are preprocessed utilizing a standard pipeline. To achieve better tissue contrast, T2 is selected for neonate, and T1 is selected for 1 year old and 2 years old. T2 images are resampled into $1 \times 1 \times 1$ mm^3. Nonbrain tissues (such as skull and dura) are stripped with a dedicated learning based algorithm [69], followed by manual editing in ITK–SNAP software [70] to ensure accurate removal. Bias correction is performed in all images with N3 method [71] to reduce the impact of intensity inhomogeneity and thus improve the performance of the subsequent segmentation and registration.

We employ the strategy proposed in [45] to first segment the last time-point image, and then take advantage of the longitudinal follow-up time-point to build a subject-specific tissue probabilistic atlas including WM, GM, and CSF, to guide the earlier time-point segmentation, which has much lower tissue contrast. In particular, the T1 image of 2 years old subjects has shown the early adult pattern, and tissue structures can be well segmented with fuzzy segmentation technique such as adaptive K-means algorithm [72]. Then the tissue probability maps of 2 years old subjects are warped into neonate and 1 year old subjects separately and serve as prior to guide their tissue segmentations. The segmentation results are used to refine the registration to better warp the probability maps of 2 years old subjects to the current time-point. With better prior, the performance of the segmentation can be improved. This joint registration-segmentation iterates until convergence. This technique can substantially improve the tissue segmentation accuracy of infant brain images, especially for neonates. After this procedure, the tissue probability maps for all images are obtained.

Next, we build the average-shape atlas for each age group, including the intensity model and the probability maps for WM, GM, and CSF. The conventional atlas building algorithm selects a subject image from or out of this population to be the template. The atlas constructed is anatomically similar with the selected template and is hence biased. Unbiased registration is more preferable here for determining an atlas which is able to better represent the anatomy of the whole population. We employ the groupwise registration method proposed in [41] for unbiased groupwise atlas building. This groupwise registration algorithm utilizes the attribute vector as the morphological signature to robustly identify the anatomical correspondences. Therefore, more accurate registration results can be achieved compared to the intensity-based algorithms.

We show the constructed average-shape atlases for 0, 1, and 2 years in Figure 5.12. The anatomical proportion of 0–1–2 years is preserved and can be observed from the figure. With these constructed

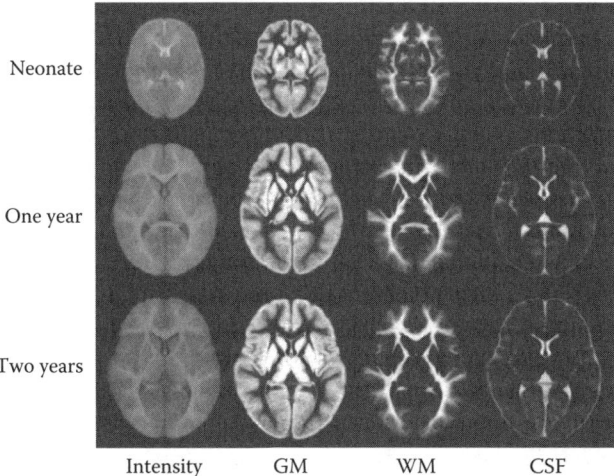

FIGURE 5.12 Illustration of the average-shape atlases of 0–1–2 years. The intensity model and tissue probability maps of WM, GM, and CSF are shown, respectively.

atlases, we now have the tissue probability for the specific age range of infants. We can use these atlases for guiding the segmentation of neonates with missing longitudinal data in the 1 year old or 2 years old, as we did in [65]. The atlases are freely available to the research community at http://bric.unc.edu/idea-group/free-softwares/.

5.6 Summary

In past decades, image registration has been proven to be important for effective medical image analysis. By normalizing an image population to the same space by image registration, qualitative and quantitative analysis on brain anatomies and morphologies can be performed. Plenty of applications have been explored, ranging from brain development study to early disease diagnosis. To meet the booming requirement for the unbiased group analysis, a relatively new family of registration methods, called as groupwise registration has come to the stage. As demonstrated in various applications, groupwise registration algorithms generally demonstrate superior performance over their pairwise counterparts, and thus becomes a hot topic in the field of medical image analysis.

References

1. E. M. Haacke, R. F. Brown, M. Thompson, and R. Venkatesan, *Magnetic Resonance Imaging: Physical Principles and Sequence Design*. New York: J. Wiley & Sons, 1999.
2. J. B. A. Maintz and M. A. Viergever, A survey of medical image registration. *Medical Image Analysis*, 2, 1–36, 1998.
3. B. Zitová and J. Flusser, Image registration methods: A survey. *Image and Vision Computing*, 21, 977–1000, 2003.
4. W. R. Crum, T. Hartkens, and D. L. G. Hill, Non-rigid image registration: Theory and practice. *British Journal of Radiology*, 77, S140–S153, 2004.
5. R. P. Woods, S. T. Grafton, C. J. Holmes, S. R. Cherry, and J. C. Mazziotta, Automated image registration: I. General methods and intrasubject, intramodality validation. *Journal of Computer Assisted Tomography*, 22, 139–152, 1998.
6. R. P. Woods, S. T. Grafton, J. D. G. Watson, N. L. Sicotte, and J. C. Mazziotta, Automated image registration: II. Intersubject validation of linear and nonlinear models. *Journal of Computer Assisted Tomography*, 22, 153–165, 1998.
7. S. Joshi and M. I. Miller, Landmark matching via large deforamtion diffeomorphisms. *IEEE Transactions on Medical Imaging*, 9, 1357–1370, 2000.
8. Z. Xue, D. Shen, and C. Davatzikos, Determining correspondence in 3D MR brain images using attribute vectors as morphological signatures of voxels. *Medical Imaging, IEEE Transactions on*, 23, 1276–1291, 2004.
9. P. J. Besl and H. D. McKay, A method for registration of 3-D shapes. *Pattern Analysis and Machine Intelligence, IEEE Transactions on*, 14, 239–256, 1992.
10. T. Vercauteren, X. Pennec, A. Perchant, and N. Ayache, Diffeomorphic demons: Efficient non-parametric image registration. *NeuroImage*, 45, S61–S72, 2009.
11. D. Rueckert, L. I. Sonoda, C. Hayes, D. L. G. Hill, M. O. Leach, and D. J. Hawkes, Nonrigid registration using free-form deformations: Application to breast MR images. *Medical Imaging, IEEE Transactions on*, 18, 712–721, 1999.
12. J. P. Thirion, Image matching as a diffusion process: An analogy with Maxwell's demons. *Medical Image Analysis*, 2, 243–260, 1998.
13. M. I. Miller, Computational anatomy: Shape, growth, and atrophy comparison via diffeomorphisms. *NeuroImage*, 23, S19–S33, 2004.
14. J. Ashburner, A fast diffeomorphic image registration algorithm. *NeuroImage*, 38, 95–113, 2007.

15. G. E. Christensen and H. J. Johnson, Consistent image registration. *Medical Imaging, IEEE Transactions on*, 20, 568–582, 2001.

16. D. Shen, Image registration by local histogram matching. *Pattern Recognition*, 40, 1161–1172, 2007.

17. D. Shen and C. Davatzikos, HAMMER: Hierarchical attribute matching mechanism for elastic registration. *Medical Imaging, IEEE Transactions on*, 21, 1421–1439, 2002.

18. D. Shen and C. Davatzikos, Very high-resolution morphometry using mass-preserving deformations and HAMMER elastic registration. *NeuroImage*, 18, 28–41, 2003.

19. G. Wu, P.-T. Yap, M. Kim, and D. Shen, TPS-HAMMER: Improving HAMMER registration algorithm by soft correspondence matching and thin-plate splines based deformation interpolation. *NeuroImage*, 49, 2225–2233, 2010.

20. C. H. Lo and H. S. Don, 3-D moment forms: Their construction and application to object identification and positioning. *IEEE Transactions on Pattern Analysis and Machine Intelligence*, 11, 1053–1064, 1989.

21. S. M. Resnick, A. F. Goldszal, C. Davatzikos, S. Golski, M. A. Kraut, E. J. Metter, R. N. Bryan, and A. B. Zonderman, One-year age changes in MRI brain volumes in older adults. *Cerebral Cortex*, 10, 464–472, 2000.

22. Z. Lao, D. Shen, Z. Xue, B. Karacali, S. M. Resnick, and C. Davatzikos, Morphological classification of brains via high-dimensional shape transformations and machine learning methods. *NeuroImage*, 21, 46–57, 2004.

23. A. W. Toga and P. M. Thompson, The role of image registration in brain mapping. *Image and Vision Computing*, 19, 3–24, 2001.

24. H. Park, P. H. Bland, A. O. Hero, and C. R. Meyer, Least biased target selection in probabilistic atlas construction, in *Medical Image Computing and Computer-Assisted Intervention—MICCAI 2005*, Palm Springs, California, pp. 419–426, 2005.

25. D. Seghers, E. D'Agostino, F. Maes, D. Vandermeulen, and P. Suetens, Construction of a brain template from MR images using state-of-the-art registration and segmentation techniques, in *Medical Image Computing and Computer-Assisted Intervention—MICCAI 2004*, Saint-Malo, France, pp. 696–703, 2004.

26. S. Joshi, B. Davis, M. Jomier, and G. Gerig, Unbiased diffeomorphic atlas construction for computational anatomy. *NeuroImage*, 23, S151–S160, 2004.

27. J. Hamm, C. Davatzikos, and R. Verma, *Efficient Large Deformation Registration Via Geodesics on a Learned Manifold of Images—MICCAI 2009*, London, UK, 2009.

28. E. G. Learned-Miller, Data driven image models through continuous joint alignment. *Pattern Analysis and Machine Intelligence, IEEE Transactions on*, 28, 236–250, 2006.

29. L. Zöllei, E. Learned-Miller, E. Grimson, and W. Wells, Efficient population registration of 3D data, in *Computer Vision for Biomedical Image Applications (ICCV)*, Beijing, China, pp. 291–301, 2005.

30. S. K. Balci, P. Golland, M. Shenton, and W. M. Wells, Free-form B-spline deformation model for groupwise registration, in *Medical Image Computing and Computer-Assisted Intervention—MICCAI 2007*, Brisbane, Australia, pp. 23–30, 2007.

31. M. R. Sabuncu, S. K. Balci, M. E. Shenton, and P. Golland, Image-driven population analysis through mixture modeling. *Medical Imaging, IEEE Transactions on*, 28, 1473–1487, 2009.

32. H. Jia, G. Wu, Q. Wang, and D. Shen, ABSORB: Atlas building by self-organized registration and bundling, in *Proceedings of IEEE Conference on Computer Vision and Pattern Recognition*, San Francisco, CA, 2010.

33. H. Jia, G. Wu, Q. Wang, and D. Shen, ABSORB: Atlas building by self-organized registration and bundling, *NeuroImage*, 51(3), 1057–1070, 2010.

34. F. Wang, B. C. Vemuri, A. Rangarajan, and S. J. Eisenschenk, Simultaneous nonrigid registration of multiple point sets and atlas construction. *Pattern Analysis and Machine Intelligence, IEEE Transactions on*, 30, 2011–2022, 2008.

35. Q. Wang, L. Chen, and D. Shen, Group-wise registration of large image dataset by hierarchical clustering and alignment, in *Medical Imaging 2009*. Orlando, Florida, vol. 7259, SPIE, 2009.

36. Q. Wang, P.-T. Yap, G. Wu, and D. Shen, Attribute vector guided groupwise registration, in *Medical Image Computing and Computer-Assisted Intervention—MICCAI 2009*, London, UK, 2009.

37. Q. Wang, G. Wu, P.-T. Yap, and D. Shen, Attribute vector guided groupwise registration. *NeuroImage*, 50, 1485–1496, 2010.

38. S. Marsland, C. J. Twining, and C. J. Taylor, A minimum description length objective function for groupwise non-rigid image registration. *Image and Vision Computing*, 26, 333–346, 2008.

39. S. Marsland and C. J. Twining, Constructing diffeomorphic representations for the groupwise analysis of nonrigid registrations of medical images. *Medical Imaging, IEEE Transactions on*, 23, 1006–1020, 2004.

40. P. T. Fletcher, S. Venkatasubramanian, and S. Joshi, The geometric median on Riemannian manifolds with application to robust atlas estimation. *NeuroImage*, 45, S143–S152, 2009.

41. G. Wu, P.-T. Yap, Q. Wang, and D. Shen, *Groupwise registration from exemplar to group mean: Extending HAMMER to groupwise registration*, in International Symposium of Biomedical Imaging (ISBI), Rotterdam, The Netherlands, 2010.

42. B. C. Munsell, A. Temlyakov, and S. Wang, Fast multiple shape correspondence by pre-organizing shape instances, in *IEEE Conference on CVPR*, Miami, Florida, pp. 840–847, 2009.

43. Q. Wang, L. Chen, P. T. Yap, G. Wu, and D. Shen, Groupwise registration based on hierarchical image clustering and atlas synthesis. *Human Brain Mapping*, 31(8), 1128–1140, 2010.

44. E. G. Miller, N. E. Matsakis, and P. A. Viola, Learning from one example through shared densities on transforms, in *Proceedings of the IEEE Conference on Computer Vision and Pattern Recognition, 2000*. Cambridge, Massachusetts, pp. 464–471, 2000.

45. F. Shi, Y. Fan, S. Tang, J. H. Gilmore, W. Lin, and D. Shen, Neonatal brain image segmentation in longitudinal MRI studies. *NeuroImage*, 49, 391–400, 2010.

46. T. Cox and M. A. A. Cox, *Multidimensional Scaling*, second ed. London: Chapman & Hall, 2000.

47. S. Baloch and C. Davatzikos, Morphological appearance manifolds in computational anatomy: Groupwise registration and morphological analysis. *NeuroImage*, 45, S73–S85, 2009.

48. S. Baloch, R. Verma, and C. Davatzikos, An anatomical equivalence class based joint transformation-residual descriptor for morphological analysis, in *Information Processing in Medical Imaging*, The Netherlands, pp. 594–606, 2007.

49. S. Tang, Y. Fan, and D. Shen, RABBIT: Rapid alignment of brains by building intermediate templates. *NeuroImage*, 47, 1277–1287, 2009.

50. M.-J. Kim, M.-H. Kim, and D. Shen, Learning-based deformation estimation for fast non-rigid registration, in *2008 IEEE Conference on Computer Vision and Pattern Recognition Workshops*, Anchorage, Alaska, pp. 1–6, 2008.

51. J. B. Kruskal, On the shortest spanning subtree of a graph and the traveling salesman problem, *Proceedings of the American Mathematical Society*, 7, 48–50, 1956.

52. K. K. Bhatia, J. V. Hajnal, B. K. Puri, A. D. Edwards, and D.Rueckert, Consistent groupwise non-rigid registration for atlas construction, in *IEEE Int. Symp. Biomed. Imag.: Macro Nano, 2004*. vol. 1, pp. 908–911, 2004.

53. J. Lin, Divergence measures based on the shannon entropy. *Information Theory, IEEE Transactions on*, 37, 145–151, 1991.

54. R. Wolz, P. Aljabar, J. V. Hajnal, A. Hammers, and D. Rueckert, LEAP: Learning embeddings for atlas propagation. *NeuroImage*, 49, 1316–1325, 2010.

55. R. C. Knickmeyer, S. Gouttard, C. Kang, D. Evans, K. Wilber, J. K. Smith, R. M. Hamer, W. Lin, G. Gerig, and J. H. Gilmore, A structural MRI study of human brain development from birth to 2 years. *Journal of Neuroscience*, 28, 12176–12182, 2008.

56. W. Gao, H. Zhu, K. S. Giovanello, J. K. Smith, D. Shen, J. H. Gilmore, and W. Lin, Evidence on the emergence of the brain's default network from 2-week-old to 2-year-old healthy pediatric subjects,

Proceedings of the National Academy of Sciences of the United States of America, 106, 6790–6795, 2009.

57. C. Hutton, E. De Vita, J. Ashburner, R. Deichmann, and R. Turner, Voxel-based cortical thickness measurements in MRI. *NeuroImage*, 40, 1701–1710, 2008.

58. S. R. Das, B. B. Avants, M. Grossman, and J. C. Gee, Registration based cortical thickness measurement. *NeuroImage*, 45867–879, 2009.

59. ADNI, http://www.loni.ucla.edu/ADNI/, 2004.

60. P.-T. Yap, G. Wu, H. Zhu, W. Lin, and D. Shen, Fast tensor image morphing for elastic registration, in *Medical Image Computing and Computer-Assisted Intervention—MICCAI 2009*, London, UK, 2009, pp. 721–729.

61. P.-T. Yap, G. Wu, H. Zhu, W. Lin, and D. Shen, TIMER: Tensor image morphing for elastic registration. *NeuroImage*, 47, 549–563, 2009.

62. P. Hagmann, L. Cammoun, X. Gigandet, R. Meuli, C. J. Honey, V. J. Wedeen, and O. Sporns, Mapping the structural core of human cerebral cortex. *PLoS Biol*, 6, 1479–1493, 2008.

63. C. Davatzikos, Y. Fan, X. Wu, D. Shen, and S. M. Resnick, Detection of prodromal Alzheimer's disease via pattern classification of MRI. *Neurobiology of Aging*, 29, 514–523, 2008.

64. F. Shi, D. Shen, P.-T. Yap, Y. Fan, J. Cheng, H. An, L. L. Wald, G. Gerig, J. H. Gilmore, and W. lin, CENTS: Cortical enhanced neonatal tissue segmentation. *Human Brain Mapping*, 32(3), 382–396, 2011.

65. F. Shi, P.-T. Yap, J. H. Gilmore, W. Lin, and D. Shen, Construction of multi-region-multi-reference atlases for neonatal brain MRI segmentation. *NeuroImage*, 51(3), 1057–1070, 2010.

66. M. Altaye, S. K. Holland, M. Wilke, and C. Gaser, Infant brain probability templates for MRI segmentation and normalization. *NeuroImage*, 43, 721–30, 2008.

67. P. Jaccard, The distribution of the flora in the alpine zone. *New Phytologist*, 11, 37–50, 1912.

68. D. J. Blezek and J. V. Miller, Atlas stratification. *Medical Image Analysis*, 11, 443–457, 2007.

69. F. Shi, L. Wang, Y. Dai, J. H. Gilmore, W. Lin, and D. Shen, LABEL: Pediatric brain extraction using learning-based meta-algorithm, *Neuroimage*, in press, 2012. Available at: http://www.sciencedirect.com/science/article/pii/S1053811912005307?v=s5

70. P. A. Yushkevich, J. Piven, H. C. Hazlett, R. G. Smith, S. Ho, J. C. Gee, and G. Gerig, User-guided 3D active contour segmentation of anatomical structures: Significantly improved efficiency and reliability. *NeuroImage*, 31, 1116–1128, 2006.

71. J. G. Sled, A. P. Zijdenbos, and A. C. Evans, A nonparametric method for automatic correction of intensity nonuniformity in MRI data. *IEEE Trans Med Imaging*, 17, 87–97, 1998.

72. D. L. Pham and J. L. Prince, An adaptive fuzzy C-means algorithm for image segmentation in the presence of intensity inhomogeneities. *Pattern Recognition Letters*, 20, 57–68, 1999.

73. F. Shi, P.-T. Yap, G. Wu, H. Jia, J. H. Gilmore, W. Lin, and D. Shen, Infant brain atlases from neonates to 1- and 2-year-olds, *PLoS ONE*, 6, e18746, 2011.

6

Functional Optical Brain Imaging

Meltem Izzetoglu
Drexel University

6.1 Introduction

Functional imaging is typically conducted in an effort to understand the activity in a given brain region in terms of its relationship to a particular behavioral state, or its interactions with inputs from another region's activity. The advances in noninvasive functional brain monitoring technologies provide opportunities to accurately examine the living brains of large groups of subjects over long periods of time, with little impact on their well-being. Neurophysiological and neuroimaging technologies have contributed much to our understanding of normative brain function, as well as to our understanding of the neural underpinnings of various neurological and psychiatric disorders. Commonly employed techniques such as electroencephalography (EEG), event-related brain potentials (ERPs), magnetoencephalography (MEG), positron emission tomography (PET), single-positron emission computed tomography (SPECT), and functional magnetic resonance imaging (fMRI), have dramatically increased our understanding of a broad range of brain disorders. Nevertheless, there is still much unknown about these syndromes. This is due, in large part, to the inherent complexity of the neurobiological substrates of these disorders and of the mind itself. In addition, each of the research methods used to study brain function and its disorders have methodological strengths as well as their own inherent limitations. These limitations place constraints on our ability to fully explicate the neural basis of neurological and psychiatric disorders both inside and outside of the laboratory setting, and to use the information gleaned from laboratory studies for clinical applications in real-world environments. New techniques that allow data to be gathered under more diverse circumstances than is possible with extant neuroimaging systems should facilitate a more thorough understanding of brain function and its pathologies.

Functional near-infrared spectroscopy (fNIR) has been introduced as a new neuroimaging modality with which to conduct functional brain imaging studies [1–24]. fNIR technology uses specific wavelengths of light, irradiated through the scalp, to enable the noninvasive measurement of changes in the relative ratios of deoxygenated hemoglobin (deoxy-Hb) and oxygenated hemoglobin (oxy-Hb) during brain activity. This technology allows the design of portable, safe, affordable, noninvasive, and minimally intrusive monitoring systems. These qualities make fNIR suitable for the study of hemodynamic changes due to cognitive and emotional brain activity under many working and educational conditions, as well as in the field. Using this technique, several types of brain activity have been assessed, including motor activity, visual activation, auditory stimulation, and the performance of cognitive tasks (e.g., [9]). To date, the outcomes of studies utilizing fNIR compare favorably with previous fMRI and complement EEG findings [21–23].

The purpose of the present chapter is to describe an emerging neuroimaging technology, fNIR, which has several attributes that make it possible to conduct neuroimaging studies of the cortex in clinical offices and under more realistic, ecologically valid parameters. In this chapter, we will first describe general working principles of fNIR and different fNIR instrumentations based on these working principles. Then, we will review algorithms developed for fNIR data processing for artifact removal and used in the extraction of hemodynamic signals from the fNIR intensity measurements. We will discuss the results of various fNIR applications in laboratory settings and in field conditions. Finally, the merits of optical imaging in brain research will be summarized.

6.2 Working Principles

6.2.1 Physiological Principles: How Can Brain Activity Be Measured through Hemodynamic Changes?

Neural activity has a direct relation with hemodynamic changes in the brain [25]. Research on brain-energy metabolism has elucidated the close link between hemodynamic and neural activity [26,27]. Understanding the brain energy metabolism and associated neural activity is of importance for realizing principles of fNIR in assessing brain activity. The brain has small energy reserves and a great majority of the energy used by brain cells is for processes that sustain physiological functioning [28]. Ames III reviewed the studies on brain energy metabolism as related to function and reported that the oxygen (O_2) consumption of the rabbit vagus nerve increased 3.4-fold when it was stimulated at 10 Hz and O_2 consumption in rabbit sympathetic ganglia increased 40% with stimulation at 15 Hz. Furthermore, glucose utilization by various brain regions increased several fold in response to physiological stimulation or in response to pharmacological agents that affect physiological activity [28]. These studies provide clear evidence that large changes occur in brain energy metabolism in response to changes in activity. The levels of compounds involved in energy metabolism and energy metabolites can be outlined as

- Neuronal activity is fueled by glucose metabolism, so increases in neural activity result in increased glucose and oxygen consumption from the local capillary bed. Brain cells consume energy when activated and oxygen is required to metabolize the glucose. The oxygen concentration in the capillaries can support the normal oxygen consumption (about 3.5 μmol g^{-1} min^{-1}) for 2 s. [27]. For that reason, a reduction in local glucose and oxygen stimulates the brain to increase local arteriolar vasodilation, which increases local cerebral blood flow (CBF) and cerebral blood volume (CBV), a mechanism known as neurovascular coupling.
- Over a period of several seconds, the increased CBF carries both glucose and oxygen to the neural tissue in the area. Oxygen is transported via oxy-Hb in the blood. The oxygen exchange occurs in the capillary beds. As oxy-Hb gives up oxygen, it is transformed into deoxy-Hb.

- The increased oxygen transported to the area via increased CBF typically exceeds the local neuronal rate of oxygen utilization, the cerebral metabolic rate of oxygen (CMRO2), resulting in an overabundance of cerebral blood oxygenation in active areas [29]. Therefore, local blood is more oxygenated and hence less deoxy-Hb is present [30]. (Although the initial increase in neural activity is thought to result in a focal increase in deoxygenated hemoglobin in the capillary bed as oxygen is withdrawn from the hemoglobin for use in the metabolization of glucose, this feature of the vascular response has been much more difficult to measure, and more controversial, than hyperoxygenation. Please see [31,32], for a more detailed discussion of this topic.)

These changes in the hemodynamic signals occur within a few seconds after the onset of the stimulation and may take 10–20 s to evolve [33,34]. Based on the brain energy metabolism, methods and imaging modalities, such as fNIR and fMRI [35,36] for measurements of slowly changing hemodynamic signals, deoxy-Hb and/or oxy-Hb are implemented to provide correlates of brain activity through oxygen consumption by neurons.

6.2.2 Physical Principles: How Can Hemodynamic Activity Be Measured by Optics?

It is well-known that the functional state of tissue can influence its optical properties, for instance, cyanosis in hypoxia; pallor in anemia. The human brain undergoes a number of physiological changes as it responds to environmental stimuli; these changes in blood levels and electrochemical activity also affect its optical properties. Functional optical imaging capitalizes on the changing optical properties of these tissues by using light in the near-infrared range (700–900 nm) to measure physiological changes. Because oxy-Hb and deoxy-Hb have characteristic optical properties in the visible and near-infrared light range between 700 and 900 nm, the change in concentration of these molecules during neurovascular coupling can be measured using optical methods [9,37]. Most biological tissues are relatively transparent to light in the near-infrared range, largely because major components of most tissues, such as water absorb very little energy at these wavelengths (see Figure 6.1). As such, this spectral band is often referred to as the "optical window" for the noninvasive assessment of brain activation. However,

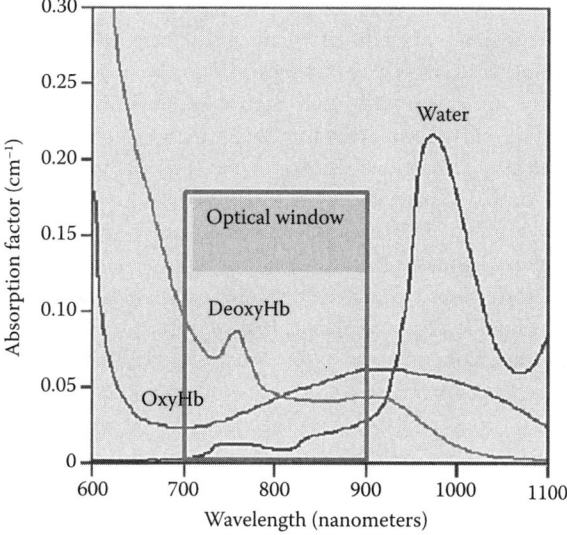

FIGURE 6.1   Absorption spectrum in near-infrared (IR) window.

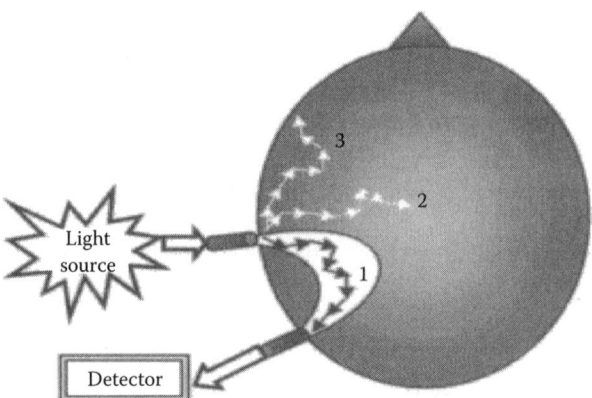

FIGURE 6.2 Photon path inside the human head. Photon 1 undergoes a number of scattering events and leaves the head at the location that the detector is placed and hence will be detected by the system. Photon 2 is absorbed by chromophores after a number of scattering events and cannot continue to travel within the tissue and hence will not be detected by the system. Photon 3 gets scattered in a different direction and leaves the head at a location where no detector is placed and hence will not be detected by the system. Changes in scattering and absorption within the banana-like shaped sampling volume will alter the amount of photons reaching the detector and hence can be monitored and quantified by the system. (From Obrig H et al. 2000. *Int. J. Psychophysiol.*, 35:125–142.)

the chromophores oxy-Hb and deoxy-Hb do absorb a fair amount of energy in this range. Fortunately, in the optical window, the absorption spectra of oxy-Hb and deoxy-Hb remain significantly different than each other as shown in Figure 6.1 allowing spectroscopic separation of these compounds to be possible using only a few sample wavelengths.

Typically, an fNIR apparatus is comprised of a light source that is coupled to the participant's head via either light-emitting diodes (LEDs) or though fiber-optical bundles (the optode), and a light detector that receives the light after it has interacted with the tissue. Photons that enter tissue undergo two different types of interaction, namely absorption and scattering [4,5,19]. When photons get absorbed by the tissue they lose their energy to the medium and hence cannot continue to travel within the tissue. After entering the tissue, photons get diffused and experience multiple scattering events. Hence, a photodetector placed 2–7 cm away from the light source can collect a relatively predictable quantity of photons that are not absorbed and traveled within the tissue along the "banana-shaped path" between the source and detector due to multiple scattering [9,38] as shown in Figure 6.2. When the distance between the source and photodetector is set at 4 cm, the fNIR signal becomes sensitive to hemodynamic changes within the top 2–3 mm of the cortex and extends laterally 1 cm to either side, perpendicular to the axis of source-detector spacing [39]. Studies have shown that at inter-optode distances as short as 2–2.5 cm, grey matter is part of the sample volume [39,40]. If wavelengths of the light sources are chosen to maximize the amount of absorption by oxy-Hb and deoxy-Hb, changes in the chromophore concentrations cause changes in the number of photons that are absorbed and the number of photons that are scattered back to the surface of the scalp. These changes in the attenuation of light measured at the surface of the scalp can be quantified using different techniques, that is, diffusion equation, modified Beer–Lambert law, and so on, and information on changes in oxy-Hb and deoxy-Hb concentrations can be assessed which will be discussed in Section 6.5.

6.3 Instrumentation

A wide variety of both commercial and custom-built fNIR instruments are currently in use [5]. These systems differ with respect to their use and system engineering, with tradeoffs between light sources, detectors, and instrument electronics that result in tradeoffs in the information available for analysis, safety, and cost. Three distinct types of fNIR implementation have been developed: time domain (TD) systems, frequency domain (FD) systems, and continuous wave (CW) spectroscopy systems, each with their own strengths and limitations [3–5]. In TD systems, also referred to as time-resolved spectroscopy (TRS), extremely short (picosecond-order) incident pulses of laser light are applied to the tissue and the temporal distribution of photons that carry the information about tissue scattering and absorption is measured. The emerging intensity is detected as a function of time (the temporal point spread function [TPSF]) with picosecond resolution [7,39,41]. Streak camera systems can provide high-temporal resolution, but they are large, expensive, and have a limited dynamic range. Time-correlated single-photon counting systems can be built with cheaper components and can provide wide dynamic range, however, they have poor temporal resolution. Even though TRS instruments offer absolute measurements of hemodynamic changes since they can be large, expensive, with limited dynamic range or poor temporal resolution, they have originally been developed as laboratory-based devices, and hence are difficult to be implemented in the clinical environment and in the field applications [5]. In FD or phase modulation spectroscopy (PM) systems, the light source is intensity modulated to the frequencies in the order of tens to hundreds of megahertz. The amplitude decay, phase shift, and modulation depth of the detected light intensity with respect to the incident light are measured to characterize the optical properties of tissue [42]. FD methods are low-cost alternatives to time-resolved methods and hence several multichannel FD instruments are now in common use [7,43].

CW systems apply either continuous or a slow-pulsed light to tissue and are limited to measuring the amplitude attenuation of the incident light [45]. These systems utilize less sophisticated detectors than time-resolved and FD systems and they cannot resolve the time-changing component of the light. As such, CW systems provide somewhat less information than time- or FD systems meaning relative measurements as opposed to absolute ones, but this tradeoff results in the capacity to design more compact, portable, easy to engineer, and affordable hardware making it advantageous for various applications [45,46]. They can be laser-based, but LEDs can also be used in CW designs to increase safety (particularly with respect to eye exposure) and comfort, and to again decrease both instrument size and cost, making it possible to deploy these systems in clinical or educational settings [5,7,32]. A detailed list of both commercially available and laboratory prototype fNIR instruments are presented in [43].

6.4 fNIR Measurements

6.4.1 Fast Neuronal Signal

Fast neuronal signal or event-related optical signal (EROS) capitalizes on the changes in the optical properties of the cell membranes themselves that occur as a function of the ionic fluxes during firing [14]. Using invasive techniques, it has been well-established that the optical properties of cell membranes change in the depolarized state relative to the resting state [32,47–49] and that optical methods can be used to detect these changes that occur within the first 200 ms of functional stimulation.

The ability to measure the actual depolarization state of neuronal tissue provides obvious advantages in that it is a direct measure of neural activity, with millisecond-level time resolution as can be measured with EEG and MEG but with the superior spatial resolution lacking in EEG/MEG. However, there are also a number of limitations to the noninvasive use of the EROS signal in humans. A primary disadvantage of the fast optical signal is the low signal-to-noise ratio (SNR) resulting from the need to image through skin, skull, and cerebral-spinal fluid. Basic sensory and motor movements such as tactile stimulation and finger tapping require between 500 and 1000 trials to establish a reliable signal [13]. There have also been failures to replicate the results of experiments reporting the fast optical signal in response to a visual stimulus among normal adult humans [32]. The low SNR may play a role in current difficulties with experimental replication; however, more cross-validation work is warranted. The final constraint is that these methods require a more expensive and cumbersome laser-based light source (vs. an LED-based light source), they are not portable, and the potential risk of inadvertent damage to the eyes is increased relative to the systems available for measuring hemodynamic responses. (LED-based near-infrared sources pose very little, if any, risk upon eye exposure [50]). In spite of these current limitations, the fast optical signal continues to be an important area of investigation because it offers glimpses of the "holy grail" of neuroimaging: the direct measurement of neuronal activity with millisecond time resolution and superior spatial resolution.

6.4.2 Slow Hemodynamic Signal

As explained in Section 6.2.1 through brain-energy metabolism, during brain activity first local oxygen consumption increases to metabolize glucose and provide energy to the activated neurons. Next, blood flow and perfusion increases in the area of activated neurons through neurovascular coupling which in turn changes the hemoglobin concentrations and oxygenation. These slow changes in hemodynamic signal occur within a few seconds after the onset of the stimulation and takes 10–20 min to take its full course to evolve [33,34] and can be measured by fNIR, PET, and fMRI as blood oxygen level dependent (BOLD) signal that is related with the changes in the concentration of deoxy-Hb.

Most fNIR applications are based upon the measurement of the slow hemodynamic responses in terms of deoxy-Hb and oxy-Hb. Typical slow hemodynamic signals together with corresponding fMRI–BOLD signal collected during a finger tapping experiment is shown in Figure 6.3a. Either the full-time course of the hemodynamic signals and/or features that can be extracted from them such as maximum amplitude, time to peak or reaction time, full width half maximum, and so on, as shown in Figure 6.3b are then used for comparison purposes in different task conditions, spatial locations or subject populations which will be discussed in detail in Sections 6.5 and 6.6.

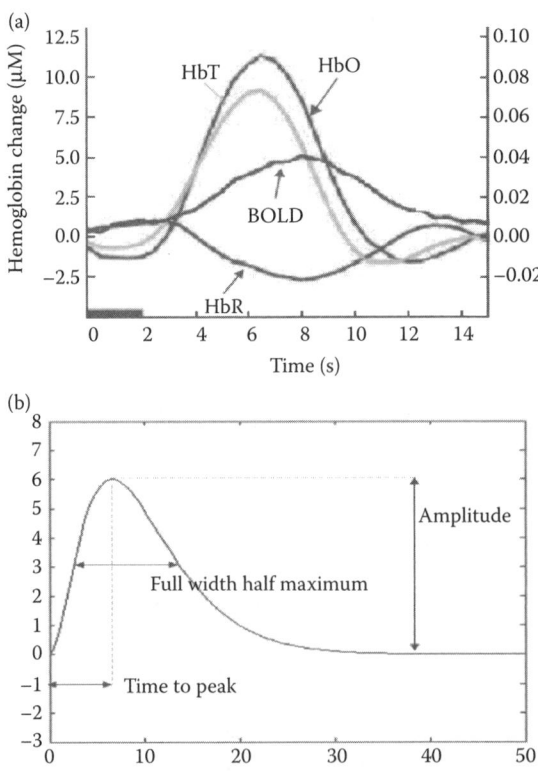

FIGURE 6.3   (a) Example hemodynamic signals. (From Boas DA, Dale AM, Francheschini MA. 2004. *Neuroimage*, 23:S275–S288.) (b) Features that can be extracted from hemodynamic responses.

6.5 fNIR Signal Processing

Analysis of fNIR measurements involves two main steps: (i) artifact and/or noise removal, and (ii) conversion of optical measurements into physiologically relevant signals and/or features. fNIR measurements can get corrupted by different sources of noise that should be suppressed in order to reliably extract information-bearing signals that are related to cognitive activity. Depending on the fNIR system used optical intensity measurements are converted to physiologically relevant signals and features for further processing using different approximations, assumptions, and algorithms. In this section, we will review different sources and characteristics of noise and existing algorithms to suppress them and the algorithms used to extract hemodynamic variables from fNIR intensity measurements.

6.5.1 Signal Separation and Noise Removal

The sources of noise in fNIR measurements can be categorized in two main groups: (i) noise of nonphysiological basis, and (ii) artifacts arise from systemic physiological origins. Noise sources that are not driven by physiological origins can happen as a result of instrumental noise, that is, electrical noise or experimental errors, that is, motion artifact, task-related errors. Since fNIR systems measure changes in hemodynamics, they measure such changes not only related with cognitive activity but also the ones that occur due to heart pulsation, respiration, and so on, resulting in systemic physiological artifacts. A detailed explanation of these noise sources and some algorithms for their suppression is presented in [52]. In this section, we will briefly explain these different sources of noise and summarize currently existing algorithms for their suppression.

Note that, noise in the optical measurements can be removed before and after the conversion of raw intensity measurements to physiological hemoglobin concentrations. The noise of nonphysiological basis such as instrument noise or experimental errors that are not related to underlying physiological changes should be removed prior to conversion of signals into hemodynamic measures. This way, errors across wavelengths will not be propagated causing additional crosstalk in the separation of oxy-Hb and deoxy-Hb. In contrast, noise of physiological origins such as blood pressure changes, heart pulsations, and so on, causes oscillations in hemoglobin concentrations together with changes related to brain activity such biological noise is better removed after the conversion of raw intensity measurements to hemodynamic variables [52].

6.5.1.1 Noise of Nonphysiological Basis

One type of noise that is not related with any physiological changes is electrical/electronic noise from the computer or other hardware in the instrument. Such electrical noise can also be generated by the use of other devices or from the surrounding space that can create interference in the measurements. This type of electrical noise is generally assumed to be white and since hemodynamic response generated by brain activity is generally slow (up to 0.1 Hz), most of the time, high frequency instrument noise are suppressed by simply low-pass filtering the data [52,53] or significantly reduced by adjusting the power of light sources within the safety limits and gain amplification at the detectors.

There can be other types of noise within fNIR measurements whose origins are not directly related with physiological changes within the underlying tissue such as artifacts that may arise as the result of subject motion or noncompliance with the experimental paradigm or the ones that are the direct results of experimental paradigm itself. This type of noise is sometimes called experimental errors [52]. Head movement can cause the fNIR detectors to shift and lose contact with the skin, exposing them to either ambient light or to light emitted directly from the fNIR sources or reflected from the skin, rather than being reflected from tissue in regions of interest. These effects cause sudden increases in the fNIR data. Another consequence of head movement is, it can cause the blood to move toward (or away from) the area that is being monitored, increasing (or decreasing) the amount of oxygen, hence result in an increase (or decrease) in the measured data. Since the dynamics of this type of motion artifact are slow, they can easily be confused with the actual hemodynamic response due to brain activation. Even though it is not as pronounced as in fMRI, motion artifacts in fNIR studies are a serious problem for real-life applications where head immobility is undesirable or untenable such as in studies involving pilots, children, and so on. Hence, cleaning the fNIR data from motion artifacts is an important and necessary task in order to deploy fNIR as a brain monitoring technology in its full potential to many real-life application areas.

The best way to deal with motion artifacts is to avoid them as much as possible which mostly depend on subject compliance, experimental design, and experimenter's expertise in the placement of the fNIR sensor. However, these conditions can be satisfied for experiments involving adults and the ones that can be carried out in the laboratory, in controlled environments or in sitting positions. Different sensor designs and placements are developed to match the requirements of the experiment and reduce dependence on experimenter's expertise for its secure placement [52]. However, such sensor designs may only eliminate motion artifacts that can arise from the shift or pop of sources and/or detectors where motion artifacts of slow nature due to blood movement may still be present if head movement occurs during data acquisition as a result of experimental design or subject incompliance. There are several different algorithms developed for the detection and elimination of motion artifacts. For motion artifacts arising from the physical displacement or movement of the optical probe, detection algorithms such as the one based on outlier detection methods was proposed in [52]. In order to suppress the motion artifact, several methods were proposed such as the ones based on principal component analysis (PCA) [52], wavelet analysis [54] or recently a combined PCA and independent component analysis (ICA) [55]. The novelty in this last method was the use of dark current measurements for the identification of the existence of motion artifacts and their removal by the use of a combined ICA/PCA-based method. This method was applied on a clinical data collected in a highly noisy environment namely operating room and shown to successfully remove motion artifacts. A comparison of algorithms in motion artifact removal based on wavelets, autoregression, adaptive filtering, and ICA are discussed in [56]. For motion artifacts that are the result of the movement of the blood within the tissue that are more slow in nature and have similar frequency spectrum as with the optical signals coming from physiological origins such as hemodynamic response to stimulus, respiration, heart pulsation, and so on, there exists different algorithms based on adaptive, Wiener and Kalman filtering. A detailed analysis of these algorithms in comparison to each other based on their ability to improve SNR on 11 subject data set where slow, medium, and high-speed head movement was tested are given in [57,58]. A sample result is shown in Figure 6.4 where motion free data, adaptive, Wiener and Kalman filtered data are presented on a medium speed head movement case. A separate study for similar type of motion artifact used the observation that motion noise may cause the measured oxy-Hb and deoxy-Hb signals, which are typically strongly negatively correlated, to become more

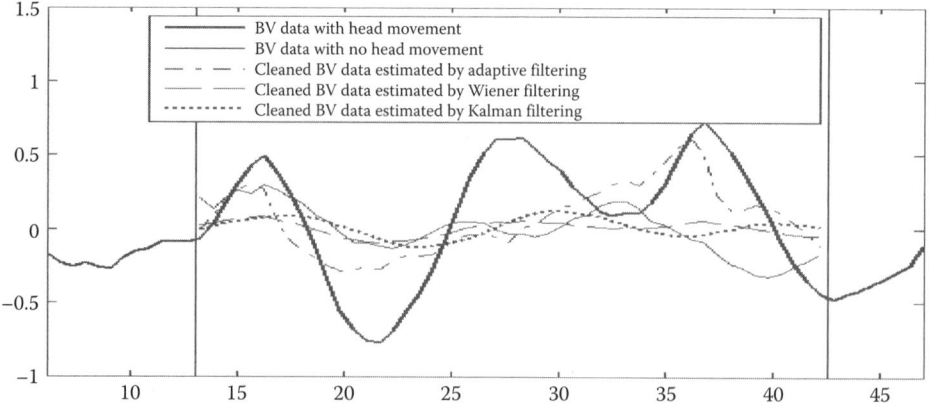

FIGURE 6.4 Comparison of different motion artifact removal algorithms on blood volume (total hemoglobin = oxy-Hb + deoxy-Hb) data.

(a)

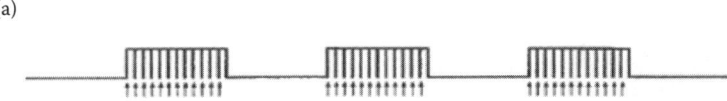

Rest for a while; do the task for a while; repeat; subtract average activity during
rest from that during task

(b)

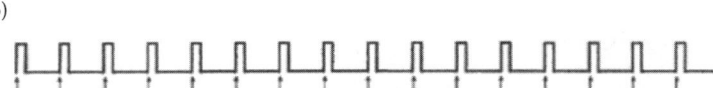

Do a single trial of the task once in a while (possibly at randomly distributed
times); record activity associated with each event; realign all recordings and
compute statistics on the average

FIGURE 6.5 Schematic diagram of (a) blocked and (b) single-trial paradigms.

positively correlated [59]. A method has been developed to reduce noise-based on the principle that the concentration changes of oxy-Hb and deoxy-Hb should be negatively correlated.

In addition to motion artifacts, experimental errors can also be introduced simply by the design of the functional task or the study itself of it being an event-related or block design or a longitudinal study, and so on. The predominant paradigms used in functional studies are the repeated single trial paradigm and the blocked trial paradigm (Figure 6.5) [60]. Usually in fNIR studies experimental designs are selected similar to the ones used in fMRI or EEG studies. However, additional care must be taken in adjusting the task or selecting data analysis methods while using fNIR. For example, since hemodynamic responses are slow in nature as compared to the fast neuronal signals as measured by EEG, improper design of the timing of an experimental paradigm can introduce errors. In general, this requires that the timing of stimulus presentation in single trial paradigms to be spaced widely apart in time to allow the evoked-hemodynamic signal to evolve completely. If a block design or a rapid event-related design is used, selection of the interstimulus interval is very important for the evoked-hemodynamic responses to still hold the linearity assumption (the assumption that repeated evoked responses will add linearly). For event-related stimulus designs or in block designs where evoked-hemodynamic responses are required to be extracted [61], the total hemodynamic responses measured may be approximated as the linear summation of evoked responses to each single stimulus, provided that the interstimulus interval is longer than around 3–4 s. Another study related error in the measurements can occur during longitudinal studies over a subject group. If the fNIR sensor is not placed on the exact same location at different recording times, the results may not reflect possible changes over time but the optical differences in different tissue area monitored [52].

6.5.1.2 Artifacts That Arise from Systemic Physiological Origins

fNIR technology measures hemodynamic changes which can be as a result of brain activity or simply due to systemic physiological variations such as cardiac pulsations, respiration, and blood pressure. In humans, the cardiac pulsation and respiration typically have a period of 0.7–1.5 s and 3–8 s, respectively. The arterial blood pressure varies on multiple time scales approximately 10 s Mayer waves and slower N50-s variation [51,52,62,63]. Note that, although often times these physiological fluctuations are considered to be artifacts because they may interfere with the evoked-functional responses, if they can be effectively and reliably separated from evoked-hemodynamic responses, it may in fact be a very valuable characteristic of fNIR to be able measure all these physiological signals with just one sensor.

In order to improve the sensitivity and interpretability of fNIR measurements to brain activation, it is necessary to separate systemic physiological signal sources spatially and temporally. There are different techniques developed to suppress or separate the systemic physiological signals from evoked-hemodynamic responses based on either (i) known approximate frequency content of signals, (ii) the spatial covariance of

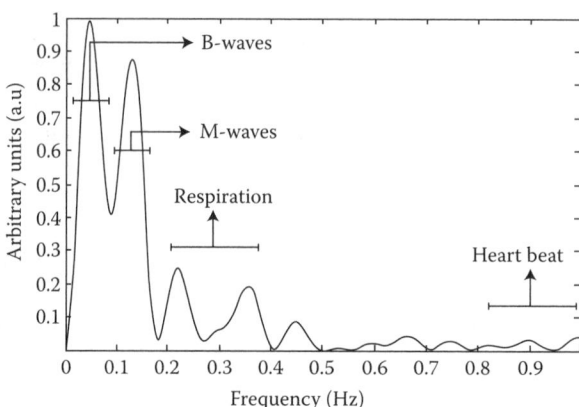

FIGURE 6.6 fNIR signal and artifacts in FD.

physiology, or (iii) the ability to remotely measure physiological signals correlated with the ones appearing in fNIR measurements of interest. Since the frequency bands of the physiological signal sources are known approximately, classical filters, that is, low-pass, band-pass, high-pass filters can effectively and efficiently be used to separate some of those signals. A classic example of the power spectral density (PSD) spectrum of the poststimulus signal segment is shown in Figure 6.6 [60]. The hemodynamic response following neural activation is embedded in the frequencies up to approximately 0.1 Hz. The 0.8 Hz and 0.2 Hz bands correspond to heart rate and respiration, respectively. The B-waves (~0.03 Hz) represent very low frequency oscillations (VLFO) generated by the various brain stem nuclei in the vasomotor tone of cerebral arterioles [64]. The Mayer waves (~0.1 Hz) represent low frequency oscillations reflecting oscillations due to blood pressure. As an example, if a band-pass filter with pass band selected to be between 0.08 and 0.12 Hz is designed, it can remove the high-frequency instrument noise, the fast cardiac oscillations, respiration, and VLFO. Note that, in such application involving band-pass filtering care should be taken to avoid removal of frequencies associated with the evoked-functional hemodynamic response. For example, bandpass filtering can generally not be used to remove Mayer waves, since their frequency band overlaps with the content of the hemodynamic response. Alternatives to conventional bandpass filtering, involve the use of curve fitting [60], adaptive, Wiener and Kalman filtering techniques [60,65,66]. In the Wiener filtering approach, the statistical changes in such physiological artifacts had been taken into account.

Other than classical filters, algorithms that use the spatial persistence nature of systemic physiological signals (specific and repeated spatial pattern across the brain) such as PCA-based physiological filtering methods have been proposed [67] similar to its use for motion correction. There also exist algorithms based on separate measurements providing correlated noise sources with the physiological signals. In these algorithms the cardiac, respiration, and blood pressure signals are separately measured by additional sensors such as with dynamic blood pressure cuff, pneumatic belt, pulse plethysmograph, pulse oximetry, or an electrocardiogram which can provide signals that are correlated with the artifacts that exist within fNIR measurements. Then, algorithm such as least squares regression algorithms [68], adaptive filtering [66], ICA [69] or RETROICOR [70] as developed for fMRI can be used to remove these signals from fNIR measurements to extract evoked-hemodynamic responses. In another technique, correlated measurements of physiological artifacts are measured by using multiple source detector separations. Since penetration depth increases with an increase in source detector separation, by measuring from detectors that are placed close enough to the source, one can guarantee penetration to only superficial tissues and not to brain. On the contrary, detectors placed farther away from the source can measure signals coming from the brain together with all the other superficial layers. Such arrangement is used in different applications to remove physiological signals [66] as well as motion artifacts [71].

6.5.2 Hemodynamic Signal Extraction from fNIR Intensity Measurements

Several different algorithms based on different mathematical models and assumptions have been developed to quantify the fNIR measurements and obtain information about the physiological/optical changes related with brain activity. Depending on the fNIR system and measurement type, appropriate algorithms can be implemented. Here, we will discuss two of the most commonly used methods (i) diffusion theory and (ii) modified Beer–Lambert law both of which are derived from linear transport theory to extract absolute or relative measurements of hemodynamic signals. Within each category, we will describe the mathematical model used, assumptions needed to meet for the algorithm to be applicable, and existing analytical and experimental solutions.

6.5.2.1 Diffusion Theory

Propagation of light in highly diffusive media such as tissue is usually modeled by using linear transport theory (radiative transport or Boltzman transport theory) [7,72–74]. However, analytical solutions to radiative transport equation can only be obtained for very simple geometries. Much simpler approximation can be derived from radiative transport equation based on diffusion theory [7,72–77] under certain assumptions such as (i) scattering coefficient is much greater than the absorption coefficient, (ii) scattering is isotropic, (iii) source detector separations are not too small, and (iv) measurement times are apart from the input times [72,77]. TD diffusion equation is given as [7,72–74]

$$\frac{1}{c}\frac{\partial \Phi(r,t)}{\partial t} - \nabla[D(r)\nabla\Phi(r,t)] + \mu_a(r)\Phi(r,t) = S(r,t), \quad D = [3(\mu_a + (1-g)\mu_s)]^{-1} \tag{6.1}$$

where $\Phi(r,t)$ is the diffuse photon fluence rate at position r and time t, $S(r,t)$ is the photon source, c is the speed of light in the tissue, D is the diffusion coefficient, μ_a is the linear absorption coefficient, μ_s is the linear scattering coefficient, and g is the mean cosine of the scattering angle.

Analytical solutions to diffusion equation as a forward problem (derivation of the resulting measurement given the distribution of light sources and detectors, tissue parameters, and boundaries) can be obtained using Green's function which provides the photon distribution when the source is an impulsive function. Green's function solutions to diffusion approximation have been driven for slab, cylindrical, and spherical geometries. For a semi-infinite half-space geometry one such solution for an impulse input is found as [7,78]

$$R(\rho,t) = \frac{z_o\exp(-\mu_a ct)}{(4\pi Dc)^{3/2}t^{5/2}}\exp\left[-\frac{\rho^2 + z_o^2}{4Dct}\right] \tag{6.2}$$

where $R(\rho,t)$ is the reflected light intensity, $z_o = 1/\mu_s'$ and $\mu_s' = (1-g)\mu_s$ is the reduced scattering coefficient. Solutions to diffusion equation in TD and FD can also be found in [77].

Experimentally, as an inverse problem (derivation of the distribution of tissue optical parameters given the distribution of light sources and measurements [72]), in TD systems the time course of the measured light intensities at different wavelengths are fitted to the solution equation and hence the absolute absorption and scattering parameters of the underlying tissue of interest are estimated [7]. Note that, since information contained in temporal profile of the measured light will also be present in FD, similar approaches to TD techniques can be applied to FD systems to extract optical parameters as an inverse problem.

Optical properties of the tissue such as absorption and scattering coefficients are wavelength dependent. Furthermore, absorption parameter of the tissue changes with the change in the concentrations of underlying tissue chromophores. Since within the optical window (700–900 nm) the dominant tissue chromophores are the oxy-Hb and deoxy-Hb, their absolute concentrations can be calculated using the absorption coefficient estimated at multiple wavelengths [51] using:

$$\mu_a(\lambda) = \varepsilon_{HBO2}(\lambda)C_{HbO2} + \varepsilon_{HB}(\lambda)C_{HB} \tag{6.3}$$

where λ is the photon wavelength, ε is the wavelength and chromophore-dependent extinction coefficients (experimental values are tabulated in [19]) and C_{HBO2} and C_{HB} are the concentrations of oxy-Hb and deoxy-Hb, respectively.

Solutions to diffusion equation cannot be obtained analytically for more complex inhomogeneous geometries. For such cases, numerical solutions are studied based on numerical integral and differential approximation methods such as finite difference methods (FDM), finite element methods (FEM), or perturbative approaches using truncated series approximations such as Born and Rytov approximations and their higher order extensions [72,73]. These numerical solutions suffer from extensive computational cost. Another numerical method used for the solution of the forward problem to study the light propagation in tissue is the Monte Carlo modeling (MCM) [73]. In MCM, photons are assumed to have certain probability of scattering and absorption where many photons are injected into the medium at every source, treated separately and at the end statistical maps of a combination of photons collected at the detectors are obtained.

6.5.2.2 Modified Beer–Lambert Law

Under various simplifying assumptions [79], radiative transport equation can be reduced to the Beer–Lambert Law which states that the attenuation of an absorbing compound dissolved in a nonabsorbent compound is proportional to the concentration of the compound and the optical path length [2,4]. In a purely absorbing medium, the transmitted light I can be expressed in terms of the input light I_o as follows:

$$I = I_o e^{-\mu_a L} \tag{6.4}$$

where μ_a is the absorption coefficient of the homogeneous medium and L is the optical path length. Since absorption coefficient is related to concentration of the absorbing compound C and the extinction coefficient ε as $\mu_a = \varepsilon C$, the absorbance or attenuation (A) in terms of optical density (OD) units can be written as

$$A = OD = \ln\left(\frac{I_o}{I}\right) = \varepsilon CL \tag{6.5}$$

If there is more than one absorbing compound within the medium then the attenuation can be given by

$$A = [\varepsilon_1 C_1 + \varepsilon_2 C_2 + \cdots + \varepsilon_N C_N]L \tag{6.6}$$

In a scattering medium where there is no absorption, the light will still be attenuated since the photons will be deflected from their path [80]. Hence similar to absorbing case, in a medium having only one scattering compound with a scattering coefficient μ_s the transmitted light intensity I can be written as

$$I = I_o e^{-\mu_s L} \tag{6.7}$$

Note that when multiple scattering occurs and the light gets diffuse, then isotropic scattering is often assumed and the reduced scattering coefficient $\mu_s' = (1 - g)\mu_s$ is used instead to represent it.

Within the tissue, light attenuation happens due to absorption and scattering together. Both of these effects should be taken into account in order to correctly quantify changes in hemodynamics. Modified Beer–Lambert law (MBLL) accounts for the effects of both the absorption and multiple scattering where the attenuation is expressed as follows:

$$A = \ln\left(\frac{I_o}{I}\right) = \varepsilon CL + G \tag{6.8}$$

where G represents the light attenuation due to scattering which depends on also on measurement geometry.

MBLL relies on several assumptions such as (i) homogeneous tissue, (ii) constant scattering G, and (iii) known path length L [4,74,80]. Even though these may not be exactly met by the biological tissues, MBLL is by far the most widely used technique in calculating hemodynamic changes especially in CW systems mostly due to its simplicity and no computational cost [74]. It is discussed in [80] that scattering in brain tissue occurs mostly due to cell and subcellular membranes and that scattering due to red blood cells is low. Hence, in functional optical imaging studies, the attenuation due to scattering can be assumed to be constant since even though the concentration of oxy-Hb and deoxy-Hb changes due to brain activity their contribution to scattering can be negligible.

The mean path length (L) that light travels in a highly scattering medium such as tissue is larger than the direct path or geometrical path length (d) between light source and detector. This increase in path length due to tissue scattering is corrected by using a differential path length factor (DPF). Then the mean path length is found as

$$L = \text{DPF} \cdot d \tag{6.9}$$

The DPF for tissues at different anatomical regions such as head (forehead, somatosensory, and occipital regions), calf, fore arm, and so on, for adult and infant populations have been both experimentally (using TD and FD systems) and numerically (using Monte Carlo simulations) studied and the values are tabulated [81–83]. It is noted that DPF is wavelength dependent and there can be subject to subject differences based on gender, age, and so on [83,84].

Even though the DPF can be measured or taken from published values assuming small across subject differences, the absolute quantification of chromophore concentrations cannot be possible since G is unknown. If G is assumed to be constant during the measurement period, then by measuring the A at two or more wavelengths, the relative change in tissue chromophores ΔC such as oxy-Hb and deoxy-Hb versus time can be obtained from relative changes in attenuation ΔA to an arbitrary time as follows:

$$\Delta A = \varepsilon \cdot \Delta C \cdot d \cdot \text{DPF} \tag{6.10}$$

By measuring attenuation change at two distinct wavelengths and using Equation 6.10, changes in oxy-Hb (HbO2) and deoxy-Hb (Hb) can be calculated as follows:

$$\begin{bmatrix} \Delta C_{HbO2} \\ \Delta C_{Hb} \end{bmatrix} = \frac{1}{d \cdot \text{DPF}} \begin{bmatrix} \varepsilon_{\lambda 1,HbO2} & \varepsilon_{\lambda 1,Hb} \\ \varepsilon_{\lambda 2,HbO2} & \varepsilon_{\lambda 2,Hb} \end{bmatrix}^{-1} \begin{bmatrix} \Delta A_{\lambda 1} \\ \Delta A_{\lambda 2} \end{bmatrix} \tag{6.11}$$

The MBLL has been widely used in CW systems for the quantification of hemodynamic changes. However, care should be taken in the selection of the wavelengths of the light sources implemented in order to correctly extract relative changes in tissue chromophores while reducing crosstalk between them [51].

6.6 fNIR Studies

Since the first *in vivo* application of fNIR on cat brain by Jobsis [1], there has been a growing interest in this exciting noninvasive, safe, affordable and portable technology and hence many different applications involving healthy and diseased groups in adult and children populations for laboratory and field conditions had been studied. Here, we will summarize some clinical applications and further give some specific examples of some of the basic research and clinical application studies that have been mainly carried out by the Optical Brain Imaging group at Drexel University within the Cognitive Neuroengineering and Quantitative Experimental Research (CONQUER) Collaborative.

6.6.1 Summary of Basic Research and Clinical Application Studies

In the past decade, brain activation studies employing fNIR have been conducted on the visual system [8], the somatosensory system [10], the auditory system [17,16], and the language system [6], and during motor tasks [5]. fNIR studies have also been used to examine a number of cognitive tasks [6,21–23,53]. In general, these studies have reported localized increases in oxy-Hb in response to functional challenge, and the results have largely been in agreement with corollary fMRI studies.

The first clinical applications of fNIR have been in the investigation of fetal, neonatal, and infant cerebral oxygenation and functional activation. For instance, fNIR studies have revealed developmental alterations in the cerebral hemodynamic response to auditory and visual stimulation [17,85]. Neurological applications have included an evaluation of the hemodynamic response during deep brain stimulation in Parkinson's patients [86], brain activations during induced seizures in patients with intractable epilepsy [87], an exploration of the pathophysiology of seizures in childhood epilepsy [88], and an examination of Alzheimer's patients during verbal fluency and other cognitive tasks [89]. Psychiatric applications have included the comparison of prefrontal brain activations of schizophrenic patients to healthy subjects during a mirror drawing task [90], a self-face recognition test [24], and during a continuous performance task [91]. fNIR was used to predict treatment response in a study of the effects of transcranial magnetic stimulation on depression [92]. A detailed review on clinical application can be found in [93].

6.6.2 Specific Example Studies

6.6.2.1 fNIR Device

In all of the specific example studies that will be discussed in this section a portable CW–fNIR system developed by Drexel University, optical brain imaging team which was originally described by Chance et al. [46] is used. The main components of the system were: (1) the sensor that covers the entire forehead, (2) a control box with integrated power supply for sensor control and data acquisition (current sampling rate is 2 Hz), and (3) a computer for the data analysis software [49,53]. The flexible sensor consisted of four light sources with three built-in LEDs sources having peak wavelengths at 730, 805, 850 nm and 10 photodetectors designed to image cortical areas underlying the forehead (dorsolateral and inferior frontal cortices). With a fixed source-detector separation of 2.5 cm and the implemented data collection scheme, this configuration resulted in a total of 16 signal channels (voxels) as shown in Figure 6.7. Communication between the data analysis computer and the task presentation computer is established via a serial port connection to time-lock fNIR measurement to the task events. The flexible sensor design consists of three parts: (i) a reusable flexible circuit board that carries the necessary infrared sources and detectors, (ii) a replaceable cushioning material, and (iii) a disposable single-use medical-grade adhesive tape that serves to attach the sensor to the participant (see Figure 6.7). The flexible circuit provides a reliable, integrated wiring solution, as well as consistent and reproducible component spacing and alignment. Because the circuit board and cushioning materials are flexible, the components move and adapt to the various contours of the participant's head, allowing the sensor elements to maintain an orthogonal orientation to the skin surface, dramatically improving light coupling efficiency and signal strength.

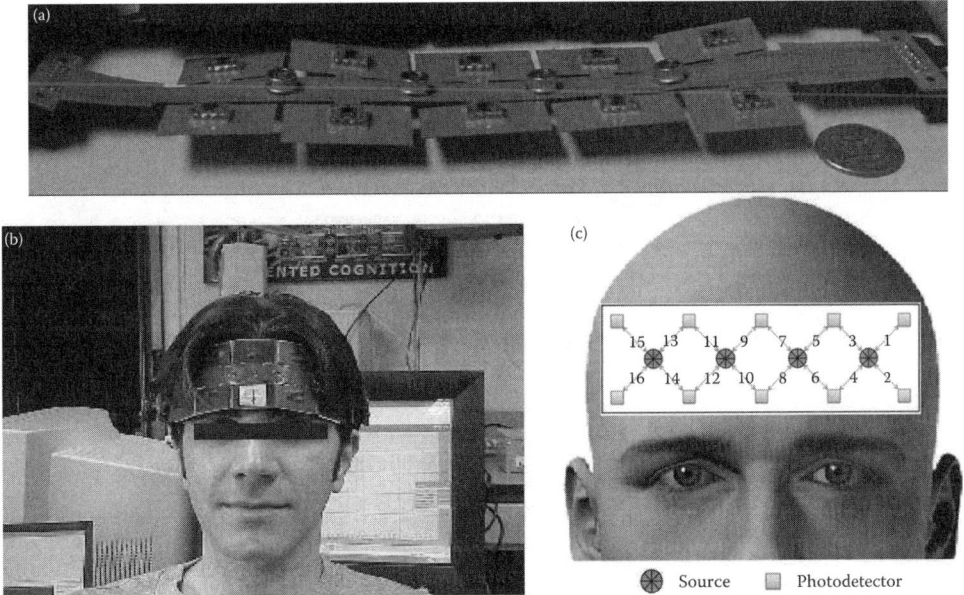

FIGURE 6.7 (a) Flexible fNIR sensor; (b) subject wearing the flexible fNIR sensor; and (c) anatomical location of fNIR measurement channels.

6.6.2.2 Basic Research Studies Targeting Different Cognitive Domains

To date, the fNIR studies of cognition and emotion have focused on functions associated with Brodman's areas BA9, BA10, BA46, BA45, BA47, and BA44. Recent PET and fMRI studies have shown that these areas play a critical role in sustained attention, both the short term storage and the executive process components of working memory, episodic memory, problem solving, response inhibition, and the perception of smell [for a recent review, see 94,95]. In addition, word recognition and the storage of verbal materials activate Broca's area and left hemisphere supplementary and premotor areas [94,96,97]. Some examples of fNIR applications and their results targeting different cognitive domains will be summarized in this section.

6.6.2.2.1 Attention

The protocol used in this study [49,53] to measure attention is a common visual oddball paradigm modified for use with fMRI by McCarthy et al. [98]. The stimuli were two strings of white letters (XXXXX and OOOOO) presented against the center of a dark background. A total of 516 stimuli were presented, 480 context stimuli (OOOOO) and 36 targets (XXXXX). Stimulus duration was 500 ms, with an interstimulus interval of 1500 ms. Target stimuli were presented randomly with respect to context stimuli with a minimum of 12 context stimuli between successive targets to allow the hemodynamic response an opportunity to return to baseline between target presentations. Fifteen right-handed participants (4 females and 11 males with age 20.8 ± 4.2) were required to press one of two buttons on a response pad after each stimulus, while both fNIR and EEG were recorded simultaneously. One button was pressed in response to targets (X's), and another button was pressed in response to context stimuli (O's).

The results for the ERPs were consistent with the literature [99]; targets elicited a pronounced P3 component with an average peak at 365 ms for both electrodes Cz and Pz (see Figure 6.8a for Pz results). The peak amplitude response to target stimuli was larger than the response to context stimuli at both Cz ($t(14) = 7.58; p < 0.001$) and Pz ($t(14) = 7.81; p < 0.001$). These ERP results confirm that the task parameters and participant responses were comparable to other ERP studies. Repeated-measures ANOVA computed on the fNIR oxygenation data (Oxy = oxy-Hb − deoxy-Hb) revealed that oxygenation values were

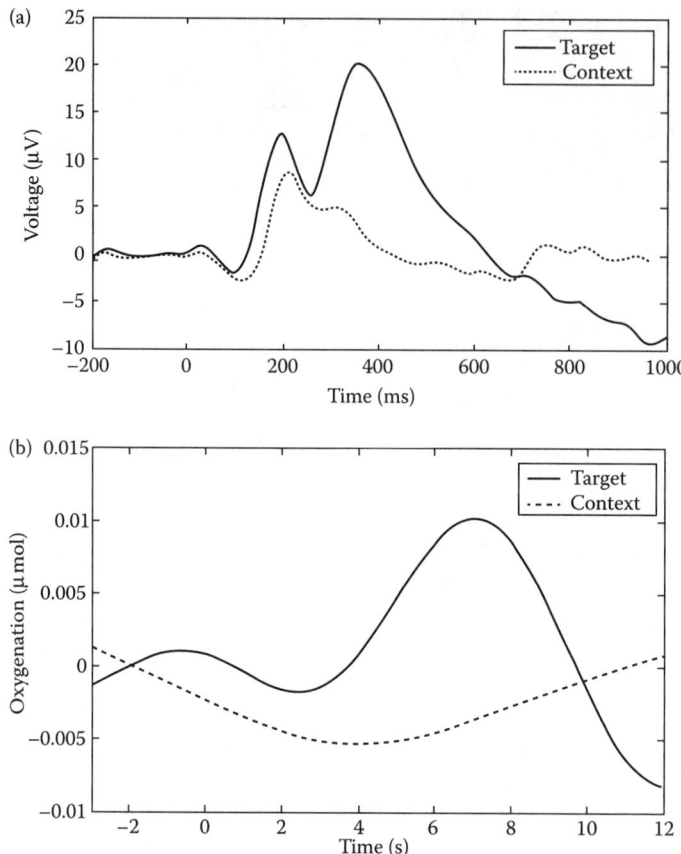

FIGURE 6.8   Averaged (a) ERP from Pz; (b) fNIR data for targets and contexts on voxel 11.

greater in response to targets than to controls in voxel 11, located over middle frontal gyrus of the right. Differentiation occurred between 6 and 9 s poststimulus as shown in Figure 6.8b. These results are consistent with the fMRI literature for visual target categorization with respect to increased oxygenation in response to targets, cortical location, and time course [98,100]. This study also demonstrated the utility of the combined EEG–fNIR system for studies of event-related designs that tap into ubiquitous cognitive functions such as attention [49].

6.6.2.2.2 Working Memory

In order to assess the working memory, the n-back task which is a sequential letter task with varied workload conditions that has frequently been used in working memory studies by cognitive psychologists and neuroscientists is used [95,96]. The stimuli are single consonants presented centrally, in pseudorandom sequences, on a computer monitor. Stimulus duration is 500 ms, with a 2500 ms interstimulus interval. Four conditions were used to incrementally vary working memory load from zero to three items. In the 0-back condition, subjects respond to a single prespecified target letter (e.g., "X") with their dominant hand (pressing a button to identify the stimulus). In the 1-back condition, the target is defined as any letter identical to the one immediately preceding it (i.e., one trial back). In the 2-back and 3-back conditions, the targets were defined as any letter that was identical to the one presented two or three trials back, respectively. Subjects pressed one button for targets (approximately 33% of trials) and another for nontargets. This strategy incrementally increased working memory load from the 0-back to the 3-back condition. Each n-back block contained 20 letters whether target

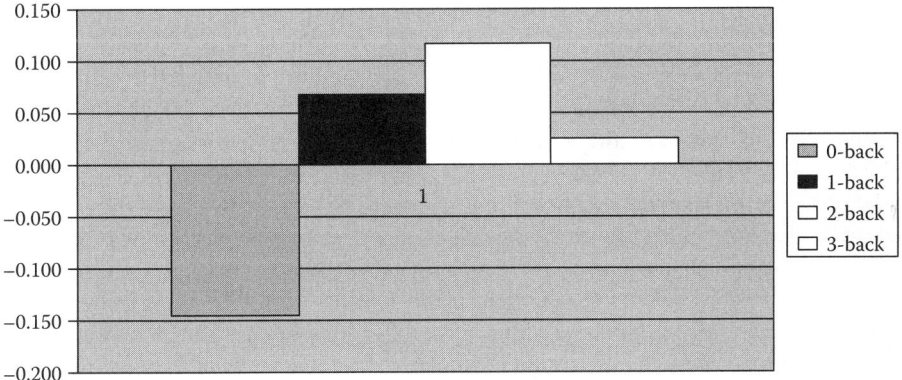

FIGURE 6.9 Averaged mean oxygenation for all subjects for four n-back conditions.

or nontarget and lasted for 60 s with 15 s of rest periods between n-back blocks. Total test included 7 trials of each of the 4 n-back conditions (hence total of 28 n-back blocks) ordered in such a way that within one trial all 4 of the n-back conditions are presented; however, their order is changed randomly from trial to trial.

In the analysis performed on 9 subjects (with age between 18 and 25), statistically significant differences between the n-back conditions in fNIR measurements are obtained on the fourth voxel located on left dorsolateral prefrontal cortex (DLPFC) [53] which is in agreement with the fMRI literature [97]. Statistical analysis revealed that the 0-back condition differed from 1- and 2-back conditions; 1-back > 0-back, $t = 3.21$, $p = .012$; 2-back > 0-back, $t = 2.58$, $p = .032$. After outlier elimination, 1- and 2-back differed from each other; 2-back > 1-back, $t = 2.77$, $p = 0.0275$. No difference was found between 2- and 3-back conditions. A positive relationship between increasing workload and the oxygenation is observed in DLPFC as shown in Figure 6.9, again in agreement with fMRI studies [97]. The drop in the oxygenation values in the most difficult condition (3-back) can be interpreted using a hypothesis similar to the human performance study discussed in Section 6.6.3.1 where subjects get overwhelmed and lost their concentration.

6.6.2.2.3 Learning and Memory

This study focused on the physiological effects of repetition on learning and working memory using an adaptation of Luria's Memory Word-Task (LMWT) [101]. The hemodynamic response in DLPFC of 13 healthy subjects (9 female), ranging in age from 23 to 43 while completing LMWT is recorded using fNIR. In LMWT, a list of 10 completely unrelated words is read aloud to the subject for he or she to memorize. This procedure is repeated 10 times. Free word recalls were acquired at the beginning, middle, and end of the task. Behavioral results showed that all subjects could recall the complete word list by the tenth trial, which was considered as successful task accomplishment. In terms of hemoglobin concentrations, it was hypothesized that there will be an increase in oxy-Hb and a decrease in deoxy-Hb in the DLPFC, reflecting activation of this area [102,103], during task learning phase, that is, when the subject is not yet able to recall the complete word list. Conversely, a significant drop in the regional-DLPFC oxy-Hb concentration, along with a significant increase in regional deoxy-Hb, is also expected, reflecting deactivation of the region of interest.

Oxy-Hb and deoxy-Hb results showed significant main effects in periods with ($F[1,12] = 6.31$, $p = 0.027$) and ($F[1,12] = 20.68$, $p < 0.001$), respectively. Post-hoc analyses showed a higher level of oxy-Hb concentration during the first period of LMWT ($M = 0.044\,\mu M$) than during the second ($M = -0.069\,\mu M$). Conversely, a lower level of deoxy-Hb concentration during the first period of the test ($M = -0.037\,\mu M$; corrected $p < 0.01$) than during the second ($M = 0.037\,\mu M$) was found in post-hoc analyses. Significant interactions between channels and period were also detected for oxy-Hb ($F[15,180] = 2.01$; $p = 0.016$) and deoxy-Hb ($F[15,180] = 1.81$; $p = 0.036$). Post-hoc analyses also showed that channels with significant highest differences between the first and second period of the test were left hemisphere channels 2, 3, 4 and right hemisphere channels 13, 14, 15, and 16 (all p's < 0.05) corresponding to BA 45, 46, 9, and 10 bilaterally. These channels also showed a lower deoxy-Hb concentration during the first period of the test (all p's < 0.05).

Correlation analyses showed significant positive correlations between oxy-Hb and memory performance in channels 1–4 and 12–16 for the first period (Spearmann's ρ's ranging from 0.54 to 0.73; p's ranging from 0.03 to 0.005). In these channels, significant negative correlations were found between memory performance and deoxy-Hb (ρ's ranging from −0.59 to −0.78; p's ranging from 0.02 to 0.003). On the contrary, for the second period, significant negative correlations were found between oxy-Hb and memory performance in channels 1–3 and 11–15 (ρ's ranging from −0.51 to −0.66; p's ranging from 0.04 to 0.013). Positive correlations between deoxy-Hb and memory performance were also detected for this period in channels 1–4 and 12–16 (ρ's ranging from 0.54 to 0.61; p's ranging from 0.03 to 0.014).

The comparison of DLPFC hemodynamic activation pattern produced during the first period of word list learning by repetition with that produced during the second period when the list was already learned but the words were still being repeated suggested an attenuation of stimulus-evoked neural activity in prefrontal neurons. These findings indicate that the temporal integration of efficient verbal learning is mediated by a mechanism known as neural repetition suppression (NRS). This mechanism facilitates cortical deactivation in DLPFC once learning is successfully completed. This cortical reorganization is interpreted as a progressive optimization of neural responses to produce a more efficient use of neural circuits. NRS could be considered one of the natural mechanisms involved in the processes of memory learning.

6.6.2.2.4 Problem Solving

The protocol used in this study involved presentation of anagram blocks on a computer screen that contains sequences of three letter (3L), four letter (4L), and five letter (5L) anagrams starting from minimal (3L anagrams) proceeding to the maximal level of difficulty (5L anagrams), and then back down again to the starting point of 3L anagrams [61,104]. Between each anagram block session, there is a rest period of 30 s. Each anagram block is displayed for approximately 1 min containing as many anagrams within depending on the number of processed anagrams by the subject. The decision of the subjects on each anagram processed and its timing is recorded on a text file for further analysis.

Since most subjects solve the anagrams within 2–5 s and since hemodynamic response takes 10–20 s period to fully evolve [33] for each anagram stimulus, hemodynamic responses overlap in time which present challenges for data analysis. In order to evaluate the subject's evoked-response times or brain activation for single anagram presentation within a block for graded difficulty analysis, a novel single trial hemodynamic response estimation algorithm was developed [61]. In this algorithm, each event-related hemodynamic response was estimated on the basis of two postulates that: (1) each single-trial hemodynamic response follows a gamma function, $hf_i = A_i t_i^{\alpha_i} e^{\beta_i t_i}$ as given in Figure 6.3b, and (2) the total oxygenation data can be modeled by the summation of individual hemodynamic responses evoked by rapidly presented stimuli, $\text{Oxy} = \sum_{i=1}^{N} hf_i$. Each single trial was estimated by optimizing the error between the total oxygenation data from fNIR measurements and the linear model: $\varepsilon = \min_{A,\alpha,\beta}\left(\text{Oxy} - \sum_{i=1}^{N} hf_i\right)^2$.

All calculations are applied to the data gathered from the left hemisphere of the prefrontal cortex on voxel 5. In block anagram study based on 14 participants (age between 18 and 23), the averaged recorded behavioral response times, the extracted rise times or time to peak (min), and the maximum amplitudes (as given in Figure 6.3b) from the estimated evoked-hemodynamic responses with respect

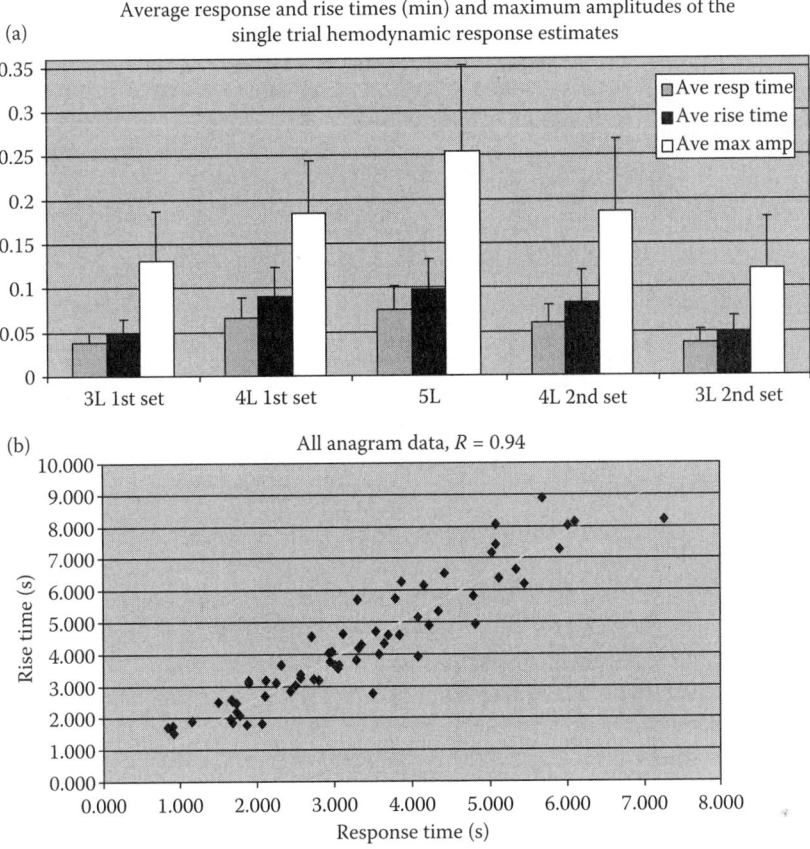

FIGURE 6.10 (a) Subject averages of rise and response times (min) and maximum amplitude; (b) scatter plot of rise time versus response time averages.

to the 3L, 4L, and 5L anagram sets are presented in Figure 6.10a. The estimated rise time which is the time required for the evoked-hemodynamic response to reach its maximum amplitude follows the same pattern as the behavioral (true) response time of the subjects having a correlation of $R = 0.94$ as presented in the scatter plot of the rise time versus response time in Figure 6.10b. Similarly, the estimated maximum amplitudes are correlated with the true response times ($R = 0.73$). The rise times and the maximum amplitude values increase as the difficulty level of the anagram solution increases, meaning that subjects need more time and more oxygen to solve difficult anagrams. Estimation of the event-related signals in a block design allows more precise analysis of the brain's function during a cognitive/problem solving task.

6.6.2.2.5 Emotion

Two affective dimensions have been studied extensively in neuroimaging research on emotional stimuli: arousal (exciting or calming) and valence (positive or negative). In this work, a new paradigm in the study of emotional processes through functional neuroimaging is introduced where the influence of the valence and arousal of visual stimuli on the neuroimaging of the evoked-hemodynamic changes are demonstrated [105]. Using fNIR, evoked-cerebral blood oxygenation (CBO) changes in DLPFC during direct exposure to different emotion-eliciting stimuli ("on" period), and during the period directly following stimulus cessation ("off" period) is investigated. It is hypothesized that the evoked-CBO, rather than return to baseline after stimulus cessation, would show either overshoot or undershoot. The study includes 30 healthy subjects (15 female) between the ages of 19 and 51 and a total of 9 stimuli, which consist of video-clips of moderate length (~20 s) with different emotional content (ranging from violence to cartoons) that can ensure that the stimuli will provoke strong lasting responses. The total sample of trials studied (270) is classified according to the valence and arousal ratings given by the subjects.

A significant negative correlation was found between valence and arousal dimensions ($r = -0.58$; $p < 0.001$). That is to say, the lower the value in valence dimension, the higher the ratings in arousal. The four-way ANOVA for repeated measures revealed significant main effects for exposure condition ($F[1,234] = 27.4$; $p < 0.001$) and the grouping factors valence ($F[2,234] = 3.93$; $p < 0.05$) and arousal ($F[1,234] = 6.94$; $p < 0.01$). A Student t-test for repeated measures between mean oxy-Hb during "on" and "off" periods revealed a significant mean difference of -0.11 µM ($t[239] = -2.98$; $p < 0.01$). Comparisons between valence groups revealed a significant difference in oxygenation of 0.33 µM in unpleasant trials compared to neutral trials ($t[125] = 3.28$; $p < 0.01$); a significant difference of 0.4 µM was found when compared to pleasant trials ($t[167] = 3.84$; $p < 0.001$). No statistically significant differences were found between the oxy-Hb levels in neutral versus pleasant trials ($t[182] = 0.94$; $p = 0.35$). A Student t-test for independent measures between arousing and nonarousing trials revealed a significant mean difference of 0.33 µM ($t(238) = -4.11$; $p < 0.001$). There was no main effect for the prefrontal cortex (PFC) region variable ($F[1,234] = 1.03$; $p = 0.31$) and no significant interactions with this variable. A significant interaction was found between arousal category and exposure condition ($F[1,234] = 16.14$; $p < 0.001$): in arousing trials, a significant difference of -0.4 µM existed between "on" and "off" conditions ($t[68] = -4.56$; $p < 0.001$), while no significant differences were detected in nonarousing trials ($t[170] = 0.23$; $p = 0.82$).

As a result, one of the main findings of this study is that when the subjective degree of arousal is high, the representation of the stimulus remains in the prefrontal cortex, even when the stimulus is no longer present. The persistence of sources of DLPFC activation during the "off" period is closely related to the degree of arousal that the subject assigns to the stimulus. Furthermore, these results show that valence alone does not determine the persistence of activation in PFC beyond the "on" period, except when the valence is unpleasant. The new and principle finding of this study is that there is an overshoot related to level of arousal in the DLPFC that persists even when the arousing stimulus has disappeared. Data also confirms that valence and arousal have different effects on the course of evoked-CBO response in DLPFC. Significant differences between "on" and "off" periods of DLPFC activation based on valence ratings was not found, but significant poststimulus overshoot related to arousal ratings was observed. These findings provide the first fNIR evidence showing that an increment in subjective arousal leads to activation in DLPFC which persists after stimulus cessation and does not occur with nonarousing stimuli. Note that since arousing stimuli produce longer periods of brain activation than nonarousing stimuli, neuroimaging studies must consider the duration and affective dimensions of the stimulus as well as the duration of the scanning. Not accounting for this difference may contribute to misinterpretation of the data.

6.6.3 Studies Involving Complex Tasks, Field, and Clinical Applications

6.6.3.1 Cognitive Performance Assessment

In this study, the deployment of fNIR for the purpose of cognitive state assessment while the user performs a complex task is presented [21]. This work is based on data collected during the DARPA Augmented Cognition-Technical Integration Experiment session participated by a total of 8 healthy subjects, 3 females and 5 males, ranging in age from 18 to 50. The experimental protocol for this session used a complex task resembling a videogame called the Warship Commander Task (WCT). The WCT was designed and developed by Pacific Science & Engineering Group under the direction of Space and Naval Warfare Systems Center to simulate naval air warfare management [106]. A sample screen shot during WCT is as shown in Figure 6.11a.

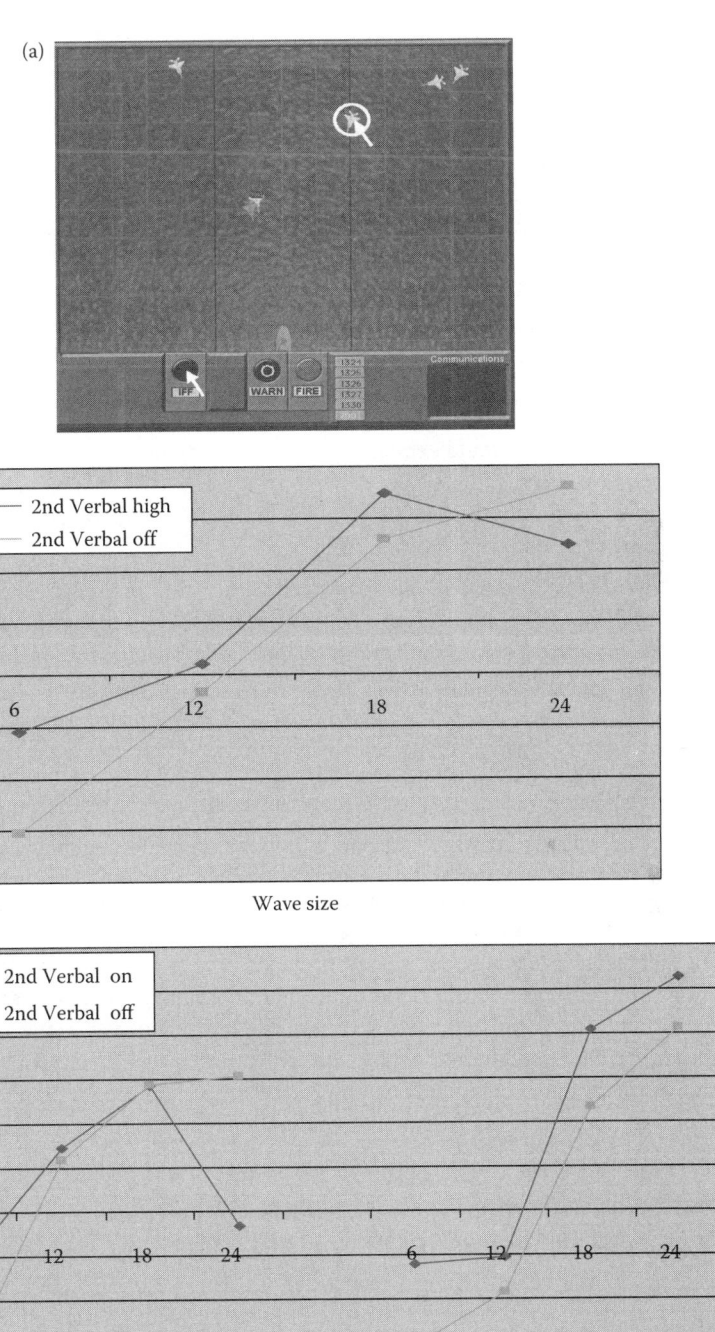

FIGURE 6.11 (a) A snapshot during WCT where air warfare management required the user to monitor "waves" of incoming airplanes, to identify the identity of the unknown ones as friendly or hostile, and to warn and then destroy hostile airplanes using rules of engagement; (b) mean oxygenation change versus wave size ($n = 8$) by secondary verbal task; (c) mean oxygenation change as a function of wave size, secondary verbal task, and average percentage of game score.

Task load and task difficulty were manipulated by changing (i) the number of airplanes that had to be managed at a given time (6, 12, 18, and 24 plane waves), (ii) the number of unknown versus known airplane identities (two levels of difficulty, *low*: 33% of the planes were unknown, and *high*: 67% of the planes were unknown), and (iii) the presence or absence of a verbal memory task (a secondary task causing divided attention). Each participant completed four sets of WCT. Each set was comprised of 3 repetitions of each of the 4 wave sizes (in the order of 6, 18, 12, and 24 planes) where each wave lasted 75 s. The factors of 4 different wave sizes, 2 different task difficulties (*high* vs. *low* percentage of unknown airplanes), and *full* versus *divided* attention (secondary verbal memory task On or Off) were crossed to create a $4 \times 2 \times 2$ repeated-measures design.

The fNIR data analysis explored (1) the relationships among cognitive workload, the participant's performance and changes in blood oxygenation levels of the dorsolateral prefrontal cortex, and (2) the effect of divided attention as elicited by the secondary component of the WCT (the auditory task). The primary hypothesis was that blood oxygenation in the prefrontal cortex, as assessed by fNIR, would rise with increasing task load and would exhibit a positive correlation with performance measures. In support of the primary hypothesis, the results indicated that the rate of change in blood oxygenation was significantly sensitive across both hemispheres ($F = 16.24$, $p < 0.001$) to task load (wave size) changes (see Figure 6.11b when secondary verbal was off).

When attention is divided by the secondary verbal task, the primary effect occurred in the 24-plane wave (the most difficult condition) causing the mean oxygenation for this case to drop below that of the 18-plane wave (see Figure 6.11c). In line with the stated hypothesis, a preliminary interpretation of this finding was that a number of participants had reached their maximal level of performance in this most difficult task level and lost their concentration/effort resulting in a drop in blood oxygenation. The hypothesis also predicts that individuals who were able to stay on task and continue to perform in this difficult condition should demonstrate increased oxygenation relative to both: (1) their own oxygenation levels in the 18-plane wave and (2) individuals who became overwhelmed and disengaged. Because sustained concentration and engagement in the task should result in increased performance, a positive correlation between performance and blood oxygenation would provide support for this interpretation. A Pearson's product-moment correlation indicated a very strong positive relationship between blood oxygenation and performance in the 24-plane condition (Pearson's $r = .89$, $p = .003$).

A median split on the Percentage Game Score provided further evidence of the hypothesized relationship between cognitive effort and the blood oxygenation response. As can be seen in Figure 6.11c, the mean levels of oxygenation were higher for both high and low performers in the 24-plane wave than the 18-plane wave when the secondary verbal task was off. However, when the secondary verbal task was on, the more difficult condition, the individuals who performed well on the 24-plane wave showed a higher mean level of oxygenation for the 24-plane wave than for the 18-plane wave, whereas those who performed poorly showed a decrease in oxygenation relative to the 18-plane wave.

6.6.3.2 Brain–Computer Interface

Brain–computer interface (BCI) is defined as a system that translates neurophysiological signals detected from the brain to supply input to a computer or to control a device. BCI research largely targets to eliminate the need for motor movement and develop mechanisms to relay information directly from the brain to a computer which, in turn, can be used to control or communicate with outside world. Development of alternative communication strategies are a recognized need for clinical applications involving patients with complete paralysis, locked-in syndrome, spinal cord injury, or muscular dystrophy. A technique that bypasses muscles and acquires signals directly from brain would be a notable help. Moreover, this technique should be minimally intrusive, noninvasive, accessible, and safe to be used continuously. In addition to their use in neuroprosthetics, noninvasive BCI systems also have potential applications for healthy individuals especially for enhancing or accelerating the learning process, or in entertainment domains such as in computer games and multimedia applications as a neurofeedback mechanism.

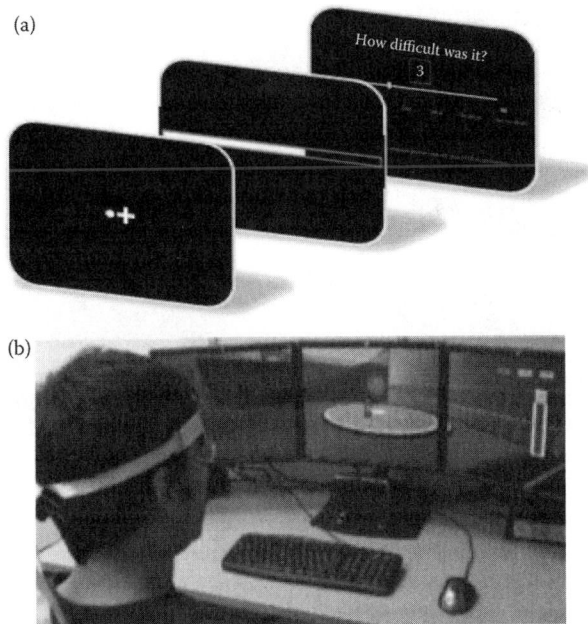

FIGURE 6.12 (a) Bar-size-control task; (b) gaming application.

The purpose of this research is to develop a new fNIR-based BCI to allow communication directly from the brain to a computer. A bar-size-control task based on a closed-loop system was designed and tested with 5 healthy subjects across two days [107]. In a single trial, subjects are first asked to rest for 20 s with a blank screen, after which a vertical or horizontal bar will appear (see Figure 6.12a). Initially, the bar is at 50% size and is mapped to the oxygenation data calculated from fNIR data that is updated at a frequency of 2 Hz. The subject is asked to concentrate on the bar for up to 120 s. Finally, the subject is asked to rate their effort on scale from 0 to 10 with 0 lowest and 10 highest effort/difficulty [108]. The subject has 30 s to complete this effort rating activity. Each trial lasts a maximum of 170 s. Comparisons of the average task and rest period oxygenation changes are significantly different ($p < 0.01$). The average task completion time (reaching + 90%) decreases with practice: day1 (mean 52.3 s) and day2 (mean 39.1 s). These preliminary results suggest that a closed-loop fNIR-based BCI can allow for a human–computer interaction with a mind switch task. Very preliminary studies incorporated fNIR technology into various 3D gaming environments that were built by student teams from Drexel University Digital Media (Figure 6.12b). Use of fNIR in this field is still an ongoing research, however preliminary results suggested that fNIR can allow participants to interact with virtual objects within the 3D environment by their thoughts.

6.6.3.3 Enhancement of Unmanned Aerial Vehicle Operator Training, Evaluation, and Interface Development

As the use of unmanned aerial vehicle (UAV) expand to near-earth applications and force-multiplying scenarios, current methods of operating UAVs and evaluating pilot performance need to expand as well. Research on human factors of UAV flight has identified several reasons underlying mishaps in UAV operations [109]. First, UAV operators have limited situational awareness due to the disembodied nature of UAV flight where operators need to fly UAVs by relying on limited camera angles. Since commands are transmitted over satellite links, UAVs are less responsive to operator input as compared to manned aircraft. In addition to this, typical UAV missions take long durations of time that require transitions

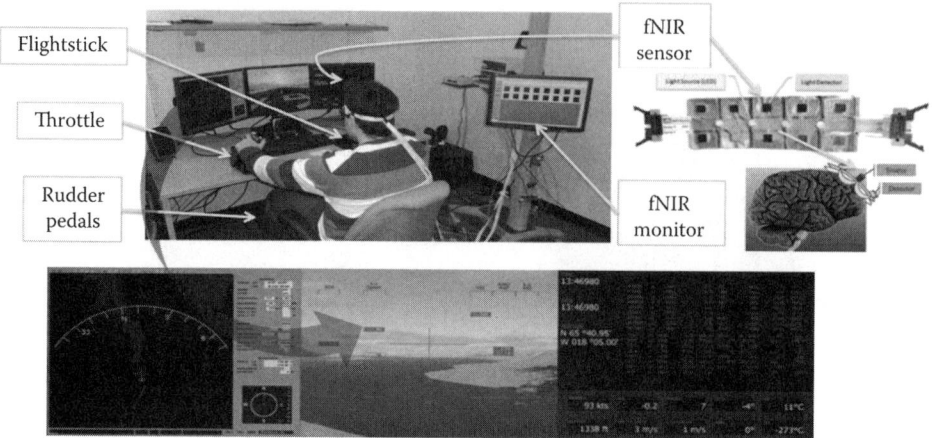

Flightstick

Throttle

Rudder
pedals

fNIR
sensor

fNIR
monitor

FIGURE 6.13 Computerized flight simulation and data collection environment.

from long periods of dull flight mode to critical moments where operators need to stay alert to engage with a target or to attend to a contingency. Many human factor studies on UAV operations rely on self-reporting surveys to assess the situational awareness and cognitive workload of an operator during a particular task which can make comparisons between operators subjective. In short, physically and cognitively taxing aspects of UAV flight have resulted in a large number of mishaps during military and civilian use. Therefore, devising reliable indices for assessing cognitive load and level of expertise are of critical importance for evaluating training regiments and interface designs, and ultimately for improving the safety and success of UAV operations.

In this project, fNIR is utilized to monitor UAV operator's cognitive workload and situational awareness during simulated missions [110]. The simulation platform is based on Microsoft's Flight Simulator X with the Predator UAV add-on by Firstclass Simulations. Using a complete joystick, throttle, and rudder pedal controller set, this simulation environment approximates an actual MQ-1 Predator user interface (Figure 6.13). After completing a demo session, each subject completes a total of 8 two-hour long training missions within 3 weeks. During each session subjects fly variants of the same mission, where they are asked to successfully take off, locate a submarine in a specified geographical area, pass over it to allow identification photographs to be taken, navigate back to an airfield with given coordinates, fly within 500 ft of the ground en route to the airfield over mountainous terrain, and successfully land after following a contingency maneuver revealed toward the end of the mission. These aspects, as well as other factors such as crosswinds, are added to the simulation to create realistic cognitive and physical demands, similar to those experienced by a real UAV pilot. This simulation environment allows replay of each session. In addition to the flight video, brain activation data is being collected by fNIR, as well as additional parameters such as pitch, roll, yaw, altitude, longitude, latitude, and air speed from within the simulation to aid in the assessment of performance (Figure 6.13).

In this ongoing study, both quantitative and qualitative methods to monitor the progress of each subject will be employed. Critical aspects of the mission that are likely to increase or decrease cognitive load (e.g., actively searching for a target, navigating toward a set of coordinates, and so on), will be identified through video analysis and the flight data. Once critical moments are identified and sampled, fNIR data collected at those moments can be correlated with operator performance to identify cognitive markers indicating expertise development and cognitive workload.

6.6.3.4 Cognitive Workload Assessment of Air Traffic Operators

The Next Generation Air Transportation System, developed by the Joint Planning and Development Office (JPDO), outlines a series of transformations designed to increase the capacity, safety, and security of air traffic operations in the United States [111]. A critical element in achieving this vision for future air-traffic management involves augmenting the current auditory-based communications between air traffic control (ATC) and the flight deck with text-based messaging, or DataComm systems. DataComm systems are expected to allow ATC to manage more air traffic at a lower level of cognitive load, thereby increasing both the capacity of the national airspace system and the safety of passengers. Although self-report measures of workload suggest that DataComm systems require less cognitive effort than voice-based systems to manage the same amount of traffic [112], to date this has not been tested using measures of neural function. The purpose of this research is to provide objective, brain-based measures of neural activity, and to determine the relative cognitive workload of DataComm versus voice-based communications systems (VoiceComm) during realistic simulations using fNIR.

In this study, fNIR has been incorporated into ongoing studies at the federal aviation administration (FAA) William J. Hughes Technical Center's (WJHTC) Research, Development, and Human Factors Laboratory, where 24 certified professional controllers (CPC) between the ages of 24 and 55 who had actively controlled traffic in an Air Route Traffic Control Center between 3 and 30 years were monitored with fNIR while they (i) performed a classic working memory (n-back) task as explained before [95,96] and (ii) managed realistic ATC scenarios under typical and emergent conditions [113]. The primary objective of this study was to use neurophysiological measures to assess cognitive workload during completion of controlled complex cognitive tasks: n-back and ATC.

For the ATC part-task, each CPC controlled traffic on workstations with a high-resolution (2048×2048), 29″ radarscope, keyboard, trackball, and direct access keypad for 10 min. To display the air traffic, the DESIREE ATC simulator and the TGF systems that were developed by software engineers at the WJHTC were used. Six simulation pilots were used within scenarios by supporting one sector or two sectors and entering data at their workstations to maneuver aircraft, all based on controller clearances. Two types of communications, either voice (VoiceComm) or data (DataComm) communications were used in separate sessions in a pseudo-random order. For each communication type, task difficulty was varied by the number of aircraft in each sector containing 6, 12, or 18 aircraft.

For the n-back fNIR data, repeated measures ANOVA showed that average oxygenation changes occurred only at voxel 2, that is, close to AF7 in the International 10–20 System, located within the left inferior frontal gyrus in the dorsolateral prefrontal cortex, was significant ($F_{3,69} = 4.37$, $p < 0.05$), see Figure 6.14a. Post-hoc analyses confirmed the differences in oxygenation changes as a function of task difficulty with 3-back is larger than the 0- and 1-back tasks (q0.05/2, 69 = 3.72, $p < 0.05$). For the ATC data, a 2 (Communication: DataComm, VoiceComm) X 2 (Prefrontal Hemisphere: right, left) X 3 (Task Difficulty: 6, 12, 18 aircrafts) ANOVA with repeated measures on all factors was calculated on mean oxygenation. Two subjects (#10, #11) were excluded from the analyses because of high-motion artifact and low signal-to-noise ratios. There were only two significant main effects: (i) task difficulty denoted by number of aircraft [$F_{2,42} = 4.39$, $p < 0.05$] and (ii) communication [$F_{1,21} = 5.09$, $p < 0.05$], which is depicted in Figure 6.14b. Tukey post-hoc tests for task difficulty ($q_{0.05/2, 42} = 3.44$, $p < 0.05$) showed than the 18 aircrafts condition (M + SD; 0.272 + 0.586 μmol) had significantly higher oxygenation change than the 12 aircrafts condition (−0.015 + 0.409 μmol). There were no other significant differences between aircraft conditions.

As a summary, fNIR results were sensitive to task difficulty specifically at left inferior frontal gyrus in the n-back test. These are in line with the earlier results [21] and with the results of fMRI studies that have used the n-back task [114]. The main hypothesis of this project is that VoiceComm would require more cognitive resources than the DataComm condition. Hence, higher activation for VoiceComm would be expected. The fNIR results from the main effect of communication type ($p < 0.05$) confirms this hypothesis with a small to moderate effect size ($d = 0.36$). These fNIR results are also in line with subjective assessments of operators as reported in earlier studies. This study indicated that operator's cognitive effort for different types of tasks can be objectively assessed by comparing fNIR results. One of the major advantages of using fNIR in this study is that it allowed monitoring brain activity of the ground operators in realistic settings.

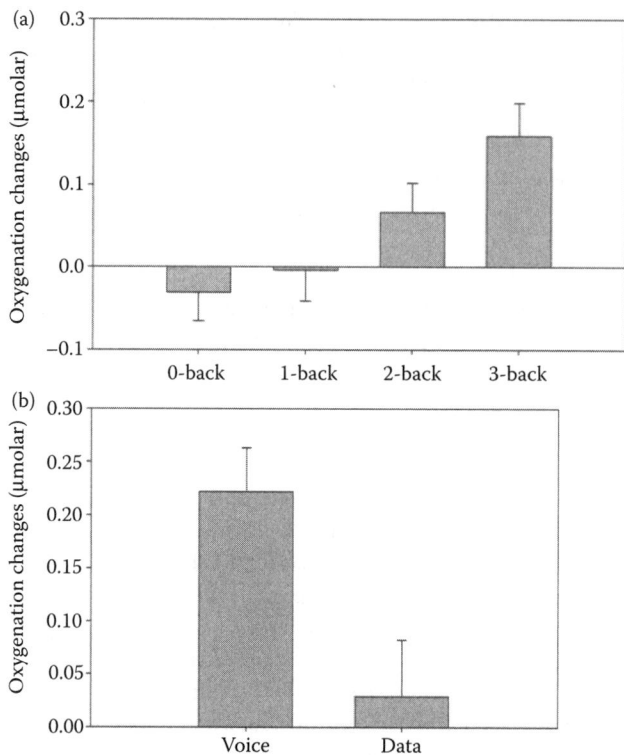

FIGURE 6.14 (a) Average oxygenation changes of all subjects (24 subjects, and 160 trials for each condition) with increasing task difficulty (n-back tasks). (b) Average oxygenation changes for DataComm and VoiceComm ($N = 22$). Error bars are SEM.

6.6.3.5 Cognitive Activity Assessment Following Traumatic Brain Injury on Attention Domain

A commonly observed consequence of traumatic brain injury (TBI) is cognitive impairment, whose assessment represents a considerable challenge. Additionally, the choice of a successful treatment among the many existing neurorehabilitation strategies still relies on behavioral observation, and little information is available about the physiological changes produced at the brain level by the specific intervention. The integration of neuroimaging and electrophysiological measures may be more objective and effective in the evaluation of cognitive impairments. This study evaluates the applicability of fNIR for assessment of TBI-induced impairments of attention [115]. Participants included five male TBI patients between 18 and 37 years old. Brain activation measures were collected during a target categorization (oddball) task as explained before. The pattern of the hemodynamic response elicited by the two classes was in agreement with previous studies that investigated the applicability of fNIR to the study of attention-related tasks. The changes in the concentration of oxy-Hb and deoxy-Hb differ between target-locked and nontarget-locked responses: target stimuli elicited in fact a more marked activation in the areas of the prefrontal cortex monitored by fNIR. This pilot study suggests the potential for fNIR to be applied to the monitoring of attention in the TBI population.

6.6.3.6 Cognitive Activity Assessment Following TBI on Working Memory Domain

Behavioral observation and neuropsychological tests have guided the planning of cognitive rehabilitation and the assessment of its effectiveness. However, the information about the actual changes that rehabilitation interventions induce at the brain level is still limited. The availability of this information would, instead, prove useful for a more objective and individualized approach to the evaluation of a treatment efficacy. To this end, the integration of functional neuroimaging in the evaluation of cognitive impairments could offer a more objective monitoring of rehabilitation outcomes.

The aim of this study is to demonstrate the applicability of fNIR, to the assessment of working memory after TBI [116]. Participants included four TBI and ten healthy controls. Neuropsychological evaluation of attention and working memory was based on the WAIS-III Digit Span and WAIS-III Letter-Number Sequencing. Brain activation measurements were collected through fNIR during a visual n-back task as explained before. Physiologically irrelevant data and noise were eliminated from fNIR measurements and the maximum change in oxy-Hb and deoxy-Hb concentration was obtained for the left and right dorsolateral prefrontal areas.

On the basis of the performance in the neuropsychological tests, the TBI group revealed impaired learning performance as compared to the group of healthy controls. Evaluation of fNIR data revealed a pattern in the hemodynamic activity that was significantly different between the healthy controls and the TBI patients in the DLPFC, known to be involved in the working memory processes. The results obtained in this preliminary study show that fNIR is a promising neuroimaging tool that can prove to be clinically useful to investigate and identify the neurological underpinnings of cognitive functioning after TBI. In particular, fNIR offers to neurorehabilitation some unique advantages over other conventional neuroimaging techniques: fNIR is in fact portable, low-cost, noninvasive, and allows a reasonably flexible task design.

6.6.3.7 Depth of Anesthesia Monitoring

Awareness is an unintended mental state during general anesthesia. An accurate, objective measure of return to consciousness would provide an important safeguard for patients and physicians alike. This exploratory investigation on predicting awareness under general anesthesia examines the hypothesis that the transition from deep to light anesthetic stages is associated with reliable changes in oxygenated, deoxygenated, and total hemoglobin in frontal cortex. Hemodynamic changes during deep and light anesthesia were examined in 26 nonbrain surgery patients [55]. fNIR recordings are collected in the operating room before, during, and after subjects were receiving their scheduled anesthetic and surgical procedures. The results suggest that the rate of deoxygenated hemoglobin change can be used as a descriptive neuromarker to differentiate between deep and light anesthesia stages ($F = 7.61$, $p < 0.01$). This marker is proposed for further development as an index of the depth of anesthesia for the purpose of monitoring awareness under general anesthesia.

In addition to the neuropsychological findings, this research demonstrates engineering and signal processing solutions in the form of customized algorithms and procedures that allow fNIR to measure usable signals under field conditions. ICA and PCA were combined in a novel procedure that employed dark current (i.e., signal from noncortical sources) as a reference measurement. This method provided improved signal-to-noise ratio for the hemodynamic measurements acquired in the operating room, and can be used to increase the signal quality of fNIR for many other applications and field situations.

6.6.4 Future Directions

Since fNIR technology is still relatively new in comparison with other neuroimaging technologies, the research published to date has been relatively conservative—focusing on establishing fNIR as a valid and reliable neuroimaging technology. Furthermore clinical investigations have also been very limited. As a result, the majority of published fNIR studies have not capitalized on the unique capabilities of the technique because of the need to validate the results with known technologies such as fMRI. We believe that the studies explained in the previous section represent examples of how fNIR can be used in research and clinical paradigms that may not be feasible with other neuroimaging technologies and may facilitate research by acquainting clinicians and researchers with the unique merits of fNIR as a brain-imaging technology.

There are several types of clinical applications that could benefit from the unique attributes of fNIR neuroimaging technology in the future:

- Populations that may not be able to readily tolerate the confines of an fMRI magnet, or be able to remain sufficiently still, for example, schizophrenics, autistic children, and neonates
- Populations that require the long-term monitoring of cerebral oxygenation, for example, premature and other high-risk infants
- Studies that require repeated, low-cost neuroimaging, for example, treatment studies that image the cortex for efficacy
- Applications where an fMRI system would be too expensive or cumbersome, for example, for use in a clinical office
- Applications that require ecological validity, for example, working at a computer, or in an educational setting

6.7 Conclusion

fNIR is an emerging technology that uses near-infrared light to measure changes in the concentration of oxygenated and deoxygenated hemoglobin in the cortex. The use of fNIR technology has increased in recent years as a means to measure hemodynamic changes in the cortex in response to cognitive activity. Although fNIR imaging is limited to the outer cortex, it provides neuroimaging that is safe, portable, and very affordable relative to other neuroimaging technologies that can be applied in the laboratory as well as field conditions. Moreover, it is a noninvasive and negligibly intrusive optical imaging modality. It is also relatively robust to movement artifacts, and can readily be integrated with other technologies such as EEG. Current state-of-the-art technologies include portable and wireless fNIR systems, data processing algorithms, and end-user software.

In this chapter, an overview of basis of optical imaging, fNIR instrumentation and signal analysis and cognitive studies carried out in the literature are summarized. In these studies, fNIR has been demonstrated to have adequate validity in the measurement of functional brain activity during a variety of cognitive, emotional, and motor tasks in healthy and diseased subject groups of both adult and children populations, and has the potential to provide a flexible neuroimaging tool for clinicians and researchers alike. The findings are in agreement with the results in current EEG and fMRI literature. The portable and wireless instrumentations, combined with robust analysis algorithms and end-user software, make fNIR a viable option for the study of cognition- and emotion-related hemodynamic changes in both adults and children, under either stationary or ambulant conditions.

Acknowledgments

The author would like to thank Drs. Banu Onaral, Kambiz Pourrezaei, Scott Bunce, Patricia Shewokis, Kurtulus Izzetoglu, Hasan Ayaz, Anna Merzagora, Britton Chance, Shoko Nioka, Jose Leon-Carrion, Murat Cakir, Ajit Devaraj, and Mr. Justin Menda and Mr. Adrian Curtin for their advice and help in the preparation of this chapter and sharing their work and results.

References

1. Jobsis FF. 1977. Noninvasive infrared monitoring of cerebral and myocardial sufficiency and circulatory parameters. *Science,* 198:1264–1267.
2. Cope M, Delpy, D. T. 1988. System for long-term measurement of cerebral blood flow and tissue oxygenation on newborn infants by infra-red transillumination. *Med. Biol. Eng. Comput.,* 26:289–294.

3. Luo Q, Zeng S, Chance B, Nioka S. 2002. Monitoring of brain activation with near infrared spectroscopy. Chapter 8 in *Handbook of Optical Biomedical Diagnostics*, Editor: Valery V. Tuchin, Press Monograph PM107, Bellingham, WA.

4. Rolfe P. 2000. *In vivo* near-infrared spectroscopy. *Annu. Rev. Biomed. Eng.*, 02:715–754.

5. Strangman G, Boas DA, Sutton JP. 2002. Non-invasive neuroimaging using near-infrared light. *Biol. Psychiatry*, 52(7):679–693.

6. Hoshi Y, Tamura M. 1993. Dynamic multichannel near-infrared optical imaging of human brain activity. *J. Appl. Phys.*, 75:1842–1846.

7. Hoshi Y. 2003. Functional near-infrared optical imaging: Utility and limitations in human brain mapping. *Psychophysiology*, 40:511–520.

8. Villringer A, Planck J, Hock C, Schleinkofer L, Dirnagl U. 1993. Near infrared spectroscopy (NIRS): A new tool to study hemodynamic changes during activation of brain function in human adults. *Neurosci. Lett.*, 154:101–104.

9. Villringer A, Chance B. 1997. Non-invasive optical spectroscopy and imaging of human brain function. *Trends Neurosci.*, 20:435–442.

10. Suto T, Ito M, Uehara T, Ida I, Fukuda M, Mikuni M. 2002. Temporal characteristics of cerebral blood volume change in motor and somatosensory cortices revealed by multichannel near infrared spectroscopy. *Int. Congress Series*, 1232:383–388.

11. Maki A, Yamashita Y, Ito Y, Watanabe E, Mayanagi Y, Koizumi H. 1995. Spatial and temporal analysis of human motor activity by using noninvasive NIR topography. *J. Neurosci.*, 11:1458–1469.

12. Gratton E, Toronov V, Wolf U, Wolf M, Webb A. 2005. Measurement of brain activity by near infrared light. *J. Biol. Optics,* 10(1)011008-1-13.

13. Franceschini MA, Boas DA. 2004. Noninvasive measurement of neuronal activity with near-infrared optical imaging. *Neuroimage*, 21:372–386.

14. Gratton G, Corballis PM, Cho E, Fabiani M, Hood DC. 1995. Shades of gray matter: Noninvasive optical images of human brain responses during visual stimulation. *Psychophysiology*, 32:505–509.

15. Heekeren HR, Obrig H, Wenzel R, Eberle K, Ruben J, Villringer K, Kurth R, Villringer A. 1997. Cerebral haemoglobin oxygenation during sustained visual stimulation—A near infrared spectroscopy study. *Physiol. Trans. Biol. Sci.*, 352:743–750.

16. Sato, H, Takeuchi T, Sakai K. 1999. Temporal cortex activation during speech recognition: An optical topography study. *Cognition*, 40:548–560.

17. Zaramella P, Freato F, Amigoni A, Salvadori S, Marangoni P, Suppjei A. 2001. Brain auditory activation measured by near-infrared spectroscopy. *Ped. Res.*, 49:213–219.

18. Son Il-Y, Guhe M, Yazici B. 2005. Human performance assessment using fNIR. *Proc. SPIE*, 5797:158–169.

19. Cope M. 1991. *The Development of a Near-Infrared Spectroscopy System and Its Application for Noninvasive Monitoring of Cerebral Blood and Tissue Oxygenation in the Newborn Infant*. Ph.D. thesis. University College London, London.

20. Bunce SC, Devaraj A, Izzetoglu M, Onaral B, Pourrezaei K. 2005a. Detecting deception in the brain: A functional near-infrared spectroscopy study of neural correlates of intentional deception. *Nondest. Detection Meas. Homeland Security III, Proc. SPIE*, 5769:24–32.

21. Izzetoglu K, Bunce S, Onaral B, Pourrezaei K, Chance B, 2004. Functional optical brain imaging using near-infrared during cognitive tasks. *Int. J. Human-Comp. Int.*, 17(2):211–227.

22. Izzetoglu K, Yurtsever G, Bozkurt A, Yazici B, Bunce S, Pourrezaei K, Onaral B. 2003a. NIR spectroscopy measurements of cognitive load elicited by GKT and target categorization. *Proceedings of 36th Hawaii International Conference on System Sciences*, Philadelphia, PA.

23. Izzetoglu M, Izzetoglu K, Bunce S, Ayaz H, Devaraj A, Onaral B, Pourrezaei K. 2005b. Functional near-infrared neuroimaging. *IEEE Trans. Neural Sys. Rehab. Eng.*, 13(2):153–159.

24. Platek SM, Fonteyn LCM, Izzetoglu M, Myers TE, Ayaz H, Li C, Chance B. 2005. Functional near infrared spectroscopy reveals differences in self-other processing as a function of schizotypal personality traits. *Schizophrenia Res.* 73(1):125–127.

25. Rajapakse JC, Kruggel F, Maisog JM, Von Cramon DY. 1998. Modelin hemodynamic response for analysis of functional MRI time series. *Hum. Brain Mapp.*, 6:283–300.
26. Magistretti PR, Pellerin L. 1999. Cellular mechanisms of brain energy metabolism and their relevance to functional brain imaging. *Phil. Trans. R. Soc. Lond. B*, 354(1387):1155–1163.
27. Magistretti PR. 2000. Cellular bases of functional brain imaging: Insights from neuron-glia metabolic coupling. *Brain Res.*, 886(1–2):108–112.
28. Ames A III. 2000. CNS energy metabolism as related to function. *Brain Res. Brain Res. Rev.* 34:42–68.
29. Fox PT, Raichle ME, Mintun MA, Dence C. 1988. Nonoxidative glucose consumption during focal physiologic neural activity. *Science*, 241:462–464.
30. Buxton RB, Uludag K, Dubowitz DJ, Liu TT. 2004. Modeling the hemodynamic response to brain activation. *Neuroimage*, 23(Suppl. 1):S220–233.
31. Buxton RB. 2001. The elusive initial dip. *Neuroimage*, 13: 953–958.
32. Obrig H, Villringer A. 2003. Beyond the visible—Imaging the human brain with light. *J. Cereb. Blood Flow Metab.*, 23:1–18.
33. Miezin FM, Maccotta L, Ollinger JM, Petersen SE, Buckner RL. 2000. Characterizing the hemodynamic response: Effects of presentation rate, sampling procedure, and the possibility of ordering brain activity based on relative timing. *NeuroImage*, 11:735–759.
34. Haensse D, Szabo P, Brown D, Fauchère JC, Niederer P, Bucher HU, Wolf M. 2005. A new multichannel near infrared spectrophotometry system for functional studies of the brain in adults and neonates. *Optics Exp.*, 13(12):4525–4538.
35. Ogawa S, Lee TM, Nayak AS, Glynn P. 1990. Oxygenation-sensitive contrast in magnetic resonance image of rodent brain at high magnetic fields. *Magn. Reson. Med.*, 14:68–78.
36. Kwong KK, Belliveau JW, Chesler DA, Goldberg IE, Weisskoff RM, Poncelet BP, Kennedy DN. et al. 1992. Dynamic magnetic resonance imaging of human brain activity during primary sensory stimulation. *PNAS*, 89:5951–5955.
37. Chance B, Cope M, Gratton E, Ramanujam N, Tromberg B. 1998. Phase measurement of light absorption and scatter in human tissue. *Rev. Sci. Instrum.*, 69:3457–3482.
38. Gratton G, Maier JS, Fabiani M, Mantulinm WW, Gratton E. 1994. Feasibility of intracranial near-infrared optical scanning. *Psychophysiology*, 31:211–215.
39. Chance B, Leig JS, Miyake H, Smith DS, Nioka S, Greenfeld R, Finander M, Kaufmann K, Levy W. et al. 1988. Comparison of time-resolved and un-resolved measurements of deoxyhemoglobin in brain. *PNAS*, 85:4971–4975.
40. Firbank M, Okada E, Delpy DT. 1998. A theoretical study of the signal contribution of regions of the adult head to near infrared spectroscopy studies of visual evoked responses. *NeuroImage*, 8:69–78.
41. Delpy DT, Cope M, van der Zee P, Arridge S, Wray S, Wyatt J. 1988. Estimation of optical pathlength through tissue from direct time of flight measurement. *Phys. Med. Biol*, 33:1433–1442.
42. Lakowicz, J. R, Berndt, K. 1990. Frequency domain measurement of photon migration in tissues. *Chem. Phys. Lett.*, 166:246–252.
43. Wolf M, Ferrari M, Quaresima V. 2007. Progress of near-infrared spectroscopy and topography for brain and muscle clinical applications. *J. Biomed. Optics*, 12(6):062104-1–14.
44. Obrig H, Wenzel R, Kohl M, Horst S, Wobst P, Steinbrink J, Thomas F, Villringer A. 2000. Near-infrared spectroscopy: Does it function in functional activation studies of the adult brain? *Int. J. Psychophysiol.*, 35:125–142.
45. Boas DA, Franceschini MA, Dunn AK, Strangman G. 2002. *Non-Invasive Imaging of Cerebral Activation with Diffuse Optical Tomography. In-Vivo Optical Imaging of Brain Function*. Boca Raton: CRC Press. pp. 193–221.
46. Chance B, Anday E, Nioka S, Zhou S, Hong L, Worden K, Li C, Murray T, Ovetsky Y, Pidikiti D, Thomas R. 1998. A novel method for fast imaging of brain function, non-invasively, with light. *Optics Exp.*, 2(10):411–423.

47. Rector DM, Poe GR, Kristensen MP, Harper RM. 1997. Light scattering changes follow evoked potentials from hippocampal Schaeffer collateral stimulation. *J. Neurophysiol.*, 78:1707–1713.

48. Stepnoski RA, LaPorta A, Raccuia-Behling F, Blonder GE, Slusher RE, Kleinfeld D. 1991. Noninvasive detection of changes in membrane potential in cultured neurons by light scattering. *PNAS*, 88:9382–9386.

49. Bunce S, Izzetoglu M, Izzetoglu K, Onaral B, Pourrezaei K, 2006. Functional near infrared spectroscopy: An emerging neuroimaging modality. *IEEE Engineering in Medicine and Biology Magazine, Special issue on Clinical Neuroengineering*, 25(4):54–62.

50. Bozkurt A, Onaral B. 2004. Safety assessment of near infrared light emitting diodes for diffuse optical measurements. *Biomed. Eng. Online*, 3(9):1–10.

51. Boas DA, Dale AM, Francheschini MA. 2004. Diffuse optical imaging of brain activation: Approaches to optimizing image sensitivity, resolution, and accuracy. *Neuroimage*, 23:S275–S288.

52. Huppert TJ, Diamond SG, Franceschini MA, Boas DA. 2009. HomER: A review of timeseries analysis methods for near-infrared spectroscopy of the brain. *Appl. Opt.*, 48(10):280–298.

53. Izzetoglu M, Bunce S, Izzetoglu K, Onaral B, Pourrezaei K. 2007. Functional brain imaging using near infrared technology for cognitive activity assessment. *IEEE Engineering in Medicine and Biology Magazine, Special issue on on the Role of Optical Imaging in Augmented Cognition*, 26(4):38–46.

54. Sato H, Tanaka N, Uchida M, Hirabayashi Y, Kanai M, Ashida T, Konishi I, Maki A. 2006. Wavelet analysis for detecting body-movement artifacts in optical topography signals. *Neuroimage*, 33:580–587.

55. Izzetoglu K. 2008. *Neural Correlates of Cognitive Workload and Anesthetic Depth: fNIR Spectroscopy Investigation in Humans*. Ph.D. thesis, Drexel University, Philadelphia, PA.

56. Robertson FC, Douglas TS, Meintjes EM. 2010. Motion artefact removal for functional near infrared spectroscopy: A comparison of methods. *IEEE Trans. Biomed. Eng.*, 57(6):1377–1387.

57. Izzetoglu M, Devaraj A, Bunce S, Onaral B. 2005. Motion artifact cancellation in NIR spectroscopy using Wiener filtering. *IEEE Trans. Biomed. Eng.*, 52(5):934–938.

58. Izzetoglu M, Chitrapu P, Bunce S, Onaral B. 2010. Motion artifact cancellation in NIR spectroscopy using discrete Kalman filtering. *Biomed. Eng. Online*, 9(16):1–10.

59. Cui X, Bray S, Reiss AL. 2010. Functional near infrared spectroscopy (NIRS) signal improvement based on negative correlation between oxygenated and deoxygenated hemoglobin dynamics. *Neuroimage*, 49:3039–3046.

60. Devaraj A. 2005. *Signal Processing for Functional Near Infrared Neuroimaging*. Master's thesis, Drexel University, Philadelphia, PA.

61. Izzetoglu M, Nioka S, Chance B, Onaral B. 2005. Single trial hemodynamic response estimation in a block anagram solution study using fNIR spectroscopy. *Proceedings of ICASSP Conference*, Vol. 5, pp: 633–636.

62. Obrig H, Neufang M, Wenzel R, Kohl M, Steinbrink J, Einhaupl K, Villringer A. 2000. Spontaneous low frequency oscillations of cerebral hemodynamics and metabolism in human adults. *Neuroimage*, 12:623–639.

63. Mayhew J, Askew S, Zheng Y, Porrill J, Westby GWM, Redgrave P, Rector DM, Harper RM. 1996. Cerebral vasomotion: A 0.1 hz oscillation in refleted light imaging of neural acitvity, *Neuroimage*, 4:183–193.

64. Lundberg N. 1960. Continuous recordings and control of ventricular fluid pressure in neurosurgical practice. *Acta Psychiatrica et Neurologica Scandinavica*, 149:1–193.

65. Diamond SG, Huppert TJ, Kolehmainen V, Franceschini MA, Kaipio JP, Arridge SR, Boas DA. 2005. Physiological system identification with the Kalman filter in diffuse optical tomography. *Lecture Notes in Computer Science*, 3750:649–656.

66. Zhang Q, Strangman GE, Ganis G. 2009. Adaptive filtering to reduce global interference in non-invasive NIRS measures of brain activation: How well and when does it work? *Neuroimage*, 45:788–794.

67. Zhang Y, Brooks DH, Francheschini MA, Boas DA. 2005. Eigenvector-based spatial filtering for reduction of physiological interference in diffuse optical imaging. *J. Biomed. Opt.*, 10(1):011014.

68. Gratton G, Corballis PM. 1995. Removing the heart from the brain: Compensation for the pulse artifact in the photon migration signal. *Psychophysiology*, 32:292–299.

69. Morren G, Wolf U, Lemmerling P, Wolf M, Choi JH, Gratton E, De Lathauwer L, Van Huffel S. 2004. Detection of fast neuronal signals in the motor cortex from functional near infrared spectroscopy measurements using independent component analysis. *Med. Biol. Eng. Comput.*, 42(1):92–99.

70. Glover GH, Li TQ, Ress D. 2000. Image-based method for retrospective correction of physiological motion effects in fMRI: RETROICOR. *Magn. Reson. Med.*, 44:162–167.

71. Yamada T, Umeyama S, Matsuda K. 2009. Multidistance probe arrangement to eliminate artifacts in functional near-infrared spectroscopy. *J. Biomed. Opt.*, 14(6):064034.

72. Arridge SR, Schweiger M. 1997. Image reconstruction in optical tomography. *Phil. Trans. R. Soc. Lond. B*, 352:717–726.

73. Boas DA, Brooks DH, Miller EL, DiMarzio CA, Kilmer M, Gaudette RJ, Zhang Q. 2001. Imaging the body with diffuse optical tomography. *IEEE Sign. Proc. Mag.*, 18:57–75.

74. Son IY, Yazici B. 2006. Near infrared imaging and spectroscopy for brain activity monitoring. Advances in Sensing with Security Applications, pp: 341–372, NATO Advanced Study Institute, NATO Security through Science Series-A: Chemistry and Biology, Springer, Edited by J. Byrnes.

75. Ishimaru A. 1997. *Wave Propagation and Scattering in Random Media*. New York: IEEE Press.

76. Tromberg BJ, Svaasand LO, Tsay T, Haskell RC. 1993. Properties of photon density waves in multiple-scattering media. *Appl. Optics*, 32:607–616.

77. Hillman E. 2002. *Experimental and Theoretical Investigations of Near Infrared Tomographic Imaging Methods and Clinical Applications*. Ph.D. thesis, University College London, London.

78. Patterson MS, Chance B, Wilson BC. 1989. Time resolved reflectance and transmittance for the non-invasive measurement of tissue optical properties. *Appl. Optics*, 28(12):2331–2336.

79. Sassaroli A, Fantini S. 2004. Comment on the modified Beer–Lambert law for scattering media. *Phys. Med. Biol.*, 49:N255–N257.

80. Tachtsidis I. 2005. *Experimental Measurements of Cerebral Haemodynamics and Oxygenation and Comparisons with a Computational Model: A Near-Infrared Spectroscopy Investigation*. Ph.D. thesis, University College London, London.

81. Duncan A, Meek JH, Clemence M, Elwell CE, Tyszczuk L, Cope M, Delpy DT. 1995. Optical pathlength measurements on adult head, calf and forearm and the head of the newborn infant using phase resolved optical spectroscopy. *Phys. Med. Biol.*, 40:295–304.

82. Hiraoka M, Firbank M, Essenpreis M, Cope M, Arridge SR, van der Zee P, Delpy DT. 1993. A Monte Carlo investigation of optical pathlength in inhomogeneous tissue and its application to near-infrared spectroscopy. *Phys. Med. Biol.*, 38:1859–1876.

83. Kohl M, Nolte C, Heekeren HR, Horst S, Scholz U, Obrig H, Villringer A. 1998. Determination of the wavelength dependence of the differential pathlength factor from near-infrared pulse signals. *Phys Med Biol.*, 43(6):1771–1782.

84. Duncan A, Meek JH, Clemence M, Elwell CE, Fallon P, Tyszczuk L, Cope M, Delpy DT. 1996. Measurement of cranial optical path length as a function of age using phase resolved near infrared spectroscopy. *Pediatr. Res.*, 39(5):889–894.

85. Meek JH, Firbank M, Elwell CE, Atkinson J, Braddick O, Wyatt JS. 1998. Regional hemodynamic responses to visual stimulation in awake infants. *Pediatr. Res.*, 43:840–843.

86. Sakatani K, Katayama Y, Yamamoto T, Suzuki S. 1999. Changes in cerebral blood oxygenation of the frontal lobe induced by direct electrical stimulation of thalamus and globus pallidus: A near infrared spectroscopy study. *J. Neurol. Neurosurg. Psych.*, 67:769–773.

87. Watanabe E, Maki A, Kawaguchi F, Yamashita Y, Koizumi H, Mayanagi Y. 2000. Noninvasive cerebral blood volume measurement during seizures using multichannel near infrared spectroscopic topography. *J. Biomed. Opt.*, 5:287–290.

88. Haginoya K, Munakata M, Kato R, Yokoyama H, Ishizuka M, Iinuma K. 2002. Ictal cerebral haemodynamics of childhood epilepsy measured with nearinfrared spectrophotometry. *Brain*, 125(9):1960–1971.

89. Hock C, Villringer K, Muller-Spahn F, Hofmann H, Heekeren H, Schuh-Hofer S. 1996. Near infrared spectroscopy in the diagnosis of Alzheimer's disease. *Ann. N.Y. Acad. Sci.*, 777:22–29.

90. Okada F, Tokumitsu Y, Hoshi Y, Tamura M. 1994. Impaired interhemispheric integration in brain oxygenation and hemodynamics in schizophrenia. *Eur. Arch. Psych. Clin. Neurosci.*, 244:17–25.

91. Fallgatter AJ, Strik WK. 2000. Reduced frontal functional asymmetry in schizophrenia during a cued continuous performance test assessed with nearinfrared spectroscopy. *Schizophr. Bull*, 26(4):913–919.

92. Eschweiler GW, Wegerer C, Schlotter W, Spandl C, Stevens A, Bartels M. 2000. Left prefrontal activation predicts therapeutic effects of repetitive transcranial magnetic stimulation (rTMS) in major depression. *Psych. Res.*, 99:161–172.

93. Irani F, Platek SM, Bunce S, Ruocco AC, Chute D. 2007. Functional near infrared spectroscopy (fNIRS): An emerging neuroimaging technology with important applications for the study of brain disorders. *Clin. Neuropsychol.*, 21:9–37.

94. Cabeza R, Nyberg L. 2000. "Imaging Cognition II: An empirical Review of 275 PET and fMRI Studies." *J. Cogn. Neurosci.*, 12:1–47.

95. Smith EE, Jonides J. 1997. "Working Memory: A View from Neuroimaging," *Cogn. Psychol.* 33:5–42.

96. Smith EE, Jonides J. 1999. Storage and executive processes in the frontal lobes. *Science*, 283:1657–1661.

97. Braver TS, Cohen JD, Nystrom LE, Jonides J. Smith EE, Noll DC. 1997. A parametric study of prefrontal cortex involvement in human working memory. *NeuroImage*, 5:49–62.

98. McCarthy G, Luby M, Gore J, Goldman-Rakic P. 1997. Infrequent events transiently activate human prefrontal and parietal cortex as measured by functional MRI. *J. Neurophysiol.*, 77:1630–1634.

99. Polich J, Kok A. 1995. Cognitive and biological determinants of P300: An integrative review. *Biol. Psychol.*, 41:103–146.

100. Ardekani BA, Choi SJ, Hossein-Zadeh G, Porjesz B, Tanabe JL, Lim KO, Bilder R, Helpern JA, Begleiter H. 2002. Functional magnetic resonance imaging of brain activity in the visual oddball task. *Cogn. Brain Res.*, 14:347–356.

101. Leon-Carrion J, Izzetoglu M, Izzetoglu K, Martin-Rodriguez JF, Damas-Lopez J, Martin JM, Dominguez-Morales MR. 2010. Efficient learning produces spontaneous neural repetition suppression in prefrontal cortex. *Behav. Brain Res.*, 208(2):502–508.

102. Strangman G, Franceschini MA, Boas DA. 2003. Factors affecting the accuracy of near-infrared spectroscopy concentration calculations for focal changes in oxygenation parameters. *Neuroimage*, 18:865–879.

103. Huppert TJ, Hoge RD, Diamond SG, Franceschini MA, Boas DA. 2006. A temporal comparison of BOLD, ASL, and NIRS hemodynamic responses to motor stimuli in adult humans. *Neuroimage*, 29:368–382.

104. Chance B., Nioka S., Sadi S., Li C. 2003. Oxygenation and blood concentration changes in human subject prefrontal activation by anagram solutions. *Adv. Exp. Med. Biol.*, 510:397–401.

105. Leon-Carrion J, Martin-Rodriguez JF, Damas-Lopez J, Pourrezai K, Izzetoglu K, Martin JM, Dominguez-Morales MR, 2007. A lasting post-stimulus activation on dorsolateral prefrontal cortex is produced when processing valence and arousal in visual affective stimuli. *Neurosci. Lett.*, 422(3):147–152.

106. John M, Kobus DA et al. 2002. A multi-tasking environment for manipulating and measuring neural Correlates of cognitive workload". *Proceedings of the IEEE 7th Conference on Human Factors and Power Plants*, 7:10–14.

107. Ayaz H, Shewokis P, Bunce S, Schultheis M, Onaral B. 2009. Assessment of Cognitive Neural Correlates for a Functional Near Infrared-based Brain Computer Interface System. Dylan D. Schmorrow at al. (eds.): Augmented Cognition, HCII 2009, Lecture Notes on Artificial Intelligence, 2009, vol. 5638:699–708, Berlin, Heidelberg: Springer-Verlag (presented at the 13th International Conference on Human-Computer Interaction, July 19–24 2009, San Diego, CA).

108. Paas FGWC, Van Merriënboer JJG. 1993. The efficiency of instructional conditions: An approach to combine mental effort and performance measures. human factors. *J. Hum. Fact. Ergon. Soc.*, 35:737–743.

109. Cooke NJ, Pringle H, Pederson H, Connor O, Salas E. 2006. *Human Factors of Remotely Operated Vehicles*. The Netherlands: Elsevier.

110. Cakir MP, Ayaz H, Menda J, Izzetoglu K, Onaral B. 2010. Connecting brain and learning sciences: An optical brain imaging approach to monitoring development of expertise in UAV piloting. *Proceedings of ICLS2010 Conference*, June 29–July 2 2010, Chicago, IL.

111. JPDO. 2004. Next Generation Air Transportation System Integrated Plan. Retrieved from http://www.jpdo.gov/library/NGATS_v1_1204r.pdf.

112. Hah S, Willems B, Phillips R. 2006. The effect of air traffic increase on controller workload. *Proceedings of the Human Factors and Ergonomics Society Annual Meeting San Francisco*, CA.

113. Ayaz H, Willems B, Bunce S, Shawokis PA, Izzetoglu K, Hah S, Deshmukh AR, Onaral B. 2010. Cognitive workload assessment of air traffic Controllers Using Optical Brain Imaging Sensors. *Proceedings of AHFE2010 Conference*, July 17–20 2010, Miami, FL.

114. Owen AM, McMillan KM, Laird AR, Bullmore E. 2005. N-back working memory paradigm: A meta-analysis of normative functional neuroimaging studies. *Hum. Brain Mapp.*, 25(1):46–59.

115. Merzagora AC., Izzetoglu M., Onaral B., Schultheis M. 2010. "fNIRS as a useful tool for cognitive evaluation following traumatic brian injury", *8th World Congress on Brian Injury*, March 10–14, 2010, Washington, DC.

116. Merzagora A.C, Martin-Rodriguez J.F, Longo Perez A, Leon-Dominguez U, Izzetoglu K, Schultheis M, Onaral B, Leon-Carrion J. 2010. "Applicability of fNIRS to the TBI population: Demonstration on an attention task", *8th World Congress on Brian Injury*, March 10–14, 2010, Washington, DC.

7

Causality Analysis of Multivariate Neural Data

Maciej Kamiński
University of Warsaw

Hualou Liang
Drexel University

7.1 Introduction

With the rapid advances in multielectrode recording and brain-imaging techniques that have occurred in recent years, multichannel data sets have become increasingly obtainable. While standard signal-processing techniques such as crosscorrelations in the time domain and coherence in the frequency domain remain the main statistics for assessing interactions among these multichannel data, it is increasingly felt that these symmetric interdependence measures are no longer sufficient for many intended applications, and further partitioning of relationships among a set of simultaneously recorded signals is needed to parcel out the functional connectivity of complex neural networks. Recent work has begun to explore a class of techniques called Granger causality as a potentially useful addition to the current analytical repertoire in the attempt to add directionality to neural interactions.

In this chapter, we want to give an overview of specific issues concerning multivariate data analysis, present available tools and give a few examples of their applications. The functions will be presented from practical point of view, which means that some technical and mathematical details will not be elaborated here. Instead, for further reading there will be bibliography references. We start with the standard symmetric measures for evaluating the statistical interdependence between two time series. We then discuss practical issues concerning how to estimate such measures from time series data with special emphasis on multivariate autoregressive (MAR) model, from which the Granger causality and its partial measures can be derived. Key technical issues of the causal measures concerning stationarity/nonstationarity, bivariate/multivariate, linearity/nonlinearity, and statistical significance are specifically addressed. Finally, we present several selected applications in the analysis of spike trains, EEG, and fMRI BOLD data, each representing a major recording modality used in neuroscience research, followed by a demonstration of clinical application in seizure localization in epilepsy patients. These applications together demonstrate that causality measures can reveal insights that are not possible with traditional analytical techniques.

7.2 Cross-Estimators, Time, and Frequency Domain

The most important part of multichannel data analysis is estimation of the influence of one signal from the set on the other signal(s). In the case of simultaneous recordings of many quantities, we implicitly record as well relations between these quantities of our multichannel set. To expose these properties we must apply special functions, able to reveal joint properties of multiple signals.

The best-known estimator of that type is covariance or correlation. For two signals $X = \{\ldots, x(0), x(1), x(2),\ldots\} = \{x(t)\}$ and $Y = \{y(t)\}$ covariance R and correlation C are defined as follows (E$[\cdot]$ denotes expectation, μ_x, μ_y are mean values of X and Y, respectively):

$$R_{xy}(s) = \mathrm{E}\big[x(t) - \mathrm{E}[x(t)]\big] \cdot \mathrm{E}\big[y(t+s) - \mathrm{E}[y(t)]\big] = \mathrm{E}\big[x(t) - \mu_x\big] \cdot \mathrm{E}\big[y(t+s) - \mu_y\big]$$

$$C_{xy}(s) = \frac{R_{xy}(s)}{R_{xy}(0)} = \frac{R_{xy}(s)}{\sqrt{R_{xx}(0)R_{yy}(0)}} \tag{7.1}$$

The value of covariance $R_{xy}(s)$ or correlation $C_{xy}(s)$ tells how much the two signals X and Y change together. Correlation may be treated as a normalized version of covariance: its value, unlike covariance, is limited to the $[-1, 1]$ range. Big absolute values of these functions indicate that changes in signal X and changes in signal Y appear in common. Negative values of covariance or correlation indicate that the changes in Y coincide with changes in X, but are in opposite direction. The covariance (correlation) defined above is in fact the covariance (correlation) function. The argument s of these functions, called a time lag, tells us about common changes (of the signals) which are delayed by the value of the time lag (positive or negative). If R is calculated for two different signals it is called cross-covariance function; if $X = Y$ we call R autocovariance function.

The covariance and correlation operate in the time domain; it means that we apply them directly to values of time series and the result is a function over time. In biomedical data analysis area, we are often interested in spectral properties of the recorded signals. A function similar to correlation, but operating in frequency domain is called coherence

$$K_{xy}(f) = \frac{S_{xy}(f)}{\sqrt{S_{xx}(f)S_{yy}(f)}} \tag{7.2}$$

which is constructed from cross-spectrum S_{xy} between signals X and Y normalized by spectra of signals X and Y called here as autospectra (the definition of cross- and autospectra will be given later). This function operates in frequency domain and tells how much common of the signal component of frequency f appear in both signals.

The coherence is a complex number and can be represented in the form

$$K_{ij}(f) = M_{ij}(f)e^{i\Phi_{ij}(f)} \tag{7.3}$$

where

$$M_{ij}(f) = \sqrt{\mathrm{Re}(K_{ij}(f))^2 + \mathrm{Im}(K_{ij}(f))^2} \tag{7.4}$$

is a modulus and

$$\Phi_{ij}(f) = \arctan \frac{\mathrm{Im}(K_{ij}(f))}{\mathrm{Re}(K_{ij}(f))} \tag{7.5}$$

is a phase of the coherence. These quantities are often more handy in presenting the values of analysis and are commonly used to measure similarity of signals in the frequency domain. For two signals in order to be considered coherent their phase difference must be constant which produces high value of coherence modulus and the coherence phase equal to the phase difference of that signals. Sometimes it is said that coherence describes linear phase coupling.

7.3 Practical Realizations of Cross-Measures

7.3.1 Linear Modeling

One successful technique in analysis of biomedical time series is application of linear models, and in particular of autoregressive (AR) model. The linear methods belong to the group of parametric approach in spectral analysis. We assume a model of data generation and then we fit that model to our data. The analysis is then done on the model parameters, not on the data samples. If the model describes our data well, the conclusions from the model can be translated to the properties of the original signals.

Parametric approach in spectral analysis gives us an opportunity to create advanced measures of relations between signals of multichannel set. Most importantly, perhaps, it allows defining causal estimators, which are based on certain models of influence between signals. Nonparametric approach (namely: Fourier analysis) does not give so many possibilities in that area.

In general, signals like EEG or MEG are of stochastic nature—they contain components of specific frequency ranges (rhythms) over a noisy background. This property fits well the theoretical shape of AR model spectrum and that is why the AR model can describe that type of data well and is so popular in the field of biomedical data analysis.

7.3.2 AR Model Introduction

AR model expresses the current value of a process as a linear combination of the previous values of the process. In a multivariate case, the current value $X(t)$ of a process is a vector containing values of all channels of the system.

$$\mathbf{X}(t) = (X_1(t), X_2(t), \ldots, X_k(t))^{\mathrm{T}}$$
$$\mathbf{X}(t) = \sum_{j=1}^{p} \mathbf{A}(j)\mathbf{X}(t-j) + \mathbf{E}(t) \tag{7.6}$$

or, by assuming $\mathbf{A}(0) = \mathbf{I}$ and changing sign of the rest of $\mathbf{A}(j)$:

$$\mathbf{E}(t) = \sum_{j=0}^{p} \mathbf{A}(j)\mathbf{X}(t-j) \tag{7.7}$$

By applying the Z transform we get

$$\mathbf{E}(Z) = \mathbf{A}(Z)\mathbf{X}(Z), \quad \text{where}$$

$$\mathbf{A}(Z) = 1 + \mathbf{A}(1)Z^{-1} + \mathbf{A}(2)Z^{-2} + \cdots + \mathbf{A}(p)Z^{-p} = \sum_{m=0}^{p} \mathbf{A}(m)Z^{-m} \tag{7.8}$$

Equation 7.8 can be expressed as depending on frequency by substituting $z = \exp(2\pi i f \Delta t)$, where Δt is the inverse of sampling frequency [67,62]:

$$\mathbf{E}(f) = \mathbf{A}(f)\mathbf{X}(f)$$
$$\mathbf{X}(f) = \mathbf{A}^{-1}(f)\mathbf{E}(f) = \mathbf{H}(f)\mathbf{E}(f)$$
$$\mathbf{H}(f) = \left(\sum_{m=0}^{p} \mathbf{A}(m)\exp(-2\pi i m f \Delta t) \right)^{-1} \tag{7.9}$$

The matrix $\mathbf{H}$ is called the transfer matrix of the system.

The power spectrum of the signal $\mathbf{X}$ is defined by the formula:

$$\mathbf{S}(f) = \mathbf{X}(f)\mathbf{X}^*(f) = \mathbf{H}(f)\mathbf{E}(f)\mathbf{E}^*(f)\mathbf{H}^*(f) = \mathbf{H}(f)\mathbf{V}\mathbf{H}^*(f) \tag{7.10}$$

In a multivariate case, the spectrum is a matrix containing autospectra of every channel on the diagonal and cross-spectra off the diagonal. The matrix $\mathbf{V}$ contains variance of model residual error $\mathbf{E}$, which can be interpreted as $\mathbf{X}(t)$ prediction error. From the spectral matrix elements, we can calculate for instance coherences. The values of $\mathbf{A}(f)$, $\mathbf{H}(f)$, and $\mathbf{V}$ (Equations 7.9 and 7.10) will be later utilized to construct various measures describing properties of the original dataset.

7.3.3 Model Parameters Estimation

The procedures of fitting of AR model to the data are described in signal analysis handbooks and in our opinion there is no need to present them here. It is rather a technical problem; even a beginner in data analysis using a data processing software package (from wide offer available) can successfully apply that technique, not knowing the implementation particulars. In fact, there are many possible algorithms differing in certain details of their performance on different kind of input data. Probably, the first algorithm was proposed by Yule and Walker. That algorithm is based on solving a set of linear equations constructed from values of correlations between data channels for different time lags.

The other algorithms (like Burg, LWR (Levinson, Wiggins, Robinson), covariance, etc.) are based on slightly different assumptions and are better suited to find sinusoidal components in the stochastic background. On the other hand, Bayesian algorithms estimate specific confidence ranges for the most probable values of the model parameters [14,70]. Application of a particular algorithm in most cases is not a crucial choice; the results obtained by different algorithms can be similar. Discussions about AR model application can be found in the literature [51,52,66,79,82,84,94], and in signal processing textbooks listed at the end of this chapter.

One very important issue concerning the model fitting is the problem of the optimal model order selection. It may seem that the bigger the model order the better the fit, but it is not the case. The number of maxima in the AR model spectrum is related to the model order. For too high orders, the model is likely to create false signal components, typically by splitting the existing "true" spectral maxima. To avoid such situations, certain statistical criteria of model order selection have been developed. Among the most popular ones are Akaike information criterion (AIC), final prediction error (FPE), criterion for AR transfer function (CAT), Bayesian information criterion (BIC) (called also the Schwarz criterion SC) or Hannan–Quinn criterion HQC, and several others. Their descriptions can be found in textbooks and articles [59,62]. Many of the criteria try to balance the variance of the residual error of the model (which gets lower with increasing order) with a penalty term, producing a minimum at certain order value p. Examples of the criteria definitions are given in Equation 7.11: P is the number of parameters, n is the number of data time points, $\mathbf{V}$ is the residual k-signal model variance matrix of order p ($\mathbf{V}_j$ for order j), and vertical bars denote determinant.

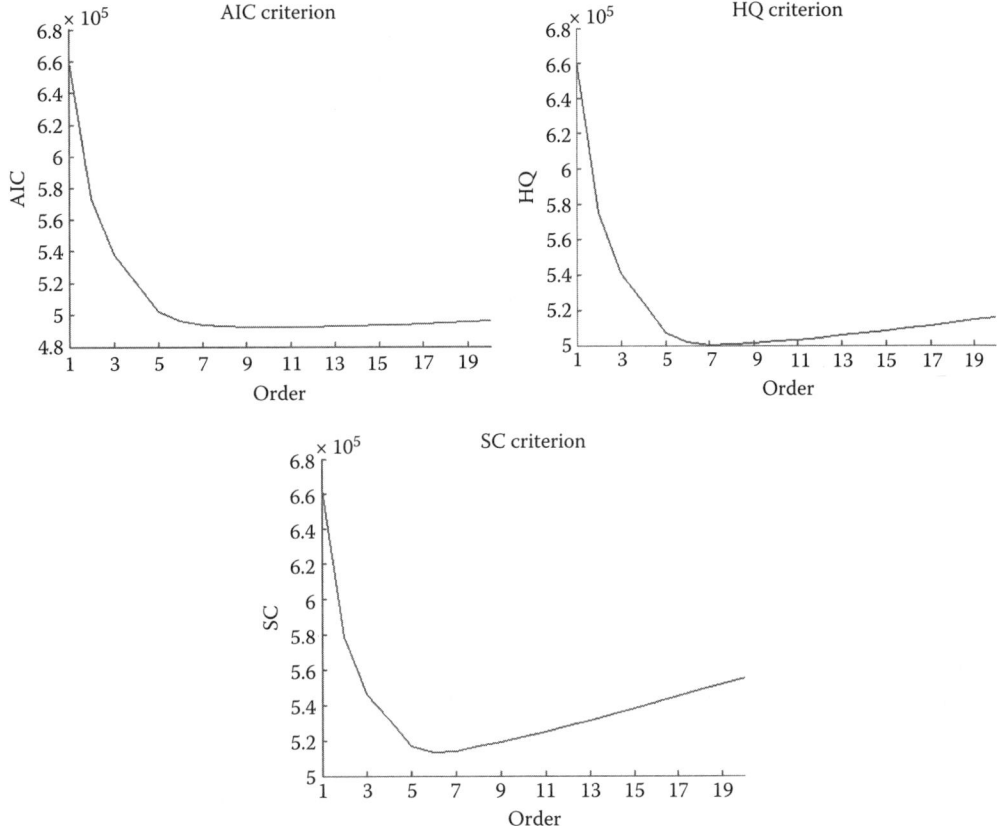

FIGURE 7.1 Example of optimal model order selection criteria. Model orders on horizontal axes, criteria value on vertical axes.

$$\text{AIC}(p) = n \log |\mathbf{V}| + 2P$$
$$\text{SC}(p) = n \log |\mathbf{V}| + 2P \log(n)$$
$$\text{HQC}(p) = n \log |\mathbf{V}| + P \log(\log(n))$$

(7.11)

$$\text{FPE}(p) = |\mathbf{V}| \left(\frac{n+P}{n-P} \right)$$

$$\text{CAT}(p) = \frac{1}{n^2} \sum_{j=1}^{p-1} \frac{n-j}{|\mathbf{V}_j|} - \frac{n-p}{(n-1)|\mathbf{V}|}$$

Typically, we calculate criterion values for a range of model orders and look for the first minimum of the obtained function. Although we can encounter slightly different definitions of that criterion in handbooks, the differences in formulas do not change the position of the minimum of those functions. The order at the minimum value is considered the "optimal" one, according to that criterion (Figure 7.1).

7.3.4 Concept of Granger Causality

Very often we are interested in knowing how the elements of the investigated system work together; for instance, we would like to know how the brain areas communicate with each other. That problem can be expressed as the question: which areas are sources of activity or how the signal propagates in our system? Finding sources of activity is sometimes a problem of primary importance and to resolve it; we must define a proper measure utilizing information about relations between signals.

When one area is the source of a signal which propagates and influences another signal, we say that the first signal is *causal* for the second one. For the mathematical purposes, we need a stricter definition of causality. The popular definition, widely adopted in that field, is the definition presented by Granger [34] (derived from a general idea given by Wiener [93]), which is based on predictability of time series.

Let us imagine we have two time series $X = \{x(t)\}$ and $Y = \{y(t)\}$. If we try to predict the current value of time series X using its own previous samples we get a value with certain error ε:

$$X(t) = \sum_{i=1}^{\infty} A_{11}(i)X(t-i) + \varepsilon(t) \tag{7.12}$$

We may add previous values of signal Y to the prediction of the current sample of signal X. In that case the prediction error ε' may be different:

$$X(t) = \sum_{i=1}^{\infty} A'_{11}(i)X(t-i) + \sum_{i=1}^{\infty} A'_{12}(i)Y(t-i) + \varepsilon'(t) \tag{7.13}$$

If the variance of the error ε' is lower than the variance of ε, we say that signal Y is causal for the signal X or signal Y Granger-causes X. Note that this property can be reciprocal, for example, Y can be causal for X and at the same time X may (or may not) be causal for Y.

The formalism presented above is defined for a pair of signals, but can be extended for a multivariate case. First, we try to predict a value of signal X_1 using all available signals except for X_m. We get a prediction error η:

$$X_1(t) = \sum_{\substack{i=1 \\ i \neq m}}^{k} \sum_{j=1}^{p_i} A_{1i}(j)X_i(t-j) + \eta(t) \tag{7.14}$$

Another prediction error η' we get when we use all signals including X_m in the prediction of channel X_1:

$$X_1(t) = \sum_{i=1}^{k} \sum_{j=1}^{p_i} A_{1i}(j)X_i(t-j) + \eta'(t) \tag{7.15}$$

If the variance of η' is smaller than the variance of η, we say that the signal X_m can be called causal for the signal X_1 in the multivariate case. These observations may be used to construct measures of causal influence between signals.

7.3.5 Directional Measures

It may seem straightforward to estimate the direction of influence between signals by analyzing the phase of coherence [33]. However, in practice that approach is possible only for certain simple cases. For biomedical multivariate stochastic data, typically of spectrum rich of components, the coherence phase analysis does not give satisfactory results.

AR model gives us an opportunity to make use of the Granger causality concept directly. We may look at the model equation as it is a prediction of the value $X(t)$. This is what we in fact do during fitting of the model—we try to find the model coefficients in a way which predicts the value of $X(t)$ with the smallest error ε. If we use previous values of many signals in the prediction, we get different set of parameters and different error values. After fitting the multivariate AR model, we get a set of model parameters $\mathbf{A}(i)$ and a matrix of the so-called residual error variance $\mathbf{V}$ which contains estimates of the prediction error variances of every signal from the investigated set. These values may be a basis for the construction of causality estimators based on the Granger causality concept.

7.3.5.1 Measures Derived from Granger Causality

In the literature, there are estimators derived directly from Granger causality definition. In Reference 31, the measure of linear feedback is defined:

$$F_{y \to x} = \ln\left(\frac{V_x}{V_{xy}}\right) \tag{7.16}$$

where variances of errors are taken from residual variances of the AR models fitted to the data: V_x is the variance of error ε and V_{xy} is the variance of error ε' (see Equations 7.12 and 7.13). Similar idea was used to define Granger causality index (GCI):

$$\mathrm{GCI}_{y \to x} = 1 - \frac{V_{xy}}{V_y} \tag{7.17}$$

This measure can be extended to a multivariate case:

$$\mathrm{GCI}_{y \to x} = 1 - \frac{V_k}{V_{k-1}} \tag{7.18}$$

Here V_k is the variance of error η' (in the case when signal Y is included into the set) and V_{k-1} is the variance of error η (cf. Equations 7.14 and 7.15) of the system containing all the signals except for the signal Y.

By its construction the value of GCI is in [0,1] range. When there is no influence on the X_1 signal, no improvement in prediction of the variance should be seen; the variance ratio is equal to 1 and the GCI measures (as well as the linear feedback measure) vanish.

The above-defined measures tell us just if the relation exists, and how strong it may be. We are often interested in frequency relations of causal influence, so we will need another estimator, able to produce results dependent on frequency. In Reference 16, there is a proposition of Granger causality spectrum estimator, based on ideas from Reference 31. It is defined in the form:

$$I_{y \to x}(f) = -\ln\left(1 - \frac{\left(V_{22} - V_{12}^2/V_{11}\right)\left|H_{12}(f)\right|^2}{S_{11}(f)}\right) \tag{7.19}$$

As we see, it utilizes information from power spectrum S, noise variance V, and model transfer function H. More details about these measures can be found in [19,20,32,35,69,81,92].

The Granger causality spectrum is defined for a pair of signals. One of the propositions for a truly multivariate measure (arbitrary number of signals) is the directed transfer function (DTF) introduced in Reference 43. Originally that quantity was presented in the normalized form given by the formula:

$$\text{DTF}_{j \to i}(f) = \frac{\left| H_{ij}(f) \right|^2}{\sum\limits_{m=1}^{k} \left| H_{im}(f) \right|^2} \tag{7.20}$$

DTF($j \to i$) describes influence of channel j to channel i at frequency f. More precisely, normalized DTF is a ratio between inflow from channel j to i and inflows from all channels of the set to the channel i at frequency f. This property assures normalization of this quantity in the form:

$$\sum_{j=1}^{k} \text{DTF}_{j \to i}(f) = \frac{\sum\limits_{j=1}^{k} \left| H_{ij}(f) \right|^2}{\sum\limits_{m=1}^{k} \left| H_{im}(f) \right|^2} = 1 \tag{7.21}$$

The values of the normalized DTF are numbers from [0, 1] range; 0 means no transmission.

Often we are interested in absolute transmission value and in that case the nonnormalized version can be helpful. It is defined as

$$\text{NDTF}_{j \to i}(f) = \left| H_{ij}(f) \right|^2 \tag{7.22}$$

The value of the nonnormalized DTF is directly related to the connection strength between signals [44]. This quantity allows for comparison between transmission values and is used for construction of the dynamical extension of DTF, which will be described later.

The value of $\text{DTF}_{j \to i}(f)$ is typically different than $\text{DTF}_{i \to j}(f)$, so we can distinguish the direction of influence by comparing these two values. There may be the case when both values of DTF are big, which means that both signals can be considered causal for each other or the relation is reciprocal. We would not be able to detect such a situation by coherence phase analysis.

7.3.6 Concept of Partial Measures

In systems containing more than two signals, we can observe not only influences between one signal on another, but more complex interactions between signals are possible. To investigate specific properties of such data sets special functions were introduced.

The concept of partialization of relations in a three-channel set can be presented in a following way: we want to measure only the influence of channel 1 on channel 2 with influence of channel 3 removed. In the time domain, we may partialize the covariance $R_{12}(s)$ by subtracting covariations with the third signal:

$$R_{12|3}(s) \sim R_{12}(s) - R_{13}(s)R_{32}(s) \tag{7.23}$$

Precisely, the partial correlation is given by such a formula supplemented by a normalization term:

$$R_{12|3}(s) = \frac{R_{12}(s) - R_{13}(s)R_{32}(s)}{\sqrt{(1 - R_{13}^2(s))(1 - R_{32}^2(s))}} \tag{7.24}$$

In the frequency domain, this concept can be translated to the so-called partial coherence. For a three-channel set, we get a formula for coherence between signals 1 and 2 partialized against signal 3:

$$C_{12|3}(f) = \frac{S_{12}(f) - S_{13}(f)S_{32}(f)}{\sqrt{\left(1 - |S_{13}(f)|^2\right)\left(1 - |S_{32}(f)|^2\right)}} \tag{7.25}$$

where S_{ij} are elements of the spectral matrix of the process.

In a general (multivariate) case, the partial coherence is defined as

$$C_{ij}(f) = \frac{\mathbf{M}_{ij}(f)}{\sqrt{\mathbf{M}_{ii}(f)\mathbf{M}_{jj}(f)}} \tag{7.26}$$

and describes only "direct" connections between channels i and j, with all linear combinations of influences of other channels removed. In the above formula $\mathbf{M}_{ij}$ is a minor (determinant) of matrix $\mathbf{S}$ with i-th row and j-th column removed. It can be shown that the Equation 7.26 may be presented using d_{ij}—elements of the inverse of the matrix $\mathbf{S}$

$$C_{ij}(f) = (-1)^{i+j} \frac{d_{ji}(f)}{\sqrt{d_{jj}(f)d_{ii}(f)}} \tag{7.27}$$

Values of partial coherence modulus are in [0,1] range.

Another possibility in a three or more channel set is a situation when several channels contain common signal component. To evaluate if a channel is similar to any other channel of the set we use the multiple coherence:

$$G_i(f) = \sqrt{1 - \frac{\det(\mathbf{S}(f))}{S_{ii}(f)\mathbf{M}_{ii}(f)}} \tag{7.28}$$

This quantity tells us if channel i is similar to any other channel from the set. The modulus of multiple coherence takes values from [0,1] range, where zero means that channel i is not coherent with any other channel of the set.

In order to distinguish the different coherence functions, the quantity given by Equation 7.26 is often called the *ordinary* coherence function.

The need to define partial measures in the area of causal influence estimators is expressed by construction of measures able to detect only direct transmissions. DTF detects the fact of signal transmission between channel i and channel j, no matter how that signal was transferred between these locations. The signal could be transferred directly, but in systems of more than two channels, the signal can be transmitted through several other channels before it appears at the destination channel. In order to resolve that problem several functions were proposed in the literature.

Baccalá and Sameshima [7] introduced partial directed coherence (PDC), defined by formula:

$$\gamma_{ij}(f) = \frac{A_{ij}(f)}{\sqrt{\sum_{m=1}^{k} |A_{mj}(f)|^2}} \tag{7.29}$$

$A(f)$ is the Fourier transformed model coefficient (Equations 7.8 and 7.9). The PDC is a normalized function and takes values from [0,1] range. It presents a ratio between influence of channel i on channel *j* and all outflows from channel *j*. This type of normalization makes the PDC more focused on sinks of activity than on sources. Recently, the modification of PDC called generalized partial directed coherence (GPDC) was proposed [8], according to the formula (for transmission from channel *j* to *i*):

$$\pi_{ij}(f) = \frac{A_{ij}(f)\frac{1}{\sigma_i}}{\sqrt{\sum_{m=1}^{k}\left|A_{mj}(f)\frac{1}{\sigma_m}\right|^2}} \tag{7.30}$$

where $\sigma_i^2 = V_{ii}$, the *i*-th diagonal element of the model noise variance matrix **V**.

Yet another proposition for a direct causal estimator can be found in Korzeniewska et al. [54]. The direct DTF (dDTF) function presented there is based on a concept of combining DTF with partial coherence. In practical realization it utilizes a modification of the original DTF function, which makes the normalization term independent of frequency.

$$\chi_{ij}^2(f) = F_{ij}^2(f)C_{ij}^2(f) \tag{7.31}$$

dDTF has a nonzero value when both functions simultaneously are nonzero; that situation indicates a presence of transmission while the relation is direct (Figure 7.2).

Various comparisons of performance of different causal estimators can be found in the literature (e.g., [80,94]). Here we present a picture from Reference 56 where a comparison of selected estimators applied to the real EEG was made. The 21-channels EEG signal was recorded from scalp electrodes (10–20 system [76]) from an adult human subject resting awake with eyes closed. Under such a condition, the alpha rhythm was generated in posterior areas and it was spread toward other derivations to the front of the head. Given the 20-s-long epoch of data (highpass forward and backward filtered above 3 Hz), a MVAR model of order 4 was fitted. DTF, dDTF, and PDC functions were calculated. For presentation purposes integrals of the functions in the range of 7–15 Hz were calculated. Results are plotted in the form of arrows pointing from the source to the destination channels, and the connection of strength (integrated function) is coded in a shade of gray. Only 40 strongest flows are shown.

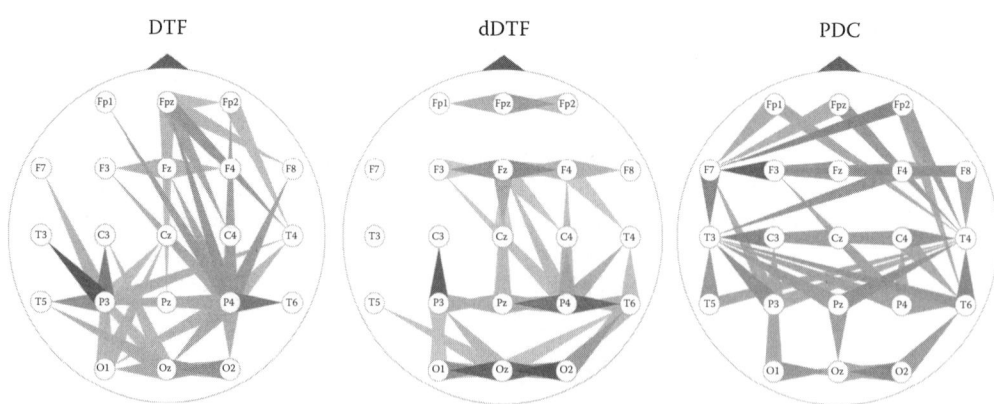

FIGURE 7.2 Comparison of DTF, dDTF, and PDC function applied to 21-channel human EEG sleep data record. Flows are represented by arrows pointing from the source to the destination electrode. Intensity of transmission is coded in shade of gray (black = the strongest). Only 40 strongest flows are shown for each function. (Reprinted from Kuś R, Kamiński M, Blinowska KJ. *IEEE Trans Biomed Eng* 51:1501–1510 © 2004 IEEE.)

In the DTF pattern, we may observe main sources of alpha activity located around P3 and P4 electrodes transmitting their activity in many directions. The dDTF picture lacks most long-distance connections indicating that the direct ones are only the relations between neighbors. The PDC shows quite different pattern. Although the sources at P3 and P4 electrodes are still visible, we see additional sites acting like sources and some sites seem to be sinks of activity.

7.3.7 Dynamical (Nonstationary) Data

When we described the principles of AR model, we said that the model expresses the current value of a process by a linear combination of its previous values with certain constant coefficients $A(i)$. Such a definition implies that we analyze stationary data epochs, where properties of the signals do not vary over time and can be described by the constant model parameters. However, very often we deal with dynamical phenomena with changing patterns of relations. We would like to analyze such processes with AR methodology as well. The solutions present in the literature can be basically divided in two general groups.

The first approach assumes that the model parameters can change over time. This so-called adaptive approach is typically realized by means of Kalman filter methodology, considered to be an optimal linear recursive estimator [83]. During the procedure, we process the nonstationary data and in each step we expand the analyzed epoch of the next sample(s) trying to make corrections to the model in order to improve the fit and minimizing the prediction error. The improvement is done by changing the values of model parameters. In that approach, we need to adjust certain variable controlling the speed of adaptation process; if the speed is too fast the model will follow every fluctuation of the data, if it is too slow the adaptation will not reveal details of changing patterns of relations. The descriptions of practical realizations of the Kalman filter for MVAR modeling can be found in literature [2,9,39,64].

The other possibility is called the short sliding window method [23]. Its application is possible when multiple repetitions (N_T) of an experiment and data recording are available. In that case, we assume that the repetitions of the experiment can be treated as different realizations of the same stochastic process (or, in other words, the process of the same origin and properties). Based on that assumption, we exchange averaging of signal properties over time (as we do in the case of long epochs of stationary data) with averaging over realizations (shorter epochs, multiple trials). This approach makes possible dividing the overall recording epoch into shorter time windows, possibly short enough to treat the data in each window as stationary. During model fitting, we do not average the data; we estimate the correlation matrix for each realization and average these estimates. The averaged correlation matrix is then used to estimate one final MVAR model for that window. Finally, from the model parameters all the interesting quantities: spectrum, coherences and causal estimators can be calculated. The time windows can overlap each other to get smoother results.

The short time window procedure contains certain preprocessing steps and, like in the case of adaptive approach, may need certain adjustments. The most important is the window size (N) selection. A shorter window can better track the dynamics of fast-changing phenomena but choosing the window size too short may compromise the quality of the fit of the model. Although there is no strict rule about the number of data points ($N \cdot N_T \cdot k$) and number of model parameters ($k^2 p$), researchers agree that there should be at least several times more data points than the parameters. It means that having only a few realizations we cannot use too short windows.

If we analyze the signal of evoked response type, where a slower wave appears over ongoing background activity of lower amplitude and higher frequency, it may be advisable to subtract the averaged response (ARP, average over realizations) from each realization. Although it may seem like removing the important information from the signal in fact that step assures better stationarity of the signal, especially for those windows which could contain raising ARP slope, and affects only the lowest part of the signal spectrum.

The results of evaluation of dynamics of spectra, coherences or causal estimators have a form of a matrix of time–frequency maps, so to present them we need to visualize connection between channel *i* and channel *j* over time and frequency. They are called short-time versions of the estimators, like short-time directed transfer function (SDTF) presented in Reference 58.

7.3.8 Statistical Significance

The coherences and causal estimators, especially in the short-time or adaptive versions, are quantities of distributions rather difficult to describe analytically. The asymptotic distribution for DTF in lack of flow case was recently given by Eichler [26]. However, in most cases the statistical properties can be estimated using methods of resampling statistics and surrogate data, depending on the case. The surrogate data technique is a concept of constructing a dataset based on the original dataset, but modified to lack certain property. For instance, we may think of surrogate data where all interrelations between channels have been cancelled. The practical realizations of such data may adapt random shuffling of each channel samples [44]. The other approach, based on idea given in Reference 87, involves Fourier transforming the data, randomization of their phases and transforming it back to the time domain. This procedure preserves amplitude spectrum of the data while canceling any phase couplings.

Resampling techniques are used to experimentally estimate the distribution of investigated functions. The functions calculated repeatedly for different datasets produce different values. Multiple generations of surrogate datasets can be used to get the distribution and significance levels for baseline (zero-level) value.

The bootstrap method [24,25,95] is especially useful for multiple repetitions case. In that approach, we randomly draw a pool of realizations (data from repetitions of the experiment) for which we calculate the results obtaining the distribution for the given case. For that empirical distribution, we get the desired significance levels.

7.3.9 Bivariate versus Multivariate

The fact that in a more than two-channel system certain channels can be common sources of signal for several other channels have important consequences in analysis of such data. Let us consider a three-channel system where channel 1 transmits its signal to channel 2 with delay of one sample and to channel 3 with delay of two samples. If we analyze every pair of channels (1–2, 1–3, and 2–3), we will get strong relations in each case. However, the relation found between channels 2 and 3 comes only from the fact that they both have a "common driver" signal, they may be independent in all other aspects. To get the correct pattern of relations, we must include all signals into the analysis and use a truly multivariate method of analysis. That so-called pair-wise approach may lead to results that will be difficult to interpret. Figure 7.3 presents results of DTF analysis of three-channel system constructed in a way described above (simulations are reprinted from Reference 10). Signal from channel 1 was transmitted to channels 2 and 3 with different delays. Nevertheless, the DTF analysis reveals true pattern of connections, with no transmission $1 \to 3$.

In Figure 7.4, we observe that channel 5 becomes a "sink of activity," the surprising effect which is an artifact of the applied method.

In general, the problem arises when we did not include all possible sources of signal in our dataset. Because we cannot detect such a situation my means of any mathematical analysis, the careful experiment planning may be essential to understand the obtained results and the investigated system well.

Many methods for cross-quantities analysis, especially nonlinear ones, are designed for a pair of channels only. One must be aware that the difference between pair-wise and multivariate analysis lies not in flaws of the method itself, but is an inherent property of multivariate systems (Figure 7.5).

7.3.10 Linear versus Nonlinear

All the methods described in this chapter, including MVAR, are considered *linear* which means that they can detect linear relations between signals. What can happen when the signals are connected in a

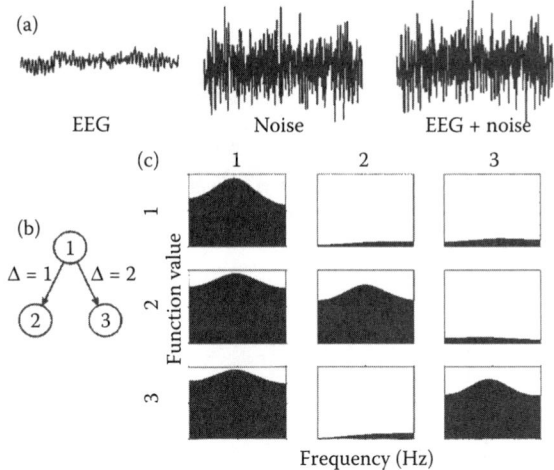

FIGURE 7.3 (a) Simulated signals. (b) Simulation scheme. (c) In each box DTF as functions of frequency (0–25 Hz); the numbers above the columns indicate output channels, the numbers on the left of the rows indicate destination channels. In the next example, we see a five-channel set, where signal from channel 1 appears in the rest of the channels with increasing delays. (Reprinted from Blinowska KJ, Kuś R, Kamiński M. *Phys Rev E* 2004; 70:050902.)

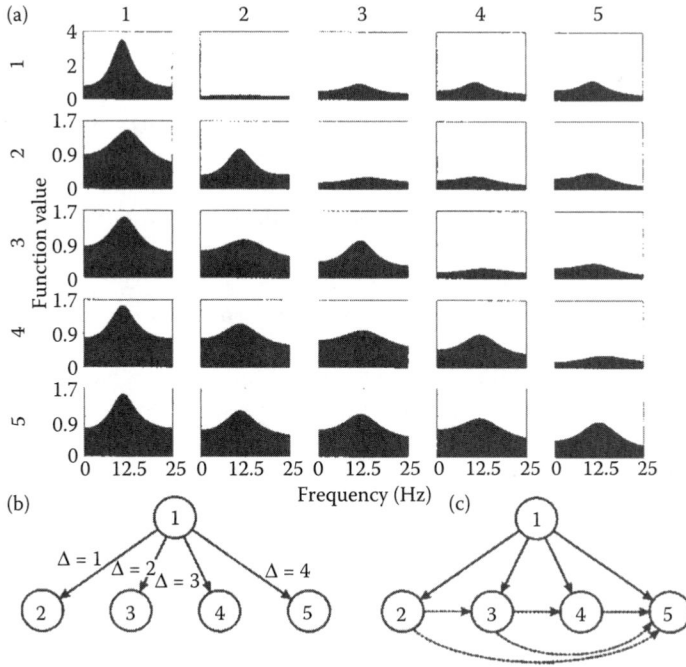

FIGURE 7.4 (a) Granger causality calculated pairwise; each graph represents the function describing transmission from the channel marked above the row to the channel marked on the left of the row. Granger causality in arbitrary units on vertical axes; graphs on the diagonal contain power spectra; frequency on horizontal axes (0–25 Hz range). (b) Simulation scheme. (c) Resulting flow scheme. The black arrows represent true (simulated) flows; the dotted arrows represent false flows found by the applied method. (Reprinted from Blinowska KJ, Kuś R, Kamiński M. *Phys Rev E* 2004; 70:050902.)

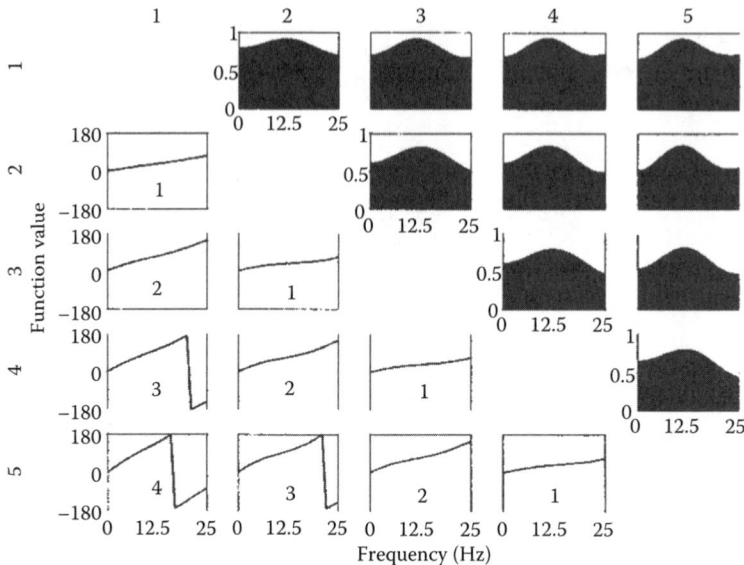

FIGURE 7.5 Pairwise coherences and resulting flows. Top: Coherence amplitude (black graphs above diagonal) and coherence phase (graphs below diagonal); each graph represents the function for the pair of channels marked on the left of the row and above the column; on the horizontal axes frequency (0–25 Hz); on vertical axes coherence amplitudes (0–1 range) or phases (−π–π range); delay values (in samples) estimated from phases, marked by the numbers shown over the phase graphs. Bottom left: Simulation scheme. Bottom right: Resulting flow scheme. The same convention in drawing arrows as in Figure 7.2. (Reprinted from Blinowska KJ, Kuś R, Kamiński M. *Phys Rev E* 2004; 70:050902.)

nonlinear way? Do we need a nonlinear measure of relations between signals? It of course depends on the character of the relation. This question is especially important in the case of brain activity research. Several systematic studies of that type were performed, where linear and nonlinear methods were compared. David et al. [22] compared several measures on the simulated data generated by populations of neurons using different connection patterns, types, and strengths. The conclusion from that work is that in most cases the coupling can be detected not only by a nonlinear but by a linear method too; the sensitivity may be lower in that case, which sometimes may lead to missing a flow. On the other hand, we should not see nonexistent flows.

The problem of detecting of nonlinearity in biomedical time series is present in the literature for many years [29,68,85]. Researchers generally agree that in the case of EEG the most pronounced nonlinear effects can be observed during certain stages of epilepsy. In different conditions there is no definite answer to that question. A comparison between performance of linear and nonlinear approach in forecasting of EEG time series was presented in Reference 12. The presented results show that the linear approach is not worse than the nonlinear one and sometimes it performs better in that case.

In Reference 65, another comparison of linear and nonlinear estimators on simulated examples with noise was presented. The study showed again the power of linear methods in revealing even weak couplings.

Summarizing, we may say that the nonlinear measures should be used only when it is really necessary. Moreover, nonlinear methods are often defined for pairs of signals, which is prone to interpretation difficulties. Considering the fact that nonlinear estimation requires more difficult calculations and the results are often very sensitive to noise, it is advisable to analyze the system with a linear method first to get the overall picture of connections. Such results would be more robust even for noisy signals, which is typical for biomedical data. If some parts of the analysis would require special treatment, the nonlinear analysis can be applied only to that part of the system. Similar conclusions can be found in Reference 94.

A few examples of nonlinear methods and their applications can be found in References 20, 46, 72, 73, 91.

7.4 Examples of Applications in Various Situations

7.4.1 Spike Train Data Analysis

The MVAR methodology cannot be applied directly to analysis of spike train time series. That type of data is characterized by long periods of "silence" (when values of the process do not change or change very little) and fast bursts of activity of high amplitude [15]. The "silent" periods may not have stochastic character at all. However, even spike train data can be adapted to MVAR analysis. The proposition of the procedure can be found in Reference 50.

In the referred paper, the origin of theta rhythm was investigated in specific structures of the nervous system of rats, namely supramamillary nucleus (SUM), septum (SEP), and hippocampus. It is known that in urethane-anesthetized rats neurons in the SUM fire in synchrony with hippocampal theta rhythm. These neurons project to the septum and hippocampus and it is assumed that they may drive the theta rhythm in the hippocampus. However, the connections between SUM and septohippocampal system are reciprocal and there is evidence that theta rhythm may remain in hippocampus after a lesion of SUM. To investigate connections between these structures, local field potentials (LFP) signals from electrodes implanted in hippocampus and spike trains from SUM neurons were recorded.

To make the MVAR analysis of spike trains possible, a preprocessing procedure was performed. The recording has a form of point process—at the moments of neuron firings the signal has high value and in other time points its value is zero. As the first step, the signal was lowpass filtered. The filter has to preserve the phase of the original signal; it was assured by filtering the data in both directions over time. The cutoff frequency of the filter was at 10% of the Nyquist frequency. Because MVAR model operates on stochastic signals, a small amount (10%) of a noise (uncorrelated with the signal) was added. The signals after the preprocessing steps are presented in Figure 7.6.

To the analysis, 500 samples long (2 s) epochs were selected. Theta oscillations appear around 4 Hz, so the 0–20 Hz frequency range was analyzed. In order to see changes in propagations, the short-time window formalism was used, here applied to the single realization of the experiment; in that study the 2 s long

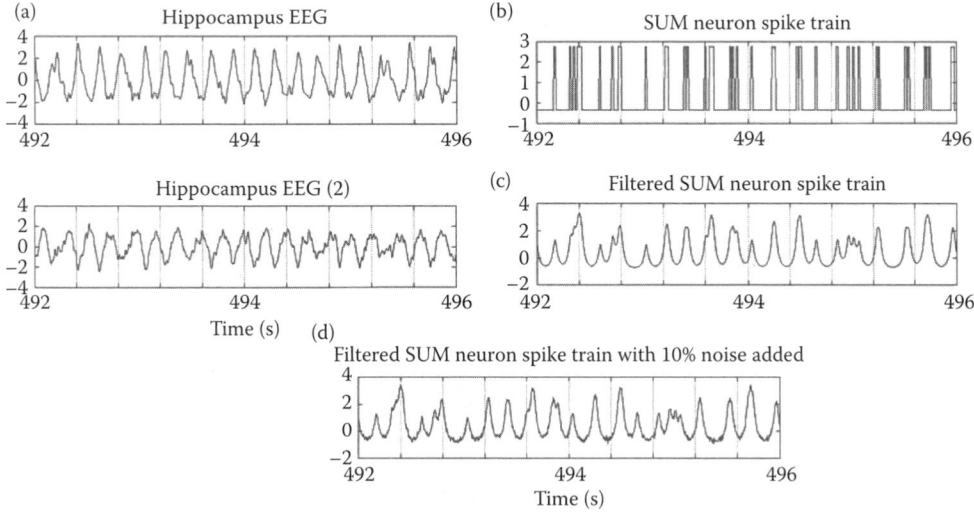

FIGURE 7.6 Preprocessing of signals for DTF. (a) Hippocampal field potentials recorded from hippocampus using two electrodes with a vertical tip separation of 1.5 mm. (b) Standardized spike train from the SUM. (c) Low-pass-filtered spike train. (d) Low-pass-filtered spike train with 10% of noise added. (Reprinted from Kocsis B, Kaminski M. *Hippocampus* 2006; 16(6):531–540.)

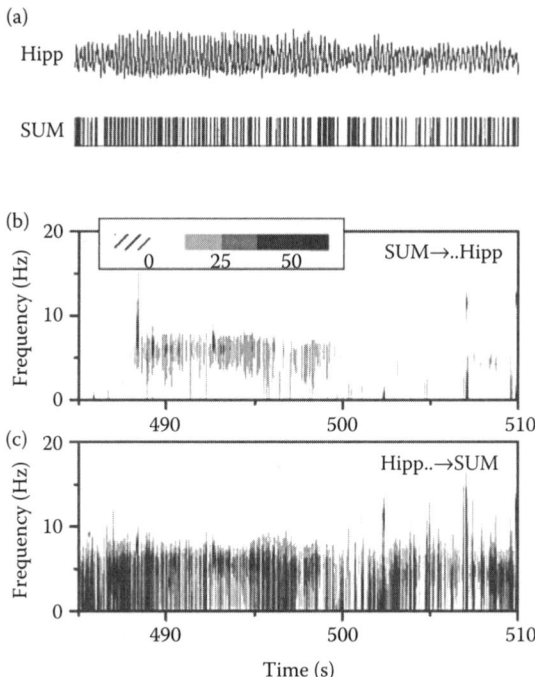

FIGURE 7.7 Activation of the theta drive directed from SUM to hippocampus during sensory stimulation. (a) Traces of rhythmic hippocampal EEG and SUM spike train. Note increase in theta frequency and amplitude during tail pinch between 488 and 499 s. (b) Temporal dynamic of the SUM → Hippocampus DTF. (c) Temporal dynamics of the hippocampus → SUM DTF. (Reprinted from Kocsis B, Kaminski M. *Hippocampus* 2006; 16(6):531–540.)

windows were shifted by 40 ms and in each window the DTF function was calculated. During the experiment the spontaneous theta rhythm was observed. After introducing a stimulus (pinch of the rat's tail), a change in the theta rhythm frequency and amplitude appeared. In Figure 7.7, we see a period of tail pinch and SDTF analysis of that epoch of data. The SUM → hippocampus transmission is low (white color) except for the period of sensory stimulation, when we see higher SDTF values around theta frequency (dark shade).

One of the results of the SDTF study was the conclusion that during sensory stimulation the theta rhythm originates in the SUM while spontaneous theta rhythm seems to be driving neurons in SUM.

7.4.2 Connectivity of Active Areas Found by fMRI Data Analysis

The work of Sato et al. [77] shows that linear modeling can be as well adapted to estimate causal connectivity for the fMRI data. The fMRI technique became popular because of its noninvasive character and high-spatial resolution; however, time resolution of fMRI scans is of the order of seconds. The images typically contain information about concentration of oxygenated blood in brain areas (the quantity called BOLD—blood oxygenated level dependent). Certain methods proposed to assess connectivity between areas identified in fMRI experiments can be found in literature [18,30,37,63]. The problem is that these methods need some *a priori* knowledge about the investigated system and its connections. MVAR modeling is free of such limitations (see also Reference 61). In the presented paper, fMRI images were collected during a language-related task. Incomplete sentences were presented on screen for 2.5 s followed by a blank screen. After 700 ms the missing word appeared and subject had to respond if that word completed the sentence or not. Eighty sentences were presented to the subjects. During the experiment, gradient echo-planar images were acquired at the Maudsley Hospital, Institute of Psychiatry,

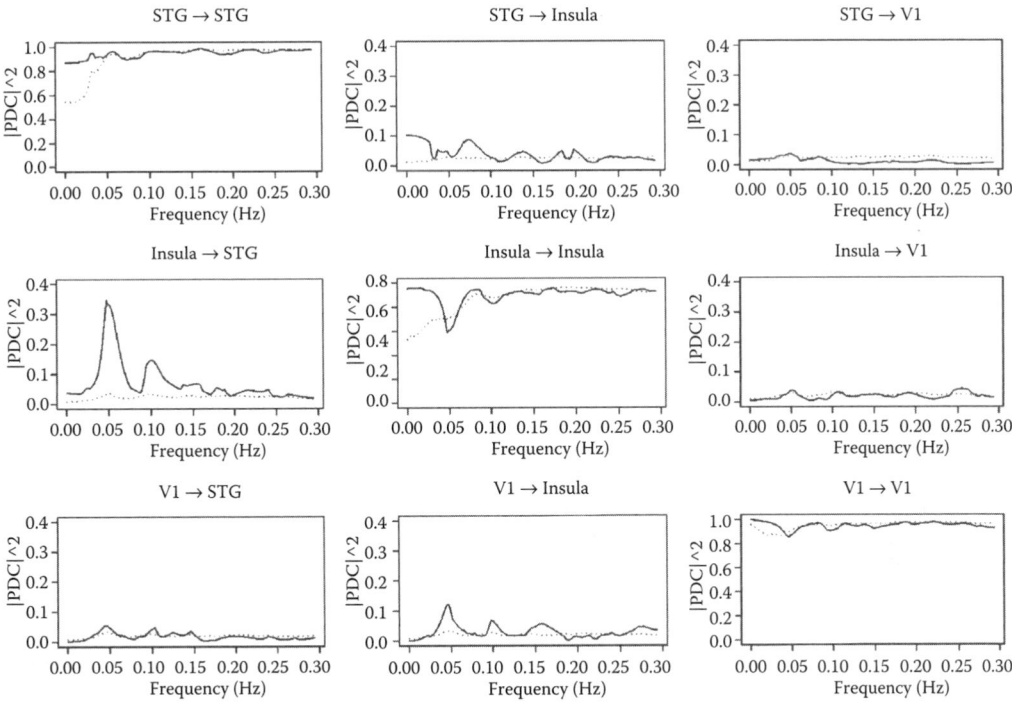

FIGURE 7.8   ROIs' multisubject median PDC. The dotted line shows the 95% confidence upper bound under the hypothesis of no connectivity between the nodes. (Reprinted from Sato JR et al. *Hum Brain Mapp* 2009; 30:452–461.)

King's College, London. The fMRI data was preprocessed by using head motion realignment, slice time correction, spatial smoothing, and normalization to Talaraich and Tournoux space [86]. Brain group activation maps were calculated and based on them primary visual cortex (V1), superior temporal gyrus (STG), and Insula were selected as regions of interest (ROI). For the connectivity analysis the GPDC function was used. The time series were constructed from averaged BOLD data from selected ROIs, normalized to zero mean, and unit variance. Spectral analysis of the ROI time series shows significant power at 0.049 Hz frequency and its harmonic, which is equal to the stimulation frequency. During GPDC analysis data from multiple subjects were incorporated. The authors proposed a complete algorithm for assessing statistical significance of the results in that case, based on the bootstrap method.

Significant connectivity was found around the maximum power frequencies, as it is shown on the graph (Figure 7.8). One can notice strong information flow from the Insula to STG and also from V1 to the Insula. The conclusion is that the information is first transmitted from visual cortex (V1) to the Insula and to the STG. These results were compared with coherence analysis which agrees with the GPDC results but was unable to show the detailed pattern of transmissions. Although fMRI experiments do not provide information about what, where, and how the information is processed during a task, the method introduced in the presented paper was able to show existence of connectivity networks based on the collected data (see also [90]) (Figure 7.9).

7.4.3 Dynamics of Transmissions during a Cognitive Task: Scalp EEG Data Analysis

Another example of MVAR model application is estimation of general dynamical pattern of connectivity from scalp EEG. In the paper [11], the continuous attention test (CAT [89]) was investigated.

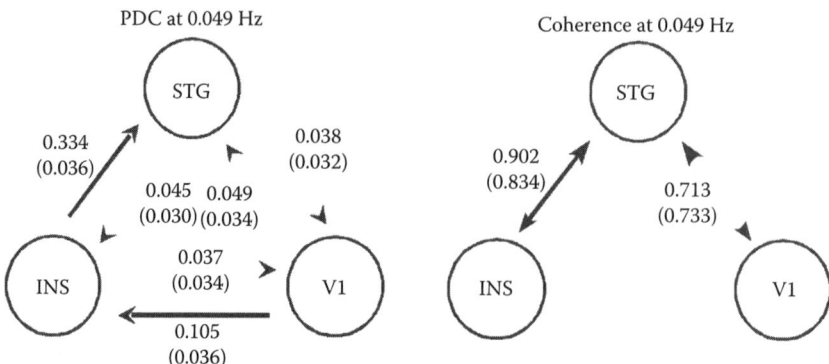

FIGURE 7.9 Multisubject median PDC at 0.049 Hz, simple coherence at 0.049 Hz (using the same bootstrap algorithm). The frequency of stimulation in the language paradigm was 0.049 Hz. The thick solid lines describe the links with relevant intensity of information flow. The critical regions at 5% of significance are values greater than the shown in parentheses. (Reprinted from Sato JR et al. *Hum Brain Mapp* 2009; 30:452–461.)

The experiment was performed at Department of Biomedical Physics, University of Warsaw, Poland. Visual stimuli (small checkerboards type) were presented on screen in random time intervals for human subjects. The subjects were asked to react (by pressing a switch) when two consecutive pictures were identical ("target" situation). Each of 16 young human male subjects observed 720 patterns, 120 of them were identical to preceding ones. EEG was collected during the experiment from 23 scalp electrodes with locations conforming to 10–20 standard [76]. After artifact-removal procedure, nine subjects were left for analysis. The data were filtered in the range of 15–45 Hz. Epochs from 0.5 s before to 1 s after the stimulus presentation were selected. The analysis was done by means of the SDTF function. Because the experiment was performed many times, multiple repetitions of the datasets were available. This allowed using the short-time methodology with windows short enough to capture changes in the relations between signals. A set of 12 selected channels was used in calculations. The sliding window of 20 samples (160 ms) was used, shifted each time by 2 samples (8 ms, overlapped windows). Trials were synchronized according to the motor reaction. The first 0.5 s at the beginning of the considered record was used as a reference to assess significant changes of transmissions during the test.

For statistical testing of the differences between the flows during the CAT test performance and the reference period, the methodology presented in Reference 53 was used. It assumes that the nonstationary SDTF consists of a smooth trend and a noise component. The smooth trend was estimated and its values are considered different for a certain time value if they are different for every value of the reference period at a given frequency. The details can be found in Reference 53.

The statistically significant changes of flow were analyzed for "target" (the switch was pressed when it should be) and "nontarget" (the switch was not pressed when it should not be) situations. For better visualization purposes, the SDTF values were integrated over frequency values of interest: beta (15–25 Hz) and gamma (25–45 Hz). The integrated values were presented in forms of arrows on an image of the head. The value of flow change was coded in color and transparence of an arrow (Figure 7.10).

Certain consistent patterns of transmissions were observed for multiple subjects. During the first stage, connected with the mental comparison of displayed pattern and decision making, the propagation from prefrontal electrodes was visible. The next stage was "silent" for target condition while for the nontarget condition propagation from electrode F8 to electrode C3 was observed, interpreted as active inhibition from right inferior cortex to hand motor area. In the third stage in target condition propagation from C3 appeared, connected with performing the hand movement (pressing the switch).

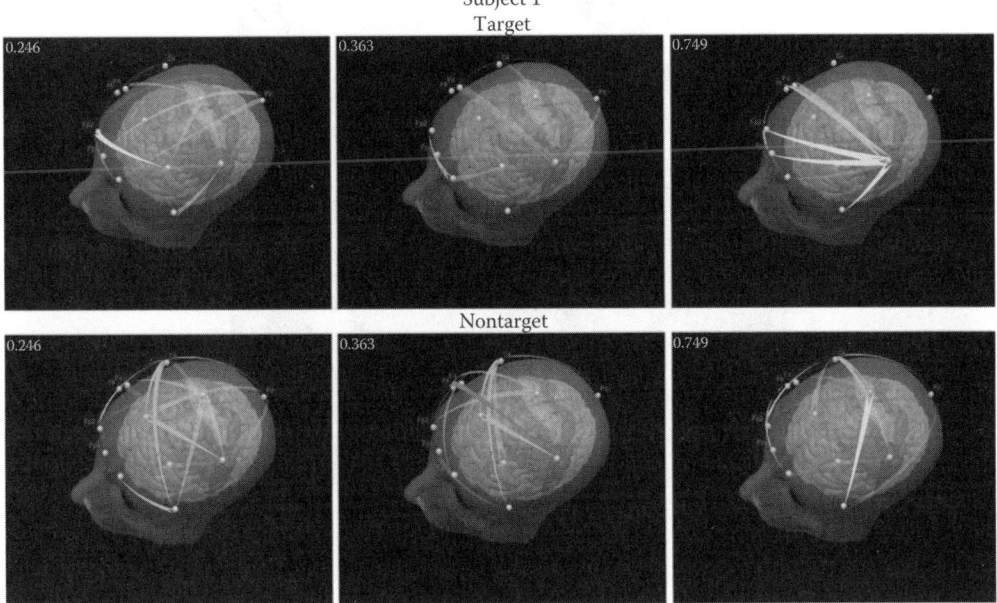

FIGURE 7.10 Snapshots from the movie presenting significant changes in transmissions in one subject, for target (upper) and nontarget (lower part). Intensity of flow changes for increase: from pale yellow to red, for decrease: from light to dark blue. In the right upper corner the time after cue presentation (in seconds). (Reprinted from Blinowska K et al. *Brain Topogr* 2010; 23:205–213.)

Another version of data analysis in that experiment, with trials aligned according to the stimulus presentation time, can be found in Reference 55.

The method of estimation of EEG signal propagation based on SDTF gives information on processes acting in the scale of milliseconds and allows for understanding the dynamical interactions between brain structures, even during tasks involving complex brain functions.

This section showed straightforward analysis of scalp EEG recordings. An interesting extension of scalp EEG research is presented in References 3–5 or 6. The authors record scalp EEG data and but before the analysis they perform regularized linear inverse source evaluation of cortical current density which estimates currents at the chosen ROIs from the values at the recording electrodes. The further analysis of functional cortical connectivity is done by computing the DTF or PDC on the estimated cortical current density waveforms in the ROIs. That way the results concern the precisely chosen locations. Together with the EEG analysis other types of data (fMRI, MEG) are simultaneously processed showing validity of the estimates.

7.4.4 Localization of Epileptic Foci: LFP Data Analysis

An important ability of multivariate causal estimators is locating sources of activity. This property can be used, for instance, to trace a localization of an epileptogenic focus. It is known that certain types of epilepsy are originated from an area of pathologically functioning tissue called a focus. In cases of seizures refractory to medical therapy, a possible treatment is to find and resect such a focus. Before that, electrodes are implanted in selected structures of the nervous system in order to provide recordings which are visually inspected by neurologists. In the presented paper ([28], see also [27]) cases of three patients were reanalyzed (after the actual surgery) using the DTF method. The data from patients were recorded at University of Maryland at Baltimore, USA. 32-contact subdural grid array was placed over the lateral temporal lobe and one or two 8-contact depth electrode arrays were placed in mesial temporal

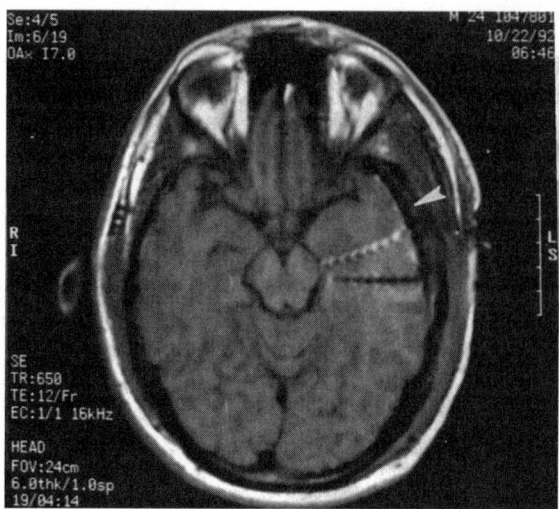

FIGURE 7.11   T1-weighted axial MRI image revealing two depth electrode arrays passing through 32-contact subdural grid array (arrow). The subdural grid array overlies the lateral temporal surface. The deepest contacts of the depth electrode array are in the amygdala and hippocampus, respectively. (Reprinted from Franaszczuk PJ, Bergey GK, Kamiński M. *Electroenceph Clin Neurophys* 1994; 91:413–427.)

structures as it was shown in the MRI image (Figure 7.11). Total of 64 channels of data during several seizures were collected with sapling frequency of 200 Hz.

To the analysis 16-channel segments of 200 samples (1 s) were selected. In the case of highly nonstationary signals longer epochs with more channels were analyzed. The results were calculated in 1–25 Hz frequency range; above 25 Hz the spectral power was low. Because both surface and depth electrodes were implanted, it was possible to see activity spreading from deeper structures to the cortex surface. For the first patient the epileptic activity was identified around 18 Hz. The DTF and autospectra graphs for the selected set of depth electrodes are shown in Figure 7.12. We see spectral peak at 18 Hz and at the same frequency high values of H2 → H1 and H2 → H3 transmissions and transmissions from H1 electrode to several others, suggesting the location of the source around H2 depth electrode. In that case epileptogenic focus was indeed located in deep mesial structures.

In the paper all three cases are discussed. We present only the analysis of the first patient case. As the conclusion, we see that MVAR formalism can be applied even for seizure recordings, when the nonlinear character of signal generation is probably most prominent for all EEG recordings. Selecting stationary fragment of such data from different parts of a seizure allows determining the patterns of seizure onset and propagation. In addition, the DTF method can provide evidence regarding patterns of flow of seizure activity that are not readily apparent from visual inspection. Moreover, we can determine if the initial focus continues to be the source of a given frequency or whether other areas become secondary generators.

7.5 Summary

Simultaneous recording from many different neurons and/or neural assemblies offers a window into how neurons work in concert to generate specific brain functions. Yet, it also presents important signal processing challenges that must be resolved to answer questions about how the brain works. Multivariate time series analysis provides the basic framework for analyzing the patterns of neural interactions in these data. Without substantial methodological development, our ability to understand the brain functions will be significantly hampered because the traditional methods fall short of what ultimately required for the analysis of multivariate neural data.

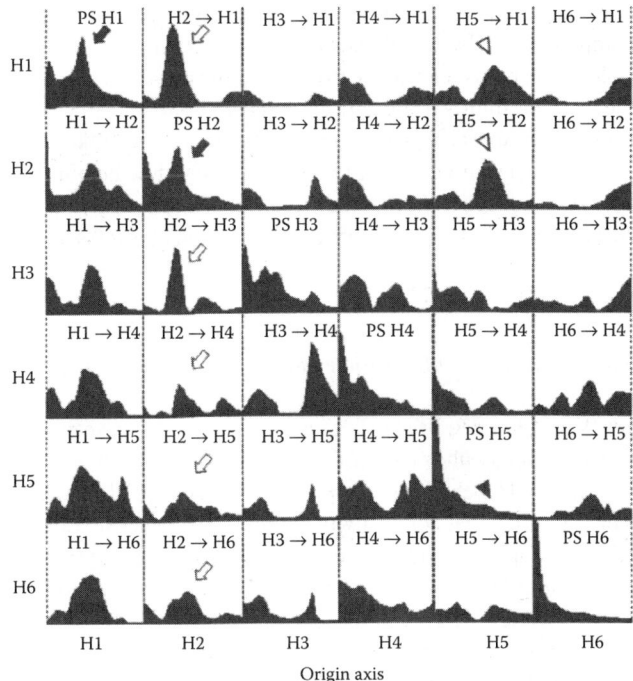

FIGURE 7.12 DTF for the seizure activity recorded from the hippocampal depth electrode during the third second of the seizure. The power spectra for each depth electrode contact are on the diagonal. The peak on the power spectra at 18 Hz is best seen in the deepest contact (H1, H2: solid arrows) but is also seen in the intermediate contacts (H3, H4). The open arrows identify prominent peaks in the DTF graphs corresponding to this peak in the power spectra (column H2). The most important peaks in the DTF graphs are those that have corresponding peaks in the power spectra. Peaks can be identified in the H5 column (open arrowheads) but there is no prominent peak at this frequency in the power spectrum for H5: only a small peak is seen (closed arrowhead). Each individual DTF is labeled to reflect the pattern of flow shown (e.g., H1 → H2). The model order was 5. The horizontal scale for each box is 0.5–50 Hz. The vertical scale for the DTF is 0–1 (full scale). The power spectra are normalized to unit power. (Reprinted from Franaszczuk PJ, Bergey GK, Kamiński M. *Electroenceph Clin Neurophys* 1994; 91:413–427.)

Therefore, in this chapter we have reviewed recent advances of causal influence measures for analyzing multivariate neural data under the framework of MAR modeling. Practical technical issues including stationarity/nonstationarity, bivariate/multivariate, linearity/nonlinearity, and statistical significance are specifically discussed. A variety of applications ranging from basic neuroscience research to clinical relevance are presented. For basic applications, we have stressed the typical applications in the analysis of spike trains, EEG, and fMRI BOLD data, each representing a major recording modality used in neuroscience research. For clinical applications, we have selected the epileptogenic seizure localization as a direct demonstration. We believe that Granger causality analysis offers a new outlook for examining patterns of neural interactions in complex brain networks, and should be a useful addition to the current analytical repertoire in revealing causal influences and directions of driving among multiple neural signals.

We should stress here that by analyzing biomedical data, especially EEG, MEG, or others (fMRI) in order to find interrelations between nervous system structures, we estimate the so-called *functional connectivity* [17]. That term refers to fact, that we observe and record acts of influence between measured regions, as it is realized in the moment of recordings. On the other hand, we may want to know *anatomical connectivity* between these regions. That knowledge comes from anatomical and histological research rather than data analysis. We may note that revealed paths of functional connectivity should be realized over existing paths of possible anatomical connections. However, as we have seen in this chapter, some connections may not be direct and signal may travel from its source to the destination (where it was recorded) by a more complex path. The actual transmission may be realized only over some paths, not every potentially possible. Some paths may be reciprocal and the direction of influence is what we want to reveal, and that is the place for multivariate data analysis methods.

We did not cover all possible approaches in biomedical data analysis, like graph theory or mutual information analysis, but the issues discussed in this chapter should be helpful in all typical problems possible to encounter in research practice. For further reading, there are many signal analysis handbooks [1, 13,21,36,38,42,47,49,60,62,71,74, 75,81] and overview articles available [40,41,45,48,51,52,78,79,84,88].

References

1. Anderson TW. *An Introduction to Multivariate Statistical Analysis.* New York: John Wiley & Sons, 1984.
2. Arnold M, Miltner WHR, Bauer R, Braun C. Multivariate autoregressive modeling of nonstationary time series by means of Kalman filtering. *IEEE Trans Biomed Eng* 1998; 45:553–62.
3. Astolfi L, Cincotti F, Mattia D, Babiloni C, Carducci F, Basiliasco A, Rossini PM, Salinari S, Ding L, Ni Y. Assessing cortical functional connectivity by linear inverse estimation and directed transfer function: Simulations and application to real data. *Clin Neurophysiol* 2005; 116(4):920–932.
4. Astolfi L, Cincotti F, Mattia D, Marciani MG, Baccala LA, de Vico Fallani F, Salinari S, Ursino M, Zavaglia M, Babiloni F. Assessing cortical functional connectivity by partial directed coherence: Simulations and application to real data. *IEEE Trans Biomed Eng* 2006; 53(9):1802–1812.
5. Babiloni F, Cincotti F, Babiloni C, Carducci F, Mattia D, Astolfi L, Basiliasco A et al. Estimation of the cortical functional connectivity with the multimodal integration of high-resolution EEG and fMRI data by directed transfer function. *Neuroimage* 2005; 24(1):118–131.
6. Babiloni F, Mattia D, Babiloni C, Astolfi L, Salinari S, Basilisco A, Rossini PM, Marciani MG, Cincotti F. Multimodal integration of EEG, MEG and fMRI data for the solution of the neuroimage puzzle (Proceedings of the International school on magnetic resonance and brain function—Frontiers of brain functional MRI and electrophysiological methods). *Magn Reson Imaging* 2004; 22(10):1471–1476.
7. Baccalá LA, Sameshima K. Partial directed coherence: A new concept in neural structure determination. *Biol Cybern* 2001; 84:463–474.
8. Baccala LA, Takahashi, YD, Sameshima K. Generalized partial directed coherence. *Proc. of the 2007, 15th International Conference on Digital Signal Processing. IEEE,* 2006; 1:162–166.
9. Benveniste A, Metivier M, Priouret P. *Adaptive Algorithms and Stochastic Approximations.* Berlin: Springer-Verlag, 1990.
10. Blinowska KJ, Kuś R, Kamiński M. Granger causality and information flow in multivariate processes. *Phys Rev E* 2004; 70:050902.
11. Blinowska K, Kus R, Kaminski M, Janiszewska J. Transmission of brain activity during cognitive task. *Brain Topogr* 2010; 23:205–213.
12. Blinowska KJ, Malinowski M. Non-linear and linear forecasting of the EEG time series. *Biol Cybern* 1991; 66:159–165.
13. Box G, Jenkins GM, Reinsel G. *Time Series Analysis: Forecasting and Control.* Englewood Cliffs, NJ: Prentice-Hall, 1994.
14. Box GEP, Tiao GC. *Bayesian Inference in Statistical Analysis.* New York: John Wiley, 1992.
15. Brillinger DR. Comparative aspects of the study of ordinary time series and point processes. *Dev Stat* 1978; 5:33–133.
16. Brovelli A, Ding M, Ledberg A, Chen Y, Nakamura R, Bressler SL. Beta oscillations in a large-scale sensorimotor cortical network: Directional influences revealed by Granger causality. *Proc Natl Acad Sci* 2004; 101(26):9849–9854.
17. Büchel C, Friston K. Characterizing functional integration. In: Frackowiak RSJ, Friston KJ, Frith CD, Dolan RJ, Mazziotta JC, (eds.). *Human Brain Function.* New York: Academic Press, 1997; pp. 127–140.

18. Büchel C, Friston K. Modulation of connectivity in visual pathways by attention: Cortical interactions evaluated with structural equation modeling and fMRI. *Cereb Cortex* 1997; 7:768–778.

19. Chen Y, Bressler SL, Ding M. Frequency decomposition of conditional Granger causality and application to multivariate neural field potential data. *J Neurosci Meth* 2006; 150:228–237.

20. Chen Y, Rangarajan G, Feng J, Ding M. Analyzing multiple nonlinear time series with extended Granger causality. *Phys Lett A* 2004; 324:26–35.

21. Dahlhaus R, Kurths J, Maass P, Timmer J (eds.). *Mathematical Methods in Time Series Analysis and Digital Image Processing (Understanding Complex Systems)*, Berlin: Springer, 2008.

22. David O, Cosmelli D, Friston KJ. Evaluation of different measures of functional connectivity using a neural mass model. *NeuroImage* 2004; 21:659–673.

23. Ding M, Bressler SL, Yang W, Liang H. Short-window spectral analysis of cortical event-related potentials by adaptive multivariate autoregressive modeling: Data preprocessing, model validation, and variability assessment. *Biol Cybern* 2000; 83:35–45.

24. Efron B. Bootstrap methods: Another look at the jackknife. *Ann Stat* 1979; 7:1–26.

25. Efron B, Tibshirani RJ. *An Introduction to the Bootstrap*. London: Chapman & Hall, 1993.

26. Eichler M. On the evaluation of information flow in multivariate systems by the directed transfer function. *Biol Cybern* 2006; 94(6):469–482.

27. Franaszczuk PJ, Bergey GK. Application of the directed transfer function method to mesial and lateral onset temporal lobe seizures. *Brain Topogr* 1998; 11:13–21.

28. Franaszczuk PJ, Bergey GK, Kamiński M. Analysis of mesial temporal seizure onset and propagation using the directed transfer function method. *Electroenceph Clin Neurophys* 1994; 91:413–427.

29. Freiwald WA, Valdes P, Bosch J, Biscay R, Jimenez JC, Rodriguez LM, Rodriguez V, Kreiter AK, Singer W. Testing non-linearity and directedness of interactions between neural groups in the macaque inferotemporal cortex. *J Neurosci Meth* 1999; 94:105–119.

30. Friston KJ, Harrison L, Penny W. Dynamic causal modeling. *Neuroimage* 2003; 19:1273–1302.

31. Geweke J. Measurement of linear dependence and feedback between multiple time series. *J Am Stat Assoc* 1982; 77:304–324.

32. Geweke J. Measures of conditional linear dependence and feedback between time series. *J Am Stat Assoc* 1984; 79:907–915.

33. Govindan RB, Raethjen J, Kopper F, Claussen JC, Deuschl G. Estimation of time delay by coherence analysis. *Physica A* 2005; 350:277–295.

34. Granger CWJ. Investigating causal relations in by econometric models and cross-spectral methods. *Econometrica* 1969; 37:424–438.

35. Guo S, Seth AK, Kendrick KM, Zhou C, Feng J. Partial Granger causality—Eliminating exogenous inputs and latent variables. *J Neurosci Meth* 2008;172:79–93.

36. Hamilton JD. *Time Series Analysis*. Princeton, NJ: Princeton University Press.

37. Harrison L, Penny WD, Friston K. Multivariate autoregressive modeling of fMRI time series. *NeuroImage* 2003; 19:1477–1491.

38. Hayes MH. *Statistical Digital Signal Processing and Modeling*. New York: Wiley & Sons, 1996.

39. Hesse W, Möller E, Arnold M, Schack B. The use of time-variant EEG Granger causality for inspecting directed interdependencies of neural assemblies. *J Neurosci Meth* 2003; 124:27–44.

40. Isaksson A, Wennberg A, Zetterberg LH. Computer analysis of EEG signals with parametric models. *Proc IEEE* 1981; 69:451–61.

41. Jansen BH. Analysis of biomedical signals by means of linear modeling. *CRC Crit Rev Biomed Eng* 1985; 12(4):343–392.

42. Jenkins GM, Watts DG. *Spectral Analysis and its Applications*. SF: Holden-Day, 1968.

43. Kamiński M, Blinowska KJ. A new method of the description of the information flow in brain structures. *Biol Cybern* 1991; 65:203–210.

44. Kamiński M, Ding M, Truccolo W, Bressler S. Evaluating causal relations in neural systems: Granger causality, directed transfer function and statistical assessment of significance. *Biol Cybern* 2001; 85:145–157.
45. Kaminski M., Liang H. Causal influence: Advances in neurosignal analysis. *Crit Rev Biomed Eng* 2005; 33(4):347–430.
46. Kantz H, Schreiber T. *Nonlinear Time Series Analysis*. Cambridge: Cambridge University Press, 2004.
47. Kay SM. *Modern Spectral Estimation*. Englewood Cliffs, NJ: Prentice-Hall, 1988.
48. Kelly EF, Lenz JE, Franaszczuk PJ, Truong YK. A general statistical framework for frequency-domain analysis of EEG topographic structure. *Comput Biomed Res* 1997; 30:129–164.
49. Kemp B, Lopes da Silva FH. Model-based analysis of neurophysiological signals. In: Weitkunat R, (ed.). *Digital Biosignal Processing*. Amsterdam: Elsevier, 1991; pp. 129–155.
50. Kocsis B, Kaminski M. Dynamic changes in the direction of the theta rhythmic drive between supra-mammillary nucleus and the septohippocampal system. *Hippocampus* 2006; 16(6):531–540.
51. Korhonen I, Mainardi L, Baselli G, Bianchi A, Loula P, Carrault G. Linear multivariate models for physiological signal analysis: Applications. *Comput Meth Prog Biomedic* 1996; 51:121–30.
52. Korhonen I, Mainardi L, Loula P, Carrault G, Baselli G, Bianchi A. Linear multivariate models for physiological signal analysis: Theory. *Comput Meth Prog Biomedic* 1996; 51:85–94.
53. Korzeniewska A, Crainiceanu C, Kus R, Franaszczuk PJ, Crone NE. Dynamics of event-related causality (ERC) in brain electrical activity. *Hum Brain Mapp* 2008; 29:1170–1192.
54. Korzeniewska A, Mańczak M, Kamiński M, Blinowska KJ, Kasicki S. Determination of information flow direction between brain structures by a modified Directed Transfer Function method (dDTF). *J Neurosci Meth* 2003; 125:195–207.
55. Kus R, Blinowska KJ, Kaminski M, Basinska-Starzycka A. Transmission of information during Continuous Attention Test. *Acta Neurobiol Exp* 2008; 68:103–112.
56. Kuś R, Kamiński M, Blinowska KJ. Determination of EEG activity propagation: Pair-wise versus multichannel estimate. *IEEE Trans Biomed Eng* 2004; 51:1501–1510.
57. Liang H, Bressler SL, Ding M, Desimone R, Fries P. Temporal dynamics of attention-modulated neuronal synchronization in macaque V4. *Neurocomputing* 2003; 52–54:481–487.
58. Liang H, Ding M, Nakamura R, Bressler SL. Causal influences in primate cerebral cortex during visual pattern discrimination. *Neuroreport* 2000; 11:2875–2880.
59. Lutkepohl H. Comparison of criteria for estimating the order of a vector autoregressive process. *J Time Ser Anal* 1985; 6(1):35–52.
60. Lutkepohl H. *Introduction to Multiple Time Series Analysis*. New York: Springer, 1993.
61. Mader W, Feess D, Lange R, Saur D, Glauche V, Weiller C, Timmer J, Schelter B. On the detection of direct directed information flow in fMRI. *IEEE J Sel Top Sig Proc* 2008; 2(6):965–974.
62. Marple SL. *Digital Spectral Analysis with Applications Prentice-Hall Signal Processing Series*. New Jersey: Simon & Schuster, 1987.
63. McIntosh AR, Gonzalez-Lima F. Structural equation modeling and its application to network analysis of functional brain imaging. *Hum Brain Map* 1994; 2:2–22.
64. Möller E, Schack B, Arnold M, Witte H. Instantaneous multivariate EEG coherence analysis by means of adaptive high-dimensional autoregressive models. *J Neurosci Meth* 2001; 105:143–158.
65. Netoff TI, Caroll L, Pecora LM, Schiff SJ. Detecting coupling in the presence of noise and nonlinearity. In: Scheleter B, Winterhalder M, Timmer J. (eds.). *Handbook of Time Series Analysis*. Weinheim: Wiley VCH, 2006.
66. Neumaier A, Schneider T. Estimation of parameters and eigenmodes of multivariate autoregressive models. *ACM Trans Math Software* 2001; 27(1):27–57.
67. Oppenheim AV, Schafer RW. *Discrete-time Signal Processing*. Englewood Cliffs, NJ: Prentice-Hall, 1989.
68. Paluš M. Detecting nonlinearity in multivariate time series. *Phys Lett A* 1996; 213:138.

69. Pascual-Marqui RD. Instantaneous and lagged measurements of linear and nonlinear dependence between groups of multivariate time series: Frequency decomposition. arXiv:0711.1455 [stat.ME], 2007; http://arxiv.org/abs/0711.1455.

70. Penny WD, Roberts SJ. Bayesian multivariate autoregressive models with structured priors. *IEE Proc Vision Image Sig Proc* 2002; 149:33–41.

71. Percival DB, Walden AT. *Spectral Analysis for Physical Applications*. Cambridge, UK: Cambridge University Press, 1993.

72. Pereda E, Quiroga RQ, Bhattacharya J. Nonlinear multivariate analysis of neurophysiological signals. *Prog Neurobiol* 2005; 77:1–37.

73. Pereda E, Rial R, Gamundi A, Gonzalez J. Assessment of changing interdependences between human electroencephalograms using nonlinear methods. *Physica D* 2001; 148:147–158.

74. Priestley MB. *Spectral Analysis and Time Series*. London: Academic Press, 1981.

75. Proakis JG, Manolakis DG. *Digital Signal Processing: Principles, Algorithms and Applications*. Englewood Cliffs, NJ: Prentice-Hall, 1996.

76. Rechtschaffen A, Kales A. A manual: Standardized terminology, techniques and scoring system for sleep stages of human subjects. *Brain Information Service. Brain Research Institute, UCLA*, 1968.

77. Sato JR, Takahashi DY, Arcuri SM, Sameshima K, Morettin PA, Baccala LA. Frequency domain connectivity identification: An application of partial directed coherence in fMRI. *Hum Brain Mapp* 2009; 30:452–461.

78. Seth AK. Causal networks in simulated neural systems. *Cogn Neurodyn* 2008; 2:49–64.

79. Schneider T, Neumaier A. Estimation of parameters and eigenmodes of multivariate autoregressive models. *ACM Trans Math Soft* 2001; 27:27–57, 58–65.

80. Schelter B, Winterhalder M, Eichler M, Peifer M, Hellwig B, Guschlbauer B, Lücking HC, Dahlhaus R, Timmer J. Testing for directed influences among neural signals using partial directed coherence. *J Neurosci Meth* 2005; 152:210–219.

81. Schelter B, Winterhalder M, Timmer J (eds.). *Handbook of Time Series Analysis*. Berlin: Wiley-VCH, 2006.

82. Schlögl A. A comparison of multivariate autoregressive estimators. *Signal Processing* 2006; 86:2426–2429.

83. Simon D. *Optimal State Estimation: Kalman, H Infinity, and Nonlinear Approaches*. Hoboken, NJ: Wiley-Interscience, 2006.

84. Spyers-Ashby JM, Bain PG, Roberts SJ. A comparison of fast Fourier transform (FFT) and autoregressive (AR) spectral estimation techniques for the analysis of tremor data. *J Neurosci Meth* 1998; 83:35–43.

85. Stam C, Pijn JPM, Suffczyński P, Lopes da Silva FH. Dynamics of the human alpha rhythm: Evidence for non-linearity? *Clin Neurophys* 1999; 110:1801–1813.

86. Talairach J, Tournoux P. *Co-planar Stereotaxic Atlas of the Human Brain*. New York: Thieme, 1988.

87. Theiler J, Eubank S, Longtin A, Galdrikian B, Farmer D. Testing for nonlinearity in time series: The method of surrogate data. *Physica D* 1992; 58:77–94.

88. Thomson DJ. Spectrum estimation and harmonic analysis. *Proc IEEE* 1982; 70:1055–1096.

89. Tiplady B. Continuous attention: Rationale and discriminant validation of a test designed for the use in psychopharmacology. *Behav Res Methods Instrum Compt* 1992; 24:16–21.

90. Valdés-Sosa PA, Sánchez-Bornot JM, Lage-Castellanos A, Vega-Hernández M, Bosch-Bayard J, Melie-García L, Canales-Rodríguez E. Estimating brain functional connectivity with sparse multivariate autoregression. *Phil Trans R Soc B* 2005; 360:969–981.

91. Veeramani B, Narayanan K, Prasad A, Iasemidis LD, Spanias AS, Tsakalis K. Measuring the direction and the strength of coupling in nonlinear systems—A modeling approach in the state space. *IEEE Sig Proc Lett* 2004; 11:617–620.

92. Verdes PF. Assessing causality from multivariate time series. *Phys Rev E* 2005; 72:026222.

93. Wiener N. The theory of prediction. In: Beckenbach EF, (ed.). *Modern Mathematics for Engineers*. New York: McGraw-Hill, 1956.

94. Winterhalder M, Schelter B, Hesse W, Schwab K, Leistritz L, Klan D, Bauer R, Timmer J, Witte H. Comparison of linear signal processing techniques to infer directed interactions in multivariate neural systems. *Signal Process* 2005; 85:2137–2160.

95. Zoubir AM, Boashash B. The bootstrap and its application in signal processing. *IEEE Sig Proc Mag* 1998; 15:56–76.

II

Medical Imaging

Mostafa Analoui
The Livingston Group

Preface

While the discovery of x-ray is commonly considered as a pivotal event, ushering in modern medical imaging, there have been various optical-based *in vitro* and *in vivo* modalities routinely used for centuries. Owing to the exponential technological innovations of the late nineteenth and twentieth centuries, imaging had an explosive growth, primarily in the emergence of new modalities and associated tools. During this period, a number of emerging technologies played key roles in advances in biomedical engineering and clinical practice. The contribution of these technologies can be summarized into (1) enabling objective and quantitative measurement of *in vivo* phenomena, (2) enhancing our understanding of disease process and interaction with therapeutic agents, and (3) new discoveries in the pathophysiology of disease and new diagnosis. Medical imaging is among the technologies that have strongly influenced all these three aspects and beyond. The discovery of x-ray, as a landmark event, enabled us to see the "invisible," opening a new era in medical diagnostics. More important, it opened up the thinking around the interaction of electromagnetic signal with human tissue and the utility of its selective absorption, scattering, diffusion, and reflection as a tool for understanding the physiology, evolution of disease, and therapy.

It is based on such a fundamental concept that all imaging modalities developed and utilized, that is, interaction of internal/external energy and its differential behavior in healthy and diseased tissues. X-ray initiated this journey, which has led to a broad range of solutions for 2-D and 3-D visualization of anatomic structures and functions. *In vitro* utilization of such tools in biomedical research has been even broader compared to clinical applications.

This section offers (1) a selective review of key imaging modalities focusing on those with established clinical utilization and (2) examples of quantitative tools for image analysis, modeling, and interpretation. The first two chapters provide a detailed overview of x-ray imaging and computed tomography. Projectional radiography and computed tomography cover a large portion of clinical imaging in practice. Although the fundamentals are quite similar to its early discovery, significant and evolutionary changes have been made in the past 115 years, which are reflected in these two chapters.

Magnetic resonance imaging (MRI) covers a broad range of tools and instrumentations based on differential magnetic properties of tissue and its relaxivity. MRI and its associated techniques have become one of the fastest-growing modalities since the last quarter of the twentieth century. The chapter on MRI covers fundamental concepts in signal acquisition and processing, followed by an overview of functional MRI (fMRI) and chemical shift imaging. Considering the depth of technical materials, an additional chapter covers topics in magnetic resonance microscopy.

While the concept of making the patient radioactive for diagnostic purposes seemed counterintuitive for a number of years, this is the basic concept behind nuclear imaging. The physics of instrumentation and signal collection have been covered in the chapter on nuclear medicine, along with their application in clinical practice.

Chapter 15 deals with electrical impedance tomography (EIT). EIT is among a number of promising emerging technologies that are identifying their unique application for *in vivo* imaging, along with the challenges for gaining clinical and regulatory acceptance.

The second half of the section covers selective topics on quantitative tools and approaches for analysis and interpretation of images acquired primarily by MRI and PET. In Chapter 16, the authors offer an overview of recent developments in the use of MRI for vascular imaging and its key advantages over ultrasound-based approaches. Chapter 17 covers dynamic contrast-enhanced MRI (DCE-MRI), a critical method for the analysis of oncologic tumor and its response to antiangiogenic class of therapeutics. The focus of Chapter 18 is modeling of myocardial deformation toward better understanding of cardiac function and associated anomalies. Perhaps one of the most promising utilities of MR in joint disease is in osteoarthritis (OA), which is covered in depth in Chapter 19. This chapter offers a comprehensive overview of OA, various MR approaches for imaging knee, and methods for quantitative image analysis. Chapter 20 offers a unique perspective in the utilization of quantitative PET for its applications in drug discovery and development, which is rapidly becoming an indispensable tool for clinical and research applications. Chapter 21 addresses the key issues around organizing and searching multimodality imaging data set, which is becoming increasingly important yet a challenging issue in clinical imaging. This chapter is intended to highlight complexities associated with high-volume data management, access, and sharing.

It must be noted that this section offers a selective overview of medical imaging and a comprehensive coverage perhaps requires multiple volumes. The editor hopes that these selected topics will provide readers the depth and breadth of this field and the challenges lying ahead of the technical and clinical community of researchers and practitioners.

8

Mammography

Martin J. Yaffe
Sunnybrook Health Sciences Centre
University of Toronto

8.1 Introduction

Mammography is an x-ray imaging procedure for examination of the breast. It is used primarily not only for the detection and diagnosis of breast cancer, but also for presurgical localization of suspicious areas and in the guidance of needle biopsies.

Breast cancer is a major killer of women. Approximately 254,650 women were diagnosed with breast cancer in the United States in 2009 and 40,170 women died of this disease (ACS, 2009). Its cause is not currently known; however, it has been demonstrated that *survival* is greatly improved if disease is detected at an *early stage* (Smart et al., 1993; Tabar et al., 1993). Mammography is at present the most effective means of detecting early-stage breast cancer. It is used both for investigating symptomatic patients (diagnostic mammography) and for *screening* of asymptomatic women in selected age groups.

Breast cancer is detected on the basis of four types of signs on the mammogram:

1. The characteristic morphology of a tumor mass
2. Certain presentations of mineral deposits as specks called microcalcifications
3. Architectural distortion of normal tissue patterns caused by the disease
4. Asymmetry between corresponding regions of images of the left and right breast

8.2 Principles of Mammography

The mammogram is an x-ray shadowgram formed when x-rays from a quasi-point source irradiate the breast and the transmitted x-rays are recorded by an *image receptor*. Because of the spreading of the x-rays from the source, structures are magnified as they are projected onto the image receptor. The signal is a result of differential attenuation of x-rays along paths passing through the structures of the breast.

The essential features of image quality are summarized in Figure 8.1. This is a one-dimensional profile of x-ray transmission through a simplified computer model of the breast (Fahrig et al., 1992), illustrated in Figure 8.2. A region of reduced transmission corresponding to a structure of interest such as a tumor, a calcification or normal *fibroglandular* tissue is shown. The imaging system must have sufficient *spatial resolution* to delineate the edges of fine structures in the breast. Structural detail as small as 50 μm must be adequately resolved. Variation in x-ray attenuation among tissue structures in the breast gives rise to *contrast*. The detectability of structures providing subtle contrast is impaired, however, by an overall random fluctuation in the profile, referred to as mottle or *noise*. Because the breast is sensitive to ionizing radiation, which at least for high doses is known to cause breast cancer, it is desirable to use the lowest radiation dose compatible with excellent image quality. The components of the imaging system will be described and their design will be related to the imaging performance factors discussed in this section.

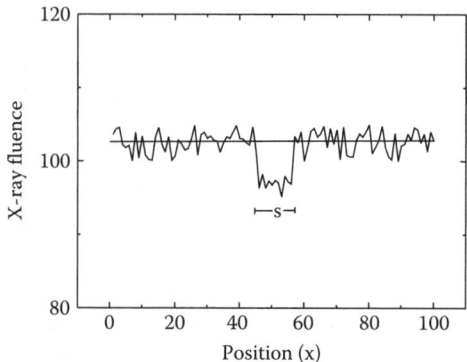

FIGURE 8.1   Profile of a simple x-ray projection image, illustrating the role of contrast, spatial resolution, and noise in mammographic image quality.

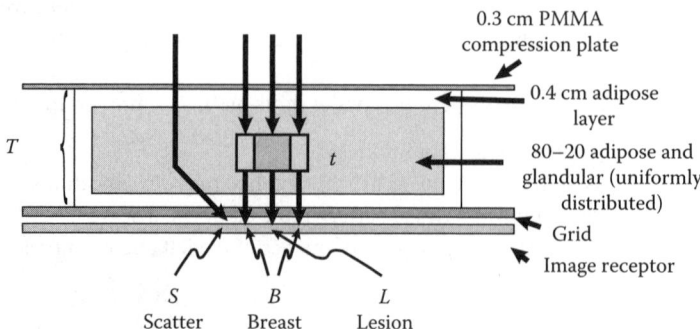

FIGURE 8.2   Simplified computer model of the mammographic image acquisition process.

8.3 Physics of Image Formation

In the model of Figure 8.2, an "average" breast composed of 80% adipose tissue and 20% fibroglandular tissue is considered (Yaffe et al., 2009). For the simplified case of monoenergetic x-rays of energy, E, the number of x-rays recorded in a fixed area of the image is proportional to

$$N_B = N_0(E)e^{-\mu T} \tag{8.1}$$

in the "background" and

$$N_L = N_0(E)e^{-[\mu(T - t) + \mu't]} \tag{8.2}$$

in the shadow of the lesion or other structure of interest. In Equations 8.1 and 8.2, $N_0(E)$ is the number of x-rays that would be recorded in the absence of tissue in the beam, μ and μ' are the attenuation coefficients of the breast tissue and the lesion, respectively, T is the thickness of the breast, and t is the thickness of the lesion.

The difference in x-ray transmission gives rise to *subject* contrast which can be defined as

$$C_0 = \frac{N_B - N_L}{N_B + N_L} \tag{8.3}$$

$$\frac{1 - e^{-[\mu' - \mu t]}}{1 + e^{-[\mu' - \mu t]}} \tag{8.4}$$

For the case of monoenergetic x-rays and temporarily ignoring scattered radiation, contrast would depend only on the thickness of the lesion and the difference between its attenuation coefficient and that of the background material. These are not valid assumptions; x-ray beams are polyenergetic and some scattered radiation is always recorded by the image receptor, so in actuality, contrast also depends to some extent on μ and T.

Shown in Figure 8.3 are x-ray attenuation coefficients measured versus energy on samples of three types of materials found in the breast: adipose tissue, normal fibroglandular breast tissue, and infiltrating ductal carcinoma (one type of breast tumor) (Johns and Yaffe, 1987). Both the attenuation coefficients themselves and their difference ($\mu' - \mu$) decrease with increasing E. As shown in Figure 8.4, which is based on Equation 8.4, this causes C_s to fall as x-ray energy increases. Note that the subject contrast of even small calcifications in the breast is greater than that for a tumor because of the greater difference in attenuation coefficient between calcium and breast tissue.

For a given image recording system (also referred to as the detector), a proper exposure requires a specific value of x-ray energy transmitted by the breast and incident on the receptor, that is, a specific value of N_B. The breast entrance air kerma required to produce an image is, therefore, proportional to

$$N_0 = N_B(E)e^{+\mu T} \tag{8.5}$$

Because μ decreases with energy, the required entrance air kerma for constant signal at the image receptor, N_B, will increase if E is reduced to improve image contrast. A better measure of the risk of radiation-induced breast cancer than air kerma is the mean glandular dose (MGD) (BEIR, 1990). MGD is calculated as the product of the entrance air kerma and a factor, obtained experimentally or by Monte Carlo radiation transport calculations, which converts from incident air kerma to dose (Wu et al., 1991, 1994; Boone, 1999; Dance et al., 2000). The conversion factor increases with E so that MGD does not fall

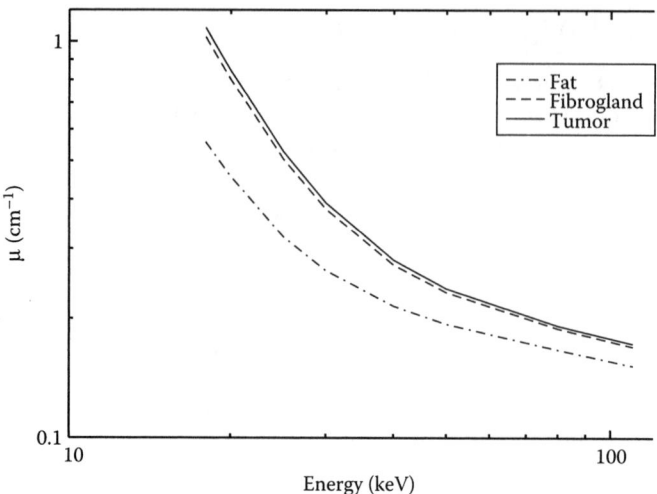

FIGURE 8.3   Measured x-ray linear attenuation coefficients of breast fibroglandular tissue, breast fat, and infiltrating ductal carcinoma plotted versus x-ray energy.

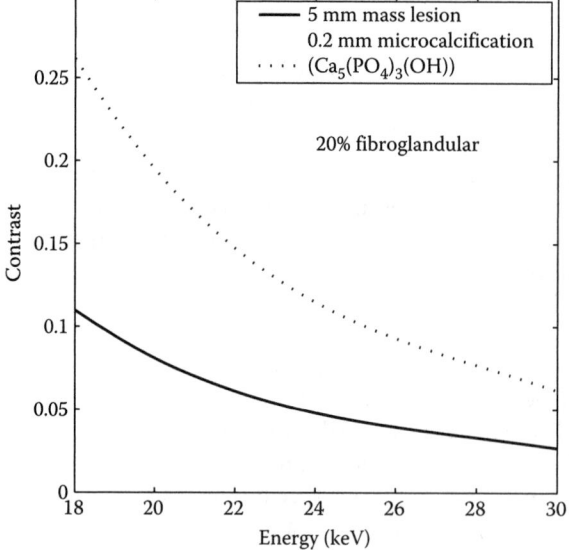

FIGURE 8.4   Dependence of mammographic subject contrast on x-ray energy.

as quickly with energy as does entrance air kerma. The trade-off between image contrast and radiation dose necessitates important compromises in establishing mammographic operating conditions.

8.4 Equipment

In a mammography unit, an x-ray tube and an image receptor are mounted on opposite sides of a mechanical assembly or gantry. Because the breast must be imaged from different aspects and to accommodate patients of different height, the assembly can be adjusted in a vertical axis and rotated about a horizontal axis as shown in Figure 8.5.

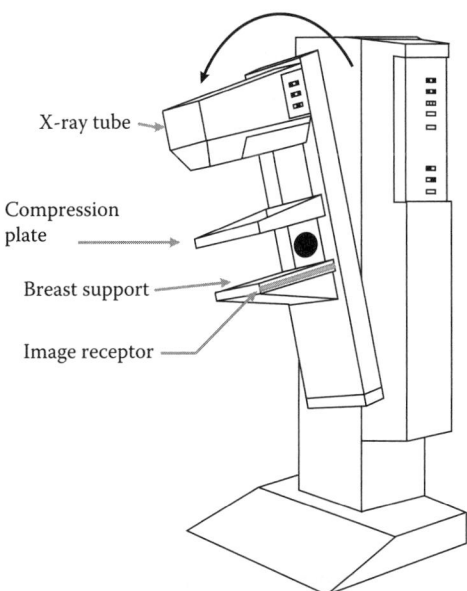

X-ray tube

Compression plate

Breast support

Image receptor

FIGURE 8.5　Schematic diagram of a dedicated mammography machine.

Most general radiography equipment is designed such that the image field is centered below the x-ray source. In mammography, the system's geometry is arranged as in Figure 8.6a where a vertical line from the x-ray source grazes the chest wall of the patient and intersects orthogonally with the edge of the image receptor closest to the patient. If the x-ray beam were centered over the breast as in Figure 8.6b, some of the tissue near the chest wall would be projected inside of the patient where it could not be recorded.

Radiation leaving the x-ray tube passes through a metallic spectral-shaping filter, a beam-defining aperture, and a plate which compresses the breast. Those rays transmitted through the breast are incident on an antiscatter "grid." The x-rays that successfully pass through the grid then strike the image receptor, where they interact, and deposit most of their energy locally. A fraction of the x-rays pass through the receptor without interaction and impinge upon a sensor which is used to activate the automatic exposure control mechanism of the unit.

8.4.1 X-Ray Source

Practical monoenergetic x-ray sources are not available and the x-rays used in mammography arise from bombardment of a metal target by electrons in a hot-cathode vacuum tube. The x-rays are emitted from the target over a spectrum of energies, ranging up to the peak kilovoltage applied to the x-ray tube. Typically, the x-ray tube employs a rotating anode design in which electrons from the cathode strike the anode *target* material at a small angle (0–16°) from normal incidence (Figure 8.7). Over 99% of the energy from the electrons is dissipated as heat in the anode. The angled surface and the distribution of the electron bombardment along the circumference of the rotating anode disk allows the energy to be spread over a larger area of target material while presenting a much smaller effective *focal spot* as viewed from the imaging plane. On modern equipment, the typical "nominal" focal spot size for normal contact mammography is 0.3 mm while the smaller spot used primarily for magnification is 0.1 mm. The specifications for x-ray focal spot size tolerance, established by NEMA (National Electrical Manufacturers Association) in their standard, NEMA XR 5-1992 (R1999), or the IEC (International Electrotechnical Commission) allow the *effective focal spot size* to be considerably larger than these nominal sizes. For example, the NEMA specification allows the effective focal spot size to be 0.45 mm in width and 0.65 mm in length for a nominal 0.3 mm spot and 0.15 mm in each dimension for a nominal 0.1 mm spot.

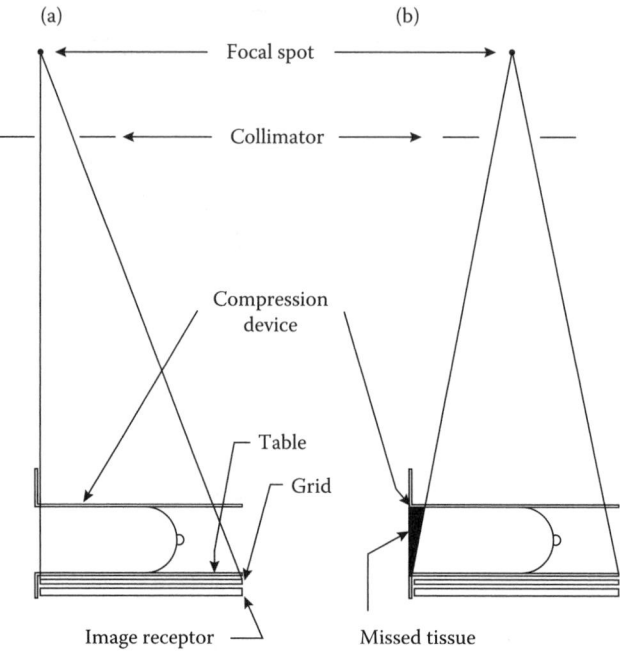

FIGURE 8.6 Geometric arrangement of system components in mammography. (a) Correct alignment provides good tissue coverage; (b) incorrect alignment causes tissue near the chest wall not to be imaged.

The nominal focal spot size is defined relative to the effective spot size at a "reference axis." As shown in Figure 8.7, this reference axis, which may vary from manufacturer to manufacturer, is normally specified at some mid-point in the image. The effective size of the focal spot will monotonically increase from the anode side to the cathode side of the imaging field. Normally, x-ray tubes are arranged such that the cathode side of the tube is adjacent to the patient's chest wall, since the highest intensity of x-rays is available at the cathode side, and the attenuation of x-rays by the patient is generally greater near the chest wall of the image.

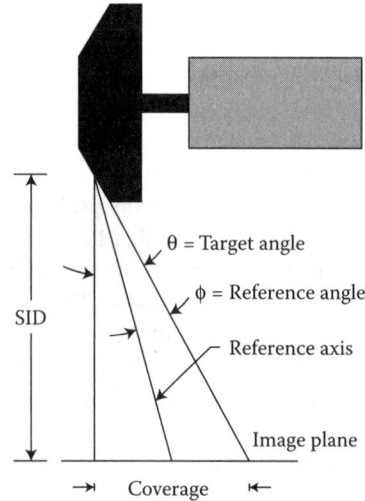

FIGURE 8.7 Angled-target x-ray source provides improved heat loading but causes effective focal spot size to vary across the image.

The spatial resolution capability of the imaging system is partially determined by the effective size of the focal spot and by the degree of magnification of the anatomy at any plane in the breast. This is illustrated in Figure 8.8 where, by similar triangles, the unsharpness region due to the finite size of the focal spot is linearly related to the effective size of the spot and to the ratio of OID to SOD, where SOD is the source–object distance and OID is the object–image receptor distance. Because the breast is a three-dimensional structure, this ratio and, therefore, the unsharpness will vary for different planes within the breast.

The size of the focal spot determines the heat loading capability of the x-ray tube target. For smaller focal spots, the current through the x-ray tube must be reduced, necessitating increased exposure times and the possibility of loss of resolution due to motion of anatomical structures. Loss of geometric resolution can be controlled in part by minimizing OID/SOD, that is, by designing the equipment with greater source–breast distances, by minimizing space between the breast and the image receptor and by compressing the breast to reduce its overall thickness.

Magnification is often used intentionally to improve the signal-to-noise ratio (SNR) or, in the case of digital mammography, the resolution of the image. This is accomplished by elevating the breast above the image receptor, in effect reducing SOD and increasing OID. Under these conditions, resolution is invariably limited by focal spot size and use of a small spot for magnification imaging (typically a nominal size of 0.1 mm) is critical.

Because monoenergetic x-rays are not available, one attempts to define a spectrum providing energies which give a reasonable compromise between radiation dose and image contrast. The spectral shape can be controlled by adjustment of the kilovoltage, choice of the target material, and the type and thickness of metallic filter placed between the x-ray tube and the breast.

Based on models of the imaging problem in mammography, it has been suggested that the optimum energy for imaging lies between 18 and 23 keV, depending on the thickness and composition of the breast (Beaman and Lillicrap, 1982). It has been found that for the breast of typical thickness and composition, the characteristic x-rays from molybdenum at 17.4 and 19.6 keV provide good

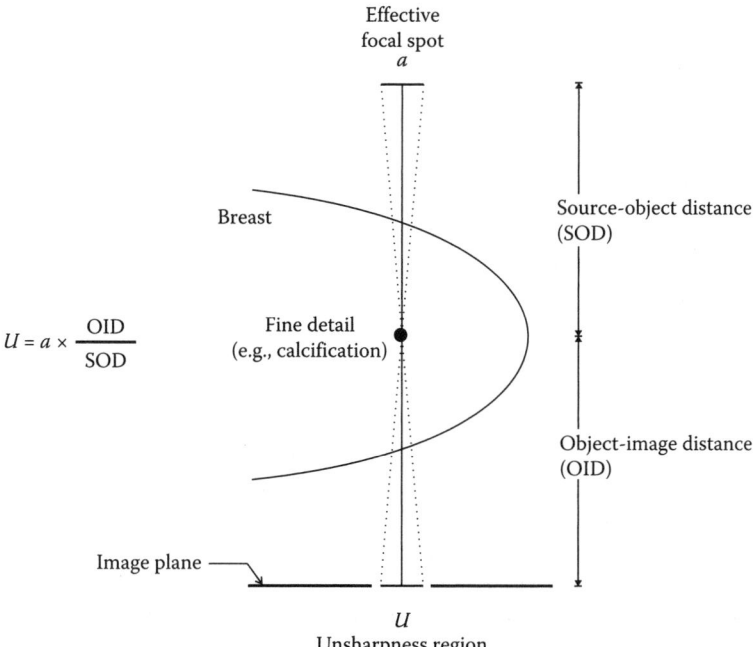

FIGURE 8.8 Dependence of focal spot unsharpness on focal spot size and magnification factor.

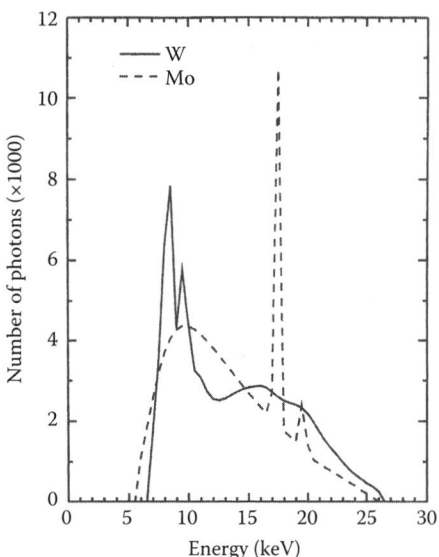

FIGURE 8.9   Comparison of tungsten and molybdenum target x-ray spectra.

imaging performance. For this reason, molybdenum target x-ray tubes are used on the vast majority of mammography machines.

Most mammography tubes use beryllium exit windows between the evacuated tube and the outside world as glass or other metals used in general-purpose tubes would provide excessive attenuation of the useful energies for mammography. Figure 8.9 compares tungsten target and molybdenum target spectra for beryllium window x-ray tubes. Under some conditions, tungsten may provide appropriate image quality for mammography; however, it is essential that the intense emission of L radiation from tungsten be filtered from the beam before it is incident upon the breast, because extremely high doses to the skin would result from this radiation without useful contribution to the mammogram.

8.4.2 Filtration of X-Ray Beam

In conventional radiology, filters made of aluminum or copper are used to provide selective removal of low x-ray energies from the beam before it is incident upon the patient. In mammography, particularly when a molybdenum anode x-ray tube is employed, a molybdenum filter 20–35 μm thick is generally used. This filter attenuates x-rays both at low energies and those above its own K-absorption edge allowing the molybdenum characteristic x-rays from the target to pass through the filter with relatively high efficiency. As illustrated in Figure 8.10, this K-edge filtration results in a spectrum enriched with x-ray energies in the range of 17–20 keV.

Although this spectrum is relatively well suited for imaging the breast of average attenuation, slightly higher energies are desirable for imaging dense thicker breasts. Because the molybdenum target spectrum is so heavily influenced by the characteristic x-rays, an increase in the kilovoltage alone does not substantially change the shape of the spectrum. The beam can be "hardened," however, by employing filters of higher atomic number than molybdenum. For example, rhodium (atomic no. 45) has a K absorption edge at 23 keV, providing strong attenuation both for x-rays above this energy and for those at substantially lower energies. Used with a molybdenum target x-ray tube and slightly increased kV, it provides a spectrum with increased penetration (reduced dose) compared to the Mo/Mo combination.

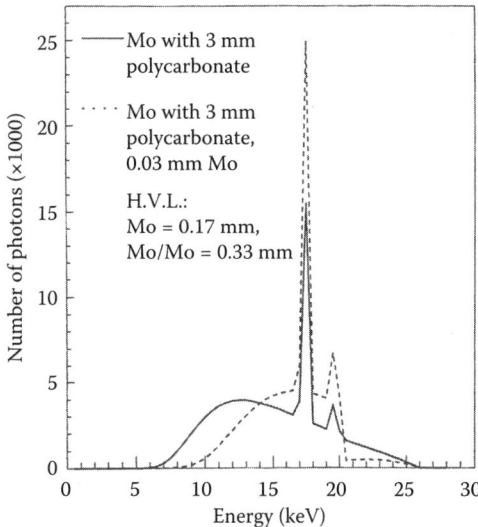

FIGURE 8.10 Molybdenum target spectrum unfiltered (solid line) and filtered by 0.03 mm Mo foil (dashed line).

It is possible to go further in optimizing imaging performance, by "tuning" the effective spectral energy by using other target materials in combination with appropriate K-edge filters (Jennings et al., 1993). One manufacturer employs an x-ray tube incorporating both molybdenum and rhodium targets, where the electron beam can be directed toward one or the other of these materials (Heidsieck et al., 1991). With this system, the filter material (rhodium, molybdenum, etc.) can be varied to suit the target which has been selected. Similarly, work has been reported on K-edge filtration of tungsten spectra (Desponds et al., 1991), where the lack of pronounced K characteristic peaks provides more flexibility in spectral shaping with filters. With the increasing use of digital mammography and tomosynthesis (described below), the optimization shifts toward the use of more penetrating beams, for example, rhodium target with a rhodium filter or tungsten target with an aluminum or silver filter.

8.4.3 Compression Device

There are several reasons for applying firm (but not necessarily painful) compression to the breast during the examination. Compression causes the different tissues to be spread out, minimizing superposition from different planes, and thereby improving a conspicuity of structures. As will be discussed later, scattered radiation can degrade contrast in the mammogram. The use of compression decreases the ratio of scattered to directly transmitted radiation reaching the image receptor. Compression also decreases the distance from any plane within the breast to the image receptor (i.e., OID) and in this way reduces geometric unsharpness. The compressed breast provides lower overall attenuation to the incident x-ray beam, allowing radiation dose to be reduced. The compressed breast also provides more uniform attenuation over the image. This reduces the exposure range that must be recorded by the imaging system, allowing more flexibility in choice of films to be used. Finally, compression provides a clamping action which reduces anatomical motion during the exposure reducing this source of image unsharpness.

It is important that the compression plate allows the breast to be compressed parallel to the image receptor, and that the edge of the plate at the chest wall be straight and aligned with both the focal spot and image receptor to maximize the amount of breast tissue which is included in the image (see Figure 8.6).

8.4.4 Antiscatter Grid

Lower x-ray energies are used for mammography than for other radiological examinations. At these energies, the probability of photoelectric interactions within the breast is significant. Nevertheless, the probability of Compton scattering of x-rays within the breast is still quite high. Scattered radiation recorded by the image receptor has the effect of creating a quasi-uniform haze on the image and causes the subject contrast to be reduced to

$$C_S = \frac{C_0}{1 + \text{SPR}} \tag{8.6}$$

where C_0 is the contrast in the absence of scattered radiation, given by Equation 8.4 and SPR is the scatter-to-primary (directly transmitted) x-ray ratio at the location of interest in the image.

In the absence of an antiscatter device, 37–50% of the total radiation incident on the image receptor would have experienced a scattering interaction within the breast, that is, the scatter to primary ratio would be 0.6–1.0. In addition to contrast reduction, the recording of scattered radiation uses up part of the dynamic range of the image receptor (a limiting factor primarily in film mammography) and adds statistical noise to the image.

Antiscatter *grids* have been designed for mammography. These are composed of linear lead (Pb) septa separated by a rigid interspace material. Generally, the grid septa are not strictly parallel but focused (toward the x-ray source). Because the primary x-rays all travel along direct lines from the x-ray source to the image receptor while the scatter diverges from points within the breast, the grid presents a smaller acceptance aperture to scattered radiation than to primary and thereby discriminates against scattered radiation. Grids are characterized by their *grid ratio* (ratio of the path length through the interspace material to the interseptal width) which typically ranges from 3.5:1 to 5:1. When a grid is used, the SPR typically is reduced by a factor of about 5, leading in most cases to a substantial improvement in image contrast (Wagner, 1991).

On modern mammography equipment, the grid is an integral part of the system, and during x-ray exposure, is moved to blur the image of the grid septa to avoid a distracting pattern in the mammogram. It is important that this motion be uniform and of sufficient amplitude to avoid nonuniformities in the image, particularly for short exposures that occur when the breast is relatively lucent.

Because of absorption of primary radiation by the septa and by the interspace material, part of the primary radiation transmitted by the patient does not arrive at the image receptor. In addition, by removing some of the scattered radiation, the grid causes the overall radiation fluence to be reduced from that which would be obtained in its absence. In film mammography, to obtain a radiograph of proper optical density (blackness), the entrance air kerma to the patient must be increased by a factor known as the *Bucky factor* to compensate for these losses. Typical Bucky factors are in the range of 2–3.

A linear grid does not provide scatter rejection for those quanta traveling in planes parallel to the septa. One manufacturer employs a crossed grid that consists of septa that run in orthogonal directions to address this limitation. The improved scatter rejection is accomplished at doses comparable to those required with a linear grid, because the interspace material of the crossed grid is air rather than a solid. To avoid artifacts, the grid is moved in a very precise way during the exposure to ensure a uniform blurring of the image of the grid itself.

8.4.5 Screen-Film Mammography

8.4.5.1 Fluorescent Screens

When first introduced, mammography was carried out using direct exposure radiographic film in order to obtain the high spatial resolution required. Since the mid-1970s, high-resolution fluorescent screens have been used to convert the x-ray pattern from the breast into an optical image. These screens are used

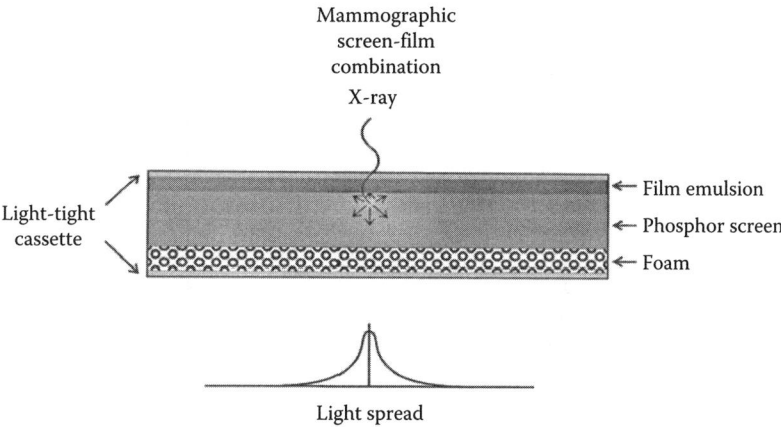

FIGURE 8.11 Design of a screen-film image receptor for mammography.

in conjunction with single-coated radiographic film, and the configuration is shown in Figure 8.11. With this arrangement, the x-rays pass through the cover of a light-tight cassette and the film to impinge upon the screen. Absorption is exponential, so that a large fraction of the x-rays are absorbed near the entrance surface of the screen. The phosphor crystals, which absorb the energy, produce light in an isotropic distribution. Because the film emulsion is pressed tightly against the entrance surface of the screen, the majority of the light quanta have only a short distance to travel to reach the film. Light quanta traveling longer distances have an opportunity to spread laterally (see Figure 8.11), and in this way degrade the spatial resolution. To discriminate against light quanta traveling along these longer oblique paths, the phosphor material of the screen is generally treated with a dye which absorbs much of this light, giving rise to a sharper image. A typical phosphor used for mammography is gadolinium oxysulfide (Gd_2O_2S). Although the K-absorption edge of gadolinium occurs at too high an energy to be useful in mammography, the phosphor material is dense (7.44 g/cm^3) so that the *quantum efficiency* (the fraction of incident x-rays which interact with the screen) is good (about 60%). The signal produced by the detector (in a phosphor, the amount of light produced) is related to the number of x-rays that interact with it (the product of the number of incident x-rays and the quantum efficiency) and the gain provided by the detector. In a phosphor, this gain results from the conversion of the kinetic energy of relatively high energy interacting x-ray quanta into much lower energy optical quanta. For example, one x-ray quantum at 24 keV carries enough kinetic energy to liberate about 8000 light quanta. The process is <100% efficient. At 15% *conversion efficiency*, about 1200 light quanta are emitted per interacting x-ray.

8.4.5.2 Film

The photographic film emulsion for mammography is designed with a characteristic curve such as that shown in Figure 8.12 which is a plot of the optical density (blackness) provided by the processed film versus the logarithm of the x-ray exposure to the screen. Film provides nonlinear input–output transfer characteristics. The local gradient of this curve controls the display contrast presented to the radiologist. Where the curve has a shallow gradient, a given increment of kerma provides little change in optical density, rendering structures imaged in this part of the curve difficult to visualize. Where the curve is steep, the film provides excellent image contrast. The range of kerma over which contrast is appreciable is referred to as the *latitude* of the film. Because the film is constrained between two optical density values, the *base ± fog* density of the film, where no intentional x-ray exposure has resulted, and the maximum density provided by the emulsion, there is a compromise between maximum gradient of the film and the latitude which it provides. For this reason, some regions of the mammogram will generally be underexposed or overexposed, that is, rendered with suboptimal contrast.

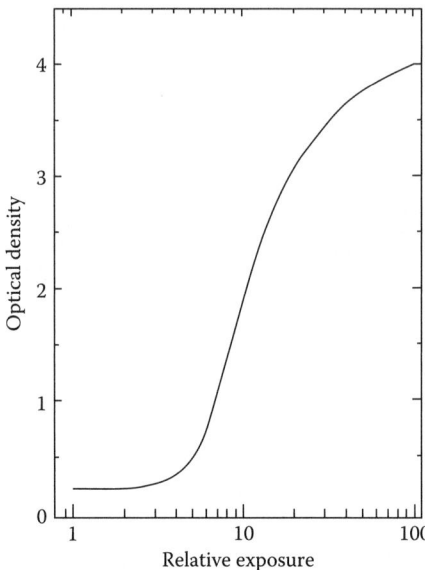

FIGURE 8.12   Characteristic curve of a mammographic screen-film image receptor.

8.4.5.3 Film Processing

Mammography film is processed in an automatic processor similar to that used for general radiographic films. It is important that the development temperature, time, and rate of replenishment of the developer chemistry be compatible with the type of film emulsion used and be designed to maintain good contrast of the film.

8.4.6 Digital Mammography

There are several technical factors associated with screen-film mammography which limit the ability to display the finest or most subtle details, and produce images with the most efficient use of radiation dose to the patient. In screen-film mammography, the film must act as an image acquisition detector as well as a storage and display device. Because of its sigmoidal shape, the range of x-ray exposures over which the film display gradient is significant, that is, the image latitude, is limited. If a tumor is located in either a relatively lucent or more opaque region of the breast, then the contrast displayed to the radiologist may be inadequate because of the limited gradient of the film. This is particularly a concern in patients whose breasts contain large amounts of fibroglandular tissue, the so-called dense breast.

Another limitation of film mammography is the effect of structural noise due to the granularity of the film emulsion used to record the image. This impairs the detectibility of microcalcifications and other fine structures within the breast. While Poisson's quantum noise is unavoidable, it should be possible to virtually eliminate structural noise by technical improvements. Existing screen-film mammography also suffers because of the inefficiency of grids in removing the effects of scattered radiation and with compromises in spatial resolution versus quantum efficiency inherent in the screen-film image receptor.

Many of the limitations of conventional mammography can be effectively overcome with a *digital mammography* imaging system, in which image acquisition, display, and storage are performed independently, allowing optimization of each. For example, acquisition can be performed with low noise, highly linear x-ray detectors, while since the image is stored digitally, it can be displayed with contrast independent of the detector properties and defined by the needs of the radiologist. Whatever image processing techniques are found useful, ranging from simple contrast enhancement to histogram modification and spatial frequency filtering, they could conveniently be applied.

The first commercial digital mammography systems were introduced in 2000 and at the time of writing over 80% of mammography systems in the United States have been converted to digital. The key technical elements that differ from screen-film mammography are the x-ray detector and the display device. The detector should have the following characteristics:

1. Efficient absorption of the incident radiation beam
2. Linear response over a wide range of incident radiation intensity
3. Low intrinsic noise
4. Spatial resolution on the order of 10 cycles/mm (50 μm sampling)
5. Can accommodate at least an 18 × 24 cm and preferably a 24 × 30 cm field size
6. Acceptable imaging time and heat loading of the x-ray tube
7. Robust and stable performance over environmental conditions and time

Two main approaches have been taken in detector development—area detectors and slot detectors. In the former, the entire image is acquired simultaneously, while in the latter only a portion of the image is acquired at one time and the full image is obtained by scanning the x-ray beam and detector across the breast. Area detectors offer convenient fast image acquisition and could be used with conventional x-ray machines, but may still require a grid, while slot systems are slower, require a scanning x-ray beam, but use relatively simple detectors and have excellent intrinsic efficiency at scatter rejection.

In addition, detectors can be distinguished by the x-ray absorber material, by the process with which the x-ray signal is converted to electronic charge and by the readout mechanism. Four designs now in clinical use will be described.

8.4.6.1 Phosphor Flat Panel Detector

In this type of detector system, x-rays are absorbed by a cesium iodide (CsI) phosphor layer and produce light. The phosphor crystal is evaporated to form needle-like structures and these tend to channel the light through the phosphor while reducing lateral spreading. The phosphor is deposited directly on a matrix of about 2000^2 photodiodes with thin film transistor (TFT) switches fabricated on a large area amorphous silicon plate (Figure 8.13) (Shaw et al., 2004). Each photodiode/TFT combination forms a detector element (del) generally corresponding to one pixel of the digital image. The electronic signal is read out on a series of data lines as the switches in each column of the array are activated. The signals from those lines are then multiplexed and digitized to form the image.

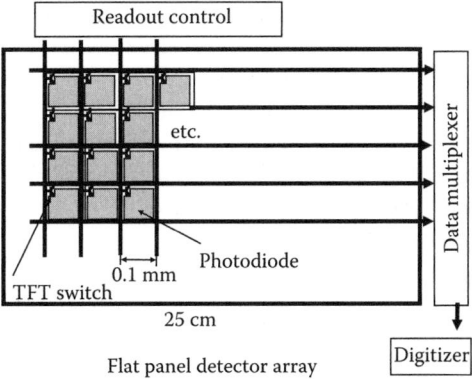

FIGURE 8.13 Schematic representation of a flat-panel phosphor-based digital mammography system. The readout assembly is shown here. A thallium-activated CsI phosphor is evaporated on this surface to serve as the x-ray absorber.

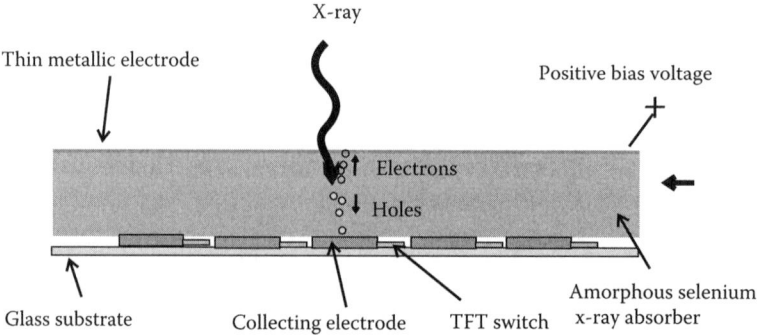

FIGURE 8.14   Cross-sectional view of an amorphous selenium flat panel detector system. The readout array is similar to that illustrated in Figure 8.13.

8.4.6.2 Amorphous Selenium Flat Panel Detector

Here, as in the previous system, the detector is based on large-area flat plate containing a matrix of TFT readout switches. In this case, however, a layer of amorphous selenium is evaporated onto the plate and a thin metal electrode is evaporated over the selenium (Figure 8.14). A bias field of a few volts per μm of detector thickness is applied across the detector. When x-rays are absorbed in the selenium, the energetic photoelectrons and Compton recoil electrons liberated in the material lose their energy by interacting with neighboring atoms and creating about 20 electron-hole pairs for each keV of energy deposited. These drift across the electric field and charges are deposited on landing electrodes that form the dels and replace the photodiodes that were employed in the flat-panel phosphor detector (Yorker et al., 2002). The charge signal from each del is read out in the same manner as described for that system. One potential advantage of this detector technology is that unlike phosphors where the light spreads between the point of creation and where it is detected, here the electrical charge is guided by the applied external field so that it the blurring due to spreading can be minimized. This allows the construction of a detector that is thick enough to have high x-ray absorption efficiency without the loss of spatial resolution that would occur as the thickness of the absorber in phosphor detectors is increased.

8.4.6.3 Photostimulable Phosphor Detector

In these systems, the x-ray absorber is a flat plate formed of a photostimulable phosphor material. When exposed to x-rays, electrons that are liberated during deceleration of the photoelectrons and Compton recoil electrons can become trapped in the phosphor. The number of electron traps filled is directly related to the total x-ray energy absorbed in the phosphor. The plate is placed in a reader device and scanned with a red HeNe laser beam which stimulates the traps to release the electrons (Fetterly and Schueler, 2003). The transition of these electrons through energy levels in the phosphor crystal results in the emission of blue light, which is measured as a function of the laser position on the plate to form the image signal as illustrated schematically in Figure 8.15.

Photostimulable phosphor detectors often have limited spatial resolution because the light from the readout laser scatters and discharges signal from traps that are laterally displaced from the point where the laser beam enters the phosphor. In addition, there is a fundamental compromise required in setting the electron trapping efficiency of the phosphor and this leads to a reduction in signal formation sensitivity. If the trapping efficiency is low, the electrons freed by the x-ray interaction will not be trapped and there will be loss of signal. On the other hand, if it is increased, then electrons that are detrapped during readout will be retrapped rather than creating the light.

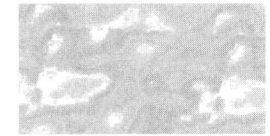

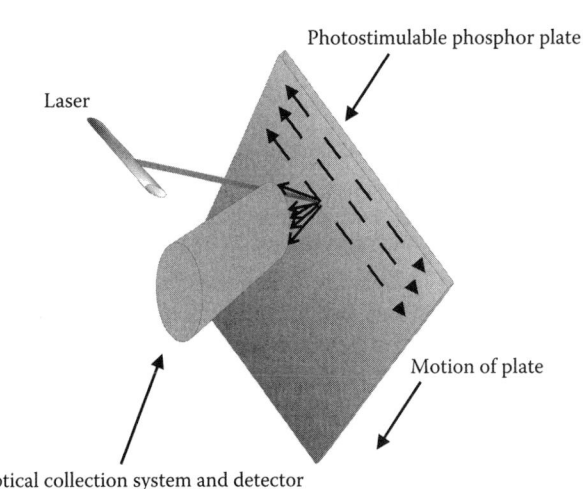

Laser

Photostimulable phosphor plate

Motion of plate

Optical collection system and detector

FIGURE 8.15 Readout system for photostimulable phosphor plates. The laser beam scans across the plate in one dimension as the plate is gradually moved through the reader in the orthogonal dimension. Typically red light is used to detrap electrons and blue light is emitted and collected to form the image.

8.4.6.4 X-Ray Quantum Counting Detectors

The detectors described previously all produce their signal by integrating the charge produced by many x-rays. Even if the x-rays were monoenergetic, there would be a statistical variation in the amount of charge deposited per quantum. Furthermore, these x-rays span an energy distribution, again causing fluctuation in the charge produced per quantum (Swank, 1973). These two sources of fluctuation form a type of image noise over and above the fundamental Poisson noise associated with the random interaction of x-rays in the detector. (Noise is discussed in the next section.) Additionally, when the detector responds to a spectrum of x-rays, the lower energy x-rays produce more contrast, but those at higher energy produce more charge. So the detector implicitly weights the signal with quanta that contain less diagnostic information. Quantum counting detectors are designed to produce one pulse of charge per x-ray quantum absorbed and that pulse is simply counted by the detector circuitry (Åslund et al., 2007). In this way, an equal signal (i.e., one count) is produced, regardless of the actual energy deposited by the quantum. A potential advantage of this design is an improvement in SNR per radiation dose or a dose reduction without loss of SNR.

A more thorough review of detectors for digital mammography is given in Yaffe (2010) and of detectors for digital x-ray imaging in Yaffe and Rowlands (1997).

8.4.7 Noise and Dose

Noise in mammography results primarily from two sources—the random absorption of x-rays in the detector and structural or electronic noise associated with the detector. The first, commonly known as quantum noise, is governed by Poisson's statistics so that for a given area of image the standard deviation in the number of x-rays recorded, σ_N is equal to the square root of the mean number, N, recorded. In other words, the noise in the image is dependent on both the amount of radiation striking the imaging system per unit area and the quantum efficiency of the imaging system. The SNR, $N/\sigma_N = N^{1/2}$, increases as the number of quanta used to form the image increases.

Structural noise is associated with the inherent granularity of the film emulsion in film imaging or the spatial nonuniformity of the detector sensitivity in digital systems. In digital systems other than CR systems, much of the structural noise, also referred to as fixed-pattern noise, can be removed from the image by correction. This is accomplished by producing a low-noise image (large exposure) of a uniform x-ray attenuator to record the pattern of detector sensitivity and any other nonuniformities in the x-ray field and then using this as a "flat-field" mask to correct subsequent images of the breast. Electronic noise arises from the circuitry employed to read out digital images.

For phosphor-based systems as used in screen-film mammography and in some digital mammography systems, in order to maintain high spatial resolution, the screen must be made relatively thin to avoid lateral diffusion of light and this limits the quantum efficiency that can be achieved. The loss of gain could be offset by increasing the conversion efficiency or, in film imaging, by employing a more sensitive film. In film mammography, both the brightness and contrast of the image are closely linked with the light exposure to the film. Therefore, there is a desired degree of exposure to the film. Increasing the gain by increasing the conversion efficiency could result in a film of the required optical density, but obtained using an insufficient number of x-rays to ensure adequate SNR. Similarly, the structural noise due to film granularity increases as more sensitive films are used, so that again film speed must be limited to maintain high image quality. For current high-quality mammographic imaging employing an antiscatter grid, with films exposed to a mean optical density of at least 1.6, the mean glandular dose to a 5.3 cm thick compressed breast is approximately 2.4 milligray. A full examination (two views of each breast) then yields a dose of approximately 4.8 mGy to each breast. For CR systems, it has been found in many cases that doses should be comparable to those used in screen-film mammography. For other types of digital mammography systems, the doses can typically be reduced by about 25–30% (Hendrick et al., 2010). For quantum counting detector systems, a greater dose decrease is often possible.

8.4.8 Automatic Control of Exposure Parameters

It is difficult for the technologist to estimate the attenuation of the breast by inspection, and, therefore, modern mammography units are equipped with automatic exposure control (AEC). For screen-film mammography, the AEC radiation sensors are located behind the image receptor so that they do not cast a shadow on the image. The sensors measure the x-ray fluence transmitted through both the breast and the receptor and provide a signal which can be used to discontinue the exposure when a certain preset amount of radiation has been received by the image receptor. The location of the sensor must be adjustable so that it can be placed behind the appropriate region of the breast in order to obtain proper image density. For film systems, the AEC devices must be calibrated so that approximately constant image optical density results independent of variations in breast attenuation, kilovoltage setting, or field size. With modern equipment, automatic exposure control is generally microprocessor-based so that relatively sophisticated corrections can be made during the exposure for the above effects and for *reciprocity law* failure of the film.

On digital mammography systems other than those using photostimulable phosphor detectors, the detector itself is generally employed as the sensor for automatic control. This provides much more flexibility as algorithms can be used to apply different weightings to signals from different areas of the image field and to ignore regions that are not relevant to the diagnosis. In digital mammography, brightness and contrast can be adjusted while viewing the image at a workstation. Therefore, the automatic control is often configured to terminate the exposure when a given SNR is obtained at a particular location in the image field (e.g., the most attenuating part of the breast).

8.4.8.1 Automatic Control of Kilovoltage and Target/Filter Combination

Many modern mammography units also incorporate automatic control of the filter/kilovoltage combination or, on systems with multitarget x-ray tubes, the target/filter/kilovoltage combination. Penetration through the breast depends on both breast thickness and composition. For a breast that is dense, it is possible that a very long exposure time would be required to achieve adequate film blackening or detector SNR. This results in high dose to the breast and possibly blur due to anatomical motion. It is possible to sense the compressed breast thickness and the transmitted exposure rate and to employ an algorithm to automatically choose the x-ray target and/or beam filter as well as the kilovoltage.

8.5 Quality Control

Mammography is one of the most technically demanding radiographic procedures, and in order to obtain optimal results, all components of the system must be operating properly. Recognizing this, many jurisdictions have implemented and administered mammography accreditation programs. These should evaluate not only the technical performance, but also the qualifications and continuing education of personnel in facilities performing mammography.

In order to verify proper operation, a rigorous quality control program should be in effect. As an example, a program of tests (summarized in Table 8.1) and methods for performing them are contained in the quality control manuals for screen-film mammography published by the American College of

TABLE 8.1 Mammographic Quality Control Minimum Test Frequencies

Test	Performed by	Minimum Frequency
Darkroom cleanliness	Radiologic technologist	Daily
Processor quality control		Daily
Screen cleanliness		Weekly
Viewboxes and viewing conditions		Weekly
Phantom images		Weekly
Visual check list		Monthly
Repeat analysis		Quarterly
Analysis of fixer retention in film		Quarterly
Darkroom fog		Semiannually
Screen-film contact		Semiannually
Compression		Semiannually
Mammographic unit assembly evaluation	Medical physicist	Annually
Collimation assessment		Annually
Focal spot size performance		Annually
kVp accuracy/reproducibility		Annually
Beam quality assessment (half-value layer)		Annually
Automatic exposure control (AEC) system performance assessment		Annually
Uniformity of screen speed		Annually
Breast entrance exposure and mean glandular dose		Annually
Image quality—phantom evaluation		Annually
Artifact assessment		Annually
Radiation output rate		Annually
Viewbox luminance and room illuminance		Annually
Compression release mechanism		Annually

Source: Hendrick RE et al. 1999. *Mammography Quality Control Manuals (Radiologist, Radiologic Technologist, Medical Physicist).* American College of Radiology, Reston, VA. With permission.

Radiology (Hendrick et al., 1999). Programs for quality assurance in digital mammography have been or are being developed by The National Health Service in the United Kingdom, the European Community, the Flemish Screening Program in Belgium, the Norwegian government, The International Atomic Energy Agency (IAEA, 2011), and The American College of Radiology.

8.6 Breast CT, Digital Breast Tomosynthesis, and Contrast Imaging

All mammography, film or digital, is based on projection of x-rays through the three-dimensional breast onto a two-dimensional detector. Superposition of structures in some cases creates complex images in which cancers can be missed; conversely, the superposition can create the appearance of cancers in the projection image where no cancer actually exists. This is a fundamental limitation in all projection radiography and has been overcome in other parts of the body by creating three-dimensional images (sets of tomographic slices) by reconstruction from projections. Systems for dedicated breast computed tomography (CT) are beginning to appear (Boone et al., 2006; Ning et al., 2006). These are based on a table in which the woman lies prone with the breast pendant through an aperture. An x-ray tube and detector array rotate about the breast below the table to acquire image projections.

Another approach, called digital breast tomosynthesis (DBT), illustrated in Figure 8.16, employs the platform of the digital mammography system with one major modification; the x-ray source can rotate over a limited angular range about the stationary compressed breast and detector. By acquiring a set of from 9 to 30 low-dose projection images over a limited angular range of between ±10° and ±20° about the normal to the breast, either iterative techniques or filtered back projection algorithms can be used to reconstruct a set of tomographic slice images (Wu et al., 2003). These slices through the breast can be viewed as a movie loop. While tomosynthesis images do contain artifacts associated with the limited-angle data set, the images provide high spatial resolution in the x-ray plane and moderate (~1 mm) resolution in the z (depth in the breast) plane at doses only slightly higher than those employed for two-dimensional mammography.

Some breast cancers will not be seen on mammography, CT, or DBT because they lack the physical differences in attenuation properties that give rise to x-ray contrast. In such cases, it is possible that an

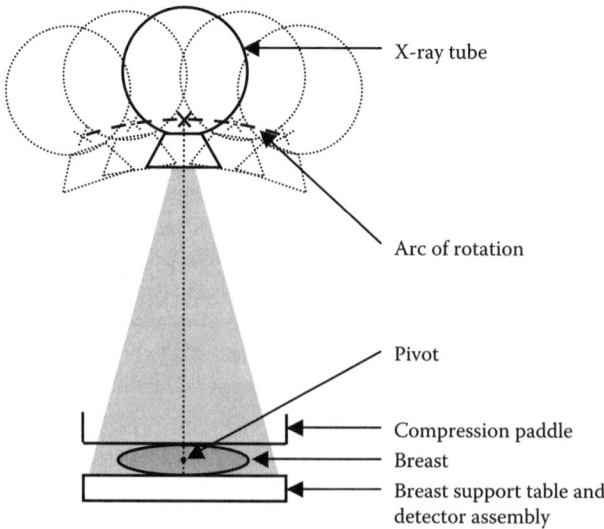

FIGURE 8.16 Concept of tomosynthesis. Tomographic images through the breast are reconstructed from a set of two-dimensional angulated x-ray projection images.

x-ray imaging technique that exploits the phenomenon of tumor angiogenesis, the development of new blood vessels to supply a tumor, may provide a signal that can reveal the presence and extent of the cancer. Angiogenic vessels tend to be poorly formed and leaky. If an iodinated contrast agent is injected into a vein in the arm, the contrast agent will leak and pool near the tumor and then will be washed out. The iodine signals are easily picked up in the mammographic image to reveal the abnormality. Because of the high atomic number of iodine, this type of imaging provides good contrast even at relatively high energies, where the x-rays easily penetrate the noniodinated areas, allowing doses to be kept low. Conspicuity of the lesion can be further enhanced by acquiring images before and after injection of the agent and displaying the result subtraction of the logarithms of the two images (Skarpathiotakis et al., 2002; Jong et al., 2003) or by acquiring images at energies below and above the K edge of iodine, and performing the appropriate weighted subtraction (Lewin et al., 2003; Dromain et al., 2006, 2009). In both cases, the iodine signal is largely isolated from that due to soft tissues in the breast, facilitating visualization of the tumor.

8.7 Stereotactic Biopsy Devices

Stereoscopic x-ray imaging techniques are currently used for the guidance of needle "core" biopsies. These procedures can be used to investigate suspicious mammographic or clinical findings without the need for surgical excisional biopsies, resulting in reduced patient risk, discomfort, and cost. In these stereotactic biopsies, the gantry of a mammography machine is modified to allow angulated views of the breast (typically ±15° from normal incidence) to be achieved. From measurements obtained from these images, the three-dimensional location of a suspicious lesion is determined and a needle equipped with a spring-loaded cutting device can be accurately placed in the breast to obtain the tissue samples. While this procedure can be performed on an upright mammography unit, special dedicated systems are available to allow its performance with the patient lying prone on a table. The accuracy of sampling the appropriate tissue depends critically on the alignment of the system components and the quality of the images produced. A thorough review of stereotactic imaging, including recommended quality control procedures, is given by Hendrick and Parker (1994).

8.8 Summary

Mammography is a technically demanding imaging procedure which can help reduce mortality from breast cancer. To be successful at this purpose, both the technology and technique used for imaging must be optimized. This requires careful system design and attention to quality control procedures. Digital mammography is gradually replacing screen-film mammography and three-dimensional techniques for mammography may provide improved accuracy for breast cancer detection and diagnosis.

Defining Terms

Conversion efficiency: The efficiency of converting the energy from x-rays absorbed in a phosphor material into that of emitted light quanta.

Fibroglandular tissue: A mixture of tissues within the breast composed of the functional glandular tissue and the fibrous supporting structures.

Focal spot: The area of the anode of an x-ray tube from which the useful beam of x-rays is emitted. Also known as the target.

Grid: A device consisting of evenly spaced lead strips which functions like a venetian blind in preferentially allowing x-rays traveling directly from the focal spot without interaction in the patient to pass through, while those whose direction has been diverted by scattering in the patient strike the slats of the grid and are rejected. Grids improve the contrast of radiographic images at the price of increased dose to the patient.

Image receptor: A device which records the distribution of x-rays to form an image. In mammography, the image receptor is generally composed of a light-tight cassette containing a fluorescent screen, which absorbs x-rays and produces light, coupled to a sheet of photographic film.

Quantum efficiency: The fraction of incident x-rays which interact with a detector or image receptor.

Screening: Examination of asymptomatic individuals to detect disease.

Survival: An epidemiological term giving the fraction of individuals diagnosed with a given disease alive at a specified time after diagnosis, for example, "10-year survival."

References

ACS American Cancer Society. Breast Cancer Facts and Figures 2009/2010. http://www.acsevents.org/downloads/STT/F861009_final%209-08-09.pdf accessed May 25, 2010.

Åslund M, Cederström B, Lundqvist M, and Danielsson M. 2007. Physical characterization of a scanning photon counting digital mammography system based on Si-strip detectors. *Med. Phys.* 34(6):1918–1925.

Beaman SA and Lillicrap SC. 1982. Optimum x-ray spectra for mammography. *Phys. Med. Biol.* 27:1209–1220.

BEIR. 1990. *Health Effects of Exposure to Low Levels of Ionizing Radiation (BEIR V).* National Academy Press, Washington DC, pp. 163–170.

Boone JM. 1999. Glandular breast dose for monoenergetic and high-energy x-ray beams: Monte Carlo assessment. *Radiology* 213:23–37.

Boone JM, Nelson T, Kwan A et al. 2006. Computed tomography of the breast: Design, fabrication, characterization, and initial clinical testing. *Med. Phys.* 33:2185.

Dance DR, Skinner CL, Young KC, Beckett JR, and Kotre CJ. 2000. Additional factors for the estimation of mean glandular breast dose using the UK mammography dosimetry protocol. *Phys. Med. Biol.* 45:3225–3240.

Desponds L, Depeursinge C, Grecescu M et al. 1991. Image of anode and filter material on image quality and glandular dose for screen-film mammography. *Phys. Med. Biol.* 36:1165–1182.

Dromain C, Balleyguier C, Adlera G et al. 2009. Contrast-enhanced digital mammography. *Eur. J. Radiol.* 69:34–42.

Dromain C, Balleyguier C, Muller S et al. 2006. Evaluation of tumor angiogenesis of breast carcinoma using contrast-enhanced digital mammography. *AJR Am. J. Roentgenol.* 187(5):W528–37.

Fahrig R, Maidment ADA, and Yaffe MJ. 1992. Optimization of peak kilovoltage and spectral shape for digital mammography. *Proc. SPIE* 1651:74–83.

Fetterly KA and Schueler BA. 2003. Performance evaluation of a dual-side read dedicated mammography computed radiography system. *Med. Phys.* 30:1843–1853.

Heidsieck R, Laurencin G, Ponchin A et al. 1991. Dual target x-ray tubes for mammographic examinations: Dose reduction with image quality equivalent to that with standard mammographic tubes. *Radiology* 181(P):311.

Hendrick RE et al. 1994. *Mammography Quality Control Manuals (Radiologist, Radiologic Technologist, Medical Physicist).* American College of Radiology, Reston, VA.

Hendrick RE et al. 1999. *Mammography Quality Control Manuals (Radiologist, Radiologic Technologist, Medical Physicist).* American College of Radiology, Reston, VA.

Hendrick RE and Parker SH. 1994. Stereotaxic imaging. In *A Categorical Course in Physics: Technical Aspects of Breast Imaging.* 3rd Edition, eds. A.G. Haus and M.J. Yaffe, pp. 263–274. RSNA Publications, Oak Brook, IL.

Hendrick RE, Pisano ED, Averbuch A et al. 2010. Technical comparison of digital mammography to screen-film mammography in the American College of Radiology Imaging Network (ACRIN) Digital Mammographic Imaging Screening Trial (DMIST). *AJR Am. J. Roentgenol.* 194(2):362–369.

IAEA Quality Assurance Programme for Digital Mammography. 2011. IAEA Human Health Series No.17 International Atomic Energy Agency, Vienna.

Jennings RJ, Quinn PW, Gagne RM, and Fewell TR. 1993. Evaluation of x-ray sources for mammography. *Proc. SPIE* 1896:259–268.

Johns PC and Yaffe MJ. 1987. X-ray characterization of normal and neoplastic breast tissues. *Phys. Med. Biol.* 32:675–695.

Jong RA, Yaffe MJ, Skarpathiotakis M et al. 2003. Contrast-enhanced digital mammography: Initial clinical experience. *Radio. Sep.* 228(3):842–850.

Lewin JM, Isaacs PK, Vance V, and Larke FJ. 2003. Dual-energy contrast-enhanced digital subtraction mammography: Feasibility. *Radiology* 229(1):261–268.

Ning R, Conover D, Yu Y et al. 2006. A novel cone beam breast CT scanner: Preliminary system evaluation. *Proc. SPIE* 6142:614211.

Shaw J, Albagli D, Wei C-Y, and Granfors P. 2004. Enhanced a-Si/CsI–based flat panel x-ray detector for mammography. In *Medical Imaging: Physics of Medical Imaging*, eds. M.J. Yaffe and M.J. Flynn, pp. 370–378. *Proceedings of SPIE* Vol. 5368 SPIE, Bellingham, WA, 2004.

Skarpathiotakis M, Yaffe MJ, Bloomquist AK et al. 2002. Development of contrast digital mammography. *Med. Phys.* 29(10):2419–26.

Smart CR, Hartmann WH, Beahrs OH et al. 1993. Insights into breast cancer screening of younger women: Evidence from the 14-year follow-up of the Breast Cancer Detection Demonstration Project. *Cancer* 72:1449–1456.

Swank RK. 1973. Absorption and noise in x-ray phosphors. *J. Appl. Phys.* 44:4199–4203.

Tabar L, Duffy SW, and Burhenne LW. 1993. New Swedish breast cancer detection results for women aged 40–49. *Cancer* 72(Suppl):1437–1448.

Wagner AJ. 1991. Contrast and grid performance in mammography. In *Screen Film Mammography: Imaging Considerations and Medical Physics Responsibilities*, eds. G.T. Barnes and G.D. Frey, pp. 115–134. Medical Physics Publishing, Madison, WI.

Wu T, Stewart A, Stanton M et al. 2003. Tomographic mammography using a limited number of low-dose cone-beam projection images. *Med. Phys.* 30:365.

Wu X, Barnes GT, and Tucker DM. 1991. Spectral dependence of glandular tissue dose in screen-film mammography. *Radiology* 179:143–148.

Wu X, Gingold EL, Barnes GT, and Tucker DM. 1994. Normalized average glandular dose in molybdenum target-rhodium filter and rhodium target-rhodium filter mammography. *Radiology* 193:83–89.

Yaffe MJ. Detectors for digital mammography. 2010. In: *Digital Mammography Series: Medical Radiology Subseries: Diagnostic Imaging Bick*, Ulrich; Diekmann, Felix (Eds), Springer, XVI, 220 p.

Yaffe MJ and Rowlands JA. 1997. X-ray detectors for digital radiography. *Phys Med Biol.* 42:1–39.

Yaffe MJ, Boone JM, Packard N et al. 2009. The myth of the 50–50 breast. *Med. Phys.* 36:5437–5443.

Yorker JG, Jeromin LS, Lee DL et al. 2002. Characterization of a full-field digital mammography detector based on direct x-ray conversion in selenium. *Proc. SPIE* 4682:21.

Further Information

Barnes GT and Frey GD (eds). 1991. *Screen Film Mammography: Imaging Considerations and Medical Physics Responsibilities*. Medical Physics Publishing, Madison, WI. Considerable practical information related to obtaining and maintaining high quality mammography is provided here.

Haus AG (ed). 1993. *Film Processing in Medical Imaging*. Medical Physics Publishing. Madison, WI. This book deals with all aspects of medical film processing with particular emphasis on mammography.

Haus AG and Yaffe MJ. 1994. *A Categorical Course in Physics: Technical Aspects of Breast Imaging*. RSNA Publications, Oak Brook, IL. In this syllabus to a course presented at the Radiological Society of North America, all technical aspects of mammography are addressed by experts and a clinical overview is presented in language understandable by the physicist or biomedical engineer.

Yaffe MJ et al. 1993. *Recommended Specifications for New Mammography Equipment: ACR-CDC Cooperative Agreement for Quality Assurance Activities in Mammography*. ACR Publications, Reston VA.

9

Computed Tomography

Ian A. Cunningham
University of Western Ontario

Philip F. Judy
Harvard Medical School

9.1 Instrumentation

Ian A. Cunningham

The development of **computed tomography (CT)** in the early 1970s revolutionized medical radiology. For the first time, physicians were able to obtain high-quality tomographic (cross-sectional) images of internal structures of the body. Over the next ten years, 18 manufacturers competed for the exploding world CT market. Technical sophistication increased dramatically, and even today, CT continues to mature, with new capabilities being researched and developed.

Computed tomographic images are reconstructed from a large number of measurements of **x-ray transmission** through the patient (called **projection data**). The resulting images are tomographic "maps" of the x-ray linear **attenuation** coefficient. The mathematical methods used to **reconstruct** CT images from projection data are discussed in the next section. In this section, the hardware and instrumentation in a modern scanner are described.

The first practical CT instrument was developed in 1971 by **Dr. G.N. Hounsfield** in England and was used to image the brain (Hounsfield, 1980). The projection data were acquired in approximately 5 min, and the tomographic image was reconstructed in approximately 20 min. Since then, CT technology has developed dramatically, and CT has become a standard imaging procedure for virtually all parts of the body in thousands of facilities throughout the world. Projection data are typically acquired in approximately 1 sec, and the image is reconstructed in 3 to 5 sec. One special-purpose scanner described below acquires the projection data for one tomographic image in 50 msec. A typical modern CT scanner is shown in Figure 9.1, and typical CT images are shown in Figure 9.2.

The fundamental task of CT systems is to make an extremely large number (approximately 500,000) of highly accurate measurements of x-ray transmission through the patient in a precisely controlled geometry. A basic system generally consists of a **gantry**, a patient table, a **control console**, and a

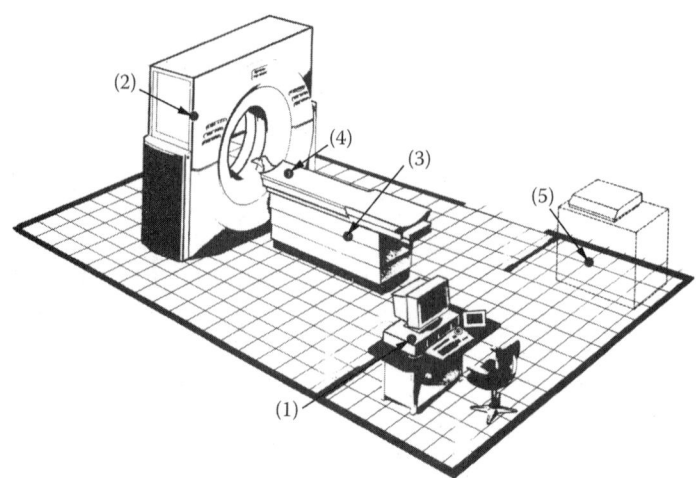

FIGURE 9.1 Schematic drawing of a typical CT scanner installation, consisting of (1) control console, (2) gantry stand, (3) patient table, (4) head holder, and (5) laser imager. (Courtesy of Picker International, Inc.)

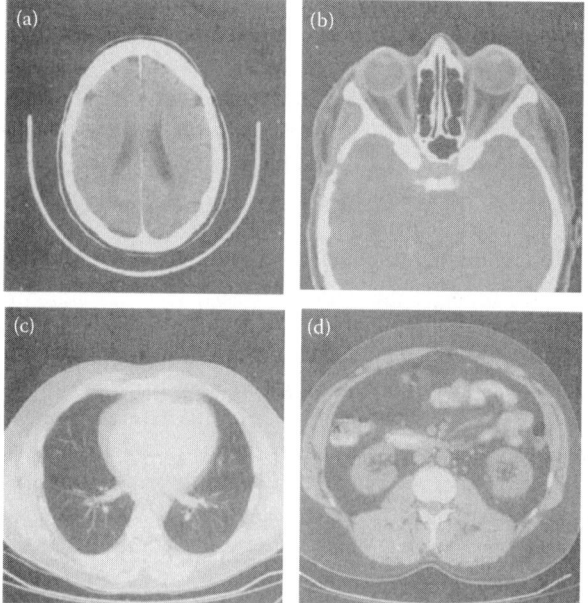

FIGURE 9.2 Typical CT images of (a) brain, (b) head showing orbits, (c) chest showing lungs, and (d) abdomen.

computer. The gantry contains the **x-ray source**, **x-ray detectors**, and the **data-acquisition system (DAS)**.

9.1.1 Data-Acquisition Geometries

Projection data may be acquired in one of several possible geometries described below, based on the scanning configuration, scanning motions, and detector arrangement. The evolution of these geometries

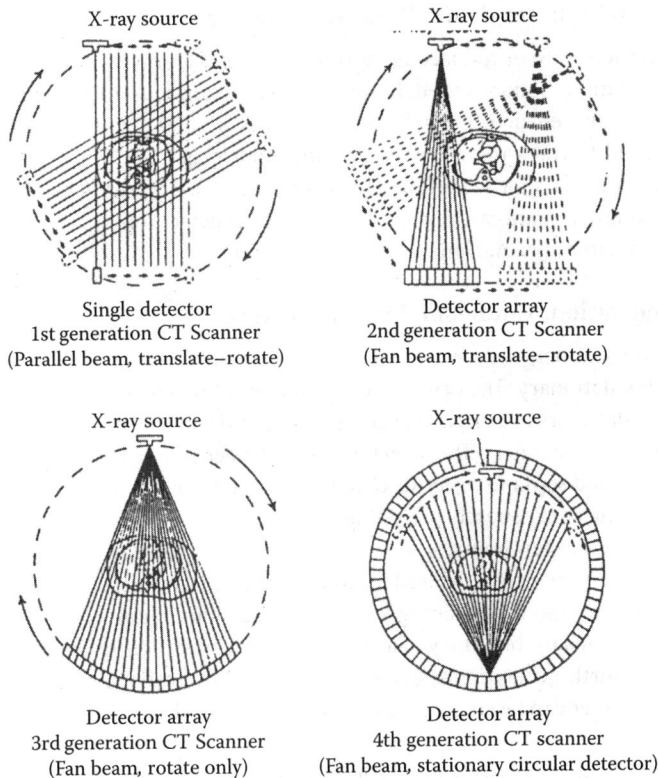

FIGURE 9.3 Four generations of CT scanners illustrating the parallel- and fan-beam geometries. (Adapted from Robb R.A. 1982. CRC *Crit. Rev. Biomed. Eng.* 7: 265.)

is descried in terms of "generations," as illustrated in Figure 9.3, and reflects the historical development (Newton and Potts, 1981; Seeram, 1994). Current CT scanners use either third-, fourth-, or fifth-generation geometries, each having their own pros and cons.

9.1.1.1 First Generation: Parallel-Beam Geometry

Parallel-beam geometry is the simplest technically and the easiest with which to understand the important CT principles. Multiple measurements of x-ray transmission are obtained using a single highly collimated x-ray **pencil beam** and detector. The beam is translated in a linear motion across the patient to obtain a projection profile. The source and detector are then rotated about the patient isocenter by approximately 1 degree, and another projection profile is obtained. This translate-rotate scanning motion is repeated until the source and detector have been rotated by 180 degrees. The highly collimated beam provides excellent rejection of radiation scattered in the patient; however, the complex scanning motion results in long (approximately 5-min) **scan times**. This geometry was used by Hounsfield in his original experiments (Hounsfield, 1980) but is not used in modern scanners.

9.1.1.2 Second Generation: Fan Beam, Multiple Detectors

Scan times were reduced to approximately 30 sec with the use of a **fan beam** of x-rays and a linear **detector array**. A translate-rotate scanning motion was still employed; however, a larger rotate increment could be used, which resulted in shorter scan times. The reconstruction algorithms are slightly more complicated than those for first-generation algorithms because they must handle fan-beam projection data.

9.1.1.3 Third Generation: Fan Beam, Rotating Detectors

Third-generation scanners were introduced in 1976. A fan beam of x-rays is rotated 360 degrees around the isocenter. No translation motion is used; however, the fan beam must be wide enough to completely contain the patient. A curved detector array consisting of several hundred independent detectors is mechanically coupled to the x-ray source, and both rotate together. As a result, these rotate-only motions acquire projection data for a single image in as little as 1 sec. Third-generation designs have the advantage that thin tungsten septa can be placed between each detector in the array and focused on the x-ray source to reject **scattered radiation**.

9.1.1.4 Fourth Generation: Fan Beam, Fixed Detectors

In a fourth-generation scanner, the x-ray source and fan beam rotate about the isocenter, while the detector array remains stationary. The detector array consists of 600 to 4800 (depending on the manufacturer) independent detectors in a circle that completely surrounds the patient. Scan times are similar to those of third-generation scanners. The detectors are no longer coupled to the x-ray source and hence cannot make use of **focused septa** to reject scattered radiation. However, detectors are calibrated twice during each rotation of the x-ray source, providing a self-calibrating system. Third-generation systems are calibrated only once every few hours.

Two detector geometries are currently used for fourth-generation systems (1) a rotating x-ray source inside a fixed detector array and (2) a rotating x-ray source outside a nutating detector array. Figure 9.4 shows the major components in the gantry of a typical fourth-generation system using a fixed-detector array. Both third- and fourth-generation systems are commercially available, and both have been highly successful clinically. Neither can be considered an overall superior design.

9.1.1.5 Fifth Generation: Scanning Electron Beam

Fifth-generation scanners are unique in that the x-ray source becomes an integral part of the system design. The detector array remains stationary, while a high-energy electron beams is electronically swept along a semicircular tungsten strip **anode**, as illustrated in Figure 9.5. X-rays are produced at the point where the electron beam hits the anode, resulting in a source of x-rays that rotates about the patient with no moving parts (Boyd et al., 1979). Projection data can be acquired in approximately 50 msec, which is fast enough to image the beating heart without significant motion artifacts (Boyd and Lipton, 1983).

An alternative fifth-generation design, called the dynamic spatial reconstructor (DSR) scanner, is in use at the Mayo Clinic (Ritman, 1980, 1990). This machine is a research prototype and is not available commercially. It consists of 14 x-ray tubes, scintillation screens, and video cameras. **Volume CT** images can be produced in as little as 10 msec.

9.1.1.6 Spiral/Helical Scanning

The requirement for faster scan times, and in particular for fast multiple scans for **three-dimensional imaging**, has resulted in the development of spiral (**helical**) scanning systems (Kalendar et al., 1990). Both third- and fourth-generation systems achieve this using self-lubricating slip-ring technology (Figure 9.6) to make the electrical connections with rotating components. This removes the need for power and signal cables which would otherwise have to be rewound between scans and allows for a continuous rotating motion of the x-ray fan beam. Multiple images are acquired while the patient is translated through the gantry in a smooth continuous motion rather than stopping for each image. Projection data for multiple images covering a volume of the patient can be acquired in a single breath hold at rates of approximately one **slice** per second. The reconstruction algorithms are more sophisticated because they must accommodate the spiral or helical path traced by the x-ray source around the patient, as illustrated in Figure 9.7.

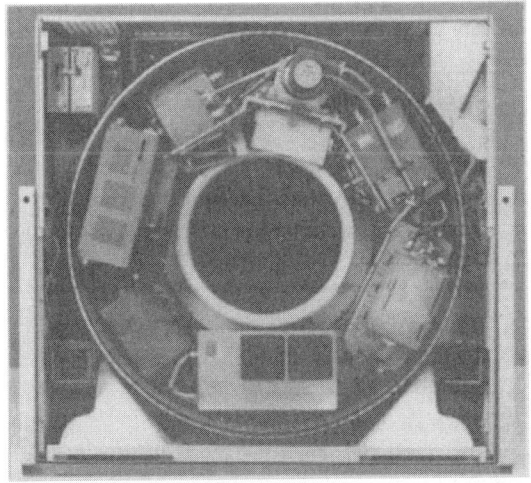

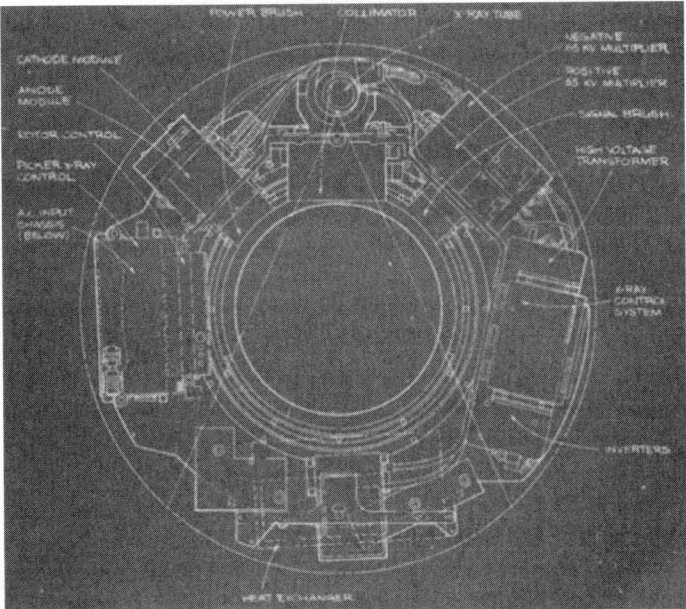

FIGURE 9.4 The major internal components of a fourth-generation CT gantry are shown in a photograph with the gantry cover removed (upper) and identified in the line drawing (lower). (Courtesy of Picker International, Inc.)

9.1.2 X-Ray System

The x-ray system consists of the x-ray source, detectors, and a data-acquisition system.

9.1.2.1 X-Ray Source

With the exception of one fifth-generation system described above, all CT scanners use bremsstrahlung x-ray tubes as the source of radiation. These tubes are typical of those used in diagnostic imaging and produce x-rays by accelerating a beam of electrons onto a target anode. The anode area from which x-rays are emitted, projected along the direction of the beam, is called the **focal spot**. Most systems have two possible focal spot sizes, approximately 0.5×1.5 mm and 1.0×2.5 mm. A collimator assembly is

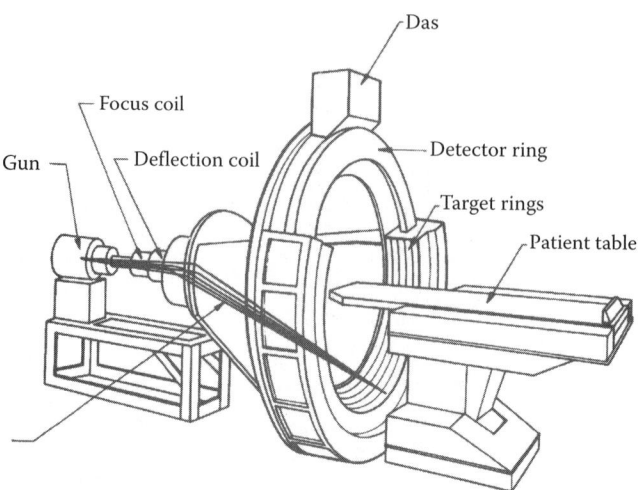

FIGURE 9.5   Schematic illustration of a fifth-generation ultrafast CT system. Image data are acquired in as little as 50 msec, as an electron beam is swept over the strip anode electronically. (Courtesy of Imatron, Inc.)

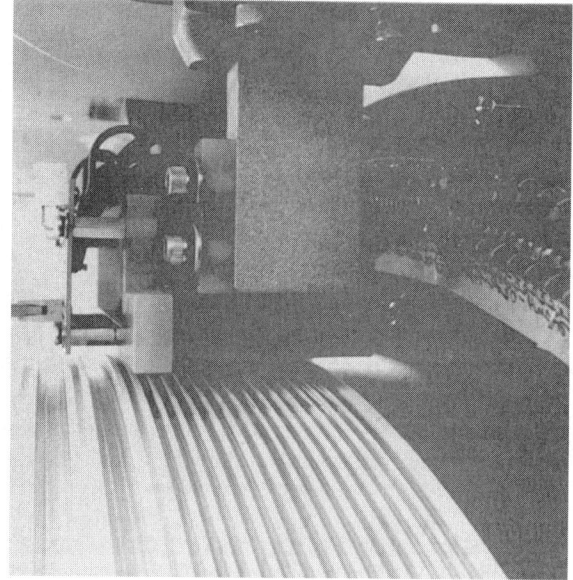

FIGURE 9.6   Photograph of the slip rings used to pass power and control signals to the rotating gantry. (Courtesy of Picker International, Inc.)

used to control the width of the fan beam between 1.0 and 10 mm, which in turn controls the width of the imaged slice.

The power requirements of these tubes are typically 120 kV at 200 to 500 mA, producing x-rays with an energy spectrum ranging between approximately 30 and 120 keV. All modern systems use high-frequency generators, typically operating between 5 and 50 kHz (Brunnett et al., 1990). Some spiral systems use a stationary generator in the gantry, requiring high-voltage (120-kV) slip rings, while others use a rotating generator with lower-voltage (480-V) slip rings. Production of x-rays in bremsstrahlung tubes is an inefficient process, and hence most of the power delivered to the tubes results in heating

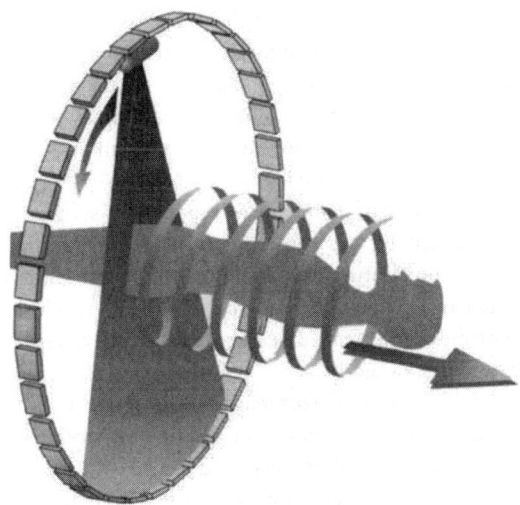

FIGURE 9.7 Spiral scanning causes the focal spot to follow a spiral path around the patient as indicated. (Courtesy of Picker International, Inc.)

of the anode. A heat exchanger on the rotating gantry is used to cool the tube. **Spiral scanning**, in particular, places heavy demands on the heat-storage capacity and cooling rate of the x-ray tube.

The intensity of the x-ray beam is attenuated by **absorption** and scattering processes as it passes through the patient. The degree of attenuation depends on the energy spectrum of the x-rays as well as on the average atomic number and mass density of the patient tissues. The transmitted intensity is given by

$$I_t = I_o e^{-\int_0^L \mu(x)dx} \tag{9.1}$$

where I_o and I_t are the incident and transmitted beam intensities, respectively; L is the length of the x-ray path; and $m(x)$ is the **x-ray linear attenuation coefficient**, which varies with tissue type and hence is a function of the distance x through the patient. The integral of the attenuation coefficient is therefore given by

$$\int_0^L \mu(x)dx = -\frac{1}{L}\ln(I_t/I_0) \tag{9.2}$$

The reconstruction algorithm requires measurements of this integral along many paths in the fan beam at each of many angles about the isocenter. The value of L is known, and I_o is determined by a system calibration. Hence values of the integral along each path can be determined from measurements of I_t.

9.1.2.2 X-Ray Detectors

X-ray detectors used in CT systems must (a) have a high overall efficiency to minimize the patient radiation dose, have a large dynamic range, (b) be very stable with time, and (c) be insensitive to temperature variations within the gantry. Three important factors contributing to the detector efficiency are geometric efficiency, quantum (also called capture) efficiency, and conversion efficiency (Villafanaet et al., 1987). Geometric efficiency refers to the area of the detectors sensitive to radiation as a fraction of the total exposed area. Thin septa between detector elements to remove scattered radiation, or other insensitive regions, will degrade this value. Quantum efficiency refers to the fraction of incident x-rays on the detector that are absorbed and contribute to the measured signal. Conversion efficiency refers to the ability to accurately convert the absorbed x-ray signal into an electrical signal (but is not the same as the energy conversion efficiency). Overall efficiency is the product of the three, and it generally lies between 0.45 and 0.85. A value of less than 1 indicates a nonideal detector system and results in a required increase in patient radiation dose if image quality is to be maintained. The term dose efficiency sometimes has been used to indicate overall efficiency.

Modern commercial systems use one of two detector types: solid-state or gas ionization detectors.

Solid-State Detectors. Solid-state detectors consist of an array of scintillating crystals and photodiodes, as illustrated in Figure 9.8. The scintillators generally are either cadmium tungstate (CdWO4) or a ceramic material made of rare earth oxides, although previous scanners have used bismuth germanate crystals with photomultiplier tubes. Solid-state detectors generally have very high quantum and conversion efficiencies and a large dynamic range.

Gas Ionization Detectors. Gas ionization detectors, as illustrated in Figure 9.9, consist of an array of chambers containing compressed gas (usually xenon at up to 30 atm pressure). A high voltage is applied to tungsten septa between chambers to collect ions produced by the radiation. These detectors have excellent stability and a large dynamic range; however, they generally have a lower quantum efficiency than solid-state detectors.

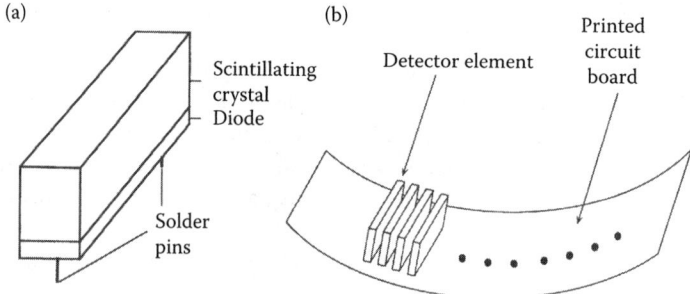

FIGURE 9.8   (a) A solid-state detector consists of a scintillating crystal and photodiode combination. (b) Many such detectors are placed side by side to form a detector array that may contain up to 4800 detectors.

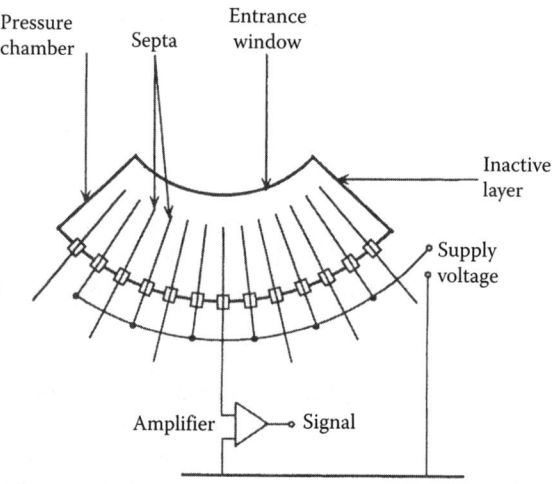

FIGURE 9.9   Gas ionization detector arrays consist of high-pressure gas in multiple chambers separated by thin septa. A voltage is applied between alternating septa. The septa also act as electrodes and collect the ions created by the radiation, converting them into an electrical signal.

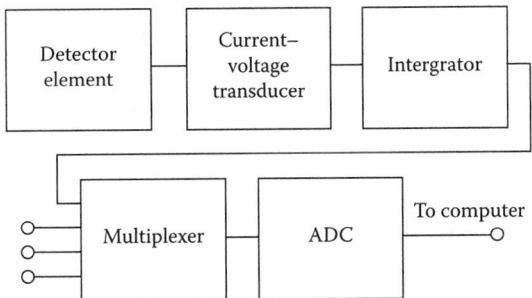

FIGURE 9.10 The data-acquisition system converts the electrical signal produced by each detector to a digital value for the computer.

9.1.2.3 Data-Acquisition System

The transmitted fraction I_t/I_o in Equation 9.2 through an obese patient can be less than 10 to 4. Thus it is the task of the data-acquisition system (DAS) to accurately measure I_t over a dynamic range of more than 104, encode the results into digital values, and transmit the values to the system computer for reconstruction. Some manufacturers use the approach illustrated in Figure 9.10, consisting of precision preamplifiers, current-to-voltage converters, analog integrators, multiplexers, and analog-to-digital converters. Alternatively, some manufacturers use the preamplifier to control a synchronous voltage-to-frequency converter (SVFC), replacing the need for the integrators, multiplexers, and analog-to-digital converters (Brunnett et al., 1990). The logarithmic conversion required in Equation 9.2 is performed with either an analog logarithmic amplifier or a digital lookup table, depending on the manufacturer.

Sustained data transfer rates to the computer are as high as 10 Mbytes/sec for some scanners. This can be accomplished with a direct connection for systems having a fixed detector array. However, third-generation slip-ring systems must use more sophisticated techniques. At least one manufacturer uses optical transmitters on the rotating gantry to send data to fixed optical receivers (Siemens, 1989).

9.1.2.4 Computer System

Various computer systems are used by manufacturers to control system hardware, acquire the projection data, and reconstruct, display, and manipulate the tomographic images. A typical system is illustrated in Figure 9.11, which uses 12 independent processors connected by a 40-Mbyte/sec multibus. Multiple custom array processors are used to achieve a combined computational speed of 200 MFLOPS (million floating-point operations per second) and a reconstruction time of approximately 5 sec to produce an image on a 1024 × 1024 pixel display. A simplified UNIX operating system is used to provide a multitasking, multiuser environment to coordinate tasks.

9.1.3 Patient Dose Considerations

The patient dose resulting from CT examinations is generally specified in terms of the CT dose index (CTDI) (Felmlee et al., 1989; Rothenberg and Pentlow, 1992), which includes the dose contribution from radiation scattered from nearby slices. A summary of CTDI values, as specified by four manufacturers, is given in Table 9.1.

9.1.4 Summary

Computed tomography revolutionized medical radiology in the early 1970s. Since that time, CT technology has developed dramatically, taking advantage of developments in computer hardware and detector technology. Modern systems acquire the projection data required for one tomographic image in approximately 1 sec and present the reconstructed image on a 1024 × 1024 matrix display within a few seconds.

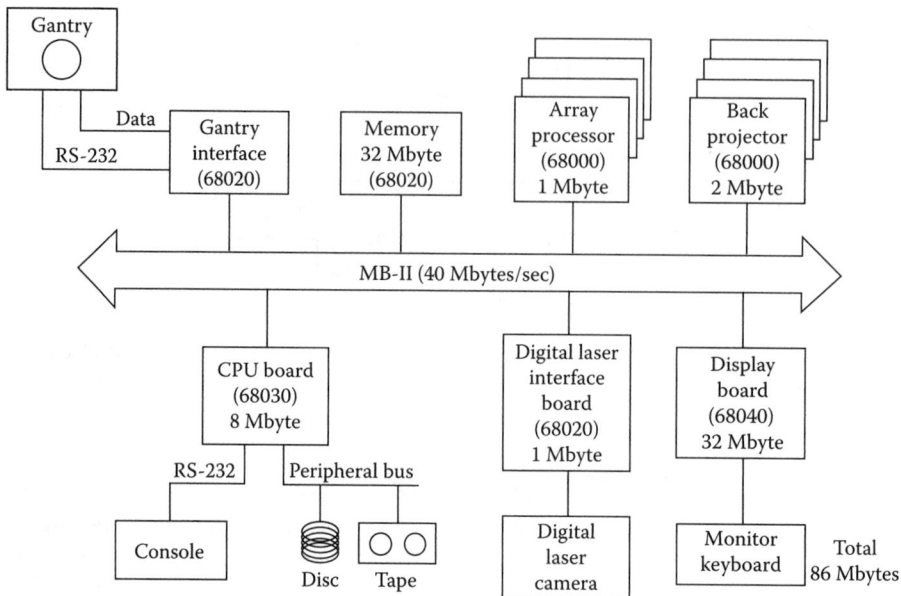

FIGURE 9.11 The computer system controls the gantry motions, acquires the x-ray transmission measurements, and reconstructs the final image. The system shown here uses 1,268,000-family CPUs. (Courtesy of Picker International, Inc.)

TABLE 9.1 Summary of the CT Dose Index (CTDI) Values at Two Positions (Center of the Patient and Near the Skin) as Specified by Four CT Manufacturers for Standard Head and Body Scans

Manufacturer	Detector	kVp	mA	Scan Time (sec)	CTDI, Center (mGy)	CTDI, Skin (mGy)
A, head	Xenon	120	170	2	50	48
A, body	Xenon	120	170	2	14	25
A, head	Solid state	120	170	2	40	40
A, body	Solid state	120	170	2	11	20
B, head	Solid state	130	80	2	37	41
B, body	Solid state	130	80	2	15	34
C, head	Solid state	120	500	2	39	50
C, body	Solid state	120	290	1	12	28
D, head	Solid state	120	200	2	78	78
D, body	Solid state	120	200	2	9	16

The images are high-quality tomographic "maps" of the x-ray linear attenuation coefficient of the patient tissues.

Defining Terms

Absorption: Some of the incident x-ray energy is absorbed in patient tissues and hence does not contribute to the transmitted beam.

Anode: A tungsten bombarded by a beam of electrons to produce x-rays. In all but one fifth-generation system, the anode rotates to distribute the resulting heat around the perimeter. The anode heat-storage capacity and maximum cooling rate often limit the maximum scanning rates of CT systems.

Attenuation: The total decrease in the intensity of the primary x-ray beam as it passes through the patient, resulting from both scatter and absorption processes. It is characterized by the linear attenuation coefficient.

Computed tomography (CT): A computerized method of producing x-ray tomographic images. Previous names for the same thing include computerized tomographic imaging, computerized axial tomography (CAT), computer-assisted tomography (CAT), and reconstructive tomography (RT).

Control console: The control console is used by the CT operator to control the scanning operations, image reconstruction, and image display.

Cormack, Dr. Allan MacLeod: A physicist who developed mathematical techniques required in the reconstruction of tomographic images. Dr. Cormack shared the Nobel Prize in Medicine and Physiology with Dr. G.N. Hounsfield in 1979 (Cormack, 1980).

Data-acquisition system (DAS): Interfaces the x-ray detectors to the system computer and may consist of a preamplifier, integrator, multiplexer, logarithmic amplifier, and analog-to-digital converter.

Detector array: An array of individual detector elements. The number of detector elements varies between a few hundred and 4800, depending on the acquisition geometry and manufacturer. Each detector element functions independently of the others.

Fan beam: The x-ray beam is generated at the focal spot and so diverges as it passes through the patient to the detector array. The thickness of the beam is generally selectable between 1.0 and 10 mm and defines the slice thickness.

Focal spot: The region of the anode where x-rays are generated.

Focused septa: Thin metal plates between detector elements which are aligned with the focal spot so that the primary beam passes unattenuated to the detector elements, while scattered x-rays which normally travel in an altered direction are blocked.

Gantry: The largest component of the CT installation, containing the x-ray tube, collimators, detector array, DAS, other control electronics, and the mechanical components required for the scanning motions.

Helical scanning: The scanning motions in which the x-ray tube rotates continuously around the patient while the patient is continuously translated through the fan beam. The focal spot therefore traces a helix around the patient. Projection data are obtained which allow the reconstruction of multiple contiguous images. This operation is sometimes called spiral, volume, or three-dimensional CT scanning.

Hounsfield, Dr. Godfrey Newbold: An engineer who developed the first practical CT instrument in 1971. Dr. Hounsfield received the McRobert Award in 1972 and shared the Nobel Prize in Medicine and Physiology with Dr. A.M. Cormack in 1979 for this invention (Hounsfield, 1980).

Image plane: The plane through the patient that is imaged. In practice, this plane (also called a slice) has a selectable thickness between 1.0 and 10 mm centered on the image plane.

Pencil beam: A narrow, well-collimated beam of x-rays.

Projection data: The set of transmission measurements used to reconstruct the image.

Reconstruct: The mathematical operation of generating the tomographic image from the projection data.

Scan time: The time required to acquire the projection data for one image, typically 1.0 sec.

Scattered radiation: Radiation that is removed from the primary beam by a scattering process. This radiation is not absorbed but continues along a path in an altered direction.

Slice: See Image plane.

Spiral scanning: See Helical scanning.

Three-dimensional imaging: See Helical scanning.

Tomography: A technique of imaging a cross-sectional slice.

Volume CT: See Helical scanning.

X-ray detector: A device that absorbs radiation and converts some or all of the absorbed energy into a small electrical signal.

X-ray linear attenuation coefficient *m*: Expresses the relative rate of attenuation of a radiation beam as it passes through a material. The value of *m* depends on the density and atomic number of the material and on the x-ray energy. The units of *m* are cm^{-1}.

X-ray source: The device that generates the x-ray beam. All CT scanners are rotating-anode bremsstrahlung x-ray tubes except one-fifth generation system, which uses a unique scanned electron beam and a strip anode.

X-ray transmission: The fraction of the x-ray beam intensity that is transmitted through the patient without being scattered or absorbed. It is equal to I_t/I_o in Equation 9.2, can be determined by measuring the beam intensity both with (I_t) and without (I_o) the patient present, and is expressed as a fraction. As a rule of thumb, n^2 independent transmission measurements are required to reconstruct an image with an $n \times n$ sized pixel matrix.

References

Body D.P. et al. 1979. A proposed dynamic cardiac 3D densitometer for early detection and evaluation of heart disease. *IEEE Trans. Nucl. Sci.* 26: 2724–2727.

Boyd D.P. and Lipton M.J. 1983. Cardiac computed tomography. *Proc. IEEE* 71: 198–307.

Brunnett C.J., Heuscher D.J., Mattson R.A., and Vrettos C.J. 1990. CT Design Considerations and Specifications. Picker International, CT Engineering Department, Ohio.

Cormack A.M. 1980. Nobel award address: early two-dimensional reconstruction and recent topics stemming from it. *Med. Phys.* 7(4): 277.

Felmlee J.P., Gray J.E., Leetzow M.L., and Price J.C. 1989. Estimated fetal radiation dose from multislice CT studies. *Am. Roent. Ray. Soc.* 154: 185.

Hounsfield G.N. 1980. Nobel award address: computed medical imaging. *Med. Phys.* 7(4): 283.

Kalendar W.A., Seissler W., Klotz E. et al. 1990. Spiral volumetric CT with single-breath-hold technique, continuous transport, and continuous scanner rotation. *Radiology* 176: 181.

Newton T.H. and Potts D.G. (eds). 1981. *Radiology of the Skull and Brain: Technical Aspects of Computed Tomography.* St. Louis, Mosby.

Picker. 1990. *Computed Dose Index PQ2000 CT Scanner.* Ohio, Picker International.

Ritman E.L. 1980. Physical and technical considerations in the design of the DSR, and high temporal resolution volume scanner. *AJR* 134: 369.

Ritman E.L. 1990. Fast computed tomography for quantitative cardiac analysis—state of the art and future perspectives. *Mayo Clin. Proc.* 65: 1336.

Robb R.A. 1982. X-ray computed tomography: an engineering synthesis of multiscientific principles. *CRC Crit. Rev. Biomed. Eng.* 7: 265.

Rothenberg L.N. and Pentlow K.S. 1992. Radiation dose in CT. *RadioGraphics* 12: 1225.

Seeram E. 1994. *Computed Tomography: Physical Principles, Clinical Applications and Quality Control.* Philadelphia, Saunders.

Siemens. 1989. *The Technology and Performance of the Somatom Plus.* Erlangen, Germany, Siemens Aktiengesellschaft, Medical Engineering Group.

Villafana T., Lee S.H., and Rao K.C.V.G. (eds). 1987. *Cranial Computed Tomography.* New York, McGraw-Hill.

Further Information

A recent summary of CT instrumentation and concepts is given by E. Seeram in *Computed Tomography: Physical Principles, Clinical Applications and Quality Control.* The author summarizes CT from the perspective of the nonmedical, nonspecialist user. A summary of average CT patient doses is described by

Rothenberg and Pentlow (1992) in *Radiation Dose in CT*. Research papers on both fundamental and practical aspects of CT physics and instrumentation are published in numerous journals, including *Medical Physics, Physics in Medicine and Biology, Journal of Computer Assisted Tomography, Radiology, British Journal of Radiology*, and the IEEE Press. A comparison of technical specifications of CT systems provided by the manufacturers is available from ECRI to help orient the new purchaser in a selection process. Their Product Comparison System includes a table of basic specifications for all the major international manufactures.

9.2 Reconstruction Principles

Philip F. Judy

Computed tomography (CT) is a two-step process: (1) the transmission of an x-ray beam is measured through all possible straight-line paths as in a plane of an object, and (2) the attenuation of an x-ray beam is estimated at points in the object. Initially, the transmission measurements will be assumed to be the results of an experiment performed with a narrow monoenergetic beam of x-rays that are confined to a plane. The designs of devices that attempt to realize these measurements are described in the preceding section. One formal consequence of these assumptions is that the logarithmic transformation of the measured x-ray intensity is proportional to the line integral of attenuation coefficients. In order to satisfy this assumption, computer processing procedures on the measurements of x-ray intensity are necessary even before image reconstruction is performed. These linearization procedures will reviewed after background.

Both analytical and iterative estimations of linear x-ray attenuation have been used for transmission CT reconstruction. Iterative procedures are of historic interest because an iterative reconstruction procedure was used in the first commercially successful CT scanner (EMI, Mark I, Hounsfield, 1973). They also permit easy incorporation of physical processes that cause deviations from the linearity. Their practical usefulness is limited. The first EMI scanner required 20 min to finish its reconstruction. Using the identical hardware and employing an analytical calculation, the estimation of attenuation values was performed during the 4.5-min data acquisition and was made on a 160×160 matrix. The original iterative procedure reconstructed the attenuation values on an 80×80 matrix and consequently failed to exploit all the spatial information inherent in transmission data.

Analytical estimation, or direct reconstruction, uses a numerical approximation of the inverse Radon transform (Radon, 1917). The direct reconstruction technique (convolution-backprojection) presently used in x-ray CT was initially applied in other areas such as radio astronomy (Bracewell and Riddle, 1967) and electron microscopy (Crowther et al., 1970; Ramachandran and Lakshminarayana, 1971). These investigations demonstrated that the reconstructions from the discrete spatial sampling of band-limited data led to full recovery of the cross-sectional attenuation. The random variation (noise) in x-ray transmission measurements may not be bandlimited. Subsequent investigators (Herman and Rowland, 1973; Shepp and Logan, 1974; Chesler and Riederer, 1975) have suggested various bandlimiting windows that reduce the propagation and amplification of noise by the reconstruction. These issues have been investigated by simulation, and investigators continue to pursue these issues using a computer phantom (e.g., Guedon and Bizais, 1994, and references therein) described by Shepp and Logan. The subsequent investigations of the details of choice of reconstruction parameters has had limited practical impact because real variation of transmission data is bandlimited by the finite size of the focal spot and radiation detector, a straightforward design question, and because random variation of the transmission tends to be uncorrelated. Consequently, the classic precedures suffice.

9.2.1 Image Processing: Artifact and Reconstruction Error

An artifact is a reconstruction defect that is obviously visible in the image. The classification of an image feature as an artifact involves some visual criterion. The effect must produce an image feature that is greater than the random variation in image caused by the intrinsic variation in transmission measurements. An artifact not recognized by the physician observer as an artifact may be reported as a lesion. Such false-positive reports could lead to an unnecessary medical procedure, for example, surgery to remove an imaginary tumor. A reconstruction error is a deviation of the reconstruction value from its expected value. Reconstruction errors are significant if the application involves a quantitative measurement, not a common medical application. The reconstruction errors are characterized by identical material at different points in the object leading to different reconstructed attenuation values in the image which are not visible in the medical image.

Investigators have used computer simulation to investigate artifact (Herman, 1980) because image noise limits the visibility of their visibility. One important issue investigated was required spatial sampling of transmission slice plane (Crawford and Kak, 1979; Parker et al., 1982). These simulations provided a useful guideline in design. In practice, these aliasing artifacts are overwhelmed by random noise, and designers tend to oversample in the slice plane. A second issue that was understood by computer simulation was the partial volume artifact (Glover and Pelc, 1980). This artifact would occur even for mononergetic beams and finite beam size, particularly in the axial dimension. The axial dimension of the beams tend to be greater (about 10 mm) than their dimensions in the slice plane (about 1 mm). The artifact is created when the variation of transmission within the beam varies considerably, and the exponential variation within the beam is summed by the radiation detector. The logarithm transformation of the detected signal produces a nonlinear effect that is propagated throughout the image by the reconstruction process. Simulation was useful in demonstrating that isolated features in the same cross-section act together to produce streak artifacts. Simulations have been useful to illustrate the effects of patient motion during the data-acquisition streaks off high-contrast objects.

9.2.2 Projection Data to Image: Calibrations

Processing of transmission data is necessary to obtain high-quality images. In general, optimization of the projection data will optimize the reconstructed image. Reconstruction is a process that removes the spatial correlation of attenuation effects in the transmitted image by taking advantage of completely sampling the possible transmissions. Two distinct calibrations are required: registration of beams with the reconstruction matrix and linearization of the measured signal.

Without loss of generalization, a projection will be considered a set of transmissions made along parallel lines in the slice plane of the CT scanner. Without loss of generalization means that essential aspects of all calibration and reconstruction procedures required for fan-beam geometries are captured by the calibration and reconstruction procedures described for parallel projections. One line of each projection is assumed to pass through the center of rotation of data collection. Shepp et al. (1979) showed that errors in the assignment of that center-of-rotation point in the projections could lead to considerable distinctive artifacts and that small errors (0.05 mm) would produce these effects. The consequences of these errors have been generalized to fan-beam collection schemes, and images reconstructed from 180-degree projection sets were compared with images reconstructed from 360-degree data sets (Kijewski and Judy, 1983). A simple misregistration of the center of rotation was found to produce blurring of image without the artifact. These differences may explain the empirical observation that most commercial CT scanners collect a full 360-degree data set even though 180 degree of data will suffice.

The data-acquisition scheme that was designed to overcome the limited sampling inherent in third-generation fan-beam systems by shifting detectors a quarter sampling distance while opposite 180-degree projection is measured, has particularly stringent registration requirements. Also, the fourth-generation scanner does not link the motion of the x-ray tube and the detector; consequently, the center of rotation is determined as part of a calibration procedure, and unsystematic effects lead to artifacts that mimic noise besides blurring the image.

Misregistration artifacts also can be mitigated by feathering. This procedure requires collection of redundant projection data at the end of the scan. A single data set is produced by linearly weighting the redundant data at the beginning and end of the data collection (Parker et al., 1982). These procedures have be useful in reducing artifacts from gated data collections (Moore et al., 1987).

The other processing necessary before reconstruction of project data is linearization. The formal requirement for reconstruction is that the line integrals of some variable be available; this is the variable that ultimately is reconstructed. The logarithm of x-ray transmission approximates this requirement. There are physical effects in real x-ray transmissions that cause deviations from this assumption. X-ray beams of sufficient intensity are composed of photons of different energies. Some photons in the beam interact with objects and are scattered rather than absorbed. The spectrum of x-ray photons of different attenuation coefficients means the logarithm of the transmission measurement will not be proportional to the line integral of the attenuation coefficient along that path, because an attenuation coefficient cannot even be defined. An effective attenuation coefficient can only be defined uniquely for a spectrum for a small mass of material that alters that intensity. It has to be small enough not to alter the spectrum (McCullough, 1979).

A straightforward approach to this nonunique attenuation coefficient error, called hardening, is to assume that the energy dependence of the attenuation coefficient is constant and that differences in attenuation are related to a generalized density factor that multiplies the spectral dependence of attenuation. The transmission of an x-ray beam then can be estimated for a standard material, typically water, as a function of thickness. This assumption is that attenuations of materials in the object, the human body, differ because specific gravities of the materials differ. Direct measurements of the transmission of an actual x-ray beam may provide initial estimates that can be parameterized. The inverse of this function provides the projection variable that is reconstructed. The parameters of the function are usually modified as part of a calibration to make the CT image of a uniform water phantom flat.

Such a calibration procedure does not deal completely with the hardening effects. The spectral dependence of bone differs considerably from that of water. This is particularly critical in imaging of the brain, which is contained within the skull. Without additional correction, the attenuation values of brain are lower in the center than near the skull.

The detection of scattered energy means that the reconstructed attenuation coefficient will differ from the attenuation coefficient estimated with careful narrow-beam measurements. The x-rays appear more penetrating because scattered x-rays are detected. The zero-ordered scatter, a decrease in the attenuation coefficient by some constant amount, is dealt with automatically by the calibration that treats hardening. First-order scattering leads to a widening of the x-ray beam and can be dealt with by a modification of the reconstruction kernel.

9.2.3 Projection Data to Image: Reconstruction

The impact of CT created considerable interest in the formal aspects of reconstruction. There are many detailed descriptions of direct reconstruction procedures. Some are presented in textbooks used in graduate courses for medical imaging (Barrett and Swindell, 1981; Cho et al., 1993). Herman (1980) published a textbook that was based on a two-semester course that dealt exclusively with reconstruction principles, demonstrating the reconstruction principles with simulation.

The standard reconstruction method is called convolution-backprojection. The first step in the procedure is to convolve the projection, a set of transmissions made along parallel lines in the slice plane, with a reconstruction kernel derived from the inverse Radon transform. The choice of kernel is dictated by bandlimiting issues (Herman and Rowland, 1973; Shepp and Logan, 1974; Chesler and Riederer, 1975). It can be modified to deal with the physical aperture of the CT system (Bracewell, 1977), which might include the effects of scatter. The convolved projection is then backprojected onto a two-dimensional image matrix. Backprojection is the opposite of projection; the value of the projection is added to each point along the line of the projection. This procedure makes sense in the continuous description, but in the discrete world of the computer, the summation is done over the image matrix.

Consider a point of the image matrix; very few, possibly no lines of the discrete projection data intersect the point. Consequently, to estimate the projection value to be added to that point, the procedure must interpolate between two values of sampled convolve projection. The linear interpolation scheme is a significant improvement over nearest project nearest to the point. More complex schemes get confounded with choices of reconstruction kernel, which are designed to accomplish standard image processing in the image, for example, edge enhancement.

Scanners have been developed to acquire a three-dimensional set of projection data (Kalender et al., 1990). The motion of the source defines a spiral motion relative to the patient. The spiral motion defines an axis. Consequently, only one projection is available for reconstruction of the attenuation values in the plane. This is the back-projection problem just discussed; no correct projection value is available from the discrete projection data set. The solution is identical: a projection value is interpolated from the existing projection values to estimate the necessary projections for each plane to be reconstructed. This procedure has the advantage that overlapping slices can be reconstructed without additional exposure, and this eliminates the risk that a small lesion will be missed because it straddles adjacent slices. This data-collection scheme is possible because systems that continuously rotate have been developed. The spiral scan motion is realized by moving the patient through the gantry. Spiral CT scanners have made possible the acquisition of an entire data set in a single breath hold.

References

Barrett H.H. and Swindell W. 1981. *Radiological Imaging: The Theory and Image Formation, Detection, and Processing*, Vol. 2. New York, Academic Press.

Bracewell R.N. and Riddle A.C. 1967. Inversion of fan-beam scans in radio astronomy. *The Astrophys. J.* 150: 427–434.

Chesler D.A. and Riederer S.J. 1975. Ripple suppression during reconstruction in transverse tomography. *Phys. Med. Biol.* 20(4): 632–636.

Cho Z., Jones J.P., and Singh M. 1993. *Foundations of Medical Imaging*. New York, Wiley & Sons, Inc.

Crawford C.R. and Kak A.C. 1979. Aliasing artifacts in computerized tomography. *Appl. Opt.* 18: 3704–3711.

Glover G.H. and Pelc N.J. 1980. Nonlinear partial volume artifacts in x-ray computed tomography. *Med. Phys.* 7: 238–248.

Guedon J.-P. and Bizais. 1994. Bandlimited and harr filtered back-projection reconstruction. *IEEE Trans. Med. Imag.* 13(3): 430–440.

Herman G.T. and Rowland S.W. 1973. Three methods for reconstruction objects for x-rays—a comparative study. *Comp. Graph. Imag. Process.* 2: 151–178.

Herman G.T. 1980. *Image Reconstruction from Projection: The Fundamentals of Computerized Tomography*. New York, Academic Press.

Hounsfield G.N. 1973. Computerized transverse axial scanning (tomography): Part I. *Brit. J. Radiol.* 46: 1016–1022.

Kalender W.A., Seissler W., Klotz E. et al. 1990. Spiral volumetric CT with single-breath-hold technique, continuous transport, and continuous scanner rotation. *Radiology* 176: 181–183.

Kijewski M.F. and Judy P.F. 1983. The effect of misregistration of the projections on spatial resolution of CT scanners. *Med. Phys.* 10: 169–175.

McCullough E.C. 1979. Specifying and evaluating the performance of computed tomographic (CT) scanners. *Med. Phys.* 7: 291–296.

Moore S.C., Judy P.F., Garnic J.D. et al. 1983. The effect of misregistration of the projections on spatial resolution of CT scanners. *Med. Phys.* 10: 169–175.

10

Steven Conolly
Stanford University

Albert Macovski
Stanford University

John Pauly
Stanford University

John Schenck
General Electric Corporate Research and Development Center

Kenneth K. Kwong
Massachusetts General Hospital

David A. Chesler
Massachusetts General Hospital

Xiaoping Hu
University of Minnesota Medical School

Wei Chen
University of Minnesota Medical School

Maqbool Patel
University of Minnesota Medical School

Kamil Ugurbil
University of Minnesota Medical School

Magnetic Resonance Imaging

10.1 Acquisition and Processing

Steven Conolly, Albert Macovski, and John Pauly

Magnetic resonance imaging (MRI) is a clinically important medical imaging modality due to its exceptional soft-tissue contrast. MRI was invented in the early 1970s [1]. The first commercial scanners appeared about 10 years later. Noninvasive MRI studies are now supplanting many conventional invasive procedures. A 1990 study [2] found that the principal applications for MRI are examinations of the head (40%), spine (33%), bone and joints (17%), and the body (10%). The percentage of bone and joint studies was growing in 1990.

Although typical imaging studies range from 1 to 10 min, new fast imaging techniques acquire images in less than 50 msec. MRI research involves fundamental tradeoffs between resolution, imaging time, and signal-to-noise ratio (SNR). It also depends heavily on both gradient and receiver coil hardware innovations.

In this section we provide a brief synopsis of basic nuclear magnetic resonance (NMR) physics. We then derive the *k*-**space** analysis of MRI, which interprets the received signal as a scan of the Fourier transform of the image. This powerful formalism is used to analyze the most important imaging sequences. Finally, we discuss the fundamental contrast mechanisms for MRI.

10.1.1 Fundamentals of MRI

Magnetic resonance imaging exploits the existence of induced nuclear magnetism in the patient. Materials with an odd number of protons or neutrons possess a weak but observable nuclear magnetic moment. Most commonly protons (^{1}H) are imaged, although carbon (^{13}C), phosphorous (^{31}P), sodium (^{23}Na), and fluorine (^{19}F) are also of significant interest. The nuclear moments are normally randomly oriented, but they align when placed in a strong magnetic field. Typical field strengths for imaging range between 0.2 and 1.5 T, although spectroscopic and functional imaging work is often performed with higher field strengths. The nuclear **magnetization** is very weak; the ratio of the induced magnetization to the applied fields is only 4×10^{-9}. The collection of nuclear moments is often referred to as magnetization or **spins**.

The static nuclear moment is far too weak to be measured when it is aligned with the strong static magnetic field. Physicists in the 1940s developed resonance techniques that permit this weak moment to be measured. The key idea is to measure the moment while it oscillates in a plane perpendicular to the static field [3,4]. First one must tip the moment away from the static field. When perpendicular to the static field, the moment feels a torque proportional to the strength of the static magnetic field. The torque always points perpendicular to the magnetization and causes the spins to oscillate or precess in a plane perpendicular to the static field. The frequency of the rotation ω_0 is proportional to the field:

$$\omega_0 = -\gamma B_0$$

where γ, the **gyromagnetic ratio**, is a constant specific to the nucleus, and B_0 is the magnetic field strength. The direction of B_0 defines the *z*-axis. The **precession** frequency is called the **Larmor frequency**. The negative sign indicates the direction of the precession.

Since the precessing moments constitute a time-varying flax, they produce a measurable voltage in a loop antenna arranged to receive the *x* and *y* components of induction. It is remarkable that in MRI we are able to directly measure induction from the precessing nuclear moments of water protons.

Recall that to observe this precession, we first need to tip the magnetization away from the static field. This is accomplished with a weak rotating radiofrequency (RF) field. It can be shown that a rotating RF field introduces a fictitious field in the *z* direction of strength ω/γ. By tuning the frequency of the RF field to ω_0, we effectively delete the B_0 field. The RF slowly nutates the magnetization away from the *z*-axis. The Larmor relation still holds in this "rotating frame," so the frequency of the nutation is γB_1, where B_1 is the amplitude of the RF field. Since the coils receive *x* and *y* (transverse) components of induction, the signal is maximized by tipping the spins completely into the transverse plane. This is accomplished by a $\pi/2$ RF pulse, which requires $\gamma B_1 \tau = \pi/2$, where τ is the duration of the RF pulse. Another useful RF pulse rotates spins by π radians. This can be used to invert spins. It also can be used to refocus transverse spins that have dephased due to B_0 field inhomogeneity. This is called a **spin echo** and is widely used in imaging.

NMR has been used for decades in chemistry. A complex molecule is placed in a strong, highly uniform magnetic field. Electronic shielding produces microscopic field variations within the molecule so that geometrically isolated nuclei rotate about distinct fields. Each distinct magnetic environment produces a peak in the spectra of the received signal. The relative size of the spectral peaks gives the ratio of nuclei in each magnetic environment. Hence the NMR spectrum is extremely useful for elucidating molecular structure.

The NMR signal from a human is due predominantly to water protons. Since these protons exist in identical magnetic environments, they all resonate at the same frequency. Hence the NMR signal is simply proportional to the volume of the water. They key innovation for MRI is to impose spatial variations on the magnetic field to distinguish spins by their location. Applying a magnetic field gradient causes each region of the volume to oscillate at a distinct frequency. The most effective nonuniform field is a linear gradient where the field and the resulting frequencies vary linearly with distance along the object being studied. Fourier analysis of the signal obtains a map of the spatial distribution of spins. This argument is formalized below, where we derive the powerful k-space analysis of MRI [5,6].

10.1.1.1 k-Space Analysis of Data Acquisition

In MRI, we receive a volume integral from an array of oscillators. By ensuring that the phase, "signature" of each oscillator is unique, one can assign a unique location to each spin and thereby reconstruct an image. During signal reception, the applied magnetic field points in the z direction. Spins precess in the xy plane at the Larmor frequency. Hence a spin at position $\mathbf{r} = (x,y,z)$ has a unique phase θ that describes its angle relative to the y axis in the xy plane:

$$s(t) \propto \frac{d}{dt} \int_V M(\mathbf{r}) e^{-i\theta(\mathbf{r},t)/dr} \tag{10.1}$$

where $B_z(\mathbf{r},t)$ is the z component of the instantaneous, local magnetic flux density. This formula assumes there are no x and y field components.

A coil large enough to receive a time-varying flux uniformly from the entire volume produces an EMF proportional to

$$\theta(\mathbf{r},t) = -\gamma \int_0^t B_z(\mathbf{r},\tau) d\tau \tag{10.2}$$

where $M(\mathbf{r})$ represents the equilibrium moment density at each point $\mathbf{r}$.

The key idea for imaging is to superimpose a linear field gradient on the static field B_0. This field points in the direction z, and its magnitude varies linearly with a coordinate direction. For example, an x gradient points in the z direction and varies along the coordinate x. This is described by the vector field $x G_x \hat{\mathbf{z}}$, where $\hat{\mathbf{z}}$ is the unit vector in the z direction. In general, the gradient is $(x G_x + y G_y + z G_z)\hat{\mathbf{z}}$, which can be written compactly as the dot product $\mathbf{G} \cdot \mathbf{r}\hat{\mathbf{z}}$. These gradient field components can vary with time, so the total z field is

$$B_z(\mathbf{r},t) = B_0 + \mathbf{G}(t) \cdot \mathbf{r} \tag{10.3}$$

In the presence of this general time-varying gradient, the received signal is

$$s(t) \propto \frac{d}{dt} \int_V e^{i\gamma B_0 t} M(\mathbf{r}) e^{-i\gamma \int_0^t \mathbf{G}(\tau) \cdot \mathbf{r} d\tau} dr \tag{10.4}$$

The center frequency γB_0 is always much larger than the bandwidth of the signal. Hence the derivative operation is approximately equivalent to multiplication by $-i\omega_0$. The signal is demodulated by the waveform $e^{i\gamma B_0 t}$ to obtain the "baseband" signal:

$$s(t) \propto -i\omega_0 \int_V M(\mathbf{r}) e^{-i\gamma \int_0^t \mathbf{G}(\tau) \cdot \mathbf{r} d\tau} dr \tag{10.5}$$

It will be helpful to define the term $\mathbf{k}(t)$:

$$\mathbf{k}(t) = \gamma \int_0^t \mathbf{G}(\tau)\,d\tau \tag{10.6}$$

Then we can rewrite the received baseband signal as

$$S(t) \propto \int_V M(\mathbf{r})e^{-i\mathbf{k}(t)\cdot\mathbf{r}}\,dr \tag{10.7}$$

which we can now identify as the spatial Fourier transform of $M(\mathbf{r})$ evaluated at $\mathbf{k}(t)$. That is, $S(t)$ scans the spatial frequencies of the function $M(\mathbf{r})$. This can be written explicitly as

$$S(t) \propto M(\mathbf{k}(t)) \tag{10.8}$$

where $M(\mathbf{k})$ is the three-dimensional Fourier transform of the object distribution $M(\mathbf{r})$. Thus we can view MRI with linear gradients as a "scan" of k-space or the spatial Fourier transform of the image. After the desired portion of k-space is scanned, the image $M(\mathbf{r})$ is reconstructed using an inverse Fourier transform.

10.1.1.1.1 2D Imaging

Many different gradient waveforms can be used to scan k-space and to obtain a desired image. The most common approach, called *two-dimensional Fourier transform imaging* (**2D FT**), is to scan through k-space along several horizontal lines covering a rectilinear grid in 2D k-space. See Figure 10.1 for a schematic of the k-space traversal. The horizontal grid lines are acquired using 128 to 256 excitations separated by a time TR, which is determined by the desired contrast, RF flip angle, and the T_1 of the desired components of the image. The horizontal-line scans through k-space are offset in k_y by a variable area y-gradient pulse, which happens before data acquisition starts. These variable offsets in k_y are

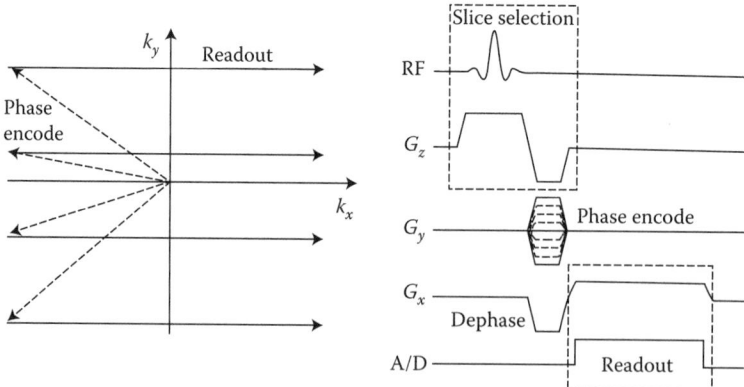

FIGURE 10.1 The drawing on the left illustrates the scanning pattern of the 2D Fourier transform imaging sequence. On the right is a plot of the gradient and RF waveforms that produce this pattern. Only four of the N_y horizontal k-space lines are shown. The phase-encode period initiates each acquisition at a different k_y and at—k_x(max). Data are collected during the horizontal traversals. After all N_y k-space lines have been acquired, a 2D FFT reconstructs the image. Usually 128 or 256 k_y lines are collected, each with 256 samples along k_x. The RF pulse and the z gradient waveform together restrict the image to a particular slice through the subject.

called *phase encodes* because they affect the phase of the signal rather than the frequency. Then for each k_y phase encode, signal is acquired while scanning horizontally with a constant x gradient.

10.1.1.1.2 Resolution and Field of View

The fundamental image characteristics of resolution and field of view (FOV) are completely determined by the characteristics of the k-space scan. The extent of the coverage of k-space determines the resolution of the reconstructed image. The resolution is inversely proportional to the highest spatial frequency acquired:

$$\frac{1}{\Delta x} = \frac{k_x(\max)}{\pi} = \frac{\gamma G_x T}{2\pi} \tag{10.9}$$

$$\frac{1}{\Delta y} = \frac{k_y(\max)}{\pi} = \frac{\gamma G_y T_{\text{phase}}}{\pi} \tag{10.10}$$

where G_x is the readout gradient amplitude and T is the readout duration. The time T_{phase} is the duration of the phase-encode gradient G_y. For proton imaging on a 1.5-T imaging system, a typical gradient strength is $G_x = 1$ G/cm. The signal is usually read for about 8 msec. For water protons, $\gamma = 26,751$ rad/sec/G, so the maximum excursion in k_x is about 21 rad/mm. Hence we cannot resolve an object smaller than 0.3 mm in width. From this one might be tempted to improve the resolution dramatically using very strong gradients or very long readouts. But there are severe practical obstacles, since higher resolution increases the scan time and also degrades the image SNR.

In the phase-encode direction, the k-space data are sampled discretely. This discrete sampling in k-space introduces replication in the imaqge domain [7]. If the sampling in k-space is finer than 1/FOV, then the image of the object will not fold back on itself. When the k-space samling is coarser than 1/FOV, the image of the object does fold back over itself. This is termed *aliasing*. Aliasing is prevented in the readout dirction by the sampling filter.

10.1.1.1.3 Perspective

For most imaging systems, diffraction limits the resolution. That is, the resolution is limited to the wavelength divided by the angle subtended by the receiver aperture, which means that the ultimate resolution is approximately the wavelength itself. This is true for imaging systems based on optics, ultrasound, and x-rays (although there are other important factors, such as quantum noise, in x-ray).

MRI is the only imaging system for which the resolution is independent of the wavelength. In MRI, the wavelength is often many meters, yet submillimeter resolution is routinely achieved. The basic reason is that no attempt is made to focus the radiation pattern to the individual pixel or voxel (volume element), as is done in all other imaging modalities. Instead, the gradients create spatially varying magnetic fields so that individual pixels emit unique waveform signatures. These signals are decoded and assigned to unique positions. An analogous problem is isolating the signals from two transmitting antenna towers separated by much less than a wavelength. Directive antenna arrays would fail because of diffraction spreading. However, we can distinguish the two signals if we use the a priori knowledge that the two antennas transmit at different frequencies. We can receive both signals with a wide-angle antenna and then distinguish the signals through frequency-selective filtering.

10.1.1.1.4 SNR Considerations

The signal strength is determined by the EMF induced from each voxel due to the processing moments. The magnetic moment density is proportional to the polarizing field B_0. Recall that the EMF is proportional to the rate of change of the coil flux. The derivative operation multiples the signal by the Larmor frequency, which is proportional to B_0, so the received signal is proportional to B_0^2 times the volume of the voxel V_v.

In a well-designed MRI system, the dominant noise source is due to thermally generated currents within the conductive tissues of the body. These currents create a time-varying flux which induces noise voltages in the receiver coil. Other noise sources include the thermal noise from the antenna and from the first amplifier. These subsystems are designed so that the noise is negligible compared with the noise from the patient. The noise received is determined by the total volume seen by the antenna pattern V_n and the effective resistivity and temperature of the conductive tissue. One can show [8] that the standard deviation of the noise from conductive tissue varies linearly with B_0. The noise is filtered by an integration over the total acquisition time T_{acq}, which effectively attenuates the noise standard deviation by $\sqrt{T_{acq}}$. Therefore, the SNR varies as

$$\text{SNR} \propto \frac{B_0^2 V_v}{B_0 V_n / \sqrt{T_{acq}}} = B_0 \sqrt{T_{acq}} \, (V_v / V_n) \tag{10.11}$$

The noise volume V_n is the effective volume based on the distribution of thermally generated currents. For example, when imaging a spherical object of radius r, the noise standard deviation varies as $r^{5/2}$ [9]. The effective resistance depends strongly on the radius because currents near the outer radius contribute more to the noise flux seen by the receiver coil.

To significantly improve the SNR, most systems use *surface coils*, which are simply small coils that are just big enough to see the desired region of the body. Such a coil effectively maximizes the voxel-volume to noise-volume ratio. The noise is significantly reduced because these coils are sensitive to currents from a smaller part of the body. However, the field of view is somewhat limited, so "phased arrays" of small coils are now being offered by the major manufacturers [10]. In the phased array, each coil sees a small noise volume, while the combined responses provide the wide coverage at a greatly improved SNR.

10.1.1.1.5 Fast Imaging

The 2D FT scan of k-space has the disadvantage that the scan time is proportional to the number of phase encodes. It is often advantageous to trade off SNR for a shorter scan time. This is especially true when motion artifacts dominate thermal noise. To allow for a flexible tradeoff of SNR for imaging time, more than a single line in k-space must be covered in a single excitation. The most popular approach, called echo-planar imaging (EPI), traverses k-space back and forth on a single excitation pulse. The k-space trajectory is drawn in Figure 10.2.

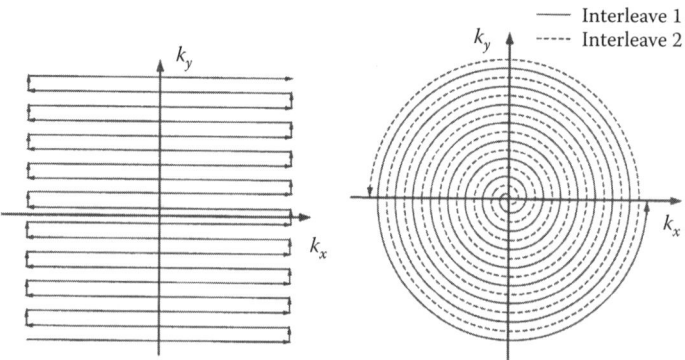

FIGURE 10.2 Alternative methods for the rapid traversal of k-space. On the left is the echo planar trajectory. Data are collected during the horizontal traversals. When all N_y horizontal lines in k-space have been acquired, the data are sent to a 2D FFT to reconstruct the image. On the right is an interleaved spiral trajectory. The data are interpolated to a 2D rectilinear grid and then Fourier transformed to reconstruct the image. These scanning techniques allow for imaging within a breathhold.

It is important that the tradeoff be flexible so that you can maximize the imaging time given the motion constraints. For example, patients can hold their breath for about 12 sec. So a scan of 12 sec duration gives the best SNR given the breath-hold constraint. The EPI trajectory can be interleaved to take full advantage of the breath-hold interval. If each acquisition takes about a second, 12 interleaves can be collected. Each interleaf acquires every twelfth line in *k*-space.

Another trajectory that allows for a flexible tradeoff between scan time and SNR is the spiral trajectory. Here the trajectory starts at the origin in *k*-space and spirals outward. Interleaving is accomplished by rotating the spirals. Figure 10.2 shows two interleaves in a spiral format. Interleaving is very helpful for reducing the hardware requirements (peak amplitude, peak slew rate, average dissipation, etc.) for the gradients amplifiers. For reconstruction, the data are interpolated to a 2D rectilinear grid and then Fourier-transformed. Our group has found spiral imaging to be very useful for imaging coronary arteries within a breath-hold scan [11]. The spiral trajectory is relatively immune to artifacts due to the motion of blood.

10.1.2 Contrast Mechanisms

The tremendous clinical utility of MRI is due to the great variety of mechanisms that can be exploited to create image contrast. If magnetic resonance images were restricted to water density, MRI would be considerably less useful, since most tissues would appear identical. Fortunately, many different MRI contrast mechanisms can be employed to distinguish different tissues and disease processes.

The primary contrast mechanisms exploit *relaxation* of the magnetization. The two types of relaxations are termed **spin–lattice relaxation**, characterized by a relaxation time T_1, and **spin–spin relaxation**, characterized by a relaxation time T_2.

Spin–lattice relaxation describes the rate of recovery of the *z* component of magnetization toward equilibrium after it has been disturbed by RF pulses. The recovery is given by

$$M_z(t) = M_0(1 - e^{-t/T_1}) + M_z(0)e^{-t/T_1} \tag{10.12}$$

where M_0 is the equilibrium magnetization. Differences in the T_1 time constant can be used to produce image contrast by exciting all magnetization and then imaging before full recovery has been achieved. This is illustrated on the left in Figure 10.3. An initial π/2 RF pulse destroys all the longitudinal

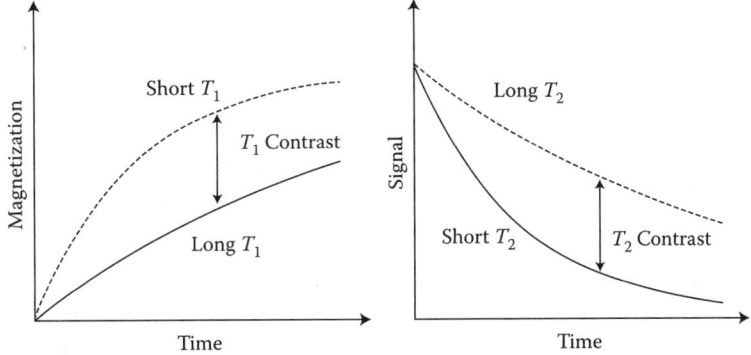

FIGURE 10.3 The two primary MRI contrast mechanisms, T_1 and T_2. T_1, illustrated on the left, describes the rate at which the equilibrium M_{zk} magnetization is restored after it has been disturbed. T_1 contrast is produced by imaging before full recovery has been obtained. T_2, illustrated on the right, describes the rate at which the MRI signal decays after it has been created. T_2 contrast is produced by delaying data acquisition, so shorter T_2 components produce less signal.

magnetization. The plots show the recovery of two different T_1 components. The short T_1 component recovers faster and produces more signal. This gives a T_1-weighted image.

Spin–spin relaxation describes the rate at which the NMR signal decays after it has been created. The signal is proportional to the transverse magnetization and is given by

$$M_{xy}(t) = M_{xy}(0)e^{-t/T_2} \tag{10.13}$$

Image contrast is produced by delaying the data acquisition. The decay of two different T_2 species is plotted on the right in Figure 10.3. The signal from the shorter T_2 component decays more rapidly, while that of the longer T_2 component persists. At the time of data collection, the longer T_2 component produces more signal. This produces a T_2-weighted image.

Figure 10.4 shows examples of these two basic types of contrast. These images are of identical axial sections through the brain of a normal volunteer. The image of the left was acquired with an imaging method that produces T_1 contrast. The very bright ring of subcutaneous fat is due to its relatively short T_1. White matter has a shorter T_1 than gray matter, so it shows up brighter in this image. The image on the right was acquired with an imaging method that produces T_2 contrast. Here the cerebrospinal fluid in the ventricles is bright due to its long T_2. White matter has a shorter T_2 than gray matter, so it is darker in this image.

There are many other contrast mechanisms that are important in MRI. Different chemical species have slightly different resonant frequencies, and this can be used to image one particular component. It is possible to design RF and gradient waveforms so that the image shows only moving spins. This is of great utility in MR angiography, allowing the noninvasive depiction of the vascular system. Another contrast mechanism is called T_2. This relaxation parameter is useful for functional imaging. It occurs when there is a significant spread of Larmor frequencies within a voxel. The superposition signal is attenuated faster than T_2 due to destructive interference between the different frequencies.

In addition to the intrinsic tissue contrast, artificial MRI contrast agents also can be introduced. These are usually administered intravenously or orally. Many different contrast mechanisms can be exploited, but the most popular agents decrease both T_1 and T_2. One agent approved for clinical use is gadolinium DPTA. Decreasing T_1 causes faster signal recovery and a higher signal on a T_1-weighted image. The contrast-enhanced regions then show up bright relative to the rest of the image.

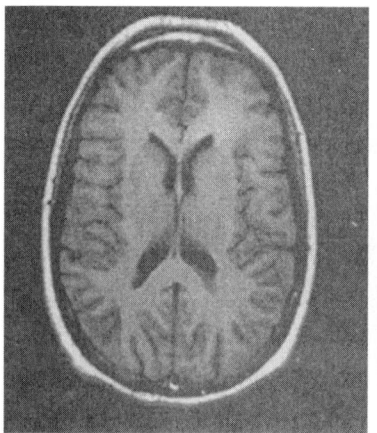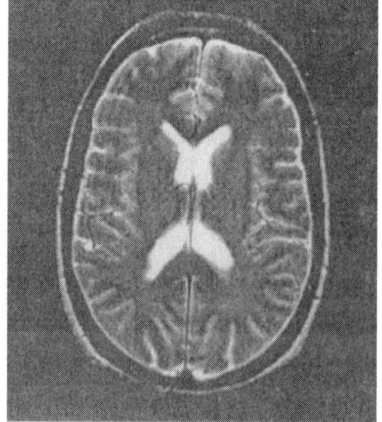

FIGURE 10.4 Example images of a normal volunteer demonstrating T_1 contrast on the left and T_2 contrast on the right.

Defining Terms

D FT: A rectilinear trajectory through *k*-space. This popular acquisition scheme requires several (usually 128 to 256) excitations separated by a time *TR*, which is determined by the desired contrast,
RF flip angle, and the T_1 of the desired components of the image.

Gyromagnetic ratio γ: An intrinsic property of a nucleus. It determines the Larmor frequency through
the relation $\omega_0 = -\gamma B_0$.

***k*-space**: The reciprocal of object space, *k*-space describes MRI data acquisition in the spatial Fourier
transform coordinate system.

Larmor frequency ω_0: The frequency of precession of the spins. It depends on the product of the applied
flux density B_0 and on the gyromagnetic ratio γ. The Larmor frequency is $\omega_0 = -\gamma B_0$.

Magnetization M: The macroscopic ensemble of nuclear moments. The moments are induced by an
applied magnetic field. At body temperatures, the amount of magnetization is linearly proportional ($M_0 = 4 \times 10^{-9}\, H_0$) to the applied magnetic field.

Precession: The term used to describe the motion of the magnetization about an applied magnetic field.
The vector locus traverses a cone. The precession frequency is the frequency of the magnetization
components perpendicular to the applied field. The precession frequency is also called the *Larmor
frequency ω_0*.

Spin echo: The transverse magnetization response to a π RF pulse. The effects of field inhomogeneity are
refocused at the middle of the spin echo.

Spin–lattice relaxation T_1: The exponential rate constant describing the decay of the *z* component of
magnetization toward the equilibrium magnetization. Typical values in the body are between 300
and 3000 msec.

Spin–spin relaxation T_2: The exponential rate constant describing the decay of the transverse components of magnetization (M_x and M_y).

Spins M: Another name for magnetization.

References

1. Lauterbur P.C. 1973. *Nature* 242: 190.
2. Evens R.G. and Evens J.R.G. 1991. *AJR* 157: 603.
3. Bloch F., Hansen W.W., and Packard M.E. 1946. *Phys. Rev.* 70: 474.
4. Bloch F. 1946. *Phys. Rev.* 70: 460.
5. Twieg D.B. 1983. *Med. Phys.* 10: 610.
6. Ljunggren S. 1983. *J. Magn. Reson.* 54: 338.
7. Bracewell R.N. 1978. *The Fourier Transform and Its Applications*. New York, McGraw-Hill.
8. Hoult D.I. and Lauterbur P.C. 1979. *J. Magn. Reson.* 34: 425.
9. Chen C.N. and Hoult D. 1989. *Biomedical Magnetic Resonance Technology*. New York, Adam Hilger.
10. Roemer P.B., Edelstein W.A., Hayes C.E. et al. 1990. *Magn. Reson. Med.* 16: 192.
11. Meyer C.H., Hu B.S., Nishimura D.G., and Macovski A. 1992. *Magn. Reson. Med.* 28: 202.

10.2 Hardware/Instrumentation

John Schenck

This section describes the basic components and the operating principles of MRI scanners. Although
scanners capable of making diagnostic images of the human internal anatomy through the use of **magnetic resonance imaging** (MRI) are now ubiquitous devices in the radiology departments of hospitals
in the United States and around the world, as recently as 1980 such scanners were available only in a
handful of research institutions. Whole-body superconducting magnets became available in the early

1980s and greatly increased the clinical acceptance of this new imaging modality. Market research data indicate that between 1980 and 1996 more than 100 million clinical MRI scans were performed worldwide. By 1996 more than 20 million MRI scans were being performed each year.

MRI scanners use the technique of **nuclear magnetic resonance (NMR)** to induce and detect a very weak radio frequency signal that is a manifestation of **nuclear magnetism**. The term *nuclear magnetism* refers to weak magnetic properties that are exhibited by some materials as a consequence of the nuclear **spin** that is associated with their atomic nuclei. In particular, the proton, which is the nucleus of the hydrogen atom, possesses a nonzero nuclear spin and is an excellent source of NMR signals. The human body contains enormous numbers of hydrogen atoms—especially in water (H_2O) and lipid molecules. Although biologically significant NMR signals can be obtained from other chemical elements in the body, such as phosphorous and sodium, the great majority of clinical MRI studies utilize signals originating from protons that are present in the lipid and water molecules within the patient's body.

The patient to be imaged must be placed in an environment in which several different magnetic fields can be simultaneously or sequentially applied to elicit the desired NMR signal. Every MRI scanner utilizes a strong static field magnet in conjunction with a sophisticated set of **gradient coil**s and radiofrequency coils. The gradients and the radiofrequency components are switched on and off in a precisely timed pattern, or **pulse sequence**. Different pulse sequences are used to extract different types of data from the patient. MR images are characterized by excellent contrast between the various forms of soft tissues within the body. For patients who have no ferromagnetic foreign bodies within them, MRI scanning appears to be perfectly safe and can be repeated as often as necessary without danger (Shellock and Kanal, 1998). This provides one of the major advantages of MRI over conventional x-ray and computed tomographic (CT) scanners. The NMR signal is not blocked at all by regions of air or bone within the body, which provides a significant advantage over ultrasound imaging. Also, unlike the case of nuclear medicine scanning, it is not necessary to add radioactive tracer materials to the patient.

10.2.1 Fundamentals of MRI Instrumentation

Three types of magnetic fields—main fields or static fields (B_2), gradient fields, an radiofrequency (RF) fields (B_1)—are required in MRI scanners. In practice, it is also usually necessary to use coils or magnets that produce shimming fields to enhance the spatial uniformity of the static field B_0. Most MRI hardware engineering is concerned with producing and controlling these various forms of magnetic fields. The ability to construct NMR instruments capable of examining test tube-sized samples has been available since shortly after World War II. The special challenge associated with the design and construction of medical scanners was to develop a practical means of scaling these devices up to sizes capable of safely and comfortably accommodating an entire human patient. Instruments capable of human scanning first became available in the late 1970s. The successful implementation of MRI requires a two-way flow of information between analog and digital formats (Figure 10.5). The main magnet, the gradient and RF coils, and the gradient and RF power supplies operate in the analog domain. The digital domain is centered on a general-purpose computer (Figure 10.6) that is used to provide control information (signal timing and amplitude) to the gradient and RF amplifiers, to process time-domain MRI signal data returning from the receiver, and to drive image display and storage systems. The computer also provides miscellaneous control functions, such as permitting the operator to control the position of the patient table.

10.2.2 Static Field Magnets

The main field magnet (Thomas, 1993) is required to produce an intense and highly uniform, **static magnetic field** over the entire region to be imaged. To be useful for imaging purposes, this field must be extremely uniform in space and constant in time. In practice, the spatial variation of the main field of a whole-body scanner must be less than about 1 to 10 parts per million (ppm) over a region approximately 40 cm in diameter. To achieve these high levels of homogeneity requires careful attention to magnet

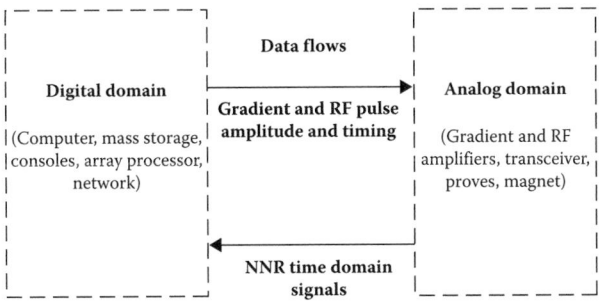

FIGURE 10.5 Digital and analog domains for MRI imaging. MRI involves the flow of data and system commands between these two domains. (Courtesy of W.M. Leue. Reprinted with permission from Schenck, J.F., and W.M. Leue, Instrumentation: Magnets, coils, and hardware, in S.W. Atlas (Ed.), *Magnetic Resonance Imaging of the Brain and Spine*, 2nd ed., pp. 1–27, Lippincott-Raven, Philadelphia, 1996.)

design and to manufacturing tolerances. The temporal drift of the field strength is normally required to be less than 0.1 ppm/h.

Two units of magnetic field strength are now in common use. The gauss (G) has a long historical usage and is firmly embedded in the older scientific literature. The tesla (T) is a more recently adopted unit, but is a part of the SI system of units and, for this reason, is generally preferred. The tesla is a much larger unit than the gauss—1 T corresponds to 10,000 G. The magnitude of the earth's magnetic field is about

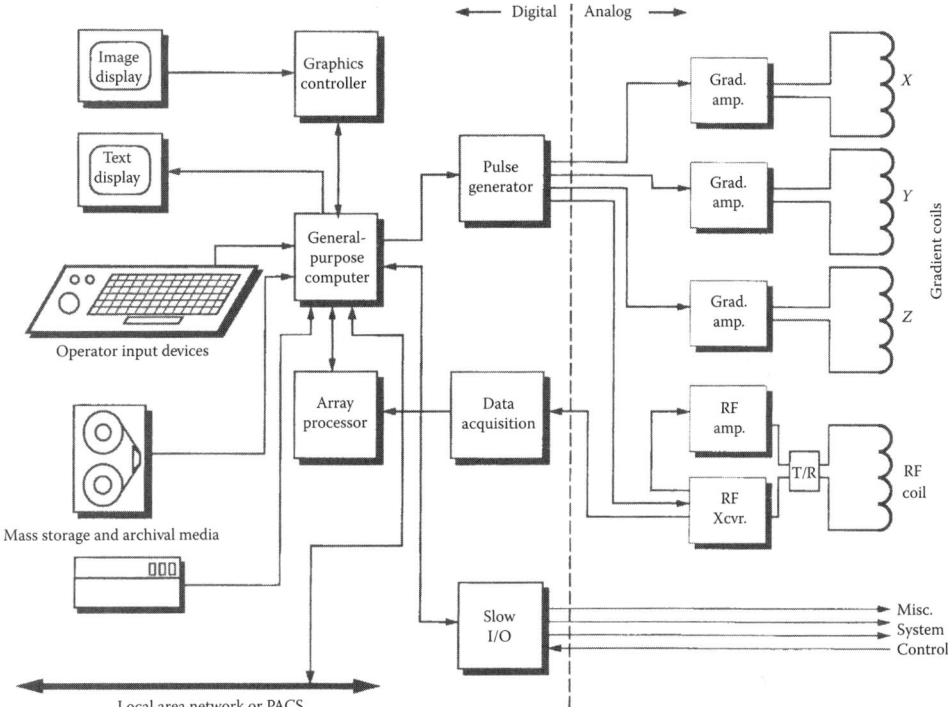

FIGURE 10.6 Block diagram for an MRI scanner. A general-purpose computer is used to generate the commands that control the pulse sequence and to process data during MR scanning. (Courtesy of W.M. Leue. Reprinted with permission from Schenck, J.F., and W.M. Leue, Instrumentation: Magnets, coils, and hardware, in S.W. Atlas (Ed.), *Magnetic Resonance Imaging of the Brain and Spine*, 2nd ed., pp. 1–27, Lippincott-Raven, Philadelphia, 1996.)

0.05 mT (5000 G). The static magnetic fields of modern MRI scanners arc most commonly in the range of 0.5 to 1.5 T; useful scanners, however, have been built using the entire range from 0.02 to 8 T. The signal-to-noise ratio (SNR) is the ratio of the NMR signal voltage to the ever-present noise voltages that arise within the patient and within the electronic components of the receiving system. The SNR is one of the key parameters that determine the performance capabilities of a scanner. The maximum available SNR increases linearly with field strength. The improvement in SNR as the field strength is increased is the major reason that so much effort has gone into producing high-field magnets for MRI systems.

Magnetic fields can be produced by using either electric currents or permanently magnetized materials as sources. In either case, the field strength falls off rapidly away from the source, and it is not possible to create a highly uniform magnetic field on the outside of a set of sources. Consequently, to produce the highly uniform field required for MRI, it is necessary to more or less surround the patient with a magnet. The main field magnet must be large enough, therefore, to effectively surround the patient; in addition, it must meet other stringent performance requirements. For these reasons, the main field magnet is the most important determinant of the cost, performance, and appearance of an MRI scanner. Four different classes of main magnets—(1) permanent magnets, (2) electromagnets, (3) resistive magnets, and (4) superconducting magnets—have been used in MRI scanners.

10.2.2.1 Permanent Magnets and Electromagnets

Both these magnet types use magnetized materials to produce the field that is applied to the patient. In a permanent magnet, the patient is placed in the gap between a pair of permanently magnetized pole faces. Electromagnets use a similar configuration, but the pole faces are made of soft magnetic materials, which become magnetized only when subjected to the influence of electric current coils that are wound around them. Electromagnets, but not permanent magnets, require the use of an external power supply. For both types of magnets, the magnetic circuit is completed by use of a soft iron yoke connecting the pole faces to one another (Figure 10.7). The gap between the pole faces must be large enough to contain the patient as well as the gradient and RF coils. The permanent magnet materials available for use in MRI scanners include high-carbon iron, alloys such as Alnico, ceramics such as barium ferrite, and rare earth alloys such as samarium cobalt.

Permanent magnet scanners have some advantages: they produce a relatively small fringing field and do not require power supplies. However, they tend to be very heavy (up to 100 T) can produce only

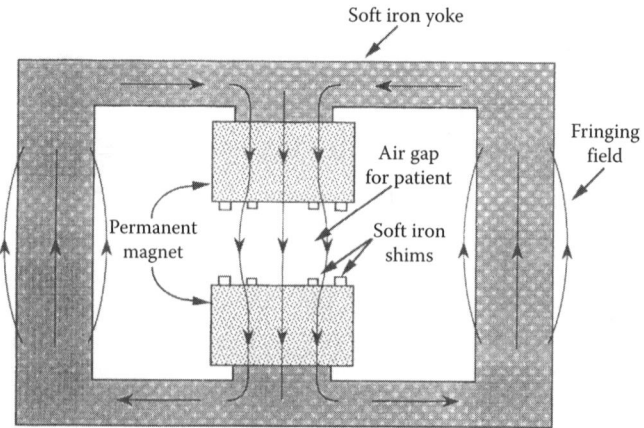

FIGURE 10.7 Permanent magnet. The figure shows a schematic cross-section of a typical permanent magnet configuration. Electromagnets have a similar construction but are energized by current-carrying coils wound around the iron yoke. Soft magnetic shims are used to enhance the homogeneity of the field. (Reprinted with permission from Schenck, J.F., and W.M. Leue, Instrumentation: Magnets, coils, and hardware, in S.W. Atlas (Ed.), *Magnetic Resonance Imaging of the Brain and Spine*, 2nd ed., pp. 1–27, Lippincott-Raven, Philadelphia, 1996.)

relatively low fields—on the order of 0.3 T or less. They are also subject to temporal field drift caused by temperature changes. If the pole faces are made from an electrically conducting material, eddy currents induced in the pole faces by the pulsed gradient fields can limit performance as well. A recently introduced alloy of neodymium, boron, and iron (usually referred to as *neodymium iron*) has been used to make lighter-weight permanent magnet scanners.

10.2.2.2 Resistive Magnets

The first whole-body scanners, manufactured in the late 1970s and early 1980s, used four to six large coils of copper or aluminum wire surrounding the patient. These coils are energized by powerful (40–100 kW) direct-current (dc) power supplies. The electrical resistance of the coils leads to substantial joule heating, and the use of cooling water flowing through the coils is necessary to prevent overheating. The heat dissipation increases rapidly with field strength, and it is not feasible to build resistive magnets operating at fields much higher than 0.15–0.3 T. At present, resistive magnets are seldom used except for very low field strength (0.02–0.06 T) applications.

10.2.2.3 Superconducting Magnets

Since the early 1980s, the use of cryogenically cooled superconducting magnets (Wilson, 1983) has been the most satisfactory solution to the problem of producing the static magnet field for MRI scanners. The property of exhibiting absolutely no electrical resistance near absolute zero has been known as an exotic property of some materials since 1911. Unfortunately, the most common of these materials, such as lead, tin, and mercury, exhibit a phase change back to the normal state at relatively low magnetic field strengths and cannot be used to produce powerful magnetic fields. In the 1950s, a new class of materials (type II superconductors) was discovered. These materials retain the ability to carry loss-free electric currents in very high fields. One such material, an alloy of niobium and titanium, has been used in most of the thousands of superconducting whole-body magnets that have been constructed for use in MRI scanners (Figure 10.8). The widely publicized discovery in 1986 of another class of materials which remain superconducting at much higher temperatures than any previously known material has not yet lead to any material capable of carrying sufficient current to be useful in MRI scanners.

Figure 10.9 illustrates the construction of a typical superconducting whole-body magnet. In this case, six coils of superconducting wire are connected in a series and carry an intense current—on the order of 200 A—to produce the 1.5-T magnetic field at the magnet's center. The diameter of the coils is about

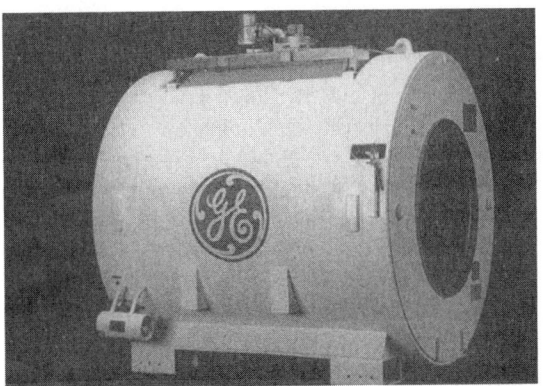

FIGURE 10.8 Superconducting magnet. This figure shows a 1.5-T whole-body superconducting magnet. The nominal warm bore diameter is 1 m. The patient to be imaged, as well as the RF and gradient coils, are located within this bore. (Courtesy of General Electric Medical Systems. Reprinted with permission from Schenck, J.F., and W.M. Leue, Instrumentation: Magnets, coils, and hardware, in S.W. Atlas (Ed.), *Magnetic Resonance Imaging of the Brain and Spine*, 2nd ed., pp. 1–27, Lippincott-Raven, Philadelphia, 1996.)

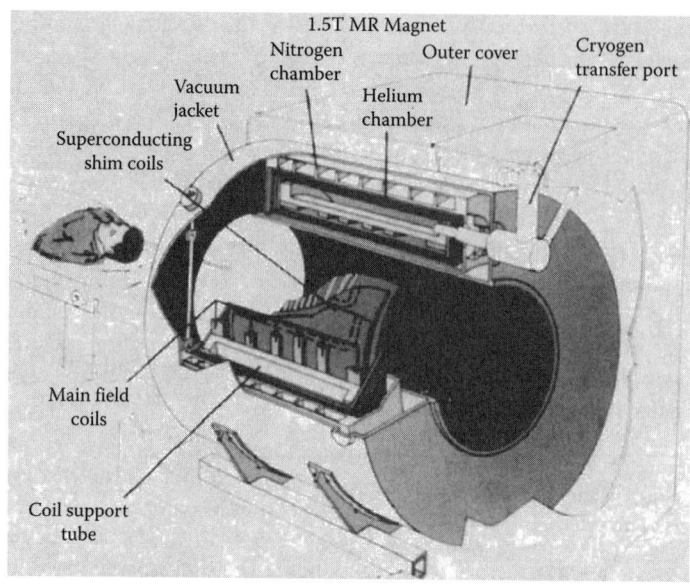

FIGURE 10.9 Schematic drawing of a superconducting magnet. The main magnet coils and the superconducting shim coils are maintained at liquid helium temperature. A computer-controlled table is used to advance the patient into the region of imaging. (Reprinted with permission from Schenck, J.F., and W.M. Leue, Instrumentation: Magnets, coils, and hardware, in S.W. Atlas (Ed.), *Magnetic Resonance Imaging of the Brain and Spine*, 2nd ed., pp. 1–27, Lippincott-Raven, Philadelphia, 1996.)

1.3 m, and the total length of wire is about 65 km (40 miles). The entire length of this wire must be without any flaws—such as imperfect welds—that would interrupt the superconducting properties. If the magnet wire has no such flaws, the magnet can be operated in the persistent mode—that is, once the current is established, the terminals may be connected together, and a constant persistent current flow indefinitely so long as the temperature of the coils is maintained below the superconducting transition temperature. This temperature is about 10 K for niobium–titanium wire. The coils are kept at this low temperature by encasing them in a double-walled cryostat (analogous to a Thermos bottle) that permits them to be immersed in liquid helium at a temperature of 4.2 K. The gradual boiling of liquid helium caused by inevitable heat leaks into the cryostat requires that the helium be replaced on a regular schedule. Many magnets now make use of cryogenic refrigerators that reduce or eliminate the need for refilling the liquid helium reservoir. The temporal stability of superconducting magnets operating in the persistent mode is truly remarkable—magnets have operated for years completely disconnected from power supplies and maintained their magnetic field constant to within a few parts per million. Because of their ability to achieve very strong and stable magnetic field strengths without undue power consumption, superconducting magnets have become the most widely used source of the main magnetic fields for MRI scanners.

10.2.2.4 Magnetic Field Homogeneity

The necessary degree of spatial uniformity of the field can be achieved only by carefully placing the coils at specific spatial locations. It is well known that a single loop of wire will produce, on its axis, a field that is directed along the coil axis and that can be expressed as a sum of spherical harmonic fields. The first term in this sum is constant in space and represents the desired field that is completely independent of position. The higher-order terms represent contaminating field inhomogeneities that spoil the field uniformity. More than a century ago, a two-coil magnet system—known as the *Helmholtz pair*—was developed which produced a much more homogeneous field at its center than is produced by a single current loop. This design is based on the mathematical finding that when two coaxial coils of the same radius are separated by a distance equal to their radius, the first nonzero contaminating term in the harmonic expansion is of the fourth order. This results in an increased region of the field homogeneity, which, although it is useful in many applications, is far too small to be useful in MRI scanners. However, the principle of eliminating low-order harmonic fields can be extended by using additional coils. This is the method now used to increase the volume of field homogeneity to values that are useful for MRI. For example, in the commonly used six-coil system, it is possible to eliminate all the error fields through the twelfth order.

In practice, manufacturing tolerances and field perturbations caused b extraneous magnetic field sources—such as steel girders in the building surrounding the magnet—produce additional inhomogeneity in the imaging region. These field imperfections are reduced by the use of shimming fields. One approach—*active shimming*—uses additional coils (either resistive coils, superconducting coils, or some of each) which are designed to produce a magnetic field corresponding to a particular term in the spherical harmonic expansion. When the magnet is installed, the magnetic field is carefully mapped, and the currents in the shim coils are adjusted to cancel out the terms in the harmonic expansion to some prescribed high order. The alternative approach—*passive shimming*—utilizes small permanent magnets that are placed at the proper locations along the inner walls of the magnet bore to cancel out contaminating fields. If a large object containing magnetic materials—such as a power supply—is moved in the vicinity of superconducting magnets, it may be necessary to reset the shimming currents or magnet locations to account for the changed pattern of field inhomogeneity.

10.2.2.5 Fringing Fields

A large, powerful magnet produces a strong magnetic field in the region surrounding it as well as in its interior. This fringing field can produce undesirable effects such as erasing magnetic tapes (and credit cards). It is also a potential hazard to people with implanted medical devices such as cardiac pacemakers. For safety purposes, it is general practice to limit access to the region where the fringing field becomes intense. A conventional boundary for this region is the "5-gaussline," which is about 10 to 12 m from the center of an unshielded 1.5-T magnet. Magnetic shielding—in the form of iron plates (passive shielding) or external coils carrying current in the direction opposite to the main coil current (active shielding)—is frequently used to restrict the region in which the fringing field is significant.

10.2.3 Gradient Coils

Three gradient fields, one each for the x, y, and z directions of a Cartesian coordinate system, are used to code position information into the MRI signal and to permit the imaging of thin anatomic slices (Thomas, 1993). Along with their larger size, it is the use of these gradient coils that distinguishes MRI scanners from the conventional NMR systems such as those used in analytical chemistry. The direction of the static field, along the axis of the scanner, is conventionally taken as the z direction, and it is only the Cartesian component of the gradient field in this direction that produces a significant contribution to the resonant behavior of the nuclei. Thus, the three relevant gradient fields are $B_z = G_x X$, $B_z = G_y X$, and $B_z = G_z X$. MRI scans are carried out by subjecting the spin system to a sequence of pulsed gradient and RF fields. Therefore, it is necessary to have three separate coils—one for each of the relevant gradient fields—each with its own power supply and under independent computer control. Ordinarily, the most practical method for constructing the gradient coils is to wind them on a cylindrical coil form that surrounds the patient and is located inside the warm bore of the magnet. The z gradient field can be produced by sets of circular coils wound around the cylinder with the current direction reversed for coils on the opposite sides of the magnet center ($z = 0$). To reduce deviations from a perfectly linear B_z gradient field, a spiral winding can be used with the direction of the turns reversed at $z = 0$ and the spacing between windings decreasing away from the coil center (Figure 10.10). A more complex current pattern is required to produce the transverse (x and y) gradients. As indicated in Figure 10.11, transverse gradient fields are produced by windings which utilize a four-quadrant current pattern.

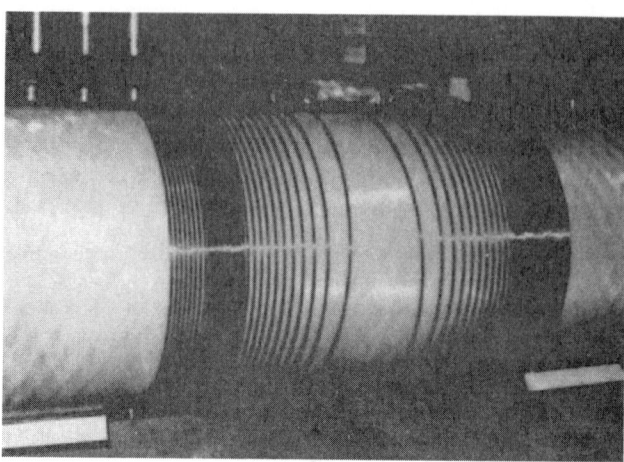

FIGURE 10.10   *Z*-gradient coil. The photograph shows a spiral coil wound on a cylindrical surface with an over-widing near the end of the coil. (Courtesy of R.J. Dobberstein, General Electric Medical Systems. Reprinted with permission from Schenck, J.F., and W.M. Leue, Instrumentation: Magnets, coils, and hardware, in S.W. Atlas (Ed.), *Magnetic Resonance Imaging of the Brain and Spine*, 2nd ed., pp. 1–27, Lippincott-Raven, Philadelphia, 1996.)

The generation of MR images requires that a rapid sequence of time-dependent gradient fields (on all three axes) be applied to the patient. For example, the commonly used technique of **spin-warp imaging** (Edelstein et al., 1980) utilizes a slice-selection gradient pulse to select the spins in a thin (3–10 mm) slice of the patient and then applies readout and phase-encoding gradients in the two orthogonal directions to encode two-dimensional spatial information into the NMR signal. This, in turn, requires that the currents in the three gradient coils be rapidly switched by computer-controlled power supplies. The rate at which gradient currents can be switched is an important determinant of the imaging capabilities of a scanner. In typical scanners, the gradient coils have an electrical resistance of about 1 Ω and an inductance of about 1 mH, and the gradient field can be switched from 0 to 10 mT/m (1 G/cm) in about

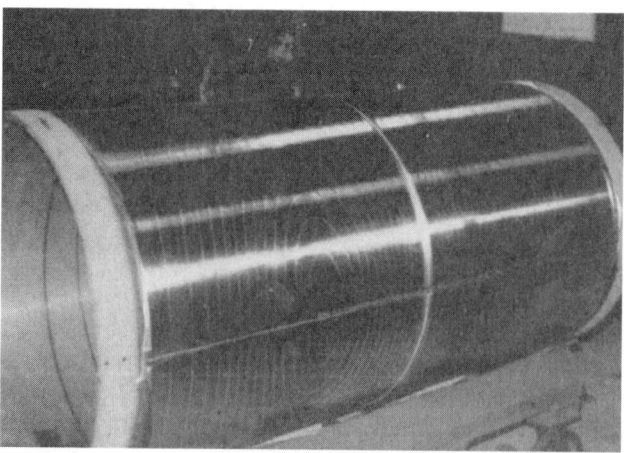

FIGURE 10.11   Transverse gradient coil. The photograph shows the outer coil pattern of an actively shielded transverse gradient coil. (Courtesy of R.J. Dobberstien, General Electric Medical Systems. Reprinted with permission from Schenck, J.F., and W.M. Leue, Instrumentation: Magnets, coils, and hardware, in S.W. Atlas (Ed.), *Magnetic Resonance Imaging of the Brain and Spine*, 2nd ed., pp. 1–27, Lippincott-Raven, Philadelphia, 1996.)

0.5 msec. The current must be switched from 0 to about 100 A in this interval, and the instantaneous voltage on the coils, $L di/dt$, is on the order of 200 V. The power dissipation during the switching interval is about 20 kW. In more demanding applications, such as are met in cardiac MRI, the gradient field may be as high as 4–5 mT/m and switched in 0.2 msec or less. In this case, the voltage required during gradient switching is more than 1 kV. In many pulse sequences, the switching duty cycle is relatively low, and coil heating is not significant. However, fast-scanning protocols use very rapidly switched gradients at a high duty cycle. This places very strong demands on the power supplies, and it is often necessary to use water cooling to prevent overheating the gradient coils.

10.2.4 Radiofrequency Coils

Radiofrequency (RF) coils are components of every scanner and are used for two essential purposes—transmitting and receiving signals at the resonant frequency of the protons within the patient (Schenck, 1993). The precession occurs at the **Larmor frequency** of the protons, which is proportional to the static magnetic field. At 1T this frequency is 42.58 MHz. Thus in the range of field strengths currently used in whole-body scanners, 0.02 to 4 T, the operating frequency ranges from 0.85 to 170.3 MHz. For the commonly used 1.5-T scanners, the operating frequency is 63.86 MHz. The frequency of MRI scanners overlaps the spectral region used for radio and television broadcasting. As an example, the frequency of a 1.5-T scanner is within the frequency hand 60 to 66 MHz, which is allocated to television channel 3. Therefore, it is not surprising that the electronic components in MRI transmitter and receiver chains closely resemble corresponding components in radio and television circuitry. An important difference between MRI scanners and broadcasting systems is that the transmitting and receiving antennas of broadcast systems operate in the far field of the electromagnetic wave. These antennas are separated by many wavelengths. On the other hand, MRI systems operate in the near field, and the spatial separation of the sources and receivers is much less than a wavelength. In far-field systems, the electromagnetic energy is shared equally between the electric and magnetic components of the wave. However, in the near field of magnetic dipole sources, the field energy is almost entirely in the magnetic component of the electromagnetic wave. This difference accounts for the differing geometries that are most cost effective for broadcast and MRI antenna structures.

Ideally, the RF field is perpendicular to the static field, which is in the z direction. Therefore, the RF field can be linearly polarized in either the x or y direction. However, the most efficient RF field results from quadrature excitation, which requires a coil that is capable of producing simultaneous x and y fields with a 90-degree phase shift between them. Three classes of RF coils—body coils, head coils, and surface coils—are commonly used in MRI scanners. These coils are located in the space between the patient and the gradient coils. Conducting shields just inside the gradient coils are used to prevent electromagnetic coupling between the RF coils and the rest of the scanner. Head and body coils are large enough to surround the legion being imaged and are designed to produce an RF magnetic field that is uniform across the region to be imaged. Body coils are usually constructed on cylindrical coil forms and have a large enough diameter (50 to 60 cm) to entirely surround the patient's body. Coils are designed only for head imaging (Figure 10.12) have a smaller diameter (typically 28 cm). Surface coils are smaller coils designed to image a restricted region of the patient's anatomy. They come in a wide variety of shapes and sizes. Because they can be closely applied to the region of interest, surface coils can provide SNR advantages over head and body coils for localized regions, but because of their asymmetric design, they do not have uniform sensitivity.

A common practice is to use separate coils for the transmitter and receiver functions. This permits the use of a large coil—such as the body coil—with a uniform excitation pattern as the transmitter and a small surface coil optimized to the anatomic region—such as the spine—being imaged. When this two-coil approach is used, it is important to provide for electronically decoupling of the two coils because they are tuned at the same frequency and will tend to have harmful mutual interactions.

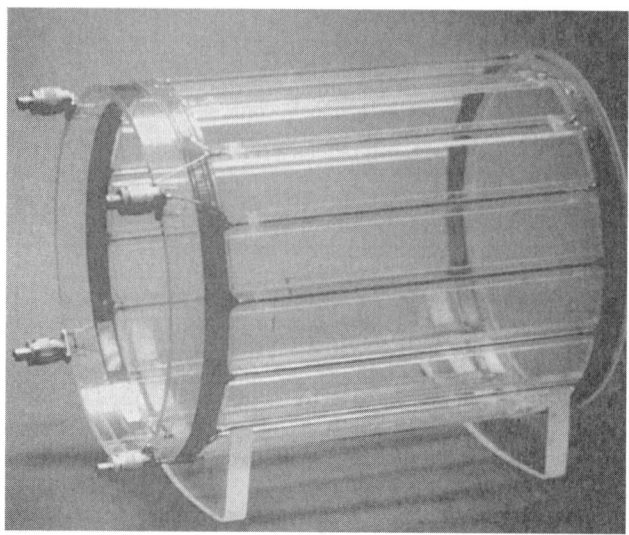

FIGURE 10.12 Birdcage resonator. This is a head coil designed to operate in a 4-T scanner at 170 MHz. Quadrature excitation and receiver performance are achieved by using two adjacent ports with a 90-degree phase shift between them. (Reprinted with permission from Schenck, J.F., and W.M. Leue, Instrumentation: Magnets, coils, and hardware, in S.W. Atlas (Ed.), *Magnetic Resonance Imaging of the Brain and Spine*, 2nd ed., pp. 1–27, Lippincott-Raven, Philadelphia, 1996.)

10.2.5 Digital Data Processing

A typical scan protocol calls for a sequence of tailored RF and gradient pulses with duration controlled in steps of 0.1 msec. To achieve sufficient dynamic range in control of pulse amplitudes, 12- to 16-bit digital-to-analog converters are used. The RF signal at the Larmor frequency (usually in the range from 1 to 200 MHz) is mixed with a local oscillator to produce a baseband signal which typically has a **bandwidth** of 16–32 kHz. The data-acquisition system must digitize the baseband signal at the Nyquist rate, which requires sampling the detected RF signal at a rate one digital data point every 5–20 msec. Again, it is necessary to provide sufficient dynamic range. Analog-to-digital converters with 16–18 bits are used to produce the desired digitized signal data. During the data acquisition, information is acquired at a rate on the order of 800 kilobytes per second, and each image can contain up to a megabyte of digital data. The array processor (AP) is a specialized computer that is designed for the rapid performance of specific algorithms, such as the **fast Fourier transform (FFT)**, which are used to convert the digitized time-domain data to image data. Two-dimensional images are typically displayed as 256×128, 256×256, or 512×512 **pixel** arrays. The images can be made available for viewing within about 1 sec after data acquisition. Three-dimensional imagining data, however, require more computer processing, and this results in longer delays between acquisition and display.

A brightness number, typically containing 16 bits of gray-scale information, is calculated for each pixel element of the image, and this corresponds to the signal intensity originating in each **voxel** of the object. To make the most effective use of the imaging information, sophisticated display techniques, such as multi-image displays, rapid sequential displays (cine loop), and three-dimensional renderings of anatomic surfaces, are frequently used. These techniques are often computationally intensive and require the use of specialized computer hardware. Interfaces to microprocessor-based workstations are frequently used to provide such additional display and analysis capabilities. MRI images are available as digital data; therefore, there is considerable utilization of local area networks (LANs) to distribute information throughout the hospital, and long-distance digital transmission of the images can be used for purposes of teleradiology.

10.2.6 Current Trends in MRI

At present, there is a substantial effort directed at enhancing the capabilities and cost-effectiveness of MR imagers. The activities include efforts to reduce the cost of these scanners, improve image quality, reduce scan times, and increase the number of useful clinical applications. Examples of these efforts include the development of high-field scanners, the advent of MRI-guided therapy, and the development of niche scanners that are designed for specific anatomical and clinical applications. Scanners have been developed that are dedicated to low-field imaging of the breast and other designs are dedicated to orthopedic applications such as the knees, wrists, and elbows. Perhaps the most promising incipient application of MRI is to cardiology. Scanners are now being developed to permit studies of cardiac wall motion, cardiac perfusion, and the coronary arteries in conjunction with cardiac stress testing. These scanners emphasize short magnet configurations to permit close monitoring and interaction with the patient, and high strength rapidly switched gradient fields.

Conventional spin-warp images typically require several minutes to acquire. The fast spin echo (FSE) technique can reduce this to the order of 20 sec, and gradient-echo techniques can reduce this time to a few seconds. The echo-planar technique (EPI) (Wehrli, 1990; Cohen and Weisskoff, 1991) requires substantially increased gradient power and receiver bandwidth but can produce images in 40 to 60 msec. Scanners with improved gradient hardware that are capable of handling higher data-acquisition rates are now available.

For most of the 1980s and 1990s, the highest field strength commonly used in MRI scanners was 1.5 T. To achieve better SNRs, higher-field scanners, operating at fields up to 4 T, were studied experimentally. The need for very high-field scanners has been enhanced by the development of functional brain MRI. This technique utilizes magnetization differences between oxygenated and deoxygenated hemoglobin, and this difference is enhanced at higher field strengths. It has now become possible to construct 3- and 4-T and even 8-T (Robitaille et al., 1998), whole-body scanners of essentially the same physical size (or footprint) as conventional 1.5-T systems. Along with the rapidly increasing clinical interest in functional MRI, this is resulting in a considerable increase in the use of high-field systems.

For the first decade or so after their introduction, MRI scanners were used almost entirely to provide diagnostic information. However, there is now considerable interest in systems capable of performing image-guided, invasive surgical procedures. Because MRI is capable of providing

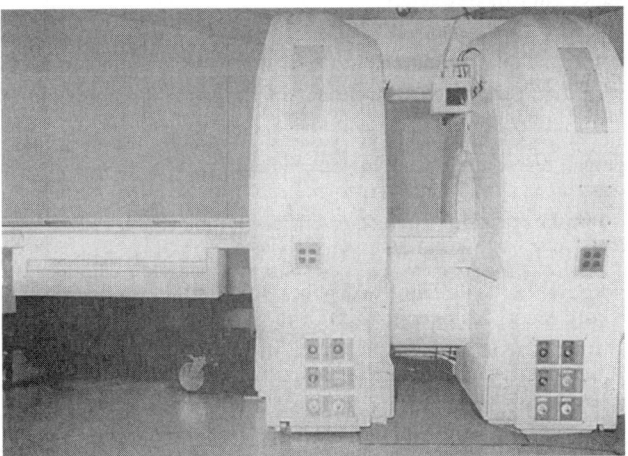

FIGURE 10.13 Open magnet for MEI-guided therapy. This open-geometry superconducting magnet provides a surgeon with direct patient access and the ability to interactively control the MRI scanner. This permits imaging to be performed simultaneously with surgical interventions.

excellent soft-tissue contrast and has the potential for providing excellent positional information with submillimeter accuracy, it can be used for guiding biopsies and stereotactic surgery. The full capabilities of MRI-guided procedures can only be achieved if it is possible to provide surgical access to the patient simultaneously with the MRI scanning. This has lead to the development of new system designs, including the introduction of a scanner with a radically modified superconducting magnet system that permits the surgeon to operate at the patient's side within the scanner (Figure 10.13) (Schenck et al., 1995; Black et al., 1997). These systems have lead to the introduction of magnetic field-compatible surgical instruments, anesthesia stations, and patient monitoring equipment (Schenck, 1996).

Defining Terms

Bandwidth: The narrow frequency range, approximately 32 kHz, over which the MRI signal is transmitted. The bandwidth is proportional to the strength of the readout gradient field.

Echo-planar imaging (EPI): A pulse sequence used to produce very fast MRI scans. EPI times can be as short as 50 msec.

Fast Fourier transform (FFT): A mathematical technique used to convert data sampled from the MRI signal into image data. This version of the Fourier transform can be performed with particular efficiency on modern array processors.

Gradient coil: A coil designed to produce a magnetic field for which the field component B: varies linearly with position. Three gradient coils, one each for the x, y, and z directions, are required MRI. These coils are used to permit slice selection and to encode position information into the MRI signal.

Larmor frequency: The rate at which the magnetic dipole moment of a particle precesses in an applied magnetic field. It is proportional to the field strength and is 42.58 MHz for protons in a 1-T magnetic field.

Magnetic resonance imaging (MRI): A technique for obtaining images of the internal anatomy based on the use of nuclear magnetic resonance signals. During the 1980s, it became a major modality for medical diagnostic imaging.

Nuclear magnetic resonance (NMR): A technique for observing and studying nuclear magnetism. It is based on partially aligning the nuclear spins by use of a strong, static magnetic field, stimulating these spins with a radiofrequency field oscillating at the Larmor frequency, and detecting the signal that is induced at this frequency.

Nuclear magnetism: The magnetic properties arising from the small magnetic dipole moments possessed by the atomic nuclei of some materials. This form of magnetism is much weaker than the more familiar form that originates from the magnetic dipole moments of the atomic electrons.

Pixel: A single element or a two-dimensional array of image data.

Pulse sequence: A series of gradient and radiofrequency pulses used to organize the nuclear spins into a pattern that encodes desired imaging information into the NMR signal.

Quadrature excitation and detection: The use of circularly polarized, rather than linearly polarized, radio frequency fields to excite an detect the NMR signal. It provides a means of reducing the required excitation power by 1/2 and increasing the signal-to-noise ratio by 2.

Radiofrequency (RF) coil: A coil designed to excite and/or detect NMR signals. These coils can usually be tuned to resonate at the Larmor frequency of the nucleus being studied.

Spin: The property of a particle, such as an electron or nucleus, that leads to the presence of an intrinsic angular momentum and magnetic moment.

Spin-warp imagining: The pulse sequence used in the most common method of MRI imaging. It uses a sequence of gradient field pulses to encode position information into the NMR signal and applies Fourier transform mathematics to this signal to calculate the image intensity value for each pixel.

Static magnetic field: The field of the main magnet that is used to magnetize the spins and to drive their Larmor precession.

Voxel: The volume element associated with a pixel. The voxel volume is equal to the pixel area multiplied by the slice thickness.

References

Black P.Mc.L., Moriarty T., Alexander E. III. et al. 1997. Development and implementation of intraoperative magnetic resonance imaging and its neurosurgical applications. *Neurosurgery* 41: 831.

Cohen M.S. and Weisskoff R.M. 1991. Ultra-fast imaging. *Magn. Reson. Imag.* 9: 1.

Edelstein W.A., Hutchinson J.M.S., Johnson G., and Redpath T.W. 1980. Spin-warp NMR imaging and applications to human whole-body imaging. *Phys. Med. Biol.* 25: 751.

Robitaille P.-M.L., Abdujalil A.M., Kangarlu A. et al. 1998. Human magnetic resonance imaging at 8 T. *NMR Biomed.* 11: 263.

Schenck J.F. 1993. Radiofrequency coils: types and characteristics. In M.I. Bronskill and P. Sprawls (Eds.), *The Physics of MRI, Medical Physics Monograph No. 21*, pp. 98–134. Woodbury, NY, American Institute of Physics.

Schenck J.F. 1996. The role of magnetic susceptibility in magnetic resonance imaging: magnetic field compatibility of the first and second kinds. *Med. Phys.* 23: 815.

Schenck J.F. and Leue W.M. 1996. Instrumentation: magnets coils and hardware. In S.W. Atlas (Ed.), *Magnetic Resonance Imaging of the Brain and Spine*, 2nd ed., pp. 1–27. Philadelphia, Lippincott-Raven.

Schenck J.F., Jolesz A., Roemer P.B. et al. 1995. Superconducting open-configuration MR imaging system for image-guided therapy. *Radiology* 195: 805.

Shellock F.G. and Kanal E. 1998. *Magnetic Resonance: Bioeffects, Safety and Patient Management*, 2nd ed. Philadelphia, Saunders.

Thomas S.R. 1993. Magnet and gradient coils: types and characteristics. In M.J. Bronskill and P. Sprawls (Eds.), *The Physics of MRI, Medical Physics Monograph No. 21*, pp. 56–97. Woodbury, NY, American Institute of Physics.

Wehrli F.W. 1990. Fast scan magnetic resonance: principles and applications. *Magn. Reson. Q.* 6: 165.

Wilson M.N. 1983. *Superconducting Magnets*. Oxford, Clarendon Press.

Further Information

There are several journals devoted entirely to MR imaging. These include *Magnetic Resonance in Medicine, JMRI—Journal of Magnetic Resonance Imaging*, and *NMR in Biomedicine*, all three of which are published by Wiley-Liss, 605 Third Avenue, New York, NY 10158. Another journal dedicated to this field is *Magnetic Resonance Imaging* (Elsevier Publishing, 655 Avenue of the Americas, New York, NY 10010). The clinical aspects of MRI are covered extensively in *Radiology* (Radiological Society of North America, 2021 Spring Road, Suite 600, Oak Brook, IL 60521), *The American Journal of Radiology* (American Roentgen Ray Society, 1891 Preston White Drive, Reston, VA 20191), as well as in several other journals devoted to the practice of radiology. There is a professional society, now known as the International Society for Magnetic Resonance in Medicine (ISMRM), devoted to the medical aspects of magnetic resonance. The main offices of this society are at 2118 Milvia, *Suite* 201, Berkeley, CA 94704. This society holds an annual meeting that includes displays of equipment and the presentation of approximately 2800 technical papers on new developments in the field. The annual *Book of Abstracts* of this meeting provides an excellent summary of current activities in the field. Similarly, the annual meeting of the Radiological Society of North America (RSNA) provides extensive coverage of MRI that is particularly strong on the clinical applications. The RSNA is located at 2021 Spring Road, Suite 600, Oak Brook, IL 60521.

Several book-length accounts of MRI instrumentation and techniques are available. *Biomedical Magnetic Resonance Technology* (Adam Higler, Bristol, 1989) by Chen and D.I. Hoult, *The Physics of MRI* (Medical Physics Monograph 21, American Institute of Physics, Woodbury, NY, 1993), edited by M.J. Bronskill and P. Sprawls, and *Electromagnetic Analysis and Design in Magnetic Resonance Imaging* (CRC Press, Boca Raton, FL, 1998) by J.M. Jin each contain thorough accounts of instrumentation and the physical aspects of MRI. There are many books that cover the clinical aspects of MRI. Of particular interest are *Magnetic Resonance Imaging*, 3rd edition (Mosby, St. Louis, 1999), edited by D.D. Stark and W.G. Bradley, Jr., and *Magnetic Resonance Imaging of the Brain and Spine*, 2nd ed. (Lipincott-Raven, Philadelphia, 1996), edited by S.W. Atlas.

10.3 Functional MRI

Kenneth K. Kwong and David A. Chesler

Functional magnetic resonance imaging (fMRI), a technique that images intrinsic blood signal change with magnetic resonance (MR) imagers, has in the last 3 years become one of the most successful tools used to study blood flow and perfusion in the brain. Since changes in neuronal activity are accompanied by focal changes in cerebral blood flow (CBF), blood volume (CBV), blood oxygenation, and metabolism, these physiologic changes can be used to produce functional maps of mental operations.

There are two basic but completely different techniques used in fMRI to measure CBF. The first one is a classic steady-state perfusion technique first proposed by Detre et al. [1], who suggested the use of saturation or inversion of incoming blood signal to quantify absolute blood flow [1–5]. By focusing on blood flow *change* and not just steady-state blood flow, Kwong et al. [6] were successful in imaging brain visual functions associated with quantitative perfusion change. There are many advantages in studying blood flow change because many common baseline artifacts associated with MRI absolute flow techniques can be subtracted out when we are interested only in changes. And one obtains adequate information in most functional neuroimaging studies with information of flow change alone.

The second technique also looks at change of a blood parameter—blood oxygenation *change* during neuronal activity. The utility of the change of blood oxygenation characteristics was strongly evident in Turner's work [7] with cats with induced hypoxia. Turner et al. found that with hypoxia, the MRI signal from the cats' brains went down as the level of deoxyhemoglobin rose, a result that was an extension of an earlier study by Ogawa et al. [8,9] of the effect of deoxyhemoglobin on MRI signals in animals' veins. Turner's new observation was that when oxygen was restored, the cats' brain signals climbed up and went *above* their baseline levels. This was the suggestion that the vascular system overcompensated by bringing more oxygen, and with more oxygen in the blood, the MRI signal would rise beyond the baseline.

Based on Turner's observation and the perfusion method suggested by Detre et al., movies of human visual cortex activation utilizing both the perfusion and blood oxygenation techniques were successfully acquired in May of 1991 (Figure 10.14) at the Massachusetts General Hospital with a specially equipped superfast 1.5-T system known as an *echo-planar imaging* (EPI) MRI system [10]. fMRI results using intrinsic blood contrast were first presented in public at the Tenth Annual Meeting of the Society of Magnetic Resonance in Medicine in August of 1991 [6,11]. The visual cortex activation work was carried out with flickering goggles, a photic stimulation protocol employed by Belliveau et al. [12] earlier to acquire the MRI functional imaging of the visual cortex with the injection of the contrast agent gadolinium-DTPA. The use of an external contrast agent allows the study of change in blood volume. The intrinsic blood contrast technique, sensitive to blood flow and blood oxygenation, uses no external contrast material. Early model calculation showed that signal due to blood perfusion change would only be around 1% above baseline, and the signal due to blood oxygenation change also was quite small. It was quite a pleasant surprise that fMRI results turned out to be so robust and easily detectable.

The blood oxygenation–sensitive MRI signal change, coined *blood oxygenation level dependent* (BOLD) by Ogawa et al. [8,9,13], is in general much larger than the MRI perfusion signal change during

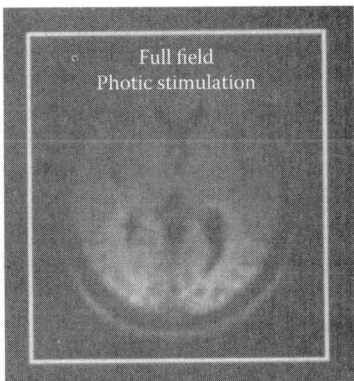

FIGURE 10.14 Functional MR image demonstrating activation of the primary visual cortex (V1). Image acquired on May 9, 1991 with a blood oxygenation–sensitive MRI gradient-echo (GE) technique.

brain activation. Also, while the first intrinsic blood contrast fMRI technique was demonstrated with a superfast EPI MRI system, most centers doing fMRI today are only equipped with conventional MRI systems, which are really not capable of applying Detre's perfusion method. Instead, the explosive growth of MR functional neuroimaging [14–33] in the last three years relies mainly on the measurement of blood oxygenation change, utilizing a MR parameter called T_2. Both high speed echo planar (EPI) and conventional MR have now been successfully employed for functional imaging in MRI systems with magnet field strength ranging from 1.5 to 4.0 T.

10.3.1 Advances in Functional Brain Mapping

The popularity of fMRI is based on many factors. It is safe and totally noninvasive. It can be acquired in single subjects for a scanning duration of several minutes, and it can be repeated on the same subjects as many times as necessary. The implementation of the blood oxygenation sensitive MR technique is universally available. Early neuroimaging, work focused on time-resolved MR topographic mapping of human primary visual (VI) (Figures 10.15 and 10.16), motor (MI), somatosensory (S1), and auditory (A1) cortices during task activation. Today, with BOLD technique combined with EPI, one can acquire 20 or more contiguous brain slices covering the whole head (3 × 3 mm in plane and 5 mm slice thickness) every 3 sec for a total duration of several minutes. Conventional scanners can only acquire a couple of slices at a time. The benefits of whole-head imaging are many. Not only can researchers identify and test their hypotheses on known brain activation centers, they can also search for previous unknown or unsuspected sites. High resolution work done with EPI has a resolution of 1.5 × 1.5 mm in plane and a slice thickness of 3 mm. Higher spatial resolution has been reported in conventional 1.5-T MR systems [34].

Of note with Figure 10.16 is that with blood oxygenation–sensitive MR technique, one observers an undershoot [6,15,35] in signal in V1 when the light stimulus is turned off. The physiologic mechanism underlying the undershoot is still not well understood.

The data collected in the last 3 years have demonstrated that fMRI maps of the visual cortex correlate well with known retinotopic organization [24,36]. Higher visual regions such as V5/MT [37] and motor-cortex organization [6,14,27,38] have been explored successfully. Preoperative planning work (Figure 10.17) using motor stimulation [21,39,40] has helped neurosurgeons who attempt to preserve primary areas from tumors to be resected. For higher cognitive functions, several fMRI language studies have already demonstrated known language-associated regions [25,26,41,42] (Figure 10.18). There is more detailed modeling work on the mechanism of functional brain mapping by blood-oxygenation change [43–46]. Postprocessing techniques that would help to alleviate the serious problem of motion/displacement artifacts are available [47].

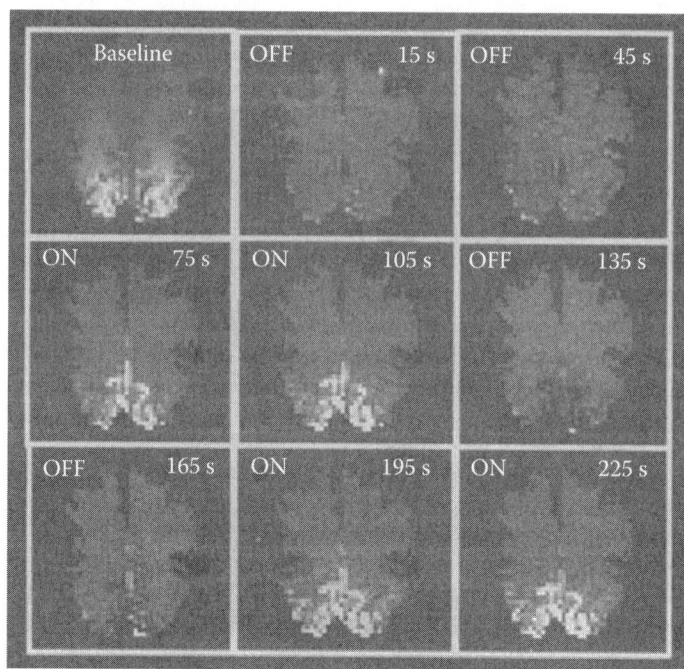

FIGURE 10.15 Movie of fMRI mapping of primary visual cortex (V1) activation during visual stimulation. Images are obliquely aligned along the calcarie fissures with the occipital pole at the bottom. Images were acquired at 3-sec intervals using a blood oxygenation–sensitive MRI sequence (80 images total). A baseline image acquired during darkness (*upper left*) was subtracted from subsequent images. Eight of these subtraction images are displayed, chosen when the image intensities reached a steady-state signal level during darkness (OFF) and during 8-Hz photic stimulation (ON). During stimulation, local increases in signal intensity are detected in the postero-medial regions of the occipital lobes along the calcarine fissures.

10.3.2 Mechanism

Flow-sensitive images show increased perfusion with stimulation, while blood oxygenation–sensitive images show changes consistent with an increase in venous blood oxygenation. Although the precise biophysical mechanisms responsible for the signal changes have yet to be determined, good hypotheses exist to account for our observations.

Two fundamental MRI relaxation rates, T_1 and T_2, are used to describe the fMRI signal. T_1 is the rate at which the nuclei approach thermal equilibrium, and perfusion change can be considered as an additional T_1 change. T_2 represents the rate of the decay of MRI signal due to magnetic field inhomogeneities, and the change of T_2 is used to measure blood-oxygenation change.

T_2 changes reflect the interplay between changes in cerebral blood flow, volume, and oxygenation. As hemoglobin becomes deoxygenated, it becomes more paramagnetic than the surrounding tissue [48] and thus creates a magnetically inhomogeneous environment. The observed *increased* signal on T_2-weighted images during activation reflects a decrease in deoxyhemoglobin content, that is, an increase in venous blood oxygenation. Oxygen delivery, cerebral blood flow, and cerebral blood volume all increase with neuronal activation. Because CBF (and hence oxygen-delivery) changes exceed CBV changes by 2 to 4 times [49], while blood–oxygen extraction increases only slightly [50,51], the total paramagnetic blood deoxyhemoglobin content within brain tissue voxels will decrease with brain activation. The resulting decrease in the tissue-blood magnetic susceptibility difference leads to less intravoxel dephasing

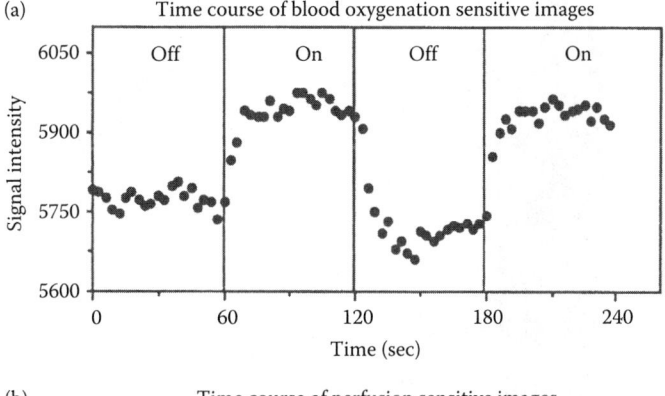

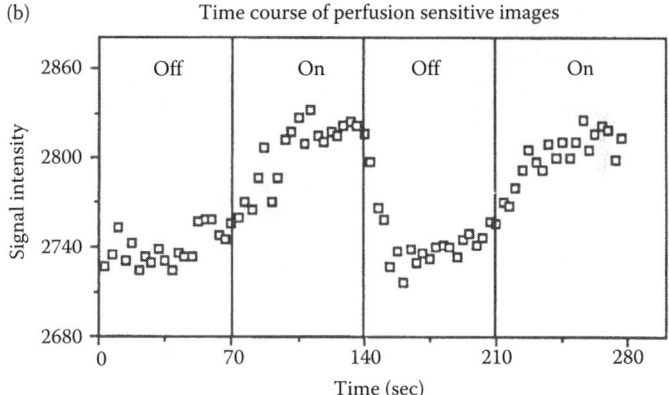

FIGURE 10.16 Signal intensity changes for a region of interest (~60 mm²) within the visual cortex during darkness and during 8-Hz photic stimulation. Results using oxygenation–sensitive (a) and flow-sensitive (b) techniques are shown. The flow-sensitive data were collected once every 3.5 sec, and the oxygenation-sensitive data were collected once every 3 sec. Upon termination of photic stimulation, an undershoot in the oxygenation-sensitive signal intensity is observed.

within brain tissue voxels and hence *increased* signal on T_2-weighted images [6,14,15,17]. These results independently confirm PET observations that activation-induced changes in blood flow and volume are accompanied by little or no increases in tissue oxygen consumption [50–52].

Since the effect of volume susceptibility difference $\Delta\chi$ is more pronounced at high field strength [53], higher-field imaging magnets [17] will increase the observed T_2 changes.

Signal changes can also be observed on T_1-weighted MR images. The relationship between T_1 and regional blood flow was characterized by Detre et al. [1]:

$$\frac{\mathrm{d}M}{\mathrm{d}t} = \frac{M_0 - M}{T_1} + fM_b - \frac{f}{\lambda}M \qquad (10.14)$$

where M is tissue magnetization and M_b is incoming blood signal. M_0 is proton density, f is the flow in mL/gm/unit time, and λ is the brain–blood partition coefficient of water (~0.95 mL/g). From this equation, the brain tissue magnetization M relaxes with an apparent T_1 time constant T_{1app} given by

$$\frac{f}{\lambda} = \frac{1}{T_{1app}} - \frac{1}{T_1} \qquad (10.15)$$

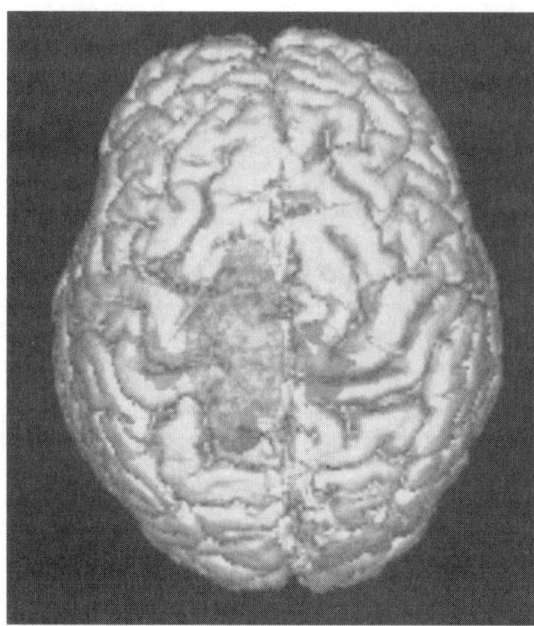

FIGURE 10.17 Functional MRI mapping of motor cortex for preoperative planning. This three-dimensional rendering of the brain represents fusion of functional and structural anatomy. Brain is viewed from the top. A tumor is shown in the left hemisphere, near the midline. The other areas depict sites of functional activation during movement of the right hand, right foot, and left foot. The right foot cortical representation is displaced by tumor mass effect from its usual location. (Courtesy of Dr. Brad Buchbinder.)

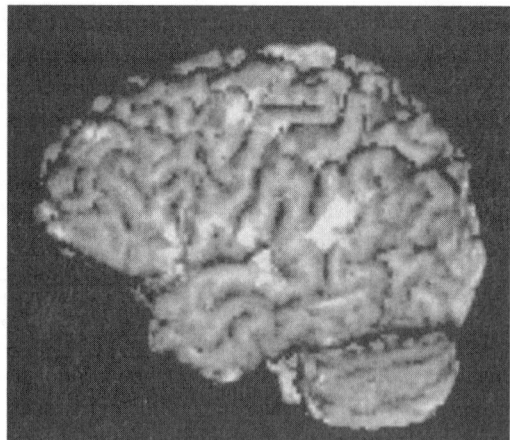

FIGURE 10.18 Left hemisphere surface rendering of functional data (EPI, gradient-echo, ten oblique coronal slices extending to posterior sylvian fissure) and high-resolution anatomic image obtained on a subject (age 33 years) during performance of a same-different (visual matching) task of pairs of words or nonwords (false font strings). Foci of greatest activation for this study are located in dominant perisylvian cortex, that is, inferior frontal gyrus (Broca's area), superior temporal gyrus (Wernicke's area), and inferior parietal lobule (angular gyrus). Also active in this task are sensorimotor cortex and prefrontal cortex. The perisylvian sites of activation are known to be key nodes in a left hemisphere language network. Prefrontal cortex probably plays a more general, modulatory role in attentional aspects of the task. Sensorimotor activation is observed in most language studies despite the absence of overt vocalization. (Courtesy of Dr. Randall Benson.)

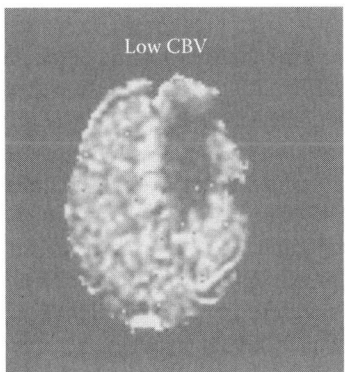
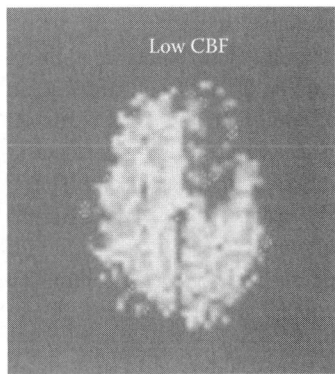

FIGURE 10.19 Functional MRI cerebral blood flow (CBF) index (*right*) of a low-flow brain tumor (dark region right of the midline) generated by the subtraction of a flow-nonsensitive image from a flow-sensitive image. This low-flow region matches well with a cerebral blood volume (CBV) map (*left*) of the tumor region generated by the injection of a bolus of MRI contrast agent Gd-DTPA, a completely different and established method to measure hemodynamics with MRI.

where the T_{1app} is the observed (apparent) longitudinal relaxation time with flow effects included. T_1 is the true tissue longitudinal relaxation time in the absence of flow. If we assume that the true tissue T_1 remains constant with stimulation, a change in blood flow Δf will lead to a change in the observed T_{1app}:

$$\Delta \frac{1}{T_{1app}} = \Delta \frac{f}{\lambda} \tag{10.16}$$

Thus the MRI signal change can be used to estimate the change in blood flow.

From Equation 10.14, if the magnetization of blood and tissue always undergoes a similar T_1 relaxation, the flow effect would be minimized. This is a condition that can be approximated by using a flow-nonsensitive T_1 technique inverting *all* the blood coming into the imaged slice of interest. This flow-nonsensitive sequence can be subtracted from a flow-sensitive T_1 technique to provide an index of CBF without the need of external stimulation [54,55] (Figure 10.19). Initial results with tumor patients show that such flow-mapping techniques are useful for mapping out blood flow of tumor regions [55].

Other flow techniques under investigation include the continuous inversion of incoming blood at the carotid level [1] or the use of a single inversion pulse at the carotid level (EPIstar) inverting the incoming blood [56,57]. Compared with the flow-nonsensitive and flow-sensitive methods, the blood-tagging techniques at the carotid level are basically similar concepts except that the MRI signal of tagged blood is expected to be smaller by a factor that depends on the time it takes blood to travel from the tagged site to the imaged slice of interest [55]. The continuous-inversion technique also has a significant problem of magnetization transfer [1] that contaminates the flow signal with a magnetization transfer signal that is several times larger. On the other hand, the advantage of the continuous inversion is that it can under optimal conditions provide a flow contrast larger than all the other methods by a factor of e [55].

10.3.3 Problem and Artifacts in fMRI: The Brain–Vein Problem? The Brain-Inflow Problem?

The artifacts arising from large vessels pose serious problems to the interpretation of oxygenation sensitive fMRI data. It is generally believed that microvascular changes are specific to the underlying region of neuronal activation. However, MRI gradient echo (GE) is sensitive to vessels of all dimensions [46,58], and there is concern that macrovascular changes distal to the site of neuronal activity can be induced [20]. This has been known as the *brain–vein problem*. For laboratories not equipped with EPI, gradient echo (GE) sensitive to variations in T_2 and magnetic susceptibility are the only realistic sequences available for fMRI acquisition, so the problem is particularly acute.

In addition, there is a non-deoxyhemoglobin-related problem, especially acute in conventional MRI. This is the inflow problem of fresh blood that can be time-locked to stimulation [28,29,59]. Such non-parenchymal and macrovascular responses can introduce error in the estimate of activated volumes.

10.3.4 Techniques to Reduce the Large Vessel Problems

In dealing with the inflow problems, EPI has special advantages over conventional scanners. The use of long repetition times (2 to 3 sec) in EPI significantly reduces the brain-inflow problem. Small-flip-angle methods in conventional MRI scanners can be used to reduce inflow effect [59]. Based on inflow modeling, one observes that at an angle smaller than the Ernst angle [60], the inflow effect drops much faster than the tissue signal response to activation. Thus one can effectively remove the inflow artifacts with small-flip-angle techniques.

A new exciting possibility is to add small additional velocity-dephasing gradients to suppress slow in-plane vessel flow [60,61]. Basically, moving spins lose signals, while stationary spins are unaffected. The addition of these velocity-dephasing gradients drops the overall MRI signal (Figure 10.20). The hypothesis that large vessel signals are suppressed while tissue signals remain intact is a subject of ongoing research.

Another advantage with EPI is that another oxygenation-sensitive method such as the EPI T_2-weighted spin-echo (T2SE) is also available. T2SE methods are sensitive to the MRI parameter T_2, which is affected by microscopic susceptibility and hence blood oxygenation. Theoretically, T2SE methods are far less sensitive to large vessel signals [1,6,46,58]. For conventional scanners, T2SE methods take too long to perform and therefore are not practical options.

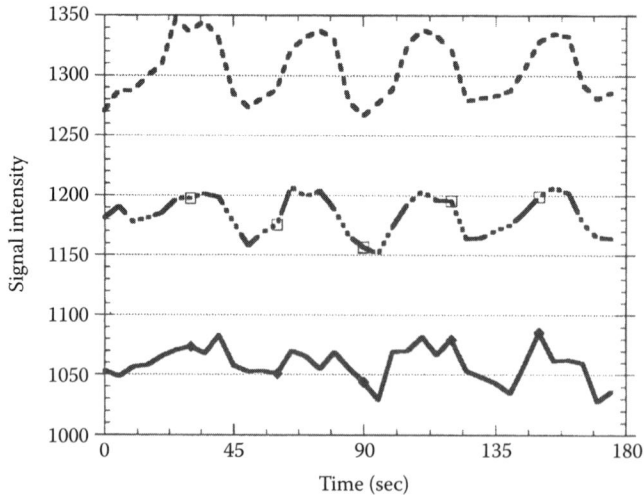

FIGURE 10.20 The curves represent time courses of MRI response to photic stimulation (off-on-off-on …) with different levels of velocity-dephasing gradients turned on to remove MRI signals coming from the flowing blood of large vessels. The top curve had no velocity-dephasing gradients turned on. The bottom curve was obtained with such strong velocity-dephasing gradients turned on that all large vessel signals were supposed to have been eliminated. The middle curve represents a moderate amount of velocity-dephasing gradients, a tradeoff between removing large vessel signals and retaining a reasonable amount of MRI signal to noise.

The flow model [1] based on T_1-weighted sequences and independent of deoxyhemoglobin is also not so prone to large vessel artifacts, since the T_1 model is a model of perfusion at the tissue level.

Based on the study of volunteers, the average T_2-weighted GE signal percentage change at V1 was $2.5 \pm 0.8\%$. The average oxygenation-weighted T2SE signal percentage change was $0.7 \pm 0.3\%$. The average perfusion-weighted and T_1-weighted MRI signal percentage change was $1.5 \pm 0.5\%$. These results demonstrate that T2SE and T_1 methods, despite their ability to suppress large vessels, are not competitive with T_2 effect at 1.5 T. However, since the microscopic effect detected by T2SE scales up with field strength [62], we expect the T2SE to be a useful sequence at high field strength such as 3 or 4 T. Advancing field strength also should benefit T_1 studies due to better signal-to-noise and to the fact that T_1 gets longer at higher field strength.

While gradient-echo sequence has a certain ambiguity when it comes to tissue versus vessels, its sensitivity at current clinical field strength makes it an extremely attractive technique to identify activation sites. By using careful paradigms that rule out possible links between the primary activation site and secondary sites, one can circumvent many of the worries of "signal from the primary site draining down to secondary sites." A good example is as follows: photic stimulation activates both the primary visual cortex and the extrastriates. To show that the extrastriates are not just a drainage from the primary cortex, one can utilize paradigms that activate the primary visual cortex but not the extrastriate, and vice versa. There are many permutations of this [37]. This allows us to study the higher-order functions umambiguously even if we are using gradient-echo sequences.

The continuous advance of MRI mapping techniques utilizing intrinsic blood-tissue contrast promises the development of a functional human neuroanatomy of unprecedented spatial and temporal resolution.

References

1. Detre J., Leigh J., Williams D., and Koretsky A. 1992. *Magn. Reson. Med.* 23: 37.
2. Williams D.S., Detre J.A., Leigh J.S., and Koretsky A.P. 1992. *Proc. Natl Acad. Sci. USA* 89: 212.
3. Zhang W., Williams D.S., and Detre J.A. 1992. *Magn. Reson. Med.* 25: 362.
4. Zhang W., Williams D.S., and Koretsky A.P. 1993. *Magn. Reson. Med.* 29: 416.
5. Dixon W.T., Du L.N., Faul D. et al. 1986. *Magn. Reson. Med.* 3: 454.
6. Kwong K.K., Belliveau J.W., Chesler D.A. et al. 1992. *Proc. Natl Acad. Sci. USA* 89: 5675.
7. Turner R., Le Bihan D., Moonen C.T. et al. 1991. *Magn. Reson. Med.* 22: 159.
8. Ogawa S., Lee T.M., Kay A.R., and Tank D.W. 1990. *Proc. Natl Acad. Sci. USA* 87: 9868.
9. Ogawa S. and Lee T.M. 1990. *Magn. Reson. Med.* 16: 9.
10. Cohen M.S. and Weisskoff R.M. 1991. *Magn. Reson. Imag.* 9: 1.
11. Brady T.J. 1991. *Society of Magnetic Resonance in Medicine*, San Francisco, CA Vol. 2.
12. Belliveau J.W., Kennedy D.N. Jr, McKinstry R.C. et al. 1991. *Science* 254: 716.
13. Ogawa S., Lee T.M., Nayak A.S., and Glynn P. 1990. *Magn. Reson. Med.* 14: 68.
14. Bandettini P.A., Wong E.C., Hinks R.S. et al. 1992. *Magn. Reson. Med.* 25: 390.
15. Ogawa S., Tank D.W., Menon R. et al. 1992. *Proc. Natl Acad. Sci. USA* 89: 5951.
16. Frahm J., Bruhn H., Merboldt K., and Hanicke W. 1992. *J. Magn. Reson. Imag.* 2: 501.
17. Turner R., Jezzard P., Wen H. et al. 1992. *Society of Magnetic Resonance in Medicine Eleventh Annual Meeting*, Berlin.
18. Blamire A., Ogawa S., Ugurbil K. et al. 1992. *Proc. Natl Acad. Sci. USA* 89: 11069.
19. Menon R., Ogawa S., Tank D., and Ugurbil K. 1993. *Magn. Reson. Med.* 30: 380.
20. Lai S., Hopkins A., Haacke E. et al. 1993. *Magn. Reson. Med.* 30: 387.
21. Cao Y., Towle V.L., Levin D.N. et al. 1993. *Society of Magnetic Resonance in Medicine Meeting*.
22. Connelly A., Jackson G.D., Frackowiak R.S.J. et al. 1993. *Radiology* 188: 125.
23. Kim S.G., Ashe J., Georgopouplos A.P. et al. 1993. *J. Neurophys.* 69: 297.

24. Schneider W., Noll D.C., and Cohen J.D. 1993. *Nature* 365: 150.
25. Hinke R.M., Hu X., Stillman A.E. et al. 1993. *Neurol. Rep.* 4: 675.
26. Binder J.R., Rao S.M., Hammeke T.A. et al. 1993. *Neurology* (suppl. 2): 189.
27. Rao S.M., Binder J.R., Bandettini P.A. et al. 1993. *Neurology* 43: 2311.
28. Gomiscek G., Beisteiner R., Hittmair K. et al. 1993. *MAGMA* 1: 109.
29. Duyn J., Moonen C., de Boer R. et al. 1993. *Society of Magnetic Resonance in Medicine, th Annual Meeting*, New York.
30. Hajnal J.V., Collins A.G., White S.J. et al.. 1993. *Magn. Reson. Med.* 30: 650.
31. Hennig J., Ernst T., Speck O. et al. 1994. *Magn. Reson. Med.* 31: 85.
32. Constable R.T., Kennan R.P., Puce A. et al. 1994. *Magn. Reson. Med.* 31: 686.
33. Binder J.R., Rao S.M., Hammeke T.A. et al. 1994. *Ann. Neurol.* 35: 662.
34. Frahm J., Merboldt K., and Hänicke W. 1993. *Magn. Reson. Med.* 29: 139.
35. Stern C.E., Kwong K.K., Belliveau J.W. et al. 1992. *Society of Magnetic Resonance in Medicine Annual Meeting*, Berlin, Germany.
36. Belliveau J.W., Kwong K.K., Baker J.R. et al. 1992. *Society of Magnetic Resonance in Medicine Annual Meeting*, Berlin, Germany.
37. Tootell R.B.H., Kwong K.K., Belliveau J.W. et al. 1993. *Investigative Ophthalmology and Visual Science*, p. 813.
38. Kim S.-G., Ashe J., Hendrich K. et al. 1993. *Science* 261: 615.
39. Buchbinder B.R., Jiang H.J., Cosgrove G.R. et al. 1994. *ASNR* 162.
40. Jack C.R., Thompson R.M., Butts R.K. et al. 1994. *Radiology* 190: 85.
41. Benson R.R., Kwong K.K., Belliveau J.W. et al. 1993. *Soc. Neurosci.*
42. Benson R.R., Kwong K.K., Buchbinder B.R. et al. 1994. *Society of Magnetic Resonance*, San Francisco.
43. Ogawa S., Menon R., Tank D. et al. 1993. *Biophys. J.* 64: 803.
44. Ogawa S., Lee T.M., and Barrere B. 1993. *Magn. Reson. Med.* 29: 205.
45. Kennan R.P., Zhong J., and Gore J.C. 1994. *Magn. Reson. Med.* 31: 9.
46. Weisskoff R.M., Zuo C.S., Boxerman J.L., and Rosen B.R. 1994. *Magn. Reson. Med.* 31: 601.
47. Bandettini P.A., Jesmanowicz A., Wong E.C., and Hyde J.S. 1993. *Magn. Reson. Med.* 30: 161.
48. Thulborn K.R., Waterton J.C., Matthews P.M., and Radda G.K. 1982. *Biochim. Biophys. Acta* 714: 265.
49. Grubb R.L., Raichle M.E., Eichling J.O., and Ter-Pogossian M.M. 1974. *Stroke* 5: 630.
50. Fox P.T. and Raichle M.E. 1986. *Proc. Natl Acad. Sci. USA* 83: 1140.
51. Fox P.T., Raichle M.E., Mintun M.A., and Dence C. 1988. *Science* 241: 462.
52. Prichard J., Rothman D., Novotny E. et al. 1991. *Proc. Natl Acad. Sci. USA* 88: 5829.
53. Brooks R.A. and Di Chiro G. 1987. *Med. Phys.* 14: 903.
54. Kwong K., Chesler D., Zuo C. et al. 1993. *Society of Magnetic Resonance in Medicine, th Annual Meeting*, New York, p. 172.
55. Kwong K.K., Chesler D.A., Weisskoff R.M., and Rosen B.R. 1994. *Society of Magnetic Resonance*, San Francisco.
56. Edelman R., Sievert B., Wielopolski P. et al. 1994. *JMRI* 4 (P): 68.
57. Warach S., Sievert B., Darby D. et al. 1994. *JMRI* 4: S8.
58. Fisel C.R., Ackerman J.L., Buxton R.B. et al. 1991. *Magn. Reson. Med.* 17: 336.
59. Frahm J., Merboldt K., and Hanicke W. 1993. *Society of Magnetic Resonance in Medicine, th Annual Meeting*, New York, p. 1427.
60. Kwong K.K., Chesler D.A., Boxerman J.L. et al. 1994. *Society of Magnetic Resonance*, San Francisco.
61. Song W., Bandettini P., Wong E., and Hyde J. 1994. Personal communication.
62. Zuo C., Boxerman J., and Weisskoff R. 1992. *Society of Magnetic Resonance in Medicine, th Annual Meeting*, Berlin, p. 866.

10.4 Chemical-Shift Imaging: An Introduction to Its Theory and Practice

Xiaoping Hu, Wei Chen, Maqbool Patel, and Kamil Ugurbil

Over the past two decades, there has been a great deal of development in the application of nuclear magnetic resonance (NMR) to biomedical research and clinical medicine. Along with the development of magnetic resonance imaging [1], *in vivo* magnetic resonance spectroscopy (MRS) is becoming a research tool for biochemical studies of humans as well as a potentially more specific diagnostic tool, since it provides specific information on individual chemical species in living systems. Experimental studies in animals and humans have demonstrated that MRS can be used to study the biochemical basis of disease and to follow the treatment of disease.

Since biologic subjects (e.g., humans) are heterogeneous, it is necessary to spatially localize the spectroscopic signals to a well-defined volume or region of interest (VOI or ROI, respectively) in the intact body. Toward this goal, various localization techniques have been developed (see Reference 2 for a recent review). Among these techniques, chemical-shift imaging (CSI) or spectroscopic imaging [3–6] is an attractive technique, since it is capable of producing images reflecting the spatial distribution of various chemical species of interest. Since the initial development of CSI in 1982 [3], further developments have been made to provide better spatial localization and sensitivity, and the technique has been applied to numerous biomedical problems.

In this section we will first present a qualitative description of the basic principles of chemical-shift imaging and subsequently present some practical examples to illustrate the technique. Finally, a summary is provided in the last subsection.

10.4.1 General Methodology

In an NMR experiment, the subject is placed in a static magnetic field B_0. Under the equilibrium condition, nuclear spins with nonzero magnetic moment are aligned along B_0, giving rise to an induced bulk magnetization. To observe the bulk magnetization, it is tipped to a direction perpendicular to B_0 (transverse plane) with a radiofrequency (RF) pulse that has a frequency corresponding to the resonance frequency of the nuclei. The resonance frequency is determined by the product of the gyromagnetic ratio of the nucleus γ and the strength of the static field, that is, γB_0, and is called the *Larmor frequency*. The Larmor frequency also depends on the chemical environment of the nuclei, and this dependency gives rise to chemical shifts that allow one to identify different chemical species in an NMR spectrum. Upon excitation, the magnetization in the transverse plane (perpendicular to the main B_0 field direction) oscillates with the Larmor frequencies of all the different chemical species and induces a signal in a receiving RF coil; the signal is also termed the *free induction decay (FID)*. The FID can be Fourier transformed with respect to time to produce a spectrum in frequency domain.

In order to localize an NMR signal from an intact subject, spatially selective excitation and/or spatial encoding are usually utilized. Selective excitation is achieved as follows: in the excitation, an RF pulse with a finite bandwidth is applied in the presence of a linear static magnetic field gradient. With the application of the gradient, the Larmor frequency of spins depends linearly on the spatial location along the direction of the gradient. Consequently, only the spins in a slice whose resonance frequency falls into the bandwidth of the RF pulse are excited.

The RF excitation rotates all or a portion of the magnetization to the transverse plane, which can be detected by a receiving RF coil. Without spatial encoding, the signal detected is the integral of the signals over the entire excited volume. In CSI based on Fourier imaging, spatial discrimination is achieved by phase encoding. Phase encoding is accomplished by applying a gradient pulse after the excitation and before the data acquisition. During the gradient pulse, spins precess at Larmor frequencies that vary linearly along the direction of the gradient and accrue a phase proportional to the position along the phase-encoding gradient as well as the strength and the duration of the gradient pulse. This acquired spatially encoded phase is typically expressed as $\vec{k} \cdot \vec{r} = \int \gamma \vec{g}(t) \cdot \vec{r} dt$, where γ is the gyromagnetic ratio; $\vec{r}$ is the vector designating spatial location; $\vec{g}(t)$ defines the magnitude, the direction, and the time dependence of the magnetic field gradient applied during the phase-encoding; and the integration is performed over time when the phase-encoding gradient is on. Thus, in one-dimensional phase encoding, if the phase encoding is along, for example, the y axis, the phase acquired becomes $k \times y = \int \gamma g_y(t) \times y\, dt$. The acquired signal $S(t)$ is the integral of the spatially distributed signals modulated by a spatially dependent phase, given by the equation

$$S(t) = \int \rho(\vec{r},t)e^{(i\vec{k}\cdot\vec{r})}d^3r \tag{10.17}$$

where ρ is a function that describes the spatial density and the time evolution of the transverse magnetization of all the chemical species in the sample. This signal mathematically corresponds to a sample of the Fourier transform along the direction of the gradient. The excitation and detection process is repeated with various phase-encoding gradients to obtain many phase-encoded signals that can be inversely Fourier-transformed to resolve an equal number of pixels along this direction. Taking the example of one-dimensional phase-encoding along the y axis to obtain a one-dimensional image along this direction of n pixels, the phase encoding gradient is incremented n times so that n FIDs are acquired, each of which is described as

$$S(t,n) = \int \rho^*(y,t)e^{(1nk_0 y)}dy \tag{10.18}$$

where ρ^* is already integrated over the x and z directions, and k_0 is the phase-encoding increment; the latter is decided on using the criteria that the full field of view undergo a 360-degree phase difference when $n = 1$, as dictated by the sampling theorem. The time required for each repetition (*TR*), which is dictated by the longitudinal relaxation time, is usually on the order of seconds.

In CSI, phase encoding is applied in one, two, or three dimensions to provide spatial localization. Meanwhile, selective excitation also can be utilized in one or more dimensions to restrict the volume to be resolved with the phase encodings. For example, with selective excitation in two dimensions, CSI in one spatial dimension can resolve voxels within the selected column. In multidimensional CSI, all the phase-encoding steps along one dimension need to be repeated for all the steps along the others. Thus, for three dimensions with M, N, and L number of phase encoding steps, one must acquire $M \times N \times L$ number of FIDS:

$$S(t,m,n,l) = \int \rho(\vec{r},t)e^{i(mkx_0 x + nky_0 y + lkz_0 z)}d^3\vec{r} \tag{10.19}$$

where m, n, and l must step through M, N, and L in integer steps, respectively. As a result, the time needed for acquiring a chemical-shift image is proportional to the number of pixels desired and may be very long. In practice, due to the time limitation as well as the signal-to-noise ratio (SNR) limitation, chemical-shift imaging is usually performed with relatively few spatial encoding steps, such as 16×16 or 32×32 in a two-dimensional experiment.

The data acquired with the CSI sequence need to be properly processed before the metabolite information can be visualized and quantitated. The processing consists of spatial reconstruction and spectral processing. Spatial reconstruction is achieved by performing discrete inverse Fourier transformation, for each of the spatial dimensions, with respect to the phase-encoding steps. The spatial Fourier transform is applied for all the points of the acquired FID. For example, for a data set from a CSI in two spatial dimensions with 32×32 phase-encoding steps and 1024 sampled data points for each FID, a 32×32 two-dimensional inverse Fourier transform is applied to each of the 1024 data points. Although the nominal spatial resolution achieved by the spatial reconstruction is determined by the number of phase-encoding steps and the field of view (FOV), it is important to note that due to the limited number of phase-encoding steps used in most CSI experiments, the spatial resolution is severely degraded by the truncation artifacts, which results in signal "bleeding" between pixels. Various methods have been developed to reduce this problem [7–14].

The localized FIDs derived from the spatial reconstruction are to be further processed by spectral analysis. Standard procedures include Fourier transformation, filtering, zero-filling, and phasing. The localized spectra can be subsequently presented for visualization or further processed to produce quantitative metabolite information. The presentation of the localized spectra in CSI is not a straightforward task because there can be thousands of spectra. In one-dimensional experiments, localized spectra are usually presented in a stack plot. In two-dimensional experiments, localized spectra are plotted in small boxes representing the extent of the pixels, and the plots can be overlaid on corresponding anatomic image for reference. Spectra from three-dimensional CSI experiments are usually presented slice by slice, each displaying the spectra as in the two-dimensional case.

To derive metabolite maps, peaks corresponding to the metabolites of interest need to be quantified. In principle, the peaks can be quantified using the standard methods developed for spectral quantification [15–17]. The most straightforward technique is to calculate the peak areas by integrating the spectra over the peak of interest if it does not overlap with other peaks significantly. In integrating all the localized spectra, spectral shift due to B_0 inhomogeneity should be taken into account. A more robust approach is to apply spectral fitting programs to each spectrum to obtain various parameters of each peak. The fitted area for the peak of interest can then be used to represent the metabolite signal. The peak areas are then used to generate metabolite maps, which are images with intensities proportional to the localized peak area. The metabolite map can be displayed by itself as a gray-scale image or color-coded image or overlaid on a reference anatomic image.

10.4.2 Practical Examples

To illustrate the practical utility of CSI, we present two representative CSI studies in this section. The sequence for the first study is shown in Figure 10.21. This is a three-dimensional sequence in which phase encoding is applied in all three directions and no slice selection is used. Such a sequence is usually used with a surface RF coil whose spatial extent of sensitivity defines the field of view. In this sequence, the FID is acquired immediately after the application of the phase-encoding gradient to minimize the decay of the transverse magnetization, and the sequence is suitable for imaging metabolites with short transverse relaxation time (e.g., ATP).

With the sequence shown in Figure 10.21, a phosphorus-31 CSI study of the human brain was conducted using a quadrature surface coil. A nonselective RF pulse with an Ernest angle (40 degrees) optimized for the repetition time was used for the excitation. Phase-encoding gradients were applied for a duration of 500 μ sec; the phase-encoding gradients were incremented according to a FOV of $25 \times 25 \times 20$ cm³. Phase-encoded FIDs were acquired with 1024 complex data points over a sampling window of 204.8 msec; the corresponding spectral width was 5000 Hz. To reduce intervoxel signal contamination, a technique that utilizes variable data averaging to introduce spatial filtering during the data acquisition for optimal signal-to-noise ratio is employed [7–10], resulting in spherical voxels with diameter of 3 cm (15 cc volume). The data were acquired with a *TR* of 1 sec, and the total acquisition time was approximately 28 min.

The acquired data were processed to generate three-dimensional voxels, each containing a localized phosphorus spectrum, in a $17 \times 13 \times 17$ matrix. In Figure 10.22a–c, spectra in three slices of the

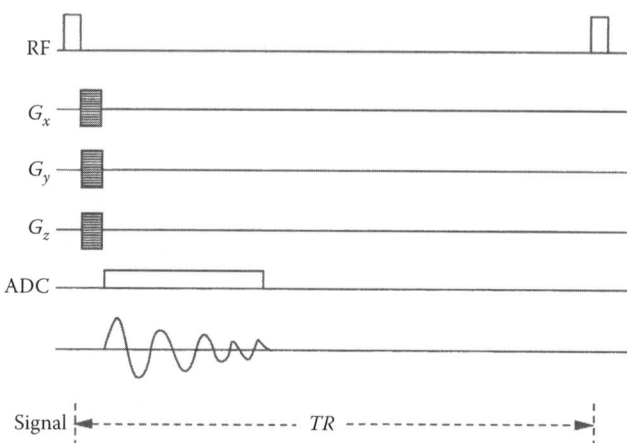

FIGURE 10.21   Sequence diagram for a three-dimensional chemical shift imaging sequence using a nonselective RF pulse.

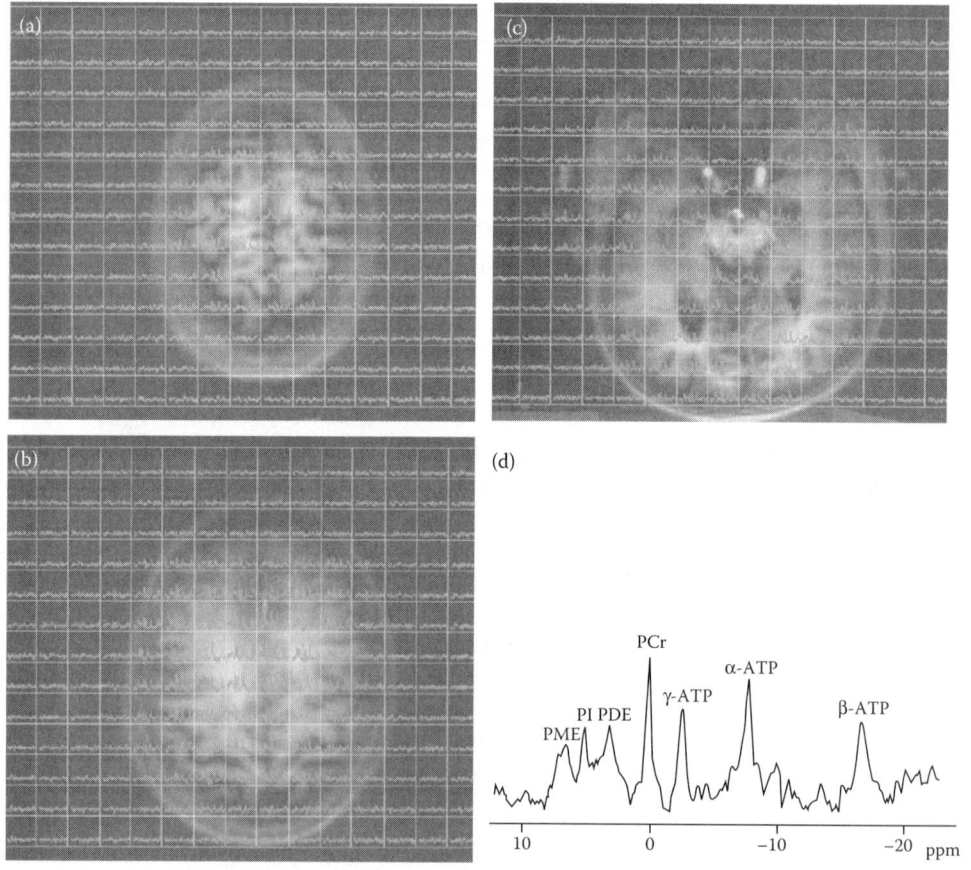

FIGURE 10.22   (a–c) Boxed plot of spectra in three slices from the three-dimensional ^{31}P CSI experiment overload on corresponding anatomic images. The spectral extent displayed is from 10 to 20 ppm. A 20-Hz line broadening is applied to all the spectra. (d) Representative spectrum from the three-dimensional ^{31}P CSI shown in (b). Metabolite peaks are labeled.

three-dimensional CSI are presented; these spectra are overlaid on the corresponding anatomic images obtained with a T_1-weighted imaging sequence. One representative spectrum of the brain is illustrated in Figure 10.22d, where the peaks corresponding to various metabolites are labeled. It is evident that the localized phosphorus spectra contain a wealth of information about several metabolites of interest, including adenosine triphosphate (ATP), phosphocreatine (PCr), phosphomonoester (PME), inorganic phosphate (P$_i$), and phosphodiester (PDE). In pathologic cases, focal abnormalities in phosphorus metabolites have been detected in patients with tumor, epilepsy, and other diseases [18–25].

The second study described below is performed with the sequence depicted in Figure 10.23. This is a two-dimensional spin-echo sequence in which a slice is selectively excited by a 90-degree excitation pulse. The 180-degree refocusing pulse is selective with a slightly broader slice profile. Here the phase-encoding gradients are applied before the refocusing pulse; they also can be placed after the 180-degree pulse or split to both sides of the 180-degree pulse. This sequence was used for a proton CSI experiment. In proton CSI, a major problem arises from the strong water signal that overwhelms that of the metabolites. In order to suppress the water signal, many techniques have been devised [26–29]. In this study, a three-pulse CHESS [26] technique was applied before the application of the excitation pulse as shown in Figure 10.23. The CSI experiment was performed on a 1.4-cm slice with 32×32 phase encodings over a 22×22 cm^2 FOV. The second half of the spin-echo was acquired with 512 complex data points over a sampling window of 256 msec, corresponding to a spectral width of 2000 Hz. Each phase-encoding FID was acquired twice for data averaging. The repetition time (*TR*) and the echo time (*TE*) used were 1.2 sec and 136 msec, respectively. The total acquisition time was approximately 40 min.

Another major problem in proton CSI study of the brain is that the signal from the subcutaneous lipid usually is much stronger than those of the metabolites, and this strong signal leaks into pixels within the brain due to truncation artifacts. To avoid lipid signal contamination, many proton CSI studies of the brain are performed within a selected region of interest excluding the subcutaneous fat [30–34]. Recently, several techniques have been proposed to suppress the lipid signal and consequently suppress the lipid signal contamination. These include the use of WEFT [27] and the use of outer-volume signal suppression [34]. In the example described below, we used a technique that utilizes the spatial location of the lipid to extrapolate data in the k-space to reduce the signal contamination due to truncation [35].

In Figure 10.24, the results from the proton CSI study are presented. In panel (a), the localized spectra are displayed. Note that the spectra in the subcutaneous lipid are ignored because they are all off the scale. The nominal spatial resolution is approximately 0.66 cc. A spectrum from an individual pixel in this study is presented in Figure 10.24b with metabolite peaks indicated. Several metabolite peaks, such as those corresponding to the *N*-acetyl aspartate (NAA), creatine/phosphocreatine (Cr/PCr), and choline (Cho), are readily identified. In addition, there is still a noticeable amount of residual lipid signal

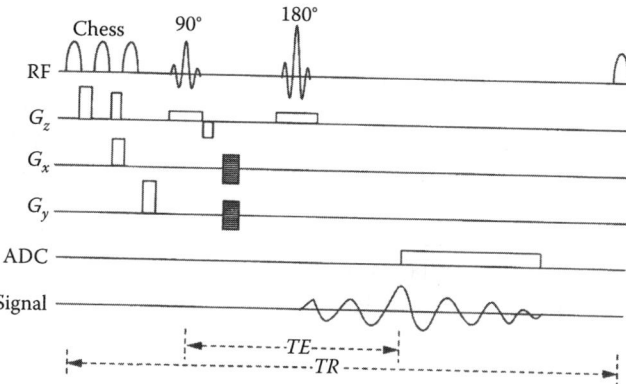

FIGURE 10.23 A two-dimensional spin-echo CSI sequence with chemical selective water suppression (CHESS) for proton study.

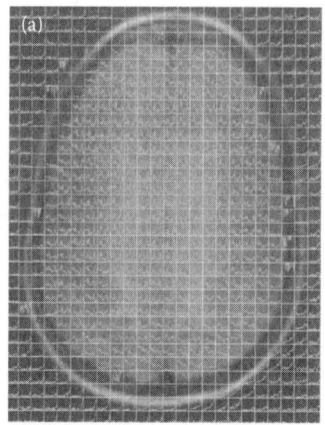

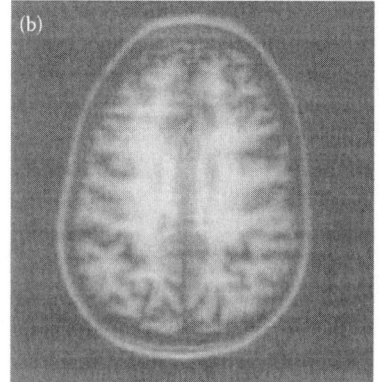
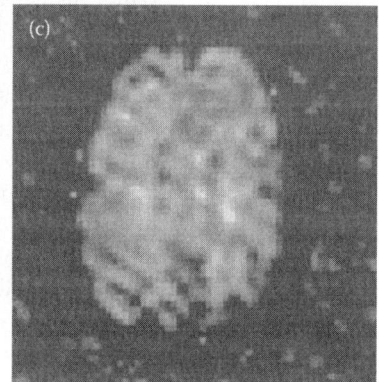

T_1 weighted image   NAA map

FIGURE 10.24 (a) Boxed plot of spectra for the two-dimensional proton study overlaid on the anatomic image. A spectral range of 1.7 to 3.5 ppm is used in the plot to show Cho, PCr/Cr, and NAA. A 5-Hz line broadening is applied in the spectral processing. (b) A representative spectrum from the two-dimensional CSI in panel (a). Peaks corresponding to Cho, PCr/Cr, and NAA are indicated. (c) A map of the area under the NAA peak obtained by spectral fitting. The anatomic image is presented along with the metabolite map for reference. The spatial resolution of the metabolite image can be appreciated from the similarities between the two images. The lipid suppression technique has successfully eliminated the signal contamination from the lipid in the skull.

contamination despite the use of the data extrapolation technique. Without the lipid suppression technique, the brain spectra would be severely contaminated by the lipid signal, making the detection of the metabolite peaks formidable. The peak of NAA in these spectra is fitted to generate the metabolite map shown in panel (c). Although the metabolite map is not corrected for coil sensitivity and other factors and only provides a relative measure of the metabolite concentration in the brain, it is a reasonable measure of the NAA distribution in the brain slice. The spatial resolution of the CSI study can be appreciated from the brain structure present in the map. In biomedical research, proton CSI is potentially the most promising technique, since it provides best sensitivity and spatial resolution. Various *in vivo* applications of proton spectroscopy can be found in the literature [36].

10.4.3 Summary

CSI is a technique for generating localized spectra that provide a wealth of biochemical information that can be used to study the metabolic activity of living system and to detect disease associated biochemical changes. This section provides an introduction to the technique and illustrates it by two representative examples. More specific topics concerning various aspects of CSI can be found in the literature.

Acknowledgments

The authors would like to thank Dr. Xiao-Hong Zhu for assisting data acquisition and Mr. Gregory Adriany for hardware support. The studies presented here are supported by the National Institute of Health (RR08079).

References

1. Lauterbur P.C. 1973. Image formation by induced local interactions: examples employing nuclear magnetic resonance. *Nature* 242: 190.
2. Alger J.R. 1994. Spatial localization for in vivo magnetic resonance spectroscopy: concepts and commentary. In R.J. Gillies (ed.), *NMR in Physiology and Biomedicine*, pp. 151–168. San Diego, CA, Academic Press.
3. Brown T.R., Kincaid M.B., and Ugurbil K. 1982. NMR chemical shift imaging in three dimensions. *Proc. Natl Acad. Sci. USA* 79: 3523.
4. Maudsley A.A., Hilal S.K., Simon H.E., and Perman W.H. 1983. Spatially resolved high resolution spectroscopy by "four dimensional" NMR. *J. Magn. Reson.* 51: 147.
5. Haselgrove J.C., Subramanian V.H., Leigh J.S. Jr. et al. 1983. in vivo one-dimensional imaging of phosphorous metabolites by phosphorus-31 nuclear magnetic resonance. *Science* 220: 1170.
6. Maudsley A.A., Hilal S.K., Simon H.E., and Wittekoek S. 1984. in vivo MR spectroscopic imaging with P-31. *Radiology* 153: 745.
7. Garwood M., Schleich T., Ross B.D. et al. 1985. A modified rotating frame experiment based on a Fourier window function: application to in vivo spatially localized NMR spectroscopy. *J. Magn. Reson.* 65: 239.
8. Garwood M., Robitalle P.M., and Ugurbil K. 1987. Fourier series windows on and off resonance using multiple coils and longitudinal modulation. *J. Magn. Reson.* 75: 244.
9. Mareci T.H. and Brooker H.R. 1984. High-resolution magnetic resonance spectra from a sensitive region defined with pulsed gradients. *J. Magn. Reson.* 57: 157.
10. Brooker H.R., Mareci T.H., and Mao J.T. 1987. Selective Fourier transform localization. *Magn. Reson. Med.* 5: 417.
11. Hu X., Levin D.N., Lauterbur P.C., and Spraggins T.A. 1988. SLIM: spectral localization by imaging. *Magn. Reson. Med.* 8: 314.
12. Liang Z.P. and Lauterbur P.C. 1991. A generalized series approach to MR spectroscopic imaging. *IEEE Trans. Med. Imag.* MI-10: 132.
13. Hu X. and Stillman A.E. 1991. Technique for reduction of truncation artifact in chemical shift images. *IEEE Trans. Med. Imag.* MI-10 3: 290.
14. Hu X., Patel M.S., and Ugurbil K. 1993. A new strategy for chemical shift imaging. *J. Magn. Reson.* B103: 30.
15. van den Boogaart A., Ala-Korpela M., Jokisaari J., and Griffiths J.R. 1994. Time and frequency domain analysis of NMR data compared: an application to 1D 1H spectra of lipoproteins. *Magn. Reson. Med.* 31: 347.
16. Ernst T., Kreis R., and Ross B. 1993. Absolute quantification of water and metabolites in human brain: I. Compartments and water. *J. Magn. Reson.* 102: 1.
17. Kreis R., Ernst T., and Ross B. 1993. Absolute quantification of water and metabolites in human brain. II. Metabolite concentration. *J. Magn. Reson.* 102: 9.
18. Lenkinski R.E., Holland G.A., Allman T. et al. 1988. Integrated MR imaging and spectroscopy with chemical shift imaging of P-31 at 1.5 T: Initial clinical experience. *Radiology* 169: 201.

19. Hugg J.W., Matson G.B., Twieg D.B. et al. [31]P MR spectroscopic imaging of normal and pathological human brains. *Magn. Reson. Imag.* 10: 227.

20. Vigneron D.B., Nelson S.J., Murphy-Boesch J. et al. 1990. Chemical shift imaging of human brain: axial, sagittal, and coronal ^{31}P metabolite images. *Radiology* 177: 643.

21. Hugg J.W., Laxer K.D., Matson G.B. et al. 1992. Lateralization of human focal epilepsy by ^{31}P magnetic resonance spectroscopic imaging. *Neurology* 42: 2011.

22. Meyerhoff D.J., Maudsley A.A., Schafer S., and Weiner M.W. 1992. Phosphorous-31 magnetic resonance metabolite imaging in the human body. *Magn. Reson. Imag.* 10: 245.

23. Bottomley P.A., Hardy C., and Boemer P. 1990. Phosphate metabolite imaging and concentration measurements in human heart by nuclear magnetic resonance. *J. Magn. Reson. Med.* 14: 425.

24. Robitaille P.M., Lew B., Merkle H. et al. 1990. Transmural high energy phosphate distribution and response to alterations in workload in the normal canine myocardium as studied with spatially localized ^{31}P NMR spectroscopy. *Magn. Reson. Med.* 16: 91.

25. Ugurbil K., Garwood M., Merkle H. et al. 1989. Metabolic consequences of coronary stenosis: transmurally heterogeneous myocardial ischemia studied by spatially localized ^{31}P NMR spectroscopy. *NMR Biomed.* 2: 317.

26. Hasse A., Frahm J., Hanicker H., and Mataei D. 1985. ^{1}H NMR chemical shift selective (CHESS) imaging. *Phys. Med. Biol.* 30: 341.

27. Patt S.L. and Sykes B.D. 1972. T_1 water eliminated Fourier transform NMR spectroscopy. *Chem. Phys.* 56: 3182.

28. Moonen C.T.W. and van Zijl P.C.M. 1990. Highly effective water suppression for in vivo proton NMR spectroscopy (DRYSTEAM). *J. Magn. Reson.* 88: 28.

29. Ogg R., Kingsley P., and Taylor J.S. 1994. WET: A T_1 and B_1 insensitive water suppression method for in vivo localized [1]H. *NMR Spectroscopy* B104: 1.

30. Lampman D.A., Murdoch J.B., and Paley M. 1991. In vivo proton metabolite maps using MESA 3D technique. *Magn. Reson. Med.* 18: 169.

31. Luyten P.R., Marien A.J.H., Heindel W. et al. 1990. Metabolic imaging of patients with intracranial tumors: [1]H MR spectroscopic imaging and PET. *Radiology* 176: 791.

32. Arnold D.L., Matthews P.M., Francis G.F. et al. 1992. Proton magnetic resonance spectroscopic imaging for metabolite characterization of demyelinating plaque. *Ann. Neurol.* 31: 319.

33. Duijin J.H., Matson G.B., Maudsley A.A. et al. 1992. Human brain infarction: proton MR spectroscopy. *Radiology* 183: 711.

34. Duyn J.H., Gillen J., Sobering G. et al. 1993. Multisection proton MR spectroscopic imaging of the brain. *Radiology* 188: 277.

35. Patel M.S. and Hu X. 1994. Selective data extrapolation for chemical shift imaging. *Soc. Magn. Reson. Abstr.* 3: 1168.

36. Rothman D.L. 1994. ^{1}H NMR studies of human brain metabolism and physiology. In R.J. Gillies (ed.), *NMR in Physiology and Biomedicine*, pp. 353–372. San Diego, CA, Academic Press.

11

Nuclear Medicine

Barbara Y. Croft
*National Institutes of
Health*

Benjamin M.W. Tsui
Johns Hopkins University

11.1 Instrumentation

Barbara Y. Croft

Nuclear medicine can be defined as the practice of making patients radioactive for diagnostic and therapeutic purposes. The radioactivity is injected intravenously, rebreathed, or ingested. It is the internal circulation of radioactive material that distinguishes nuclear medicine from diagnostic radiology and radiation oncology in most of its forms. This section will examine only the diagnostic use and will concentrate on methods for detecting the radioactivity from outside the body without trauma to the patient. Diagnostic nuclear medicine is successful for two main reasons: (1) it can rely on the use of very small amounts of materials (picomolar concentrations in chemical terms) thus usually not having any effect on the processes being studied, and (2) the radionuclides being used can penetrate tissue and be detected outside the patient. Thus the materials can trace processes or "opacify" organs without affecting their function.

11.1.1 Parameters for Choices in Nuclear Medicine

Of the various kinds of emanations from radioactive materials, photons alone have a range in tissue great enough to escape so that they can be detected externally. Electrons or beta-minus particles of high energy can create bremsstrahlung in interactions with tissue, but the radiation emanates from the site of the interaction, not the site of the beta ray's production. Positrons or beta-plus particles annihilate with electrons to create gamma rays so that they can be detected. For certain radionuclides, the emanation being detected is x-rays, in the 50- to 100-keV energy range.

The half-lives of materials in use in nuclear medicine range from a few minutes to weeks. The half-life must be chosen with two major points in mind: the time course of the process being studied and the radiation dose to the target organ, that is, that organ with the highest concentration over the longest

TABLE 11.1 Gamma Ray Detection

Type of Sample	Activity (μCi)	Energy (keV)	Type of Instrument
Patient samples, for example, blood, urine	0.001	0–5000	Gamma counter with annular NaI(TI) detector, 1 or 2 PMTs, external Pb shielding
Small organ function <30 cm field of view at 60 cm distance	5–200	20–1500	2–4-in. NaI(TI) detector with flared Pb collimator
Static image of body part, for example, liver, lung	0.2–30	50–650	Rectilinear scanner with focused Pb collimator
Dynamic image of body part, for example, xenon in airways	2–30	80–300	Anger camera and parallel-hole Pb collimator
Static tomographic image of body part	See Section 11.1		

time (the cumulated activity or area underneath the activity versus time curve). In general, it is desired to stay under 5 **rad** to the target organ.

The choice of the best energy range to use is also based on two major criteria: the energy that will penetrate tissue but can be channeled by heavy metal shielding and collimation and that which will interact in the detector to produce a pulse. Thus the ideal energy is dependent on the detector being used and the kind of examination being performed. Table 11.1 describes the kinds of gamma-ray detection, the activity and energy ranges, and an example of the kind of information to be gained. The lesser amounts of activity are used in situations of lesser spatial resolution and of greater sensitivity. Positron imaging is omitted because it is treated elsewhere.

Radiation dose is affected by all the emanations of a radionuclide, not just the desirable ones, thus constricting the choice of nuclide further. There can be no alpha radiation used in diagnosis; the use of materials with primary beta radiation should be avoided because the beta radiation confers a radiation dose without adding to the information being gained. For imaging, in addition, even if there is a primary gamma ray in the correct energy window for the detector, there should be no large amount of radiation, either of primary radiation of higher energy, because it interferes with the image collimation, or of secondary radiation of a very similar energy, because it interferes with the perception of the primary radiation emanating from the site of interest.

For imaging using heavy-metal collimation, the energy range is constrained to be that which will emanate from the human body and which the collimation can contain, or about 50 to 500 keV.

Detectors must be made from materials that exhibit some detectable change when ionizing radiation is absorbed and that are of a high enough atomic number and density to make possible stopping large percentages of those gamma rays emanating (high sensitivity). In addition, because the primary gamma rays are not the only rays emanating from the source—a human body and therefore a distributed source accompanied by an absorber—there must be energy discrimination in the instrument to prevent the formation of an image of the scattered radiation. To achieve pulse size proportional to energy, and therefore to achieve identification of the energy and source of the energy, the detector must be a proportional detector. This means that Geiger-Muller detection, operating in an all-or-none fashion, is not acceptable.

Gaseous detectors are not practical because their density is not great enough. Liquid detectors (in which any component is liquid) are not practical because the liquid can spill when the detector is positioned; this problem can be compensated for if absolutely necessary, but it is better to consider it from the outset. Another property of a good detector is its ability to detect large numbers of gamma rays per time unit. With detection capabilities to separate 100,000 counts per second or a dead time of 2 msec, the system is still only detecting perhaps 1,000 counts per square centimeter per second over a 10×10 cm area. The precision of the information is governed by **Poisson statistics**, so the imprecision in information collected for 1 sec in a square centimeter is ±3% at the 1 standard deviation level. Since we would hope for better spatial resolution than 1 cm², the precision is obviously worse than this. This points to the need for fast detectors, in addition to the aforementioned sensitivity. The more detector that

TABLE 11.2 Ways of Imaging Using Lead Collimation

Moving probe; rectilinear scanner

Array of multiple crystals; autofluoroscope, "fly-eye" camera

Two moving probes: dual-head rectilinear scanner

Large single-crystal system: Anger camera

Two crystals on opposite sides of patient for two views using Anger logic

Large multiple-crystal systems using Anger logic SPECT

Other possibilities

surrounds the patient, the more sensitive the system will be. Table 11.2 lists in order from least sensitive to most sensitive some of the geometries used for imaging in nuclear medicine. This generally is also a listing from the older methods to the more recent.

For the purposes of this section, we shall consider that the problems of counting patient and other samples and of detecting the time course of activity changes in extended areas with probes are not our topic and confine ourselves to the attempts made to image distributions of gamma-emitting radionuclides in patients and research subjects. The previous section treats the three-dimensional imaging of these distributions; this section will treat detection of the distribution in a planar fashion or the image of the projection of the distribution onto a planar detector.

11.1.2 Detection of Photon Radiation

Gamma rays are detected when atoms in a detector are ionized and the ions are collected either directly as in gaseous or semiconductor systems or by first conversion of the ionized electrons to light and subsequent conversion of the light to electrons in a photomultiplier tube (P-M tube or PMT). In all cases there is a voltage applied across some distance that causes a pulse to be created when a photon is absorbed.

The gamma rays are emitted according to Poisson statistics because each decaying nucleus is independent of the others and has an equal probability of decaying per unit time. Because the uncertainty in the production of gamma rays is therefore on the order of magnitude of the square root of the number of gamma rays, the more gamma rays that are detected, the less the proportional uncertainty will be. Thus sensitivity is a very important issue for the creation of images, since the rays will be detected by area. To get better resolution, one must have the numbers of counts and the apparatus to resolve them spatially. Having the large numbers of counts also means the apparatus must resolve them temporally.

The need for **energy resolution** carries its own burden. Depending on the detector, the energy resolution may be easily achieved or not (Table 11.3). In any case, the attenuation and scattering inside the body means that there will be a range of gamma rays emitted, and it will be difficult to tell those scattered through very small angles from those not scattered at all. This affects the spatial resolution of the instrument.

TABLE 11.3 Detector Substances and Size Considerations, Atomic Number of the Attenuator, Energy Resolution Capability

PMT connected

   NaI(TI): up to 50 cm across; 63; 5–10%

   Plastic scintillators: unlimited; 6; only Compton absorption for gamma rays used in imaging

   CsI(TI): < 3 × 3 cm; 53, 55; poorer than NaI(TI)

   BiGermanate: < 3 × 3 cm; 83; poorer than NaI(TI)

Semiconductors: Liquid nitrogen operation and liquid nitrogen storage

   GeLi: < 3 × 3 cm; 32; < 1%

   SiLi: < 3 × 3 cm; 14; < 1%

TABLE 11.4 Calculation of Number of Counts Achieved with Anger Camera

	Cpm	Cps
Activity	0.001	
mCi/cm^3		
counts/sec		3.7×10^7
counts/min	2.22×10^9	
2π geometry	1.11×10^9	1.85×10^7
Attenuated by tissue of 0.12/cm attenuation and 3 cm thick	7.44×10^8	1.29×10^7
X Camera efficiency of 0.0006	4.64×10^5	7744
Good uptake in liver = 5 mCi/1000 g = 0.005 mCi/g	2.32×10^6	3.8×10^4
Thyroid uptake of Tc-99m = (2 mCi/37 g)	4.6×10^5	7.7×10^3
2% = 0.001 mCi/G		

The current practice of nuclear medicine has defined the limits of the amount of activity that can be administered to a patient by the amount of radiation dose. Since planar imaging with one detector allows only 2 pi detection at best and generally a view of somewhat less because the source is in the patient and the lead collimation means that only rays that are directed from the decay toward the crystal will be detected, it is of utmost importance to detect every ray possible. To the extent that no one is ever satisfied with the resolution of any system and always wishes for better, there is the need to be able to get spatial resolution better than the intrinsic 2 mm currently achievable. Some better collimation system, such as envisioned in a coincidence detection system like that used in PET, might make it possible to avoid stopping so many of the rays with the collimator.

We have now seen that energy resolution, sensitivity and resolving time of the detector are all bound up together to produce the spatial resolution of the instrument as well as the more obvious temporal resolution. The need to collimate to create an image rather than a blush greatly decreases the numbers of counts and makes Poisson statistics a major determinant of the appearance of nuclear medical images.

Table 11.4 shows a calculation for the NaI(TI)-based Anger camera showing 0.06% efficiency for the detection system. Thus the number of counts per second is not high and so is well within the temporal resolving capabilities of the detector system. The problem is the 0.06% efficiency, which is the effect of both the crystal thickness being optimized for imaging rather than for stopping all the gamma rays, and the lead collimation. Improvements in nuclear medicine imaging resolution can only come if both these factors are addressed.

11.1.3 Various Detector Configurations

The detectors in clinical nuclear medicine are NaI(TI) crystals. In research applications, other substances are employed, but the engineering considerations for the use of other detectors are more complex and have been less thoroughly explored (Table 11.3).

The possibilities for configuring the detectors have been increasing, although the older methods tend to be discarded as the new ones are exploited (see Table 11.2). This is in part because each laboratory cannot afford to have one of every kind of instrument, although there are tasks for which each one is ideally suited.

The first instruments possible for plane-projection imaging consisted of a moving single crystal probe, called a rectilinear scanner. The probe consisted of a detector (beginning with NaI(TI) but later incorporating small semiconductors) that was collimated by a focused lead collimator of appreciable thickness (often 2 in. of lead or more) with hole sizes and thicknesses of septa consonant with the intended energy and organ size and depth to be imaged. The collimated detector was caused to move across the patient at a constant speed; the pulses from the detector were converted to visible signals either by virtue of markings on a sheet or of light flashes exposing a film. This detector could see only one spot at a time, so only slow temporal changes in activity could be appreciated. A small organ such as the thyroid could be imaged in this fashion very satisfactorily. Bone imaging also could be done with the later versions of this instrument.

To enlarge the size of the detector, several probes, each with its own photomultiplier tube and collimator, could be used. Versions of this idea were used to create dual-probe instruments to image both sides of the patient simultaneously, bars of probes to sweep down the patient and create a combined image, etc.

To go further with the multiple crystals to create yet larger fields of view, the autofluoroscope (Figure 11.1) combined crystals in a rectangular array. For each to have its own photomultiplier tube required too many PMTs, so the instrument was designed with a light pipe to connect each crystal with a PMT to indicate its row and a second one to indicate its column. The crystals are separated by lead septa to prevent scattered photons from one crystal affecting the next. Because of the large number of crystals and PMTs, the instrument is very fast, but because of the size of the crystals, the resolution is coarse. To improve the resolution, the collimator is often jittered so that each crystal is made to see more than one field of view to create a better resolved image. For those dynamic examinations in which temporal resolution is more important than spatial resolution, the system has a clear advantage. It has not been very popular for general use, however. In its commercial realization, the field of view was not large enough to image either lungs or livers or bones in any single image fashion.

As large NaI(TI) crystals became a reality, new ways to use them were conceived. The Anger camera (Figure 11.2) is one of the older of these methods. The idea is to use a single crystal of diameter large enough to image a significant part of the human body and to back the crystal by an array of

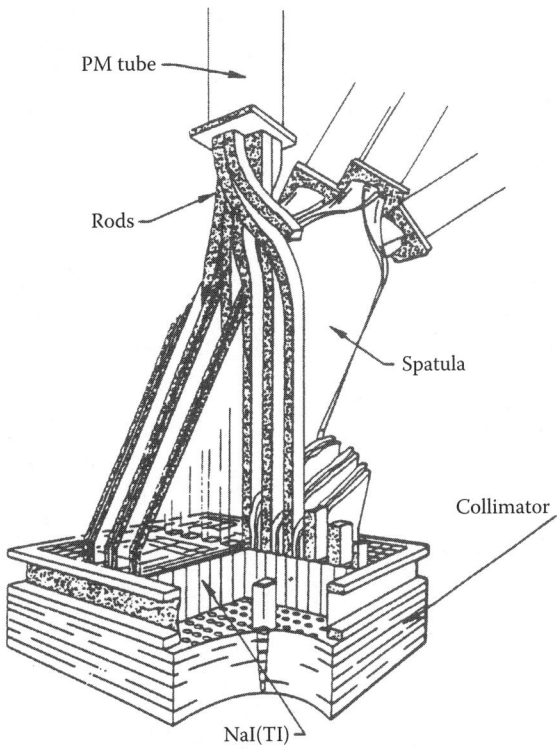

FIGURE 11.1 The Bender–Blau autofluoroscope is a multicrystal imager with a rectangular array of crystals connected to PMTs by plastic light guides. There is a PMT for each row of crystals and a PMT for each column of crystals, so an N by M array would have $(N + M)$ PMTs.

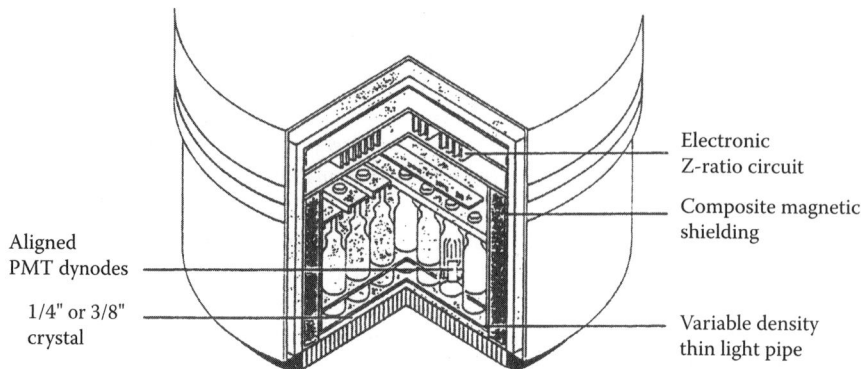

FIGURE 11.2 Anger camera detector design. This figure shows a cross section through the camera head. The active surface is pointed down. Shielding surrounds the assembly on the sides and top.

photomultiplier tubes to give positional sensitivity. Each PMT is assigned coordinates (Figure 11.3). When a photon is absorbed by the crystal, a number of PMTs receive light and therefore emit signals. The X and Y signal values for the emanation are determined by the strength of the signal from each of the tubes and its x and y position, and the energy of the emanation (which determines if it will be used to create the image) is the sum of all the signals (the Z pulse). If the discriminator passes the Z pulse, then the X and Y signals are sent to whatever device is recording the image, be it an oscilloscope and film recording system or the analog-to-digital (A/D) converters of a computer system. More recently, the A/D conversion is done earlier in the system so that the X and Y signals are themselves digital. The Anger camera is the major instrument in use in nuclear medicine today. It has been optimized for use with the 140-keV radiation from Tc-99m, although collimators have been designed for lower and higher energies, as well as optimized for higher sensitivity and higher resolution. The early systems used circular crystals, while the current configuration is likely to be rectangular or square.

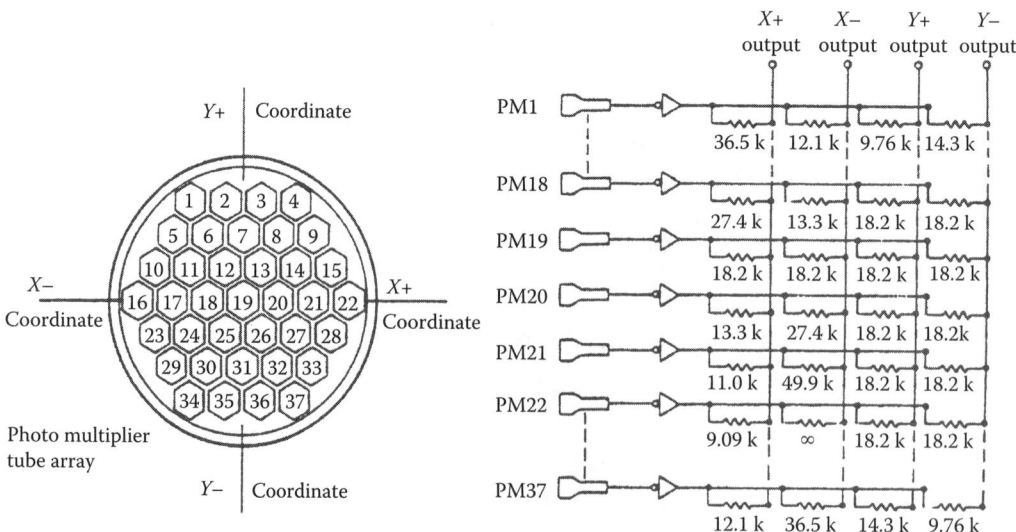

FIGURE 11.3 An array of PMTs in the Anger camera showing the geometric connection between the PMTs and the X and Y output.

A combination of the Anger positional logic and the focused collimator in a scanner produced the PhoCon instrument, which, because of the design of its collimators, had planar tomographic capabilities (the instrument could partially resolve activity in different planes, parallel to the direction of movement of the detector).

11.1.4 Ancillary Electronic Equipment for Detection

The detectors used in nuclear medicine are attached to preamplifiers, amplifiers, and pulse shapers to form a signal that can be examined for information about the energy of the detected photon (Figure 11.4). The energy discriminator has lower and upper windows that are set with reference radionuclides so that typically the particular nuclide in use can be dialed in along with the width of the energy window. A photon with an energy that falls in the selected range will cause the creation of a pulse of a voltage that falls in between the levels; all other photon energies will cause voltages either too high or too low. If only gross features are being recorded, any of the instruments may be used as probe detectors and the results recorded on strip-chart recordings of activity vs. time.

The PMT "multiplies" photons (Figure 11.5) because it has a quartz entrance window which is coated to release electrons when it absorbs a light photon and there is a voltage drop; the number of electrons released is proportional to the amount of light that hits the coating. The electrons are guided through a hole and caused to hit the first dynode, which is coated with a special substance to allow it to release electrons when it is hit by an electron. There are a series of dynodes each with a voltage that pulls the electrons from the last dynodes toward it. The surface coating not only releases electrons but also multiplies the electron shower. In a cascade through 10–12 dynodes, there is a multiplication of approximately 106, so that pulses of a few electrons become currents of the order of 10–12 A. The PMTs must be protected from other influences, such as stray radioactivity or strong magnetic fields, which might cause extraneous electron formation or curves in the electron path. Without the voltage drop from one dynode to the next, there is no cascade of electrons and no counting.

For imaging, the x and y positions of those photons in the correct energy range will be recorded in the image because they have a Z pulse. Once the pulse has been accepted and the position determined, that position may be recorded to make an image either in analog or digital fashion; a spot may be made on an oscilloscope screen and recorded on film or paper, or the position may be digitized and stored in a computer file for later imaging on an oscilloscope screen and/or for photography. In general, the computers required are very similar to those used for other imaging modalities, except for the hardware that allows the acceptance of the pulse. The software is usually specifically created for nuclear medicine because of the unique needs for determination of function.

The calibration of the systems follows a similar pattern, no matter how simple or complex the instrument. Most probe detectors must be "peaked," which means that the energy of the radioactivity must be connected with some setting of the instrument, often meant to read in kiloelectronvolts. This is accomplished by counting a sample with the instrument, using a reasonably narrow energy window, while varying the high voltage until the count rate reading is a maximum. The window is then widened for counting samples to encompass all the energy peak being counted. The detector is said to be liner if it can be set with one energy and another energy can be found where it should be on the kiloelectronvolt scale.

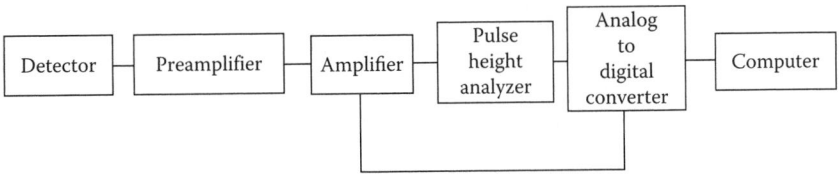

FIGURE 11.4 Schematic drawing of a generalized detector system. There would be a high-voltage power supply for the detector in an NaI(Tl)-PMT detector system.

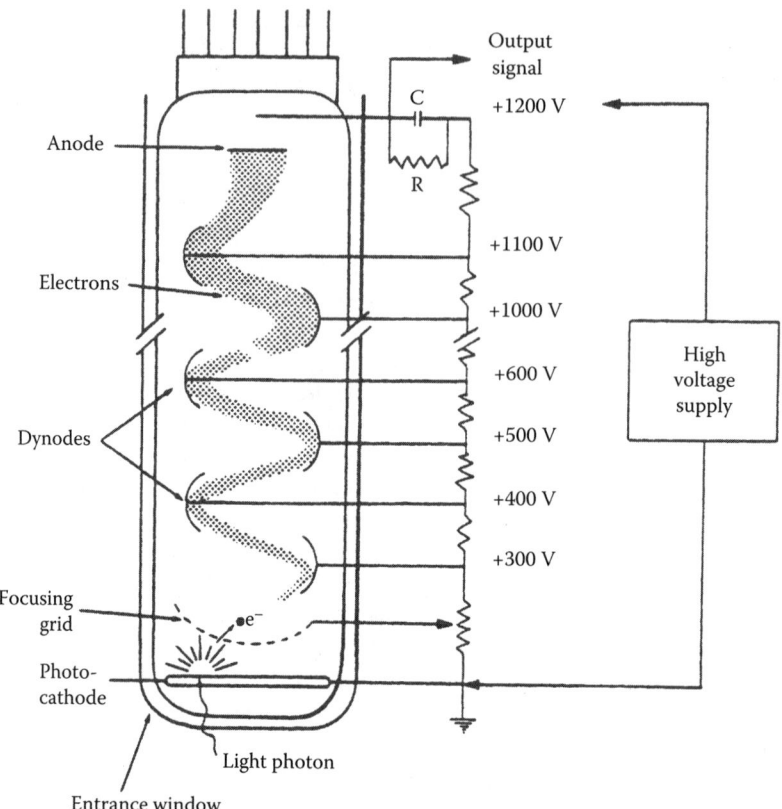

FIGURE 11.5 Schematic drawing of a photomultiplier tube (PMT). Each of the dynodes and the anode is connected to a separate pin in the tube socket. The inside of the tube is evacuated of all gas. Dynodes are typically copper with a special oxidized coating for electron multiplication.

To ensure that the images of the radioactivity accurately depict the distribution in the object being imaged, the system must be initialized correctly and tested at intervals. The several properties that must be calibrated and corrected are sensitivity, uniformity, energy pulse shape, and linearity.

These issues are addressed in several ways. The first is that all the PMTs used in an imaging system must be chosen to have matched sensitivities and energy spectra. Next, during manufacture, and at intervals during maintenance, the PMTs' response to voltage is matched so that the voltage from the power supply causes all the tubes to have maximum counts at the same voltage. The sensitivities of all the tubes are also matched during periodic maintenance. Prior to operation, usually at the start of each working day, the user will check the radioactive peak and then present the instrument with a source of activity to give an even exposure over the whole crystal. This uniform "flood" is recorded. The image may be used by the instrument for calibration; recalibration is usually performed at weekly intervals. The number of counts needed depends on the use the instrument is to be put to, but generally the instrument must be tested and calibrated with numbers of counts at least equal to those being emitted by the patients and other objects being imaged.

Because the PMT placement means that placement of the x and y locations is not perfect over the face of the crystal but has the effect of creating wiggly lines that may be closer together over the center of the PMT and farther apart at the interstices between tubes, the image may suffer from spatial nonlinearity. This can be corrected for by presenting the system with a lead pattern in straight-line bars or holes in rows and using a hard-wired or software method to position the X and Y signals correctly. This is called a linearity correction. In addition, there may be adjustments of the energy spectra of each tube to make them match each other so that variations in the number of kiloelectronvolts included in the window (created by varying the discriminator settings) will not create variations in sensitivity. This is called an energy correction.

11.1.5 Place of Planar Imaging in Nuclear Medicine Today: Applications and Economics

There are various ways of thinking about diagnostic imaging and nuclear medicine. If the reason for imaging the patient is to determine the presence of disease, then there are at least two possible strategies. One is to do the most complicated examination that will give a complete set of results on all patients. The other is to start with a simple examination and hope to categorize patients, perhaps into certain abnormals and all others, or even into abnormals, indeterminates, and normals. Then a subsequent, more complex examination is used to determine if there are more abnormals, or perhaps how abnormal they are. If the reason for imaging the patient is to collect a set of data that will be compared with results from that patient at a later time and with a range of normal results from all patients, then the least complex method possible for collecting the information should be used in a regular and routine fashion so that the comparison are possible.

In the former setting, where the complexity of the examination may have to be changed after the initial results are seen, in order to take full advantage of the dose of radioactive material that has been given to the patient, it is sensible to have the equipment available that will be able to perform the more complex examination and not to confine the equipment available to that capable of doing only the simple first examination. For this reason and because for some organs, such as the brain, the first examination is a SPECT examination, the new Anger cameras being sold today are mostly capable of doing rotating SPECT. The added necessities that SPECT brings to the instrument specifications are of degree: better stability, uniformity, and resolution. Thus they do not obviate the use of the equipment for planar imaging but rather enhance it. In the setting of performing only the examination necessary to define the disease, the Anger SPECT camera can be used for plane projection imaging and afterward for SPECT to further refine the examination. There are settings in which a planar camera will be purchased because of the simplicity of all the examinations (as in a very large laboratory that can have specialized instruments, a thyroid practice, or in the developing countries), but in the small- to medium-sized nuclear medicine practice, the new cameras being purchased are all SPECT-capable.

Nuclear medicine studies are generally less expensive than x-ray computed tomography or magnetic resonance imaging and more so than planar x-ray or ultrasound imaging. The general conduct of a nuclear medicine laboratory is more complex than these others because of the radioactive materials and the accompanying regulations. The specialty is practice both in clinics and in hospitals, but again, the complication imposed by the presence of the radioactive materials tips the balance of the practices toward the hospital. In that setting the practitioners may be imagers with a broad range of studies offered or cardiologists with a concentration on cardiac studies. Thus the setting also will determine what kind of instrument is most suitable.

Defining Terms

Energy resolution: Full width at half maximum of graph of detected counts vs. energy, expressed as a percentage of the energy.

Poisson statistics: Expresses probability in situations of equal probability for an event per unit of time, such as radioactive decay or cosmic-ray appearance. The standard deviation of a mean number of counts is the square root of the mean number of counts, which is a decreasing fraction of the number of counts when expressed as a fraction of the number of counts.

rad: The unit of radiation energy absorption (dose) in matter, defined as the absorption of 100 ergs per gram of irradiated material. The unit is being replaced by the gray, an SI unit, where 1 gray (Gy) = 100 rad.

Further Information

A good introduction to nuclear medicine, written as a text for technologists, is *Nuclear Medicine Technology and Techniques*, edited by D.R. Bernier, J.K. Langan, and L.D. Wells. A treatment of many of the nuclear medicine physics issues is given in L.E. Williams' *Nuclear Medicine Physics*, published in three volumes. Journals that publish nuclear medicine articles include the monthly *Journal of Nuclear Medicine, the European Journal of Nuclear Medicine, Clinical Nuclear Medicine, IEEE Transactions in Nuclear Science, IEEE Transactions in Medical Imaging*, and *Medical Physics*. Quarterly and annual publications include *Seminars in Nuclear Medicine, Yearbook of Nuclear Medicine*, and *Nuclear Medicine Annual*.

The Society of Nuclear Medicine holds an annual scientific meeting that includes scientific papers, continuing education which could give the novice a broad introduction, poster sessions, and a large equipment exhibition. Another large meeting, devoted to many radiologic specialties is the Radiologic Society of North America's annual meeting, held just after Thanksgiving.

11.2 SPECT (Single-Photon Emission Computed Tomography)

Benjamin M.W. Tsui

During the last three decades, there has been much excitement in the development of diagnostic radiology. The development is fueled by inventions and advances made in a number of exciting new medical imaging modalities, including ultrasound (US), x-ray CT (computed tomography), PET (positron emission tomography), SPECT (single-photon emission computed tomography), and MRI (magnetic resonance imaging). These new imaging modalities have revolutionized the practice of diagnostic radiology, resulting in substantial improvement in patient care.

Single-photon emission computed tomography (SPECT) is a medical imaging modality that combines conventional nuclear medicine (NM) imaging techniques and CT methods. Different from x-ray CT, SPECT uses radioactive-labeled pharmaceuticals, that is, radiopharmaceuticals, that distribute in different internal tissues or organs instead of an external x-ray source. The spatial and uptake distributions of the radiopharmaceuticals depend on the biokinetic properties of the pharmaceuticals and the normal or abnormal state of the patient. The gamma photons emitted from the radioactive source are detected by radiation detectors similar to those used in conventional nuclear medicine. The CT method requires projection (or planar) image data to be acquired from different views around the patient. These projection data are subsequently reconstructed using image reconstruction methods that generate cross-sectional images of the internally distributed radiopharmaceuticals. The SPECT images provide much improved contrast and detailed information about the radiopharmaceutical distribution as compared with the planar images obtained from conventional nuclear medicine methods.

As an emission computed tomographic (ECT) method, SPECT differs from PET in the types of radionuclides used. PET uses radionuclides such as C-11, N-13, O-15, and F-18 that emit positrons with subsequent emission of two coincident 511 keV annihilation photons. These radionuclides allow studies of biophysiologic functions that cannot be obtained from other means. However, they have very short half-lives, often requiring an on-site cyclotron for their production. Also, detection of the annihilation photons requires expensive imaging systems. SPECT uses standard radionuclides normally found in nuclear medicine clinics and which emit individual gamma-ray photons with energies that are much lower than 511 keV. Typical examples are the 140-keV photons from Tc-99m and the ~70-keV photons from TI-201. Subsequently, the costs of SPECT instrumentation and of performing SPECT are substantially less than PET.

Furthermore, substantial advances have been made in the development of new radiopharmaceuticals, instrumentation, and image processing and reconstruction methods for SPECT. The results are much improved quality and quantitative accuracy of SPECT images. These advances, combined with the relatively lower costs, have propelled SPECT to become an increasingly more important diagnostic tool in nuclear medicine clinics.

This section will present the basic principles of SPECT and the instrumentation and image processing and reconstruction methods that are necessary to reconstruct SPECT images. Finally, recent advances and future development that will continue to improve the diagnostic capability of SPECT will be discussed.

11.2.1 Basic Principles of SPECT

Single-photon emission computed tomography (SPECT) is a medical imaging technique that is based on the conventional nuclear medicine imaging technique and tomographic reconstruction methods. General review of the basic principles, instrumentation, and reconstruction technique for SPECT can be found in a few review articles (Jaszczak et al., 1980; Jaszczak and Coleman, 1985a; Barrett, 1986; Jaszczak and Tsui, 1994).

11.2.1.1 SPECT Imaging Process

The imaging process of SPECT can be simply depicted as in Figure 11.6. Gamma-ray photons emitted from the internal distributed radiopharmaceutical penetrate through the patient's body and are detected by a single or a set of collimated radiation detectors. The emitted photons experience interactions with the intervening tissues through basic interactions of radiation with matter (Evans, 1955). The photoelectric effect absorbs all the energy of the photons and stops their emergence from the patient's body. The other major interaction is Compton interaction, which transfers part of the photon energy to free electrons. The original photon is scattered into a new direction with reduced energy that is dependent on the scatter angle. Photons that escape from the patient's body include those that have not experienced any interactions and those which have experienced Compton scattering. For the primary photons from the commonly used radionuclides in SPECT, for example, 140-keV of TC-99m and ~70-keV of TI-201, the probability of pair production is zero.

Most of the radiation detectors used in current SPECT systems are based on a single or multiple NaI(TI) scintillation detectors. The most significant development in nuclear medicine is the scintillation camera (or Anger camera) that is based on a large-area (typically 40 cm in diameter) NaI(TI) crystal

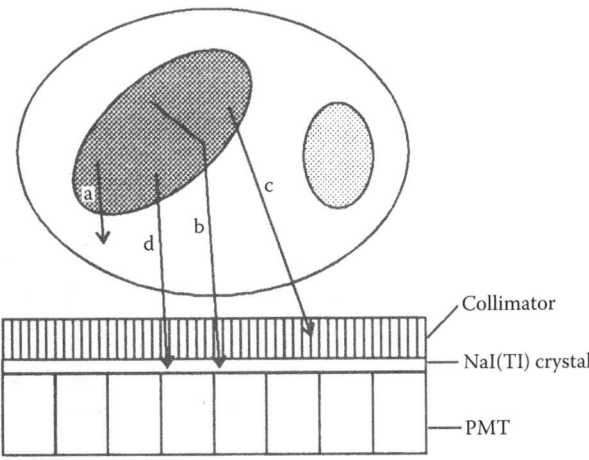

FIGURE 11.6 The conventional nuclear medicine imaging process. Gamma-ray photons emitted from the internally distributed radioactivity may experience photoelectric (a) or scatter (b) interactions. Photons that are not traveling in the direction within the acceptance analog of the collimator (c) will be intercepted by the lead collimator. Photons that experience no interaction and travel within the acceptance angle of the collimator will be detected (d).

(Anger, 1958, 1964). An array of photomultiplier tubes (PMTs) is placed at the back of the scintillation crystal. When a photon hits and interacts with the crystal, the scintillation generated will be detected by the array of PMTs. An electronic circuitry evaluates the relative signals from the PMTs and determines the location of interaction of the incident photon in the scintillation crystal. In addition, the scintillation cameras have built-in energy discrimination electronic circuitry with finite energy resolution that provides selection of the photons that have not been scattered or been scattered within a small scattered angle. The scintillation cameras are commonly used in commercial SPECT systems.

Analogous to the lens in an optical imaging system, a scintillation camera system consists of a collimator placed in front of the NaI(TI) crystal for the imaging purpose. The commonly used collimator is made of a large number of parallel holes separated by lead septa (Anger, 1964; Keller, 1968; Tsui, 1988). The geometric dimensions, that is, length, size, and shape of the collimator apertures, determine the directions of photons that will be detected by the scintillation crystals or the geometric response of the collimator. The width of the geometric response function increases (or the spatial resolution worsens) as the source distance from the collimator increases. Photons that do not pass through the collimator holes properly will be intercepted and absorbed by the lead septal walls of the collimator. In general, the detection efficiency is approximately proportional to the square of the width of the geometric response function of the collimator. This tradeoff between detection efficiency and spatial resolution is a fundamental property of a typical SPECT system using conventional collimators.

The amount of radioactivity that is used in SPECT is restricted by the allowable radiation dose to the patient. Combined with photon attenuation within the patient, the practical limit on imaging time, and the tradeoff between detection efficiency and spatial resolution of the collimator, the number of photons that are collected by a SPECT system is limited. These limitations resulted in SPECT images with relatively poor spatial resolution and high statistical noise fluctuations as compared with other medical imaging modalities. For example, currently a typical brain SPECT image has a total of about 500K counts per image slice and a spatial resolution in the order of approximately 8 mm. A typical myocardial SPECT study using TI-201 has about 150K total count per image slice and a spatial resolution of approximately 15 mm.

In SPECT, projection data are acquired from different views around the patient. Similar to x-ray CT, image processing and reconstruction methods are used to obtain transaxial or cross-sectional images from the multiple projection data. These methods consist of preprocessing and calibration procedures before further processing, mathematical algorithms for reconstruction from projections, and compensation methods for image degradation due to photon attenuation, scatter, and detector response.

The biokinetics of the radiopharmaceutical used, anatomy of the patient, instrumentation for data acquisition, preprocessing methods, image reconstruction techniques, and compensation methods have important effects on the quality and quantitative accuracy of the final SPECT images. A full understanding of SPECT cannot be accomplished without clear understanding of these factors. The biokinetics of radiopharmaceuticals and conventional radiation detectors have been described in the previous section on conventional nuclear medicine. The following subsections will present the major physical factors that affect SPECT and a summary review of the instrumentation, image reconstruction techniques, and compensation methods that are important technological and engineering aspects in the practice of SPECT.

11.2.1.2 Physical and Instrumentation Factors That Affect SPECT Images

There are several important physical and instrumentation factors that affect the measured data and subsequently the SPECT images. The characteristics and effects of these factors can be found in a few review articles (Jaszczak et al., 1981; Jaszczak and Tsui, 1994; Tsui et al., 1994a,b). As described earlier, gamma-ray photons that emit from an internal source may experience photoelectric absorption within the patient without contributing to the acquired data, Compton scattering with change in direction and loss of energy, or no interaction before exiting the patient's body. The exiting photons will be further selected by the geometric response of the collimator–detector. The photoelectric and Compton interactions and the characteristics of the collimator–detector have significant effects on both the quality and quantitative accuracy of SPECT image.

Photon attenuation is defined as the effect due to photoelectric and Compton interactions resulting in a reduced number of photons that would have been detected without them. The degree of attenuation is determined by the linear attenuation coefficient, which is a function of photon energy and the amount and types of materials contained in the attenuating medium. For example, the attenuation coefficient for the 140-keV photon emitted from the commonly used Tc-99m in water or soft tissue is 0.15 cm^{-1}. This gives rise to a half-valued-layer, the thickness of material that attenuates half the incident photons, or 4.5 cm H$_2$O for the 140-keV photon. Attenuation is the most important factor that affects the quantitative accuracy of SPECT images.

Attenuation effect is complicated by the fact that within the patient the attenuation coefficient can be quite different in various organs. The effect is most prominent in the thorax, where the attenuation coefficients range from as low as 0.05 cm^{-1} in the lung to as high as 0.18 cm^{-1} in the compact bone for the 140-keV photons. In x-ray CT, the attenuation coefficient distribution is the target for image reconstruction. In SPECT, however, the wide range of attenuation coefficient values and the variations of attenuation coefficient distributions among patients are major difficulties in obtaining quantitative accurate SPECT images. Therefore, compensation for attenuation is important to ensure good image quality and quantitatively high accuracy in SPECT. Review of different attenuation methods that have been used in SPECT is a subject of discussion later in this chapter.

Photons that have been scattered before reaching the radiation detector provide misplaced spatial information about the origin of the radioactive source. The results are inaccurate quantitative information and poor contrast in the SPECT images. For radiation detectors with perfect energy discrimination, scattered photons can be completely rejected. In a typical scintillation camera system, however, the energy resolution is in the order of 10% at 140 keV. With this energy resolution, the ratio of scattered to scattered total photons detected by a typical scintillation detector is about 20–30% in brain and about 30–40% in cardiac and body SPECT studies for 140-keV photons. Furthermore, the effect of scatter depends on the distribution of the radiopharmaceutical, the proximity of the source organ to the target organ, and the energy window used in addition to the photon energy and the energy resolution of the scintillation detector. The compensation of scatter is another important aspect of SPECT to ensure good image quality and quantitative accuracy.

The advances in SPECT can be attributed to simultaneous development of new radiopharmaceuticals, instrumentation, reconstruction methods, and clinical applications. Most radiopharmaceuticals that are developed for conventional nuclear medicine can readily be used in SPECT, and review of these developments is beyond the scope of this chapter. Recent advances include new agents that are labeled with iodine and technetium for blood perfusion for brain and cardiac studies. Also, the use of receptor agents and labeled antibiotics is being investigated. These developments have resulted in radiopharmaceuticals with improved uptake distribution, biokinetics properties, and potentially new clinical applications. The following subsections will concentrate on the development of instrumentation and image reconstruction methods that have made substantial impact on SPECT.

11.2.2 SPECT Instrumentation

Review of the advances in SPECT instrumentation can be found in several recent articles (Jaszczak et al., 1980; Rogers and Ackermann, 1992; Jaszczak and Tsui, 1994). A typical SPECT system consists of a single or multiple units of radiation detectors arranged in a specific geometric configuration and a mechanism for moving the radiation detector(s) or specially designed collimators to acquire data from different projection views. In general, SPECT instrumentation can be divided into three general categories (1) arrays of multiple scintillation detectors, (2) one or more scintillation cameras, and (3) hybrid scintillation detectors combining the first two approaches. In addition, special collimator designs have been proposed for SPECT for specific purposes and clinical applications. The following is a brief review of these SPECT systems and special collimators.

11.2.2.1 Multidetector SPECT System

The first fully functional SPECT imaging acquisition system was designed and constructed by Kuhl and Edwards (Kuhl and Edwards, 1963, 1964, 1968) in the 1960s, well before the conception of x-ray CT. As shown in Figure 11.7a, the MARK IV brain SPECT system consisted of four linear arrays of eight discrete NaI(TI) scintillation detectors assembled in a square arrangement. Projection data were obtained by rotating the square detector array around the patient's head. Although images from the pioneer MARK IV SPECT system were unimpressive without the use of proper reconstruction methods that were developed in later years, the multidetector design has been the theme of several other SPECT systems that were developed. An example is the Gammatom-1 developed by Cho et al. (1982). The design concept also was used in a dynamic SPECT system (Stokely et al., 1980) and commercial multidetector SPECT systems marketed by Medimatic, A/S (Tomomatic-32). Recently, the system design was extended to a multislice SPECT system with the Tomomatic-896, consisting of eight layers of 96 scintillation detectors. Also, the system allows both body and brain SPECT imaging by varying the aperture size.

Variations of the multiple-detectors arrangement have been proposed for SPECT system designs. Figure 11.7b shows the Headtome-II system by Shimadzu Corporation (Hirose et al., 1982), which consists of a stationary array of scintillation detectors arranged in a circular ring. Projection data are obtained by a set of collimator vanes that swings in front of the discrete detectors. A unique Cleon brain SPECT system (see Figure 11.7c), originally developed by Union Carbide Corporation in the 1970s, consists of 12 detectors that scan both radially and tangentially (Stoddart and Stoddart, 1979). Images from the original system were unimpressive due to inadequate sampling, poor axial resolution, and a reconstruction algorithm that did not take full advantage of the unique system design and data acquisition strategy. A much improved version of the system with a new reconstruction method (Moore et al., 1984) is currently marketed by Strichman Corporation.

The advantages of multidetector SPECT systems are their high sensitivity per image slice and high counting rate capability resulting from the array of multidetectors fully surrounding the patient. However, disadvantages of multidetector SPECT systems include their ability to provide only one or a few noncontiguous cross-sectional image slices. Also, these systems are relatively more expensive compared with camera-based SPECT systems described in the next section. With the advance of multi-camera SPECT systems, the disadvantages of multidetector SPECT systems outweigh their advantages. As a result, they are less often found in nuclear medicine clinics.

11.2.2.2 Camera-Based SPECT Systems

The most popular SPECT systems are based on single or multiple scintillation cameras mounted on a rotating gantry. The successful design was developed almost simultaneously by three separate groups

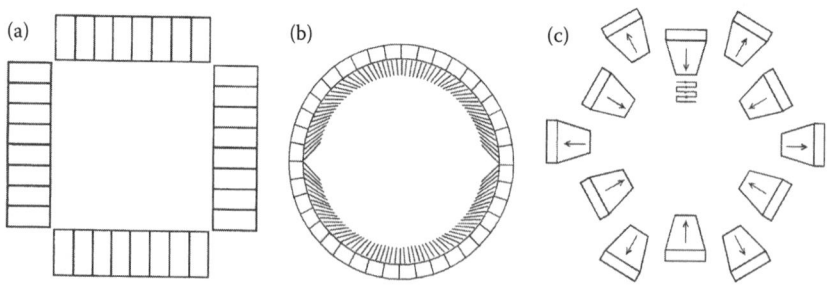

FIGURE 11.7 Examples of multidetector-based SPECT systems. (a) The MARK IV system consists of four arrays of eight individual NaI(TI) detectors arranged in a square configuration. (b) The Headtome-II system consists of a circular ring of detectors. A set of collimator vanes that swings in front of the discrete detector is used to collect projection data from different views. (c) A unique Cleon brain SPECT system consists of 12 detectors that scan both radially and tangentially.

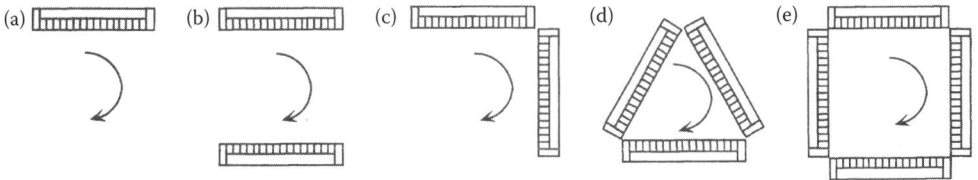

FIGURE 11.8 Examples of camera-based SPECT systems. (a) Single-camera system. (b) Dual-camera system with the two cameras placed at opposing sides of patient during rotation. (c) Dual-camera system with the two cameras placed at right angles. (d) Triple-camera system. (e) Quadruple-camera system.

(Budinger and Gullberg, 1977; Jaszczak et al., 1977; Keyes et al., 1977). In 1981, General Electric Medical Systems offered the first commercial SPECT system based on a single rotating camera and brought SPECT to clinical use. Today, there are over ten manufacturers (e.g., ADAC, Elscint, General Electric, Hitachi, Picker, Siemens, Sopha, Toshiba, and Trionix) offering an array of commercial SPECT systems in the marketplace.

An advantage of camera-based SPECT systems is their use of off-the-shelf scintillation cameras that have been widely used in conventional nuclear medicine. These systems usually can be used in both conventional planar and SPECT imaging. Also, camera-based SPECT systems allow truly three-dimensional (3D) imaging by providing a large set of contiguous transaxial images that cover the entire organ of interest. They are easily adaptable for SPECT imaging of the brain or body by simply changing the radius of rotation of the camera.

A disadvantage of a camera-based SPECT system is its relatively low counting rate capability. The dead time of a typical state-of-the-art scintillation camera gives rise to a loss of 20% of its true counts at about 80K counts per second. A few special high-count-rate systems give the same count rate loss at about 150K counts per second. For SPECT systems using a single scintillation camera, the sensitivity per image slice is relative low compared with a typical multidetector SPECT system.

Recently, SPECT systems based on multiple cameras became increasingly more popular. Systems with two (Jaszczak et al., 1979a), three (Lim et al., 1980, 1985), and four cameras provide increased sensitivity per image slice that is proportional to the number of cameras. Figure 11.8 shows the system configurations of these camera-based SPECT systems. The dual-camera systems with two opposing cameras (Figure 11.8b) can be used for both whole-body scanning and SPECT, and those with two right-angled cameras (Figure 11.8c) are especially useful for 180-degree acquisition in cardiac SPECT. The use of multicameras has virtually eliminated the disadvantages of camera-based SPECT systems as compared with multidetector SPECT systems. The detection efficiency of camera-based SPECT systems can be further increased by using converging-hole collimators such as fan, cone, and astigmatic collimators at the cost of a smaller field of view. The use of converging-hole collimators in SPECT will be described in a later section.

11.2.2.3 Novel SPECT System Designs

There are several special SPECT systems designs that do not fit into the preceding two general categories. The commercially available CERESPECT (formerly known as ASPECT) (Genna and Smith, 1988) is a dedicated brain SPECT system. As shown in Figure 11.9a, it consists of a single fixed-annular NaI(TI) crystal that completely surrounds the patient's head. Similar to a scintillation camera, an array of PMTs and electronics circuitry are placed behind the crystal to provide positional and energy information about photons that interact with the crystal. Projection data are obtained by rotating a segmented annular collimator with parallel holes that fits inside the stationary detector. A similar system is also being developed by Larsson et al. (1991) in Sweden.

Several unique SPECT systems are currently being developed in research laboratories. They consist of modules of small scintillation cameras that surround the patient. The hybrid designs combine

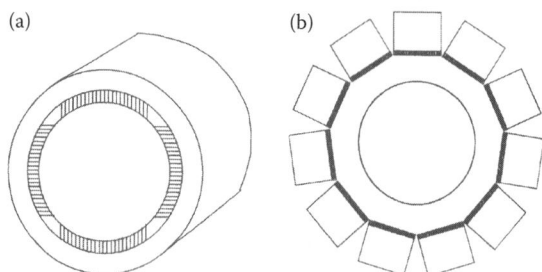

FIGURE 11.9 Examples of novel SPECT system designs. (a) The CERESPECT brain SPECT system consists of a single fixed annular NaI(TI) crystal and a rotating segmented annular collimator. (b) The SPRINT II brain SPECT system consists of 11 detector modules and a rotating lead ring with slit opening.

the advantage of multidetector and camera-based SPECT systems with added flexibility in system configuration. An example is the SPRINT II brain SPECT system developed at the University of Michigan (Rogers et al., 1988). As shown in Figure 11.9b, the system consists of 11 detector modules arranged in a circular ring around the patient's head. Each detector module consists of 44 one-dimensional (1D) bar NaI(TI) scintillation cameras. Projection data are required through a series of narrow slit openings on a rotating lead ring that fits inside the circular detector assemblies. A similar system was developed at the University of Iowa (Chang et al., 1990) with 22 detector modules, each consisting of four bar detectors. A set of rotating focused collimators is used to acquire projection data necessary for image reconstruction. At the University of Arizona, a novel SPECT system is being developed that consists of 20 small modular scintillation cameras (Milster et al., 1990) arranged in a hemispherical shell surrounding the patient's head (Rowe et al., 1992). Projection data are acquired through a stationary hemispherical array of pinholes that are fitted inside the camera array. Without moving parts, the system allows acquisition of dynamic 3D SPECT data.

11.2.2.4 Special Collimator Designs for SPECT Systems

Similar to conventional nuclear medicine imaging, parallel-hole collimators (Figure 11.10a) are commonly used in camera-based SPECT systems. As described earlier, the tradeoff between detection efficiency and spatial resolution of parallel-hole collimator is a limiting factor for SPECT. A means to improve SPECT system performance is to improve the tradeoff imposed by the parallel-hole collimation.

To achieve this goal, converging-hole collimator designs that increase the angle of acceptance of incoming photons without sacrificing spatial resolution have been developed. Examples are fan-beam (Jaszczak et al., 1979b; Tsui et al., 1986), cone-beam (Jaszczak et al., 1987), astigmatic (Hawman and Hsieh, 1986), and more recently varifocal collimators. As shown in Figure 11.10b, the collimator holes converge to a line that is oriented parallel to the axis of rotation for a fan-beam collimator, to a point for a cone-beam collimator, and to various points for a varifocal collimator, respectively. The gain in detection efficiency of a typical fan-beam and cone-beam collimator is about 1.5 and 2 times of that of a parallel-hole collimator with the same spatial resolution. The anticipated gain in detection efficiency and corresponding decrease in image noise are the main reasons for the interest in applying converging-hole collimators in SPECT.

Despite the advantage of increased detection efficiency, the use of converging-hole collimators in SPECT poses special problems. The tradeoff for increase in detection efficiency as compared with parallel-hole collimators is a decrease in field of view (see Figure 11.10). Consequently, converging-hole collimators are restricted to imaging small organs or body parts such as the head (Jaszczak et al., 1979b; Tsui et al., 1986) and heart (Gullberg et al., 1991). In addition, the use of converging-hole collimators requires special data-acquisition strategies and image reconstruction algorithms. For example, for cone-beam tomography using a conventional single planar orbit, the acquired projection data become

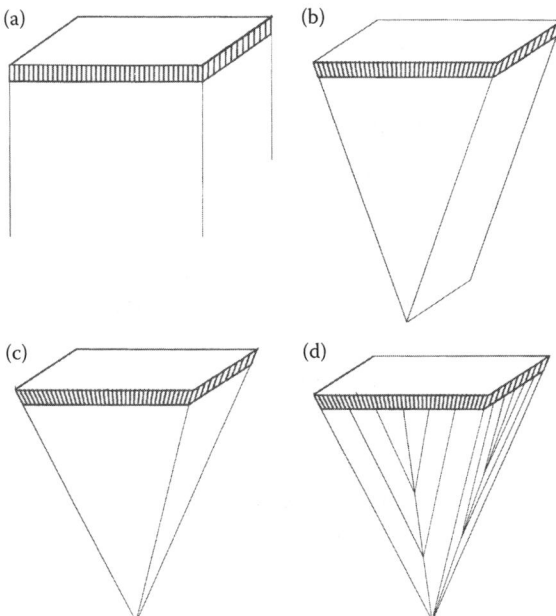

FIGURE 11.10 Collimator designs used in camera-based SPECT systems. (a) The commonly used parallel-hole collimator. (b) The fan-beam collimator, where the collimator holes are converged to a line that is parallel to the axis of rotation. (c) The cone-beam collimator, where the collimator holes are converged to a point. (d) A varifocal collimator, where the collimator holes are converged to various focal points.

increasingly insufficient for reconstructing transaxial image sections that are further away from the central plane of the cone-beam geometry. Active research is underway to study special rotational orbits for sufficient projection data acquisition and 3D image reconstruction methods specific for cone-beam SPECT.

11.2.3 Reconstruction Methods

As discussed earlier, SPECT combines conventional nuclear medicine image techniques and methods for image reconstruction from projections. Aside from radiopharmaceuticals and instrumentation, image reconstruction methods are another important engineering and technological aspect of the SPECT imaging technique.

In x-ray CT, accurate transaxial images can be obtained through the use of standard algorithms for image reconstruction from projections. The results are images of attenuation coefficient distribution of various organs within the patient's body. In SPECT, the goal of image reconstruction is to determine the distribution of administered radiopharmaceutical in the patient. However, the presence of photon attenuation affects the measured projection data. If conventional reconstruction algorithms are used without proper compensation for the attenuation effects, inaccurate reconstructed images will be obtained. Effects of scatter and the finite collimator–detector response impose additional difficulties on image reconstruction in SPECT.

In order to achieve quantitatively accurate images, special reconstruction methods are required for SPECT. Quantitatively accurate image reconstruction methods for SPECT consist of two major components. They are the standard algorithms for image reconstruction from projections and methods that compensate for the image-degrading effects described earlier. Often, image reconstruction algorithms are inseparable from the compensation methods, resulting in a new breed of reconstruction method not found in other tomographic medical imaging modalities. The following sections will present the reconstruction problem and a brief review of conventional algorithms for image reconstruction from projections. Then quantitative SPECT reconstruction methods that include additional compensation methods will be described.

11.2.3.1 Image Reconstruction Problem

Figure 11.11 shows a schematic diagram of the two-dimensional (2D) image reconstruction problem. Let $f(x, y)$ represent a 2D object distribution that is to be determined. A 1D detector array is oriented at an angle q with respect to the x-axis of the laboratory coordinates system (x, y). The data collected into each detector element at location t, called the projection data $p(t, q)$, is equal to the sum of $f(x, y)$ along a ray that is perpendicular to the detector array and intersects the detector at position t; that is,

$$p(t,\theta) = c \int_{-\alpha}^{\alpha} f(x,y)\,ds \tag{11.1}$$

where (s, t) represents a coordinate system with s along the direction of the ray sum and t parallel to the 1D detector array, and c is the gain factor of the detection system. The angle between the s and x-axes is θ. The relationship between the source position (x, y), the projection angle θ, and the position of detection on the 1D detector array is given by

$$t = y\cos\theta - x\sin\theta \tag{11.2}$$

In 2D tomographic imaging, the 1D detector array rotates around the object distribution $f(x, y)$ and collects projection data from various projection data from various projection angles θ. The integral transform of the object distribution to its projections given by Equation 11.1 is called the Radon transform (Radon, 1917). The goal of image reconstruction is to solve the inverse Radon transform. The solution is the reconstructed image estimate $\hat{f}(x, y)$ of the object distribution $f(x, y)$.

In x-ray CT, the measured projection data is given by

$$p'(t,\theta) = c_t I_o \exp\left[-\int_{-\alpha}^{+\alpha} \mu(x,y)\,ds\right] \tag{11.3}$$

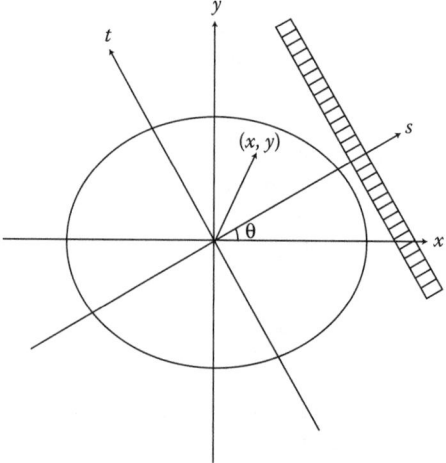

FIGURE 11.11 Schematic diagram of the two-dimensional image reconstruction problem. The projection data are line integrals of the object distribution along rays that are perpendicular to the detector. A source point (x, y) is projected onto a point $p(t, \theta)$, where t is a position along the projection and θ is the projection angle.

where I_o is the intensity of the incident x-ray, $\mu(x, y)$ is the 2D attenuation coefficient, and c_t is the gain factor which transforms x-ray intensity to detected signals. The reconstruction problem can be rewritten as

$$p(t,\theta) = \ln\left[\frac{I_o}{p'(t,\theta)}\right] = \int_{-\alpha}^{+\alpha} \mu(x,y)\,ds \qquad (11.4)$$

with the goal to solve for the attenuation coefficient distribution $\mu(x, y)$. Also, in x-ray CT, if parallel rays are used, the projection data at opposing views are the same, that is, $p(t, \theta) = p(\theta + p)$, and projection data acquired over 180 degrees will be sufficient for reconstruction. The number of linear samples along the 1D projection array and angular samples, that is, the number of projection views, over 180 degrees must be chosen carefully to avoid aliasing error and resolution loss in the reconstructed images.

In SPECT, if the effects of attenuation, scatter, and collimator–detector response are ignored, the measured projection data can be written as the integral of radioactivity along the projection rays; that is,

$$p(t,\theta) = c_e \int_{-\alpha}^{+\alpha} \rho(x,y)\,ds \qquad (11.5)$$

where $\rho(x,y)$ is the radioactivity concentration distribution of the object, and C_e is the gain factor which transforms radioactivity concentration to detected signals. Equation 11.5 fits in the form of the Radon transform, and similar to x-ray CT, the radioactivity distribution can be obtained by solving the inverse Radon transform problem.

If attenuation is taken into consideration, the attenuated Radon transform (Gullberg, 1979) can be written as

$$p(t,\theta_i) = c_e \int_{-\alpha}^{+\alpha} \rho(x,y) \exp\left[-\int_{(x,y)}^{+\alpha} \mu(u,v)\,ds'\right]ds \qquad (11.6)$$

where $\mu(u,v)$ is the 2D attenuation coefficient distribution, and $\int_{x,y}^{+\alpha} \mu(u,v)\,ds$ is the attenuation factor for photons that originate from (x, y), travel along the direction perpendicular to the detector array, and are detected by the collimator–detector. A major difficulty in SPECT image reconstruction lies in the attenuation factor, which makes the inverse problem given by Equation 11.6 difficult to solve analytically. However, the solution is important in cardiac SPECT, where the widely different attenuation coefficients are found in various organs within the thorax. Also, due to the attenuation factor, the projection views at opposing angles are different. Hence full 360-degree projection data are usually necessary for image reconstruction in SPECT.

Different from x-ray CT, small differences in attenuation coefficient are not as important in SPECT. When the attenuation coefficient in the body region can be considered constant, the attenuated Radon transform given by Equation 11.6 can be written as (Tretiak and Metz, 1980)

$$p(t,\theta) = c_e \int_{-\alpha}^{+\alpha} \rho(x,y) \exp[-\mu l(x,y)]\,ds \qquad (11.7)$$

where μ is the constant attenuation coefficient in the body region, and $l(x, y)$ is the path length between the point (x, y) and the edge of the attenuator (or patient's body) along the direction of the projection ray. The solution of the inverse problem with constant attenuator has been a subject of several investigations. It forms the basis for analytical methods for compensation of uniform attenuation described later in this chapter.

When scatter and collimator–detector response are taken into consideration, the assumption that the projection data can be represented by line integrals given by Equation 11.1 to Equation 11.7 will no longer be exactly correct. Instead, the integration will have to include a wider region covering the field of view of the collimator–detector (or the collimator–detector response function). The image reconstruction problem is further complicated by the nonstationary properties of the collimator–detector and scatter response functions and their dependence on the size and composition of the patient's body.

11.2.3.2 Algorithms for Image Reconstruction from Projections

The application of methods for image reconstruction from projections was a major component in the development of x-ray CT in the 1970s. The goal was to solve for the inverse Radon transform problem given in Equation 11.1. There is an extensive literature on these reconstruction algorithms. Reviews of the applications of these algorithms to SPECT can be found in several articles (Budinger and Gullberg, 1974; Brooks and Di Chiro, 1975, 1976; Barrett, 1986).

Simple backprojection: An intuitive image reconstruction method is simple backprojection. Here, the reconstructed image is formed simply by spreading the values of the measured projection data uniformly along the projection ray into the reconstructed image array. By backprojecting the measured projection data from all projection views, an estimate of the object distribution can be obtained. Mathematically, the simple backproject operation is given by

$$\hat{f}(x,y) = \sum_{j=1}^{m} p(y\cos\theta_j - x\sin\theta_j, \theta_j)\Delta\theta \tag{11.8}$$

where θ_j is the *j*th projection angle, *m* is the number of projection views, and $\Delta\theta$ is the angular spacing between adjacent projections. The simple backprojected image $\hat{f}(x,y)$ is a poor approximation of the true object distribution $f(x, y)$. It is equivalent to the true object distribution blurred by a blurring function in the form of $1/r$.

There are two approaches for accurate image reconstruction, and both have been applied to SPECT. The first approach is based on direct analytical methods and is widely used in commercial SPECT systems. The second approach is based on statistical criteria and iterative algorithms. They have been found useful in reconstruction methods that include compensation for the image-degrading effects.

Analytical reconstruction algorithms: filtered backprojection: The most widely used analytical image-reconstruction algorithm is the filtered backprojection (FBP) method, which involves backprojecting the filtered projections (Bracewell and Riddle, 1967; Ramachandran and Lakshminarayanan, 1971). The algorithm consists of two major steps:

1. Filter the measured projection data at different projection angles with a special function
2. Backproject the filtered projection data to form the reconstructed image

The first step of the filtered backprojection method can be implemented in two different ways. In the spatial domain, the filter operation is equivalent to convolving the measured projection data using a special convolving function $h(t)$; that is,

$$p'(t,\theta) = p(t,\theta) * h(t) \tag{11.8a}$$

where * is the convolution operation. With the advance of FFT methods, the convolution operation can be replaced by a more efficient multiplication in the spatial frequency domain. The equivalent operation consists of three steps:

1. Fourier-transform the measured projection data into spatial frequency domain using the FFT method, that is, $P(v, \theta) = FT\{p(t, \theta)\}$, where FT is the Fourier transform operation.
2. Multiply the Fourier-transformed projection data with a special function that is equal to the Fourier transform of the special function used in the convolution operation described above, that is, $P'(v, \theta) = P(v, \theta) \cdot H(v)$, where $H(v) = FT\{h(x)\}$ is the Fourier transform of $h(x)$.
3. Inverse Fourier transform the product $P'(v, \theta)$ into spatial domain.

Again, the filtered projections from different projection angles are backprojected to form the reconstructed images.

The solution of the inverse Radon transform given in Equation 11.1 specifies the form of the special function. In the spatial domain, the special function h(x) used in the convolution operation in Equation 11.8 is given by

$$h(x) = \frac{1}{2(\Delta x)^2}\left\{\text{sinc}\left[\frac{x}{(\Delta x)}\right]\right\} - \frac{1}{4(\Delta x)^2}\left\{\text{sinc}^2\left[\frac{x}{2(\Delta x)}\right]\right\} \tag{11.9}$$

where Δx is the linear sampling interval, and sinc(z) = [sin(z)]/z. The function $h(x)$ consists of a narrow central peak with high magnitude and small negative side lobes. It removes the blurring from the $1/r$ function found in the simple backprojected images.

In the frequency domain, the special function $H(v)$ is equivalent to the Fourier transform of $h(x)$ and is a truncated ramp function given by

$$H(v) = |v| \cdot \text{rect}(v) \tag{11.10}$$

where $|v|$ is the ramp function, and

$$\text{rect}(v) = \begin{cases} 1, & |v| \le 0.5 \\ 0, & v < 0.5 \end{cases} \tag{11.11}$$

that is, the rectangular function rect (v) has a value of 1 when the absolute value of v is less than the Nyquist frequency at 0.5 cycles per pixel.

For noisy projection data, the ramp function tends to amplify the high-frequency noise. In these situations, an additional smoothing filter is often applied to smoothly roll off the high-frequency response of the ramp function. Examples are Hann and Butterworth filters (Huesman et al., 1977). Also, deconvolution filters have been used to provide partial compensation of spatial resolution loss due to the collimator-detection response and noise smoothing. Examples are the Metz and Wiener filters (see later).

Iterative reconstruction algorithms: Another approach to image reconstruction is based on statistical criteria and iterative algorithms. They were investigated for application in SPECT before the development of analytical image reconstruction methods (Kuhl and Edwards, 1968; Gordon et al., 1970; Gilbert, 1972; Goitein, 1972). The major drawbacks of iterative reconstruction algorithms are the extensive computations and long processing time required. For these reasons, the analytical reconstruction methods have gained widespread acceptance in clinical SPECT systems. In recent years, there has been renewed interest in the use of iterative reconstruction algorithms in SPECT to achieve accurate quantitation by compensating for the image-degrading effects.

A typical iterative reconstruction algorithm starts with an initial estimate of the object source distribution. A set of projection data is estimated from the initial estimate using a projector that models the imaging process. The estimated projection data are compared with the measured projection data at the same projection angles, and their differences are calculated. Using an algorithm derived from specific statistical criteria, the differences are used to update the initial image estimate. The updated image estimate is then used to recalculate a new set of estimated projection data that are again compared with the measured projection data. The procedure is repeated until the difference between the estimated and measured projection data are smaller than a preselected small value. Statistical criteria that have been used in formulating iterative reconstruction algorithms include the minimum mean squares error (MMSE) (Budinger and Gullberg, 1977), weighted least squares (WLS) (Huesman et al., 1977), maximum entropy (ME) (Minerbo, 1979), maximum likelihood (ML) (Shepp and Vardi, 1982), and maximum a posteriori approaches (Geman and McClure, 1985; Barrett, 1986; Levitan and Herman, 1987; Liang and Hart, 1987; Johnson et al., 1991). Iterative algorithms that have been used in estimating the reconstructed images include the conjugate gradient (CG) (Huesman et al., 1977) and expectation maximization (EM) (Lange and Carson, 1984).

Recently, interest in the application of iterative reconstruction algorithms in SPECT has been revitalized. The interest is sparked by the need to compensate for the spatially variant and/or nonstationary image-degrading factors in the SPECT imaging process. The compensation can be achieved by modeling the imaging process that includes the image-degrading factors in the projection and backprojection operations of the iterative steps. The development is aided by advances made in computer technology and custom-dedicated processors. The drawback of long processing time in using these algorithms is substantially reduced. Discussion of the application of iterative reconstruction algorithms in SPECT will be presented in a later section.

11.2.3.3 Compensation Methods

For a typical SPECT system, the measured projection data are severely affected by attenuation, scatter, and collimator–detector response. Direct reconstruction of the measured projection data without compensation of these effects produces images with artifacts, distortions, and inaccurate quantitation. In recent years, substantial efforts have been made to develop compensation methods for these image-degrading effects. This development has produced much improved quality and quantitatively accurate reconstructed images. The following sections will present a brief review of some of these compensation methods.

Compensation for attenuation: Methods for attenuation compensation can be grouped into two categories (1) methods that assume the attenuation coefficient is uniform over the body region, and (2) methods that address situations of nonuniform attenuation coefficient distribution. The assumption of uniform attenuation can be applied to SPECT imaging of the head and abdomen regions. The compensation methods seek to solve for the inverse of the attenuated Radon transform given in Equation 11.7. For cardiac and lung SPECT imaging, nonuniform attenuation compensation methods must be used due to the very different attenuation coefficient values in various organs in the thorax. Here, the goal is to solve the more complicated problem of the inverse of the attenuated Radon transform in Equation 11.6.

There are several approximate methods for compensating uniform attenuation. They include methods that preprocess the projection data or postprocess the reconstructed image. The typical preprocess methods are those which use the geometric or arithmetic mean (Sorenson, 1974) of projections from opposing views. These compensation methods are easy to implement and work well with a single, isolated source. However, they are relatively inaccurate for more complicated source configurations. Another method achieves uniform attenuation compensation by processing the Fourier transform of the sinogram (Bellini et al., 1979). The method provides accurate compensation even for complicated source configurations.

A popular compensation method for uniform attenuation is that proposed by Chang (1978). The method requires knowledge of the body contour. The information is used in calculating the average attenuation factor at each image point from all projection views. The array of attenuation factors is used to multiply the reconstructed image obtained without attenuation compensation. The result is the attenuation-compensated image. An iterative scheme also can be implemented for improved accuracy. In general, the Chang method performs well for uniform attenuation situations. However, the noise level in the reconstructed images increases with iteration number. Also, certain image features tend to fluctuate as a function of iteration. For these reasons, no more than one or two iterations are recommended.

Another class of methods for uniform attenuation compensation is based on analytical solution of the inverse of the attenuation Radon transform given in Equation 11.7 for a convex-shaped medium (Tretiak and Metz, 1980; Gullberg and Budinger, 1981). The resultant compensation method involves multiplying the projection data by an exponential function. Then the FBP algorithm is used in the image reconstruction except that the ramp filter is modified such that its value is zero in the frequency range between 0 and $\mu/2\pi$, where μ is the constant attenuation coefficient. The compensation method is easy to implement and provides good quantitative accuracy. However, it tends to amplify noise in the resulting image, and smoothing is required to obtain acceptable image quality (Gullberg and Budinger, 1981).

An analytical solution for the more complicated inverse attenuated Radon transform with nonuniform attenuation distribution (Equation 11.6) has been found difficult (Gullberg, 1979). Instead, iterative approaches have been used to estimate a solution of the problem. The application is especially important in cardiac and lung SPECT studies. The iterative methods model the attenuation distribution in the projection and backprojection operations (Manglos et al., 1987; Tsui et al., 1989). The ML criterion with the EM algorithm (Lange and Carson, 1984) has been used with success (Tsui et al., 1989). The compensation method requires information about the attenuation distribution of the region to be imaged. Recently, transmission CT methods are being developed using existing SPECT systems to obtain attenuation distribution from the patient. The accurate attenuation compensation of cardiac SPECT promises to provide much improved quality and quantitative accuracy in cardiac SPECT images (Tsui et al., 1989, 1994a).

Compensation for scatter: As described earlier in this chapter, scattered photons carry misplaced positional information about the source distribution resulting in lower image contrast and inaccurate quantitation in SPECT images. Compensation for scatter will improve image contrast for better image quality and images that will more accurately represent the true object distribution. Much research has been devoted to develop scatter compensation methods that can be grouped into two general approaches. In the first approach, various methods have been developed to estimate the scatter contribution in the measured data. The scatter component is then subtracted from the measured data or from the reconstructed images to obtain scatter-free reconstructed images. The compensation method based on this approach tends to increase noise level in the compensated images.

One method estimates the scatter contribution as a convolution of the measured projection data with an empirically derived function (Axelsson et al., 1984). Another method models the scatter component as the convolution of the primary (or unscattered) component of the projection data with an exponential function (Floyd et al., 1985). The convolution method is extended to 3D by estimating the 2D scatter component (Yanch et al., 1988). These convolution methods assume that the scatter response function is stationary, which is only an approximation.

The scatter component also has been estimated using two energy windows acquisition methods. One method estimates the scatter component in the primary energy window from the measured data obtained from a lower and adjacent energy window (Jaszczak et al., 1984, 1985b). In a dual photopeak window (DPW) method, two nonoverlapping windows spanning the primary photopeak window are used (King et al., 1992). This method provides more accurate estimation of the scatter response function.

Multiple energy windows also have been used to estimate the scatter component. One method uses two satellite energy windows that are placed directly above and below the photopeak window to estimate the scatter component in the center window (Ogawa et al., 1991). In another method, the energy spectrum detected at each image pixel is used to predict the scatter contribution (Koral et al., 1988). An energy-weighted acquisition (EWA) technique acquires data from multiple energy windows. The images reconstructed from these data are weighted with energy-dependent factors to minimize scatter contribution to the weighted image (DeVito et al., 1989; DeVito and Hamill, 1991). Finally, the holospectral imaging method (Gagnon et al., 1989) estimates the scatter contribution from a series of eigenimages derived from images reconstructed from data obtained from a series of multiple energy windows.

In the second approach, the scatter photons are utilized in estimating the true object distribution. Without subtracting the scatter component, the compensated images are less noisy than those obtained from the first approach. In one method, an average scatter response function can be combined with the geometric response of the collimator–detector to form the total response of the imaging system (Gilland et al., 1988; Tsui et al., 1994a). The total response function is then used to generate a restoration filter for an approximate geometric and scatter response compensation (see later).

Another class of methods, characterizes the exact scatter response function and incorporates it into iterative reconstruction algorithms for accurate compensation for scatter (Floyd et al., 1985; Frey and Tsui, 1992). Since the exact scatter response functions are nonstationary and are asymmetric in shape, implementation of the methods requires extensive computations. However, efforts are being made to parameterize the scatter response function and to optimize the algorithm for substantial reduction in processing time (Frey and Tsui, 1991; Frey et al., 1993).

Compensation for collimator–detector response: As described earlier, for a typical collimator–detector, the response function broadens as the distance from the collimator face increases. The effect of the collimator–detector response is loss of spatial resolution and blurring of fine detail in SPECT images. Also, the spatially variant detector response function will cause nonisotropic point response in SPECT images (Knesaurek et al., 1989; Maniawski et al., 1991). The spatially variant collimator–detector response is a major difficulty in its exact compensation.

By assuming an average and stationary collimator–detector response function, restoration filters can be used to provide partial and approximate compensation for the effects of the collimator–detector. Examples are the Metz (King et al., 1984, 1986) and Wiener (Penney et al., 1990) filters, where the inverse of the average collimator–detector response function is used in the design of the restoration filters. Two-dimensional compensation is achieved by applying the 1D restoration filters to the 1D projection data, and 3D compensation by applying the 2D filters to the 2D projection images (Tsui et al., 1994b).

Analytical methods have been developed for compensation of the spatially variant detector response. A spatially variant filtering method has been proposed which is based on the frequency distance principle (FDP) (Edholm et al., 1986; Lewitt et al., 1989). The method has been shown to provide an isotropic point response function in phantom SPECT images (Glick et al., 1993).

Iterative reconstruction methods also have been used to accurately compensate for both nonuniform attenuation and collimator–detector response by modeling the attenuation distribution and spatially variant detector response function in the projection and backprojection steps. The compensation methods have been applied in 2D reconstruction (Tsui et al., 1988; Formiconi et al., 1990), and more recently in 3D reconstruction (Zeng et al., 1991; Tsui et al., 1994b). It has been found that the iterative reconstruction methods provide better image quality and more accurate quantitation when compared with the conventional restoration filtering techniques. Furthermore, 3D compensation outperforms 2D compensation at the expense of more extensive computations (Tsui et al., 1994b).

11.2.4 Sample SPECT Images

This section presents sample SPECT images to demonstrate the performance of various reconstruction and compensation methods. Two data sets were used. The first set was acquired from a 3D physical phantom that mimics a human brain perfusion study. The phantom study provided knowledge of the true radioactivity distribution for evaluation purposes. The second data set was obtained from a patient myocardial SPECT study using thallium-201.

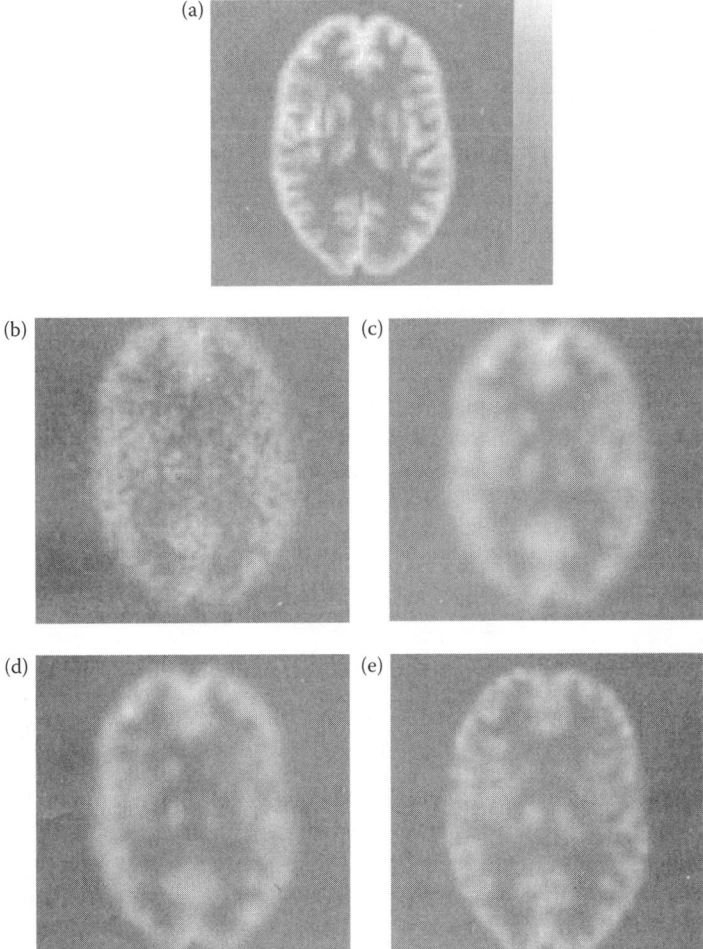

FIGURE 11.12 Sample images from a phantom SPECT study. (a) Radioactivity distribution from a selected slice of a 3D brain phantom. (b) Reconstructed image obtained from the FBP algorithm without any compensation. (c) Reconstructed image obtained with the application of noise-smoothing filter and compensation for uniform attenuation and scatter. (d) Similar to (c) except for an additional application of a Metz filter to partially compensate for the collimator–detector blurring. (e) Reconstructed image similar to that obtained from the iterative ML-EM algorithm that accurately models the attenuation and spatially variant detector response. (From Tsui B.M.W., Frey E.C., Zhao X.-D. et al. 1994. *Phys. Med. Biol.* 39: 509. Reprinted with permission.)

Figure 11.12a shows the radioactivity distribution from a selected slice of a 3D brain phantom manufactured by the Data Spectrum Corporation. The phantom design was based on PET images from a normal patient to simulate cerebral blood flow (Hoffman et al., 1990). The phantom was filled with water containing 74 mBq of Tc-99m. A single-camera-based GE 400AC/T SPECT system fitted with a high-resolution collimator was used for data collection. The projection data were acquired into 128 × 128 matrices at 128 views over 360 degrees. Figure 11.12b shows the reconstructed image obtained from the FBP algorithm without any compensation. The poor image quality is due to statistical noise fluctuations, effects of attenuation (especially at the central portion of the image), loss of spatial resolution due to the collimator–detector response, and loss of contrast due to scatter.

Figure 11.12c shows the reconstructed image obtained with the application of a noise-smoothing filter and compensation for the uniform attenuation and scatter. The resulting image has lower noise level, reduced attenuation effect, and higher contrast as compared with the image shown in Figure 11.12b. Figure 11.12d is similar to Figure 11.12c except for an additional application of a Metz filter to partially compensate for the collimator–detector blurring. Figure 11.12e shows the reconstructed image obtained from the iterative ML-EM algorithm that accurately modeled the attenuation and spatially variant detector response. The much superior image quality is apparent.

Figure 11.13a shows a selected FBP reconstructed transaxial image slice from a typical patient myocardial SPECT study using thallium-201. Figure 11.13b shows the reconstructed image obtained from the Chang algorithm for approximate nonuniform attenuation compensation and 2D processing

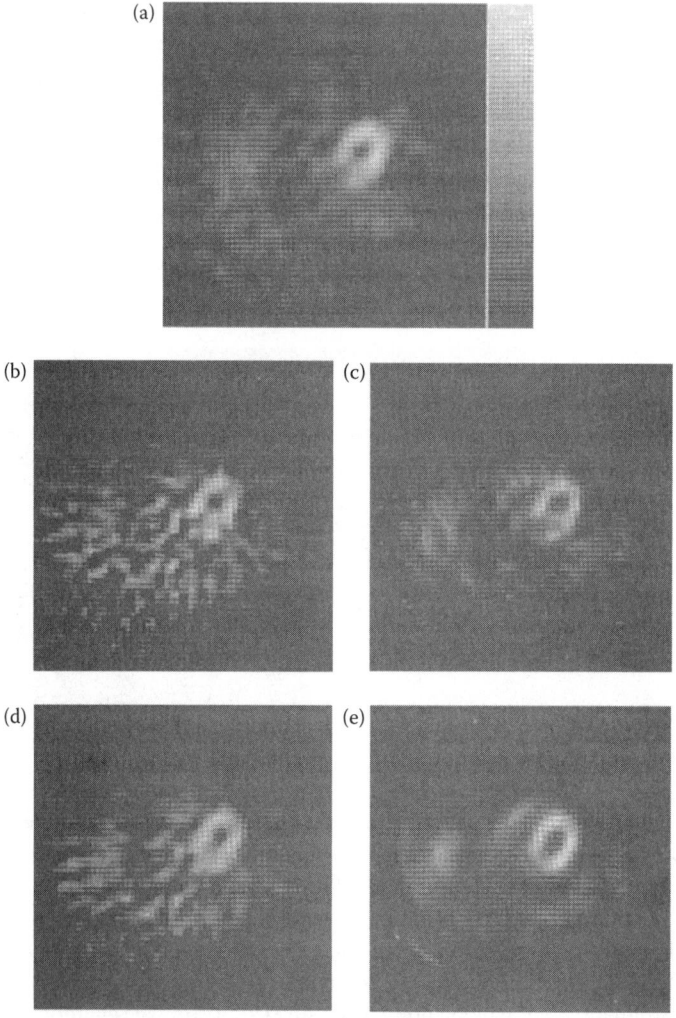

FIGURE 11.13 Sample images from a patient myocardial SPECT study using TI-201. (a) A selected transaxial image slice from a typical patient myocardial SPECT study using TI-201. The reconstructed image was obtained with the FBP algorithm without any compensation. (b) Reconstructed image obtained from the Chang algorithm for approximate nonuniform attenuation compensation and 2D processing using a Metz filter for approximate compensation for collimator–detector response. (c) Reconstructed image obtained from the iterative ML-EM algorithm using a measured transmission CT image for accurate attenuation compensation and 2D model of the collimator–detector response for accurate collimator–detector response compensation. (d) Similar to (b) except that the Metz filter was implemented in 3D. (e) Similar to (c) except that a 3D model of the collimator–detector response is used.

using a Metz filter for approximate compensation for collimator–detector response. Figure 11.13c shows the reconstructed image obtained from the iterative ML-EM algorithm using a measured transmission CT image for accurate attenuation compensation and a 2D model of the collimator–detector response for accurate collimator–detector response compensation. The reconstructed image in Figure 11.13d is similar to that in Figure 11.13b except that the Metz filter was implemented in 3D. Finally, the reconstructed image in Figure 11.13e is similar to that in Figure 11.13c except that a 3D model of the collimator–detector response is used. The superior image quality obtained from using an accurate 3D model of the imaging process is evident.

11.2.5 Discussion

The development of SPECT has been a combination of advances in radiopharmaceuticals, instrumentation, image processing and reconstruction methods, and clinical applications. Although substantial progress has been made during the last decade, there are many opportunities for contributions from biomedical engineering in the future.

The future SPECT instrumentation will consist of more detector area to fully surround the patient for high detection efficiency and multiple contiguous transaxial slice capability. Multicamera SPECT systems will continue to dominate the commercial market. The use of new radiation detector materials and detector systems with high spatial resolution will receive increased attention. Continued research is needed to investigate special converging-hole collimator design geometries, fully 3D reconstruction algorithms, and their clinical applications.

To improve image quality and to achieve quantitatively accurate SPECT images will continue to be the goals of image processing and image reconstruction methods for SPECT. An important direction of research in analytical reconstruction methods will involve solving the inverse Radon transform, which includes the effects of attenuation, the spatially variant collimator–detector response function, and scatter. The development of iterative reconstruction methods will require more accurate models of the complex SPECT imaging process, faster and more stable iterative algorithms, and more powerful computers and special computational hardware.

These improvements in SPECT instrumentation and image reconstruction methods, combined with newly developed radiopharmaceuticals, will bring SPECT images with increasingly higher quality and more accurate quantitation to nuclear medicine clinics for improved diagnosis and patient care.

References

Anger H.O. 1958. Scintillation camera. *Rev. Sci. Instrum.* 29: 27.

Anger H.O. 1964. Scintillation camera with multichannel collimators. *J. Nucl. Med.* 5: 515.

Axelsson B., Msaki P., and Israelsson A. 1984. Subtraction of Compton-scattered photons in single-photon emission computed tomography. *J. Nucl. Med.* 25: 490.

Barrett H.H. 1986. Perspectives on SPECT. *Proc. SPIE* 671: 178.

Bellini S., Piacentini M., Cafforio C. et al. 1979. Compensation of tissue absorption in emission tomography. *IEEE Trans. Acoust. Speech Signal Process.* ASSP 27: 213.

Bracewell R.N. and Riddle A.C. 1967. Inversion of fan-beam scans in radio astronomy. *Astrophys. J.* 150: 427.

Brooks R.A. and Di Chiro G. 1975. Theory of image reconstruction in computed tomography. *Radiology* 117: 561.

Brooks R.A. and Di Chiro G. 1976. Principles of computer assisted tomography (CAT) in radiographic and radioisotopic imaging. *Phys. Med. Biol.* 21: 689.

Budinger T.F. and Gullberg G.T. 1974. Three-dimensional reconstruction in nuclear medicine emission imaging. *IEEE Trans. Nucl. Sci.* NS 21: 2.

Budinger T.F. and Gullberg G.T. 1977. Transverse section reconstruction of gamma-ray emitting radio-nuclides in patients. In M.M. Ter-Pogossian, M.E. Phelps, G.L. Brownell et al. (Eds), *Reconstruction Tomography in Diagnostic Radiology and Nuclear Medicine.* Baltimore, University Park Press.

Chang L.T. 1978. A method for attenuation correction in radionuclide computed tomography. *IEEE Trans. Nucl. Sci. NS* 25: 638.

Chang W., Huang G., and Wang L. 1990. A multi-detector cylindrical SPECT system for phantom imaging. In *Conference Record of the 1990 Nuclear Science Symposium*, Vol. 2, pp. 1208–1211. Piscataway, NJ, IEEE.

Cho Z.H., Yi W., Jung K.J. et al. 1982. Performance of single photon tomography system-Gamma-tom-1. *IEEE Trans. Nucl. Sci. NS* 29: 484.

DeVito R.P. and Hamill J.J. 1991. Determination of weighting functions for energy-weighted acquisition. *J. Nucl. Med.* 32: 343.

DeVito R.P., Hamill J.J., Treffert J.D., and Stoub E.W. 1989. Energy-weighted acquisition of scintigraphic images using finite spatial filters. *J. Nucl. Med.* 30: 2029.

Edholm P.R., Lewitt R.M., and Lindholm B. 1986. Novel properties of the Fourier decomposition of the sinogram. *Proc. SPIE* 671: 8.

Evans R.D. 1955. *The Atomic Nucleus.* Malabar, FL, Robert E. Krieger.

Floyd C.E., Jaszczak R.J., Greer K.L., and Coleman R.E. 1985. Deconvolution of Compton scatter in SPECT. *J. Nucl. Med.* 26: 403.

Formiconi A.R., Pupi A., and Passeri A. 1990. Compensation of spatial system response in SPECT with conjugate gradient reconstruction technique. *Phys. Med. Biol.* 34: 69.

Frey E.C., Ju Z.-W., and Tsui B.M.W. 1993. A fast projector-backprojector pair modeling the asymmetric, spatially varying scatter response function for scatter compensation in SPECT imaging. *IEEE Trans. Nucl. Sci. NS* 40: 1192.

Frey E.C. and Tsui B.M.W. 1991. Spatial properties of the scatter response function in SPECT. *IEEE Trans. Nucl. Sci. NS* 38: 789.

Frey E.C. and Tsui B.M.W. 1992. A comparison of scatter compensation methods in SPECT: subtraction-based techniques versus iterative reconstruction with an accurate scatter model. In *Conference Record of the 1992 Nuclear Science Symposium and the Medical Imaging Conference*, October 27–31, Orlando, FL, pp. 1035–1037.

Gagnon D., Todd-Pokropek A., Arsenault A., and Dupros G. 1989. Introduction to holospectral imaging in nuclear medicine for scatter subtraction. *IEEE Trans. Med. Imag.* 8: 245.

Geman S. and McClure D.E. 1985. Bayesian image analysis: an application to single photon emission tomography. In *Proceedings of the Statistical Computing Section.* Washington, American Statistical Association.

Genna S. and Smith A. 1988. The development of ASPECT, an annular single crystal brain camera for high efficiency SPECT. *IEEE Trans. Nucl. Sci. NS* 35: 654.

Gilbert P. 1972. Iterative methods for the three-dimensional reconstruction of an object from projections. *J. Theor. Biol.* 36: 105.

Gilland D.R., Tsui B.M.W., Perry J.R. et al. 1988. Optimum filter function for SPECT imaging. *J. Nucl. Med.* 29: 643.

Glick S.J., Penney B.C., King M.A., and Byrne C.L. 1993. Non-iterative compensation for the distance-dependent detector response and photon attenuation in SPECT imaging. *IEEE Trans. Med. Imag.* 13: 363.

Goitein M. 1972. Three-dimensional density reconstruction from a series of two-dimensional projections. *Nucl. Instrum. Meth.* 101: 509.

Gordon R. 1974. A tutorial on ART (Algebraic reconstruction techniques). *IEEE Trans. Nucl. Sci.* 21: 78.

Gordon R., Bender R., and Herman G.T. 1970. Algebraic reconstruction techniques (ART) for three-dimensional electron microscopy and x-ray photography. *J. Theor. Biol.* 29: 471.

Gullberg G.T. 1979. The attenuated Radon transform: theory and application in medicine and biology. Ph.D. dissertation, University of California at Berkeley.

Gullberg G.T. and Budinger T.F. 1981. The use of filtering methods to compensate for constant attenuation in single-photon emission computed tomography. *IEEE Trans. Biomed. Eng. BME* 28: 142.

Gullberg G.T., Christian P.E., Zeng G.L. et al. 1991. Cone beam tomography of the heart using single-photon emission-computed tomography. *Invest. Radiol.* 26: 681.

Hawman E.G. and Hsieh J. 1986. An astigmatic collimator for high sensitivity SPECT of the brain. *J. Nucl. Med.* 27: 930.

Hirose Y., Ikeda Y., Higashi Y. et al. 1982. A hybrid emission CT-HEADTOME II. *IEEE Trans. Nucl. Sci. NS* 29: 520.

Hoffman E.J., Cutler P.D., Kigby W.M., and Mazziotta J.C. 1990. 3-D phantom to simulate cerebral blood flow and metabolic images for PET. *IEEE Trans. Nucl. Sci. NS* 37: 616.

Huesman R.H., Gullberg G.T., Greenberg W.L., and Budinger T.F. 1977. *RECLBL Library Users Manual, Donner Algorithms for Reconstruction Tomography*. Lawrence Berkeley Laboratory, University of California.

Jaszczak R.J., Chang L.T., and Murphy P.H. 1979. Single photon emission computed tomography using multi-slice fan beam collimators. *IEEE Trans. Nucl. Sci. NS* 26: 610.

Jaszczak R.J., Chang L.T., Stein N.A., and Moore F.E. 1979. Whole-body single-photon emission computed tomography using dual, large-field-of-view scintillation cameras. *Phys. Med. Biol.* 24: 1123.

Jaszczak R.J. and Coleman R.E. 1985. Single photon emission computed tomography (SPECT) principles and instrumentation. *Invest. Radiol.* 20: 897.

Jaszczak R.J., Coleman R.E., and Lim C.B. 1980. SPECT: single photon emission computed tomography. *IEEE Trans. Nucl. Sci. NS* 27: 1137.

Jaszczak R.J., Coleman R.E., and Whitehead F.R. 1981. Physical factors affecting quantitative measurements using camera-based single photon emission computed tomography (SPECT). *IEEE Trans. Nucl. Sci. NS* 28: 69.

Jaszczak R.J., Floyd C.E., and Coleman R.E. 1985. Scatter compensation techniques for SPECT. *IEEE Trans. Nucl. Sci. NS* 32: 786.

Jaszczak R.J., Floyd C.E., Manglos S.M. et al. 1987. Cone beam collimation for single photon emission computed tomography: Analysis, simulation, and image reconstruction using filtered backprojection. *Med. Phys.* 13: 484.

Jaszczak R.J., Greer K.L., Floyd C.E. et al. 1984. Improved SPECT quantification using compensation for scattered photons. *J. Nucl. Med.* 25: 893.

Jaszczak R.J., Murphy P.H., Huard D., and Burdine J.A. 1977. Radionuclide emission computed tomography of the head with 99 mTc and a scintillation camera. *J. Nucl. Med.* 18: 373.

Jaszczak R.J. and Tsui B.M.W. 1994. Single photon emission computed tomography. In H.N. Wagner and Z. Szabo (Eds), Principles of Nuclear Medicine, 2nd ed. Philadelphia, Saunders.

Johnson V.E., Wong W.H., Hu X., and Chen C.T. 1991. Image restoration using Gibbs priors: boundary modeling, treatment of blurring and selection of hyperparameters. *IEEE Trans. Pat.* 13: 413.

Keller E.L. 1968. Optimum dimensions of parallel-hole, multiaperture collimators for gamma-ray camera. *J. Nucl. Med.* 9: 233.

Keyes J.W., Jr, Orlandea N., Heetderks W.J. et al. 1977. The humogotron— a scintillation-camera transaxial tomography. *J. Nucl. Med.* 18: 381.

King M.A., Hademenos G., and Glick S.J. 1992. A dual photopeak window method for scatter correction. *J. Nucl. Med.* 33: 605.

King M.A., Schwinger R.B., Doherty P.W., and Penney B.C. 1984. Two-dimensional filtering of SPECT images using the Metz and Wiener filters. *J. Nucl. Med.* 25: 1234.

King M.A., Schwinger R.B., and Penney B.C. 1986. Variation of the count-dependent Metz filter with imaging system modulation transfer function. *Med. Phys.* 25: 139.

Knesaurek K., King M.A., Glick S.J. et al. 1989. Investigation of causes of geometric distortion in 180 degree and 360 degree angular sampling in SPECT. *J. Nucl. Med.* 30: 1666.

Koral K.F., Wang X., Rogers W.L., and Clinthorne N.H. 1988. SPECT Compton-scattering correction by analysis of energy spectra. *J. Nucl. Med.* 29: 195.

Kuhl D.E. and Edwards R.Q. 1963. Image separation radioisotope scanning. *Radiology* 80: 653.

Kuhl D.E. and Edwards R.Q. 1964. Cylindrical and section radioisotope scanning of the liver and brain. *Radiology* 83: 926.

Kuhl D.E. and Edwards R.Q. 1968. Reorganizing data from transverse section scans of the brain using digital processing. *Radiology* 91: 975.

Lange K. and Carson R. 1984. EM reconstruction algorithms for emission and transmission tomography. *J. Comput. Assist. Tomogr.* 8: 306.

Larsson S.A., Hohm C., Carnebrink T. et al. 1991. A new cylindrical SPECT Anger camera with a decentralized transputer based data acquisition system. *IEEE Trans. Nucl. Sci. NS* 38: 654.

Lassen N.A., Sveinsdottir E., Kanno I. et al. 1978. A fast moving single photon emission tomograph for regional cerebral blood flow studies in man. *J. Comput. Assist. Tomogr.* 2: 661.

Levitan E. and Herman G.T. 1987. A maximum a posteriori probability expectation maximization algorithm for image reconstruction in emission tomography. *IEEE Trans. Med. Imag. MI* 6: 185.

Lewitt R.M., Edholm P.R., and Xia W. 1989. Fourier method for correction of depth dependent collimator blurring. *Proc. SPIE* 1092: 232.

Liang Z. and Hart H. 1987. Bayesian image processing of data from constrained source distribution: I. Nonvalued, uncorrelated and correlated constraints. *Bull. Math. Biol.* 49: 51.

Lim C.B., Chang J.T., and Jaszczak R.J. 1980. Performance analysis of three camera configurations for single photon emission computed tomography. *IEEE Trans. Nucl. Sci. NS* 27: 559.

Lim C.B., Gottschalk S., Walker R. et al. 1985. Tri-angular SPECT system for 3-D total organ volume imaging: design concept and preliminary imaging results. *IEEE Trans. Nucl. Sci. NS* 32: 741.

Manglos S.H., Jaszczak R.J., Floyd C.E. et al. 1987. Nonisotropic attenuation in SPECT: phantom test of quantitative effects and compensation techniques. *J. Nucl. Med.* 28: 1584.

Maniawski P.J., Morgan H.T., and Wackers F.J.T. 1991. Orbit-related variations in spatial resolution as a source of artifactual defects in thallium-201 SPECT. *J. Nucl. Med.* 32: 871.

Milster T.D., Aarsvold J.N., Barrett H.H. et al. 1990. A full-field modular gamma camera. *J. Nucl. Med.* 31: 632.

Minerbo G. 1979. Maximum entropy reconstruction from cone-beam projection data. *Comput. Biol. Med.* 9: 29.

Moore S.C., Doherty M.D., Zimmerman R.E., and Holman B.L. 1984. Improved performance from modifications to the multidetector SPECT brain scanner. *J. Nucl. Med.* 25: 688.

Ogawa K., Harata Y., Ichihara T. et al. 1991. A practical method for position-dependent Compton scatter correction in SPECT. *IEEE Trans. Med. Imag.* 10: 408.

Penney B.C., Glick S.J., and King M.A. 1990. Relative importance of the errors sources in Wiener restoration of scintigrams. *IEEE Trans. Med. Imag.* 9: 60.

Radon J. 1917. Uber die bestimmung von funktionen durch ihre integral-werte langs gewisser mannigfaltigkeiten. *Ber. Verh. Sachs. Akad. Wiss.* 67: 26.

Ramachandran G.N. and Lakshminarayanan A.V. 1971. Three-dimensional reconstruction from radiographs and electron micrographs: application of convolutions instead of Fourier transforms. *Proc. Natl Acad. Sci. USA* 68: 2236.

Roger W.L. and Ackermann R.J. 1992. SPECT instrumentation. *Am. J. Physiol. Imag.* 314: 105.

Rogers W.L., Clinthorne N.H., Shao L. et al. 1988. SPRINT II: a second-generation single photon ring tomograph. *IEEE Trans. Med. Imag.* 7: 291.

Rowe R.K., Aarsvold J.N., Barrett H.H. et al. 1992. A stationary, hemispherical SPECT imager for 3D brain imaging. *J. Nucl. Med.* 34: 474.

Shepp L.A. and Vardi Y. 1982. Maximum likelihood reconstruction for emission tomography. *IEEE Trans. Med. Imag. MI* 1: 113.

Sorenson J.A. 1974. Quantitative measurement of radiation in vivo by whole body counting. In G.H. Hine and J.A. Sorenson (Eds), Instrumentation in Nuclear Medicine, Vol. 2, pp. 311–348. New York, Academic Press.

Stoddart H.F. and Stoddart H.A. 1979. A new development in single gamma transaxial tomography Union Carbide focused collimator scanner. *IEEE Trans. Nucl. Sci. NS* 26: 2710.

Stokely E.M., Sveinsdottir E., Lassen N.A., and Rommer P. 1980. A single photon dynamic computer assisted tomography (DCAT) for imaging brain function in multiple cross-sections. *J. Comput. Assist. Tomogr.* 4: 230.

Tretiak O.J. and Metz C.E. 1980. The exponential Radon transform. *SIAM J. Appl. Math.* 39: 341.

Tsui B.M.W. 1988. Collimator design, properties and characteristics. Chapter 2. In G.H. Simmons (Ed.), *The Scintillation Camera*, pp. 17–45. New York, The Society of Nuclear Medicine.

Tsui B.M.W., Frey E.C., Zhao X.-D. et al. 1994. The importance and implementation of accurate 3D compensation methods for quantitative SPECT. *Phys. Med. Biol.* 39: 509.

Tsui B.M.W., Gullberg G.T., Edgerton E.R. et al. 1986. The design and clinical utility of a fan beam collimator for a SPECT system. *J. Nucl. Med.* 247: 810.

Tsui B.M.W., Gullberg G.T., Edgerton E.R. et al. 1989. Correction of nonuniform attenuation in cardiac SPECT imaging. *J. Nucl. Med.* 30: 497.

Tsui B.M.W., Hu H.B., Gilland D.R., and Gullberg G.T. 1988. Implementation of simultaneous attenuation and detector response correction in SPECT. *IEEE Trans. Nucl. Sci. NS* 35: 778.

Tsui B.M.W., Zhao X.-D., Frey E.C., and McCartney W.H. 1994. Quantitative single-photon emission computed tomography: basics and clinical considerations. *Semin. Nucl. Med.* 24: 38.

Yanch J.C., Flower M.A., and Webb S. 1988. Comparison of deconvolution and windowed subtraction techniques for scatter compensation in SPECT. *IEEE Trans. Med. Imag.* 7: 13.

Zeng G.L., Gullberg G.T., Tsui B.M.W., and Terry J.A. 1991. Three-dimensional iterative reconstruction algorithms with attenuation and geometric point response correction. *IEEE Trans. Nucl. Sci. NS* 38: 693.

12

Ultrasound

Richard L. Goldberg
*University of North
Carolina*

Stephen W. Smith
Duke University

Jack G. Mottley
University of Rochester

K. Whittaker Ferrara
Riverside Research Institute

12.1 Transducers

Richard L. Goldberg and Stephen W. Smith

An ultrasound transducer generates acoustic waves by converting magnetic, thermal, and electrical energy into mechanical energy. The most efficient technique for medical ultrasound uses the piezoelectric effect, which was first demonstrated in 1880 by Jacques and Pierre Curie (Curie and Curie, 1880). They applied a stress to a quartz crystal and detected an electrical potential across opposite faces of the material. The Curies also discovered the inverse piezoelectric effect by applying an electric field across the crystal to induce a mechanical deformation. In this manner, a piezoelectric transducer converts an oscillating electric signal into an acoustic wave, and vice versa.

Many significant advances in ultrasound imaging have resulted from innovation in transducer technology. One such instance was the development of linear-array transducers. Previously, ultrasound systems had made an image by manually moving the transducer across the region of interest. Even the faster scanners had required several seconds to generate an ultrasound image, and as a result, only static targets could be scanned. On the other hand, if the acoustic beam could be scanned rapidly, clinicians could visualize moving targets such as a beating heart. In addition, real-time imaging would provide instantaneous feedback to the clinician of the transducer position and system settings.

To implement real-time imaging, researchers developed new types of transducers that rapidly steer the acoustic beam. Piston-shaped transducers were designed to wobble or rotate about a fixed axis to mechanically steer the beam through a sector-shaped region. Linear sequential arrays were designed to electronically focus the beam in a rectangular image region. Linear phased-array transducers were designed to electronically steer and focus the beam at high speed in a sector image format.

This section describes the application of piezoelectric ceramics to transducer arrays for medical ultrasound. Background is presented on transducer materials and beam steering with phased arrays. Array performance is described, and the design of an idealized array is presented.

12.1.1 Transducer Materials

Ferroelectric materials strongly exhibit the piezoelectric effect, and they are ideal materials for medical ultrasound. For many years, the ferroelectric ceramic lead-zirconate-titanate (PZT) has been the standard transducer material for medical ultrasound, in part because of its high electromechanical conversion efficiency and low intrinsic losses. The properties of PZT can be adjusted by modifying the ratio of zirconium to titanium and introducing small amounts of other substances, such as lanthanum (Berlincourt, 1971). Table 12.1 shows the material properties of linear-array elements made from PZT-5H.

PZT has a high dielectric constant compared with many piezoelectric materials, resulting is favorable electrical characteristics. The ceramic is mechanically strong, and it can be machined to various shapes and sizes. PZT can operate at temperatures up to 100°C or higher, and it is stable over long periods of time.

The disadvantages of PZT include its high **acoustic impedance** ($Z = 30$ MRayls) compared with body tissue ($Z = 1.5$ MRayls) and the presence of **lateral modes** in array elements. One or more acoustic matching layers can largely compensate for the acoustic impedance mismatch. The effect of lateral modes can be diminished by choosing the appropriate element dimensions or by subdicing the elements.

Other piezoelectric materials are used for various applications. Composites are made from PZT interspersed in an epoxy matrix (Smith, 1992). Lateral modes are reduced in a composite because of its inhomo-geneous structure. By combining the PZT and epoxy in different ratios and spatial distributions, one can tailor the composite's properties for different applications. Polyvinylidene difluoride (PVDF) is a ferroelectric polymer that has been used effectively in high-frequency transducers (Sherar and Foster, 1989). The copolymer of PVDF with trifluoroethylene has an improved electromechanical conversion efficiency. Relaxor ferroelectric materials, such as lead-magnesium-niobate (PMN), become piezoelectric when a large direct-current (dc) bias voltage is applied (Takeuchi et al., 1990). They have a very large dielectric constant ($\varepsilon > 20{,}000\varepsilon_0$), resulting in higher transducer capacitance and a lower electrical impedance.

12.1.2 Scanning with Array Transducers

Array transducers use the same principles as acoustic lenses to focus an acoustic beam. In both cases, variable delays are applied across the transducer aperture. With a sequential or phased array, however,

TABLE 12.1 Material Properties of Linear-Array Elements Made of PZT-5H

Parameter	Symbol	Value	Units
Density	ρ	7500	kg/m^3
Speed of sound	c	3970	m/sec
Acoustic impedance	Z	29.75	MRayls
Relative dielectric constant	$\varepsilon/\varepsilon_0$	1475	None
Electromechanical coupling coefficient	k	0.698	None
Mechanical loss tangent	$\tan \delta_m$	0.015	None
Electrical loss tangent	$\tan \delta_e$	0.02	None

the delays are electronically controlled and can be changed instantaneously to focus the beam in different regions. Linear arrays were first developed for radar, sonar, and radio astronomy (Allen, 1964; Bobber, 1970), and they were implemented in a medical ultrasound system by Somer in 1968 (Somer, 1968).

Linear-array transducers have increased versatility over piston transducers. Electronic scanning involves no moving parts, and the focal point can be changed dynamically to any location in the scanning plane. The system can generate a wide variety of scan formats, and it can process the received echoes for other applications, such as dynamic receive focusing (von Ramm and Thurstone, 1976), correction for phase aberrations (Flax and O'Donnell, 1988; Trahey et al., 1990), and synthetic aperture imaging (Nock and Trahey, 1992).

The disadvantages of linear arrays are due to the increased complexity and higher cost of the transducers and scanners. For high-quality ultrasound images, many identical array elements are required (currently 128 and rising). The array elements are typically less than a millimeter on one side, and each has a separate connection to its own transmitter and receiver electronics.

The widespread use of array transducers for many applications indicates that the advantages often outweigh the disadvantages. In addition, improvement in transducer fabrication techniques and integrated circuit technology have led to more advanced array transducers and scanners.

12.1.2.1 Focusing and Steering with Phased Arrays

This section describes how a phased-array transducer can focus and steer an acoustic beam along a specific direction. An ultrasound image is formed by repeating this process over 100 times to interrogate a two-(2D) or three-dimensional (3D) region of the medium.

Figure 12.1a illustrates a simple example of a six-element linear array focusing the transmitted beam. One can assume that each array element is a point source that radiates a spherically shaped wavefront

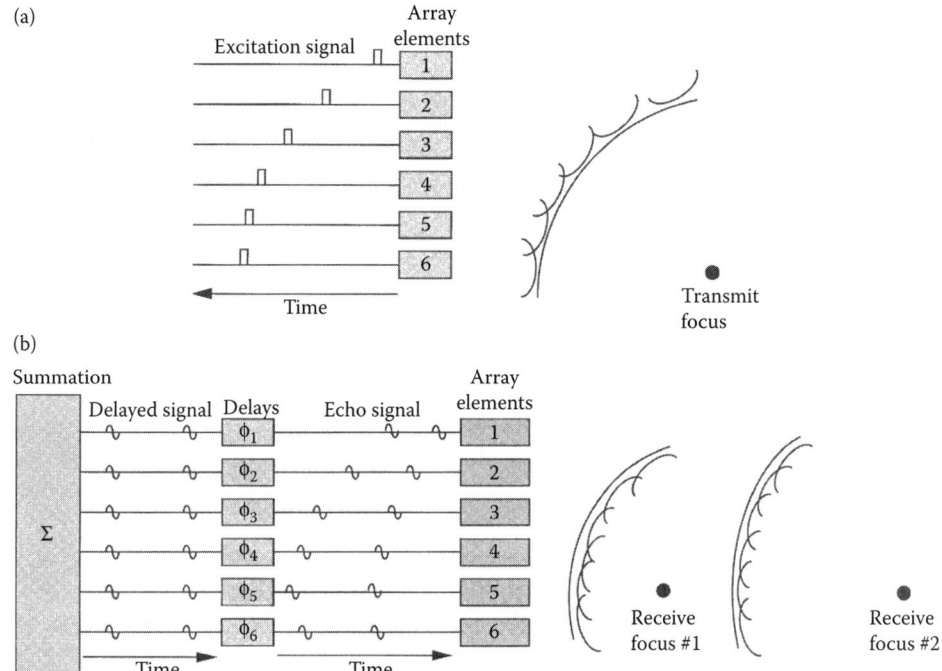

FIGURE 12.1 Focusing and steering an acoustic 1 Focusing beam using a phased array. A 6-element linear array is shown (a) in the transmit mode and (b) in the receive mode. Dynamic focusing in receive allows the scanner focus to track the range of returning echoes.

into the medium. Since the top element is farthest from the focus in this example, it is excited first. The remaining elements are excited at the appropriate time intervals so that the acoustic signals from all the elements reach the focal point at the same time. According to Huygens' principle, the net acoustic signal is the sum of the signals that have arrived from each source. At the focal point, the contributions from every element add in phase to produce a peak in the acoustic signal. Elsewhere, at least some of the contributions add out of phase, reducing the signal relative to the peak.

For receiving an ultrasound echo, the phased array works in reverse. Figure 12.1b shows an echo originating from focus 1. The echo is incident on each array element at a different time interval. The received signals are electronically delayed so that the delayed signals add in phase for an echo originating at the focal point. For echoes originating elsewhere, at least some of the delayed signals will add out of phase, reducing the receive signal relative to the peak at the focus.

In the receive mode, the focal point can be dynamically adjusted so that it coincides with the range of returning echoes. After transmission of an acoustic pulse, the initial echoes return from targets near the transducer. Therefore, the scanner focuses the phased array on these targets, located at focus 1 in Figure 12.1b. As echoes return from more distant targets, the scanner focuses at a greater depth (focus 2 in the figure). Focal zones are established with adequate depth of field so that the targets are always in focus in receive. This process is called dynamic receive focusing and was first implemented by von Ramm and Thurstone in 1976 (von Ramm and Thurstone, 1976).

12.1.2.2 Array-Element Configurations

An ultrasound image is formed by repeating the preceding process many times to scan a 2D or 3D region of tissue. For a 2D image, the scanning plane is the *azimuth dimension;* the *elevation dimension* is perpendicular to the azimuth scanning plane. The shape of the region scanned is determined by the array-element configuration, described in the paragraph below.

Linear Sequential Arrays: Sequential linear arrays have as many as 512 elements in current commercial scanners. A subaperture of up to 128 elements is selected to operate at a given time. As shown in Figure 12.2a, the scanning lines are directed perpendicular to the face of the transducer; the acoustic beam is focused but not steered. The advantage of this scheme is that the array elements have high sensitivity when the beam is directed straight ahead. The disadvantage is that the field of view is limited to the rectangular region directly in front of the transducer. Linear-array transducers have a large footprint to obtain an adequate field of view.

Curvilinear Arrays: Curvilinear or convex arrays have a different shape than sequential linear arrays, but they operate in the same manner. In both cases, the scan lines are directed perpendicular to the transducer face. A curvilinear array, however, scans a wider field of view because of its convex shape, as shown in Figure 12.2b.

Linear Phased Arrays: The more advanced linear phased arrays have 128 elements. All the elements are used to transmit and receive each line of data. As shown in Figure 12.2c, the scanner steers the ultrasound beam through a sector-shaped region in the azimuth plane. Phased arrays scan a region that is significantly wider than the footprint of the transducer, making them suitable for scanning through restricted acoustic windows. As a result, these transducers are ideal for cardiac imaging, where the transducer must scan through a small window to avoid the obstructions of the ribs (bone) and lungs (air).

1.5D Arrays: The so-called 1.5D array is similar to a 2D array in construction but a 1D array in operation. The 1.5D array contains elements along both the azimuth and elevation dimensions. Features such dynamic focusing and phase correction can be implemented in both dimensions to improve image quality. Since a 1.5D array contains a limited number of elements in elevation (e.g., 3 to 9 elements), steering is not possible in that direction. Figure 12.2d illustrates a B-scan made with a 1.5D phased array. Linear sequential scanning is also possible with 1.5D arrays.

2D Phased Arrays: A 2D phased-array has a large number of elements in both the azimuth and elevation dimensions. Therefore, 2D arrays can focus and steer the acoustic beam in both dimensions.

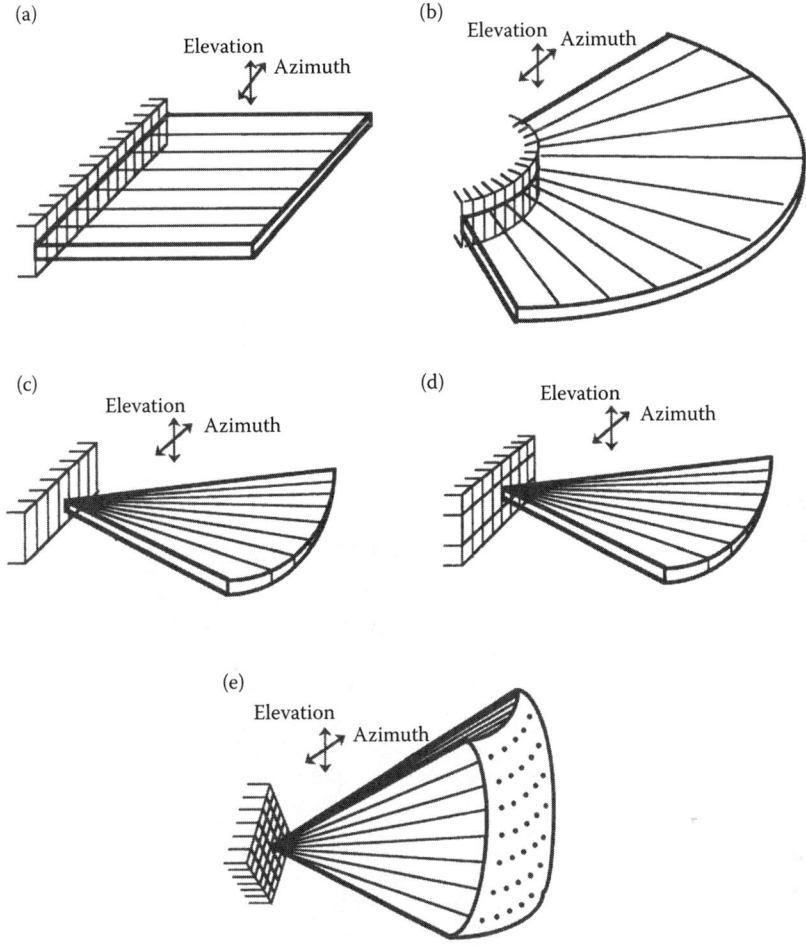

FIGURE 12.2 Array-element configurations and the region scanned by the acoustic beam. (a) A sequential linear array scans a rectangular region; (b) a curvilinear array scans a sector-shaped region; (c) a linear phased array scans a sector-shaped region; (d) a 1.5D array scans a sector-shaped region; and (e) a 2D array scans a pyramidal-shaped region.

Using parallel receive processing (Shattuck et al., 1984), a 2D array can scan a pyramidal region in real time to produce a volumetric image, as shown in Figure 12.2e (von Ramm and Smith, 1990).

12.1.3 Linear-Array Transducer Performance

Designing an ultrasound transducer array involves many compromises. Ideally, a transducer has high sensitivity or signal-to-noise ratio (SNR), good spatial resolution, and no artifacts. The individual array elements should have wide **angular response** in the steering dimensions, low cross-coupling, and an electrical impedance matched to the transmitter.

Figure 12.3a illustrates the connections to the transducer assembly. The transmitter and receiver circuits are located in the ultrasound scanner and are connected to the array elements through 1 to 2 m of coaxial cable. **Electrical matching networks** can be added to tune out the capacitance of the coaxial cable and/or the transducer element and increase the SNR.

A more detailed picture of six-transducer elements is shown in Figure 12.3b. Electrical leads connect to the ground and signal electrodes of the piezoelectric material. Acoustically, the array elements

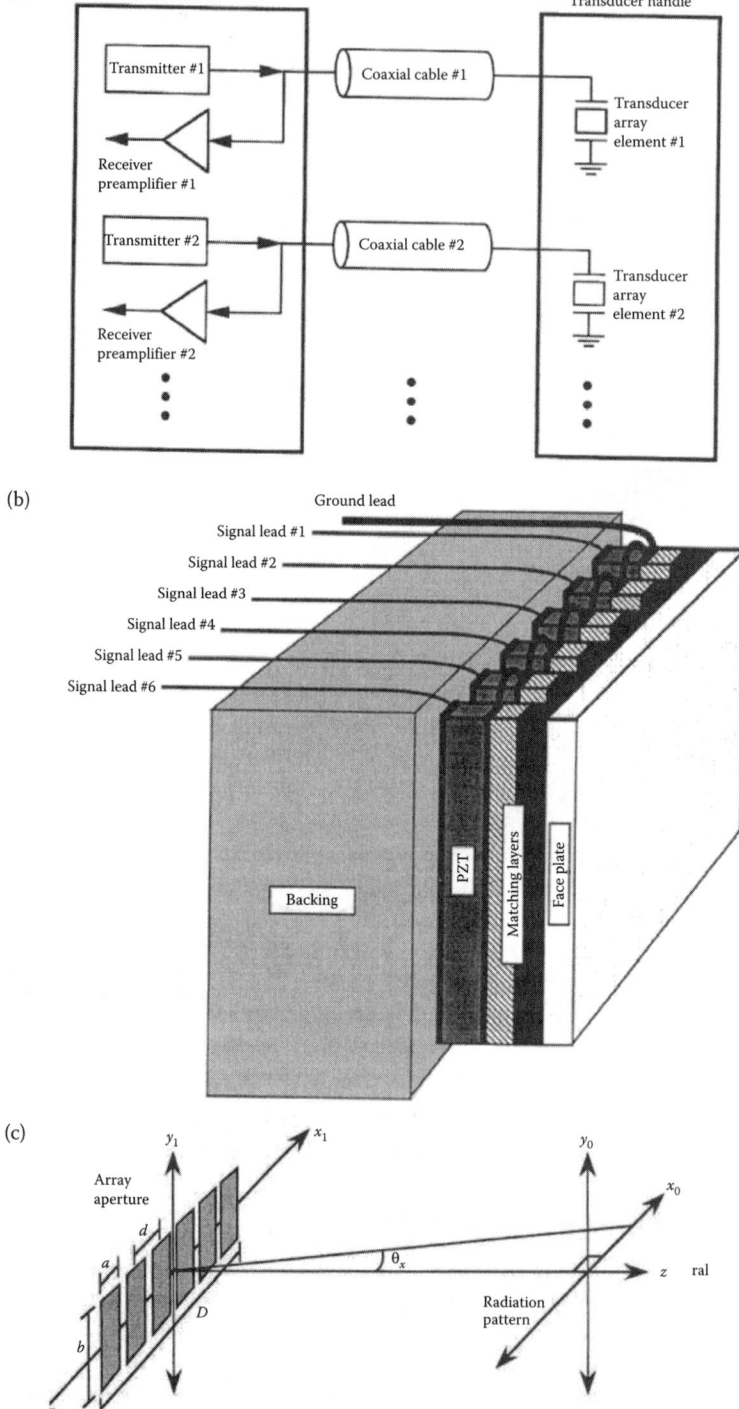

FIGURE 12.3 (a) The connections between the ultrasound scanner and the transducer assembly for two elements of an array. (b) A more detailed picture of the transducer assembly for six elements of an array. (c) Coordinate system and labeling used to describe an array transducer.

are loaded on the front side by one or two **quarter-wave matching layers** and the tissue medium. The matching layers may be made from glass or epoxy. A backing material, such as epoxy, loads the back side of the array elements. The faceplate protects the transducer assembly and also may act as an acoustic lens. Faceplates are often made from silicone or polyurethane.

The following sections describe several important characteristics of an array transducer. Figure 12.3c shows a six-element array and its dimensions. The element thickness, width, and length are labeled as t, a, and b, respectively. The interelement spacing is d, and the total aperture size is D in azimuth. The acoustic wavelength in the load medium, usually human tissue, is designated as l, while the wavelength in the transducer material is λ_t.

Examples are given below for a 128-element linear array operating at 5 MHz. The array is made of PZT-5H with element dimensions of $0.1 \times 5 \times 0.3$ mm³. The interelement spacing is $d = 0.15$ mm in azimuth, and the total aperture is $D = 128 \times 0.15$ mm $= 19.3$ mm (see Table 12.1 for the piezoelectric material characteristics). The elements have an epoxy backing of $Z = 3.25$ MRayls. For simplicity, the example array does not contain a $\lambda/4$ matching layer.

12.1.3.1 Axial Resolution

Axial resolution determines the ability to distinguish between targets aligned in the axial direction (the direction of acoustic propagation). In pulse-echo imaging, the echoes off of two targets separated by r/2 have a path length difference of r. If the acoustic pulse length is r, then echoes off the two targets are just distinguishable. As a result, the **axial resolution** is often defined as one-half the pulse length (Christensen, 1988). A transducer with a high resonant frequency and a broad bandwidth has a short acoustic pulse and good axial resolution.

12.1.3.2 Radiation Pattern

The radiation pattern of a transducer determines the insonified region of tissue. For **good lateral resolution** and sensitivity, the acoustic energy should be concentrated in a small region. The radiation pattern for a narrow-band or continuous-wave (CW) transducer is described by the Rayleigh-Sommerfeld diffraction formula (Goodman, 1986). For a pulse-echo imaging system, this diffraction formula is not exact due to the broadband acoustic waves used. Nevertheless, the Rayleigh-Sommerfeld formula is a reasonable first-order approximation to the actual radiation pattern.

The following analysis considers only the azimuth scanning dimension. Near the focal point or in the far field, the Fraunhofer approximation reduces the diffraction formula to a Fourier transform formula. For a circular or rectangular aperture, the far field is at a range of

$$z > \frac{D^2}{4\lambda} \tag{12.1}$$

Figure 12.3c shows the coordinate system used to label the array aperture and its radiation pattern. The array aperture is described by

$$\text{Array}(c_1) = \text{rect}\left(\frac{x_1}{a}\right) * \text{comb}\left(\frac{x_1}{d}\right) \cdot \text{rect}\left(\frac{x_1}{D}\right) \tag{12.2}$$

where the rect(x) function is a rectangular pulse of width x, and the comb(x) function is a delta function repeated at intervals of x. The diffraction pattern is evaluated in the x_0 plane at a distance z from the transducer, and θ_x is the angle of the point x_0 from the normal axis. With the Fraunhofer approximation, the normalized diffraction pattern is given by

$$P_x(\theta_x) = \text{sinc}\left(\frac{a\sin\theta_x}{\lambda}\right) \cdot \text{comp}\left(\frac{d\sin\theta_x}{\lambda}\right) * \text{sinc}\left(\frac{D\sin\theta_x}{\lambda}\right) \tag{12.3}$$

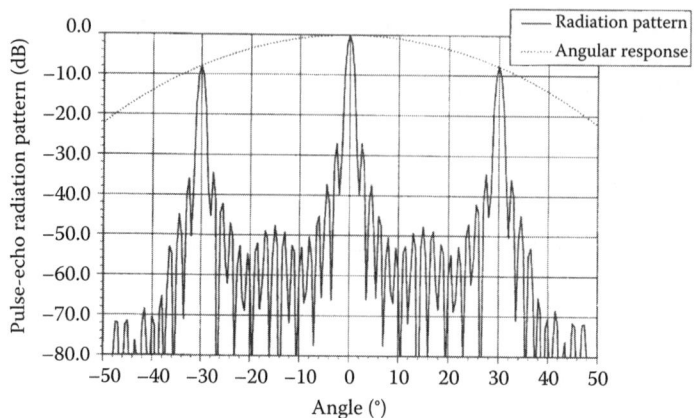

FIGURE 12.4 Radiation pattern of Equation 12.3 for a 16-element array with $a = \lambda$, $d = 2\lambda$, and $D = 32\lambda$. The angular response, the first term of Equation 12.3, is also shown as a dashed line.

in azimuth, where the Fourier transform of Equation 12.2 has been evaluated at the spatial frequency

$$f_x = \frac{x_0}{\lambda z} = \frac{\sin \theta_x}{\lambda} \tag{12.4}$$

Figure 12.4 shows a graph of Equation 12.3 for a 16-element array with $a = \lambda$, $d = 2\lambda$, and $D = 32\lambda$. In the graph, the significance of each term is easily distinguished. The first term determines the angular response weighting, the second term determines the location of **grating lobes** off-axis, and the third term determines the shape of the main lobe and the grating lobes. The significance of *lateral resolution*, angular response, and grating lobes is seen from the CW diffraction pattern.

Lateral resolution determines the ability to distinguish between targets in the azimuth and elevation dimensions. According to the Rayleigh criterion (Goodman, 1986), the lateral resolution can be defined by the first null in the main lobe, which is determined from the third term of Equation 12.3.

$$\theta_x = \sin^{-1} \frac{\lambda}{D} \tag{12.5}$$

in the **azimuth dimension**. A larger aperture results in a more narrow main lobe and better resolution.

A broad angular response is desired to maintain sensitivity while steering off-axis. The first term of Equation 12.3 determines the one-way angular response. The element is usually surrounded by a soft baffle, such as air, resulting in an additional cosine factor in the radiation pattern (Selfridge et al., 1980). Assuming transmit/receive reciprocity, the pulse-echo angular response for a single element is

$$P_x(\theta_x) = \frac{\sin^2(\pi a/\lambda \cdot \sin \theta_x)}{\pi a/\lambda \cdot \sin \theta_x} \cdot \cos^2 \theta_x \tag{12.6}$$

in the azimuth dimension. As the aperture size becomes smaller, the element more closely resembles a point source, and the angular response becomes more broad. Another useful indicator is the −6-dB angular response, defined as the full-width at half-maximum of the angular response graph.

Grating lobes are produced at a location where the path length difference to adjacent array elements is a multiple of a wavelength (the main lobe is located where the path length difference is zero). The acoustic contributions from the elements constructively interfere, producing off-axis peaks. The term grating

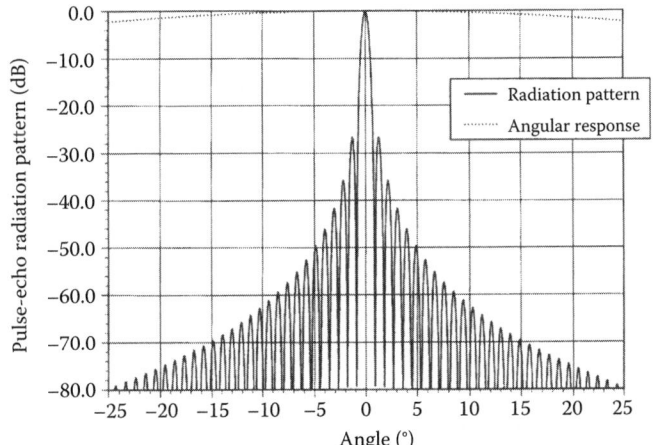

FIGURE 12.5 Radiation pattern of the example array element with $a = 0.1$ mm, $d = 0.15$ mm, $D = 19.2$ mm, and $\lambda = 0.3$ mm. The angular response of Equation 12.6 was substituted into Equation 12.3 for this graph.

lobe was originally used to describe the optical peaks produced by a diffraction grating. In ultrasound, grating lobes are undesirable because they represent acoustic energy steered away from the main lobe. From the comb function in Equation 12.3, the grating lobes are located at

$$\theta_x = \sin^{-1}\frac{i\lambda}{d} \quad i = 1,2,3,\ldots \tag{12.7}$$

in azimuth.

If d is a wavelength, then grating lobes are centered at ±90 degrees from the steering direction in that dimension. Grating lobes at such large angles are less significant because the array elements have poor angular response in those regions. If the main lobe is steered at a large angle, however, the grating lobes are brought toward the front of the array. In this case, the angular response weighting produces a relatively weak main lobe and a relatively strong grating lobe. To eliminate grating lobes at all steering angles, the interelement spacing is set to $\lambda/2$ or less (Steinberg, 1967).

Figure 12.5 shows the theoretical radiation pattern of the 128-element example. For this graph, the angular response weighting of Equation 12.6 was substituted into Equation 12.3. The lateral resolution, as defined by Equation 12.7, $\theta_x = 0.9$ degrees at the focal point. The −6-dB angular response is ±40 degrees from Equation 12.6.

12.1.3.3 Electrical Impedance

The electric impedance of an element relative to the electrical loads has a significant impact on transducer signal-to-noise ratio (SNR). At frequencies away from resonance, the transducer has electrical characteristics of a capacitor. The construction of the transducer is a parallel-plate capacitor with clamped capacitance of

$$C_0 = \varepsilon^s \frac{ab}{t} \tag{12.8}$$

where ε^s is the clamped dielectric constant.

Near resonance, equivalent circuits help to explain the impedance behavior of a transducer. The simplified circuit of Figure 12.6a is valid for transducers operating at series resonance without losses and

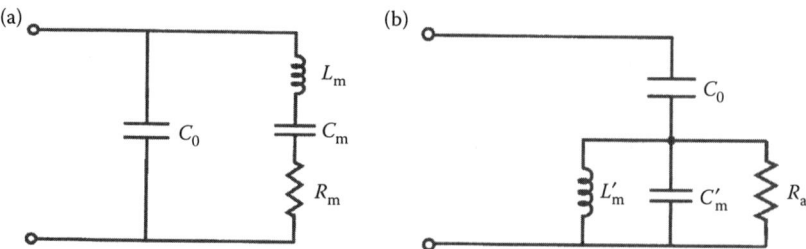

FIGURE 12.6 Simplified equivalent circuits for a piezoelectric transducer (a) near-series resonance and (b) near-parallel resonance.

with low acoustic impedance loads (Kino, 1987). The mechanical resistance R_m represents the acoustic loads as seen from the electrical terminals:

$$R_m = \frac{\pi}{4k^2\omega c_0} \cdot \frac{Z_1 + Z_2}{Z_C} \tag{12.9}$$

where k is the electromechanical coupling coefficient of the piezoelectric material, Z_C is the acoustic impedance of the piezoelectric material, Z_1 is the acoustic impedance of the transducer backing, and Z_2 is the acoustic impedance of the load medium (body tissue). The power dissipated through R_m corresponds to the acoustic output power from the transducer.

The mechanical inductance L_m and mechanical capacitance C_m are analogous to the inductance and capacitance of a mass-spring system. At the series resonant frequency of

$$f_s = \frac{1}{2\pi\sqrt{L_m C_m}} \tag{12.10}$$

the impedances of these components add to zero, resulting in a local impedance minimum.

The equivalent circuit of Figure 12.6a can be redrawn in the form shown in Figure 12.6b. In this circuit, Q is the same as before, but the mechanical impedances have values of L'_m, C'_m, and R_a. The resistive component R_a is

$$R_a = \frac{4k^2}{\pi\omega C_0} \cdot \frac{Z_C}{Z_1 - Z_2} \tag{12.11}$$

The inductor and capacitor combine to form an open circuit at the parallel resonant frequency of

$$f_p = \frac{1}{2\pi\sqrt{L'_m C'_m}} \tag{12.12}$$

The parallel resonance, which is at a slightly higher frequency than the series resonance, is indicated by a local impedance maximum.

Figure 12.7 shows a simulated plot of magnitude and phase versus frequency for the example array element described at the beginning of this subsection. The series resonance frequency is immediately identified at 5.0 MHz with an impedance minimum of $|Z| = 350\ \Omega$. Parallel resonance occurs at 6.7 MHz with an impedance maximum of $|Z| = 4000\ \Omega$. Note the capacitive behavior (approximately −90-degree phase) at frequenciess far from resonance.

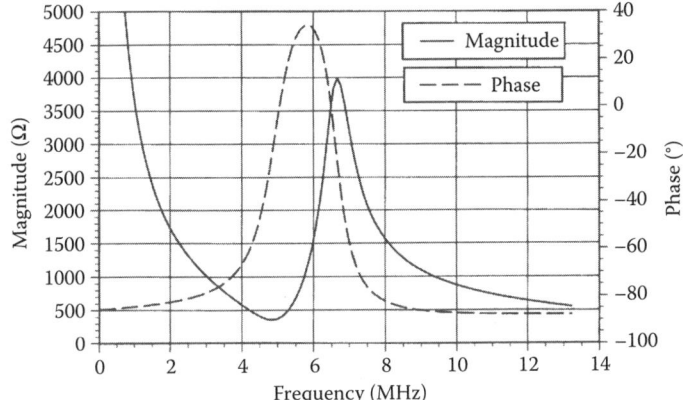

FIGURE 12.7 Complex electrical impedance of the example array element. Series resonance is located at 5.0 MHz, and parallel resonance is located at 6.7 MHz.

12.1.4 Designing a Phased-Array Transducer

In this section the design of an idealized phased-array transducer is considered in terms of the performance characteristics described above. Criteria are described for selecting array dimensions, acoustic backing and matching layers, and electrical matching networks.

12.1.4.1 Choosing Array Dimensions

The array element thickness is determined by the parallel resonant frequency. For $\lambda/2$ resonance, the thickness is

$$t = \frac{\lambda_t}{2}\frac{c_t}{2f_p} \tag{12.13}$$

where c_t is the longitudinal speed of sound in the transducer material.

There are three constraints for choosing the element width and length (1) a nearly square cross-section should be avoided so that lateral vibrations are not coupled to the thickness vibration; as a rule of thumb (Kino and DeSilets, 1979),

$$a/t = 0.6 \quad \text{or} \quad a/t = 10 \tag{12.14}$$

(2) a small width and length are also desirable for a wide angular response weighting function; and (3) an interelement spacing of $\lambda/2$ or less is necessary to eliminate grating lobes.

Fortunately, these requirements are consistent for PZT array elements. For all forms of PZT, $c_t > 2c$, where c is the speed of sound in body tissue (an average of 1540 m/sec). At a given frequency, then $\lambda_t > 2\lambda$. Also, Equation 12.13 states that $\lambda_t = 2t$ at a frequency of f_p. By combining these equations, $t > \lambda$ for PZT array elements operating at a frequency of f_p. If $d = \lambda/2$, then $a < \lambda/2$ because of the finite kerf width that separates the elements. Given this observation, then $a < t/2$. This is consistent with Equation 12.14 to reduce lateral modes.

An element having $d = \lambda/2$ also has adequate angular response. For illustrative purposes, one can assume a zero kerf width so that $a = \lambda/2$. In this case, the −6-dB angular response is $\theta_x = \pm 35$ degrees according to Equation 12.6.

The array dimensions determine the transducer's lateral resolution. In the azimuth dimension, if $d = \lambda/2$, then the transducer aperture is $D = n\lambda/2$, where n is the number of elements in a fully sampled array. From Equation 12.5, the lateral resolution in azimuth is

$$\theta_x = \sin^{-1}\frac{2}{n} \tag{12.15}$$

Therefore, the lateral resolution is independent of frequency in a fully sampled array with $d = \lambda/2$. For this configuration, the lateral resolution is improved by increasing the number of elements.

12.1.4.2 Acoustic Backing and Matching Layers

The backing and matching layers affect the transducer bandwidth and sensitivity. While a lossy, matched backing improves bandwidth, it also dissipates acoustic energy that could otherwise be transmitted into the tissue medium. Therefore, a low-impedance acoustic backing is preferred because it reflects the acoustic pulses toward the front side of the transducer. In this case, adequate bandwidth is maintained by acoustically matching the transducer to the tissue medium using matching layers.

Matching layers are designed with a thickness of $\lambda/4$ at the center frequency and an acoustic impedance between those of the transducer Z_T and the load medium Z_L. The ideal acoustic impedances can be determined from several different models (Hunt et al., 1983). Using the KLM equivalent circuit model (Desilets et al., 1978), the ideal acoustic impedance is

$$Z_1 = \sqrt[3]{Z_T Z_L^2} \tag{12.16}$$

for a single matching layer. For matching PZT-5H array elements ($Z_T = 30$ MRayls) to a water load ($Z_L = 1.5$ MRayls), a matching layer of $Z_1 = 4.1$ MRayls should be chosen. If two matching layers are used, they should have acoustic impedances of

$$Z_1 \sqrt[7]{Z_T^4 Z_L^3} \tag{12.17a}$$

$$Z_2 \sqrt[7]{Z_T Z_L^6} \tag{12.17b}$$

In this case, $Z_1 = 8.3$ MRayls and $Z_2 = 2.3$ MRayls for matching PZT-5H to a water load.

When constructing a transducer, a practical matching layer material is not always available, with the ideal acoustic impedance (Equation 12.16 or Equation 12.17). Adequate bandwidth is obtained by using materials that have an impedance close to the ideal value. With a single matching layer, for example, conductive epoxy can be used with $Z = 5.1$ MRayls.

12.1.4.3 Electrical Impedance Matching

Signal-to-noise ratio and bandwidth are also improved when electrical impedance of an array element is matched to that of the transmit circuitry. Consider the simplified circuit in Figure 12.8 with a transmitter of impedance R_0 and a transducer of real impedance R_t. The power output is proportional to the power dissipated in R_t, as expressed as

$$P_{out} = \frac{V_{out}^2}{R_t} \quad \text{where } V_{out} = \frac{R_t}{R_0 + R_t}V_{in} \tag{12.18}$$

The power available from the transmitter is

$$P_{in} = \frac{(V_{in}/2)^2}{R_0} \tag{12.19}$$

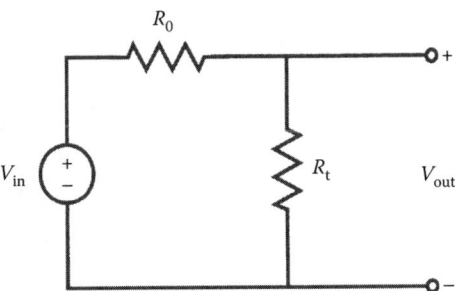

FIGURE 12.8 A transducer of real impedance R_t being excited by a transmitter with source impedance R_0 and source voltage V_{in}.

into a matched load. From the two previous equations, the power efficiency is

$$\frac{P_{out}}{P_{in}} = \frac{4R_0R_t}{(R_0 + R_t)^2} \tag{12.20}$$

For a fixed-source impedance, the maximum efficiency is obtained by taking the derivative of Equation 12.20 with respect to R_t and setting it to zero. Maximum efficiency occurs when the source impedance is matched to the transducer impedance, $R_0 = R_t$.

In practice, the transducer has a complex impedance of R_m in parallel with C_0 (see Figure 12.6), which is excited by a transmitter with a real impedance of 50 Ω. The transducer has a maximum efficiency when the imaginary component is tuned out and the real component is 50 Ω. This can be accomplished with electrical matching networks.

The capacitance C_0 is tuned out in the frequency range near Ω_0 using an inductor of

$$L_0 = \frac{1}{\omega_0^2 C_0} \tag{12.21}$$

for an inductor in shunt, or

$$L_1 \frac{1}{\omega_0^2 C_0 + 1/R_m^2 C_0} \tag{12.22}$$

for an inductor in series. The example array elements described in the preceding subsection have $C_0 = 22$ pF and $R_m = 340$ Ω at series resonance of 5.0 MHz. Therefore, tuning inductors of $L_0 = 46$ mH or $L_1 = 2.4$ mH should be used.

A shunt inductor also raises the impedance of the transducer, as seen from the scanner, while a series inductor lowers the terminal impedance (Hunt et al., 1983). For more significant changes in terminal impedance, transformers are used.

A transformer of turns ratio 1:N multiplies the terminal impedance by $1/N^2$. In the transmit mode, N can be adjusted so that the terminal impedance matches the transmitter impedance. In the receive mode, the open-circuit sensitivity varies as $1/N$ because of the step-down transformer. The lower terminal impedance of the array element, however, provides increased ability to drive an electrical load.

More complicated circuits can be used for better electrical matching across a wide bandwidth (Hunt et al., 1983). These circuits can be either passive, as above, or active. Inductors also can be used in the scanner to tune out the capacitance of the coaxial cable that loads the transducer on receive.

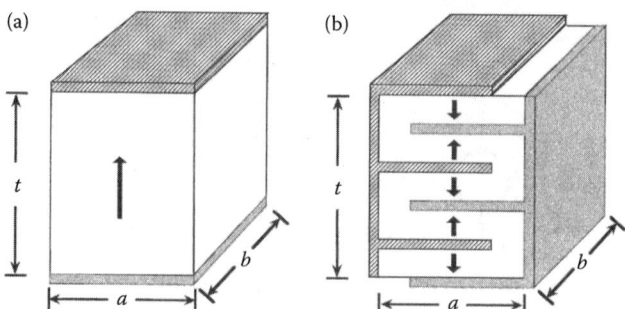

FIGURE 12.9 (a) Conventional single-layer ceramic; (b) five-layer ceramic of the same overall dimensions. The layers are electrically in parallel and acoustically in series. The arrows indicate the piezoelectric poling directions of each layer.

Another alternative for electrical matching is to use multilayer piezoelectric ceramics (Goldberg and Smith, 1994). Figure 12.9 shows an example of a single layer and a five-layer array element with the same overall dimensions of a, b, and t. Since the layers are connected electrically in parallel, the clamped capacitance of a multilayer ceramic (MLC) element is

$$C_0 = N \cdot \varepsilon^S \cdot \frac{ab}{t/N} = N^2 \cdot C_{single} \qquad (12.23)$$

where C_{single} is the capacitance of the single-layer element (Equation 12.8). As a result, the MLC impedance is reduced by a factor of N^2. Acoustically, the layers of the MLC are in series so the $\lambda/2$ resonant thickness is t, the stack thickness.

To a first order, an N-layer ceramic has identical performance compared with a 1:N transformer, but the impedance is transformed within the ceramic. MLCs also can be fabricated in large quantities more easily than hand-wound transformers. While MLCs do not tune out the reactive impedance, they make it easier to tune a low capacitance array element. By lowering the terminal impedance of an array element, MLCs significantly improve transducer SNR.

12.1.5 Summary

The piezoelectric transducer is an important component in the ultrasound imaging system. The transducer often consists of a liner array that can electronically focus an acoustic beam. Depending on the configuration of array elements, the region scanned may be sector shaped or rectangular in two dimensions or pyramidal shaped in three dimensions.

The transducer performance large determines the resolution and the signal-to-noise ratio of the resulting ultrasound image. The design of an array involves many compromises in choosing operating frequency and array-element dimensions. Electrical matching networks and quarter-wave matching layers may be added to improve transducer performance.

Further improvements in transducer performance may result from several areas of research. Newer materials, such as composites, are gaining widespread use in medical ultrasound. In addition, 1.5D arrays or 2D arrays may be employed to control the acoustic beam in both azimuth and elevation. Problems in fabrication and electrical impedance matching must be overcome to implement these arrays in an ultrasound system.

Defining Terms

Acoustic impedance: In an analogy to transmission line impedance, the acoustic impedance is the ratio of pressure to particle velocity in a medium; more commonly, it is defined as $Z = \rho c$, where ρ = density and c = speed of sound in a medium [the units are kg/(m^2 sec) or Rayls].

Angular response: The radiation pattern versus angle for a single element of an array.

Axial resolution: The ability to distinguish between targets aligned in the axial direction (the direction of acoustic propagation).

Azimuth dimension: The lateral dimension that is along the scanning plane for an array transducer.

Electrical matching networks: Active or passive networks designed to tune out reactive components of the transducer and match the transducer impedance to the source and receiver impedance.

Elevation dimension: The lateral dimension that is perpendicular to the scanning plane for an array transducer.

Grating lobes: Undesirable artifacts in the radiation pattern of a transducer; they are produced at a location where the path length difference to adjacent array elements is a multiple of a wavelength.

Lateral modes: Transducer vibrations that occur in the lateral dimensions when the transducer is excited in the thickness dimension.

Lateral resolution: The ability to distinguish between targets in the azimuth and elevation dimensions (perpendicular to the axial dimension).

Quarter-wave matching layers: One or more layers of material placed between the transducer and the load medium (water or human tissue); they effectively match the acoustic impedance of the transducer to the load medium to improve the transducer bandwidth and signal-to-noise ratio.

References

Allen J.L. 1964. Array antennas: New applications for an old technique. *IEEE Spect.* 1: 115.

Berlincourt D. 1971. Piezoelectric crystals and ceramics. In O.E. Mattiat (Ed.), *Ultrasonic Transducer Materials*. New York, Plenum Press.

Bobber R.J. 1970. *UnderwaterElectro acoustic Measurements*. Washington, Naval Research Laboratory.

Christensen D.A. 1988. *Ultrasonic Bioinstrumentation*. New York, Wiley.

Curie P. and Curie J. 1980. Development par pression de l'electricite polaire dans les cristaux hemiedres a faces enclinees. *Comp. Rend.* 91: 383.

Desilets C.S., Fraser J.D., and Kino G.S. 1978. The design of efficient broad-band piezoelectric transducers. *IEEE Trans. Son. Ultrason.* SU-25: 115.

Flax S.W. and O'Donnell M. 1988. Phase aberration correction using signals from point reflectors and diffuse scatters: Basic principles. *IEEE Trans. Ultrason. Ferroelec. Freq. Contr.* 35: 758.

Goldberg R.L. and Smith S.W. 1994. Multi-layer piezoelectric ceramics for two-dimensional array transducers. *IEEE Trans. Ultrason. Ferroelec. Freq. Contr.*

Goodman W. 1986. *Introduction to Fourier Optics*. New York, McGraw-Hill.

Hunt J.W., Arditi M., and Foster F.S. 1983. Ultrasound transducers for pulse-echo medical imaging. *IEEE Trans. Biomed. Eng.* 30: 453.

Kino G.S. 1987. *Acoustic Waves*. Englewood Cliffs, NJ, Prentice-Hall.

Kino G.S. and DeSilets C.S. 1979. Design of slotted transducer arrays with matched backings. *Ultrason. Imag.* 1: 189.

Nock L.F. and Trahey G.E. 1992. Synthetic receive aperture imaging with phase correction for motion and for tissue inhomogeneities: I. Basic principles. *IEEE Trans. Ultrason. Ferroelec. Freq. Contr.* 39: 489.

Selfridge A.R., Kino G.S., and Khuri-Yahub B.T. 1980. A theory for the radiation pattern of a narrow strip acoustic transducer. *Appl. Phys. Lett.* 37: 35.

Shattuck D.P., Weinshenker M.D.,Smith S.W., and von Ramm O.T. 1984. Explososcan: A parallel processing technique for high speed ultrasound imaging with linear phased arrays. *J. Acoust. Soc. Am.* 75:1273.

Sherar M.D. and Foster F.S. 1989. The design and fabrication of high frequency poly(vinylidene fluoride) transducers. *Ultrason. Imag.* 11: 75.

Smith W.A. 1992. New opportunities in ultrasonic transducers emerging from innovations in piezoelectric materials. In F.L. Lizzi (Ed.), *New Developments in Ultrasonic Transducers and Transducer Systems*, pp. 3–26. New York, SPIE.

Somer J.C. 1968. Electronic sector scanning for ultrasonic diagnosis. *Ultrasonics* 153.

Steinberg B.D. 1976. *Principles of Aperture and Array System Design*. New York, Wiley.

Takeuchi H., Masuzawa H., Nakaya C., and Ito Y. 1990. Relaxor ferroelectric transducers. *Proceedings of IEEE Ultrasonics Symposium*, IEEE cat no 90CH2938-9, pp. 697–705.

Trahey G.E., Zhao D., Miglin J.A., and Smith S.W. 1990. Experimental results with a real-time adaptive ultrasonic imaging system for viewing through distorting media. *IEEE Trans. Ultrason. Ferroelec. Freq. Contr.* 37: 418.

von Ramm O.T. and Smith S.W. 1990. Real time volumetric ultrasound imaging system. In *SPIE Medical Imaging IV: Image Formation,Vol* 1231, pp. 15–22. New York, SPIE.

von Ramm O.T. and Thurstone F.L. 1976. Cardiac imaging using a phased array ultrasound system: I. System design. *Circulation* 53: 258.

Further Information

A good overview of linear array design and performance is contained in von O.T. Ramm and S.W. Smith (1983), Beam steering with linear arrays, *IEEE Trans. Biomed. Eng.* 30: 438. The same issue contains a more general article on transducer design and performance: J.W. Hunt, M.' Arditi, and F.S. Foster (1983), Ultrasound transducers for pulse-echo medical imaging, *IEEE Trans. Biomed. Eng.* 30: 453.

The journal *IEEE Transactions on Ultrasonics, Ferroelectrics, and Frequency Control* frequently contains articles on medical ultrasound transducers. For subscription information, contact IEEE Service Center, 445 Hoes Lane, P.O. Box 1331, Piscataway, NJ 08855-1331, phone (800) 678-IEEE.

Another good source is the proceedings of the IEEE Ultrasonics Symposium, published each year. Also, the proceedings from *New Developments in Ultrasonics Transducers and Transducer Systems*, edited by F.L. Lizzi, was published by SPIE, Vol. 1733, in 1992.

12.2 Ultrasonic Imaging

Jack G. Mottley

It was recognized long ago that the tissues of the body are inhomogeneous and that signals sent into them, like pulses of high-frequency sound, are reflected and scattered by those tissues. **Scattering**, or redirection of some of an incident energy signal to other directions by small particles, is why we see the beam of a spotlight in fog or smoke. That part of the scattered energy that returns to the transmitter is called the **backscatter**.

Ultrasonic imaging of the soft tissues of the body really began in the early 1970s. At that time, the technologies began to become available to capture and display the echoes backscattered by structures within the body as images, at first as static **compound images** and later as real-time moving images. The development followed much the same sequence (and borrowed much of the terminology) as did radar and sonar, from initial crude single-line-of-sight displays (**A-mode**) to recording these side by side to build up recordings over time to show motion (**M-mode**), to finally sweeping the transducer either mechanically or electronically over many directions and building up two-dimensional views (**B-mode or 2D**).

Since this technology was intended for civilian use, applications had to wait for the development of inexpensive data handling, storage, and display technologies. A-mode was usually shown on

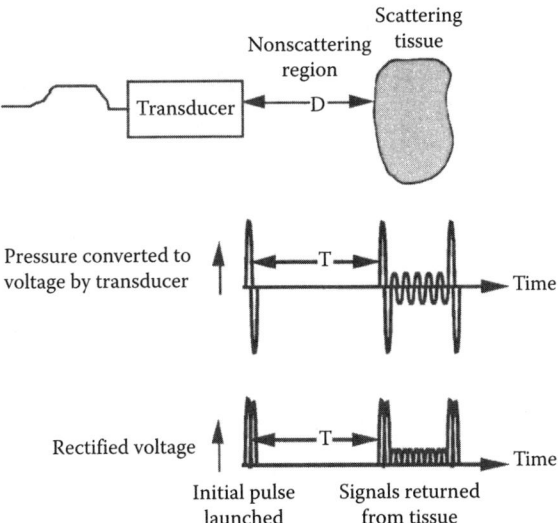

FIGURE 12.10 Schematic representation of the signal received from along a single line of sight in a tissue. The rectified voltage signals are displayed for A-mode.

oscilloscopes, M-modes were printed onto specially treated light-sensitive thermal paper, and B-mode was initially built up as a static image in analog scan converters and shown on television monitors. Now all modes are produced in real time in proprietary scan converters, shown on television monitors, and recorded either on commercially available videotape recorders (for organs or studies in which motion is a part of the diagnostic information) or as still frames on photographic film (for those cases in which organ dimensions and appearance are useful, but motion is not important).

Using commercial videotape reduces expenses and greatly simplifies the review of cases for quality control and training, since review stations can be set up in offices or conference rooms with commonly available monitors and videocassette recorders, and tapes from any imaging system can be played back. Also, the tapes are immediately available and do not have to be chemically processed.

Since the earliest systems were mostly capable of showing motion, the first applications were in studying the heart, which must move to carry out its function. A-mode and M-mode displays (see Figures 12.10 through 12.12) were able to demonstrate the motion of valves, thickening of heart chamber walls, relationships between heart motion and pressure, and other parameters that enabled diagnoses of heart problems that had been difficult or impossible before. For some valvular diseases, the preferred display format for diagnosis is still the M-mode, on which the speed of valve motions can be measured and the relations of valve motions to the electrocardiogram (ECG) are easily seen.

Later, as 2D displays became available, ultrasound was applied more and more to imaging of the soft abdominal organs and in obstetrics (Figure 12.13). In this format, organ dimensions and structural relations are seen more easily, and since the images are now made in real time, motions of organs such as the heart are still well appreciated. These images are used in a wide variety of areas from obstetrics and gynecology to ophthalmology to measure the dimensions of organs or tissue masses and have been widely accepted as a safe and convenient imaging modality.

12.2.1 Fundamentals

Strictly speaking, ultrasound is simply any sound wave whose frequency is above the limit of human hearing, which is usually taken to be 20 kHz. In the context of imaging of the human body, since frequency and wavelength (and therefore resolution) are inversely related, the lowest frequency of sound commonly used is around 1 MHz, with a constant trend toward higher frequencies in order to obtain

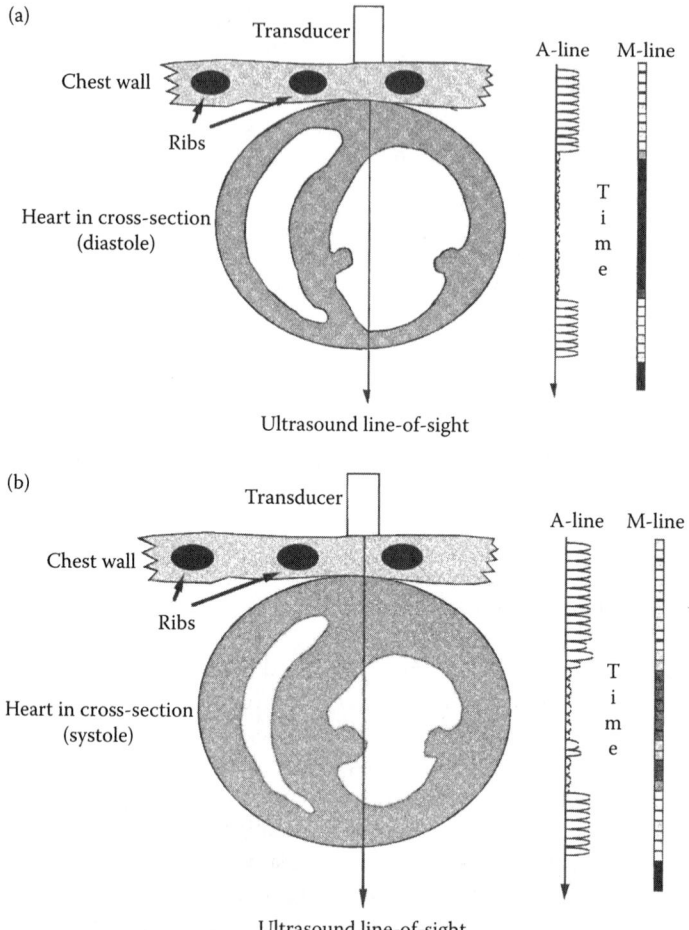

FIGURE 12.11 Example of M-mode imaging of a heart at two points during the cardiac cycle. (a) Upper panel shows heart during diastole (relaxation) with a line of sight through it and the corresponding A-line converted to an M-line. (b) The lower panel shows the same heart during systole (contraction) and the A- and M-lines. Note the thicker walls and smaller ventricular cross-section during systole.

better resolution. Axial resolution is approximately one wavelength, and at 1 MHz, the wavelength is 1.5 mm in most soft tissues, so one must go to 1.5 MHz to achieve 1-mm resolution.

Attenuation of ultrasonic signals increases with frequency in soft tissues, and so a tradeoff must be made between the depth of penetration that must be achieved for a particular application and the highest frequency that can be used. Applications that require deep penetration (e.g., cardiology, abdominal, obstetrics) typically use frequencies in the 2- to 5-MHz range, while those applications which only require shallow penetration but high resolution (e.g., ophthalmology, peripheral vascular, testicular) use frequencies up to around 20 MHz. Intra-arterial imaging systems, requiring submillimeter resolution, use even higher frequencies of 20 to 50 MHz, and laboratory applications of ultrasonic microscopy use frequencies up to 100 or even 200 MHz to examine structures within individual cells.

There are two basic equations used in ultrasonic imaging. One relates the (one-way) distance d of an object that caused an echo from the transducer to the (round-trip) time delay t and speed of sound in the medium c:

$$d = \frac{1}{2}tc$$

(12.24)

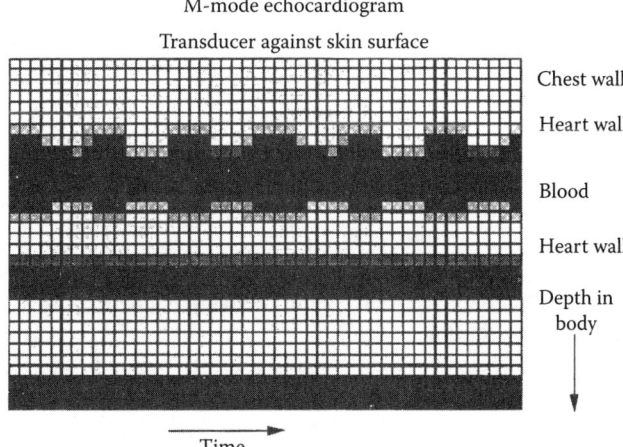

FIGURE 12.12 Completed M-mode display obtained by showing the M-lines of Figure 12.11 side by side. The motion of the heart walls and their thickening and thinning are well appreciated. Often the ECG or heart sounds are also shown in order to coordinate the motions of the heart with other physiologic markers.

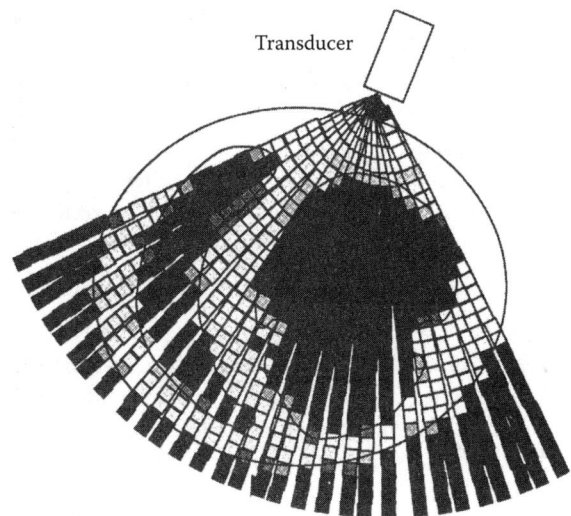

FIGURE 12.13 Schematic representation of a heart and how a 2D image is constructed by scanning the transducer.

The speed of sound in soft body tissues lies in a fairly narrow range from 1450 to 1520 m/sec. For rough estimates of time of flight, one often uses 1500 m/sec, which can be converted to 1.5 mm/μsec, a more convenient set of units. This leads to delay times for the longest-range measurements (20 cm) of 270 μsec.

To allow echoes and reverberations to die out, one needs to wait several of these periods before launching the next interrogating pulse, so pulse repetition frequencies of about a kilohertz are possible.

The other equation relates the received signal strength $S(t)$ to the transmitted signal $T(t)$, the transducer's properties $B(t)$, the attenuation of the signal path to and from the scatterer $A(t)$, and the strength of the scatterer $h(t)$:

$$S(t) = T(t) \otimes B(t) \otimes A(t) \otimes \eta(t) \tag{12.25}$$

where $\otimes$ denotes time-domain convolution. Using the property of Fourier transforms that a convolution in the time domain is a multiplication in the frequency domain, this is more often written in the frequency domain as

$$S(f) = T(f)B(f)A(f)\eta(f) \tag{12.26}$$

where each term is the Fourier transform of the corresponding term in the time-domain expression 12.25 and is written as a function of frequency f.

The goal of most imaging applications is to measure and produce an image based on the local values of the scattering strength, which requires some assumptions to be made concerning each of the other terms. The amplitude of the transmitted signal $T(f)$ is a user-adjustable parameter that simply adds a scale factor to the image values, unless it increases the returned signal to the point of saturating the receiver amplifier. Increasing the transmit power increases the strength of return from distant or faint echoes simply by increasing the power that illuminates them, like using a more powerful flashlight lets you see farther at night. Some care must be taken to not turn the transmit power up too high, since very high power levels are capable of causing acoustic cavitation or local heating of tissues, both of which can cause cellular damage. Advances in both electronics and transducers make it possible to transmit more and more power. For this reason, new ultrasonic imaging systems are required to display an index value that indicates the transmitted power. If the index exceeds established thresholds, it is possible that damage may occur, and the examiner should limit the time of exposure.

Most imaging systems are fairly narrow band, so the transducer properties $B(f)$ are constant and produce only a scale factor to the image values. On phased-array systems it is possible to change the depth of focus on both transmit and receive. This improves image quality and detection of lesions by matching the focusing characteristics of the transducer to best image the object in question, like focusing a pair of binoculars on a particular object.

As the ultrasonic energy travels along the path from transmitter to scatterer and back, attenuation causes the signal to decrease with distance. This builds up as a line integral from time 0 to time t as

$$A(f,t) = e^{-\int_0^t \alpha(f)c\,dt'}$$

An average value of attenuation can be corrected for electronically by increasing the gain of the imaging system as a function of time (variously called time gain compensation [TGC] or depth gain compensation [DGC]). In addition, some systems allow for lateral portions of the image region to have different attenuation by adding a lateral gain compensation in which the gain is increased to either side of the center region of the image.

Time gain compensation is usually set to give a uniform gray level to the scattering along the center of the image. Most operators develop a "usual" setting on each machine, and if it becomes necessary to change those settings to obtain acceptable images on a patient, then that indicates that the patient has a higher attenuation or that there is a problem with the electronics, transducer, or acoustic coupling.

12.2.2 Applications and Example Calculations

As an example of calculating the time of flight of an ultrasonic image, consider the following.

> *Example 12.1*: A tissue has a speed of sound $c = 1460$ m/sec, and a given feature is 10 cm deep within. Calculate the time it will take an ultrasonic signal to travel from the surface to the feature and back.
> *Answer*: $t = 2 \times (10 \text{ cm})/(1460 \text{ m/sec}) = 137 \text{ } \mu\text{sec}$, where the factor of 2 is to account for the round trip the signal has to make (i.e., go in and back out).

Example 12.2: Typical soft tissues attenuate ultrasonic signals at a rate of 0.5 dB/cm/MHz. How much attenuation would be suffered by a 3-MHz signal going through 5 cm of tissue and returning?
Answer: a = 3 MHz × (0.5 dB/cm/MHz)/(8.686 dB/neper) = 0.173 neper/cm, A (3 MHz, 5 cm) = $e^{(-0.173 \text{ neper/cm}) \times (5 \text{ cm}) \times 2}$ = 0.177.

12.2.3 Economics

Ultrasonic imaging has many economic advantages over other imaging modalities. The imaging systems are typically much less expensive than those used for other modalities and do not require special preparations of facilities such as shielding for x-rays or uniformity of magnetic field for MRI. Most ultrasonic imaging systems can be rolled easily from one location to another, so one system can be shared among technicians or examining rooms or even taken to patients' rooms for critically ill patients.

There are minimal expendables used in ultrasonic examinations, mostly the coupling gel used to couple the transducer to the skin and videotape or film for recording. Transducers are reusable and amortized over many examinations. These low costs make ultrasonic imaging one of the least expensive modalities, far preferred over others when indicated. The low cost also means these systems can be a part of private practices and used only occasionally.

As an indication of the interest in ultrasonic imaging as an alternative to other modalities, in 1993, the *Wall Street Journal* reported that spending in the United States on MRI units was approximately $520 million, on CT units $800 million, and on ultrasonic imaging systems $1000 million, and that sales of ultrasound systems was growing at 15% annually [1].

Defining Terms

A-mode: The original display of ultrasound measurements, in which the amplitude of the returned echoes along a single line is displayed on an oscilloscope.
Attenuation: The reduction is signal amplitude that occurs per unit distance traveled. Some attenuation occurs in homogeneous media such as water due to viscous heating and other phenomena, but that is very small and is usually taken to be negligible over the 10- to 20-cm distances typical of imaging systems. In inhomogeneous media such as soft tissues, the attenuation is much higher and increases with frequency. The values reported for most soft tissues lie around 0.5 dB/cm/MHz.
Backscatter: That part of a scattered signal that goes back toward the transmitter of the energy.
B-mode or 2D: The current display mode of choice. This is produced by sweeping the transducer from side to side and displaying the strength of the returned echoes as bright spots in their geometrically correct direction and distance.
Compound images: Images built up by adding, or compounding, data obtained from a single transducer or multiple transducers swept through arcs. Often these transducers were not fixed to a single point of rotation but could be swept over a surface of the body like the abdomen in order to build up a picture of the underlying organs such as the liver. This required an elaborate position-sensing apparatus attached to the patient's bed or the scanner and that the organ in question be held very still throughout the scanning process, or else the image was blurred.
M-mode: Followed A-mode by recording the strength of the echoes as dark spots on moving light-sensitive paper. Objects that move, such as the heart, caused standard patterns of motion to be displayed, and a lot of diagnostic information such as valve closure rates, whether valves opened or closed completely, and wall thickness could be obtained from M-mode recordings.
Real-time images: Images currently made on ultrasound imaging systems by rapidly sweeping the transducer through an arc either mechanically or electronically. Typical images might have 120 scan lines in each image, each 20 cm long. Since each line has a time of flight of 267 μsec,

a single frame takes 120×267 μsec $= 32$ msec. It is therefore possible to produce images at standard video frame rates (30 frames/sec, or 33.3 msec/frame).

Reflection: Occurs at interfaces between large regions (much larger than a wavelength) of media with differing acoustic properties such as density or compressibility. This is similar to the reflection of light at interfaces and can be either total, like a mirror, or partial, like a half-silvered mirror or the ghostlike reflection seen in a sheet of glass.

Scattering: Occurs when there are irregularities or inhomogeneities in the acoustic properties of a medium over distances comparable with or smaller than the wavelength of the sound. Scattering from objects much smaller than a wavelength typically increases with frequency (the blue-sky law in optics), while that from an object comparable to a wavelength is constant with frequency (why clouds appear white).

Reference

1. Naj A.K. 1993. Industry focus: Big medical equipment makers try ultrasound market; cost-cutting pressures prompt shift away from more expensive devices. *Wall Street J.*, November 30, B-4.

Further Information

There are many textbooks that contain good introduction to ultrasonic imaging. *Physical Principles of Ultrasonic Diagnosis*, by P. N. Wells, is a classic, and there is a new edition of another classic, *Diagnostic Ultrasound: Principles, Instruments and Exercises*, 4th ed., by Frederick Kremkau. Books on medical imaging that contain introductions to ultrasonic imaging include *Medical Imaging Systems*, by Albert Macovski; *Principles of Medical Imaging*, by Kirk Shung, Michael Smith, and Benjamin Tsui; and *Foundations of Medical Imaging*, by Zang-Hee Cho, Joie P. Jones, and Manbir Singh.

The monthly journals *IEEE Transactions on Ultrasonics, Ferroelectrics, and Frequency Control* and *IEEE Transactions on Biomedical Engineering* often contain information and research reports on ultrasonic imaging. For subscription information, contact IEEE Service Center, 445 Hoes Lane, P.O. Box 1331, Piscataway, NJ 08855-1331, phone (800) 678-4333. Another journal that often contains articles on ultrasonic imaging is the *Journal of the Acoustical Society of America*. For subscription information, contact AIP Circulation and Fulfillment Division, 500 Sunnyside Blvd., Woodbury, NY 11797-2999, phone (800) 344-6908; e-mail: elecprod\@pinet.aip.org.

There are many journals that deal with medical ultrasonic imaging exclusively. These include *Ultrasonic Imaging the Journal of Ultrasound in Medicine*, American Institute of Ultrasound of Medicine (AIUM), 14750 Sweitzer Lane, Suite 100, Laurel, MD 20707-5906, and the Journal of Ultrasound in Medicine and Biology, Elsevier Science, Inc., 660 White Plains Road, Tarrytown, NY 10591-5153, e-mail: esuk.usa@elsevier.com.

There are also specialty journals for particular medical areas, for example, the *Journal of the American Society of Echocardiography*, that are available through medical libraries and are indexed in Index Medicus, Current Contents, Science Citation Index, and other databases.

12.3 Blood Flow Measurement Using Ultrasound

K. Whittaker Ferrara

In order to introduce the fundamental challenges of blood velocity estimation, a brief description of the unique operating environment produced by the ultrasonic system, intervening tissue, and the scattering of ultrasound by blood is provided. In providing an overview of the parameters that differentiate this problem from radar and sonar target estimation problems, an introduction to the fluid dynamics of the cardiovascular system is presented, and the requirements of specific clinical applications are summarized. An overview of blood flow estimation systems and their performance limitations is then presented. Next, an overview of the theory of moving target estimation, with its roots in radar and sonar signal processing, is provided. The application of this theory to blood velocity estimation is then reviewed, and a number of signal processing strategies that have been applied to this problem are considered. Areas of new research including three-dimensional (3D) velocity estimation and the use of ultrasonic contrast agents are described in the final section.

12.3.1 Fundamental Concepts

In blood velocity estimation, the goal is not simply to estimate the mean target position and mean target velocity. The goal instead is to measure the velocity profile over the smallest region possible and to repeat this measurement quickly and accurately over the entire target. Therefore, the joint optimization of spatial, velocity, and temporal resolution is critical. In addition to the mean velocity, diagnostically useful information is contained in the volume of blood flowing through various vessels, spatial variations in the velocity profile, and the presence of turbulence. While current methods have proven extremely valuable in the assessment of the velocity profile over an entire vessel, improved *spatial resolution* is required in several diagnostic situations. Improved *velocity resolution* is also desirable for a number of clinical applications. Blood velocity estimation algorithms implemented in current systems also suffer from a velocity ambiguity due to aliasing.

12.3.1.1 Unique Features of the Operating Environment

A number of features make blood flow estimation distinct from typical radar and sonar target estimation situations. The combination of factors associated with the beam formation system, properties of the intervening medium, and properties of the target medium lead to a difficult and unique operating environment. Figure 12.14 summarizes the operating environment of an ultrasonic blood velocity estimation system, and Table 12.2 summarizes the key parameters.

12.3.1.1.1 Beam Formation—Data Acquisition System

The transducer bandwidth is limited. Most current transducers are limited to a 50 to 75% fractional bandwidth due to their finite dimensions and a variety of electrical and mechanical properties. This limits the form of the transmitted signal. The transmitted pulse is typically a short pulse with a carrier frequency, which is the center **frequency** in the spectrum of the transmitted signal.

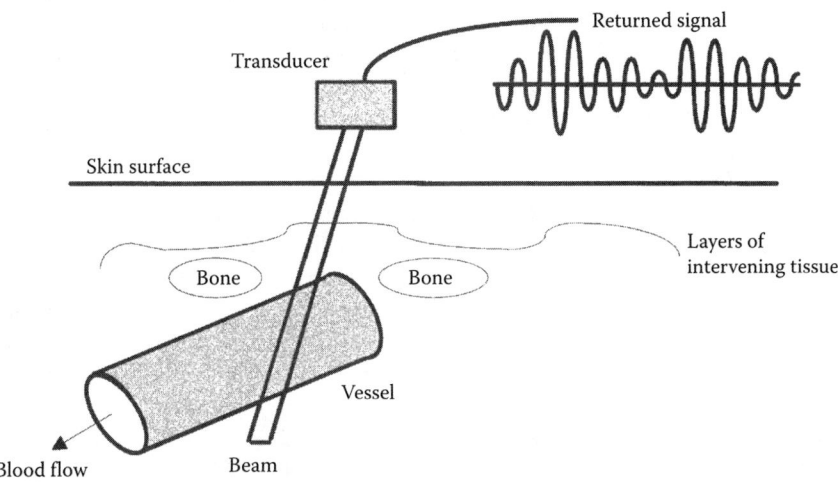

FIGURE 12.14 Operating environment for the estimation of blood velocity.

TABLE 12.2   Important Parameters

Typical transducer center frequency	2–10 MHz
Maximum transducer fractional bandwidth	50–75%
Speed of sound c	1500–1600 m/sec
Acoustic wavelength ($c = 1540$)	0.154–1.54 mm
Phased-array size	> 32·wavelength
Sample volume size	mm³
Blood velocity	Normal; up to 1 m/sec
	Pathological: up to 8 m/sec
Vessel wall echo/blood echo	20–40 dB
Diameter of a red blood cell	8.5 μm
Thickness of a red blood cell	2.4 μm
Volume of a red blood cell	87 ± 6 mm³
Volume concentration of cells (hematocrit)	45%
Maximum concentration without cell deformation	58%

Normal Adult Maximal Velocity (m/sec)		
Mitral	Flow	0.9
Tricuspid	Flow	0.5
Pulmonary	Artery	0.75
Left	Ventricle	0.9

Artery	Peak Systolic Velocity (cm/sec)	Standard Deviation
Proximal external iliac	99	22
Distal external iliac	96	13
Proximal common femoral	89	16
Distal common femoral	71	15
Proximal popliteal	53	9
Distal popliteal	53	24
Proximal peroneal	46	14
Distal peroneal	44	12

Federal agencies monitor four distinct intensity levels. The levels are TASA, TASP, TPSA, and TPSP, where T represents temporal, S represents spatial, A represents average, and P represents peak. Therefore, the use of long bursts requires a proportionate reduction in the transmitted peak power. This may limit the signal-to-noise ratio (SNR) obtained with a long transmitted burst due to the weak reflections from the complex set of targets within the body.

12.3.1.1.2 Intervening Medium

Acoustic windows, which are locations for placement of a transducer to successfully interrogate particular organs, are limited in number and size. Due to the presence of bone and air, the number of usable acoustic windows is extremely limited. The reflection of acoustic energy from bone is only 3 dB below that of a perfect reflector (Wells, 1977). Therefore, transducers cannot typically surround a desired imaging site. In many cases, it is difficult to find a single small access window. This limits the use of inverse techniques.

Intervening tissue produces acoustic refraction and reflection. Energy is reflected at unpredictable angles.

The **clutter**-to-signal ratio is very high. Clutter is the returned signal from stationary or slowly moving tissue, which can be 40 dB above the returned signal from blood. Movement of the vessel walls and valves during the cardiac cycle introduces a high-amplitude, low-frequency signal. This is typically considered to be unwanted noise, and a high-pass filter is used to eliminate the estimated wall frequencies.

The sampling rate is restricted. The speed of sound in tissue is low (~1540 m/sec), and each transmitted pulse must reach the target and return before the returned signal is recorded. Thus the sampling rate is restricted, and the aliasing limit is often exceeded.

The total observation time is limited (due to low acoustic velocity). In order to estimate the velocity of blood in all locations in a 2D field in real time, the estimate for each region must be based on the return from a limited number of pulses because of the low speed of sound.

Frequency-dependent attenuation affects the signal. Tissue acts as a low-pass transmission filter; the scattering functions as a high-pass filter. The received signal is therefore a distorted version of the transmitted signal. In order to estimate the effective filter function, the type and extent of each tissue type encountered by the wave must be known. Also, extension of the bandwidth of the transmitted signal to higher frequencies increases absorption, requiring higher power levels that can increase health concerns.

12.3.1.1.3 Target Scattering Medium (Red Blood Cells)

Multiple groups of scatterers are present. The target medium consists of multiple volumes of diffuse moving scatterers with velocity vectors that vary in magnitude and direction. The target medium is spread in space and velocity. The goal is to estimate the velocity over the smallest region possible.

There is a limited period of statistical stationarity. The underlying cardiac process can only be considered to be stationary for a limited time. This time was estimated to be 10 msec for the arterial system by Hatle and Angelsen (1985). If an observation interval greater than this period is used, the average scatterer velocity cannot be considered to be constant.

12.3.1.2 Overview of Ultrasonic Flow Estimation Systems

Current ultrasonic imaging systems operate in a pulse-echo (PE) or continuous-wave (CW) intensity mapping mode. In pulse-echo mode, a very short pulse is transmitted, and the reflected signal is analyzed. For a continuous-wave system, a lower-intensity signal is continuously transmitted into the body, and the reflected energy is analyzed. In both types of systems, an acoustic wave is launched along a specific path into the body, and the return from this wave is processed as a function of time. The return is due to reflected waves from structures along the line of sight, combined with unwanted noise. Spatial selectivity is provided by beam formation performed on burst transmission and reception. Steering of the beam to a particular angle and creating a narrow beam width at the depth of interest are accomplished by an effective lens applied to the ultrasonic transducer. This lens may be produced by a contoured material, or it may be simulated by phased pulses applied to a transducer array. The spatial weighting pattern will ultimately be the product of the effective lens on transmission and reception. The returned signal from the formed beam can be used to map the backscattered intensity into a two-dimensional gray-scale image, or to estimate target velocity. *We shall focus on the use of this information to estimate the velocity of red blood cells moving through the body.*

12.3.1.2.1 Single Sample Volume Doppler Instruments

One type of system uses the Doppler effect to estimate velocity in a single volume of blood, known as the sample volume, which is designated by the system operator. The Doppler shift frequency from a moving target can be shown to equal $2f_c v/c$, where f_c is the transducer center frequency in Hertz, c is the speed of sound within tissue, and v is the velocity component of the blood cells toward or away from the transducer. These "Doppler" systems transmit a train of long pulses with a well-defined carrier frequency and measure the Doppler shift in the returned signal. The spectrum of Doppler frequencies is proportional to the distribution of velocities present in the sample volume. The sample volume is on a cubic millimeter scale for typical pulse-echo systems operating in the frequency range of 2–10 MHz. Therefore, a thorough cardiac or peripheral vascular examination requires a long period. In these systems, 64–128 temporal samples are acquired for each estimate. The spectrum of these samples is typically computed using a fast Fourier transform (FFT) technique (Kay and Marple, 1981). The range of velocities present within the sample volume can then be estimated. The spectrum is scaled to represent velocity and plotted on the vertical axis. Subsequent spectral estimates are then calculated and plotted vertically adjacent to the first estimate.

12.3.1.2.2 Color Flow Mapping

In color flow mapping, a pseudo-color velocity display is overlaid on a 2D gray-scale image. Simultaneous amplitude and velocity information is thus available for a 2D sector area of the body. The clinical advantage is a reduction in the examination time and the ability to visualize the velocity profile as a 2D map. Figure 12.15 shows a typical color flow map of ovarian blood flow combined with the Doppler spectrum of the region indicated by the small graphic sample volume. The color flow map shows color-encoded velocities superimposed on the gray-scale image with the velocity magnitude indicated by the color bar on the side of the image. Motion toward the transducer is shown in yellow and red, and motion away from the transducer is shown in blue and green, with the range of colors representing a range of velocities to a maximum of 6 cm/sec in each direction. Velocities above this limit would produce aliasing for the parameters used in optimizing the instrument for the display of ovarian flow. A velocity of 0 m/sec would be indicated by black, as shown at the center of the color bar. Early discussions of the implementation of color flow mapping systems can be found in Curry and White (1978) and Nowicki and Reid (1981).

The lower portion of the image presents an intensity-modulated display of instantaneous Doppler components along the vertical axis. As time progresses, the display is translated along the horizontal axis to generate a Doppler time history for the selected region of interest (provided by Acuson Corporation, Mountain View, California).

Limitations of color flow instruments result in part from the transmission of a narrowband (long) pulse that is needed for velocity estimation but degrades spatial resolution and prevents mapping of the spatial-velocity profile. Due to the velocity gradient in each blood vessel, the transmission of a long pulse also degrades the velocity resolution. This is caused by the simultaneous examination of blood cells moving at different velocities and the resulting mixing of regions of the scattering medium, which can be distinctly resolved on a conventional B-mode image. Since the limited speed of acoustic propagation velocity limits the sampling rate, a second problem is aliasing of the Doppler frequency. Third, information regarding the presence of velocity gradients and turbulence is desired and is not currently available. Finally, estimation of blood velocity based on the Doppler shift provides only an estimate of the axial velocity, which is the movement toward or away from the transducer, and cannot be used to estimate movement across the transducer beam. It is the 3D velocity magnitude that is of clinical interest.

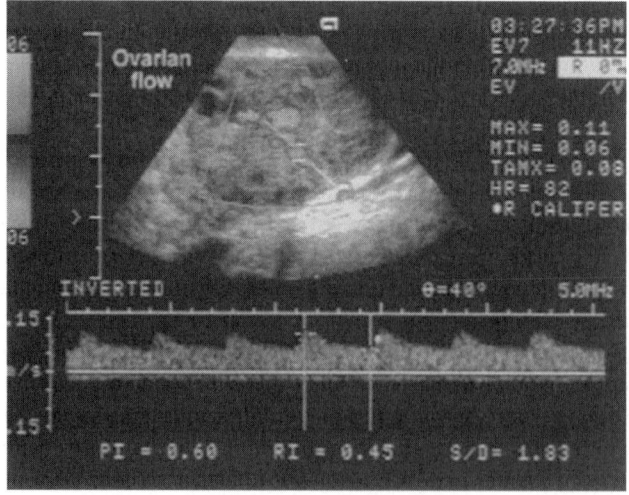

FIGURE 12.15 Flow map and Doppler spectrum for ovarian blood flow.

For a color flow map, the velocity estimation technique is based on estimation of the mean Doppler shift using signal-processing techniques optimized for rapid (real-time) estimation of velocity in each region of the image. The transmitted pulse is typically a burst of 4 to 8 cycles of the carrier frequency. Data acquisition for use in velocity estimation is interleaved with the acquisition of information for the gray-scale image. Each frame of acquired data samples is used to generate one update of the image display. An azimuthal line is a line that describes the direction of the beam from the transducer to the target. A typical 2D ultrasound scanner uses 128 azimuthal lines per frame and 30 frames per second to generate a gray-scale image. Data acquisition for the velocity estimator used in color flow imaging requires an additional 4 to 18 transducer firings per azimuthal line and therefore reduces both the number of azimuthal lines and the number of frames per second. If the number of lines per frame is decreased, spatial undersampling or a reduced examination area results. If the number of frames per second is decreased, temporal undersampling results, and the display becomes difficult to interpret.

The number of data samples available for each color flow velocity estimate is reduced to 4–18 in comparison with the 64–128 data samples available to estimate velocity in a single sample volume Doppler mode. This reduction, required to estimate velocity over the 2D image, produces a large increase in the estimator variance.

12.3.1.3 Fluid Dynamics and the Cardiovascular System

In order to predict and adequately assess blood flow profiles within the body, the fluid dynamics of the cardiovascular system will be briefly reviewed. The idealized case known as Poiseuille flow will be considered first, allowed by a summary of the factors that disturb Poiseuille flow.

A Poiseuille flow model is appropriate in a long rigid circular pipe at a large distance from the entrance. The velocity in this case is described by the equation $v/v_0 = 1 - (r/a)^2$, where v represents the velocity parallel to the wall, v_0 represents the center-line velocity, r is the radial distance variable, and a is the radius of the tube. In this case, the mean velocity is half the center-line velocity, and the volume flow rate is given by the mean velocity multiplied by the cross-sectional area of the vessel.

For the actual conditions within the arterial system, Poiseuille flow is only an approximation. The actual arterial geometry is tortuous and individualistic, and the resulting flow is perturbed by entrance effects and reflections. Reflections are produced by vascular branches and the geometric taper of the arterial diameter. In addition, spatial variations in vessel elasticity influence the amplitude and wave velocity of the arterial pulse. Several parameters can be used to characterize the velocity profile, including the Reynolds number, the Womersly number, the pulsatility index, and the resistive index. The pulsatility and resistive indices are frequently estimated during a clinical examination.

The Reynolds number is denoted Re and measures the ratio of fluid inertia to the viscous forces acting on the fluid. The Reynolds number is defined by $Re = Dv'/\mu_k$, where v' is the average cross-sectional velocity μ_k is the kinematic viscosity, and D is the vessel diameter. *Kinematic viscosity* is defined as the fluid viscosity divided by the fluid density. When the Reynolds number is high, fluid inertia dominates. This is true in the aorta and larger arteries, and bursts of turbulence are possible. When the number is low, viscous effects dominate.

The Womersly number is used to describe the effect introduced by the unsteady, pulsatile nature of the flow. This parameter, defined by $a(\omega/\mu_k)^{1/2}$, where ω represents radian frequency of the wave, governs propagation along an elastic, fluid-filled tube. When the Womersly number is small, the instantaneous profile will be parabolic in shape, the flow is viscous dominated, and the profile is oscillatory and Poiseuille in nature. When the Womersly number is large, the flow will be blunt, inviscid, and have thin wall layers (Nicholas and O'Rourke, 1990).

The pulsatility index represents the ratio of the unsteady and steady velocity components of the flow. This shows the magnitude of the velocity changes that occur during acceleration and deceleration of blood constituents. Since the arterial pulse decreases in magnitude as it travels, this index is maximum in the aorta. The pulsatility index is given by the difference between the peak systolic and minimum diastolic values divided by the average value over one cardiac cycle. The Pourcelot, or resistance, index is the peak-to-peak swing in velocity from systole to diastole divided by the peak systolic value (Nichols and O'Rourke, 1990).

12.3.1.3.1 Blood Velocity Profiles

Specific factors that influence the blood velocity profile include the entrance effect, vessel curvature, skewing, stenosis, acceleration, secondary flows, and turbulence. These effects are briefly introduced in this section.

The entrance effect is a result of fluid flow passing from a large tube or chamber into a smaller tube. The velocity distribution at the entrance becomes blunt. At a distance known as the entry length, the fully developed parabolic profile is restored, where the entry length is given by 0.06Re·(2*a*) (Nerem, 1985). Distal to this point the profile is independent of distance.

If the vessel is curved, there will also be an entrance effect. The blunt profile in this case is skewed, with the peak velocity closer to the inner wall of curvature. When the fully developed profile occurs downstream, the distribution will again be skewed, with the maximal velocity toward the outer wall of curvature. Skewing also occurs at a bifurcation where proximal flow divides into daughter vessels. The higher-velocity components, which occurred at the center of the parent vessel, are then closer to the flow divider, and the velocity distribution in the daughter vessels is skewed toward the divider.

Stenosis, a localized narrowing of the vessel diameter, dampens the pulsatility of the flow and pressure waveforms. The downstream flow profile depends on the shape and degree of stenosis. Acceleration adds a flat component to the velocity profile. It is responsible for the flat profile during systole, as well as the negative flat component near the walls in the deceleration phase.

Secondary flows are swirling components which are superimposed on the main velocity profile. These occur at bends and branches, although regions of secondary flow can break away from the vessel wall and are then known as separated flow. These regions reattach to the wall at a point downstream.

One definition of turbulent flow is flow that demonstrates a random fluctuation in the magnitude and direction of velocity as a function of space and time. The intensity of turbulence is calculated using the magnitude of the fluctuating velocities. The relative intensity of turbulence is given by $I_t = u_{rms}/u_{mean}$, where u_{rms} represents the root-mean-square value of the fluctuating portion of the velocity, and u_{mean} represents the nonfluctuating mean velocity (Hinze, 1975).

12.3.1.4 Clinical Applications and Their Requirements

Blood flow measurement with ultrasound is used in estimating the velocity and volume of flow within the heart and peripheral arteries and veins. Normal blood vessels vary in diameter up to a maximum of 2 cm, although most vessels examined with ultrasound have a diameter of 1 to 10 mm. Motion of the vessel wall results in a diameter change of 5 to 10% during a cardiac cycle.

12.3.1.4.1 Carotid Arteries (Common, Internal, External)

The evaluation of flow in the carotid arteries is of great clinical interest due to their importance in supplying blood to the brain, their proximity to the skin, and the wealth of experience that has been developed in characterizing vascular pathology through an evaluation of flow. The size of the carotid arteries is moderate; they narrow quickly from a maximum diameter of 0.8 cm. The shape of carotid flow waveforms over the cardiac cycle can be related to the pathophysiology of the circulation. Numerous attempts have been made to characterize the parameters of carotid waveforms and to compare these parameters in normal and stenotic cases. A number of indices have been used to summarize the information contained in these waveforms. The normal range of the Pourcelot index is 0.55 to 0.75. Many researchers have shown that accurate detection of a minor stenosis requires accurate quantitation of the entire Doppler spectrum and remains very difficult with current technology. The presence of a stenosis causes spectral broadening with the introduction of lower frequency or velocity components.

12.3.1.4.2 Cardiology

Blood velocity measurement in cardiology requires analysis of information at depths up to 18 cm. A relatively low center frequency (e.g., 2.5 to 3.5 MHz) typically is used in order to reduce attenuation. Areas commonly studied and the maximum rate of flow include the following (Hatle, 1985):

12.3.1.4.3 Aorta

Aortic flow exhibits a blunt profile with entrance region characteristics. The entrance length is approximately 30 cm. The vessel diameter is approximately 2 cm. The mean Reynolds number is 2500 (Nerem, 1985), although the peak Reynolds number in the ascending aorta can range from 4300 to 8900, and the peak Reynolds number in the abdominal aorta is in the range of 400 to 1100 (Nichols and O'Rourke, 1990). The maximal velocity is on the order of 1.35 m/sec. The flow is skewed in the aortic arch with a higher velocity at the inner wall. The flow is unsteady and laminar with possible turbulent bursts at peak systole.

12.3.1.4.4 Peripheral Arteries

The peak systolic velocity (Hatsukami et al., 1992) in centimeters per second and standard deviation of the velocity measurement technique are provided below for selected arteries.

Nearly all the vessels above normally show some flow reversal during early diastole. A value of the pulsatility index of 5 or more in a limb artery is considered to be normal.

12.3.2 Velocity Estimation Techniques

Prior to the basic overview of theoretical approaches to target velocity estimation, it is necessary to understand a few basic features of the received signal from blood scatterers. It is the statistical correlation of the received signal in space and time that provides the opportunity to use a variety of velocity estimation strategies. Velocity estimation based on analysis of the frequency shift or the temporal correlation can be justified by these statistical properties.

Blood velocity mapping has unique features due to the substantial viscosity of blood and the spatial limitations imposed by the vessel walls. Because of these properties, groups of redblood cells can be tracked over a significant distance. Blood consists of a viscous incompressible fluid containing an average volume concentration of red blood cells of 45%, although this concentration varies randomly through the blood medium. The red blood cells are primarily responsible for producing the scattered wave, due to the difference in their acoustic properties in comparison with plasma. Recent research into the characteristics of blood has led to stochastic models for its properties as a function of time and space (Atkinson and Berry, 1974; Shung et al., 1976, 1992; Angelson, 1980; Mo and Cobbold, 1986). The scattered signal from an insonified spatial volume is a random process that varies with the fluctuations in the density of scatterers in the insonified area, the shear rate within the vessel, and the hematocrit (Atkinson and Berry, 1974; Mo and Cobbold, 1986; Ferrara and Algazi, 1994a,b).

Since the concentration of cells varies randomly through the vessel, the magnitude of the returned signal varies when the group of scatterers being insonified changes. The returned amplitude from one spatial region is independent of the amplitude of the signal from adjacent spatial areas. As blood flows through a vessel, it transports cells whose backscattered signals can be tracked to estimate flow velocities.

Between the transmission of one pulse and the next, the scatterers move a small distance within the vessel. As shown in Figure 12.16, a group of cells with a particular concentration which are originally located at depth D_1 at time T_1 move to depth D_2 at time T_2. The resulting change in axial depth produces a change in the delay of the signal returning to the transducer from each group of scatterers. This change in delay of the radiofrequency (RF) signal can be estimated in several ways. As shown in Figure 12.17, the returned signal from a set of sequential pulses then shows a random amplitude that can be used to estimate the velocity. Motion is detected using signal-processing techniques that estimate the shift of the signal between pulses.

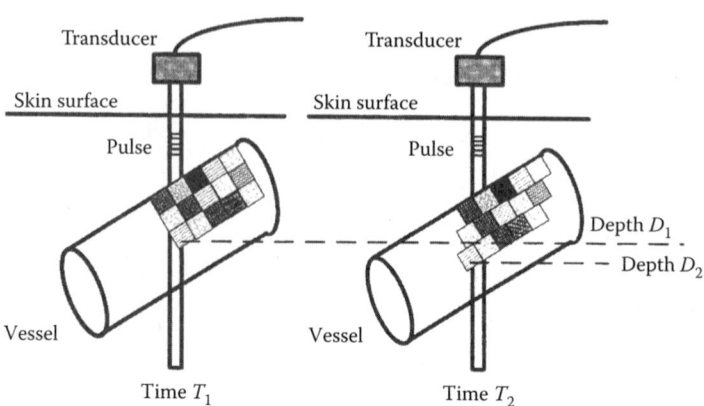

FIGURE 12.16 Random concentration of red blood cells within a vessel at times T_1 and T_2, where the change in depth from D_1 to D_2 would be used to estimate velocity.

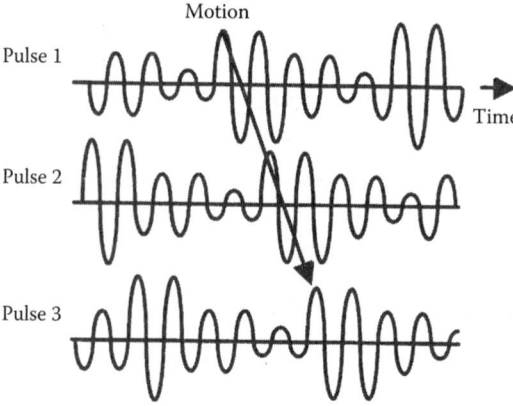

FIGURE 12.17 Received RF signal from three transmitted pulses, with a random amplitude which can be used to estimate the axial movement of blood between pulses. Motion is shown by the shift in the signal with a recognizable amplitude.

12.3.2.1 Clutter

In addition to the desired signal from the blood scatterers, the received signal contains clutter echoes returned from the surrounding tissue. An important component of this clutter signal arises from slowly moving vessel walls. The wall motion produces Doppler frequency shifts typically below 1 kHz, while the desired information from the blood cells exists in frequencies up to 15 kHz. Due to the smooth structure of the walls, energy is scattered coherently, and the clutter signal can be 40 dB above the scattered signal from blood. High-pass filters have been developed to remove the unwanted signal from the surrounding vessel walls.

12.3.2.2 Classic Theory of Velocity Estimation

Most current commercial ultrasound systems transmit a train of long pulses with a carrier frequency of 2 to 10 MHz and estimate velocity using the Doppler shift of the reflected signal. The transmission of a train of short pulses and new signal-processing strategies may improve the spatial resolution and quality of the resulting velocity estimate. In order to provide a basis for discussion and comparison of these techniques, the problem of blood velocity estimation is considered in this subsection from the view of classic velocity estimation theory typically applied to radar and sonar problems.

Important differences exist between classic detection and estimation for radar and sonar and the application of such techniques to medical ultrasound. The Van Trees (1971) approach is based on joint estimation of the Doppler shift and position over the entire target. In medical ultrasound, the velocity is estimated in small regions of a large target, where the target position is assumed to be known. While classic theories have been developed for estimation of all velocities within a large target by Van Trees and others, such techniques require a model for the velocity in each spatial region of interest. For the case of blood velocity estimation, the spatial variation in the velocity profile is complex, and it is difficult to postulate a model that can be used to derive a high-quality estimate. The theory of velocity estimation in the presence of spread targets is also discussed by Kennedy (1969) and Price (1968) as it applies to radar astronomy and dispersive communication channels.

It is the desire to improve the spatial and velocity resolution of the estimate of blood velocity that has motivated the evaluation of alternative wideband estimation techniques. Narrowband velocity estimation techniques use the Doppler frequency shift produced by the moving cells with a sample volume that is fixed in space. Wideband estimation techniques incorporate the change in delay of the returned pulse due to the motion of the moving cells. Within the classification of narrowband techniques are a number of estimation strategies to be detailed below. These include the fast Fourier transform (FFT), finite derivative estimation, the autocorrelator, and modern spectral estimation techniques, including autoregressive strategies. Within the classification of wideband techniques are cross-correlation strategies and the wideband maximum **likelihood** estimator (WMLE).

For improving the spatial mapping of blood velocity within the body, the transmission of short pulses is desirable. Therefore, it is of interest to assess the quality of velocity estimates made using narrowband and wideband estimators with transmitted signals of varying lengths. If $(2v/c)BT > 1$, where v represents the axial velocity of the target, c represents the speed of the wave in tissue, B represents the transmitted signal bandwidth, and T represents the total time interval used in estimating velocity within an individual region, then the change in delay produced by the motion of the red blood cells can be ignored (Van Trees, 1971).

This inequality is interpreted for the physical conditions of medical ultrasound in Figure 12.18. As shown in Figure 12.18, the value vT represents the axial distance traveled by the target while it is observed by the transducer beam, and $c/(2B)$ represents the effective length of the signal that is used to observe the moving cells. If $vT > c/(2B)$, the shift in the position of a group of red blood cells during their travel

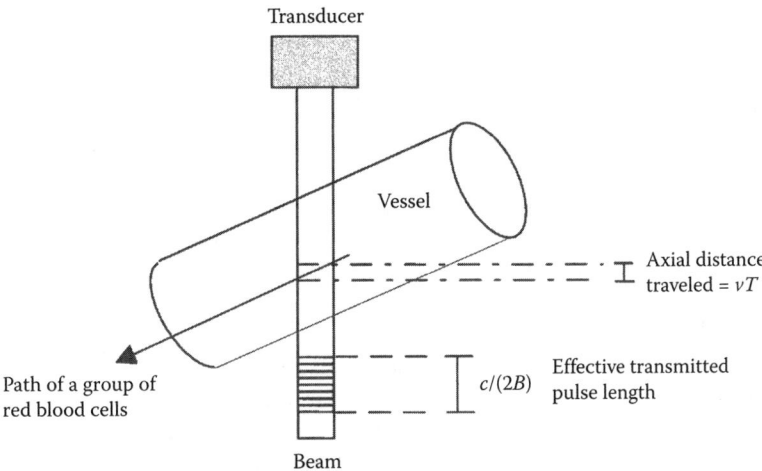

FIGURE 12.18 Comparison of the axial distance traveled and the effective length of the transmitted pulse.

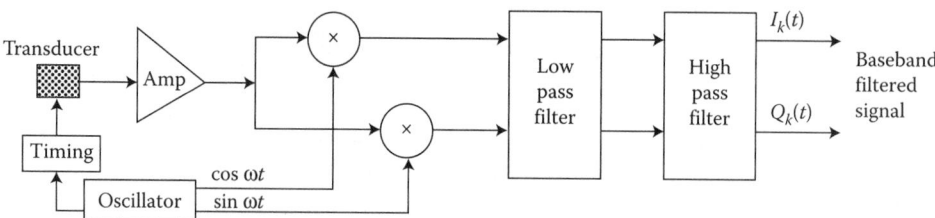

FIGURE 12.19 Block diagram of the system architecture required to generate the baseband signal used by several estimation techniques.

though the ultrasonic beam is not a detectable fraction of the signal length. This leads to two important restrictions on estimation techniques. First, under the "narrowband" condition of transmission of a long (narrowband) pulse, motion of a group of cells through the beam can only be estimated using the Doppler frequency shift. Second, if the inequality is not satisfied and therefore the transmitted signal is short (wideband), faster-moving red blood cells leave the region of interest, and the use of a narrowband estimation technique produces a biased velocity estimate. Thus two strategies can be used to estimate velocity. A long (narrowband) pulse can transmitted, and the signal from a fixed depth then can be used to estimate velocity. Alternatively, a short (wideband) signal can be transmitted in order to improve spatial resolution, and the estimator used to determine the velocity must move along with the red blood cells.

The inequality is now evaluated for typical parameters. When the angle between the axis of the beam and the axis of the vessel is 45 degrees, the axial distance traveled by the red blood cells while they cross the beam is equivalent to the lateral beam width. Using an axial distance vT of 0.75 mm, which is a reasonable lateral beam width, and an acoustic velocity of 1540 m/sec, the bandwidth of the transmitted pulse must be much less than 1.026 MHz for the narrowband approximation to be valid.

Due to practical advantages in the implementation of the smaller bandwidth required by **baseband signals**, the center frequency of the signal is often removed before velocity estimation. The processing required for the extraction of the baseband signal is shown in Figure 12.19. The returned signal from the transducer is amplified and coherently demodulated, through multiplication by the carrier frequency, and then a low-pass filter is applied to remove the signal sideband frequencies and noise. The remaining signal is the **complex envelope**. A high-pass filter is then applied to the signal from each fixed depth to remove the unwanted echoes from stationary tissue. The output of this processing is denoted as $I_k(t)$ for the in-phase signal from the kth pulse as a function of time and $Q_k(t)$ for the quadrature signal from the kth pulse.

12.3.2.3 Narrowband Estimation

Narrowband estimation techniques that estimate velocity for blood at a fixed depth are described in this subsection. Both the classic Doppler technique, which frequently is used in single-sample volume systems, and the autocorrelator, which frequently is used in color flow mapping systems, are included, as well as a finite derivative estimator and an autoregressive estimator, which have been the subject of previous research. The autocorrelator is used in real-time color flow mapping systems due to the ease of implementation and the relatively small bias and variance.

12.3.2.3.1 Classic Doppler Estimation

If the carrier frequency is removed by coherently demodulating the signal, the change in delay of the RF signal becomes a change in the phase of the baseband signal. The Doppler shift frequency from a moving target equals $2f_cv/c$. With a center frequency of 5 MHz, sound velocity of 1540 m/sec, and blood velocity of 1 m/sec, the resulting frequency shift is 6493.5 Hz. For the estimation of blood velocity, the Doppler shift is not detectable using a single short pulse, and therefore, the signal from a fixed depth and a train of pulses is acquired.

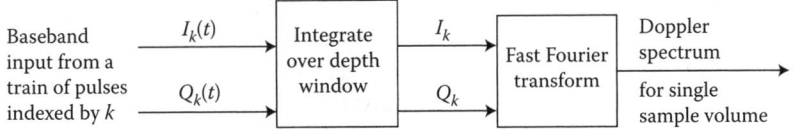

FIGURE 12.20 Block diagram of the system architecture required to estimate the Doppler spectrum from a set of baseband samples from a fixed depth.

A pulse-echo Doppler processing block diagram is shown in Figure 12.20. The baseband signal, from Figure 12.19, is shown as the input to this processing block. The received signal from each pulse is multiplied by a time window that is typically equal to the length of the transmitted pulse and integrated to produce a single data sample from each pulse. The set of data samples from a train of pulses is then Fourier-transformed, with the resulting frequency spectrum related to the axial velocity using the Doppler relationship.

Estimation of velocity using the Fourier transform of the signal from a fixed depth suffers from the limitations of all narrowband estimators, in that the variance of the estimate increases when a short pulse is transmitted. In addition, the velocity resolution produced using the Fourier transform is inversely proportional to the length of the data window. Therefore, if 64 pulses with a pulse repetition frequency of 5 kHz are used in the spectral estimate, the frequency resolution is on the order of 78.125 Hz (5000/64). The velocity resolution for a carrier frequency of 5 MHz and speed of sound of 1540 m/sec is then on the order of 1.2 cm/sec, determined from the Doppler relationship. Increasing the data window only improves the velocity resolution if the majority of the red blood cells have not left the sample volume and the flow conditions have not produced a decorrelation of the signal. It is this relationship between the data window and velocity resolution, a fundamental feature of Fourier transform techniques, that has motivated the use of autoregressive estimators. The frequency and velocity resolution are not fundamentally constrained by the data window using these modern spectral estimators introduced below.

12.3.2.3.2 Autoregressive Estimation (AR)

In addition to the classic techniques discussed previously, higher-order modern spectral estimation techniques have been used in an attempt to improve the velocity resolution of the estimate. These techniques are again narrowband estimation techniques, since the data samples used in computing the estimate are obtained from a fixed depth. The challenges encountered in applying such techniques to blood velocity estimation include the selection of an appropriate order which adequately models the data sequence while providing the opportunity for real-time velocity estimation and determination of the length of the data sequence to be used in the estimation process.

The goal in autogressive velocity estimation is to model the frequency content of the received signal by a set of coefficients which cold be used to reconstruct the signal spectrum. The coefficients $a(m)$ represent the AR parameters of the AR(p) process, where p is the number of poles in the model for the signal. Estimation of the AR parameters has been accomplished using the Burg and Levinson-Durban recursion methods. The spectrum $P(f)$ is then estimated using the following equation:

$$p(f) = k \left| 1 + \sum_{m=1}^{p} a(m) \exp[-i2\pi mf] \right|^{-2}$$

The poles of the AR transfer function which lie within the unit circle can then be determined based on these parameters, and the velocity associated with each pole is determined by the Doppler equation.

Both autoregressive and autoregressive moving-average estimation techniques have been applied to single-sample-volume Doppler estimation. Order selection for single-sample-volume AR estimators is discussed in Kaluzinski (1989). Second-order autoregressive estimation has been applied to color flow mapping by Loupas and McDicken (1990) andAhnandPark (1991). Although two poles are not sufficient to model the data sequence, the parameters of a higher-order process cannot be estimated in real time. In addition, the estimation of parameters of a higher-order process using the limited number of data points available in color flow mapping produces a large variance. Loupas and McDicken have used the two poles to model the signal returned from blood. Ahn and Park have used one pole to model the received signal from blood and the second pole to model the stationary signal from the surrounding tissue.

While AR techniques are useful in modeling the stationary tissue and blood and in providing a high-resolution estimate of multiple velocity components, several problems have been encountered in the practical application to blood velocity estimation. First, the order required to adequately model any region of the vessel can change when stationary tissue is present in the sample volume or when the range of velocity components in the sample volume increases. In addition, the performance of an AR estimate degrades rapidly in the presence of white noise, particularly with a small number of data samples.

12.3.2.3.3 Autocorrelator

Kasai et al. (1985) and Barber et al. (1985) discussed a narrowband mean velocity estimation structure for use in color flow mapping. The phase of the signal correlation at a lag of one transmitted period is estimated and used in an inverse tangent calculation of the estimated mean Doppler shift f_{mean} of the returned signal. A block diagram of the autocorrelator is shown in Figure 12.21. The baseband signal is first integrated over a short depth window. The phase of the correlation at a lag of one pulse period is then estimated as the inverse tangent of the imaginary part of the correlation divided by the real part of the correlation. The estimated mean velocity v_{mean} of the scattering medium is then determined by scaling the estimated Doppler shift by several factors, including the expected center frequency of the returned signal.

The autocorrelator structure can be derived from the definition of instantaneous frequency, from the phase of the correlation at a lag of one period, or as the first-order autoregressive estimate of the mean frequency of a baseband signal. The contributions of uncorrelated noise should average to zero in both the numerator and denominator of the autocorrelator. This is an advantage because the autocorrelation estimate is unbiased when the input signal includes the desired flow signal and noise. Alternatively, in the absence of a moving target, the input to the autocorrelator may consist only of white noise. Under these conditions, both the numerator and denominator can average to values near zero, and the resulting output of the autocorrelator has a very large variance. This estimation structure must therefore be used with a power threshold that can determine the presence or absence of a signal from blood flow and set the output of the estimator to zero when this motion is absent.

The variance of the autocorrelation estimate increases with the transmitted bandwidth, and therefore, the performance is degraded by transmitting a short pulse.

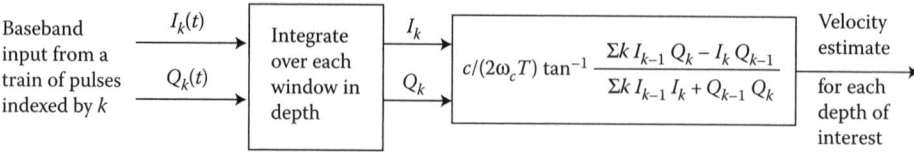

FIGURE 12.21 Block diagram of the system architecture required to estimate the mean Doppler shift for each depth location using the autocorrelator.

12.3.2.3.4 Finite Derivative Estimator (FDE)

A second approach to mean velocity or frequency estimation is based on a finite implementation of a derivative operator. The finite derivative estimator is derived based on the first and second moments of the spectrum. The basis for this estimator comes from the definition of the spectral centroid:

$$v_{mean} = \frac{\int \omega S(\omega) d\omega}{\int S(\omega) d\omega} \tag{12.27}$$

The mean velocity is given by v_{mean}, which is a scaled version of the mean frequency, where the scaling constant is given by k' and $S(\omega)$ represents the power spectral density. Letting $R_r(\cdot)$ represent the complex signal correlation and t represent the difference between the two times used in the correlation estimate, Equation 12.27 is equivalent to

$$v_{mean} = k' \frac{\left[(\partial/\partial\tau)R_r(\tau) \big|_{\tau=0} \right]}{R_r(0)} \tag{12.28}$$

Writing the baseband signal as the sum $I(t) + jQ(t)$ and letting E indicate the statistical expectation, Brody and Meindl (1974) have shown that the mean velocity estimate can be rewritten as

$$v_{mean} = \frac{k' E\{(\partial/\partial t)[I(t)]Q(t) - (\partial/\partial t)[Q(t)]I(t)\}}{E[I^2(t) + Q^2(t)]} \tag{12.29}$$

The estimate of this quantity requires estimation of the derivative of the in-phase portion $I(t)$ and quadrature portion $Q(t)$ of the signal. For an analog, continuous-time implementation, the bias and variance were evaluated by Brody and Meindl (1974). The discrete case has been studied by Kristoffersen (1986). The differentiation has been implemented in the discrete case as a finite difference or as a finite impulse response differentiation filter. The estimator is biased by noise, since the denominator represents power in the returned signal. Therefore, for nonzero noise power, the averaged noise power in the denominator will not be zero mean and will constitute a bias. The variance of the finite derivative estimator depends on the shape and bandwidth of the Doppler spectrum, as well as on the observation interval.

12.3.2.4 Wideband Estimation Techniques

It is desirable to transmit a short ultrasonic pulse in order to examine blood flow in small regions individually. For these short pulses, the narrowband approximation is not valid, and the estimation techniques used should track the motion of the red blood cells as they move to a new position over time. Estimation techniques that track the motion of the red blood cells are known as wideband estimation techniques and include cross-correlation techniques, the wideband maximum likelihood estimator and high time bandwidth estimation techniques. A thorough review of time-domain estimation techniques to estimate tissue motion is presented in Hein and O'Brien (1993).

12.3.2.4.1 Cross-Correlation Estimator

The use of time shift to estimate signal parameters has been studied extensively in radar. If the transmitted signal is known, a maximum likelihood (ML) solution for the estimation of delay has been discussed by Van Trees (1971) and others. If the signal shape is not known, the use of cross-correlation for delay estimation has been discussed by Helstrom (1968) and Knapp and Carter (1976). If information regarding the statistics of the signal and noise are available, an MLE based on cross-correlation

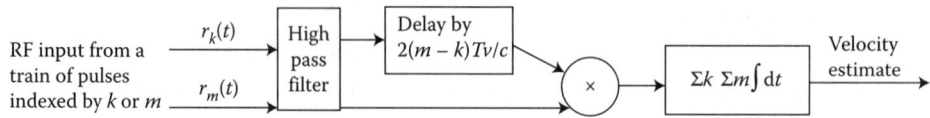

FIGURE 12.22 Block diagram of the system architecture required to estimate the velocity at each depth using a cross-correlation estimator.

has been proposed by Knapp and Carter (1976) known as the generalized correlation method for the estimation of time delay.

Several researchers have applied cross-correlation analysis to medical ultrasound. Bonnefous and Pesque (1986), Embree and O'Brien (1986), Foster et al. (1990), and Trahey et al. (1987) have studied the estimation of mean velocity based on the change in delay due to target movement. This analysis has assumed the shape of the transmitted signal to be unknown, and a cross-correlation technique has been used to estimate the difference in delay between successive pulses. This differential delay has then been used to estimate target velocity, where the velocity estimate is now based on the change in delay of the signal over an axial window, by maximizing the cross-correlation of the returned signal over all possible target velocities. Cross-correlation processing is typically performed on the radiofrequency (RF) signal, and a typical cross-correlation block diagram is shown in Figure 12.22. A high-pass filter is first applied to the signal from a fixed depth to remove the unwanted return from stationary tissue. One advantage of this strategy is that the variance is now inversely proportional to bandwidth of the transmitted signal rather than proportional.

12.3.2.4.2 Wideband Maximum Likelihood Estimator (WMLE)

Wideband maximum likelihood estimation is a baseband strategy with performance properties that are similar to cross-correlation. The estimate of the velocity of the blood cells is jointly based on the shift in the signal envelope and the shift in the carrier frequency of the returned signal. This estimator can be derived using a model for the signal that is expected to be reflected from the moving blood medium after the signal passes through intervening tissue. The processing of the signal can be interpreted as a filter matched to the expected signal. A diagram of the processing required for the wideband maximum likelihood estimator is shown in Figure 12.23 (Ferrara and Algazi, 1991). Assume that P pulses were transmitted. Required processing involves the delay of the signal from the $(P-k)$th pulse by an amount equal to $2v/ckT$, which corresponds to the movement of the cells between pulses for a specific v, followed by multiplication by a frequency which corresponds to the expected Doppler shift frequency of the baseband returned signal. The result of this multiplication is summed for all pulses, and the maximum likelihood velocity is then the velocity which produces the largest output from this estimator structure.

12.3.2.4.3 Estimation Using High-Time-Bandwidth Signals

Several researchers have also investigated the use of long wideband signals including "chirp" modulated signals and pseduo-random noise for the estimation of blood velocity. These signals are transmitted

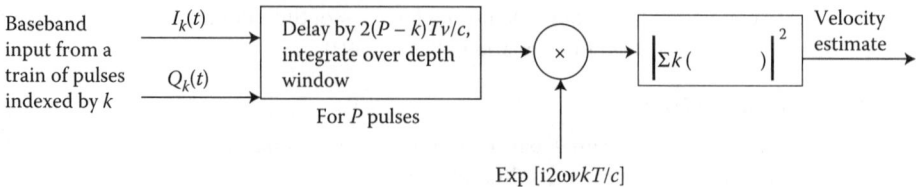

FIGURE 12.23 Block diagram of the system architecture required to estimate the velocity at each depth using the wideband MLE.

continuously (or with a short "flyback" time). Since these signals require continual transmission, the instantaneous power level must be reduced in order to achieve safe average power levels.

Bertram (1979) concluded that transmission of a "chirp" appears to give inferior precision for range measurement and inferior resolution of closely spaced multiple targets than a conventional pulse-echo system applied to a similar transducer. Multiple targets confuse the analysis. Using a simple sawtooth waveform, it is not possible to differentiate a stationary target at one range from a moving target at a different range. This problem could possibly be overcome with increasing and decreasing frequency intervals. Axial resolution is independent of the modulation rate, dependent only on the spectral frequency range (which is limited).

The limitations of systems that have transmitted a long pulse of random noise and correlated the return with the transmitted signal include reverberations from outside the sample volume which degrade the signal-to-noise ratio (the federally required reduction in peak transmitted power also reduces SNR), limited signal bandwidth due to frequency-dependent attenuation in tissue, and the finite transducer bandwidth (Cooper and McGillem, 1972; Bendick and Newhouse, 1974).

12.3.3 New Directions

Areas of research interest, including estimation of the 3D velocity magnitude, volume flow estimation, the use of high-frequency catheter-based transducers, mapping blood flow within malignant tumors, a new display mode known as color Doppler energy, and the use of contrast agents, are summarized in this subsection.

Estimation of the 3D velocity magnitude and beam vessel angle: Continued research designed to provide an estimate of the 3D magnitude of the flow velocity includes the use of crossed-beam Doppler systems (Wang and Yao, 1982; Overbeck et al., 1992) and tracking of speckle in two and three dimensions (Trahey et al., 1987). Mapping of the velocity estimate in two and three dimensions, resulting in a 3D color flow map has been described by Carson et al. (1992), Picot et al. (1993), and Cosgrove et al. (1990).

Volume flow estimation: Along with the peak velocity, instantaneous velocity profile, and velocity indices, a parameter of clinical interest is the volume of flow through vessels as a function of time. Estimation strategies for the determination of the volume of flow through a vessel have been described by Embree and O'Brien (1990), Gill (1979), Hottinger and Meindl (1979), and Uematsu (1981).

Intravascular ultrasound: It has been shown that intravascular ultrasonic imaging can provide information about the composition of healthy tissue and atheroma as well as anatomic data. A number of researchers have now shown that using frequencies of 30 MHz or above, individual layers and tissue types can be differentiated (de Kroon et al., 1991a,b; Lockwood et al., 1991). Although obvious changes in the vessel wall, such as dense fibrosis and calcification, have been identified with lower-frequency transducers, more subtle changes have been difficult to detect. Recent research has indicated that the character of plaque may be a more reliable predictor of subsequent cerebrovascular symptoms than the degree of vessel narrowing or the presence of ulceration (Merritt et al., 1992). Therefore, the recognition of subtle differences in tissue type may be extremely valuable. One signal-processing challenge in imaging the vascular wall at frequencies of 30 MHz or above is the removal of the unwanted echo from red blood cells, which is a strong interfering signal at high frequencies.

Vascular changes associated with tumors: Three-dimensional color flow mapping of the vascular structure is proposed to provide new information for the differentiation of benign and malignant masses. Judah Folkman and associates first recognized the importance of tumor vascularity in 1971 (Folkman et al., 1971). They hypothesized that the increased cell population required for the growth of a malignant tumor must be preceded by the production of new vessels. Subsequent work has shown that the walls of these vessels are deficient in muscular elements, and this deficiency results in a low impedance to flow (Gammill et al., 1976). This change can be detected by an increase in diastolic flow and a change in the resistive index.

More recently, Less et al. (1991) have shown that the vascular architecture of solid mammary tumors has several distinct differences from normal tissues, at least in the microvasculature. A type of network exists that exhibits fluctuations in both the diameter and length of the vessel with increasing branch order. Current color flow mapping systems with a center frequency of 5 MHz or above have been able to detect abnormal flow with varying degrees of clinical sensitivity from 40 to 82% (Belcaro et al., 1988; Balu-Maestro et al., 1991; Luska et al., 1992). Researchers using traditional Doppler systems have also reported a range of clinical sensitivity, with a general reporting of high sensitivity but moderate to low specificity. Burns et al., (1982) studied the signal from benign and malignant masses with 10-MHz CW Doppler. They hypothesized, and confirmed through angiography, that the tumors under study were fed by multiple small arteries, with a mean flow velocity below 10 cm/sec. Carson et al. (1992) compared 10-MHz CW Doppler to 5- and 7.5-MHz color flow mapping and concluded that while 3D reconstruction of the vasculature could provide significant additional information, color flow mapping systems must increase their ability to detect slow flow in small vessels in order to effectively map the vasculature.

Ultrasound contrast agents: The introduction of substances that enhance the ultrasonic echo signal from blood primarily through the production of microbubbles is of growing interest in ultrasonic flow measurement. The increased echo power may have a significant impact in contrast echocardiography, where acquisition of the signal from the coronary arteries has been difficult. In addition, such agents have been used to increase the backscattered signal from small vessels in masses that are suspected to be malignant. Contrast agents have been developed using sonicated albumen, saccharide microbubbles, and gelatin-encapsulated microbubbles.

Research to improve the sensitivity of flow measurement systems to low-velocity flow and small volumes of flow, with the goal of mapping the vasculature architecture, includes the use of ultrasonic contrast agents with conventional Doppler signal processing (Hartley et al., 1993), as well as the detection of the second harmonic of the transducer center frequency (Shrope and Newhouse, 1993).

Color Doppler energy: During 1993, a new format for the presentation of the returned signal from the blood scattering medium was introduced and termed color Doppler energy (CDE) or color power imaging (CPI). In this format, the backscattered signal is filtered to remove the signal from stationary tissue, and the remaining energy in the backscattered signal is color encoded and displayed as an overlay on the gray-scale image. The advantage of this signal-processing technique is the sensitivity to very low flow velocities.

Defining Terms

Baseband signal: The received signal after the center frequency component (carrier frequency) has been removed by demodulation.

Carrier frequency: The center frequency in the spectrum of the transmitted signal.

Clutter: An unwanted fixed signal component generated by stationary targets typically outside the region of interest (such as vessel walls).

Complex envelope: A signal expressed by the product of the carrier, a high-frequency component, and other lower-frequency components that comprise the envelope. The envelope is usually expressed in complex form.

Maximum likelihood: A statistical estimation technique that maximizes the probability of the occurrence of an event to estimate a parameter. ML estimate is the minimum variance, unbiased estimate.

References

Ahn Y. and Park S. 1991. Estimation of mean frequency and variance of ultrasonic Doppler signal by using second-order autoregressive model. *IEEE Trans. Ultrason. Ferroelec. Freq. Cont.* 38: 172.

Angelson B. 1980. Theoretical study of the scattering of ultrasound from blood. *IEEE Trans. Biomed. Eng.* 27: 61.

Atkinson P. and Berry M.V. 1974. Random noise in ultrasonic echoes diffracted by blood. *J. Phys. A: Math. Nucl. Gen.* 7: 1293.

Balu-Maestro C., Bruneton J.N., Giudicelli T. et al. 1991. Color Doppler in breast tumor pathology. *J. Radiol.* 72: 579.

Barber W., Eberhard J.W., and Karr S. 1985. A new time domain technique for velocity measurements using Doppler ultrasound. *IEEE Trans. Biomed. Eng.* 32: 213.

Belcaro G., Laurora G., Ricci A. et al. 1988. Evaluation of flow in nodular tumors of the breast by Doppler and duplex scanning. *Acta Chir. Belg.* 88: 323.

Bertram C.D. 1979. Distance resolution with the FM-CW ultrasonic echo-ranging system. *Ultrasound Med. Biol.* 61.

Bonnefous O. and Pesque P. 1986. Time domain formulation of pulse-Doppler ultrasound and blood velocity estimators by cross correlation. *Ultrason. Imag.* 8: 73.

Brody W. and Meindl J. 1974. Theoretical analysis of the CW Doppler ultrasonic flowmeter. *IEEE Trans. Biomed. Eng.* 21: 183.

Burns P.N., Halliwell M., Wells P.N.T., and Webb A.J. 1982. Ultrasonic Doppler studies of the breast. *Ultrasound Med. Biol.* 8: 127.

Carson P.L., Adler D.D., Fowlkes J.B. et al. 1992. Enhanced color flow imaging of breast cancer vasculature: Continuous wave Doppler and three-dimensional display. *J. Ultrasound Med.* 11: 77.

Cosgrove D.O., Bamber J.C., Davey J.B. et al. 1990. Color Doppler signals from breast tumors: Work in progress. *Radiology* 176: 175.

Curry G.R. and White D.N. 1978. Color coded ultrasonic differential velocity arterial scanner. *Ultrasound Med. Biol.* 4: 27.

de Kroon M.G.M., Slager C.J., Gussenhoven W.J. et al. 1991. Cyclic changes of blood echogenicity in high-frequency ultrasound. *Ultrasound Med. Biol.* 17: 723.

de Kroon M.G.M., van der Wal L.F., Gussenhoven W.J. et al. 1991. Backscatter directivity and integrated backscatter power of arterial tissue. *Int. J. Cardiac. Imag.* 6: 265.

Embree P.M. and O'Brien W.D. Jr. 1990. Volumetric blood flow via time-domain correlation: Experimental verification. *IEEE Trans. Ultrason. Ferroelec. Freq. Cont.* 37: 176.

Ferrara K. W and Algazi V.R. 1994a. A statistical analysis of the received signal from blood during laminar flow. *IEEE Trans. Ultrason. Ferroelec. Freq. Cont.* 41: 185.

Ferrara K.W. and Algazi V.R. 1994b. A theoretical and experimental analysis of the received signal from disturbed blood flow. *IEEE Trans. Ultrason. Ferroelec. Freq. Cont.* 41: 172.

Ferrara K.W. and Algazi V.R. 1991. A new wideband spread target maximum likelihood estimator for blood velocity estimation: I. Theory. *IEEE Trans. Ultrason. Ferroelec. Freq. Cont.* 38: 1.

Folkman J., Nerler E., Abernathy C., and Williams G. 1971. Isolation of a tumor factor responsible for angiogenesis. *J. Exp. Med.* 33: 275.

Foster S.G., Embree P.M., and O'Brien W.D. Jr. 1990. Flow velocity profile via time-domain correlation: Error analysis and computer simulation. *IEEE Trans. Ultrason. Ferroelec. Freq. Cont.* 37: 164.

Gammill S.L., Stapkey K.B., and Himmellarb E.H. 1976. Roenigenology—pathology correlative study of neovascularay. *AJR* 126: 376.

Gill R.W. 1979. Pulsed Doppler with B-mode imaging for quantitative blood flow measurement. *Ultrasound Med. Biol.* 5: 223.

Hartley C.J., Cheirif J., Collier K.R., and Bravenec J.S. 1993. Doppler quantification of echo-contrast injections *in vivo*. *Ultrasound Med. Biol.* 19: 269.

Hatle L. and Angelsen B. 1985. *Doppler Ultrasound in Cardiology*, 3rd ed. Philadelphia, Lea and Febiger.

Hatsukami T.S., Primozich J., Zierler R.E., and Strandness D.E. 1992. Color Doppler characteristics in normal lower extremity arteries. *Ultrasound Med. Biol.* 18(2): 167.

Hein I. and O'Brien W 1993. Current time domain methods for assessing tissue motion. *IEEE Trans. Ultrason. Ferroelec. Freq. Cont.* 40(2): 84.

Helstrom C.W. 1968. *Statistical Theory of Signal Detection*. London, Pergamon Press.

Hinze J.O. 1975. *Turbulence.* New York, McGraw-Hill.

Hottinger C.F. and Meindl J.D. 1979. Blood flow measurement using the attenuation compensated volume flowmeter. *Ultrason. Imag.* 1:1.

Kaluzinski K. 1989. Order selection in Doppler blood flow signal spectral analysis using autoregressive modelling. *Med. Biol. Eng. Com.* 27: 89.

Kasai C., Namekawa K., Koyano A., and Omoto R. 1985. Real-time two-dimensional blood flow imaging using an autocorrelation technique. *IEEE Trans. Sonics Ultrason.* 32.

Kay S. and Marple S.L. 1981. Spectrum analysis. A modern perspective. *Proc. IEEE* 69: 1380. Kennedy R.S. 1969. *Fading Dispersive Channel Theory.* New York, Wiley Interscience.

Knapp C.H. and Carter G.C. 1976. The generalized correlation method for estimation of time delay. *IEEE Trans. Acoust. Speech Signal Proc.* 24: 320.

Kristoffersen K. and Angelsen B.J. 1985. A comparison between mean frequency estimators for multigated Doppler systems with serial signal processing. *IEEE Trans. Biomed. Eng.* 32: 645.

Less J.R., Skalak T.C., Sevick E.M., and Jain R.K. 1991. Microvascular architecture in a mammary carcinoma: Branching patterns and vessel dimensions. *Cancer Res.* 51: 265.

Lockwood G.R., Ryan L.K., Hunt J.W., and Foster F.S. 1991. Measurement of the ultrasonic properties of vascular tissues and blood from 35-65 MHz. *Ultrasound Med. Biol.* 17: 653.

Loupas T. and McDicken W.N. 1990. Low-order AR models for mean and maximum frequency estimation in the context of Doppler color flow mapping. *IEEE Trans. Ultrason. Ferroelec. Freq. Cont.*37: 590.

Luska G., Lott D., Risch U., and von Boetticher H. 1992. The findings of color Doppler sonography in breast tumors. *Rofo Forts aufdem Gebiete derRontgens und derNeuen Bildg Verf 156:* 142.

Merritt C. and Bluth E. 1992. The future of carotid sonography. *AJR* 158: 37.

Mo L. and Cobbold R. 1986. A stochastic model of the backscattered Doppler ultrasound from blood. *IEEE Trans. Biomed. Eng.* 33: 20.

Nerem R.M. 1985. Fluid dynamic considerations in the application of ultrasound flowmetry. In S.A. Altobelli, W.F. Voyles, and E.R. Greene (Eds.), *Cardiovascular Ultrasonic Flowmetry.* New York, Elsevier.

Nichols W.W. and O'Rourke M.F. 1990. *McDonald's Blood Flow in Arteries: Theoretic, Experimental and Clinical principles.* Philadelphia, Lea and Febiger.

Nowicki A. and Reid J.M. 1981. An infinite gate pulse Doppler. *Ultrasound Med. Biol.* 7: 1.

Overbeck J.R., Beach K.W., and Strandness D.E. Jr. 1992. Vector Doppler: Accurate measurement of blood velocity in two dimensions. *Ultrasound Med. Biol.* 18: 19.

Picot P.A., Rickey D.W., and Mitchell R. et al. 1993. Three dimensional color Doppler mapping. *Ultrasound Med. Biol.* 19: 95.

Price R. 1968. Detectors for radar astronomy. In J. Evans and T. Hagfors (Eds.), *Radar Astronomy.* New York, McGraw-Hill.

Schrope B.A. and Newhouse V.L. 1993. Second harmonic ultrasound blood perfusion measurement. *Ultrasound Med. Biol.* 19: 567.

Shung K.K., Sigelman R.A., and Reid J.M. 1976. Scattering of ultrasound by blood. *IEEE Trans. Biomed. Eng.* 23: 460.

Shung K.K., Cloutier G., and Lim C.C. 1992. The effects of hematocrit, shear rate, and turbulence on ultrasonic Doppler spectrum from blood. *IEEE Trans. Biomed. Eng.* 39: 462.

Trahey G.E., Allison J.W., and Von Ramm O.T. 1987. Angle independent ultrasonic detection of blood flow. *IEEE Trans. Biomed. Eng.* 34: 964.

Uematsu S. 1981. Determination of volume of arterial blood flow by an ultrasonic device. *J. Clin. Ultrason.* 9: 209.

Van Trees H.L. 1971. *Detection, Estimation and Modulation Theory*, Part III. New York, Wiley.

Wang W. and Yao L. 1982. A double beam Doppler ultrasound method for quantitative blood flow velocity measurement. *Ultrasound Med. Biol.* 421.

Wells P.N.T. 1977. *Biomedical Ultrasonics.* London, Academic Press.

Further Information

The bimonthly journal *IEEE Transactions on Ultrasonics Ferroelectrics and Frequency* Control reports engineering advances in the area of ultrasonic flow measurement. For subscription information, contact IEEE Service Center, 445 Hoes Lane, P.O. Box 1331, Piscataway, NJ 08855-1331. Phone (800) 678-IEEE. The journal and the yearly conference proceedings of the IEEE Ultrasonic Symposium are published by the IEEE Ultrasonic Ferroelectrics and Frequency Control Society. Membership information can be obtained from the IEEE address above or from K. Ferrara, Riverside Research Institute, 330 West 42nd Street, New York, NY 10036.

The journal *Ultrasound in Medicine and Biology*, published 10 times per year, includes new developments in ultrasound signal processing and the clinical application of these developments. For subscription information, contact Pergamon Press, Inc., 660 White Plains Road, Tarrytown, NY 10591-5153. The American Institute of Ultrasound Medicine sponsors a yearly meeting which reviews new developments in ultrasound instrumentation and the clinical applications. For information, please contact American Institute of Ultrasound in Medicine, 11200 Rockville Pike, Suite 205, Rockville, MD 20852-3139; phone: (800) 638-5352.

13

Magnetic Resonance Microscopy

Xiaohong Zhou
Duke University Medical Center

G. Allan Johnson
Duke University Medical Center

Visualization of internal structures of opaque biologic objects is essential in many biomedical studies. Limited by the penetration depth of the probing sources (photons and electrons) and the lack of endogenous contrast, conventional forms of microscopy such as optical microscopy and electron microscopy require tissues to be sectioned into thin slices and stained with organic chemicals or heavy-metal compounds prior to examination. These invasive and destructive procedures, as well as the harmful radiation in the case of electron microscopy, make it difficult to obtain three-dimensional information and virtually impossible to study biologic tissues *in vivo*.

Magnetic resonance (MR) microscopy is a new form of microscopy that overcomes the aforementioned limitations. Operating in the radiofrequency (RF) range, MR microscopy allows biologic samples to be examined in the living state without bleaching or damage by ionizing radiation and in fresh and fixed specimens after minimal preparation. It also can use a number of endogenous contrast mechanisms that are directly related to tissue biochemistry, physiology, and pathology. Additionally, MR microscopy is digital and three-dimensional; internal structures of opaque tissues can be quantitatively mapped out in three dimensions to accurately reveal their histopathologic status. These unique properties provide new opportunities for biomedical scientists to attack problems that have been difficult to investigate using conventional techniques.

Conceptually, MR microscopy is an extension of magnetic resonance imaging (MRI) to the microscopic domain, generating images with spatial resolution better than 100 mm (Lauterbur, 1984). As such, MR microscopy is challenged by a new set of theoretical and technical problems (Johnson et al., 1992). For example, to improve isotropic resolution from 1 to 10 mm, signal-to-noise ratio (SNR) per voxel must be increased by a million times to maintain the same image quality. In order to do so, almost every component of hardware must be optimized to the fullest extent, pulse sequences have to be carefully designed to minimize any potential signal loss, and special software and dedicated computation facilities must be involved to handle large image arrays (e.g., 256^3). Over the past decade, development of MR microscopy has focused mainly on these issues. Persistent efforts by many researchers have recently lead to images with isotropic resolution of the order of ~10 μm (Cho et al., 1992; Johnson et al., 1992; Zhou and Lauterbur, 1992; Jacobs and Fraser, 1994). The significant resolution improvement opens up a broad range of applications, from histology to cancer biology and from toxicology to plant biology (Johnson et al., 1992). In this chapter we will first discuss the basic principles of MR microscopy, with special attention to such issues as resolution limits and sensitivity improvements. Then we will give an overview of the instrumentation. Finally, we will provide some examples to demonstrate the applications.

13.1 Basic Principles

13.1.1 Spatial Encoding and Decoding

Any digital imaging systems involve two processes. First, spatially resolved information must be encoded into a measurable signal, and second, the spatially encoded signal must be decoded to produce an image. In MR microscopy, the spatial encoding process is accomplished by acquiring nuclear magnetic resonance (NMR) signals under the influence of three orthogonal magnetic field gradients. There are many ways that a gradient can interact with a spin system. If the gradient is applied during a frequency-selective RF pulse, then the NMR signal arises only from a thin slab along the gradient direction. Thus a slice is selected from a three-dimensional (3D) object. If the gradient is applied during the acquisition of an NMR signal, the signal will consist of a range of spatially dependent frequencies given by

$$\omega(\vec{r}) = \gamma B_0 + \gamma \vec{G} \cdot \vec{r} \tag{13.1}$$

where γ is gyromagnetic ratio, B_0 is the static magnetic field, $\vec{G}$ is the magnetic field gradient, and $\vec{r}$ is the spatial variable. In this way, the spatial information along $\vec{G}$ direction is encoded into the signal as frequency variations. This method of encoding is called frequency encoding, and the gradient is referred to as a frequency-encoding gradient (or read-out gradient). If the gradient is applied for a fixed amount of time t_{pe} before the signal acquisition, then the phase of the signal, instead of the frequency, becomes spatially dependent, as given by

$$\phi(\vec{r}) = \int_0^{t_{pe}} \omega(\vec{r}) \, dt = \phi_0 + \int_0^{t_{pe}} \gamma \vec{G} \cdot \vec{r} \, dt \tag{13.2}$$

where ϕ_0 is the phase originated from the static magnetic field. This encoding method is known as phase encoding, and the gradient is called a phase-encoding gradient.

Based on the three basic spatial encoding approaches, many imaging schemes can be synthesized. For two-dimensional (2D) imaging, a slice-selection gradient is first applied to confine the NMR signal in a slice. Spatial encoding within the slice is then accomplished by frequency encoding and by phase encoding. For 3D imaging, the slice-selection gradient is replaced by either a frequency-encoding or a phase-encoding gradient. If all spatial directions are frequency-encoded, the encoding scheme is called projection acquisition, and the corresponding decoding method is called projection reconstruction (Lauterbur, 1973; Lai and Lauterbur, 1981). If one of the spatial dimensions is frequency encoded while the rest are phase encoded, the method is known as Fourier imaging, and the image can be reconstructed simply by a multidimensional Fourier transform (Kumar et al., 1975; Edelstein et al., 1980). Although other methods do exist, projection reconstruction and Fourier imaging are the two most popular in MR microscopy.

Projection reconstruction is particularly useful for spin systems with short apparent T_2 values, such as protons in lung and liver. Since the T_2 of most tissues decreases as static magnetic field increases, the advantage of projection reconstruction is more obvious at high magnetic fields. Another advantage of projection reconstruction is its superior SNR to Fourier imaging. This advantage has been theoretically analyzed and experimentally demonstrated in a number of independent studies (Callaghan and Eccles, 1987; Zhou and Lauterbur, 1992; Gewalt et al., 1993). Recently, it also has been shown that projection reconstruction is less sensitive to motion and motion artifacts can be effectively reduced using sinograms (Glover and Pauly, 1992; Gmitro and Alexander, 1993; Glover and Noll, 1993). Unlike projection reconstruction, data acquisition in Fourier imaging generates Fourier coefficients of the image in a cartesian coordinate. Since multidimensional fast Fourier transform algorithms can be applied directly to the raw data, Fourier imaging is computationally more efficient than projection reconstruction. This advantage is most evident when reconstructing 3D images with large arrays (e.g., 2563). In addition, Fourier transform imaging is less prone to image artifacts arising from various off-resonance effects and is more robust in applications such as chemical shift imaging (Brown et al., 1982) and flow imaging (Moran, 1982).

13.1.2 Image Contrast

A variety of contrast mechanisms can be exploited in MR microscopy, including spin density (r), spin–spin relaxation time (T_1), spin-lattice relaxation time (T_2), apparent T_2 relaxation time (T_2), diffusion coefficient (D), flow and chemical shift (d). One of the contrasts can be highlighted by varying data-acquisition parameters or by choosing different pulse sequences. Table 13.1 summarizes the pulse sequences and data-acquisition parameters to obtain each of the preceding contrasts.

In high-field MR microscopy (>1.5T), T_2 and diffusion contrast are strongly coupled together. An increasing number of evidences indicate that the apparent T_2 contrast observed in high-field MR microscopy is largely due to microscopic magnetic susceptibility variations (Majumdar and Gore, 1988; Zhong and Gore, 1991). The magnetic susceptibility difference produces strong local magnetic field gradients. Molecular diffusion through the induced gradients causes significant signal loss. In addition, the large external magnetic field gradients required for spatial encoding further increase the diffusion-induced signal loss. Since the signal loss has similar dependence on echo time (TE) to T_2-related loss, the diffusion contrast mechanism is involved in virtually all T_2-weighted images. This unique contrast mechanism provides a direct means to probe the microscopic tissue heterogeneities and forms the basis for many histopathologic studies (Benveniste et al., 1992; Zhou et al., 1994).

Chemical shift is another unique contrast mechanism. Changes in chemical shift can directly reveal tissue metabolic and histopathologic stages. This mechanism exists in many spin systems such as ^{1}H, ^{31}P, and ^{13}C. Recently, Lean et al. (1993) showed that based on proton chemical shifts, MR microscopy can detect tissue pathologic changes with superior sensitivity to optical microscopy in a number of tumor models. A major limitation for chemical-shift MR microscopy is the rather poor spatial resolution, since most spin species other than water protons are of considerably low concentration and sensitivity.

TABLE 13.1 Choice of Acquisition Parameters for Different Image Contrasts

Contrast	TR[a]	TE[a]	Pulse Sequences[b]
r	3–5 $T_{1,max}$	>$T_{2,max}$	SE, GE
T_1	–$T_{1,avg}$	>$T_{2,min}$	SE, GE
T_2	3–5 $T_{1,max}$	~$T_{2,avg}$	SE, FSE
T_2^*	3–5 $T_{1,max}$	~$T_{s,avg}^*$	GE
D[c]	3–5 $T_{1,max}$	>$T_{2,min}$	Diffusion-weighted SE, GE, or FSE

[a] Subscripts min, max and avg stand for minimum, maximum and average values, respectively.
[b] SE: spin-echo; GE: gradient echo; FSE: fast spin echo.
[c] A pair of diffusion weighting gradients must be used.

In addition, the long data-acquisition time required to resolve both spatial and spectral information also appears as an obstacle.

13.2 Resolution Limits

13.2.1 Intrinsic Resolution Limit

Intrinsic resolution is defined as the width of the point-spread function originated from physics laws. In MR microscopy, the intrinsic resolution arises from two sources: natural linewidth broadening and diffusion (House, 1984; Callaghan and Eccles, 1988; Cho et al., 1988).

In most conventional pulse sequences, natural linewidth broadening affects the resolution limit only in the frequency-encoding direction. In some special cases, such as fast spin echo (Hennig et al., 1986) and echo planar imaging (Mansfield and Maudsley, 1977), natural linewidth broadening also imposes resolution limits in the phase-encoding direction (Zhou et al., 1993). The natural linewidth resolution limit, defined by

$$\Delta r_{\text{n.l.w.}} = \frac{2}{\gamma G T_2} \tag{13.3}$$

is determined by the T_2 relaxation time and can be improved using a stronger gradient G. To obtain 1 mm resolution from a specimen with $T_2 = 50$ msec, the gradient should be at least 14.9 G/cm. This gradient requirement is well within the range of most MR microscopes.

Molecular diffusion affects the spatial resolution in a number of ways. The bounded diffusion is responsible for many interesting phenomena known as edge enhancements (Hills et al., 1990; Hyslop and Lauterbur, 1991; Putz et al., 1991; Callaghan et al., 1993). They are observable only at the microscopic resolution and are potentially useful to detect microscopic boundaries. The unbounded diffusion, on the other hand, causes signal attenuation, line broadening, and phase misregistration. All these effects originate from an incoherent and irreversible phase-dispersion. The root-mean-square value of the phase dispersion is

$$\sigma = \gamma \left\{ 2D \int_0^t \left[\int_t^t G(t'') dt'' \right]^2 dt' \right\}^{1/2} \tag{13.4}$$

where t' and t are pulse-sequence-dependent time variables defined by Ahn and Cho (1989). Because of the phase uncertainty, an intrinsic resolution limit along the phase encoding direction arises:

$$\Delta r_{\text{pe}} = \frac{\sigma}{\gamma \int_0^t G_{\text{pe}}(t') dt'} \tag{13.5}$$

For a rectangularly shaped phase-encoding gradient, the preceding equation can be reduced to a very simple form:

$$\Delta r_{\text{pe}} = \sqrt{\frac{2}{3} D t_{\text{pe}}} \tag{13.6}$$

This simple result indicates that the diffusion resolution limit in the phase-encoded direction is determined only by the phase-encoding time t_{pe} (D is a constant for a chosen sample). This is so because the phase uncertainty is introduced only during the phase-encoding period. Once the spins are phase-encoded, they always carry the same spatial information no matter where they diffuse to. In the frequency-encoding direction, diffusion imposes resolution limits by broadening the point-spread function. Unlike natural linewidth broadening, broadening caused by diffusion is pulse-sequence-dependent. For the simplest pulse sequence, a 3D projection acquisition using free induction decays, the full width at half maximum (Callaghan and Eccles, 1988; McFarland, 1992; Zhou, 1992) is

$$\Delta r_{fr} = 8 \left[\frac{D(\ln 2)^2}{3 \gamma G_{fr}} \right]^{1/3} \tag{13.7}$$

Compared with the case of the natural linewidth broadening (Equation 13.3), the resolution limit caused by diffusion varies slowly with the frequency-encoding gradient G_{fr}. Therefore, to improve resolution by a same factor, a much larger gradient is required. With the currently achievable gradient strength, the diffusion resolution limit is estimated to be 5 to 10 μm.

13.2.2 Digital Resolution Limit

When the requirements imposed by intrinsic resolution limits are satisfied, image resolution is largely determined by the voxel size, provided that SNR is sufficient and the amplitude of physiologic motion is limited to a voxel. The voxel size, also known as digital resolution, can be calculated from the following equations:

Frequency-encoding direction:

$$\Delta x \equiv \frac{L_x}{N_x} = \frac{\Delta v}{2\pi \gamma G_x N_x} \tag{13.8}$$

Phase-encoding direction:

$$\Delta y \equiv \frac{L_y}{N_y} = \frac{\Delta \phi}{\gamma G_y t_{pe}} \tag{13.9}$$

where L is the field of view, N is the number of data points or the linear matrix size, G is the gradient strength, Δv is the receiver bandwidth, $\Delta \phi$ is the phase range of the phase-encoding data (e.g., if the data cover a phase range from $-\pi$ to $+\pi$, then $\Delta \phi = 2\pi$), and the subscripts x and y represent frequency- and phase-encoding directions, respectively. To obtain a high digital resolution, L should be kept minimal, while N maximal. In practice, the minimal field of view and the maximal data points are constrained by other experimental parameters. In the frequency-encoding direction, decreasing field of view results in an increase in gradient amplitude at a constant receiver bandwidth or a decrease in the bandwidth for a constant gradient (Equation 13.8). Since the receiver bandwidth must be large enough to keep the acquisition of NMR signals within a certain time window, the largest available gradient strength thus imposes the digital resolution limit. In the phase-encoding direction, $\Delta \phi$ is fixed at 2π in most experiments, and the maximum t_{pe} value is refrained by the echo time. Thus digital resolution is also determined by the maximum available gradient, as indicated by Equation 13.9. It has been estimated that in order to achieve 1 mm resolution with a phase-encoding time of 4 msec, the required gradient strength is as high as 587 G/cm. This gradient requirement is beyond the range of current MR microscopes. Fortunately, the requirement is fully relaxed in projection acquisition where no phase encoding is involved.

13.2.3 Practical Resolution Limit

The intrinsic resolution limits predict that MR microscopy can theoretically reach the micron regime. To realize the resolution, one must overcome several technical obstacles. These obstacles, or practical resolution limits, include insufficient SNR, long data-acquisition times, and physiologic motion. At the current stage of development, these practical limitations are considerably more important than other resolution limits discussed earlier and actually determine the true image resolution.

SNR is of paramount importance in MR microscopy. As resolution improves, the total number of spins per voxel decreases drastically, resulting in a cubic decrease in signal intensity. When the voxel signal intensity becomes comparable with noise level, structures become unresolvable even if the digital resolution and intrinsic resolution are adequate.

SNR in a voxel depends on many factors. The relationship between SNR and common experimental variables is given by

$$\text{SNR} \propto \frac{B_1 B_0^2 \sqrt{n}}{\sqrt{4kT\Delta\nu(R_{\text{coil}} + R_{\text{sample}})}} \tag{13.10}$$

where B_1 is the RF magnetic field, B_0 is the static magnetic field, n is the number of average, T is the temperature, $\Delta\nu$ is the bandwidth, k is the Boltzmann constant, and R_{coil} and R_{sample} are the coil and sample resistance, respectively. When small RF coils are used, R_{sample} is negligible. Since R_{coil} is proportional to due to skin effects, the overall SNR increases as $B_0^{7/4}$. This result strongly suggests that MR microscopy be performed at high magnetic field. Another way to improve SNR is to increase the B_1 field. This is accomplished by reducing the size of RF coils (Peck et al., 1990; McFarland and Mortara, 1992; Schoeniger et al., 1991; Zhou and Lauterbur, 1992). Although increasing B_0 and B_1 is the most common approach to attacking the SNR problem, other methods such as signal averaging, pulse-sequence optimization, and post data processing are also useful in MR microscopy. For example, diffusion-induced signal loss can be effectively minimized using diffusion-reduced-gradient (DRG) echo pulse sequences (Cho et al., 1992). Various forms of projection acquisition techniques (Hedges, 1984; McFarland and Mortara, 1992; Zhou and Lauterbur, 1992; Gewalt et al., 1993), as well as new k-space sampling schemes (Zhou et al., 1993), also have proved useful in SNR improvements. Recently, Black et al. (1993) used high-temperature superconducting materials for coil fabrication to simultaneously reduce coil resistance R_{coil} and coil temperature T. This novel approach can provide up to 70-fold SNR increase, equivalent to the SNR gain by increasing the magnetic field strength 11 times.

Long data-acquisition time is another practical limitation. Large image arrays, long repetition times (TR), and signal averaging all contribute to the overall acquisition time. For instance, a T_2-weighted image with a 256^3 image array requires a total acquisition time of more than 18 h (assuming TR = 500 msec and $n = 2$). Such a long acquisition time is unacceptable for most applications. To reduce the acquisition time while still maintaining the desired contrast, fast-imaging pulse sequences such as echo-planar imaging (EPI) (Mansfield and Maudsley, 1977), driven equilibrium Fourier transform (DEFT) (Maki et al., 1988), fast low angle shot (FLASH) (Haase et al., 1986), gradient refocused acquisition at steady state (GRASS) (Karis et al., 1987), and rapid acquisition with relaxation enhancement (RARE) (Hennig et al., 1986) have been developed and applied to MR microscopy. The RARE pulse sequence, or fast spin-echo (FSE) (Mulkern et al., 1990), is particularly useful in high-field MR microscopy because of its insensitivity to magnetic susceptibility effects as well as the reduced diffusion loss (Zhou et al., 1993). Using fast spin-echo techniques, a 256^3 image has been acquired in less than 2 h (Zhou et al., 1993).

For *in vivo* studies, the true image resolution is also limited by physiologic motion (Hedges, 1984; Wood and Henkelman, 1985). Techniques to minimize the motion effects have been largely focused on pulse sequences and post data processing algorithms, including navigator echoes (Ehman and Felmlee, 1989), motion compensation using even echo or moment nulling gradients, projection acquisition (Glover and

Noll, 1993), and various kinds of ghost-image decomposition techniques (Xiang and Henkelman, 1991). It should be noted, however, that by refining animal handling techniques and using synchronized data acquisition, physiologic motion effects can be effectively avoided and very high quality images can be obtained (Hedlund et al., 1986; Johnson et al., 1992).

13.3 Instrumentation

An MR microscope consists of a high-field magnet (>1.5 T), a set of gradient coils, an RF coil (or RF coils), and the associated RF systems, gradient power supplies, and computers. Among these components, RF coils and gradient coils are often customized for specific applications in order to achieve optimal performance. Some general guidelines to design customized RF coils and gradient coils are presented below.

13.3.1 Radiofrequency Coils

Many types of RF coils can be used in MR microscopy (Figure 13.1). The choice of a particular coil configuration is determined by specific task and specimen size. If possible, the smallest coil size should always be chosen in order to obtain the highest SNR. For *ex-vivo* studies of tissue specimens, solenoid coils are a common choice because of their superior B_1 field homogeneity, high sensitivity, as well as simplicity in fabrication. Using a 2.9 mm solenoid coil (5 turn), Zhou and Lauterbur (1992) have achieved the highest ever reported spatial resolution at 6.4 μm^3. Solenoid coil configurations are also used by others to obtain images with similar resolution (~10 μm) (Hedges, 1984; Cho et al., 1988; Schoeniger et al., 1991; McFarland and Mortara, 1992). Recently, several researchers began to develop microscopic solenoid coils with a size of a few hundred microns (Peck et al., 1990; McFarland and Mortara, 1992). Fabrication of these microcoils often requires special techniques, such as light lithography and electron-beam lithography.

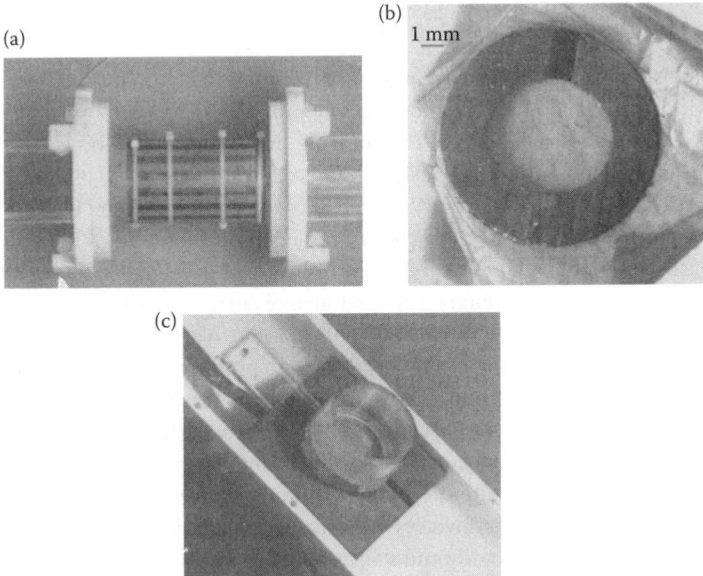

FIGURE 13.1   A range of radiofrequency coils are used in MR microscopy. (a) A quadrature birdcage coil scaled to the appropriate diameter for rats (6 cm) is used for whole-body imaging. (b) Resonant coils have been constructed on microwave substrate that can be surgically implanted to provide both localization and improved SNR. (c) MR microscopy of specimens is accomplished with a modified Helmholz coil providing good filling factors, high B homogeneity, and ease of access.

The direction of the B_1 field generated by a solenoid coil prevents the coil from being coaxially placed in the magnet. Thus accessing and positioning samples are difficult. To solve this problem, Banson et al. (1992) devised a unique Helmholtz coil that consists of two separate loops. Each loop is made from a microwave laminate with a dielectric material sandwiched between two copper foils. By making use of the distributed capacitance, the coil can be tuned to a desired frequency. Since the two loops of the coil are mechanically separated, samples can be easily slid into the gap between the loops without any obstruction. Under certain circumstances, the Helmholtz coil can outperform an optimally designed solenoid coil with similar dimensions.

For *in vivo* studies, although volume coils such as solenoid coils and birdcage coils can be employed, most high-resolution experiments are carried out using local RF coils, including surface coils (Rudin, 1987; Banson et al., 1992) and implanted coils (Hollett et al., 1987; Farmer et al., 1989; Zhou et al., 1994). Surface coils can effectively reduce coil size and simultaneously limit the field of view to a small region of interest. They can be easily adaptable to the shape of samples and provide high sensitivity in the surface region. The problem of inhomogeneous B_1 fields can be minimized using composite pulses (Hetherington et al., 1986) or adiabatic pulses (Ugurbil et al., 1987). To obtain high-resolution images from regions distant from the surface, surgically implantable coils become the method of choice. These coils not only give better SNR than optimized surface coils (Zhou et al., 1992) but also provide accurate and consistent localization. The latter advantage is particularly useful for time-course studies on dynamic processes such as the development of pathology and monitoring the effects of therapeutic drugs.

The recent advent of high-temperature superconducting (HTS) RF coils has brought new excitement to MR microscopy (Black et al., 1993). The substantial improvement, as discussed earlier, makes signal averaging unnecessary. Using these coils, the total imaging time will be solely determined by the efficiency to traverse the *k*-space. Although much research is yet to be done in this new area, combination of the HTS coils with fast-imaging algorithms will most likely provide a unique way to fully realize the potential of MR microscopy and eventually bring the technique into routine use.

13.3.2 Magnetic Field Gradient Coils

As discussed previously, high spatial resolution requires magnetic field gradients. The gradient strength increases proportional to the coil current and inversely proportional to the coil size. Since increasing current generates many undesirable effects (overheating, mechanical vibrations, eddy current, etc.), strong magnetic field gradient is almost exclusively achieved by reducing the coil diameter.

Design of magnetic field gradient coils for MR microscopy is a classic problem. Based on Maxwell equations, ideal surface current density can be calculated for a chosen geometry of the conducting surface. Two conducting surfaces are mostly used: a cylindrical surface parallel to the axis of the magnet and a cylindrical surface perpendicular to the axis. The ideal surface current density distributions for these two geometries are illustrated in Figure 13.2 (Suits and Wilken, 1989). After the ideal surface current density distribution is obtained, design of gradient coils is reduced to a problem of using discrete conductors with a finite length to approximate the continuous current distribution function. The error in the approximation determines the gradient linearity. Recent advancements in computer-based fabrication and etching techniques have made it feasible to produce complicated current density distributions. Using these techniques, nonlinear terms up to the eleventh order can be eliminated over a predefined cylindrical volume.

Another issue in gradient coil design involves minimizing the gradient rise time so that fast-imaging techniques can be implemented successfully and short echo times can be achieved to minimize signal loss for short T_2 specimens. The gradient rise time relies on three factors: the inductance over resistance ratio of the gradient coil, the time constant of the feedback circuit of the gradient power supply, and the decay rate of eddy current triggered by gradient switching. The time constant attributed to inductive resistance (L/R) is relatively short (<100 μsec) for most microscopy gradient coils, and the inductive resistance from the power supply can be easily adjusted to match the time constant of the coil. However, considering the high magnetic field gradient strength used in MR microscopy, eddy currents can be a serious problem. This problem is

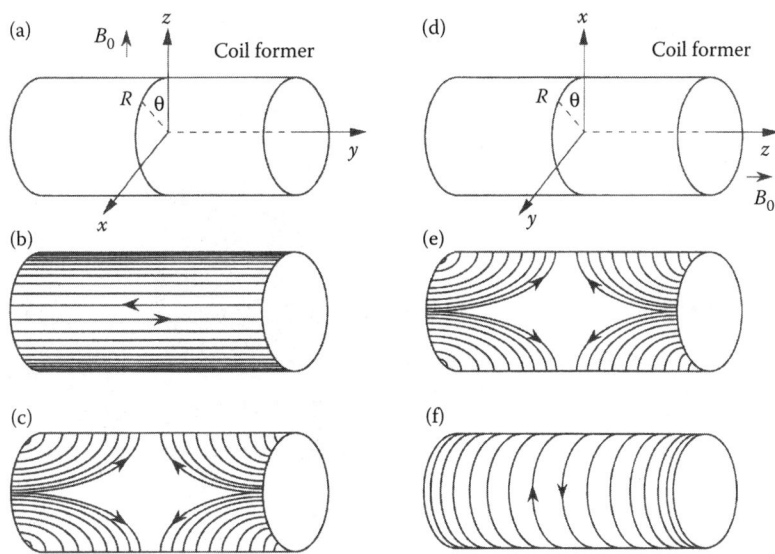

FIGURE 13.2 (a) Ideal surface current distributions to generate linear magnetic field gradients when the gradient coil former is parallel to the magnet bore: (b) for x gradient and (c) for z gradient. The analytical expressions for the current density distribution functions are $J_x = KG_x[R\cos\theta(\sin\theta i - \cos\theta j) - z\sin\theta k]$ and $J_z = KG_z Z[\sin\theta_i - \cos\theta_j]$. The y gradient can be obtained by rotating J_x 90°. (d) Ideal surface current distributions to generate linear magnetic field gradients when the gradient coil former is perpendicular to the magnet bore: (e) for x gradient and (f) for y gradient. The analytical expressions for the current density distribution functions are $J_x = KG_x R(\sin 2\theta_j)$ and $J_y = KG_y(-R\cos^2\theta_i + y\sin j + 0.5 R\sin 2\theta_k)$. The z gradient can be obtained by rotating J_x 45°. (The graphs are adapted based on Suits, B.H. and Wilken, D.E. 1989. *J. Phys. E: Sci. Instrum.* 22: 565.)

even worsened when the gradient coils are closely placed in a narrow magnet bore. To minimize the eddy currents, modern design of gradient coils uses an extra set of coils so that the eddy currents can be actively cancelled (Mansfield and Chapman, 1986). Under close to optimal conditions, a rise time of <150 µsec can be achieved with a maximum gradient of 82 G/cm in a set of 8 cm coils (Johnson et al., 1992).

Although the majority of microscopic MR images are obtained using cylindrical gradient coils, surface gradient coils have been used recently in several studies (Cho et al., 1992). Similar to surface RF coils, surface gradient coils can be easily adapted to the shape of samples and are capable of producing strong magnetic field gradient in limited areas. The surface gradient coils also provide more free space in the magnet, allowing easy access to samples. A major problem with surface gradient coils is the gradient nonlinearity. But when the region of interest is small, high-quality images can still be obtained with negligible distortions.

13.4 Applications

MR microscopy has a broad range of applications. We include here several examples. Figure 13.3 illustrates an application of MR microscopy in *ex vivo* histology. In this study, a fixed sheep heart with experimentally-induced infarct is imaged at $2T$ using 3D fast-spin-echo techniques with T_1 (Figure 13.3a) and T_2 (Figure 13.3b) contrasts. The infarct region is clearly detected in both images. The region of infarct can be segmented from the rest of the tissue and its volume can be accurately measured. Since the image is three-dimensional, the tissue pathology can be examined in any arbitrary orientation. The nondestructive nature of MR microscopy also allows the same specimen to be restudied using other techniques as well as using other contrast mechanisms of MR microscopy. Obtaining this dimension of information from conventional histologic studies would be virtually impossible.

(a)   (b)

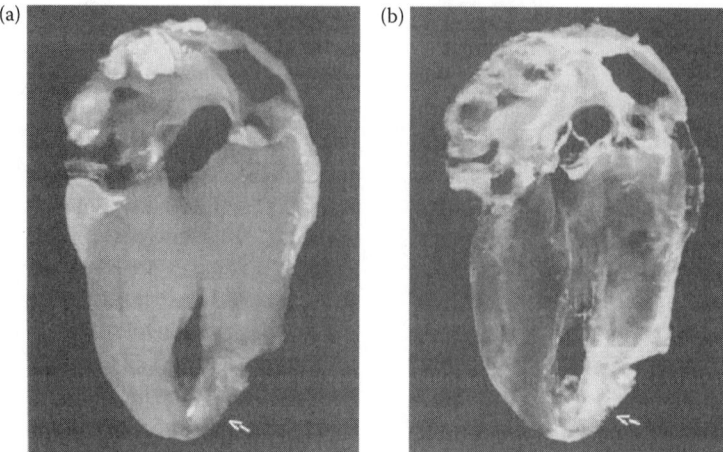

FIGURE 13.3   Selected sections of 3D isotropic images of a sheep heart with experimentally induced infarct show the utility of MRM in pathology studies. A 3D FSE sequence has been designed to allow rapid acquisition of either (a) T_1-weighted or (b) T_2-weighted images giving two separate "stains" for the pathology. Arrows indicate areas of necrosis.

The *in vivo* capability of MR microscopy for toxicologic studies is illustrated in Figure 13.4. In this study (Farmer et al., 1989), the effect of mercuric chloride in rat kidney is monitored in a single animal. Therefore, development of tissue pathology over a time period is directly observed without the unnecessary interference arising from interanimal variabilities. Since the kidney was the only region of interest in this study, a surgically implanted coil was chosen to optimize SNR and to obtain consistent localization. Figure 13.4 shows four images obtained from the same animal at different time points to show the

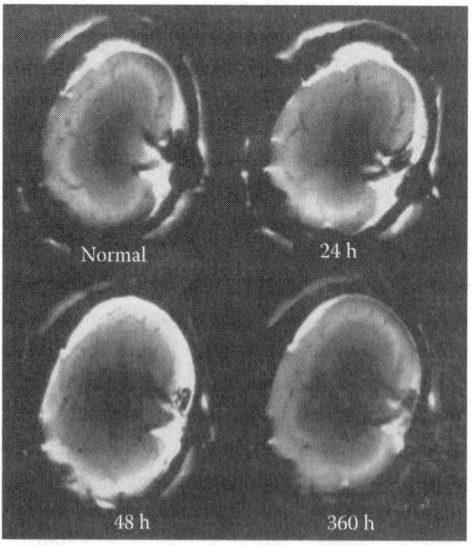

FIGURE 13.4   Implanted RF coils allow *in vivo* studies of deep structures with much higher spatial resolution by limiting the field of view during excitation and by increasing the SNR over volume coils. An added benefit is the ability to accurately localize the same region during a time course study. Shown here is the same region of a kidney at four different time points following exposure to mercuric chloride. Note the description of boundaries between the several zones of the kidney in the early part of the study followed by regeneration of the boundaries upon repair.

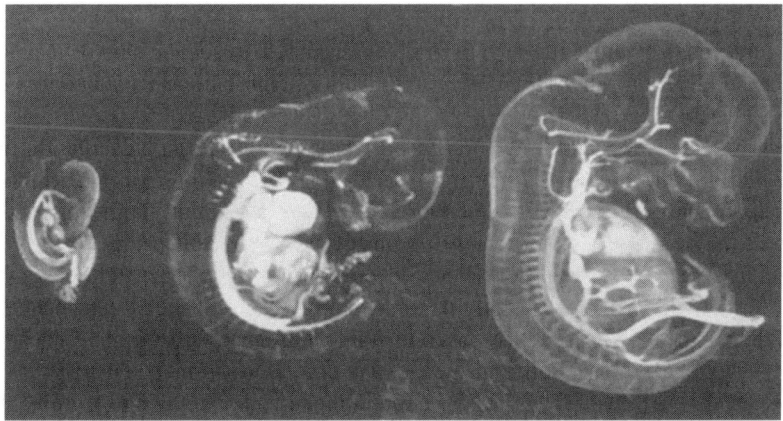

FIGURE 13.5 Isotropic 3D images of fixed mouse embryos at three stages of development have been volume rendered to allow visualization of the developing vascular anatomy.

progression and regression of the $HgCl_2$-induced renal pathology. Tissue damage is first observed 24 h after the animal was treated by the chemical, as evident by the blurring between the cortex and the outer medulla. The degree of damage is greater in the image obtained at 48 h. Finally, at 360 h, the blurred boundary between the two tissue regions completely disappeared, indicating full recovery of the organ. The capability to monitor tissue pathologic changes *in vivo*, as illustrated in this example, bodes well for a broad range of applications in pharmacology, toxicology, and pathology.

Development biology is another area where MR microscopy has found an increasing number of applications, Jacobs and Fraser (1994) used MR microscopy to follow cell movements and lineages in developing frog embryos. In their study, 3D images of the developing embryo were obtained on a time scale faster than the cell division time and analyzed forward and backward in time to reconstruct full cell divisions and cell movements. By labeling a 16-cell embryo with an exogenous contrast agent (Gd-DTPA), they successfully followed the progression from early cleavage and blastula stage through gastrulation, neurulation, and finally to tail bud stage. More important, they found that external ectodermal and internal mesodermal tissues extend at different rates during amphibian gastrulation and neurulation. This and many other key events in vertebrate embryogenesis would be very difficult to observe with optical microscopy. Another example in developmental biology is given in Figure 13.5. Using 3D high-field (9.4-T) MR microscopy with large image arrays (256^3), Smith et al. (1993) studied the early development of the circulatory system of mouse embryos. With the aid of a T_1 contrast agent made from bovine serum albumin and Gd-DTPA, vasculature such as ventricles, atria, aorta, cardinal sinuses, basilar arteries, and thoracic arteries are clearly identified in mouse embryos at between 9.5 and 12.5 days of gestation. The ability to study embryonic development in a noninvasive fashion provided great opportunities to explore many problems in transgenic studies, gene targeting, and *in situ* hybridization.

In less than 10 yr, MR microscopy has grown from a scientific curiosity to a tool with a wide range of applications. Although many theoretical and experimental problems still exist at the present time, there is no doubt that MR microscopy will soon make a significant impact in many areas of basic research and clinical diagnosis.

References

Ahn, C.B. and Cho, Z.H. 1989. A generalized formulation of diffusion effects in mm resolution nuclear magnetic resonance imaging. *Med. Phys.* 16: 22.

Banson, M.B., Cofer, G.P., Black, R.D., and Johnson, G.A. 1992a. A probe for specimen magnetic resonance microscopy. *Invest. Radiol.* 27: 157.

Banson, M.L., Cofer, G.P., Hedlund, L.W., and Johnson, G.A. 1992b. Surface coil imaging of rat spine at 7.0 T. *Magn. Reson. Imag.* 10: 929.

Benveniste, H., Hedlund, L.W., and Johnson, G.A. 1992. Mechanism of detection of acute cerebral ischemia in rats by diffusion-weighted magnetic resonance microscopy. *Stroke* 23: 746.

Black, R.D., Early, T.A., Roemer, P.B. et al. 1993. A high-temperature superconducting receiver for NMR microscopy. *Science* 259: 793.

Brown, T.R., Kincaid, B.M., and Ugurbil, K. 1982. NMR chemical shift imaging in three dimensions. *Proc. Natl Acad. Sci. USA* 79: 3523.

Callaghan, P.T. and Eccles, C.D. 1987. Sensitivity and resolution in NMR imaging. *J. Magn. Reson.* 71: 426.

Callaghan, P.T. and Eccles, C.D. 1988. Diffusion-limited resolution in nuclear magnetic resonance microscopy. *J. Magn. Reson.* 78: 1.

Callaghan, P.T., Coy, A., Forde, L.C., and Rofe, C.J. 1993. Diffusive relaxation and edge enhancement in NMR microscopy. *J. Magn. Reson. Ser. A* 101: 347.

Cho, Z.H., Ahn, C.B., Juh, S.C. et al. 1988. Nuclear magnetic resonance microscopy with 4 mm resolution: theoretical study and experimental results. *Med. Phys.* 15: 815.

Cho, Z.H., Yi, J.H., and Friedenberg, R.M. 1992. NMR microscopy and ultra-high resolution NMR imaging. *Rev. Magn. Reson. Med.* 4: 221.

Edelstein, W.A., Hutchison, J.M.S., Johnson, G., and Redpath, T. 1980. Spin warp NMR imaging and applications to human whole-body imaging. *Phys. Med. Biol.* 25: 751.

Ehman, R.L. and Felmlee, J.P. 1989. Adaptive technique for high-definition MR imaging of moving structures. *Radiology* 173: 255.

Farmer, T.H.R., Johnson, G.A., Cofer, G.P. et al. 1989. Implanted coil MR microscopy of renal pathology. *Magn. Reson. Med.* 10: 310.

Gewalt, S.L., Glover, G.H., MacFall, J.R. et al. 1993. MR microscopy of the rat lung using projection reconstruction. *Magn. Reson. Med.* 29: 99.

Glover, G.H. and Noll, D.C. 1993. Consistent projection reconstruction techniques for MRI. *Magn. Reson. Med.* 29: 345.

Glover, G.H. and Pauly, J.M. 1992. Projection reconstruction techniques for suppression of motion artifacts. *Magn. Reson. Med.* 28: 275.

Gmitro, A. and Alexander, A.L. 1993. Use of a projection reconstruction method to decrease motion sensitivity in diffusion-weighted MRI. *Magn. Reson. Med.* 29: 835.

Haase, A., Frahm, J., Matthaei, D. et al. 1986. FLASH imaging: rapid NMR imaging using low flip angle pulses. *J. Magn. Reson.* 67: 258.

Hedges, H.K. 1984. Nuclear magnetic resonance microscopy. Ph.D. dissertation, State University of New York at Stony Brook.

Hedlund, L.W., Dietz, J., Nassar, R. et al. 1986. A ventilator for magnetic resonance imaging. *Invest. Radiol.* 21: 18.

Hennig, J., Nauerth, A., and Friedburg, H. 1986. RARE imaging: a fast imaging method for clinical MR. *Magn. Reson. Med.* 3: 823.

Hetherington, H.P., Wishart, D., Fitzpatrick, S.M. et al. 1986. The application of composite pulses to surface coil NMR. *J. Magn. Reson.* 66: 313.

Hills, B.P., Wright, K.M., and Belton, P.S. 1990. The effects of restricted diffusion in nuclear magnetic resonance microscopy. *Magn. Reson. Imag.* 8: 755.

Hollett, M.D., Cofer, G.P., and Johnson, G.A. 1987. *In situ* magnetic resonance microscopy. *Invest. Radiol.* 22: 965.

House, W.V. 1984. NMR microscopy. *IEEE Trans. Nucl. Sci.* NS-31: 570.

Hyslop, W.B. and Lauterbur, P.C. 1991. Effects of restricted diffusion on microscopic NMR imaging. *J. Magn. Reson.* 94: 501.

Jacobs, R.E. and Fraser, S.E. 1994. Magnetic resonance microscopy of embryonic cell lineages and movements. *Science* 263: 681.

Johnson, G.A., Hedlund, L.W., Cofer, G.P., and Suddarth, S.A. 1992. Magnetic resonance microscopy in the life sciences. *Rev. Magn. Reson. Med.* 4: 187.

Karis, J.P., Johnson, G.A., and Glover, G.H. 1987. Signal to noise improvements in three dimensional NMR microscopy using limited angle excitation. *J. Magn. Reson.* 71: 24.

Kumar, A., Welti, D., and Ernst, R.R. 1975. NMR Fourier zeugmatography. *J. Magn. Reson.* 18: 69.

Lai, C.M. and Lauterbur, P.C. 1981. True three-dimensional image reconstruction by nuclear magnetic resonance zeugmatography. *Phys. Med. Biol.* 26: 851.

Lauterbur, P.C. 1973. Image formation by induced local interactions: examples employing nuclear magnetic resonance. *Nature* 242: 190.

Lauterbur, P.C. 1984. New direction in NMR imaging. *IEEE Trans. Nucl. Sci.* NS-31: 1010.

Lean, C.L., Russell, P., Delbridge, L. et al. 1993. Metastatic follicular thyroid diagnosed by 1H MRS. *Proc. Soc. Magn. Reson. Med.* 1: 71.

Majumdar, S. and Gore, J.C. 1988. Studies of diffusion in random fields produced by variations in susceptibility. *J. Magn. Reson.* 78: 41.

Maki, J.H., Johnson, G.A., Cofer, G.P., and MacFall, J.R. 1988. SNR improvement in NMR microscopy using DEFT. *J. Magn. Reson.* 80: 482.

Mansfield, P. and Chapman, B. 1986. Active magnetic screening of gradient coils in NMR imaging. *J. Magn. Reson.* 66: 573.

Mansfield, P. and Maudsley, A.A. 1977. Planar spin imaging by NMR. *J. Magn. Reson.* 27: 129.

McFarland, E.W. 1992. Time independent point-spread function for MR microscopy. *Magn. Reson. Imag.* 10: 269.

McFarland, E.W. and Mortara, A. 1992. Three-dimensional NMR microscopy: improving SNR with temperature and microcoils. *Magn. Reson. Imag.* 10: 279.

Moran, P.R. 1982. A flow velocity zeugmatographic interlace for NMR imaging in humans. *Magn. Reson. Imag.* 1: 197.

Mulkern, R.V., Wong, S.T.S., Winalski, C., and Jolesz, F.A. 1990. Contrast manipulation and artifact assessment of 2D and 3D RARE sequences. *Magn. Reson. Imag.* 8: 557.

Peck, T.L., Magin, R.L., and Lauterbur, P.C. 1990. Microdomain magnetic resonance imaging. *Proc. Soc. Magn. Reson. Med.* 1: 207.

Putz, B., Barsky, D., and Schulten, K. 1991. Edge enhancement by diffusion: microscopic magnetic resonance imaging of an ultrathin glass capillary. *Chem. Phys.* 183: 391.

Rudin, M. 1987. MR microscopy on rats *in vivo* at 4.7 T using surface coils. *Magn. Reson. Med.* 5: 443.

Schoeniger, J.S., Aiken, N.R., and Blackband, S.J. 1991. NMR microscopy of single neurons. *Proc. Soc. Magn. Reson. Med.* 2: 880.

Smith, B.R., Johnson, G.A., Groman, E.V., and Linney, E. 1993. Contrast enhancement of normal and abnormal mouse embryo vasculature. *Proc. Soc. Magn. Reson. Med.* 1: 303.

Suits, B.H. and Wilken, D.E. 1989. Improving magnetic field gradient coils for NMR imaging. *J. Phys. E: Sci. Instrum.* 22: 565.

Ugurbil, K., Garwood, M., and Bendall, R. 1987. Amplitude- and frequency-modulated pulses to achieve 90° plane rotation with inhomogeneous B_1 fields. *J. Magn. Reson.* 72: 177.

Wood, M.L. and Henkelman, R.M. 1985. NMR image artifacts from periodic motion. *Med. Phys.* 12: 143.

Xiang, Q.-S. and Henkelman, R.M. 1991. Motion artifact reduction with three-point ghost phase cancellation. *J. Magn. Reson. Imag.* 1: 633.

Zhong, J. and Gore, J.C. 1991. Studies of restricted diffusion in heterogeneous media containing variations in susceptibility. *Magn. Reson. Med.* 19: 276.

Zhou, X. and Lauterbur, P.C. 1992. NMR microscopy using projection reconstruction. In Blümich, B. and Kuhn, W. (eds.), *Magnetic Resonance Microscopy*, pp. 1–27. Weinheim, Germany, VCH.

Zhou, X., Cofer, G.P., Mills, G.I., and Johnson, G.A. 1992. An inductively coupled probe for MR microscopy at 7 T. *Proc. Soc. Magn. Reson. Med.* 1: 971.

Zhou, X., Cofer, G.P., Suddarth, S.A., and Johnson, G.A. 1993. High-field MR microscopy using fast spin-echoes. *Magn. Reson. Med.* 31: 60.

Zhou, X., Liang, Z.-P., Cofer, G.P. et al. 1993. An FSE pulse sequence with circular sampling for MR microscopy. *Proc. Soc. Magn. Reson. Med.* 1: 297.

Zhou, X., Maronpot, R.R., Mills, G.I. et al. 1994. Studies on bromobenzene-induced hepatotoxicity using *in vivo* MR microscopy. *Magn. Reson. Med.* 31: 619.

Zhou, Z. 1992. Nuclear magnetic resonance microscopy: new theoretical and technical developments. Ph.D. dissertation, University of Illinois at Urbana-Champaign.

Further Information

A detailed description of the physics of NMR and MRI can be found in Principles of Magnetic Resonance, by C.S., Slichter (3rd edition, Springer-Verlag, 1989), in NMR Imaging in Biology and Medicine, by P. Morris (Clarendon Press, 1986), and in Principles of Magnetic Resonance Microscopy, by P.T., Callaghan (Oxford Press, 1991). The latter two books also contain detailed discussions on instrumentation, data acquisition, and image reconstruction for conventional and microscopic magnetic resonance imaging.

Magnetic Resonance Microscopy, edited by Blümich and Kuhn (VCH, 1992), is particularly helpful to understand various aspects of MR microscopy, both methodology and applications. Each chapter of the book covers a specific topic and is written by experts in the field.

Proceedings of the Society of Magnetic Resonance (formerly Society of Magnetic Resonance in Medicine, Berkeley, California), published annually, documents the most recent developments in the field of MR microscopy. Magnetic Resonance in Medicine, Journal of Magnetic Resonance Imaging, and Magnetic Resonance Imaging, all monthly journals, contain original research articles and are good sources for up-to-date developments.

14

Positron-Emission Tomography

Thomas F. Budinger
University of California, Berkeley

Henry F. VanBrocklin
University of California, Berkeley

14.1 Radiopharmaceuticals

Thomas F. Budinger and Henry F. VanBrocklin

Since the discovery of artificial radioactivity a half century ago, radiotracers, radionuclides, and radio-nuclide compounds have played a vital role in biology and medicine. Common to all is radionuclide (radioactive isotope) production. This section describes the basic ideas involved in radionuclide production and gives examples of the applications of radionuclides. The field of radiopharmaceutical chemistry has fallen into subspecialties of positron-emission tomography (PET) chemistry and general radiopharmaceutical chemistry, including specialists in technetium chemistry, taking advantage of the imaging attributes of technetium-99m.

The two general methods of radionuclide production are neutron addition (activation) from neutron reactors to make neutron-rich radionuclides which decay to give off electrons and gamma rays and charged-particle accelerators (linacs and cyclotrons) which usually produce neutron-deficient isotopes that decay by electron capture and emission of x-rays, gamma rays, and positrons. The production of artificial radionuclides is governed by the number of neutrons or charged particles hitting an appropriate target per time, the cross section for the particular reaction, the number of atoms in the target, and the half-life of the artificial radionuclide:

$$A(t) = \frac{N\sigma\phi}{3.7 \times 10^{10}} \left(1 - e^{0.693t/T_{1/2}}\right) \tag{14.1}$$

where $A(t)$ is the produced activity in number of atoms per second, N is the number of target nuclei, σ is the cross section (probability that the neutron or charged particles will interact with the nucleus to form the artificial radioisotope) for the reaction, ϕ is the flux of charged particles, and $T_{1/2}$ is the half-life of the product. Note that N is the target mass divided by the atomic weight and multiplied by Avogadro's number (6.024×10^{23}) and σ is measured in cm^2. The usual flux is about 10^{14} neutrons per sec or, for charged particles, 10 to 100 mA, which is equivalent to 6.25×10^{13} to 6.25×10^{14} charged particles per second.

14.1.1 Nuclear Reactor-Produced Radionuclides

Thermal neutrons of the order of 10^{14} neutrons/sec/cm^2 are produced in a nuclear reactor usually during a controlled nuclear fission of uranium, though thorium or plutonium are also used. High specific activity neutron-rich radionuclides are produced usually through the (n, g), (n, p), or (n, a) reactions (Figure 14.1a). The product nuclides usually decay by b—followed by g. Most of the reactor-produced radionuclides are produced by the (n, g) reaction. The final step in the production of a radionuclide consists of the separation of the product nuclide from the target container by chemical or physical means.

An alternative method for producing isotopes from a reactor is to separate the fission fragments from the spent fuel rods. This is the leading source of ^{99}Mo for medical applications. The following two methods of ^{99}Mo production are examples of carrier-added and no-carrier-added radionuclide synthesis, respectively. In Figure 14.1a, the ^{99}Mo is production from ^{98}Mo. Only a small fraction of the ^{98}Mo nuclei will be converted to ^{99}Mo. Therefore, at the end of neutron bombardment, there is a mixture of both isotopes. These are inseparable by conventional chemical separation techniques, and both isotopes would participate equally well in chemical reactions. The ^{99}Mo from fission of ^{238}U would not contain any other isotopes of Mo and is considered carrier-free. Thus radioisotopes produced by any means having the same atomic number as the target material would be considered carrier-added. Medical tracer techniques obviate the need for carrier-free isotopes.

14.1.2 Accelerator-Produced Radionuclides

Cyclotrons and linear accelerators (linacs) are sources of beams of protons, deuterons, or helium ions that bombarded targets to produce neutron-deficient (proton-rich) radionuclides (Figure 14.1b). The neutron-deficient radionuclides produced through these reactions are shown in Table 14.1. These product nuclides (usually carrier-free) decay either by electron capture or by positron emission tomography or both, followed by g emission. In Table 14.2, most of the useful charged-particle reactions are listed.

The heat produced by the beam current on the target material can interfere with isotope production and requires efficient heat-removal strategies using extremely stable heat-conducting target materials such as metal foils, electroplates metals, metal powders, metal oxides, and salts melted on duralmin plate. All the modern targets use circulating cold deionized water and chilled helium gas to aid in

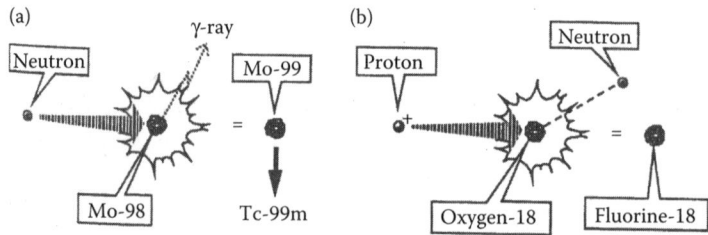

FIGURE 14.1 (a) High specific activity neutron-excess radionuclides are produced usually through the (n, g), (n, p) or (n, a) reactions. The product nuclides usually decay b—followed by g. Most of the reactor produced radionuclides are produced by the (n, g) reaction. (b) Cyclotrons and linear accelerators (linacs) are sources of beams of protons, deuterons, or helium ions which bombard targets to produce neutron-deficient radionuclides.

TABLE 14.1   Radionuclides Used in Biomedicine

Radionuclide	Half-Life	Application(s)
Arsenic-74[a]	17.9 d	A positron emitting chemical analog of phosphorus
Barium-128[a]	2.4 d	Parent in the generator system for producing the positron emitting [128]Cs, a potassium analog
Berylium-7[a]	53.37 d	Berylliosis studies
Bromine-77	57 h	Radioimmunotherapy
Bromin-82	35.3 h	Used in metabolic studies and studies of estrogen receptor content
Carbon-11[a]	20.3 min	Positron emitter for metabolism imaging
Cobalt-57[a]	270 d	Calibration of imaging instruments
Copper-62	9.8 min	Heart perfusion
Copper-64	12.8 h	Used as a clinical diagnostic agent for cancer and metabolic disorders
Copper-67	58.5 h	Radioimmunotherapy
Chromium-51	27.8 d	Used to assess red blood cell survival
Fluorine-18	109.7 min	Positron emitter used in glucose analogs uptake and neuroreceptor imaging
Gallium-68	68 min	Required in calibrating PET tomographs. Potential antibody level
Germanium-68[a]	287 d	Parent in the generator system for producing the positron emitting [68]Ga
Indium-111[a]	2.8 d	Radioimmunotherapy
Iodine-122	3.76 min	Positron emitter for blood flow studies
Iodine-123[a]	13.3 h	SPECT brain imaging agent
Iodine-124[a]	4.2 d	Radioimmunotherapy, positron emitter
Iodine-125	60.2 d	Used as a potential cancer therapeutic agent
Iodine-131	8.1 d	Used to diagnose and treat thyroid disorders including cancer
Iron-52[a]	8.2 h	Used as an iron tracer, positron emitter for bone-marrow imaging
Magnesium-28[a]	21.2 h	Magnesium tracer which decays to 2.3 in aluminum-28
Magnese-52m	5.6 d	Flow tracer for heart muscle
Mercury-195m[a]	40 h	Parent in the generator system for producing [195]mAu, which is used in cardiac blood pool studies
Molybdenum-99	67 h	Used to produce technetium-99m, the most commonly used radioisotope in clinical nuclear medicine
Nitrogen-13[a]	9.9 min	Positron emitter used as [13]NH for heart perfusion studies
Osmium-191	15 d	Decays to iridium-191 used for cardiac studies
Oxygen-15[a]	123 s	Positron emitter used for blood flow studies as H152O
Palladium-103	17 d	Used in the treatment of prostate cancer
Phosphorus-32	14.3 d	Used in cancer treatment, cell metabolism and kinetics, molecular biology, genetics research, biochemistry, microbiology, enzymology, and as a starter to make many basic chemicals and research products
Rhenium-188	17 h	Used for treatment of medullary thyroid carcinoma and alleviation of pain in bone metastases
Rubidium-82[a]	1.2 min	Positron emitter used for heart perfusion studies
Ruthemiun-97[a]	2.9 d	Hepatobiliary function, tumor and inflammation localization
Samarium-145	340 d	Treatment of ocular cancer
Samarium-153	46.8 h	Used to radiolabel various molecules as cancer therapeutic agents and to alleviate bone cancer pain
Scandium-47	3.4 d	Radioimmunotherapy
Scandium-47[a]	3.4 d	Used in the therapy of cancer

continued

TABLE 14.1 (continued) Radionuclides Used in Biomedicine

Radionuclide	Half-Life	Application(s)
Strontium-82[a]	64.0 d	Parent in the generator system for producing the positron emitting ^{82}Rb, a potassium analogue
Strontium-85	64 d	Used to study bone formation metabolism
Strontium-89	52 d	Used to alleviate metastatic bone pain
Sulfur-35	87.9 d	Used in studies of cell metabolism and kinetics, molecular biology, genetics research, biochemistry, microbiology, enzymology, and as a start to make many basic chemicals and research products
Technetium-99m	6 h	The most widely used radiopharmaceutical in nuclear medicine and produced from molybdenum-99
Thalium-201[a]	74 h	Cardiac imaging agent
Tin-117m	14.0 d	Palliative treatment of bone cancer pain
Tritium (hydrogen-3)	12.3 yr	Used to make tritiated water which is used as a starter for thousands of different research products and basic chemicals; used for life science and drug metabolism studies to ensure the safety of potential new drugs
Tungsten-178[a]	21.5 d	Parent in generator system for producing ^{178}Ta, short-lived scanning agent
Tungsten-188	69 d	Decays to rhenium-188 for treatment of cancer and rheumatoid arthritis
Vanadium-48[a]	16.0 d	Nutrition and environmental studies
Xenon-122[a]	20 h	Parent in the generator system for producing the positron emitting ^{122}I
Xenon-127[a]	36.4 d	Used in lung ventilation studies
Xenon-133	5.3 d	Used in lung ventilation and perfusion studies
Yttrium-88[a]	106.6 d	Radioimmunotherapy
Yttrium-90	64 h	Used to radiolabel various molecules as cancer therapeutic agents
Zinc-62[a]	9.13 h	Parent in the generator system for producing the positron emitting ^{62}Cu
Zirconium-89[a]	78.4 h	Radioimmunotherapy, positron emitter

[a] Produced by accelerated charged particles. Others are produced by neutron reactors.

cooling the target body and window foils. Cyclotrons used in medical studies have ^{11}C, ^{13}N, ^{15}O, and ^{18}F production capabilities that deliver the product nuclides on demand through computer-executed commands. The radionuclide is remotely transferred into a lead-shielded hot cell for processing. The resulting radionuclides are manipulated using microscale radiochemical techniques: small-scale synthetic methodology, ion-exchange chromatography, solvent extraction, electrochemical synthesis, distillation, simple filtration, paper chromatography, and isotopic carrier precipitation. Various relevant radiochemical techniques have been published in standard texts.

TABLE 14.2 Important Reactions for Cyclotron-Produced Radioisotopes

1. p, n	7. p, pn
2. $p, 2n$	8. $p, 2p$
3. d, n	9. d, p
4. $d, 2n$	10. $d, {}^4$He
5. $d, {}^4$He	11. p, d
6. $d, {}^4$Hen	12. ^{4}He, n
	13. ^{3}He, p

14.1.3 Generator-Produced Radionuclides

If the reactor, cyclotron, or natural product radionuclide of long half-life decays to a daughter with nuclear characteristics appropriate for medical application, the system is called a medical radionuclide generator. There are several advantages afforded by generator-produced isotopes. These generators represent a convenient source of short-lived medical isotopes without the need for an on-site reactor or particle accelerator. Generators provide delivery of the radionuclide on demand at a site remote from the production facility. They are a source of both gamma- and positron-emitting isotopes.

The most common medical radionuclide generator is the ^{99}Mo Æ ^{99m}Tc system, the source of ^{99m}Tc, a gamma-emitting isotope currently used in 70% of the clinical nuclear medicine studies. The ^{99}Mo has a 67-h half-life, giving this generator a useful life of about a week. Another common generator is the ^{68}Ge Æ ^{68}Ga system. Germanium (half-life is 287 d) is accelerator-produced in high-energy accelerators (e.g., BLIP, LAMPF, TRIUMF) through the alpha-particle bombardment of ^{66}Zn. The 68Ge decays to ^{68}Ga, a positron emitter, which has a 68-min half-life. Gallium generators can last for several months.

The generator operation is fairly straightforward. In general, the parent isotope is bound to a solid chemical matrix (e.g., alumina column, anionic resin, Donux resin). As the parent decays, the daughter nuclide grows in. The column is then flushed ("milked") with a suitable solution (e.g., saline, hydrochloric acid) that elutes the daughter and leaves the remaining parent absorbed on the column. The eluent may be injected directly or processed into a radiopharmaceutical.

14.1.4 Radiopharmaceuticals

^{99m}Tc is removed from the generator in the form of TcO_4^- (pertechnetate). This species can be injected directly for imaging or incorporated into a variety of useful radiopharmaceuticals. The labeling of ^{99m}Tc usually involves reduction complexation/chelation. ^{99m}Tc-Sestamibi (Figure 14.2) is a radiopharmaceutical used to evaluate myocardial perfusion or to diagnose cancer. There are several reduction methods employed, including Sn(II) reduction in $NaHCO_3$ at pH of 8 and other reduction and complexation reactions such as $S_2O_3 = HCl$, $FeCl_3$ + ascorbic acid, $LiBH_4$, Zn + HCl, HCl, Fe(II), Sn(II)F_2, Sn(II) citrate, and Sn(II) tartrate reduction and complexation, electrolytic reduction, and *in vivo* labeling of red cells following Sn(II) pyrophosphate or Sn(II) DTPA administration. ^{131}I, ^{125}I, and ^{123}I labeling requires special reagents or conditions such as chloramine-T, widely used for protein labeling at 7.5 pH;

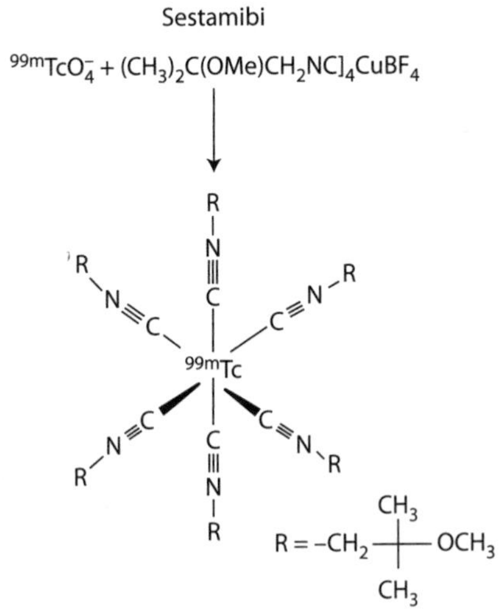

Sestamibi

$$^{99m}TcO_4^- + (CH_3)_2C(OMe)CH_2NC]_4CuBF_4$$

$$R = -CH_2 - \overset{CH_3}{\underset{CH_3}{\overset{|}{\underset{|}{C}}}} - OCH_3$$

FIGURE 14.2 ^{99m}Tc-Sestamibi is a radiopharmaceutical used to evaluate myocardial perfusion or in the diagnosis of cancer using both computed tomography and scintigraphy techniques.

peroxidase + H_2O_2 widely used for radioassay tracers; isotopic exchange for imaging tracers; excitation labeling as in ^{123}Xe Æ ^{123}I diazotization plus iodination for primary amines; conjugation labeling with Bolton Hunter agent (N-succinimidyl 3-[4-hydroxy 5-$(^{131,125,123}$I)iodophenyl] propionate); hydroboration plus iodination; electrophilic destannylation; microdiffusion with fresh iodine vapor; and other methods. Radiopharmaceuticals in common use for brain perfusion studies are N-isopropyl-p $[^{123}$I] iodoamphetamine and ^{99m}Tc-labeled hexamethylpropyleneamine.

14.1.5 PET Radionuclides

For ^{11}C, ^{13}N, ^{15}O, and ^{18}F, the modes of production of short-lived positron emitters can dictate the chemical form of the product, as shown in Table 14.3. Online chemistry is used to make various PET agents and precursors. For example, ^{11}C cyanide, an important precursor for synthesis of other labeled compounds, is produced in the cyclotron target by first bombarding N_2 + 5% H_2 gas target with 20-MeV protons. The product is carbon-labeled methane, $^{11}CH_4$, which when combined with ammonia and passed over a platinum wool catalyst at 1000°C becomes $^{11}CN^-$, which is subsequently trapped in NaOH.

Molecular oxygen is produced by bombarding a gas target of $^{14}N_2$ + 2% O_2 with deuterons (6 to 8 MeV). A number of products (e.g., $^{15}O_2$, $C^{15}O_2$, $N^{15}O_2$, $^{15}O_3$, and $H_2^{15}O$) are trapped by soda lime followed by charcoal to give $^{15}O_2$ as the product. However, if an activated charcoal trap at 900°C is used before the soda lime trap, the $^{15}O_2$ will be converted to $C^{15}O$. The specific strategies for other online PET agents is given in Rayudu (1990).

Fluorine-18 (^{18}F) is a very versatile positron emitting isotope. With a 2-h half-life and two forms (F^+ and F^-), one can develop several synthetic methods for incorporating ^{18}F into medically useful compounds (Kilbourn, 1990). Additionally, fluorine forms strong bonds with carbon and is roughly the same size as a hydrogen atom, imparting metabolic and chemical stability of the molecules without drastically altering biologic activity. The most commonly produced ^{18}F radiopharmaceutical is 2-deoxy-2-$[^{18}$F]fluoroglucose (FDG). This radiotracer mimics part of the glucose metabolic pathway and has shown both hypo- and hypermetabolic abnormalities in cardiology, oncology, and neurology. The synthetic pathway for the production of FDG is shown in Figure 14.3.

The production of positron radiopharmaceuticals requires the rapid incorporation of the isotope into the desired molecule. Chemical techniques and synthetic strategies have been developed to facilitate these reactions. Many of these synthetic manipulations require hands-on operations by a highly trained chemist. Additionally, since positrons give off 2- to 511-keV gamma rays upon annihilation, proximity to the source can increase one's personal dose. The demand for the routine production of positron radiopharmaceuticals such as FDG has led to the development of remote synthetic devices. These devices can be human-controlled (i.e., flipping switches to open air-actuated valves), computer-controlled, or

TABLE 14.3   Major Positron-Emitting Radionuclides Produced by Accelerated Protons

Radionuclide	Half-Life	Reaction
Carbon-11	20 min	^{12}C (p, pn) ^{11}C
		^{14}N (p, α) ^{11}C
Nitrogen-12	10 min	^{16}O (p, α) ^{13}N
		^{13}C (p, n) ^{13}N
Oxygen-15	2 min	^{15}N (p, n) ^{15}C
		^{14}N (d, n) ^{15}O
Fluorine-18	110 min	^{18}O (p, n) ^{18}F
		^{20}Ne (d, α) ^{18}F

Note: A(x,y)B: A is target, *x* is the bombarding particle, *y* is the radiation product, and *B* is the isotope produced.

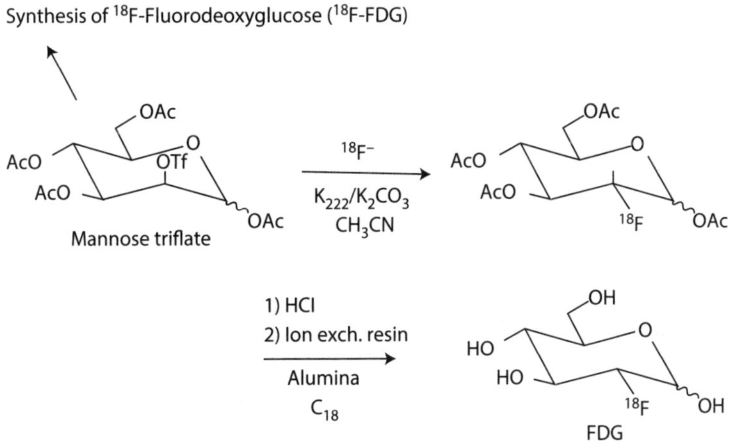

Synthesis of ^{18}F-Fluorodeoxyglucose (^{18}F-FDG)

FIGURE 14.3 Schematic for the chemical production of deoxyglucose labeled with fluorine-18. Here K_{222} refers to Kryptofix and C_{18} denotes a reverse-phase high-pressure liquid chromatography column.

robotic. A sophisticated computer-controlled chemistry synthesis unit has been assembled for the fully automated production of ^{18}FDG (Padgett, 1989). A computer-controlled robot has been programmed to produce 6a-[^{18}F]fluoroestradiol for breast cancer imaging (Brodack et al., 1986; Mathias et al., 1987). Both these types of units increase the availability and reduce the cost of short-lived radiopharmaceutical production through greater reliability and reduced need for a highly trained staff. Additionally, these automated devices reduce personnel radiation exposure. These and other devices are being designed with greater versatility in mind to allow a variety of radiopharmaceuticals to be produced just by changing the programming and the required reagents.

These PET radionuclides have been incorporated into a wide variety of medically useful radiopharmaceuticals through a number of synthetic techniques. The development of PET scanner technology has added a new dimension to synthetic chemistry by challenging radiochemists to devise labeling and purification strategies that proceed on the order of minutes rather than hours or days as in conventional synthetic chemistry. To meet this challenge, radiochemists are developing new target systems to improve isotope production and sophisticated synthetic units to streamline routine production of commonly desired radiotracers as well as preparing short-lived radiopharmaceuticals for many applications.

Acknowledgments

This work was supported in part by the Director, Office of Energy Research, Office of Health and Environmental Research, Medical Applications and Biophysical Research Division of the U.S. Department of Energy, under contract No. DE-AC03-SF00098, and in part by NIH Grant HL25840.

References

Brodack, J.W., Dence, C.S., Kilbourn, M.R., and Welch, M.J. 1988. Robotic production of 2-deoxy-2-[^{18}F] fluoro-d-glucose: aroutine method of synthesis using tetrabutylammonium [^{18}F]fluoride. *Int. J. Radiat. Appl. Instrum. Part A: Appl. Radiat. Isotopes* 39: 699.

Brodack, J.W., Kilbourn, M.R., Welch, M.J., and Katzenellenbogen, J.A. 1986. Application of robotics to radiopharmaceutical preparation: controlled synthesis of fluorine-18 16 alpha-fluoroestradiol-17 beta. *J. Nucl. Med.* 27: 714.

Hupf, H.B. 1976. Production and purification of radionuclides. In *Radiopharmacy*. New York, Wiley.

Kilbourn, M.R. 1990. *Fluorine-18 Labeling of Radiopharmaceuticals.* Washington, National Academy Press.

Lamb, J. and Kramer, H.H. 1983. Commercial production of radioisotopes for nuclear medicine. In *Radiotracers for Medical Applications,* pp. 17–62. Boca Raton, FL, CRC Press.

Mathias, C.J., Welch, M.J., Katzenellenbogen, J.A. et al. 1987. Characterization of the uptake of 16 alpha-([18F]fluoro)-17 beta-estradiol in DMBA-induced mammary tumors. *Int. J. Radiat. Appl. Instrum. Part B: Nucl. Med. Biol.* 14: 15.

Padgett, H.C., Schmidt, D.G., Luxen, A. et al. 1989. Computed-controlled radiochemical synthesis: a chemistry process control unit for the automated production of radiochemicals. *Int. J. Radiat. Appl. Instrum. Part A: Appl. Radiat. Isotopes* 40: 433.

Rayudu, G.V. 1990. Production of radionuclides for medicine. *Semin. Nucl. Med.* 20: 100.

Sorenson, J.A. and Phelps, M.E. 1987. *Physics in Nuclear Medicine.* New York, Grune & Stratton.

Steigman, J. and Eckerman, W.C. 1992. *The Chemistry of Technetium in Medicine.* Washington, National Academy Press.

Stocklin, G. 1992. Tracers for metabolic imaging of brain and heart: radiochemistry and radiopharmacology. *Eur. J. Nucl. Med.* 19: 527.

14.2 Instrumentation

Thomas F. Budinger

14.2.1 Background

The history of positron-emission tomography (PET) can be traced to the early 1950s, when workers in Boston first realized the medical imaging possibilities of a particular class of radioactive substances. It was recognized then that the high-energy photons produced by annihilation of the positron from positron-emitting isotopes could be used to describe, in three dimensions, the physiologic distribution of "tagged" chemical compounds. After two decades of moderate technological developments by a few research centers, widespread interest and broadly based research activity began in earnest following the development of sophisticated reconstruction algorithms and improvements in detector technology. By the mid-1980s, PET had become a tool for medical diagnosis and for dynamic studies of human metabolism.

Today, because of its million-fold sensitivity advantage over magnetic resonance imaging (MRI) in tracer studies and its chemical specificity, PET is used to study neuroreceptors in the brain and other body tissues. In contrast, MRI has exquisite resolution for anatomic (Figure 14.4) and flow studies as well as unique attributes of evaluating chemical composition of tissue but in the millimolar range rather

MRI   PET

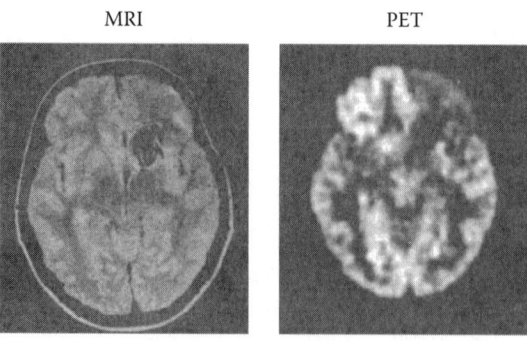

FIGURE 14.4 The MRI image shows the arteriovenous malformation (AVM) as an area of signal loss due to blood flow. The PET image shows the AVM as a region devoid of glucose metabolism and also shows decreased metabolism in the adjacent frontal cortex. This is a metabolic effect of the AVM on the brain and may explain some of the patient's symptoms.

than the nanomolar range of much of the receptor proteins in the body. Clinical studies include tumors of the brain, breast, lungs, lower gastrointestinal tract, and other sites. Additional clinical uses include Alzheimer's disease, Parkinson's disease, epilepsy, and coronary artery disease affecting heart muscle metabolism and flow. Its use has added immeasurably to our current understanding of flow, oxygen utilization, and the metabolic changes that accompany disease and that change during brain stimulation and cognitive activation.

14.2.2 PET Theory

PET imaging begins with the injection of a metabolically active tracer—a biologic molecule that carries with it a positron-emitting isotope (e.g., ^{11}C, ^{13}N, ^{15}O, or ^{18}F). Over a few minutes, the isotope accumulates in an area of the body for which the molecule has an affinity. As an example, glucose labeled with ^{11}C, or a glucose analogue labeled with ^{18}F, accumulates in the brain or tumors, where glucose is used as the primary source of energy. The radioactive nuclei then decay by positron emission. In positron (positive electron) emission, a nuclear proton changes into a positive electron and a neutron. The atom maintains its atomic mass but decreases its atomic number by 1. The ejected positron combines with an electron almost instantaneously, and these two particles undergo the process of annihilation. The energy associated with the masses of the positron and electron particles is 1.022 MeV in accordance with the energy E to mass m equivalence $E = mc^2$, where c is the velocity of light. This energy is divided equally between two photons that fly away from one another at a 180-degree angle. Each photon has an energy of 511 keV. These high-energy gamma rays emerge from the body in opposite directions, to be detected by an array of detectors that surround the patient (Figure 14.5). When two photons are recorded simultaneously by a pair of detectors, the annihilation event that gave rise to them must have occurred somewhere along the line connecting the detectors. Of course, if one of the photons is scattered, then the line of coincidence will be incorrect. After 100,000 or more annihilation events are detected, the distribution of the positron-emitting tracer is calculated by tomographic reconstruction procedures. PET reconstructs a two-dimensional (2D) image from the one-dimensional projections seen at different angles. Three-dimensional (3D) reconstructions also can be done using 2D projections from multiple angles.

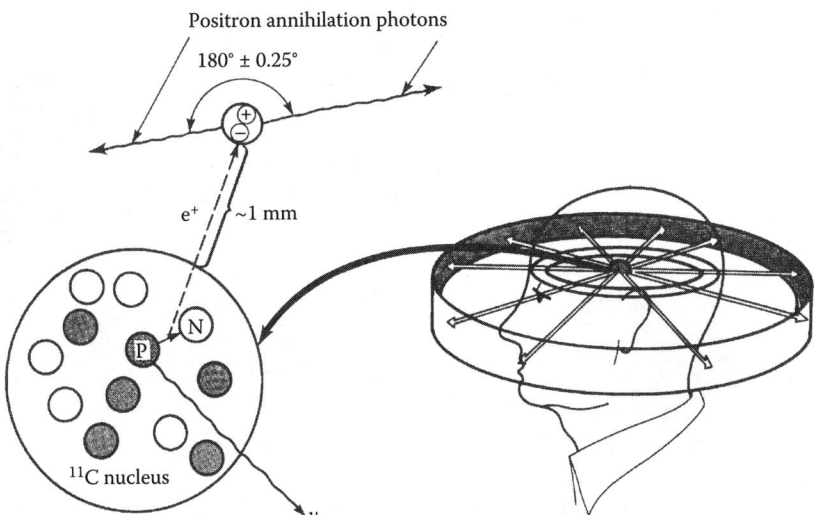

FIGURE 14.5 The physical basis of positron-emission tomography. Positrons emitted by "tagged" metabolically active molecules annihilate nearby electrons and give rise to a pair of high-energy photons. The photons fly off in nearly opposite directions and thus serve to pinpoint their source. The biologic activity of the tagged molecule can be used to investigate a number of physiologic functions, both normal and pathologic.

14.2.3 PET Detectors

Efficient detection of the annihilation photons from positron emitters is usually provided by the combination of a crystal, which converts the high-energy photons to visible-light photons, and a photomultiplier tube that produces an amplified electric current pulse proportional to the amount of light photons interacting with the photocathode. The fact that imaging system sensitivity is proportional to the square of the detector efficiency leads to a very important requirement that the detector be nearly 100% efficient. Thus other detector systems such as plastic scintillators or gas-filled wire chambers, with typical individual efficiencies of 20% or less, would result in a coincident efficiency of only 4% or less.

Most modern PET cameras are multilayered with 15 to 47 levels or transaxial layers to be reconstructed (Figure 14.6). The lead shields prevent activity from the patient from causing spurious counts in the tomograph ring, while the tungsten septa reject some of the events in which one (or both) of the 511-keV photons suffer a Compton scatter in the patient. The sensitivity of this design is improved by collection of data from cross-planes (Figure 14.6). The arrangement of scintillators and phototubes is shown in Figure 14.7.

The "individually coupled" design is capable of very high resolution, and because the design is very parallel (all the photomultiplier tubes and scintillator crystals operate independently), it is capable of very high data throughput. The disadvantages of this type of design are the requirement for many expensive photomultiplier tubes and, additionally, that connecting round photomultiplier tubes to rectangular scintillation crystals leads to problems of packing rectangular crystals and circular phototubes of sufficiently small diameter to form a solid ring.

The contemporary method of packing many scintillators for 511 keV around the patient is to use what is called a block detector design. A block detector couples several photomultiplier tubes to a bank of scintillator crystals and uses a coding scheme to determine the crystal of interaction. In the two-layer block (Figure 14.7), five photomultiplier tubes are coupled to eight scintillator crystals. Whenever one of the outside four photomultiplier tubes fires, a 511-keV photon has interacted in one of the two crystals attached to that photomultiplier tube, and the center photomultiplier tube is then used to determine whether it was the inner or outer crystal. This is known as a digital coding scheme, since each photomultiplier tube is either "hit" or "not hit" and the crystal of interaction is determined by a "digital" mapping of the hit pattern. Block detector designs are much less expensive and practical to form into a multilayer camera. However, errors in the decoding scheme reduce the spatial resolution, and since the entire block is "dead" whenever one of its member crystals is struck by a photon, the dead time is worse than with

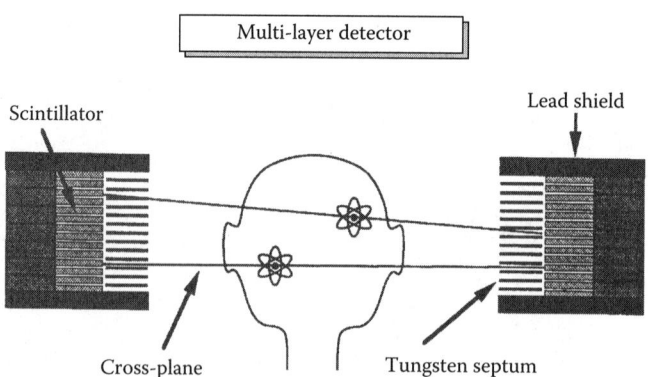

FIGURE 14.6 Most modern PET cameras are multilayered with 15 to 47 levels or transaxial layers to be reconstructed. The lead shields prevent activity from the patient from causing spurious counts in the tomograph ring, while the tungsten septa reject some of the events in which one (or both) of the 511-keV photons suffer a Compton scatter in the patient. The sensitivity of this design is improved by collection of data from cross-planes.

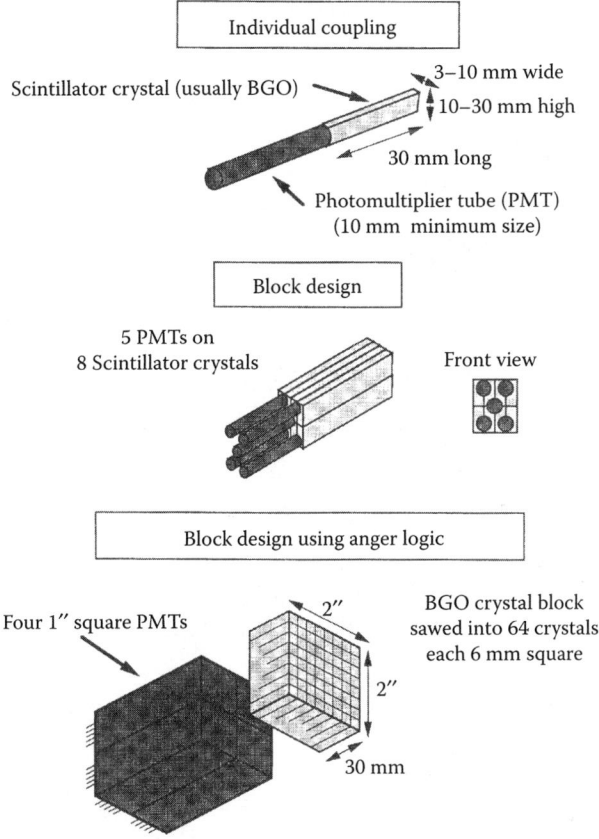

FIGURE 14.7 The arrangement of scintillators and phototubes is shown. The "individually coupled" design is capable of very high resolution, and because the design is very parallel (all the photomultiplier tubes and scintillator crystals operate independently), it is capable of very high data throughput. A block detector couples several photomultiplier tubes to a bank of scintillator crystals and uses a coding scheme to determine the crystal of interaction. In the two-layer block, five photomultiplier tubes are coupled to eight scintillator crystals.

individual coupling. The electronics necessary to decode the output of the block are straightforward but more complex than that needed for the individually coupled design.

Most block detector coding schemes use an analog coding scheme, where the ratio of light output is used to determine the crystal of interaction. In the example above, four photomultiplier tubes are coupled to a block of BGO that has been partially sawed through to form 64 "individual" crystals. The depth of the cuts are critical; that is, deep cuts tend to focus the scintillation light onto the face of a single photomultiplier tube, while shallow cuts tend to spread the light over all four photomultiplier tubes. This type of coding scheme is more difficult to implement than digital coding, since analog light ratios place more stringent requirements on the photomultiplier tube linearity and uniformity as well as scintillator crystal uniformity. However, most commercial PET cameras use an analog coding scheme because it is much less expensive due to the lower number of photomultiplier tubes required.

14.2.4 Physical Factors Affecting Resolution

The factors that affect the spatial resolution of PET tomographs are shown in Figure 14.8. The size of the detector is critical in determining the system's geometric resolution. If the block design is used, there is

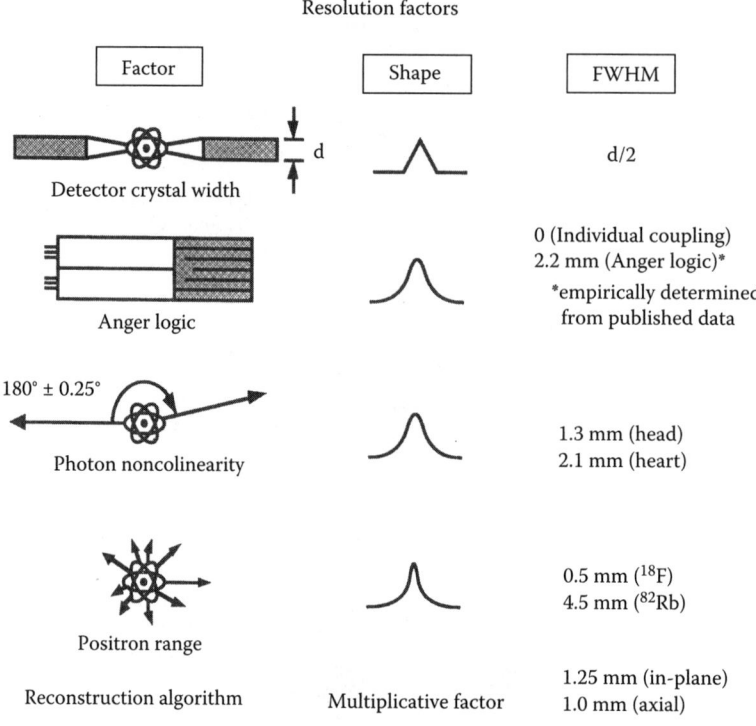

FIGURE 14.8 Factors contributing to the resolution of the PET tomograph. The contribution most accessible to further reduction is the size of the detector crystals.

a degradation in this geometric resolution by 2.2 mm for BGO. The degradation is probably due to the limited light output of BGO and the ratio of crystals (cuts) per phototube.

The angle between the paths of the annihilation photons can deviated from 180 degrees as a result of some residual kinetic motion (Fermi motion) at the time of annihilation. The effect on resolution of this deviation increases as the detector ring diameter increases so that eventually this factor can have a significant effect.

The distance the positron travels after being emitted from the nucleus and before annihilation causes a deterioration in spatial resolution. This distance depends on the particular nuclide. For example, the range of blurring for ^{18}F, the isotope used for many of the current PET studies, is quite small compared with that of the other isotopes. Combining values for these factors for the PET-600 tomograph, we can estimate a detector-pair spatial resolution of 2.0 mm and a reconstructed image resolution of 2.6 mm. The measured resolution of this system is 2.6 mm, but most commercially available tomographs use a block detector design (Figure 14.7), and the resolution of these systems is above 5 mm. The evolution of resolution improvement is shown in Figure 14.9.

The resolution evolutions discussed above pertain to results for the center or axis of the tomograph. The resolution at the edge of the object (e.g., patient) will be less by a significant amount due to two factors. First, the path of the photon from an "off-center" annihilation event typically traverses more than one detector crystal, as shown in Figure 14.10. This results in an elongation of the resolution spread function along the radius of the transaxial plane. The loss of resolution is dependent on the crystal density and the diameter of the tomograph detector ring. For a 60-cm diameter system, the resolution can deteriorate by a factor of 2 from the axis to 10 cm.

The coincidence circuitry must be able to determine coincident events with 10- to 20-nsec resolution for each crystal–crystal combination (i.e., chord). The timing requirement is set jointly by the time

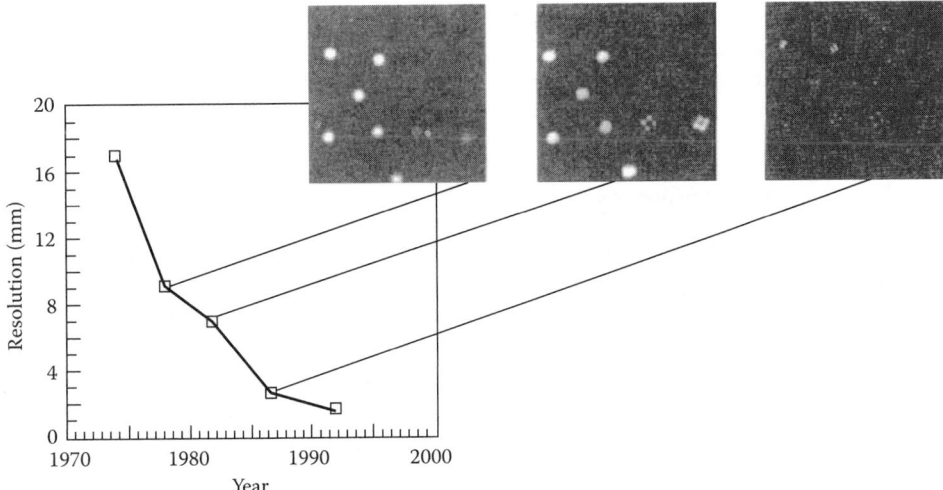

FIGURE 14.9 The evolution of resolution. Over the past decade, the resolving power of PET has improved from about 9 to 2.6 mm. This improvement is graphically illustrated by the increasing success with which one is able to resolve "hot spots" of an artificial sample that are detected and imaged by the tomographs.

of flight across the detector ring (4 nsec) and the crystal-to-crystal resolving time (typically 3 nsec). The most stringent requirement, however, is the vast number of chords in which coincidences must be determined (over 1.5 million in a 24-layer camera with septa in place and 18 million with the septa removed).

It is obviously impractical to have an individual coincidence circuit for each chord, so tomograph builders use parallel organization to solve this problem. A typical method is to use a high-speed clock (typically 200 MHz) to mark the arrival time of each 511-keV photon and a digital coincidence processor to search for coincident pairs of detected photons based on this time marker. This search can be done extremely quickly by having multiple sorters working in parallel.

The maximum event rate is also quite important, especially in septaless systems. The maximum rate in a single detector crystals is limited by the dead time due to the scintillator fluorescent lifetime

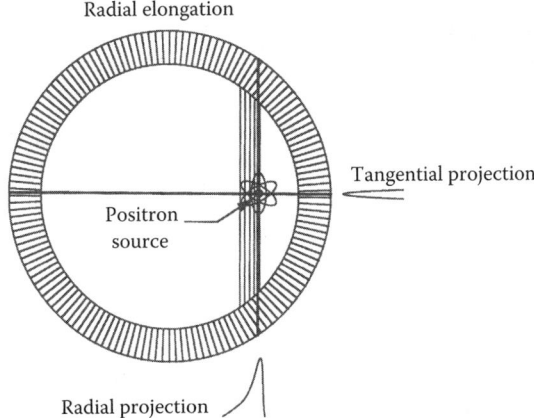

FIGURE 14.10 Resolution astigmatism in detecting off-center events. Because annihilation photons can penetrate crystals to different depths, the resolution is not equal in all directions, particularly at the edge of the imaging field. This problem of astigmatism will be taken into account in future PET instrumentation.

(typically 1 msec per event), but as the remainder of the scintillator crystals are available, the instrument has much higher event rates (e.g., number of crystals ¥ 1 msec). Combining crystals together to form contiguous blocks reduces the maximum event rate because the fluorescent lifetime applies to the entire block and a fraction of the tomograph is dead after each event.

14.2.5 Random Coincidences

If two annihilation events occurs within the time resolution of the tomograph (e.g., 10 nsec), then random coincident "events" add erroneous background activity to the tomograph and are significant at high event rates. These can be corrected for on a chord-by-chord basis. The noncoincidence event rate of each crystal pair is measured by observing the rate of events beyond the coincident timing window. The random rate for the particular chord R_{ij} corresponding to a crystal pair is

$$R_{ij} = r_i \times r_j \times 2\tau \quad R_{ij} = R_{ij} \tag{14.2}$$

where r_i and r_j are the event rates of crystal i and crystal j, and τ is the coincidence window width. As the activity in the subject increases, the event rate in each detector increases. Thus the random event rate will increase as the square of the activity.

14.2.6 Tomographic Reconstruction

Before reconstruction, each projection ray or chord receives three corrections: crystal efficiency, attenuation, and random efficiency. The efficiency for each chord is computed by dividing the observed count rate for that chord by the average court rate for chords with a similar geometry (i.e., length). This is typically done daily using a transmission source without the patient or object in place. Once the patient is in position in the camera, a transmission scan is taken, and the attenuation factor for each chord is computed by dividing its transmission count rate by its efficiency count rate. The patient is then injected with the isotope, and an emission scan is taken, during which time the random count rate is also measured. For each chord, the random event rate is subtracted from the emission rate, and the difference is divided by the attenuation factor and the chord efficiency. (The detector efficiency is divided twice because two separate detection's measurements are made—transmission and emission.) The resulting value is reconstructed, usually with the filtered backprojection algorithm. This is the same algorithm used in x-ray computed tomography (CT) and in projection MRI. The corrected projection data are formatted onto parallel- or fan-beam data sets for each angle. These are modified by a high-pass filter and backprojected.

The process of PET reconstruction is linear and shown by operators successively operating on the projection P:

$$A = \sum_\theta BPF^{-1}RF(P) \tag{14.3}$$

where A is the image, F is the Fourier transform, R is the ramp-shaped high-pass filter, F^{-1} is the inverse Fourier transform, BP is the backprojection operation, and θ denotes the superposition operation.

The alternative class of reconstruction algorithms involves iterative solutions to the classic inverse problem:

$$P = FA \tag{14.4}$$

where P is the projection matrix, A is the matrix of true data being sought, and F is the projection operation. The inverse is

$$A = F^{-1}P \qquad (14.4a)$$

which is computed by iteratively estimating the data A' and modifying the estimate by comparison of the calculated projection set P' with the true observed projections P. The expectation-maximization algorithm solves the inverse problem by updating each pixel value ai in accord with

$$a_1^{k+1} = \sum p_j \frac{a_j^k f_{ij}}{\sum_i a_l^k f_{ij}} \qquad (14.5)$$

where P is the measured projection, f_{ij} is the probability a source at pixel i will be detected in projection detector j, and k is the iteration.

14.2.7 Sensitivity

The sensitivity is a measure of how efficiently the tomograph detects coincident events and has units of count rate per unit activity concentration. It is measured by placing a known concentration of radionuclide in a water-filled 20-cm-diameter cylinder in the field of view. This cylinder, known as a phantom, is placed in the tomograph, and the coincidence event rate is measured. High sensitivity is important because emission imaging involves counting each event, and the resulting data are as much as 1000 times less than experienced in x-ray CT. Most tomographs have high individual detection efficiency for 511-keV photons impinging on the detector (>90%), so the sensitivity is mostly determined by geometric factors, that is, the solid angle subtended by the tomograph:

$$S = \frac{A\varepsilon^2\gamma \times 3.7 \times 10^4}{4\pi r^2} \text{(events/sec)/(mCi/cc)} \qquad (14.6)$$

where
    r = radius of tomograph
    A = area of detector material seen by each point in the object ($2\pi r$ ¥ axial aperture)
    ε = efficiency of scintillator
    γ = attenuation factor

For a single layer, the sensitivity of a tomograph of 90 cm diameter (2-cm axial crystals) will be 15,000 events/sec/mCi/mL for a disk of activity 20 cm in diameter and 1 cm thick. For a 20-cm-diameter cylinder, the sensitivity will be the same for a single layer with shields or septa that limit the off-slice activity from entering the collimators. However, modern multislice instruments use septa that allow activity from adjacent planes to be detected, thus increasing the solid angle and therefore the sensitivity. This increase comes at some cost due to increase in scatter. The improvement in sensitivity is by a factor of 7, but after correction for the noise, the improvement is 4. The noise equivalent sensitivity S_{NE} is given by

$$S_{NE} = \frac{(\text{true events})^2}{\text{true} \times \text{scatter} \times \text{random}} \qquad (14.7)$$

14.2.8 Statistical Properties of PET

The ability to map quantitatively the spatial distribution of a positron-emitting isotope depends on adequate spatial resolution to avoid blurring. In addition, sufficient data must be acquired to allow a statistically reliable estimation of the tracer concentration. The amount of available data depends on the biomedical accumulation, the imaging system sensitivity, and the dose of injected radioactivity. The propagation of errors due to the reconstruction process results in an increase in the noise over that expected for an independent signal, for example, by a factor proportional to the square root of the number of resolution elements (true pixels) across the image. The formula that deals with the general case of emission reconstruction (PET or SPECT) is

$$\% \text{ uncertainty} = \frac{1.2 \times 100 (\text{total no. of events})^{3/4}}{(\text{total no. of events})^{1/2}} \tag{14.8}$$

The statistical requirements are closely related to the spatial resolution, as shown in Figure 14.11.

For a given accuracy or a signal-to-noise ratio for a uniform distribution, the ratio of the number of events needed in a high-resolution system to that needed in a low-resolution system is proportional to

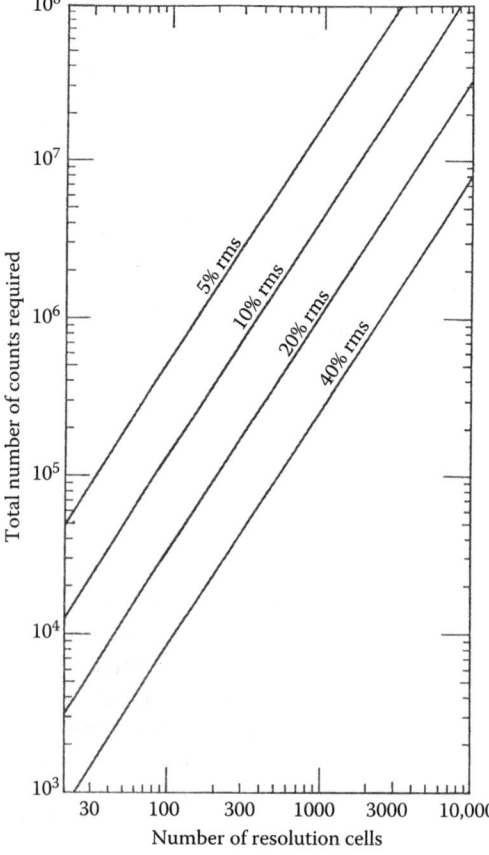

FIGURE 14.11 Statistical requirements and spatial resolution. The general relationship between the detected number of events and the number of resolution elements in an image is graphed for various levels of precision. These are relations for planes of constant thickness.

the 3/2 power of the ratio of the number of effective resolution elements in the two systems. Equation 14.8 and Figure 14.11 should be used not with the total pixels in the image but with the effective resolution cells. The number of effective resolution cells is the sum of the occupied resolution elements weighted by the activity within each element. Suppose, however, that the activity is mainly in a few resolution cells (e.g., 100 events per cell) and the remainder of the 10,000 cells have a background of 1 event per cell. The curves of Figure 14.11 would suggest unacceptable statistics; however, in this case, the effective number of resolution cells is below 100. The relevant equation for this situation is

$$\% \text{ uncertainty} = \frac{1.2 \times 100 (\text{no. of resolutiion cells})^{3/4}}{(\text{avg. no. of events per resolution cell in target})^{3/4}} \tag{14.9}$$

The better resolution gives improved results without the requirement for a drastic increase in the number of detected events is that the improved resolution increases contrast. (It is well known that the number of events needed to detect an object is inversely related to the square of the contrast.)

Acknowledgments

This work was supported in part by the Director, Office of Energy Research, Office of Health and Environmental Research, Medical Applications and Biophysical Research Division of the U.S. Department of Energy under contract No. DE-AC03-SF00098 and in part by NIH Grant HL25840. I wish to thank Drs. Stephen Derenzo and William Moses, who contributed material to this presentation.

References

1. Anger, H.O. 1963. Gamma-ray and positron scintillator camera. *Nucleonics* 21: 56.
2. Bailey, D.L. 1992. 3D acquisition and reconstruction in positron emission tomography. *Ann. Nucl. Med.* 6: 123.
3. Brownell, G.L. and Sweet, W.H. 1953. Localization of brain tumors with positron emitters. *Nucleonics* 11: 40.
4. Budinger, T.F., Greenberg, W.L., Derenzo, S.E. et al. 1978. Quantitative potentials of dynamic emission computed tomography. *J. Nucl. Med.* 19: 309.
5. Budinger, T.F., Gullberg, G.T., and Huesman, R.H. 1979. Emission computed tomography. In G.T. Herman (ed.), *Topics in Applied Physics: Image Reconstruction from Projections: Implementation and Applications*, pp. 147–246. Berlin, Springer-Verlag.
6. Cherry, S.R., Dahlbom, M., and Hoffman, E.J. 1991. 3D PET using a conventional multislice tomograph without septa. *J. Comput. Assist. Tomogr.* 15: 655.
7. Daube-Witherspoon, M.E. and Muehllehner, G. 1987. Treatment of axial data in three-dimensional PET. *J. Nucl. Med.* 28: 1717.
8. Derenzo, S.E., Huesman, R.H., Cahoon, J.L. et al. 1988. A positron tomograph with 600 BGO crystals and 2.6 mm resolution. *IEEE Trans. Nucl. Sci.* 35: 659.
9. Kinahan, P.E. and Rogers, J.G. 1989. Analytic 3D image reconstruction using all detected events. *IEEE Trans. Nucl. Sci.* 36: 964–968.
10. Shepp, L.A. and Vardi, Y. 1982. Maximum likelihood reconstruction for emission tomography. *IEEE Trans. Med. Imaging* 1: 113.
11. Ter-Pogossian, M.M., Phelps, M.E., Hoffman, E.J. et al. 1975. A positron-emission transaxial tomograph for nuclear imaging (PETT). *Radiology* 114: 89.

15

Electrical Impedance Tomography

N. Huber
University of Sussex

W. Wang
University of Sussex

D.C. Barber
Sheffield University

15.1 Electrical Impedance of Tissue

Human tissue is electrically conductive, with tissue conductivity varying significantly between different tissues. Electrical impedance tomography (EIT) is a relatively new imaging modality, first developed in Sheffield, UK in 1982 (Brown and Barber), whose purpose is to produce images from the internal conductivity distribution of an object, based on measurements collected from the surface of the object (Kohn and Vogelius, 1984a,b; Sylvester and Uhlmann, 1986). The original assumptions made were of the near-isotropic distribution of conductivity of the imaged object.

Conductivity images produced through EIT have been mostly cross-sectional, hence the association with tomography, even though this term is not entirely accurate. Moreover, it has been shown that tissue incorporates a reactive component, making it not merely conductive. Hence, it is more fitting to be referring to the *impedance* (or its inverse, the *admittance*) of tissue, rather than the conductivity or resistivity of tissue. Hence, the term *impedance* in EIT.

15.2 Conduction in Human Tissues

In short, tissue can be considered as a collection of conducting fluids (electrolytes) bound by insulating membranes, these membranes themselves existing in a conductive suspension. This, to all intents and purposes, resembles a leaky dielectric. The first model developed (Fricke, 1925) portrayed the cell as a multitude of resistances representing every minute section of the extracellular and intracellular media, and capacitances representing every minute section of the membrane. With the use of circuit theory, these elements can be combined such that an equivalent circuit is produced, as seen from the perspective

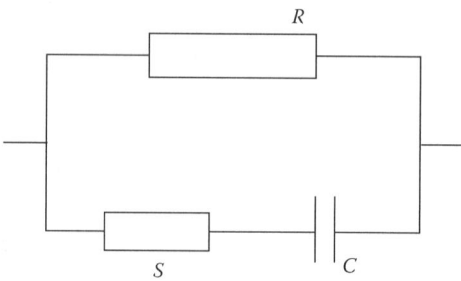

FIGURE 15.1   The Cole–Cole model of tissue impedance.

of the electrodes. It is interesting to note that, apart from a change in actual component values, both a single cell in suspension and tissue can be represented with the same electrical model.

The developed model for bulk tissue most widely in use today (Cole and Cole, 1941) consists of a resistor R in parallel with a combination of a capacitor C and a resistor S, as shown in Figure 15.1.

It is worth noting that S has also been portrayed as being in series with both R and C (for a more detailed review, refer to McAdams and Jossinet, 1995). This oversimplified model has been shown empirically to fit data well, when a term is added to represent the frequency dependence of the component values. When expressed in terms of impedance, tissue behavior with respect to frequency can be shown to be

$$Z = Z_\infty + \frac{(Z_0 - Z_\infty)}{1 + \left(j(f/f_c)\right)^{(1-\alpha)}} \tag{15.1}$$

where Z_0 is tissue impedance at very low frequency, Z_∞ the impedance at high frequency, both complex, and f_c is a characteristic frequency. Alpha (α) allows for the frequency dependency of the model components, and is found experimentally to match the particular tissue type.

Diseased tissue is known to exhibit altered R, S, and C due to structural change. By extracting the component values through complex measurements of impedance of tissue can allow for the differentiation of tissues and of different disease conditions. It is worth noting that although maximum accuracy in the determination of the model components can be obtained if both real and imaginary components are available, in principle, knowledge of the resistive component alone should enable the values to be determined, provided an adequate range of frequencies is used. This can have practical consequences for data collection, since accurate measurement of the capacitive component can prove difficult.

The prevailing assumption in EIT is that tissue is isotropic. However, this is not true in the macroscopic scale for various types of tissue due to their anistropic physical structure. The inherent anisotropy can be shown to prevent the existence of unique solutions to the conductivity distributions, since there are sets of different anisotropic conductivity distributions that give the same surface voltages, rendering them indistinguishable from each other. It is an open issue as to the degree to which tissue anisotropy affects the generation of useful images through EIT, which is actively being explored (e.g., Lionheart and Paridis, 2010).

15.3 Determination of Impedance Distribution

The distribution of electrical potential within an isotropic conducting object through which a low-frequency current is flowing is given by

$$\nabla(\sigma\nabla\varphi) = 0 \tag{15.2}$$

where φ is the potential distribution within the object and σ is the distribution of conductivity (generally admittivity) within the object (Brown and Barber, 1982). If the conductivity is uniform, this reduces to Laplace's equation. Strictly speaking, this equation is only correct for direct current, but for the frequencies of alternating current used in EIT (up to 1 MHz) and the sizes of objects being imaged, it can be assumed that this equation continues to describe the instantaneous distribution of potential within the conducting object. If this equation is solved for a given conductivity distribution and current distribution through the surface of the object, the potential distribution developed on the surface of the object may be determined. The distribution of potential will depend on several things. It will depend on the pattern of current applied and the shape of the object. It will also depend on the internal conductivity of the object, and it is this that needs to be determined. In theory, the current may be applied in a continuous and nonuniform pattern at every point across the surface. In practice, current is applied to an object through electrodes attached to the surface of the object. Theoretically, potential may be measured at every point on the surface of the object. Again, voltage on the surface of the object is measured in practice using electrodes (possibly different from those used to apply current) attached to the surface of the object. There will be a relationship, the forward solution, between an *applied current pattern* j_i, the conductivity distribution σ, and the surface potential distribution φ_i which can be formally represented as

$$\varphi_i = R(j_i, \sigma) \tag{15.3}$$

If σ and j_i are known, φ_i can be computed. For one current pattern j_i, knowledge of φ_i is not in general sufficient to uniquely determine σ. However, by applying a complete set of independent current patterns, it becomes possible to obtain sufficient information to determine σ, at least in the isotropic case. This is the inverse solution. In practice, measurements of surface potential or voltage can only be made at a finite number of positions, corresponding to electrodes placed on the surface of the object. This also means that only a finite number of independent current patterns can be applied. For N electrodes, $N - 1$ independent current patterns can be defined and $N(N - 1)/2$ independent measurements made. This latter number determines the limit of image resolution achievable with N electrodes. In practice, it may not be possible to collect all possible independent measurements. Since only a finite number of current patterns and measurements is available, the set of equations represented by Equation 15.3 can be rewritten as

$$v = A_c c \tag{15.4}$$

where v is now a concatenated vector of all voltage values for all current patterns, c is a vector of conductivity values, representing the conductivity distribution divided into uniform image *pixels*, and A_c a matrix representing the transformation of this conductivity vector into the voltage vector. Since A_c depends on the conductivity distribution, this equation is nonlinear. Although formally the preceding equation can be solved for c by inverting A_c, the nonlinear nature of this equation means that this cannot be done in a single step. An iterative procedure will therefore be needed to obtain c.

Examination of the physics of current flow shows that current tends to take the easiest path possible in its passage through the object. If the conductivity at some point is changed, the current path redistributes in such a way that the effects of this change are minimized. The practical effect of this is that it is possible to have fairly large changes in conductivity within the object which only produce relatively small changes in voltage at the surface of the object. The converse of this is that when reconstructing the conductivity distribution, small errors on the measured voltage data, both random and systematic, can translate into large errors in the estimate of the conductivity distribution. This effect forms, and

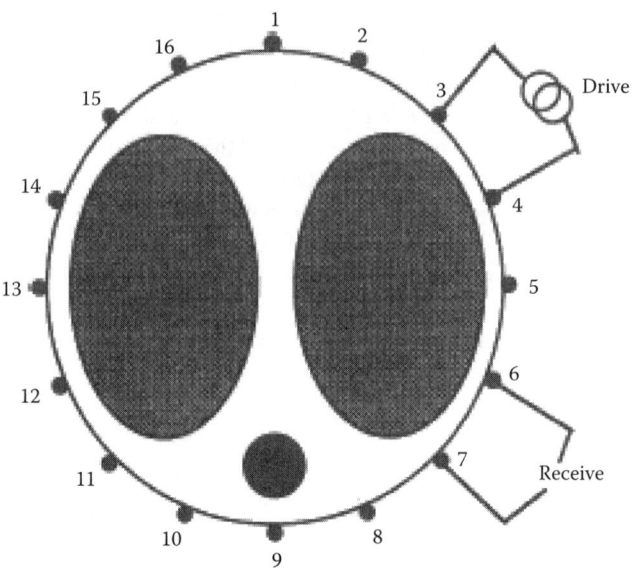

FIGURE 15.2 Idealized electrode positions around a conducting object with typical drive and measurement electrode pairs indicated.

will continue to form, a limit to the quality of reconstructed conductivity images in terms of resolution, accuracy, and sensitivity.

Any measurement of voltage must always be referred to a reference point. Usually this is one of the electrodes, which is given the nominal value of 0 V. The voltage on all other electrodes is determined by measuring the voltage difference between each electrode and the reference electrode. Alternatively, voltage differences may be measured between pairs of electrodes. A common approach is to measure the voltage between adjacent pairs of electrodes (Figure 15.2). Clearly, the measurement scheme affects the form of A_c. Choice of the pattern of applied currents and the voltage measurement scheme used can affect the accuracy with which images of conductivity can be reconstructed.

EIT is not a mature technology. However, it has been the subject of intensive research over the past few years, and this work is still continuing. Nearly all the research effort has been devoted to exploring the different possible ways of collecting data and producing images of tissue resistivity, with the aim of optimizing image reconstruction in terms of image accuracy, spatial resolution, and sensitivity.

Although the most current interest is in the use of EIT for medical imaging, there is also interest in its use in whole-body composition monitoring (Rebeyrol et al., 2010). Other applications include geophysical measurements (e.g., Marescot et al., 2003), and a comprehensive review of the applications of electrical tomography for industrial applications is given in York (2005).

15.3.1 Data Collection

15.3.1.1 Basic Requirements

Data are collected by applying a current to the object through electrodes connected to the surface of the object and then making measurements of the voltage on the object surface through the same or other electrodes. Although conceptually simple, technically this can be difficult. Great attention must be paid to the reduction of noise and the elimination of any voltage offsets on the measurements. The currents applied are alternating currents usually in the range 10 kHz to 1 MHz. Since tissue has a complex impedance, the voltage signals will contain in-phase and out-of-phase components. In principle, both of these can be measured. In practice, measurement of the out-of-phase (the capacitive) component is significantly more difficult because of the presence of unwanted (stray) capacitances between various parts of the voltage measurement system, including the leads from the data-collection apparatus to the electrodes. These stray capacitances can lead to appreciable leakage currents, especially at the higher frequencies, which translate into systematic errors on the voltage measurements. McEwan et al. (2007) offers an in-depth review of the errors affecting EIT systems, and a simplified, practical approach to measuring errors is given in Hahn et al. (2008).

The signal measured on an electrode, or between a pair of electrodes, oscillates at the same frequency as the applied current. The magnitude of this signal (usually separated into real and imaginary components) is determined, typically by demodulation and integration. The frequency of the demodulated signal is much less than the frequency of the applied signal, and the effects of stray capacitances on this signal are generally negligible. This realization has led some workers to propose that the signal demodulation and detection system be mounted as close to the electrodes as possible, ideally at the electrode site itself, and some systems have been developed that use this approach, although none with sufficient miniaturization of the electronics to be practical in a clinical setting. This solution is not in itself free of problems, but this approach is likely to be of increasing importance if the frequency range of applied currents is to be extended beyond 1 MHz, necessary if the value of the complex impedance is to be adequately explored as a function of frequency.

Various data-collection schemes have been proposed. Most data are collected from a two-dimensional (2D) configuration of electrodes, either from 2D objects or around the border of a plane normal to the principal axis of a cylindrical (in the general sense) object where that plane intersects the object surface. The simplest data-collection protocol is to apply a current between a pair of electrodes (often an adjacent pair) and measure the voltage difference between other adjacent pairs (see Figure 15.2). Although in principle voltage could be measured on electrodes through which current is simultaneously flowing, the presence of an electrode impedance, generally unknown, between the electrode and the body surface means that the voltage measured is not actually that on the body surface. Various means have been suggested for either measuring the electrode impedance in some way or including it as an unknown in the image-reconstruction process. However, in many systems, measurements from electrodes through which current is flowing are simply ignored. Electrode impedance is generally not considered to be a problem when making voltage measurements on electrodes through which current is not flowing, provided a voltmeter with sufficiently high input impedance is used, although, since the input impedance is always finite, every attempt should be made to keep the electrode impedance as low as possible. Using the same electrode for driving current and making voltage measurements, even at different times in the data-collection cycle, means that at some point in the data-collection apparatus, wires carrying current and wires carrying voltage signals will be brought close together in a switching system, leading to the possibility of leakage currents. There is a good argument for using separate sets of electrodes for driving and measuring to reduce this problem. Paulson et al. (1992) have also proposed this approach and have noted that it can aid in the modeling of the forward solution (see Section 15.3.2). Brown et al. (1994) have used this approach in making multifrequency measurements.

Clearly, the magnitude of the voltage measured will depend on the magnitude of the current applied. If a constant-current drive is used, this must be able to deliver a known current to a variety of input impedances with a stability of better than 0.1%. This is technically demanding. The best approach to this problem is to measure the current being applied, which can easily be done to this accuracy. These measurements are then used to normalize the voltage data.

The current application and data-collection regime will depend on the reconstruction algorithm used. Several EIT systems apply current in a distributed manner, with currents of various magnitudes being applied to several or all of the electrodes. These optimal currents (see Section 15.3.2) must be specified accurately, and again, it is technically difficult to ensure that the correct current is applied at each electrode. Although there are significant theoretical advantages to using distributed current patterns, the increased technical problems associated with this approach, and the higher noise levels associated with the increase in electronic complexity, may outweigh these advantages.

Although most EIT at present is 2D in the sense given above, it is intrinsically a three-dimensional (3D) imaging procedure, since current cannot be constrained to flow in a plane through a 3D object. 3D data collection does not pose any further problems apart from increased complexity due to the need for more electrodes. Whereas most data-collection systems to date have been based on 16 or 32 electrodes, 3D systems will require four times or more electrodes distributed over the surface of the object if adequate resolution is to be maintained. Technically, this will require "belts" or "vests" of electrodes that can be rapidly applied (McAdams et al., 1994). Some of these are already available, and the application of an adequate number of electrodes should not prove insuperable provided electrode-mounted electronics are not required. Metherall et al. (1996) describe a three-dimensional data-collection system and reconstruction algorithm and note the improved accuracy of three-dimensional images compared to two-dimensional images constructed using data collected from three-dimensional objects.

15.3.1.2 EIT Hardware Design Principles

The vast majority of EIT systems depend on the application of current patterns and the measurement of voltages. The architecture of systems is rather common, and at first glance straightforward (Figure 15.3).

The signal to be applied to the subject (commonly a sinusoid of known frequency) is first generated, and is fed to a voltage-to-current converter circuit. This converter can be either single- or multiple-output, providing a means of classifying EIT systems by the number of current sources used.

The number of electrodes of the system is, generally, larger than the number of sources, and hence a switching network to serve all electrodes with current is required, ordinarily implemented through multiplexers. In most cases, cables (with driven shields in most cases) supply the current to the electrodes. Measurements are taken from the electrodes in either single-ended or differential mode, demultiplexed appropriately. A differential amplifier is more frequently used to take a measurement between pairs of electrodes, both to achieve high common mode rejection and to reduce the dynamic range compared to measurements made with respect to ground. As the measurement has to be taken during the time of

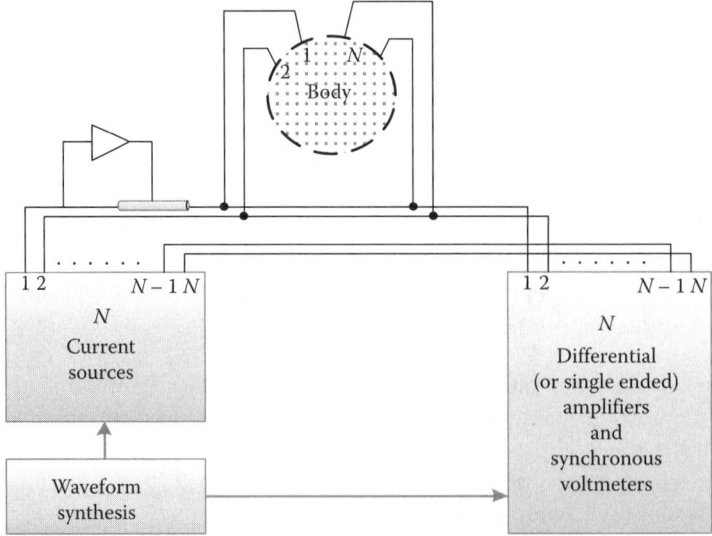

FIGURE 15.3 A typical multichannel EIT system. The number of current sources is commonly smaller than the number of electrodes, requiring multiplexing at the source and demultiplexing at the voltmeters. (Reproduced from Saulnier, G.J. 2005. *Electrical Impedance Tomography: Methods, History and Applications*, Institute of Physics Publishing, Bristol, pp. 67–104.)

application of the signal into the body under investigation, there is commonly digital synchronization between the signal generation and voltage measurement.

The challenges of EIT electronics design are not directly apparent. In simulations, current sources behave ideally, supplying constant current for a constant voltage input irrespective of load over a frequency bandwidth well beyond the medical requirements of EIT (i.e., >10 MHz). The output impedance of the current source is assumed infinite, the full current passed directly to the load. In practice, however, the output impedance of current sources is better modeled as a resistance and a capacitance in parallel. The output response of the source is, then, dependent on the load, with current actually shunted directly to ground rather than through the load, especially at higher frequencies. Stray capacitances external to the source introduced either by the PCB design/implementation or any cables used. A very thorough analysis of the techniques used in EIT instrumentation design can be found in Saulnier (2005), the author looking into every aspect of the hardware from signal generation to sampling, source design, and performance compensation.

15.3.2 Image Reconstruction

15.3.2.1 Basics of Reconstruction

Several different approaches to image reconstruction have been tried and established since 1982 (Brown and Barber, 1982; Wexler et al., 1985; Yorkey, 1986; Barber and Seagar, 1987; Kim and Woo, 1987; Hua et al., 1988; Breckon, 1990; Cheney et al., 1990; Zadehkoochak et al., 1991; Koire et al., 1992; Bayford, 1994; Morucci et al., 1994). A detailed review of reconstruction efforts can be found in work specifically on this topic by Lionheart (2004).

The most accurate approaches are based broadly on the following algorithm. For a given set of current patterns, a forward transform is set up for determining the voltages v produced from the conductivity distribution c (Equation 15.4). A_c is dependent on c, so it is necessary to assume an initial starting conductivity distribution c_0. This is usually taken to be uniform. Using A_c, the expected voltages v_0 are calculated and compared with the actual measured voltages v_m. Unless c_0 is correct (which it will not be initially), v_0 and v_m will differ. It can be shown that an improved estimate of c is given by

$$\Delta c = \left(S_c^t S_c \right)^{-1} S_c^t (v_0 - v_m) \tag{15.5}$$

$$c_1 = c_0 + \Delta c \tag{15.6}$$

where S_c is the differential of A_c with respect to c, the sensitivity matrix and S_c^t is the transpose of S_c. The improved value of c is then used in the next iteration to compute an improved estimate of v_m, that is, v_1. This iterative process is continued until some appropriate endpoint is reached. Although convergence is not guaranteed, in practice, convergence to the correct c in the absence of noise can be expected, provided a good starting value is chosen. Uniform conductivity seems to be a reasonable choice. In the presence of noise on the measurements, iteration is stopped when the difference between v and v_m is within the margin of error set by the known noise on the data.

There are some practical difficulties associated with this approach. One is that large changes in c may only produce small changes in v, and this will be reflected in the structure of S_c, making $S_c^t S_c$ very difficult to invert reliably. Various methods of regularization have been used, with varying degrees of success, to achieve stable inversion of this matrix although the greater the regularization applied, the poorer the resolution that can be achieved. A more difficult practical problem is that for convergence to be possible the computed voltages v must be equal to the measured voltages v_m when the correct conductivity values are used in the forward calculation. Although in a few idealized cases analytical solutions of the forward problem are possible, in general, numerical solutions must be used. Techniques such as the finite-element method (FEM) have been developed to solve problems of this type numerically. However, the accuracy of these methods has to be carefully examined (Paulson et al., 1992) and, while they are adequate for many applications, they may not be adequate for the EIT reconstruction problem, especially in the case of 3D objects. Accuracies of rather better than 1% appear to be required if image artifacts are to be minimized. Consider a situation in which the actual distortion of conductivity is uniform. Then the initial v should be equal to the v_m to an accuracy less than the magnitude of the noise. If this is not the case, then the algorithm will alter the conductivity distribution from uniform, which will clearly result in error. While the required accuracies have been approached under ideal conditions, there is only a limited amount of evidence at present to suggest that they can be achieved with data taken from human subjects.

15.3.2.2 Optimal Current Patterns

So far little has been said about the form of the current patterns applied to the object except that a set of independent patterns is needed. The simplest current patterns to use are those given by passing current into the object through one electrode and extracting current through a second electrode (a bipolar pattern). This pattern has the virtue of simplicity and ease of application. However, other current patterns are possible. Current can be passed simultaneously through many electrodes, with different amounts passing through each electrode. Indeed, an infinite number of patterns are possible, the only limiting condition being that the magnitude of the current flowing into the conducting object equals the magnitude of the current flowing out of the object. Isaacson (1986) has shown that for any conducting object there is a set of optimal current patterns and has provided an algorithm to compute them even if the conductivity distribution is initially unknown. Isaacson showed that by using optimal patterns, significant improvements in sensitivity could be obtained compared with simpler two-electrode current patterns. However, the additional computation and hardware required to use optimal current patterns compared with fixed, nonoptimal patterns are considerable.

Use of suboptimal patterns close to optimum will also produce significant gains. In general, the optimal patterns are very different from the patterns produced in the simple two-electrode case. The optimal patterns are often cosine-like patterns of current amplitude distributed around the object boundary rather than being localized at a pair of points, as in the two-electrode case. Since the currents are passed simultaneously through many electrodes, it is tempting to try and use the same electrodes for voltage measurements. This produces two problems. As noted above, measurement of voltage on an electrode through which an electric current is passing is compromised by the presence of electrode resistance, which causes a generally unknown voltage drop across the electrode, whereas voltage can be accurately measured on an electrode through which current is not flowing using a voltmeter of high input impedance. In addition, it has proved difficult to model current flow around an electrode through which current is flowing with sufficient accuracy to allow the reliable calculation of voltage on that electrode, which is needed for accurate reconstruction. It seems that separate electrodes should be used for voltage measurements with distributed current systems.

Theoretically, distributed (near-)optimal current systems have some advantages. As each of the optimal current patterns is applied, it is possible to determine if the voltage patterns produced contain any useful information or if they are simply noise. Since the patterns can be generated and applied in order of decreasing significance, it is possible to terminate application of further current patterns when no further information can be obtained. A consequence of this is that signal-to-noise ratios (SNR) can be maximized for a given total data-collection time. With bipolar current patterns, this option is not available. All patterns must be applied. Provided the SNR in the data is sufficiently good and only a limited number of electrodes are used, this may not be too important, and the extra effort involved in generating the optimal or near-optimal patterns may not be justified. However, as the number of electrodes is increased, the use of optimal patterns becomes more significant. It also has been suggested that the distributed nature of the optimal patterns makes the forward problem less sensitive to modeling errors. Although there is currently no firm evidence for this, this seems a reasonable assertion.

15.3.2.3 Three-Dimensional Imaging

Most published work so far on image reconstruction has concentrated on solving the 2D problem. However, real medical objects, that is, patients, are three-dimensional. Theoretically, as the dimensionality of the object increases, reconstruction should become better conditioned. However, unlike 3D x-ray images, which can be constructed from a set of independent 2D images, EIT data from 3D objects cannot be so decomposed and data from over the whole surface of the object is required for 3D reconstruction. The principles of reconstruction in 3D are identical to the 2D situation although practically the problem is quite formidable, principally because of the need to solve the forward problem in three dimensions. Some early work on 3D imaging was presented by Goble and Isaacson (1990). Metherall et al. (1996) have shown images using data collected from human subjects. Cherepenin et al. (2001) started using 3D imaging for impedance mammography, with other systems being reported since (e.g., Sze et al., 2011). With further theoretical proof of the necessity for 3D imaging over conventional 2D (Halter et al., 2007a), and lately it has been shown that the creation of patient-specific forward models through accurate knowledge of electrode positioning enhances performance of reconstruction algorithms used, and conforms more realistically with the breast geometry (Tizzard et al., 2010). Indeed, it has been stressed in recent publications that the use of accurate shape information is paramount to achieving much higher sensitivity, and works have been carried out to use *a priori* knowledge from multiple other modalities to this end (e.g., CT (Grychtol et al., 2011), MRI (Davidson et al., 2011), ultrasound (Borsic et al., 2011)), most performed for 3D EIT.

15.3.2.4 Single-Step Reconstruction

The complete reconstruction problem is nonlinear and requires iteration. However, each step in the iterative process is linear. Images reconstructed using only the first step of iteration effectively treat image formation as a linear process, an assumption approximately justified for small changes in conductivity from uniform. In the case, the functions A_c and S_c often can be precomputed with reasonable accuracy because they usually are computed for the case of uniform conductivity. Although the solution cannot be correct, since the nonlinearity is not taken into account, it may be useful, and first-step linear approximations have gained some popularity. Cheney et al. (1990) have published some results from a first-step process using optimal currents. Most, if not all, of the clinical images produced to date have used a single-step reconstruction algorithm (Barber and Seagar, 1987; Barber and Brown, 1990). The use of linearity for each reconstruction iteration has more recently been incorporated into the concerted effort of standardizing 2D pulmonary monitoring (Adler et al., 2009), evidently showing that this is the method of choice for a large number of researchers worldwide.

15.3.2.5 Differential Imaging

Ideally, the aim of EIT is to reconstruct images of the absolute distribution of conductivity (or admittivity). These images are known as absolute (or static) images. However, this requires that the forward problem can be solved to a high degree of accuracy, and this can be difficult. The magnitude of the voltage signal measured on an electrode or between electrodes will depend on the body shape, the electrode shape and position, and the internal conductivity distribution. The signal magnitude is in fact dominated by the first two effects rather than by conductivity. However, if a change in conductivity occurs within the object, then it can often be assumed that the change in surface voltage is dominated by this conductivity change. In differential (or dynamic) imaging, the aim is to image changes in conductivity rather than absolute values. If the voltage difference between a pair of (usually adjacent) electrodes before a conductivity change occurs is g_1 and the value after change occurs is g_2, then a normalized data value is defined as

$$\Delta g_n = 2\frac{g_1 - g_2}{g_1 + g_2} = \frac{\Delta g}{g_{\text{mean}}} \tag{15.7}$$

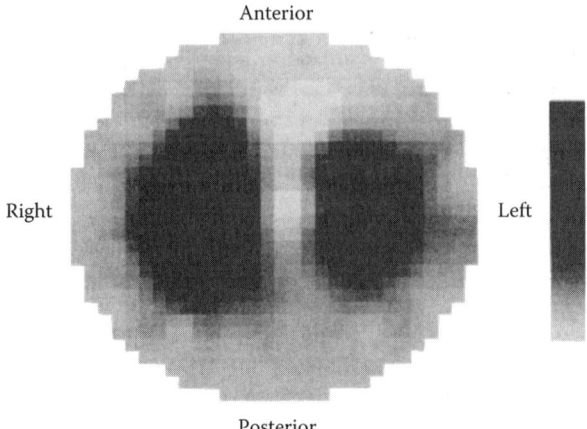

FIGURE 15.4   A differential conductivity image representing the changes in conductivity in going from maximum inspiration (breathing in) to maximum expiration (breathing out). Increasing blackness represents increasing conductivity.

Many of the effects of body shape (including interpreting the data as coming from a 2D object when in fact it is from a 3D object) and electrode placing at least partially cancel out in this definition. The values of the normalized data are determined largely by the conductivity changes. It can be argued that the relationship between the (normalized) changes in conductivity c_n and the normalized changes in boundary data g_n is given by

$$\Delta g_n = F \Delta c_n \qquad\qquad (15.8)$$

where F is a sensitivity matrix which can be shown to be much less sensitive to object shape end electrode positions than the sensitivity matrix of Equation 15.5. Although images produced using this algorithm are not completely free of artifact, that is the only algorithm which has reliably produced images using data taken from human subjects. Metherall et al. (1996) used a version of this algorithm for 3D imaging and Brown et al. (1994) for multifrequency imaging, in this case imaging changes in conductivity with frequency. The principle disadvantage of this algorithm is that it can only image changes in conductivity, which must be either natural or induced. Figure 15.4 shows a typical differential image. This represents the changes in the conductivity of the lungs between expiration and inspiration.

15.3.3 Multifrequency Measurements

Differential algorithms can only image changes in conductivity. Absolute distributions of conductivity cannot be produced using these methods. In addition, any gross movement of the electrodes, either because they have to be removed and replaced or even because of significant patient movement, makes the use of this technique difficult for long-term measurements of changes. As an alternative to changes in time, differential algorithms can image changes in conductivity with frequency. Brown et al. (1994) have shown that if measurements are made over a range of frequencies and differential images produced using data from the lowest frequency and the other frequencies in turn, these images can be used to compute parametric images representing the distribution of combinations of the circuit values in Figure 15.1. For example, images representing the ratio of S to R, a measure of the ratio of intracellular to extracellular volume, can be produced, as well as images of $f_o = 1/(2p(RC + SC))$, the tissue characteristic frequency. Although not images of the absolute distribution of conductivity, they are images of absolute tissue properties. Some cancer research has also been performed on combining these parameters in ways considered related to pathological conditions for diagnosis of an abnormality (Wang et al., 2007a), but which are also useful for enhancing the imaging performance. Since these properties are related to tissue structure, they should produce images with useful contrast. Data sufficient to reconstruct an image can be collected in a time short enough to preclude significant patient movement, which means these images are robust against movement artifacts. Changes of these parameters with time can still be observed.

15.4 Areas of Clinical Application

EIT is yet to be widely accepted in the clinical environment. The strengths and weaknesses of EIT have to be weighed so that the most appropriate applications can be identified. This modality cannot compete in spatial resolution or resemblance to real-life with other anatomic imaging methods (MRI, CT, x-ray, etc.), but is safe, relatively cheap, does not involve any ionizing radiation, and has high temporal resolution, as well as the unique capability of providing images that are directly assistive to condition diagnosis.

The advantages of EIT have spurred a large amount of research in the field, of which excellent coverage is given in Holder (2005). Some applications are highlighted here for completeness, with particular emphasis on applications that have been tested clinically.

15.4.1 Cancer Detection in Soft Tissue

15.4.1.1 Tissue Impedance Spectroscopy

Tissue impedance (often referred to as electrical impedance spectroscopy, EIS) measurements *in vitro* not only have been used as the reference point for most clinical *in vivo* studies (Surowiec et al., 1988; Tunstall et al., 1997; Jossinet and Schmitt, 1999), but also have other practical applications. In an example, impedance spectroscopy was employed for identification of cancerous mouse pancreas by taking measurements of the electrical properties of the mouse pancreas (Qiao et al., 2008). In the context of cell biology, the results of other experiments are not disturbed by the electrical impedance measurements. Through the measurement of the impedance of tissue, the time taken to locate a malignant islet could be dramatically reduced.

The standard method for bioimpedance measurements is the "four-electrode chamber," a proven stable system for such applications (Ferris and Rose, 1972; Wang et al., 2006; Grimnes and Martinsen, 2008), but recent studies have also shown that cell culture imaging is possible for monitoring of cell growth through the use of impedance tomography at the micro-scale level (Linderholm et al., 2008). There has also been effort on imaging at the cellular level, such as the system discussed in Liu et al. (2010).

With the advent of nanoparticles, the EIT group of Middlesex University have suggested the use of gold nanoparticles as contrast enhancement media for *in vivo* applications (Callaghan et al., 2010). Their research recognizes that the impedance change caused by these particles is on the almost beyond the reach of current EIT systems, but the idea of EIT contrast enhancement is a very appealing one.

15.4.1.2 Breast Cancer

Early breast cancer detection has been linked directly with a reduction in mortality rate. The golden standard of detection, x-ray mammography, is limited by low sensitivity, more pronouncedly so in dense breasts, as well as lack of diagnostic ability, requiring needle aspirations for a positive diagnosis.

Various early *in vitro* studies have shown that the electrical properties of malignant tissue of the breast differ significantly to both benign and healthy tissue. Indicatively, fat tissue is at 0.5 mS/cm conductivity, connective tissue at 0.6–0.8 mS/cm, carcinoma at 1.5–2.2 mS/cm, mastopathy tissue at 2.7–3.5 mS/cm,

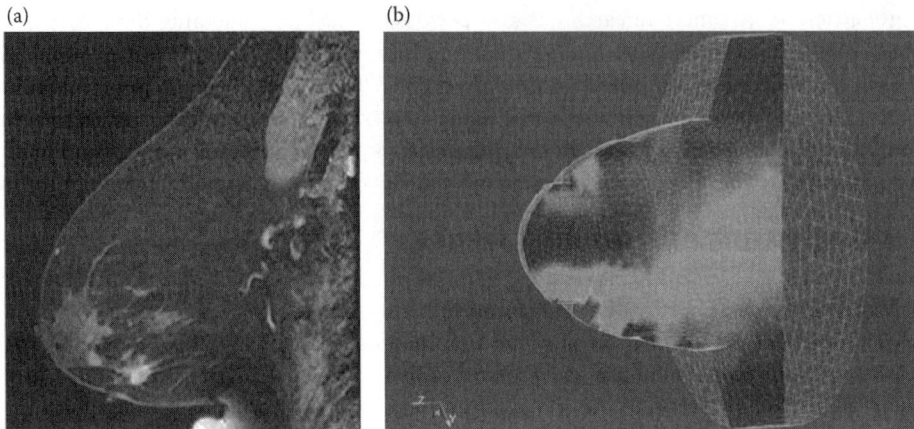

FIGURE 15.5 (a) Sagittal contrast-enhanced breast MRI images. 1.3 cm cancerous mass visible at 5 cm from nipple. (b) 3D EIT reconstruction of breast. (Adapted from Tizzard, A. et al. 2010. *J. Phys. Conf. Ser.* 224(1): 012034.)

and fibroadenoma at 3.3–4.0 mS/cm, depending on the source (e.g., Surowiec et al., 1988; Tunstall et al., 1997; Jossinet and Schmitt, 1999). Consequently, EIT has been suggested and pursued by a large number of researchers for early breast cancer detection due to its noninvasive or ionizing nature, with the application sometimes referred to as electrical impedance mammography (EIM) (Wang et al., 1996). Indeed, one of the first electrical impedance-based devices to reach the market was for EIM (Assenheimer et al., 2001), even though not strictly tomographic. A number of clinical trials have shown that EIT is a promising modality, or at least an adjunctive diagnostic method to the more established techniques (Malich et al., 2001), and has also been suggested as a real-time, noninvasive monitoring method of breast tissue thermoablation (e.g., Lukaszewicz et al., 2010). There has also been suggestion of guiding noninvasive breast cancer treatment based on high-intensity focused ultrasound (HIFU) through the combined use of EIM and ultrasound (Lobstein-Adams et al., 2011).

The two main directions followed by researchers are those of ring-electrode configurations (Wheeler et al., 2002; Halter et al., 2005; Oh et al., 2007), or of planar-array electrodes (Cherepenin et al., 2002; Tang et al., 2002), with 16 to 256, and up to thousands of electrodes (Zhao et al., 2010), hand-held or fixed in a set patient interface, with the use or not of contact media, such as through a saline bath, with physical contact (dry) with the electrodes, or with recessed (wet) electrodes (Wang et al., 2007b). Reported results vary significantly due to the different nature of each device and the reconstruction approach followed. As an example, Figure 15.5 shows the 3D model generated using the system in Halter et al. (2005). However, the same sources of errors and hurdles seem to be common between all systems: low spatial resolution, especially at a distance from the electrodes, variable contact impedance and optimization of current driving, and voltage measurement methods.

15.4.1.3 Cervical Cancer

Cervical cancer accounts for approximately 10% of cancers diagnosed in women worldwide, with much higher incidence rates found mostly in Southern Africa and Central America. Currently, an impedance-based device is on an EU multicenter trial, having shown that the device can be used as an adjunct to the gold standard, colposcopy, for the diagnosis of high-grade cervical intraepithelial neoplasia (Balasubramani et al., 2009), based on the original work by Brown et al. (1998). Further effort has been carried out by Korjenevsky et al. (2010), following a different approach borrowed by EIM, also showing promising clinical results. The main difference between the two systems is that the latter is designed to produce impedance images of the cervix, while the former returns localized impedance measurements.

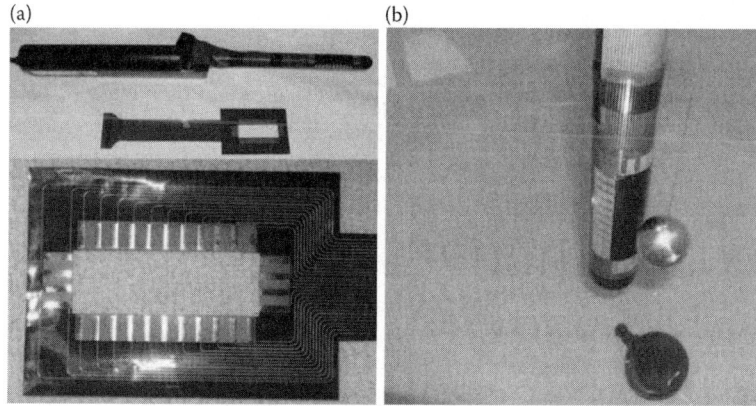

FIGURE 15.6 (a) Top: flex circuit of electrodes wrapped around the ultrasound probe. (a) Bottom: magnified view of flex circuit of electrodes laid flat. (b) Imaging configuration; an inclusion (steel ball) is placed immediately in front of the acoustic window. (Adapted from Wan, Y. et al. 2010. *J. Phys. Conf. Ser.* 224(1): 012067.)

15.4.1.4 Skin Cancer

Melanoma is rapidly becoming the fastest-growing type of cancer, with a reported 120,000 new cases per year in the United States alone. EIT was first employed in studies related to skin conditions in the work by Ollmar and Emtestam (1992), where it was deemed useful as a tool for the noninvasive detection of skin irritation. More importantly, they later demonstrated the relationship between impedance spectral changes due to irritation caused by a variety of surfactants, and the related histopathology (Nicander et al., 1996). Their recent work (Aberg et al., 2004) has shown that multifrequency EIT can be used as a screening tool for the diagnosis of skin malignancies, with very high specificity and sensitivity, leading to the development of the latest commercial device to this end. Modeling of the skin is still under investigation with some very interesting findings (Grimnes and Martinsen, 2010; Martinsen et al., 2010).

15.4.1.5 Prostate Cancer

Prostate cancer is one of the most prevalent forms of the disease to afflict men, mostly of older age. Figures provided by Cancer Research UK state that approximately 913,000 men were diagnosed with prostate cancer in 2008. By the original work done at Dartmouth College, it was shown that the conductivity of cancerous versus healthy prostatic tissue removed from patients differed significantly over the entire frequency range (1 kHz to 1 MHz) (Halter et al., 2008). The work has taken an interesting direction, as there has been study into the incorporation of an EIT system into a conventional transrectal, ultrasonic (US) probe for prostate cancer detection *in vivo* (Borsic et al., 2009). The multimodality of this approach will provide better boundary detection of the prostate, increasing the accuracy of the segmentation of the organ into EIT voxels. The probe itself has recently been presented (Wan et al., 2010), consisting of a standard transrectal probe with a set of flexible electrodes positioned around the acoustic window (Figure 15.6), and clinical trials are under way.

15.4.2 Lung Imaging

Lung pathology can be imaged by conventional radiography, x-ray computed tomography, or magnetic resonance imaging (MRI), but there are clinical situations where it would be desirable to have a portable means of imaging regional lung ventilation which could, if necessary, generate repeated images over time. EIT, being inexpensive, relatively portable, and of high temporal resolution, is ideally suited for this application, but significant challenges, of course, remain.

Lung imaging is widely recognized as one of the most viable areas of research for EIT (Barber, 2005). Over the years, EIT has been applied to the imaging of a large number of medical conditions in the thoracic region, and the techniques, algorithms, and devices developed are too varied to cover fully here. Adequate coverage is given in Smit et al. (2005), with some comparisons against other, more established techniques. From the topical review by Frerichs (2000), it is evident that the body of work is extensive and has occupied EIT experts since the technique was introduced in 1985. The studies conducted have almost exclusively used ring electrode configurations, but the conditions of the tests have varied considerably. Animal (Hahn et al., 1995; Newell et al., 1996) and human studies have taken place, the latter with subjects being either healthy or with such conditions as pulmonary embolism (PE) (Leathard et al., 1994), emphysema (Harris et al., 1987; Eyüboglu et al., 1995) bronchial carcinoma (Holder and Temple, 1993; Morice et al., 1993; Shinkarenko et al., 1997), and chronic obstructive pulmonary disease (COPD) (Eyüboglu et al., 1995; Von Noordergraaf et al., 1998), among others. Subjects in these studies were under spontaneous or mechanical ventilation, depending on the study.

Specifically for the case of patients under mechanical ventilation, pioneering work performed by a close collaboration between clinicians and EIT experts showed the viability of the use of EIT for establishing the best ventilator regime to be used in critically ill patients by the bedside. In the work by Luepschen et al. (2007), it was conclusively shown that thoracic EIT can be used to dynamically image lung ventilation, hence, leading to the individualization of protective ventilation strategies and lung recruitment maneuvers. This research, then, successfully led to the development of the first commercially available, critical-care tool for such applications (for a very interesting read, visit Dräger, website).

Neonatal lung formation has been one of the first areas of research for EIT lung imaging, owing to the fact that noninvasiveness and lack of radiation are preferred in such applications. Early on, Hampshire et al. (1995) looked into the development of the neonatal lung, drawing conclusions on their differentiation to adult lungs. Later on, similar work showed that the definition of absolute conductivity of the lung in neonates could be used to determine lung density and air volume (Brown et al., 2002), and the later work in Brown et al. (2006).

Blood volume in the thorax has also been a topic of intense study, as it could allow for the detection of PE and COPD, as the conductivity of blood is about 6.7 mS/cm, which is approximately three times that of most intrathoracic tissues. The imaged quantity will be the change in conductivity due to replacement of tissue by blood (or vice versa) as a result of the pulsatile flow through the thorax. This may be relatively large in the cardiac ventricles but will be smaller in the peripheral lung fields. If a blood clot is present in the lung, the lung beyond the clot will not be perfused, and under favorable circumstances, this may be visualized using a gated blood volume image of the lung, and PE can be diagnosed if a ventilation image of the same region shows normal ventilation. This was experimentally shown by the work of Newell et al. (1996), whereby PE was simulated in a dog in each lung separately through occlusion of a major branch of the pulmonary artery, observing that the nonperfused lung had different electrical properties.

Research is ongoing in this very promising field. It is, hence, fitting that lung imaging is possibly the only application of EIT to enjoy a linear reconstruction algorithm developed from the consensus of most of the EIT groups in the world (Adler et al., 2009), which can be modified to suit specific devices and applications (example shown in Figure 15.7). Moreover, lung EIT is used as the testing ground of new reconstruction algorithms, such as those proposed in Borsic et al. (2010), where the efficacy of a novel reconstruction algorithm in preserving sharp conductivity boundaries was proven via the use of *in vivo* thoracic measurements. EIT of the lungs is, obviously, close to becoming a clinical reality.

15.4.3 Gastrointestinal System

A priori, it seems likely that EIT could be applied usefully to the measurement of motor activity in the gut. Electrodes can be applied with ease around the abdomen, and there are no large bony structures likely to seriously violate the assumption of constant initial conductivity. During motor activity, such as gastric emptying or peristalsis, there are relatively large movements of the conducting fluids within

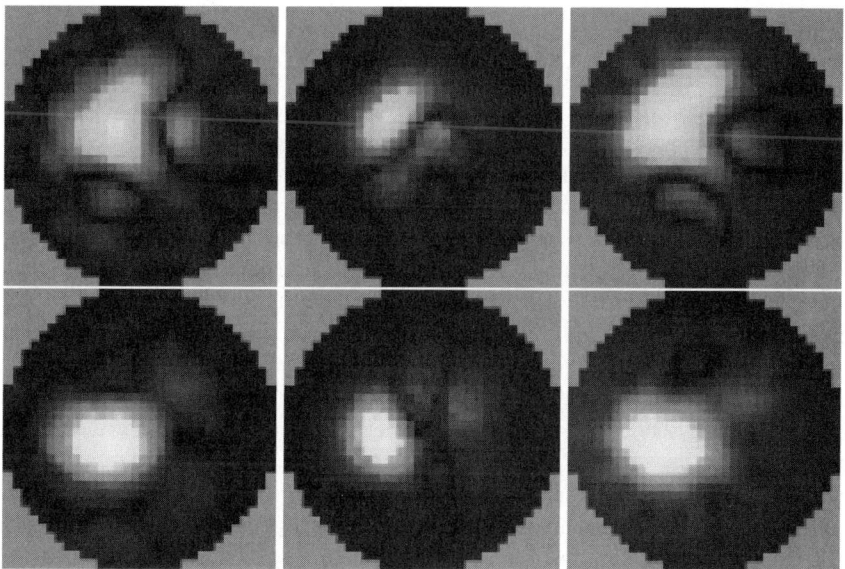

FIGURE 15.7 Images of localized (top row) pneumothorax and (bottom row) pleural effusion in an anesthetized, ventilated pig. Left: GREIT (R_{GN}), center: Gauss–Newton (R_{GN}), right: Sheffield backprojection (R_{SBP}). (Adapted from Adler, A. et al. 2009. *Physiol. Meas.* 30: S35–S55.)

the bowel. The quantity of interest is the timing of activity, for example, the rate at which the stomach empties, and the absolute impedance change and its exact location in space area of secondary importance. The principal limitations of EIT of poor spatial resolution and amplitude measurement are largely circumvented in this application (Avill et al., 1987).

Most research has concentrated on the correlation of conductivity and consistency of meals, as imaged through EIT, and at this, the Sheffield Mark I system has been used almost exclusively (Soulsby et al., 2005). The accuracy of EIT has been validated in parallel, mostly by the use of scintigraphy, and the results are generally in agreement. Wright (1995), for example, investigated gastric emptying of liquid and semisolid meals in healthy volunteers, both male and female, showing that gastric emptying was quicker for males than females on semisolids, but there was no significant difference between the groups on liquids. There has also been some interest in the measurement of other aspects of gastrointestinal function such as esophageal activity (Erol et al., 1995).

The lack of clinical acceptance of EIT for gastrointestinal studies has been largely attributed to the lack of standardization of test meals, the acceptance of EIT by clinicians, and the lack of commercially available EIT systems (Soulsby et al., 2005). This, unfortunately, seems to have limited more extensive research in this particular application of EIT.

15.4.4 Brain Imaging

Brain imaging through EIT has been the effort mostly of the University College London (UCL) group, and their work is well documented in Holder et al. (2005), where the devices, method, and reconstruction algorithms developed by the group are summarized. The applications they envisage for EIT in this field are twofold: accurate localization of epileptic foci in subjects suffering from intractable epilepsy to assist surgical intervention, and detection of cell swelling in cerebral energy failure as caused by pathological conditions such as stroke and ischemia, among others.

For the former, the subjects are monitored through EEG for a period of a week before surgery, during which time their epilepsy suppressant medication is suspended, but this technique is beneficial for superficial foci only. For deeper foci, implantable electrodes are used, with obvious dangers, and this is where EIT may prove to be of great importance as a noninvasive alternative, even though a combination of both types of electrodes has been proposed (Manwaring et al., 2010). Holder et al. (1996) performed animal studies to this effect, reporting that induced epileptic seizures as measured invasively induce conductivity changes of about 10%. However, this signal is expected to be attenuated by a factor of 10 when measured at the scalp, due to the diffusion caused by the scalp, skull, and cerebral matter. Recent work (Fabrizi et al., 2009) showed that, in phantom studies, the EIT device in use (UCH Mk2.5) produced comparable localization results to standard 31-electrode EEG. The authors, however, were cautious to state that the SNR expected in measurements of human subjects would be 50% lower, and baseline noise would be of the order of 1% (as observed clinically in Fabrizi et al. (2006, 2007)). This would imply that localization in human subjects is still a challenge. This fact is further corroborated by simulations performed on a FEM of the skull for intracerebral hemorrhage (ICH) (Tehrani et al., 2010), establishing that the required noise level for detection of a 1 mL blood clot has to be <0.005%, inclusive of all physiological and systematic error sources. This performance is at the limit of detectability of current EIT systems.

A very interesting and important application of EIT in brain monitoring would be of the imaging of neuronal depolarization, the high temporal resolution of EIT rendering it ideal for this. Early work has been performed, not only for the design of electrodes for this application (Gilad et al., 2007), but also on human subjects (Gilad and Holder, 2009). Unfortunately, the results obtained so far have not been of adequate quality for reliable imaging, due to the formidable nature of the challenge, but research is still ongoing in this exciting field.

15.5 New Directions

15.5.1 Multimodal Applications

EIT has been combined with other, more established modalities, which can benefit from its advantages. The use of EIT with ultrasound specifically for prostate cancer has already been discussed earlier. However, other applications exist where other modalities in conjunction with EIT are used, the most prominent one being that of breast cancer.

The Rensselaer group, New York, has devised a method to simultaneously scan both modalities with the use of a handheld probe (Kulkarni et al., 2010). A 6 × 6 array of electrodes, with the central two columns constructed by gold deposition on sonolucent material forms the front of a specially made housing for a standard ultrasound probe. The coupling to the patient, both electrically and acoustically, is provided through standard ultrasound gel. The impedance measurements are performed using the fourth generation of the Adaptive Current Tomograph (ACT4), developed by the same group (Saulnier et al., 2007).

The same group is also active in the combination of the golden standard for breast cancer detection, x-ray mammography, and EIT (Saulnier et al., 2007). Employing electron beam deposition, they applied thin layers of metal on Kapton to create radiolucent electrode arrays, which are subsequently adapted to the compression plates of an x-ray mammography system, performing simultaneous, dual-modality scans. Impedance measurements are again provided by the ACT4 system, with a frequency range of 3.33 kHz to 1 MHz.

15.5.2 Magnetic Resonance EIT

One of the most promising areas of research in EIT is that of magnetic resonance EIT (MREIT). During current injection into an electrically conductive medium, both a magnetic and an electric field are produced. The concept behind MREIT is to utilize the additional information derived from the magnetic field to assist in turning the ill-posed EIT reconstruction problem into a well-posed one, by effectively deducing the internal current pathways due to the resistivity distribution. The magnetic field can be detected using a conventional MRI scanner, but then the challenge remains in using this internal information in resistivity image reconstructions (Woo et al., 2005). A very thorough review of MREIT can be found in Woo and Seo (2008) and Seo and Woo (2011).

Ampère's law states that the internal current density $\mathbf{J} = (J_x, J_y, J_z)$ is related to the magnetic flux density $\mathbf{B} = (B_x, B_y, B_z)$ by $\mathbf{J} = \nabla \times (\mathbf{B}/\mu_0)$, where μ_0 is the magnetic permeability of free space. The novelty of MREIT lies in the use of an MRI scanner to measure B while actively injecting a current. However, measuring all orthogonal components of the flux density would require the subject to be rotated, a difficult task to achieve, causing problems such as pixel misalignment, which deteriorate the image quality (Woo et al., 2005). One of the most important breakthroughs in this respect was the development of the so-called harmonic B_z algorithm, developed by the Kyung Hee University, Korea, the driving force behind MREIT since its inception. The algorithm proposed (Seo et al., 2003; Oh et al., 2003) enables the reconstruction of conductivity images from a single magnetic flux component parallel to the main magnetic axis of the MRI scanner, this generally being B_z, requiring at least two data sets to be measured. However, the algorithm was found to perform poorly at boundaries of such regions with low conductivity as bones, lungs and the subject boundary, and the solution investigated currently is that of localized algorithm (Seo et al., 2008), which, interestingly, can provide scaled, regional conductivity images without knowing the conductivity distribution outside of the region. A software package (called CoReHA (Jeon et al., 2009)) now incorporates all the above algorithms for MREIT image reconstruction.

The research was limited to phantom studies (Figure 15.8) and postmortem animal tissue studies (e.g., Oh et al., 2005), but has recently been applied to *in vivo* animal and human subjects. The first experiment on a human subject was reported in Kim et al. (2009), where the human leg was imaged (Figure 15.9), and more recently, the human knee (Jeong et al., 2010). These recent images produced are encouraging, but significant challenges have been surpassed, and some are still under investigation. For example, carbon-hydrogel electrodes have been selected to minimize near-electrode artifacts, and a multiecho pulse sequence was developed to increase the SNR of MR magnitude images at lower injected current amplitudes, to be kept at 90% of subject sensation (Han et al., 2010). This latter problem has been the biggest stumbling block for human subject experiments to date. Other issues include the anisotropic nature of some tissues, and an improved electrode configuration and data-collection method (Woo et al., 2005).

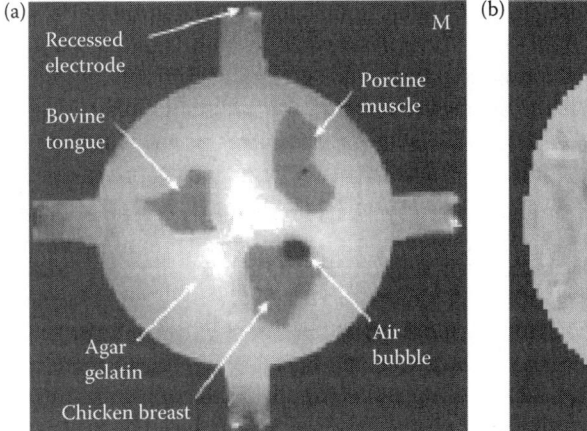 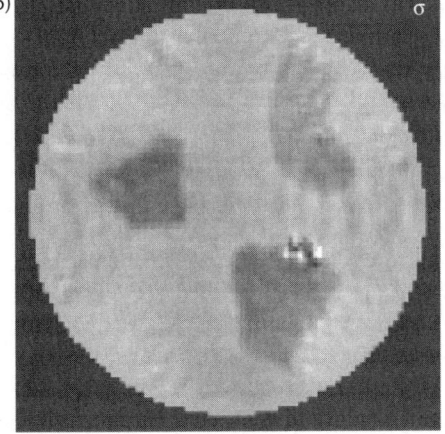

FIGURE 15.8 (a) MREIT biological test phantom, consisting of agar tissue mimicking material, with implanted animal tissue samples. (b) Results recorded from the test phantom using MREIT.

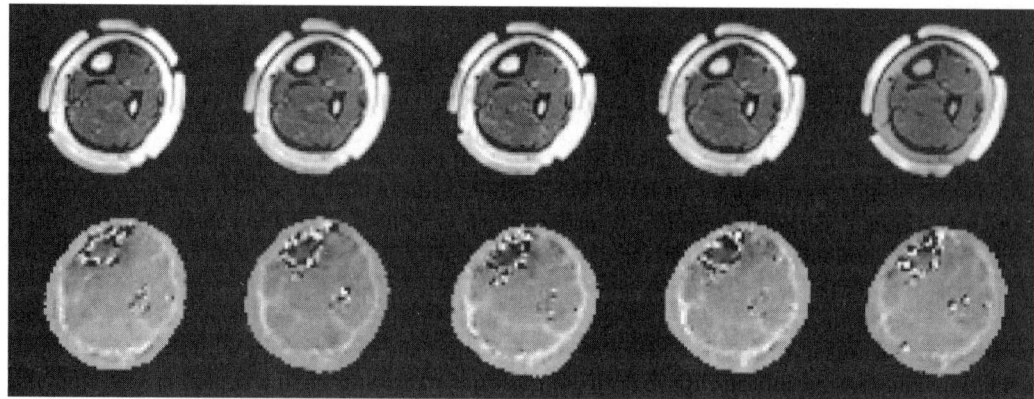

FIGURE 15.9 *In vivo* MREIT imaging experiment of a human leg using a 3 T MRI scanner. Multislice images and reconstructed equivalent isotropic conductivity images of a human leg are shown in the top and bottom rows, respectively. (Adapted from Woo, E.J. and Seo, J.K. 2008. *Physiol. Meas.* 29: R1–R26.)

MREIT is a medical imaging technique based on electrical impedance, but offering much higher resolution than conventional EIT. This advantage comes at the expense of nonportability and much higher expense due to the use of an MRI scanner, but its advantages, if put into routine clinical use, may prove it to be a new standard in medical imaging.

15.5.3 Magnetic Induction Tomography

Another newly developed technique based on the pioneering work from Sheffield Group in the 1980s, which is gaining wide interest and has seen significant advances in recent years, is magnetic induction tomography (MIT). This modality has been, somewhat arbitrarily, called "electromagnetic tomography" (EMT), "mutual inductance tomography" (again MIT), and "eddy current tomography," among others. For clarity, by MIT we are referring here to the field of study in which eddy currents are induced through the magnetic field from an excitation coil, and the magnetic fields subsequently caused by these eddy currents are then measured externally.

As described in depth in Griffiths (2005), the key advantage of MIT, compared with other electrical impedance-based modalities, is that there is no contact with the subject under investigation. This, of course, means that imaging can be performed without the need for time-consuming electrode placement. Further, contact artifacts will not affect imaging, and monitoring can be carried out over long periods of time without adverse effects to the subject.

In the sensing coil, the signal detected is a combination of the primary signal, $\mathbf{B}$, which is directly induced by the field from the excitation coil, and a much smaller, secondary signal, $\Delta\mathbf{B}$, caused by the magnetic field induced by the eddy currents in the subject. It can be shown that $\Delta\mathbf{B}$ is proportional to frequency and conductivity, and lags the primary signal by 90°, with the total detected field $(\mathbf{B} + \Delta\mathbf{B})$ lagging the primary field by an angle φ. In biological tissues, $\Delta\mathbf{B}$ is much smaller in magnitude than $\mathbf{B}$, and thus φ can be expressed as

$$\varphi \simeq \left|\frac{\Delta\mathbf{B}}{\mathbf{B}}\right| \propto \omega\sigma \tag{15.9}$$

showing that the phase angle between the total detected signal and the primary signal is proportional to the angular frequency, ω, of the primary signal, and σ is the conductivity of the sample. Hence, the electrical properties of the measured biological material can be extracted.

MIT is a promising modality, but is faced with significant challenges that so far have not allowed the production of a system with high-enough spatial resolution for clinical applications. Careful screening is required to reduce the effects of external to the system stimuli, and to minimize capacitive coupling that can swamp the wanted, inductive coupling-induced signal. Furthermore, as the primary signal is orders of magnitude larger than the secondary one, there has been interest in the elimination of the primary signal from the measurements, with varying degree of success. Other technical challenges include, among others, the limiting of the spatial resolution by the number of excitor/sensor combinations, high inherent noise figures compared to the measured signal and significant difficulties in the reconstruction algorithms akin to those of EIT (Griffiths, 2005). Further research is being carried out in confronting all the above challenges, and improved results of studies in this field are eagerly awaited.

15.6 Summary and Future Developments

EIT is still an emerging technology. In its development, several novel and difficult measurement and image-reconstruction problems have had to be addressed. Most of these have been satisfactorily solved. This is evident from the move toward standardization, especially with respect to a particular application. Furthermore, the adoption of information from other modalities into the EIT reconstruction problem has been hailed as a critical step forward that may finally see the adoption of EIT widely in clinical use.

The current generation of EIT imaging systems are multifrequency, with some capable of 3D imaging. These should be capable of greater quantitative accuracy and be less prone to image artifact and are likely to find a practical role in clinical diagnosis. Although there are still many technical problems to be answered and many clinical applications to be addressed, the technology may be close to coming of age.

What may possibly be the reason this promising modality has been hindered in its wide recognition is the need for the collaboration of individuals from different, and sometimes disparate, disciplines. Clinicians, hardware and software engineers, medical physicists, and inverse problem experts are required to collaborate with a single clinical application in mind, for any success to ever be gleaned. As EIT groups are maturing, and expertise in this field is now more widespread, it is reasonable to hope that EIT will find its way to widespread, routine clinical use in the near future.

Defining Terms

Absolute imaging: Imaging the actual distribution of conductivity.
Admittivity: The specific admittance of an electrically conducting material. For simple biomedical materials such as saline with no reactive component of resistance, this is, the same as conductivity.
Anisotropic conductor: A material in which the conductivity is dependent on the direction in which it is measured through the material.
Applied current pattern: In EIT, the electric current is applied to the surface of the conducting object via electrodes placed on the surface of the object. The spatial distribution of current flow through the surface of the object is the applied current pattern.
Bipolar current pattern: A current pattern applied between a single pair of electrodes.
Conductivity: The specific conductance of an electrically conducting material. The inverse of resistivity.
Differential imaging: An EIT imaging technique that specifically images changes in conductivity.
Distributed current: A current pattern applied through more than two electrodes.
Dynamic imaging: The same as differential imaging.
EIT: Electrical impedance tomography.
Forward transform or problem or solution: The operation, real or computational, that maps or transforms the conductivity distribution to surface voltages.
Impedivity: The specific impedance of an electrically conducting material. The inverse of admittivity. For simple biomedical materials such as saline with no reactive component of resistance, this is the same as resistivity.

Inverse transform or problem or solution: The computational operation that maps voltage measurements on the surface of the object to the conductivity distribution.

Optimal current: One of a set of current patterns computed for a particular conductivity distribution that produce data with maximum possible SNR.

Pixel: The conductivity distribution is usually represented as a set of connected piecewise uniform patches. Each of these patches is a pixel. The pixel may take any shape, but square or triangular shapes are most common.

Resistivity: The specific electrical resistance of an electrical conducting material. The inverse of conductivity.

Static imaging: The same as absolute imaging.

References

Aberg, P., Nicander, I., Hansson, J., Geladi, P., Holmgren, U., and Ollmar, S. 2004. Skin cancer identification using multifrequency electrical Impedance—A potential screening tool, *IEEE Trans. Biomed. Eng.* 51(12): 2097–2102.

Adler, A., Arnold, J.H., Bayford, R., Borsic, A., Brown, B., Dixon, P., Faes, T.J.C. et al. 2009. GREIT: A unified approach to 2D linear EIT reconstruction of lung images. *Physiol. Meas.* 30: S35–S55.

Assenheimer, M., Laver-Moskovitz, O., Malonek, D., Manor, D., Nahaliel, U., Nitzan, R., and Saad, A. 2001. The T-SCAN technology: Electrical impedance as a diagnostic tool for breast cancer detection. *Physiol. Meas.* 22(1): 1–8.

Avill, R.F., Mangnall, Y.F., Bird, N.C., Brown, B.H., Barber, D.C., Seagar, A.D., Johnson, A.G., and Read, N.W. 1987. Applied potential tomography: A new non-invasive technique for measuring gastric emptying. *Gastroenterology* 92: 1019.

Balasubramani, L., Brown, B.H., Healey, J., and Tidy, J.A. 2009. The detection of cervical intraepithelial neoplasia by electrical impedance spectroscopy: The effects of acetic acid and tissue homogeneity. *Gynecol. Oncol.* 115(2): 267–271.

Barber, D.C. 2005. EIT: The view from Sheffield. In D.S. Holder (Ed.), *Electrical Impedance Tomography: Methods, History and Applications*, Institute of Physics Publishing, Bristol, pp. 348–372.

Barber, D.C. and Brown, B.H. 1990. Progress in electrical impedance tomography. In D. Colton, R. Ewing and W. Rundell (Eds), *Inverse Problems in Partial Differential Equations*, pp. 149–162. New York: SIAM.

Barber, D.C. and Seagar, A.D. 1987. Fast reconstruction of resistive images. *Clin. Phys. Physiol. Meas.* 8: 47.

Bayford, R. 1994. Application of constrained optimization techniques in electrical impedance tomography, PhD thesis. Middlesex University, U.K.

Borsic, A., Graham, B.M., Adler, A., and Lionheart, W.R.B. 2010. *In vivo* impedance imaging with total variation regularization. *IEEE Trans. Med. Imag.* 29(1): 44–54.

Borsic, A., Halter, R., Wan, Y., Hartov, A., and Paulsen, K.D. 2009. Sensitivity study and optimization of a 3D electric impedance tomography prostate probe. *Physiol. Meas.* 30: S1–S18.

Borsic, A., Syed, H., Halter, R.J., and Hartov, A. 2011. Using ultrasound information in EIT reconstruction of the electrical properties of the prostate. In *Proceedings of the 12th International Conference in Electrical Impedance Tomography*, Bath, UK.

Breckon, W.R. 1990. Image Reconstruction in Electrical Impedance Tomography. Ph.D. thesis, School of Computing and Mathematical Sciences, Oxford Polytechnic, Oxford, UK.

Brown, B.H. and Barber, D.C. 1982. Applied potential tomography—A new in vivo medical imaging technique. In *Proceedings of Hospital Physicists' Association, Annual Conference*, Sheffield.

Brown, B.H., Barber, D.C., Wang, W., Lu, L., Leathard, A.D., Smallwood, R.H., Hampshire, A.R., Mackay, R., and Hatzigalanis, K. 1994. Multifrequency imaging and modelling of respiratory related electrical impedance changes. *Physiol. Meas.* 15: A1.

Brown, B.H., Milnes, P., and Mills, G.H. 2006. Indirect measurement of lung density and air volume from electrical impedance tomography (EIT) data. In *Proceedings of 7th Conference on Biomed. Appl. Electrical Impedance Tomography*, Seoul, pp. 85–89.

Brown, D.C. and Seagar, A.D. 1987. The Sheffield data collection system. *Clin. Phys. Physiol. Meas.* 8(suppl A): 91–98.

Brown, B.H., Tidy, J., Boston, K., Blackett, A.D., and Sharp, F. 1998. Tetrapolar measurement of cervical tissue structure using impedance spectroscopy. In *IEEE/EMBS International Conference*, pp. 2886–2889.

Brown, B.H., Primhak, R.A., Smallwood, R.H., Milnes, P., Narracott, A.J., and Jackson, M.J. 2002. Neonatal lungs—Can absolute lung resistivity be determined non-invasively? *Med. Biol. Eng.* 40: 388–394.

Callaghan, M.F., Lund, T., Hashemzadeh, P., Roitt, I.M., and Bayford, R.H. 2010. An investigation of the impedance properties of gold nanoparticles. *J. Phys. Conf. Ser.* 224(1): 012058.

Cheney, M.D., Isaacson, D., Newell, J.C., Simske, S., and Goble, J. 1990. Noser: An algorithm for solving the inverse conductivity problem. *Int. J. Imag. Syst. Tech.* 2: 66–75.

Cherepenin, V.A., Karpov, A.Y., Korjenevsky, A., Kornienko, V., Mazaletskaya, A., Mazourov, D., and Meister, D. 2001. A 3D electrical impedance tomography (EIT) system for breast cancer detection. *Physiol. Meas.* 22(1): 9–18.

Cherepenin, V.A., Karpov, A.Y., Korjenevsky, A.V., Kornienko, V.N., Kultiasov, Y.S., Ochapkin, M.B., and Trochanova, O.V. 2002. Three-dimensional EIT imaging of breast tissues: System design and clinical testing. *IEEE Trans. Med. Imag.* 21(6): 662–667.

Cole, K.S. and Cole, R.H. 1941. Dispersion and absorption in dielectrics: I. Alternating current characteristics. *J. Chem. Phys.* 9: 431.

Davidson, J.L., Little, R.A., Wright, P., Naish, J., Kikinis, R., Parker, G.J.M., and McCann, H. 2011. Co-registration and fusion of EIT images with MRI scan data. In *Proceedings of the 12th International Conference in Electrical Impedance Tomography*, Bath, UK.

Dräger. Electrical impedance tomography: The realization of regional ventilation monitoring. http://www.draeger.com/media/10/08/98/10089883/rsp_eit_booklet_9066788_en.pdf.

Erol, R.A., Smallwood, R.H., Brown, B.H., Cherian, P., and Bardham, K.D. 1995. Detecting oesophageal-related changes using electrical impedance tomography. *Physiol. Meas.* 16(suppl 3A): 143–152.

Eyüboglu, B.M., Oner, A.F., Baysal, U., Biber, C., Keyf, A.I., Yilmaz, U., and Erdogan, Y. 1995. Application of electrical impedance tomography in diagnosis of emphysema—A clinical study. *Physiol. Meas.* 16: A191–A211.

Fabrizi, L., McEwan, A., Oh, T., Woo, E.J., and Holder, D.S. 2009. A comparison of two EIT systems suitable for imaging changes in epilepsy, *Physiol. Meas.*, 30: S103–S120.

Fabrizi, L., McEwan, A., Woo, E., and Holder, D.S. 2007. Analysis of resting noise characteristics of three EIT systems in order to compare suitability for time difference imaging with scalp electrodes during epileptic seizures. *Physiol. Meas.* 28: S217–S236.

Fabrizi, L., Sparkes, M., Horesh, L., Perez-JusteAbascal, J.F., McEwan, A., Bayford, R.H., Elwes, R., Binnie, C.D., and Holder, D.S. 2006. Factors limiting the application of electrical impedance tomography for identification of regional conductivity changes using scalp electrodes during epileptic seizures in humans. *Physiol. Meas.* 27: 163–174.

Ferris, C.D. and Rose, D.R. 1972. An operational amplifier 4-electrode impedance bridge for electrolyte measurement. *Med. Biol. Eng.* 10: 647–654.

Frerichs, I. 2000. Electrical impedance tomography (EIT) in applications related to lung and ventilation: A review of experimental and clinical activities, *Physiol. Meas.* 21: R1–R21.

Fricke, H. 1925. The electrical capacity of suspensions with special reference to blood. *J. Gen. Physiol.* 9: 137–152.

Gilad, O. and Holder, D.S. 2009. Impedance changes recorded with scalp electrodes during visual evoked responses: Implications for electric impedance tomography of fast neural activity. *NeuroImage* 47: 412–522.

Gilad, O., Horesh, L., and Holder, D.S. 2007. Design of electrodes and current limits for low frequency electrical impedance tomography of the brain. *Med. Biol. Eng. Comput.* 45: 612–633.

Goble, J. and Isaacson, D. 1990. Fast reconstruction algorithms for three-dimensional electrical tomography. In *IEEE EMBS Proceedings of the 12th Annual International Conference*, Philadelphia, pp. 285–286.

Griffiths, H. 2005. Magnetic induction tomography. In D.S. Holder (Ed.), *Electrical Impedance Tomography: Methods, History and Applications*, Institute of Physics Publishing, Bristol, pp. 213–238.

Grimnes, S. and Martinsen, O.G. 2008. *Bioimpedance & Bioelectricity Basics*, 2nd Ed., Elsevier, Academic Press, Oxford, UK.

Grimnes, S. and Martinsen, O.G. 2010. Alpha dispersion in human tissue. *J. Phys. Conf. Ser.* 224(1): 012073.

Grychtol, B., Lionheart, W.R.B., Wolf, K.G., Bodenstein, M., and Adler, A. 2011. The importance of shape: Thorax models for GREIT. In *Proceedings of the 12th International Conference in EIT*, Bath, UK.

Hahn, G., Sipinková, I., Baisch, F., and Hellige, G. 1995. Changes in the thoracic impedance distribution under different ventilator conditions. *Physiol. Meas.* 16: A161–A173.

Hahn, G., Just, A., Dittmar, J., and Hellige, G. 2008. Systematic errors of EIT systems determined by easily-scalable resistive phantoms. *Physiol. Meas.* 29: S163–S172.

Halter, R., Hartov, A., and Paulsen, K.D. 2005. High frequency EIT for breast imaging. In *Conf. Biomed. Appl. Elec. Impedance Tomography, 6th*, London, UK.

Halter, R.J., Hartov, A., and Paulsen, K.D. 2007a. Experimental justification for using 3D conductivity reconstructions in electrical impedance tomography. *Physiol. Meas.* 28: S115–S127.

Halter, R., Schned, A., Heaney, J., Hartov, A., Schutz, S., and Paulson, K.D. 2007b. Electrical impedance spectroscopy of benign and malignant prostatic tissues. *J. Urol.* 4: 1580–1596.

Halter, R.J., Schned, A., Heaney, J., Hartov, A., Schutz, S., and Paulsen, K.D. 2008. Electrical impedance spectroscopy of benign and malignant prostatic tissue, *J. Urol.* 179(4): 1580–1586.

Hampshire, A.R., Smallwood, R.H., Brown, B.H., and Primhak, R.A. 1995. Multifrequency and parametric EIT images of neonatal lungs. *Physiol. Meas.* 16(suppl 3A): 175–189.

Han, Y.Q., Meng, Z.J., Jeong, W.C., Kim, Y.T., Minhas, A.S., Kim, H.J., Nam, H.S., Kwon, O., and Woo, E.J. 2010. MREIT conductivity imaging of canine head using multi-echo pulse sequence. *J. Phys. Conf. Ser.* 224(1): 012078.

Harris, N.D., Sugget, A.J., Barber, D.C., and Brown, B.H. 1987. Applications of applied potential tomography (APT) in respiratory medicine. *Clin. Phys. Physiol. Meas.* 8: 155–165.

Holder, D.S., Rao, A., and Hanquan, Y. 1996. Imaging of physiologically evoked responses by EIT tomography with cortical electrodes in the anaesthisised rabbit. *Physiol. Meas.* 17(A): 179–186.

Holder, D.S. and Temple, A.J. 1993. Effectiveness of the Sheffield EIT system in distinguishing patients with pulmonary pathology from a series of normal subjects. In D.S. Holder (Ed.), *Clinical and Physiological Applications of Electrical Impedance Tomography*, UCL Press, London, pp. 227–298.

Holder, D.S. (Ed.). 2005. *Electrical Impedance Tomography: Methods, History and Applications*, Institute of Physics Publishing, Bristol.

Hua, P., Webster, J.G., and Tompkins, W.J. 1988. A regularized electrical impedance tomography reconstruction algorithm. *Clin. Phys. Physiol. Meas.* 9(suppl A): 137–141.

Isaacson, D. 1986. Distinguishability of conductivities by electric current computed tomography. *IEEE Trans. Med. Imag.* 5: 91.

Jeon, K., Kim, H.J., Lee, C.O., Woo, E.J., and Seo, J.K. 2009. CoReHA: Conductivity reconstructor using harmonic algorithms for magnetic resonance electrical impedance tomography (MREIT). *J. Biomed. Eng. Res.* 30: 279–287.

Jeong, W.C., Kim, Y.T., Minhas, A.S., Lee, T.H., Kim, H.J., Nam, H.S., Kwon, O., and Woo, E.J. 2010. *In-vivo* conductivity imaging of human knee using 3 mA injection current in MREIT. *J. Phys. Conf. Ser.* 224(1): 012148.

Jossinet, J. and Schmitt, M. 1999. A review of parameters for the bioelectrical characterization of breast tissue. *Ann. NY Acad. Sci.* 20: 30–41.

Kim, H.J., Kim, Y.T., Minhas, A.S., Jeong, W.C., Woo, E.J., Seo, J.K., and Kwon, O.J. 2009. *In vivo* high-resolution conductivity imaging of the human leg using MREIT: The first human experiment. *IEEE. Trans. Med. Imag.* 28(11): 1681–1687.

Kim, H. and Woo, H.W. 1987. A prototype system and reconstruction algorithms for electrical impedance technique in medical imaging. *Clin. Phys. Physiol. Meas.* 8: 63.

Kohn, R.V. and Vogelius, M. 1984a. Determining the conductivity by boundary measurement. *Commun. Pure Appl. Math.* 37: 289.

Kohn, R.V. and Vogelius, M. 1984b. Identification of an unknown conductivity by means of the boundary. *SIAM-AMS Proc.* 14: 113.

Koire, C.J. 1992. EIT image reconstruction using sensitivity coefficient weighted backprojection. *Physiol. Meas.* 15(suppl 2A): 125–136.

Korjenevsky, A., Cherepenin, V., Trokhanova, O., and Tuykin, T. 2010. Gynecologic electrical impedance tomography. *J. Phys. Conf. Ser.* 224(1): 012070.

Kulkarni, R., Kao, T-J., Boverman, G., Saulnier, G.J., Isaacson, D., Szabo, T.L., and Newell J.C. 2010. A hand-held probe for combined ultrasound and electrical impedance tomography. *J. Phys. Conf. Ser.* 224(1): 012043.

Leathard, A.D., Brown, B.H., Campbell, J., Zhang, F., Morice, A.H., and Tayler, D. 1994. A comparison of ventilatory and cardiac related changes in EIT images of normal human lungs and of lungs with pulmonary embolism. *Physiol. Meas.* 15: A137.

Lindherholm, P., Marescot, L., Loke, M. H., and Renaud, P. 2008. Cell culture imaging using microimpedance tomography. IEEE. *Trans. Biomed. Eng.* 55(1): 138–145.

Lionheart, W.R.B. 2004. Review: EIT reconstruction algorithms: Pitfalls, challenges and recent developments. *Physiol. Meas.* 25(1): 125.

Lionheart, W.R.B. and Paridis, K. 2010. Finite elements and anisotropic EIT reconstruction. *J. Phys. Conf. Ser.* 224(1): 012022.

Liu, Q., Wi, H., Oh, T.I., Woo, E.J., and Seo, J.K. 2010. Development of a prototype micro-EIT system using three sets of 15 × 8 array electrodes. *J. Phys. Conf. Ser.* 224(1): 012161.

Lobstein-Adams, C., Beqo, N., and Wang, W. 2011. Electrical impedance assisted ultrasound guided focused ultrasound surgery: A comprehensive out-patient procedure? In *Proceedings of the 12th International Conference in Electrical Impedance Tomography*, Bath, UK.

Luepschen, H., Meier, T., Grossherr, M., Leibecke, T., Karsten, J., and Leonhardt, S. 2007. Protective ventilation using electrical impedance tomography, *Physiol. Meas.* 28: S247–S260.

Lukaszewicz, K., Wtorek, J., Bujnowski, A., and Skokowski, J. 2010. Monitoring of breast tissue thermoablation by means of impedance measurements. *J. Phys. Conf. Ser.* 224(1): 012136.

Malich, A., Boehm, T., Facius, M., Freesmeyer, M.G., Fleck, M., Anderson, R., and Kaiser, W.A. 2001. Differentiation of mammographically suspicious lesions: Evaluation of breast ultrasound, MRI mammography and electrical impedance scanning as adjunctive technologies in breast cancer detection. *Clin. Radiol.* 56: 278–283.

Manwaring, P.K., Halter, R.J., Borsic, A., and Hartov, A. 2010. A modified electrode configuration for brain EIT. *J. Phys. Conf. Ser.* 224(1): 012062.

Marescot, L., Loke, M.H., Chapelier, D., Delaloye, R., Lambiel, C., and Reynard, E. 2003. Assessing reliability of 2D resistivity imaging in mountain permafrost studies using the depth of investigation index method. *Near Surface Geophys.* 1: 57–68.

Martinsen, Ø.G., Grimnes, S., Lütken, C.A., and Johnsen, G.K. 2010. Memristance in human skin. *J. Phys. Conf. Ser.* 224(1): 012071.

McAdams, E.T. and Jossinet, J. 1995. Tissue impedance: A historical overview. *Physiol. Meas.* 16: A1–A13.

McAdams, E.T., McLaughlin, J.A., and Anderson, J.Mc.C. 1994. Multielectrode systems for electrical impedance tomography. *Physiol. Meas.* 15: A101.

McEwan, A., Cusick, G., and Holder, D.S., 2007. A review of errors in multi-frequency EIT instrumentation. *Physiol. Meas.* 28: S197–S215.

Metherall, P., Barber, D.C., Smallwood, R.H., and Brown, B.H. 1996. Three-dimensional electrical impedance tomography. *Physiol. Meas.* 15: A101.

Morice, A.H., Harris, N., Campbell, J., Zhang, F., and Brown, B. 1993. EIT in the investigation of chest disease. In *Clinical and Physiological Applications of Electrical Impedance Tomography*, UCL Press, London, pp. 655–677.

Morucci, J.P., Marsili, P.M., Granie, M., Dai, W.W., and Shi, Y. 1994. Direct sensitivity matrix approach for fast reconstruction in electrical impedance tomography. *Physiol. Meas.* 15(suppl 2A): 107–114.

Newell, J.C., Edic, P.M., Ren, X., Larson-Wiseman, J.L., and Danylecko, M.D. 1996. Assessment of acute pulmonary edema in dogs by electrical impedance imaging. *IEEE Trans. Biomed. Eng.* 43: 133–139.

Nicander, I., Ollmar, S., Eek, A., LundhRozell, B., and Emtestam, L. 1996. Correlation of impedance response patterns to histological findings in irritant skin reactions induced by various surfactants. *Br. J. Dermatol.* 134: 221–228.

Oh, S.H., Lee, B.I., Woo, E.J., Lee, S.Y., Kim, T-S., Kwon, O., and Seo, J.K. 2005. Electrical conductivity images of biological tissue phantoms in MREIT. *Physiol. Meas.* 26: S279–S288.

Oh, S.H., Lee, B.I., Woo, E.J., Lee, S.Y., Cho, M.H., Kwon, O., and Seo, J.K. 2003. Conductivity and current density image reconstruction using harmonic Bz algorithm in magnetic resonance electrical impedance tomography. *Phys. Med. Biol.* 48: 3101–3116.

Oh, T.I., Woo, E.J., and Holder, D. 2007. Multi-frequency EIT system with radially symmetric architecture: KHU Mark1. *Physiol. Meas.* 28: S183–S196.

Ollmar, S. and Emtestam, L. 1992. Electrical impedance applied to non-invasive detection of irritation in skin. *Contact Dermatitis* 27: 278–282.

Paulson, K., Breckon, W., and Pidcock, M. 1992. Optimal measurements in electrical impedance tomography, In *14th IEEE EMBS, Annual International Conference*, Paris.

Qiao, G., Wang, W., Sze, G., Hussain, W., Wang, L., and Al-Akaidi, M. 2008. Investigation of in-vitro bioimpedance test system for mouse pancreas. In *9th Electrical Impedance Tomography Conference*, Hanover, USA.

Rebeyrol, J., Moreno, M-V., Ribbe, E., and Vannicatte, A. 2010. Case study: Using monitoring of body composition data obtained by bioimpedance, in training of an elite male runner. In *ISEA, Proceedings of 8th*, 2, pp. 3059–3064.

Saulnier, G.J. 2005. EIT instrumentation. In D.S. Holder (Ed.), *Electrical Impedance Tomography: Methods, History and Applications*, Institute of Physics Publishing, Bristol pp. 67–104.

Saulnier, G.J., Liu, N., Tamma, C., Hongjun, X., Tzu-Jen Kao, Newell, J.C., and Isaacson, D. 2007. An electrical impedance spectroscopy system for breast cancer detection. *Proceedings of the 29th Annual International Conference on IEEE EMBS.* pp. 4154–4157.

Seo, J.K., Kim, S.W., Kim, S., Liu, J., Woo, E.J., Jeon, K., and Lee, C-O. 2008. Local harmonic B_z algorithm with domain decomposition in MREIT: Computer simulation study. *IEEE Trans. Med. Imag.* 27: 1754–1761.

Seo, J.K. and Woo, E.J. 2011. Magnetic resonance electrical impedance tomography (MREIT). *SIAM Rev.* 53(1): 40–68.

Seo, J.K., Yoon, J.R., Woo, E.J., and Kwon, O. 2003. Reconstruction of conductivity and current density images using only one component of magnetic field measurements. *IEEE Trans. Biomed. Eng.* 50: 1121–1124.

Shinkarenko, V.S., Chuchalin, A.G., Kostromina, E., Aïsanov, Z.R., Pashkova, T.L., Voloshina, N.A., and Iag'ia, T.N. 1997. Electrical impedance tomography in pulmonology. *Ter. Arkh.* 69: 48–51.

Smit, H.J., VonkNoordegraaf, A., van Genderingen, H.R., and Kunst, P.W.A. 2005. Imaging of the thorax by EIT. In D.S. Holder (Ed.), *Electrical Impedance Tomography: Methods, History and Applications*, Institute of Physics Publishing, Bristol, pp. 107–126.

Soulsby, C., Yazaki, E., and Evans, D.F. 2005. Applications of electrical impedance tomography in the gastrointestinal tract. In D.S. Holder (Ed.), *Electrical Impedance Tomography: Methods, History and Applications*, Institute of Physics Publishing, Bristol, pp. 186–206.

Surowiec, A.J., Stuchly, S.S., Barr, J.R., and Swarup, A. 1988. Dielectric properties of breast carcinoma and the surrounding tissues. *IEEE Trans. Biomed. Eng.* 35: 257–263.

Sylvester, J. and Uhlmann, G. 1986. A uniqueness theorem for an inverse boundary value problem in electrical prospection. *Commun. Pure Appl. Math.* 39: 91.

Sze, G., Wang, W., Barber, D.C., and Huber, N. 2011. Preliminary study of the sensitivity of the Sussex MK4 Electrical Impedance Mammography planar electrode system. In *Proceedings of the 12th International Conference in Electrical Impedance Tomography*, Bath, UK.

Tang, M., Wang, W., Wheeler, J., McCormick, M., and Dong, X., 2002. Effects of incompatible boundary information in EIT on the convergence behaviour of an iterative algorithm. *IEEE Trans. Biomed. Eng.* 21(6): 620–628.

Tehrani, J.N., Anderson, C., Jin, C., Van Schaik, A., Holder, D.S., and McEwan, A. 2010. Feasibility of electrical impedance tomography in heamorrhagic stroke treatment using adaptive mesh. *J. Phys. Conf. Ser.* 224(1): 012065.

Tizzard, A., Borsic, A., Halter, R., and Bayford, R. 2010. Generation and performance of patient-specific forward models for breast imaging with EIT. *J. Phys. Conf. Ser.* 224(1): 012034.

Tunstall, B., Wang, W., McCormick, M., Walker, R., and Rew, D. 1997. Preliminary *in vitro* studies of electrical impedance mammography (EIM): A future technique for non-invasive breast tissue imaging? *Breast* 6(4): 253.

Von Noordergraaf, A. A., Kunst, P.W., Janse, A., Marcus, J.T., Postmus, P.E., Faes, T.J., and deVries, P.M. 1998. Pulmonary perfusion measured by means of electrical impedance tomography. *Physiol. Meas.* 19(2): 263–273.

Wan, Y., Halter, R., Borsic, A., Manwaring, P., Hartov, A., and Paulsen, K.D. 2010. Sensitivity study of an ultrasound coupled transrectal electrical impedance tomography system for prostate imaging. *J. Phys. Conf. Ser.* 224(1): 012067.

Wang, L., Wang, W., Qiao, G., Brien, M., and Al-Akaidi, M. 2006. Preliminary report of optimisation of in-vitro studies with an in-vitro specimen measuring system. In *Proceedings of the 7th Conference on Biomedical Applications of Electrical Impedance Tomography, WC2006*, Korea.

Wang, W., Cheng, Z., and McCormick, M. 1996. Design of programmable wide bandwidth current source for an impedance tomography system. In *IEEE, EMBS 18th Annual International Conference*, Amsterdam, the Netherlands.

Wang, W., Wang, L., Huang, T., Tunstall, B., Gu, D-W., and Sze, G. 2007a. Parametric image: A step forward for virtual biopsy by EIT? In *IFMBE Proceedings 2007*. 17(1): 432–435.

Wang, W., Wang, L., Qiao, G., Prickett, P., Bramer, B., Tunstall, B., and Al-Akaidi, M. 2007b. Study into the repeatability of the electrode-skin interface utilizing electrodes commonly used in electrical impedance tomography. *In IFMBE Proceedings* 2007, 17(10): 336–339.

Wexler, A., Fry, B., and Neuman, M.R. 1985. Impedance-computed tomography: Algorithm and system. *Appl. Opt.* 24: 3985.

Wheeler, J., Wang, W., and Tang, M. 2002. A comparison of methods for measurement of spatial resolution in two-dimensional circular EIT images. *Physiol. Meas.* 23(1): 169–176.

Woo, E.J. and Seo, J.K. 2008. Magnetic resonance electrical impedance tomography (MREIT) for high-resolution conductivity imaging. *Physiol. Meas.* 29: R1–R26.

Woo, E.J., Seo, J.K., and Lee, S.Y. 2005. Magnetic resonance electrical impedance tomography (MREIT). In D.S. Holder (Ed.), *Electrical Impedance Tomography: Methods, History and Applications*, Institute of Physics Publishing, Bristol, pp. 239–294.

Wright, J.W. 1994. The effect of intraluminal content on gastrointestinal motility in man, PhD thesis, Nottingham, UK.

York, T. 2005. Electrical tomography for industrial applications. In D.S. Holder (Ed.), *Electrical Impedance Tomography: Methods, History and Applications*, Institute of Physics Publishing, Bristol, pp. 105–209.

Yorkey, T.J. 1986. Comparing Reconstruction Algorithms for Electrical Impedance Imaging. Ph.D. thesis, University of Wisconsin, Madison, WI.

Zadehkoochak, M., Blott, B.H., Hames, T.K., and George, R.E. 1991. Spectral expansion analysis in electrical impedance tomography. *J. Phys. D: Appl. Phys.* 24: 1911–1916.

Zhao, M., Liu, Q., Oh, T.I., Woo, E.J., and Seo, J.K. 2010. Development of a trans-admittance mammography (TAM) using 60×60 electrode array. *J. Phys. Conf. Ser.* 224(1): 012045.

16
Magnetic Resonance Imaging of Atherosclerosis

Chun Yuan
University of Washington

William S. Kerwin
University of Washington

Gador Canton
University of Washington

Jinnan Wang
Philips Research North America

Huijun Chen
University of Washington

Niranjan Balu
University of Washington

16.1 Introduction

Despite new drug therapies and increasing research, deaths from heart disease and stroke remain the leading causes of death in the United States, the developed world, and are increasingly prevalent in the developing world. Clinically, the majority of these deaths are attributed to atherosclerosis, literally meaning "hardening of the arteries" (Ross et al. 1999). Although the outcomes of the disease are clear, the exact process and biological mechanisms that lead to death or a clinical event by atherosclerosis remain an intensively studied area.

It has been thought that heart attack, stroke, and other clinical events from atherosclerosis are caused by vessel occlusion; a buildup of plaque which eventually blocks the artery, removing the blood supply. Thus, extensive medical imaging techniques have been developed that focus on identifying narrowing of blood vessels (stenosis). In medical terminology, these techniques are referred to as angiographic methods. Angiographic methods, with ultrasound, x-ray, computed tomography (CT), and magnetic resonance imaging (MRI), remain the standard methodology for clinical assessment of the severity of atherosclerotic disease, and are used as criteria for surgical decision making (Achenbach et al. 2010).

However, as indicated by the continued high rates of mortality, assessment of luminal narrowing provides an incomplete picture of the severity of atherosclerosis. In part, this is due to the phenomenon of arterial remodeling (Glagov et al. 1987)—the vessel wall is a responsive organ and atherosclerotic plaques may develop without infringing on the vessel lumen by pushing the vessel wall outward. It is the disease within the vessel wall that contributes to the progression and clinical complication of atherosclerosis. Recently, the concept of "vulnerable plaque" (VP) was introduced defining a series of different types of atherosclerotic plaques with higher risk of causing clinical events such as heart attack and stroke (Naghavi et al. 2003). Most of these plaque types involve plaque tissue compositions and distributions which lead to plaque rupture and subsequent clinical events. Vessel wall imaging (VWI) has also undergone rapid development, in parallel with the realization of the importance of VP.

VWI is defined as using imaging means to characterize atherosclerotic plaques of the vessel wall *in vivo*. Figure 16.1 shows a typical atherosclerotic plaque excised intact from the human carotid artery during a surgical procedure called carotid endarterectomy. It highlights the complexity of an advanced plaque and outlines the need for VWI, including ways to measure the size of an atherosclerotic plaque (volume, cross-sectional area, thickness), identify and quantify plaque tissue composition, determine inflammatory activity, and plaque–lumen interface condition such as ulcers and surface disruption.

This chapter provides an overview of MRI-based techniques for VWI and the basic hardware requirements and acquisition techniques, image processing tools which enable qualitative and quantitative data analysis, and advanced and developing techniques such as dynamic contrast imaging (DCE), and biomechanics.

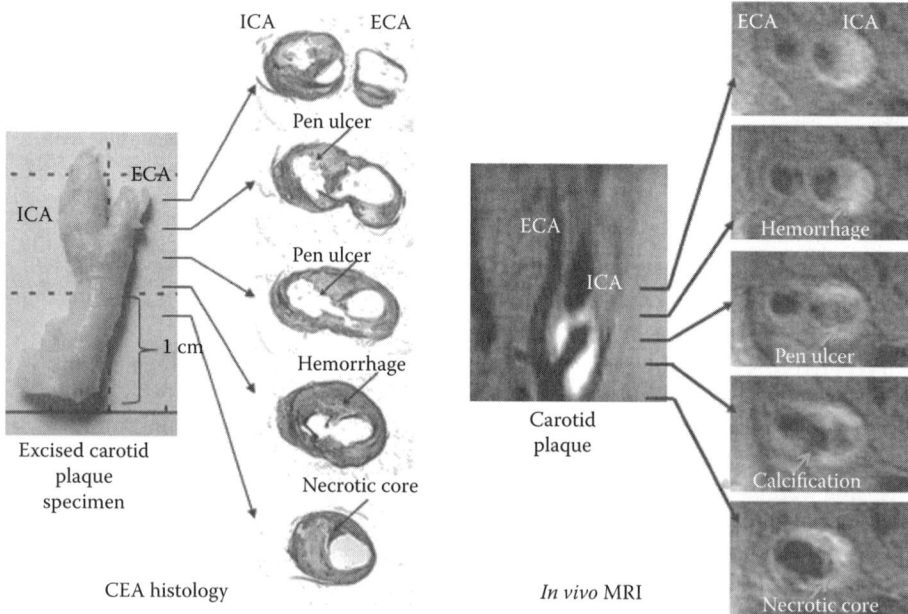

FIGURE 16.1 Two examples of carotid atherosclerotic plaque visualization. On the left is a photograph of a carotid endarterectomy (CEA) specimen measuring 2 cm in length. Serial sections of the specimen show the components of the plaque: intraplaque hemorrhage; necrotic core; calcification; and penetrating ulcer. The blue stain is a Mallory's trichrome. On the right are *in vivo* MRI images showing the common carotid bifurcation which separates into the external carotid (ECA) and internal carotid arteries (ICA). The longitudinal scan reveals a large bright plaque that almost occludes the lumen in the internal carotid. The cross-sectional images show the complexity of the lesion. Hemorrhage, calcification, necrotic core, and a penetrating ulcer are clearly visible.

16.2 Vessel Wall MRI Acquisition Techniques

VWI using MRI within a clinical feasible time frame is a demanding task that presents a number of technical challenges. Atherosclerotic lesions in the vessel wall with small but complicated plaque structures require high signal-to-noise ratio (SNR) imaging with high spatial resolution and good lumen-to-wall contrast. A high spatial resolution of 0.5–0.8 mm in the wall thickness direction is generally needed to image major arteries in the human body. Even higher resolutions may be needed when smaller or more peripheral arteries are to be imaged. To achieve this resolution, specially designed radiofrequency (RF) coils are needed to improve the SNR of the acquired images. Signal due to flowing blood and motion of surrounding soft tissues must also be considered in vessel wall MRI. Effective blood suppression is required for lumen boundary identification. Additionally, to detect and accurately quantify the various tissue components found in the atherosclerotic plaques, imaging techniques also need to be specifically optimized for certain types of tissue contrast. In addition to the above considerations, blood vessels are often surrounded by fat, and fat suppression is required to better define the margins of the outer wall. Techniques for motion artifact suppression can also help improve vessel wall boundary identification on images.

Recent developments in vessel wall MR imaging have successfully addressed many of the above-mentioned challenges, allowing VWI in clinical environments. These technical advancements will be discussed in detail throughout the section. The carotid arteries are frequent sites of atherosclerosis and several MR imaging techniques have been developed for carotid imaging. Since histological confirmation of image findings is best performed in the carotid artery using surgical endarterectomy specimens, many imaging techniques have been first developed in carotid arteries and then migrated to other arterial beds. In this section, we focus on carotid imaging techniques and their extension to other arterial beds.

16.2.1 Hardware

16.2.1.1 Field Strength

A whole-body clinical scanner can be used for VWI if it is equipped with dedicated RF coils to provide high SNR while maintaining the high spatial resolution required for discerning small plaque components. While field strengths from 1.5 T have been used for vessel wall MRI, higher main magnetic field strengths provide increased SNR and thereby higher increase contrast-to-noise ratio (CNR) in VWI (Figure 16.2). Compared to 1.5 T, black-blood carotid MRI at 3 T provides a 1.4–2.4 times higher CNR (Yarnykh et al. 2006). While plaque morphological measurements and identification of plaque components are similar at 1.5 and 3 T field strengths, appearance of some tissue components may differ at 3 T and higher field strengths due to increased susceptibility.

Moving to even higher field strengths such as 7 T can theoretically improve carotid VWI further, and a 3 times SNR gain at 7 T over 3 T has been demonstrated (Wiggins et al. 2009). However, the potential increase in SNR from high field imaging is outweighed by other issues at high field strengths, such as higher susceptibility, and B_0 and B_1 inhomogeneities. Furthermore, MR techniques based on balanced steady-state gradient echo imaging cannot be applied at 7 T fields due to higher field inhomogeneities. For these reasons, VWI is currently best performed at 3 T. 3 T VWI is capable of visualizing all major arterial beds, including carotid, aorta, femoral, and coronary. 3 T MR scanners are also widely available and used in clinical practice, making it possible to transition even advanced 3 T techniques to clinical practice. In the future, as MR techniques to mitigate effects of susceptibility and field inhomogeneities become available, VWI may become practical at higher field strengths.

16.2.1.2 Coils

Body coil transmission is used for VWI and is useful for uniform excitation and large coverage needed for spatial blood suppression sequences. However, body coil reception does not provide high-enough

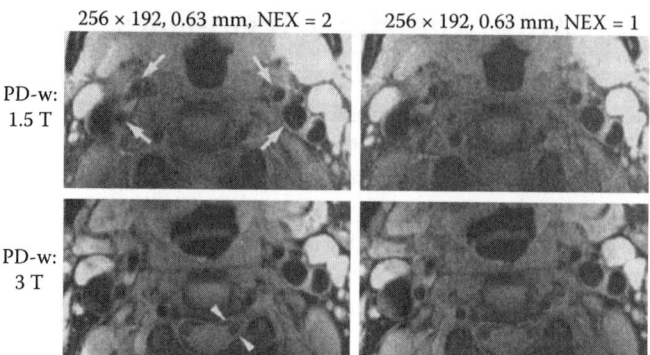

FIGURE 16.2   Axial carotid MRI sequences obtained at 1.5 and 3 T using the same sequence parameters. Note the improved SNR at 3 T with NEX = 1 showing improved vessel wall delineation (arrow) and appearance of small structures as nerve roots (arrowheads). With NEX = 2 at 1.5 T, some of the SNR loss can be offset but comes at the expense of increased scan time. (Adapted from Yarnykh VL et al. 2006. *J Magn Reson Imaging.* 5:691–698.)

SNR for visualizing the vessel wall. Surface coils can be applied close to the area of interest and pick up signal from a limited region of interest with high sensitivity. For example, the carotid bifurcation is a frequent location for atherosclerosis and is located close to the surface. Phased-array surface coils designed for carotid artery imaging provide improved SNR at the carotid bifurcation compared to body coil reception. Increasing the number of coil elements can provide improved coverage coupled with the inherent high SNR of surface coil imaging. Four- and eight-element bilateral phased-array carotid coils are now commercially available. Figure 16.3 shows an 8-element coil design and its commercial available design. The 8-element phased-array provides 1.7-fold SNR increase and increased longitudinal coverage compared to its 4-channel predecessor (Balu et al. 2009b). While these coils can be used for parallel imaging, VWI is often SNR limited. Therefore, parallel imaging in VWI is not preferred since it can decrease SNR. Thoracic vessels can be imaged with cardiac coils and peripheral vessels can be imaged with general-purpose surface coils.

16.2.2 Black-Blood Imaging Techniques

Effective suppression of the blood signal in the vessel wall is critical for accurate atherosclerotic plaque burden measurements because residual blood signal, commonly referred to as plaque-mimicking artifacts, can often be confused as part of the vessel wall, thus leading to inaccurate lumen/wall boundary segmentation. In addition, the effective suppression of the blood signal also allows for more prominent vessel wall visualization. *Black-blood (BB) imaging* indicates special MRI techniques in which the blood signal is suppressed. The suppression of blood signal generally takes the advantage of one or multiple of the following properties of the blood: the *inflow effect*, the unique magnetic relaxation values (T_1 and T_2 times) of the blood, and the diamagnetic nature of the blood. These properties are fairly unique to blood and therefore could be used to differentiate blood from surrounding tissues like the vessel wall.

16.2.2.1 Inflow-Suppression Technique

The *inflow-suppression* (IS) technique (Edelman et al. 1990) uses only the inflow effect for blood suppression. As shown in Figure 16.4, the essence of the IS technique is very straightforward: suppressing the upstream blood signal before it enters the imaging volume and acquiring the image once the imaging volume is filled with nullified blood.

In the IS technique, the upstream blood is usually suppressed by applying an excitation pulse (usually 90°) to flip all the spins and then the signal is suppressed with a spoiler gradient. With a certain

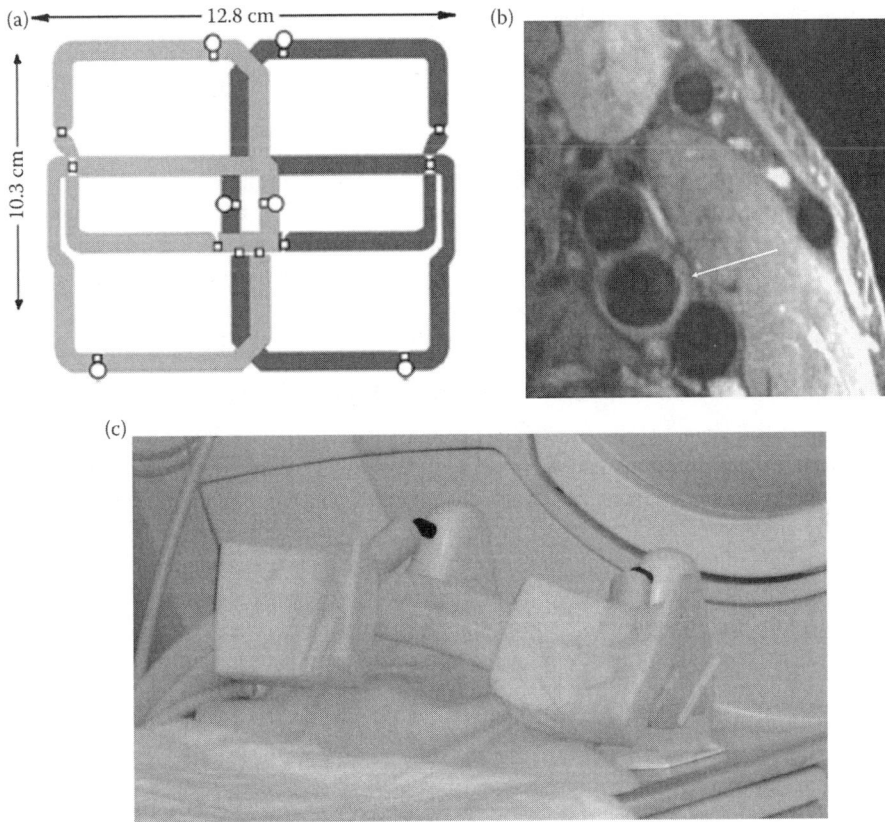

FIGURE 16.3 The 8-element carotid coil is made of bilateral coils of four elements each. The four elements of one side are shown in (a) with resistors and capacitors. High resolution (0.27 mm² in-plane resolution T_1w MRI) (b) obtained with the coil shows excellent delineation of the thin carotid walls. (c) A commercial version of the coil design in (a) showing the bilateral carotid "paddles" and integrated head rest. (Adapted from Balu N et al. 2009a. *ISMRM*, April, pp. 18–24, Honolulu, Hawaii.)

amount of delay time, after all prepared blood in the imaging volume is completely replaced by the nullified blood, a black-blood image can be acquired. The module itself usually takes no more than tens of milliseconds and can usually be combined with any kind of sequence (spin echo, gradient echo, etc.) for data acquisition. The delay time between the IS and acquisition modules is usually very short to avoid the blood signal increase due to the T_1 relaxation.

Compared to the other BB techniques, the advantage of the IS technique is the ease of implementation and directional selectivity. It is typically available in clinical MR scanners and no special optimization

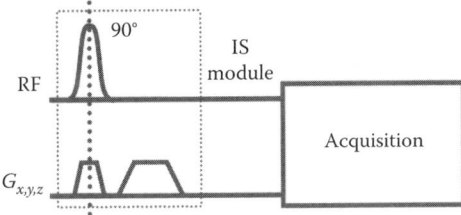

FIGURE 16.4 Pulse sequence diagram of the inflow-suppression technique.

is needed. Benefiting from the flexibility of placing the suppression bands, the blood from different directions can be selectively suppressed as long as the suppression bands are properly placed. The IS technique is therefore also frequently used to suppress only the arterial (or venous) flows without affecting flow in the other direction.

A major disadvantage of the IS technique is insufficient blood suppression. Owing to the short delay between the IS and acquisition modules, slow-flowing blood and/or blood flow without a through-plane velocity usually cannot be effectively replenished by the nullified blood, leading to an insufficient BB effect. The IS technique is therefore not frequently used for quantitative vessel wall MR applications; rather, it is more frequently used as an auxiliary tool to suppress blood signal when other imaging goals are explored, for example, to help maintain a black-blood contrast in perfusion MRI.

16.2.2.2 Double Inversion Recovery Technique and Its Variations

The *Double Inversion Recovery (DIR) technique* (Edelman et al. 1991) suppresses blood signal by using both the inflow effect and the T_1 relaxation time of the blood. Compared to the IS technique, the DIR technique can suppress blood more efficiently, especially in regions where slow and/or recirculating flow exists.

The pulse sequence of the DIR sequence is shown in Figure 16.5. It comprises two inversion pulses, where the first one is a nonselective RF pulse and the second is a selective RF pulse that covers only the imaging volume. The two RF pulses are usually placed as close as possible to minimize the magnetization perturbation for the spins inside the imaging volume. The net effect after the application of both pulses is that the magnetizations of all spins outside the imaging volume will be inverted while the magnetizations of the spins inside the imaging volume remain untouched. Since all blood magnetizations outside the imaging volume have been inverted, the images will be acquired after a delay time TI, at which time the blood signal reaches zero magnetization through T_1 relaxation.

The selection of the TI time is determined by both the T_1 relaxation time of the blood and the particular sequence used in acquisition. For example, if a standard spin echo sequence is used, the optimal TI is determined by

$$\mathrm{TI} = -T_1 \ln \frac{1 + e^{-\mathrm{TR}/T_1}}{2} \tag{16.1}$$

where T_1 is the blood relaxation time and TR is the repetition time of the sequence. Due to the relatively long T_1 time of the blood, the optimal TI time is usually a few hundred milliseconds.

Similar to the IS technique, the DIR technique also requires the blood in the imaging volume to be completely replenished by the inverted blood to achieve the best black-blood imaging effect. Due to the longer delay (TI) time, the DIR sequence allows for even slow flow in the imaging volume to be replenished. It therefore greatly relaxes the flow velocity requirement to achieve satisfactory BB effect.

However, DIR is still limited in a number of ways: (1) it still depends on the complete outflow of the blood to achieve satisfactory BB effect, which could be an issue for large-coverage three-dimensional (3D) imaging and in-plane blood flow suppression; (2) it is essentially a single-slice imaging scheme

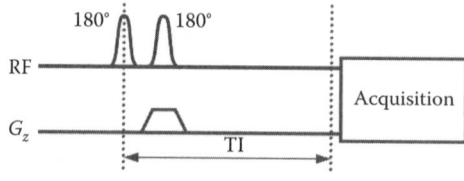

FIGURE 16.5 Pulse sequence diagram of the double inversion recovery technique.

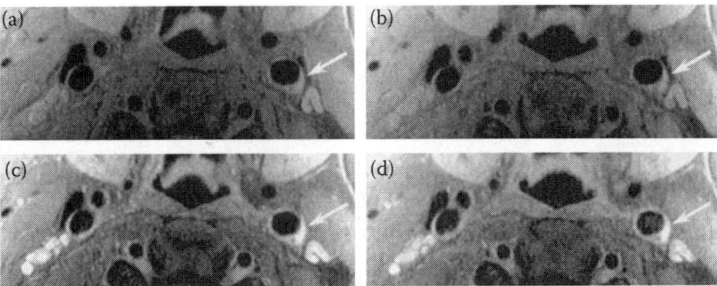

FIGURE 16.6 (a) and (b) Pre- and (c) and (d) postcontrast T_1-weighted black-blood images of carotid arteries: (a) and (c) images acquired with the QIR preparation; (b) and (d) images acquired with the DIR sequence. Note marked enhancement in the lesion and incomplete flow suppression in the left common carotid artery on (d) the postcontrast DIR image. Blood suppression is markedly improved postcontrast by use of the QIR preparation. (Adapted from Yarnykh VL and Yuan C. 2002. *Magn Reson Med.* 5:899–905.)

so it is usually very time consuming if a large volume of tissue is to be covered; and (3) it relies on the blood T_1 value for parameter optimization so the BB effect will become suboptimal or completely ineffective after the contrast agent is administered. To address these issues, a number of techniques have been proposed to improve the acquisition efficiency (Parker et al. 2002; Yarnykh and Yuan 2003; Itskovich et al. 2004), to improve lumen/wall contrast (Abd-Elmoniem et al. 2010), and to remove T_1 sensitivity (Yarnykh and Yuan 2002). As shown in Figure 16.6, the quadruple inversion recovery (QIR) technique has been shown to be very insensitive to the blood T_1 change and therefore maintains very good blood suppression efficiency even for postcontrast BB imaging when blood T_1 times are much lower than precontrast values. These solutions, however, usually come at a price of reduced blood suppression efficiency.

16.2.2.3 Motion-Sensitized-Driven Equilibrium Technique

Unlike IS and DIR, the *motion-sensitized-driven equilibrium (MSDE) technique* suppresses blood with no direct dependence on the inflow effect from the blood; rather, it suppresses blood based on phase dispersion of magnetization among moving spins (Koktzoglou and Li 2007; Wang et al. 2007). As shown in Figure 16.7, the MSDE sequence utilizes the motion-sensitizing gradient pulses to induce phase dispersions among spins with different velocities. For static tissues, no phase dispersion will be introduced by the gradient pairs. For flowing blood, however, different phases will be introduced for spins with different velocity vectors. If the phase variation is significant enough within a pixel, the signal will be dephased and black-blood contrast will be achieved.

Because the MSDE sequence does not directly rely on the flow replenishing rate for blood suppression, it provides more effective blood suppression compared to the IS and DIR techniques. As shown in Figure 16.8A, when different BB techniques were applied to image the carotid bulb, where stagnant flow tends to be found, only the MSDE technique completely removed the flow artifacts. For the same reason, the MSDE technique is also more suitable for tortuous arteries, in-plane flow suppression and

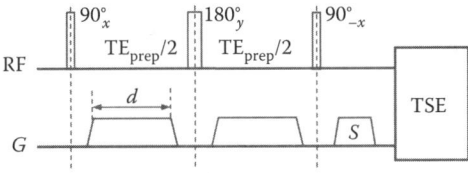

FIGURE 16.7 Pulse sequence diagram of the motion-sensitized-driven equilibrium (MSDE) sequence.

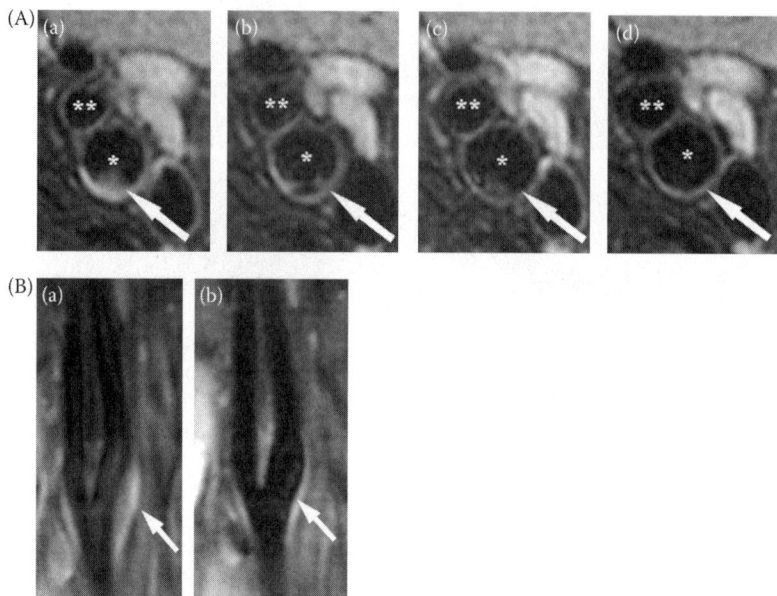

FIGURE 16.8   (A) Sample images illustrating the flow suppression capability of different BB imaging techniques: (a) IS, (b) DIR, (c) multislice DIR, and (d) MSDE. The residual flow signal is eliminated by the MSDE sequence but is visible for other techniques (arrows). All images are presented using the identical window settings. *, internal carotid lumen; **, external carotid lumen. (Adapted from Wang J et al. 2007. *Magn Reson Med.* 58(5):973–981.) (B) Sample sagittal carotid bifurcation images illustrating the improved flow suppression capability of MSDE for in-plane flows. Plaque-mimicking artifacts (arrows) can be observed on the multislice DIR images (a) but were completely removed on the MSDE images (b).

large-coverage 3D imaging, as shown in Figure 16.8B. The MSDE technique can also be used for post-contrast imaging since it does not rely on the blood T_1 time for blood suppression.

One limitation of the MSDE sequence is the signal drop caused by the inherent T_2/diffusion decay and/or system imperfection like magnetic field inhomogeneity and eddy current effects. In a typical clinical environment, this may cause ~12% of signal loss. An improved MSDE sequence (Wang et al. 2010b) has also been proposed to compensate for the signal loss caused by the RF transmission field inhomogeneity and eddy current effects. In the improved MSDE version, a second refocusing pulse is added reducing effects of field inhomogeneity.

16.2.2.4 Other Black-Blood Imaging Techniques

In addition to the BB techniques mentioned above, other black-blood imaging techniques based on different mechanisms have also been proposed. The T_2-IR technique achieves black-blood contrast by taking advantage of the longer T_1 and T_2 values of the blood compared to other tissues (Brown et al. 2010). In this technique, when a T_2 preparation module is combined with an inversion RF pulse, the black-blood effect can be achieved if the TI value is properly selected. Compared to the other techniques, the advantage of the T_2-IR technique is that it poses no reliance on the blood flow to achieve the black-blood effect. It can therefore usually achieve satisfactory blood suppression in even the most challenging regions. The T_2-IR technique, however, is still limited by the fact that it heavily relies on the blood T_1 and T_2 values for BB effect and therefore may need to be individually optimized for postcontrast imaging. Besides, it is also limited by the fact that it is a single slice imaging technique and therefore may have to be acquired at reduced time efficiency. Besides the inflow effect and blood relaxation properties, the difference in *diamagnetism* between blood and vessel wall has been used for VWI. The *susceptibility weighted imaging (SWI)* technique has been shown to demonstrate a distinct lumen/wall separation when used for peripheral artery plaque burden imaging (Yang et al. 2009). Since no flow velocity requirement is needed for this technique, the SWI image is also expected to achieve satisfactory lumen/wall separation in most circumstances. A current limitation of the technique is that no uniform phase enhancement maybe achieved for complicated plaque components where different tissues with various diamagnetic effect may present. This inhomogeneous phase shift may cause impaired lumen and/or outer wall boundaries segmentation (Yang et al. 2009).

16.2.3 Plaque Composition and Multicontrast MRI

The atherosclerotic plaque can contain several components such as calcification, lipid-rich necrotic core (LRNC), and intraplaque hemorrhage (IPH). Relaxation properties of tissues comprising each plaque component provide an indication of the type of plaque component. By varying pulse sequence parameters, multicontrast images of each component can be obtained and analyzed to identify the particular plaque component. For example, Figure 16.9 shows the appearance of IPH using a multicontrast MRI protocol. The area identified as IPH on MRI can be seen to agree well with IPH on histology. Appearance of LRNC and calcification on multicontrast MRI is shown in Figure 16.10A and B, respectively. Knowledge of the histological and chemical constituents of plaque components are important in choosing optimal pulse sequence parameters for plaque imaging and are considered next.

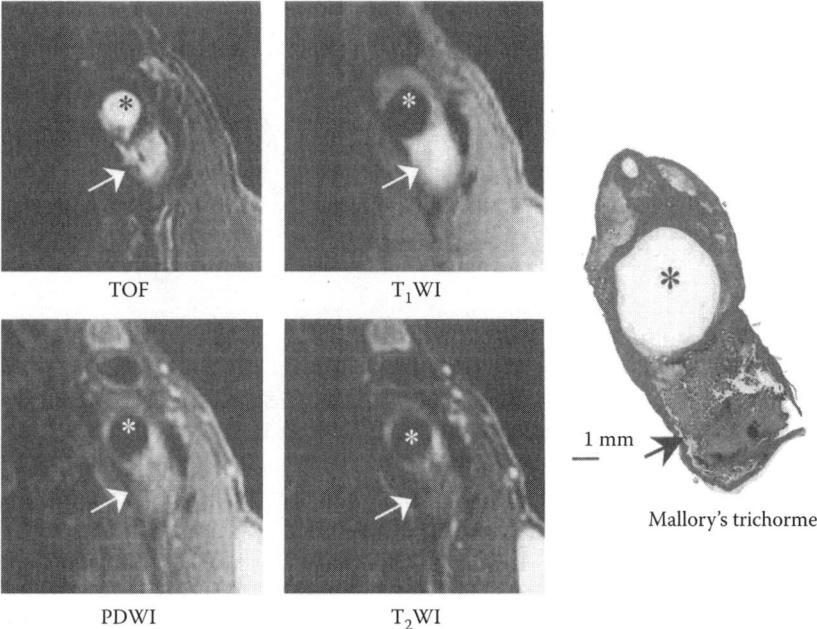

FIGURE 16.9 Multicontrast carotid MRI protocol with 3D-TOF, T_1-weighted, PD-weighted, and T_2-weighted images compared to histology (Mallory's trichrome stain). IPH is bright on T_1-weighted sequences such as TOF and T_1w. Corresponding area on histology verifies IPH (arrow). (Adapted from Cai J et al. 2002. *Circulation.* 106:1368–1373.)

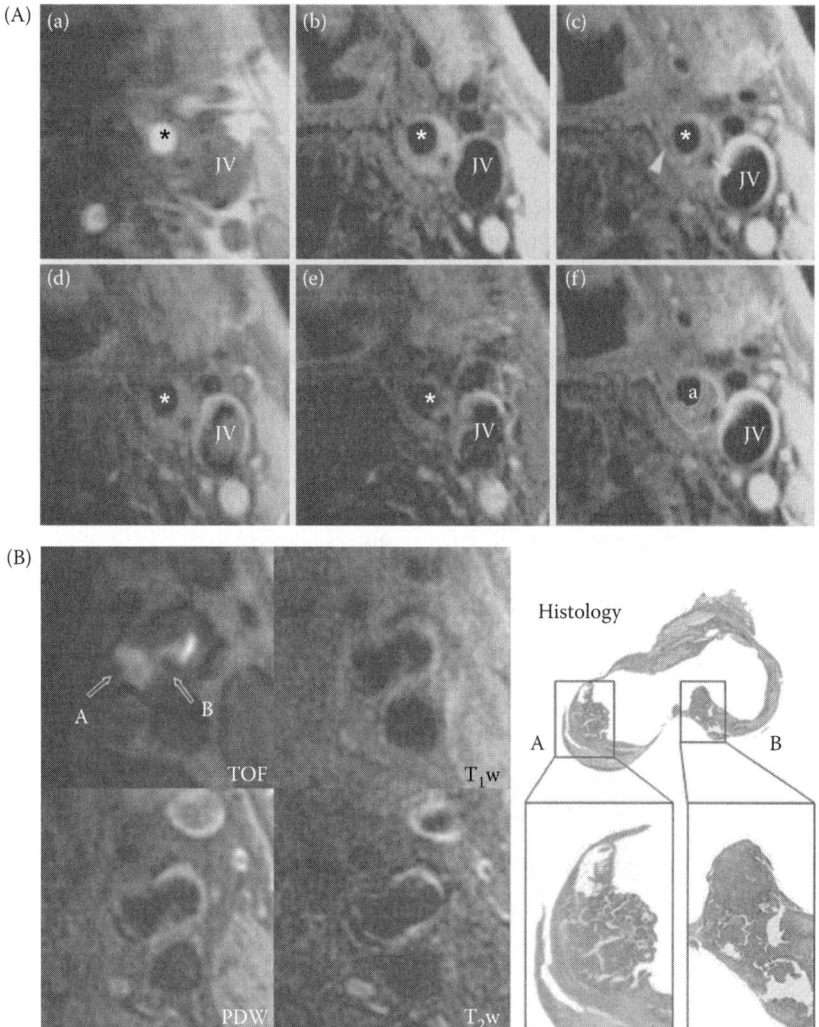

FIGURE 16.10 (A) Multicontrast MRI showing identification of LRNC. Comparing postcontrast T_1w (CE-T_1w) to precontrast T_1w (T_1w), nonenhancement of LRNC postcontrast (arrow) is clearly visible. (Adapted from Cai J et al. 2005. *Circulation.* 22:3437–3444.) (B) Calcification (arrows on TOF) appears hypointense on all contrast weightings. Boxes A and B on histology correspond to arrows on TOF. The juxtaluminal location of calcification marked by arrow B on TOF makes interpretation on dark blood images difficult but is well appreciated on the bright-blood TOF. (From Chu B et al. 2009. *J Am Coll Cardiol Img.* 2009(2):883–896.)

16.2.3.1 Intraplaque Hemorrhage and Thrombus

In advanced stages of atherosclerosis, there may be bleeding into the plaque from either the lumen after the surface is disrupted or the *vasa vasorum* which supplies blood to both the normal and abnormal parts of the vessel wall. Such bleeding into the plaque is termed intraplaque hemorrhage (IPH). Evolution of IPH signal over time is not yet fully understood but findings have been extrapolated to IPH from known characteristics of brain hemorrhage. Immediately after hemorrhage into the brain, intracellular hemoglobin from the red blood cells gets deoxygenated to deoxyhemoglobin and then oxidized to methemoglobin. The five unpaired electrons in methemoglobin render it paramagnetic with short T_1 relaxation times. After cell lysis, the paramagnetic methemoglobin becomes extracellular until it is reabsorbed by reparative processes. The high signal from methemoglobin on T_1-weighted images is also seen in IPH. Both acute IPH (intracellular methemoglobin) and older IPH (extracellular methemoglobin) are seen as hyperintense signals on T_1-weighted sequences such as black-blood T_1 turbo spin echo or bright-blood 3D time-of-flight sequences. Both sequences are used for IPH identification in a multi-contrast review. However, highly T_1-weighted sequences such as magnetization-prepared rapid gradient echo (MP-RAGE) are more sensitive and specific for IPH detection (Ota et al. 2010).

In the MP-RAGE technique, additional T_1 weighting is imparted by a nonselective inversion pulse applied before a slice-selective gradient echo readout. Optimization of the inversion time is required for good blood suppression while at the same time providing high contrast for methemoglobin (Zhu et al. 2008). A sequence diagram of MP-RAGE is given in Figure 16.11. At 3 T, the T_1 of blood is around 1500 ms and of vessel wall is around 1000 ms. However, the T_1 relaxation times of methemoglobin in plaque is not fully characterized. If T_1 of methemoglobin is assumed to be 500 ms, Zhu et al. (2008) showed that the optimal sequence parameters that minimized blood signal while maximizing IPH contrast depended on TI. Short T_1 times provide the best contrast between vessel wall and intraluminal blood while at the same time providing good contrast for methemoglobin in IPH. However, longer TI times may be needed to improve overall signal. A range of TI times varying from 300 to 600 ms are used for IPH imaging at 3 T depending on scan time, coverage, and SNR constraints. Imaging parameters guided by Bloch simulation and adjusted by scanning subjects with IPH are usually used. Optimized MP-RAGE parameters show IPH as hyperintense regions while most tissues including vessel wall are not visible (Figure 16.11). Increased TI times can be used to show vessel wall and surrounding muscle/fibrous tissue but this comes at the expense of lowered contrast between IPH and the fibrous tissue of plaque. Long TI times can reduce the sensitivity to detect small IPH. Alternatively, increasing the number of averages can be used to visualize the vessel wall in addition to IPH but it comes at the expense of increased scan time or lowered resolution.

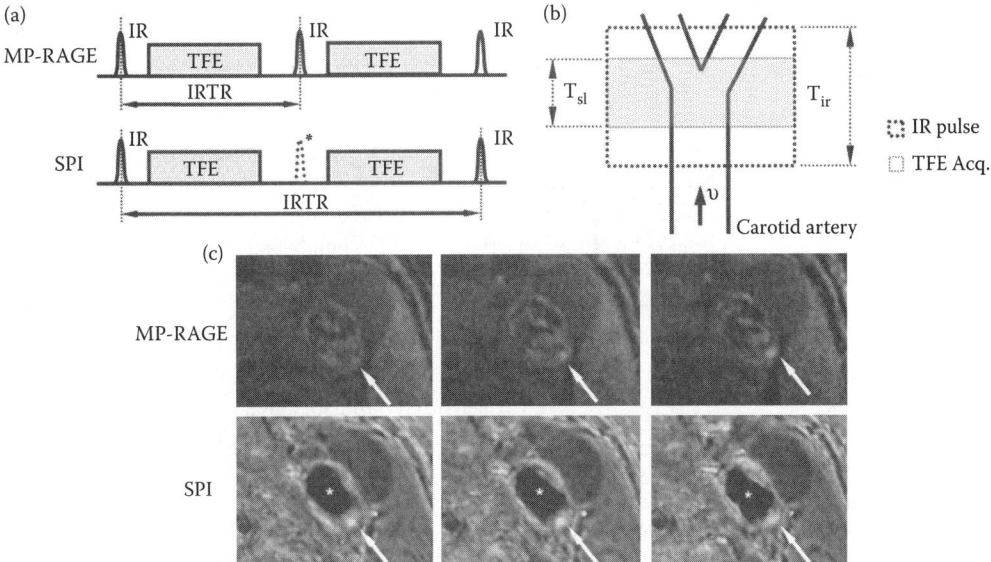

FIGURE 16.11 (a) The MP-RAGE sequence has repeated nonselective inversion pulses applied. SPI has a slab-selective inversion followed by a similar acquisition (noted with a *) to obtain a PDw image for phase correction thus doubling scan time compared to MP-RAGE. (b) The inversion slab thickness (T_{ir}) is larger than the imaging slab (T_{sl}). IPH signal is bright on both MP-RAGE and SPI (arrow in c). However note the better lumen delineation (*) by SPI. Corresponding MP-RAGE images show flow artifacts that can interfere with detection of *juxtaluminal* IPH. (Adapted from Wang J et al. 2010a. *Magn Reson Med.* 64(5):1332–1340.)

Optimization of MP-RAGE TI is difficult since both blood signal suppression and methemoglobin signal enhancement have to be balanced by choosing TI. Phase-sensitive reconstruction combined with slab-selective inversion instead of the nonselective inversion of MP-RAGE can be used to suppress blood signal relative to the vessel wall. This allows more room in the adjustment of TI for improving contrast of IPH relative the vessel wall. This technique called slab-selective phase-sensitive inversion recovery (SPI) (Wang et al. 2010a) is compared to MP-RAGE in Figure 16.11. Phase-sensitive correction requires an additional PD-weighted image for phase correction of the SPI image. Thus, phase correction doubles scan time over MP-RAGE but provides improved CNR for IPH and blood suppression. In MP-RAGE, blood inflow into the imaging slab is reinverted multiple times by the nonselective inversion pulse. However, in SPI, the slab thickness of the inversion pulse (T_{ir}) is optimized such that inflowing blood is only inverted once before image acquisition. The "inverted" blood in SPI provides "negative" blood signal compared to the vessel wall signal, whereas in MP-RAGE, blood signal is saturated by repetitive reinversion thereby reducing the vessel wall-blood CNR. The T_{ir} in SPI is governed by the following two equations:

$$\frac{T_{ir} - T_{sl}}{2} \rangle TI \times v_{max}$$

$$\frac{T_{ir} - T_{sl}}{2} \langle (TI + IRTR) \times v_{min}$$

where IRTR is the time interval between two consecutive IR pulses and v_{min} and v_{max} are the minimum and maximum velocities of inflowing blood, respectively. TI of SPI is adjusted to maximize IPH-vessel wall CNR. Figure 16.11 shows the improved IPH contrast and blood suppression of SPI compared to MP-RAGE.

Thrombus is a blood clot usually covering the rupture site. Thrombi can cause transient ischemic symptoms or stroke through emboli. The intracellular methemoglobin within a thrombus can be seen on T_1-weighted sequences especially MP-RAGE, which is also referred to as direct thrombus imaging (Moody et al. 2003). Use of SPI over MP-RAGE is also advantageous for thrombus imaging because of better blood suppression.

16.2.3.2 Lipid-Rich Necrotic Core

The hallmark of atherosclerosis is the accumulation of lipid within the vessel wall. It has been suggested that lipid may exist in several forms within the atherosclerotic plaque contributing to its varied appearance on T_1- and T_2-weighted MRI. Lipid rarely exists as a pure lipid pool in advanced atherosclerotic plaques. Instead, it is usually mixed with cells and cellular debris and presents a heterogeneous appearance on MRI. Such advanced lipid collections are called LRNC to emphasize their necrotic and varied contents. Fat suppression used in VWI does not suppress LRNC signal in contrast to subcutaneous fat. LRNC appears isotense to surrounding muscle on T_1-weighted sequences such as T_1w TSE and TOF images but are hypointense on T_2-weighted images. The shorter T_2 of LRNC compared to the vessel wall makes T_2-weighted images more reliable for identification of LRNC. Administration of gadolinium contrast agents such as Magnevist can improve the sensitivity and specificity for detection of LRNC. Compared to the normal vessel wall, uptake of contrast by LRNC is low. Thus, LRNC can be identified by its hypointensity on postcontrast T_1w compared to the precontrast T_1w (Figure 16.10A). Delineation of the LRNC boundaries also helps define the thickness of the overlying fibrous cap. Contrast-enhanced T_1w images have been shown to improve measurement reproducibility of LRNC (Takaya et al. 2006) and allow fibrous cap length measurements (Cai et al. 2005). Use of the QIR black-blood preparation allows the same sequence parameters to be used between pre- and postcontrast T_1w images, thereby simplifying both the image acquisition and image review. The low diffusivity of LRNC has also been used for its detection using *diffusion weighted imaging* (DWI). DWI images using reduced field-of-view echo planar imaging show lipid core as dark regions on the apparent diffusion coefficient (ADC) maps (Kim et al. 2009). However, due to challenging requirements of DWI, it is difficult to obtain ADC maps in the carotids with high SNR. Hence unlike IPH, LRNC is still best detected using a combination of weightings rather than a single sequence. Use of contrast-enhanced T_1w MRI provides the most reliable measurement of LRNC.

16.2.3.3 Loose Matrix

The fibrous tissue of plaque consists primarily of organized collagen fibers in the intact plaque. When there are reparative processes secondary to rupture, reabsorption of lipid, and so on, a loose fibrous tissue is laid down. Several different proteins, including hyaluronan, proteoglycans, and so on, can form a loose framework collectively referred to as "loose matrix." Although loose matrix in carotid plaque has not been shown to have any risk associated with it, loose matrix is often found in advanced plaques and may be a sign of tissue repair. Due to the high water content of loose matrix, it appears hyperintense on T_2-weighted images. Loose matrix has high permeability and therefore has high uptake of gadolinium contrast agents and is hyperintense on postcontrast T_1-weighted images compared to precontrast T_1-weighted images, where it is, in general, similar to other fibrous tissues.

16.2.3.4 Calcification

Calcification is a frequent finding in atherosclerotic plaques but its implications are not well understood. Calcification has been implicated in both plaque rupture and plaque stability. Calcification can serve as a measure of disease burden, especially in arterial beds that are difficult to image such as coronary arteries. Calcification has a very short T_2 relaxation time and appears hypointense on all traditional MRI contrast weightings such as T_1w, T_2w, and PDw. Size measurements of calcification using gradient echo techniques tend to overestimate the size due to effect of magnetic field inhomogeneity. This effect however is advantageous for visualizing small plaque components. Thus, spin echo images may be preferable for calcification size estimation but gradient echo sequences for detection of calcification. Identification of calcium may be difficult due to its negative contrast in two situations: (1) in SNR limited images and (2) when calcium is juxtaluminal and black-blood images are acquired. For the latter case, 3D-time-of-flight is often preferred since dark juxtaluminal calcification is easily identified against the bright-blood lumen. A better approach is to acquire images where calcium has positive contrast. Ultrashort echo time (UTE) MRI, a gradient echo technique, provides "positive contrast" for calcium by rapid image readout immediately following the excitation RF pulse. In UTE imaging, an ultrashort echo and a regular echo are acquired for each excitation RF pulse. Subtracting the regular echo image from the ultrashort echo image highlights short T_2 components such as calcifications (Herzka et al. 2008). Short echo times also reduce susceptibility issues and may provide a better size measurement of calcification. Since the readout must immediately follow the excitation RF, radial or spiral readouts are preferred over Cartesian phase encoding. Applications of UTE in plaque imaging are still under investigation.

16.2.4 Cardiac Gating and Motion Compensation

While all major blood vessels are subject to pulsation with each cardiac cycle, the effects on vessel wall images differ depending on the arterial beds. Use of motion compensation techniques such as cardiac or respiratory gating can prolong image acquisition time. Therefore, use of such techniques should consider both the necessity for motion compensation and image acquisition time to obtain high-quality images with short scan times. Coronary arteries, thoracic aorta, and abdominal aorta require vector cardiographic gating for image acquisition fully synchronized with the heartbeat. They also require diaphragmatic respiratory navigator to be applied every TR to reduce the incidence of motion artifacts from the abdominal wall and reduce motion artifacts of the heart. Alternatively, respiratory bellows may also be used for thoracic or abdominal aorta MRI. Carotid VWI has been known to be affected by cardiac, respiratory, and swallowing motion (Boussel et al. 2006). Swallowing motion had the largest effect with respiratory and cardiac motion having lesser effect. Swallowing motion is unique to carotid artery imaging and is difficult to correct for owing to its nonperiodic nature. Navigators positioned on the posterior pharyngeal wall can be used for detecting the motion of the pharynx with swallowing. Although these techniques for detecting swallowing are useful, they have not been widely adopted in carotid VWI. Plaque volume measurements in the carotids have been shown to not benefit from cardiac gating (Mani et al. 2005) and most carotid MRI protocols are not cardiac gated. Peripheral artery imaging in general also does not require cardiac gating for vessel wall measurements. In addition, motion artifacts are also less common with peripheral artery imaging than other arterial beds making peripheral artery imaging relatively straightforward.

16.2.5 Protocols for Vessel Wall Imaging

Plaque morphology, such as lumen and outer wall boundaries, must be visualized clearly for accurate plaque burden measurement. Plaque components such as IPH, LRNC, loose matrix, and calcification should also be assessed for identification of plaque at risk of rupture. Direct assessment of plaque rupture or fibrous cap thickness is an area of research interest in plaque imaging. Proper assessment of plaque thus requires high-resolution images with high SNR obtained without motion degradation. VWI protocols are optimized to address these requirements in a short scan time to avoid excessive subject discomfort and motion artifacts. Recent advances in VWI have addressed these challenges to provide high-quality vessel wall images in multiple vascular beds. Imaging techniques developed for the carotid arteries can be extended to other arterial beds with proper attention to cardiac and respiratory gating requirements. DIR, multislice DIR, and MSDE have been used for aortic imaging. DIR, T_2-IR, and SPACE have been shown useful for peripheral artery imaging. Due to lower blood velocities in the peripheral arteries, T_2-IR can provide better blood suppression than other flow velocity-dependent methods. Coronary VWI has been demonstrated with DIR and MSDE. Special modifications of DIR such as pencil beam reinversion and oblique reinversion slab can also be used for the coronaries. Gating requirements are very stringent for coronary VWI. Methods to reduce scan time such as radial trajectories and subject-specific trigger delays are often used for coronary MRI. Due to the small size of the coronary vessels, resolution requirements are also higher. This, coupled with their position deep within the thorax, has prompted research into better ways to improve coronary vessel wall SNR such as post-contrast imaging.

16.2.6 New Trends in Vessel Wall MRI Techniques

Although the two-dimensional (2D) acquisition schemes for atherosclerotic vessel wall MRI remain the mainstay of many VWI sequences, 3D imaging provides a number of advantages that may represent the future of vessel wall MRI. The utilization of a second phase encoding direction in 3D acquisition schemes provides dramatic SNR advantages as the imaging volume expands in the third dimension. This SNR gain can also be used to improve the spatial resolution in that direction, typically the slice selection direction on the 2D images, to achieve isotropic voxel size in all directions. In addition, 3D dataset and isotropic voxel size can also potentially provide advantages in reducing registration and segmentation errors for quantitative and longitudinal vessel wall measurements.

3D black-blood MR VWI, however, represents significant technical challenges for IS- and DIR-based techniques. Although feasibility of DIR-based 3D BB MRI has been demonstrated (Balu et al. 2008), such techniques are significantly limited by the blood replenishing requirements posed by IS and DIR. In 3D imaging, the blood in a large volume, compared to a thin slice in the 2D case, needs to be replaced to achieve a satisfactory BB effect. This requirement can be very challenging when the image volume is extended. To address this issue, 3D turbo spin echo with variable-flip-angle refocusing RF pulses (SPACE) technique was proposed as a candidate for effective blood suppression when imaging a large-coverage 3D volume (Zhang et al. 2009). The multiple IR pulses used by the SPACE saturate blood signal thus provide automatic blood signal suppression.

Although the SPACE technique provides some black-blood effect, its blood suppression efficiency is still limited due to the lack of a dedicated BB module. The utilization of MSDE-based BB techniques provides an ideal solution for 3D imaging due to its effective, large-volume, flow-direction-independent blood suppression. The blood efficiency has also been shown to be superior than simply relying on the SPACE sequence (Fan et al. 2010). MSDE has been combined with different acquisition schemes, that is, spin echo (Wang et al. 2007; Fan et al. 2010), gradient echo (Balu 2011), steady-state free procession (Koktzoglou and Li 2007), and so on, for large-volume 3D acquisitions. They have also been applied in a number of vascular beds such as carotid, peripheral, and coronary arteries. The elimination of flow replenishing requirements of MSDE technique also allows the imaging volume to be planned in parallel to (as opposed to only perpendicular to) the targeted artery so that more time-efficient acquisition can be achieved.

As shown in Figure 16.12, a 3D MSDE-prepared rapid gradient echo (MERGE) sequence was used to acquire high-resolution carotid artery images. With the SNR benefit from 3D acquisition and efficient black-blood effect from the MSDE sequence, high spatial resolution ($0.7 \times 0.7 \times 0.7$ mm³) and large-coverage (250 mm foot–head direction) imaging volume was acquired in only 2 min. Owing to its time efficiency, 3D-MERGE is highly suitable for applications such as carotid disease screening.

A remaining challenge of the 3D vessel wall MRI is its vulnerability to potential motion artifacts. Unlike in 2D acquisition where the motion-corrupted data impacts only individual images, any corrupted data in 3D volumes contributes to the whole volume. Potential solutions for such issues include switching to motion robust k-space acquisition schemes like radial or spiral acquisition, and combining with special motion compensation schemes. 3D acquisition schemes have not only been applied to plaque burden measurement but also for detecting plaque components such as hemorrhages and/or calcifications. MP-RAGE, SPI, and UTE imaging techniques for IPH and calcium detection described earlier are essentially 3D imaging techniques and have been successfully applied in patient studies. With the advent of fast and robust 3D VWI with good blood suppression, large coverage high-resolution imaging of atherosclerotic lesions that can be applied for patient imaging directly in the clinic is gaining traction. While such techniques for carotid MRI are mature and are being applied in clinical studies, their translation to the coronaries remains challenging and is an active area of research.

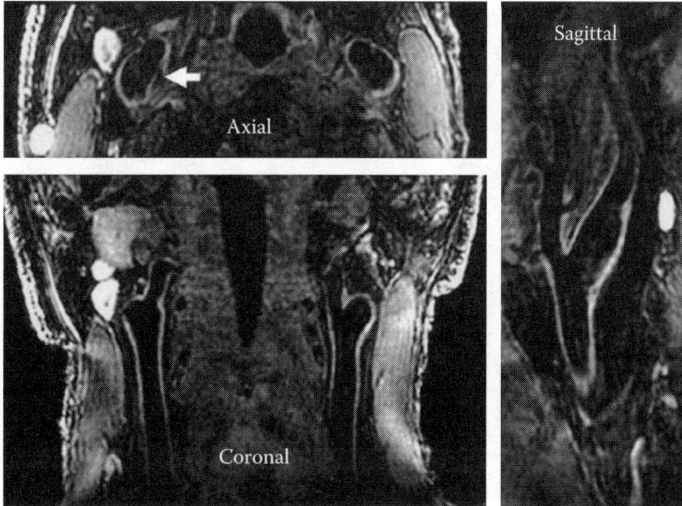

FIGURE 16.12 3D isotropic high-resolution ($0.7 \times 0.7 \times 0.7$ mm³) carotid artery image acquired with 3D MERGE sequence. Arrow on axial reformat shows a small piece of calcification. Vessel wall boundaries are clearly visible on all reformats. (From Balu N et al. 2011. *Magn. Reson. Med.* 65:627–637.)

16.3 Image Processing in Vessel Wall MRI

The end goal of vessel wall MRI is to extract qualitative and quantitative descriptors of the atherosclerotic plaque that can be used for diagnostic risk assessment, monitoring of therapy, or scientific studies of plaque pathophysiology. The volume and complexity of available imaging information—characterized by multiple contrast weightings and multiple, high-resolution image cross sections—mandates the use of image processing tools for robust and efficient analysis. This section describes the major goals and methods for image processing of vessel wall MRI.

Typically, vessel wall MRI yields serial cross-sectional images perpendicular to the axis of the vessel. Other useful views include longitudinal cross sections and reformatted images, such as curviplanar reformats, and maximum intensity projections (MIPs). These basic image formats are illustrated in Figure 16.13. All are useful for aspects of vessel wall image processing.

A major advantage of MRI for VWI is the availability of multiple contrast weightings and techniques for both flow enhancement and suppression. As illustrated in Figure 16.9, this permits image contrasts with both bright and dark vessel lumens, and with varying intensities for internal components of the atherosclerotic plaque. Utilization of the multiple contrast data is both an advantage and a challenge for image processing of vessel wall MRI.

This section is organized as follows. First, methods for assessment of plaque burden are presented, where burden refers to the general size and shape of the vessel wall and lumen. Second, methods for assessing plaque composition are presented, in which the internal structure of the plaque itself is determined. Finally, the section closes with a description of emerging 3D techniques in image processing for vessel wall MRI.

16.3.1 Plaque Burden

The term "plaque burden" is used to denote the severity of atherosclerosis as measured by the size of the plaque. As such, it is used interchangeably to denote a variety of measurements, including thickness, cross-sectional area, volume, or ratios of these measurements. All of these measurements share

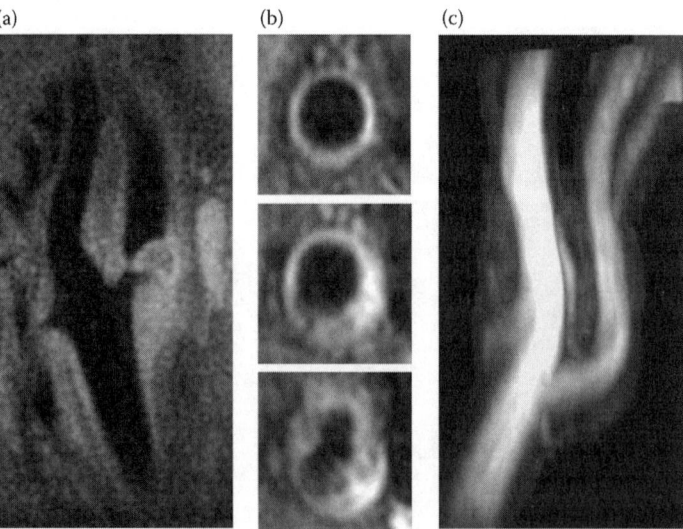

FIGURE 16.13 Useful image viewing options include (a) longitudinal cuts along the vessel axis, (b) axial cuts perpendicular to the vessel axis, and (c) reformatted images, such as maximum intensity projections (MIPs) of 3D image volumes.

TABLE 16.1   Common Plaque Burden Measurements

Measurement	Description
Max NWI	Maximal value of normalized wall index over all slices
Mean NWI	Mean value of normalized wall index over all slices
Max thickness	Maximal thickness over all slices
Max wall area	Maximal wall area over all slices
Wall volume	Total volume of wall over all slices
Max eccentricity	Maximal value of eccentricity over all slices

the common need to determine the inner (lumen) and/or outer boundaries of the vessel wall. When discussing plaque burden, it is important to be explicit regarding which measurement is being made. Common examples are summarized in Table 16.1.

16.3.1.1 Common Burden Measurements

Stenosis, which is the standard clinical assessment of disease severity, can also be viewed as a measure of plaque burden. Stenosis is defined as the difference between the normal and most narrowed vessel diameters divided by the normal diameter, and expressed as a percentage

$$\text{Stenosis} = 100\% \times (d_{\text{normal}} - d_{\text{min}})/d_{\text{normal}}$$

Stenosis of 0% indicates an apparently normal artery, whereas highly diseased arteries approach stenosis of 100%. Most commonly, the normal diameter is measured distal to the point of maximal narrowing, but can also be estimated from the point of maximal narrowing by estimating the apparent original diameter. In the carotid artery, these two approaches are referred to as the "NASCET" and "ACAS" criteria, respectively (ACAS et al. 1995, Barnett et al. 1998). To a lesser extent, "area stenosis" may also be used, in which the diameter measurements are replaced by cross-sectional area measurements.

A limitation of stenosis measurements is that they often fail to accurately depict the severity of disease, in part due to a phenomenon known as "Glagovian remodeling" in which the vessel wall expands with plaque growth (Glagov et al. 1987). As a result, large plaques have been reported even in vessels with 0% stenosis (Dong et al. 2010a). To address this shortcoming, the "normalized wall index" (NWI) was introduced, which is defined as the ratio of the vessel wall area to the total vessel (wall plus lumen) area

$$\text{NWI} = A_{\text{wall}}/(A_{\text{lumen}} + A_{\text{wall}})$$

NWI appears similar in definition to stenosis, but studies have shown little association between maximal NWI and stenosis. Values of NWI range from 0.4 or less in apparently normal arteries to approaching 1.0 for nearly occluded arteries. NWI has also been called "plaque index," "wall/outer wall ratio," and "percent atheroma."

16.3.1.1.1 Thickness

Vessel wall thickness has also emerged as an important indicator of plaque burden. Ultrasound studies have established that intima-media thickness (IMT) along with proximal segments of the carotid arteries reflects global atherosclerosis risk (Lorenz et al. 2007). MRI techniques for thickness measurement have been shown to agree closely with ultrasound measurements (Underhill et al. 2006). Furthermore, MRI provides omnidirectional thickness measurements throughout the carotid bulb and into the internal carotid artery. Thickness measurement does, however, present some challenges in advanced plaques due to the lack of an objective definition of thickness.

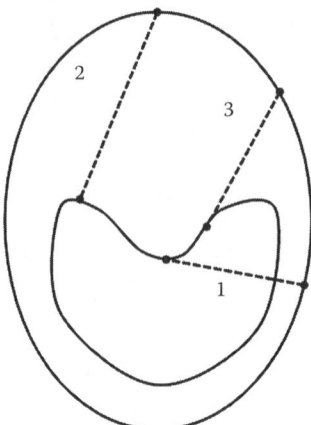

FIGURE 16.14 Challenges for thickness measurement encountered in vessel wall imaging with three approaches: (1) closest point on outer contour, (2) closest point on inner contour, and (3) radial rays from inner contour centroid.

In general, thickness can be defined as the length of a line connecting corresponding points on the inner and outer boundaries. Additionally, the set of lines of thickness circumscribing the vessel wall does not cross one another and each line of thickness should be as close to perpendicular to the vessel wall boundaries as possible. Simple thickness measurement techniques have been proposed based on casting rays from the centroid of the lumen or identifying the closest point on the second contour for each point on the first contour. These approaches work well for relatively normal arteries, but for more complicated shapes in highly diseased arteries, the methods break down (Figure 16.14).

More robust thickness measurement algorithms have been developed that provide appropriate results on any encountered morphology. One approach identifies points of mutual correspondence where each point is mutually closest to the other point on the opposite contour. For points where mutual correspondence is not achieved, corresponding points are identified via interpolation. A second approach is to identify a contour midway between the inner and outer contours. Then, lines of thickness are cast perpendicular to this midline. Finally, an approach using Delaunay triangulation has been proposed that ensures nearly perpendicular lines of thickness through the angle maximization property of Delaunay triangulation (Kerwin et al. 2007).

16.3.1.2 Eccentricity

Another useful but undefined concept for characterizing plaque burden is eccentricity, which captures the extent to which the plaque differentially accumulates along only one portion of the vessel circumference. One method to characterize eccentricity is to compute the ratio of the maximal and minimal lesion thickness. However, the minimal thickness is sensitive to error making the measurement unstable. For nondiseased vessels, this sensitivity can lead to erroneously high eccentricity indices. A better index, based on the centroids c_{wall} and c_{lumen} of the two contours, is given by

$$\text{Eccentricity} = \frac{\sqrt{\pi}}{A_{lumen} + A_{wall}} \|c_{wall} - c_{lumen}\|$$

where the multiplier out front normalizes the difference in centroids by the effective radius of the vessel wall.

16.3.1.3 Boundary Detection

The preceding discussion of measurements of plaque burden presumes that contours have been drawn defining the inner and outer boundaries of the vessel wall. Boundary detection is thus the central image processing concern for plaque burden analysis. In general, detection of the lumen boundary is comparatively easier than detection of the outer wall boundary.

Typically, the lumen exhibits a reasonably uniform signal with a sharp contrast with the vessel wall. This contrast can be either the result of flow enhancement in time-of-flight acquisitions or black blood in flow-suppressed images. Strategies for detecting the boundary of this region generally depend on region growing techniques and/or active contours.

One such active contour approach that has been used is a B-spline snake (Kerwin et al. 2007). In this approach, the boundary is represented as a contour with x and y components given by closed B-splines

$$c_x(u) = \sum_{k=1}^{K} \xi_k \beta\left(\lfloor u - k \rfloor_K\right)$$

$$c_y(u) = \sum_{k=1}^{K} \psi_k \beta\left(\lfloor u - k \rfloor_K\right)$$

where ξ_k and ψ_k are spline coefficients, K is the number of control points in the spline

$$\lfloor u \rfloor_K = \begin{cases} u + K & u < 2 - K \\ u - K & u > K - 2 \\ u & \text{otherwise} \end{cases}$$

and

$$\beta(u) = \begin{cases} \dfrac{3}{4}|u|^3 - \dfrac{2}{3}u^2 + 1 & 0 \le |u| < 1 \\ \dfrac{1}{4}(2 - |u|)^3 & 1 \le |u| < 2 \\ 0 & \text{otherwise} \end{cases}$$

The optimal boundary contour minimizes an energy functional based on the underlying image, such as

$$E = \frac{1}{l(C)} \int_0^K \left\| \frac{dC(u)}{du} \right\| (n(u) \cdot \nabla I(C(u))) du$$

where $C(u) = [c_x(u), c_y(u)]$, $l(C)$ is the total length of the contour, $n(u)$ is the unit normal to the contour at the point u, and ∇I is the image gradient. The contour that minimizes this energy can be found by gradient descent given an initial estimate of the contour.

For the outer boundary of the vessel, boundary detection can be substantially more challenging. Contrast of the vessel wall with surrounding tissues can be minimal. Furthermore, the vessel wall does not have a uniform intensity, which can range from hypointense calcified plaque to hyperintense. Finally, both within and adjacent to the plaque, additional boundaries can lead a boundary detection algorithm to converge to the wrong boundary. To overcome these challenges, shape-based constraints, such as an elliptical prior or active shape model, are advisable (Kerwin et al. 2007).

16.3.1.4 Measurement Accuracy Considerations

The fundamental concern in the accuracy of plaque burden measurements is the accuracy with which an edge can be located. In this regard, the edges are the inner and outer boundaries of the vessel wall. Surprisingly, accuracy of edge detection is not strongly dependent on image resolution. The standard deviation of the estimated location of a step edge can be shown to be approximated by

$$\sigma_d = \frac{p}{\text{CNR}}$$

where p is the fundamental pixel size (resolution) and CNR is the CNR of the edge. Notably, CNR scales with p, so any attempt to reduce σ_d by improving resolution is counteracted by a corresponding reduction of CNR. Furthermore, imaging at higher resolutions increases acquisition time, whereas that time could alternatively be used to acquire more signal averages and reduce σ_d by increasing CNR.

The resolution should, however, be set high enough to ensure the salient features of the vessel wall are captured. For plaque burden measurements, this requires that any Gibbs ringing from one edge does not significantly impinge upon the other. In general, a resolution of at most half the minimum thickness of the vessel wall will ensure any bias in plaque burden measurements is negligible.

MRI scanners also offer two features that should be considered in obtaining accurate measurements of plaque burden: magnitude detection and zero-filled interpolation. Magnitude detection is a standard step used on all scanners for MR image formation in order to eliminate random phase variations. For edges adjacent to a low-signal region, however, magnitude detection slightly perturbs the apparent location of the edge. Zero-filled interpolation is used to reconstruct images with pixel dimensions smaller than the fundamental resolution. Although zero-filled interpolation does not add information, its use does improve accuracy of edge detection based on subsequent linear interpolation and eliminates bias due to magnitude detection. The effects of zero-filled interpolation and magnitude detection on edge position errors are illustrated in Figure 16.15.

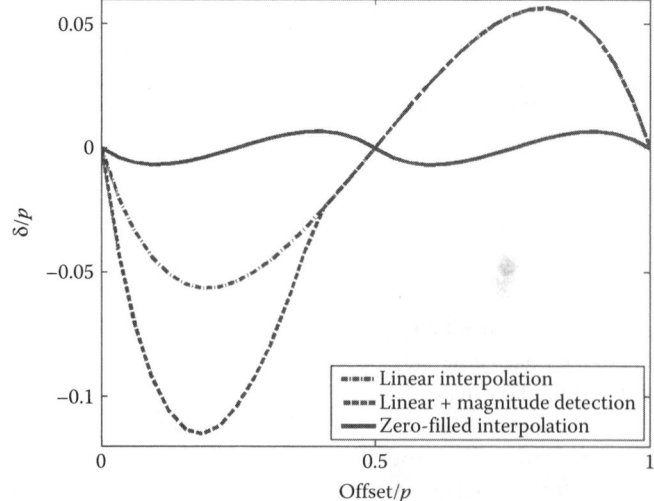

FIGURE 16.15 Measurement error due to interpolation and magnitude detection. Plot shows the error encountered relative to the fundamental image resolution p versus the location of the edge relative to the location of the pixels (i.e., zero and one are the locations of adjacent pixels and 0.5 is midway between).

16.3.2 Plaque Composition

Although plaque burden appears to provide additional clinical insight over and above stenosis, still further insight is provided by examining the components of the plaques themselves. Stable morphologies include greater amounts of fibrous tissue and possibly calcification, whereas components of the soft necrotic core appear to increase risk of clinical events as they increase in size. In particular, IPH within the necrotic core has recently been implicated as a leading marker of risk in carotid atherosclerosis. These components can be further subdivided as illustrated by the hierarchy in Figure 16.16. Notably, fibrous tissue may be subdivided into both dense fibrous tissue and loose matrix. Hemorrhage has been differentiated into type I with intact red blood cells and older type II with lysed red blood cells.

Numerous studies have shown that regions consisting of these different components can be identified by human interpretation of the relative image intensity levels on MRI. These studies have also shown the importance of using multiple contrast weightings. Given the need to integrate information from multiple contrast weightings, this is an especially attractive application for multicontrast segmentation algorithms.

16.3.2.1 Image Registration

Before information can be shared among contrast weightings, the images must be coregistered to account for movement of the patient between multiple contrast acquisitions. VWI poses some challenges for registration in that arteries of interest, such as the carotid arteries, are embedded in soft, deformable tissues in highly mobile areas of the body. Furthermore, adjacent structures can undergo independent motions, such as compression of the jugular veins. Because of these complications, registration techniques that rely on alignment of rigid landmarks or smoothness of the deformation field tend to fail for vessel wall image registration.

Fortunately, the hardening of the arteries in atherosclerosis lends the arteries themselves substantial rigidity. Therefore, in-plane translations are usually sufficient for image registration of the vessel wall itself. This has been successfully accomplished by optimizing the alignment of the previously identified lumen and wall boundaries with the edge features in the images (Kerwin et al. 2007). Simple, in-plane shifts are also conducive to human adjustment of the registration results, if needed.

16.3.2.2 Plaque Segmentation

The central function of segmentation is to estimate the probability of a given pixel being tissue type T_i given the set of observed intensities x in the multiple contrast-weighted images. Using Bayes' rule, this probability can be expressed as

$$\Pr(T_i|x) = \frac{p(x|T_i)\Pr(T_i)}{\Sigma p(x|T_j)\Pr(T_j)}$$

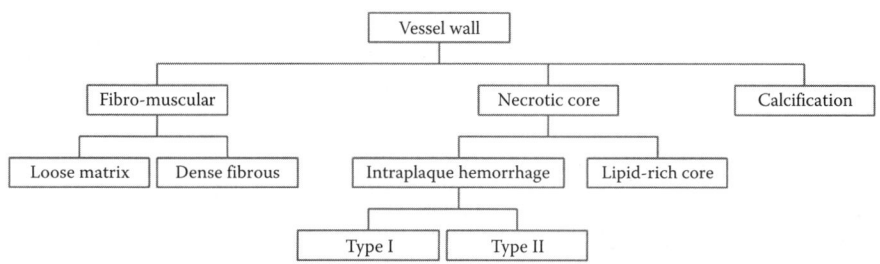

FIGURE 16.16 Hierarchy of common plaque components targeted for segmentation.

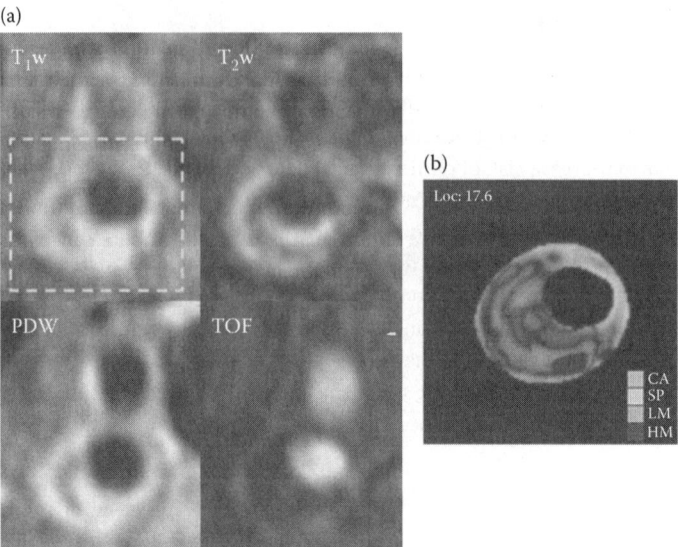

FIGURE 16.17 Segmentation based on multiple contrast-weighting MRI: (a) carotid artery immediately after bifurcation obtained with four indicated contrast weightings; (b) probabilities (high probabilities are dark) for each tissue type: fibrous tissue (Fib), calcification (CA), loose matrix (LM), hemorrhage (Hem), and lipid-rich core (LC). Final contours are shown on the T_1w image.

where the sum is carried out over all tissue types *j*. This probabilistic framework has been further expanded based on the observation that there are morphological cues regarding the likelihood of a given tissue being present. Specifically, this likelihood is dependent on the local thickness *t* of the vessel wall and the depth *d* of the pixel relative to the lumen. Under an assumption of conditional independence, these factors are entered into the morphology-enhanced probabilistic plaque segmentation (MEPPS; Liu et al. 2006) algorithm as

$$\Pr(T_i|t,d,x) = \frac{p(t,d|T_i)p(x|T_i)\Pr(T_i)}{\sum_{j=1}^{4} p(t,d|T_j)p(x|T_j)\Pr(T_j)}$$

For any pixel in the image, this model is able to determine the probability that it is any of the available tissue types (Figure 16.17). The probability distributions are trained based on a histological gold standard.

Once the probabilities for each pixel are available, the final step is to classify each pixel, which can be based on a maximum *a posteriori* assignment to the highest probability tissue class. Alternatively, regions of each tissue type can be captured by competing active contours in order to facilitate editing of the contour regions. In the MEPPS approach, this is done by maximizing the total probability contained within the set of contours, subject to the constraints that each pixel is classified as a single tissue and the contours are smooth.

16.3.3 Three-Dimensional Image Processing

The preceding descriptions of image processing adhere to the common approach of treating 2D cross-sectional images as mutually independent when, in reality, they correspond to closely spaced slices of the same anatomical structures. Thus, a subsequent consideration in VWI is how to account for and take advantage of the 3D information in the images.

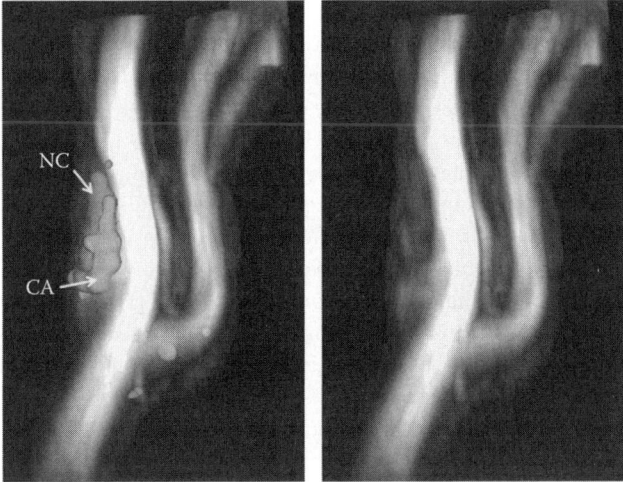

FIGURE 16.18 Three-dimensional rendering of plaque components in relationship to MIP view of angiogram.

16.3.3.1 Angular Measurement

One advantage of a 3D approach to VWI is that additional morphology metrics become available. One set of such metrics has been introduced for describing lumen morphology. By defining geometric positions using a series of maximal inscribed spheres, a scale-independent geometry is introduced. The center of each enumerated sphere is located on the surface of its preceding sphere. Then, metrics are defined based on specific sphere combinations on the set. Example metrics include bifurcation angle, planarity of the bifurcation, and tortuosity (Thomas et al. 2005).

16.3.3.2 Mesh Modeling

A common theme of these 3D approaches is a need to accurately reconstruct the 3D geometry of the vessel, often from sequential 2D contour data. For this, common approaches yield either tetrahedral volume meshes or surface patch models. Applications include mechanical analysis (see below) and rendering of plaque structures in relationship to traditional MRA visualizations (Figure 16.18).

16.3.3.3 3D Imaging

Finally, MRI methods are enabling high-resolution isotropic data to be obtained in 3D. This has the potential to allow image processing to account not only for in-plane information, but also through-plane continuity and smoothness. Image processing techniques to directly extract 3D surfaces corresponding to vessel wall features, as opposed to serial 2D contours, should be forthcoming.

16.4 Contrast Agent Application in Atherosclerosis

As we have established, MRI is a modality that is capable of providing structural as well as functional information on the human body. For VWI, MRI can provide high-resolution imaging of vessel lumen, outer wall boundary, and plaque components. Such information, however, tells only part of the story of the atherosclerotic plaque. Functional and active processes, such as angiogenesis and inflammation, also have significant effects in the initiation, progression, and rupture of plaque (Ross et al. 1999, Libby 2002). Fortunately, MRI has the ability to assess such processes through the use of contrast agents.

Currently, most MRI contrast agents utilize gadolinium, which can shorten T_1 and T_2 times. Accumulation of the gadolinium-based agent can be characterized as bright and dark regions in T_1- and T_2-weighted images, respectively. Chelates of gadolinium, such as Gd-DTPA, are currently available for clinical use. Except for MR angiography, techniques utilizing such agents in plaque imaging include late enhancement imaging (Wasserman et al. 2002, Yuan et al. 2002), which characterizes the agent diffused into the extracellular space of the tissue, and dynamic imaging, which observes the transfer of the agent from the blood stream to the tissue over time. The contrast agent delivery mainly takes place through leaky microvessels in the atherosclerotic plaque—a feature thought to be associated with inflammation. As a result, these techniques can quantify the angiogenesis and inflammation of the atherosclerotic plaque, as well as provide structural information with improved image contrast.

While established MRI contrast agents have proven valuable in plaque imaging, the development of new contrast agents with specific enhancements is a rapidly expanding research area. In plaque imaging, agents that bind to specifically targeted cells or molecules can provide functional information on atherosclerotic plaques (such as the plaque inflammation and angiogenesis), or better identification of key compositional features in atherosclerotic plaque (such as the thrombus), providing a way to better study and understand atherosclerotic disease.

This section describes the state of the art in contrast-enhanced MRI of atherosclerosis. It begins with description of late enhanced MRI and applications in plaque imaging. The majority of this section will cover quantitative techniques for dynamic contrast-enhanced imaging of plaque. Finally, a brief overview of other contrast agents used in plaque imaging, including blood pool and tissue-specific agents, will be presented.

16.4.1 Contrast-Enhanced MRI

Using clinically available contrast agents, such as Gd-DTPA, Lin et al. (1997) and Aoki et al. (1999) observed that atherosclerotic plaques showed significant enhancement in contrast-enhanced (CE) T_1-weighted MR images. The angiogenesis of the vessel wall and endothelial permeability are likely related to the mechanisms of the enhancement. Wasserman et al. (2002), Weiss et al. (2001), Yuan et al. (2002), and Cai et al. (2005) have all shown that CE-MRI can provide unique information regarding plaque composition, function, and vulnerability.

16.4.1.1 CE Imaging Techniques

Blood signal suppression is a common requirement for VWI MRI because black-blood imaging techniques provide excellent vessel wall contrast. As covered in Section 16.2, typically, spatial saturation bands and DIR techniques (Shen et al. 1993) are used to suppress the blood signal by dephasing the magnetization of inflowing blood.

However, as covered in Section 16.2.2.2, with gadolinium-based contrast agents, the DIR technique has a number of limitations, and Yarnykh and Yuan (2002) proposed the QIR technique to overcome them. QIR technique contains two double inversion recovery pulse set to introduce nearly perfect blood suppression over a wide range of T_1 values. Figure 16.6 shows the blood suppression comparison between QIR and DIR before and after contrast agent injection, clearly showing the advantages of QIR for CE-MRI of atherosclerotic plaque.

As covered in Section 16.2.2.3, Wang et al. (2007) recently proposed an improved motion-sensitized-driven equilibrium (iMSDE) sequence, in which the blood signal suppression is T_1 independent. This provides another potential option for blood suppression in CE-MRI.

16.4.1.2 Tissue-Specific Characteristic

By analyzing the enhancement patterns in T_1-weighted CE-MRI, several researchers have demonstrated a relationship between enhancement and plaque characteristics. Both Yuan et al. (2002) and Wasserman et al. (2002) found higher enhancement associated with fibrous tissue in CE-MRI, suggesting that the contrast-enhanced images have the potential to improve differentiation of necrotic core from fibrous tissue. Cai et al. (2005) further proved that *in vivo* high-resolution CE-MRI is capable of quantitatively

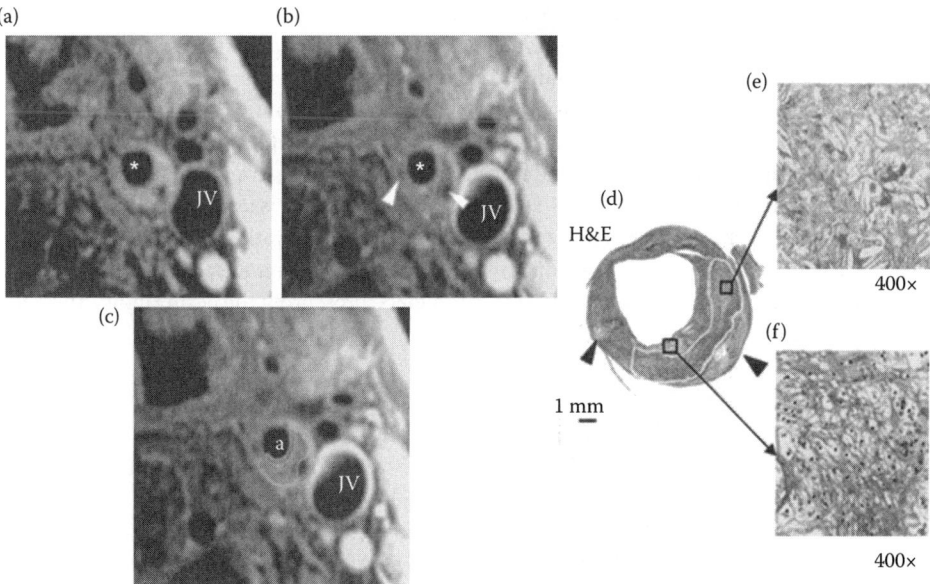

FIGURE 16.19 Corresponding precontrast and postcontrast MR and histological images, showing delineation of the fibrous cap (green contour) and lipid rich/necrotic core (yellow contour) in the left carotid artery. (a) Precontrast T_1-weighted image. (b) Postcontrast T_1-weighted image. (c) Illustration of the measurement method for length of fibrous cap (orange line a). The fibrous cap shows strong enhancement. Histology image (d) shows a matched section with green and yellow contours. High-power photomicrograph shows necrotic debris and cholesterol clefts taken from an area in the lipid rich/necrotic core (e) with no enhancement and loose matrix taken from an area in the fibrous cap (f) with corresponding strong enhancement in postcontrast MR images (b) and (c). Calcification is visible on all images (arrow head). * indicates lumen; JV, jugular vein; H&E, hemotoxylin–eosin staining. (From Cai J et al. 2005. *Circulation.* 22:3437–3444.)

measuring the dimensions of intact LRNC and evaluating the status of fibrous cap, both important parameters to evaluate plaque vulnerability (Underhill et al. 2010). Figure 16.19 shows an example of corresponding CE-MRI and histological images to present how CE-MRI are used in quantitatively measuring the lipid-rich/necrotic core and fibrous cap.

Many researchers have also demonstrated the values of CE-MRI in evaluating plaque inflammation. Inflammation is thought to play an important role in atherosclerotic plaque initiation, progression, and disruption, and is currently a major target in atherosclerosis research and treatment. Yuan et al. (2002) found that contrast-enhanced MRI can identify high neovascularization—thought to be a feature of inflammation and a contributor to plaque destabilization (Ross et al. 1999). Weiss et al. (2001) found that contrast-enhanced MRI characteristics were associated with elevated serum marker of inflammation, likewise suggesting the value CE-MRI for evaluating plaque inflammation. Also, in a study using a rabbit model, Hur et al. (2010) found that the macrophage area and microvessel density were associated with enhancement ratio in CE-MRI, further indicating the CE-MRI may be an efficient method to detect plaque inflammation.

16.4.2 Dynamic Contrast-Enhanced Imaging

Although CE-MRI has been shown to provide useful information for evaluation of the plaque inflammation, it is mainly used in characterizing the plaque composition. CE-MRI is not suitable for quantitative assessment of plaque inflammation because the enhancement of CE-MRI only provides limited information on the amount of remaining contrast agent within the tissue. Furthermore, the amount of enhancement varies depending on factors such as dose, scanning parameter, and timing. Dynamic contrast-enhanced (DCE) MRI, which acquires images over the course of contrast agent injection, can provide detailed information on the transfer of the contrast agent from plasma into tissue. Compared with CE-MRI, DCE-MRI has the advantage of showing not just "what" enhances but also "how" it enhances. For example, both neovasculature and loose matrix have strong enhancement patterns in CE-MRI. However, in DCE-MRI, the enhancement of neovasculature is faster than that of loose matrix because the contrast agent transfer in loose matrix relies on diffusion rather than direct perfusion from vascular system as in neovasculature. To quantitatively assess the enhancement pattern of DCE-MRI, kinetic modeling is used to generate quantitative parameters, presenting the permeability and perfusion characteristics of the plaque.

16.4.2.1 DCE Imaging Technique

DCE-MRI typically utilizes multiple T_1-weighted image acquisitions over a period of time. The imaging sequence of DCE-MRI requires a short acquisition time to capture the rapidly changing enhancement patterns. Quantitative DCE-MRI of atherosclerotic plaque also differs from CE-MRI in that it requires bright-blood imaging. Bright-blood imaging is useful for DCE because the blood signal can be used to extract the changes of contrast agent concentration in the blood, also referred as the arterial input function (AIF), a key function for kinetic modeling (see Section 16.4.2.3). To acquire an accurate AIF, the requirement of the DCE-MRI sequence then is to generate a T_1-dependent blood signal which should be proportional to contrast agent concentration.

The most commonly used imaging technique in bright-blood DCE-MRI of atherosclerotic plaque is the 2D spoiled gradient-recalled echo (SPGR) T_1-weighted sequence (Kerwin et al. 2003). Images usually need to be obtained at 15 time points or more, for a duration of about 4 min. Coincident with the second image in the sequence, the gadolinium-based contrast agent (0.1 mmol/kg for human carotid imaging) should be injected at a constant rate (2 mL/s for human carotid imaging) by a power injector. Spatial saturation bands should be placed at the proximal and distal ends of the imaging block to induce a T_1-dependent blood signal by suppressing the effect of untipped inflowing blood, resulting in dark blood on images prior to contrast bolus arrival. See Figure 16.20.

Although bright-blood DCE-MRI has some advantages, such as the availability of AIF, it creates difficulty in separating the signal in the vessel wall from the adjacent signal in the lumen. Consequently, bright-blood is only suitable for imaging moderate and advanced plaques, which are thick enough to negate the signal influence from a bright lumen. To overcome this challenge, Calcagno et al. (2008) proposed a black-blood DCE-MRI protocol for small lesion imaging. The requirements of black-blood DCE-MRI are similar to CE-MRI of plaque, except for a higher temporal resolution. The previously described DIR, QIR, and MSDE sequences (see Section 16.2) can fulfill the requirements for black-blood DCE-MRI by limiting acquisition coverage to reduce the scan time. To further minimize acquisition time, Yarnykh and Yuan (2006) proposed a small field of view quadruple inversion recovery (sfQIR) technique, which allows rapid dynamic imaging and black-blood preparation without wrap-around artifacts. Figure 16.21 shows an example of black-blood DCE-MRI of rabbit aorta obtained by using sfQIR.

16.4.2.2 DCE Image Processing

To generate quantitative parameters from DCE-MRI, kinetic modeling of enhancement pattern is necessary. To accurately carry out kinetic modeling, image processing of the dynamic images is essential. The main goal of the image processing is to correct image misalignment in the sequence caused by patient motion during the scan. This is very important for kinetic modeling as even small shifts can cause severe bias in the generated quantitative parameter due to the small size of the vessel wall. Additionally, image processing may correct for noise attenuation. Kerwin et al. (2002) proposed a Kalman filtering registration and smoothing (KFRS) algorithm to simultaneously automatically register and reduce the

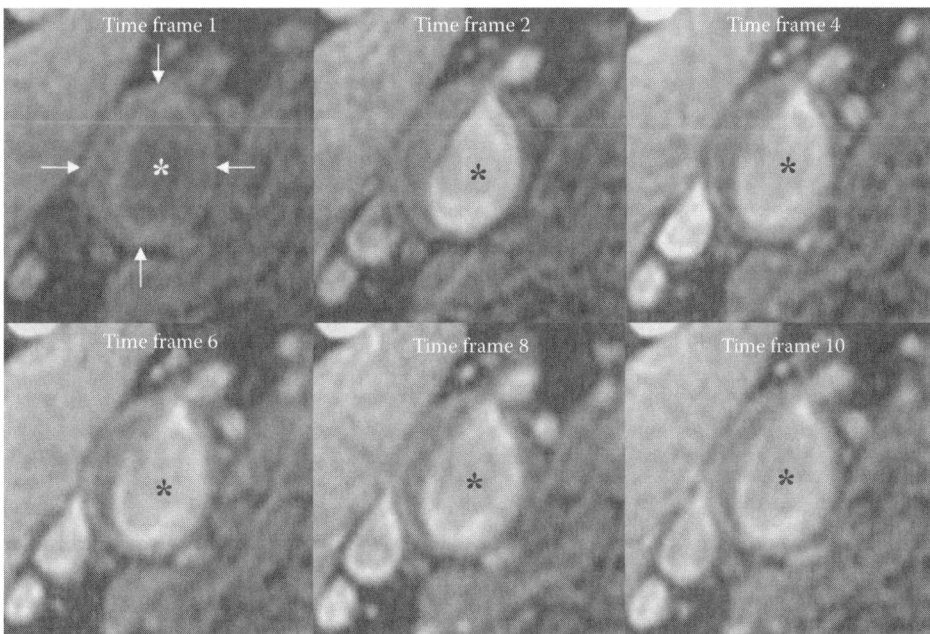

FIGURE 16.20 An example of bright-blood DCE-MRI of a human carotid artery near bifurcation, showing images at six different time points. The time frame 1 shows the precontrast image. * indicates the carotid lumen. The arrows show the outer wall boundary of carotid artery.

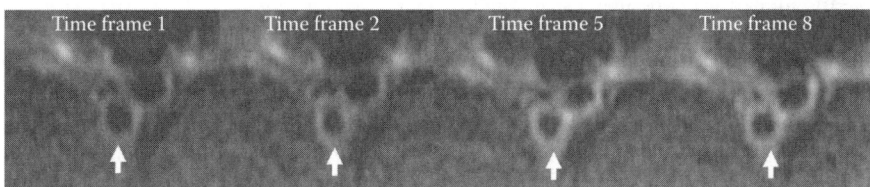

FIGURE 16.21 An example of black-blood DCE-MRI of an injured rabbit aorta, showing images at four time points in the dynamic sequence. Time frame 1 is the precontrast image. The arrows indicate the aorta.

noise for DCE-MRI of atherosclerotic vessels. Registration is performed by searching for displacement of the image at time frame j ($\mathbf{d}_j$) in a user-defined range of displacement that minimizes the cost function:

$$\sum_{\mathbf{x}}[I_j(\mathbf{x} + \mathbf{d}_j) - I_{j-1}(\mathbf{x})]^2$$

where I_j is the image at time frame j. This registration method attempts to find relative movement that minimizes the difference between adjacent time frames. It is also suitable for most DCE-MRI studies. The Kalman filtering method is based on a state model that estimates the true state of a linear dynamic system from a series of noisy observations over time. The Kalman filtering method can also denoise a series of DCE-MRI images by modeling the image with Gaussian noise.

Figure 16.22 shows an example of the processing result of KFRS algorithm. Detailed information of the KFRS algorithm can be found in Kerwin et al. (2002).

After registration and noise attenuation, the change in contrast concentration needs to be extracted from the processed serial images of DCE-MRI. First, change in contrast concentration can be converted

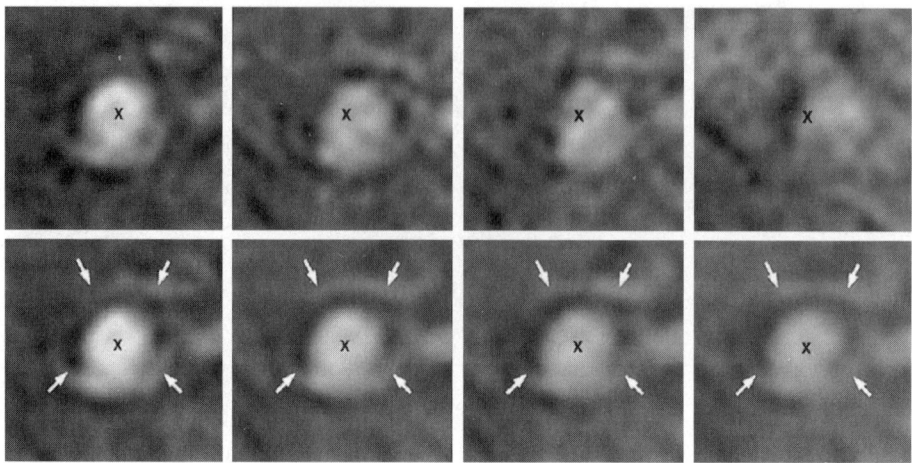

FIGURE 16.22   Four misaligned images in a DCE-MRI series with poor initial image quality before (top) and after (bottom) application of the KFRS algorithm. The filtered images show less motion relative to the fixed "X" and the presence of an enhancing outer wall (arrow). (Adapted from Kerwin W, Cai J, and Yuan C. 2002. *Magn Reson Med.* 47:1211–1217.)

from the MR intensity curves (Cron et al. 1999) based on an obtained precontrast T_1 map and the relationship between intensity and concentration known for the specific imaging sequence. This conversion conforms to the assumption of kinetic modeling and is widely used for relatively large tissues. However, this technique requires additional T_1 mapping, resulting in a longer acquisition time and more image processing and modeling challenges, especially for small tissues prone to motion. Alternately, an intensity curve can be used as a surrogate for the concentration curves for kinetic modeling because the linear relationship between the contrast agent concentration and the MR intensity can be assumed for low contrast concentrations in most DCE-MRI sequences. This technique simplifies both the acquisition and analysis, but can introduce bias in the kinetic modeling because its assumptions are not valid for high contrast concentrations.

16.4.2.3 Kinetic Modeling of DCE

The goal of kinetic modeling is to extract biologically relevant parameters from the contrast agent concentration curves. The contrast concentration change in the tissue of interests is dependent on the blood supply and permeability of the neovasculature. By properly modeling the contrast agent transfer in the targeted tissue after agent injection, the parameters can be calculated by fitting the mathematical model to reflect tissue permeability and blood supply.

The two-compartment model is the most popular model for kinetic modeling of DCE-MRI. As shown in Figure 16.23, this model describes the kinetic transfer of clinically available gadolinium extravascular extracellular agents from the plasma to extravascular extracellular space (EES), but not through the cellular membrane. The tissue in contrast kinetic can therefore be considered to be composed of two compartments: plasma and EES. There are several models proposed based on two-compartment model by multiple researcher groups.

A commonly used two-compartment model is the Kety/Tofts model (Tofts 1997). This model only considers the contrast agent in EES. Also, the bidirectional transfer of contrast agent between the plasma and EES is assumed. The equation of the Kety/Tofts model is

$$C_t(t) = K^{\text{trans}} \int_0^t C_p(\tau) e^{-\frac{K^{\text{trans}}}{v_e}(t-\tau)} d\tau \qquad (16.2)$$

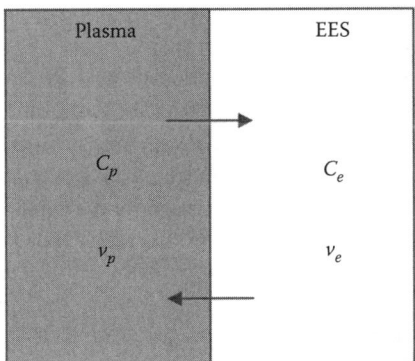

FIGURE 16.23 Illustration of the two-compartment model. Tissue concentration is composited by plasma and EES, v_p and v_e are the fractional volumes of plasma and EES, and C_p and C_e are the contrast agent concentrations in the plasma and EES. Contrast transfer from plasma to EES and can efflux from EES back to plasma.

where K^{trans} is the transfer constant, v_e is the fractional volumes of EES, and C_p and C_t are the contrast agent concentrations in the plasma and tissue. Based on this model, a modified Kety/Tofts model (Tofts, 1997) has been proposed that includes the contrast agent in plasma into consideration. The equation is

$$C_t(t) = v_p C_p(t) + K^{\text{trans}} \int_0^t C_p(\tau) e^{-\frac{K^{\text{trans}}}{v_e}(t-\tau)} d\tau \qquad (16.3)$$

where v_p is the fractional volumes of plasma.

Another popular two-compartment model is the Patlak model (Patlak et al. 1983), which assumes that the efflux of the contrast agent from the EES back to plasma is negligible. The equation is

$$C_t(t) = v_p C_p(t) + K^{\text{trans}} \int_0^t C_p(\tau) d\tau \qquad (16.4)$$

By mathematically analyzing the relationship between the modified Kety/Tofts model (Equation 16.3) and the Patlak model (Equation 16.4), an extended graphical model was proposed by partially modeling the contrast efflux effect from EES back to plasma (Chen et al. 2011):

$$C_t(t) = v_p C_p(t) + K^{\text{trans}} \int_0^t C_p(\tau) d\tau - \frac{K^{\text{trans}^2}}{v_e} \int_0^t \int_0^t C_p(\tau_2) d\tau_2 d\tau_1 \qquad (16.5)$$

In these models, K^{trans}, v_e, and v_p are the parameters related to the physiology of the tissue. Usually, the transfer constant K^{trans} is considered important because it is associated with blood flow, capillary surface area, and permeability, making it a good indicator of blood supply and neovasculature permeability in the tissue.

As we can see from these models, given temporal measurements of C_p and C_t, physiology-related parameters can be estimated that provide the best fit between the observed measurements and the model. C_t can be easily extracted from the tissue of interest. However, extraction of C_p, which is also known as arterial input function (AIF), is typically difficult due to the high concentration of contrast agent in blood and the high temporal resolution requirement. In kinetic modeling of black-blood DCE-MRI, this is more challenging because the blood signal has been suppressed.

As a result, many studies fall back on calculating nonmodel-based parameters instead of the model-based parameters, such as the area under enhancement curve (AUC) (Patlak et al. 1983, Calcagno et al. 2008). These model-free parameters are easily calculated. However, their relationship to the physiological properties is neither intuitive nor obvious.

Many researchers have made efforts to develop kinetic modeling methods without the knowledge of the AIF. A population-derived AIF (Tofts et al. 1999) has been proposed to standardize AIF for an entire study population. However, to determine this population-derived AIF, extra experiments are needed, which increases the study cost. Also, the assumption that all individuals have the same AIF may introduce bias in the analysis. An alternative approach is to use the reference region model (Yankeelov et al. 2005). This technique can calculate the AIF by using the reverse function of the kinetic model from a reference region. For example, the reverse function of Patlak model is

$$C_p(t) = \frac{1}{v_{PRR}} C_{RR}(t) - \frac{K^{\text{trans}}_{RR}}{v^2_{PRR}} \int_0^t C_{RR}(\tau) e^{-\frac{K^{\text{trans}}_{RR}}{v_{PRR}}(t-\tau)} d\tau \qquad (16.6)$$

With the concentration curve C_{RR} and known parameters K^{trans}_{RR}, v_{pRR} of the reference region, the AIF can be calculated. Then, the parameters of the tissue of interest (ROI) can be computed by fitting Equation 16.4. Furthermore, by substituting Equation 16.6 into Equation 16.4, we can get

$$C_t(t) = \alpha C_{RR}(t) - \alpha\beta \int_0^t C_{RR}(t) e^{-\beta(t-\tau)} d\tau + \gamma \int_0^t C_{RR}(\tau) d\tau - \gamma\beta \int_0^t \int_0^{\tau_1} C_{RR}(\tau) e^{-\beta(t-\tau)} d\tau d\tau_1 \qquad (16.7)$$

where $\alpha = \frac{v_p}{v_{PRR}}$, $\beta = \frac{k^{\text{trans}}_{RR}}{v_{PRR}}$, $\gamma \frac{k^{\text{trans}}}{v_{PRR}}$. In this manner, K^{trans}_{RR} and v_{pRR} are not necessarily preknown. They can be estimated together with K^{trans} and v_p by fitting Equation 16.7 with measured C_{RR} and C_t. However, the complicated integer and the nonlinearity of the equation in these two methods increase the complexity of the estimate, resulting in higher noise sensitivity and poor stability of the fitting algorithm.

Alternatively, instead of directly using the reversion function, the AIF can be eliminated to generate an equation allowing linearized fitting algorithm (Wu 2008):

$$v_{PRR} C_t(t) + K^{\text{trans}}_{RR} \int_0^t C_t(\tau) d\tau = v_p C_{RR}(t) + K^{\text{trans}} \int_0^t C_{RR}(\tau) d\tau \qquad (16.8)$$

The reference region model for the original and modified Kety/Tofts model can be found in Yankeelov et al. (2005) and Faranesh and Yankeelov (2008).

16.4.2.4 DCE-MRI Studies of Arterial Atherosclerosis

By utilizing the previously described MRI, image processing, and kinetic modeling techniques, many studies have proven that the DCE-MRI can provide unique information on revascularization and inflammation of atherosclerotic plaque.

Kerwin et al. conducted serial studies (Kerwin et al. 2003, 2006, 2008) to investigate quantitative evaluation of the plaque vascularity and inflammation using bright-blood DCE-MRI acquired by SPGR sequence and quantitative parameters derived from Patlak model (v_p and K^{trans}). In the first study (Kerwin et al. 2003), by analyzing 16 patients, v_p was found to be correlated ($r = 0.80$, $p < 0.001$) with neovessel area obtained in histological sections, indicating that v_p was an effective marker of plaque vascularities. In a subsequent study (Kerwin et al. 2006) involving 30 patients, measurements of K^{trans} and v_p were found to have a high correlation with macrophage (K^{trans}: $r = 0.75$, $p < 0.001$; v_p: $r = 0.54$,

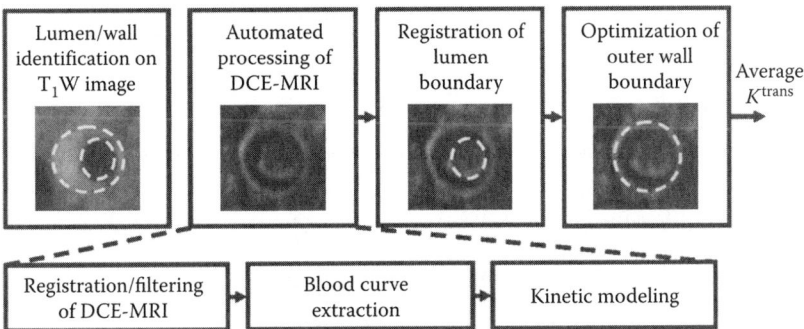

FIGURE 16.24   Illustration of the steps in creating a vasa vasorum image: boundaries drawn on a conventional contrast (T_1-weighted) define a region of interest for processing. Within this region, DCE-MRI images are run through the KFRS algorithm, then a blood curve (AIF) is automatically extracted and used for kinetic modeling. Finally, the boundaries are mapped to the resulting vasa vasorum image and K^{trans} is measured in the wall. (From Kerwin W et al. 2006. *Radiology*. 241:459–468.)

$p < 0.004$) and neovasculature (K^{trans}: $r = 0.71$, $p < 0.001$; v_p: $r = 0.68$, $p < 0.001$) content in 27 patients with analyzable MR images and histological results. Additionally, K^{trans} was significantly correlated with high-density lipoprotein levels ($r = -0.66$, $p < 0.001$) and was elevated in smokers compared with nonsmokers (mean, 0.134 min^{-1} vs. 0.074 min^{-1}; $p < 0.01$). Another study (Kerwin et al. 2008) has shown that K^{trans} measurements of the adventitial region of the carotid were significantly correlated with serum markers of inflammation. In 20 patients with moderate carotid lesions, adventitial K^{trans} was significantly correlated with the log of C-reactive protein (CRP) levels ($r = 0.57$; $p = 0.01$) and was elevated in active smokers compared to nonsmokers (0.141 vs. 0.111 min^{-1}; $p = 0.02$). This study also proposed a complete processing chain that produces colorized parametric images called "vasa vasorum images" (V-V image) (Figure 16.24). In V-V image, v_p are presented in red and K^{trans} is presented in green, a convenient and intuitive way to present the Patlak model-derived parameters. Based on this image acquisition and processing protocol, Chen et al. (2010) further showed that bright-blood DCE-MRI can exhibit differences in kinetic parameters within different plaque components, indicating the DCE-MRI can differentiate plaque components. More significantly, this study suggests that DCE-MRI has the potential to assess the inflammatory burden in specific regions.

By using a rabbit model, Calcagno et al. (2008) investigated the relationship between DCE-MRI-derived model-free parameter AUC and plaque vascularization. In this study, a DIR sequence was used for black-blood DCE-MRI acquisition. AUC was found to have a positive correlation between neovessels count in atherosclerotic plaques ($r = 0.89$, $p = 0.016$). In a following study, good reproducibility of the black-blood DCE-MRI-based AUC analysis was reported.

Table 16.2 is a summary of the significant findings from these studies. As we can see, these studies establish the basis for *in vivo* quantitative assessment of plaque neovasculature and inflammation using DCE-MRI. Inflammation is thought to play an important role in atherosclerotic plaque initiation, progression, and rupture, and there is a strong interest in treatments with anti-inflammatory effects. Recent studies have assessed the effectiveness of anti-inflammatory, antiatherosclerotic treatments using DCE-MRI. By using black-blood DCE-MRI, Lobatto et al. (2010) successfully revealed early changes in plaque permeability after liposomal glucocorticoid treatment with anti-inflammation effect in a rabbit model.

16.4.3 Other Contrast Agents

Small molecular extravascular extracellular gadolinium contrast agents have been the major agents used in clinical MRI research of arterial atherosclerosis. Currently, many researchers have put efforts

TABLE 16.2 Summary of Associations between DCE-MRI Parameters and Inflammation-Related Factors

Study	v_p Association with Neovessel	v_p Association with Macrophage	K^{trans} Association with Neovessel	K^{trans} Association with Macrophage	Smoking	HDL	Log CRP	AUC Association with Neovessel
Kerwin 03	0.80[a]							
Kerwin 06	0.68[a]	0.54[a]	0.71[a]	0.75[a]	0.13 vs. 0.07[a]	−0.66[a]		
Kerwin 08			0.41[a]	0.49[a]	0.14 vs. 0.11[a]		0.57[a]	
Calcagno 08								0.89[a]

[a] Indicates statistical significance, $p < 0.05$.

into developing new contrast agents sensitive to specific tissues, cells, and even molecules to detect vulnerable atherosclerotic plaque in preclinical or clinical studies.

The challenge of developing new specific agents to target specific molecules or cells is that often these cells are present in very small numbers (Briley-Saebo et al. 2007). To be visible on MRI, contrast agents may be designed so that the agent has a high payload of the magnetic entity (Winter et al. 2003a), or high concentration when interacting with the targets (Sirol et al. 2009), or specify a target with a large number of cells or molecules in the diseased vessel wall (Winter et al. 2003a, Botnar et al. 2004a,b). There are two major nanoparticle platforms for new MR contrast agents development: first, the use of amphiphiles possessing both hydrophilic and lipophilic properties that can self-assemble into larger nanoparticles to deliver large payloads of magnetic entity, such as microemulsions (Briley-Saebo et al. 2007), micelles (Briley-Saebo et al. 2008, Howarth et al. 2009), liposomes (Briley-Saebo et al. 2007), and lipoproteins (Briley-Saebo et al. 2007); second, ultrasmall superparamagnetic iron oxide particles (USPIOs) (Johansson et al. 2001, Kooi et al. 2003, Trivedi et al. 2006, Howarth et al. 2009) with a size of 18–30 nm.

16.4.3.1 Gadolinium-Based Agents

Many new agents are still gadolinium based but possess unique characteristics that facilitate VWI, such as the ability to bind to blood albumin. Gadofosveset is an agent that binds to albumin with an 80–96% bound fraction in human plasma, resulting in a dramatic increase in both relaxivity and elimination half-life (Lauffer et al. 1998). The increased relaxivity can be characterized by signal enhancement in T_1-weighted images. By binding with the albumin, Gadofosveset should be restricted in the blood pool in normal vessels. However, in atherosclerosis, increased content of microvessel and permeability of the microvessel, enable albumin-bound Gadofosveset to enter the vessel wall. Therefore, Gadofosveset accumulation inside the vessel wall is a sign of atherosclerosis (Lobbes et al. 2009). Another albumin-binding agent under intensive investigation for atherosclerotic plaque MR imaging is the Gadoflurine M. Gadoflurine M is a lipophilic, water-soluble gadolinium chelate complex with a perfluorinated side chain (Meding et al. 2007). Besides binding to albumin, it can also bind to collagens, proteoglycans, and tenascin inside the plaque (Meding et al. 2007). As a result, Gadoflurine M can enter the atherosclerotic plaque by increased highly permeable neovasculature. Gadoflurine M can also accumulate inside the fibrous parts of the plaque containing collagens, proteoglycans, and tenascin. In preclinical studies, Barkhausen et al. (2003) found this accumulation in the aortic wall of Watanabe heritable hyperlipidemic (WHHL) rabbits at 48 h after injection. Gadoflurine M accumulation was also found to be related to degree of inflammation and extent of core neovascularization in atherosclerotic plaque (Sirol et al. 2009). Other gadolinium-based contrast agents have relative large molecules. They cannot be transferred easily inside normal vessel walls, but will enhance in diseased vessel walls with leaky microvessels. Carboxymethyl-dex-tran derivative CMD-A2-Gd-DOTA (P717) is a contrast agent with large molecules and has been investigated in a mouse model of atherosclerosis (Chaabane et al. 2004). This kind of macromolecular agent may be useful in kinetic modeling of DCE-MRI because the slow transfer rate of the large molecular agents reduces the need for rapid imaging (Pradel et al. 2003).

16.4.3.2 Iron-Based Agents

Another important type of the specific contrast agent are the iron-based agents, such as USPIOs. USPIOs are composed of an iron crystalline core and a biocompatible coating. Unlike gadolinium-based contrast agents which create bright signal in MR images, USPIOs usually are called negative contrast agents because they can significantly enhance T_2^* relaxation, resulting in signal void in T_2^*-weighted images (Hofmann-Amtenbrink et al. 2010). USPIOs can be taken up by macrophages in the whole body because of their long half-life in blood. In atherosclerotic plaque imaging, this nature of USPIOs has made them good contrast agents specific to inflammation, featured with macrophages infiltration inside the vessel wall. Kooi et al. (2003) found that USPIO accumulation in human aortic atherosclerotic vessel walls can be observed *in vivo* 24 h after administration, and ruptured and rupture-prone plaque showed more accumulation than stable lesions. Trivedi et al. (2006) showed that signal loss induced by USPIOs corresponded to macrophage uptake in the fibrous cap of human carotid artery. Howarth et al. (2009) investigated the role of *in vivo* inflammation detection in risk assessment of vulnerable plaque using USPIOs. They found symptomatic patients had more quadrants with signal drop than asymptomatic patients, indicating more inflammatory regions in symptomatic patients.

16.4.3.3 Molecular Imaging Agents

Although the previously mentioned gadolinium-based agents and USPIOs are macrophage or tissue specific, these agents are not targeted to specific molecules or receptors. Application of specifically targeted molecular contrast agents is a promising technique that allows molecular imaging of MRI to study the functional process of atherosclerosis.

The most popular goals in molecular imaging of plaque are plaque inflammation and angiogenesis. Inflammation is a complicated process in plaque which has not been fully defined, although it typically means inflammatory cells, such as macrophages, infiltrate the plaque. This infiltration process is accompanied by angiogenesis and endothelium dysfunction, which reinforces the infiltration of the inflammatory cells. To image inflammation in plaque, an immunomicelle targeted to the mouse macrophage scavenger receptor (MSR) A has been proposed for atherosclerotic plaque imaging of apoE − /− mouse aorta (Lipinski et al. 2006). The oxidized low-density lipoprotein, which can stimulate the process of inflammation and atherosclerosis, has been visualized with molecular MR imaging (Briley-Saebo et al. 2008) by using an agent that binds unique oxidation-specific epitopes. The matrix metalloproteinases (MMPs) produced in macrophages and released into plaque in macrophage apoptosis are considered to contribute to plaque rupture (Libby 2002) and to be viable targets in VWI. MMPs-targeted agent has been successfully applied for plaque MMPs MRI (Lancelot et al. 2008). Also, MR contrast agents targeting cell apoptosis can also be used in VWI (Strijkers et al. 2010). The dysfunctional endothelium of atherosclerotic lesions has also been characterized with MRI by contrast agent targeting VCAM-1, which is expressed by dysfunctional endothelium (Kelly et al. 2005). For angiogenesis MR imaging, Winter et al. (2003b) proposed an agent targeting $\alpha_v\beta_3$-integrin, which accompanies the process of angiogenesis. They found significantly greater enhancement in the aorta wall with expanded vasa vasorum in a rabbit model after injection of the new agent.

Another target of molecular plaque imaging is the thrombus. Thrombus may lead to a total occlusion of the vessel or lethal ischemia events. Therefore, early detection of thrombus in atherosclerosis has significant diagnostic value. USPIOs with a cyclic arginine–glycine–aspartic acid (RGD-USPIO) specific for the $\alpha_{IIb}\beta_3$-integrin, which is expressed on activated platelets, have been used to image the thrombus (Johansson et al. 2001). Small-molecule gadolinium-based contrast agents have also been proposed and successfully applied in the evaluation of acute and subacute coronary thrombus (Botnar et al. 2004a,b).

Winter et al. (2003a) also proposed a fibrin-targeted agent with larger molecule for thrombus imaging based on a different gadolinium formulation.

Another goal of molecular imaging is to improve the detection of plaque morphology. Recently, an elastin-specific MR contrast agent was proposed to assess the atherosclerotic plaque burden (Makowksi et al. 2011). Elastin is a key extracellular matrix protein in plaque. The authors showed the new agent can provide strong signal for accurate quantification of the plaque burden in a mouse model of atherosclerosis. This kind of contrast agent may be useful in the VWI of certain small but important arteries, which are difficult to image using traditional agents and MR imaging techniques, such as the coronary artery.

16.5 Imaging-Based Biomechanical Analysis of Atherosclerotic Plaques

The arterial wall must regenerate and remodel continuously to maintain its integrity and function while withstanding the hemodynamic stresses imposed by the pulsatile blood flow upon it. In fact, this remodeling process is the result of the response of the endothelial cells lining the luminal wall to those stresses. These biomechanical stimuli include blood flow-induced frictional stress or shear stress, pressure-induced cyclic stress or tensile stress, and a normal stress due to hydrostatic pressure differential across the wall. Unfortunately, the complex interrelationship between the endothelial response and the biomechanical stimuli might be altered, inducing endothelial dysfunction that will trigger pathophysiological processes leading to cardiovascular disease (Ku 1997, Taber 2001).

In particular, it is well accepted that the reaction of endothelial cells to the low and oscillatory shear stress resulting from the distinct complex patterns of blood flow in arterial bifurcations and bends (Figure 16.25) is responsible for the local susceptibility to atherosclerosis initiation in vessels such as the carotid or coronary arteries (Taber 2001, Ku 1997, Slager et al. 2005, Lee et al. 2008). Hypertension has also been identified as a risk factor in atherosclerosis. Increased pressure induces endothelial dysfunction increasing the mass transport from the lumen to the vessel wall, as well as endothelial cell proliferation and apoptosis (VanEpps and Vorp 2007). Several studies have indicated that the biomechanical stimuli also contribute to the lipid accumulation and inflammatory cell recruitment and adhesion occurring in atherogenesis (VanEpps and Vorp 2007).

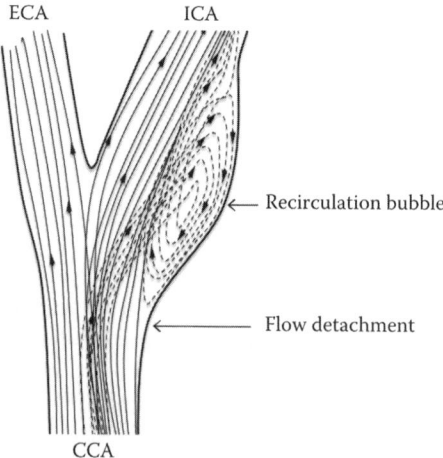

FIGURE 16.25 Depiction of some of the flow features developing with pulsatile flow through the common carotid artery (CCA) bifurcation into the external and internal carotid arteries (ECA and ICA, respectively). (Modified from Dong L et al. 2010a. *AJNR Am J Neuroradiol.* 31:311–316.)

Even though the hemodynamic stresses involved in the initiation of the disease and the pathological processes that they trigger have been extensively described in the literature, their role in plaque growth and rupture has not yet been established. Endothelial cells react to shear stress modifying the balance between fibrous cap-reinforcing extracellular matrix synthesis by smooth muscle cells and extracellular matrix degradation by metalloproteinases secreted by infiltrating macrophages (Cheng et al. 2006, Clowes and Berceli 2000). This imbalance seems to be a major contributor to plaque rupture. Focal regions of high strain in the fibrous cap are linked to the location of plaque rupture (Li et al. 2006) indicating that the failure of the wall biological tissues to compensate the effect of the increased tensile (pressure-induced) stress (Arroyo and Lee 1999) could also be a major factor in plaque rupture.

As mentioned in previous sections, current criteria to identify plaques at risk of rupture mainly rely on morphological and compositional factors, and do not take into consideration the biomechanical factors. Thus, plaque vulnerability assessment could be considerably improved by incorporating hemodynamic stress information.

MRI has successfully been used to characterize the atherosclerotic plaques in terms of their morphological and compositional features. This unique quality of MRI is currently used to determine the patient-specific hemodynamic stress distributions that could be responsible for, or the result of patient-specific, atherosclerotic plaque features. This section will examine the combined use of MRI and mechanical engineering tools to obtain a comprehensive characterization of the atherosclerotic lesion in terms of both its morphological and compositional features, as well as of its hemodynamic factors. This comprehensive evaluation of the atherosclerotic vessels would allow advancing the knowledge of the role of biomechanics in plaque progression and rupture and would lead, in turn, to a more precise assessment of plaque vulnerability.

16.5.1 Image-Based Numerical Models to Characterize Hemodynamic Stresses in Atherosclerosis

The ability of MRI to define the vessel lumen has allowed reconstructing the geometry of atherosclerotic plaques to analyze the flow features present in the diseased vessel with the aid of computational fluid dynamics (CFD) models.

16.5.1.1 Computational Fluid Dynamics Models

The luminal boundary obtained from the segmentation of MR images is used to render a 3D surface that is discretized into a finite-element mesh constituting the fluid domain as shown in Figure 16.26. The size and distribution of the mesh elements is set by the compromise between the accuracy of the computed velocity field and the computational expense. Unstructured meshes with varying mesh density are most commonly used when dealing with atherosclerotic vessels for adequately resolving the complex velocity field that develops in those bent and/or bifurcating vessels.

16.5.1.1.1 Boundary Conditions and Assumptions Needed to Solve for Flow

Once the fluid domain is defined, special attention should be paid to specifying the physical properties and boundary conditions needed to solve the equations that govern blood flow. Due to the complexity of the problem, image-based CFD models have traditionally made simplifying assumptions regarding both blood properties and flow boundary conditions.

Blood is known to be non-Newtonian, that is, it exhibits a nonlinear relationship between shear stress and shear strain rate. However, the behavior of blood can be described as Newtonian (constant viscosity at all rates of shear) at the high shear strain rates present in large arteries, such as the ones where atherosclerosis is most often found (Ku 1997). Thus, in image-based CFD modeling of flow in atherosclerosis, blood is commonly assumed to be Newtonian. This assumption is even more reasonable after considering that the uncertainty of geometry reconstruction has a greater effect on the distribution of wall shear stresses (Lee and Steinman 2007).

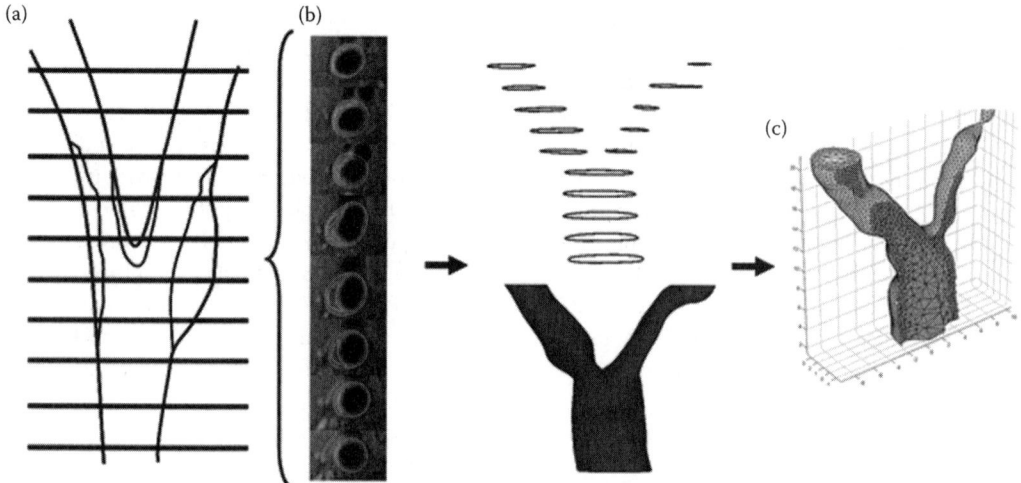

FIGURE 16.26 Summary of typical steps required for the reconstruction of a finite-element mesh from serial MR images. (a) Segmentation of the stack of cross-sectional MR images along the bifurcation; (b) three-dimensional reconstruction of the luminal volume from the extracted lumen contours; (c) three-dimensional computational mesh of the luminal volume or fluid domain.

The equations governing the flow of a Newtonian viscous fluid are known as the Navier–Stokes equations, which are the result of applying Newton's second law to fluid motion. Assuming that blood is an incompressible fluid, these equations are simplified to

$$\rho \frac{Du}{Dt} = \rho X - \frac{\partial p}{\partial x} + \mu \nabla^2 u$$

$$\rho \frac{Dv}{Dt} = \rho Y - \frac{\partial p}{\partial y} + \mu \nabla^2 v$$

$$\rho \frac{Dw}{Dt} = \rho Z - \frac{\partial p}{\partial z} + \mu \nabla^2 w$$

where ρ is the density of blood, normally set at 1045 kg/cm³; u, v, and w are the velocity components along the x-, y-, and z-axis directions, respectively; X, Y, and Z are the body force per unit mass components along the x-, y-, and z-axis directions, respectively; p denotes pressure; and μ is the dynamic viscosity of blood, a typically chosen value is 0.0035 Pa · s.

Blood flow must also satisfy the continuity equation, derived from the conservation of mass. For an incompressible fluid, the equation of continuity becomes

$$\frac{\partial u}{\partial x} + \frac{\partial v}{\partial y} + \frac{\partial w}{\partial z} = 0$$

These equations are solved using finite-element methods to obtain the velocity profile. However, in order to solve these equations, boundary conditions must be specified. Blood flow is not constant, but varies with the cardiac cycle. The importance of the unsteady forces resulting from the flow pulsatility is characterized by the dimensionless Womersley number (α), which accounts for the relationship between unsteady inertial forces and viscous forces (Womersley 1955):

$$\alpha = R\sqrt{\frac{w}{v}}$$

where R is the arterial radius, ω is the angular frequency, and v is the kinematic viscosity (μ/ρ). In the case of a healthy carotid bifurcation, α is approximately 4, indicating that the viscous forces dominate the flow (Ku 1997). Womersley analytical solution for fully developed flow is usually imposed as inlet boundary condition to account for the pulsatile nature of blood flow (Womersley 1955). This analytical solution for pulsatile flow in a straight or tapered tube expands the physiologic pressure or flow waveform as a Fourier series, and the harmonic components of the velocity are summed to yield the unsteady velocity profiles. The flow waveform used to obtain the Fourier coefficients is often determined from cine phase-contrast images or ultrasound centerline velocity measurements. However, this inflow velocity assumption should be accompanied by a sufficient entrance length to allow the flow to adapt to the specific vessel geometry, which might not always be straight, so that the results are not that dependent on the inlet condition, guarantying nonnegligible errors in the prediction of the distribution of hemodynamic stresses. At least three diameters of common carotid artery length prior to the bifurcation have been proposed when considering carotid atherosclerosis (Hoi et al. 2010). Again, a compromise is needed since the additional entrance length would require more 2D axial slices for the geometry reconstruction, and thus more scanning time. An alternate solution is to measure the time-varying axial velocity using cine phase-contrast MRI (PC-MRI) at the slice corresponding to the inlet surface of the computational mesh and interpolate the image grid onto the inlet CFD nodes (Figure 16.27). This solution is still not fully adopted since it requires high-quality cine PC-MR images at the expense of scan time. Approaches similar to the inlet boundary condition definition have been used for the outlet conditions. In the case of the carotid bifurcation, where there are two outlets, a combination of velocity profile and zero normal traction is normally prescribed as outlet boundary conditions.

Flow in a normal healthy carotid is considered to be laminar. In fact, the mean Reynolds number (dimensionless number that measures the ratio between inertia and viscous forces) in this artery is

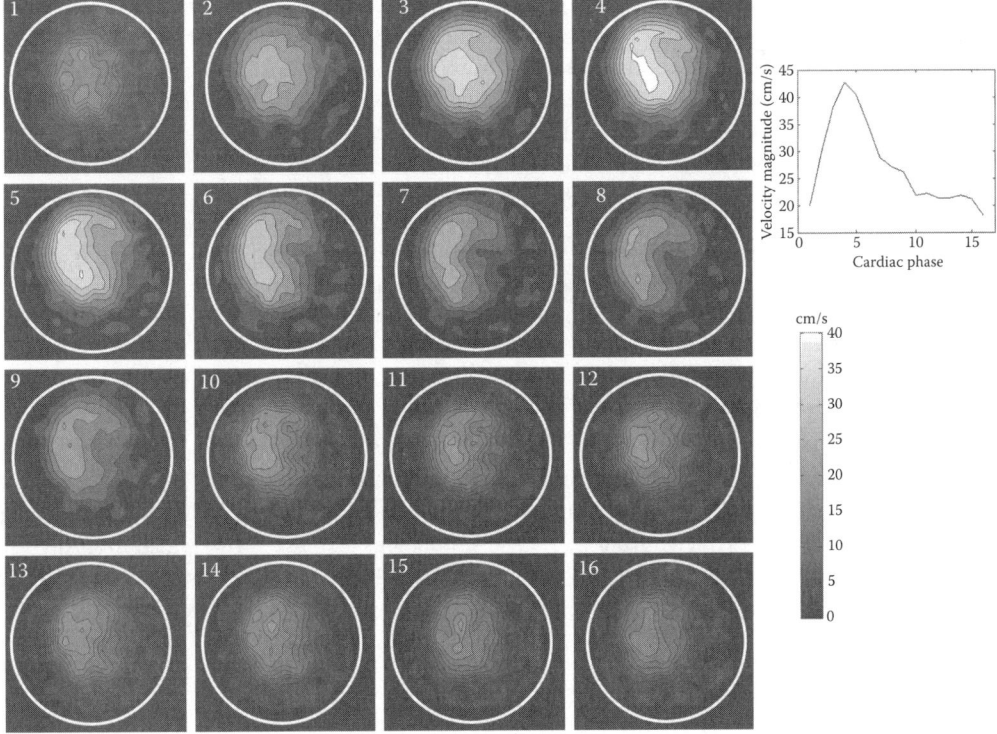

FIGURE 16.27 Flow field calculated from three-directional encoding cine PC-MR images of a cross-sectional plane of a human healthy common carotid artery (16 cardiac phases).

approximately 300, a value too low to be considered as turbulent. However, the stenosis can lead to an altered chaotic flow that could be described as in transition to turbulence or even as turbulent flow in most severe stenotic cases. Still, there is controversy in the literature on which model best describes the flow downstream of the stenosis (Banks and Bressloff 2007, Tan et al. 2008).

Another typical assumption made in image-based CFD simulations is the use of rigid-walled models; thus, no-slip boundary condition is applied to the rigid walls. Most numerical studies targeted to determine the distribution of wall shear stress make this assumption. Though it results in a modest overestimation of wall shear stress distribution compared to a compliant wall model, it is considered an appropriate approximation when analyzing atherosclerotic vessels due to their small wall motion. However, this approximation can be avoided by performing simulations of the fluid–structure interaction (FSI) between the flowing blood and vessel wall.

16.5.1.2 Fluid–Structure Interaction Models: Flow and Solid Mechanics Involved in Atherosclerosis

FSI models require solving the equations of motion for the flow and the wall simultaneously. The solution of these equations provides both the velocity profile as well as the distribution of tensional stresses, achieving a more comprehensive evaluation of the hemodynamic stresses present at the diseased vessel. The computational mesh includes both the fluid and solid domains; thus, it is built from segmenting the lumen, outer-wall, and wall components.

The 3D geometry reconstructed from MRI needs to be shrunk axially and circumferentially *a priori* to obtain the no-load starting geometry for the computational simulation that accounts for the fact that, under *in vivo* conditions, arteries are axially stretched and pressurized. This shrinkage is determined guarantying conservation of the mass of the vessel and that the loaded vessel geometry after the stretch underwent with pressurization matches the MRI-reconstructed geometry.

Although the arterial wall exhibits a viscoelastic behavior, FSI models usually assume the artery wall to be hyperelastic. Other assumptions commonly made are considering the wall to be isotropic, incompressible, and homogeneous. The effects of these assumptions on the resulting hemodynamic stresses have not been analyzed in the same detail as in the case of the approximations made in CFD modeling.

The nonlinear stress/strain dependency of the wall tissue is accounted for by describing the material properties of the vessel wall with a Mooney–Rivlin hyperelastic model using material parameters estimated from *in vitro* models of the wall and plaque tissues to define the strain-energy function. Several strain-energy functions have been proposed for the vessel wall (Fung 1994) and used in various FSI models of carotid atherosclerosis (Kock et al. 2008, Tang et al. 2009, Gao et al. 2009, Leach et al. 2010).

The arbitrary Lagrangian–Eulerian formulation is often used for modeling the fluid–solid coupling. Inlet and outlet are often fixed in the axial direction, but allowed to expand/contract in response to the pulsatile flow.

16.5.1.3 Hemodynamic Stresses: Wall Shear Stress and Tensile Stress

The hemodynamic stresses are extracted from the solution of the numerical model. In the case of only solving for the blood flow, the focus is on the distribution of wall shear stress (WSS). WSS is a vector ($\vec{\tau}_w$) proportional to the gradient of the velocity at the wall and blood viscosity. However, the challenge in analyzing the WSS data extracted from numerical simulations is to determine which WSS-derived parameters are most closely linked to the underlying pathology. The parameters most often reported are the peak systole and cycle-averaged WSS magnitude, and the oscillatory shear index (OSI):

$$\text{OSI} = \frac{1}{2}\left(1 - \frac{\left\|\int_0^T \vec{\tau}_w dt\right\|}{\int_0^T |\vec{\tau}_w| dt}\right)$$

where *T* is the period of the cardiac cycle (inverse of hear rate); this index describes the temporal change in direction of the shear stress vector with respect to its mean direction.

Tensile stress results can be extracted together with WSS when using an FSI technique. The first principal stress, representing the circumferential component of the stress tensor, is chosen to represent the wall tensile stress. As in the case of WSS, different quantities can be derived from the distribution of wall tensile stress. The relevance of each one with respect to the response of the endothelium and other wall cellular components is still to be determined. The tensile stress distribution and its temporal gradients resulting from the pulsatile nature of blood flow (normally defined in FSI models as the fibrous tissue covering the lipid region) are commonly considered to be closely related to plaque rupture, not only for the cellular response but also for the fatigue damage that could cause on the fibrous cap.

The challenge of image-based modeling is to assess how restricting assumptions on blood rheology, boundary conditions, vessel wall material properties, or blood–vessel interactions (among others) may affect the accuracy of the results. Recent advances in MRI technology are allowing MRI to be used as a tool to overcome the limitations of the numerical models by either improving the boundary conditions and assumptions on material properties by *in vivo* measurements, or estimating the hemodynamic stresses acquiring *in vivo* blood flow and vessel wall deformation measurements. The use of MRI in this direction is discussed in the following section.

16.5.2 *In Vivo* MR Quantification of Blood Flow (4D Flow MRI) and Wall Properties of Atherosclerotic Vessels

Cine phase contrast MRI (PC-MRI) provides flow rate wave forms measured at the inlet and outlet sections as boundary conditions for image-based CFD models. However, there is an increasing interest in advancing this and other MR sequences to provide *in vivo* information of blood flow and flow-derived parameters, as well as material properties and deformation data of the arterial wall.

16.5.2.1 WSS Estimation from 4D Flow MRI

Time-resolved gated cine PC-MRI with three-directional encoding, known as 4D flow MRI, is emerging as a tool to provide full hemodynamic information on 3D blood flow in large arteries.

The accuracy of the estimations of WSS is constrained by the limitations in time and spatial resolutions, partial volume artifacts and the numerical derivation of WSS from discrete velocity data. Indeed, the major challenge of 4D flow MRI is to obtain detailed measurement of the time-varying velocity near the wall in the branching and curved arteries where atherosclerosis develops, where the flow can be highly skewed; or in stenotic regions where the lumen is not circular. However, current advances in cine PCMRI indicate that the results can be sufficient to characterize pathological spatiotemporal distributions of WSS and OSI in atherosclerotic prone arteries, or at regions of atherosclerotic arteries other than the highly stenotic, where WSS estimations will suffer from large numerical errors due to the above-mentioned technical limitations.

Deriving WSS from the velocity data measured in atherosclerotic arteries needs to take into consideration the complexity of the flow through those arteries were atherosclerosis occurred. The secondary flow developing in branching and curved arteries, such as helical flow, can lead to shear stresses along the lumen circumference in addition to stresses along the main flow. Therefore, the 3D paraboloid model initially proposed to estimate WSS from cine PC-MRI velocity data (Oyre et al. 1998) does not seem accurate enough when studying the hemodynamics in atherosclerotic vessels. Markl and collaborators proposed to obtain an analytical expression for the velocity derivatives using a cubic B-spline interpolation that compensates for the limited spatial resolution of the PCMR data (Stalder et al. 2008, Markl et al. 2010).

16.5.2.2 Evaluation of Biomechanical Properties of Tissue Components in Atherosclerotic Plaques

The arterial wall is composed of three layers: the intima, composed of a monolayer of endothelial cells covering a layer of connective tissue, elastic fibril, and collagenous fibers; the media, consisting of a number of elastic sheets and fibrils and collagenous fibers and accounting for the elasticity of the wall; and the adventitia, formed mainly by ground substances, collagen fibers, nerves, and small blood vessels (vasa vasorum). The thickness, structure, and composition of these layers change with age and also with disease.

Release of nitric oxide due to endothelial dysfunction produces vasoconstriction that, in turn, increases stiffness. The arterial elasticity is further decreased as the media layer thickens with atherosclerosis progression. Risk factors associated to atherosclerosis such as hypertension and diabetes also accelerate arterial stiffness. This increase of stiffness in atherosclerotic arteries leads to a reduction of the pressure-driven cyclic stretching or strain.

Current imaging techniques are not able to monitor the changes in cellular function and structure that occur with aging and lead to alterations in the biomechanical properties of the wall (i.e., increase in stiffness). However, they can detect and characterize the strain (deformation resulting from the hemodynamic forces) and measure the biomechanical properties.

Displacement encoding with stimulated echoes (DENSE) pulse sequence can measure the 2D displacement vectors of the arterial wall and surrounding tissue. The circumferential strain distribution is computed from the tissue deformation matrix derived from linear regression of the displacement vectors (Lin et al. 2008).

Gated cine imaging MRI is used to measure the arterial wall distensibility by assessing the maximal change in luminal diameter during systole and diastole and calculating the distensibility coefficient, DC:

$$DC = \frac{2 \times \Delta d / d_D}{\Delta P}$$

where Δd is the change in luminal diameter, d_D is the end diastolic diameter, and ΔP is the pulse pressure, calculated as the difference between maximal systolic and diastolic blood pressures.

Although the higher field strength of 3 T scanners have been shown to be a promising tool to measure strain and distensibility due to its substantially increase of the signal-to-noise, further increase of spatial and temporal resolution is needed to provide reliable measurements of distensibility in diseased carotid arteries (Harloff et al. 2009).

16.5.2.3 Concluding Remarks

MRI has shown its potential as a tool able to provide a comprehensive characterization of hemodynamic stresses and plaque features. In particular, MRI techniques are currently used in the evaluation of atherosclerotic plaque vulnerability by noninvasively characterizing the plaque in terms of its morphology and composition. Recently, hemodynamic stress information provided mainly by image-based computational models is being investigated to advance the knowledge of the hemodynamic stress role in plaque progression and rupture. Cine PC-MRI has emerged as a promising tool in the estimation of the hemodynamic stresses by either providing improved boundary conditions to numerical models, or on its own evaluation of WSS, wall strain, and vessel wall material properties. However, much research is still needed to improve current spatiotemporal resolution to reliably calculate WSS and wall strain and in highly stenotic or slow recirculation flow regions where few pixels are available for WSS estimation.

Furthermore, prospective studies are still warranted to investigate in depth the complex interplay of hemodynamic stresses and pathological processes underlying the morphological and compositional changes that occur as the disease progresses. Still, it is undoubtful that plaque assessment would

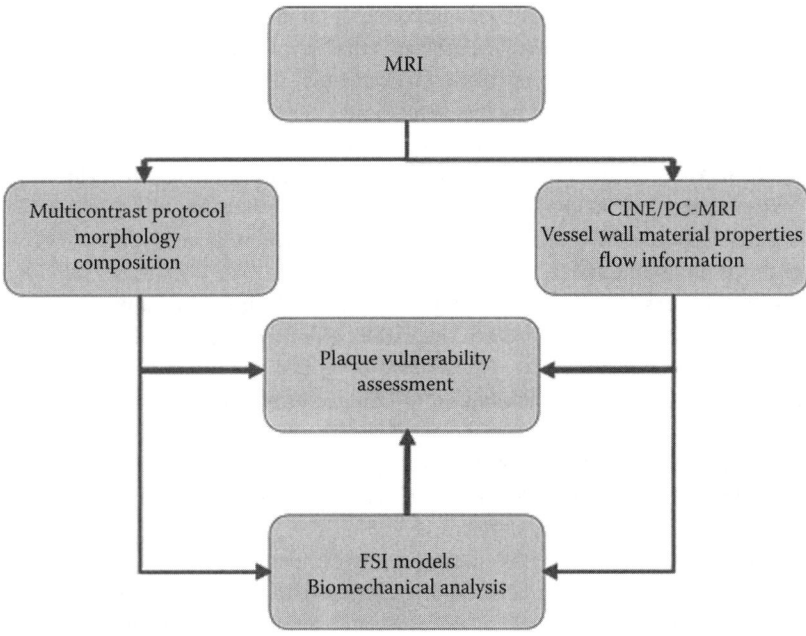

FIGURE 16.28 Integration of hemodynamic stress and morphological and compositional features in the assessment of atherosclerotic plaque vulnerability.

extremely benefit by considering the multifactorial nature of the disease integrating morphological and compositional features and hemodynamic factors (Figure 16.28).

16.6 Summary of the Chapter

VWI and VWI have gone through rapid technical development and validation in recent years. These technologies are used in many ways: for atherosclerotic disease risk assessment, in understanding the vascular pathophysiology, in monitoring the effects of atherosclerotic lesions under medical treatment, and in assessing the hemodynamical effects of plaque progression. These techniques are likely to be applied in clinical applications to present comprehensive evaluations of all aspects of atherosclerosis and improve cardiovascular risk assessment and guide treatment options. As discussed in this chapter, VWI also provides a unique opportunity in technological advancement in imaging hardware software, especially for the ultimate goal of coronary imaging.

Defining Terms

AIF: Abbreviation of arterial input function. In DCE-MRI, it refers to the contrast agent concentration curve over time inside plasma and is essential input function for kinetic modeling.

Angiogenesis: A physiological process involving the growth of new blood vessels from preexisting vessels. In atherosclerosis, it usually refers to the growth of new microvessel inside the vessel wall. It is also considered to accompany with plaque inflammation process.

AUC: Area under enhancement curve, a nonmodel-based parameter used in quantification of DCE-MRI.

Black-blood (BB) imaging: An image acquisition technique that suppresses the usually bright-blood signal for improved vessel wall visualization. It is frequently used in vessel wall imaging applications.

CE-MRI: Abbreviation of contrast-enhanced MRI, refers to an MR technique to acquire image after contrast agent injection, characterizing the agent diffused into the tissue.

CFD: Computational fluid dynamics (CFD) is a branch of fluid mechanics that uses numerical methods and algorithms to solve and analyze problems that involve fluid flows.

DCE-MRI: Abbreviation of dynamic contrast-enhanced MRI, refers to the MR imaging technique to consequently acquire series of images before and after the contrast agent injection, observing the contrast agent transfer process into the tissue over time.

Diamagnetic effect: An effect used to describe an object that causes a magnetic field in opposition to the external magnetic field.

Diffusion-weighted imaging: MRI technique to detect incoherent motion of water molecules by use of large diffusion gradients.

Double inversion recovery (DIR): A black-blood imaging technique that suppresses the blood signal by taking the advantage of both the inflow effect and the blood's unique T_1 relaxation time.

Finite-element method: A numerical technique for finding approximate solutions of partial differential equations.

FSI: Fluid–structure interactions (FSI) refer to the coupling of fluid and solid.

Image registration: A process of transforming different set of image into one coordinate system. In DCE-MRI of atherosclerosis, it refers to the process of correcting the relative movement between images obtained at different time due to patient motion.

Inflow effect: An effect that describes the blood flowing nature in vascular imaging: the blood segment at the start of an MR sequence is usually different from the blood segment at the time of image acquisition. Inflow effect a major cause of flow artifact in vessel wall imaging but it has also been used to achieve black-blood contrast.

Inflow suppression: A black-blood imaging technique that suppresses the blood signal by taking the advantage of the inflow effect.

Juxtaluminal: Close to the lumen of the vessel. IPH and calcification may both be found in juxtaluminal locations.

Kinetic modeling: A mathematical modeling technique for predicting the absorption, distribution, metabolism, and excretion of synthetic or natural chemical substances in humans and other animal species. In atherosclerotic plaque imaging, it is used to characterize the blood supply and permeability of the targeted tissue from DCE-MRI images.

K^{trans}: Transfer constant, a parameter in two-compartment model. In atherosclerotic plaque imaging, it is considered to characterize the blood supply and permeability.

Motion-sensitized-driven equilibrium (MSDE): A black-blood imaging technique that suppresses the blood signal by using the flow-dephasing effect in flowing blood.

Navier–Stokes equations: Named after Claude-Louis Navier and George Gabriel Stokes, describes the motion of fluid substances. These equations arise from applying Newton's second law to fluid motion of a Newtonian viscous fluid.

Neovasculature or microvessel: In atherosclerosis, it refers to the small vessels grown from vasa vasorum, providing blood supply to the plaque.

Strain: normalized measure of deformation representing the displacement of particle in the body relative to a reference length.

Strain rate: rate of change in strain.

Stress: Force exerted per unit area.

Susceptibility: The degree of magnetization of an object in response to the external magnetic field.

Susceptibility-weighted imaging (SWI): An MR imaging technique that creates unique imaging contrast by using the susceptibility differences between tissues.

Tensile stress: Force per unit area exerted normal to the body and results in compression or expansion.

Vasa vasorum: Blood vessels of small caliber that supply oxygen to the vessel wall. They may arise from surrounding vessels or from the lumen of the same vessel.

v_e: Fractional volumes of extravascular extracellular space (EES).

v_p: Fractional volumes of plasma, a parameter in two-compartment model. In atherosclerotic plaque imaging, it is considered to characterize the blood supply.

Wall shear stress: Force per unit area exerted in the direction tangential to the body. In fluid mechanics, it depends on the fluid viscosity and flow velocity profile.

References

Abd-Elmoniem KZ, Weiss RG, and Stuber M. 2010. Phase-sensitive black-blood coronary vessel wall imaging. *Magn Reson Med*. 4:1021–1030.

ACAS. 1995. Endarterectomy for asymptomatic carotid artery stenosis. Executive Committee for the Asymptomatic Carotid Atherosclerosis Study. *JAMA*. 273(18):1421–1428.

Achenbach S, Kramer CM, Zoghbi WA, and Dilsizian V. 2010. The year in coronary artery disease. *JACC Cardiovasc Imaging*. 10:1065–1077.

Aoki S, Aoki K, Ohsawa S, Nakajima H, Kumagai H, and Araki T. 1999. Dynamic MR imaging of the carotid wall. *J Magn Reson Imaging*. 9:420–427.

Arroyo LH and Lee RT. 1999. Mechanisms of plaque rupture: Mechanical and biologic interactions. *Cardiovasc Res*. 41:369–375.

Balu N, Chu B, Hatsukami TS, Yuan C, and Yarnykh VL. 2008. Comparison between 2D and 3D high-resolution black-blood techniques for carotid artery wall imaging in clinically significant atherosclerosis. *J Magn Reson Imaging*. 4:918–924.

Balu N, Yarnykh V, Chu B, Wang J, and Yuan C. 2009a. Carotid plaque assessment using fast 3D isotropic-resolution black-blood MRI. Poster presentation. *ISMRM*, April, pp. 18–24, Honolulu, Hawaii.

Balu N, Yarnykh VL, Scholnick J, Chu BC, Yuan C, and Hayes CE. 2009b. Improvements in carotid plaque imaging using a new eight-element phased array coil at 3T. *J Magn Reson Imaging*. 30(5):1209–1214.

Balu N, Yarnykh VL, Chu B, Wang J, Hatsukami T, and Yuan C. 2011. Carotid plaque assessment using fast 3D isotropic resolution black-blood MRI. *Magn. Reson. Med*. 65:627–637.

Banks J and Bressloff NW. 2007. Turbulence modeling in three-dimensional stenosed arterial bifurcations. *J Biomech Eng—Trans ASME*. 129:40–50.

Barkhausen J, Ebert W, Heyer C, Debatin Jf, and Weinmann HJ. 2003. Detection of atherosclerotic plaque with gadofluorine-enhanced magnetic resonance imaging. *Circulation*. 108:605–609.

Barnett HJ, Taylor DW, Eliasziw M et al. 1998. Benefit of carotid endarterectomy in patients with symptomatic moderate or severe stenosis. North American Symptomatic Carotid Endarterectomy Trial Collaborators. *N Engl J Med*. 339:1415–1425.

Botnar RM, Buecker A, Wiethoff AJ et al. 2004a. *In vivo* magnetic resonance imaging of coronary thrombosis using a fibrin-binding molecular magnetic resonance contrast agent. *Circulation*. 110:1463–1466.

Botnar RM, Perez AS, Witte S et al. 2004b. *In vivo* molecular imaging of acute and subacute thrombosis using a fibrin-binding magnetic resonance imaging contrast agent. *Circulation*. 109:2023–2029.

Boussel L, Herigault G, De La Vega A, Nonent M, Douek PC, and Serfaty JM. 2006. Swallowing, arterial pulsation, and breathing induce motion artifacts in carotid artery MRI. *J Magn Reson Imaging*. 3:413–415.

Briley-Saebo KC, Mulder WJ, Mani V et al. 2007. Magnetic resonance imaging of vulnerable atherosclerotic plaques: Current imaging strategies and molecular imaging probes. *J Magn Reson Imaging*. 26:460–479.

Briley-Saebo KC, Shaw PX, Mulder WJ et al. 2008. Targeted molecular probes for imaging atherosclerotic lesions with magnetic resonance using antibodies that recognize oxidation-specific epitopes. *Circulation*. 117:3206–3215.

Brown R, Nguyen TD, Spincemaille P et al. 2010. Effect of blood flow on double inversion recovery vessel wall MRI of the peripheral arteries: Quantitation with T_2 mapping and comparison with flow-insensitive T_2-prepared inversion recovery imaging. *Magn Reson Med*. 3:736–744.

Cai J, Hatsukami T, Ferguson M, Small R, Polissar N, and Yuan C. 2002. Classification of human carotid atherosclerotic lesions with *in vivo* multicontrast magnetic resonance imaging. *Circulation*. 106:1368–1373.

Cai J, Hatsukami TS, Ferguson MS et al. 2005. *In vivo* quantitative measurement of intact fibrous cap and lipid-rich necrotic core size in atherosclerotic carotid plaque—Comparison of high-resolution, contrast-enhanced magnetic resonance imaging and histology. *Circulation.* 22:3437–3444.

Calcagno C, Cornily J, Hyafil F et al. 2008. Detection of neovessels in atherosclerotic plaques of rabbits using dynamic contrast enhanced MRI and 18f-fdg pet. *Arterioscler Thromb Vasc Biol.* 28:1311–1317.

Chaabane L, Pellet N, Bourdillon MC et al. 2004. Contrast enhancement in atherosclerosis development in a mouse model: *In vivo* results at 2 tesla. *MAGMA.* 17:188–195.

Chen H, Cai J, Zhao X et al. 2010. Localized measurement of atherosclerotic plaque inflammatory burden with dynamic contrast-enhanced MRI. *Magn Reson Med.* 64:567–573.

Chen H, Li F, Zhao X, Yuan C, Rutt B, and Kerwin WS. 2011. Extended graphical model for analysis of dynamic contrast-enhanced MRI. *Magn Reson Med.* 66:868–878.

Cheng C, Tempel D, Van Haperen R et al. 2006. Atherosclerotic lesion size and vulnerability are determined by patterns of fluid shear stress. *Circulation.* 113:2744–2753.

Chu B, Ferguson MS, Chen H, Hippe DS, Kerwin WS, Canton G, Yuan C, and Hatsukami TS. 2009. Cardiac magnetic resonance features of the disruption-prone and the disrupted carotid plaque. *J Am Coll Cardiol Img.* 2009(2):883–896.

Clowes AW and Berceli SA. 2000. Mechanisms of vascular atrophy and fibrous cap disruption. *Ann. N. Y. Acad. Sci.* 902(1):153–162.

Cron GO, Santyr G, and Kelcz F. 1999. Accurate and rapid quantitative dynamic contrast-enhanced breast MR imaging using spoiled gradient-recalled echoes and bookend t(1) measurements. *Magn Reson Med.* 42:746–753.

Dong L, Underhill HR, Yu W et al. 2010a. Geometric and compositional appearance of atheroma in an angiographically normal carotid artery in patients with atherosclerosis. *AJNR Am J Neuroradiol.* 31:311–316.

Dong L, Wang JN, Yarnykh VL et al. 2010b. Efficient flow suppressed MRI improves interscan reproducibility of carotid atherosclerosis plaque burden measurements. *J Magn Reson Imaging.* 32:452–458.

Edelman RR, Mattle HP, Wallner B et al. 1990. Extracranial carotid arteries: Evaluation with "black blood" MR angiography. *Radiology.* 1:45–50.

Edelman RR, Chien D, and Kim D. 1991. Fast selective black blood MR imaging. *Radiology.* 3:655–660.

Fan Z, Zhang Z, Chung YC et al. 2010. Carotid arterial wall MRI at 3T using 3D variable-flip-angle turbo spin-echo (TSE) with flow-sensitive dephasing (FSD). *J Magn Reson Imaging.* 3:645–654.

Faranesh AZ and Yankeelov TE. 2008. Incorporating a vascular term into a reference region model for the analysis of DCE-MRI data: A simulation study. *Phys Med Biol.* 53:2617–2631.

Fung YC. 1994. *A First Course in Continuum Mechanics.* New Jersey: Prentice Hall.

Gao H, Long Q, Sadat U, Graves M, Gillard JH, and Li ZY. 2009. Stress analysis of carotid atheroma in a transient ischaemic attack patient using the MRI-based fluid-structure interaction method. *Br J Radiol.* 82:S46–S54.

Glagov S, Weisenberg E, Zarins CK, Stankunavicius R, and Kolettis GJ. 1987. Compensatory enlargement of human atherosclerotic coronary arteries. *N Engl J Med.* 22:1371–1375.

Harloff A, Zech T, Frydrychowicz A, Schumacher M, Schollhorn J, Hennig J, Weiller C, and Markl M. 2009. Carotid intima-media thickness and distensibility measured by MRI at 3 T versus high-resolution ultrasound. *Eur Radiol.* 19:1470–1479.

Herzka DA, Nezafat R, Chan R, Liu W, and Boernert P. 2008. high-resolution ultra-short TE imaging of ex vivo human carotid plaques correlates with CT. Proceedings 16th ISMRM Scientific Meeting and Exhibition, Toronto.

Hofmann-Amtenbrink M, Hofmann H, and Montet X. 2010. Superparamagnetic nanoparticles—A tool for early diagnostics. *Swiss Med Wkly.* 140:w13081.

Hoi Y, Wasserman BA, Lakatta EG, and Steinman DA. 2010. Carotid bifurcation hemodynamics in older adults: Effect of measured versus assumed flow waveform. *J Biomech Eng—Trans ASME.* 132 (7):071006.

Howarth S, Tang T, Trivedi R, Weerakkody R, U-King-Im J, Gaunt M, Boyle J, Li Z, Miller S, Graves M, and Gillard J. 2009. Utility of USPIO-enhanced MR imaging to identify inflammation and the fibrous cap: A comparison of symptomatic and asymptomatic individuals. *Eur J Radiol.* 70:555–560.

Hur J, Park J, Kim YJ, Lee HJ, Shim HS, Choe KO, and Choi BW. 2010. Use of contrast enhancement and high-resolution 3D black-blood MRI to identify inflammation in atherosclerosis. *JACC Cardiovasc Imaging.* 3:1127–1135.

Itskovich VV, Mani V, Mizsei G, Aguinaldo JG et al. 2004. Parallel and nonparallel simultaneous multislice black-blood double inversion recovery techniques for vessel wall imaging. *J Magn Reson Imaging.* 4:59–67.

Johansson LO, Bjørnerud A, Ahlström HK, Ladd DL, and Fujii DK. 2001. A targeted contrast agent for magnetic resonance imaging of thrombus: Implications of spatial resolution. *J Magn Reson Imaging.* 13:615–618.

Kelly KA, Allport JR, Tsourkas A, Shinde-Patil VR, Josephson L, and Weissleder R. 2005. Detection of vascular adhesion molecule-1 expression using a novel multimodal nanoparticle. *Circ Res.* 96:327–336.

Kerwin W, Cai J, and Yuan C. 2002. Noise and motion correction in dynamic contrast-enhanced MRI for analysis of atherosclerotic lesions. *Magn Reson Med.* 47:1211–1217.

Kerwin W, Hooker A, Spilker M et al. 2003. Quantitative magnetic resonance imaging analysis of neovasculature volume in carotid atherosclerotic plaque. *Circulation.* 107:851–856.

Kerwin W, O'Brien K, Ferguson M, Polissar N, Hatsukami T, and Yuan C. 2006. Inflammation in carotid atherosclerotic plaque: A dynamic contrast-enhanced MR imaging study. *Radiology.* 241:459–468.

Kerwin W, Xu D, Liu F et al. 2007. Magnetic resonance imaging of carotid atherosclerosis: Plaque analysis. *Top Magn Reson Imaging.* 18(5):371–378.

Kerwin W, Oikawa M, Yuan C, Jarvik G, and Hatsukami T. 2008. MR imaging of adventitial vasa vasorum in carotid atherosclerosis. *Magn Reson Med.* 59:507–514.

Kim SE, Jeong EK, Shi XF, Morrell G, Treiman GS, and Parker DL. 2009. Diffusion-weighted imaging of human carotid artery using 2D single-shot interleaved multislice inner volume diffusion-weighted echo planar imaging (2D ss-IMIV-DWEPI) at 3T: Diffusion measurement in atherosclerotic plaque. *J Magn Reson Imaging.* 5:1068–1077.

Kock SA, Nygaard JV, Eldrup N et al. 2008. Mechanical stresses in carotid plaques using MRI-based fluid-structure interaction models. *J Biomech.* 41:1651–1658.

Koktzoglou I and Li D. 2007. Diffusion-prepared segmented steady-state free precession: Application to 3D black-blood cardiovascular magnetic resonance of the thoracic aorta and carotid artery walls. *J Cardiovasc Magn Reson.* 1:33–42.

Kooi M, Cappendijk V, Cleutjens K et al. 2003. Accumulation of ultrasmall superparamagnetic particles of iron oxide in human atherosclerotic plaques can be detected by *in vivo* magnetic resonance imaging. *Circulation.* 107:2453–2458.

Ku DN. 1997. Blood flow in arteries. *Annu Rev Fluid Mech.* 29:399–434.

Lancelot E, Amirbekian V, Brigger I et al. 2008. Evaluation of matrix metalloproteinases in atherosclerosis using a novel noninvasive imaging approach. *Arterioscler Thromb Vasc Biol.* 28:425–432.

Lauffer RB, Parmelee DJ, Dunham SU et al. 1998. Ms-325: Albumin-targeted contrast agent for MR angiography. *Radiology.* 207:529–538.

Leach JR, Rayz VL, Soares B et al. 2010. Carotid atheroma rupture observed *in vivo* and FSI-predicted stress distribution based on pre-rupture imaging. *Ann Biomed Eng.* 38:2748–2765.

Lee SW, Antiga L, Spence JD, and Steinman DA. 2008. Geometry of the carotid bifurcation predicts its exposure to disturbed flow. *Stroke.* 39:2341–2347.

Lee SW and Steinman DA. 2007. On the relative importance of rheology for image-based CFD models of the carotid bifurcation. *J Biomech Eng—Trans ASME.* 129:273–278.

Li ZY, Howarth S, Trivedi RA et al. 2006. Stress analysis of carotid plaque rupture based on *in vivo* high resolution MRI. *J Biomech.* 39:2611–2622.

Libby P. 2002. Inflammation in atherosclerosis. *Nature.* 420:868–874.

Lin AP, Bennett E, Wisk LE, Gharib M, Fraser SE, and Wen H. 2008. Circumferential strain in the wall of the common carotid artery: Comparing displacement-encoded and cine MRI in volunteers. *Magn Reson Med.* 60:8–13.

Lin W, Abendschein DR, and Haacke EM. 1997. Contrast-enhanced magnetic resonance angiography of carotid arterial wall in pigs. *J Magn Reson Imaging.* 7:183–190.

Lipinski MJ, Amirbekian V, Frias JC et al. 2006. MRI to detect atherosclerosis with gadolinium-containing immunomicelles targeting the macrophage scavenger receptor. *Magn Reson Med.* 56:601–610.

Liu F, Xu D, Ferguson MS, Chu B et al. 2006. Automated *in vivo* segmentation of carotid plaque MRI with morphology-enhanced probability maps. *Magn Reson Med.* 55:659–668.

Lobatto ME, Fayad ZA, Silvera S et al. 2010. Multimodal clinical imaging to longitudinally assess a nanomedical anti-inflammatory treatment in experimental atherosclerosis. *Mol Pharm.* 7:2020–2029.

Lobbes MB, Miserus RJ, Heeneman S et al. 2009. Atherosclerosis: Contrast-enhanced mr imaging of vessel wall in rabbit model—Comparison of gadofosveset and gadopentetate dimeglumine. *Radiology.* 250:682–691.

Lorenz MW, Markus HS, Bots ML, Rosvall M, and Sitzer M. 2007. Prediction of clinical cardiovascular events with carotid intima-media thickness: A systematic review and meta-analysis. *Circulation.* 115(4):459–467.

Makowski MR, Wiethoff AJ, Blume U et al. 2011. Assessment of atherosclerotic plaque burden with an elastin-specific magnetic resonance contrast agent. *Nat Med.* 17:383–388.

Mani V, Itskovich VV, Aguiar SH et al. 2005. Comparison of gated and nongated fast multislice black-blood carotid imaging using rapid extended coverage and inflow/outflow saturation techniques. *J Magn Reson Imaging.* 5:628–633.

Markl M, Wegent F, Zech T et al. 2010. *In vivo* wall shear stress distribution in the carotid artery effect of bifurcation geometry, Internal carotid artery stenosis, and recanalization therapy. *Circulation—Cardiovasc Imaging.* 3:647–655.

Meding J, Urich M, Licha K et al. 2007. Magnetic resonance imaging of atherosclerosis by targeting extracellular matrix deposition with gadofluorine m. *Contrast Media Mol Imaging.* 2:120–129.

Moody AR, Murphy RE, Morgan PS et al. 2003. Characterization of complicated carotid plaque with magnetic resonance direct thrombus imaging in patients with cerebral ischemia. *Circulation.* 24:3047–3052.

Naghavi M, Libby P, Falk E et al. 2003. From vulnerable plaque to vulnerable patient: A call for new definitions and risk assessment strategies: Part I. *Circulation.* 14:1664–1672.

Ota H, Yarnykh VL, Ferguson MS et al. 2010. Carotid intraplaque hemorrhage imaging at 3.0-T MR imaging: Comparison of the diagnostic performance of three T_1-weighted sequences. *Radiology.* 2:551–563.

Oyre S, Ringgaard S, Kozerke S et al. 1998. Accurate noninvasive quantitation of blood flow, cross-sectional lumen vessel area and wall shear stress by three-dimensional paraboloid modeling of magnetic resonance imaging velocity data. *J Am College Cardiol.* 32:128–134.

Parker DL, Goodrich KC, Masiker M, Tsuruda JS, and Katzman GL. 2002. Improved efficiency in double-inversion fast spin-echo imaging. *Magn Reson Med.* 5:1017–1021.

Patlak C, Blasberg R, and Fenstermacher J. 1983. Graphical evaluation of blood-to-brain transfer constants from multiple-time uptake data. *J Cereb Blood Flow Metab.* 3:1–7.

Pradel C, Siauve N, Bruneteau G et al. 2003. Reduced capillary perfusion and permeability in human tumour xenografts treated with the vegf signalling inhibitor zd4190: An *in vivo* assessment using dynamic MR imaging and macromolecular contrast media. *Magn Reson Imaging.* 21:845–851.

Ross R. 1999. Atherosclerosis—An inflammatory disease. *N Engl J Med.* 2:115–126.

Shen Jf and Saunders JK. 1993. Double inversion recovery improves water suppression *in vivo*. *Magn Reson Med.* 29:540–542.

Sirol M, Moreno PR, Purushothaman KR et al. 2009. Increased neovascularization in advanced lipid-rich atherosclerotic lesions detected by gadofluorine-m-enhanced MRI: Implications for plaque vulnerability. *Circ Cardiovasc Imaging.* 2:391–396.

Slager CJ, Wentzel JK, Gijsen FJH et al. 2005. The role of shear stress in the generation of rupture-prone vulnerable plaques. *Nat Clin Pract Cardiovasc Med.* 2:401–407.

Stalder AF, Russe MF, Frydrychowicz A, Bock J, Hennig J, and Markl M. 2008. Quantitative 2D and 3D phase contrast MRI: Optimized analysis of blood flow and vessel wall parameters. *Magn Reson Med.* 60:1218–1231.

Strijkers GJ, Van Tilborg GA, Geelen T, Reutelingsperger CP, and Nicolay K. 2010. Current applications of nanotechnology for magnetic resonance imaging of apoptosis. *Methods Mol Biol.* 624:325–342.

Taber LA. 2001. Biomechanics of cardiovascular development. *Annu Rev Biomed Eng.* 3:1–25.

Takaya N, Cai J, and Ferguson MS. 2006. Intra- and interreader reproducibility of magnetic resonance imaging for quantifying the lipid-rich necrotic core is improved with gadolinium contrast enhancement. *J Magn Reson Imaging.* 1:203–210.

Tan FPP, Soloperto G, Bashford S et al. 2008. Analysis of flow disturbance in a stenosed carotid artery bifurcation using two-equation transitional and turbulence models. *J Biomech Eng—Trans ASME.* 130(6):061008-1-12.

Tang DL, Teng ZZ, Canton G et al. 2009. Sites of rupture in human atherosclerotic carotid plaques are associated with high structural stresses an *in vivo* MRI-based 3D fluid-structure interaction study. *Stroke.* 40:3258–3263.

Thomas JB, Antiga L, Che SL et al. 2005. Variation in the carotid bifurcation geometry of young versus older adults: Implications for geometric risk of atherosclerosis. *Stroke.* 36:2450–2456.

Tofts P. 1997. Modeling tracer kinetics in dynamic gd-dtpa MR imaging. *J Magn Reson Imaging.* 7:91–101.

Tofts P, Brix G, Buckley D et al. 1999. Estimating kinetic parameters from dynamic contrast-enhanced t(1)-weighted MRI of a diffusable tracer: Standardized quantities and symbols. *J Magn Reson Imaging.* 10:223–232.

Trivedi R, Mallawarachi C, U-King-Im J et al. 2006. Identifying inflamed carotid plaques using *in vivo* USPIO-enhanced MR Imaging to label plaque macrophages. *Arterioscler Thromb Vasc Biol.* 26:1601–1606.

Underhill HR, Hatsukami TS, Cai J et al. 2010. A noninvasive imaging approach to assess plaque severity: The carotid atherosclerosis score. *AJNR Am J Neuroradiol.* 31:1068–1075.

Underhill HR, Kerwin WS, Hatsukami TS, and Yuan C. 2006. Automated measurement of mean wall thickness in the common carotid artery by MRI: A comparison to intima-media thickness by B-mode ultrasound. *J Magn Reson Imaging.* 24:379–387.

Vanepps JS and Vorp DA. 2007. Mechanopathobiology of atherogenesis: A review. *J Surgical Res.* 142:202–217.

Wang J, Ferguson MS, Balu N, Yuan C, Hatsukami TS, and Börnert P. 2010a. Improved carotid intraplaque hemorrhage imaging using a slab-selective phase-sensitive inversion-recovery (SPI) sequence. *Magn Reson Med.* 64(5):1332–1340.

Wang J, Yarnykh VL, Hatsukami T, Chu B, Balu N, and Yuan C. 2007. Improved suppression of plaque-mimicking artifacts in black-blood carotid atherosclerosis imaging using a multislice motion-sensitized driven-equilibrium (MSDE) turbo spin-echo (TSE) sequence. *Magn Reson Med.* 58(5):973–981.

Wang J, Yarnykh VL, and Yuan C. 2010b. Enhanced image quality in black-blood MRI using the improved motion-sensitized driven-equilibrium (iMSDE) sequence. *J Magn Reson Imaging.* 31:1256–1263.

Wasserman BA, Smith WI, Trout HH, Cannon RO, Balaban RS, and Arai AE. 2002. Carotid artery atherosclerosis: *In vivo* morphologic characterization with gadolinium-enhanced double-oblique MR imaging initial results. *Radiology.* 223:566–573.

Weiss CR, Arai AE, Bui MN et al. 2001. Arterial wall MRI characteristics are associated with elevated serum markers of inflammation in humans. *J Magn Reson Imaging.* 14:698–704.

Wiggins G, Duan Q, Lattanzi R, Biber S, Stoeckel B, Mcgorty K, and Sodickson DK. 2009. 7 Tesla transmit-receive array for carotid imaging: Simulation and experiment. Proceedings of the 17th ISMRM Scientific Meeting and Exhibition, Honolulu.

Winter PM, Caruthers SD, Yu X et al. 2003a. Improved molecular imaging contrast agent for detection of human thrombus. *Magn Reson Med.* 50:411–416.

Winter PM, Morawski AM, Caruthers SD et al. 2003b. Molecular imaging of angiogenesis in early-stage atherosclerosis with alpha(v)beta3-integrin-targeted nanoparticles. *Circulation.* 108:2270–2274.

Womersley JR. 1955. Method for the calculation of velocity, rate of flow and viscous drag in arteries when the pressure gradient is known. *J Physiol—London.* 127:553–563.

Wu YG. 2008. Noninvasive quantification of local cerebral metabolic rate of glucose for clinical application using positron emission tomography and 18f-fluoro-2-deoxy-d-glucose. *J Cereb Blood Flow Metab.* 28:242–250.

Yang Q, Liu J, Barnes SR et al. 2009. Imaging the vessel wall in major peripheral arteries using susceptibility-weighted imaging. *J Magn Reson Imaging.* 2:357–365.

Yankeelov T, Luci J, Lepage M et al. 2005. Quantitative pharmacokinetic analysis of DCE-MRI data without an arterial input function: A reference region model. *Magn Reson Imaging.* 23:519–529.

Yarnykh VL, Terashima M, Hayes CE et al. 2006. Multicontrast black-blood MRI of carotid arteries: Comparison between 1.5 and 3 tesla magnetic field strengths. *J Magn Reson Imaging.* 5:691–698.

Yarnykh VL and Yuan C. 2002. T_1-insensitive flow suppression using quadruple inversion-recovery. *Magn Reson Med.* 5:899–905.

Yarnykh VL and Yuan C. 2003. Multislice double inversion-recovery black-blood imaging with simultaneous slice reinversion. *J Magn Reson Imaging.* 4:478–483.

Yarnykh VL and Yuan C. 2006. Simultaneous outer volume and blood suppression by quadruple inversion-recovery. *Magn Reson Med.* 55:1083–1092.

Yuan C, Kerwin WS, Ferguson MS et al. 2002. Contrast-enhanced high resolution MRI for atherosclerotic carotid artery tissue characterization. *J Magn Reson Imaging.* 15:62–67.

Zhang Z, Fan Z, Carroll TJ et al. 2009. Three-dimensional T_2-weighted MRI of the human femoral arterial vessel wall at 3.0 Tesla. *Invest Radiol.* 9:619–626.

Zhu DC, Ferguson MS, and Demarco JK. 2008. An optimized 3D inversion recovery prepared fast spoiled gradient recalled sequence for carotid plaque hemorrhage imaging at 3.0 T. *Magn Reson Imaging.* 10:1360–1366.

Further Information

The following review papers provide more information about utilizing contrast agents in atherosclerotic plaque imaging:

Calcagno C, Mani V, Ramachandran S, and Fayad ZA. 2010. Dynamic contrast enhanced (DCE) magnetic resonance imaging (MRI) of atherosclerotic plaque angiogenesis. *Angiogenesis.* 13:87–99.

Cormode DP, Skajaa T, Fayad ZA, and Mulder WJ. 2009. Nanotechnology in medical imaging: Probe design and applications. *Arterioscler Thromb Vasc Biol.* 29:992–1000.

Wickline SA, Neubauer AM, Winter PM, Caruthers SD, and Lanza GM. 2007. Molecular imaging and therapy of atherosclerosis with targeted nanoparticles. *J Magn Reson Imaging.* 25:667–680.

Winter PM, Caruthers SD, Lanza GM, and Wickline SA. 2010. Quantitative cardiovascular magnetic resonance for molecular imaging. *J Cardiovasc Magn Reson.* 12:62.

For biomechanical analysis of atherosclerotic plaque, David Steinman and the members of the Biomedical Simulation Laboratory of the University of Toronto (http://www.mie.utoronto.ca/labs/bsl/) have provided over the years a thorough analysis of the effect of the various simplifying assumptions commonly made in image-based CFD simulations of the flow through atherosclerotic vessels. They have also characterized extensively the patterns of WSS and OSI in athero-prone regions of the carotid artery.

Serial MRI has been used to build FSI models to track the changes in the distribution of hemodynamic stresses as atherosclerosis evolves with time. The reader is referred to the work of Dalin Tang from the Department of Mathematical Sciences of Worcester Polytechnic Institute.

Michael Markl from the Department of Radiology, Medical Physics, of the University Hospital Freiburg and his team are one of the leading groups in advancing 4D flow MR technology.

The following review papers provide more information on the role of hemodynamic forces in atherosclerosis:

Makris GC, Nicolaides AN, Xu XY, and Geroulakos G. 2010. Introduction to the biomechanics of carotid plaque pathogenesis and rupture: Review of the clinical evidence. *Br J Radiol.* 83:729–735.

Slager CJ, Wentzel JJ, Gijsen FJH, Thury A, Van der Wal AC, Schaar JA, and Serruys PW. 2005. The role of shear stress in the destabilization of vulnerable plaques and related therapeutic implications. *Nat Clin Pract Cardiovasc Med.* 2:456–464.

Slager CJ, Wentzel JJ, Gijsen FJH, Schuurbiers JCH, Van der Wal AC, Van der Steen AFW, and Serruys PW. 2005. The role of shear stress in the generation of rupture-prone vulnerable plaques. *Nat Clin Pract Cardiovasc Med.* 2: 401–407.

Vanepps JS and Vorp DA. 2007. Mechanopathobiology of atherogenesis: A review. *J Surgical Res.* 142:202–217.

17

Dynamic Contrast-Enhanced Magnetic Resonance Imaging

Edward Ashton
VirtualScopics, Inc.

Vijay Shah
VirtualScopics, Inc.

17.1 Introduction

Dynamic contrast-enhanced magnetic resonance imaging (DCE-MRI) is a specialized technique for both imaging and quantitatively measuring changes in vascular function using standard magnetic resonance imaging systems as described in the previous chapter. DCE-MRI involves the periodic acquisition of T_1-weighted images before, during, and after injection of a gadolinium-labeled contrast agent such as gadopentetate dimeglumine. Contrast agents used in MRI affect the observed image signal by shortening the longitudinal (T_1) and transverse (T_2) relaxation time for protons that are in the vicinity of the contrast agent. The change over time in signal intensity in a voxel or region of interest in this time series can then be related to contrast agent concentration in that tissue. The observed enhancement curves in tissue and plasma can then be used to estimate various physiological parameters [1–4]. Figure 17.1 shows a typical time course for contrast agent uptake in sample tissue and in arterial plasma. Generally, contrast agents used with MRI are classified based on the effects they have on different compartments, including intravascular space (arterial-capillary and venous spaces), extracellular extravascular space (EES), the recticuloendothelial system, and the parenchymal cells of various organs [5]. In this chapter, we restrict our discussion to imaging and analysis techniques used for gadolinium-based contrast agents that distribute within the intravascular space and then rapidly diffuse to the EES of perfused tissues. A representative sampling of FDA-approved contrast agents available for clinical use in the United States is summarized in Table 17.1.

A number of models have been proposed for the derivation of useful parameters from DCE-MRI data. The most commonly used at this time was first proposed by Tofts and Kermonde [6] and is based on the Kety equations [7]. This model, like most others, assumes that the tumor vascular bed can be

(a) (b)

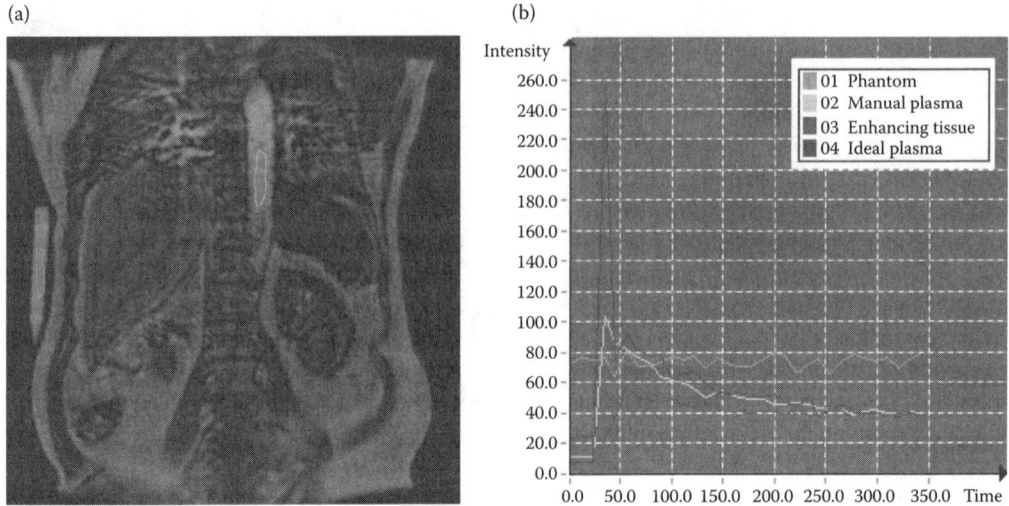

FIGURE 17.1 (a) MR image with contrast agent and (b) typical time course for enhancing tissue and plasma. Note that the y-axis shows signal intensity. This is generally converted to millimolar concentration of gadolinium prior to parameter estimation.

TABLE 17.1 FDA-Approved MRI Contrast Agents

Commercial Name	Active Ingredients	Vendor
Magnevist	Gadopentetate dimeglumine	Bayer HealthCare Pharmaceuticals, Wayne, NJ, USA
Eovist	Gadoxetate disodium	
Gadavist	Gadobutrol	
Optimark	Gadoversetamide	Covidien, Inc. Hazelwood, MO, USA
Omniscan	Gadodiamide	GE Healthcare, AS Oslo, Norway
Multihance	Gadobenate dimeglumine	Bracco Diagnostics, Milan, Italy
Prohance	Gadoteridol	

modeled as two compartments—intravascular plasma and EES. Gadolinium-based contrast agents do not cross cellular membranes, so intracellular space is ignored. A linear system model is assumed, with the input given by the contrast agent concentration in arterial plasma and the output given by the contrast agent concentration in tumor tissue. The transfer function $h(t)$ is parameterized by K^{Trans} and k_{ep}, where K^{Trans} is the volume transfer constant between arterial plasma and EES, k_{ep} is the volume transfer constant between EES and arterial plasma, and v_e is the fractional volume of EES. Both K^{Trans} and k_{ep} are composite parameters, which are affected by both blood flow and vascular permeability. Given these assumptions, it is a simple matter to fit an appropriately parameterized transfer function to any given set of plasma and tissue time–concentration curves. This model is described schematically in Figure 17.2.

The most common application of DCE-MRI currently is in the assessment of treatment effect for antiangiogenic and antivascular cancer therapies [8,9]. The technique is well suited to this task, as these therapies are generally designed to affect both blood flow and vascular permeability through a variety of biological mechanisms, including inhibition of vascular endothelial growth factor (VEGF) [8], inhibition of platelet-derived growth factor (PDGF) [10], and direct disruption of the cytoskeletons of tumor endothelial cells [9]. DCE-MRI and related techniques are able to directly assess the mechanistic effects of these therapies, allowing a rapid and precise estimate

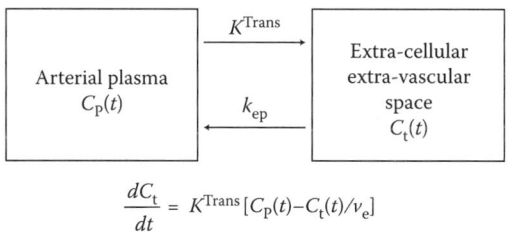

$$\frac{dC_t}{dt} = K^{Trans}[C_p(t) - C_t(t)/v_e]$$

FIGURE 17.2 Two-compartment model for the analysis of DCE-MRI data.

of pharmacodynamic (though not necessarily clinically significant) drug effect. Other clinical applications of DCE-MRI include the assessment of bone edema and synovial inflammation in rheumatoid arthritis patients [11,12], where observed changes are more likely related to changes in blood volume and flow rather than vascular permeability, and the assessment of neurological disorders such as multiple sclerosis, where observed changes are related primarily to disruptions in the blood–brain barrier which result in large changes in vascular permeability with limited effect on blood flow or volume.

The following sections will provide a detailed discussion of the various imaging techniques used to acquire DCE-MRI data, the analysis models that have been employed to derive biologically meaningful parameters from these images, and the clinical and experimental uses of this technique.

17.2 Imaging Techniques

17.2.1 Dynamic Contrast-Enhanced MRI

DCE-MRI refers specifically to techniques which make use of T_1-weighted images to measure changes in concentration of contrast agent in plasma and tissue over time. Time–concentration curves for contrast agent in arterial plasma (generally referred to as the arterial input function or AIF) and tissue are extracted from the image data. Modeling is then used to estimate biologically meaningful parameters such as blood flow, blood volume, and vascular permeability surface area product based on these curves. The development of an imaging protocol for DCE-MRI requires a complex trade-off among several competing priorities. In particular, as with many MRI protocols, DCE-MRI requires that the imager exchange both signal-to-noise ratio (SNR) and spatial coverage for acquisition speed.

Precisely how much speed will be required is heavily dependent on the analysis model that will be used to convert the observed time–concentration curves in arterial plasma and tissue into biologically meaningful parameters such as blood flow, blood volume, or vascular permeability–surface area product. These requirements will be discussed in detail in a subsequent section, but in general the temporal resolution required to extract meaningful information regarding tracer kinetics ranges from a minimum of 2 s/volume to a maximum of 15 s/volume. Protocol design is further constrained by the following requirements:

- Spatial coverage: The imaged volume for a DCE-MRI acquisition must be large enough to contain both the tissue of interest (target tumor, inflamed joint, brain lesion, etc.) and preferably one or more major arteries that can be used in the derivation of an AIF.
- 3-D acquisition: Because it is necessary to estimate changes in contrast concentration in arterial plasma, it is very desirable to minimize inflow and other artifacts. This is most easily done by prescribing a 3-D acquisition with the plane of imaging aligned as nearly as possible with the direction of flow in the target artery.
- Motion correction: Because images are acquired continuously over a period of several minutes, DCE-MRI protocols generally do not recommend breath-holding, opting instead for a so-called quiet breathing technique. As a result, there may be substantial movement of organs such as the

liver due to respiratory motion between acquisitions. This motion is most easily corrected if it is confined to the plane of imaging rather than between images. DCE-MRI of the chest and abdomen are therefore best acquired in either the coronal or sagittal planes.

• Conversion from signal delta to contrast concentration: We wish to extract the change over time in millimolar concentration of contrast agent in tissue from DCE-MRI images. However, this information cannot be directly measured, but must rather be inferred from observed changed in signal intensity in the images. This requirement limits both the selection of pulse sequence and the selection of acquisition coil in ways that will be discussed in detail in a subsequent section.

The most commonly used MR sequences are gradient-echo, turboFLASH, or echoplanar sequences. This choice is driven largely by the necessity for rapid acquisition time. For similar reasons, echo time (T_E) and repetition time (T_R) are typically kept as short as is practically possible, with flip angle (α) set to 20°–30°. Typical DCE-MRI sequence implementations for General Electric and Siemens 1.5 T systems are given in Table 17.2. Figure 17.3 provides sample MR images for both manufacturers.

If these sequence options are used in conjunction with a 3-D acquisition, a 256 × 192 in-plane acquisition matrix, and a slab thickness of 96 mm, they will yield a temporal resolution on the order of 6–9 s per volume. As will be seen in subsequent sections, this resolution will be adequate for some models but far too slow for others. If faster acquisition is required, it is possible to trade spatial coverage, spatial resolution, and SNR in this protocol for additional speed. Reducing the repetition time and echo time to the minimum allowable, for example, may reduce acquisition time substantially on more advanced systems. Reducing the in-plane acquisition matrix to 128 × 128 or even 64 × 64 and/or reducing the thickness of the acquired slab will further accelerate the acquisition.

TABLE 17.2 Differences between GE and Siemens Implementations of a Basic DCE-MRI Protocol

Parameter	GE	Siemens
Sequence type	SPGR	SPGR
Sequence variants	SS\SP\SK	SP\OSP
Sequence options	FAST\VB\EDR\MP\PFF	PFP
T_R/T_E/FA	4.62/1.05/30	5.00/1.57/30

(a) (b)

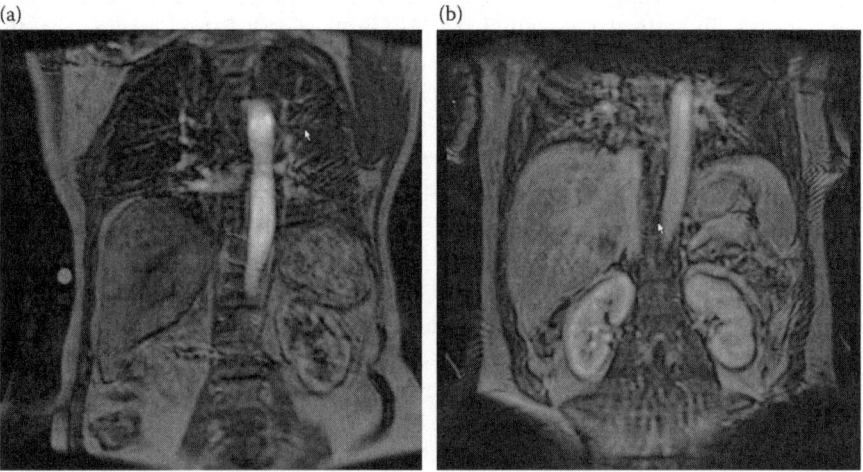

FIGURE 17.3 Image acquired using 3D-squences on 1.5 T scanners: (a) GE Signa (SP/SK with PFF option), slice thickness of 8 mm, T_R = 5.9 ms, T_E = 1.2 ms. (b) Seimens Espree scanner with slice thickness 5 mm, T_R = 5 ms, T_E = 1.69 ms. Both images have inplane resolution of 1.56 × 1.56 mm and FA = 30.

In addition to the methods outlined above, higher temporal resolution in T_1-weighted imaging can be achieved through switching to a small number (typically 1–3) of 2-D slices, switching to a so-called semi-keyhole acquisition [13,14], or a combination of the two [15]. Each of these approaches has significant drawbacks, however, and should be undertaken with caution.

Issues associated with 2-D acquisition are fairly obvious. Because the resulting acquired volume is very thin, it will often not contain the entirety of the target tissue. As an example, a target tumor that is well-suited to DCE-MRI analysis will typically be between 3 and 7 cm in diameter. A 3-slice acquisition with 8 mm slice thickness will only be able to capture the central portion of such a tumor, and repeating the precise positioning of the slices at later acquisitions may be very difficult. As a result, pretreatment and posttreatment images may in fact cover substantially different portions of the tumor. Additionally, as mentioned previously, 2-D acquisitions are frequently subject to severe artifacts within large arteries due to varying flow rates as individual slices are acquired at different points in the cardiac cycle. This makes it very difficult to accurately characterize the AIF using 2-D acquisitions. Comparison of images acquired with 2-D and 3-D acquisition techniques is shown in Figure 17.4.

The issues associated with semi-keyhole acquisition are less obvious and less well established, but are significant enough that the imaging community has generally been wary of this technique. Semi-keyhole acquisition techniques achieve improved acquisition speed through some combination of sub-sampling k-space in frequency and time. As a result, images acquired using this technique are subject to cross-talk between pixels and between volumes. The pixel values observed at a given time, therefore, may include signal contribution from prior times as well as the current one. As a result, contrast concentrations observed in arterial plasma during the period of first bolus passage, when concentration levels are changing very rapidly, are likely to be inaccurate. Because accurate characterization of the AIF during the first bolus passage is critical for most high-speed models, this acquisition technique is not an ideal one for these applications.

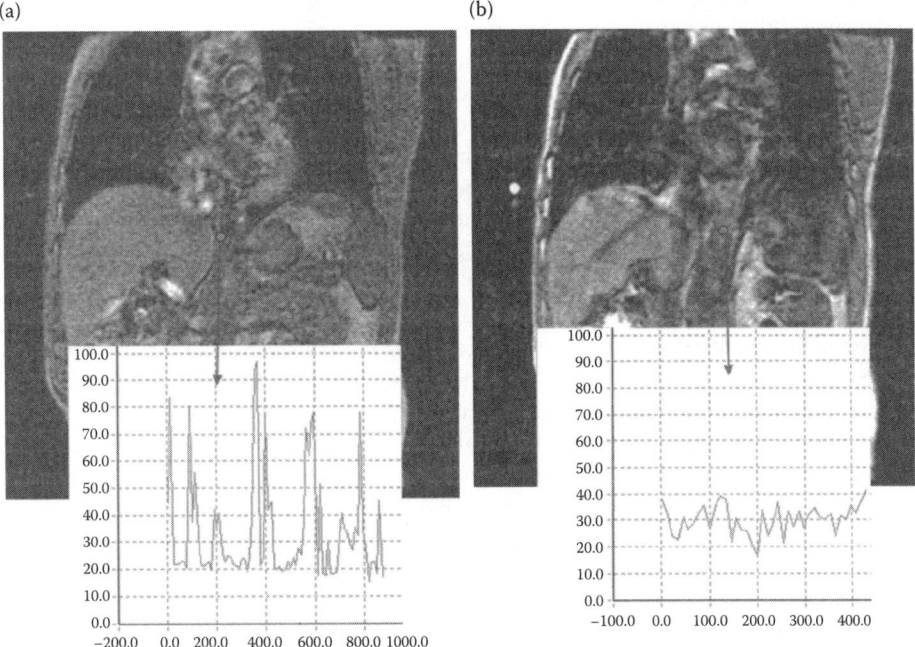

FIGURE 17.4 Comparison of images acquired using 2D (a) and 3D (b) techniques. The given plots show signal intensity changes due to flow artifacts in the descending aorta. Note that artifacts are much more severe in the 2D image.

As will be seen, many analysis models require temporal resolution of 2 s per volume. This is achievable with sufficient trade-offs along the lines described above. However, it must be understood that the loss of information on a per-volume basis in terms of coverage, spatial resolution, and SNR will be significant, and that these losses will translate directly into increased variability in the measured parameters which are the output of this process. High-speed models should therefore only be implemented with T_1-weighted acquisition protocols in cases where the more detailed parameter sets available with these models will provide information that is critical to the experiment being conducted. This issue will be addressed in greater detail in a later section.

17.2.2 Dynamic Susceptibility Contrast-Enhanced MRI

As we have seen, acquisition time is a severely limiting factor when working with T_1-weighted images. However, gadolinium-based contrast agents also affect both T_2- and T_2^*-weighted images. T_2^*-weighted images in particular are an attractive option due to their potential for high acquisition speed relative to T_1-weighted images. Acquisition times of 0.2 s/slice for T_2^*-weighted images are easily achievable using echo-planar imaging (EPI) techniques. As should be expected, however, there are a number of differences in the way contrast concentration changes affect T_2^*-weighted images that must be understood if this technique is to be used for perfusion assessment.

First and most obviously, the presence of intravascular contrast in T_2^*-weighted images causes a reduction in observed signal intensity (darkening) rather than increased signal intensity (brightening) as in T_1-weighted images [16]. From a modeling perspective, this is not particularly relevant as long as methods are available to convert observed changes in signal intensity into millimolar concentration of contrast in tissues. These methods will be discussed in a later section.

More significantly, the induced change in signal relative to background noise levels at a given contrast concentration is substantially lower in T_2^*-weighted images than it is in T_1-weighted images. As a result, the contrast agent dose administered for a DSC-MRI acquisition is higher than that for a DCE-MRI acquisition [17]. Typical values are 0.1 mmol/kg for T_1-weighted images versus 0.2–0.3 mmol/kg for T_2^*-weighted images. Until 2006, this limitation was seen primarily as a cost issue. However, in that year Marckmann et al. identified gadolinium-based contrast agents as a causative factor in nephrogenic systemic fibrosis (NSF), a potentially serious disease affecting patients with renal failure [18]. While the occurrence of NSF is very rare (the original paper identified only 13 cases) and has been seen only in patients with severe preexisting kidney disease, these findings do raise some concerns about administering high doses of gadolinium without significant medical justification.

The most intractable issue associated with DSC-MRI, however, is that echo-planar imaging sequences are very strongly affected by magnetic susceptibility artifacts [19,20]. They are therefore ill-suited for use in regions of the body containing significant amounts of air space, such as the chest or abdomen. They are also ill-suited for use with extravascular contrast. This is a severe drawback insofar as gadolinium-labeled contrast agents generally are able to cross from the capillary bed into EES even in normal tissues—and even more so in tumors, whose capillaries typically have poorly formed and highly permeable endothelia. Gadolinium-labeled contrast agents are generally not, however, able to cross an intact blood–brain barrier, with the result that they are essentially intravascular agents within the brain.

As a result of these limitations, despite the apparent attractiveness of this technique from a speed standpoint, DSC-MRI is used almost exclusively for assessing perfusion within the brain at this time.

17.3 Analysis Methods

17.3.1 Arterial Input Function Estimation

One of the primary challenges in estimating perfusion parameters is identifying an accurate arterial input function (AIF)—defined as the time–concentration curve for contrast agent in arterial plasma and given by $C_p(t)$ in Figure 17.2. One common approach is to avoid this problem by making use of a general concentration–time curve such as that utilized by Weinmann et al. [21]. However, using a theoretical AIF ignores differences in injection rate and cardiac output, which may vary from subject to subject and even with a single subject over time [22]. These differences can greatly reduce measurement reproducibility. Galbraith et al. have reported thresholds for statistically significant change over time in K^{Trans} in a single tumor using this method of −45% and +83% [23].

A second option is for an analyst to draw a manual ROI within an artery, and use the mean enhancement curve within that ROI as the subject-specific AIF (see Figures 17.1 and 17.5), as described by Vonken et al. [24]. This approach is complicated by the fact that the MR signal in arteries is frequently corrupted by flow artifacts, with the result that regions of interest at different points in the same artery or in other nearby vessels can provide grossly different enhancement curves. It should be noted that these artifacts are sequence dependent, and are worse for 2D methods than for central regions of 3D methods.

Several groups have described methods for the automated or semiautomated identification of a patient-specific arterial input function using either information from large arteries present in the scan [25–27] or a model-based derived AIF using information taken from normal tissues such as muscle [28]. Scan–rescan variability data on these various methods is not widely available in the literature. However, available evidence indicates that systems using automated, patient-specific AIF derivation generally show lower variability, as would be expected [22,23,26,29,30].

Sampling the AIF from large blood vessels presents some challenges, as a result of both artifacts present in vessels due to flow effects and the lack of availability of suitable large vessels in some commonly scanned anatomical regions such as the pelvis or extremities. In order to avoid sampling of the AIF from blood vessels, an alternative approach has been proposed using a reference region model (RRM) [31]. This approach was expanded by Yang et al. to use two different reference tissues. They showed that despite the use of two potential error sources, the double-reference tissue method provided a reliable estimate of the AIF [32]. Currently, efforts are also being made to incorporate a vascular term into a reference region analysis to study its effect on the accuracy of the model in estimating tissue kinetics using systematic computer simulations. Faranesh et al. showed that the vascular term may have a significant effect on parameter estimation, but was inconclusive about the effect of the sampling period [33]. Hsiao et al. studied the effect of the AIF onset-time shift and the injection duration under various

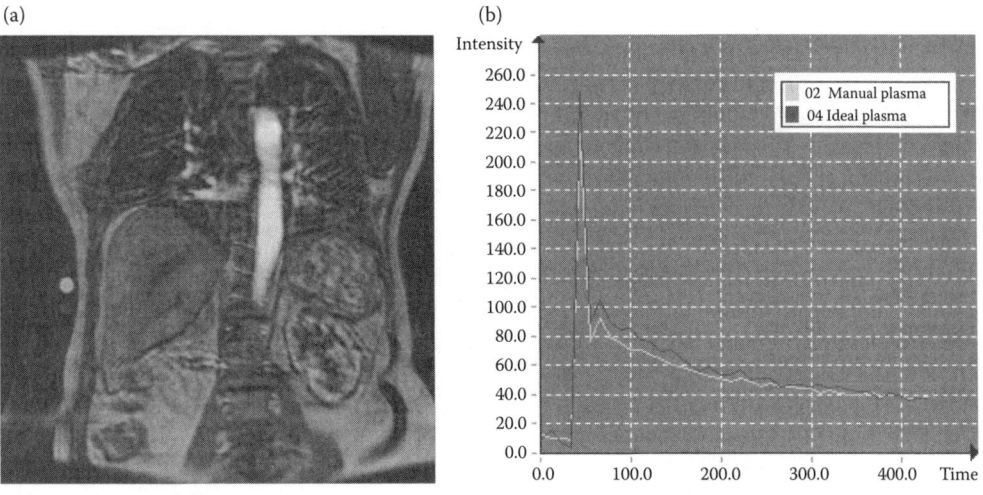

FIGURE 17.5 (a) Sample location for selection of the AIF in the descending aorta and (b) the resulting time-intensity plot.

sampling intervals, on physiological parameter estimation, using both the GKM and RRM. Their results suggested that with compromised temporal resolution, the RRM was relatively less sensitive to the AIF onset-time shift and the injection duration compared with GKM, but the coefficient of variance was higher because of lower SNR in the reference region [34].

The major limitations of the RRM approach are that it requires K^{Trans} and v_e (fractional volume of EES) for the reference region, and so inclusion of an additional parameter such as the vascular term v_p (fractional intravascular volume) means that it is a requirement to know this *a priori*. Additionally, the RRM method works well only when the reference region and tissue of interest share the same AIF. In practice, the measured concentration curves are noisy, and because of the dispersion effects, AIFs of the two tissues are not exactly the same and thus could produce errors in the AIF estimate [32].

17.3.2 Conversion from Signal Delta to Contrast Concentration

17.3.2.1 Conversion Using a Look-Up Table

As has been mentioned previously, most (though not all) DCE-MRI parameter calculation schemes are dependent first on the conversion of observed changes in signal intensity in individual image voxels or larger volumes of interest into millimolar concentrations of contrast agent. The simplest way to do this is to make use of a phantom-generated look-up table [35]. This method requires that a phantom containing a range of concentrations of gadolinium and a range of baseline T_1 values (generally obtained via different concentrations of copper sulfate or a similar compound) is scanned using the dynamic protocol on each scanner that will be used for the study. Data from these phantoms can then be used to construct a look-up table relating baseline T_1, signal delta, and gadolinium concentration (see Figure 17.6). This look-up table can then be used during the analysis process to directly convert signal delta to gadolinium concentration prior to parameter calculation.

This approach has the advantage of simplicity. Additionally, by avoiding the use of complex modeling, each step of which carries its own variability and therefore adds to the noise level in the calculated parameters, it holds the promise of improved measurement precision. This method does have some drawbacks, however. First, it requires a uniform set of suitable phantoms. Such phantoms are not commercially available, and can be difficult and expensive to design and build. Second, it assumes that the available phantom data are representative of the data being analyzed. This may not be valid unless a separate phantom

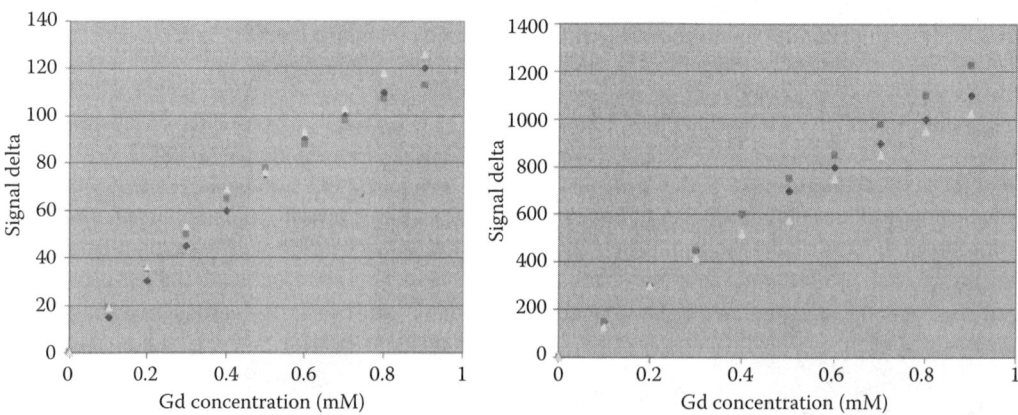

FIGURE 17.6 Plot of signal change versus gadolinium concentration for GE (l) and Siemens (r) systems. Baseline T_1 values were 90 ms (yellow), 300 ms (pink), and 700 ms (blue). Note that the Siemens system shows roll-off in signal response at significantly longer T_1 than the GE system.

scan is acquired with each patient scan, since software or hardware upgrades may potentially change the relationship between signal and contrast concentration that the phantoms are designed to assess.

17.3.2.2 Conversion Using a Signal Formation Model

The more common approach to the problem of conversion from signal delta to gadolinium concentration is to make use of a signal formation model. The most frequently used model requires knowledge of the relaxivity of the contrast agent being used, as well as the baseline T_1 value at each voxel in the image, the baseline signal value at each voxel, and the postcontrast signal value at each voxel and at each postcontrast volume. Baseline T_1 must be calculated using a T_1 mapping sequence. There are a number of options for generating a T_1 map. However, many of them (e.g., acquiring sequences with multiple inversion recovery times) are very time consuming and so poorly suited for this application. A popular approach is to acquire two or more sequences with different flip angles, preferably covering a broad range above and below the Ernst angles for the acquired T_R and range of T_1 values expected in the human body. A typical protocol might call for five sequences with flip angles ranging from 5° to 30°. These images should be prescribed identically to the dynamic series so that the resulting T_1 map can be conveniently coregistered with the dynamic data, and should be acquired immediately prior to the dynamic series. The T_1 values at each voxel can then be calculated as follows:

1. Create a vector x containing the signal intensity at each flip angle divided by the tangent of the flip angle.
2. Create a vector y containing the signal intensity at each flip angle divided by the sine of the flip angle.
3. For the n acquired flip angles, create a set of points $(x_0,y_0)\cdots(x_{n-1},y_{n-1})$.
4. Fit a line with slope s to the set of points defined in Step 3.
5. $T_1 = -T_R/\log(s)$.

Given the resulting T_1 map, the gadolinium concentration at each image voxel at time t is given by

$$C(t) = \left(\frac{1}{T_1} - \frac{1}{T_{10}} \right) \Big/ R_1$$

In this equation, T_{10} is taken from the T_1 map calculated above. R_1 is the relaxivity of the contrast agent, and T_1 is given by

$$\frac{1}{T_1} = \left(\frac{-1}{T_R} \right) * \log\left(\frac{1-(A+B)}{1-\cos(\alpha)*(A+B)} \right)$$

here T_R is the repetition time for the dynamic series, α is the flip angle for the dynamic series, and A and B are given by

$$A = (S(t) - S_0)/(M_0 * \sin(\alpha))$$
$$B = (1 - E_{10})/(1 - \cos(\alpha) * E_{10})$$

17.3.3 Subjective and Semiquantitative Analysis Methods

Because DCE-MRI images are inherently four-dimensional, they are not in their raw form particularly well suited to visual interpretation. As a result, a number of heuristically selected characteristics of the observed time–signal intensity curves have been used to color-code DCE-MRI images for visual inspection (see Section 17.3.4.6). Most common among these are maximum slope and peak enhancement. These parameters help to characterize the shape of the uptake curve, which may differ between, for example, malignant and benign breast lesions. False-coloring images according to these parameters, therefore, can provide a useful visual cue to an examining radiologist. These parameters are not well suited, however, to quantitative analysis.

A more common semiquantitative approach is to make use of some variation of the initial area under the tumor uptake curve (IAUC)—"initial" generally referring to the first 30, 60, 90, or 120 s postinjection. IAUC is not in itself biologically meaningful. It is dependent on the fractional volume of EES in addition to blood flow and endothelial permeability–surface area product. It is in general highly correlated with K^{Trans} (see Section 17.3.4.1), but is not dependent on any physiological model, and is therefore in some cases less sensitive to noise and data irregularities. IAUC has been used frequently as a marker of drug effect [3,36]. There is no generally agreed-upon definition for precisely what IAUC should refer to, however, so any use of this parameter should include as explicit a definition as possible. In particular, it is important to specify

- Duration: How many seconds postinjection will be analyzed? Shorter times will emphasize flow effects, while longer times place more emphasis on permeability effects.
- Signal type: Will the data be corrected to gadolinium concentration prior to analysis? Some investigators have designated this parameter taken from corrected data as IAUGC in order to distinguish it from the area under the signal intensity curve IAUC. However, this usage is not consistent.
- Normalization: One of the primary weaknesses of this parameter is that it is strongly affected by differences in injection volume or cardiac output. Some investigators have attempted to correct for this by dividing the IAUC or IAUGC for the tissue of interest by the IAUC or IAUCG for the arterial input function. The resulting parameter is generally referred to as IAUC_{BN}, where BN refers to blood normalization. This usage is also somewhat inconsistent.

These parameters are sometimes used in isolation. However, more commonly, they are used in conjunction with some subset of the more physiologically meaningful parameters described in Section 17.3.4.

17.3.4 Quantitative Analysis Methods

17.3.4.1 Generalized Kinetic Model

As was mentioned previously, the most commonly used model for analysis of DCE-MRI data at this time is the generalized kinetic model (GKM), frequently referred to as the standard Tofts model, first proposed by Tofts and Kermonde [6]. Nomenclature and usage for this model were standardized by Tofts et al. in 1999 [37]. This model is described schematically in Figure 17.2. There are several critical points which distinguish this model from those that will be described subsequently. First, relative to most other proposed models, the standard Tofts model is minimally parameterized. It assumes that the vascular bed can be modeled as a linear system in which the AIF (usually referred to as $C_p(t)$) can be related to the time–concentration curve in the tissue of interest (usually referred to as $C_t(t)$) via the transfer function $h(t)$, given by

$$h(t) = K^{\text{Trans}} \cdot e^{-(k_{\text{ep}} \cdot t)}$$

where K^{Trans} is the volume transfer constant between arterial plasma and EES, and k_{ep} is the volume transfer constant between EES and arterial plasma (both in units of 1/min). Given $C_p(t)$ and $C_t(t)$, which can be derived directly from the dynamic images, estimation of K^{Trans} and k_{ep} is an optimization problem, frequently carried out using the alternating estimation (AE) or another similar energy minimization scheme. Parameter estimation will be discussed in detail in a later section. The third parameter associated with this model, v_e, the fractional volume of EES, is given by K^{Trans}/k_{ep}. Because of this relatively straightforward formulation, parameter calculation using this model is computationally inexpensive relative to other models in this class.

A second distinguishing aspect of this model is that it does not attempt to separate changes in contrast uptake due to blood flow or blood volume from those due to vascular permeability. Both K^{Trans} and k_{ep} are composite parameters which are related to both flow and permeability. This is in some respects a weakness of this model, in that therapies which produce differential effects on flow and permeability may not produce a distinguishable signal using this model. Certain PDGF inhibitors, as an example, have been shown to selectively prune smaller, more tortuous and immature vessels within tumors. As a result, these therapies induce a regularization of the tumor vascular bed, which results in a net decrease in vascular permeability coupled with a net decrease in tumor interstitial pressure and corresponding increase in blood flow. These changes may manifest as either an increase or decrease in K^{Trans}, depending largely on whether the contrast uptake in the tumor pretherapy was more heavily dependent on flow or permeability. As a result, K^{Trans} calculated using this model is not a particularly useful measure of drug effect for this class of therapies.

Interestingly, however, this same property is also one of the primary strengths of this model. The information which allows a model to distinguish between flow effects and permeability effects is entirely contained in the first contrast bolus passage, when contrast agent concentration in the arterial plasma is both very high and rapidly changing (see Figure 17.7). Total injected contrast volume for a DCE-MRI examination is generally between 10 and 15 cc. This volume is followed with a saline flush of roughly 20 cc. Contrast is administered with a power injector at a rate of ~3 cc/s. As a result, the period between injection, when contrast concentration in plasma rises rapidly to a peak of 3 mM or more, and the end of first bolus passage, when contrast concentration reaches a "shoulder value" of approximately 0.5 mM and the rate of decline drops rapidly, is no more than 15 s. Distinguishing between flow effects and permeability effects requires an accurate characterization of both $C_p(t)$ and $C_t(t)$ during this period, and

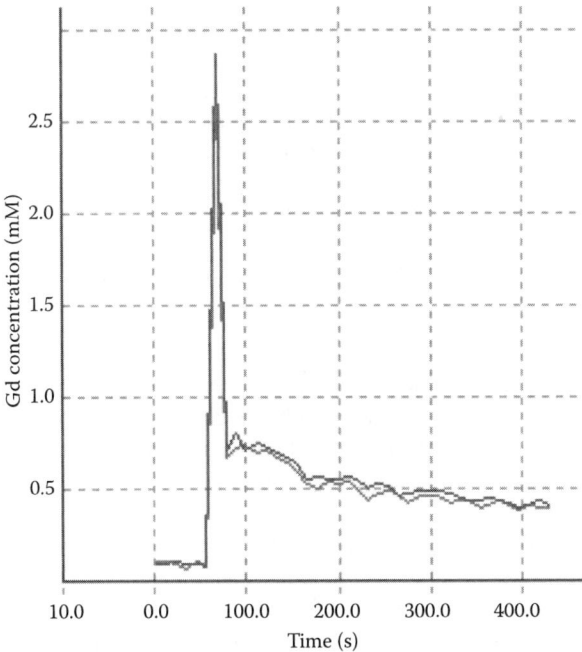

FIGURE 17.7 Typical AIF obtained using T_1-weighted imaging with a 0.1 mmol/kg contrast injection and 6 s temporal resolution.

therefore requires that these curves must be sampled at their Nyquist rate or better [38]—in this case roughly 2 s per sample.

Because this model does not attempt to make this distinction, it can be implemented with sampling rates of 6 s per sample or slower. This allows the use of acquisition protocols (like that described previously) with relatively high SNR, spatial resolution, and spatial coverage. As a result, with other factors held constant, this model can be expected to provide higher precision than those requiring more rapid sampling. It can be argued (as detailed in the following section) that this increased precision is coupled with a systematic bias in estimation of K^{Trans}. However, in most applications, precision is in fact more important than absolute accuracy. If the intent of an experiment is to determine whether a particular antivascular therapy induces a 50% decline in K^{Trans}, for example, it makes no difference whether the absolute values measured for K^{Trans} are biased 20% high or 20% low, as long as an identical bias is applied to both pre- and posttherapy measurements.

In other applications, where the critical factor is not changed over time but rather the absolute value of K^{Trans} at a single time, however, this model may be a poor choice. An example of this is the use of K^{Trans} measurement to determine malignancy in breast lesions [39]. Such applications require one of the more biologically accurate models described below.

17.3.4.2 Extended Tofts Model

In the standard Tofts model described above, it is implicitly assumed that all observed signal changes are a result of contrast agent in the EES—contrast agent that remains within the vasculature is ignored. It should be clear that this assumption will lead to an overestimation of both K^{Trans} and k_{ep}, since the model will treat any contrast that remains intravascular during its passage through the capillary bed as if it had passed into the EES and back into the plasma compartment, thus contributing inappropriately to both K^{Trans} and k_{ep}. This observation has been confirmed experimentally [40].

The extended Tofts model [2] compensates for this error by separating $C_t(t)$ into two components—one intravascular and one extravascular, such that

$$C_t(t) = v_e C_e(t) + v_p C_p(t)$$

where v_e is the fractional extracellular extravascular volume, v_p is the fractional intravascular volume, $C_e(t)$ is the contrast concentration in EES, and $C_p(t)$ is the AIF. This yields a revised relationship between $C_p(t)$ and $C_t(t)$:

$$C_t(t) = K^{\text{Trans}} \int_0^t C_p(t') e^{-(k_{\text{ep}}(t-t'))} dt' + v_p C_p(t)$$

Given an observed $C_p(t)$ and $C_t(t)$, the vascular parameters K^{Trans}, k_{ep}, and v_p can be estimated using similar methods to those used for the standard Tofts model. This model is an improvement over the standard Tofts model insofar as it provides a more biologically accurate estimate of K^{Trans} and k_{ep}. It may also provide greater insight into the effects of therapies that induce differential effects on flow, blood volume, and vascular permeability.

The primary drawback of this model is that it does require temporal resolution of roughly 2 s per volume or better. When this model is applied to data which was acquired at a lower rate, the resulting aliasing manifests as parameter instability in K^{Trans} and v_p. In this case, given a particular $C_p(t)$ and $C_t(t)$, multiple equally valid solutions can often be obtained by increasing one parameter and decreasing the other, yielding nearly identical results when the resulting transfer function is convolved with $C_p(t)$. Because of the previously described difficulty in achieving the temporal resolution necessary for this model, it should be used only in applications where there is a reasonable expectation that the improved biological accuracy will compensate for the necessary decrease in SNR, spatial resolution, and spatial coverage.

17.3.4.3 Distributed Parameter Model

The distributed parameter model was developed by Ting-Yim Lee and others [41], originally for analysis of DCE-CT data of the brain. This model is also the most common one used to analyze DSC-MRI data of the brain. Because this model is heavily dependent on an accurate characterization of the first bolus passage, like the extended Tofts model, it requires temporal resolution of 2 s/volume or better. It is a two-compartment model, similar conceptually to the GKM described previously. Rather than assuming a parameterized transfer function as described in Section 17.3.4.1, however, the distributed parameter model attempts to estimate the transfer function directly through deconvolution of $C_p(t)$ and $C_t(t)$, such that

$$C_t(t) = \text{rBF}(C_p(t) * h(t))$$

where rBF is the regional blood flow. It is assumed that $h(t)$ will have a roughly biexponential form, with an early maximum followed by a rapid decline to a shoulder value, an increase to a second peak representing recirculation, and a much slower roll-off from there. From this function, we extract the maximum value M_1, the maximum value of the second peak M_2, and the area under the first peak A. We are then able to calculate the extraction fraction (E), representing the portion of contrast agent entering the EES on first pass, the mean transit time (MTT), regional blood flow (rBF), regional blood volume (rBV), and permeability–surface area product (PS) according to the following equations:

$$E = M_2/M_1$$
$$\text{MTT} = A/M_1$$
$$\text{rBF} = M_1/(1.0 - E)$$
$$\text{rBV} = A/(1.0 - E)$$
$$\text{PS} = -\text{rBF} * \log(1.0 - E)$$

Results obtained using this model have been shown to correlate reasonably well with K^{Trans}, and to correlate with drug exposure in some clinical trials [42]. This model is attractive in that it provides the most biologically meaningful measures of any described here. The major drawbacks associated with this model are that (1) it requires very high speed imaging and (2) it is reliant on deconvolution, which is both computationally expensive and very noise sensitive. For these reasons, this model has not been used extensively with T_1-weighted images in the body.

17.3.4.4 Shutter Speed Model

The standard GKM described previously yields pharmacokinetic parameters with the assumption that equilibrium transcytolemmal water exchange is effectively infinitely fast. Recent studies have shown that consideration of the transmembrane water exchange affects the accuracy of the tissue contrast agent concentration estimates [43–45]. These studies compared the accuracy of the standard GKM and shutter-speed model (SSM) to differentiate malignant and benign breast lesions, and found that K^{Trans} in malignant tumors is generally underestimated by the standard GKM model, while the estimation for benign tumors was similar. However, this model is still controversial, and needs to be evaluated in one or more large clinical trials to determine whether its application yields any significant benefits over older methods.

17.3.4.5 Computational Methods for Parameter Estimation

Quantitative estimates of tissue physiological parameters such as perfusion, capillary permeability, and the volume of extravascular–extracellular space (EES) as described above are obtained by curve-fitting and compartmental modeling, where the minimization of a merit function yields the "best fit" of model to data. The two most popular curve-fittings methods are Levenberg–Marquardt and Minpack-1. Ahearn et al. have investigated these methods with respect to the search start points, and found that both algorithms return unreliable results with a single starting point. This is a result of the fact that both of these methods are gradient-descent techniques, which are known to be vulnerable to local minima. Their experimental analysis showed that with multiple start points, both algorithms returned reliable parameters. Additionally, they also showed that the Minpack-1 method generally outperformed the Levenberg–Marquardt method [46].

In order to increase the speed of parameter estimation, several groups have proposed the use of linear-least square (LLSQ) estimation approaches by using the differential equation for kinetic behavior of contrast agents in tissue [4,47]. Computer simulation showed that in comparison with the nonlinear least-squares (NLSQ) method, the LLSQ approach is much quicker and more accurate than the NLSQ method at an SNR of <10 [4]. Horsfield et al. proposed more sophisticated schemes for data processing for a sparsely sampled AIF using three discrete approximation schemes that include the dirac delta function, piecewise constant, and piecewise linear to quantify the errors involved in estimating parameters. They concluded that more sophisticated schemes gave more accurate parameter estimates, with the piecewise constant representation of the AIF giving the best results when data are sparsely sampled [47]. However, the LLSQ approach has a severe limitation in that it does not provide any bounding condition to the estimated dataset. Hence, it is possible that the estimated parameters might not have any physiological meaning. Some examples are a negative plasma volume fraction for a three parameter fit, or an EES volume fraction that is >1. Such limitations should be accounted for when developing parametric maps from DCE-MRI data.

Recent studies have shown that incorporation of additional parameters such as bolus arrival delay and mean transit time can increase the accuracy of estimated parameters in some cases. Experimental results show that unless the AIF initial bolus passage sampling is accurate, more robust parameter estimates are achieved simply by a more slowly sampled biexponential fit. Small values of K^{Trans} can be accurately estimated, but this approach may underestimate blood volume [48].

17.3.4.6 Presentation of Analysis Results

As we have seen, calculation of a DCE-MRI parameter set requires time–concentration curves in both arterial plasma ($C_p(t)$ – the AIF) and in the tissue of interest ($C_t(t)$). Generally the AIF is defined on either a per-scan or population basis as described above. $C_t(t)$ can also be defined in one of two ways: by averaging the uptake curves for all pixels within a user-defined volume of interest (VOI), yielding a single $C_t(t)$ which can be used to calculate a single parameter set for that region, or on a voxel-by-voxel basis, yielding a unique parameter set for each voxel in the image. The VOI-based technique has the advantage of simplicity. Parameter estimation using energy minimization techniques is computationally expensive, and can be extremely so when the process must be carried out for every voxel in a large image. VOI-based estimation avoids this problem, but it does not help to visualize the heterogeneity in the target tissue. Tumors in particular are typically highly heterogeneous. Because they often have very high interstitial pressure, enhancement is generally much more rapid around the periphery of tumors and slower in the interior. As a result, parameter estimation using a single $C_t(t)$ averaged across a VOI may lead to erroneous results [49].

Several groups have proposed the use of voxel-by-voxel analysis to generate parametric images to overcome this shortcoming. With this approach, parametric kinetic enhancement maps are coregistered with high-resolution anatomic images to visualize the spatially heterogeneous distributions of kinetic parameters in tumors [50–52]. However, use of this approach provides significant challenges in terms of both data acquisitions and analysis. Because each voxel has a low SNR, signal quality becomes increasingly important. Furthermore, because $C_t(t)$ is estimated on a per-voxel basis, registration between volumes must be accurate to within a single pixel. This can be challenging in areas such as the chest and abdomen that have significant physiologic motion [53,54]. Development of specialized data acquisition techniques and postprocessing algorithms designed to reduce between-volume motion is an active area of research [55,56].

No uniform consensus is available on quantification methodology to understand the heterogeneity of parametric maps. The most common approach is to report out the mean and/or median value for a VOI for each estimated parameter. Recommendations have been made to use summary statistics, histogram analysis, and pixel scatter plots derived from the parameters. However, all these approaches still require clinical validation [43,57–60]. It is more challenging to analyze the heterogeneity changes in physiologic parameters that occur after therapeutic intervention. It is impractical to obtain voxel-by-voxel match between different visits of the same subject, so comparison is performed using histograms obtained from the parametric maps [26]. Recent efforts also include the use of texture analyses and analytic methods to generate functional response maps for use in monitoring the response to therapy [61,62].

Recently, nonphysiological approaches have been evaluated to analyze the high-dimensional data such as DCE-MRI datasets for visual exploration. Varini et al. have compared established data-reduction algorithms such as principal component analysis (PCA), self-organizing maps (SOM), and locally linearly embedded (LLE). They showed that LLE achieves higher separation between the benign and malignant data points compared to PCA, but that SOM provided the best separation. In another study, Twellmann et al. showed that image fusion can be performed using kernel-principal component analysis (KPCA) for gray or color image visualization for discrimination of malignant, benign, and normal tissues [63,64]. However, the accuracy of nonlinear algorithms such as KPCA and SOM depends on the initial set parameters, which may make its tuning difficult. This is a significant limiting factor for their use in clinical applications.

Another nonpharmacokinetic-based approach very commonly used involves categorizing kinetic curves based on different patterns such as nonenhancing, persistently enhancing (progressive), plateau type, and washout type [65–67]. With this approach, each voxel is color-coded based on uptake curve type for display. Such methods may be useful for visualization of DCE-MRI data to differentiate different types of regions in the tissue. However, their application to determine the effects of therapeutic intervention is still unknown.

17.4 Clinical Utility: Connection to Response in Clinical Trials

The most common practical use of DCE-MRI at this time is in clinical trials of cancer therapeutics which are designed to affect the tumor microvasculature. There are numerous cancer therapeutics either approved or currently in development that are either antiangiogenic or vascular disruptive agents [8,9,68]. The ability to accurately and precisely estimate parameters related to blood flow and vascular permeability is critical to the early evaluation of these compounds, as this gives the most direct window into their targeted biological effects (see Figure 17.8). DCE-MRI has been used frequently in Phase I trials of antiangiogenic and vascular disruptive agents [8,9,69] as a screen to determine whether the expected mechanistic changes in tumor microvasculature are being observed in study patients. In order for this technique to progress to later phase trials, however, two conditions must be met:

- It must be demonstrated that a DCE-MRI protocol can be implemented consistently and accurately across a large number of clinical sites in a single trial.
- It must be demonstrated that there is a significant connection between changes observed using DCE-MRI and other clinically significant endpoints such as changes in tumor size.

Adherence to a consistent protocol and a strict quality control process can largely address the first concern [70]. Numerous multisite clinical trials using DCE-MRI as a mechanistic biomarker have

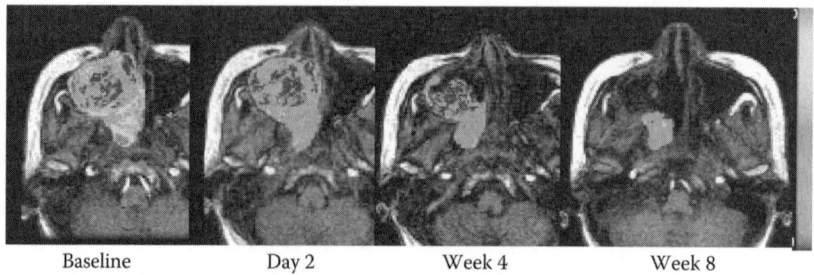

| Baseline | Day 2 | Week 4 | Week 8 |

FIGURE 17.8 Overlay of the pharmacokinetic parameter K^{Trans} on a target tumor. Note the large reduction observed in K^{Trans} at Day 2, which precedes the morphological changes observed by Week 8.

been carried out successfully in the past several years using some variation of this approach [8,9,69,71]. However, in order to have serious utility in Phase II and beyond, changes detected using DCE-MRI must be predictive of clinical changes that might be used to obtain approval in Phase III. A number of studies have attempted to address this question, with somewhat mixed results. Flaherty et al. have shown early changes seen with DCE-MRI to be predictive of progression-free survival in renal cell carcinoma patients [72]. These results are contradicted by those of Hahn et al., who show no such relationship in a study of 44 renal cell carcinoma patients [73]. A meta-analysis of 13 Phase I and II clinical trials comprising a total of 156 subjects has shown that early DCE-MRI changes are highly predictive of later changes in tumor burden measured using CT [74]. These divergent results are most easily explained by differences in acquisition and analysis techniques, which can cause measurement variability (and thus predictive power) to vary widely among studies [26,75]. A useful overview of studies comparing DCE-MRI changes to clinical endpoints has been provided by O'Connor et al. [76].

17.5 Summary and Conclusions

DCE-MRI has demonstrated considerable utility over the past 20+ years in both the clinic and in the clinical trials arena. This technique provides information about blood flow, blood volume, and vascular perfusion *in vivo*, providing insight into the mechanistic effects of numerous therapeutic interventions as well as helping to identify viable tissue and to distinguish in some cases between benign and malignant lesions. While a great deal of work has gone into the standardization of nomenclature and general classification of acquisition and analysis techniques, there is not as yet any single widely accepted approach to either the appropriate imaging protocol or the optimal analysis method for DCE-MRI data. In part, this is a necessary consequence of the nature of MRI in general and DCE-MRI in particular, in that gains in one area typically must be balanced by sacrifices in another. So, improvements in acquisition speed allow the use of more biologically relevant analysis models, permitting the separation of flow and permeability effects. However, this comes at the price of a reduction in spatial coverage and/or SNR, decreasing the final reliability of measured parameters. Any DCE-MRI protocol, whether for use in the clinic or in a clinical trial, must therefore be designed with the specific application in mind, and with an understanding of the necessary trade-offs between precision and absolute accuracy outlined above.

References

1. Jackson A, Haroon H, Zhu X, Li K, Thacker N, Jayson G: Breath-hold perfusion and permeability mapping of hepatic malignancies using magnetic resonance imaging and a first-pass leakage profile model. *NMR Biomed* 2002; 15:164.
2. Tofts P: Modeling tracer kinetics in dynamic Gd-DTPA MR Imaging. *J Magn Reson Imag* 1997; 7:91.

3. Evelhoch J: Key factors in the acquisition of contrast kinetic data for oncology. *J Magn Reson Imag* 1999; 10:254.

4. Taylor J, Tofts P, Port R et al.: MR imaging of tumor microcirculation: Promise for the new millennium. *J Magn Reson Imag* 1999; 10:903.

5. Mitchell D, Cohen M: In: *MRI Principles II* (Ed.). Philadelphia, Pennsylvania, Saunders, 2003; p. 275.

6. Tofts P, Kermonde A: Measurement of the blood-brain barrier permeability and leakage space using dynamic MR imaging. 1. Fundamental Concepts. *Magn Reson Med* 1991; 17:357.

7. Kety S: Peripheral blood flow measurement. In: *Methods in Medical Research*, vol. 8. (Potter, VR ed.), Chicago, Year Book Medical Publishers 1960; p. 223.

8. Liu G, Rugo H, Wilding G et al.: Dynamic contrast-enhanced magnetic resonance imaging as a pharmacodynamic measure of response after acute dosing of AG-013736, an oral angiogenesis inhibitor, in patients with advanced solid tumors: Results from a phase I study. *J Clin Oncol* 2005; 23:5464.

9. Anderson H, Yap J, Miller M, Robbins A, Jones T, Price P: Assessment of pharmacodynamic vascular response in a phase I trial of combretastatin A4 phosphate. *J Clin Oncol* 2003; 21:2823.

10. Jayson G, Parker G, Mullamitha S et al.: Blockade of platelet-derived growth factor receptor-beta by CDP860, a humanized, PEGylated di-Fab', leads to fluid accumulation and is associated with increased tumor vascularized volume. *J Clin Oncol* 2005; 23:973.

11. Hodgson R, Grainger A, O'Connor P, Barnes T, Connolly S, Moots R: Dynamic contrast enhanced MRI of bone marrow oedema in rheumatoid arthritis. *Ann Rheum Dis* 2008; 67:270.

12. Malattia C, Damasio M, Basso C, Verri A, Magnaguangno F, Viola S, Gattorno M, Ravelli A, Toma P, Martini A: Dynamic contrast-enhanced magnetic resonance imaging in the assessment of disease activity in patients with juvenile idiopathic arthritis. *Rheumatology* 2010; 49:178.

13. Medic J, Tomazic S, Sersa I, Demsar F: Fast frequency selective keyhole MRI. In: *Proceedings of the 7th Annual Meeting of ISMRM*, Philadelphia, Pennsylvania, 1999 (abstract 2139).

14. McGrath D, Bradley D, Tessier J, Lacey T, Taylor C, Parker G: Comparison of model-based arterial input functions for dynamic contrast-enhanced MRI in tumor bearing rats. *Magn Reson Med* 2009; 61(5):1173.

15. Ashton E, Remick S, Tolcher A et al.: Assessment of pharmacodynamic effect in a phase I study of MN-029, and IV administered vascular disruptive agent, using dynamic contrast-enhanced MRI. In: *Proceedings of ECCO*, Barcelona, Spain, 2007 (abstract 1001).

16. Sorensen A, Tievsky A, Ostergaard L, Weisskoff R, Rosen B: Contrast agents in functional MR imaging. *J Magn Reson Imag* 1997; 7(1):47.

17. Bruening R: Effects of three different doses of a bolus injection of gadodiamide: Assessment of regional cerebral blood volume maps in a blinded reader study. *Am J Neuroradiol* 2000; 21(9):1603.

18. Marckmann P, Skov L, Rossen K et al.: Nephrogenic systemic fibrosis: Suspected causative role of gadodiamide used for contrast-enhanced magnetic resonance imaging. *J Am Soc Nephrol* 2006; 17:2359.

19. Rausch M, Scheffler K, Rudin M, Radu E: Analysis of input functions from different arterial branches with gamma variate functions and cluster analysis for quantitative blood volume measurements. *Magn Reson Imag* 2000; 18(10):1235–1243.

20. Collins D, Padhani A: Dynamic magnetic resonance imaging of tumor perfusion—Approaches and biomedical challenges. *IEEE Eng Med Bio Mag* 2004; 65–83.

21. Weinmann HJ, Laniado M, Mutzel W: Pharmacokinetics of Gd-DTPA/dimeglumine after intravenous injection into healthy volunteers. *Physiol Chem Phys Med NMR* 1984; 16:167.

22. Padhani A, Hayes C, Landau S, Leach M: Reproducibility of quantitative dynamic MRI of normal human tissues. *NMR Biomed* 2002; 15:143.

23. Galbraith S, Lodge M, Taylor N et al.: Reproducibility of dynamic contrast-enhanced MRI in human muscle and tumours: Comparison of quantitative and semi-quantitative analysis. *NMR Biomed* 2002; 15:132.

24. Vonken E, Osch M, Bakker C, Viergever M: Measurement of cerebral perfusion with dual-echo multi-slice quantitative dynamic susceptibility contrast MRI. *J Magn Reson Imag* 1999; 10:109.

25. Ashton E, McShane T, Evelhoch J: Inter-operator variability in perfusion assessment of tumors in MRI using automated AIF detection. *LNCS* 2005; 3749:451.

26. Rijpkema M, Kaanders J, Joosten F, Van Der Kogel A, Heerschap A: Method for quantitative mapping of dynamic MRI contrast agent enhancement in human tumors. *J Magn Reson Imag* 2001; 14:457.

27. Shah V, Turkbey B, Pang Y, Liu W, Choyke P, Bernardo M: Population-averaged arterial input function for dynamic-contrast enhanced MRI obtained with inflow suppression and B1 correction. In *In vivo Studies & Development/Novel Use of Imaging Probes*, World Molecular Imaging Congress, Kyoto Japan, September 8, 2010.

28. Walker-Samuel S, Leach M, Collins D: Reference tissue quantification of DCE-MRI data without a contrast agent calibration. *Phys Med Biol* 2007; 52:589.

29. Ashton E: Quantitative medical imaging. *J Imag Sci Technol* 2007; 51:117.

30. Ashton E, Raunig D, Ng C, Kelcz F, McShane T, Evelhoch J: Scan-rescan variability in perfusion assessment of tumors in MRI using both model and data-derived arterial input functions. *J Magn Reson Imag* 2008; 28:791.

31. Kovar D, Lewis M, Karczmar G: A new method for imaging perfusion and contrast extraction fraction: Input functions derived from reference tissues. *J Magn Reson Imag* 1998; 8(5):1126.

32. Yang C, Karczmar G, Medved M, Stadler W: Estimating the arterial input function using two reference tissues in dynamic contrast-enhanced MRI studies: Fundamental concepts and simulations. *Magn Reson Med* 2004; 52:1110.

33. Faranesh A, Yankeelov T: Incorporating a vascular term into a reference region model for the analysis of DCE-MRI data: A simulation study. *Phys Med Biol* 2008; 53:2617.

34. Hsiao I, Liao Y, Liu H: Study of onset time-shift and injection duration in DCE-MRI: A comparison of a reference region model with the general kinetic model. *NMR Biomed* 2010; 23(4):375.

35. Ashton E, Durkin E, Kwok E, Evelhoch J: Conversion from signal intensity to Gd concentration may be unnecessary for perfusion assessment of tumors using DCE-MRI. In: *Proceedings of the 15th Annual Meeting of ISMRM*, Berlin, 2007. (abstract 2813).

36. Leach M, Brindle K, Evelhoch J et al.: The assessment of antiangiogenic and antivascular therapies in early-stage clinical trials using magnetic resonance imaging: Issues and recommendations. *Br J Cancer* 2005; 92:1599.

37. Tofts P, Brix G, Buckley D et al.: Estimating kinetic parameters from dynamic contrast-enhanced T_1-weighted MRI of a diffusable tracer: Standardized quantities and symbols. *J Magn Reson Imag* 1999; 10:223.

38. Landau H: Sampling, data transmission, and the Nyquist rate. *Proc IEEE* 1967; 55:1701.

39. Huang W, Carney P, Tudorica L et al.: Approaching complete separation of benign and malignant breast lesions by DCE-MRI: Impact on healthcare costs. In: *Proceedings of the 18th Annual Meeting of ISMRM*, Stockholm, 2010. (abstract 987).

40. Buckley D: Uncertainty in the analysis of tracer kinetics using dynamic contrast-enhanced T1-weighted MRI. *Magn Reson Med* 2002; 47(3):601.

41. Koh T, Tan C, Cheong L, Lim C: Cerebral perfusion mapping using a robust and efficient method for deconvolution analysis of dynamic contrast-enhanced images. *NeuroImage* 2006; 32:643.

42. Thng C, Hartono S, Koh T et al.: Dynamic contrast enhanced MRI (DCE MRI) for Phase I anti-angiogenic tiral: Comparison of the transfer constant (Ktrans) to blood flow and permeability derived by a distributed parameter model. *J Clin Oncol* 2008; 26 (May 20 suppl; abstr 3514).

43. Li K, Wilmes L, Henry R et al.: Heterogeneity in the angiogenic response of a BT474 human breast cancer to a novel vascular endothelial growth factor-receptor tyrosine kinase inhibitor: Assessment by voxel analysis of dynamic contrast-enhanced MRI. *J Magn Reson Imag* 2005; 22:511.

44. Huang W, Lid X, Morris E, Tudorica L, Seshan V, Rooney W, Tagged I, Wang Y, Xu J, Springer, Jr. C: The magnetic resonance shutter speed discriminates vascular properties of malignant and benign breast tumors in vivo. *PNAS* 2008; 105(46):17,947.

45. Lowry M, Zelhof B, Liney G, Gibbs P, Pickles M, Turnbull L: Analysis of prostate DCE-MRI: Comparison of fast exchange limit and fast exchange regimen pharmacokinetic models in the discrimination of malignant from normal tissue. *Investigative Radiol* 2009; 44(9):577.

46. Ahearn T, Staff R, Redpath T, Semple S: The use of the Levenberg-Marquardt curve-fitting algorithm in pharmacokinetic modeling of DCE-MRI data. *Phys Med Biol* 2005; 50:85.

47. Horsfield M, Morgan B: Algorithms for calculation of kinetic parameters from T1-weighted dynamic contrast-enhanced magnetic resonance imaging. *J Magn Reson Imag* 2004; 20:723.

48. Cheng H: Investigation and optimization of parameter accuracy in dynamic contrast-enhanced MRI. *J Magn Reson Imag* 2008; 28:736.

49. Gribbestad I, Nilsen G, Fjosne H et al.: Comparative signal intensity measurements in dynamic gadolinium-enhanced MR mammography. *J Magn Reson Imag* 1994; 4:477.

50. Teifke A, Behr O, Schmidt M et al.: Dynamic MR imaging of breast lesions: correlation with microvessel distribution pattern and histological characteristics of prognosis. *Radiology* 2006; 239:351.

51. Gaustad J, Benjaminsen I, Graff B et al.: Intratumor heterogeneity in blood perfusion in orthotopic human melanoma xenografts assessed by dynamic contrast-enhanced magnetic resonance imaging. *J Magn Reson Imag* 2005; 21:792.

52. Jackson A, Kassner A, Annesley-Williams D et al.: Abnormalities in the recirculation phase of contrast agent bolus passage in cerebral gliomas: Comparison with relative blood volume and tumor grade. *Am J Neuroradiol* 2002; 23:7.

53. Jackson A, O'Connor JP, Parker GJ et al.: Imaging tumor vascular heterogeneity and angiogenesis using dynamic contrast-enhanced magnetic resonance imaging. *Clin Cancer Res* 2007; 13:3449.

54. Gribbestad I, Gjesdal K, Nilsen G et al.: An introduction to dynamic contrast-enhanced MRI in oncology. In: *Dynamic Contrast-Enhanced MRI in Oncology* (Jackson A, Buckley DL, Parker GJ, eds.), 1st edition. Berlin/Heidelberg (NY): Springer; 2005; 1:3.

55. Orton M, Miyazaki K, Koh D, Collins D, Hawkes D, Atkinson D, Leach M: Optimizing functional parameter accuracy for breath-hold DCE-MRI of liver tumors. *Phys Med Biol* 2009; 54:2197.

56. Melbourne A, Atkinson D, White M, Collins D, Leach M, Hawkes D: Registration of dynamic contrast-enhanced MRI using a progressive principal component registration (PPCR). *Phys Med Biol* 2007; 52:5147.

57. Parker G, Suckling J, Tanner S et al.: MRI: Parameteric analysis software for contrast-enhanced dynamic MR imaging in cancer. *Radiographics* 1998; 18:497.

58. Parker G, Buckley D: Tracer kinetic modeling for T1-weighted DCE-MR imaging. In: *Dynamic Contrast-Enhanced Magnetic Resonance Imaging in Oncology* (Jackson A, Parker GJ, Buckley DL, eds.), 1st Edition. Berlin/Heidelberg (NY): Springer; 2005; 1:81.

59. de Lussanet Q, Backes W, Griffioen A et al.: Dynamic contrast-enhanced magnetic resonance imaging of radiation therapy-induced microcirculation changes in rectal cancer. *Int J Radiat Oncol Biol Phys* 2005; 63:1309.

60. Rose C, Mills S, O'Connor J et al.: Quantifying heterogeneity in dynamic contrast-enhanced MRI parameter maps. In: *Lecture Notes in Computer Science* (Ayache N, Ourselin A, Maeder A, eds.), Verlag/Berlin/Heidelberg (NY): Springer; 2007; 4792:376.

61. Rose C, Mills S, O'Connor J: Quantifying spatial heterogeneity in dynamic contrast-enhanced MRI parameter maps. *Magn Reson Med* 2009; 62:488.

62. Moffat B, Chenevert T, Lawrence T et al.: Functional diffusion map: a noninvasive MRI biomarker for early stratification of clinical brain tumor response. *Proc Natl Acad Sci USA* 2005; 102:5524.

63. Twellmann T, Saalbach A, Gerstung O, Leach M, Nattkemper T: Image fusion for dynamic contrast enhanced magnetic resonance imaging. *BioMedical Eng Online* 2004; 3:35.

64. Twellmann T, Meyer-Baese A, Lange O, Foo S, Nattkemper T: Model–free visualization of suspicious lesions in breast MRI based on supervised and unsupervised learning. *Eng Appl Artif Intell* 2008; 21(2):129.

65. Khouli R, Macura K, Jacobs M, Khalil T, Kamel I, Dwyer A, Bluemke D: Dynamic contrast-enhanced MRI of the breast: Quantitative method for kinetic curve type assessment. *Am J Radiol* 2009; 193:295.

66. Leinsinger G, Schlossbauer T, Scherr M, Lange O, Reiser M, Wismuller A: Cluster analysis of signal-intensity time course in dynamic breast MRI: Does unsupervised vector quantization help to evaluate small mammographic lesions? *Eur Radiol* 2006; 16:1138.

67. Kubassova O, Boesen M, Boyle R, Cimmino M, Jensen K, Bliddal H, Radjenovic A: Fast and robust analysis of dynamic contrast enhanced MRI datasets. *Med Image Comput Comput Assist Interv* 2007; 10(2):261.

68. Herbst R, Onn A, Sandler A: Angiogenesis and lung cancer: Prognostic and therapeutic implications. *J Clin Oncol* 2005; 23:3243.

69. Mross K, Drevs J, Muller M, Medinger M, Marme D, Hennig J, Morgan B, Lebwohl D, Masson E, Ho Y: Phase I clinical and pharmacokinetic study of PTK/ZK, a multiple VEGF receptor inhibitor, in patients with liver metastases from solid tumors. *Eur J Cancer* 2005; 41:1291.

70. Ashton E: Quantitative MR in multi-center clinical trials. *J Magn Reson Imag* 2010; 31:279.

71. Collins J: Imaging and other biomarkers in early clinical studies: Ones step at a time or re-engineering drug development? *J Clin Oncol* 2005; 23:5417.

72. Flaherty K, Rosen M, Heitjan D, Gallagher M, Schwartz B, Schnall M, O'Dwyer P: Pilot study of DCE-MRI to predict progression-free survival with Sorafenib therapy in renal cell carcinoma. *Cancer Biol Therapy* 2008; 7:496.

73. Hahn O, Yang C, Medved M, Karczmar G, Kistner E, Karrison T, Manchen E, Mitchell M, Ratain M, Stadler W: Dynamic contrast-enhanced magnetic resonance imaging pharmacodynamic biomarker study of Sorafenib in metastatic renal carcinoma. *J Clin Oncol* 2008; 26:4572.

74. Ashton E: Early DCE-MRI findings predict tumor volume changes. In: *Proceedings of the 17th Annual Meeting of ISMRM*, Honolulu, 2009. (abstract 806).

75. Ashton E, Raunig D, Ng C, Kelcz F, McShane T, Evelhoch J: Scan-rescan variability in perfusion assessment of tumors in MRI using both model and data-derived arterial input functions. *J Magn Reson Imag* 2008; 28:791.

76. O'Connor J, Jackson A, Parker G, Jayson G: DCE-MRI biomarkers in the clinical evaluation of anti-angiogenic and vascular disrupting agents. *Br J Cancer* 2007; 96:189.

18

MRI of Myocardial Deformations: Imaging and Modeling

Hui Wang
University of Louisville

Amir A. Amini
University of Louisville

Globally, cardiovascular diseases (CVD) are the number one cause of death and are projected to remain so. An estimated 17 million people died from CVD in 2005, representing 30% of all global deaths. Among these deaths, 7.2 million were due to heart attacks and 5.7 million were due to stroke. If current trends continue, by 2030, an estimated 23.6 million people will die from CVD in the world [138]. In America, an estimated 80 million adults (more than one in three) have one or more types of CVD. In 2005, about 864,000 people died of CVD, accounting for 35.3% of all deaths [8].

Heart disease, such as myocardial ischemia, secondary to coronary artery disease, may be identified and localized through the analysis of the cardiac deformation. Early efforts for quantifying ventricular wall motion used surgical implantation and tracking of radiopaque markers with x-ray imaging in canine hearts [47]. Such techniques are invasive and affect the regional motion pattern of the ventricular wall during the marker tracking process and, clearly are not feasible clinically. Noninvasive imaging techniques are vital and have been widely applied to clinical use. Magnetic resonance imaging (MRI) is a noninvasive imaging technique with the capability to monitor and assess the progression of CVD so that effective procedures for the care and treatment of patients can be developed by physicians and researchers. MRI can provide three-dimensional (3D) analysis of global and regional cardiac function with great accuracy and reproducibility [23]. In the past few years, numerous efforts have been devoted to cardiac imaging techniques for deformation recovery. Many approaches have been proposed for tracking cardiac motion and for computing deformation parameters and mechanical properties of the heart from a variety of cardiac MR imaging techniques.

There are many techniques available nowadays for cardiac imaging which provide qualitative and quantitative measurements of cardiac function. MRI is a highly advanced and sophisticated imaging modality for cardiac motion assessment and quantitative analysis. In the realm of MRI, cardiac cine MRI is considered as the standard technique for measuring global function parameters, for example, ejection fraction, cavity volume, and myocardial mass [23]. It also can reveal important regional function parameters, such as wall thickness. MR tagging [17,145] is a well-known method to track local deformations. Local parameters such as twist, strain, and strain rate can be derived from tagged MRI. Other techniques, such as phase contrast MRI (PCMRI), displacement encoding with stimulated echoes imaging (DENSE), and strain encoding (SENC), can also reveal regional properties of the heart. Several review papers have previously been published in the field of deformation recovery from cardiac MR imaging [18,23,40,153]. This chapter describes cardiac MR image acquisition techniques as well as image analysis techniques for recovery of ventricular deformations from the acquired images.

The organization of this chapter is as follows. Section 18.1 gives a review of cardiac cine MRI pulse sequences and motion analysis techniques from cine MR images. Section 18.2 gives an overview of tagged MRI techniques and the associated image analysis methods. A novel acquisition technique, termed Orthogonal CSPAMM, is included in this section. Section 18.3 summarizes phase contrast MRI for cardiac deformation recovery. Sections 18.4 and 18.5 introduce two more recent techniques: DENSE and SENC. Strain is an important kinematic index, revealing fractional change in length of a continuously deforming body. Section 18.6 provides a review of prior work on strain analysis from cardiac MRI. Conclusions and future research trends are provided in Section 18.7.

18.1 Cine MRI

Cardiac cine MRI is widely used clinically due to its high soft-tissue contrast. The temporal resolution is also high enough to do motion tracking over the cardiac cycle. It is the gold standard for noninvasively quantifying global *in vivo* heart function and for measuring ejection fraction, cavity volume, and mass.

18.1.1 Cine MR Imaging

Cine gradient echo sequences, often known as bright blood sequences, are commonly used for evaluating cardiac function. Blood appears bright in these sequences due to the contrast properties of blood and its rapid flow. The technique can discriminate between blood and myocardium very well. Two imaging pulse sequences are most commonly used for acquiring cine MRI: spoiled gradient echo (GRE) and balanced steady-state free precession (b-SSFP). b-SSFP can yield better signal-to-noise ratio (SNR) and contrast-to-noise ratio (CNR) than spoiled GRE and is less sensitive to motion-induced signal loss. Therefore, cine MR images using b-SSFP appear more uniform within the blood and are darker in the myocardium. b-SSFP gradient echo sequences have largely replaced spoiled gradient echo sequences for this purpose. Different trade names for these b-SSFP sequences are TrueFISP (True Fast Imaging with Steady-State Precession; Siemens), FIESTA (Fast Imaging Employing Steady-State Acquisition; GE), and b-FFE (Balanced Fast-Field Echo; Phillips). These sequences are typically used in conjunction with segmented *k*-space acquisition. Segmented acquisition is the process of dividing the cardiac cycle into multiple segments (phases) to produce a series of images that can be displayed as a movie (cine). Each image in the cine is typically constructed from information gathered over several heart beats—within a breath hold of 10–20 s depending on the sequence. Figures 18.1 and 18.2 show a sequence of short-axis (SA) and long-axis (LA) cine images, respectively. Thirty frames were required using a b-FFE sequence on a Philips 3T Achieva scanner showing the contraction wave during the cardiac cycle. One-third of them have been displayed here. The first row shows systolic images and the second row shows diastolic images.

In cine MRI, there are multiple cardiac phases in one cardiac cycle, usually between 20 and 30, depending on the temporal resolution (30–50 ms per frame). Although it is possible to image the heart in real time with cine MRI, the resulting image quality is poor. Instead, most sequences use electrocardiogram

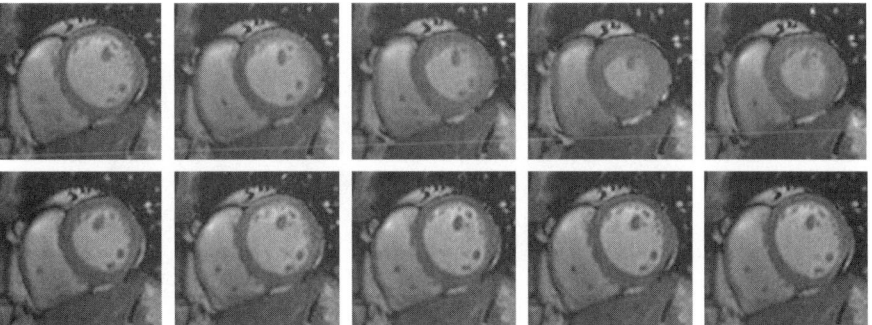

FIGURE 18.1 A sequence of short-axis cine images acquired with b-FFE on a Philips Achieva 3T scanner. Ten out of thirty phases are shown from the top left to bottom right. The first row shows systolic images and the second row shows the diastolic images. Imaging parameters were as follows: TE = 1.603 ms, slice thickness = 8 mm, spatial resolution = 1.25×1.25 mm^2, acquisition matrix = 160×187, flip angle = 45°. A phased-array thoracic coil with 16 elements was used.

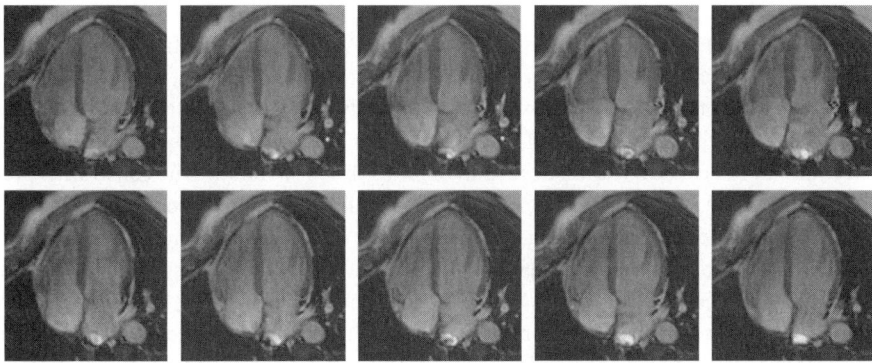

FIGURE 18.2 A sequence of long-axis cine images acquired with b-FFE on a Philips Achieva 3T scanner in the same volunteer whose short-axis images were shown in Figure 18.1. Ten out of thirty phases are shown from the top left to bottom right. The first row shows systolic images and the second row shows diastolic images. Imaging parameters were as follows: TE = 1.737 ms, slice thickness = 8 mm, spatial resolution = 1.21×1.21 mm^2, acquisition matrix = 176×211, flip angle = 45°. A phased-array thoracic coil with 16 elements was used.

(ECG) gating to acquire images at each stage of the cardiac cycle over several heart beats. This technique is the primary basis for functional assessment by cine MRI. During one cardiac cycle, ECG-gated cine MRI acquires one segment of image raw data for each cardiac phase, as shown in Figure 18.3. Multiple segments comprising the complete k-space raw data are acquired in multiple heartbeats. With the help of a phased-array radio frequency (RF) receiver coil and parallel image acquisition and reconstruction techniques, typical scan times of 6–7 heartbeats per slice are now routine. The in-plane spatial resolution of cine MRI is on the order of 1.5×2 mm^2. The slice thickness is between 5 and 10 mm [40]. Multiple 2D-imaged slices may be stacked to construct a 3D volume for each cardiac phase.

18.1.2 Deformation Recovery from Cine MR Images

Since to a large extent the myocardium appears homogeneous in cine MR images, cine MRI cannot directly provide information on myocardial motion patterns, for example, relative rotation of the endocardial layer relative to the epicardial layer (transmural shear), or of basal slices with respect to apical slices (torsion) [128]. The most commonly used features in cine MRI are endocardial and epicardial

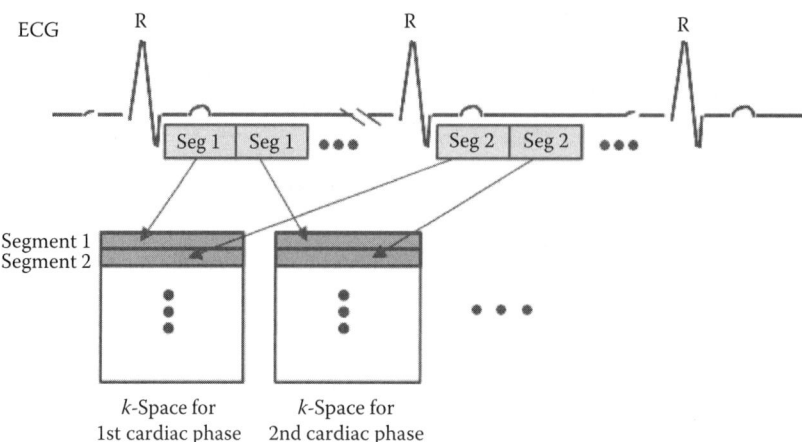

FIGURE 18.3 Schematic diagram of ECG-gated breath-hold cine MRI. There are multiple cardiac phases in one cardiac cycle. For each phase, a segment is acquired in one heart beat.

contours, or specific feature points on these contours. For motion analysis from cine MRI, a useful model that could be utilized is its incompressibility. One strategy for motion tracking may be to first track sparse feature points on the contours and subsequently perform dense motion field reconstruction. Reconstruction of the dense motion field from a sparse set of landmarks is an ill-posed problem and therefore additional constraints are needed to obtain a unique solution. The constraints previously proposed in the literature are either mathematical or mechanical, enforcing smoothness of the deformation field subject to additional requirements [20,21,140]. The other strategy is to use image registration [97,124,130,131], either for the whole image or for some feature points. Due to the substantial challenges in deformation recovery from cine MRI, including significant modeling needs, it is reasonable to assume that the accuracy of cine MRI deformation recovery techniques is not on par with the methods that will be described later in this chapter. In the rest of this section, a detailed review of cardiac motion tracking methods based on cine MRI is provided.

18.1.2.1 Incompressible Deformable Models

Aside from the effect of blood perfusion, which will alter myocardial volume, the myocardium is nearly incompressible. The common conclusion regarding myocardial volume change is that it is no more than 4% during the cardiac cycle [20]. Song et al. [121] were the first in applying divergence-free and incompressibility constraints to construct 3D velocity field inside the heart though utilizing 3D CT data. Based on the assumptions that myocardium is almost incompressible and that there is no transmural bending during myocardial movement, Bistoquet et al. [20] proposed an incompressible deformable model to recover the motion of the left ventricle from cine MRI data. The main contribution was that this method modeled the deformation using a new transformation which was the displacements of middle surface nodes between the reference frame and current frame. The framework was extended to biventricular model in Reference 21. Different from the model in Reference 20, the new model had the ability to represent the deformation of structures with arbitrary topologies. The nodes were approximately uniformly spaced over the left ventricle (LV) and right ventricle (RV) wall middle surfaces. A divergence-free matrix-valued radial basis function scheme was used to interpolate the displacements at the nodes.

18.1.2.2 Registration-Based Methods

Veress et al. [130,131] proposed a deformable registration technique, called hyperelastic warping, to determine left ventricular strains from mid-diastole to end-diastole using multiple slices SA cine MR images. A finite element (FE) model was deformed by the difference in image intensities as a body force and a hyperelastic strain energy based on continuum mechanics as the regularization force. The boundaries of the LV were manually segmented for both epicardium and endocardium. The myocardium was represented as transversely isotropic hyperelastic with fiber angles varying from −90° at the epicardial surface to 90° at the endocardial surface. Phatak et al. [98] validated hyperelastic warping for LV strain measurement during systole, by comparing circumferential and radial strains with results obtained from HARP [83]. Image-based forces driving deformations were combined with a computational model which included estimated myocardial material properties, fiber direction, and active fiber contraction. Different from diastole, where the forces acting on the myocardium are passive and are associated with diastolic filling, the forces in systole are active and are generated by myofiber contraction, making the model more complicated. A transversely isotropic hyperelastic constitutive model was utilized to represent the myocardium.

Shen and Sundar et al. [117,124] used a 4D image registration method to estimate cardiac motion. This framework considered registering the first frame to all other frames simultaneously. An attribute vector for every point in the image was used to contain information about intensity, boundary, and geometric moment invariants. Perperidis et al. [97] proposed two B-spline-based free-form registration methods for the spatiotemporal alignment of cardiac MR image sequences. It extended Ruckert's framework [108] to 4D B-spline tensor products and enabled comparison between corresponding anatomy at different temporal positions in the cardiac cycle. These two B-splines methods used the same transformation. The difference between them was the order of the optimization process. One performed a combined optimization with spatial and temporal components. The other optimized each component separately. Chenuoune et al. [30] proposed a method to assess relative circumferential shortening strain of endocardium by segmenting endocardial contours of a 2D + t SA cine MR data set using a level set method and then matched these contours using a morphing registration method. This method only tracked the endocardial contours for 2D SA images.

18.1.2.3 Feature-Based Tracking Methods

This category is usually involved in segmenting the ventricular wall first followed by tracking the movement of feature points, such as epicardial and endocardial boundaries [30], geometric measure as tracking tokens [66,67,120,140]. Quantifying the boundary motion of nonrigid body from feature points is often treated as a two-step process: first establishing correspondence between sampled points on the boundaries at two time points, then finding the transformation for every point on the boundaries according to the feature point correspondences.

Amini and Duncan [11] used principal surface curvatures to track local bending and stretching of the left ventricular endocardial wall. Surface patches around geometrically significant landmark points were modeled as thin plates. Subsequently, a smoothing procedure was employed to generate a dense motion field. McEachen et al. [74] proposed a method to track the LV endocardial contour. Presegmented endocardial contours at each frame were the input to this method. Correspondence of tokens with geometric properties on the contours were determined by shape-based tracking. An adaptive filtering scheme was used to produce a set of sinusoidal parameters that represent quantified motion trajectories. Three-dimensional motion trajectory of the endocardial surface can be recovered by locating and matching differential surface properties [120]. These trajectories were then used to deform a mesh that represented the left ventricular myocardial surfaces.

Lin et al. proposed a generalized robust point matching (G-RPM) framework [67] to track the motion of left ventricle and extended this framework using extended free-form deformation (EFFD) as regularization model [66]. Different from free-form deformation (FFD) which uses parallelepipedical lattice, the EFFD model employed an arbitrarily shaped lattice. Feature points were extracted according to the curvatures. Under G-RPM framework, Pan et al. [140] proposed a new regularization model based on the boundary element method (BEM) to estimate dense displacement fields and strains from 3D cine MRI sequences of the LV. This method was also applicable to 4D echocardiographic image sequences. The most attractive feature of BEM over FEM is that it only requires discretization of the surface rather than the volume. In order to automatically obtain the endocardial and epicardial contours and feature points, Zhu et al. [149,152] proposed an integrated Bayesian framework to segment LV and estimate its motion. The feature points were extracted from the narrowband of segmented contours and the motion estimation was accomplished by BEM-GRPM algorithm [140].

Shi et al. [119] used both image-derived information from myocardial surfaces and the mid-wall from phase contrast MRI. This method combined image-derived information and mechanical modeling of the myocardium, using FEM to solve for deformations. Papademetris et al. [90] validated strains derived from 3D cine MRI and 3D echocardiography images using shape-based tracking. The dense motion field was obtained from integrating a transversely linear elastic model and sparse displacements using a shape-tracking method. Papademetris et al. [91] utilized a symmetric nearest neighbor algorithm for initialization in the shape-tracking step, instead of nearest neighbor [120].

Remme et al. [105] proposed a modality-independent method to analyze LV motion from anatomic modalities, using fiducial marker fitting in conjunction with a parameter distribution model. A FEM mesh was constructed according to the geometry of the myocardium and deformed by optimizing the nodal parameters to the motion of a sparse number of manually tracked fiducial markers. In order to overcome the sparsity of the fiducial markers, *a priori* information from tagged MRI database on the probability distribution of possible LV motion was incorporated.

18.2 Tagged MRI

18.2.1 Acquisition

Myocardial tagging was first introduced by Zerhouni et al. [145] and Axel et al. [17] in 1988 and 1989, respectively. It uses spin tagging prepulses to produce noninvasive markers in the myocardial tissues. The main reason why tagged MRI can image motion is that when the local magnetization of a material point is altered, the material point maintains the altered magnetization when it moves within the limits of the T_1 relaxation time. The process of MR tagging uses a special pulse sequence to spatially modulate the longitudinal magnetization, prior to image acquisition using conventional imaging, as shown in Figure 18.4. The varying magnetization produces alternating light and dark pattern on the image. Spatial modulation of magnetization (SPAMM) [17] is the most commonly used technique to produce sinusoidal tag patterns. Optimal tagging and acquisition of MR images for cardiac motion analysis were investigated by Nguyen et al. [81]. Pai and Axel [87] gave a thorough review of tagged cardiac MR imaging methods, including advances in pulse sequence development, image acquisition, high temporal and spatial resolution imaging, high field strength imaging, and 3D whole heart tagging. A review covering the current clinical applications of myocardial tagging can be found in Reference 116.

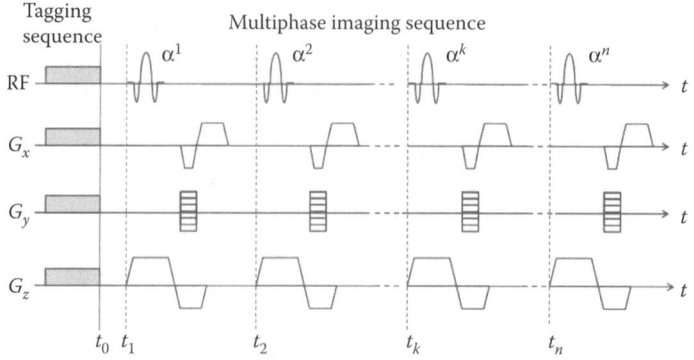

FIGURE 18.4 Timing diagram of a typical tagging experiment. A tagging sequence is followed by a standard multiphase imaging sequence. t_i corresponds to the start of the *i*th phase in the cardiac cycle.

18.2.1.1 Spatial Modulation of Magnetization

The SPAMM myocardial tagging technique is widely available commercially [17,145] and is the most commonly used technique for producing sinusoidal tag patterns. Figure 18.5 (left) shows a one-dimensional 1–1 SPAMM sequence with two 90° RF pulses, an interspersed tagging gradient in the readout direction, and a spoiler gradient. Before the first RF pulse, magnetization in rotating frame is initially all polarized along the main magnetic field (in the z direction) (Figure 18.5a). The first RF pulse flips the initial longitudinal magnetization into the transverse plane (Figure 18.5b). The gradient G_t produces a periodic spatial modulation of the phase of the transverse magnetization along the gradient direction (Figure 18.5c). The second RF pulse produces modulated longitudinal magnetization (Figure 18.5d). A tag grid can be produced by following the second RF pulse with a second gradient in the direction orthogonal to the first gradient and then with another RF pulse. Some tagged and untagged images from a canine are shown in Figure 18.6. In the subsequent imaging step, the spatially modulated longitudinal magnetization is made visible by the RF pulse which flips it to the transverse plane, followed with phase-encoding and read-out. The tag lines are not sharp, but have sinusoidal variation of intensity in the image (Figure 18.5d). Sharper tagging stripes can be obtained by using more binomially distributed RF pulses that are each separated by dephasing gradients [16]. The effect of the SPAMM pulse sequence is to produce a series of stripes in the acquired images. As shown in Figure 18.7, the tag lines fade at the end of the cardiac cycle.

18.2.1.2 Complementary Spatial Modulation of Magnetization

Complementary SPAMM (CSPAMM) was introduced by Fischer et al. to improve tagging contrast in later phases of the cardiac cycle [42]. CSPAMM is based on the subtraction of two images with complementary signed tagging modulation. Compared to SPAMM, CSPAMM has the ability to eliminate the DC interference of the off-center peaks, resulting in significant improvement of tagging contrast in later phases of the cardiac cycle [42]. The diagram for the CSPAMM pulse sequence is shown in Figure 18.8. The tagging pulses in (a) and (b) are out of phase by 180°. By subtracting them, CSPAMM reduces tagline intensity fading and consequently allows longer net tag persistence throughout the heart cycle.

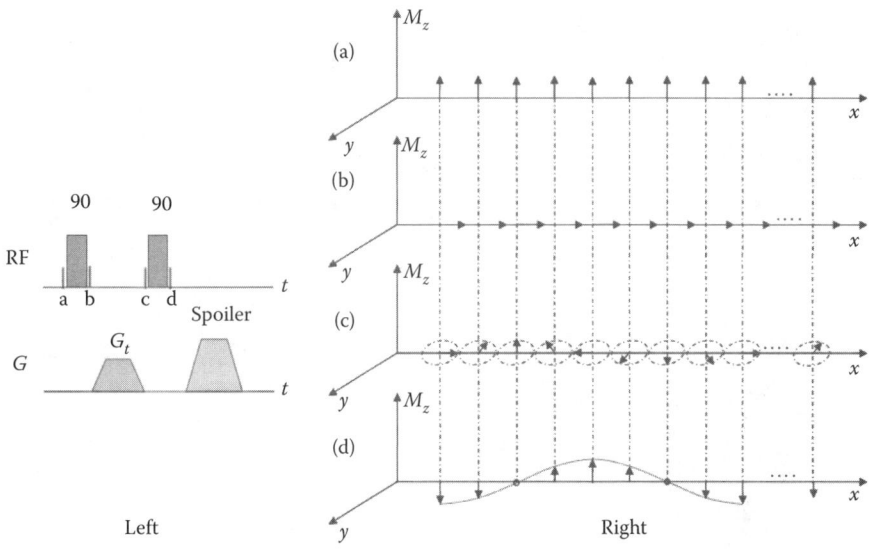

FIGURE 18.5 SPAMM pulse sequence. Left: Timing diagram for SPAMM. RF = nonselective radio-frequency excitation, t = time, G_t = wrap gradient for production of modulation. Letters a–d indicate corresponding time points in the right figures. Right: State of magnetization at different times. (a) Magnetization prior to initiation of the modulation sequence. (b) Magnetization after the first RF pulse. (c) Magnetization after wrap (modulating) gradient pulse. (d) Longitudinal magnetization after second RF pulse.

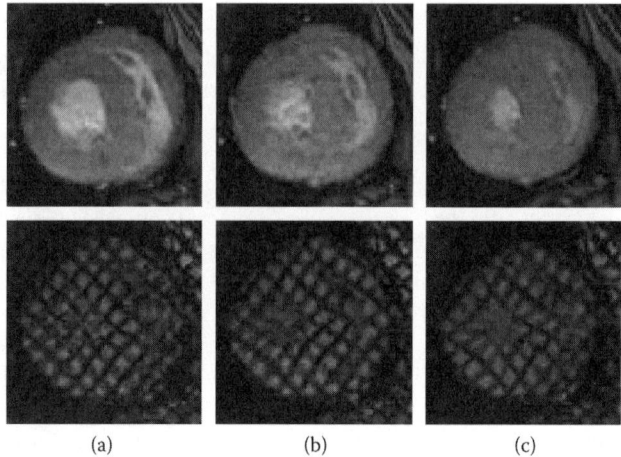

(a)   (b)   (c)

FIGURE 18.6 The top row shows a sequence of short-axis mid-ventricular untagged images acquired in a dog at three different time points in the cardiac cycle. (a) End-diastole, (b) mid-systole, and (c) end-systole. The bottom row shows tagged images at corresponding times and locations. Imaging parameters were as follows: TR/TE = 32/2.8 ms, slice thickness = 8 mm, spatial resolution = 1.17×1.17 mm², flip angle = 20°.

In CSPAMM, the longitudinal magnetization M_z is decomposed into two terms: one for tagging information Q_T, the other for the relaxation part Q_R. A timing diagram of a typical tagging experiment is shown in Figure 18.4. At time t_0 right after the SPAMM tagging sequence, the modulated longitudinal magnetization is

$$M_z(t_0) = M_{ss}TAG(x, y) \tag{18.1}$$

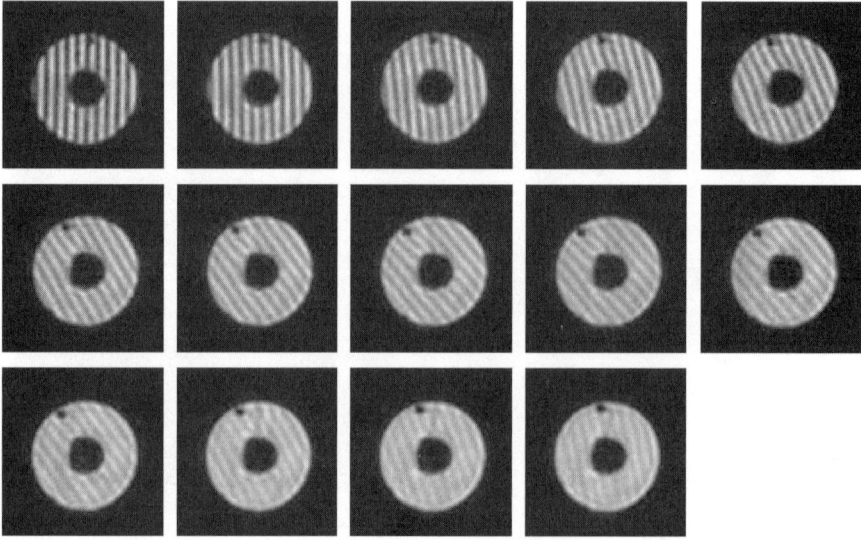

FIGURE 18.7 Fourteen cardiac phases for a rotating phantom imaged during an entire "cardiac cycle" (see Figure 18.15) using the SPAMM pulse sequence: starting at the top left and to the right and bottom. As may be seen, the tags fade as a function of time due to the T_1 effect. Imaging parameters were as follows: TR/TE = 7.9/4.0 ms, slice thickness = 8 mm, spatial resolution = 1.17×1.17 mm², acquisition matrix = 102×112, tag spacing = 6.22 mm, flip angle = 10°.

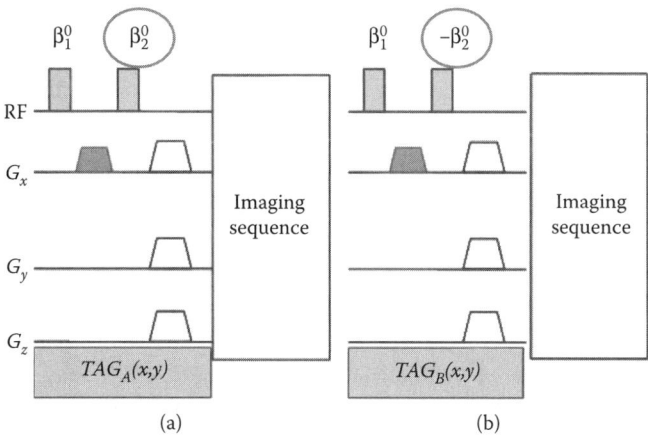

FIGURE 18.8 Timing diagram of a 1–1 CSPAMM sequence. (a) Measurement with positive tagging pattern $TAG_A(x,y)$. (b) Measurement with negative tagging pattern $TAG_B(x,y)$.

where M_{ss} is the steady-state magnetization before tagging and $TAG(x,y)$ represents the spatial modulation of magnetization introduced by tagging sequence. At time t_1

$$
\begin{aligned}
M_z(t_1) &= (M_z(t_0) - M_0)e^{-t_1/T_1} + M_0 \\
&= (M_{ss}TAG(x,y) - M_0)e^{-t_1/T_1} + M_0 \\
&= \underline{M_{ss}TAG(x,y)e^{-t_1/T_1}} + \underline{M_0(1 - e^{-t_1/T_1})} \\
&= Q_{T_1} + Q_{R_1}
\end{aligned}
\tag{18.2}
$$

where M_0 is the equilibrium magnetization and T_1 is the longitudinal relaxation time. At time t_k

$$
\begin{aligned}
M_z(t_k) &= (M_z(t_{k-1}) - M_0)e^{-(t_k-t_{k-1})/T_1} + M_0 \\
&= [(Q_{T_{k-1}} + Q_{R_{k-1}})\cos\alpha_{k-1} - M_0]e^{-(t_k-t_{k-1})/T_1} + M_0 \\
&= (Q_{T_{k-1}}\cos\alpha_{k-1} + Q_{R_{k-1}}\cos\alpha_{k-1} - M_0)e^{-(t_k-t_{k-1})/T_1} + M_0 \\
&= \underline{Q_{T_{k-1}}\cos\alpha_{k-1}e^{-(t_k-t_{k-1})/T_1}} + \underline{(Q_{R_{k-1}}\cos\alpha_{k-1} - M_0)e^{-(t_k-t_{k-1})/T_1} + M_0} \\
&= Q_{T_k} + Q_{R_k}
\end{aligned}
\tag{18.3}
$$

Therefore, the two components of the longitudinal magnetization just before the kth RF pulse are

$$
\begin{aligned}
Q_{T_k} &= Q_{T_{k-1}}\cos\alpha_{k-1}e^{-(t_k-t_{k-1})/T_1} \\
&= (Q_{T_{k-2}}\cos\alpha_{k-2}e^{-(t_{k-1}-t_{k-2})/T_1}\cos\alpha_{k-1}e^{-(t_k-t_{k-1})/T_1} \\
&= \dots \\
&= M_{ss}TAG(x,y)e^{-t_k/T_1}\prod_{j=0}^{k-1}\cos\alpha_j \\
Q_{R_k} &= (Q_{R_{k-1}}\cos\alpha_{k-1} - M_0)e^{-(t_k-t_{k-1})/T_1} + M_0
\end{aligned}
\tag{18.4}
$$

where Q_{T_k} is the tagging component, while Q_{R_k} is the relaxed term. After the kth RF imaging pulse of flip angle α_k, the longitudinal magnetization is rotated to the xy plane which contributes to the kth image.

$$I_k = M_z(t_k)\sin\alpha_k e^{-TE/T_2^*} = (Q_{T_k} + Q_{R_k})\sin\alpha_k e^{-TE/T_2^*} \tag{18.5}$$

The basic idea of CSPAMM is to eliminate the relaxation term Q_{R_k} while only keeping the tagging information term Q_{T_k} by acquiring two images A_k and B_k using the same parameters except for their respective tagging patterns $TAG_A(x,y)$ and $TAG_B(x,y)$ (see Figure 18.8). The subtraction of the kth pair of images leads to

$$A_k - B_k = M_{ss}[TAG_A(x,y) - TAG_B(x,y)]e^{-t_k/T_1}\left(\prod_{j=0}^{k-1}\cos\alpha_j\right)\sin\alpha_k e^{-TE/T_2^*} \tag{18.6}$$

In order to obtain the maximum grid amplitude, the tagging pattern $TAG_A(x,y)$ and $TAG_B(x,y)$ should satisfy the following condition:

$$TAG_A(x,y) + TAG_B(x,y) = 0 \tag{18.7}$$

which will produce the kth tagged image

$$I_k = 2Q_{T_k}\sin\alpha_k e^{-TE/T_2^*} \tag{18.8}$$

Visualization of k-space for an image modulated by a cosine tagging function in the horizontal direction is shown in Figure 18.9 and for the vertical direction is shown in Figure 18.10. In both figures,

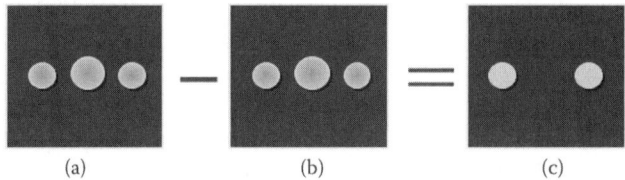

FIGURE 18.9   Visualization of k-space for an image modulated by a cosine in the horizontal direction. (a) k-Space for one SPAMM with positive tagging pattern. (b) k-Space for the other SPAMM with negative tagging pattern. (c) k-Space for CSPAMM.

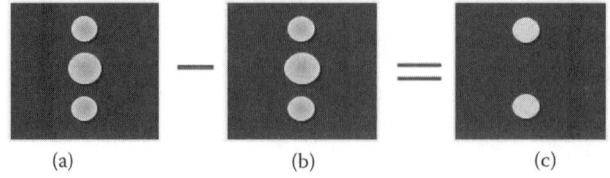

FIGURE 18.10   Visualization of k-space for an image modulated by a cosine in the vertical direction. (a) k-Space for one SPAMM with positive tagging pattern. (b) k-Space for the other SPAMM with negative tagging pattern. (c) k-Space for CSPAMM.

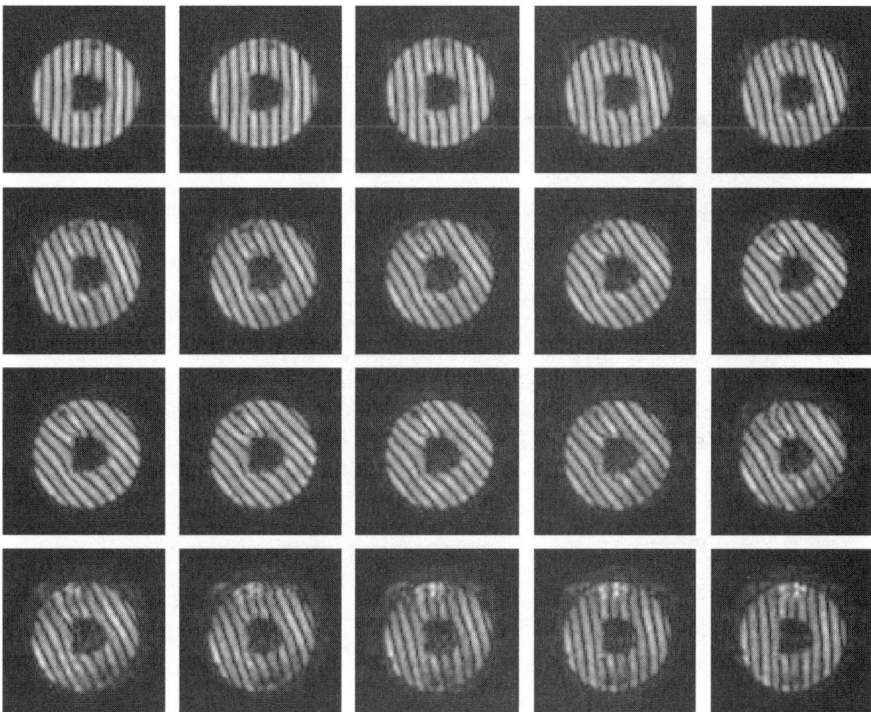

FIGURE 18.11 Twenty cardiac phases during an entire cardiac cycle imaged for a rotating phantom (see Figure 18.15) using CSPAMM pulse sequence. Starting at the top left and traversing to the right and bottom. Imaging parameters were as follows: TR/TE = 12/6.5 ms, slice thickness = 8 mm, spatial resolution = 1.17 × 1.17 mm^2, acquisition matrix = 102 × 112, tag spacing = 6.22 mm, flip angle = 10°.

(a) shows the k-space for the SPAMM with positive tagging pattern, (b) shows the k-space for the other SPAMM with negative tagging pattern, and (c) is the k-space for CSPAMM which is the subtraction of (b) from (a). Figure 18.11 shows a cine sequence of vertical CSPAMM tagging lines on a rotating phantom for the entire cardiac cycle.

18.2.1.3 Orthogonal CSPAMM

In this section, a new tagging pulse sequence, Orthogonal CSPAMM (OCSPAMM), is proposed which acquires tagged data in two orthogonal directions within the same time as the common SPAMM acquisition procedure for creating grid tags. However, relative to SPAMM, OCSPAMM has the advantage of eliminating the DC peak which contributes significantly to the loss of tag-myocardium contrast.

As seen in Figure 18.8, in CSPAMM, two SPAMM tagging sequences 180° out of phase are placed in the same direction, either in frequency encoding or in phase encoding direction, resulting in the need for four separate acquisitions. In the proposed OCSPAMM sequence, the second SPAMM tag orientation is rotated 90° relative to the first so that tag lines in two directions are combined (through subtraction) after only two acquisitions, therefore achieving removing of the central DC peak in k-space. The OCSPAMM sequence timing diagram is shown in Figure 18.12. As may be seen in this figure, the first tagging gradient is in G_x direction, while the second tagging gradient is in G_y direction. A TFE-EPI sequence is used to image the modulated magnetization, as shown in Figure 18.13.

Visualization of k-space for OCSPAMM sequence is shown in Figure 18.14. Similar to the CSPAMM sequence of Figure 18.9, two SPAMM images are subtracted, but unlike the original CSPAMM technique, the second tagged acquisition is orthogonal to the first one. This approach eliminates the DC

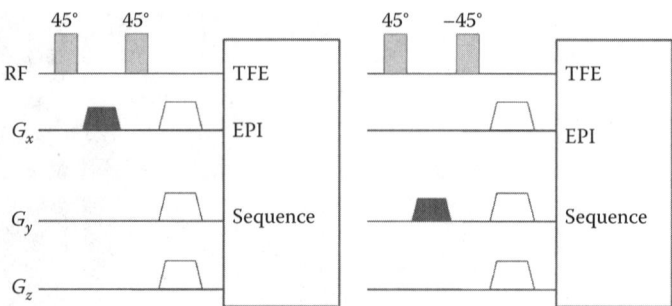

FIGURE 18.12 Timing diagram for the OCSPAMM sequence. The first pair of 45° RF pulses with an interspersed tagging gradient are used to define the tags in G_x direction. The second pair of 45° RF pulses with an interspersed tagging gradient orthogonal to the first tagging gradient are used to define the tags in G_y direction. A TFE-EPI sequence is used for imaging as shown in Figure 18.13.

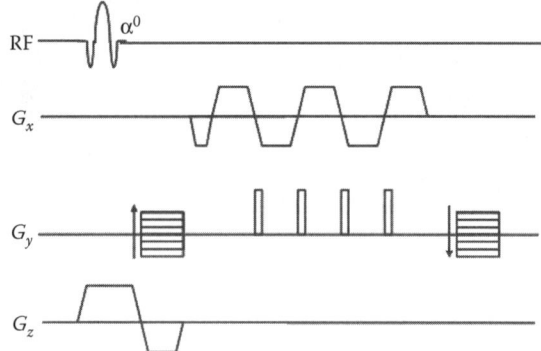

FIGURE 18.13 Timing diagram for the TFE-EPI sequence used for imaging the modulated magnetization with EPI factor 5. After each RF pulse, five k-space profiles are acquired with the help of the blip gradients in phase encoding direction.

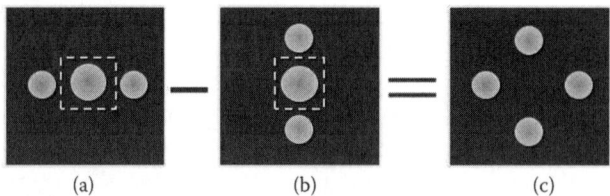

FIGURE 18.14 Visualization of k-space for the OCSPAMM sequence. (a) k-Space for tagged image with positive tagging pattern. (b) k-Space for tagged image with negative tagging pattern in orthogonal direction to (a). (c) k-Space for OCSPAMM.

component while leaving the off-center peaks in k-space intact and reduces the acquisition time by a factor of two when compared to the original CSPAMM technique.

All imaging experiments were conducted on a 3T Achieva MR scanner (Philips Healthcare, Best, NL) using a two-element receive coil. The tag line distance is 7 mm. The phantom was imaged using a turbo field echo-echo planar imaging (TFE-EPI) cine pulse sequence (Figure 18.13) with the following parameters: TR/TE = 9.1/4.7 ms, 10° flip angle, turbo factor 7, FOV 225 × 225 mm², in-plane voxel size 2 × 2 mm², reconstruction resolution 1.25 × 1.25 mm², slice thickness 8 mm, 14 heart phases, 112 × 85

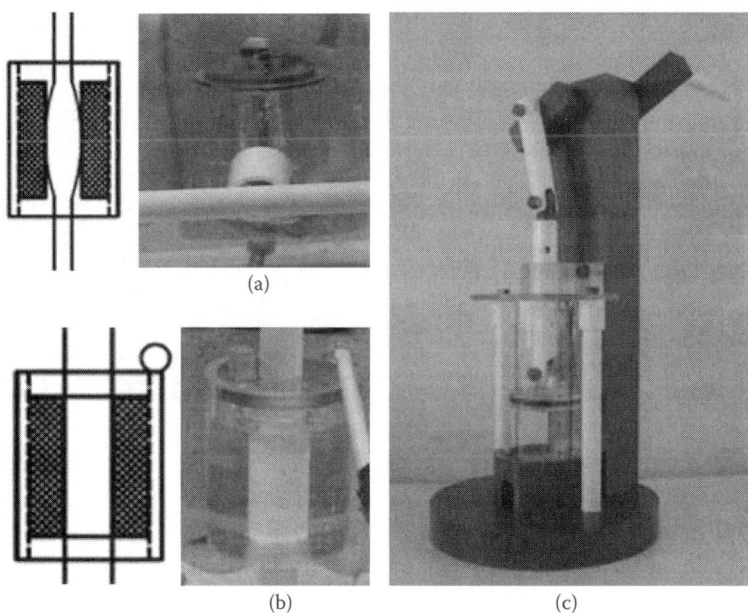

FIGURE 18.15 Phantom components. (a) Contraction motion phantom. (b) Rotation motion phantom. (c) Air pump.

acquired matrix, EPI factor 5. The cardiac cycle was approximately 1000 ms and T_1 of dielectric gel in the phantom was 728 ms (similar to myocardial tissue, *in vivo*).

A cardiac motion phantom, which independently models myocardial wall thickening and rotation in the human heart, was utilized to test the proposed OCSPAMM pulse sequence. The main elements of the LV motion phantom are the air pump, two phantoms within a common enclosure, trigger circuit, and rotation motion actuator. The two phantoms and the air pump are shown in Figure 18.15. Other than the triggering circuit, all materials used in construction of the phantom were nonferromagnetic and MR compatible (polycarbonate, wood, latex, sponge, dielectric gel) [41].

Two experiments were conducted on the cardiac phantom to validate the proposed OCSPAMM tagging sequence: one for rotation as shown in Figure 18.16 and the other for contraction as shown in Figure 18.17. The OCSPAMM tagged images showed good image quality and persistent tag contrast for the entire duration of the cardiac cycle. For comparison to SPAMM sequence, Figure 18.18 shows a cine sequence of SPAMM tagging on the same rotation phantom during an entire cardiac cycle. Notice that there are some artifacts in the upper and lower portion of the last frame in Figure 18.17. These were due to susceptibility from the air inside the center of the phantom and are unrelated to the OCSPAMM pulse sequence.

18.2.2 Analysis of Tagged MR Images

Although MR tagging provides visually interesting data reflecting myocardial motion, fast and accurate image analysis methods are required before tagged MRI data can be used for routine quantitative analysis. Since the development of tagged MRI, many methods have been developed to detect tag features and track the heart motion. This should be seen in the backdrop of more recent work on frequency-based analysis of tagged data (such as HARP and SinMod), or DENSE, and SENC techniques which will be presented later in this chapter, all of which present the possibility for more automated analysis. In the rest of this section, different image analysis methods using tagged MRI are discussed.

There are two different categories of cardiac motion analysis methods using tagged MRI. The first category is feature-based motion tracking methods, that is, those that measure the deformations by tracking

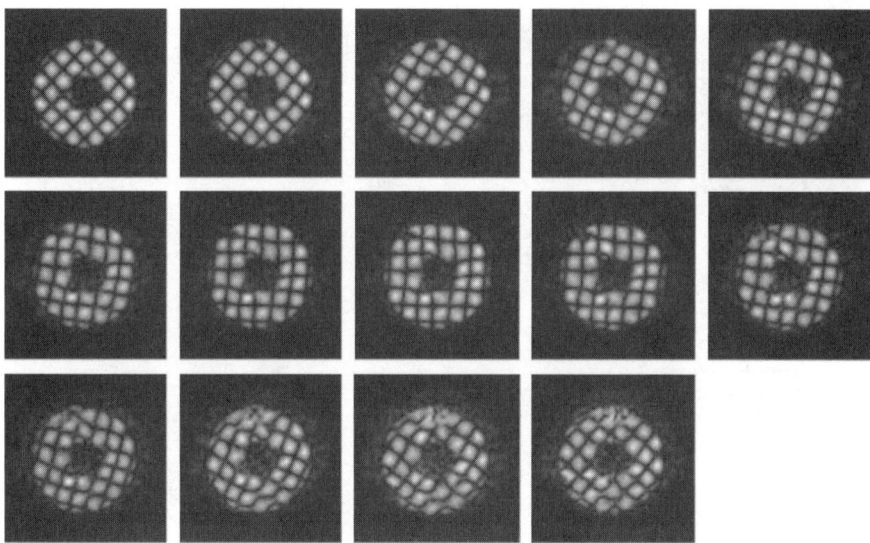

FIGURE 18.16   Fourteen cardiac phases imaged for a rotating phantom (see Figure 18.15) using OCSPAMM pulse sequence. Starting at the top left and traversing to the right and bottom. Imaging parameters were as follows: TR/TE = 9.1/4.7 ms, slice thickness = 8 mm, spatial resolution = 1.17×1.17 mm², acquisition matrix = 85×112, tag spacing = 10 mm, flip angle = 10°.

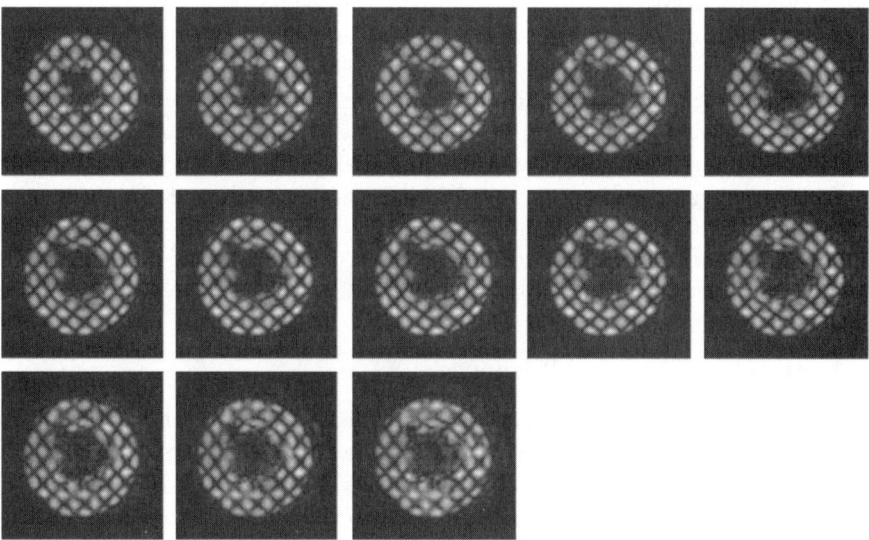

FIGURE 18.17   Thirteen cardiac phases imaged for a contraction phantom (see Figure 18.15) using OCSPAMM pulse sequence. Starting at the top left and traversing to the right and bottom. Imaging parameters were as follows: TR/TE = 9.1/4.7 ms, slice thickness = 8 mm, spatial resolution = 1.17×1.17 mm², acquisition matrix = 85×112, tag spacing = 10 mm, flip angle = 10°.

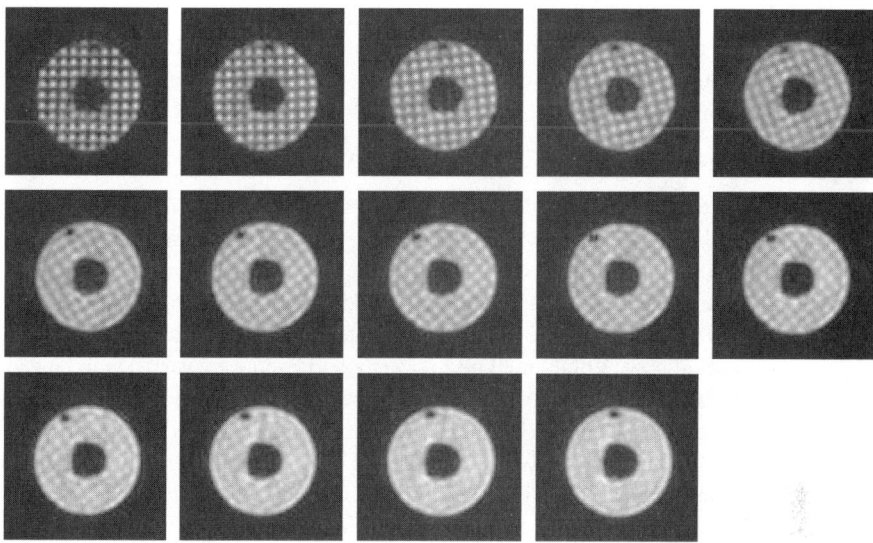

FIGURE 18.18 Fourteen cardiac phases during an entire cardiac cycle imaged for a rotating phantom (see Figure 18.15) using SPAMM pulse sequence. Starting at the top left and traversing to the right and bottom. TR/TE = 11/5.4 ms, slice thickness = 8 mm, spatial resolution = 1.25×1.25 mm^2, acquisition matrix = 144×160, tag spacing = 7 mm, flip angle = 10°.

the movement of tagging features. The most commonly used features are sparse tag lines, geometrically salient land markers, tag line intersections, as well as epicardial and endocardial contours. A number of papers have been published on how to detect tag lines and contours [26,37,48]. For tracking, two sets of techniques have emerged. One set of techniques is to track the features without constructing a dense motion field. The other set constructs a dense motion field from the sparse motion field obtained by tracking the tag features. The accuracy of feature-based image analysis methods using tagged MRI depends highly on the quality of the image and the spacing of tag lines. Tagged MR images with higher spatial resolution will provide more information and constraints on the models. Any advances and improvements in MR imaging, tagging techniques, tag detecting methods, and modeling methods will have impact on another. The second category aims to obtain the deformation field directly from tagged MR images, without extracting tag features. Three different types of methods fall in this category: optical flow methods, registration-based methods [25,107], and frequency-based methods, for example, HARP [83] and SinMod [14].

18.2.2.1 Tracking Myocardial Beads/Landmark-Based Methods

Myocardial beads, defined as the intersection points of orthogonal tagging planes, can be used as non-invasive markers [10]. Compared to physical implanted markers, tagged MRI offers a larger number of MR markers in the myocardium, with the clear advantage that they are placed noninvasively. Tracking beads is based on the fact that intersections encode a unique 3D position in the myocardium which move along with the deforming tissue during the cardiac cycle. Because in MRI imaging planes are fixed relative to the magnet's coordinate system throughout the cardiac cycle, as the myocardial tissue deforms, the intersections in the reference frame may move in and out of the imaging plane.

Kerwin and Prince [59] proposed a method for measuring 3D material points displacements by tracking the intersection points of a 3D grid of applied tag surfaces. Amini et al. [10] proposed a fast method to track myocardial beads by utilizing the B-spline surface to represent tag planes in 3D explicitly. The parametric representation of the tag surfaces leads to an easy way to compute the position of 3D myocardial beads by minimizing the summation of distances between any two reconstructed tag surfaces. Instead of extracting MR beads by reconstructing tag planes, Sampath et al. [114] proposed an automatic 3D cardiac beads tracking method. A true 3D trajectories (instead of apparent motion) of the tag beads were obtained by combining two 2D pathlines that were computed on both SA and LA image planes using 2D HARP tracking techniques. The slice-following CSPAMM technique was used to take through-plane motion into account.

18.2.2.2 Optical Flow Methods

Optical flow is a motion tracking technique first proposed in computer vision. The fundamental assumption is that image intensity remains constant along a motion trajectory. However, in tagged MR images, the intensity constancy condition is not satisfied because of the relaxation of the magnetization of the spins throughout the cardiac cycle, which causes the intensity and contrast to change from image to image. There are different ways to deal with the variable intensity in tagged MRI. Prince and McVeigh [100] used a variable brightness optical flow (VBOF) method to overcome the intensity variation in tagged MRI by introducing a term which accounts for the variable brightness of the stripes using the MR parameters T_1, T_2, and initial magnetization M_0. Dougherty et al. [38] utilized a Laplacian filter to compensate for intensity and contrast loss in myocardial tags. Xu et al. proposed a 3D optical flow method to extract tissue displacements from 3D tagged images [139]. For harmonic phase images (which will be introduced later) the phase of each material point undergoing motion is preserved—the idea is based on phase-based optical flow proposed by Fleet and Jepson [44]. Harmonic images are produced by filtering the spectral peaks in Fourier domain and extracting the spatial phase information from the inverse Fourier transform of the filtered images. Florack et al. [45] applied a multiscale optical flow framework using HARP images. A spatiotemporal Gaussian filter was applied as a preprocessing step. It can simultaneously capture 0th- and 1st-order structure of the motion field. LV rotational analysis was performed using this method [129].

18.2.2.3 Deformable Models

In the deformable modeling approach, a model deforms to fit the data using energy minimization or based on classical physics-based equation of motion [75]. How to deform models and apply constraints to the deformable model vary with application. The force to drive the model deformation can originate from tag intersections, tag lines, or tag surfaces. Because of the sparsity of feature information, vector field interpolation is needed to be incorporated to obtain a dense motion field for every point within the myocardial region. Interpolation methods used to date include mathematical regularization [120], FEM [118,136], BEM [140], deformable model with parameter functions [92], B-splines [10,127], incompressibility assumptions [20], and continuum-mechanics-based energy minimization [91].

Clarysse et al. [31] proposed a cosine series-based model to get a mathematical expression of the reconstructed displacement field for 2D + *t* series of tagged MR images. The coefficients of cosine model were obtained by minimizing the Euclidean distances between projection of deformed tag lines and undeformed ones.

Park et al. proposed a surface deformable model with parameter functions for mid-wall analysis [94] and volumetric deformable model with parameter functions [92]. Continuously varying functions of parameters were used, instead of fixed parameters. Reference 92 was one of the first papers that used 3D FEMs (prismatic FEMs) and converted the FEM nodal deformations into parameter functions. It used tag intersection points in the image plane (three orthogonal sets) and boundary points to estimate the volumetric deformation of the LV. The tag line intersections were automatically computed and were used to deform the model's tagging lines. In order to study the cardiac motion in its complete cycle, Park et al. were the first to use cascaded SPAMM data acquisition within a deformable model framework to avoid the problem of SPAMM tags not lasting throughout the entire cardiac cycle [93]. Haber et al. [49] modified this framework to estimate the motion and deformation of right ventricular free wall and septum. It used volumetric FEMs and tag line intersections in the plane, as well as points within the tag intersections. The 3D motion was reconstructed by constructing a volumetric FEM model from the tag lines and the estimated boundaries of the RV and the LV. A physics-based FEM approach with Poisson's ratio 0.05 and Young's modulus 0.02 was used to estimate the strains throughout the LV and the RV.

However, in this work, the focus was on RV disease. In addition, an *in vivo* validation method was first proposed based on the agreement between the model's tagging lines and the imaging-based tagging lines. Hu et al. [51] presented a statistical model to estimate *in vivo* material properties and strain and stress distributions in both ventricles, using the displacements calculated from tagged MRI data based on Haber's work [49]. It investigated both kinematics and material properties.

Amini et al. [9] proposed an efficient thin-plate spline warp method that warped an area in the plane such that two embedded snake grids from two tagged frames were brought into registration, interpolating a dense displacement vector field. A major problem for techniques relying on 2D short-axis data [9,135] is that in general they do not take into account the through-plane motion. Extended to 3D and 4D (3D B-spline solid plus 1D B-spline interpolation over time), B-spline cubic deformable models [52,103] were introduced for analysis of cardiac motion. Tustison [127] improved the 4D B-spline model framework in Reference 52 by using an internal energy function and enabling inserting additional control points. Ozturk and McVeigh [86] also used the 4D B-spline model to analyze cardiac motion for both ventricles. In Reference 126, Tustison extended the 4D B-spline models proposed in References 127 and 52 to NonUniform Rational B-spline (NURBS) models. The proposed NURBS models were implemented in both polar and cylindrical coordinates and were restricted to the ventricular wall. Due to the spatial resolution of MRI tags, only sparse displacement information in both short and long axis images can be used. In order to make use of more information, Chen [28] extended Tustison's work [126] by introducing dense virtual tag lines obtained from phase-based displacement estimates. In References 132 and 133, a multilevel B-spline (MBS) model was used to integrate displacement information obtained from tagged images in the spatial domain with displacement information obtained from spectral peaks in the frequency domain in order to improve the accuracy of motion tracking. MBS uses both real and virtual tag intersections to derive motion fields and has several advantages: First, B-spline inherent characteristics guarantee the smoothness of the recovered motion fields. Second, it results in fast, accurate fitting. Third, incorporation of phase information (see the section on frequency-based methods) helps overcome the sparsity of real tag intersections.

Instead of B-spline models parameterizing the Cartesian space, Deng and Denney [35,36] proposed a 3D B-spline cylindrical parameterized model. This was further improved on by Tustison and Amini [126] who showed that Cartesian-based cylindrical and prolate-spheroidal B-spline parameterization improves on accuracy of circumferential strains. Young [141] proposed a FEM model to reconstruct 3D myocardial motion from tagged MRI. As with other methods using deformable models and tag lines, for example, References 49 and 92, the model deformation was driven by the distance between model stripe points and image stripe points in the direction orthogonal to the tags. Wang et al. [136] proposed a method to determine the passive diastolic mechanics. The 3D deformation field was constructed from tagged MRI data and material properties were estimated by matching the observed deformations with the FE model.

18.2.2.4 Registration-Based Methods

Cardiac motion tracking can also be considered as a 4D intramodality registration problem [69]. In general, image registration is a process to find the optimal transformation that can transform one image to the other, maximizing a similarity metric between them. The advantages of registration methods are: (1) tag detection and extraction steps are not required and (2) they are automatic without the need for user supervision. The disadvantages of the method involve getting stuck in local minima and potential misalignment due to image noise and artifacts. Additionally, the computational time for the registration-based approaches in general is long.

Numerous methods have been proposed for image registration, for example, nonrigid registration using FFD. In Rueckert's approach [108], global motion was modeled by an affine transformation, while local motion was described by an FFD based on multilevel B-splines. Registration was achieved by optimizing a cost function measuring the similarity between two images as well as the smoothness of the deformation needed to align the images. Chandrashekara et al. [25] made use of the nonrigid registration algorithm first proposed in Reference 108 and applied it to the analysis of myocardial deformations. The algorithm in Reference 108 can only be applied to either SA or LA images, which means that through-plane motion could not be accounted for. In order to obtain complete 3D motion of the myocardium, the cost function was modified to be the sum of the normalized mutual information (NMI) between the registered SA and LA images. The main advantage of this method is that tag localization and deformation field reconstruction were performed simultaneously. Another advantage is that no assumptions about the nature of the tag pattern are made so that the proposed method could potentially be applicable to untagged cine MR images or ultrasound images. However, the fact that no tag position information is incorporated could be considered a limitation. Rougon et al. [107] extended the similarity measure based on NMI to generalized information measures in order to quantitatively assess ventricular wall function from tagged MRI. Different from Chandrashekara's method, Ali-Silvey class of generalized information measures was used, which is a superset of mutual information (MI) and NMI. For more information about medical image registration, refer to the survey paper [68,69].

18.2.2.5 Frequency-Based Methods

18.2.2.5.1 Harmonic Phase Imaging

Harmonic phase imaging (HARP) is a phase-based technique for rapid analysis of tagged cardiac MR images [83]. Rather than working on tagged images directly, HARP uses phase information in the frequency domain. It is based on the fact that the Fourier transform of a SPAMM tag image has a collection of distinct spectral peaks, each of which contains motion information in a certain direction. After bandpass filtering, one spectral peak can be extracted and an inverse Fourier transform applied, yielding the harmonic image. A harmonic image is a complex image that has magnitude and phase images, as given by Equation 18.9. This process is illustrated in Figure 18.19 for simulated data from a 3D solid model (Figure 18.20) and in Figure 18.21 for real dog data. The HARP method uses $\Phi_k(y,t)$, the phase of the harmonic image, which is called harmonic phase image or simply HARP image. The harmonic phase image is linearly related to a directional component of the true motion.

$$I_k(y,t) = D_k(y,t)e^{j\Phi_k(y,t)} \tag{18.9}$$

The principle of HARP tracking is that the harmonic phase of a point remains constant as it moves during the cardiac cycle. For a given material point (x,y) at image slice s at time t, which takes on

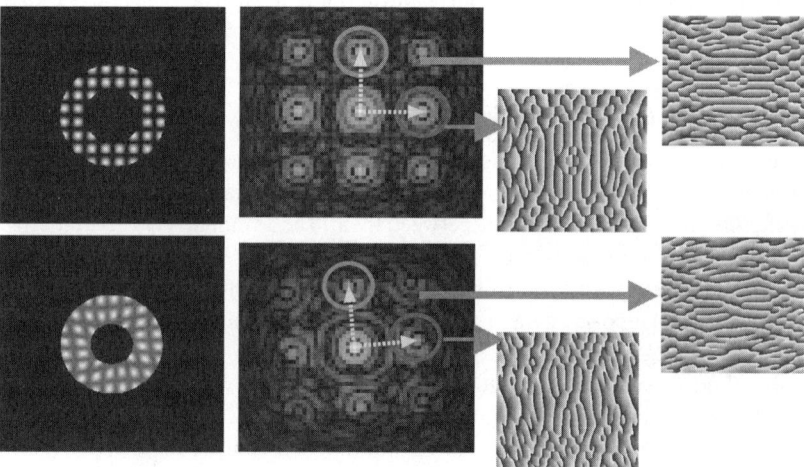

FIGURE 18.19 Tagged images, their Fourier peaks, and their corresponding phase images.

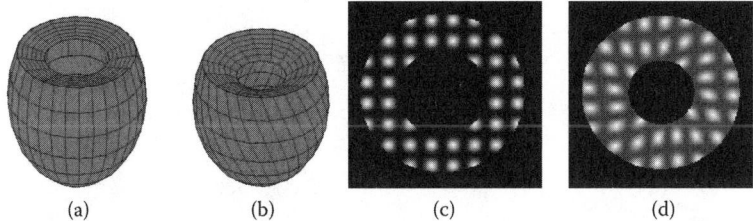

FIGURE 18.20 A realistic simulation. A 3D solid model of the heart from Arts' 13-parameter kinematic model [13] at (a) end-diastole and (b) end-systole. Corresponding mid-ventricular short-axis simulated images at (c) end-diastole and (d) end-systole.

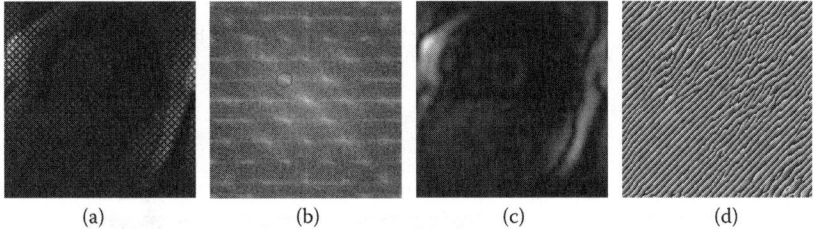

FIGURE 18.21 (a) A tagged MR image. (b) The magnitude of its Fourier transform. By extracting the spectral peak inside the circle in (b), a complex image is produced with a magnitude (c) and a phase (d).

position (x',y') in the same slice at time $t + 1$, the phase time-invariance condition is expressed as follows:

$$\begin{cases} P^h(x',y',s,t+1) = P^h(x,y,s,t), \\ P^v(x',y',s,t+1) = P^v(x,y,s,t) \end{cases} \tag{18.10}$$

where x, y, s, and t stand for x and y coordinates of a point in image plane, the short-axis image slice location, and the time frame, respectively.

Although HARP is fast in postprocessing tagged MR images, the time needed to acquire a cine sequence of tagged images is on the order of 8–20 heartbeats during a breath-hold. The reason for long acquisition time is that traditional tagged MR imaging approach is to use the segmented k-space method with breath-hold [15]. The segmented k-space technique acquires the entire k-space over several cardiac cycle, where each cycle yields a part of the k-space. Based on the fact that only two spectral peaks are needed to compute 2D deformation, Sampath et al. proposed a pulse sequence to only acquire the region of k-space corresponding to the application of the selected spectral peaks, thereby reducing the acquisition time [112]. The region of k-space acquired for both a full k-space acquisition and a partial k-space acquisition are shown in Figures 18.22 and 18.23, respectively. The timing diagram for partial k-space acquisition is shown in Figure 18.24. Gradient B compensates for the dephasing of the gradients in the EPI read-out and the tagging gradient. The purpose of gradient B is to center the acquisition matrix on the frequency of one of the spectral peaks, and the sign of gradient B determines which peak is acquired. The pulse sequence used by Sampath was based on SPAMM and suffered from low spatial resolution. We have developed a partial k-space acquisition based on CSPAMM with the ability to remove the DC component in order to improve the spatial resolution compared to SPAMM (see Figure 18.8) [134]. Using the partial acquisition based on CSPAMM, a larger acquisition matrix was possible when compared to Reference 112 (60×56 compared to 32×32), thus allowing for higher spatial resolution (5×5 mm^2 compared to 9×9 mm^2) and larger deformations to be tracked within the larger acquisition window in k-space. Eight odd number frames out of 15 cardiac phases are displayed in Figure 18.25 for the rotation

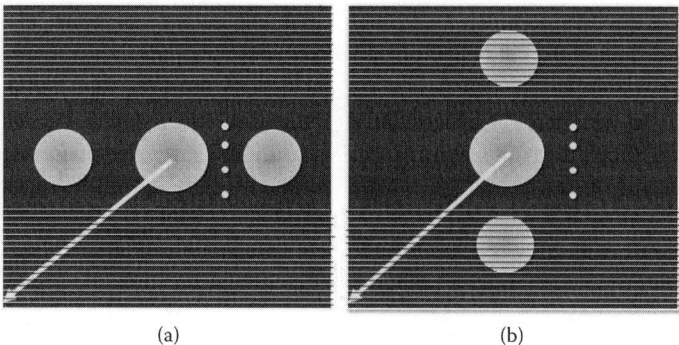

FIGURE 18.22   Full k-space acquisition for data acquisition in MR tagging. The arrow points to the k-space trajectory. (a) Tagging in horizontal direction and (b) tagging in vertical direction.

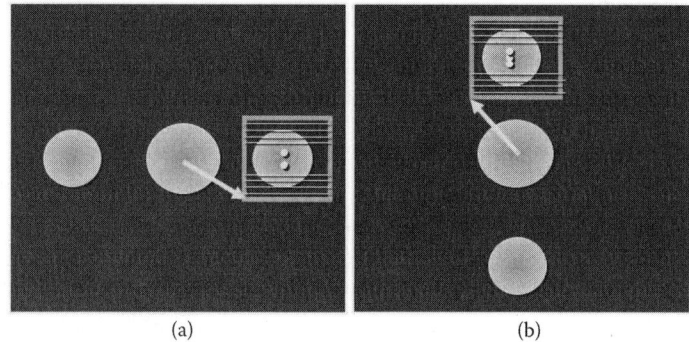

FIGURE 18.23   Partial k-space acquisition of off-center spectral peak. The arrow points to the k-space trajectory. (a) Tagging in horizontal direction and (b) tagging in vertical direction.

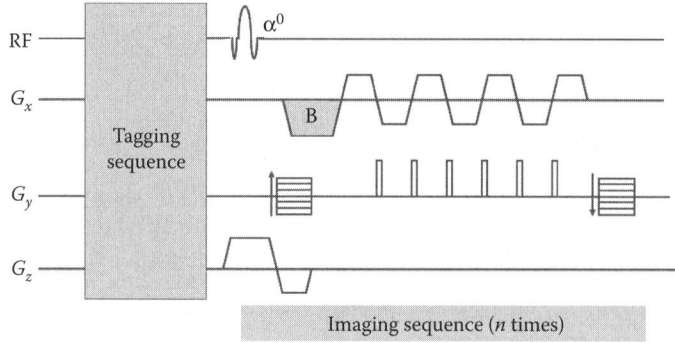

FIGURE 18.24   Timing diagram for partial k-space acquisition utilized in acquisition of images in Figure 18.25 [134]. A modified TFE-EPI sequence is used as the imaging sequence. Gradient B compensates for the dephasing of the gradients in the EPI read-out and the tagging gradient.

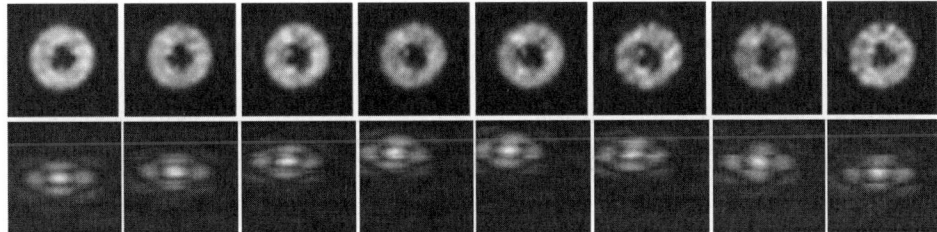

FIGURE 18.25 Eight temporal frames acquired with partial k-space acquisition using CSPAMM in the rotating phantom of Figure 18.15b [134]. Top row: magnitude images. Bottom row: corresponding k-space magnitude data. The imaging parameters were as follows: TR/TE = 7.2/3.8 ms, flip angle = 10°, turbo factor = 8, FOV = 300 × 300 mm², acquired voxel size = 5 × 5 mm², recon resolution = 5 × 5 mm², slice thickness = 8 mm, heart phases = 15, acquisition matrix = 60 × 56, EPI factor = 7, total scan duration = 2 s.

experiment. The top row displays the magnitude images which are blurred versions of the phantom anatomy. Since only the off-center peak is acquired, there are no tag lines visible on these images. The bottom row displays the corresponding k-space data. We can see clearly that the off-center peak rotates from the center to the upper-left corner and then back to the center, in conformance with the rotation of the moving phantom. The phases of the acquired data contain motion information and therefore can be utilized as part of frequency-based motion tracking techniques. Additionally, acquisition time decreases dramatically when compared to full k-space tagged MRI acquisition with CSPAMM.

Using the fast-HARP pulse sequence, real-time myocardial strains were computed in 2D by Abdelmoneim et al. [2]. By using chirp inverse Fourier transform, myocardial ROI was cropped from the raw k-space data so that image reconstruction and cardiac strain map computation could be accomplished in 11 ms. It was shown that fast-HARP can produce the same results as original HARP with a four times speedup.

By manipulating harmonic peaks, more desirable tag patterns from conventional SPAMM, CSPAMM, and fast-HARP tagged images can be synthesized [84]. In order to correct errors in harmonic phase images, Ryf et al. [111] employed both negative and positive peaks from CSPAMM to produce more accurate harmonic phase images. The main advantage of HARP is that it is fast and automatic with no need for extracting tag lines in a preprocessing step.

One limitation of HARP and fast-HARP is that they can only estimate the in-plane motion, typically using 2D SA tagged MR images. Several solutions for including the out-plane component of motion have been proposed. Pan et al. [88] extended the traditional HARP method for 3D cardiac motion tracking. A stack of SA images with tagging grid as well as LA images with one horizontal set of tags were used. Similar to 2D HARP, phase invariant condition was used to track the motion. A material mesh model was used for interpolation from sparse phase information. In this study, only a single layer mesh inside the myocardium was created and tracked according to 3D phase invariant condition. The use of CSPAMM led to improved myocardial strain maps with HARP analysis which was achieved through the suppression of the center peak [64]. Using a true 3D tagging technique followed by a conventional fast 3D gradient echo imaging sequence, Ryf et al. [110] extended HARP from 2D to 3D. The phase invariant property in three directions was utilized after extracting spectral peaks in 3D Fourier space. True 3D motion can be captured, but the scan time was quite long and demanded a sophisticated breath-holding technique. Rutz et al. proposed a fast method for acquiring 3D CSPAMM data using localized tagging preparation and a hybrid multishot, segmented echo planar imaging sequence [109]. Abd-Elmoniem et al. [1] developed a new method, zHARP pulse sequence, which can track both in-plane and through-plane motion from a single image plane. It is similar to slice-following CSPAMM [43] and combines tagged MRI with through-plane displacement phase encoding without affecting the image acquisition time. A z-encoding gradient is added to the refocusing lobe of the slice-selection gradient and produces a phase term depending on the displacement in through-plane direction in the final data. From two or more images in one orientation, 3D strain can be calculated [3]. zHARP can compute 3D strain tensor over the whole LV with no spatial interpolation. Another method to obtain through-plane strain as well as in-plane strain is to combine fast-HARP with SENC which will be discussed later [113]. Using the HARP-SENC pulse sequence, a single slice of SA image can be acquired in six heartbeats and multiple slices can be acquired in a sequential fashion.

18.2.2.5.2 Local Sine Wave Modeling

SinMod is also a frequency-based method to analyze the heart displacement and deformation from tagged MRI sequences using phase information [14]. The main difference between SinMod and HARP is that SinMod detects both local spatial phase shift and local spatial frequency from band-pass filtered images, while HARP uses the phase invariant condition and tracks local spatial phase. The speed of SinMod method is as fast as HARP but SinMod method has advantages in accuracy, noise reduction, and lack of artifacts [14]. In SinMod, the intensity distribution around each pixel (p, q) is modeled as a cosine wave front:

$$I_1(p,q) = A_1 \cos\left(\omega_p\left(p + \frac{u}{2}\right) + \varphi\right) + n_1(p,q)$$

$$I_2(p,q) = A_2 \cos\left(\omega_p\left(p - \frac{u}{2}\right) + \varphi\right) + n_2(p,q)$$

(18.11)

where ω_p and φ are the spatial frequency and phase of the wave, respectively. A_1 and A_2 are wave magnitudes for the first image I_1 and the second image I_2, while n_1 and n_2 are additive noise. u is the displacement between these two images at position (p, q) along the p direction.

The flow chart of SinMod algorithm is shown in Figure 18.26. The principle behind SinMod tracking is that both phase and frequency for each pixel are determined directly from the frequency analysis and the displacement is calculated from the quotient of phase difference and local frequency. After obtaining the Fourier Transform of the input images $I_1(p, q)$ and $I_2(p,q)$ (temporal frames at time t and time $t + 1$), the same band-pass filter is applied to both (similar to HARP) isolate corresponding spectral peaks and produce a pair of complex images in the Fourier domain (since the Fourier Transform will be complex to begin with). Let us refer to the two complex images in Fourier domain following band-pass filtering $I_{bf1}(\omega_p, \omega_q)$ and $I_{bf2}(\omega_p, \omega_q)$. Applying a low-frequency band-pass filter and a high-frequency one to both I_{bf1} and I_{bf2} followed by an inverse Fourier transform leads to four complex images $I_{bfLf1}(p,q)$, $I_{bfHf1}(p,q)$, $I_{bfHf2}(p,q)$, and $I_{bfHf2}(p,q)$. The reasoning behind application of an LPF and a HPF to I_{bf1} and I_{bf2} is to determine the local spatial frequency by power spectra. Then the displacement is the local quotient of

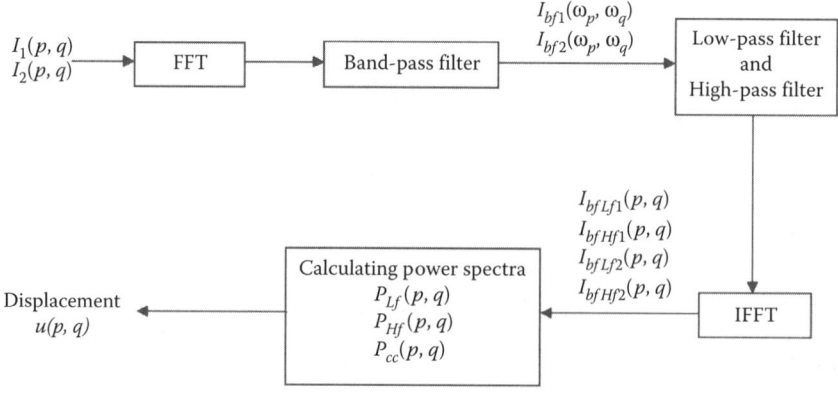

FIGURE 18.26 Flow chart for the SinMod method.

phase difference and local frequency at that position. The power spectra and cross power spectrum are given by

$$
\begin{aligned}
P_{Lf}(p,q) &= \mid I_{bfLf1} \mid^2 + \mid I_{bfLf2} \mid^2 \\
P_{Hf}(p,q) &= \mid I_{bfHf1} \mid^2 + \mid I_{bfHf2} \mid^2 \\
P_{cc}(p,q) &= I_{bfLf1}\overline{I}_{bfLf2} + I_{bfHf1}\overline{I}_{bfHf2}
\end{aligned}
\tag{18.12}
$$

where $\overline{I}$ is the complex conjugation of I.

The local frequency ω_p and local displacement u can then be estimated from

$$
\omega_p(p,q) = \omega_c \sqrt{\frac{P_{Hf}}{P_{Lf}}} \qquad u(p,q) = \frac{\arg(P_{cc})}{\omega_p}
\tag{18.13}
$$

where ω_c is the band-pass center-frequency.

18.2.2.5.3 Gabor Filter Banks

Gabor filter is a band-pass filter, with the form of a Gaussian multiplied by a complex sinusoid in the spatial domain, or equivalently, a shifted Gaussian in the spatial frequency domain. By choosing appropriate parameters, the magnitude response of the Gabor filter can be used to remove tags in the myocardium, and the phase response can be used to track tags. Once again, utilizing phase-based optical flow, the phase response of Gabor filter bank for a material point is assumed to be constant during the deformation [27].

A Gabor filter bank is a set of 2D Gabor filters with tunable parameters that represent the variable spacing and orientation of tag lines. By finding optimal parameters that maximize the Gabor filter response, Montillo et al. [77] extracted deformation information in a 2D simulated model. Qian et al. [101] extended the 2D Gabor filter bank method to 3D in order to extract and track deformed tag surfaces. Chen et al. [27] used the phase information from Gabor filters to track tag lines. To increase the accuracy of tag tracking, a combination of the response of Gabor filters, gradient information of original images, an intensity probabilistic model, and a spatiotemporal smoothness constraint was used in the deformable model. Chen et al. [29] proposed a three-step process for 3D cardiac motion tracking: extract tag intersections based on local phase analysis using Gabor filter bank, robust point matching (RPM) method to track the intersections movement, and meshless deformable modeling to generate a dense displacement field.

Instead of calculating the strain values in terms of gradient of the displacement by tracking the tag pattern, Qian et al. [102] developed a nontracking-based strain estimation method for tagged MRI. It is based on the extraction of tag's deformation gradient using Gabor filter, instead of tracking displacement prior to strain calculation. Subsequently, 2D strains can be obtained by using the strain formula in terms of the deformation gradient tensor.

18.3 Phase Contrast MRI

Another approach for cardiac motion tracking is through phase contrast MR imaging (PCMRI) of myocardium. PCMRI is based on the idea that the motion of tissue on blood produces a change in the MR signal phase that is proportion to the velocity of the tissue [96]. Therefore, PCMRI is also called velocity-encoded MRI.

18.3.1 Phase Contrast MR Imaging

Phase contrast methods are based on the fact that moving spins accumulate a different phase offset than static spins in the presence of a magnetic field gradient. The phase shift is proportional to the product

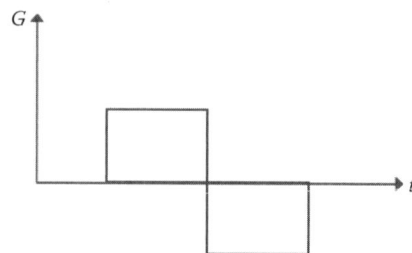

FIGURE 18.27 A bipolar gradient lobe.

of tissue velocity and the first moment of the magnetic field gradient in the direction of motion (see Equation 18.16). PCMRI sequence uses a bipolar gradient as shown in Figure 18.27, which is first positive at a particular amplitude and duration and then negative for an equal amplitude and duration to encode the velocity. For static spins, the accumulated phase under the bipolar gradient is zero. However, for spins that move at a constant velocity, there is an accumulated phase shift. The accumulated phase at time TE is

$$\Phi = \gamma \int_0^{TE} G(t) r(t) dt \qquad (18.14)$$

where $G(t)$ is the gradient, $r(t)$ is the position in the direction of $G(t)$, and γ is the gyromagnetic ratio. The Taylor expansion of position vector $r(t)$ on initial position r_0 is

$$r(t) = r_0 + vt + a\frac{t^2}{2} \cdots \qquad (18.15)$$

Under the condition that there are no phase shifts from initial position r_0 (which is the case for bipolar gradient) and the phase shifts due to higher-order terms are small, Equation 18.14 becomes

$$\Phi = v(\gamma M_1) \qquad (18.16)$$

where M_1 is the first moment of the gradient waveform evaluated at TE.

$$M_1 = \int_0^{TE} G(t) t dt \qquad (18.17)$$

This forms the foundation for PCMRI. In deriving this expression, we have assumed that the velocity is constant during the time (0,TE).

Unfortunately, the phase can be affected by many other factors, including magnetic field inhomogeneity, tissue magnetic susceptibility, pulse sequence tuning, and eddy currents due to gradient switching. Therefore, to accurately extract the motion of interest, phase shift due to these sources have to be eliminated. In order to do that, the procedure in PCMRI consists of a reference scan without velocity encoding, followed by two or three further acquisitions with velocity encoding along different directions [95,96]. The reference scan is used to correct undesired phase offsets of the second acquisition with velocity encoding. Since the phase of each pixel is modulated by velocity, one can obtain functional data with maximum resolution, the same spatial and temporal resolution as the underlying anatomical images. Velocity information in PCMRI can be used directly to calculate strain rate. The motion of the myocardium (i.e., displacements) may be found by integration with respect to time. Gradient system performance is critical in accurately extracting velocity information with phase contrast methods.

18.3.2 Analysis Techniques for Phase Contrast MR Images

Meyer et al. [76] used a deformable mesh guided by a Kalman filter to obtain myocardial deformation. Zhu et al. [147] developed a Fourier tracking algorithm which modeled trajectories as composed of Fourier harmonics and integrated the velocity data in the frequency domain. Deformation gradient tensor and strain can be calculated using a least-squares fit of the trajectory data to a local deformation model [148]. The accuracy of the forward-backward [33] and Fourier tracking methods was analyzed using a computer-controlled deformable phantom in Reference 39. The Fourier tracking algorithm in Reference 147 was extended to 3D volumetric data analysis [151]. Compared to method in Reference 147, a dynamic spatiotemporal FEM model was proposed to calculate deformation by taking into account all velocity information from the entire analyzed region [150].

Masood et al. [73] presented a B-spline-based deformable model, named virtual tagging framework, to track cardiac motion and deformation from PCMRI. The intersections of virtual tag lines served as control points which were determined by minimizing the difference between calculated velocity field from B-spline-based deformable model and the velocity field measured from PCMRI. The mass conservation constraint was incorporated into the proposed framework to ensure that the derived strain complied with physical constraints. Selskog et al. [115] proposed a method to calculate 4D strain rate from 3D PCMRI data by weighting of a forward and a backward difference and a 3D strain tensor visualization method using ellipsoids where the three axes of the ellipsoid denoted the directions of the strain rate and the length of the axes denoted the magnitude. Bergvall et al. [19] fitted a spatiotemporal spline model to track cardiac motion and deformation from PCMRI data. It extended the spatiotemporal model first proposed in Reference 150 by using TPS and Navier splines as spatial elements.

Reese et al. [104] developed a single-shot 3D PCMRI data acquisition sequence by acquiring two contiguous 2D images in k-space in a single echo train of an EPI readout. Markl et al. [72] developed a fast 2D PCMRI protocol based on a black blood k-space segmented gradient echo imaging. The in-plane velocity information can be obtained within a single breath-hold measurement by choosing optimal number of k-space lines and view-sharing technique. Jung et al. [58] proposed a high-temporal-resolution phase contrast MRI acquisition method using a prospective respiratory gating technique with two navigators in each cardiac cycle. The usage of dual navigator gating and view sharing [71] increased the temporal resolution to 13.8 ms. This method was applied to investigate details in LV motion patterns [56,57]. A schematic visualization model and correlation analysis on myocardial velocities in different segments and slices were done to a large number of 58 normal subjects in three different age groups and one patient with dilated cardiomyopathy [46].

18.4 Displacement Encoding with Stimulated Echoes

DENSE is a quantitative imaging technique that encodes tissue displacement in the phase of the acquired signal. In order to overcome the low resolution limit of tagged MRI and bypass the integration required in PCMRI in order to obtain displacements, Aletras et al. [5] were the first to apply stimulated echo techniques for quantification of myocardial strain, named DENSE, which combines many of the advantages of both tagging and phase velocity mapping. DENSE is a high-resolution myocardial displacement mapping method. Similar to PCMRI, it uses a bipolar gradient to encode motion of spins into the phase of the MRI signal. Figure 18.28 shows a timing diagram of DENSE in readout direction. Using stimulated echo, the phase is modulated and demodulated by the gradients applied between the first two RF pulses G_1 and the one after the third RF pulse G_2. The displacements occurring during the mix time TM (time between the second and third RF pulses) is recorded in the phase of stimulated echo image. Similar to PCMRI, in order to eliminate the phase contributions from other sources, the sequence is repeated once more with a different gradient (shown in red dots in Figure 18.28) and subtracted from the first acquisition. In other words, the phase of DENSE images is proportional to the displacement, therefore strain can be obtained by computing the derivatives of the phase. This technique encodes motion over

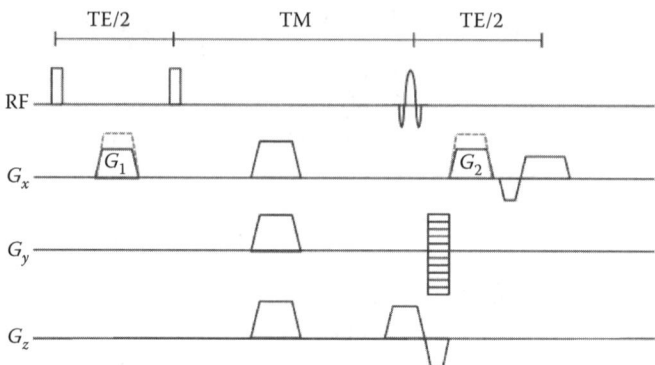

FIGURE 18.28 Timing diagram for DENSE in readout direction. Phase wrapping happens through the application of G_1, G_2 unwraps the phase. (From A. H. Aletras et al. *Journal of Magnetic Resonance*, 137(1):247–252, March 1999.)

long time intervals. The encoded displacements are large; therefore, improved phase contrast is obtained with moderate gradient strength. For more details of this technique, refer to Reference 5.

DENSE has also been used in detecting small focal regions of abnormal contraction in patients, in characterizing mouse ischemia models, and in tissue tracking of human hearts via 2D breath-hold imaging. In Reference 4, DENSE was combined with a segmented echo-planar imaging readout (fast-DENSE) and applied to normal volunteers. In order to improve SNR and reduce breath-hold time, mixed echo train acquisition DENSE (meta-DENSE) was proposed in [6]. Aletras et al. [7] accelerated the image acquisition process by incorporating SENSE into DENSE. This method can reduce the breath-hold time by a factor of two.

Initial DENSE sequence in Reference 5 imaged the heart at a single cardiac phase; Kim et al. [61] developed a cine DENSE imaging sequence to sample 2D DENSE images at multiple phases of the cardiac cycle. A SPAMM sequence was used to encode the magnetization at end-diastole, then the displacement was presented as the phase shift between position encoding and readout. Cine DENSE data provide a way to track every material point in myocardium through time in the cardiac cycle. In order to improve the SNR for cine DENSE [61], a signal-averaged DENSE (sav-DENSE) was proposed [60], which extracted a pair of DENSE images with uncorrelated noise from CSPAMM image, and combined them during image reconstruction. In order to decrease the phase shifts from sources other than the encoded displacement, a general *n*-dimensional balanced multipoint encoding strategy was used in DENSE [146]. Spatiotemporal phase unwrapping methods were used to process cine DENSE images in Reference 122. In Reference 123, slice following was incorporated into cine DENSE to track 3D cardiac motion. An adaptive phase-unwrapping and spatial filtering techniques were developed to process cine DENSE data and compared with conventional phase-unwrapping and spatial filtering techniques [137]. The novelty of this technique is that it incorporates the location of the myocardial wall into the quality map.

Since DENSE is based on stimulated echo, there is an inherent 50% signal loss. Although DENSE and HARP may seem to be quite different at first glance, these two techniques turn out to be different implementations of phase displacement encoding. A thorough comparison of these two techniques was given in Reference 63.

18.5 Strain Encoding MRI

Strain encoding, or SENC, is a relatively new MRI technique that can measure regional contraction, or relaxation, of the heart's myocardium. SENC pulse sequence was first developed by Osman et al. [85] to image longitudinal strain from short-axis images. SENC is built on the concept of MR tagging, but it uses tag planes parallel to the image plane. Strain is calculated from two images with different frequency modulation in the slice-selection direction. Longitudinal strain can be computed by measuring the local tag frequency components from SA images, while circumferential strain can be measured from the LA images. The unique advantage of SENC is that it directly encodes the regional strain of the heart into the acquired image without measuring the displacement or velocity first. Using SENC imaging, the existence of stiff masses can be detected in the acquired MR images without postprocessing [82]. Pan et al. [89] proposed a fast-SENC pulse sequence which can reduce the strain image acquisition time to one heartbeat by combining localized SENC, interleaved tuning, and spiral imaging. Youssef et al. [144] used SENC to estimate the circumferential strain of the RV free wall.

Ibrahim et al. [53] combined SENC with slice-following to correct for the through-plane motion in real time. SENC imaging with and without slice-following can result in significantly different strain values as expected with tagged MRI [53]. Ibrahim et al. [54] proposed a composite-SENC (C-SENC) pulse sequence which adjusted the tunings such that an additional image was acquired at zero frequency. Three consecutive SENC images can be obtained which contain both strain information and myocardial viability information. C-SENC produces three images: no-tuning (NT), low-tuning (LT), and high tuning (HT). Adding LT and HT images will result in an anatomical (ANAT) image of the myocardium. According to different intensity distribution in this NT-ANAT-HT 3D space, different tissue types can be classified using an unsupervised, multistage fuzzy clustering technique [55].

SENC is a 1D out-of-plane strain encoding method. In order to obtain 3D strain, Sampath et al. [113] integrated SENC with HARP, which can produce 2D in-plane strain. In this way, 3D strains can be obtained from a single slice of SA image. Hess et al. [50] combined DENSE and SENC to obtain 3D strain map in a single slice of the myocardium.

SENC has some limitations versus MR tagging and DENSE. First, it is not capable of tracking the motion of the heart. Because it only encodes the strain (contractility), the exact motion of the tissue cannot be followed. Therefore, it cannot be directly used to calculate quantities such as rotation and twisting. Second, SENC provides strain measurements only in the through-plane direction, and not the in-plane directions. The advantages of SENC include its simplicity, as images of strain can be directly produced in real time. It does not require image postprocessing. Also, SENC has higher in-plane resolution of strain than MR tagging, which can be very useful in assessing regional function of the RV free wall [65].

18.6 Strain Pattern Analysis

An important application of MRI motion-imaging methods such as tagging is in providing a better definition of the normal patterns of motion. Similarly, the effects of heart diseases such as hypertrophy, infarction, failure, and dyssynchrony can be well characterized and quantified with tagging.

Regional myocardial strains have direct or indirect relationship with cardiac diseases. Most of the motion tracking methods aim to extract strains in the heart, for the reason that strain encapsulates the basic mechanical function of the myocardium and has clinical potential. There are different types of strains. Normal strain is defined as the ratio of the length of the deformed line element to its original length. Due to the geometry of the ventricle, normal strains are usually calculated in radial, circumferential, and longitudinal directions. Shear strain is defined as the angular change between any two originally mutually orthogonal line elements that occurs as a result of a continuous deformation. These can be defined in terms of the off-diagonal terms of the Lagrangian strain tensor [12].

In order to analyze regional strain patterns in the myocardium, the LV and RV are typically divided into segments and each of the directional strains (e.g., radial, circumferential, and/or longitudinal) is averaged over the segment. Ideally, in 3D, the 16 segment and 17 segment models as recommended by the American Society of Echocardiography should be used [24]. In the 16 segment model, the LV is divided into six basal, six mid-ventricular, and four apical regions. In the 17 segment model, the apex comprises the 17th segment [35,78,79,88,126,127,139]. In 3D, the RV can be divided into three layers in the long-axis direction and each layer further divided into three segments [62,126]. However other finer

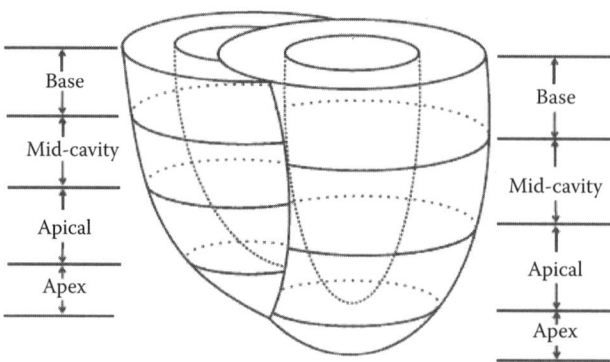

FIGURE 18.29 Geometrical representation of the regional divisions for strain analysis for both the left and right ventricles in the LA view. (From N. J. Tustison. *Biventricular Myocardial Strains with Anatomical NURBS Models from Tagged MRI*. PhD thesis, Washington University in St. Louis, August 2004.)

or sparser partitions have also been utilized. For 2D analysis, typically, mid-ventricular strains for four to eight regions are reported [102,112–114].

In Reference 125, the division along the long-axis consisted of four layers: basal, mid-cavity, apical, and apex as shown in Figure 18.29. Based on the location of the LV/RV junctions, the basal and mid-cavity portions of the left ventricle were each further divided into six regions in the short-axis view: antero-septal (AS), anterior (A), lateral (L), posterior (P), inferior (I), and inferoseptal (IS) as shown in Figure 18.30. Similar to the left ventricle, the right ventricle was divided into basal, mid-cavity, and apical layers and each layer was further divided into anterior, mid, and inferior regions. Tustison et al. [125] calculated both the Eulerian and Lagrangian strain values for LV data sets from three species: canine data, human data, and porcine data. The strain values from the RV for two canine data sets were also included. Results showed that across normal species, radial strains remain positive for most of the regions indicative of systolic thickening of the left ventricle while the circumferential and the longitudinal strains are negative. Circumferential shortening during left ventricular contraction results in the negative strain values in the circumferential direction while compression in the longitudinal direction results in negative longitudinal strains.

Strain analysis can also be done based on extracted model parameter functions [92] where quantitative differences between normal and abnormal hearts with hypertrophic cardiomyopathy (htcm) were extracted. Park et al. [92] showed that the contraction and the twisting deformation are more significant

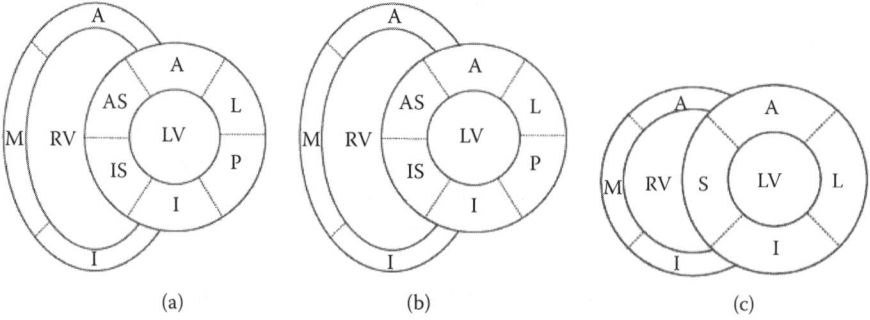

FIGURE 18.30 Geometrical representation of the regional divisions for strain analysis for both the left and right ventricles in the SA view. Illustrated are (a) the basal region, (b) the mid-cavity region, and (c) the apical region. (From N. J. Tustison. *Biventricular Myocardial Strains with Anatomical NURBS Models from Tagged MRI*. PhD thesis, Washington University in St. Louis, August 2004.)

on the endocardial wall compared to the epicardial wall. Due to the complexity of RV geometry, Haber et al. [49] utilized coordinate-system-independent principal strains and directions to describe regional deformations, which were derived by calculating the eigenvalues and eigenvectors of the Lagrangian strain tensor. The strains in normal hearts and the hearts with right ventricular hypertrophy (RVH) diseases were compared. Maximum and minimum principal strains were used to quantify normal sheep left ventricular functions [139].

Normal strains have been widely used, in radial, circumferential, and longitudinal directions, though the circumferential strain values have been reported most [29,83,88,112,126,127]. In Reference 114, circumferential strains were computed, not for every material points, but based on the percent change in the distance between every set of two adjacent markers with respect to the reference time frame. In [113], radial, circumferential, and longitudinal strains (in-plane and out-of-plane strains) were obtained simultaneously within a mid-ventricular SA slice. In Reference 35, circumferential, radial, and longitudinal strains for a normal volunteer and a patient with an antero-septal myocardial infarction were computed. In Reference 14, circumferential strains of the LV in five slices from apex to base and the mid-wall circumferential strain for a patient with LBBB and infarction in the lateral LV-free wall were investigated.

Moore et al. [78,79] reported 3D displacement and strain evolution of the normal LV in humans determined from tagged MRI. Such data can serve as a database of strain in normal hearts. Clarysse et al. [32] proposed a framework for analysis of spatiotemporal deformation parameters of the myocardium throughout the systolic phase from tagged MR data. After strain calculation, a functional data analysis method was applied to healthy subjects, which provided a normal contraction reference model. Pathological cases were then compared with the reference model. Statistical analysis of regional wall motion performance parameters in normals relative to disease processes was done in Reference 142. After the deformation was reconstructed based on FEM models fitted to tagged MR images [143], the deformation of LV can be decomposed into separate deformation modes such as longitudinal shortening, wall thickening, and twisting [106]. By doing this, healthy and diseased cardiac deformation patterns can be distinguished.

Cupps et al. [34] estimated LV wall stress distribution at rest in patients with chronic aortic insufficiency and normal ejection fraction within a FEM formulation. Differences in regional LV systolic stress in normal subjects and patients with aortic insufficiency were given. Moustakidis et al. [80] estimated 3D strain distribution at rest and with inotropic stimulation in patients with ischemic cardiomyopathy using tagged MR imaging and FE analysis. Similar studies were performed in a group of normal volunteers for comparison. Further study showed that circumferential strains at rest and with low-dose dobutamine could discriminate viable and nonviable myocardium in patients with ischemic cardiomyopathy [22]. Maniar et al. [70] compared circumferential strain in patients before and after 3 months after coronary artery bypass grafting using tagged MRI. Strain analysis from dobutamine-stressed tagged MRI was shown to be feasible to quantitatively predict myocardial recoverability after coronary artery bypass grafting [99]. Chen et al. [29] assessed the differences in myocardial strain distributions between hearts with left ventricular hypertrophy and normal hearts. They calculated statistics of 17 different variables related to the circumferential strain distribution in the LVH patients and the normal control.

18.7 Conclusions and Research Trends

In this chapter, we reviewed different imaging and image analysis methods to evaluate cardiac function from MRI. Cine MRI is critical in imaging the anatomy of the heart and calculating global indices, but with limited ability to track local motion. Traditional cardiac motion imaging pulse sequences, that is, tagged MRI, PCMRI, contain more information about the regional myocardial motion than cine MRI. It is felt that tagged MRI will continue to play an important role in cardiac motion analysis. Among different tagging methods, SPAMM is the most commonly used sequence. Given the current advances in gradient technology, image reconstruction techniques, and data analysis algorithms, MR tagging has become the reference modality for calculating strain in the heart [116]. Data in tagged MRI provides information with respect to muscle deformation, but suffers from low spatial resolution. Spatial resolution of phase contrast MR images is 1–3 mm, while the distance between tags in tagged MRI is around 4–8 mm [57]. In recent years, several new pulse sequences have been proposed to image cardiac motion, such as HARP, DENSE, and SENC, which have characteristics of high spatial resolution, and direct encoding of displacement or strain. HARP is largely limited to 2D in-plane strain computation, while SENC is for 1D through-plane strain calculation. A comparison between DENSE and HARP imaging may be found in [63]. Both SENC and HARP use tagging. The difference is the tagging in HARP is orthogonal to the image plane, while the tagging in SENC is parallel to the image plane. Thanks to the fast tagging and imaging method for cardiac motion tracking, deformation throughout the entire cardiac cycle can be tracked, instead of only systole or diastole.

The motion of heart is 3D and nonrigid. There are several strategies to capture its 3D motion. One way is to use a stack of SA images. Another one is to use multiview planar images, both in SA and in LA directions. For tagged MRI, the tag planes only provide information about motion in the direction perpendicular to the initial tag planes, three mutually perpendicular tag planes are necessary. For the fact that MR imaging plane is fixed, pixels in 2D images are not always the same material points in myocardium. Slice-following technique can overcome this limitation. Slice-following images a thicker slice which encompasses a thinner tagged slice to ensure imaging the same tagged slice throughout the cardiac cycle, despite tissue displacement in the through-plane direction. Slice-following (SF) technique is also used in other sequences, for example, SF-SENC [53] and SF-DENSE [123]. Another way is to use 3D imaging and analysis approaches to recover true motion [110].

Cardiac analysis has focused mostly on the myocardium of the left ventricle, since LV, as the primary heart chamber, controls systemic perfusion and is responsible for pumping blood throughout the entire body. Compared to LV, RV has thinner wall and more complex geometry. Besides, RV can have a large through-plane motion near the base of the ventricle, about 15 mm, which is more than two short-axis image planes [49]. All these factors increase the difficulty in motion analysis. But in recent years, RV function has also been investigated [21,126].

Better understanding of pathological mechanism of the heart can be achieved due to increasing performance of medical imaging techniques. Strain is considered to have more potential for clinical diagnosis. Researchers have already investigated alterations of strain patterns in diseased populations. Most analysis methods end up obtaining strains in different directions. Most commonly reported are radial, circumferential, and longitudinal strains. After strains are obtained, strain analysis approaches are emerging.

The trends in cardiac MR imaging and image analysis methods are as follows:

- Phase- and frequency-based methods, for example, SinMod [14], HARP [83]
- Integration of frequency-based and spatial analysis for improved measurement of myocardial strains [28,132,133]
- Direct displacement or strain imaging, for example, DENSE (Section 18.4) and SENC (Section 18.5)
- Real-time imaging (one heartbeat), for example, fast-HARP [112] and fast-SENC [89]
- Approaches to analysis of both LV and RV [21,51,126]
- 3D tagging and imaging [110]
- High resolution PCMRI [46,56]
- Clinically useful strain analysis methods [22,29,32,99,106,126,127,142]

The literature on cardiac motion analysis based on MRI has grown rapidly in the past decade. Cardiac motion analysis is continuing to be a hot and challenging research area. Research efforts on cardiac motion analysis are devoted to quantitative methods for automatic, fast, and robust image analysis. The trend in image analysis is toward phase-based methods. With the development of more advanced MR imaging techniques and progress in hardware, research in this area will continue to grow.

Acknowledgments

We are grateful to the following individuals for their help in various aspects of this work: Melanie Kotys and Stefan Fischer for useful discussions, and Mehmet Ersoy and Randy Setser for providing the cardiac phantom used in Section 18.2.1.3.

References

1. K. Z. Abd-Elmoniem, N. F. Osman, J. L. Prince, and M. Stuber. Three-dimensional magnetic resonance myocardial motion tracking from a single image plane. *Magnetic Resonance in Medicine*, 58(1):92–102, July 2007.

2. K. Z. Abd-Elmoniem, S. Sampath, N. F. Osman, and J. L. Prince. Real-time monitoring of cardiac regional function using fastHARP MRI and region-of-interest reconstruction. *IEEE Transactions on Biomedical Engineering*, 54(9):1650–1656, September 2007.

3. K. Z. Abd-Elmoniem, M. Stuber, and J. L. Prince. Direct three-dimensional myocardial strain tensor quantification and tracking using zHARP. *Medical Image Analysis*, 12(6):778–786, December 2008.

4. A. H. Aletras, R. S. Balaban, and W. Han. High-resolution strain analysis of the human heart with fast-DENSE. *Journal of Magnetic Resonance*, 140(1):41–57, September 1999.

5. A. H. Aletras, S. Ding, R. S. Balaban, and W. Han. DENSE: Displacement encoding with stimulated echoes in cardiac functional MRI. *Journal of Magnetic Resonance*, 137(1):247–252, March 1999.

6. A. H. Aletras and W. Han. Mixed echo train acquisition displacement encoding with stimulated echoes: An optimized DENSE method for *in vivo* functional imaging of the human heart. *Magnetic Resonance in Medicine*, 46(3):523–534, September 2001.

7. A. H. Aletras, W. P. Ingkanisorn, C. Mancini, and A. E. Arai. DENSE with SENSE. *Journal of Magnetic Resonance*, 176(1):99–106, September 2005.

8. American Heart Association. Heart disease and stroke statistics—2009 update (at-a-glance version). http://www.americanheart.org/presenter.jhtml?identifier=3037327.

9. A. A. Amini, Y. Chen, R. W. Curwen, V. Mani, and J. Sun. Coupled B-snake grids and constrained thin-plate splines for analysis of 2-D tissue deformations from tagged MRI. *IEEE Transactions on Medical Imaging*, 17(3):344–356, June 1998.

10. A. A. Amini, Y. Chen, M. Elayyadi, and P. Radeva. Tag surface reconstruction and tracking of myocardial beads from SPAMM-MRI with parametric B-spline surfaces. *IEEE Transactions on Medical Imaging*, 20(2):94–103, February 2001.

11. A. A. Amini and J. S. Duncan. Bending and stretching models for LV wall motion analysis from curves and surfaces. *Image and Vision Computing*, 10(6):418–430, July–August 1992.

12. A. A. Amini and J. L. Prince. *Measurement of Cardiac Deformations from MRI: Physical and Mathematical Models*. Kluwer Academic Publishers, Dordrecht, The Netherlands, 2001.

13. T. Arts, W. C. Hunter, A. Douglas, A. M. Muijtjens, and R. S. Reneman. Description of the deformation of the left ventricle by a kinematic model. *Journal of Biomechanics*, 25(10):1119–1127, 1992.

14. T. Arts, F. W. Prinzen, T. Delhaas, J. Milles, A. Rossi, and P. Clarysse. Mapping displacement and deformation of the heart with local sine wave modeling. *IEEE Transactions on Medical Imaging*, 29(5):1114–1123, May 2010.

15. D. J. Atkinson and R. R. Edelman. Cineangiography of the heart in a single breath hold with a segmented turboFLASH sequence. *Radiology*, 178(2):357–360, February 1991.

16. L. Axel and L. Dougherty. Heart wall motion: Improved method of spatial modulation of magnetization for MR imaging. *Radiology*, 172(2):349–350, 1989.

17. L. Axel and L. Dougherty. MR imaging of motion with spatial modulation of magnetization. *Radiology*, 171(3):841–845, June 1989.

18. L. Axel, A. Montillo, and D. Kim. Tagged magnetic resonance imaging of the heart: A survey. *Medical Image Analysis*, 9(4):376–393, August 2005.

19. E. Bergvall, E. Hedstrom, K. M. Bloch, H. Arheden, and G. Sparr. Spline-based cardiac motion tracking using velocity-encoded magnetic resonance imaging. *IEEE Transactions on Medical Imaging*, 27(8):1045–1053, August 2008.

20. A. Bistoquet, J. Oshinshi, and O. Skrinjar. Left ventricular deformation recovery from cine MRI using an incompressible model. *IEEE Transactions on Medical Imaging*, 26(9):1136–1153, September 2007.

21. A. Bistoquet, J. Oshinshi, and O. Skrinjar. Myocardial deformation recovery from cine MRI using a nearly incompressible biventricular model. *Medical Image Analysis*, 12(1):69–85, February 2008.

22. D. Bree, J. R. Wollmuth, B. P. Cupps, M. D. Krock, A. Howells, J. Rogers, N. Moazami, and M. K Pasque. Low-dose dobutamine tissue-tagged MRI with 3D strain analysis allows assessment of myocardial viability in patients with ischemic cardiomyopathy. *Circulation*, 114(1 Suppl):I33–I36, July 2006.

23. E. Castillo, A. C. Lima, and D. A. Bluemke. Regional myocardial function: Advances in MR imaging and analysis. *Radiographics*, 23:S127–S140, October 2003.

24. M. D. Cerqueira, N. J. Weissman, V. Dilsizian, A. K. Jacobs, S. Kaul, W. K. Laskey, D. J. Pennell, J. A. Rumberger, T. Ryan, and M. S. Verani. Standardized myocardial segmentation and nomenclature for tomographic imaging of the heart: A statement for healthcare professionals from the cardiac imaging committee of the council on clinical cardiology of the American Heart Association. *Circulation*, 105:539–542, 2002.

25. R. Chandrashekara, R. H. Mohiaddin, and D. Rueckert. Analysis of 3-D myocardial motion in tagged MR images using nonrigid image registration. *IEEE Transactions on Medical Imaging*, 23(10):1245–1250, October 2004.

26. Y. Chen and A. A. Amini. A MAP framework for tag line detection in SPAMM data using Markov random fields on the B-spline solid. *IEEE Transactions on Medical Imaging*, 21(9):1110–1122, September 2002.

27. T. Chen and L. Axel. Using Gabor filter banks and temporal-spatial constraints to compute 3D myocardium strain. In *Proceedings of IEEE 2006 International Conference of the Engineering in Medicine and Biology Society*, Volume 1, pp. 4755–4758, August 2006.

28. J. Chen, N. J. Tustison, and A. A. Amini. Accurate recovery of 4-D left ventricular deformations using volumetric B-splines incorporating phase based displacement estimates. In *Proceedings of SPIE Medical Imaging*, Volume 6143, February 2006.

29. T. Chen, X. Wang, S. Chung, D. Metaxas, and L. Axel. Automated 3D motion tracking using Gabor filter bank, robust point matching, and deformable models. *IEEE Transactions on Medical Imaging*, 29(1):1–11, January 2010.

30. Y. Chenoune, E. Delechelle, E. Petit, T. Goissen, J. Garot, and A. Rahmouni. Segmentation of cardiac cine-MR images and myocardial deformation assessment using level set methods. *Computerized Medical Imaging and Graphics*, 29(8):607–616, December 2005.

31. P. Clarysse, C. Basset, L. Khouas, P. Croisille, D. Friboulet, C. Odet, and I. E. Magnin. Two-dimensional spatial and temporal displacement and deformation field fitting from cardiac magnetic resonance tagging. *Medical Image Analysis*, 4(3):253–268, September 2000.

32. P. Clarysse, M. Han, P. Croisille, and I. E. Magnin. Exploratory analysis of the spatio-temporal deformation of the myocardium during systole from tagged MRI. *IEEE Transactions on Biomedical Engineering*, 49(11):1328–1339, November 2002.

33. R. T. Constable, K. M. Rath, A. J. Sinusas, and J. C. Gore. Development and evaluation of tracking algorithms for cardiac wall motion analysis using phase velocity MR imaging. *Magnetic Resonance in Medicine*, 32(1):33–42, June 1994.

34. B. P. Cupps, P. Moustakidis, B. J. Pomerantz, G. Vedala, R. P. Scheri, N. T. Kou-choukos, V. G. Davila-Roman, and M. K. Pasque. Severe aortic insufficiency and normal systolic function: Determining regional left ventricular wall stress by finite-element analysis. *Annals of Thoracic Surgery*, 76(3):668–675, September 2003.

35. X. Deng and T. S. Denney, Jr. Three-dimensional myocardial strain reconstruction from tagged MRI using a cylindrical B-spline model. *IEEE Transactions on Medical Imaging*, 23(7):861–867, July 2004.

36. X. Deng and T. S. Denney, Jr. Combined tag tracking and strain reconstruction from tagged cardiac MR images without user-defined myocardial contours. *Journal of Magnetic Resonance Imaging*, 21(1):12–22, January 2005.

37. T. S. Denney, Jr. Estimation and detection of myocardial tags in MR image without user-defined myocardial contours. *IEEE Transactions on Medical Imaging*, 18(4):330–344, April 1999.

38. L. Dougherty, J. C. Asmuth, A. S. Blom, L. Axel, and R. Kumar. Validation of an optical flow method for tag displacement estimation. *IEEE Transactions on Medical Imaging*, 18(4):359–363, April 1999.

39. M. Drangova, B. Bowman, Y. Zhu, and N. J. Pelc. *In vitro* verification of myocardial motion tracking from phase-contrast velocity data. *Magnetic Resonance Imaging*, 16(8):863–870, October 1998.

40. F. H. Epstein. MRI of left ventricular function. *Journal of Nuclear Cardiology*, 14(5):729–744, September/October 2007.

41. M. Ersoy, M. Kotys, X. Zhou, and R. M. Setser. A left ventricular motion phantom for cardiac MRI. In *BMES 2010 Annual Meeting*, October 2010.

42. S. E. Fischer, G. C. McKinnon, S. E. Maier, and P. Boesiger. Improved myocardial tagging contrast. *Magnetic Resonance in Medicine*, 30(2):191–200, August 1993.

43. S. E. Fischer, G. C. McKinnon, M. B. Scheidegger, W. Prins, D. Maier, and P. Boesiger. True myocardial motion tracking. *Magnetic Resonance in Medicine*, 31(4):401–413, April 1994.

44. D. Fleet and A. Jepson. Computation of component image velocity from local phase information. *International Journal of Computer Vision*, 5:77–104, 1990.

45. L. Florack, H. V. Assen, and A. Suinesiaputra. Dense multiscale motion extraction from cardiac cine MR tagging using HARP technology. In *ICCV Workshop on MMBIA*, pp. 372–375, October 2007.

46. D. Föll, B. Jung, F. Staehle, E. Schilli, C. Bode, J. Hennig, and M. Markl. Visualization of multidirectional regional left ventricular dynamics by high-temporal-resolution tissue phase mapping. *Journal of Magnetic Resonance Imaging*, 29(5):1043–1052, May 2009.

47. J. B. Garrison, W. L. Ebert, R. E. Jenkins, S. M. Yionoulis, H. Malcom, G. A. Heyler, A. A. Shoukas, W. L. Maughan, and K. Sagawa. Measurement of three-dimensional positions and motions of large numbers of spherical radiopaque markers from biplane cineradiograms. *Computers and Biomedical Research*, 15(1):76–96, February 1982.

48. M. A. Guttman, J. L. Prince, and E. R. McVeigh. Tag and contour detection in tagged MR images of the left ventricle. *IEEE Transactions on Medical Imaging*, 13(1):74–88, 1994.

49. I. Haber, D. Metaxas, and L. Axel. Three-dimensional motion reconstruction and analysis of the right ventricle using tagged MRI. *Medical Image Analysis*, 4(4):335–355, December 2000.

50. A. T. Hess, X. Zhong, B. S. Spottiswoode, F. H. Epstein, and E. M. Meintjes. Myocardial 3D strain calculation by combining cine displacement encoding with stimulated echoes (DENSE) and cine strain encoding (SENC) imaging. *Magnetic Resonance in Medicine*, 62(1):77–84, July 2009.

51. Z. Hu, D. Metaxas, and L. Axel. *In vivo* strain and stress estimation of the heart left and right ventricles from MRI images. *Medical Image Analysis*, 7(4):435–444, December 2003.

52. J. Huang, D. Abendschein, V. G. Davila-Román, and A. A. Amini. Spatio-temporal tracking of myocardial deformations with a 4-D B-spline model from tagged MRI. *IEEE Transactions on Medical Imaging*, 18(10):957–972, October 1999.

53. E. H. Ibrahim, M. Stuber, A. S. Fahmy, K. Z. Abd-Elmoniem, T. Sasano, M. R. Abraham, and N. F. Osman. Real-time MR imaging of myocardial regional function using strain-encoding (SENC) with tissue through-plane motion tracking. *Journal of Magnetic Resonance Imaging*, 26(6):1461–1470, December 2007.

54. E. H. Ibrahim, M. Stuber, D. L. Kraitchman, R. G. Weiss, and N. F. Osman. Combined functional and viability cardiac MR imaging in a single breathhold. *Magnetic Resonance in Medicine*, 58(4):843–849, October 2007.

55. E. H. Ibrahim, R. G. Weiss, M. Stuber, A. E. Spooner, and N. F. Osman. Identification of different heart tissues from MRI C-SENC images using an unsupervised multi-stage fuzzy clustering technique. *Journal of Magnetic Resonance Imaging*, 28(2):519–526, August 2008.

56. B. Jung, D. Fooll, P. Boottler, S. Petersen, J. Hennig, and M. Markl. Detailed analysis of myocardial motion in volunteers and patients using high-temporal-resolution MR tissue phase mapping. *Journal of Magnetic Resonance Imaging*, 24(5):1033–1039, November 2006.

57. B. Jung, M. Markl, D. Föll, and J. Hennig. Investigating myocardial motion by MRI using tissue phase mapping. *European Journal of Cardio-Thoracic Surgery*, 29S(1):S150–S157, April 2006.

58. B. Jung, M. Zaitsev, J. Hennig, and M. Markl. Navigator gated high temporal resolution tissue phase mapping of myocardial motion. *Magnetic Resonance in Medicine*, 55(4):937–942, April 2006.

59. W. S. Kerwin and J. L. Prince. Cardiac material markers from tagged MR images. *Medical Image Analysis*, 2(4):339–353, December 1998.

60. D. Kim, F. H. Epstein, W. D. Gilson, and L. Axel. Increasing the signal-to-noise ratio in DENSE MRI by combining displacement-encoded echoes. *Magnetic Resonance in Medicine*, 52(1):188–192, July 2004.

61. D. Kim, W. D. Gilson, C. M. Kramer, and F. H. Epstein. Myocardial tissue tracking with two-dimensional cine displacement encoded MR imaging: Development and initial evaluation. *Radiology*, 230(3):862–871, March 2004.

62. S. S. Klein, T. P. Graham, Jr., and C. H. Lorenz. Noninvasive delineation of normal right ventricular contractile motion with magnetic resonance imaging myocardial tagging. *Annals of Biomedical Engineering*, 26(5):756–763, September–October 1998.

63. J. P. Kuijer, M. B. Hofman, J. J. Zwanenburg, J. T. Marcus, A. C. van Rossum, and R. M Heethaar. DENSE and HARP: Two views on the same technique of phase-based strain imaging. *Journal of Magnetic Resonance Imaging*, 24(6):1432–1438, December 2006.

64. J. P. Kuijer, E. Jansen, J. T. Marcus, A. C. van Rossum, and R. M. Heethaar. Improved harmonic phase myocardial strain maps. *Magnetic Resonance in Medicine*, 46(5):993–999, November 2001.

65. Medical Imaging & Image Processing Lab. Strain encoded MRI (SENC). http://miip.nileu.edu.eg/senc.

66. N. Lin and J. S. Duncan. Generalized robust point matching using an extended free-form deformation model: Application to cardiac images. In *IEEE International Symposium on Biomedical Imaging: Nano to Macro*, pp. 320–323, April 2004.

67. N. Lin, X. Papademetris, A. Sinusas, and J. S. Duncan. Analysis of left ventricular motion using a general robust point matching algorithm. In *Medical Image Computing and Computer-Assisted Intervention*, pp. 556–563, November 2003.

68. J. B. A. Maintz and M. A. Viergever. A survey of medical image registration. *Medical Image Analysis*, 2(1):1–36, March 1998.

69. T. Mäkelä, P. Clarysse, O. Sipilä, N. Pauna, Q. C. Pham, T. Katila, and I. E. Magnin. A review of cardiac image registration methods. *IEEE Transactions on Medical Imaging*, 21(9):1011–1021, September 2002.

70. H. S. Maniar, B. P. Cupps, D. D. Potter, P. Moustakidis, C. J. Camillo, C. M Chu, M. K. Pasque, and T. M. Sundt, 3rd. Ventricular function after coronary artery bypass grafting: Evaluation by magnetic resonance imaging and myocardial strain analysis. *Journal of Thoracic and Cardiovascular Surgery*, 128(1):76–82, July 2004.

71. M. Markl and J. Hennig. Phase contrast MRI with improved temporal resolution by view sharing: k-space related velocity mapping properties. *Magnetic Resonance Imaging*, 19(5):669–676, June 2001.

72. M. Markl, B. Schneider, and J. Hennig. Fast phase contrast cardiac magnetic resonance imaging: Improved assessment and analysis of left ventricular wall motion. *Journal of Magnetic Resonance Imaging*, 15(6):642–653, June 2002.

73. S. Masood, J. Gao, and G. Yang. Virtual tagging: Numerical considerations and phantom validation. *IEEE Transactions on Medical Imaging*, 21(9):1123–1131, September 2002.

74. J. C. McEachen, A. Nehorai, and J. S. Duncan. Multiframe temporal estimation of cardiac nonrigid motion. *IEEE Transactions on Image Processing*, 9(4):651–665, April 2000.

75. T. McInerney and D. Terzopoulos. Deformable models in medical image analysis: A survey. *Medical Image Analysis*, 1(2):91–108, June 1996.

76. F. G. Meyer, R. T. Constable, A. J. Sinusas, and J. S. Duncan. Tracking myocardial deformation using phase contrast MR velocity fields: A stochastic approach. *IEEE Transactions on Medical Imaging*, 15(4):453–465, 1996.

77. A. Montillo, D. N. Metaxas, and L. Axel. Extracting tissue deformation using Gabor filter banks. In *Proceedings of SPIE Medical Imaging 2004: Physiology, Function, and Structure from Medical Images*, Volume 5369, February 2004.

78. C. C. Moore, C. H. Lugo-Olivieri, E. R. McVeigh, and E. A. Zerhouni. Three-dimensional systolic strain patterns in the normal human left ventricle: Characterization with tagged MR imaging. *Radiology*, 214(2):453–466, February 2000.

79. C. C. Moore, E. R. McVeigh, and E. A. Zerhouni. Quantitative tagged magnetic resonance imaging of the normal human left ventricle. *Top Magnetic Resonance Imaging*, 11(6):359–371, 2000.

80. P. Moustakidis, B. P. Cupps, B. J. Pomerantz, R. P. Scheri, H. S. Maniar, A. M. Kates, R. J. Gropler, M. K. Pasque, and T. M. Sundt, 3rd. Noninvasive, quantitative assessment of left ventricular function in ischemic cardiomyopathy. *Journal of Surgical Research*, 116(2):187–196, February 2004.

81. T. D. Nguyen, S. J. Reeves, and T. S. Denney, Jr. On the optimality of magnetic resonance tag patterns for heart wall motion estimation. *IEEE Transactions on Image Processing*, 12(5):524–532, 2003.

82. N. F. Osman. Detecting stiff masses using strain-encoded (SENC) imaging. *Magnetic Resonance in Medicine*, 49(3):605–608, March 2003.

83. N. F. Osman, W. S. Kerwin, E. R. McVeigh, and J. L. Prince. Cardiac motion tracking using CINE harmonic phase (HARP) magnetic resonance imaging. *Magnetic Resonance in Medicine*, 42(6):1048–1060, December 1999.

84. N. F. Osman and J. L. Prince. Regenerating MR tagged images using harmonic phase (HARP) methods. *IEEE Transactions on Biomedical Engineering*, 51(8):1428–1433, August 2004.

85. N. F. Osman, S. Sampath, E. Atalar, and J. L. Prince. Imaging longitudinal cardiac strain on short-axis images using strain-encoded MRI. *Magnetic Resonance in Medicine*, 46(2):324–334, August 2001.

86. C. Ozturk and E. R. McVeigh. Four-dimensional B-spline based motion analysis of tagged MR images: Introduction and *in vivo* validation. *Physics in Medicine and Biology*, 45(6):1683–1702, June 2000.

87. V. M. Pai and L. Axel. Advances in MRI tagging techniques for determining regional myocardial strain. *Current Cardiology Reports*, 8(1):53–58, 2006.

88. L. Pan, J. L. Prince, J. A. C. Lima, and N. F. Osman. Fast tracking of cardiac motion using 3D-HARP. *IEEE Transactions on Biomedical Engineering*, 52(8):1425–1435, August 2005.

89. L. Pan, M. Stuber, D. L. Kraitchman, D. L. Fritzges, W. D. Gilson, and N. F. Osman. Real-time imaging of regional myocardial function using fast-SENC. *Magnetic Resonance in Medicine*, 55(2):386–395, February 2006.

90. X. Papademetris, A. J. Sinusas, D. P. Dione, R. T. Constable, and J. S. Duncan. Estimating 3D strain from 4D cine-MRI and echocardiography: *In-vivo* validation. In *Medical Image Computing and Computer-Assisted Intervention*, pp. 196–205, October 2000.

91. X. Papademetris, A. J. Sinusas, P. Dione, R. T. Constable, and J. S. Duncan. Estimation of 3-D left ventricular deformation from medical images using biomechanical models. *IEEE Transactions on Medical Imaging*, 21(7):786–800, July 2002.

92. J. Park, D. Metaxas, and L. Axel. Analysis of left ventricular wall motion based on volumetric deformable models and MRI-SPAMM. *Medical Image Analysis*, 1(1):53–71, March 1996.

93. J. Park, D. Metaxas, L. Axel, Q. Yuan, and A. S. Blom. Cascaded MRI-SPAMM for LV motion analysis during a whole cardiac cycle. *International Journal of Medical Informatics*, 55(2):117–126, August 1999.

94. J. Park, D. Metaxas, A. A. Young, and L. Axel. Deformable models with parameter functions for cardiac motion analysis from tagged MRI data. *IEEE Transactions on Medical Imaging*, 15(3):278–289, June 1996.

95. N. J. Pelc, R. J. Herfkens, A. Shimakawa, and D. R. Enzmann. Phase contrast cine magnetic resonance imaging. *Magnetic Resonance Quarterly*, 7(4):229–254, October 1991.

96. N. J. Pelc, F. G. Sommer, K. C. Li, T. J. Brosnan, R. J. Herfkens, and D. R. Enzmann. Quantitative magnetic resonance flow imaging. *Magnetic Resonance Quarterly*, 10(3):125–147, September 1994.

97. D. Perperidis, R. H. Mohiaddin, and D. Rueckert. Spatio-temporal free-form registration of cardiac MR image sequences. *Medical Image Analysis*, 9(5):441–456, October 2005.

98. N. S. Phatak, S. A. Mass, A. I. Veress, N. A. Pack, E. V. R. Di Bella, and J. A. Weiss. Strain measurement in the left ventricle during systole with deformable image registration. *Medical Image Analysis*, 13(2):354–361, April 2009.

99. D. D. Potter, P. A. Araoz, K. P. McGee, W. S. Harmsen, J. N. Mandrekar, and T. M. Sundt, 3rd. Low-dose dobutamine cardiac magnetic resonance imaging with myocardial strain analysis predicts myocardial recoverability after coronary artery bypass grafting. *Journal of Thoracic and Cardiovascular Surgery*, 135(6):1342–1347, June 2008.

100. J. L. Prince and E. R. McVeigh. Motion estimation from tagged MR image sequences. *IEEE Transactions on Medical Imaging*, 11(2):238–249, 1992.

101. Z. Qian, D. N. Metaxas, and L. Axel. Extraction and tracking of MRI tagging sheets using a 3D Gabor filter bank. In *Proceedings of IEEE 2006 International Conference of the Engineering in Medicine and Biology Society*, Volume 1, pp. 711–714, August 2006.

102. Z. Qian, D. N. Metaxas, and L. Axel. Non-tracking-based 2D strain estimation in tagged MRI. In *IEEE International Symposium on Biomedical Imaging: Nano to Macro*, Volume 1, pp. 711–714, May 2008.

103. P. Radeva, A. A. Amini, and J. Huang. Deformable B-solids and implicit snakes for 3D localization and tracking of SPAMM MRI data. *Computer Vision and Image Understanding*, 66(2):163–178, May 1997.

104. T. G. Reese, D. A. Feinberg, J. Dou, and V. J. Wedeen. Phase contrast MRI of myocardial 3D strain by encoding contiguous slices in a single shot. *Magnetic Resonance in Medicine*, 47(4):665–676, April 2002.

105. E. W. Remme, K. F. Augenstein, A. A. Young, and P. J. Hunter. Parameter distribution models for estimation of population based left ventricular deformation using sparse fiducial markers. *IEEE Transactions on Medical Imaging*, 24(3):381–388, March 2005.

106. E. W. Remme, A. A. Young, K. F. Augenstein, B. Cowan, and P. J. Hunter. Extraction and quantification of left ventricular deformation modes. *IEEE Transactions on Biomedical Engineering*, 51(11):1923–1931, November 2004.

107. N. Rougon, C. Petitjean, F. Preteux, P. Cluzel, and P. Grenier. A non-rigid registration approach for quantifying myocardial contraction in tagged MRI using generalized information measures. *Medical Image Analysis*, 9(4):353–375, August 2005.

108. D. Rueckert, L. I. Sonoda, C. Hayes, D. L. G. Hill, M. O. Leach, and D. J. Hawkes. Nonrigid registration using free-form deformations: Application to breast MR images. *IEEE Transactions on Medical Imaging*, 18(8):712–721, August 1999.

109. A. K. Rutz, S. Ryf, S. Plein, P. Boesiger, and S. Kozerke. Accelerated whole-heart 3D CSPAMM for myocardial motion quantification. *Magnetic Resonance in Medicine*, 59(4):755–763, April 2008.

110. S. Ryf, M. A. Spiegel, M. Gerber, and P. Boesiger. Myocardial tagging with 3D-CSPAMM. *Journal of Magnetic Resonance Imaging*, 16(3):320–325, September 2002.

111. S. Ryf, J. Tsao, J. Schwitter, A. Stuessi, and P. Boesiger. Peak-combination HARP: A method to correct for phase error in HARP. *Journal of Magnetic Resonance Imaging*, 20(5):874–880, November 2004.

112. S. Sampath, J. A. Derbyshire, E. Atalar, N. F. Osman, and J. L. Prince. Real-time imaging of two-dimensional cardiac strain using a harmonic phase magnetic resonance imaging (HARP-MRI) pulse sequence. *Magnetic Resonance in Medicine*, 50(1):154–163, July 2003.

113. S. Sampath, N. F. Osman, and J. L. Prince. A combined harmonic phase and strain-encoded pulse sequence for measuring three-dimensional strain. *Magnetic Resonance Imaging*, 27(1):55–61, January 2009.

114. S. Sampath and J. L. Prince. Automatic 3D tracking of cardiac material markers using slice-following and harmonic-phase MRI. *Magnetic Resonance Imaging*, 25(2):197–208, February 2007.

115. P. Selskog, E. Heiberg, T. Ebbers, L. Wigstrom, and M. Karlsson. Kinematics of the heart: Strain-rate imaging from time-resolved three-dimensional phase contrast MRI. *IEEE Transactions on Medical Imaging*, 21(9):1105–1109, September 2002.

116. M. L. Shehata, S. Cheng, N. F. Osman, D. A. Bluemke, and J. A. Lima. Myocardial tissue tagging with cardiovascular magnetic resonance. *Journal of Cardiovascular Magnetic Resonance*, 11(55):1–12, December 2009.

117. D. Shen, H. Sundar, Z. Xue, Y. Fan, and H. Litt. Consistent estimation of cardiac motions by 4D image registration. In *Medical Image Computing and Computer-Assisted Intervention (MICCAI)*, Volume 3750, pp. 902–910, October 2005.

118. P. Shi and H. Liu. Stochastic finite element framework for simultaneous estimation of cardiac kinematic functions and material parameters. *Medical Image Analysis*, 7(4):445–464, December 2003.

119. P. Shi, A. J. Sinusas, R. T. Constable, and J. S. Duncan. Volumetric deformation analysis using mechanics-based data fusion: Applications in cardiac motion recovery. *International Journal of Computer Vision*, 35(1):87–107, November 1999.

120. P. Shi, A. J. Sinusas, R. T. Constable, E. Ritman, and J. S. Duncan. Point-tracked quantitative analysis of left ventricular surface motion from 3-D image sequences. *IEEE Transactions on Medical Imaging*, 19(1):36–50, January 2000.

121. S. M. Song and R. M. Leahy. Computation of 3D velocity fields from 3D cine CT images of a human heart. *IEEE Transactions on Medical Imaging*, 10(3):295–306, 1992.

122. B. S. Spottiswoode, X. Zhong, A. T. Hess, C. M. Kramer, E. M. Meintjes, B. M. Mayosi, and F. H. Epstein. Tracking myocardial motion from cine DENSE images using spatiotemporal phase unwrapping and temporal fitting. *IEEE Transactions on Medical Imaging*, 26(1):15–30, January 2007.

123. B. S. Spottiswoode, X. Zhong, C. H. Lorenz, B. M. Mayosi, E. M. Meintjes, and F. H. Epstein. 3D myocardial tissue tracking with slice followed cine DENSE MRI. *Journal of Magnetic Resonance Imaging*, 27(5):1019–1027, May 2008.

124. H. Sundar, H. Litt, and D. Shen. Estimating myocardial motion by 4D image warping. *Pattern Recognition*, 42(11):2514–2526, November 2009.

125. N. J. Tustison. *Biventricular Myocardial Strains with Anatomical NURBS Models from Tagged MRI*. PhD thesis, Washington University in St. Louis, August 2004.

126. N. J. Tustison and A. A. Amini. Biventricular myocardial strains via nonrigid registration of anatomical NURBS models. *IEEE Transactions on Medical Imaging*, 25(1):94–112, January 2006.

127. N. J. Tustison, V. G. Davila-Román, and A. A. Amini. Myocardial kinematics from tagged MRI based on a 4-D B-spline model. *IEEE Transactions on Biomedical Engineering*, 50(8):1038–1040, August 2003.

128. S. W. J. Ubbink, P. H. M. Bovendeerd, T. Delhaas, T. Arts, and F. N. van de Vosse. Towards model-based analysis of cardiac MR tagging data: Relation between left ventricular shear strain and myofiber orientation. *Medical Image Analysis*, 10(4):632–641, August 2006.

129. H. C. van Assen, L. M. J. Florack, J. J. M. Westenberg, and B. M. ter Haar Romeny. Tuple image multiscale optical flow for detailed cardiac motion extraction: Application to left ventricle rotation analysis. In *Proceedings of the MICCAI Workshop on Analysis of Functional Medical Images*, pp. 73–80, September 2008.

130. A. I. Veress, G. T. Gullberg, and J. A. Weiss. Measurement of strain in the left ventricle during diastole with cine-MRI and deformable image registration. *Journal of Biomechanical Engineering*, 127(7):1195–1207, December 2005.

131. A. I. Veress, J. A. Weiss, R. D. Rabbitt, J. N. Lee, and G. T. Gullberg. Measurement of 3D of left ventricular strains during diastole using image warping and untagged MRI images. *Computers in Cardiology*, 28:165–168, 2001.

132. H. Wang and A. A. Amini. Accurate 2-D cardiac motion tracking using scattered data fitting incorporating phase information from MRI. In *Proceedings of SPIE Medical Imaging 2010: Biomedical Applications in Molecular, Structural, and Functional Imaging*, Volume 7626, February 2010.

133. H. Wang and A. A. Amini. Cardiac motion tracking approach with multilevel B-splines and SinMod from tagged MRI. In *Proceedings of SPIE Medical Imaging 2011: Biomedical Applications in Molecular, Structural, and Functional Imaging*, February 2011.

134. H. Wang and A. A. Amini. A partial *k*-space acquisition pulse sequence for tagged MRI using CSPAMM. Technical report, Medical Imaging Lab, Electrical and Computer Engineering Department, University of Louisville, 2011.

135. Y. Wang, Y. Chen, and A. A. Amini. Fast LV motion estimation using subspace approximation techniques. *IEEE Transactions on Medical Imaging*, 20(6):499–513, June 2001.

136. V. Y. Wang, H. I. Lam, D. B. Ennis, B. R. Cowan, A. A. Young, and M. P. Nash. Modelling passive diastolic mechanics with quantitative MRI of cardiac structure and function. *Medical Image Analysis*, 13(5):773–784, October 2009.

137. H. Wen, K. A. Marsolo, E. E. Bennett, K. S. Kutten, R. P. Lewis, D. B. Lipps, N. D. Epstein, J. F. Plehn, and P. Croisille. Adaptive postprocessing techniques for myocardial tissue tracking with displacement-encoded MR imaging. *Radiology*, 246(1):229–240, January 2008.

138. World Health Organization. Cardiovascular diseases. http://www.who.int/entity/nmh/publications/fact_sheet_cardiovascular_en.pdf.

139. C. Xu, J. J Pilla, G. Isaac, J. H Gorman, A. S. Blom, R. C. Gorman, Z. Ling, and L. Dougherty. Deformation analysis of 3D tagged cardiac images using an optical flow method. *Journal of Cardiovascular Magnetic Resonance*, 12(19), March 2010.

140. P. Yan, A. Sinusas, and J. S. Duncan. Boundary element method-based regularization for recovering of LV deformation. *Medical Image Analysis*, 11(6):540–554, December 2007.

141. A. A. Young. Model tags: Direct three-dimensional tracking of heart wall motion from tagged magnetic resonance images. *Medical Image Analysis*, 3(4):361–372, December 1999.

142. A. A. Young. Assessment of cardiac performance with magnetic resonance imaging. *Current Cardiology Reviews*, 2(4):271–282, November 2006.

143. A. A. Young, D. L. Kraitchman, L. Dougherty, and L. Axel. Tracking and finite-element analysis of stripe deformation in magnetic resonance tagging. *IEEE Transactions on Medical Imaging*, 14(5):413–421, 1995.

144. A. Youssef, E. H. Ibrahim, G. Korosoglou, M. R. Abraham, R. G. Weiss, and N. F. Osman. Strain-encoding cardiovascular magnetic resonance for assessment of right-ventricular regional function. *Journal of Cardiovascular Magnetic Resonance*, 10(33):1–12, July 2008.

145. E. A. Zerhouni, D. M. Parish, W. J. Rogers, A. Yang, and E. P. Shapiro. Human heart: Tagging with MR imaging–a method for noninvasive assessment of myocardial motion. *Radiology*, 169(1):59–63, October 1988.

146. X. Zhong, P. A. Helm, and F. H. Epstein. Balanced multipoint displacement encoding for DENSE MRI. *Magnetic Resonance in Medicine*, 61(6):981–988, April 2009.

147. Y. Zhu, M. Drangova, and N. J. Pelc. Fourier tracking of myocardial motion using cine-PC data. *Magnetic Resonance in Medicine*, 35(4):471–480, April 1996.

148. Y. Zhu, M. Drangova, and N. J. Pelc. Estimation of deformation gradient and strain from cine-PC velocity data. *IEEE Transactions on Medical Imaging*, 16(6):840–851, December 1997.

149. Y. Zhu, X. Papademetris, A. J. Sinusas, and J. S. Duncan. Integrated segmentation and motion analysis of cardiac MR images using a subject-specific dynamical model. In *IEEE Computer Society Conference on Computer Vision and Pattern Recognition Workshops*, pp. 1–8, June 2008.

150. Y. Zhu and N. J. Pelc. A spatiotemporal model of cyclic kinematics and its application to analyzing non-rigid motion with MR velocity images. *IEEE Transactions on Medical Imaging*, 18(7):557–569, July 1999.

151. Y. Zhu and N. J. Pelc. Three-dimensional motion tracking with volumetric phase contrast MR velocity imaging. *Journal of Magnetic Resonance Imaging*, 9(1):111–118, January 1999.

152. Y. Zhu, P. Yan, X. Papademetris, A. J. Sinusas, and J. S. Duncan. Integrated segmentation and deformation analysis of 4-D cardiac MR images. In *IEEE International Symposium on Biomedical Imaging: Nano to Macro*, pp. 1437–1440, May 2008.

153. H. Wang and A. Amini. Cardiac motion and deformation recovery from MRI: A review. *IEEE Transactions on Medical Imaging*, 31(2):487–503, Feburary 2012.

19

MRI for OA Diagnosis and Drug Development

Saara Totterman
Qmetrics Technologies, LLC

José G. Tamez-Peña
Tec de Monterrey

19.1 Introduction to Osteoarthritis

Saara Totterman

19.1.1 What Is Osteoarthritis?

Osteoarthritis (OA), a degenerative disease of the joint, is loosely divided into different groups based on the joints involved. The form which includes multiple joints, hands, knees, hips, and spine, is considered to be hereditary; the form which includes only peripheral joints or a single joint such as knee or hip is not considered to be hereditary [1–4]. OA can be primary, purely degenerative, or secondary, typically to trauma, rheumatoid arthritis, or to infection [3]. In this chapter, we will concentrate on degenerative joint disease. Since many of the histopathological changes and other disease features in OA are similar in different joints; for the sake of simplicity, we will concentrate on the knee joint.

19.1.2 Etiology of Knee Osteoarthritis

One of the causes of OA is joint injury; however, in cases without clear injury, the etiology of OA is not well understood. Therefore, there are several schools of thoughts regarding the underlying cause

[1–4]. Since cartilage fractures heal through fibrocartilage formation and the cartilage is not able to produce new cartilage to fill the fracture site, joints with either chondral or osteochondral fracture have a very high risk of developing OA. Anterior cruciate ligament tears have high risk regardless of treatment to lead to the development of OA. Whether the underlying cause is changed in the knee biomechanics due to the tear itself or the acute cartilage injury caused by the impact of the femur on tibia cartilage is not clear [5].

There are different thoughts about the etiology. One is heavily leaning toward the changes in biomechanics either due to the microinjuries in the supporting structures or due to the microinjuries in the bone or cartilage itself. In these cases, the cartilage and/or bone fails to heal the repeated microinjury leading to the development of OA [3].

19.1.3 Anatomy of Knee

The anatomic structures of the knee include three bones, their articulating cartilage, two menisci, and four main ligaments [6]. The knee joint itself has three different components, the medial tibio-femoral joint, lateral tibio-femoral joint, and patello-femoral joint. The articulating components for the medial tibio-femoral joint are the medial tibial plateau and the medial femoral condyle; in the lateral tibio-femoral joint, they include the lateral tibial plateau and the lateral femoral condyle. In the patello-femoral joint, they include the patella and the femoral trochlea [6]. The articulating bone surfaces are covered by smooth hyaline cartilage. The medial and lateral tibial plateaus have their own separate hyaline articular cartilage plates. The lateral and medial femoral condyle cartilage plates are connected via the trochlear cartilage, which contributes to the patello-femoral joint [6].

The two menisci, the medial meniscus, and the lateral meniscus in their corresponding knee joint compartments are wedged between the articulating cartilage surfaces. The main ligaments include the anterior cruciate ligament (ACL) extending from the medio-posterior part of the lateral femoral condyle to the anterolateral part of the medial tibial spine and the posterior cruciate ligament (PCL) extending from the anterolateral part of the medial femoral condyle to the posterior part of the tibia and crossing in the middle of the knee. In addition, the joint is supported by the medial collateral ligament extending from the medial surface of the medial femoral condyle to the medial surface of the tibia and the lateral collateral ligament extending from the lateral surface of the lateral femoral condyle to the fibular head [6].

19.1.4 Histology and Magnetic Resonance Image Appearance of Knee Structures

In magnetic resonance image (MRI), signal behavior of the anatomic structures in MR images depends on the microscopic anatomy, structural architecture, and composition. The following will discuss the histology of the knee structures and then their MRI appearance. The discussion includes bones, articular cartilage, menisci, and the main knee joint ligaments.

19.1.4.1 Normal Bone Histology

The tibia and femur are long bones while the patella is a sesamoid bone. Histologically, the articulating surfaces are composed of the hyaline cartilage and its underlying bone. The subchondral bone, the bone adjacent to the cartilage, is comprised of the subchondral bone plate followed deeper by the trabecular bone, where the trabecular network is filled by hematogenous bone marrow and bone marrow fat (Figure 19.1) [7]. The cartilage is tightly connected, anchored to the subchondral bone plate by a zigzagging osteochondral junction. The deep layer of cartilage, the thin layer adjacent to the bone plate, is calcified cartilage; the much thicker superficial layer is noncalcified cartilage (Figure 19.1). These two are separated from each other by a very thin tidemark [8]. Superficial cartilage is covered by a very thin lamina splendum.

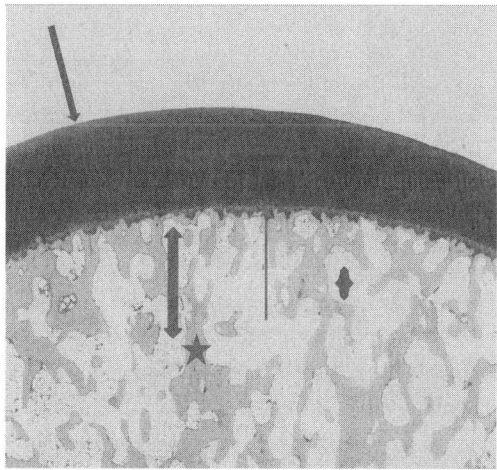

FIGURE 19.1 Histology section of cartilage showing dark blue noncalcified cartilage (thick arrow), light blue calcified cartilage underneath it (thin arrow), tide mark, a thin line between two cartilage types, subchondral bone plate underneath the calcified cartilage (double ended arrow), trabecular bone (star), and bone marrow space (cross) between them. The dark blue color of the cartilage indicates normal cartilage with high proteoglycan concentration.

19.1.4.2 MRI Appearance of Normal Bones

Regardless of used pulse sequence, bones in MR images are outlined by a very low-signal-intensity structure. In peripheral bone, this is cortical bone. Underneath the cartilage, this is subchondral bone plate. The calcified cartilage due to its high calcium concentration is seen as part of the bone plate. In the trabecular bone, the trabeculae appear as a low-signal-intensity network separated by high-signal-intensity fatty marrow and/or medium-signal-intensity hematogenous marrow (Figure 19.2). In most MR imaging sequences, only the thickest trabecular structures can be appreciated.

19.1.4.3 Normal Articular Cartilage Histology

The knee hyaline cartilage is a well-organized structure, which is composed of a matrix with proteoglycans (PG) which have a glycosaminoglycan (GAG) component, well-organized collagen fibers, and well-organized chondrocytes all covered by lamina splendum. In normal cartilage, the collagen fibers are attached to the subchondral bone plate from where they radiate upwards toward the articular surface. The collagen orientation varies from perpendicular to the subchondral bone closest to the bone (the deep layer) to parallel to the articular surface closest to the articular surface (superficial layer).

19.1.4.4 MRI Features of Normal Hyaline Cartilage

The normal cartilage has three signal intensity zones: the thin high-signal-intensity zone, the intermediate-signal-intensity middle zone, and the low-signal-intensity deep zone with some correlation to the histology (Figure 19.3) [9–12]. The well-organized collagen bundles are a major component affecting the signal behavior of the cartilage in MR images. The tightly knit well-organized collagen fibers in the normal knee are reflected in low T2 values, especially in the lower cartilage layers [13]. The variance of the normal cartilage T2 values in normal population is small as is the intrasubject variance.

19.1.4.5 Behavior of Cartilage in dGEMRIC Images

Toluidine blue staining is used to histologically evaluate cartilage GAG (Figure 19.1). Those studies have shown that GAG concentration is high in normal cartilage [14]. In MRI, the cartilage GAG

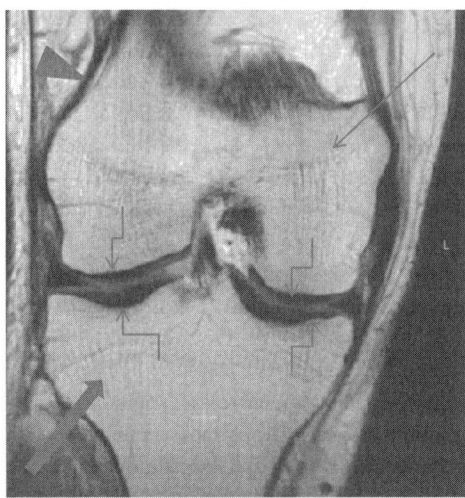

FIGURE 19.2 Proton density spin echo image of knee shows femur bone (thin arrow) and tibia bone (thick arrow) and the cartilage covering their ends (zigzag arrows). Note the low signal intensity of the deeper and high signal intensity of the superficial layers of the cartilage. The thin lines inside the bones are part of the trabecular network. Note the high signal intensity inside the bone coming from bone marrow fat and the low signal intensity of the enveloping cortical bone (triangles).

concentration is evaluated by measuring the delayed gadolinium-enhanced T1 relaxation time after an intravenous injection of an anionic paramagnetic contrast agent: gadolinium diethylene triamine penta-acid Gd(DPTA)2, Magnevist. This MRI study of GAG concentration is called delayed gadolinium-enhanced MR imaging of cartilage (dGEMRIC). Because the anionic agent, Magnevist, is repelled by the negatively charged GAG, it will concentrate in GAG-depleted areas. Furthermore, gadolinium concentration lowers T1. Therefore, T1 relaxation time is directly related to the cartilage GAG concentration in dGEMRIC studies [12]. Those studies have shown that, in normal knees, GAG concentration in normal population is age and physical activity dependent [15].

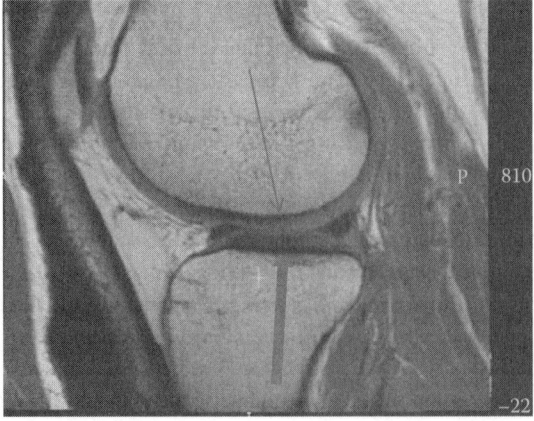

FIGURE 19.3 Sagittal proton density spin echo image shows femur (thin arrow) and tibia (thick arrow) cartilage plates. Note the low signal intensity in the deeper layers of tibia cartilage and the high signal intensity in the superficial layer.

19.1.4.6 Normal Menisci Histology

The lateral and medial menisci are fibrocartilagenous wedge-shaped crescents between the periphery of the articulating tibial and femoral cartilage surfaces. Their ends have ligamentous attachments to the tibia outside the articular cartilage. The anterior ends attach at the anterior edge of anterior tibia anterior to the tibial spines and the posterior ends to the posterior intercondylar fossa of tibia, posterior to the tibial spines. The menisci have ligamentous attachments to each other, to the corresponding collateral ligaments, to other small knee ligaments, and to the femur and tibia. Both menisci are divided based on the anatomical location into anterior horn, body, and posterior horn [6,16].

19.1.4.7 MRI Appearance of Normal Menisci

Most of the MR pulse sequences show menisci as very low-signal-intensity structures, which have high-signal-intensity lines traveling close to the periphery; these represent their vascular structures (Figure 19.4). Their ligamentous attachments to the tibia have more ligamentous appearance, higher SI (signal intensity), and parallel low-signal-intensity lines. Based on their appearance, they can be easily identified in MR images. The connecting meniscus to meniscus ligaments are well seen in MRI images. The higher-resolution images also show their smaller ligamentous attachments to the tibia and femur and to other knee ligaments [17].

19.1.4.8 Histology and MRI Appearance of Main Knee Ligaments

The main ligaments of the knee joint ACL, PCL, medial collateral ligament (MCL), and lateral collateral ligament (LCL) all have very different structures (Figure 19.5). ACL has two different components or bundles, the anteromedial (AM) and the posterolateral (PL) bundles [18,19]. The anterior bundle is more ligamentous and more vascular, while the posterior bundle is stronger and is composed of thicker, more tightly knit collagen bundles. In MR images, the AM bundle appears as a flatter higher-signal-intensity structure with parallel lower-signal-intensity lines, and the PL bundle appears with rounder well-defined low-SI structure [20]. The relative position of the two bundles is flexion dependent being parallel in full extension and being more and more crossed with increasing flexion. MCL and LCL are important for knee functions but are not discussed in detail in this chapter.

19.1.5 Functions of Knee Joint Structures

All anatomic structures of the knee have the following functions: load bearing, load distribution, stabilization, motion guiding, supporting, and geometry forming [21–23]. Although many of them have

(a)   (b)   (c)

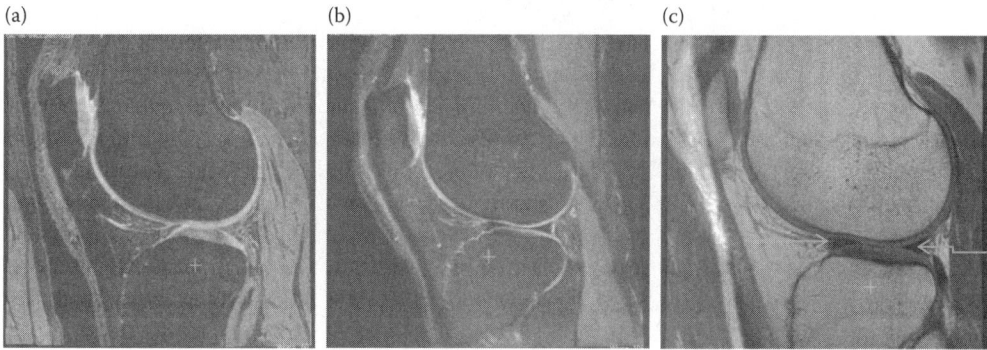

FIGURE 19.4 Anterior (thin straight arrow in c) and posterior (thin zigzag arrow in c) horn of lateral meniscus in (a) 3D water-exited DESS, (b) in fat-suppressed proton density spin echo, and (c) in proton density spin echo. Note the low signal intensity of bones in water-exited and fat-suppressed images. Also note the signal behavior of cartilage in different pulse sequences images.

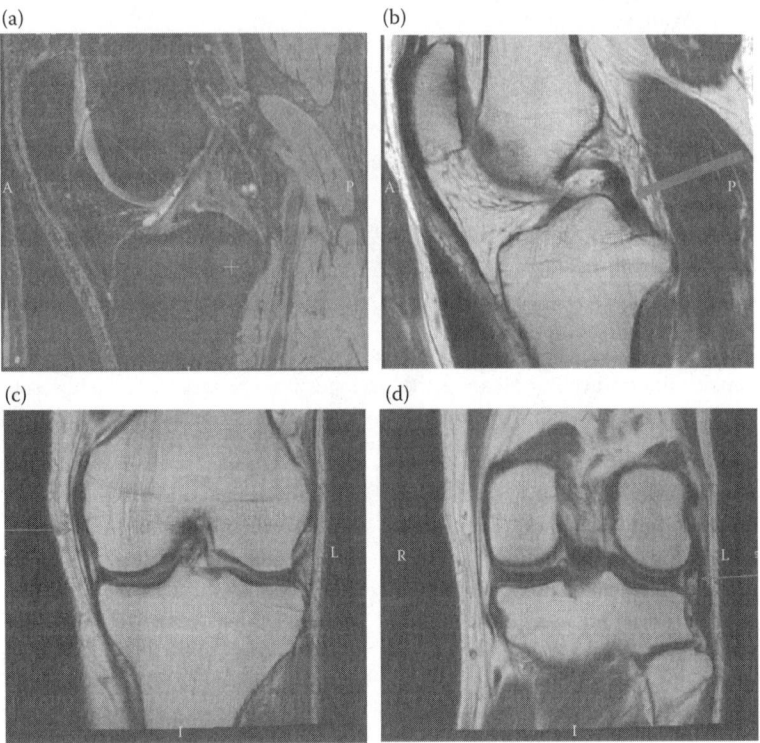

FIGURE 19.5 (a) ACL (thin arrow) in sagittal water-exited DESS and (b) PCL (thick arrow) in proton density spin echo. (c) MCL (thin arrow) and (d) LCL (thin arrow) in coronal proton density spin echo.

multiple functions, one is their primary function. The bones are the main supporting structures and form the structural platform of the joint, on which all other structures are built. Their shape forms the joint geometry, which provides the basis for the function of the joint and defines the path of the movements [21,23]. The articulating cartilage plates have their own geometry and they are guiding components of the movement mechanism (Figure 19.6). They are softer than bone and contribute to the load

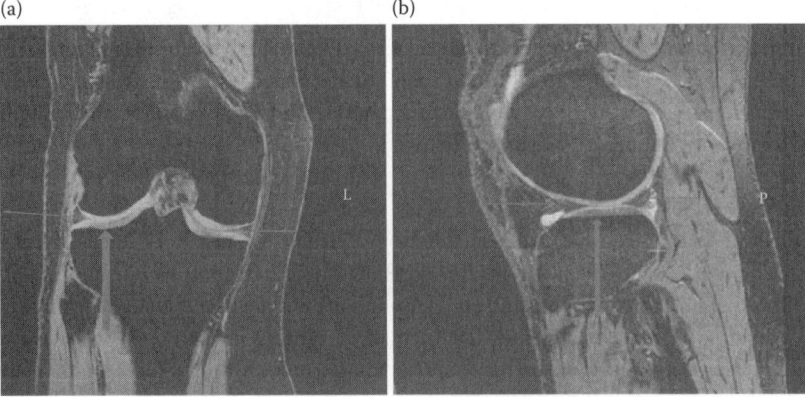

FIGURE 19.6 Images demonstrate the smoothness and geometry of the articulating cartilage surfaces (thick arrow in a and b). Also note that the curvature of the underlying bone is different from the curvature of the superficial surface of the corresponding cartilage. They also show how the geometry of the menisci (thin arrows in a and b) accommodates the shape of the cartilage plates.

bearing and load transmission and distribution to the tibial bone [22,23]. For smooth gliding motions, the articulating cartilage plates are lubricated by joint fluid.

The main function of all soft tissue structures of the joint is to stabilize the joint. In a normal knee, the smooth wedge shape of the menisci matches perfectly with the shape of the underlying tibia cartilage and the overlying femoral cartilage [24]. Their smooth surfaces and concave shapes contribute to the geometry of the articulating surfaces (Figure 19.6). As cushions between tibial and femoral cartilage, their main functions are load bearing, load transmission, and load distribution [25,26]. They are important components of the knee stabilization and their motion during knee flexion/extension guides and allows the rotation of the tibia [27–29]. The main ligaments, ACL, PCL, MCL, and LCL, are the primary knee stabilizers; the cruciate ligaments stabilize and limit the anteroposterior motion of the knee [30]. However, one important function of ACL is to guide and limit the rotation of the tibia during the knee flexion/extension. Even collateral ligaments also serve as anterior/posterior stabilizers; their main function is to provide varus valgus stability.

19.1.6 Knee OA Histopathology and MRI Findings

The knee OA can involve any or all of the three compartments of the knee joint. In the past, most of the studies have concentrated in the medial tibio-femoral joint; even the incidence in both lateral tibio-femoral OA and patello-femoral OA is relatively frequent.

Even though cartilage degeneration leading to cartilage loss is an important component of the knee OA, the use of MR imaging has shown that OA is a whole-joint disease. As such, it involves all soft tissue structures of the affected joint, not just cartilage and bone. Therefore, the next sections will describe the pathological OA changes in cartilage and bone as well as in menisci and ligaments. The picture of a knee with end-stage OA is very well known and understood. It is a knee with severe cartilage loss where two opposing bones are in contact with each other, forming the articulating surfaces. The articulating bones themselves have rough borders and, the articulating surfaces are wider and flattened, and the surface may also have attritions. The articulating bones have large peripheral and varying degrees of central osteophytes. The menisci are severely torn or totally macerated (Figure 19.7). The tibia and femur are malaligned and are either in varus or in valgus angulation (Figure 19.8). The following will try to describe the partially understood path from normal knee to knee with severe OA.

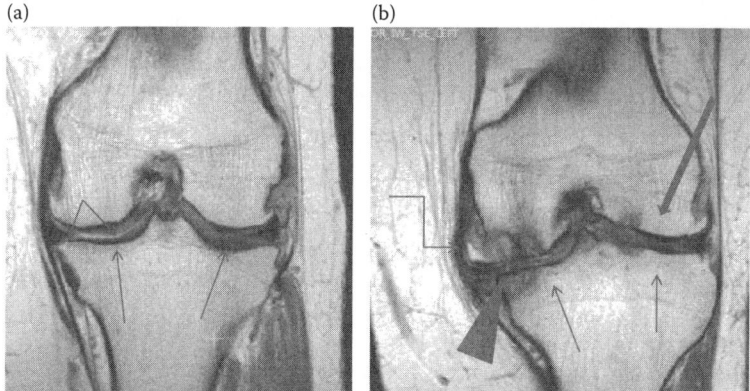

(a)   (b)

FIGURE 19.7 (a) Moderate and (b) an advanced OA MR images. Note the wide and flat ends of tibia in both cases (thin arrows), the flattened femur (thick arrow in b) and large osteophytes (zigzag arrow in b). There is advanced tibial cartilage thinning in a (dual arrows) and total cartilage loss and macerated meniscus in medial compartment in b (triangle in b).

(a)   (b)

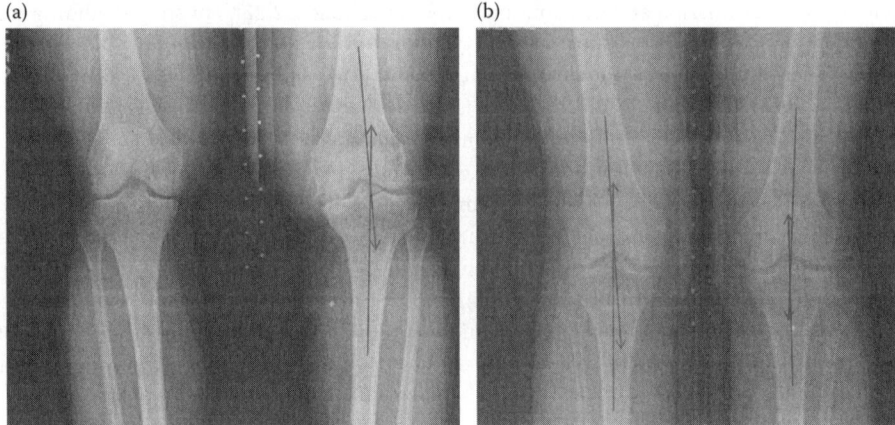

FIGURE 19.8   Plain film shows (a) varus alignment in left knee and (b) valgus alignment in both knees.

19.1.7 Bones

19.1.7.1 Histological OA Changes in Bones

19.1.7.1.1 Changes in Bone–Cartilage Interface

In the very early phase of the disease, far before cartilage defects appear, both the bone–cartilage interface and the osteochondral junction go through several changes [31].

19.1.7.1.2 Enchondral Ossification Leading to Cartilage Thinning and Subchondral Bone Thickening

Enchondral ossification, new bone formation at the bone–cartilage interface, causes many of OA-related changes. Their relationship to other cartilage changes and even the order of those changes are not well understood. Whether they are triggered by structural or compositional changes in other soft tissue structures, which alter the biomechanics or biochemical environments of the joint, or whether these changes are in the cartilage, is presently not well understood. In either case, in early OA, neurovascular bundles from the bone marrow located in the adjacent trabecular bone grow into the subchondral bone and calcified cartilage and advances further through the tidemark into noncalcified cartilage [32]. This phenomenon leads to enchondral ossification, resulting in multiple tidemarks as well as tidemark movement toward the cartilage surface. This leads to subchondral bone thickening from above and cartilage thinning from below (Figure 19.9) [33,34]. This phenomenon is probably at least partly responsible for the widening of the articulating surfaces of the bones (Figure 19.7), a common OA phenomenon seen also in plain films (Figure 19.9) [35–38].

19.1.7.1.3 Central Osteophytes

Enchondral ossification also leads to the formation of the so-called central osteophytes, where osteophyte seems to be growing from the underlying bone and slowly protruding through the cartilage into the joint space (Figure 19.10). Whether these bone–cartilage interface changes precede cartilage degeneration, occur simultaneously, or are a response to the biomechanical changes caused by cartilage deterioration is not clear.

19.1.7.1.4 Bone Shape Changes

The advancement of the tidemarks related to the enchondral ossification is not a global phenomenon. Both in the femur and in the tibia, it is more common at the periphery of the articulating surfaces but can also be seen in the middle of the cartilage, where it seems to favor certain anatomic locations. Central osteophytes are the most advanced form of that phenomenon (Figure 19.10). The local advancement of tidemark changes both the global and the local shape of the articulating bone surfaces.

(a) (b)

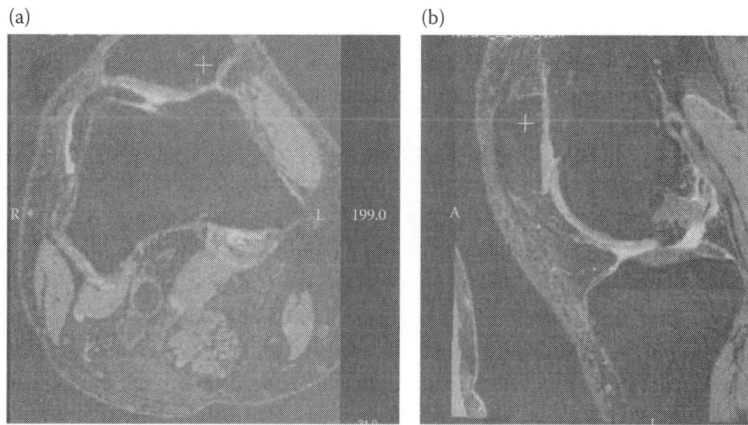

FIGURE 19.9 Axial (a) and Sagittal (b) slices showing the enchondral bone formation in patellar cartilage (cross-hair), which has led to irregular bone–cartilage interface where the bone advances into the cartilage. Also note the subsequent shape changes in the articulating surface of the patella.

The change of the shape of femoral condyles was noticed by Kellgren in 1957 [35]; however, it was ignored and forgotten for decades. During the last decade, MRI showed the widened tibial plateau in OA subjects and the widening of the plateau in increasing severity of the disease (Figure 19.7) [36,37]. More recently, besides widening articulating tibial plateaus, femoral condyles and trochlea were shown to be flattened in more advanced MRI study analysis (Figure 19.7) [38]. The articulating bone surfaces can also experience attrition in very advanced stages of OA.

19.1.7.1.5 Bone Marrow Lesions

Bone marrow edema lesions (BMEL), which were first identified as high-signal-intensity regions in T2-weighted fat-suppressed spin echo images [39], are located in the trabecular bone adjacent to the articular cartilage (Figure 19.11). Histologically, they are partly necrotic bone with vascularized fibrotic components; however, they do not have edema [40,41]. Their etiology is not yet clear.

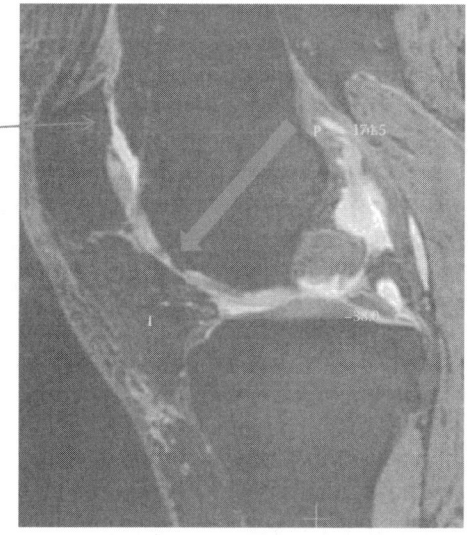

FIGURE 19.10 Central osteophyte in trochlea (thick arrow) and new bone formation in patella (thin arrow) have replaced the overlying cartilage and caused shape changes in corresponding articulating bone surfaces.

(a)   (b)   (c)

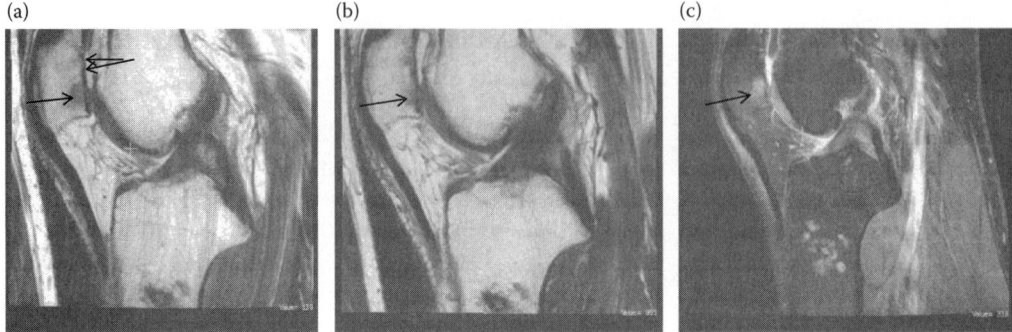

FIGURE 19.11   Bone marrow edema lesion (thin arrow) in proton density (a), in T2 (b), and in fat-suppressed proton density-weighted (c) image. In the fat-suppressed image, the lesion is well visualized while in the T2-weighted image, it blends with the surrounding tissue. Also note the advanced cartilage loss (two thin arrows) and shape changes in patella.

19.1.7.1.6 Trabecular Bone Architecture

The architecture of subchondral trabecular bone adjacent to the subchondral bone plate, to which it is directly connected, changes in OA. In OA, the subchondral bone plate itself may thicken or get thinner. Furthermore, the trabecular network is partially interrupted and the trabeculae themselves are thinner than in the contralateral normal knee [42–43].

19.1.8 Cartilage

19.1.8.1 Histological OA Cartilage Changes

Experimental animal studies and MR imaging in animals and in humans have indicated that local compositional cartilage changes precede the structural cartilage changes, cartilage thinning, and defects [44–48]. Histological cartilage studies in early OA have shown cartilage cell death and hypertrophy, edema, disappearance of lamina splendum, cartilage surface fibrillation, and decrease in cartilage GAG (Figure 19.12) [7]. The cell death and hypertrophy continue to the deeper layers and surface defects start appearing. This continues until there is full thickness defect extending to the underlying bone [7]. However, longitudinal MR studies have also shown that new areas will appear simultaneously in other regions of the same compartment or in other compartments; initially, as cartilage hypertrophy evolving into development of defects [46]. As a result, the same cartilage can have multiple hypertrophied areas and multiple defects with varying degrees of severity [46].

Collagen fibers, which are an integral part of the cartilage structure and play a significant role in the biomechanical properties of the cartilage, degenerate in OA. The degeneration changes the integrity of the collagen bundles and consequently the integrity of the cartilage [47]. This in turn changes the biomechanical properties of the cartilage [26]. The degeneration also leads to an increase in the water content of the cartilage [45].

19.1.9 MRI Findings in OA

19.1.9.1 Bones

The enchondral ossification, new bone formation at the bone–cartilage interface as mentioned before, causes many of the OA-related changes. The advancing tidemark can be seen in MRI as heterogeneity of signal intensity in the bone–cartilage interface, and later this leads to irregularity of the otherwise smooth bone–cartilage interface (Figure 19.10) [48]. The most advanced local case is a central osteophyte, which penetrates through the cartilage. The widening of the articulating ends of the bones has

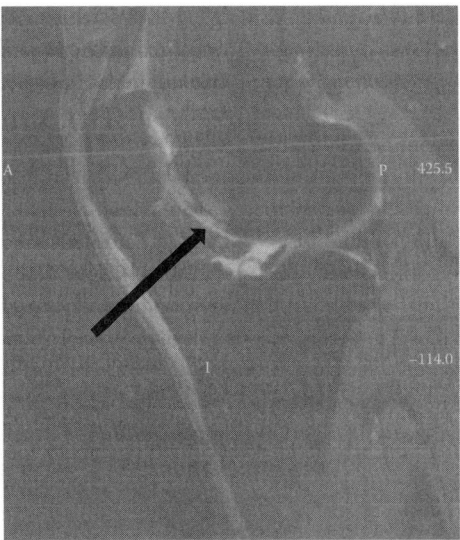

FIGURE 19.12 Fat-suppressed proton density spin echo image shows high-signal-intensity T2 cartilage lesion in trochlea cartilage (thick arrow). Note the underlying bone marrow edema lesion.

been shown by MRI (Figure 19.7) [36,37]. Besides widening of articulating tibial plateaus, femoral condyles and trochlea flatten in advanced OA [38]. The articulating bone surfaces can also experience attrition in very advanced stages of OA.

The MRI changes related to the changes in subchondral bone trabecular architecture have so far been studied only in research environment. However, there is promising research showing that the thinning of the trabeculae and disruption of the trabecular network is also identified in high-resolution MR images [43].

19.1.9.1.1 Bone Marrow Lesions

BMEL, which were first identified as high-signal-intensity regions in T2-weighted fat-suppressed spin echo images [49], are located in the trabecular bone adjacent to the articular cartilage (Figure 19.11). They are observed in all phases of OA. Small BMLs can be seen in any phase of the diseases and they have a tendency to come and go. Larger ones have a tendency to stay but their volume can fluctuate [39]. They are not specific to OA and can result from a multitude of other factors, including trauma, inflammation, infection, tumor, or osteonecrosis [39]. They can be transient and are also commonly seen in rheumatoid and psoriatic arthritis. Bone marrow lesions in OA are histologically partly necrotic bone with vascularized fibrotic components; however they do not have edema. Even though large bone marrow lesions predict disease progression and have been associated with pain, their role in early OA is not clear [40,41]. Nor do we know their temporal relationship to early cartilage changes or what leads to their disappearance.

19.1.9.2 Articular Cartilage

19.1.9.2.1 Compositional Changes

Cartilage changes in MR images can be divided into compositional and structural. The changes in GAG content, edema, and collagen degeneration are part of the compositional changes of the cartilage. The compositional changes change the MRI properties of the tissue, its signal behavior, T2 behavior and T1 values, and the dGEMRIC index. The increase in water content due to either edema or degeneration of collagen bundles changes cartilage signal intensity in MR images. This is well seen in proton density and in T2-weighted images and most probably is the source of the so-called T2 lesions (Figure 19.13), the high-signal-intensity areas in the deep layer of the cartilage with high T2 values [50,51]. In the same way, the

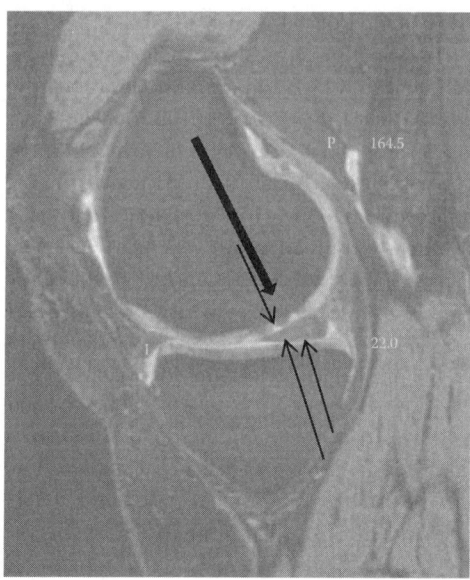

FIGURE 19.13   3D water-exited DESS image shows small very focal cartilage defects adjacent to each other. Note the good contrast between cartilage (thick arrow) and the adjacent high signal fluid (thin arrow) and meniscus (two thin arrows).

fibrillation of the cartilage surface will increase the water content and the signal intensity of the affected part of cartilage. The degeneration of collagen fibers per se affects the T2 of the cartilage; the decrease of well-organized tightly knit collagen fibers increases the cartilage T2 and increases its signal intensity [45,46]. The signal behavior of the cartilage is also affected by the enchondral ossification where the signal of the deeper layers due to the vascular invasion increases and later decreases due to the calcification of the noncalcified cartilage during the process of new bone formation as shown by advancing tidemark [48].

19.1.9.2.2 Structural Changes

The structural changes at the superficial surface of cartilage include surface fibrillation, fissures, and cartilage defects and thinning [7]. At the early phase of the disease, the superficial surface changes are detected in high-resolution MR images. In those images, the fibrillation caused distinct borders of the cartilage to disappear [44,45]. Since cartilage defects are filled by joint fluid, which has its own MRI SI, different from that of cartilage, the contrast between the cartilage and joint fluid allows their detection in MR images (Figure 19.13) [44]. In the same way, the small fissures are filled by fluid and can be seen in the early phase zigzagging inside the cartilage and in finally reaching the bone [44]. In later studies, those have led to cartilage defects and dislodged free pieces of cartilage in the joint space.

Cartilage hypertrophy or swelling and cartilage loss caused by thinning of the cartilage, either from below as a result of enchondral ossification or from above as a result of focal or larger cartilage defects, lead to changes in local cartilage thickness. Both of these phenomena also change the shape of cartilage plates and the smoothness of the corresponding surface.

19.1.9.3 Menisci

The lateral and medial menisci are crescent-shaped fibrocartilagenous structures between the periphery of the articulating tibial and femoral cartilage surfaces [6]. The menisci cushions between the tibial and the femoral cartilage bear part of the load. Their smooth surfaces and concave shapes contribute to the geometry of the articulating surfaces [24,25]. Their ends are attached to the tibia in front of and posterior to the tibial spines and have ligamentous attachments to the femur, controlling the path of

(a)   (b)   (c)

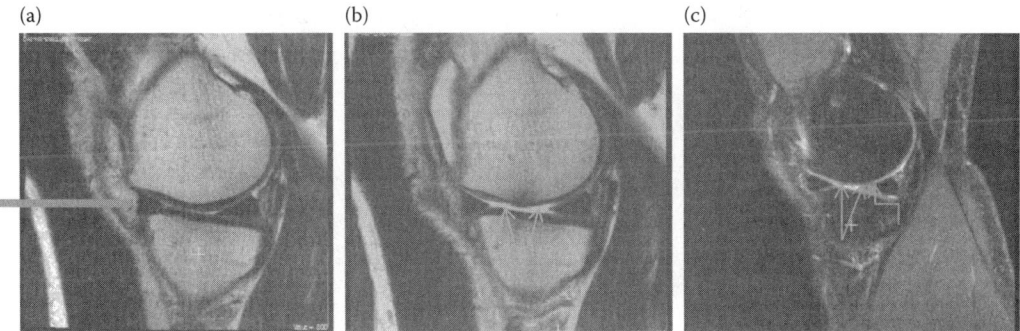

FIGURE 19.14 Low-signal-intensity anterior and posterior horn of medial meniscus (thick arrow) in proton density (a), in T2-weighted (b), and in fat-suppressed proton density spin echo (c) images. Note a tear seen in posterior horn in (c) (zigzag arrow). Note the high-signal-intensity of joint fluid in T2W and in fat-suppressed image (dual arrow).

movement during knee flexion. The end-stage OA is very much an end stage also for that compartment's meniscus; it is either severely torn, or macerated or entirely absent (Figures 19.14 and 19.15) [52]. Any structural change in meniscus will affect all of its functions [27,28,53]. Meniscus tears are common in advanced OA in the affected compartment, but they are less common in the early phase of the disease. They can affect any or all parts of the meniscus [54]. Tears in the meniscal body can extend to the anterior and/or posterior horn and vice versa. Meniscus tears change the hoop forces in the meniscus altering meniscus' load-absorbing ability and in thus changing the loading conditions in the knee [27,28]. On the other hand, the tears also affect the joint geometry and the ability of the meniscus to contribute to knee joint flexion. The meniscectomy, which also changes the geometry of the articulating surfaces and the load distribution over the joint, is known to lead to the development of knee OA [27,28,53]. Meniscus subluxation, where part of the meniscus is extruded outside the articulating tibia cartilage surface, changes the geometry of the articulating surface and the distribution of the load (Figure 19.15) [53]. Advanced meniscus tears have predicted the progression of the disease, defined as cartilage loss [54,55]. Meniscus subluxation has been associated with OA and has also correlated to and

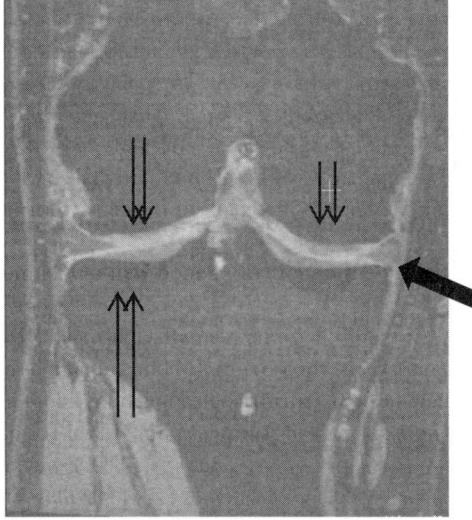

FIGURE 19.15 Coronal water-suppressed 3D DESS image shows subluxation of the body of medial meniscus (thick arrow). Also note the widened and flattened articulating bone surfaces of femur (two short arrows) and tibia (two long arrows).

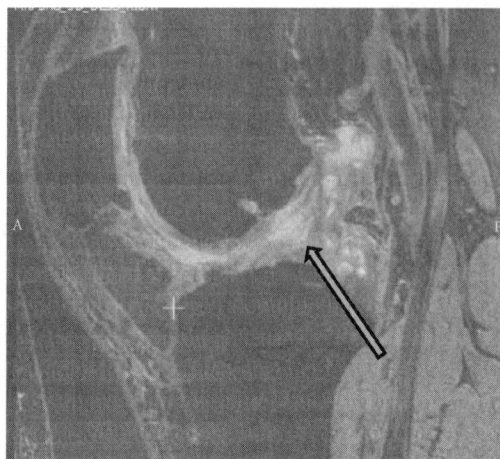

FIGURE 19.16   Sagittal image of knee with torn ACL (thick arrow).

predicted disease progression [56]. However, since meniscus tears are not as common in earlier OA, it is not clear how they are associated with the development of OA.

19.1.9.4 Knee Alignment

Changes in knee alignment, defined as the angle between the long axis of the distal tibia to the long axis of the distal femur at the level of knee joint, have been associated with the development of OA [57]. Several studies have shown that many knees with medial compartment OA have a greater degree of varus than normal knees and many knees with lateral compartment OA have a greater degree of valgus. These findings have led to an interpretation that varus or valgus malalignment is either associated with or is a risk factor for OA [57]. The change in knee alignment is considered to affect the biomechanics of the knee; the increase in varus or valgus is considered to change the load balance between the medial and lateral compartment. However, whether the malalignment is a result of OA or a result of changes in knee supporting structures leading to OA is not clear.

19.1.9.5 Ligaments

Acute ACL tears lead to a very high incidence of later OA regardless of the type of treatment.

On the other hand, an ACL tear can be a complication/consequence of the OA. Enlarging osteophytes at the edges of the intercondylar femoral notch can physically wear and consequently cause a rupture of weakened ACL. A torn ACL appears in MR as an ill-defined, greatly enlarged structure with a higher-SI band at the location of the ACL (Figure 19.16) [58].

In the acute post-ACL tear phase, the MR images have revealed bone marrow edema lesions and local compression fractures both in the lateral femur and in the tibia [59]. Even if all these injuries by themselves can lead to secondary OA, the changes in knee biomechanics are considered to be an equally important factor in the development of post-ACL tear OA [59,60].

19.2 MR Imaging of Osteoarthritis

Saara Totterman

MRI is currently the best imaging modality for musculoskeletal structures. It visualizes bones, including cortex and trabecular bone, bone marrow, cartilage, ligamentous structures, menisci, fat, muscles, tendons, vascular structures, and larger nerves in great detail.

Clinically, MR imaging is a diagnostic tool for different knee diseases and conditions. Both in late and acute post-traumatic phases, it is used for meniscal tears, ligament tears and injuries, cartilage and cartilage bone fractures, and ruptures and tears of tendon and muscles. Perhaps the most common indication for MR imaging outside of trauma is diagnosing the source of knee pain. Even if MR imaging is not used to make the OA diagnosis, it is now widely used by the medical device industry to develop patient-specific treatment options and tools to guide surgical procedures.

Since MR imaging shows the soft tissue structures of the knee in great detail, it is extensively used in cross-sectional and longitudinal OA progression studies to better understand the disease itself [61]. The hope is that this will lead to the discovery of new measurable OA MR imaging findings which are sensitive to disease progression. Their use in OA drug discovery should then facilitate more efficient and less costly development of new OA therapies.

The following will discuss the imaging sequences used for imaging bone and soft tissue structures in knee OA subjects, their MR image findings, and how to image them for quantitative measurements. The following discussion will concentrate on cartilage, bones, menisci, and ligaments.

19.2.1 MR Imaging of Cartilage in OA

19.2.1.1 MR Imaging Sequences for Cartilage

The most common cartilage imaging MR pulse sequences are: T1-weighted (T1W), proton density (PD), T2-weighted (T2W), spin echo (SE), multiecho SE sequences, and their fat-saturated or water-suppressed counterparts, 3D spoiled gradient recall echo (SPGR), 3D gradient recall echo (GRE), and fat-saturated or water-excited counterparts with newer faster modifications, all with their manufacturer-dependent variances, and 3D dual echo steady-state gradient recall echo sequence (DESS) [62,63]. Since the detection of changes, including small cartilage defects and local SI changes, greatly depends on the image resolution, many new pulse sequences have emerged with better signal-to-noise ratios and high isotropic resolution. Examples are the 3D fast spin echo (FSE) and the 3D FSE-Cube sequences [64,65]. To better evaluate the cartilage–bone interface considering the very short T2 time of calcified cartilage, new ultra-short-echo time imaging (UTE) sequences have been applied in cartilage imaging with and without fat saturation.

19.2.1.2 Imaging Planes

The MR images can be acquired in any of the three orthogonal planes or any in oblique modifications of them (Figure 19.17). The most qMRI studies evaluating tibio-femoral joint cartilage plates have acquired images in sagittal and/or in coronal planes. The 3D WE DESS imaging in the sagittal plane used for OAI data is more sensitive for cartilage loss than the 3D fat-saturated T1W SPGR sequence acquired in the coronal plane. Cartilage in the patello-femoral joint can also be seen in sagittal plane images [66]. However, axial plane imaging is better for knee cartilage due to its curved anatomy. The newer isotropic high-resolution sequences may make future imaging plane selection more or less irrelevant [64,65].

19.2.1.3 Cartilage in Different Pulse Sequences

MR appearance of cartilage depends on the pulse sequence used and the resolution. In highly T1-weighted (T1W) images like 3D spoiled gradient recall echo (SPGR) images, it has an almost homogenously high signal intensity (Figure 19.17a); in proton density (PD) images, for example, proton density SE images and proton density-weighted (PDW) 3D gradient recall echo (GRE) images, its SI changes gradually from lower signal intensity in deep layers to high signal intensity in the superficial layer [66,67]. In T2-weighted (T2W) images like T2W spin echo images and T*-weighted (T2*W) GRE images, the cartilage has lower SI (Figure 19.18). Higher-resolution images like 3D GRE and 3D DESS reveal more intricate inner structures of the normal cartilage, including a columnar appearance of normal cartilage whose origin is not well understood (Figure 19.19).

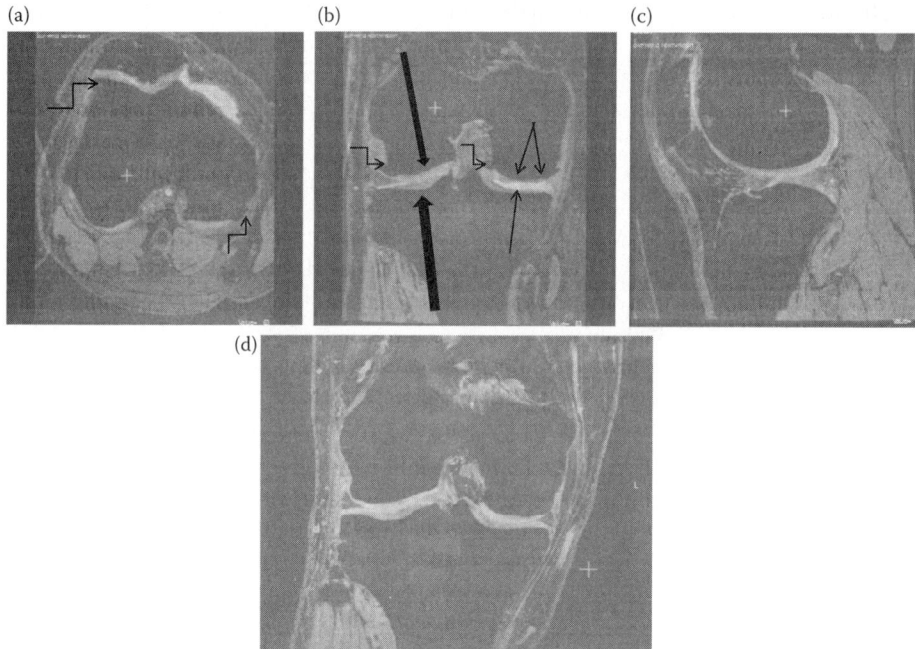

FIGURE 19.17 MR images of the osteoarthritic knee in three orthogonal planes, axial (a), coronal (b), and sagittal (c). The crosshair shows the same anatomic location in each plane. Note the widening and flattening of the tibial and femoral articulating surfaces (thick arrows), thinning and defect in lateral tibia and femur cartilage (thin arrows), and osteophytes (zigzag arrows). (d) 3D spoiled gradient recall echo (SPGR) images.

What imaging sequences and what planes are used depend on the purpose of the imaging. The purpose of clinical imaging is making a diagnosis and generally staging the disease. Progression studies have multiple purposes, including to detect how the diseased joint is different from a normal joint; in other words which MR findings reflect the existence of the disease, which show the progression of the disease, which predict disease progression, and which change most over time or are most sensitive to the progression. The clinical trials have predefined MR image findings, or imaging biomarkers, for which

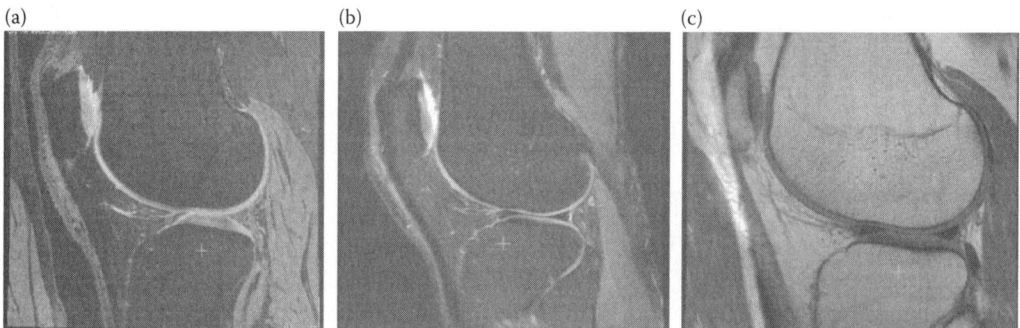

FIGURE 19.18 Cartilage signal behavior in water-exited 3D DESS (a), in fat-suppressed proton density spin echo (b), and in proton density spin echo (c) images. Note the good contrast between low-signal-intensity bone and high-signal-intensity cartilage in the water-exited 3D DESS image and the contrast between the low-signal-intensity deep layer and the higher-signal-intensity superficial layer in the spin echo images. The signal intensity difference is accentuated by fat suppression.

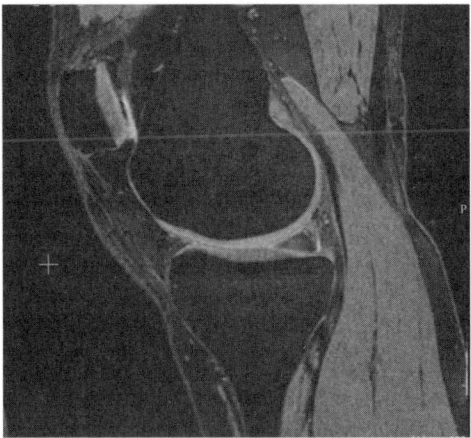

FIGURE 19.19 This high-resolution water-exited 3D DESS image demonstrates the columnar appearance of normal tibial cartilage.

the knee is imaged over the trial period. The image findings are then either scored or quantitatively measured to determine therapeutic efficacy.

19.2.2 Imaging of Structural Cartilage Changes

19.2.2.1 Quantitative Magnetic Resonance Imaging

Quantitative magnetic resonance imaging (qMRI) is widely used for cartilage, and less for bones, menisci, or muscles. The purpose of quantitative MRI is to provide numerical measurements for different OA-related structural changes. For that purpose, the cartilage, bones, menisci, and or muscles are segmented either by manual tracing or by semiautomated or automated segmentation methods (Figure 19.20) [67–70]. The segmentation provides a basis for both simple thickness and volume or more advanced curvature or other shape parameters' calculations. For visualization purposes, the segmented structures need to be surface rendered to create their 3D models (Figure 19.21) [71–74]. For complex measurements, the segmentations are treated as physical objects and all their physical parameters like

(a) (b)

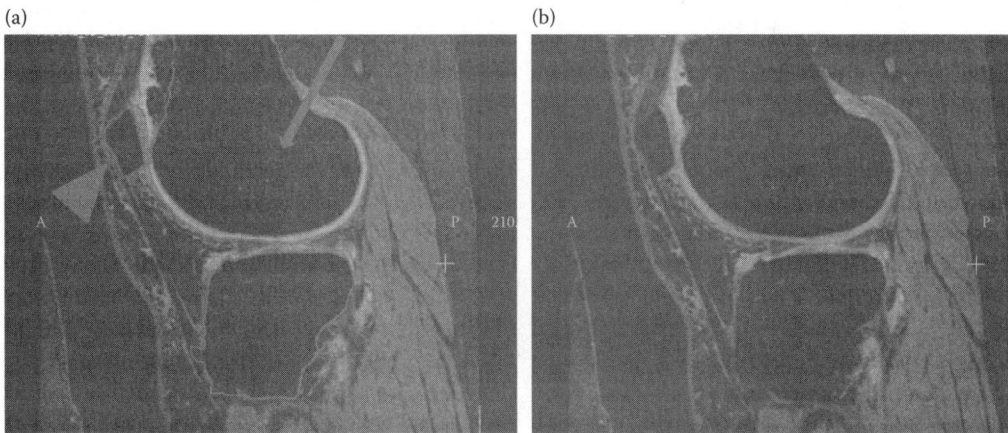

FIGURE 19.20 Segmented femur (thick arrow), tibia (thin arrows), and patella (triangle) bones and their cartilage in (a). These were automatically segmented from water-exited 3D DESS image series. The corresponding slice location is shown in (b).

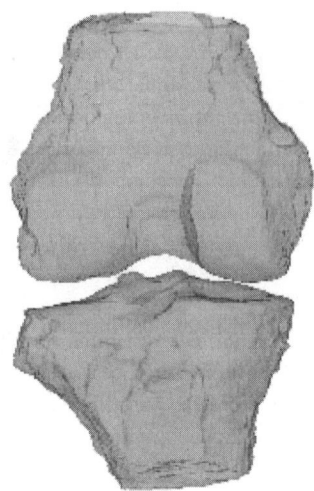

FIGURE 19.21 A surface rendering of automatically segmented femur and tibia bones seen from behind. Note the widened and flattened tibia and femur in this OA knee.

thickness, curvature, and so on can be calculated (Figure 19.22) [38,75]. Information, for example, thickness, can be also visualized and displayed as a thickness map that visualizes the thickness measured at each point on the cartilage surface (Figure 19.23) [72–74]. Parameter maps such as thickness for different time points can be compared to create difference/change maps. Since the thickness maps calculate thickness for each surface point on the structure's surface, change maps calculate and visualize the change in thickness over time, either increase or decrease, for every surface point [72–74]. Newer, more advanced methods calculate numeric values representing the local or whole volume of cartilage lost due to defects and/or thinning or that gained in hypertrophic regions [73,74].

19.2.2.2 Cartilage Thickness and Volume Changes

Structural cartilage changes are caused by loss or gain [76]. Cartilage loss in OA is caused by degenerative defects and/or thinning from above or by advancing calcifying cartilage with an advancing tidemark from below [77–80]. Both of these lead to a decrease in cartilage thickness and volume. Cartilage hypertrophy and swelling, noted in the early phase of the disease, increase both thickness and volume [80].

In the OA knee, qMRI using manual, semiautomated, or automated segmentation is mostly used to study cartilage volume and thickness and corresponding changes in longitudinal and cross-sectional

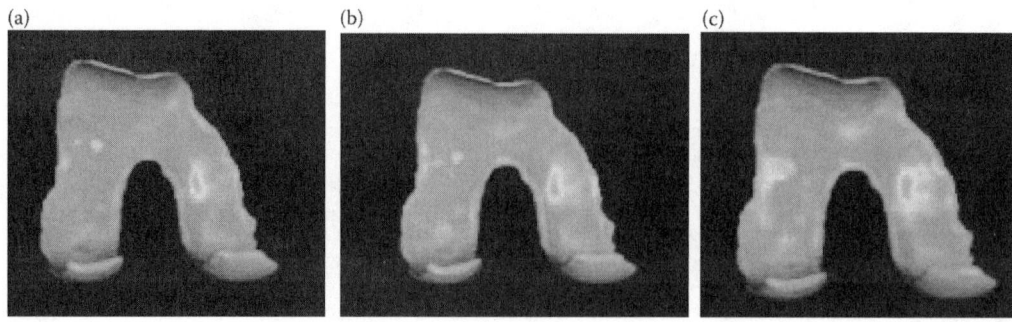

FIGURE 19.22 Femur cartilage thickness maps derived from automatically segmented image sets for baseline (a), 12 months (b), and for 24 months (c) follow up. The maps are seen from above. The yellow to red indicates areas of increasingly thinner cartilage.

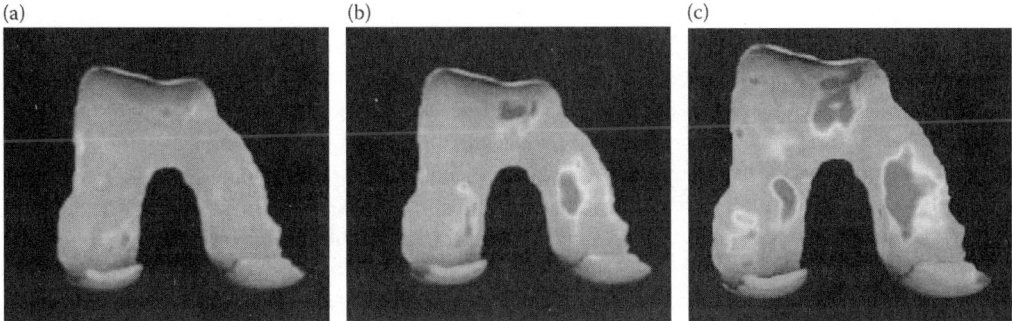

FIGURE 19.23 Results of mapping the cartilage thickness maps from Figure 19.6 to the reference atlas. The maps are seen from above. The baseline cartilage thickness (a) is compared to the 24 month follow-up visit (b) to compute the change in cartilage thickness over time (c). Note the locality of the changes; the defects are local and the local defects are getting deeper and bigger. However, at the same time, new local areas of defects as well as thickening appear.

OA studies. However, since cartilage swelling and hypertrophy as well as cartilage defects are often colocated in the same cartilage regions, their combined effects on such gross measurements can obscure longitudinal change. The thickness maps capture the local bidirectionality of the changes with greater sensitivity (Figures 19.22 and 19.23) [71–74]. Therefore, particularly in early OA studies, thickness change maps are gaining more interest. Their use has improved the medical communities' understanding of the events related to the progression of the disease. Existing studies have shown that bidirectional changes continue through the different stages of the disease; they do not progress in the same location on a continuous scale, and instead new areas in different regions get involved and progress more rapidly [80]. This heterogeneity in the location and rate of progression makes it very difficult to follow disease progression with average thickness and volume measurements [80]. Therefore, more advanced algorithms have been developed to quantify changes related only to cartilage lost or gained from the thickness difference maps [72–74]. These will be discussed in detail in the following section.

Cartilage qMRI studies use mainly fat-saturated 3D SPGR, water-excited (WE) 3D DESS, and their fast counterparts (Figure 19.24) [62–66]. One group used both fat-saturated 3D SPGR and 3D GRE sequences, which they are coregistered and fused for segmentation [70]. The fat-saturated 3D SPGR provides good contrast between the saturated low-SI bone marrow fat and the high-SI cartilage [14].

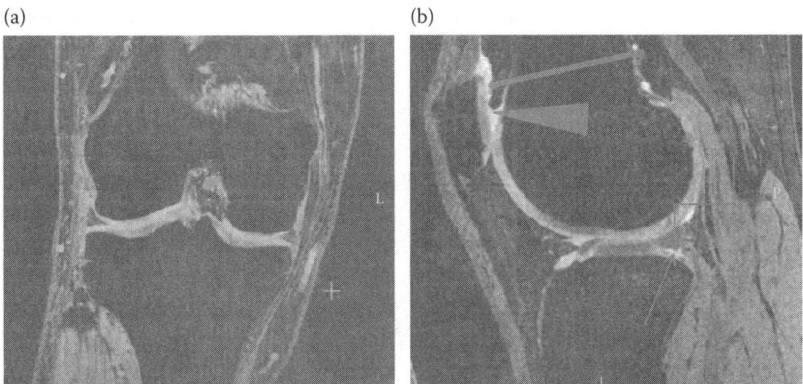

FIGURE 19.24 The two most common qMR images, a fat-saturated 3D SPGR (a) in coronal plane, and a water-exited 3D DESS in sagittal plane (b). Note the good contrast between bones and the cartilage in both images. Also note the good contrast in DESS series between the high signal intensity fluid (zigzag arrow) and a small cartilage defect in lateral tibia cartilage (thin arrow) and between fluid (triangle) and patella cartilage irregularities (thick arrow in b).

However, the contrast between the fluid and cartilage and between degenerated cartilage and degenerated menisci is not good [62–66]. When appropriate imaging parameters are used, the WE 3D DESS series provides good contrast between the medium-SI cartilage and the high-SI fluid (Figure 19.24) [62–66]. Both pulse sequences have problems separating the degenerating cartilage from the inflamed synovial tissue and separating the cartilage from the degenerated menisci.

The most important factor in early OA cartilage imaging besides tissue contrast is image resolution. In-plane resolution is crucial for detection of small cartilage defects and fissures, while slice thickness is important for accurately reflecting the thickness and MR properties of the curved cartilage [62–66]. The higher performance of the newer 3D pulse sequences and the newer receiver coil technology has considerably improved the odds of detecting earlier cartilage, bone–cartilage interface, and even bone changes [64,65].

19.2.3 Imaging of Compositional Cartilage Changes

19.2.3.1 T2 and Signal Intensity Changes

As mentioned before, osteoarthritic changes lead to cartilage T2 relaxation time (T2) and SI changes, and changes in GAG content of the cartilage. T2 is evaluated using both dual and multiecho spin echo sequences with 4–11 echoes [81,82]. Although the fast spin echo (FSE) dual echo sequences, due to stimulated echo, were not considered to provide reliable measurements, their fat-suppressed counterpart has performed satisfactorily well [62]. T1rho has also been used to evaluate compositional changes; however, since it requires special pulse sequences, it has not yet been widely applied in research [83]. The newer approach is to measure T2*, where the use of UTE T2 mapping has provided promising results to evaluate T2 changes in deep layers of cartilage [84]. The change is considered to reflect degeneration of the collagen bundles.

The signal intensity measurements have mainly used 3D fat-suppressed SPGR and 3D WE DESS sequences [85]. In T1W images, SI changes have roughly correlated to the K-L scores; in 3D WE DESS images, the correlation has been higher [85]. Due to the heterogeneity of OA pathology and that of its locations, both T2 and SI changes vary from local through multiple local to global changes [85]. The conventional 2D T2 measurements from one to two slices provided new information on OA. However, to fully understand the local and global changes during disease progression, studies require T2 information across the entire cartilage plates. Therefore, newer methods use a 3D approach by segmenting the cartilage either manually from T2 image sets or by coregistering the segmented 3D structural images to the T2 image sets and extracting the T2 values (Figure 19.25) as discussed in the following section. In OA populations, the 3D T2 measurements have proven to be reproducible. Even though they correlate to K-L scores, they are not in wide clinical use for diagnosis or for staging of the disease. However, there is a concerted effort by using the data collected in the NIH Osteoarthritis Initiative (OAI) to validate its utility as an early-phase diagnostic tool and its predictive value for disease progression.

Heterogeneity of cartilage SI is reflected in the variance of cartilage plate SI values. Cartilage SI changes are also reflected in the contrast between subchondral bone and the deep layers of cartilage. Normal cartilage has high contrast values; however, the vascularization of the subchondral bone plate, advancement of the tidemark, and increase in cartilage water content in osteoarthritic cartilage decrease the contrast. Since the nature of such changes in cartilage SI behavior is very sequence dependent, there is much less information available about local or global cartilage SI behavior in OA.

19.2.3.2 Cartilage dGEMRIC

Cartilage GAG content is measured using delayed gadolinium-enhanced MR imaging (dGEMRIC) [14]. Even though dGEMRIC images showed that cartilage T1 decreases in advancing OA, several confounding factors make defining the significance of the measurement and its change problematic. For example, body mass index (BMI), a known predictor and risk factor for OA, is directly related to the dGEMRIC index. Further, hypertrophic cartilage changes in degenerating cartilage may increase GAG content, also increasing the index. For that reason, though dGEMRIC is useful in cartilage research, it has less value in longitudinal progression studies or clinical trials.

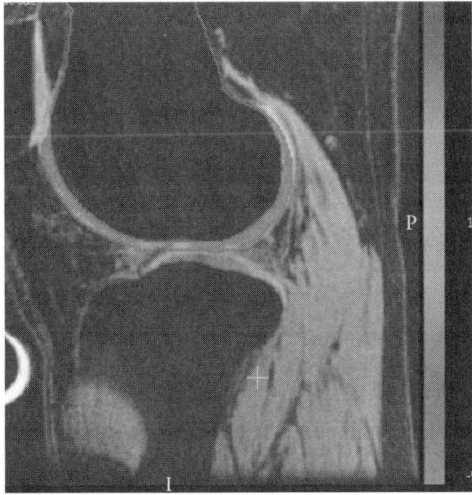

FIGURE 19.25 T2 map of segmented femoral cartilage.

19.2.4 MR Imaging of Bones in OA

19.2.4.1 Bones in Different Pulse Sequences

As mentioned before, bones are composed of two structurally different components, the very tightly woven cortical bone and the loosely connected trabecular network of inner trabecular, cancellous bone. Cortical bone envelops the inner trabecular bone and is directly connected to it. Due to the lack of water protons, cortical bone has very low signal intensity in all pulse sequences. Trabecular bone is seen as a low SI network visualized especially in more T2*W 3D GRE image series against the higher-SI red marrow and the high-signal-intensity fatty marrow, which fill the spaces in the trabecular network [79].

The commonly used qMRI sequences are suitable for segmenting the bones using both manual and automated approaches. The osteochondral junctions in tibia, femur, and patella are best seen in T1W fat saturated and WE 3D SPGR series, but can be easily seen in the other common qMR imaging series, WE 3D DESS series (Figure 19.26) [62–66]. In both of these series, the high-signal-intensity cartilage is well contrasted against the low-signal-intensity saturated/suppressed bone marrow fat. In

(a)   (b)

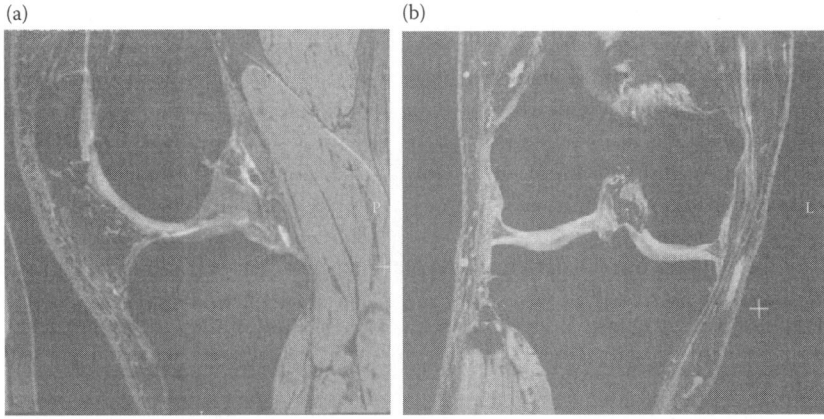

FIGURE 19.26 Water-exited 3D DESS (a) and fat-suppressed 3D SPGR (b) images. Both show good contrast between cartilage and bone. Cartilage to cartilage separation is not clear in SPGR sequence in (b).

these images, the cortical bone in the shaft, which is bone outside the articulating surfaces, is not as easily distinguished from the surrounding low-SI fat. Therefore, some groups have chosen to use both a fat-suppressed 3D SPGR sequence and a 3D GRE sequence, then coregister and fuse them and use the combined data for bone segmentation [70,73]. Automated atlas-based segmentation algorithms perform well in qMRI sequences [74].

19.2.4.2 Imaging of Structural Bone Changes

The structural bone changes induced by OA include flattening of the subchondral bone plate, widening of the cartilage–bone interface and the articulating ends of the bones, and emergence of peripheral and central osteophytes (Figure 19.27). All of these change the shape of the articulating end of the bones. Flattening of the subchondral bone plate changes the curvature and the spatial location of the bone–cartilage interface; widening of the articulating end of the bones increases the surface area of the subchondral bone plate and the curvature; the central osteophytes make the bone–cartilage interface irregular and bumpy; and formation of peripheral osteophytes widens the bone ends [71,75,86,87].

19.2.4.2.1 Curvature Changes

As mentioned above, flattening and widening of the subchondral bone plate in OA changes the curvature of the articulating bone surfaces [75,87]. Measuring the curvature or the bone–cartilage interfaces of the tibia, femur, or patella per se do not require segmenting the bones (Figure 19.20). The curvature can be evaluated from the segmented cartilage image data sets which are created during the routine articular cartilage qMRI processes. However, it does require surface rendering of the segmented cartilage and evaluating the bone-facing surface (Figure 19.28). Since the cartilage-only segmentation approaches do not include the cartilage at the osteophytes, this portion of bone–cartilage interface is excluded from surface area and curvature calculations. Many of the segmentation approaches divide the femur cartilage into medial and lateral weight-bearing regions, and medial and lateral posterior condyle and trochlea regions, and this enables the curvature change calculations to be performed on a per-region basis [75,89]. The commonly used measurement is average curvature; however, the standard deviation of curvature measurements reflects the variability of the local curvature measurements, indicating irregularity, the presence of central osteophytes, or other local changes in curvature [75].

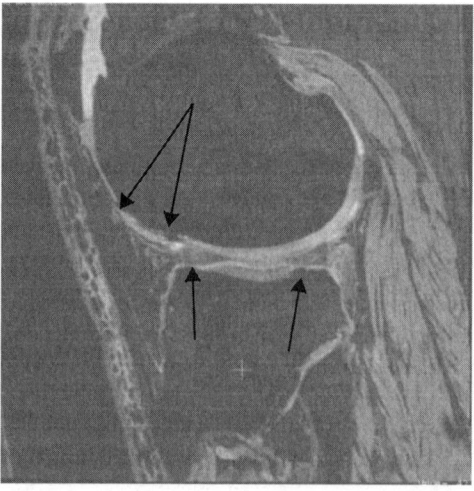

FIGURE 19.27 A sagittal 3D DESS image of advanced knee OA. Also note how the advancing bone in the form of central osteophytes and the lateral tibia and femoral trochlea (thin arrows) is changing the shape of the articulating surface of the lateral tibia and that of the femoral trochlea.

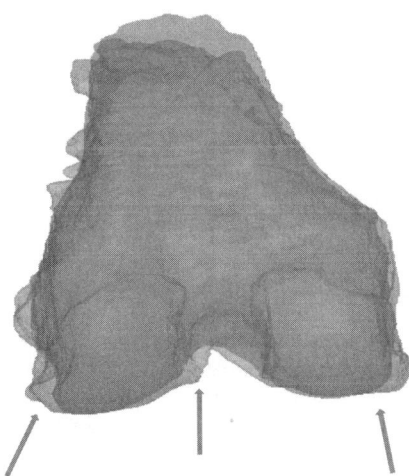

FIGURE 19.28 Surface-rendered results of mapping the segmented femur of the OA subject (green) to the segmented femur of the reference atlas (red). Note the flattened and widened articulating surfaces in the subject's femur (thick arrows).

19.2.4.2.2 Increase in Bone–Cartilage Interface Surface Area

The processed qMRI cartilage data can also be used to compute the bone–cartilage interface surface area. Similar to curvature calculations, the bone-facing surface needs to be identified in the image set. The increase in bone–cartilage surface area is primarily caused by widening of the articulating ends of tibia and femur. The widening of the entire tibial end, including the proximal end of the shaft and formation of osteophytes, is easily identified in MR images. This phenomenon can be evaluated from processed cartilage qMRI image sets, in cases where the bone segmentation is part of the cartilage qMRI process. The surface-rendered segmented bone image data can also be used to create shape change maps to visualize the nature, location, and the degree of the widening either from time point to time point or in correlation to the normal population reference map. These maps can also be used to investigate the changes. These methods are explained in the following section.

19.2.4.3 Osteophytes

Peripheral osteophytes cannot be evaluated from segmented cartilage image data. Their evaluation requires segmenting the bones themselves. That could be done manually, semimanually, or using automated methods. The automated segmentation methods are considerably faster and more reproducible than the others. Most of the automated cartilage segmentation methods include bone segmentation as part of the process. Many of the methods also divide the bones into anatomic regions, which enables following local changes in the resulting numerical data. Using the same method employed for following cartilage and bone surface features, the segmented bone image sets can also be used to create osteophyte maps and osteophyte change maps. Those have shown a measureable increase in osteophytes volume over a 1-year period of time.

The bone and bone–cartilage segmentations from research subjects' and OA patients' MR images are commonly used by the medical device industry. For years, the industry used research subjects' image segmentations in total and partial knee prosthesis product development. Now, as the medical device industry is moving toward patient-specific device development, it uses patient-based bone and cartilage segmentations from MR images for surgical planning and for developing patient-specific guides for surgery or for developing patient-specific prostheses.

19.2.4.4 Imaging of Compositional Bone Changes

19.2.4.4.1 Bone Marrow Edema Lesions

Bone marrow edema lesions and changes in trabecular architecture are considered compositional bone changes. Bone marrow edema lesions are seen as high-signal-intensity areas in T2-weighted (T2W), fat-suppressed (FS), and water-excited (WE) spin echo (SE) images (Figure 19.29) [88]. However, due to their watery content, they are also seen in both PD and intermediate-weighted FS and WE spin echo images and PD and IW inversion recovery image series. However, the FS and WE gradient echo (GRE) images, either SPGR or GRASS or the WE 3D DESS series, do not visualize them well. Partially, this is caused by the magnetic susceptibility effects of the trabecular bone [88].

Quantitative BME lesion measurements require their segmentation [90]. Since the BME lesions can be located in any or all knee compartments or regions and since they have high variability, reliable clinically useful information of BML changes in volume, T2, and/or location requires also segmentation of all knee bones.

In theory, that could be accomplished just by manual segmentation of BME lesions and bones from T2 image sets. However, automated segmentation using the T2 image sets or coregistering automatically segmented structural image sets with T2 images and then segmenting the lesions and calculating their values is much faster and more reproducible [90]. In addition, the segmented data can be used to create local BME lesions' change maps. Furthermore, it can be used to correlate their spatial relationship to local cartilage defects and local compositional cartilage changes [90].

19.2.4.5 Changes in Trabecular Bone Architecture

The architectural changes in trabecular bone seen in OA have mostly been evaluated using fractal analysis and connectivity in CT and fractal analysis in plain films. However, since the high-resolution higher-field MR images show the trabecular bone structures in great detail, there is a growing interest and effort to extract the same parameters, bone volume fraction, trabecular bone thickness, number, and connectivity also from MR images and to develop more sensitive methods to detect the change [91].

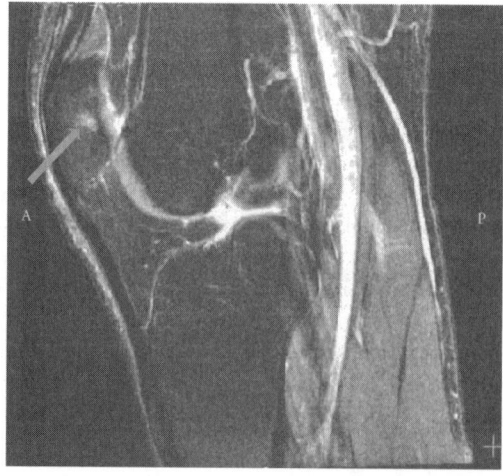

FIGURE 19.29   A bone marrow edema (thick arrow) in the patella seen in a fat-suppressed proton density spin echo image.

19.2.5 MR Imaging of Menisci in OA

19.2.5.1 Menisci in Different Pulse Sequences

The MR imaging appearance of menisci reflects their inner architecture of dense, mainly unidirectional tightly bound collagen bundles. This leads to their very low signal intensity in most of the pulse sequences, traversed by peripheral higher-signal-intensity vascular structures. Meniscus degeneration, tears, and maceration disturb or disrupt that architecture. Degeneration leads to local high-SI areas located in the middle of the meniscus; tears are seen as irregular lines traversing from the upper or lower surface into the meniscus or being contained inside the meniscus [92]. Commonly used pulse sequences for diagnosing meniscus tears are T1W, PDW spin echo (SE), sequences, T1W and PDW fast spin echo (SE) sequences and PD fat-suppressed (FS), or water-excited (WE) FSE, sequences. Cross-sectional and longitudinal OA studies use PD FSE or FS PD FSE sequences to score the meniscus changes [92]. The 3D WE SPGR qMRI cartilage sequence, which is heavily T1W, is not good for meniscus imaging. In those images, the higher-signal-intensity menisci blend with the surrounding structures. On the other hand, 3D WE DESS sequence demonstrates menisci well and, due to the high resolution, shows tears better than the SE sequences.

19.2.5.2 Imaging Composition and Volume of Meniscus

Since meniscus tears and degeneration eventually decrease the size of the menisci, some groups have developed methods to segment them for volume calculations [93,94]. Other groups use dGEMRIC, T2, or T1rho to detect the early degenerative meniscus changes or correlate the changes to the OA stage [95]. Meniscus subluxation has been shown to be a risk factor and/or predictor for OA progression. Most groups score the changes, even though some groups have developed methods to quantify subluxation. Much still needs to be done before those methods will be in common use.

19.2.6 Knee Alignment

Knee alignment measurements have long relied on plain films, where varus/valgus angulation between the long axis of the tibia and femur has been measured [96,97]. Flattening and widening of tibia and femur as well as changes in cartilage thickness changes the geometry of the articulating surfaces [96–98]. Furthermore, meniscus degeneration, tears, and maceration cause considerable changes to the location and amount of the local physical loads [99]. All of these factors have the potential to cause changes in the 3D spatial relationship between the bones by rotating, translating, and/or angulating them in different degrees. Therefore, it is highly likely that OA, which affects the geometry of all joint structures, will change the alignment of the bones three-dimensionally not only in plain film plane. Furthermore, both plain films and MR images show that in OA changes, the spatial relationship between the tibia and femur and between patella and femur has changed. Visually, the femur in OA knees has translated medially. Furthermore, for two decades, radiologists have used the posterior translation of the femur over the tibia as secondary for ACL tear diagnosis. As mentioned before, the segmentation of structures generates anatomically accurate 3D objects, whose physical parameters and their relationships to each other can then be evaluated [89]. Different groups have already used that approach to compute the distance between the closest point of femur and tibia and femur and patella [89]. Furthermore, they have computed and visualized the location for tibia and femur cartilage contact areas and calculated the size for the contact area [101]. Newer algorithms are in development to calculate the translational and rotational differences between normal and ACL-deficient knees and evaluate whether and to what degree the 3D spatial relationship in OA knees is different from that in normal knees (Figure 19.30) [101]. One reason, which has greatly increased the interest in 3D spatial relationship between the articulating bones in the knee joint, is the fact that anterior cruciate tears in the majority of cases lead to OA regardless of whether they are treated conservatively or surgically and regardless of the surgical method. That realization has led to a series of studies to develop methods to

(a)   (b)

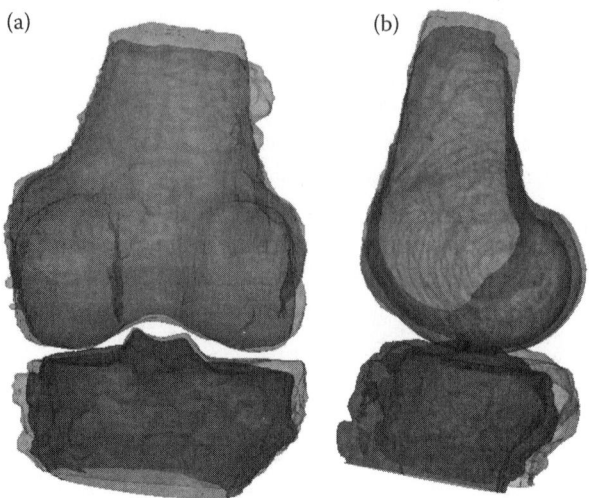

FIGURE 19.30 Posterior (a) and lateral (b) views of the 3D relationships. The 3D relationship between the subject's tibia and atlas' tibia. The subject's segmented tibia and femur were coregistered to the atlas' tibia and femur. The images show subject's tibia as green and the location of atlas tibia as blue. The atlas femur is red and the subject's femur is green.

investigate how the tibio-femoral contact points and their movement during knee flexion are different in normal and ACL-deficient knees and how the ACL tear has changed their 3D relationship [100–103].

Some semiautomated and all automated segmentation methods used for cartilage qMRI studies segment both bones and their cartilage from the MR images. Thus, they already provide the basic data needed to process their 3D relationship. The segmented bones need to be surface rendered, after which they can be treated as 3D objects and their 3D spatial relationship can be calculated (Figure 19.30). The direction and the degree of the translation and possible rotation in OA are still under investigation. Furthermore, how these changes are associated or correlated to the progression of other OA changes or can serve as predictors for the disease progression still needs to be evaluated.

19.3 Quantitative MRI-Based Evaluation of OA: Procedures and Algorithms

José G. Tamez-Peña

19.3.1 Analytical Procedures for Use of Quantitative MRI in OA

During the last couple of decades, the progression of the OA has been studied using MRI and it has been found that the annual degree of cartilage loss is very small (Figure 19.31) [104–109]. These results and others indicate that precise measurements are required from the MRI analysis in order to achieve a good understanding of the OA progression. Not just good precision is required, but accurate measurements are required to compare results from different studies and to make valid conclusions from multicenter data. The desired accuracy and precision necessary in OA analysis require a good understanding of the process involved in getting the quantitative results. Therefore, it is important to map all the process in getting a quantitative measurement from patient preparation to the final calibrated measurement. This section will map the process involved in an OA measurement using a standardized approach that can be used to create robust operating procedures aimed to get valid OA measurements from current MRI equipment. Furthermore, this section will describe the different approaches

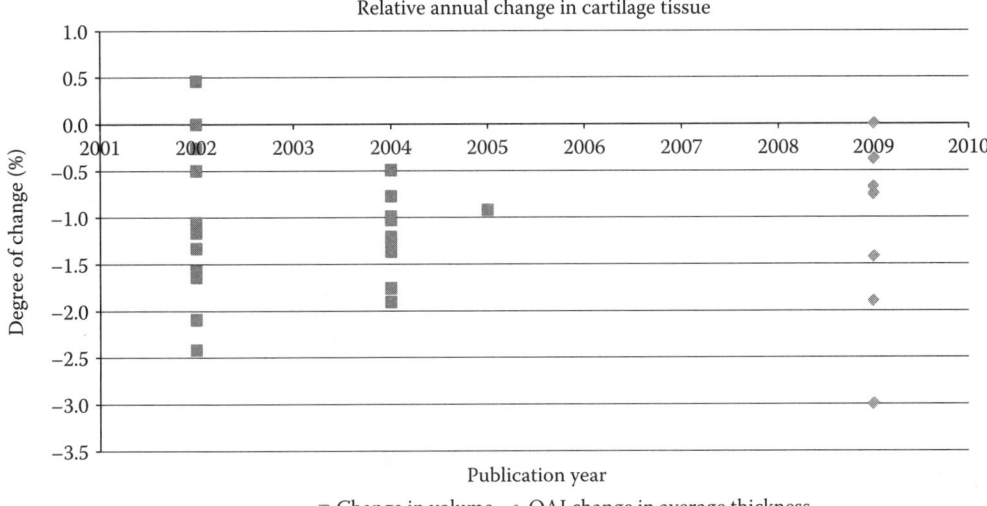

FIGURE 19.31 The slow progression of cartilage loss. The reported degree of cartilage loss by different studies (Eckstein et al. 2006) has been on average similar across time (1%). Therefore, the qMRI system must be able to measure small amounts of changes for year-long studies.

that have been used in getting quantitative information from MR images. Figure 19.32 shows a block diagram of the different processes involved in getting a measurement from the MRI system. These processes are

- Subject preparation
- Image acquisition
- Image analysis
- Quantification
- Phantom scanning
- MRI calibration

To get a valid measurement, each one of these processes must be standardized and the proper documentation must be created to aid in reproducibility of the results. Although all major OA studies have been following this recommendation, sometimes they miss taking into account some aspects that may affect the interpretation of the results. To mitigate the introduction of unwanted errors in the quantitative measurements, it is important to systematically map all the processes that may affect the measurements. In the following sections, we will summarize the different aspects involved in the quantification of the different OA features that can be analyzed in an MRI system. We will place special attention to the validity and reproducibility of the results in light of the nature of the OA progression: a slow degenerative disease.

By considering the quantitative MRI system as an analytical procedure for OA evaluation, the sources of variability and the uncertainties present in the measurement process can be mapped using current guidances. The mapping of uncertainties used in this chapter was done using the EURACHEM/CITAC Guide [110] or the National Institute of Standards and Technology (NIST) Technical note 1297 [111]. Once the variables that can affect the interpretation of the results have been identified, the quantitative procedures must be validated and it is recommended to follow the guidance on valid analytical procedures by the International Conference on Harmonization of Technical Requirements for Registration of Pharmaceuticals for Human Use (ICH) [112,113] and to use the philosophy of the Valid Analytical Methodology Programme of the UK (VAM: http://www.nmschembio.org.uk/).

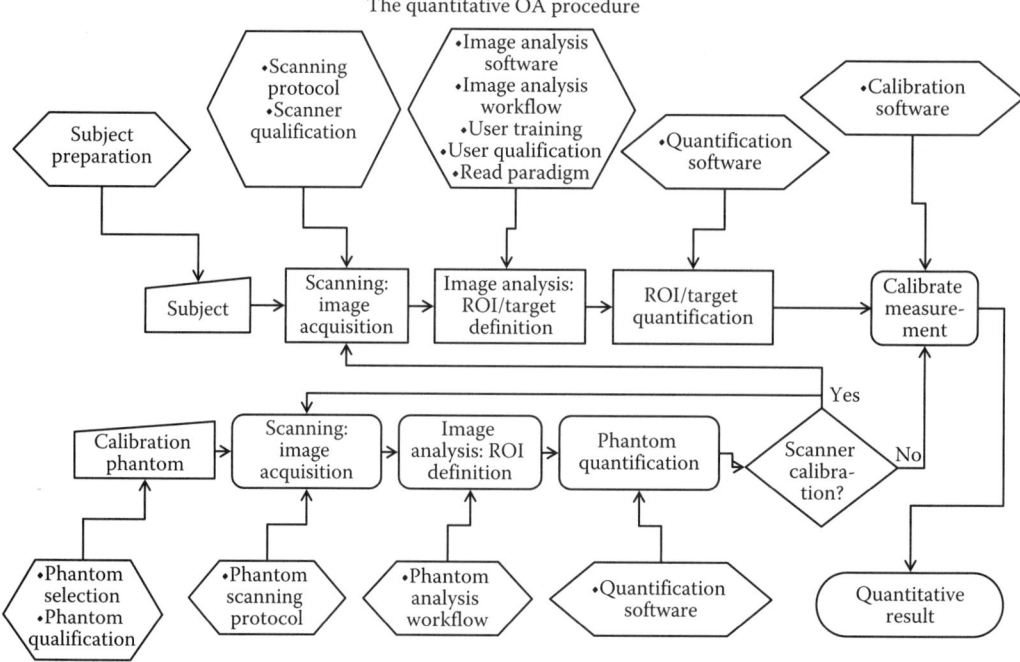

FIGURE 19.32   Procedures involved in obtaining a valid OA quantitative measure from an MRI equipment.

19.3.1.1 Uncertainties of OA Measurement

The mapping of uncertainties in OA is based on the EURACHEM/CITAC Guide CG 4 on the quantification of uncertainty in analytical measurements and the NIST Technical Note 1297 on the Guidelines for Evaluating and Expressing the Uncertainty of NIST Measurement Results [114]. The EURACHEM guide recommends drawing a cause–effect diagram to identify the major components of the system. Figure 19.33 shows a simple cause–effect diagram required to start mapping the possible sources of uncertainties that may play a role in the performance and accuracy of an OA quantitative measurement. The cause–effect diagram places the final measurement in the main horizontal axis and the diagonal arrows indicate different aspects of the quantitative process that may affect the measure via systematic errors (bias) or random errors. Figure 19.34 shows some of the aspects that may affect the quantitative measurements of OA systematically or randomly. As the diagram

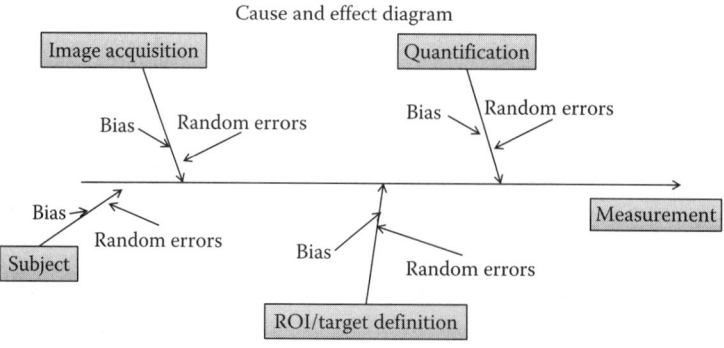

FIGURE 19.33   The identification of the sources of variation in an MRI-based quantitative system starts by drawing the cause–effect diagram of the different processes involved.

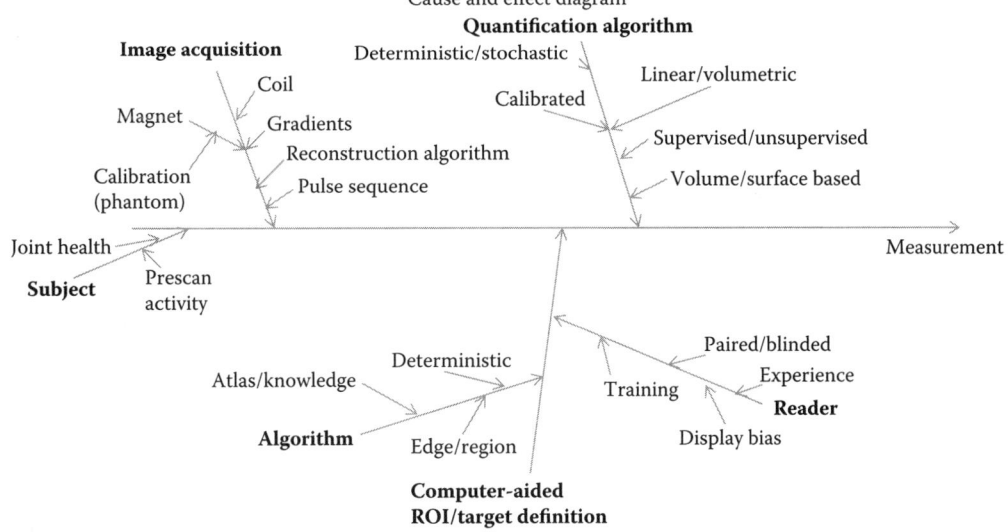

FIGURE 19.34 Different sources of systematic and random noise are present in the quantification of OA features. This fish-bone diagram identifies the different sources of errors that can affect the OA measurements.

shows, we have to consider the following aspects when evaluating the validity of an OA structural measurement:

- Subject:
  - Joint degradation stage: attrition, fibrillation, cartilage lesions, bone lesions
  - Prescan activity: anxiety, standing, walking, running, climbing stairs, and so on
  - magnetic susceptibility: tattoos, metal implants, blood clots, and so on

- Image acquisition:
  - Global distortions: B_0 drift, shim calibration, calibration phantoms
  - Local distortions and spatial sampling: gradient coils, pulse sequence
  - Signal: receiving coil, B_1 inhomogeneity, pulse sequence, flow, patient motion, truncation, partial volumes, and so on
  - Image reconstruction: reconstruction algorithm, geometric reconstruction algorithm, calibrations

- Image analysis—ROI definition:

  - Algorithm type:
    - Supervised
    - Edge/contour-based
    - Region-based
    - Unsupervised
    - Atlas-based: training set
    - Statistical knowledge-based
    - Stochastic/deterministic

  - Reader:
    - Expertise
    - Level of education
    - Years of experience

- Reading paradigm:
  - Blinded
  - Unblinded

- Graphical user interface and hardware:
  - Input device
  - Display

- Quantitation:
  - Preprocessing steps
  - Volume/voxel-based
  - 3D surface reconstructed
  - Stochastic/deterministic
  - Parametric model-based:
    - Linear/nonlinear
    - Fitting algorithm
  - Parameter calibration procedure

The former are some of the steps/issues involved in getting a measurement from an MRI image. Evaluating their individual impact on the final quantitative measurement will be a daunting task, but determining if the effect of each step is random or systemic is not. The systematic errors can be calibrated or randomly controlled and the stochastic errors can be controlled by increasing the number of samples. In the following sections, we will describe the most common algorithms used for the extraction of OA features, but first we will introduce the characteristics of a valid OA measure.

19.3.1.2 Quantitative Validation Characteristics

The quantitative OA measurement may be affected by any of the aspects described in the previous section; therefore, an OA/qMRI manual (imaging charter) will be required to treat the complex imaging procedure as a simple measurement unit that can be described with a unique validation characteristic. The OA/MRI manual procedure refers to the way of performing the quantitative analysis. It should describe the steps necessary to perform each test in detail. This may include but is not limited to the subject cohort, the phantoms, subject preparation, site preparations, use of the imaging equipment, generation of the calibration procedures, image analysis work-stream, and use of the algorithms for the calculation, among others.

We list the validation characteristics of a measurement in Table 19.1. Based on that, we recommend the quantification and documentation of the characteristics in order to have confidence in the final OA quantitative result. The characteristics are

- *Specificity:* The ability of the system to unequivocally assess the imaging endpoint in the presence of components which may be expected to be present. Typically, this may include imaging artifacts, lesions, and so on. The lack of specificity of an individual imaging endpoint can be compensated by other supporting imaging procedures. This definition has strong implications in the pulse sequence selection in OA studies: Not all OA characteristics can be evaluated in a single pulse sequence. Therefore, for structural cartilage evaluation, 3D high-resolution pulse sequences with fat suppression are preferred over 2D sequences. On the other hand, T1 and T2 cartilage evaluation requires sequences that have good SNR; therefore, 2D sequences are preferred over 3D sequences. At the end, the pulse sequence specificity plays an important role in the overall system specificity.
- *Accuracy:* Expresses the closeness of the agreement between the value which is accepted as either the conventional truth or an accepted reference value and the value found.

TABLE 19.1 ICH Q2A Requirements for the Identification of the Validation Characteristics of Any Analytical Procedure

Type of Image Analysis	Semiquantitative	Quantitative Continuous
Accuracy	NA[a]	+
Precision		
• Repeatability	+	+
• Intermediate precision	+	+
Specificity	+	+
Detection limit	−	−
Quantitation limit	−	−
Linearity	−	+
Range	−	+

Note: The quantitative analysis of OA can be seen as an analytical procedure.

[a] NA, not applicable.

The accuracy of a given measurement is composed by the bias and the precision.

- *Bias/linearity:* Expresses the average deviation between the value which is accepted as either the conventional true value or an accepted reference value and the value found using a series of measurements obtained from multiple sampling of the same subject(s) under the prescribed conditions.
- *Precision:* Expresses the closeness of agreement between a series of measurements obtained from multiple sampling of the same subject(s) under the prescribed conditions.
  - *Repeatability:* Expresses the precision under the same operating conditions over a short period of time. When a human observer is involved in the analysis process, this is also known as the short-term intraoperator precision.
  - *Intermediate precision:* Expresses the variability of the whole system under different analysts, different equipment, and so on. When only human observers are involved, this is known as the interobserver variability.
  - *Reproducibility:* Expresses the precision among laboratories (collaborative studies usually applied to standardization of methodology).

The specificity, accuracy, and precision in OA have been determined using pilot experiments usually involving TKA or cadaver studies [115–117]. Volume accuracy has been determined by water displacement, while area evaluation has been done using thin foil analysis [118,119]. The proper method to evaluate and report accuracy and precision is the one recommended by Bland and Altman. Bland and Altman define the statistical instruments to measure the agreement between the new method and the reference standard. Most of the time the pulse sequence defines the sensitivity of the OA measurements, the magnet/hardware calibration dominates the accuracy and the image analysis method is a key player in the precision [106,120,121]. The quantification algorithm also may play a role in the accuracy/precision of the measurement and this is especially true in indirect measurements, like area, thickness, T1, and T2 [122–125]. Therefore, the reported accuracy and precision reported in the literature must be then interpreted carefully to readily identify the source of the measured bias/accuracy/precision in the OA measurement. The specification of the specificity, accuracy, and precision should be accompanied by the following characteristics:

- *Linearity:* The ability (within a given range) to obtain test results which are directly proportional to the accurate value of the measurement.
- *Range:* The interval between the upper and lower value (amount) of the measurement for which it has been demonstrated that system has a suitable level of precision, accuracy, and linearity.

In OA, the linearity/range is important in all T2 and T1 measurements. The pulse sequence selection and the fitting algorithm will determine either the range at which the T1 measurements have a linear relationship between the T1 value and the GAG concentration or if the T2 measurement has this linear relationship to the true T2 relaxation.

For structural measurements, the range is also a very important parameter. Due to the volumetric sampling characteristics of the MRI, the volume precision is not homoscedastic as seen in Figure 19.35a. Therefore, it is important to specify the tested range of the volume, or apply the proper mathematical transform that may remove the dependency of the variance to the measurement level. For volume and area measurements, the cubic root and the square root transforms make a decent job in removing the dependency of the sampling variance from the measurement level as seen in Figure 19.35b and c.

Besides linearity and range, the following characteristics are useful in defining rules for removing questionable OA measurements.

- *Detection limit*: The detection limit is not usually reported or measured, but when reported, it represents the smallest size, signal, or amount in an individual subject that can be imaged by the acquisition device, but not necessarily quantitated as an exact value. In qMRI, the minimum detection limit is governed by the Nyquist–Shannon sampling theorem. Therefore, we can use this theorem to estimate the detection limit in all structural measurements. It is important to remember that the sampling rate will be given by the sampled voxel resolution, not the reconstructed voxel. It will be safe to set the detection limit to twice the acquisition slice thickness. Structures that are smaller than two slice thicknesses will not be properly measured and quantitative measurements from those structures cannot be trusted. For signal-based measurements, the detection limit can be placed at 3.3 standard deviations of the precision error [113].
- *Quantitation limit*: As well as in the detection limit, the quantitation limit is not usually reported or measured, but this characteristic represents the smallest size, signal, or amount that will be quantitated with the desired accuracy. For OA, the quantitation limit can be safely placed at 10

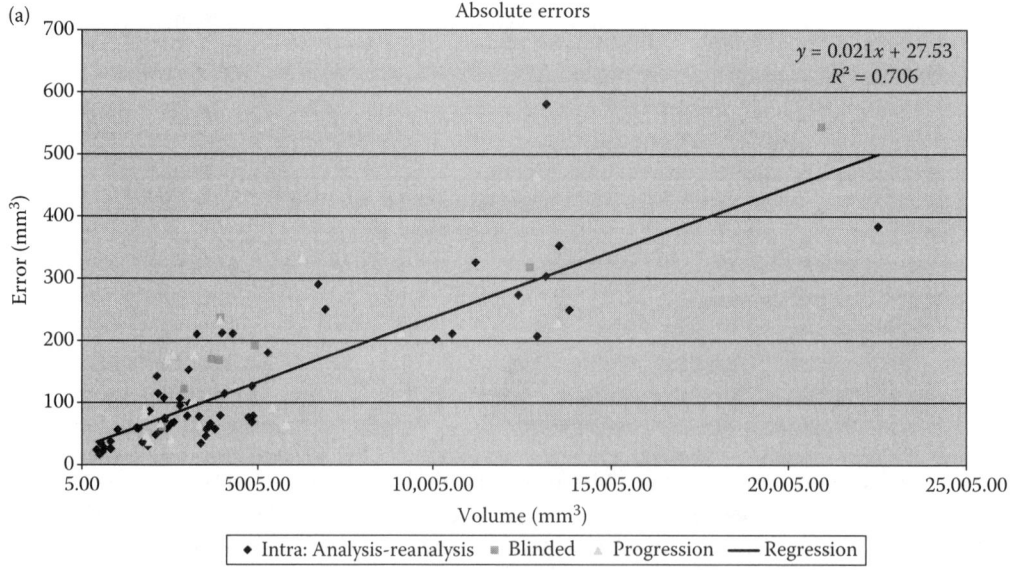

FIGURE 19.35 Reported random errors in the measurement of cartilage tissue. (a) The error in the quantification of cartilage volume from MRI is highly associated with the volume itself. This is not a desired characteristic of a measurement. (b) The reported CV values are also associated with the size of the cartilage tissue. There is a nonlinear relationship between CV values and cartilage size. (c) After transforming the cartilage volumes by a cubic root transform, the CV values of the measurements do not show a dependency to cartilage size. This transformation allows the cross-comparison of reported CV values across studies.

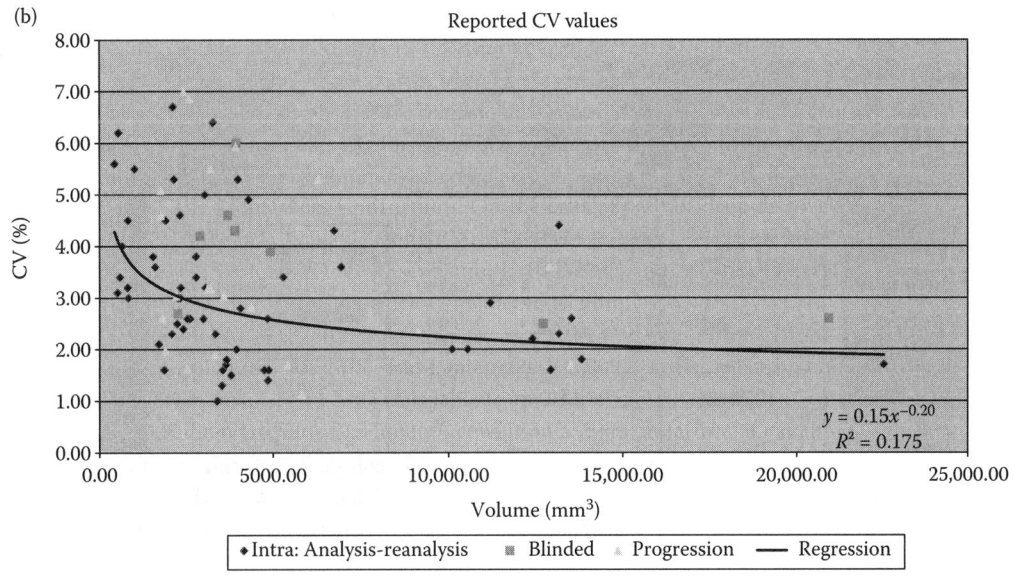

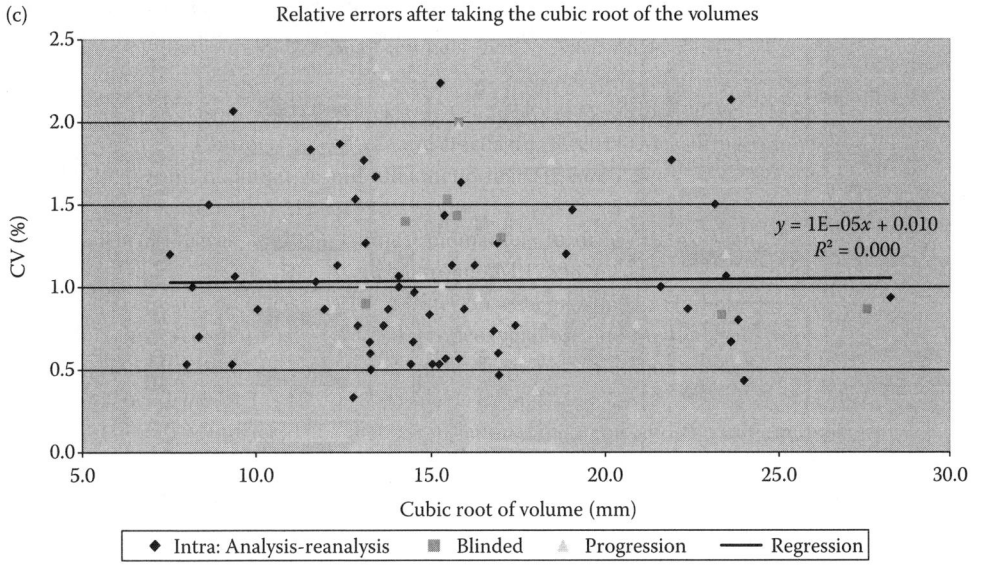

FIGURE 19.35 (Continued.)

standard deviations of the observed absolute measurement precision [113]. Knowing the signal quantitation limit is also very important in all T1 and T2 measurements especially when fitting the signal data to the nonlinear models of the signal formation.

Finally, it is recommended the whole system be tested for

- *Robustness or ruggedness:* It is a measure of the ability to remain unaffected by small but deliberate variations in method parameters and provides an indication of its reliability during normal usage. Ruggedness tests are used to determine the parameters that can affect the measurement.

Therefore, for any quantitative OA measurement, it is important to evaluate the roughness of the measure to Image Reader expertise, Paired-Read Order, Display Contrast, Image Analysis Algorithm Parameters, and so on.

19.3.1.3 Valid Quantitative Image Analysis Method in OA

The knowledge of the measurement characteristics of the MRI-based OA quantitative system does not guarantee that the system is producing valid measurements. The UK VAM Programme identified six principles of a valid analytical measurement (http://www.nmschembio.org.uk). We took the freedom to adjust them to fit the OA quantitative imaging requirements. Those principles are

1. Image measurements should be made to satisfy an agreed requirement.
2. Image measurements should be made using methods and equipment which have been tested to ensure that they are fit for purpose.
3. Staff making image measurements should be both qualified and competent to undertake the task.
4. There should be a regular independent assessment of the technical performance of the system.
5. Image measurements made in one location should be consistent with others made elsewhere.
6. Organizations making image measurements should have well-defined quality control and quality assurance procedures.

These principles are in line with the ICH2Qa guidance in validated analytical methods and in line with the FDA draft guidance in the use of statistical analysis plans, independent review charters (imaging charters or MRI manuals). The main purpose of the principles is to remind us that a good measurement device does not necessarily guarantee valid results. Quality control steps are required to guarantee that the numbers provided can be reproduced. Taking that recommendation into account, the simple OA procedure described in Figure 19.31 can be expanded to add the quality control and quality assurance procedures.

For example, in the OAI observational trail, there is an MRI manual that describes all the quality control steps [126,127]. The magnet is carefully monitored using special OA phantoms seen in Figure 19.36. These phantoms are quantitated using specific procedures and the result has been published. Figure 19.37a and b shows how one of the phantoms measurements slightly changes over time. These changes may have an impact on the measurement, especially when the expected degree of change in the measurements is in the order of magnitude of the natural drift of the magnet.

19.3.1.4 Revalidation

Revalidation of an OA measurement system may be necessary in the following circumstances:

- Changes in the composition of the system, that is,
  - Subject preparation guidelines
  - Imaging device
  - Changes in imaging phantoms and/or calibration criteria
  - Imaging protocol/pulse sequences
  - Change in readers
  - Reading paradigm: paired, blinded, sequential, and so on
- Image quantification algorithms
- Changes in the software versions

The degree of revalidation required depends on the nature of the changes. The most dramatic change will be modifications in the system itself. Changes in software versions must be carefully monitored because they can introduce new analysis algorithms, or may change the way a system performs. Careful software design controls will be required to verify that the changes in software meet the requirements. Do no change validated and calibrated image analysis algorithms in the middle of the study.

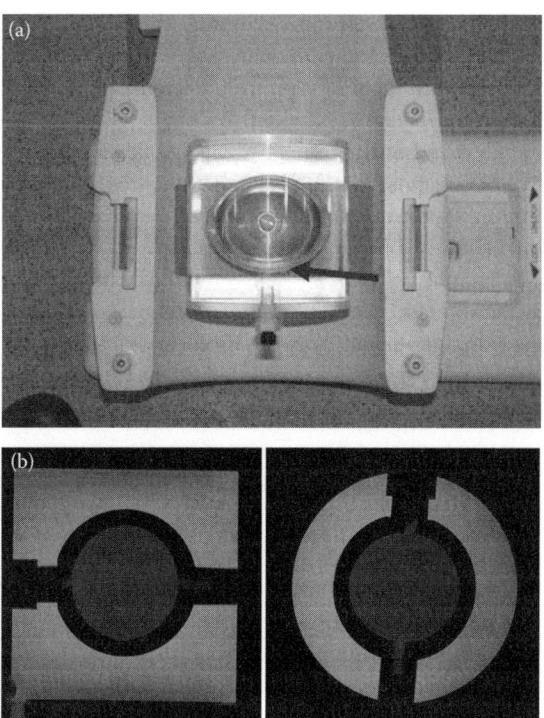

FIGURE 19.36 (a) The OIA using a cartilage phantom to monitor any deviation from the quantitation requirements of all the OAI equipment. (b) MRI imaging of the OAI phantom. (Courtesy of the OAI.)

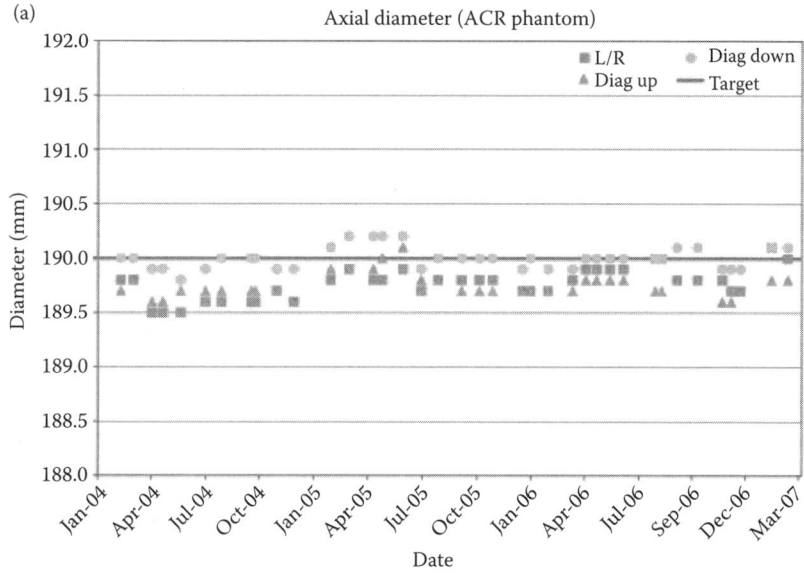

FIGURE 19.37 Quantitative analysis of the ACR and OAI phantom. (a,b) The ACR and OAI show small oscillations from the expected values. These variations are not large enough to drift measurements, but they show how the random variations of the MRI magnetic field are a source of linear noise on the order of 0.25%. (c) Example of longitudinal variation in OAI phantom spherical volume (b). The volume drift is from 210 to 211 mm^3. This 0.5% drift can yield to progression misinterpretations if ignored in the volumetric analysis of cartilage tissue.

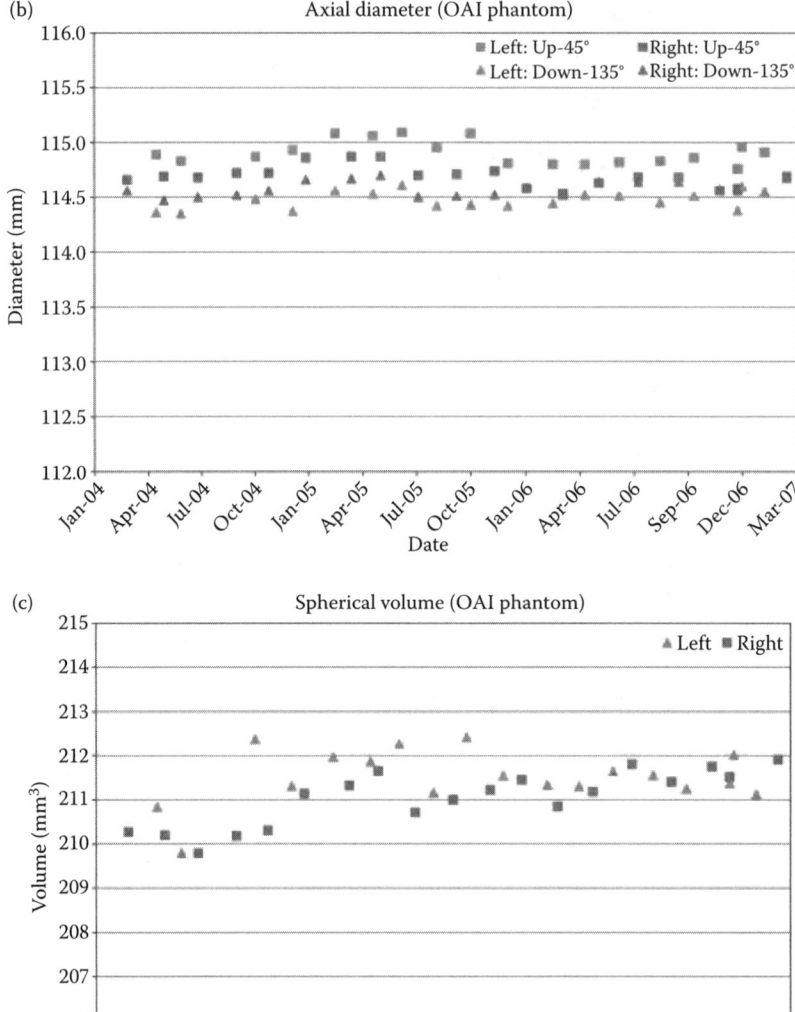

FIGURE 19.37 (Continued.)

19.3.2 MRI Image Analysis Algorithms in OA

As we have described in the former sections, an image analysis procedure is required to get quantitative data from the MRI. The most common algorithms used in OA are segmentation algorithms, registration algorithms, and quantification algorithms.

19.3.2.1 OA Segmentation Algorithms

As seen in Table 19.2, the OA segmentation algorithms can be classified into three major categories: supervised, atlas-based, and hybrid algorithms. Most of the OA quantitative work done up to date is based on supervised segmentation methods [120,125,128–131]. The reason behind this is the difficulty in accurately separating cartilage tissue from bone, synovium, or fat in MRI images with OA. The task

TABLE 19.2 Segmentation Methods with Different Sources of Random and Systematic Noise

Tissue Region of Interest	Reference Standard	Segmentation Method	Sources of Bias	Bias Control	Sources of Random Error
Cartilage	Expert manual trace	Manual/ semiautomated	Reader expertise Order of analysis	Training Blinding	Reader + acquisition noise
		Atlas	Atlas set	Multiple atlas	Acquisition noise/ registration
		Voxel classification	Training set/pulse sequence shift	Pulse sequence/ coil control	Acquisition noise
Bone marrow lesion	Expert manual trace	Manual/ semiautomated	Reader expertise Order of analysis	Training Blinding	Reader + acquisition noise
		Atlas/outlier detection	Outlier rules	Parameter calibration	Acquisition noise/ registration
		Voxel classification	Classification rules	Parameter calibration	Acquisition noise

Note: The degree of bias can be controlled by different procedures, but still, the human observer is considered the gold standard in all cartilage segmentation procedures.

is so challenging that even semiautomated approaches require trained users to properly identify the tissues. The nature of OA also makes the unsupervised segmentation methods fairly complex [132–134]. They are based in the use of anatomical atlases that are used to seed either a more complex classification algorithm or knowledge-based [135–141]. Figure 19.38 shows one of the early attempts in getting a fully automated segmentation from MRI images, and Figure 19.39 shows a more recent development of the use of multiple atlases to get accurate segmentations from MRI images. The main limitation of the fully automated approaches is the large variety of OA abnormalities that can be present in the joints: bone marrow lesions, synovities, inflammation, cartilage defect, full thickness defects, flow artifacts, and so on. Therefore, most of the fully automated approaches are limited to early stages of OA.

19.3.2.2 OA Registration Algorithms

The registration algorithms in OA are commonly used in atlas-based approaches to align the atlas to the incoming data set. These registration algorithms must accommodate to the articulating nature of

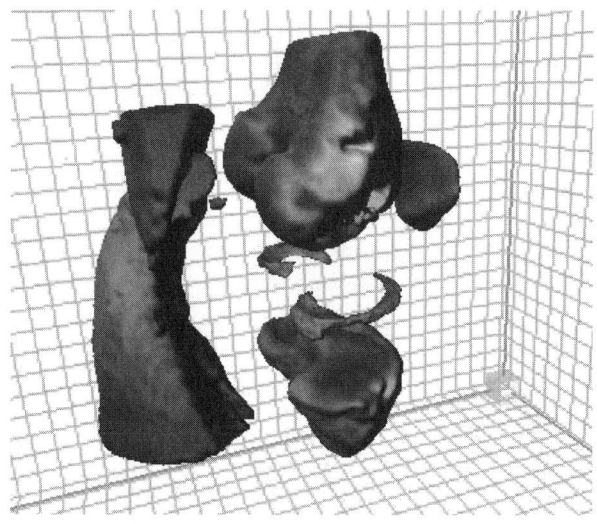

FIGURE 19.38 The normal knee anatomy can be automatically segmented from MRI data sets using advanced statistical analysis tools.

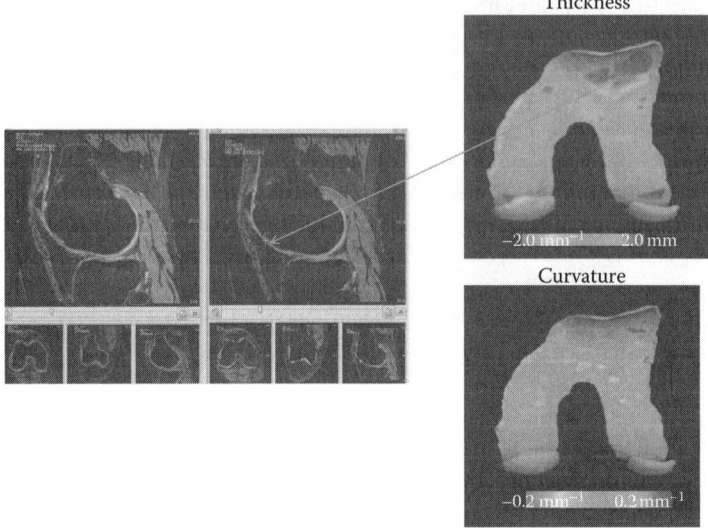

FIGURE 19.39 In the presence of OA, atlas-based approaches are a practical alternative to the segmentation of thousands of MRI images. Left, slice through the DESS images. (Courtesy of OAI.) Top right, 3D reconstruction of the cartilage thickness in the atlas space. Red values represent areas of cartilage loss. Bottom right, the curvature of the cartilage surface can be computed and measured. Drastic changes in cartilage topography can be measured by the curvature values and are seen as red and blue spots in the curvature map.

the joints [142,143]. Therefore, masks are required to isolate each articulating bone from each other. Besides masks, the registration algorithms must deal with large deformations due to the development of bone deformities and osteophyte formation. The other challenge of an OA registration algorithm is the use of surface coils in joint imaging. These coils make the signal intensity fairly nonuniform across the imaging plane; therefore, robust algorithms are required to deal with signal fading or, preprocessing is required to mitigate the change in signal intensity.

A second use of image registration in OA is the intrasubject alignment of the different pulse sequences either for T1/T2 computations or for MRI pulse-sequence fusion required for multispectral-based segmentation. Although intraalignment is an easier task than interpatient alignment, it is still a challenge in OA analysis. Subjects tend to move between pulse sequence acquisitions. That movement may include a change in the relative position of bones, tendons, ligaments, and muscles. Therefore, articulated registration is required for the proper alignment of intrasubject MRI series. The final use of image registration algorithms in OA is the alignment of segmented data to get statistical maps of changes. This last registration algorithm is usually a surface-to-surface method, but atlas dense motion flow can be used to get the statistical maps. Once the surfaces are aligned, spatial statistics analysis can be done in the aligned surfaces [125,144]. Figure 19.40 shows an example of statistical maps generated after registering the quantitative thickness data.

19.3.2.3 Quantitation Algorithms

The final classes of algorithms used in OA analysis are quantitation algorithms as those listed in Table 19.3. Those algorithms can be as simple as voxel counting or as complex as the generation of statistical parametric maps that describe the voxel-by-voxel behavior of cartilage tissue. The three mayor classes of quantitation algorithms used in OA are the algorithms used for the estimation of cartilage thickness, the algorithms required to get T1 and T2 measurements, and the algorithms required to get statistical maps of the point-by-point measurements of thickness, curvature, T1, T2, and so on.

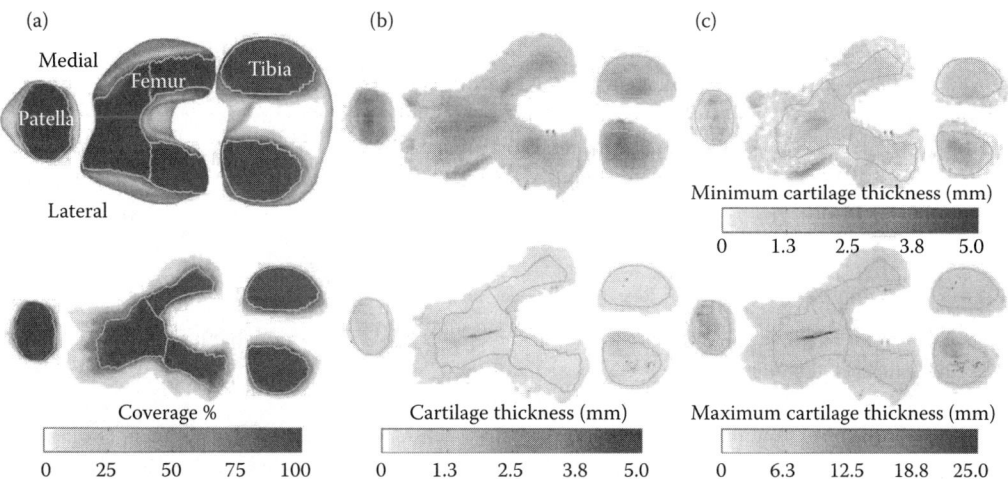

FIGURE 19.40 Statistical maps of changes in cartilage thickness. The thickness maps are a very useful tool for the visualization of the localized changes and heterogeneity in the patterns of cartilage loss in subjects with OA. (a) Top, 3D rendering of knee bones with coverage analysis. (b) Mean (top) and standard deviation (bottom) of cartilage thickness. (c) Minimum and Maximum of the thickness. (This picture has copyrights by the IEEE TMI.)

TABLE 19.3 Quantification Procedures Calibrated to Avoid the Introduction of Biases into the Measurements

Quantitative Measurement	Reference Standard	Quantitation Method	Sources of Bias	Bias Control	Sources of Random Error
Volume	Phantom/ synthetic or real	Voxel count Surface volume	B_0 shift/gradients B_0 shift/gradients + surface reconstruction algorithm	Calibration	B_0 heterogeneties
Thickness	Phantom/ synthetic or real	Euclidian distance Laplacian distance Mid-surface	B_0 shift/ gradients + algorithm	Calibration	B_0 heterogeneties
Area	Phantom/ synthetic or real	Surface reconstruction Voxel edge count	B_0 shift/gradients + algortihm	Calibration	B_0 heterogeneties
T2	Phantom/ synthetic or real	Spin echo monoexponential fitting Constrained spin echo monoexponential fitting	B_1/pulse sequence + algorithm	Calibration	B_1 Heterogeneities + flow + partial volume
T1	Phantom/ synthetic or real	Nonlinear IR fitting Nonlinear multiple flip angle fitting	B_1/pulse sequence + registration + algorithm	Calibration	B_1 Heterogeneities + registration + flow + patial volume
T1 dGEMRIC	Phantom/ synthetic or real	Nonlinear IR fitting Nonlinear multiple flip angle fitting	B_1/pulse sequence + registration + algorithm	Calibration	B_1 heterogeneities + registration + flow + partial volume + Gd-DTPA(2−)/ subject

Note: The degree of bias depends heavily on the algorithm used to compute the measurement. Calibration and characterization in the range of the measurement are essential to avoid using those quantification algorithms outside the specification range.

The main issue in the quantitative algorithms is the validation and calibration of the quantitative data. To isolate image segmentation and image registration issues from the validation and calibration procedures, it is recommended to use synthetic phantoms or real phantoms for the calibration. Real phantoms are very important in the calibration of T1/T2 algorithms while synthetic phantoms are very useful in the validation of structural measurement algorithms [145]. The advantage of the synthetic phantoms is that the ground truth is known and that they can be designed to represent the whole range of conditions present in real life.

19.3.3 OA Image-Based Biomarkers

The FDA website (www.FDA.gov) states: "Biomarker, or biological marker, A characteristic that is objectively measured and evaluated as an indicator of normal biologic processes, pathogenic processes, or pharmacologic responses to a therapeutic intervention."

The final goal of the quantitative data generated from an MRI is to develop surrogated endpoints to stage the progression of the disease. The road to get image-based surrogated markers is very challenging and it requires the consensus of the OA community in a clear definition of a useful clinical endpoint for clinical diagnosis, for treatment decision-making, or for treatment monitoring. Presently, the most common criteria to stage the disease is the radiological evaluation of OA via the use of KL scores or radiological atlases like OARSIs. MRI-based evaluation of OA is still under development. In the meantime, WORMS and BLOCKS are used as tools to evaluate the findings and severity of OA-related features [146,147]. The other alternative is to use clinical evaluations via the use of either WOMAC scores or KOOS scores [148–150]. Both approaches are ill-defined and have not shown clear sensitivity or objectivity to the progression of OA.

Regardless of the state of the clinical endpoint in the OA community, the OA MRI-based biomarkers can be classified into structural biomarkers and imaging biomarkers. Structural biomarkers are single measurements of a specific tissue or region of interest, that is, total femoral cartilage volume, average medial tibia area, total bone marrow lesion volume, and so on. On the other hand, imaging biomarkers are maps or quantitative images of cartilage thickness, cartilage curvature, T1 dGEMRIC values, T2, and so on. Because the imaging biomarkers create maps or quantitative images, the imaging biomarkers can be described by statistical descriptors like mean, standard deviations, skewness, and so on. Therefore, there is an endless count of possible statistical descriptors that can be used as surrogated endpoints coming from the imaging biomarkers. Figure 19.41 shows an example of an interjoint distance map generated using MRI data. The map can be interpreted as an imaging biomarker of the distance between the tibia and the femur. On the other hand, functional biomarkers of the cartilage and surrounding tissues are possible with the use of loading devices as seen in Figure 19.42. The loading device

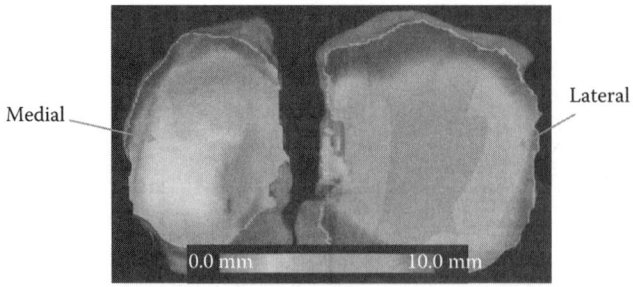

Femur-tibia inter-bone distance map

FIGURE 19.41 The MRI images can be used to compute the interjoint distance. Distance maps can automatically be computed and they are an indirect measurement of changes in the soft tissues in joint anatomy.

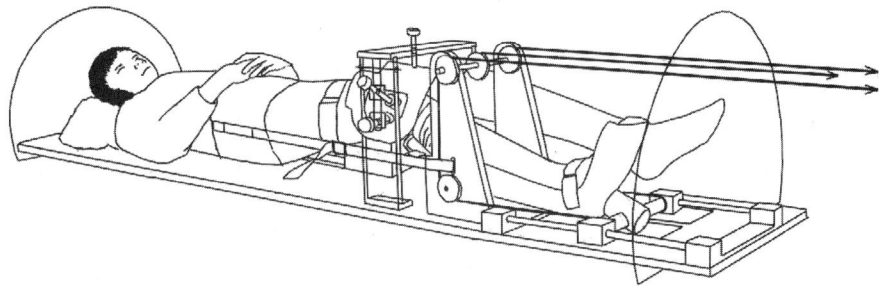

FIGURE 19.42 Functional joint analysis can be done by using lading devices. These devices allow the application of dynamic loads into the knee while the person is being imaged. The changes in cartilage deformation may be an indication of early cartilage degeneration.

places a load into the knee that allows the computation of stress and strain in the cartilage and meniscus. Therefore, early stages of joint degradation can be inferred by changes in the mechanical properties estimated from those functional experiments.

Regardless of the type of image-based biomarker, the ideal image-based OA biomarker must predict the stage of the disease and must have good responsiveness to either disease progression or treatment intervention. The search of this biomarker has produced hundreds of candidates, some of them with good responsiveness but not clear association to the ill-defined OA stage. Others have a good association to some OA definition, but they do not show clear change over time, which makes them weak candidates for monitoring OA progression. At this stage of the OA biomarker development, only a few measurements have been able to be associated with the established radiological OA evaluation or clinical indexes [151–153].

A very important point in the validation of OA biomarker is the proper design and its association to disease stage and change responsiveness. Statistical models must be used to do these tasks and several time points (at least three) must be included to evaluate the responsiveness. The use of only two time points to evaluate biomarker progression rate has yielded many false estimations of progression rate. One of the main factors is that investigators forget to take into account that some biomarker or image analysis procedures are biased toward positive change even in the lack of real progression. The most common source of analysis bias is unblinded pair reading. Paired evaluation is biased by the natural expectation of the human observer toward symptoms worsening in OA. Besides analysis bias, there are biased biomarkers. Biased biomarkers are those which may have a nonzero value between repeated measurements. Order values, percentile analysis, and detection analysis are samples of biomarkers that will have that behavior in the presence of random noise. The estimation of the right rate of progression of those biased biomarkers is the inclusion of at least three time points and the use of a statistical model with bias term. Once the statistical model is fitted to the data, the bias and the time responsiveness can be estimated. The beta coefficient of the time-dependent variable can be used to estimate the rate of progression.

The number of biomarkers that is generated from imaging is very large, and the analysis of this data is very complex. Therefore, bioinformatics tools (see Figure 19.43) may be required to establish surrogated biomarker candidates that in a near future may be accepted by the OA community to be used as a diagnosis criteria, disease staging, or treatment monitoring.

19.3.4 Conclusion

The MRI has provided the OA community with an invaluable tool to observe and understand the progression of this chronic disease. Magnets, coils, and pulse sequences coupled with image analysis algorithms have made the quantitation of the OA phenomena possible. This has been very useful in understanding and redefining the disease progression. The final goal is to obtain a surrogate biomarker of OA that can be used to first diagnose the disease clinically, and then used to monitor treatment

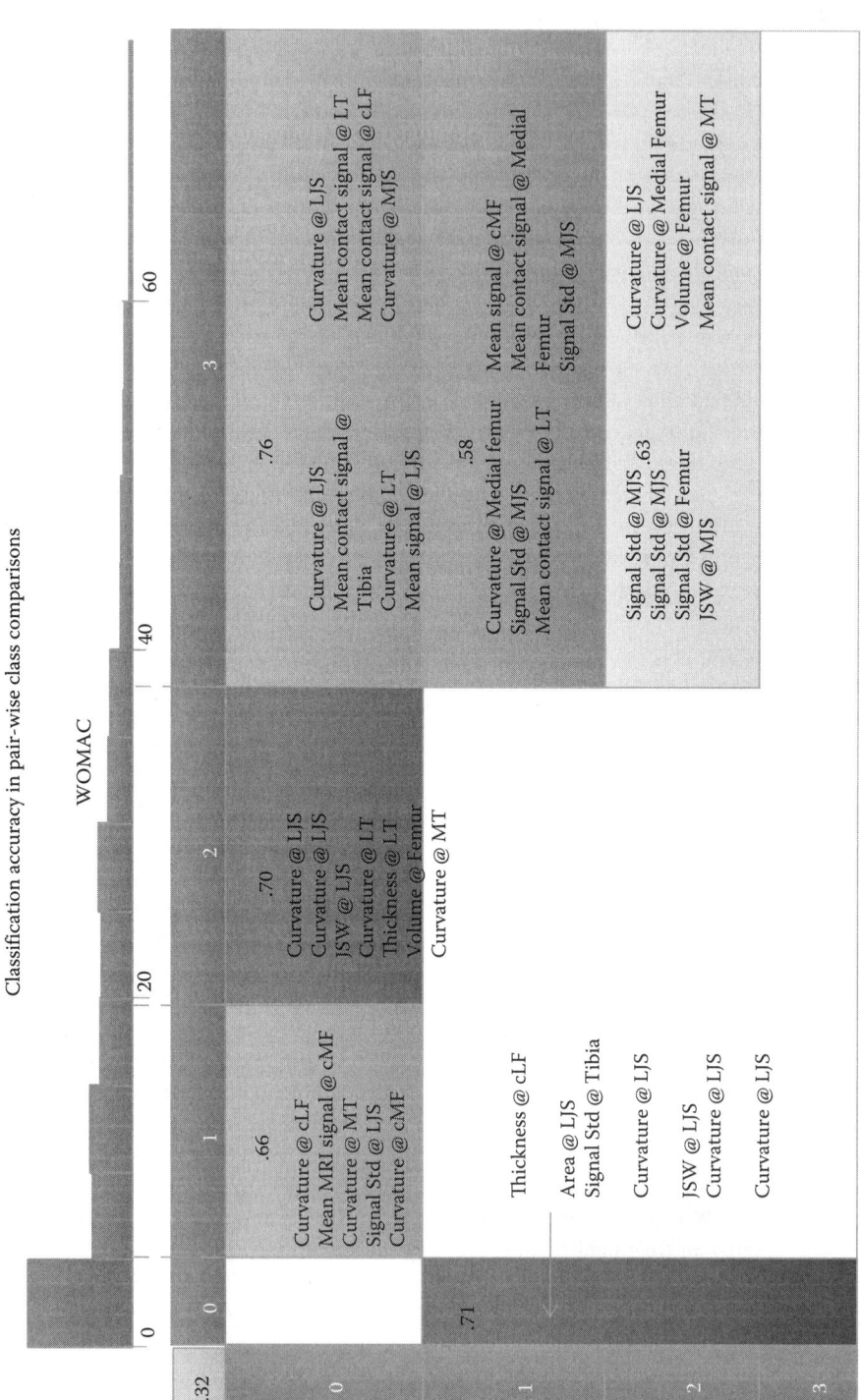

FIGURE 19.43 Advanced bioinformatic tools can be used to explore hundreds of variables and their association to clinical outcomes. In this example, GALGO was used to explore associations between MRI measurements and the total WOMAC score.

Classes 0, 1, 2, and 3 contain 0–25%, 25–50%, 50–75% and 75–100%, respectively of the WOMAC population.

efficacy. We are not there yet, but this desire of the ultimate biomarker has pushed the scientific, pharmaceutical device, and regulatory community to work together to develop OA studies, algorithms, and standard methodologies aimed to get the biomarker that will enable the development of effective OA therapies.

Acknowledgment

The OAI is a public–private partnership comprised of five contracts (N01-AR-2-2258; N01-AR-2-2259; N01-AR-2-2260; N01-AR-2-2261; N01-AR-2-2262) funded by the National Institutes of Health, a branch of the Department of Health and Human Services, and conducted by the OAI Study Investigators. Private funding partners include Merck Research Laboratories, Novartis Pharmaceuticals Corporation, GlaxoSmithKline, and Pfizer, Inc. Private sector funding for the OAI is managed by the Foundation for the National Institutes of Health. This manuscript was prepared using an OAI public use data set and does not necessarily reflect the opinions or views of the OAI investigators, the NIH, or the private funding partners.

References

1. Brandt KD, Dieppe P, and Radin EL. Etiopathogenesis of osteoarthritis. *Rheum Dis Clin North Am.* 2008;34:531–559.
2. Brandt KD, Dieppe P, and Radin EL. Commentary: Is it useful to subset "primary" osteoarthritis? A critique based on evidence regarding the etiopathogenesis of osteoarthritis. *Semin Arthritis Rheum.* 2009;39:81–95.
3. Brandt K. Defining osteoarthritis: What it is and what it is not. *J Musculoskel Med.* 2010;27:338–350.
4. Felson DT, Lawrence RC, Dieppe PA, Hirsch R, Helmick CG, Jordan JM, Kington RS et al. Osteoarthritis: New insights. Part 1: The disease and its risk factors. [Review] [120 refs]. *Ann Internal Med.* 2000;133(8):635–646.
5. Frobell RB, Roos EM, Roos HP, Ranstam J, and Lohmander LS. A randomized trial of treatment for acute anterior cruciate ligament tears. *N Engl J Med.* 2010;363(4):331–342.
6. Hansen JT, and Lambert DR. *Netters Clinical Anatomy*, Saunders Elsevier, Philadelphia, PA, 2008: pp. 234–239.
7. Pritzker KPH, Gay S, Jimenez SA, Ostergaard K, Pelletier JP, Revell PA, Salter D, and van den Berg WB. Osteoarthritis cartilage histopathology: Grading and staging. *Osteoarthritis Cartilage.* 2006;14:13–29.
8. Jiang J, Leong NL, Mung JC, Hidaka C, and Lu HH. Interaction between zonal populations of articular chondrocytes suppresses chondrocyte mineralization and this process is mediated by PTHrP. *Osteoarthritis Cartilage.* 2008;16:70–82.
9. Modl JM, Sether LA, Haughton VM, and Kneeland JB. Articularcartilage: Correlation of histologiczones with signal intensity at MR imaging. *Radiology.* 1991;181(3):853–855.
10. Uhl M, Ihling C, Allmann KH, Laubenberger J, Tauer U, Adler CP, and Langer M. Human articular cartilage: *In vitro* correlation of MRI and histologic findings. *Eur Radiol.* 1998;8(7):1123–1129.
11. Minns RJ, and Steven FS. The collagen fibril organization in human articular cartilage. *J Anat.* 1977;123:437–457.
12. Xia Y, Moody JB, Burton-Wurster N, and Lust G. Quantitative *in situ* correlation between microscopic MRI and polarized light microscopy studies of articular cartilage. *Osteoarthritis Cartilage.* 2001;9:393–406.
13. Nieminen MT, Rieppo J, Töyräs J, Hakumäki JM, Silvennoinen J, Hyttinen MM, Helminen HJ, and Jurvelin JS. T2 relaxation reveals spatial collagen architecture in articular cartilage: A comparative quantitative MRI and polarized light microscopic study. *Magn Reson Med.* 2001;46(3):487–493.
14. Bashir A, Gray ML, Boutin RD, and Burstein D. Glycosaminoglycan in articular cartilage: *In vivo* assessment with delayed Gd(DTPA)(2-)-enhanced MR imaging. *Radiology.* 1997;205(2):551–558.

15. Van Ginckel A, Baelde N, Almqvist KF, Roosen P, McNair P, and Witvrouw E. Functional adaptation of knee cartilage in asymptomatic female novice runners compared to sedentary controls. A longitudinal analysis using delayed Gadolinium Enhanced Magnetic Resonance Imaging of Cartilage (dGEMRIC). *Osteoarthritis Cartilage*. 2010;18(12):1564–1569.

16. Hauch KN, Villegas DF, and Haut Donahue TL. Geometry, time dependent and failure properties of human meniscal attachments. *J Biomech*. 201010;43(3):463.

17. Kaplan PA, Nelson NL, Garvin KL, and Brown DE. MR of the knee: The significance of high signal in the meniscus that does not clearly extend to the surface. *AJR Am J Roentgenol*. 1991;156(2):333–336.

18. Giuliani JR, Kilcoyne KG, and Rue JP. Anterior cruciate ligament anatomy: A review of the anteromedial and posterolateral bundles. *J Knee Surg*. 2009;22(2):148–154.

19. Chhabra A, Starman JS, Ferretti M, Vidal AF, Zantop T, and Fu FH. Anatomic, radiographic, biomechanical, and kinematic evaluation of the anterior cruciate ligament and its two functional bundles. *J Bone Joint Surg Am*. 2006;88 Suppl 4:2–10.

20. Roberts CC, Towers JD, Spangehl MJ, Carrino JA, and Morrison WB. Advanced MR imaging of the cruciate ligaments. *Magn Reson Imaging Clin N Am*. 2007;15(1):73–86.

21. Johal P, Williams A, Wragg P, Hunt D, and Gedroyc W. Tibio-femoral movement in the living knee. A study of weight bearing and non-weight bearing knee kinematics using "interventional" MRI. *J Biomech*. 2005;38(2):269–276.

22. Burr DB. Anatomy and physiology of the mineralized tissues: Role in the pathogenesis of osteoarthrosis. *Osteoarthritis Cartilage*. 2004;12:S20–S30.

23. Bullough PG. The role of joint architecture in the etiology of arthritis. *Osteoarthritis Cartilage*. 2004;12:S2–S9.

24. Walker PS, and Erkman MJ. The role of the menisci in force transmission across the knee. *Clin Orthop Relat Res*. 1975;109:184–192.

25. Fukuda Y, Takai S, Yoshino N, Murase K, Tsutsumi S, Ikeuchi K, and Hirasawa Y. Impact load transmission of the knee joint-influence of leg alignment and the role of meniscus and articular cartilage. *Clin Biomech (Bristol, Avon)*. 2000;15(7):516–521.

26. Hasler EM, Herzog W, Wu JZ, Müller W, and Wyss U. Articular cartilage biomechanics: Theoretical models, material properties, and biosynthetic response. *Crit Rev Biomed Eng*. 1999;27(6):415–488. Review.

27. Greis PE, Bardana DD, Holmstrom MC, and Burks RT. Meniscal injury: I. Basic science and evaluation. *Am Acad Orthop Surg*. 2002;10(3):168–176.

28. Aagaard H, and Verdonk R. Function of the normal meniscus and consequences of meniscal resection. *Scand J Med Sci Sports*. 1999;9(3):134–140.

29. Musahl V, Citak M, O'Loughlin PF, Choi D, Bedi A, and Pearle AD. The effect of medial versus lateral meniscectomy on the stability of the anterior cruciate ligament-deficient knee. *Am J Sports Med*. 2010;38(8):1591–1597.

30. Moglo KE, and Shirazi-Adl A. Biomechanics of passive knee joint in drawer: Load transmission in intact and ACL-deficient joints. *Knee*. 2003;10(3):265–276.

31. Burr DB, and Schaffler MB. The involvement of subchondral mineralized tissues in osteoarthrosis: Quantitative microscopic evidence. *Microsc Res Tech*. 1997;37(4):343–357.

32. Lane LB, Villacin A, and Bullough PG. The vascularity and remodelling of subchondral bone and calcified cartilage in adult human femoral and humeral heads. An age- and stress-related phenomenon. *J Bone Joint Surg Br*. 1977;59:272–278.

33. Muir P, McCarthy J, Radtke CL, Markel MD, Santschi EM, Scollay MC, and Kalscheur VL. Role of endochondral ossification of articular cartilage and functional adaptation of the subchondral plate in the development of fatigue microcracking of joints. *Bone*. 2006;38:342–349.

34. Suri S, Gill SE, Massena de Camin S, Wilson D, McWilliams DF, and Walsh DA. Neurovascular invasion at the osteochondral junction and in osteophytes in osteoarthritis. *Ann Rheum Dis*. 2007;66:1423–1508.

35. Kellgren JH, and Lawrence JS. Radiological assessment of osteo-arthrosis. *Ann Rheum Dis*. 1957;16:494–502.

36. Wluka AE, Wang Y, Davis SR, and Cicuttini FM. Tibial plateau size is related to grade of joint space narrowing and osteophytes in healthy women and in women with osteoarthritis. *Ann Rheum Dis.* 2005;64:1033–1037.

37. Eckstein F, Hudelmaier M, Cahue S, Marshall M, and Sharma L. Medial-to-lateral ratio of tibio-femoral subchondral bone area is adapted to alignment and mechanical load. *Calcif Tissue Int.* 2009;84(3):186–194.

38. Bowes MA, Vincent GR, Williams TC, Hutchinson CE, Lacey T, and Brett A. Statistical shape models show differences in bone shape between progressors and non-progressors in OAI progression cohort. *Osteoarthritis Cartilage.* 2008;16(S4):S26–S27.

39. Roemer FW, Frobell R, Hunter DJ, Crema MD, Fischer W, Bohndorf K, and Guermazi A. MRI-detected subchondral bone marrow signal alterations of the knee joint: Terminology, imaging appearance, relevance and radiological differential diagnosis. *Osteoarthritis Cartilage.* 2009;17(9):1115–1131.

40. Davies-Tuck ML, Wluka AE, Forbes A, Wang Y, English DR, Giles GG, O'Sullivan R, and Cicuttini FM. Development of bone marrow lesions is associated with adverse effects on knee cartilage while resolution is associated with improvement—A potential target for prevention of knee osteoarthritis: A longitudinal study. *Arthritis Res Ther.* 2010;12(1):R10.

41. Wluka AE, Hanna F, Davies-Tuck M, Wang Y, Bell RJ, Davis SR, Adams J, and Cicuttini FM. Bone marrow lesions predict progression of cartilage defects and loss of cartilage volume in healthy middle-aged adults without knee pain over 2 yrs. *Rheumatology (Oxford).* 2008;47(9):1392–1396.

42. Messent EA, Ward RJ, Tonkin CJ, and Buckland-Wright C. Tibial cancellous bone changes in patients with knee osteoarthritis. A short-term longitudinal study using Fractal Signature Analysis. *Osteoarthritis Cartilage.* 2005;13(6):463–470.

43. Lindsey CT, Narasimhan A, Adolfo JM, Jin H, Steinbach LS, Link T, Ries M, and Majumdar S. Magnetic resonance evaluation of the interrelationship between articular cartilage and trabecular bone of the osteoarthritic knee. *Osteoarthritis Cartilage.* 2004;12(2):86–96.

44. Peterfy CG, Guermazi A, Zaim S, Tirman PF, Miaux Y, White D, Kothari M et al. Whole-Organ Magnetic Resonance Imaging Score (WORMS) of the knee in osteoarthritis. *Osteoarthritis Cartilage.* 2004;12(3):177–190.

45. Huebner JL, Williams JM, Deberg M, Henrotin Y, and Kraus VB. Collagen fibril disruption occurs early in primary guinea pig knee osteoarthritis. *Osteoarthritis Cartilage.* 2010;18(3):397–405. Epub 2009, October 1.

46. Calvo E, Palacios I, Delgado E, Sánchez-Pernaute O, Largo R, Egido J, and Herrero-Beaumont G. Histopathological correlation of cartilage swelling detected by magnetic resonance imaging in early experimental osteoarthritis. *Osteoarthritis Cartilage.* 2004;12:878–886.

47. Watson PJ, Carpenter TA, Hall LD, and Tyler JA. Cartilage swelling and loss in a spontaneous model of osteoarthritis visualized by magnetic resonance imaging. *Osteoarthritis Cartilage.* 1996;4:197–207.

48. Thambyah A, and Broom N. On new bone formation in the pre-osteoarthritic joint. *Osteoarthritis Cartilage.* 2009;17:456–463.

49. Bi X, Yang X, Bostrom MP, Bartusik D, Ramaswamy S, Fishbein KW, Spencer RG, and Camacho NP. Fourier transform infrared imaging and MR microscopy studies detect compositional and structural changes in cartilage in a rabbit model of osteoarthritis. *Anal Bioanal Chem.* 2007;387:1601–1612.

50. David-Vaudey E, Ghosh S, Ries M, and Majumdar S. T2 relaxation time measurements in osteoarthritis. *Magn Reson Imaging.* 2004;22:673–682.

51. Hannila I, Nieminen MT, Rauvala E, Tervonen, and Ojala, O. Patellar cartilage lesions: Comparison of magnetic resonance imaging and T2 relaxation-time mapping. *Acta Radiol.* 2007;48:444–448.

52. Ding C, Garnero P, Cicuttini F, Scott F, Cooley H, and Jones G. Knee cartilage defects: Association with early radiographic osteoarthritis, decreased cartilage volume, increased joint surface area and type II collagen breakdown. *Osteoarthritis Cartilage.* 2005;13:198–205.

53. McDermott ID, and Amis AA. The consequences of meniscectomy. *J Bone Joint Surg Br.* 2006;88(12):1549–1556.

54. Englund M, Guermazi A, and Lohmander SL. The role of the meniscus in knee osteoarthritis: A cause or consequence? *Radiol Clin North Am.* 2009;47(4):703–712.

55. Bhattacharyya T, Gale D, Dewire P, Totterman S, Gale ME, McLaughlin S, Einhorn TA, and Felson DT. The clinical importance of meniscal tears demonstrated by magnetic resonance imaging in osteoarthritis of the knee. *J Bone Joint Surg Am.* 2003;85-A:4–9.

56. Crema MD, Guermazi A, Li L, Nogueira-Barbosa MH, Marra MD, Roemer FW, Eckstein F, Le Graverand MP, Wyman BT, and Hunter DJ. The association of prevalent medial meniscalpathology with cartilage loss in the medial tibiofemoral compartment over a 2-year period. *Osteoarthritis Cartilage.* 2010;18(3):336–343.

57. Wang Y, Wluka AE, Pelletier JP, Martel-Pelletier J, Abram F, Ding C, and Cicuttini FM. Meniscal extrusion predicts increases in subchondral bone marrow lesions and bone cysts and expansion of subchondral bone in osteoarthritic knees. *Rheumatology (Oxford).* 2010;49(5):997–1004.

58. Roberts CC, Towers JD, Spangehl MJ, Carrino JA, and Morrison WB. Advanced MR imaging of the cruciate ligaments. *Magn Reson Imaging Clin N Am.* 2007;15(1):73–86.

59. Frobell RB, Le Graverand MP, Buck R, Roos EM, Roos HP, Tamez-Pena J, Totterman S, and Lohmander LS. The acutely ACL injured knee assessed by MRI: Changes in joint fluid, bone marrow lesions, and cartilage during the first year. *Osteoarthritis Cartilage.* 2009;17(2):161–167.

60. Li G, Moses JM, Papannagari R, Pathare NP, DeFrate E, and Gill TJ. Anterior cruciate ligament deficiency alters the *in vivo* motion of the tibiofemoral cartilage contact points in both the anteroposterior and mediolateral directions. *J Bone Joint Surg Am.* 2006;88:1826–1834.

61. Fernandez-Madrid F, Karvonen RL, Teitge RA, Miller PR, and Negendank WG. MR features of osteoarthritis of the knee. *Magn Reson Imaging.* 1994;12:703–709.

62. Crema MD, Roemer FW, Marra MD, Burstein D, Gold GE, Eckstein F, Baum T, Mosher TJ, Carrino JA, and Guermazi A. Articular cartilage in the knee: Current MR imaging techniques and applications in clinical practice and research. *Radiographics.* 2011;31(1):37–61.

63. Roemer FW, Eckstein F, and Guermazi A. Magnetic resonance imaging-based semiquantitative and quantitative assessment in osteoarthritis. *Rheum Dis Clin North Am.* 2009;35(3):521–555.

64. Tyler DJ, Robson MR, Henkelman M, Young IR, and Bydder GM. Magnetic resonance imaging with ultrashort TE (UTE) PULSE sequences: Technical considerations. *J Magn Reson Imaging.* 2007;25:279–289.

65. Chen CA, Kijowski R, Shapiro LM, Tuite MJ, Kirkland W, Davis KW, Klaers JL, Block WF, Reeder SB, and Gold GE. Cartilage morphology at 3.0T: Assessment of three-dimensional magnetic resonance imaging techniques. *J Magn Reson Imaging.* 2010;32:173–183.

66. Wirth W, Nevitt M, Hellio Le Graverand MP, Benichou O, Dreher D, Davies RY, Lee J et al. OAI investigators: Sensitivity to change of cartilage morphometry using coronal FLASH, sagittal DESS, and coronal MPR DESS protocols—Comparative data from the Osteoarthritis Initiative (OAI). *Osteoarthritis Cartilage.* 2010;18(4):547–554.

67. Eckstein F, Maschek S, Wirth W, Hudelmaier M, Hitzl W, Wyman B, Nevitt M, and Le Graverand MP. OAI Investigator Group: One year change of knee cartilage morphology in the first release of participants from the Osteoarthritis Initiative progression subcohort: Association with sex, body mass index, symptoms and radiographic osteoarthritis status. *Ann Rheum Dis.* 2009;68(5):674–679.

68. Cashman PM, Kitney RI, Gariba MA, and Carter ME. Automated techniques for visualization and mapping of articular cartilage in MR images of the osteoarthritic knee: A base technique for the assessment of microdamage and submicro damage. *IEEE Trans Nanobiosci.* 2002;1(1):42–51.

69. Hunter DJ, Li L, Zhang YQ, Totterman S, Tamez J, Kwoh CK, Eaton CB, Hellio Le Graverand M-P, and Beals CR. Region of interest analysis: By selecting regions with denuded areas can we detect greater amounts of change? *Osteoarthritis Cartilage.* 2010;18:175–183.

70. Frobell RB, Le Graverand MP, Buck R, Roos EM, Roos HP, Tamez-Pena J, Totterman S, and Lohmander LS. The acutely ACL injured knee assessed by MRI: Changes in joint fluid, bone marrow lesions, and cartilage during the first year. *Osteoarthritis Cartilage.* 2009;17(2):161–167.

71. Williams TG, Holmes AP, Waterton JC, Maciewicz RA, Hutchinson CE, Moots RJ, Nash AF, and Taylor CJ. Anatomically corresponded regional analysis of cartilage in asymptomatic and osteoarthritic knees by statistical shape modeling of the bone. *IEEE Trans Med Imaging.* 2010;29(8):1541–1559.

72. Williams TG, Holmes AP, Bowes M, Vincent G, Hutchinson CE, Waterton JC, Maciewicz RA, and Taylor CJ. Measurement and visualization of focal cartilage thickness change by MRI in a study of knee osteoarthritis using a novel image analysis tool. *Br J Radiol.* 2010;83(995):940–948.

73. Tamez-Pena JG, Jackson R, Yu J, Eaton CB, Schneider E, and Totterman S. Thickness delta maps: Methodology for the spatial detection and quantification longitudinal changes in cartilage thickness. *Osteoarthritis Cartilage.* 2007;15(Suppl C):C180–C181.

74. Tamez-Peña JG, Gonzalez PC, Schreyer EH, Farber JM, and Totterman SM. Atlas based standardized quantification of cartilage thickness maps: Data from osteoarthritis Initiative. *Osteoarthritis Cartilage.* 2010;18(Suppl 2):S64–S65.

75. Tamez-Peña J, González PC, Schreyer EH, Farber JM, and Totterman SM. Detection of early changes in subchondral bone plate curvature in OA: Data from Osteoarthritis initiative. *Osteoarthritis Cartilage.* 2010;18 S 2:60–61.

76. Wirth W, Buck R, Nevitt M, Le Graverand MP, Benichou O, Dreher D, Davies RY et al. MRI-based extended ordered values more efficiently differentiate cartilage loss in knees with and without joint space narrowing than region-specific approaches using MRI or radiography—Data from the OA initiative. *Osteoarthritis Cartilage.* 2011;19(6):689–699.

77. Muir P, McCarthy J, Radtke CL, Markel MD, Santschi EM, Scollay MC, and Kalscheur VL. Role of endochondral ossification of articular cartilage and functional adaptation of the subchondral plate in the development of fatigue microcracking of joints. *Bone.* 2006;38:342–349.

78. Thambyah A, and Broom N. On new bone formation in the pre-osteoarthritic joint. *Osteoarthritis Cartilage.* 2009;17:456–63.

79. Pritzker KPH, Gay S, Jimenez SA, Ostergaard K, Pelletier J-P, Revell PA, Salter D, and van den Berg WB. Osteoarthritis cartilage histopathology: Grading and staging. *Osteoarthritis Cartilage.* 2006;14:13–29.

80. Wirth W, Larroque S, Davies RY, Nevitt M, Gimona A, Baribaud F, Lee JH et al. OA Initiative Investigators Group: Comparison of 1-year vs 2-year change in regional cartilage thickness in osteoarthritis results from 346 participants from the Osteoarthritis Initiative. *Osteoarthritis Cartilage.* 2011;19(1):74–83.

81. David-Vaudey E, Ghosh S, Ries M, and Majumdar S. T2 relaxation time measurements in osteoarthritis. *Magn Reson Imaging.* 2004;22(5):673–682.

82. Riek JK, and Zhang. A comparison of T2 mapping sequences at 1.5 Tesla for use in clinical trial. *Osteoarthritis Cartilage.* 2009;17(Suppl 1):S231–S232.

83. Li X, Benjamin Ma C, Link TM, Castillo DD, Blumenkrantz G, Lozano J, Carballido-Gamio J, Ries M, and Majumdar S. *In vivo* T(1rho) and T(2) mapping of articular cartilage in osteoarthritis of the knee using 3 T MRI. *Osteoarthritis Cartilage.* 2007;15(7):789–797.

84. Williams A, Qian Y, and Chu CR. UTE-T2* mapping of human articular cartilage in vivo: A repeatability assessment. *Osteoarthritis Cartilage.* 2011;19(1):84–88.

85. Qazi AA, Dam EB, Nielsen M, Karsdal MA, Pettersen PC, and Christiansen C. Separation of healthy and early osteoarthritis by automatic quantification of cartilage homogeneity. *Osteoarthritis Cartilage.* 2007;15(10):1199–1206.

86. Kellgren JH, and Lawrence JS. Radiological assessment of osteo-arthrosis. *Ann Rheum Dis.* 1957;16:494–502.

87. Wluka AE, Wang Y, Davis SR, and Cicuttini FM. Tibial plateau size is related to grade of joint space narrowing and osteophytes in healthy women and in women with osteoarthritis. *Ann Rheum Dis.* 2005;64:1033–1037.

88. Roemer FW, Frobell R, Hunter DJ, Crema MD, Fischer W, Bohndorf K, and Guermazi A. MRI-detected subchondral bone marrow signal alterations of the knee joint: Terminology, imaging appearance, relevance and radiological differential diagnosis. *Osteoarthritis Cartilage.* 2009;17(9):1115–1131.

89. Tamez-Peña J, Farber J, González P, Schreyer E, and Totterman S. Unsupervised segmentation and quantification of knee features: Data from the osteoarthritis initiative, *IEEE Transactions on Biomedical Engineering.* 2012;59(4):1177–1186.

90. Frobell RB, Le Graverand MP, Buck R, Roos EM, Roos HP, Tamez-Pena J, Totterman S, and Lohmander LS. The acutely ACL injured knee assessed by MRI: Changes in joint fluid, bone marrow lesions, and cartilage during the first year. *Osteoarthritis Cartilage.* 2009;17(2):161–167.

91. Folkesson J, Goldenstein J, Carballido-Gamio J, Kazakia G, Burghardt AJ, Rodriguez A, Krug R, de Papp AE, Link TM, and Majumdar S. Longitudinal evaluation of the effects of alendronate on MRI bone microarchitecture in postmenopausal osteopenic women. *Bone.* 2011;48(3):611–621.

92. Peterfy CG, Guermazi A, Zaim S, Tirman PF, Miaux Y, White D, Kothari M et al. Whole-organ magnetic resonance imaging score (WORMS) of the knee in osteoarthritis. *Osteoarthritis Cartilage.* 2004;12(3):177–190.

93. Swanson MS, Prescott JW, Best TM, Powell K, Jackson RD, Haq F, and Gurcan MN. Semi-automated segmentation to assess the lateral meniscus in normal and osteoarthritic knees. *Osteoarthritis Cartilage.* 2010;18(3):344–353.

94. Wirth W, Frobell RB, Souza RB, Li X, Wyman BT, Le Graverand MP, Link TM, Majumdar S, and Eckstein F. A three-dimensional quantitative method to measure meniscus shape, position, and signal intensity using MR images: A pilot study and preliminary results in knee osteoarthritis. *Magn Reson Med.* 2010;63(5):1162–1171.

95. Zarins ZA, Bolbos RI, Pialat JB, Link TM, Li X, Souza RB, and Majumdar S. Cartilage and meniscus assessment using T1rho and T2 measurements in healthy subjects and patients with osteoarthritis. *Osteoarthritis Cartilage.* 2010;18(11):1408–1416.

96. Kraus VB, Vail TP, Worrell T, and McDaniel G. A comparative assessment of alignment angle of the knee by radiographic and physical examination methods. *Arthritis Rheum.* 2005;52(6):1730–1735.

97. Hsu RW, Himeno S, Coventry MB, and Chao EY. Normal axial alignment of the lower extremity and load-bearing distribution atthe knee. *Clin Orthop.* 1990;255:215–227.

98. Hunter DJ, Zhang Y, Niu J, Tu X, Amin S, Goggins J, Lavalley M, Guermazi A, Gale D, and Felson DT. Structural factors associated with malalignment in knee osteoarthritis: The Boston osteoarthritis knee study. *J Rheumatol.* 2005;32:2192–2199.

99. Allaire R, Muriuki M, Gilbertson L, Harner CD, Allaire R, Muriuki M, Gilbertson L, and Harner CD. Biomechanical consequences of a tear of the posterior root of the medial meniscus. Similar to total meniscectomy. *J Bone Joint Surg Am.* 2008;90(9):1922–1931.

100. Li G, Moses JM, Papannagari R, Pathare NP, DeFrate E, and Gill TJ. Anterior cruciate ligament deficiency alters the *in vivo* motion of the tibiofemoral cartilage contact points in both the anteroposterior and mediolateral directions. *J Bone Joint Surg Am.* 2006;88:1826–1834.

101. Papannagari R, Gill TJ, Defrate LE, Moses JM, Petruska AJ, and Li G. *In vivo* kinematics of the knee after anterior cruciate ligament reconstruction: A clinical and functional evaluation. *Am J Sports Med.* 2006;34(12):2006–2012.

102. Van de Velde SK, Gill TJ, and Li G. Evaluation of kinematics of anterior cruciate ligament-deficient knees with use of advanced imaging techniques, three-dimensional modeling techniques, and robotics. *J Bone Joint Surg Am.* 2009;91 Suppl 1:108–114.

103. Van de Velde SK, Bingham JT, Hosseini A, Kozanek M, DeFrate LE, Gill TJ, and Li G. Increased tibiofemoral cartilage contact deformation in patients with anterior cruciate ligament deficiency. *Arthritis Rheum.* 2009;60(12):3693–3702.

104. Eckstein F, Burstein D, and Link TM. Quantitative MRI of cartilage and bone: Degenerative changes in osteoarthritis. *Nmr in Biomed.* 2006; 19:822–854.

105. Burstein D. MRI for development osteoarthritis drugs of disease-modifying. *NMR Biomed.* 2006;19:669–680.

106. Wirth W, Nevitt M, Le Graverand MPH, Benichou O, Dreher D, Davies RY et al. Sensitivity to change of cartilage morphometry using coronal FLASH, sagittal DESS, and coronal MPR DESS protocols—Comparative data from the osteoarthritis initiative (OAI). *Osteoarthritis Cartilage.* 2010;18:547–554.

107. Eckstein F, Guermazi A, and Roemer FW. Quantitative MR Imaging of cartilage and trabecular bone in osteoarthritis. *Radiol Clin North Am.* 2009;47:655–+.

108. Hunter DJ, Niu J, Zhang Y, Totterman S, Tamez J, Dabrowski C et al. Change in cartilage morphometry: A sample of the progression cohort of the Osteoarthritis Initiative. *Ann Rheum Dis.* 2009;68:349–356.

109. Eckstein F, Wyman BT, Buck RJ, Wirth W, Maschek S, Hudelmaier M et al. Longitudinal quantitative MR imaging of cartilage morphology in the presence of gadopentetate dimeglumine (Gd-DTPA). *Magn Reson Med.* 2009;61:975–980.

110. Ellison SLR, Rosslein M, and Williams A. Quantifying uncertainty in analytical measurement. s.l; *Eurachem.* ii, 2000.

111. Taylor BN, and Kuyatt CE. Guidelines for Evaluating and Expressing the Uncertainty of NIST Measurement Results. In: NIST: NIST 1994.

112. FDA. ICH-Q2A: Text on Validation of Analytical Procedures. In: FDA CDER 1995.

113. FDA. ICH-Q2B: Validation of Analytical Procedures: Methodology. In: FDA CDER 1996.

114. Taylor BN, and Kuyatt CE. Technical Note 1297: Guidelines for Evaluating and Expressing the Uncertainty of NIST Measurement Results. In: NIST: NIST 1994.

115. Eckstein F, Sittek H, Milz S, Putz R, and Reiser M. The morphology of articular-cartilage assessed by magnetic-resonance-imaging (MRI)—Reproducibility and anatomical correlation. *Surgical Radiologic Anatomy.* 1994;16:429–438.

116. Schnier M, Eckstein F, Priebsch J, Haubner M, Sittek H, Becker C et al. Three-dimensional thickness and volume measurements of knee joint cartilage with MRI: Validation in anatomical specimens via CT arthrography. *Rofo-Fortschritte Auf Dem Gebiet Der Rontgenstrahlen Und Der Bildgebenden Verfahren.* 1997;167:521–526.

117. Eckstein F, Schnier M, Haubner M, Priebsch J, Glaser C, Englmeier KH et al. Accuracy of cartilage volume and thickness measurements with magnetic resonance imaging. *Clin Orthopaedics Related Res.* 1998:137–148.

118. Muensterer OJ, Eckstein F, Hahn D, and Putz R. Computer-aided three dimensional assessment of knee-joint cartilage with magnetic resonance imaging. *Clin Biomech.* 1996;11:260–266.

119. Hohe J, Ateshian G, Reiser M, Englmeier KH, and Eckstein F. Surface size, curvature analysis, and assessment of knee joint incongruity with MRI in vivo. *Magn Reson Med.* 2002;47:554–561.

120. Eckstein F, Westhoff J, Sittek H, Maag KP, Haubner M, Faber S, Englmeier KH, and Reiser M. In vivo reproducibility of three-dimensional cartilage volume and thickness measurements with MR imaging. *Am J Roentgenol.* 1998; 170:593–597.

121. Eckstein F, Buck RJ, Burstein D, Charles HC, Crim J, Hudelmaier M et al. Precision of 3.0 Tesla quantitative magnetic resonance imaging of cartilage morphology in a multicentre clinical trial. *Ann Rheum Dis.* 2008;67:1683–1688.

122. McKenzie CA, Williams A, Prasad PV, and Burstein D. Three-dimensional delayed gadolinium-enhanced MRI of cartilage (dGEMRIC) at 1.5T and 3.0T. *J Magn Reson Imaging.* 2006;24:928–933.

123. Williams A, Gillis A, McKenzie C, Po B, Sharma L, Micheli L et al. Glycosaminoglycan distribution in cartilage as determined by delayed gadolinium-enhanced MRI of cartilage (dGEMRIC): Potential clinical applications. *Am J Roentgenol.* 2004;182:167–172.

124. Liang ZR, Macfall JR, and Harrington DP. Parameter-estimation and tissue segmentation from multispectral MR-images. *IEEE Trans Med Imaging.* 1994;13:441–449.

125. Williams TG, Holmes AP, Waterton JC, Maciewicz RA, Hutchinson CE, Moots RJ et al. Anatomically corresponded regional analysis of cartilage in asymptomatic and osteoarthritic knees by statistical shape modelling of the bone. *IEEE Trans Med Imaging.* 2010;29:1541–1559.

126. Nevit MC, Felson DT, and Lester G. Protocol for the Cohort study. In: OAI 2002.

127. Synarc. MRI Procedure manual for examinations of the knee and thigh. In: OAI 2006.

128. Williams TG, Holmes AP, Waterton JC, Maciewicz RA, Nash AFP, Taylor CJ. Regional quantitative analysis of knee cartilage in a population study using MRI and model based correspondences. *In Proceedings of the 3rd IEEE International Symposium on Biomedical Imaging: From Nano to Macro.* Arlington, VA. 2006:311–314.

129. Raynauld JP, Kauffmann C, Beaudoin G, Berthiaume MJ, de Guise JA, Bloch DA et al. Reliability of a quantification imaging system using magnetic resonance images to measure cartilage thickness and volume in human normal and osteoarthritic knees. *Osteoarthritis Cartilage.* 2003;11:351–360.

130. Raynauld JP, Martel-Pelletier J, Berthiaume MJ, Beaudoin G, Choquette D, Haraoui B, Tannenbaum H et al. Long term evaluation of disease progression through the quantitative magnetic resonance imaging of symptomatic knee osteoarthritis patients: Correlation with clinical symptoms and radiographic changes. *Arthritis Res Therap.* 2006; 8:R21, Available at http://0-www.scopus.com. millenium.itesm.mx/inward/record.url?eid=2-s2.0-34247551198&partnerID=40&md5=412d7bb1 fe07eaaae886387cac70501b

131. Wirth W, and Eckstein F. A technique for regional analysis of femorotibial cartilage thickness based on quantitative magnetic resonance Imaging. *IEEE Trans Med Imaging.* 2008;27:737–744.

132. Hudelmaier M, Wirth W, Wehr B, Kraus V, Wyman BT, Le Graverand MPH et al. Femorotibial cartilage morphology: Reproducibility of different metrics and femoral regions, and sensitivity to change in disease. *Cells Tissues Organs.* 2010;192:340–350.

133. Guermazi A, Burstein D, Conaghan P, Eckstein F, Le Graverand-Gastineau MPH, Keen H et al. Imaging in osteoarthritis. *Rheum Dis Clin North Am.* 2008; 34:645–+.

134. Eckstein F, Mosher T, and Hunter D. Imaging of knee osteoarthritis: Data beyond the beauty. *Curr Opin Rheumatol.* 2007;19:435–443.

135. Tamez-Pena JG, Gonzalez PC, Schreyer EH, Farber JM, and Totterman SM. Atlas-based standardized quantification of cartilage thickness maps: Data from the osteoarthritis initiative. *Osteoarthritis Cartilage.* 2010;18:S64–S65.

136. Pakin SK, Tamez-Pena JG, Totterman S, and Parker KJ. Segmentation, surface extraction and thickness computation of articular cartilage. *Medical Imaging 2002: Image Processing Vol 1–3* 2002; 4684:155–166.

137. Tamez-Pena JG, Barbu-McInnis M, and Totterman S. Knee cartilage extraction and bone-cartilage interface analysis from 3D MRI data sets. *Medical Imaging 2004: Image Processing,* Pts, 2004;5370:1774–1784.

138. Dodin P, Pelletier JP, Martel-Pelletier J, and Abram F. Automatic human knee cartilage segmentation from 3-D magnetic resonance images. *IEEE Trans Biomed Eng.* 2010;57:2699–2711.

139. Bowers ME, Trinh N, Tung GA, Crisco JJ, Kimia BB, and Fleming BC. Quantitative MR imaging using "LiveWire" to measure tibiofemoral articular cartilage thickness. *Osteoarthritis Cartilage.* 2008;16:1167–1173.

140. Folkesson J, Dam EB, Olsen OF, Pettersen PC, and Christiansen C. Segmenting articular cartilage automatically using a voxel classification approach. *IEEE Trans Med Imaging.* 2007;26:106–115.

141. Baldwin MA, Langenderfer JE, Rullkoetter PJ, and Laz PJ. Development of subject-specific and statistical shape models of the knee using an efficient segmentation and mesh-morphing approach. *Computer Methods Programs Biomed.* 2010;97:232–240.

142. Tamez-Pena JG, Parker KJ, and Totterman S. The integration of automatic segmentation and motion tracking for 4D reconstruction and visualization of musculoskeletal structures. In: Vemuri B Ed. *IEEE Workshop on Biomedical Image Analysis.* IEEE, Santa Barbara, CA, 1998: pp. 154–163.

143. Tamez-Pena JG, Totterman S, and Parker KJ. Kinematic analysis of musculoskeletal structures via volumetric MRI and unsupervised segmentation. *Medical Imaging 1999: Physiology and Function from Multidimensional Images.* 1999;3660:488–499.

144. Tamez-Pena JG, Barbu-McInnis M, and Totterman S. Structural quantification of cartilage changes using statistical parametric mapping—Art. no. 651248. In: Pluim JPW, Reinhardt JM Eds. *Medical Imaging 2007 Conference*. San Diego, CA, 2007: pp. 51248–51248.

145. Kauffmann C, Gravel P, Godbout B, Gravel A, Beaudoin G, Raynauld JP et al. Computer-aided, method for quantification of cartilage thickness and volume changes using MRL: Validation study using a synthetic model. *IEEE Trans Biomed Eng*. 2003;50:978–988.

146. Peterfy CG, Guermazi A, Zaim S, Tirman PFJ, Miaux Y, White D et al. Whole-organ magnetic resonance imaging score (WORMS) of the knee in osteoarthritis. *Osteoarthritis Cartilage*. 2004;12:177–190.

147. Felson DT, Lynch J, Guermazi A, Roemer FW, Niu J, McAlindon T et al. Comparison of BLOKS and WORMS scoring systems part II. Longitudinal assessment of knee MRIs for osteoarthritis and suggested approach based on their performance: Data from the Osteoarthritis Initiative. *Osteoarthritis Cartilage*. 2010;18:1402–1407.

148. Wolfe F, and Kong SX. Rasch analysis of the Western Ontario MacMaster Questionnaire (WOMAC) in 2205 patients with osteoarthritis, rheumatoid arthritis, and fibromyalgia. *Ann Rheum Dis*. 1999;58:563–568.

149. Thumboo J, Chew LH, and Soh CH. Validation of the Western Ontario and McMaster University Osteoarthritis Index in Asians with osteoarthritis in Singapore. *Osteoarthritis Cartilage*. 2001;9:440–446.

150. Roos EM, Roos HP, Lohmander LS, Ekdahl C, and Beynnon BD. Knee injury and osteoarthritis outcome score (KOOS)—Development of a self-administered outcome measure. *J Orthopaedic Sports Physical Therapy*. 1998;28:88–96.

151. Tamez-Pena JG, Gonzalez PC, Schreyer E, Farber J, Trevino V, and Totterman S. Advanced MRI-based measurements as surrogate markers of KOOS pain and KOOS other knee symptoms: Data from the osteoarthritis initiative. *Osteoarthritis Cartilage*. 2010;18:S187–S187.

152. Eckstein F, Wirth W, Hunter DJ, Guermazi A, Kwoh CK, Nelson DR et al. Magnitude and regional distribution of cartilage loss associated with grades of joint space narrowing in radiographic osteoarthritis—Data from the Osteoarthritis Initiative (OAI). *Osteoarthritis Cartilage*. 2010;18:760–768.

153. Eckstein F, Wirth W, Hudelmaier MI, Maschek S, Hitzl W, Wyman BT et al. Relationship of compartment-specific structural knee status at baseline with change in cartilage morphology: A prospective observational study using data from the osteoarthritis initiative. *Arthritis Res Therapy*. 2009; 11(3):R90, Available at http://0-www.scopus.com.millenium.itesm.mx/inward/record.url?eid=2-s2.0-67650095293&partnerID=40&md5=de3cf28d340df0839ad7c6919ff32767

154. Tamez-Pena JG, Lerner AL, Yao J, Salo AD, Totterman S. Evaluation of distance maps from fast GRE MRI as a tool to study the knee joint space. *Medical Imaging 2003: Physiology and Function: Methods, Systems, and Applications*. 2003;5031:551–562.

20

Utility of PET in Pharmaceutical Development

R. Boellaard
VU University Medical Center

M. Lubberink
Uppsala University

R.P. Maguire
Novartis Institutes for Biomedical Research

20.1 Introduction

Noninvasive imaging is a critical biotechnology tool for efficient pharmaceutical development. Precise measurement of pharmaceutical effects *in vivo*, in man, allows detailed study of target interaction and effects on pathology. Positron emission tomography (PET) enables measurement of uptake, distribution, and binding with high specificity. Optimal application of the technology requires critical selection of spatial and temporal resolution to optimize the sensitivity for the specific clinical question. From knowledge of the pharmacokinetics of the PET tracer and the statistical properties of the measurement system, data analysis methods for each radiotracer and application have been developed. In this way, the measurement sensitivity to radioligands and targets has been maximized and the signal response to potential confounding effects minimized. Both scientifically and from an operational and regulatory standpoint, PET imaging in pharmaceutical development has matured. Further research and work will be necessary to refine the technology, in order to reduce the number of study subjects required and increase the sensitivity to small changes.

PET may be useful in several different ways for clinical trials:

1. Longitudinal outcome biomarker. Changes in uptake are used as an index for treatment response.
2. Target engagement biomarker. Receptor expression or receptor occupancy studies using a specific radiotracer.
3. Staging and inclusion criteria for patient participation in clinical trials.
4. Stratification, that is, based on the PET findings patients may be assigned to a specific arm of the trial (e.g., high-risk vs. low-risk groups).
5. Biodistribution of a radiolabeled pharmaceutical.

Application of molecular imaging for receptor occupancy measurement and tumor metabolism is well understood in the pharmaceutical industry. The opportunity to derisk development programs by proving pathway engagement and efficacy early in clinical trials provides a critical advantage in pharmaceutical projects. Molecular imaging has also been used to study preclinical disease and therapy models. The main advantage of noninvasive measurement is clear, but it may not deliver the best sensitivity. Other methods such as *ex vivo* autoradiography may in fact be more appropriate to study pharmaceuticals in detail. The main advantages of *in vivo* translational imaging are the within-subject, longitudinal study designs allowing better precision, the ability to study processes *in vivo*, *in situ*, and the potential to reduce subject numbers, especially for precious animal models. Development of specific ligands for other organs and receptor systems will understandably increase the number of applications. As protein and antibody therapies are developed, PET imaging will be available to confirm biodistribution. Novel combined modality PET-MR devices will enable the measurement of function (pharmacodynamics) and target simultaneously. Development of noninvasive techniques, such as amyloid imaging in Alzheimer's disease, will permit earlier diagnosis and treatment. This chapter concentrates on current advances in technology that will permit advances in the next generation of vital treatments.

20.2 Phases of Pharmaceutical Development

As a pharmaceutical is developed from an initial concept and a pathway target, it is tested first in *in vitro* models and preclinical models to understand its interaction with the biological system in detail. The first clinical studies are designed to confirm the pharmacokinetic properties and safety profile of the pharmaceutical. As the new treatment moves into clinical trials in larger cohorts of patients, the clinical science, safety, and efficacy of the pharmaceutical will have more emphasis than the basic science of the pathway (Figure 20.1).

Molecular imaging can make contributions in all these phases. However, since it is related to the target, it is in the translational phase of early clinical development where the most obvious contribution can be made. Molecular imaging allows the noninvasive study of receptor and molecular level effects *in vivo* in man. This allows a more precise measurement and selection of dose, depending on the expected effect at the receptor/pathway level. In later stages of pharmaceutical development, the molecular imaging signal will be more directly related to disease outcome and the use of *non invasive* imaging can be used to monitor treatment effects on the disease. In this respect, the linkage between imaging signal change and the disease needs to be established and this will likely require that the imaging signal has been closely associated with disease outcome in previous treatment trials.

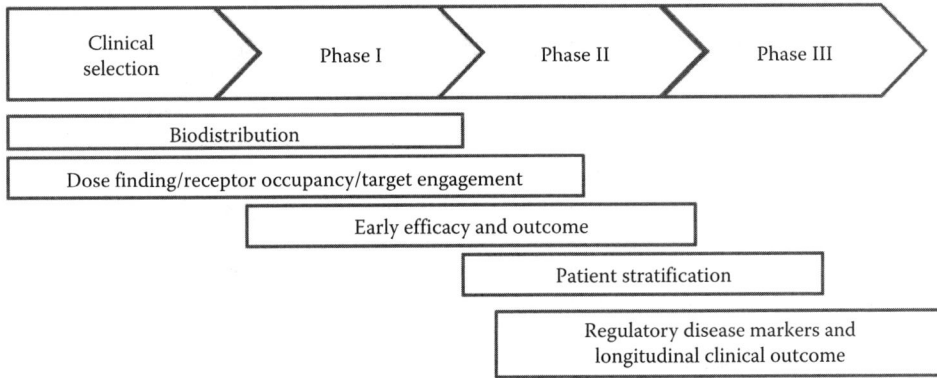

FIGURE 20.1   Applications of PET in different phases of pharmaceutical development.

20.3 State-of-the-Art Instrumentation for Clinical Trials

In this section, a brief summary of PET imaging principles, acquisition, and image reconstruction is given (Townsend 2004). Interested readers are referred to Townsend part 1 (Townsend 2004) for a more detailed explanation of PET imaging fundamentals.

20.3.1 Principles of PET

PET is a molecular imaging technique, which measures the distribution of a radioactive tracer *in vivo*. Upon administration of very small amounts (pico- or nanomoles) of a radiotracer to the patient, it distributes in the central compartment and in organs. The radioactive atom of the radiotracer (e.g., [F-18] FDG) emits positrons. The emitted positron combines with an electron after traveling a distance up to several mm in tissue. The positron and electron are then converted into two photons, each with an energy of 511 keV, which are emitted into near opposite directions. PET image acquisition is based on the simultaneous (coincidence) detection of these two photons. A PET scanner consists of many photon detectors surrounding the patient. A line connecting any two detectors that have detected two annihilation photons simultaneously is called the line of response (LOR) and ideally indicates the line along which a positron emission took place. In practice, a time window of a couple of ns (4–10 ns) is usually applied for the "simultaneous" detection of the annihilation photons. During a PET scan, millions of coincidence detections along LORs are being collected, providing information about the distribution of the radiotracer in tissue.

Unfortunately, not all coincidences contribute to the signal, that is, the "true" 3D distribution of the tracer. Background noise is added to the signal due to photons that are scattered before detection or by coincidence detection of two uncorrelated photons, that is, the so-called random coincidences. True coincidences arise from the simultaneous (coincident) detection of two annihilation photons generated by one positron emission. Ideally, only true counts are detected. A large fraction of the emitted photons (up to 50%) is scattered, mainly by Compton scattering, before leaving the patient. When one of the photons has been scattered, it will result in a dislocation of the "true" coincidence detection. Moreover, when two photons from two different positron emissions are accidentally (randomly) detected simultaneously, that is, within the duration of the time window (while the others are undetected), the PET camera will notice a random coincidence detection. It may be clear that these random coincidences result in image distortions (appears as an addition of a smooth background). Finally, multiple detections can occur when three or more photons are detected at the same time. These multiples are usually discarded.

In PET studies, it is necessary to account for the contribution of scattered and random coincidences. In most modern PET systems, scatter correction is usually performed using the single scatter simulation (SSS) method developed by Watson (2000). Randoms are usually measured by the so-called delayed coincidence time window technique. It is beyond the scope of this chapter to address these corrections in detail. Yet, it should be realized that especially accurate and precise scatter correction is one of the most challenging issues in quantitative PET imaging.

Moreover, due to attenuation (scatter and absorption) of photons in the patient, a large fraction of the emitted photons are not detected. Fortunately in PET, attenuation does not depend on the location of the positron emission along the LOR, but is determined by the total "radiological," or attenuating, thickness of the patient along the LOR. Consequently, by making specific (low dose) CT scans, the transmission through the subject along all LORs can be measured and thus correct exactly for the effects of attenuation. CT scans made for attenuation correction purposes are usually acquired using a low beam current (e.g., 30–70 mAs) to minimize the radiation dose for the patient. The (average) energy of the photons generated by the x-ray tube of the CT scanner is usually about 80 keV (actually it is a spectrum). In order to use these CT scans for attenuation correction of 511 keV annihilation photon, the CT image first needs to be converted into a 511 keV attenuation coefficient map. The latter step usually involves automated segmentation of the CT image in various tissue classes (lung, soft tissue, and bone) followed by (bi-)linear rescaling functions. After these conversions, an accurate attenuation correction can be derived from the CT images. In practice, however, attenuation correction is somewhat hampered by patient motion (e.g., breathing). An overview of potential pitfalls or artifacts when using CT-based attenuation correction is given by Sureshbabu and Mawlawi (2005).

Finally, with current state-of-the-art PET detectors, it is possible to measure the difference in arrival time of the two emitted annihilation photons with an accuracy of 300–600 ps. The technology that measures and uses this difference in arrival time is called "time of flight (TOF)." At present, with TOF (300–600 ps), it is possible to determine the location of the positron emission along the LOR with a spatial accuracy of about 5–10 cm. Clearly, this spatial accuracy is not high enough to exactly (within 1 mm) indicate the location of the positron emission. Yet, by taking TOF into account during image reconstruction, the image quality is improved and specifically the detection of small tumors nearby large high uptake organs (liver, heart, brain, and bladder) is enhanced.

20.3.2 Reconstruction Algorithms

PET or PET/CT systems measure are based on the coincidence detection of annihilation photons that are emitted from the patient; thus, a PET or PET/CT system measures coincident photons or projection data outside and around the patient. These projection or "raw" data are then used to calculate a 3D PET image representing the distribution of the radiotracer in the patient. The process that calculates the 3D PET image from the raw projection data while including all necessary corrections, such as, for example, scatter, randoms, and attenuation corrections, is called PET image reconstruction.

Up to the late 1990s, raw PET data were primarily reconstructed using the so-called filtered backprojection (FBP). The latter method is linear and quantitatively accurate but suffers from noise and streak artifacts. Nowadays, iterative reconstructions are almost exclusively used and PET/CT systems are equipped with dedicated reconstruction computer clusters to deal with the higher computational demand of iterative versus FBP reconstruction. Most commercially available iterative reconstruction methods are based on the maximum likelihood expectation maximization (MLEM) algorithm described by Shepp and Vardi (1982). Later, Hudson and Larkin (1994) invented a faster implementation of MLEM by taking the so-called ordered subsets of the raw data during the reconstruction process resulting in the ordered subset expectation maximization (OSEM) method. The main advantage of iterative reconstructions is that they provide enhanced image quality compared to FBP and thereby improving diagnostic accuracy. Another advantage is that various corrections can be applied or implemented more easily and/or in a more sophisticated way.

Recently, two new technologies have been introduced into PET image reconstruction technology. First of all, TOF information can be incorporated in the reconstruction process. By using TOF, the recovery of signal from small lesions, especially when located to larger high-uptake regions, is improved and this technique therefore enhances the detectability of small lesions. Secondly, PET/CT systems suffer from a relatively low resolution. Typically, the spatial resolution of a clinical PET system is about 4–6 mm FWHM. Yet, the PET system's point spread function can be measured and taken into account during the iterative image reconstruction process, the so-called recovery corrected image reconstruction (Brix et al. 1997). There are several terminologies being used for this reconstruction technique, such as resolution recovery, resolution modeling, "high definition," and PVC-OSEM reconstruction. Use of resolution recovery during reconstruction improves the spatial resolution of the reconstructed images, but the quantitative robustness of this technique has not yet been fully validated.

20.3.3 Multimodality Imaging Systems Useful for Clinical Trials

20.3.3.1 PET/CT

Nowadays, most PET systems are combined multimodality PET/CT systems. An excellent overview on PET/CT technology was recently published in the *European Journal of Nuclear Medicine and Molecular Imaging* by Mawlawi and Townsend (2009). To the best knowledge of these authors, there are at present five vendors offering PET/CT systems: Philips Healthcare, Siemens Medical Solutions, Hitachi Medical, Toshiba Medical Corporation, and GE Healthcare. All PET/CT systems have a sequential, but integrated, system design in which the CT scanner is placed in front of the PET part either within one large enclosure or in two separate enclosures, allowing the two systems to be moved apart. The latter may allow for a more easy patient access and/or improve patient comfort (e.g., claustrophobia). The main advantage of combined PET/CT image is the spatial correlation of functional information obtained with PET with the anatomical information collected with CT. The latter allows for more accurate localization of the PET tracer distribution, for example, the localization of PET tracer avid lesions. Yet, an important application for clinical trials may be the (near) simultaneous collection of structural and functional information. Specifically, the use of contrast-enhanced dynamic CT imaging may allow for assessment of (tumor or organ) perfusion, which can then be used in combination with both structural information (from the CT) and functional or metabolic information from the PET. Use of multimodality imaging may thus be helpful to understand to what extent changes in tracer uptake because of therapy may have been caused by changes in perfusion and/or structural changes. Finally, tumor response can now be assessed based on anatomical (tumor size) criteria as indicated by RECIST 1.1, and also on the basis of metabolic responses using PET at the same time (Wahl et al. 2009). In all causes, multimodality imaging may provide a more complete picture of (tumor) response to therapy.

20.3.3.2 PET/MR

At present, the first clinical PET/MRI systems are being built and/or have been installed. There are now PET/MRI systems with different designs: (a) A PET insert placed within the MRI thereby allowing for true simultaneous PET and MR acquisitions, but restricting its application to brain imaging due to the small FOV/gantry opening of the PET insert. (b) A fully integrated whole-body PET/MRI system in which a 3D PET system is fully integrated within the MRI system. (c) A design in which the MRI and PET are placed side by side, that is, in a similar arrangement as used for PET/CT systems. In the latter case, acquisitions will be near but not exact simultaneous, but these systems also allow for whole-body acquisitions. A possible advantage of this setup is that the PET system is distant (about 3–5 m) from the MRI system, thereby avoiding difficulties associated with the sensitivity of conventional PET detectors for the high magnetic fields. In other words, a "regular" state-of-the-art PET system can be used in such a sequential system design. Major challenges for integrated MRI/PET systems are the development of PET detectors that are insensitive to the magnetic field of the MR and, for any PET/MR system, use of MR data for attenuation (and scatter) correction of the PET data. High count rate capable detectors with good timing resolution (required for TOF acquisitions) that are insensitive to the magnetic field may allow for a fully integrated PET/MRI design for which the PET acquisition can be made while applying TOF technology to enhance the image quality. Much progress has been made and reported to address these issues (Pichler et al. 2008). Despite the technical challenges for optimizing PET/MR design and PET image quality and quantification, there may be several promising advantages for PET/MR. First, MR provides images with better soft tissue contrast, thereby enhancing the localization of areas with unusual tracer uptake. Moreover, MR can be used to provide various types of functional information, such as perfusion by use of contrast-enhanced or arterial spin labeling MR, MR spectroscopy to determine presence of specific molecules in tissue, and changes in blood flow by functional MRI.

20.4 Quantitation

PET is a clinical tool and radiological evaluation of PET images is important in clinical trial application. For subject inclusion and evaluation, this may be the most appropriate analysis approach. PET data also has critical spatial, temporal, and specific uptake and binding data and it is often appropriate to use quantitiative analysis.

20.4.1 Pharmacokinetics

The uptake and distribution of the PET ligand in the central blood compartment and side compartments, including the target organ, is called pharmacokinetics. In most PET applications, the tracer is given as an intravenous injection, although it can be given as an intravenous infusion. The ligand rapidly distributes itself in the blood and is taken up generally more slowly into other organs. In the target organ, the uptake is usually described in two phases—(1) extraction and nonspecific distribution into the organ and (2) binding (perhaps after enzymatic conversion). The binding phase can either be clearly reversible—for example, receptor binding—or irreversible—for example, trapping after incorporation.

Pharmacokinetic models for PET data analysis have been developed to address the irreversible and reversible-binding situations. A full kinetic analysis of the PET study might require extensive measurement of both the blood and the organ concentrations of the radiotracer. That requires PET measurement from the time of injection and during the uptake phase, which might take an hour or longer. At the same time, blood, venous, or arterial samples need to be measured. Nonlinear compartmental analysis to compute the kinetic rate constants of all exchange processes is one approach to estimate parameters (Gunn et al. 2001). In clinical trials, it is critical to minimize the patient burden whenever possible and it is often possible to fulfill the study objectives using simpler quantification approaches.

For [F-18]FDG and other irreversible tracers, the multiple time graphical analysis approach of Gjedde (Gjedde et al. 1985) and Patlak (Patlak et al. 1983) allows computation of the metabolic or incorporation rate K_m. This approach is a linearization which permits linear regression to compute the incorporation rate. The standardized uptake value is an even simpler methodology which only requires PET measurement of the organ activity at the end of the uptake phase.

Radiotracers which show reversible binding can best be analyzed by considering the partition between free and bound radiotracer at equilibrium. Although the equilibrium conditions are difficult to achieve in a PET clinical trial, it is possible to use the measured image and blood concentration data to compute the partition ratio. The partition ratio between free and bound is directly related to the affinity (K_d) and the available receptor density (B_{avail}). At least two methods, the simplified reference tissue method (SRTM) and the Logan plot, can be used to analyze PET data from reversible tracers. A standardized nomenclature associated with these concepts has been published (Innis et al. 2007).

20.5 Oncology Imaging

The application of PET in the clinic is most widespread in oncology. The glucose analog tracer [F-18]FDG is avidly metabolized by many tumor types because of their increased metabolism, and also because of changes in the metabolic pathways and transporters. The combination of functional PET and structural CT has allowed clinical imaging and staging of soft tissue tumors and has been a major driver for the expansion of PET technology in the clinic.

20.5.1 Oncology Quantitation

There are several degrees of quantification. To date, the most common method for quantifying tracer (mostly FDG) uptake is the use of standardized uptake values (SUV). This represents uptake in a tumor or organ at a fixed time after tracer administration, corrected for net injected dose of the tracer per patient weight. Limitations of SUV include its dependency on patient preparation, scanning procedure, image reconstruction, and image analysis procedures (Boellaard 2009; Weber 2005). These limitations, however, can to a large extent be overcome by proper standardizing procedures (Boellaard 2009; Boellaard et al. 2010; Shankar et al. 2006).

Apart from SUV, various other more complex and/or accurate quantitative measures can be used for the analysis of FDG-PET studies. Hoekstra et al. (2000, 2002) reviewed and compared various methods for quantifying FDG uptake in nonsmall-cell lung cancer (NSCLC). Nonlinear regression (NLR) of the data using a pharmacokinetic model could be used as gold standard. Yet, Patlak's analysis and various simplified methods, such as the simplified kinetic method (SKM) (Hunter et al. 1996), SUV normalized by body surface area and corrected for glucose (SUVBSAg), and SadatoBSA (Sadato et al. 1998), correlated well with NLR (R2 > 0.95). Lammertsma (Lammertsma et al. 2006) discussed the relationship between these simplified methods and full kinetic analysis for monitoring response to classic cytotoxic medicines. Both authors emphasized that care should be taken in using simplified methods (i.e., SUV-based methods) for evaluation of new medicines.

Potential discrepancies between SUV and full kinetic analysis results may be caused by changes in plasma glucose levels, changes in perfusion, or differences in FDG plasma clearance among scans (Cheebsumon et al. 2011). Therefore, full kinetic approaches are considered most quantitative as they use the entire (measured) arterial input and (tumor or organ) time–activity curves in combination with a tracer kinetic model to derive a more quantitative measure of tracer uptake or binding. However, one of the main limitations of full quantitative studies is the need for a dynamic scanning protocol as it requires information of tracer uptake as a function of time after tracer injection (typically up to 60–90 min or most tracers), thereby limiting the data acquisition to one bed position, that is, a restricted axial field of view or anatomical coverage. In addition, full quantitative kinetic analysis requires an input function, that is, the concentration of the radiotracer in plasma over time. The input function can be measured invasively by taking several or continuous arterial samples during the PET study. The latter procedure is invasive and causes patient discomfort. Therefore, when feasible, use of image-derived input function (IDIF) should be considered. IDIFs may be derived directly from the dynamic PET images in case large blood pool structures, such as the left ventricle or aorta ascendens, are in the field of view of the PET scanner. For some brain studies, an alternative approach is the use of reference tissue kinetic modeling, for which the time course of tracer uptake in a reference region in the brain can be used as input function. Typically, use of reference regions requires the presence of an anatomical region that does not show any specific uptake or binding of the radiotracer. Due to the various limitations of full kinetic analysis, simplified semiquantitative indices are preferred in a clinical setting and thus for larger clinical trials (phase 3), as they allow for whole-body scanning and require less complex scanning and data analysis procedures. On the other hand, they may be less accurate for reasons listed above.

20.6 Brain Imaging

20.6.1 Receptor Occupancy

PET using radiotracers that bind (reversibly) to a neuroreceptor can be used to assess the occupancy of a new drug as function of drug dosage (Figure 20.2). At the same time, it can be used to determine the optimal drug administration or intake schedule. The principle of measuring drug neuroreceptor occupancy is based on receptor availability. Usually, PET studies are performed by administering tracer (picomolar) amounts of a radiopharmaceutical. At these tracers levels, only a few percent of all available neuroreceptors in a brain region are occupied by the radiotracer and nearly 100% of neuroreceptors are freely available for radiotracer binding. Performing a PET study under tracer conditions thus results in highest uptake or (specific) binding of that tracer. Drug receptor occupancy can be measured when drug and radiotracer are binding to the same receptor. By giving a drug at various doses to a subject, different levels of neuroreceptors are occupied by that drug and consequently, the amount of freely available neuroreceptors for radiotracer binding is reduced. As a result, radiotracer uptake or binding measured by PET will be lower at increasing dosages of the drug. By quantifying tracer uptake or specific binding at various drug dosage levels, it is possible to determine the percentage neuroreceptor occupancy by that drug. For example, for an antagonist, when the PET signal is 50% of that measured under tracer conditions, 50% of the neuroreceptors are occupied by the drug. A drug-receptor occupancy of about 50–80% is usually considered to provide a (sufficient possible) therapeutic effect. Likewise, by making several PET studies after administration of a drug, the neuroreceptor occupancy by the drug can be measured as function of the postinjection time interval, which provides useful information for optimizing the drug dosage scheduling.

20.6.2 Amyloid Imaging

In the past decade, various tracers have been developed that bind to amyloid in the brain. Amyloid is a protein that accumulates in the brain of Alzheimer's disease (AD) patients. Already before clinical symptoms are present, increased levels of amyloid may be present in the brain. PET is a very sensitive technique that can detect the presence of amyloid in the brain at very low levels (Figure 20.3). Amyloid imaging by PET may thus be helpful for early identification of subjects with increasing levels of amyloid

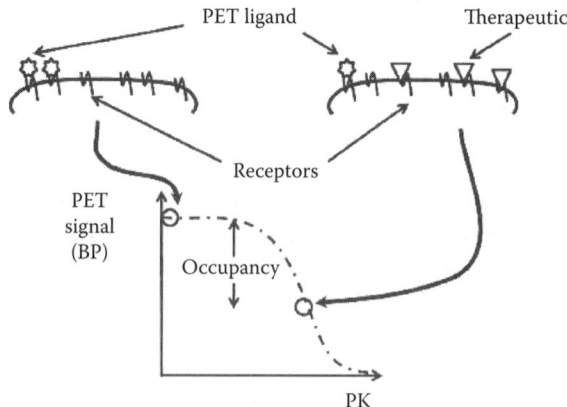

FIGURE 20.2 Receptor occupancy. Upper left shows a cell membrane with receptors crossing it. The PET ligand (stars) occupies the receptors in proportion to their availability. On the upper right, as the receptors are occupied by pharmaceutical (triangles), the PET ligand concentration reduces in proportion. The two conditions are plotted on a binding potential versus pharmaceutical concentration (PK) curve at the bottom. The receptor occupancy is the proportional change in binding potential.

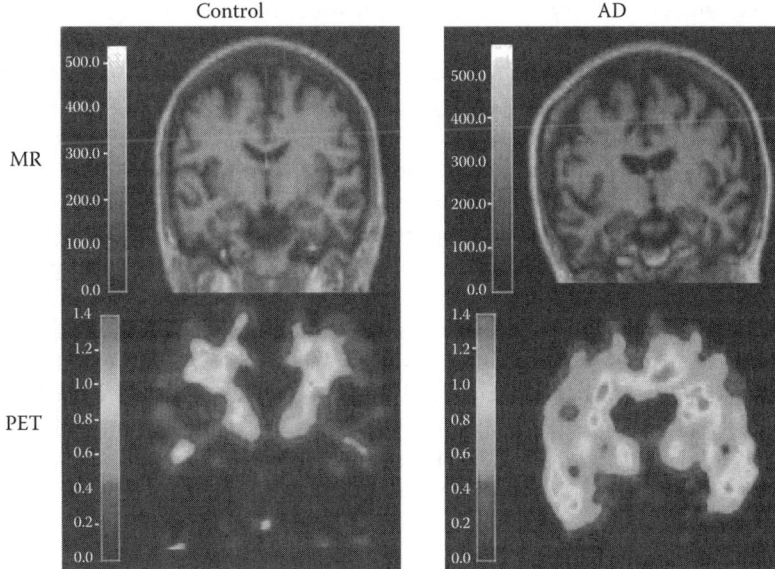

FIGURE 20.3 MRI (top row) and PET tracer-binding images obtained with the amyloid tracers [11C]-PIB (bottom) row for a healthy control (first column) and AD patient (second column). A clear increase in tracer binding is seen in the AD subject compared to the healthy control.

in their brain, even before they show symptoms of dementia. Moreover, amyloid accumulation is characteristic for AD and PET can thus be supportive for improved differential diagnosis. Identification of Alzheimer's disease patients early in the disease spectrum is very important for clinical trials. Amyloid PET imaging could be used as an inclusion criterion in order to correctly identify AD subject eligible for trial participation. At present, the first response assessment studies using changes in PET tracer amyloid binding as index for drug efficacy are ongoing.

20.7 Cardiac PET

PET has been used in cardiology since the late 1970s, with its main application in the measurement of myocardial blood flow (MBF) and viability, but it has also been used extensively in basic research in the area of myocardial substrate metabolism. Since molecular cardiac imaging with PET is aimed at diagnosis at the earliest stage of disease, its use can be valuable in drug development. It provides well-defined end-points for clinical trials, for example, when measuring myocardial efficiency after therapies for heart failure or when imaging the effects of metabolic interventions (Bengel et al. 2009).

The advantage of using PET to measure MBF compared to other methods is that MBF can not only be visualized but also quantified, giving absolute MBF values in ml blood per gram tissue per minute. Several different tracers have been suggested for measuring MBF with PET, of which ^{13}N-ammonia, ^{82}Rb (rubidium), and ^{15}O-water have been used most widely. ^{15}O-Water is considered the gold standard for flow measurements because it is freely diffusible, metabolically inert, and has a 100% extraction. The extraction of ^{13}N-ammonia and ^{82}Rb is flow dependent and decreases for high flow levels. ^{13}N-Ammonia and ^{15}O-water require the presence of an onsite cyclotron because of the 9 and 2 min half-lives of both tracers, whereas ^{82}Rb is generator produced and hence more easily available where it has been approved for clinical use. ^{13}N-Ammonia and ^{82}Rb can give qualitative images showing the distribution of flow over the myocardium, whereas this is not possible with ^{15}O-water. Recent developments in scanner technology and image processing methods, however, have also enabled generation of quantitative MBF images with ^{15}O-water, showing MBF at the voxel level (Harms et al. 2011).

All of these three tracers have a very short radioactive half-life, but a number of promising F-18-labeled tracers are currently under development. One of these is ^{18}F-BMS747158, a novel pyridaven derivative which has a first-pass extraction of 94% and a myocardial uptake that is proportional to MBF up to high flow values (Nekolla et al. 2009). This compound is currently being tested in clinical studies and may allow for a more widespread use of MBF imaging with PET. The introduction of integrated PET-CT scanners allows for acquisition of functional data, CT angiography, and calcium score within a single session with quantitative MBF PET imaging (Knaapen et al. 2010).

FDG is considered the gold standard for imaging myocardial viability, with viable areas showing a mismatch with reduced MBF but normal FDG. Another marker of myocardial viability is the perfusable tissue index (PTI), measured using ^{15}O-water in the same procedure as MBF (Iida et al. 1995). Oxygen gas labeled with ^{15}O, as well as ^{11}C-acetate, can provide quantitative measures of myocardial oxygen consumption. ^{11}C-Palmitate can be used to measure fatty acid metabolism (Schelbert et al. 1986). Myocardial sympathetic innervation has been assessed with ^{11}C-hydroxyephidrine (HED) (Schäfers et al. 1998). A mismatch between MBF and HED retention is thought to be a predictor of ventricular arrhythmia in patients with previous heart failure. Recently, there has been an increased interest in the development of imaging markers for aortic aneurisms and especially vulnerable plaques before rupture.

20.8 Other Therapeutic Areas

20.8.1 Use of [F-18]FDG in Inflammatory Disease

The most common PET tracer, [F-18]FDG is used to measure the metabolism through the glucose pathway. Utilization of glucose for cellular energy metabolism means that this signal can be found in many cells and depends not only on the energy metabolism rate, but also on the density of cells. In brain, for example, a reduced [F-18]FDG uptake in a certain area of the brain can be indicative of either reduced glucose metabolism (e.g., due to a reduction in neuronal activity) or a loss of neurons, depending on the circumstances. In inflammation, the invasion of tissues by neutrophils increases the density (cells per unit volume) of high-energy-demand cells. This results in a strong PET signal which can be used as a marker of inflammation, for example, in COPD (Schuster 2007) and gastrointestinal disorders (Jacene et al. 2009).

20.8.2 Other Tracers for Inflammatory Disease

Joint inflammation is a complex process, which can be studied using functional markers. Leucocytes labeled with Tc-99m outside the body and reinjected to concentrate at the site of inflammation are a standard technique in nuclear medicine with SPECT (Basu et al. 2009). Because of the shorter half-life of the common PET isotopes, which is much shorter than the distribution time of labeled cells, this technique has not translated well to the PET technology. Tracers (Gotthardt et al. 2010; van der Bruggen et al. 2010) such as Ga-67-citrate have been used to study inflammation through perfusion changes. In the future, Ga-68-labeled peptides may provide a means for distribution of highly specific ligands to enable study of inflammatory pathways with PET (Rizzello et al. 2009). Gastrointestinal imaging with SPECT using Tc-99m and In-111 is well established (Wilding et al. 2001). These techniques have been used to study gastric emptying and gut motility.

20.9 Qualification of PET as a Biomarker

Processes and methods for qualification of imaging and other biomarkers are an area of current active development. Health authorities have an active interest in advancing new imaging tools that will allow testing of safe and effective medicines at all stages in development (Goodsaid and Mendrick 2010). Imaging biomarkers that are being used to understand pathway and receptor interactions can aid in advancing the basic science of programs and can be enabling tools to discover new targets to advance treatments for unmet medical needs.

20.9.1 Qualification of PET as Fit-for-Purpose

In qualifying a biomarker, the specific context and purpose of use have to be defined clearly. For example, use of PET imaging to monitor treatment-related change in a clinical study will have to be considered differently from a screening tool to select patients with rapidly progressing disease for inclusion in trials of neuroprotective agents. Both the FDA in the United States and the EMA in Europe are engaged in biomarker qualification initiatives and have invited interested parties to submit dossiers outlining potential biomarkers to be qualified for application. For PET imaging biomarkers, it will be critical to establish the technical validation of the instrument, outlining the minimum standards required to ensure instrument calibration. The performance of the specific PET tracer will also be important; What is the target? How is this related to the disease, pathology, or target? The promise of the validation process is that, having established a marker for a particular purpose with the health authority, a user can be confident that the health authority will accept the marker for this purpose. In this way, PET imaging biomarker investment can be derisked.

20.9.2 Using PET as a Surrogate Biomarker

In order to develop surrogate biomarker tools for late-stage development, we need to establish the linkage (Frank and Hargreaves 2003) between the signal and the disease outcome further, the change in signal under effective treatments needs to be established and correlated with outcome. This is a big hurdle. The number of PET techniques which can be considered to be surrogate markers is very limited. Some examples of previous use in this context are the use of F-18-FDOPA to measure dopaminergic neurodegeneration in Parkinson's disease (Oertel et al. 2006) and the use of F-18-FDG in Lymphoma oncology trials (Kelloff et al. 2007).

20.10 Antibody Imaging

There has been a large advance in the design of medicines targeting molecular targets on tumor cells, such as those involved in proliferation, differentiation, apoptosis, angiogenesis, and so on. Monoclonal antibodies (MAbs) form the largest category of targeted medicines. Targeted therapies are challenging to develop and will generally be beneficial to a subgroup of patients, depending, for example, on overexpression of the target and variability and heterogeneity of tumor uptake. The efficacy of a targeted medicine in an individual patient has to be evaluated by assessing its uptake in tumor and normal tissue during a scouting procedure prior to start of therapy or immediately upon onset of therapy to avoid unnecessary expensive treatments and delayed onset of effective treatment. Response, however, as addressed using RECIST criteria is usually not visible during earlier stages of therapy, and even the use of FDG-PET for response monitoring requires one or two cycles of therapy before efficacy can be evaluated.

Labeling of the targeted pharmaceutical with a positron-emitting nuclide, however, may provide a predictor of treatment efficacy even before the onset of therapy. Quantitative PET can image the distribution of the pharmaceutical both prior to and during therapy. Since the radioactive half-lives of the most common PET isotopes F-18 and C-11 are too short to measure the kinetics of MAbs, isotopes with longer half-lives such as I-124 (100 h) and Zr-89 (78 h) have been used for labeling MAbs. Methods for large-scale production of highly pure Zr-89 and I-24I, and for facile and stabling coupling of these isotopes with MAbs, have been developed (Perk et al. 2010; Vosjan et al. 2010, 2011), and the radioactive half-life of Zr-89 and I-124 allows for their worldwide supply.

A microdosing PET study with a labeled targeted medicine can be used to understand the biodistribution and target engagement before starting the treatment. This, of course, assumes that target organ distribution of the pharmaceutical is a good predictor for treatment efficacy, and that a tracer study is representative of the uptake of the medicine at efficacious concentrations. In pharmaceutical development, quantitative imaging of labeled-targeted pharmaceuticals with PET can provide information on optimal dosage, uptake in critical organs, and interpatient variations in kinetics and targeting. Pharmaceutical imaging provides this information in an efficient and safe way, with fewer patients treated at suboptimal doses. This approach is especially attractive when the pharmaceutical of interest is directed against a novel tumor target that has not been previously validated. Thus, use of labeled pharmaceuticals allows for early selection of promising pharmaceutical candidates and reduction of development costs.

20.11 Precompetitive Consortia

Health authorities have recognized (Altar 2008; Hunter 2008; Kamel et al. 2008; Woodcock 2009) the need to advance imaging and other biomarkers as decision-making tools in pharmaceutical development and a number of interconnected public–private consortia partnerships have been established in order to tackle these issues. The Innovative Medicines Initiative (IMI) is a partnership between European Pharmaceutical Industry partners represented by EFPIA and the European Union. Two of the current projects involve molecular imaging: IMIDIA which is studying Beta-cell demise in diabetes and NEWMEDS which is developing novel biomarkers for psychiatry. The Foundation of the National Institutes of Health Biomarkers Consortium has a broad stakeholder base of for-profit and nonprofit organizations, including the health agency and the pharmaceutical industry. The FNIH biomarkers consortium has identified multiple projects with a molecular imaging component: I-SPY 2 studying personalized medicine in oncology; ADNI developing imaging biomarkers, including amyloid imaging for Alzheimer's disease; and OAI, which has studied imaging technologies in osteoarthritis.

This is an opportunity to bring academic and industry scientists closer, where there is potential impact of a new technology on pharmaceutical development. The framework for these consortia provides a practical way to work on precompetitive projects and share resources and expertise.

One area which is perhaps underutilized in the current consortia is the development of novel radiopharmaceuticals for all disease areas. Although there are focused and fruitful efforts within specific consortia, this is such a critical area in molecular medicine with specific challenges on intellectual property and licensing that it is in need of a focused consortium activity.

20.12 Future Outlook

PET will continue to be a valuable tool to understand the *in vivo* action of pharmaceuticals on target, mechanisms, and disease outcomes. The contribution of PET imaging in oncology and neurology will continue and the use in decision making in clinical trials will be even clearer and more refined. At the same time, there is scope to consider how to develop PET agents and techniques as readouts that can be used in personalized medicine paradigms to select the treatments most appropriate for specific patients and to monitor the treatment efficacy. The use of PET technology in other disease areas and organ systems is gaining ground. Focused broad scientific understanding of the specific contributions PET can bring in decision making is critical to ensuring that the method is used efficiently.

Rapid development and characterization of specific radiotracers for target engagement are one area which would benefit from new methods and clear selection process, for example, high specific activity ligand synthesis techniques and microfluidic systems may improve radiochemical process yields. However, early *in vitro* test systems and screening tools to quickly identify the *in vivo* clinical performance of PET ligands would be an important step.

Further interdisciplinary integration of research and development of PET for clinical trials across disciplines combined with standardization of instrumentation and methods will increase future efficient application. Precompetitive consortia will allow academic and industry collaboration to develop an appropriate set of tools and to establish the validation of those methods for clinical trial application.

The application of PET in clinical trials has reached a stage of maturity that will now allow more refined early-development trial designs. This will enable the next generation of treatments to be selected and advanced in clinical development.

References

Altar, C.A. 2008. The Biomarkers Consortium: On the critical path of drug discovery. *Clin. Pharmacol. Ther.*, 83, (2) 361–364. Available from: PM:18183037.

Basu, S., Zhuang, H., Torigian, D.A., Rosenbaum, J., Chen, W., and Alavi, A. 2009. Functional imaging of inflammatory diseases using nuclear medicine techniques. *Semin. Nucl. Med.*, 39, (2) 124–145. Available from: PM:19187805.

Bengel, F.M., Higuchi, T., Javadi, M.S., and Lautamaki, R. 2009. Cardiac positron emission tomography. *J. Am. Coll. Cardiol.*, 54, (1) 1–15. Available from: PM:19555834.

Boellaard, R. 2009. Standards for PET image acquisition and quantitative data analysis. *J. Nucl. Med.*, 50 Suppl 1, 11S–20S. Available from: PM:19380405.

Boellaard, R., O'Doherty, M.J., Weber, W.A., Mottaghy, F.M., Lonsdale, M.N., Stroobants, S.G., Oyen, W.J. et al. 2010. FDG PET and PET/CT: EANM procedure guidelines for tumour PET imaging: Version 1.0. *Eur. J. Nucl. Med. Mol. Imaging*, 37, (1) 181–200. Available from: PM:19915839.

Brix, G., Doll, J., Bellemann, M.E., Trojan, H., Haberkorn, U., Schmidlin, P., and Ostertag, H. 1997. Use of scanner characteristics in iterative image reconstruction for high-resolution positron emission tomography studies of small animals. *Eur. J. Nucl. Med.*, 24, (7) 779–786. Available from: PM:9211765.

Cheebsumon, P., Velasquez, L.M., Hoekstra, C.J., Hayes, W., Kloet, R.W., Hoetjes, N.J., Smit, E.F., Hoekstra, O.S., Lammertsma, A.A., and Boellaard, R. 2011. Measuring response to therapy using FDG PET: Semi-quantitative and full kinetic analysis. *Eur. J. Nucl. Med. Mol. Imaging.*, 38, (5) 832–842. Available from: PM:21210109.

Frank, R. and Hargreaves, R. 2003. Clinical biomarkers in drug discovery and development. *Nat. Rev. Drug Discov.*, 2, (7) 566–580. Available from: PM:12838269.

Gjedde, A., Wienhard, K., Heiss, W.D., Kloster, G., Diemer, N.H., Herholz, K., and Pawlik, G. 1985. Comparative regional analysis of 2-fluorodeoxyglucose and methylglucose uptake in brain of four stroke patients. With special reference to the regional estimation of the lumped constant. *J. Cereb. Blood Flow Metab.*, 5, (2) 163–178. Available from: PM:3872872.

Goodsaid, F.M. and Mendrick, D.L. 2010. Translational medicine and the value of biomarker qualification. *Sci. Transl. Med.*, 2, (47) 47–44. Available from: PM:20811041.

Gotthardt, M., Bleeker-Rovers, C.P., Boerman, O.C., and Oyen, W.J. 2010. Imaging of inflammation by PET, conventional scintigraphy, and other imaging techniques. *J. Nucl. Med.*, 51, (12) 1937–1949. Available from: PM:21078798.

Gunn, R.N., Gunn, S.R., and Cunningham, V.J. 2001. Positron emission tomography compartmental models. *J. Cereb. Blood Flow Metab.*, 21, (6) 635–652. Available from: PM:11488533.

Harms, H.J., Knaapen, P., de, H.S., Halbmeijer, R., Lammertsma, A.A., and Lubberink, M. 2011. Automatic generation of absolute myocardial blood flow images using [(15)O]H (2)O and a clinical PET/CT scanner. *Eur. J. Nucl. Med. Mol. Imaging*, 38, (5) 930–939. Available from: PM:21271246.

Hoekstra, C.J., Hoekstra, O.S., Stroobants, S.G., Vansteenkiste, J., Nuyts, J., Smit, E.F., Boers, M., Twisk, J.W.R., and Lammertsma, A.A. 2002. Methods to monitor response to chemotherapy in non-small cell lung cancer with F-18-FDG PET. *J. Nucl. Med.*, 43, (10) 1304–1309. Available from: ISI:000178393900011.

Hoekstra, C.J., Paglianiti, I., Hoekstra, O.S., Smit, E.F., Postmus, P.E., Teule, G.J.J., and Lammertsma, A.A. 2000. Monitoring response to therapy in cancer using [F-18]-2-fluouo-2-deoxy-D-glucose and positron emission tomography: An overview of different analytical methods. *Eur. J. Nucl. Med.*, 27, (6) 731–743. Available from: ISI:000087883200017.

Hudson, H.M. and Larkin, R.S. 1994. Accelerated image reconstruction using ordered subsets of projection data. *IEEE Trans. Med. Imaging*, 13, (4) 601–609. Available from: PM:18218538.

Hunter, A.J. 2008. The Innovative Medicines Initiative: A pre-competitive initiative to enhance the biomedical science base of Europe to expedite the development of new medicines for patients. *Drug Discov. Today.*, 13, (9–10) 371–373. Available from: PM:18468553.

Hunter, G.J., Hamberg, L.M., Alpert, N.M., Choi, N.C., and Fischman, A.J. 1996. Simplified measurement of deoxyglucose utilization rate. *J. Nucl. Med.*, 37, (6) 950–955. Available from: PM:8683318.

Iida, H., Takahashi, A., Tamura, Y., Ono, Y., and Lammertsma, A.A. 1995. Myocardial blood flow: Comparison of oxygen-15-water bolus injection, slow infusion and oxygen-15-carbon dioxide slow inhalation. *J. Nucl. Med.*, 36, (1) 78–85. Available from: PM:7799088.

Innis, R.B., Cunningham, V.J., Delforge, J., Fujita, M., Gjedde, A., Gunn, R.N., Holden, J. et al. 2007. Consensus nomenclature for *in vivo* imaging of reversibly binding radioligands. *J. Cereb. Blood Flow Metab.*, 27, (9) 1533–1539. Available from: PM:17519979.

Jacene, H.A., Ginsburg, P., Kwon, J., Nguyen, G.C., Montgomery, E.A., Bayless, T.M., and Wahl, R.L. 2009. Prediction of the need for surgical intervention in obstructive Crohn's disease by 18F-FDG PET/CT. *J. Nucl. Med.*, 50, (11) 1751–1759. Available from: PM:19837758.

Kamel, N., Compton, C., Middelveld, R., Higenbottam, T., and Dahlen, S.E. 2008. The Innovative Medicines Initiative (IMI): A new opportunity for scientific collaboration between academia and industry at the European level. *Eur. Respir. J.*, 31, (5) 924–926. Available from: PM:18448501.

Kelloff, G.J., Sullivan, D.M., Wilson, W., Cheson, B., Juweid, M., Mills, G.Q., Zelenetz, A.D. et al. 2007. FDG-PET lymphoma demonstration project invitational workshop. *Acad. Radiol.*, 14, (3) 330–339. Available from: PM:17307666.

Knaapen, P., de Haan, S., Hoekstra, O.S., Halbmeijer, R., Appelman, Y.E., Groothuis, J.G., Comans, E.F. et al. 2010. Cardiac PET-CT: Advanced hybrid imaging for the detection of coronary artery disease. *Neth. Heart J.*, 8, (2) 90-8. PubMed PMID: 20200615; PubMed Central PMCID: PMC2828569.

Lammertsma, A.A., Hoekstra, C.J., Giaccone, G., and Hoekstra, O.S. 2006. How should we analyse FDG PET studies for monitoring tumour response?. *Eur. J. Nucl. Med. Mol. Imaging.*, 33 Suppl 1, 16–21. Available from: PM:16763817.

Mawlawi, O. and Townsend, D.W. 2009. Multimodality imaging: An update on PET/CT technology. *Eur. J. Nucl. Med. Mol. Imaging.*, 36 Suppl 1, S15–S29. Available from: PM:19104808.

Nekolla, S.G., Reder, S., Saraste, A., Higuchi, T., Dzewas, G., Preissel, A., Huisman, M. et al. 2009. Evaluation of the novel myocardial perfusion positron-emission tomography tracer 18F-BMS-747158-02: Comparison to 13N-ammonia and validation with microspheres in a pig model. *Circulation*, 119, (17) 2333–2342. Epub 2009 Apr 20. PubMed PMID: 19380625.

Oertel, W.H., Wolters, E., Sampaio, C., Gimenez-Roldan, S., Bergamasco, B., Dujardin, M., Grosset, D.G. et al. 2006. Pergolide versus levodopa monotherapy in early Parkinson's disease patients: The PELMOPET study. *Mov. Disord.*, 21, (3) 343–353. Available from: PM:16211594.

Patlak, C.S., Blasberg, R.G., and Fenstermacher, J.D. 1983. Graphical evaluation of blood-to-brain transfer constants from multiple-time uptake data. *J. Cereb. Blood Flow Metab.*, 3, (1) 1–7. Available from: PM:6822610.

Perk, L.R., Vosjan, M.J., Visser, G.W., Budde, M., Jurek, P., Kiefer, G.E., and van Dongen, G.A. 2010. p-Isothiocyanatobenzyl-desferrioxamine: A new bifunctional chelate for facile radiolabeling of monoclonal antibodies with zirconium-89 for immuno-PET imaging. *Eur. J. Nucl. Med. Mol. Imaging.*, 37, (2) 250–259. Available from: PM:19763566.

Pichler, B.J., Judenhofer, M.S., and Wehrl, H.F. 2008. PET/MRI hybrid imaging: Devices and initial results. *Eur. Radiol.*, 18, (6) 1077–1086. Available from: PM:18357456.

Rizzello, A., Di, P.D., Lodi, F., Trespidi, S., Cicoria, G., Pancaldi, D., Nanni, C. et al. 2009. Synthesis and quality control of 68Ga citrate for routine clinical PET. *Nucl. Med. Commun.*, 30, (7) 542–545. Available from: PM:19424101.

Sadato, N., Tsuchida, T., Nakaumra, S., Waki, A., Uematsu, H., Takahashi, N., Hayashi, N., Yonekura, Y., and Ishii, Y. 1998. Non-invasive estimation of the net influx constant using the standardized uptake value for quantification of FDG uptake of tumours. *Eur. J. Nucl. Med.*, 25, (6) 559–564. Available from: PM:9618569.

Schäfers, M., Lerch, H., Wichter, T., Rhodes, C.G., Lammertsma, A.A., Borggrefe, M., Hermansen, F., Schober, O., Breithardt, G., Camici, P.G. 1998. Cardiac sympathetic innervation in patients with idiopathic right ventricular outflow tract tachycardia. *J. Am. Coll. Cardiol.*, 32, (1) 181–186. PubMed PMID: 9669268.

Schelbert, H.R., Henze, E., Sochor, H., Grossman, R.G., Huang, S.C., Barrio, J.R., Schwaiger, M., Phelps, M.E. 1986. Effects of substrate availability on myocardial C-11 palmitate kinetics by positron emission tomography in normal subjects and patients with ventricular dysfunction. *Am. Heart J.*, 111, (6) 1055–1064. PubMed PMID: 3487240.

Schuster, D.P. 2007. The opportunities and challenges of developing imaging biomarkers to study lung function and disease. *Am. J. Respir. Crit Care Med.*, 176, (3) 224–230. Available from: PM:17478617.

Shankar, L.K., Hoffman, J.M., Bacharach, S., Graham, M.M., Karp, J., Lammertsma, A.A., Larson, S., Mankoff, D.A., Siegel, B.A., den Abbeele, A., Yap, J., and Sullivan, D. 2006. Consensus recommendations for the use of F-18-FDG PET as an indicator of therapeutic response in patients in national cancer institute trials. *J. Nucl. Med.*, 47, (6) 1059–1066. Available from: ISI:000238104800028.

Shepp, L.A. and Vardi, Y. 1982. Maximum likelihood reconstruction for emission tomography. *IEEE Trans. Med. Imaging.*, 1, (2) 113–122. Available from: PM:18238264.

Sureshbabu, W., and Mawlawi, O. 2005. PET/CT imaging artifacts. *J. Nucl. Med. Technol.*, 33, (3) 156–161. Available from: PM:16145223.

Townsend, D.W. 2004. Physical principles and technology of clinical PET imaging. *Ann. Acad. Med. Singapore.*, 33, (2) 133–145. Available from: PM:15098626.

van der Bruggen, W., Bleeker-Rovers, C.P., Boerman, O.C., Gotthardt, M., and Oyen, W.J. 2010. PET and SPECT in osteomyelitis and prosthetic bone and joint infections: A systematic review. *Semin. Nucl. Med.*, 40, (1) 3–15. Available from: PM:19958846.

Vosjan, M.J., Perk, L.R., Roovers, R.C., Visser, G.W., Stigter-van, W.M., van Bergen En Henegouwen, P.M., and van Dongen, G.A. 2011. Facile labelling of an anti-epidermal growth factor receptor Nanobody with 68Ga via a novel bifunctional desferal chelate for immuno-PET. *Eur. J. Nucl. Med. Mol. Imaging.*, 38, (4) 753–763. Available from: PM:21210114.

Vosjan, M.J., Perk, L.R., Visser, G.W., Budde, M., Jurek, P., Kiefer, G.E., and van Dongen, G.A. 2010. Conjugation and radiolabeling of monoclonal antibodies with zirconium-89 for PET imaging using the bifunctional chelate p-isothiocyanatobenzyl-desferrioxamine. *Nat. Protoc.*, 5, (4) 739–743. Available from: PM:20360768.

Wahl, R.L., Jacene, H., Kasamon, Y., and Lodge, M.A. 2009. From RECIST to PERCIST: Evolving Considerations for PET response criteria in solid tumors. *J. Nucl. Med.*, 50 Suppl 1, 122S-150S. Available from: PM:19403881.

Watson, C.C. 2000. New, faster, image-based scatter correction for 3D PET. *IEEE Trans. Nucl. Sci.*, 47, (4) 1587–1594. Available from: ISI:000089576400009.

Weber, W.A. 2005. PET for response assessment in oncology: Radiotherapy and chemotherapy. *Br. J. Radiol.*, 78, 42–49. Available from: ISI:000234894100006.

Wilding, I.R., Coupe, A.J., and Davis, S.S. 2001. The role of gamma-scintigraphy in oral drug delivery. *Adv. Drug Deliv. Rev.*, 46, (1–3) 103–124. Available from: PM:11259836.

Woodcock, J. 2009. Chutes and ladders on the critical path: Comparative effectiveness, product value, and the use of biomarkers in drug development. *Clin. Pharmacol. Ther.*, 86, (1) 12–14. Available from: PM:19536116.

21

Medical Image Search

Thomas Deserno
Aachen University

21.1 Introduction

The search for images is a well-known problem to all of us using digital cameras: while image data is usually ordered on your hard disk by trips, events, or dates (alphanumerical metainformation), you rather remember a certain landscape, scene, or person shown in an image (pattern and content). In this chapter, we will explore the state of the art in medical image search by image content. While image mining denotes the analysis of (often large) observational data sets in order to find unsuspected relationships and to summarize the data in ways that are better understandable to human observers (Hand et al. 2001), content-based image retrieval (CBIR) or content-based visual image retrieval (CBVIR) aims at searching image databases for specific images that are similar to a given query image (Smeulders et al. 2000, Müller and Deserno 2011).

21.1.1 Relevance of Images

Images are the main carriers of information as processed in the human brain. It has been estimated that more than 90% of experience and knowledge of humans are learned via visual perception. This may also explain that best-working mnemonics are those where the numbers or words to remember are mapped to images, and their order is learned by composing a story as a virtual moving picture. For many of us,

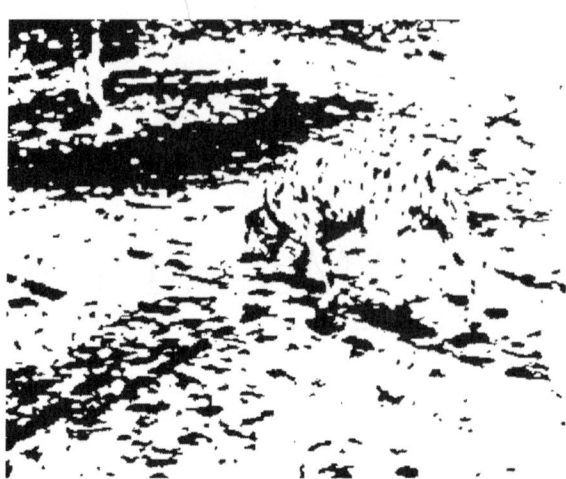

FIGURE 21.1   Image pattern. (From Gordon IE. *Theories of Visual Perception*. 1989. Copyright Wiley-VCH Verlag GmbH & Co. KGaA.)

a face is recognized much easier than a name, although the visual pattern is by far more complex than a couple of letters.

In the beginning of the twentieth century, scientists discovered the steps of image pattern reception and perception in the human brain. According to the Gestalt theory (Wertheimer 1925), edges and color/texture information are extracted locally, and image components are formed, grouped, and recognized with access to the mind and its memory. Two of the gestalt paradigms are worth mentioning:

- *Emergence* is the process of complex pattern formation from simpler rules. However, objects are recognized as a whole, and not by parts. For example, Figure 21.1 depicts a Dalmatian dog sniffing the ground in the shade of overhanging trees. The dog is perceived as a whole, all at once, and is not recognized by first identifying its parts (feet, ears, nose, tail, etc.), and then inferring the dog from those component parts.
- *Reification* is the constructive or generative aspect of perception, by which the experienced percept contains more explicit spatial information than the sensory stimulus on which it is based. Again referring to the dog in Figure 21.1, the dog's shape is clearly seen as closed contour, although several parts of this imaginary line are not present in the image at all. Obviously, illusory contours are composed and treated by the human visual system as real contours.

Since then, computer vision aims at finding algorithms for segmentation and pattern recognition that are capable of performing like humans. When referring to Figure 21.1, a human may immediately recognize the "dog" or "Dalmatian" on a conceptual level, while today's computer programs are far away from responding to such words when fed by the binary pattern of Figure 21.1.

21.1.2 Relevance of Medical Images

Starting with the discovery of x-rays by Wilhelm Conrad Röntgen in 1896, images have been established in the medical domain as the main resource of diagnostics, therapy planning, and intervention. In the first part of this book, the most relevant imaging modalities have been described, such as radiography (plain x-ray imaging), computed tomography (CT), magnetic resonance imaging (MRI), positron emission tomography (PET), single photon emission computed tomography (SPECT), and ultrasound

(US). Furthermore, optical imaging as used in endoscopy and microscopy is frequently applied in medicine.

Nowadays, almost all of these imaging modalities are operated direct digitally. Picture archiving and communication systems (PACS) are installed in a hospital to manage (store, retrieve, and communicate) the image information. Easily, several terabytes of pixel data are acquired in a hospital each year (Müller and Deserno 2011). And again, however, this huge amount of data is managed solely by alphanumerical metainformation such as the patient's name, the date of exposure, or additional study information. The same holds for the radiologists reading images. He reports a diagnosis in natural language, which is coded additionally, for instance, using the international classification of diseases (ICD) nomenclature as nonvisual, that is, textual metainformation.

21.1.3 Idea of Content-Based Image Retrieval

Contrarily, CBIR aims at managing images by pattern and retrieving images from an (PACS) archive by means of visual similarity rather than comparing the alphanumerical metainformation. The advantages of this paradigm arise directly from the limitations of describing pictures by words. The saying "A picture is worth a thousand words" depicts the inherent incompleteness of any natural language description of an image—a problem well known in the medical field too.

Hence, any system for content-based image data mining usually is composed of the following four steps:

- *Feature extraction*: based on the image pattern, numerical features, which are also referred to as signature, are extracted. The features may describe color, texture, and shape of the entire image or image parts. They are stored separately to the image in a feature database.
- *Similarity computation*: According to the signature, appropriate similarity measures are defined to quantify the visual distance of two images or image patterns.
- *Signature indexing*: Assuming a large number of images hosted in the archive, processing a request requires many feature comparisons. Hence, the feature vectors are indexed to speed up the response time of the CBIR system.
- *Image retrieval*: On time of retrieval, a pattern is presented to the system, and its signature is extracted and compared to those indexed in the CBIR archive. According to the most similar signatures, the corresponding set of response images is presented to the user.

In this chapter, we focus on medical image search by means of CBIR. We will briefly discover the history of medical and nonmedical CBIR techniques and discuss its potential in medical use in general regarding diagnostics, research, and medical teaching. In Section 21.4, we explore the engineering fields in medical CBIR, and a state of the art of all important techniques is given in Section 21.5. As an example, three outstanding systems and ideas of medical CBIR applications are presented in Section 21.6, before we conclude this chapter with a prospective view on future developments.

21.2 History of CBIR

The emerging development of the World Wide Web holding millions of images has majorly influenced the development of visual image retrieval technologies. The first CBIR systems had already been discussed in the early 1980s (Chang and Kunii 1981). Hence, this section briefly reports on the nonmedical CBIR systems and discusses the fundamental differences when retrieving medical imaging data by content. A more comprehensive review on nonmedical CBIR approaches is given by Smeulders et al. (2000).

21.2.1 Nonmedical CBIR

In the early 1990s, the query by image content (QBIC) system of IBM was one of the first approaches to CBIR (Niblack et al. 1993). The QBIC signature is composed of color, texture, and edge orientation. In particular, the three-dimensional (3D) average color vector of an object or the whole image is computed. The texture features used in QBIC are modified versions of the coarseness, contrast, and directionality, as they have been proposed by Tamura et al. (1978). The shape features consist of shape area, circularity, eccentricity, major axis orientation, and a set of algebraic moment invariants. They are based on a reduced binary map of edge points, which is obtained applying a Canny edge detector to the gray-scale image (Canny 1986).

The query by image example (QBE) paradigm has also been proposed by the authors. QBIC allows queries based on (i) example images, (ii) user-constructed sketches, and (iii) color and texture patterns selected from a sampler. In the latter cases, the percentage of a desired color in the QBE is adjusted manually by moving sliders.

Since color has been identified as most relevant structure for CBIR, the *semantic gap* has been recognized within the first approaches to CBIR systems. It describes the differences between image similarity on the high level of human perception, which is based on emergence and reification (cf. Section 21.1.1), and on the low level of a few numerical numbers describing a mean color. Accordingly, first approaches to bridge the semantic gap are based on local image signatures.

The Blobworld system was one of the first CBIR systems that applied a local concept of image representation (Belongie et al. 1998, Carson et al. 2002). Again, color, texture, and edge features were extracted from the images. Then, the expectation-maximization (EM) algorithm was applied for clustering the feature space. The image pixel coordinates were added to the feature space representing the local connectedness. Prominent regions were described by best-fitting Gaussians and visualized with ellipses, which have been called "blobs" (Figure 21.2).

Proving its value for image search, nonmedical CBIR systems have already been commercialized. For instance, MICHELscope identifies stamps using CBIR technology (Siggelkow 2002). The first edition of the software product was released in 2002. At that time, it was based on a reference dataset of 12,000 scanned stamps from Germany. Nowadays, commercial CBIR products are also available for paintings, industrial components, textile patterns, and catalogs in general.

21.2.2 Differences to Medical Images

Images from the Internet or large sets of photographs or scans (e.g., stamps) are rather unstructured image collections, usually containing color as a most discriminate feature and usually differing significantly in

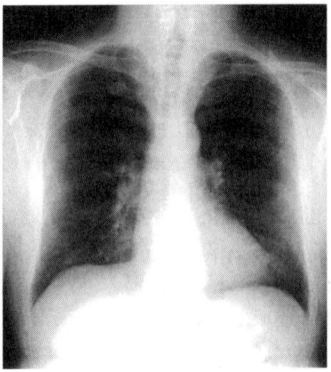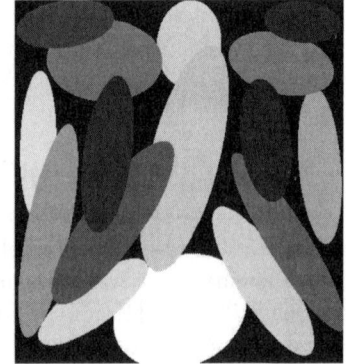

FIGURE 21.2 Blob representation of a chest radiograph. (From Greenspan H and Pinhas AT. *IEEE Trans Inf Technol Biomed.* 11(2): 190–202 © 2007 IEEE.)

their visual content. Hence, simple signatures may be suitable to describe them. However, the characteristic of medical images differs substantially:

- *Noncolor*: In medical imaging modalities, color is less relevant. For instance, x-ray imaging (radiography, fluoroscopy), CT, MRI, ultrasound, and nuclear medicine all form gray-scale images. Hence, color cannot be used to describe the images appropriately.
- *Structure*: The pathology that is visualized in medical images may result from only subtle or small alterations in the image pattern—if a history of images is available for comparison at all. Usually, intraindividual differences in size, shape, and appearance of biological tissue are more prominent than the diagnostically relevant alterations.
- *Multidimensionality*: Medical images are often 3D, for example, representing a volume composed of two-dimensional (2D) slices or a temporal sequence of 2D images (moving picture), or even four-dimensional (4D), such as MRI sequences of the beating heart. Hence, more complex features must be used in the medical domain.
- *Mutlimodality*: Furthermore, medical diagnostics frequently is based on more than only one set of image data, and imaging data is usually obtained from different modalities. Comparing ultrasound with radiography or MRI exemplifies that the different nature of medical modalities does not support representing all such images using the same numerical features.
- *Metainformation*: Medical images are only a part of the information that is relevant in a medical case. Gender, age, and other data are required to compare diagnostics in medical cases. Consequently, combining CBIR with natural language processing (NLP) is superior to medical document retrieval.

Anyway, in this chapter, we will focus on 2D gray-scale images. Starting in 2000, medical CBIR systems have been described in the literature. A brief history is given in the next section.

21.2.3 Medical CBIR Systems

A comprehensive review of CBIR systems in medical applications is given by Müller et al. (2004a). From the previous section, it is obvious that medical CBIR systems have been focused on certain imaging modalities, body regions, and diagnostic tasks (Table 21.1). The ASSERT system, for instance, is a physician-in-the-loop content-based retrieval system for high-resolution CT (HRCT) data. The gap of lacking appropriate signatures and similarity measures for such complex semantics is bridged with user interaction: the physician manually marks pathology-bearing regions of interest (ROIs) in selected 2D

TABLE 21.1 Various Images Types and the Medical CBIR Systems That are Using These Images

Images Used	Names of the Systems
HRCTs of the Lung	ASSERT
Functional PET	FICBDS
Spine x-rays	CBIR2, MIRS
Pathologic images	IDEM, I-Browse, PathFinder, PathMaster
CTs of the head	MIMS
Mammographies	APKS
Images from biology	BioImage, BIRN
Dermatology	MELDOQ, MEDS
Breast cancer biopsies	BASS
Varied images	I²C, IRMA, KMed, COBRA, MedGIFT, ImageEngine

Source: Adapted from Müller H et al. *Int J Med Inform.* 2004a; 73(1): 1–23.

slices (Shyu et al. 1999). Some approaches, however, try to address the medical imagery in general. Two of these approaches are depicted in the following sections.

21.2.3.1 MedGIFT

The MedGIFT project aims at providing an open-source framework of reusable components for a variety of medical applications. It is based strongly on the GNU image finding tool (GIFT)[*] as its central piece. Main developments are on the integration of various new components to create a domain-specific search and navigation tool (Müller et al. 2003, 2005).

GIFT supports retrieval of images by their visual content. Scripts permit indexing entire directory trees of images and build inverted file indices. Supported visual features are aimed at color photography, such as color histograms applied on the entire image and on block partitions at various scales. Gabor texture features are also computed and stored. Query and retrieval are done using a specialized extensible markup language (XML)-type language called multimedia retrieval markup language (MRML), which facilitates communication between the query interface and the retrieval engine.

MedGIFT supports some basic keyword-based retrieval by including search of patient records along with images. It should be noted that MedGIFT is not a fixed system but rather a framework upon which to base various image retrieval systems/experiments. For feature selection, MedGIFT applies general concepts from information retrieval and text mining:

- *Term frequency (TF)*: a feature frequent in an image describes this image well.
- *Inverse document frequency (IDF)*: a feature frequent in the collection is a weak indicator to distinguish images.

A weighted TF-IDF function is used to determine the feature weight, which is then applied to each feature computing an overall similarity score. The images are segmented to the extent of background removal and some object localization through thresholding or other high-level methods. Simple relevance feedback is also implemented.

21.2.3.2 IRMA

The Image Retrieval in Medical Applications (IRMA) project aims at developing and implementing high-level methods for CBIR, including prototypical application to medico-diagnostic tasks on a radiological image archive (Lehmann et al. 2000, 2004). The IRMA team wants to perform semantic and formalized queries on the medical image database, which includes intra- and interindividual variance and diseases. Three levels of image content similarity are modeled:

- *Global* features are linked to the entire images and used to automatically classify an image according to the (a) anatomic region and (b) biosystem that is captured, the imaging modality (c, creation) that is used, and the relative (d) direction of imaging device and patient, including the pose (ABCD code) (Lehmann et al. 2003).
- *Local* features are linked to prominent image regions and used for object recognition.
- *Structural* features are linked to spatial and/or temporal relations between the objects. They are used for high-level image interpretation.

A pipeline of image processing is suggested. Iterative region merging builds up a hierarchical attributed region adjacency graph (HARAG), the data structure that is used to represent images. Hence, image retrieval is converted to graph matching. Object comparison operates on the HARAG nodes, while scenes are modeled by rather structural graph to subgraph comparison.

The system is set up on a Unix platform, with a central server, relational database, and shared computing in the cluster of connected workstations for distributed computing. All interfaces are based

---

[*] Available at http://www.gnu.org/software/gift.

on HTML and recorded in the database too. The coupling of CBIR and PACS is based on the Digital Imaging and Communications in Medicine (DICOM) protocol.

21.3 Medical Use of CBIR

Using such generic frameworks, medical CBIR applications have been explored and developed recently. They cover a wide range of applications, from medical education to clinical routine and research. In this section, we will describe in general the possible use of CBIR in medicine.

Figure 21.3 emphasizes the radiological process (Greenes 1989). The outer loop refers to diagnostics, while quality assessment and performance monitoring are rather research-oriented. The third complex in using medical imagery addresses medical education and training.

21.3.1 Diagnostics

As mentioned before, medical images are acquired primarily for diagnostics, and hence CBIR systems are designed to assist diagnosis. In any case, the major goal is to retrieve similar images from the archive, since these images are annotated with metainformation that is stored in the medical record and may be helpful for the current case.

- *Case-based reasoning (CBR)*, broadly construed, is the process of solving new problems based on the solutions of similar past problems (Macura and Macura 1997). According to the radiological process, The CBR cycle (retrieve, reuse, revise, retain, Figure 21.4) requires access to previous cases (Aamodt and Plaza 1994). Usually, such cases are retrieved from textbooks and medical atlases (general knowledge). In particular, the radiologist may easily recognize an irregular structure in

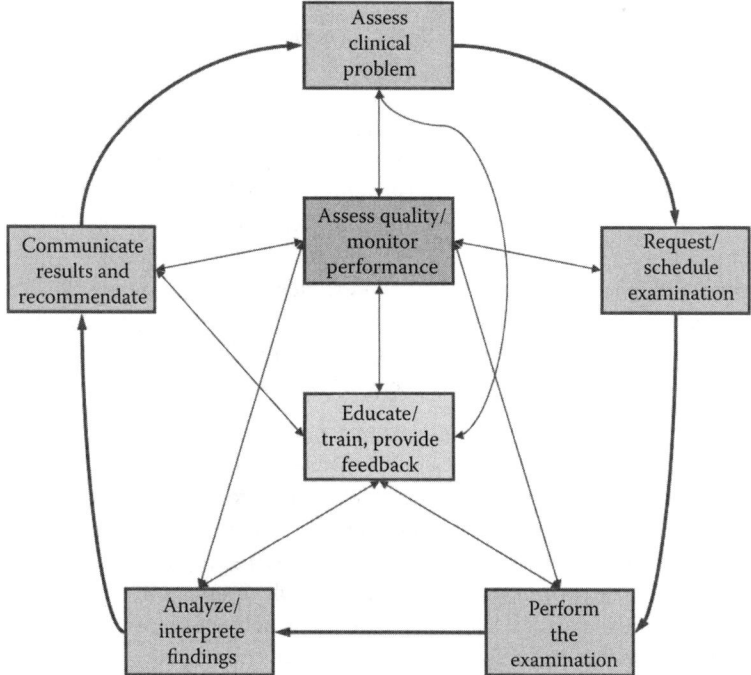

FIGURE 21.3 The radiological process of diagnostics, research, and education. (From Lehmann TM. Digitale Bildverarbeitung für Routineanwendungen. Evaluierung und Integration am Beispiel der Medizin. Deutscher Universitäts-Verlag, Wiesbaden 2005. ISBN 3-8244-2191-7 (in German).)

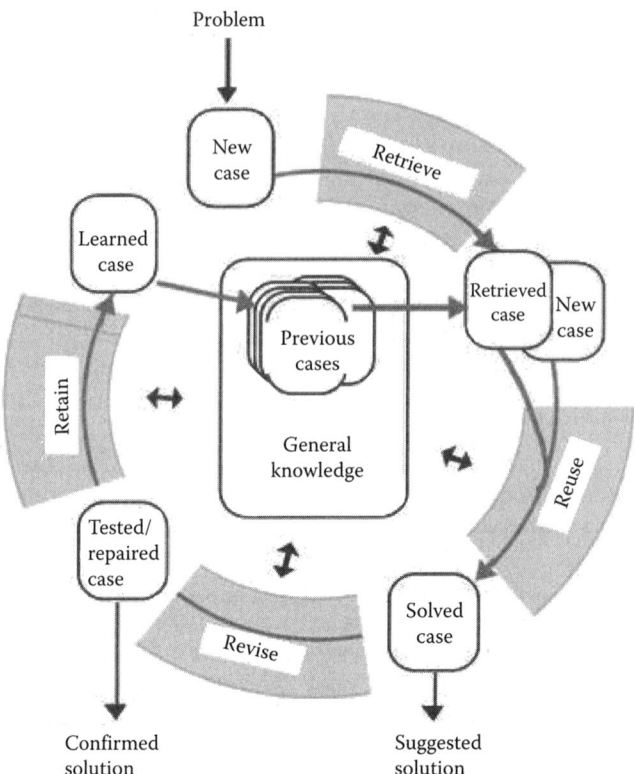

FIGURE 21.4 The CBR cycle transforms a problem into a confirmed solution. (From Aamodt A and Plaza E. *AICom—Artif Intell Commun.* 1994; 7(1): 39–59.)

an image, but deciding on its reason is more challenging. Using his knowledge, he may form some hypotheses, which are then evaluated step by step. For each hypothesis, corresponding images are sought in the printed resources by textual labels rather than image pattern. If the actual pathology is not among the initial hypotheses, relevant images will not be compared to the current case and the CBR process may fail. Within a CBIR-based CBR scenario, the physician may mark the ROI in the image, and the selected pattern is used to retrieve similar images by contained pattern. In a second step, the radiologist is put into the loop again, when selecting relevant images from the CBIR response. Accessing the medical records that are linked to these cases may expose the correct diagnosis even if this particular hypothesis has not been within the initial guess of the radiologist.

- *Computer-aided diagnosis*: The CBR process may be further automated by taking the physician out of the loop. This, however, requires a more reliable ground truth associated with the reference images in the archive. In a certain context, for example, for tumor staging, each class of diagnostics (e.g., benign vs. malignant) is represented by several images. Again, the current examination forms the QBE, and a set of similar images is retrieved automatically from the archive. Using appropriate features and similarity measures, which of course must be carefully selected and parameterized, which is still a field of ongoing research, the set of returned images is majorly composed of a particular diagnostic class, which is then transferred automatically to the current case. More sophisticated methods may construct a measurement automatically using similarity scores and ordinal measurements that are linked to the retrieved images in their accompanying metadata (ground truth).

21.3.2 Research

- *Evidence-based medicine (EBM)* aims at applying the best available evidence gained from the scientific method to clinical decision making (Guyatt et al. 1992, Sackett et al. 1996). It seeks to assess the strength of evidence of the risks and benefits of treatments (including lack of treatment) and diagnostic tests. The quality of evidence can range from meta-analyses and systematic reviews of double-blind, placebo-controlled clinical trials at the top end, down to conventional wisdom at the bottom. In contrast to CBR, EBM usually refers to more than only one similar case, and content-based methods may be applied to retrieve such cases. However, EBM rather implies image mining (identifying classes of images) than image retrieval (identifying images from a given class or type).

- *Drug development*: Another field of research-driven CBIR applications is the development process of drugs. Here, clinical trials are performed in order to assess safety and efficacy of a new drug:
  - *Phase I* trials are the first stage of testing in human subjects. A small group of up to 100 healthy volunteers is selected to assess the tolerability and safety (pharmacovigilance), pharmacokinetics, and pharmacodynamics of a drug.
  - *Phase II* trials are performed on larger groups of up to 300 subjects and designed to assess how well the drug is working, for example, determining dosing requirements (*Phase IIa*) and efficacy (*Phase IIb*).
  - *Phase III* trials are randomized controlled multicenter trials on large patient groups (3000 or more) aiming at assessing effectiveness of the drug in comparison to the current gold standard treatment.
  - *Phase IV* trials (postmarketing surveillance trial) involve safety surveillance (pharmacovigilance) and technical support after the drug has received permission to be sold. Involving up to a million of individuals, they may also aim at finding a new market or indication for the drug.

In each phase, a so-called endpoint is defined reflecting how a subject feels, functions, or survives. Based on a hypothetical new drug for treating congestive heart failure (CHF), Figure 21.5 emphasizes the four different phases of clinical trials and it is corresponding clinical endpoints.

Sometimes, however, the endpoint in a clinical trial cannot be assessed that easily by a simple parameter as, for instance, the heart's ejection rate. Then, a surrogate may be used. A surrogate endpoint is defined as a biomarker (objectively measured and evaluated indicator of normal biological processes,

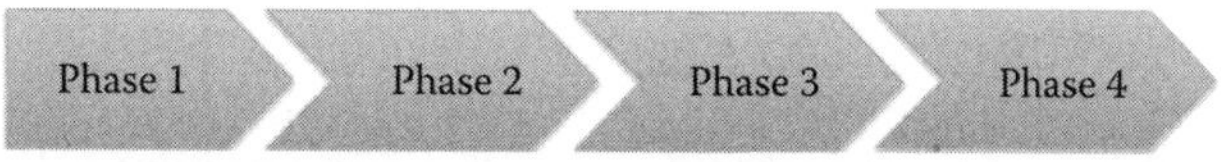

	Phase 1	Phase 2	Phase 3	Phase 4
Stage of Development	Phase 1	Phase 2	Phase 3	Phase 4
End point	Safety	Efficacy	Efficacy	Efficacy
Specific end point	Safety profile	Cardiac output	Reduction in mortality rate	Reduction in mortality rate
Types of studies	Different indications; single or multiple dose	Placebo controlled; dose escalation	Placebo controlled; long-term follow up	Comparative; new indications

FIGURE 21.5 Specific endpoints in clinical trials for drug development. (From Silverman M. Clinical trial end points at different phases of clinical development. Technical Report, BioStrategics Consulting Ltd, 2011.)

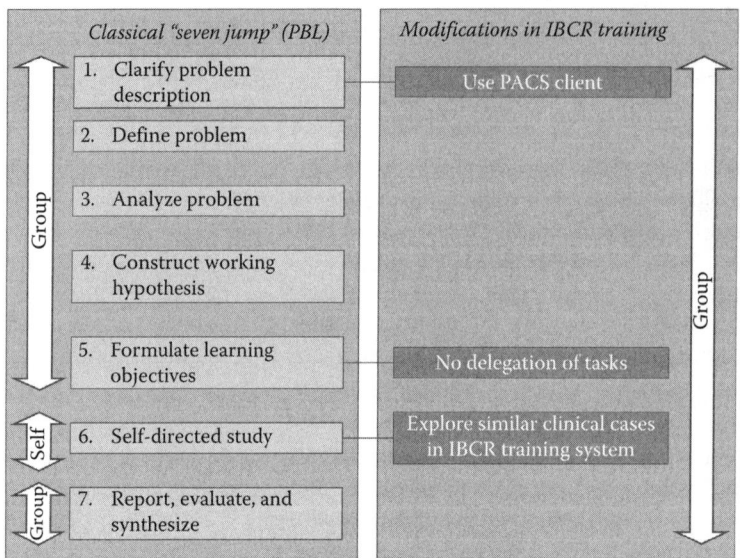

FIGURE 21.6 The Seven Jumps for PBL (left) and IBCR support (right). (From Welter P et al. *BMC*. 2011a; 11(68).)

pathogenic processes, or pharmacologic responses to a therapeutic intervention) that is intended to substitute for a clinical endpoint. Image-based surrogates, for instance, are computed from almost all of the imaging modalities that have been addressed in this book, including ultrasound (de Groot et al. 2004), CT (Jaffe 2008), MRI (Warach 2001), or molecular imaging methods such as PET (de Geus-Oei et al. 2007). It is obvious that image-based biomarkers require comprehensive evaluation (Analoui 2011), which shall rely on a large set of images. Hence, CBIR may become the key technology in further developments of surrogate endpoints.

21.3.3 Education

Medical education relies on practical experience within healthcare institutions such as hospitals. The majority of problems physicians have to deal with are directly concerning the patient. Therefore, the presentation of clinical cases in medical education is essential. Problem-based learning (PBL) is known to provide positive effects on medical education, especially pertaining to social and cognitive aspects (Koh et al. 2008). A clinical case is a stimulus for learning, while fostering the acquisition of knowledge related to the problem together with an improvement of problem-solving skills.

More formalized, a seven-step procedure usually is applied in PBL, which is referred to as Seven Jump (Gijselaers 1995, Wood and Diana 2003). Access to the case collection supports all of the steps but is essentially required at least in Steps 1 and 6. It is eased by integrating CBIR technology with the PACS (Welter et al. 2011a). If image-based case retrieval (IBCR) is applied to PBL, the PACS client is used to select the learning material, to clarify the problem description, and to explore similar cases in a self-directed study (Figure 21.6).

21.4 Engineering Fields of Medical CBIR Systems

Within the broad scope of CBIR in medical diagnosis, education, and research, there are plenty of problems that still have to be addressed by biomedical engineers. For instance, in Section 21.2.1, we have already discussed the semantic gap between simple numerical features that are applied to represent the meaning of an image for the human observer, and engineers are trying to bridge this gap defining advanced features, for instance, a HARAG (Fischer et al. 2004).

However, there are more essential gaps still hindering the clinical application of content-based image search (Deserno et al. 2009a). Figure 21.7 visualizes a classification scheme for such gaps and additional characteristics of medical CBIR systems. According to this scheme, the most relevant fields of medical CBIR engineering are addressed in the following sections.

21.4.1 Content and Features

The content gaps address the level of image understanding (semantic gap) as well as the imaging and/ or clinical context in which a CBIR system may be used (use context gap). Obviously, designing a medical CBIR system for a broad use is more challenging, since the level of image details relevant for the retrieval, the type of image data (modality) to handle, and other system preferences are highly variable.

The feature gaps address the automation of feature extraction (extraction gap), the granularity of structure of image objects recognized by the system (structure gap), the granularity of visual details in the image processed by the system (scale gap), the dimensionality of spatial and time inputs actually used to compute the signature (space and time dimension gap), and the dimensionality of channel inputs actually used to compute the signature (channel dimension gap).

Biomedical engineers trying to establish clinical CBIR systems must face these problems. Signatures must be developed that are calculated automatically rather than manually from the entire dimensions and range of image data: 3D and 4D image data cannot be represented appropriately by features that have been extracted from 2D slices, and multichannel data (e.g., true color) cannot be completely represented using only singular channel (e.g., gray scale). Also, local and structural signatures must become available for clinical applications of CBIR.

21.4.2 Performance

Another field requiring customized engineering approaches is the performance of CBIR systems. In the medical field, images, and especially digital images, are produced in an ever-increasing quantity. For instance, the Radiology Department of the University Hospitals of Geneva (HUG), Geneva, Switzerland has produced more than 114,000 images a day in 2009, risen form 12,000 in 2002. Large hospital groups such as Kaiser Permanente that manage several hospitals have reported about 700 TB of data stored in the institutional archives by early 2009, and very large hospitals such as the University Hospital of Vienna, Austria currently produce more than 100 GB of image data per day (Müller and Deserno 2011).

For CBIR, numerous comparisons are required, and hence, the response time of a retrieval system becomes a serious parameter. The level of support for fast database searching must be increased to bridge the indexing gap. Hardware and software solutions are engineered, including parallel computing and extensive use of field programmable gate arrays (FPGAs) and graphics processing units (GPUs) (Scholl et al. 2011).

Currently, performance engineering also addresses the efficiency of medical CBIR systems. When applied in clinical routine, the performance of CBIR turns out to be rather low. Frequently, the images returned may be inappropriate with respect to the query semantics or even wrong. This fact results from insufficient evaluation of the algorithms, and the evaluation gap addresses the level to which the system validity of retrieval has been evaluated. Unavailability of large image repositories reliably annotated with ground truth information is one of the major problems to face.

21.4.3 Usability

However, deploying a valid and well-performing CBIR system does not guarantee its successful establishment in clinical practice. Graphical user interfaces (GUIs) and input/output (I/O) devices must

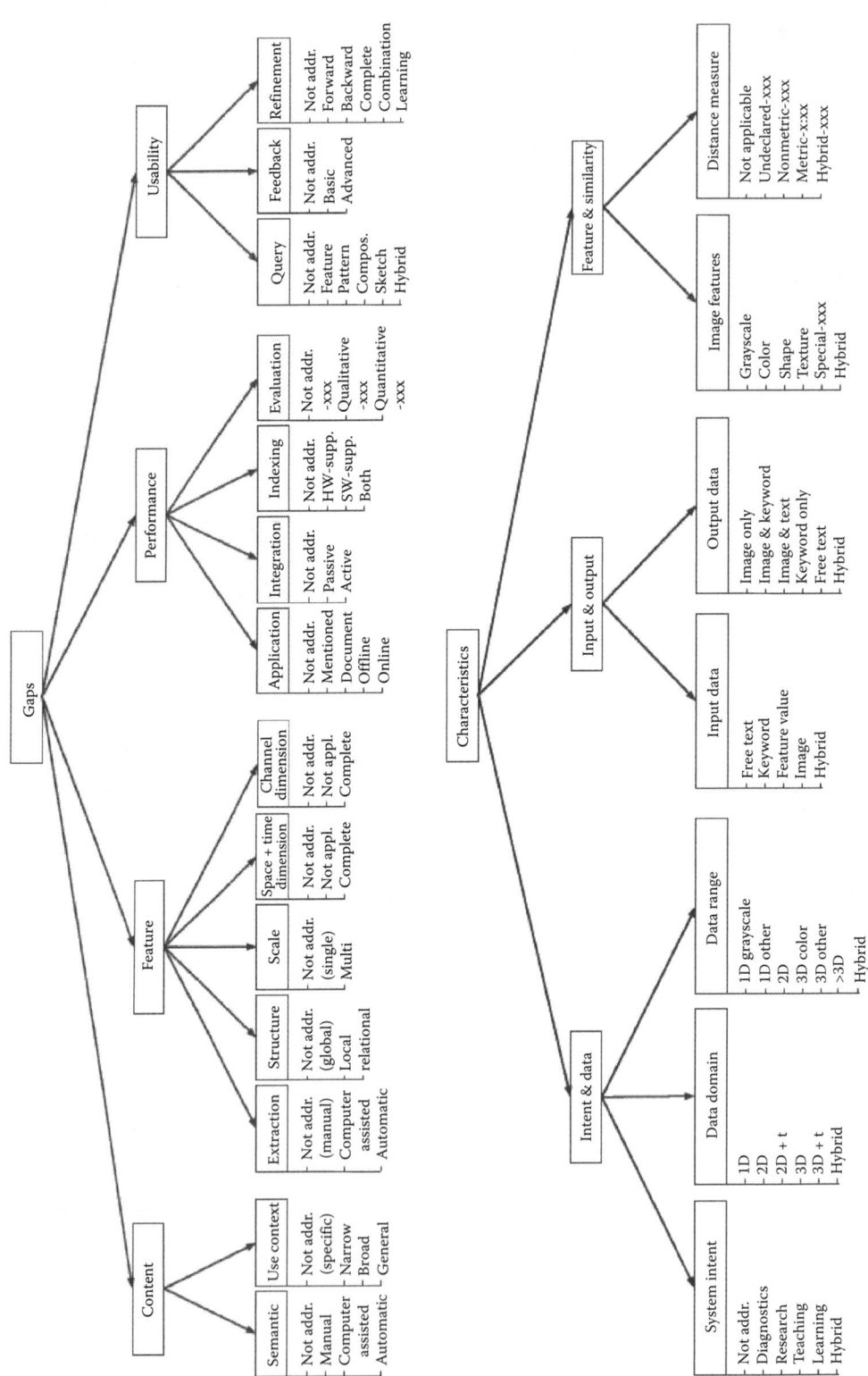

FIGURE 21.7 Gaps and characteristics of medical CBIR systems. (From Deserno TM, Antani S, and Long R. *J Digit Imaging*. 2009; 22(2): 202–215.)

be carefully designed, and the workflow within the application must be intuitive and easy to follow. Relevant fields of engineering address the levels to which a user may use and combine visual as well as textual (alphanumerical) queries (query gap), to which the system helps the user to understand the query results (feedback gap), and to which the system helps the user to refine and improve the query results (refinement gap).

Engineering approaches to bridge the visual query gap include 3D interaction such as marking a partial volume of interest (VOI). While in 2D, a surface may be sketched quickly upon an image, annotating a 3D surface into a voxel-based volume is challenging. Obviously, the 2D mouse is inappropriate. 3D input devices such as the gloves or optical scanners may be useful. Furthermore, the image data must be positioned appropriately in 3D space, which may require two rather than only one sophisticated input device. Even more difficult is user interaction for retrieval of volume sequences over time (4D data).

21.4.4 Integration

In Figure 21.7, the integration gap is defined within the group of performance gaps (see Section 21.4.2). However, integration of medical image processing technology into the clinical workflow is of fundamental prominence to justify paying a special attention.

More than 10 years ago, Eakins and Graham have already stated that the experience of all commercial vendors of CBIR software is that system acceptability is heavily influenced by the extent to which image retrieval capabilities can be embedded within user's overall work tasks (Eakins and Graham 1999). Such work tasks in medicine have already been visualized in Figure 21.3. They require seamless integration on different levels (Leisch et al. 1997, Winter et al. 2010):

- *Data integration* is achieved if any data stored in the modules must not be entered more than once.
- *Functional integration* is obtained if any services provided by a certain module can be used from any other module requiring this particular service within the entire system.
- *Presentation integration* is obtained if different modules present their data in a unified way and style.
- *Context integration* is present if specific setting such as the selection of a certain patient or image, which is done in one module, is passed automatically to another module when this is called.

This short list emphasizes the challenges of integration of CBIR technology into medical diagnosis, research, and education. Accordingly, research and development in medical image search must include communication interfaces such as DICOM and Health Level Seven (HL7).

21.5 State of the Art in Medical CBIR Technology

In this section, we will briefly describe the state of the art in medical content-based image search regarding features and similarity measures, user interfaces, workflow integration, combined visual and textual retrieval, and evaluation.

21.5.1 Features Extraction and Selection

As mentioned before, features or signatures may be computed on different levels. The following description of global and local features is according to Müller and Deserno (2011).

21.5.1.1 Global Features

Visual features have been classified into (i) primitive features such as color or shape, (ii) logical features such as identity of objects shown, and (iii) abstract features such as significance of depicted scenes

(Eakins and Graham 1999). However, basically, all currently available systems exclusively rely on primitive features, such as

- *Color*: In stock photography (large, varied databases used by artists, advertisers, and journalists), color has been the most effective feature. The red, green, blue (RGB) color space is only rarely used, as it does not correspond sufficiently with human color perception. Other color models such as hue, saturation, value (HSV), or the International Commission on Illumination (Commission internationale de l'éclairage, CIE) Lab and Luv spaces perform superiorly because a metric distance in such a color model is more similar to the difference between the colors that a human observer perceives. Much effort has also been spent on creating color spaces that are optimal with respect to lighting conditions or that are invariant to shades and other influences such as viewing position (Geusebroek et al. 2001).
- *Texture*: Texture measures try to capture the characteristics of the image with respect to changes in certain directions and the scale of the changes. This is most useful for images with homogeneous texture. Some of the most common measures are wavelets and Gabor filters. Invariances with respect to rotation, shift, or scale can be included into the feature space but information on the texture may get lost in this process (Milanese and Cherbuliez 1999). Other popular texture descriptors contain features derived from co-occurrence matrices (Haralick et al. 1973, Kuo et al. 2002), the Fourier transform (Milanese and Cherbuliez 1999), and the so-called wold features, which represent image texture combining wavelets that have been certainly tuned to various scales and rotations (deterministic component) with an autoregressive model (nondeterministic component) (Lu and Chung 1998).

21.5.1.2 Local Features

Both color and texture features can also be used on a local or regional level, that is, on parts of the image, disregarding whether such parts have been obtained from image-driven segmentation or geometric partitioning. The easiest way to employing regional features is to produce blocks of fixed size. However, such blocks do not reflect any semantics in the image (Squire et al. 2000). When allowing the user to choose ROIs (Comaniciu et al. 1998), or when segmenting the image into areas with similar properties (Winter and Nastar 1999), local features may capture more information about relevant image structures. The following local features are commonly used:

- *Shape*: Fully automated segmentation of images into objects itself is an unsolved problem. Even in fairly specialized domains, automated segmentation causes many problems. In image retrieval, several systems attempt to perform an automatic segmentation for feature extraction (Lucchese and Mitra 1999). The segmentation process should be based on color and texture properties of the image regions. Then, the segments can be described by shape features, usually being invariant to shift, rotation, and scaling (Loncaric 1998). Medical image segmentation for browsing large image repositories is frequently addressed in the literature (Lapeer et al. 2002).
- *Salient points*: In recent years, salient point-based features have best performed in most of the image retrieval and object classification tasks (Mikolajczyk and Schmid 2005). The idea is to find representative points (or points that attract visual attention) in the images and then analyze the relationships of the points. This permits to extract features that possess several invariants such as invariance to shift, rotation, scale, and even the point of view. A large number of such techniques exist for detecting as well as extracting features from the salient points. A prominent example is the scale-invariant feature transform (SIFT) (Lowe 2004).
- *Patches and visual words*: Patches and visual words are closely linked to salient point-based features, because they are usually extracted from regions in the images that were identified as salient point. Then, features are extracted regionally from these regions. Alternatively, a regular grid is placed in the image and the patches are extracted around the center points of the grid. The term "visual word" stems from text retrieval. Visual features are clustered into a limited number

of homogeneous characteristics that can have distributions similar to the distribution of words in text. This allows us to apply techniques that are well known from text retrieval (Sivic and Zisserman 2006). The image annotation task in the cross-language evaluation forum (CLEF) (Deselaers et al. 2007, 2008) has shown that x-ray categorization and retrieval on the organ and pathology level is performed best using patch-based visual words (Avni et al. 2011).

On the one hand, all of these features provide benefits and have confirmed application domains, but on the other hand, all of them are low-level visual features not corresponding to semantic categories. For this reason, text, whenever available, should be used additionally for medical image search, as semantic information is conveyed inherently with natural language. All benchmarks show that text has a superior performance compared to visual characteristics, but is complemented effectively by visual retrieval.

21.5.1.3 Structural Features

In medical image processing, scene-based approaches are used successfully for segmentation (Deserno 2011). For instance, the commercial software BoneXpert® (http://www.bonexpert.com) for automated determination of skeletal maturity is segmenting the relevant bones from left hand's radiographs using an active shape model (Thodberg et al. 2009).

The use of structural features for image retrieval is even more advanced and has not yet been implemented in any system that is used in routine. The challenging idea is to capture not only the relevant objects in an image but also their constellation in a spatial and/or temporal scene. Fischer et al. (2008) have published an approach where the so-called structural prototypes are trained from reference images. The prototypes are attributed relational graphs (ARG), where nodes and edges capture the object and relation properties, respectively (Figure 21.8). To cope with the variety in shape, appearance, and constellation of living biological tissue, node and edge annotations are represented by unimodal Gaussian distributions of the corresponding feature. On time of retrieval, graph matching is computed to assess

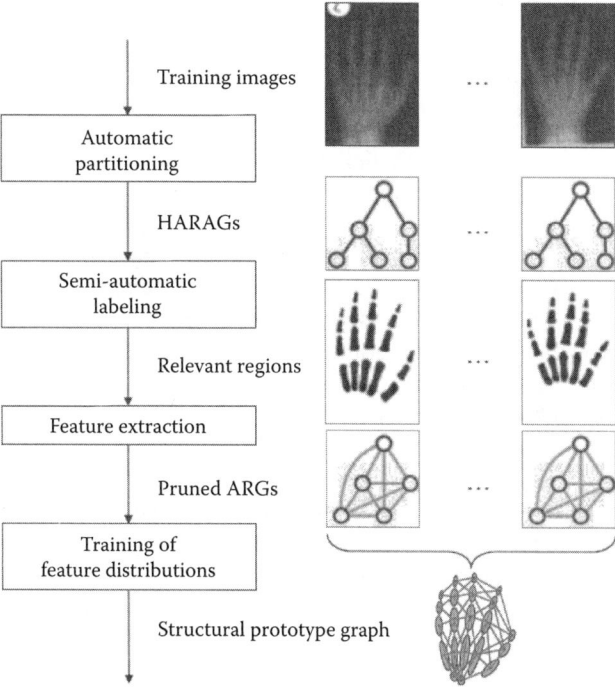

FIGURE 21.8 Structural prototypes for scene-based image retrieval. (From Fischer B et al. *Proc SPIE.* 2008; 6914: 1X1–1X9.)

the similarity of two scenes that can cope with missing objects. The similarity computed based on the signature is discussed in detail in the next section.

21.5.2 Distance and Similarity Measures

To perform a similarity query, we can define in general two main operators for comparison (Traina et al. 2011):

- *Range query*: Given a dataset, a query center, and a radius, each element is selected for which the distance between the query center and the element is below the radius; for example, retrieve all images that differ five units of similarity to the QBE.
- *Nearest-neighbor query*: Given a dataset, a query center, and an integer value $k \geq 1$, the k-nearest neighbor (k-NN) query selects the k elements of the dataset that are at the shortest distances from the query center; for example, retrieve the five most similar images to the QBE.

For both types of queries, one needs to define a distance or similarity measure as well as one or more reference elements (QBE), which also have been referred to as the query center. Basically, all systems for image retrieval assume equivalence of an image and its representation in the feature space, and the Euclidean vector space model is used for measuring the distances between a query image (represented by its features) and possible results representing all images as feature vectors in an n-dimensional (nD) vector space. Although such metrics have been shown to disagree with the visual perception of human (Tversky 1977), they are broadly used and formally defined in the following section.

21.5.2.1 Metrics

A metric space is defined as a pair $\mathbf{M} = \langle \mathbf{S}, d \rangle$, where $\mathbf{S}$ denotes the universe of valid elements and d is the function $d: \mathbf{S} \times \mathbf{S} \rightarrow \mathbf{R}^+$ called a metric that expresses the distance between elements in $\mathbf{S}$. To be a metric, d must satisfy the following properties for every $s_1, s_2, s_3 \in \mathbf{S}$:

1. *Symmetry*: $d(s_1, s_2) = d(s_2, s_1)$
2. *Nonnegativity*: $0 < d(s_1, s_2) < \infty$ if $s_1 \neq s_2$ and $d(s_1, s_1) = 0$
3. *Triangular inequality*: $d(s_1, s_3) \leq d(s_1, s_2) + d(s_2, s_3)$

Using a metric to compare elements, a similarity query returns the stored elements that satisfy a given similarity criterion, usually expressed in terms of query centers (QBE parameter in feature space).

In addition to the Euclidian distance, several other metrics are known for the vector space model such as the city-block distance, the Mahalanobis distance, histogram intersection, or other histogram-based metrics that can be used for histogram-based features such as SIFT (Pele and Werman 2008). However, the use of high-dimensional feature spaces bears the *curse of dimensionality* (increasing the number of features is decreasing the performance of the classifier), and appropriate features and distance measures must be selected carefully (Aggarwal et al. 2001).

21.5.2.2 Other Measures

Another approach is a probabilistic framework to measure the likelihood that an image is relevant (Jain et al. 2000). Some probabilistic approaches use the support vector machine (SVM) for grouping of images into classes of relevance and nonrelevance (de Oliveira et al. 2010). In most visual classification tasks, SVM reaches the overall best performance.

Various systems rely on methods that are well known from the field of text retrieval. Adapting them to visual features that are corresponding roughly to words in the text is based on the TF-IDF principle (cf. Section 21.2.3.1). Several weighting schemes for text retrieval have also been used in image retrieval. Accordingly, the TF-IDF method perfectly fits to features extracted from patches and visual words (cf. Section 21.5.1.2).

21.5.3 User Interaction

Designing ergonomic user interfaces is a challenging task of engineering in general, and becomes even more sophisticated if the task is complex and the desired user group is specialists from a nontechnical domain, such as in medicine and biology. Since the early 1990s, the International Organization of Standardization (ISO) is publishing a series of standards (ISO 9241) initially titled "Ergonomic requirements for office work with visual display terminals (VDTs)." Part 10 (nowadays part 110) of this series defines seven basic principles: (i) suitability for the task, (ii) self-descriptiveness, (iii) controllability, (iv) conformity with user expectation, (v) error tolerance, (vi) suitability for individualization, and (vii) suitability for learning, which in summary support (ISO 9241-11):

- *Effectiveness*: With respect to the ISO standard, effectiveness means that the software performs all the task it has been designed for, and is not interrupted by errors, malfunctions, or system failures of any kind. In addition, the results obtained using the software must have a minimum (well-defined) quality.
- *Efficiency*: All tasks can be performed with minimal efforts. In particular, required user interaction such as keyboard hits, mouse clicks, and so on must be minimized and redundancy shall be avoided.
- *User satisfaction*: In general, user satisfaction is defined as the opinion of the user about a specific computer application, which they use (Doll and Torkzadeh 1988, 1991). The user subjectively must "feel" effectiveness and efficiency, disregarding their objective measurements. We shall realize that user satisfaction is regarded as *the* general key measure of computer system success at all (de Lone and Mc Lean 1992, 2003).

With this in mind, important functionality for medical image search has been identified. In particular, mechanisms for query refinement and relevance feedback are required (Smeulders et al. 2000).

21.5.3.1 Query Refinement

Query refinement is a common task in document retrieval. For example, retrieving literature from bibliographic databases such as PubMed, the resulting set of papers matching a query is reduced in the numbers of entities by additional constraints, such as determining the language of the paper, its publication date, or simply requiring the presented key words to occur in the title of the paper rather than within its abstract. This process, called query refinement, is performed by the user until the set of retrieved documents is suitable for manual inspection.

In image retrieval, in particular, performing a range query, the user also needs to lower the query range. Here, however, the task is more sophisticated, since the range is defined by similarity rather than exact match, and the features are numerical vectors computed from color, texture, and shape as compared to simple words that are applied in text-based document retrieval. Hence, the process of query specification and display is iterated, where, in each step, the user revises the query. Considering such an interactive session in its entirety, the system updates the query space, attempting to learn the goals from the user's feedback. Accordingly, an interactive query session is defined as a sequence of query spaces Q visualized in display space $V(Q)$ (Smeulders et al. 2000):

$$\{Q^0, Q^1, ..., Q^{n-1}, Q^n\} \text{ with } A^n(q) = V(Q^n)$$

In a truly successful session, the system's answer $A^n(q)$ equals the user's search goal. The interaction process is indicated schematically in Figure 21.9. The framework is suitable to model different types of searches, such as the

- *Associative search* aiming at finding relevant images by a range or nearest-neighbor query
- *Category search* aiming at identifying a certain category the query image is belonging to, for example, in CAD applications, where each category represents a certain pathology or tumor stage
- *Target search* aiming at retrieving only a certain image

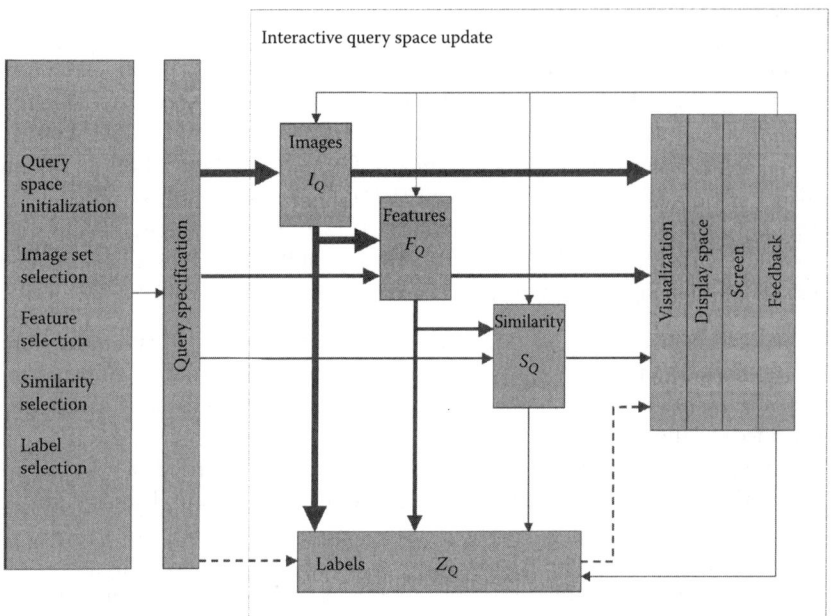

FIGURE 21.9 Framework for interactive CBIR sessions. (From Smeulders AWM et al. *IEEE Trans Pattern Anal Mach Intell.* 22(12): 1349–1380 © 2000 IEEE.)

21.5.3.2 Relevance Feedback

The interaction of the user yields a relevance feedback RF_i in every iteration i of the session. The transition from Q^i to Q^{i+1} materializes this feedback of the user. For all types of search, various ways of user feedback have been considered in the literature (Smeulders et al. 2000). All are balancing between obtaining as much information from the user as possible (cf. effectiveness) and keeping the burden on the user minimal (cf. efficiency). The simplest form of feedback is to indicate which of the retrieved images are relevant. More sophisticated approaches allow continuous-valued feedback between relevance and nonrelevance.

With respect to the framework defined in Figure 21.9, user feedback in general leads to an update of the query space

$$\{I_Q^i, F_Q^i, S_Q^i, Z_Q^i\} \to RF_i \to \{I_Q^{i+1}, F_Q^{i+1}, S_Q^{i+1}, Z_Q^{i+1}\}$$

Marking relevant images refines the query space on elements I_Q. Here, the user zooms on a target or category. More sophisticated, feedback from the user may also yield an optimization of the features used for retrieval. For instance, the user is allowed to select between color, texture, and shape-based features. Then, relevance feedback addresses the elements F_Q. For associative search, users typically interact to teach the system the right associations. Hence, the system updates the similarity function S_Q. The last set of systems operates on grouping or partitioning that is based on the similarity for each individual feature. The feedback from the user is employed to create compound groupings corresponding to a user given $z \in Z_Q$. Usually, the compound groupings are such that they include the entire positive and none of the negative examples.

21.5.3.3 User Interfaces

Aiming at full user satisfaction, the challenge in GUI engineering lies in integrating all required types of search and interaction into a simple, preferably web-based design, where medical CBIR can be used via a web browser that is already installed on the user's system. Furthermore, it cannot be assumed that query refinement is always successful, and previous query spaces Q^{n-i} shall stay available within a session. Based on only four types of interface modules, an award-winning approach has been proposed in Deserno et al. (2008):

1. *Output modules* contain all functionality regarding the visualization of information such as images, descriptions, or numerical parameters. In particular, "text," "image," "line," "shadow," "frame," and "table" are basic output modules. These modules are used to initialize the query, to visualize the query result, and to display the relevance facts.

2. *Parameter modules* allow the user to interact with the system. "Input field," "radio button," "slider," or "selection box" are some prominent examples. Furthermore, tools for selecting an ROI within an image or drawing a sketch belong to this class of modules. The parameter modules are used whenever a query is initialized or (re)submitted. In particular, they support relevance feedback.

3. *Transaction modules* include all functions that allow the user to step back and forward (UNDO or REDO functions) and to restore any "steady state" that the system has had within the current session, and also within already closed sessions (HISTORY functions). Using web-based GUIs, all output and parameter modules can be embedded in a hypertext form sheet, and the data transfer between server and client (the browser) is captured and stored. Then, previous stages are easily restored by "updating" the hypertext form with information from older stages.

4. *Process modules* are defined as union or intersection of intermediate sets of query results, which have already been refined by relevance feedback loops. The image lists and all corresponding relevant facts are stored, when process modules are activated during a session. Boolean AND/OR operations are available to operate on these lists for advanced query refinement.

Based on these module classes, Figure 21.10 diagrams the flow of a retrieval session. Parameter or function modules are used to initialize the query. After performing the search, which compares the query with all images in the system by means of the selected features, resulting images are displayed and relevance facts are given by means of the output or function modules.

In Figure 21.10, four nested loops are indicated. Without any query refinement, the straight line from start to end is followed. If the system offers relevance feedback, a central loop from output to parameter modules is added (Loop 1). The sequence of performing relevance feedback, computing a revised search, and presenting relevant facts of updated results is repeated until the user accepts the current response to his query. The transaction modules add a second inner loop to the flowchart intra-connecting the output modules (Loop 2). This loop is supported by the system's query logging, which also reads from the parameter and the output modules. Finally, a third loop is added to provide extended query refinement by combining successive but independent queries over the same database (Loop 3). If the system is currently not within a Boolean loop, such a loop can be opened to extend (OR relationship) or refine (AND relationship) the resulting image list, which is stored as pending in the database via the query logging mechanisms. The Boolean loop is closed automatically by merging the pending with the current response list of images if the user accepts the current result (Loop 4). Again, this loop can be iterated until the user agrees to the final result.

21.5.4 CBIR Workflow Integration

In Section 21.4, we have already emphasized the relevance of seamless workflow integration. In medical applications, CBIR-based CAD may assist the radiologists, and all levels of integration from data to context are equally important. In this section, we focus on data and functional integration. Data integration, however, needs to be considered in both ways, PACS to CBIR and CBIR to PACS.

21.5.4.1 CBIR-Based Access to PACS Images

Within a DICOM-based PACS, any DICOM-conformant system may be integrated and retrieves images from the PACS archive using the DICOM Query/Retrieve (Q/R) services (Onken et al. 2011).

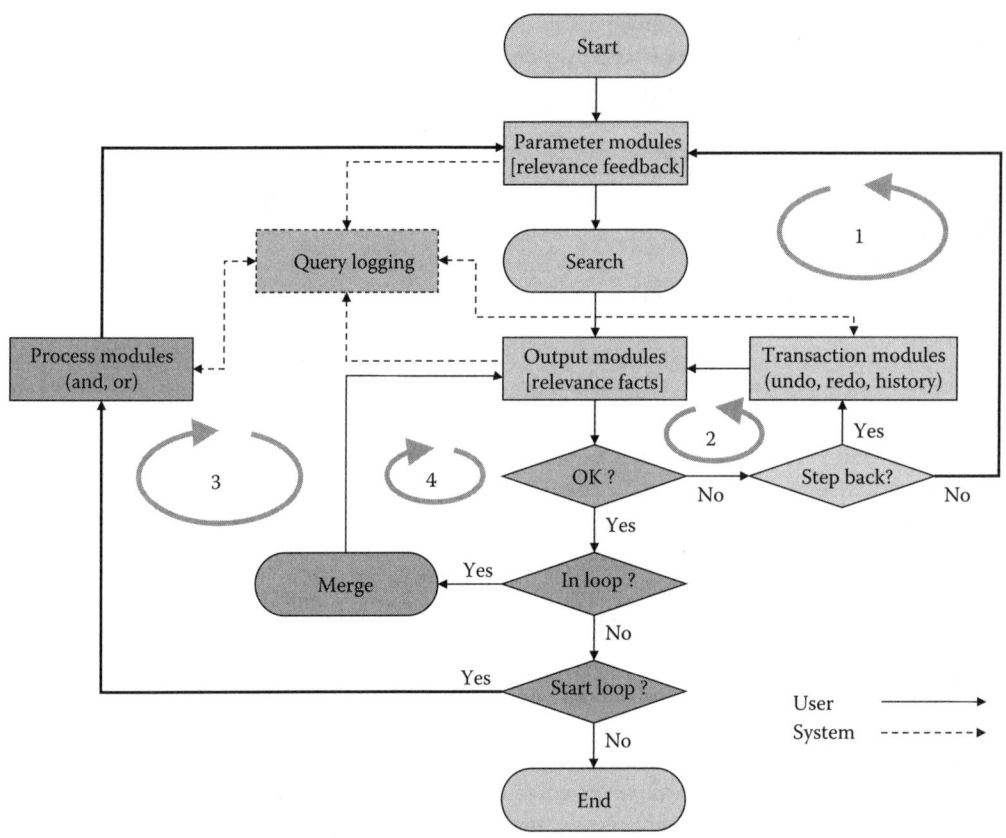

FIGURE 21.10 Flowchart of extended query refinement. (From Deserno TM et al. *J Digit Imaging.* 2008; 21(3): 280–289.)

Q/R offers different service object pair (SOP) classes for searching and retrieving, which are varying in what information can be searched and how transmission of objects is performed. In the query phase, an archive can be searched for images based on filter mechanisms, for example, it is possible to ask for a list of studies based on a defined patient name. If the service class user (SCU) decides to download any DICOM objects (retrieve phase), the Q/R protocol is used to initiate the transfer. However, the transmission itself is done via the DICOM Storage SOP classes. It is also possible for an SCU to tell the service class provider (SCP) not to transfer the DICOM objects to the SCU itself but to a third system. In this way, the reading application may also invoke a CBIR process by sending the QBE (functional integration).

The first approaches of CBIR-PACS integration based on DICOM have been proposed in 1999 (Qi and Snyder 1999). Le Bozec et al. have described new representational and retrieval models allowing hospital-wide access to the images based on demographic and procedure-type information and fostering CBIR to enhance the medical impact of image retrieval in daily practice. The approach was applied in the Gerorges Pompiduo Hospital in Paris, France (Le Bozec et al. 2000). More recently, Traina et al. have presented a novel PACS approach, called cbPACS, which provides content-based capabilities for image retrieval. The cbPACS answers range and *k*-NN similarity queries. By now, the system implemented works on features based on color distribution of the images through normalized histograms as well as metric histograms (Traina et al. 2005). Nonetheless, a recent review demonstrates the remaining gap between intensive CBIR research and development, and its effective use in clinical practice (Depeursinge et al. 2011).

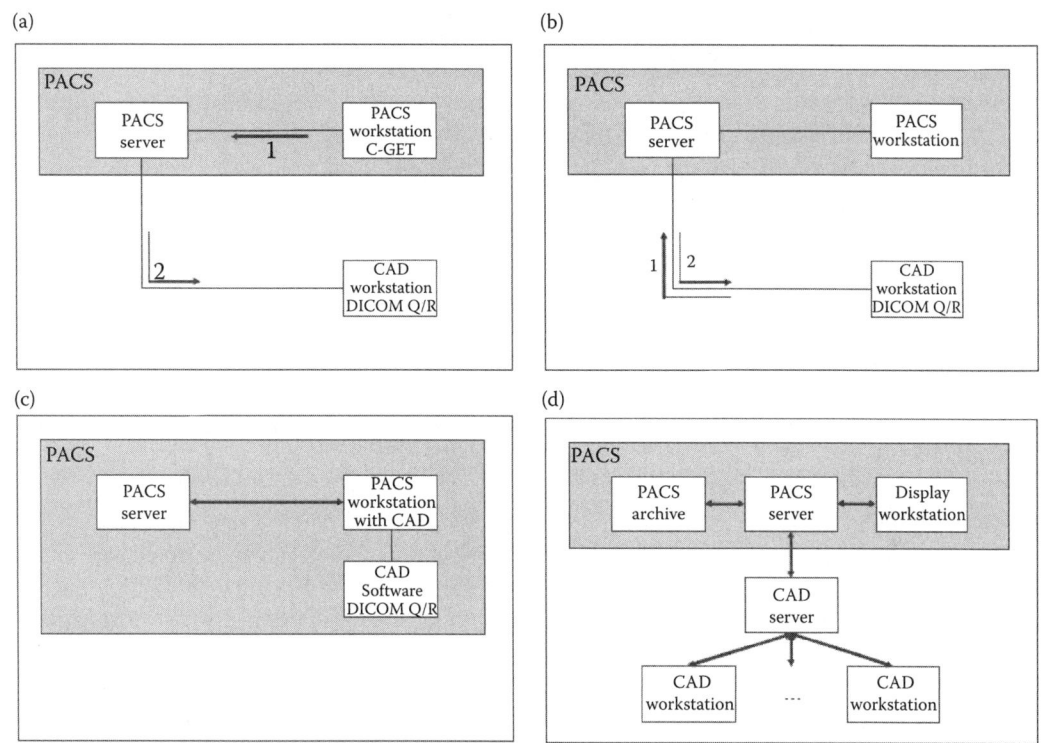

FIGURE 21.11 Conceptual methods of integration CAD with PACS. (From Huang HK et al. PACS-based computer-aided detection and diagnosis. Chapter 18 in Deserno, 2011; pp. 455–470.)

More methodically, data integration of CAD (including CBIR-based CAD) with DICOM PACS can have four approaches, which differ in the systems performing the query and retrieve commands (Huang et al. 2011). In panels (a), (b), and (c) of Figure 21.11, the CAD is connected directly to the PACS, while the fourth approach is to use a CAD server to connect with the PACS (Figure 21.11d). This is seen advantageous since DICOM must not be installed on the CBIR engine. The CAD server can automatically manage the clinical workflow of image studies to be processed and can archive the CAD results back to PACS, for the clinicians to review directly on the PACS workstation. This also eliminates the need for both the PACS and the CBIR manufacturer to open up their respective software platforms for installing an application programming interface (API).

Accordingly, a workflow management of CBIR for CAD support in PACS environments has been proposed recently by Welter et al. (2010). It is based on concepts developed by the Integrating the Healthcare Analysis (IHE) initiative, a consortium of healthcare professionals from industry and research that has been founded to establish unified and generally accepted process flows between information and communication technology (ICT) systems for medical applications improving interoperability. Information exchange is based on established standards like DICOM and Health Level 7 (HL7). IHE provides a framework that accumulates requirements in use cases and defines guidelines, called Integration Profiles, which represent scenarios and prescribe how well-known standards like DICOM shall be applied. Each scenario involves a set of actors, which represent components or modules that occur in medical information systems (MIS) such as the hospital information system (HIS).

21.5.4.2 Persistent Storing CBIR Results in PACS

However, CBIR-based CAD usually does not end up only with an image and some additional descriptive measures that have been created by the CAD software. Instead, it delivers a list of DICOM study unique

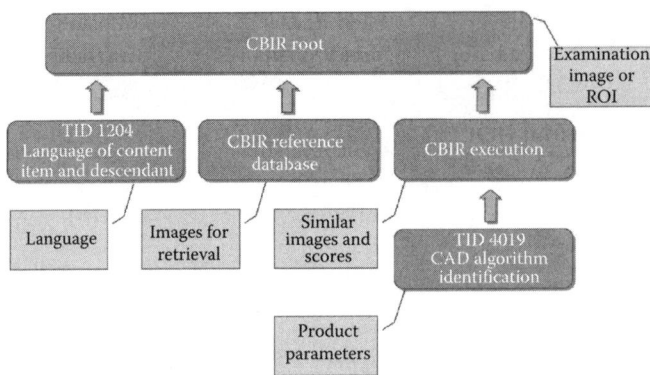

FIGURE 21.12   Composition of the CBIR SR template. (From Welter P et al. *J Am Med Informatics Assoc (JAMIA)*. 2011b; 18(4): 506–510.)

identifiers (UID) containing relevant images and pointing to relevant cases (electronic health record, EHR), which are already included within the HIS. This type of information cannot be stored back to the PACS by means of novel DICOM objects.

Here, DICOM Structured Reporting (SR) is an appropriate tool for designing persistent storage of CBIR results (Welter et al. 2011b). A CBIR-CAD DICOM-SR document is built from SR templates and includes information on the CBIR system, the QBE image or ROI of query, the reference database on which CBIR was performed, and a list of resulting image UIDs associated with similarity scores. In Figure 21.12, the template identifier (TID) refers to a predefined template from the DICOM standard.

21.5.4.3 Functional CAD-PACS Integration

In 2009, DICOM supplement 118 titled "Application Hosting" has become part of the standard. It may be regarded as the future of CAD-PACS coupling, including CBIR integration to the hospitals and clinical practice. It defines a generic API between the hosting systems and the hosted application that supports full integration on all the data, function, context, and presentation levels, since the application is now simply plugged into the clinical workstation, and all user interfaces remain from the hosting program. The API supports the entire software life cycle management. The hosting system is able to launch and terminate the hosted application. While running, hosting system and hosted application exchange input, processing, and output data, and communicate status information. This is done by the hosted application switching between several states (Onken et al. 2011), which are visualized in the state chart (Figure 21.13):

- *Idle*: waiting for a new task assignment from the hosting system. This is the initial state when the hosted application is started.
- *Inprogress*: performing the assigned task.
- *Suspended*: stopping processing and releasing as many resources as possible, while still preserving enough state to be able to continue processing.
- *Completed*: completing processing and waiting for the hosting system to access and release any output data.
- *Canceled*: stopping processing and releasing all resources giving up any chance to resume.
- *Exit*: terminating the service. This is the terminal state of the hosted application.

21.5.5 Combined Visual and Textual Retrieval

Disregarding all efforts on CBIR technology, it is important to realize that medical images are never created isolated. They are always embedded with rich annotations and metainformation, which may be

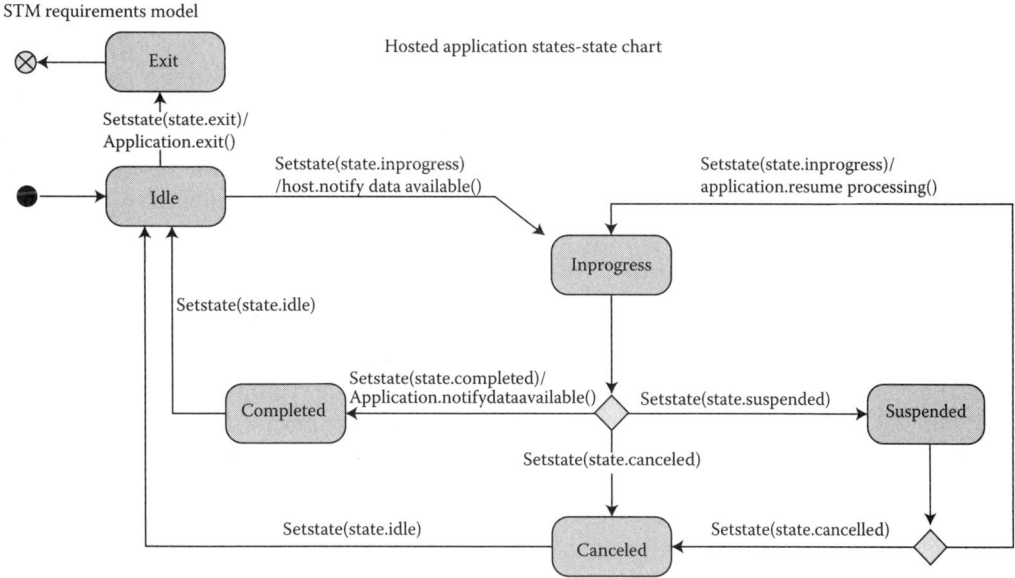

FIGURE 21.13 State chart of DICOM Application Hosting. (From DICOM Working Group 23. (ed). Digital Imaging and Communications in Medicine (DICOM) supplement 118 application hosting. Technical Report, DICOM Work Item 2004-09-E, 2010/09/30. Rosslyn, VA, USA.)

composed of either structured or unstructured text. Hence, CBIR shall always be combined with text-based retrieval methods based on either alphanumerical matches or natural language processing (NLP), respectively. Sinha et al. have reviewed methods to present imaging and associated data without causing an overload, including image study summarization using CBIR and NLP (Sinha et al. 2002).

Some examples are the works of Ruiz, combining image features, case descriptions, and unified medical language system (UMLS) concepts to improve retrieval of medical image (Ruiz 2006), and integrating this automatic classification method into the medical image retrieval process (Uwimana and Ruiz 2008). Three publicly available tools were combined: GIFT (cf. Section 21.2.3.1), a text retrieval system, and a tool for mapping free text to UMLS concepts. Data from the CLEF campaign was used for evaluation. Névéol et al. applied a set of 180 medical documents from a standard reference set in French language, combining the IRMA (cf. Section 21.2.3.2) engine with NLP and Medical Subject Heading (MeSH) mapping (Névéol et al. 2009). Another example of visual and textual combined retrieval is the cbPACS system (cf. Section 21.5.4.1). Here, the standard query language (SQL) was extended to seamlessly integrating similarity queries based on visual features resulting in a command language interpreter called Similarity Retrieval Engine (SiREn) (Barioni et al. 2009).

21.5.6 Evaluation

One of the most challenging tasks in medical image search is its comprehensive evaluation. Obviously, large databases with well-known references are required. As a response to the need for standardized test collections and evaluation forums, ImageCLEF was initiated in 2003. It has grown to become a preeminent venue today for image retrieval evaluation (Kalpathy-Cramer and Müller 2011). ImageCLEF itself also includes several subtracks dealing with various aspects of image retrieval (Müller et al. 2010).

One of these tracks is the IRMA image annotation task, where CBIR systems perform a categorization of images. In 2005 and 2006, the goal was a flat classification into 57 and 116 unique classes, respectively, and error rates based on the number of misclassified images have been used as evaluation metric (Deselaers et al. 2007). In 2007 and 2008, the hierarchical IRMA code (Lehmann et al. 2003) was used, and errors were penalized depending on the level of the hierarchy at which they occurred (Deselaers et al. 2008). Typically, participants were provided about 10,000 training images and were to submit classification for 1000 test images. All radiographs have been transferred into the IRMA system from the PACS of the Aachen University Hospital, Aachen, Germany, anonymized, and semiautomatically categorized by experienced physicians and radiologists providing the ground truth. Both secondarily scanned x-ray films and direct digitally acquired radiographs were included in the IRMA repository. In 2009, the goal was to classify 2000 test images using the different classification schemes used in 2005–2008, given a set of about 12,000 training images.

In ImageCLEF, the Medical Image Retrieval task's test collection has began with a rather small database of 8700 images as an amalgamation of several teaching case files in English, French, and German (Müller et al. 2004b). By 2007, it had grown to a collection of over 66,000 images from several teaching collections, as well as a set of topics that were known to be well suited for textual, visual, or mixed retrieval methods. The 2009 database already contained a total of 74,902 images (Kalpathy-Cramer and Müller 2011). However, such large collections cannot be annotated manually to provide a reliable ground truth. Hence, the results obtained by different CBIR methods in the campaign are merged and evaluated retrospectively by the experts. This method, however, leaves large parts of the repositories unexplored.

21.6 Examples

It is worth exemplarily describing outstanding CBIR approaches in more detail. Within the numerous fields of medical CBIR application that we have discussed already, case retrieval and CAD in diagnostics and research as well as medical document retrieval in research and education are focused in the following sections.

21.6.1 CBIR-Based Access to Medical Literature

It is self-suggesting to apply CBIR techniques to medical image repositories, and the medical literature itself is a prominent example. For instance, the 2005 volumes of (i) *New England Journal of Medicine*, (ii) *Radiology*, (iii) *Journal of Dental Research*, and (iv) *Journal of the American Medical Informatics Association* (JAMIA) in total contain about 11,753 journal pages and 11,238 figure panels (Deserno et al. 2009b).

Figure 21.14 demonstrates the variety of illustrations that can be found in the medical literature. On the top level, 12 categories have been defined:

1. *Diagnostic image*, that is, an original image as obtained from any medical imaging modality (e.g., radiography, microscopy, endoscopy, sonography) that may be color or grayscale and annotated.
2. *Diagnostic visualization*, that is, a color or grayscale computed visualization of medical image data, such as a 3D direct volume rendering of CT or MRI data.
3. *Photograph*, that is, any type of an optical static image, which, again, may be in color or grayscale and show devices, medical objects or situations, persons, or portraits.
4. *Screen shot*, that is, any illustration showing a computer screen, window, or a part thereof.
5. *Graph*, that is, any visualization of numerical data such as plots, curves, as well as block or pie charts.
6. *Diagram*, that is, any kind of functional or block diagram, scheme, or mind map.
7. *Drawing*, that is, any type of manual drawings.
8. *Multipanel figure*, that is, a composition of different parts, which may be composed of *strictly medical*.
9. *Nonmedical*, or.
10. *Mixed panels*, and may be presented in color or grayscale.
11. *Protein spot*, that is, a special type of multipanel figures, where the high number of spots (panels) frequently is ambiguous, and therefore, not countable.
12. *Other*, for instance, equations that are embedded in the PDF file as figure.

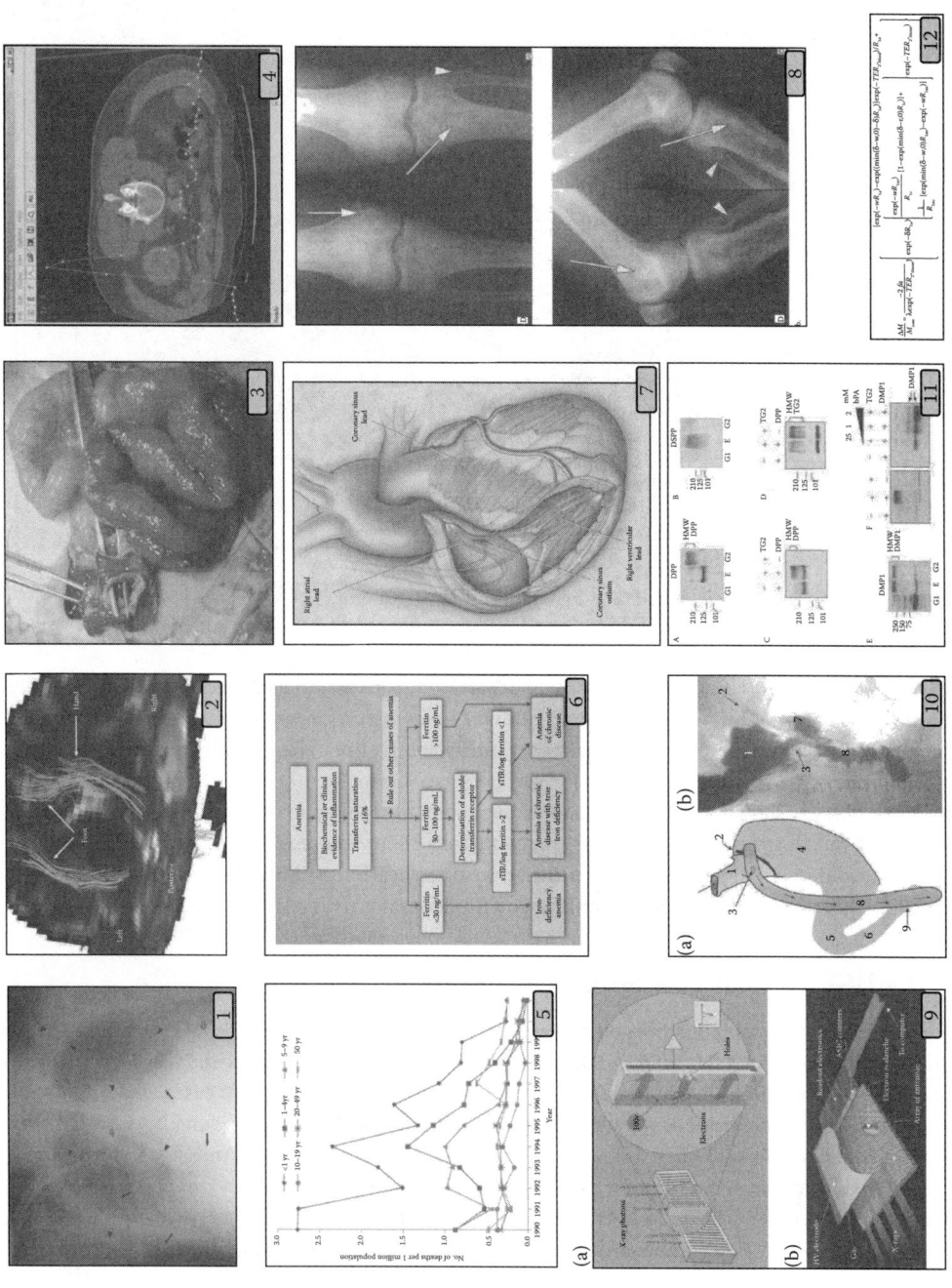

FIGURE 21.14 The 12 categories of images in medical scientific literature. (From Deserno TM, Antani S, and Long RL. *Methods Inf Med.* 2009b; 48(4): 371–380.)

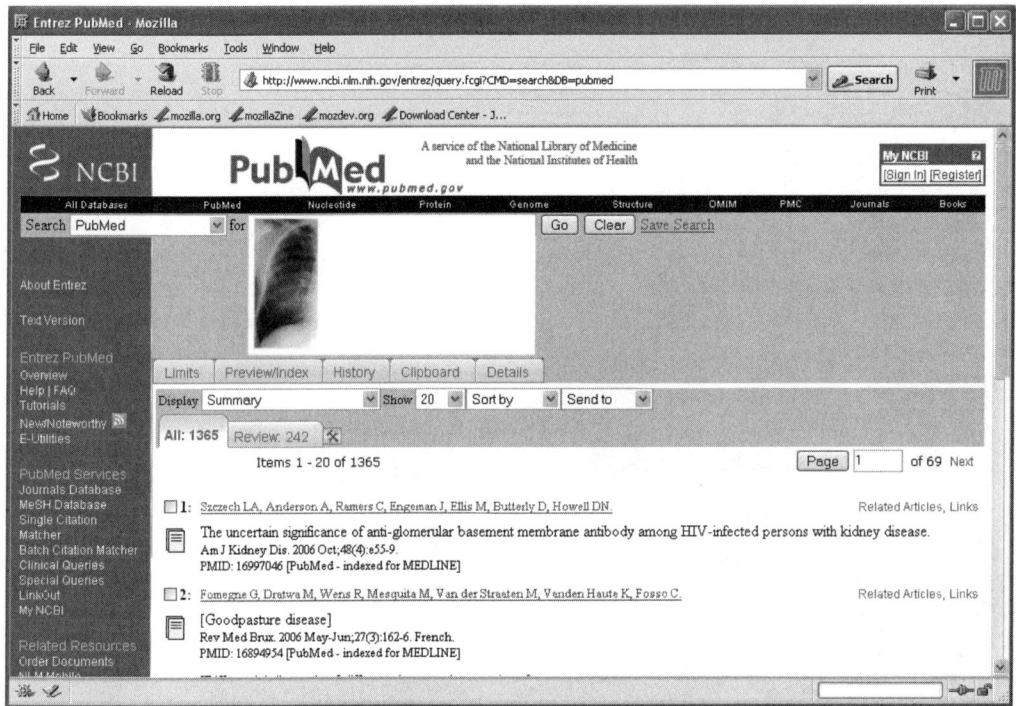

FIGURE 21.15 A vision on medical literature retrieval using CBIR technology.

Figure 21.15 visualizes the well-known PubMed Entrez screen, which has been expanded virtually to support CBIR-based queries. Deserno et al. (2009b) have shown exemplarily that combining textual and visual retrieval methods may improve the query completion when seeking scientific medical literature.

Accordingly, Müller has emphasized the enormous potential from content-based access to images in the scientific literature as physicians can directly compare a current case with similar existing cases in the peer-reviewed literature (Müller 2008). However, such applications still need to be implemented and integrated with the clinical patient record and large knowledge archives of literature.

21.6.2 CBIR-Based CBR for Surgery Planning

A case-based CBIR system for surgical planning of bone fractures has been developed at HUG (Zhou et al. 2011) and demonstrated live at the CADdemo@CARS 2010 (Depeursinge et al. 2011). It is using an image database built at the surgery department of HUG containing 2693 fracture cases associated with 43 different fracture types. Beside images, a few clinical attributes such as age, gender, implant type, and exact diagnosis are available in XML files. The fracture retrieval engine is based purely on visual information extracted from image content and the diagnosis information is used for evaluation only. Images are indexed using a bag of visual words strategy, where local descriptors based on SIFT are obtained at fixed positions (cf. Section 21.5.1.2). Finally, each image is represented by a histogram of 1000 numerical features.

Figure 21.16 shows the case-based query interface. Similarity measurements based on histogram intersection are used to rank the returned cases. Both query and results are case-based and contain multiple images. A fusion strategy based on a mix of sum and max operators is used (Zhou et al. 2011).

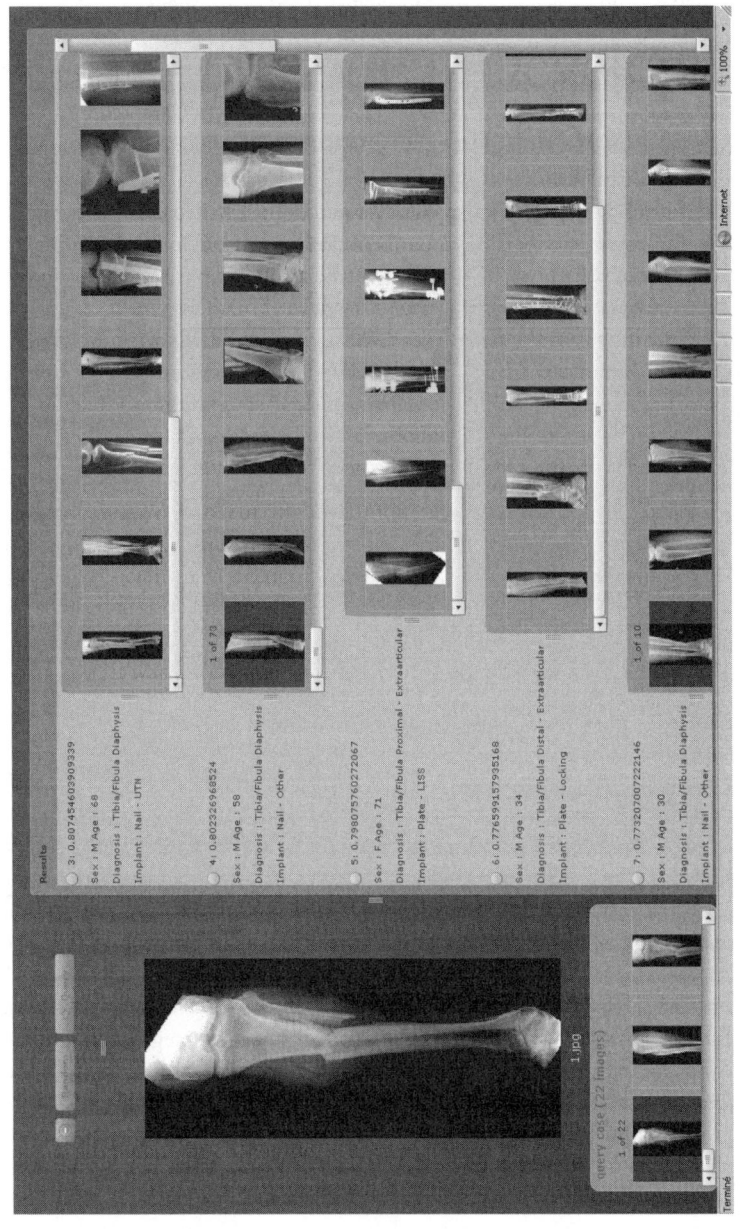

FIGURE 21.16 GUI for visual retrieval of fracture cases. (From Depeursinge A et al. *Open Med Imaging J.* 2011; 5 Suppl 1-M7: 58–72.)

21.6.3 CBIR-Based CAD for Bone Age Assessment

Recently, Depeursinge et al. have identified four CBIR-based CAD systems with a high degree of "user readiness" (Depeursinge et al. 2011). For example, with its underlying flexible structure of image processing and image retrieval algorithms, the IRMA framework has been adjusted to enrich CAD in the context of bone age assessment (BAA) (Fischer et al. 2011). Similar radiographs with validated ages are retrieved from a reference database and presented to the radiologist along with a suggested bone age. The reference database contains about 1000 hand radiographs, corresponding epiphysial ROIs, and metainformation such as gender, ethnic origin, chronological age, and the validated bone age from expert's readings.

For a new hand radiograph, the processing pipeline consists of four steps:

1. *Center localization*: At first, the centers of the epiphyses are localized. Optionally, manual and automatic methods can be applied.
2. *Region extraction*: A bounding box is adjusted automatically around these centers, scaled and extracted, yielding epiphysial ROIs in standard vertical orientation for the CBIR part of IRMA-BAA.
3. *CBIR query*: With each extracted ROI, a QBE k-NN query is performed (cf. Section 21.5.2). Similar images are returned with similarity scoring and validated bone age.
4. *Age assessment*: The overall bone age is predicted by a similarity score-weighted mean of ages associated to the response images.

The IRMA framework provides several modules for integration of CBIR into web-based interfaces (cf. Section 21.5.3.3). Using this technology, the result of CBIR-based age estimation is presented to the user (Figure 21.17). The query image and its extracted ROIs are shown at the top-most area of the interface. Their most similar counterparts retrieved from the database are shown below (scrollable) in decreasing similarity and with the validated bone age. The estimated bone age is shown below the query image. If the query image is contained in the demo database, the validated bone age is also provided. A click on one of the thumbnails opens the full-resolution image. The display mode can also be switched to show the hands belonging to the retrieved ROIs. In leaving-one-out experiments, a mean absolute error of 0.97 years and a variance of 0.63 were observed over all ages and regardless of gender (Fischer et al. 2011).

21.7 Summary and Conclusions

In this chapter, we have explored the relevance and state of the art of medical image search by means of CBIR techniques. Initially focused on nonmedical image repositories, and using color as most relevant feature, CBIR has been established in the commercial markets in the early 2000s. Deducted from the relevance of images in general and the relevance of medical images in particular, we have explored general fields of biomedical engineering, where CBIR methodology can be applied meaningfully in medical practice, including diagnostic, research, and medical education. The state of the art has been described regarding features and similarity measures, user interaction, workflow integration, combined visual and textual retrieval, and evaluation of medical CBIR systems. Exemplarily, three outstanding approaches have been described in detail, regarding CBIR-based access to medical literature, CBIR-based CBR for surgery planning, and CBIR-based CAD for maturity measurements.

Despite such user-ready implementations, CBIR technology in general has not yet been established in clinical practice. With respect to the concept of gaps that we have described in Section 21.4, current systems adequately narrow the semantic gap focusing on a particular imaging and application domain. However, this specific use context is hindering the transfer into other application domains in clinical practice. Future CBIR applications in the medical domain shall aim at more generic architectures, principles, and interfaces to support rapid prototyping and implementation in other fields of medical applications.

Nonetheless, today's prototype systems have bridged the various feature gaps, and efficiency has been proven on relatively large databases of reference and ground truth images. This can be seen as a prerequisite

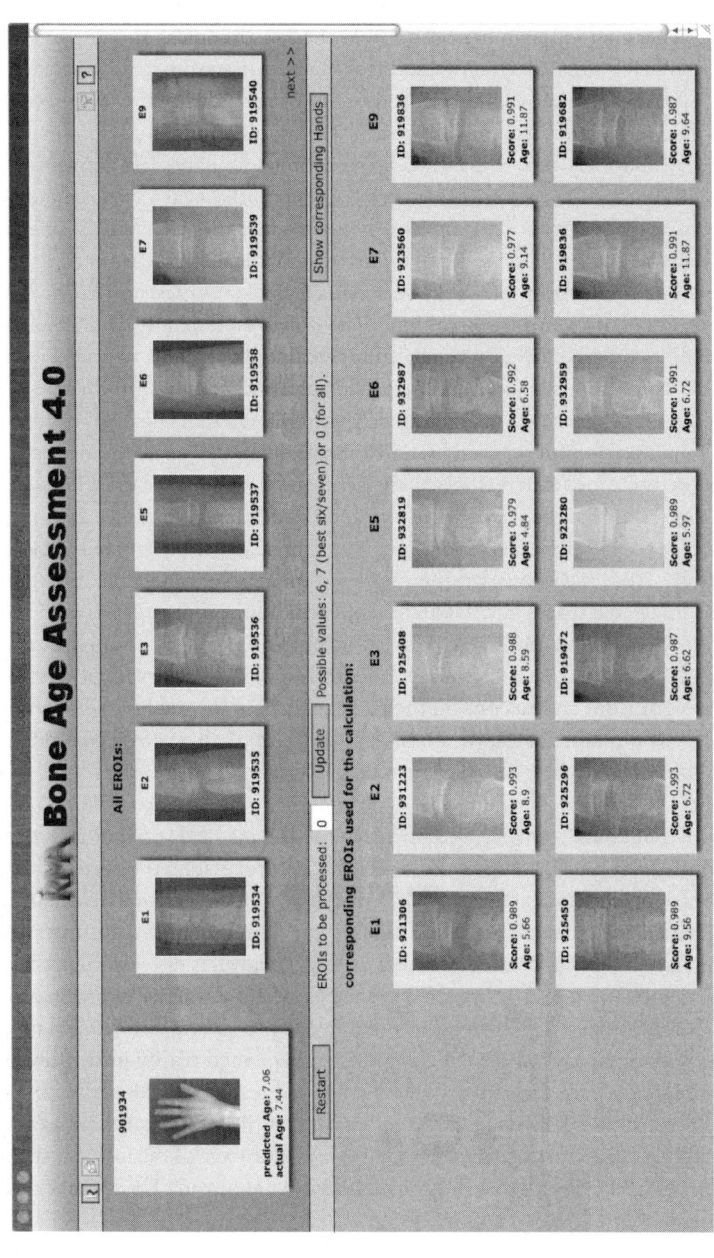

FIGURE 21.17 IRMA bone age assessment. (From Fischer B et al. *Int J Computer Assisted Radiol Surgery*. 2012; 7(3): 389–399.)

for any system in the field of CBIR-based CAD. However, user interaction and system integration still need improvement. So far, stand-alone systems are demonstrated, which are inappropriately integrated in the hospital information system environments. DICOM Hosted Application and DICOM Structured Reporting might be suitable concepts in bridging the integration gap (Welter et al. 2011b).

Müller has suggested establishing small modules or blocks, developed in open-source projects and made available to a large community free of charge, to foster the development of CBIR in medicine (Müller 2008). Plug-in technology, as it has been established in the Internet, is a good example of the impact obtained from open interfaces. Google Earth, for instance, is easily interconnected with any website, and the web browser itself offers various options to plug-in and combine other pieces of software.

However, the large reference databases that are needed for development and evaluation of medical CBIR systems are seen more crucial. Until now, sufficient data is unavailable, and the ground truth provided along with the images cannot always be trusted. Currently, legal affairs, data privacy policies, and other restrictions must be coped with laboriously to build a medical reference image database. In particular, written consent is needed for academia research if patient images are used else than personal diagnostic. On the other hand, social networks such as Facebook, Twitter, and Flickr have shown the intrinsic vigilance of the entire human population to share personal details. Soon, technology will be available to host medical images in the Internet, and educated individuals will take over the responsibility of their EHR. This will foster medical image sharing, and preparation of large medical image repositories including images and metainformation. Then, the need to navigate in databases of billions of medical images in a meaningful way, allowing efficient and effective retrieval satisfying the user, will become even more prominent. Here, it also seems necessary to better integrate visual, textual, and structured data retrieval into unique systems (Müller and Deserno 2011).

Anyway, reference annotations and reliable ground truth still need trusted establishment. For example, Horsch et al. (2011) have assessed the needs for the next-generation computer-aided mammography reference image databases and evaluation studies. The authors developed 13 recommendations concerning the construction and usage of a test database, as well as the application of statistical evaluation methods. In particular, a test database should ultimately reflect realistic clinical conditions, in order to allow for significant conclusions on the performance of the method or system under evaluation. Furthermore, a clear picture of the variability of a measure shall be given by reporting either the corresponding standard deviation or standard error, or the confidence interval, that is, the range of values which are likely.

As we have emphasized already, the 3D and 4D nature of the medical imagery is not yet sufficiently coped in both medical CBIR user interfaces and system's data processing. Interactive navigation in 3D and 4D data, its manual annotation, and the process of fast and efficient browsing according databases requires novel human machine interfaces and fast processing methods. Again, consumer industry might have a large impact on medical applications. Game industry already has developed powerful but—since huge numbers of pieces are being sold—inexpensive devices for 3D computer interaction. Parallel computing on GPU is already used successfully in medical image processing, and tablet computers (iPad) have been established in the operation theatre supporting augmented reality in surgery (Volonté et al. 2011). Furthermore, Mezzana et al. have introduced augmented reality in oculoplastic and orbit surgery through a simple iPhone application evaluating the position of the lateral canthal ligament (Mezzana et al. 2011). Such examples show how the medical field takes advantage of the lower costs of technology adaptation than technology development. The consumer has paid already for device development that is now used in medicine.

Another cost-intensive field is drug development, where a paradigm change has been noticed. Individualized medicine and personalized drug development are fostered, and medical imaging is expected to provide surrogate endpoints in clinical trials (Rosenkranz 2003). Pharmaceutical industry will face the need for large reference databases and efficient techniques for image-based data search, providing much more financial power than medical technology industry, which is reimbursed rather slowly by the public health insurance systems. 3D and 4D ultrasound visualizations in prenatal imaging or full-body CT scans are other examples emphasizing the impact of economic interests in medical imaging and image management technology.

Another point that is particular important for medical image search using CBIR technology is that medical image processing has not yet reached the level of scene interpretation. As we have emphasized in the introduction, computer-based image analysis still is by far less powerful than the human visual system. We have presented approaches for graph representations, where the nodes correspond to objects in the image and the edges in the graph describe their constellation in temporal and/or spatial domains. Such annotated graphs will form the basis of Web 2.0 technology, which is about to be delivered. Annotating hyperlinks with certain characteristics will enable search engines such as Google to retrieve information more selectively and provide a much better query completion. Such novel technologies will boost medical image search on both levels: scene analysis within an image and CBIR-based CBR within the entire medical databases.

All in all, medical image search is active field of biomedical engineering, which is expected to develop quickly by adopting technology and processing knowledge from other fields such as consumer industry, the Internet, and Web 2.0 technology.

References

Aamodt A and Plaza E. Case-based reasoning: Foundational issues, methodological variations, and system approaches. *AICom—Artif Intell Commun*. 1994; 7(1): 39–59.

Aggarwal CC, Hinneburg A, and Keim DA. On the surprising behavior of distance metrics in high dimensional space. *Lect Notes Computer Sci*. 2001; 1973: 420–434.

Analoui M. Quantitative medical image analysis for clinical development of therapeutics. Chapter 14 in Deserno, 2011; pp. 359–374.

Avni U, Greenspan H, Konen E, Sharon M, and Goldberger J. X-ray categorization and retrieval on the organ and pathology level using patch-based visual words. *IEEE Trans Med Imaging*. 2011; 30(3): 733–746.

Barioni MCN, Razente HL, Traina AJM, and Traina C, Jr. Seamlessly integrating similarity queries in SQL. *Software: Practice Experience*. 2009; 39(4): 355–384.

Belongie S, Carson C, Greenspan H, and Malik J. Color- and texture-based image segmentation using EM and its application to content-based image retrieval. *Sixth International Conference on Computer Vision (IEEE Cat. No.98CH36271)*. Narosa Publishing House, New Delhi, India, 1998; pp. 675–682.

Canny JF. A computational approach to edge detection. *IEEE Trans Pattern Anal Mach Intell*. 1986; 8(6): 679–698.

Carson C, Belongie S, Greenspan H, and Malik J. Blobworld: Image segmentation using expectation-maximization and its application to image querying. *IEEE Trans Pattern Anal Mach Intell*. 2002; 24(8): 1026–1038.

Chang SK and Kunii T. Pictorial database systems. *IEEE Comput*. 1981; 14(11): 13–21.

Comaniciu D, Meer P, Foran D et al. Bimodal system for interactive indexing and retrieval of pathology images. *Proc IEEE Workshop Appl Comput*. 1998; 76–81.

de Geus-Oei LF, van der Heijden HFM, Visser EP, Hermsen R, van Hoorn BA, Timmer-Bonte JNH, Willemsen AT, Pruim J, Corstens FHM, Krabbe PFM, and Oyen WJG. Chemotherapy response evaluation with 18F-FDG PET in patients with non-small cell lung cancer. *J Nucl Med*. 2007; 48: 1592–1598.

de Groot E, Hovingh GK, Wiegman A, Duriez P, Smit AJ, Fruchart J-C, and Kastelein JJP. Measurement of arterial wall thickness as a surrogate marker for atherosclerosis. *Circulation*. 2004; 109: 33–38.

De Lone WH and Mc Lean ER. Information systems success: The quest for the dependent variable. *Inf Syst Res*. 1992; 3(1): 60–95.

De Lone WH and Mc Lean ER. The DeLone and McLean Model of information systems success: A ten-year update. *J Manage Inf Syst*. 2003; 19(4): 9–30.

De Oliveira JEE, Machado AMC, Chavez GC et al. MammoSys: A content-based image retrieval system using breast density patterns. *Comput Methods Programs Biomed.* 2010; 99(3): 289–297.

Depeursinge A, Fischer B, Müller H, and Deserno TM. Prototypes for content-based image retrieval in clinical practice. *Open Med Imaging J.* 2011; 5 Suppl 1-M7: 58–72.

Deselaers T, Müller H, Clough P, Ney H, and Lehmann TM. The CLEF 2005 automatic medical image annotation task. *Int J Computer Vis.* 2007; 74(1): 51–58.

Deselaers T, Deserno TM, and Müller H. Automatic medical image annotation in ImageCLEF 2007. Overview, results, and discussion. *Pattern Recognit Lett.* 2008; 29(15): 1988–1995.

Deserno TM, Güld MO, Plodowski B, Spitzer K, Wein BB, Schubert H, Ney H, and Seidl T. Extended query refinement for medical image retrieval. *J Digit Imaging.* 2008; 21(3): 280–289.

Deserno TM, Antani S, and Long R. Ontology of gaps in content-based image retrieval. *J Digit Imaging.* 2009a; 22(2): 202–215.

Deserno TM, Antani S, and Long RL. Content-based image retrieval for scientific literature access. *Methods Inf Med.* 2009b; 48(4): 371–380.

Deserno TM (ed). *Biomedical Image Processing. Series 3740: Biological and Medical Physics, Biomedical Engineering.* Springer, Berlin, 2011.

Deserno TM. Fundamentals of biomedical image processing. Chapter 1 in Deserno, 2011; pp. 1–51.

DICOM Working Group 23. (ed). Digital Imaging and Communications in Medicine (DICOM) supplement 118 application hosting. Technical Report, DICOM Work Item 2004-09-E, 2010/09/30. Rosslyn, VA, USA.

Doll WJ and Torkzadeh G. The measurement of end-user computing satisfaction. *MIS Quarterly.* 1988; 12(2): 259–274.

Doll WJ and Torkzadeh G. The measurement of end-user computing satisfaction: Theoretical considerations. *MIS Quarterly.* 1991; 15(1): 5–10.

Eakins J and Graham M. Content-based image retrieval. Technical Report No 39, JISC Technology Applications Programme, University of Northumbria at Newcastle, October 1999.

Fischer B, Thies C, Güld MO, and Lehmann TM. Content-based retrieval of medical images by matching hierarchical attributed region adjacency graphs. *Procs SPIE.* 2004; 5370: 598–606.

Fischer B, Sauren M, Güld MO, and Deserno TD. Scene analysis with structural prototypes for content-based image retrieval in medicine. *Procs SPIE.* 2008; 6914: 1X1–1X9.

Fischer B, Welter P, Günther RW, and Deserno TM. Web-based bone age assessment by content-based image retrieval for case-based reasoning. *Int J Computer Assisted Radiol Surgery.* 2011; 7(3): 389–399.

Geusebroek JM, van den Boogaard R, Smeulders AWM et al. Color invariance. *IEEE Trans Pattern Anal Mach Intell.* 2001; 23(12): 1338–1350.

Gijselaers W. Perspectives on problem-based learning; Chapter 5 in Gijselaers W, Tempelaar D, Keizer P, Blommaert J, Bernard E, and Kapser H (eds). *Educational Innovation in Economics and Business Administration: The Case of Problem-Based Learning.* Kluwer, Dordrecht, 1995; pp. 39–52.

Gordon IE. *Theories of Visual Perception.* Wiley, Chichester, 1989.

Greenes RA. The radiologist as clinical activist—A time to focus outward. *Proceedings of the First International Conference on Image Management and Communication in Patient Care—Implementation and Impact.* IEEE Computer Society Press, Washington, 1989; pp. 136–140.

Greenspan H and Pinhas AT. Medical image categorization and retrieval for PACS using the GMM-KL framework. *IEEE Trans Inf Technol Biomed.* 2007; 11(2): 190–202.

Guyatt G, Cairns J, Churchill D et al. Evidence-based medicine. A new approach to teaching the practice of medicine. *J Am Med Assoc.* 1992; 268(17): 2420–2425.

Hand D, Manila H, and Smyth P. *Principles of Data Mining.* MIT Press, Cambridge, MA, 2001.

Haralick RM, Shanmugam K, and Dinstein I. Textural features for image classification. *IEEE Trans Syst Man Cybern.* 1973; 3(6): 610–621.

Horsch A, Hapfelmeier A, and Elter M. Needs assessment for next generation computer-aided mammography reference image databases and evaluation studies. *Int J CARS.* 2011; 6(6):749–767.

Huang HK, Liu BJ, Le AH, and Documet J. PACS-based computer-aided detection and diagnosis. Chapter 18 in Deserno, 2011; pp. 455–470.

Jaffe CC. Response assessment in clinical trials: Implications for sarcoma clinical trial design. *The Oncologist.* 2008; 13(Suppl 2): 14–18.

Jain AK, Duin RPW, and Mao J. Statistical pattern recognition: A review. *IEEE Trans Pattern Anal Mach Intell.* 2000; 22(1): 4–37.

Kalpathy-Cramer J and Müller H. Systematic evaluations and ground truth. Chapter 20 in Deserno, 2011; pp. 497–520.

Koh GC, Khoo HE, Wong ML, and Koh D. The effects of problem-based learning during medical school on physician competency: A systematic review. *CMAJ.* 2008; 178(1): 34–41.

Kuo WJ, Chang RF, Lee CC et al. Retrieval technique for the diagnosis of solid breast tumors on sonogram. *Ultrasound Med Biol.* 2002; 28(7): 903–909.

Lapeer RJ, Tan AC, and Aldridge R. A combined approach to 3D medical image segmentation using marker-based watersheds and active contours: The active watershed method. *Lect Notes Computer Sci.* 2002; 2488: 596–603.

Le Bozec C, Zapletal E, Jaulent MC, Heudes D, and Degoulet P. Towards content-based image retrieval in a HIS-integrated PACS. *Proc AMIA Symp.* 2000; 477–481. 1

Lehmann TM, Wein B, Dahmen J, Bredno J, Vogelsang F, and Kohnen M. Content-based image retrieval in medical applications. A novel multi-step approach. *Procs SPIE.* 2000; 3972: 312–320.

Lehmann TM, Schubert H, Keysers D, Kohnen M, and Wein BB. The IRMA code for unique classification of medical images. *Procs SPIE.* 2003; 5033: 440–451.

Lehmann TM, Güld MO, Thies C, Fischer B, Spitzer K, Keysers D, Ney H, Kohnen M, Schubert H, and Wein BB. Content-based image retrieval in medical applications. *Methods Inf Med.* 2004; 43(4): 354–361.

Lehmann TM. Digitale Bildverarbeitung für Routineanwendungen. Evaluierung und Integration am Beispiel der Medizin. Deutscher Universitäts-Verlag, Wiesbaden 2005. ISBN 3-8244-2191-7 (in German).

Leisch E, Sartzetakis S, Tsiknakis M, and Orphanoudakis SC. A framework for the integration of distributed autonomous healthcare information systems. *Medical Informatics, Special Issue.* 1997; 22(4): 325–335.

Loncaric S. A survey of shape analysis techniques. *Pattern Recognit.* 1998; 31(8): 983–1001.

Lowe DG. Distinctive image features from scale-invariant keypoints. *Int J Computer Vision.* 2004; 60(2): 91–110.

Lu CS and Chung PC. Wold features for unsupervised texture segmentation. *Proc Int Conf Pattern Recognit Lett.* 1998; 2: 1689–1693.

Lucchese L and Mitra SK. Unsupervised segmentation of color images based on k-means clustering in the chromaticity plane. *Proc Content Based Access of Image and Video Libraries.* 1999; 74–78.

Macura RT and Macura K. Case-based reasoning: Opportunities and applications in health care. *Artif Intell Med.* 1997; 9(1): 1–4.

Mezzana P, Scarinci F, and Marabottini N. Augmented reality in oculoplastic surgery: First iPhone application. *Plast Reconstr Surg.* 2011; 127(3): 57e–58e.

Mikolajczyk K and Schmid C. A performance evaluation of local descriptors. *IEEE Trans Pattern Anal Mach Intell.* 2005; 27(10): 1615–1630.

Milanese R and Cherbuliez M. A rotation, translation and scale-invariant approach to content-based image retrieval. *J Vis Commun Image Represent.* 1999; 10: 186–196.

Müller H, Fabry P, Lovis C, and Geissbuhler A. medGIFT—Retrieving medical image by their visual content, in *World Summit of the Information Society, Forum Science and Society,* 2003.

Müller H, Michoux N, Bandon D, and Geissbuhler A. A review of content-based image retrieval systems in medical applications. Clinical benefits and future directions. *Int J Med Inform.* 2004a; 73(1): 1–23.

Müller H, Rosset A, Vallée JP, Terrier F, and Geissbuhler A. A reference data set for the evaluation of medical image retrieval systems. *Comput Med Imaging Graph.* 2004b; 28(6): 295–305.

Müller H, Lovis C, and Geissbuhler A. Medical image retrieval and the medGIFT project, in *Medical Imaging and Telemedicine (MIT 2005)*, pp. 2–7, 2005.

Müller H. Medical multimedia retrieval 2.0. *Yearb Med Inform.* 2008; 55–63.

Müller H, Clough P, Deselaers T, and Caputo B (eds). *ImageCLEF: Experimental Evaluation in Visual Information Retrieval.* Springer, Berlin, 2010.

Müller H and Deserno TM. Content-based medical image retrieval. Chapter 19 in Deserno, 2011; pp. 471–494.

Névéol A, Deserno TM, Darmoni SJ, Güld MO, and Aronson AR. Natural language processing versus content-based image analysis for medical document retrieval. *J Am Soc Inf Sci Technol.* 2009; 60(1): 123–34.

Niblack W, Barber R, Equitz W, Flickner MD, Glasman EH, Petkovic D, Yanke, P, Faloutsos C, and Taubin G. The QBIC Project: Querying images by content, using color, texture, and shape. *Proc. Storage Retrieval Image Video Databases (SPIE).* 1993; 1908: 173–187.

Onken M, Eichelberg M, Riesmeier J, and Jentsch P. Digital imaging and communications in medicine. Chapter 17 in Deserno, 2011; pp. 427–454.

Pele O and Werman M. A linear time histogram metric for improved SIFT matching. *Lect Notes Computer Sci.* 2008; 5304: 495–508.

Qi H and Snyder WE. Content-based image retrieval in picture archiving and communications systems. *J Digit Imaging.* 1999; 12(2 Suppl 1): 81–83.

Rosenkranz B. Biomarkers and surrogate endpoints in clinical drug development. *Appl Clin Trials.* 2003; 7: 30–40.

Ruiz ME. Combining image features, case descriptions and UMLS concepts to improve retrieval of medical images. *AMIA Annu Symp Proc.* 2006; 674–678.

Sackett DL, Rosenberg WM, Gray JA, Haynes RB, and Richardson WS. Evidence based medicine: What it is and what it isn't. *BMJ.* 1996 13; 312(7023): 71–72.

Scholl I, Aach T, Deserno TM, and Kuhlen T. Challenges of medical image processing: From kilo- to tera-byte. *Computer Sci Res Dev.* 2011; 26(1): 5–13.

Shyu CR, Brodley CE, Kak AC et al. ASSERT: A physician-in-the-loop content-based retrieval system for HRCT image databases. *Comput Vis Image Underst.* 1999; 75(1–2): 111–132.

Siggelkow S. *Feature Histograms for Content-Based Image Retrieval.* PhD Thesis. University of Freiburg, Freiburg im Breisgau, Germany, 2002.

Silverman M. Clinical trial end points at different phases of clinical development. Technical Report, BioStrategics Consulting Ltd, 2011.

Sinha U, Bui A, Taira R, Dionisio J, Morioka C, Johnson D, and Kangarloo H. A review of medical imaging informatics. *Ann N Y Acad Sci.* 2002; 980: 168–197.

Sivic J and Zisserman A. Video Google: Efficient visual search of videos. *Lecture Notes in Computer Science* 2006; 4170: 127–14.

Smeulders AWM, Worring M, Santini S, Gupta A, and Jain R. Content-based image retrieval at the end of the early years. *IEEE Trans Pattern Anal Mach Intell.* 2000; 22(12): 1349–1380.

Squire DM, Müller W, Müller H et al. Content-based query of image databases: Inspirations from text retrieval. *Pattern Recognit Lett.* 2000; 21(13–14): 1193–1198.

Tamura H, Mori S, and Yamawaki T. Texture features corresponding to visual perception. *IEEE Trans Systems, Man Cybernetics.* 1978; 8(6): 460–473.

Thodberg HH, Kreiborg S, Juul A, and Pedersen KD. The BoneXpert method for automated determination of skeletal maturity. *IEEE Trans Med Imaging.* 2009; 28(1): 52–66.

Traina AJM, Traina C Jr, Balan AGR, Ribeiro MX, Bugatti PH, Watanabe CYVW, and Paulo M. Feature extraction and selection for decision making. Chapter 8 in Deserno, 2011; pp. 197–223.

Traina C Jr, Traina AJ, Araújo MR, Bueno JM, Chino FJ, Razente H, and Azevedo-Marques PM. Using an image-extended relational database to support content-based image retrieval in a PACS. *Comput Methods Programs Biomed.* 2005; 80(Suppl 1): S71–S83.

Tversky A. Features of similarity. *Psychol Rev.* 1977; 84(4): 327–352.

Uwimana E and Ruiz ME. Integrating an automatic classification method into the medical image retrieval process. *AMIA Annu Symp Proc.* 2008; 747–751.

Volonté F, Robert JH, Ratib O, and Triponez FA. Lung segmentectomy performed with 3D reconstruction images available on the operating table with an iPad. *Interact Cardiovasc Thorac Surg.* 2011; March 8; 12(6): 1066–1068 (Epub ahead of print).

Warach S. Use of diffusion and perfusion magnetic resonance imaging as a tool in acute stroke clinical trials. *Curr Control Trials Cardiovasc Med.* 2001; 2: 38–44.

Welter P, Hocken C, Deserno TM, Grouls C, and Günther RW. Workflow management of content-based image retrieval for CAD support in PACS environments based on IHE. *Int J Comput Assist Radiol Surg.* 2010; 5(4): 393–400.

Welter P, Spreckelsen C, Fischer B, Günther RW, and Deserno TM. Case-based medical learning in radiological decision making using content-based image retrieval. *BMC.* 2011a; 11(68).

Welter P, Riesmeier J, Fischer B, Grouls C, Kuhl C, and Deserno TM. Bridging the integration gap from imaging to information systems: A uniform data concept for content-based image retrieval in computer-aided diagnosis. *J Am Med Informatics Assoc (JAMIA).* 2011b 18(4): 506–510.

Wertheimer M. Über Gestalttheorie. Vortrag vor der Kant-Gesellschaft, Berlin am 17. Dezember 1924. Verlag der Philosophischen Akademie, Erlangen 1925, in German.

Winter A and Nastar C. Differential feature distribution maps for image segmentation and region queries in image databases. *Proc Content-Based Access of Image and Video Libraries.* 1999; 9–17.

Winter A, Haux R, Ammenwerth E, Brigl B, Hellrung N, and Jahn F. *Health Information Systems: Architectures and Strategies.* Springer, Berlin 2010.

Wood DF. ABC of learning and teaching in medicine. Problem based learning. *BMJ.* 2003; 326(7384): 328–330.

Zhou X, Stern R, and Müller H. Multi-scale salient point-based retrieval of fracture cases. *Proc SPIE.* 2011; 7967: 06.

III

Infrared Imaging

Mary Diakides
Advanced Concepts Analysis, Inc.

Preface

The evolution of technological advances in infrared sensor technology, image processing, "smart" algorithms, knowledge-based databases, and their overall system integration has resulted in new methods of research and use in medical infrared imaging. The development of infrared cameras with focal plane arrays no longer requiring cooling added a new dimension to this modality. New detector materials with improved thermal sensitivity are now available, and production of high-density focal plane arrays (640 × 480) has been achieved. Advance read-out circuitry using on-chip signal processing is now commonly used. These breakthroughs permit low-cost and easy-to-use camera systems with thermal sensitivity less than 50 mK, as well as spatial resolution of 25–50 μm, given the appropriate optics. Another important factor is the emerging interest in the development of smart image processing algorithms to enhance the interpretation of thermal signatures. In the clinical area, new research addresses the key issues of diagnostic sensitivity and specificity of infrared imaging. Increased efforts are underway to achieve quantitative clinical data interpretation in standardized diagnostic procedures. For this purpose, clinical protocols and appropriate training are emphasized.

New concepts such as dynamic thermal imaging and thermal texture mapping (thermal tomography) and thermal multispectral imaging are being commonly used in clinical environments. Other areas such as three-dimensional infrared are being investigated.

These new ideas, concepts, and technologies are covered in this section. We have assembled a set of chapters that range in content from historical background, concepts, clinical applications, standards, and infrared technology.

Chapter 22 deals with worldwide advances in and a guide to thermal imaging systems for medical applications. Chapter 23 presents a historical perspective and the evolution of thermal imaging. Chapters 24 through 26 are comprehensive chapters on technology and hardware including detectors, detector materials, un-cooled focal plane arrays, high-performance systems, camera characterization, electronics for on-chip image processing, optics, and cost-reduction designs.

Chapter 27 deals with the physiological basis of the thermal signature and its interpretation in a medical setting. It discusses the physics of thermal radiation theory and the physiology as related to infrared imaging. Chapters 28 and 29 cover innovative concepts such as dynamic thermal imaging and thermal tomography that enhance the clinical utility leading to improved diagnostic capability. Chapter 30 presents thermal texture mapping as used in a clinical environment. Chapters 31 and 32 expose the fundamentals of infrared breast imaging, equipment considerations, early detection, and the use of infrared imaging in a multimodality setting. Chapters 33 through 37 are on innovative image processing techniques for the early detection of breast cancer. Chapter 38 discusses the practical value of inspection and measurements of thermal imaging during surgical interventions. Chapter 39 presents biometrics, a novel method for facial recognition. Today, this technology is of utmost importance in the area of homeland security and other applications. Chapter 40 deals with infrared monitoring of therapies using multispectral optical imaging in Kaposi's sarcoma investigations at the National Institutes of Health (NIH). Chapters 41 through 51 deal with the use of infrared in various clinical applications: fever, surgery, dental, skeletal and neuromuscular diseases, as well as the quantification of the TAU image technique in the relevance and stage of a disease. Chapter 52 is on infrared imaging in veterinary medicine. Chapter 53 discusses the complexities and importance of standardization, calibration, and protocols for effective and reproducible results. Chapter 54 deals with databases and primarily with the storage and retrieval of thermal images. Chapter 55 addresses the ethical obligations in infrared research and clinical practice.

This section will be of interest to both the medical and biomedical engineering communities. It could provide many opportunities for developing and conducting multidisciplinary research in many areas of medical infrared imaging. These range from clinical quantification to intelligent image processing for enhancement of the interpretation of images and for further development of user-friendly high-resolution thermal cameras. These would enable the wide use of infrared imaging as a viable, noninvasive, low-cost, first-line detection modality.

22

Advances in Medical Infrared Imaging: An Update

Nicholas A. Diakides
Advanced Concepts Analysis, Inc.

Mary Diakides
Advanced Concepts Analysis, Inc.

Jasper Lupo
Applied Research Associates, Inc.

Jeffrey Paul
Applied Research Associates, Inc.

Raymond Balcerak
RSB Consulting LLC

22.1 Introduction

Since the last publication of the *Medical Infrared Imaging* handbook in 2008, our dear friend and medical infrared (IR) pioneer, Dr. Nick Diakides passed away. His wife, Mary Diakides, Advanced Concepts Analysis, continues the quest to bring thermal imaging into the forefront for medical imaging, especially the early detection of breast cancer. It is an honor to have been Nick's friends and to continue efforts to realize his goals. If we succeed, someday women and their doctors will have a new screening option to complement existing tools such as mammography.

During the intervening few years, there have been steady improvements in low cost, high-resolution thermal cameras that operate at room temperature. With the continued investment of military R&D, it is now possible to buy uncooled cameras with nearly 1.0 megapixel arrays at prices below $15,000 in a competitive industrial base. These cameras can resolve temperature differences as low as 0.035°K, thus providing exquisite detail for medical diagnostics.

IR imaging in medicine has been used in the past but without the advantage of twenty-first century technology. In 1994, under the Department of Defense (DOD) grants jointly funded by the Office of the Secretary of Defense (S&T), the Defense Advanced Research Projects Agency (DARPA) and the Army Research Office (ARO), a concerted effort was initiated to re-visit this subject. Specifically, it was to explore the potential of integrating advanced IR technology with "smart" image processing for use in medicine. The major challenges for acceptance of this modality by the medical community were investigated. It was found that the following issues were of prime importance: (1) standardization and quantification of clinical data, (2) better understanding of the pathophysiological nature of thermal signatures, (3) wider publication and exposure of medical IR imaging in conferences and leading journals, (4) characterization of thermal signatures through an interactive web-based database, and (5) training in both image acquisition and interpretation.

Over the last 10 years, significant progress has been made internationally by advancing a thrust for new initiatives worldwide for clinical quantification, international collaboration, and providing a forum for coordination, discussion, and publication through the following activities: (1) medical IR imaging symposia, workshops, and tracks at IEEE/Engineering in Medicine and Biology Society (EMBS) conferences from 1994 to 2004, (2) three EMBS, Special Issues dedicated to this topic [1–3], (3) the DOD "From Tanks to Tumors" Workshop [4]. The products of these efforts are documented in final government technical reports [5–8] and IEEE/EMBS Conference Proceedings (1994–2004).

Likewise, great technological progress has been made in camera development over the last 15 years. Early IR cameras used a small, linear array of 1×180 detectors, which used a mechanically scanned mirror to form an image, and required cryogenic cooling in order to produce a clear image. Electrical contact was made to each individual detector by means of a manually connected wire—a very laborious and expensive process. The images formed by these cameras were limited in spatial and thermal resolution. The 1990s saw the advent of 2-D thermal imaging arrays and the emergence of un-cooled thermal imaging technology. Developers focused on producing larger and larger arrays, capitalizing in large measure on the same technology that drives the commercial digital camera boom. Thermal cameras with 2-D arrays produce images without mechanical scanning in much the same way as a modern digital camera. Electrical scanning and lithographic techniques provide an elegant and simplified image readout that produces standard analog and digital video with very little external processing. New cameras mentioned above can feed imagery directly into a laptop computer or a video monitor.

Presently, IR imaging is used in many different medical applications. The most prominent of these are oncology (breast, skin, etc.), vascular disorders (diabetes DVT, etc.), pain, surgery, tissue viability, monitoring the efficacy of drugs and therapies; respiratory (recently introduced for testing of SARS).

There are various methods used to acquire IR images: Static, Dynamic, Passive and Active—Dynamic Area Telethermometry (DAT), subtraction, and so on [9], Thermal Texture Mapping (TTM), Multispectral/Hyperspectral, Multimodality, and Sensor Fusion. A list of current applications and IR imaging methods are listed in Table 22.1. Figures 22.1 and 22.2 illustrate thermal signatures of breast screening and Kaposi sarcoma.

22.2 Worldwide Use of IR Imaging in Medicine

22.2.1 United States of America and Canada

IR imaging is beginning to be reconsidered in the United States, largely due to new IR technology, advanced image processing, powerful, high-speed computers, and the promotion of research. This is evidenced by the increased number of publications available in open literature and national databases such as *Index Medicus* and *Medline* (National Library of Medicine) on this modality. Currently, there are several academic institutions with research initiatives in IR imaging. Some of the most prominent are the following: NIH, John's Hopkins University, University of Houston, University of Texas. NIH has several ongoing programs: vascular disorders (diabetes, deep-venous thrombosis), monitoring angiogenesis activity—Kaposi sarcoma, pain-reflex sympathetic dystrophy, monitoring the efficacy of radiation therapy, organ transplant—perfusion, multispectral imaging.

Johns Hopkins University carries out research on microcirculation, monitoring angiogenic activity in Kaposi sarcoma and breast screening, laparoscopic IR images—renal disease.

TABLE 22.1   Medical Applications and Methods

Applications	IR Imaging Methods
Oncology (breast, skin, etc.)	Static (classical)
Pain (management/control)	Dynamic (DAT, subtraction, etc.)
Vascular disorders (diabetes, DVT)	Dynamic (active)
Arthritis/rheumatism	TTM
Neurology	Multispectral/hyperspectral
Surgery (open heart, transplant, etc.)	Multimodality
Ophthalmic (cataract removal)	Sensor fusion
Tissue viability (burns, etc.)	
Dermatological disorders	
Monitoring efficacy of drugs and therapies	
Thyroid	
Dentistry	
Respiratory (allergies, SARS)	
Sports and rehabilitation medicine	

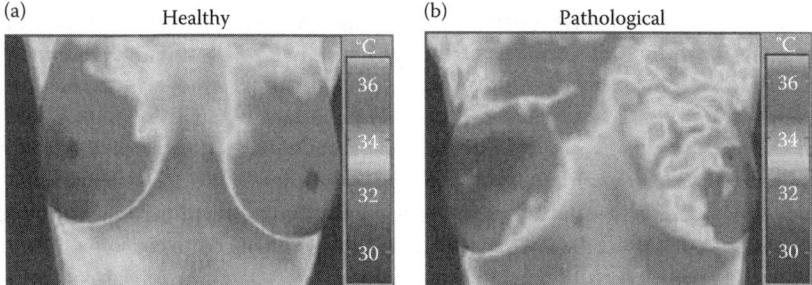

FIGURE 22.1   An application of infrared technique for breast screening: (a) healthy; (b) pathological breast. (Courtesy of Prof. Reinhold Berz, MD. Informatics, Germany.)

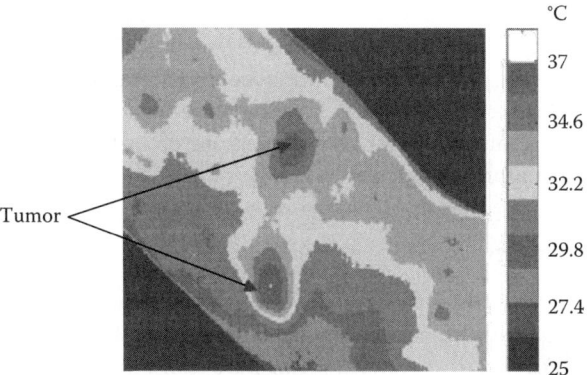

FIGURE 22.2   An application of infrared technique for cancer research. (Adapted from Hassan, M. et al., *Technology in Cancer Research and Treatment*, 3(5), 451–457, 2004.)

University of Houston just created an IR imaging laboratory to investigate using IR the facial thermal characteristics for such applications as lie detection and other behavioral issues (fatigue, anxiety, fear, etc.).

There are two medical centers specializing in breast cancer research and treatment which use IR routinely as part of their first-line detection system, which also includes mammography and clinical exam. These are: EHH Breast Cancer and Treatment Center, Baton Rouge, LA and Ville Marie Oncology Research Center, Montreal, Canada. Their centers are fully equipped with all state-of-the-art imaging equipment. These centers are members of the coalition team for the development of a "knowledge-based" database of thermal signatures of the breast with "ground-truth" validation.

22.2.2 China

China has a long-standing interest in IR imaging. More recently, the novel method Thermal Texture Mapping (TTM) has added increased specificity to static imaging. It is known that this method is widely used in this country, but unfortunately there is no formal literature about this important work. This is urgently needed in order for TTM to be exposed and accepted as a viable, effective method by the international community. The clinical results obtained through this method should be published in open literature of medical journals and international conference proceedings. Despite the lack of the availability of this documentation, introduction of TTM has been made to The National Institutes of Health (NIH). They are now using this method and its camera successfully in detection and treatment in Kaposi sarcoma (associated with AIDS patients). China has also shown interest in breast cancer detection and associated angiogenesis. There are further possibilities for high-level research for this method in the United States and abroad.

22.2.3 Japan

IR imaging is widely accepted in Japan by the government and the medical community. More than 1500 hospitals and clinics use IR imaging routinely. The government sets the standards and reimburses clinical tests. Their focus is in the following areas: blood perfusion, breast cancer, dermatology, pain, neurology, surgery (open-heart, orthopedic, dental, cosmetic), sports medicine, oriental medicine. The main research is performed at the following universities: University of Tokyo—organ transplant; Tokyo Medical and Dental University (skin temperature characterization and thermal properties); Toho University—neurological operation); Cancer Institute hospital (breast cancer). In addition, around 40 other medical institutions are using IR for breast cancer screening.

22.2.4 Korea

The involvement in IR imaging in Korea began during the early 1990s. More than 450 systems are being used in hospitals and medical centers. Primary clinical applications are neurology, back pain/treatment, surgery, oriental medicine. Yonsei College of Medicine is one of the leading institutions in medical IR imaging research along with three others.

22.2.5 United Kingdom

The University of Glamorgan is the center of IR imaging; the School of Computing has a thermal physiology laboratory which focuses in the following areas: medical IR research, standardization, training (degree offered), "SPORTI" Project funded by the European Union Organization. The objective of this effort is to develop a reference database of normal, thermal signatures from healthy subjects.

The Royal National Hospital of Rheumatic Diseases specializes in rheumatic disorders, occupational health (Raynaud's Disease, Carpal Tunnel Syndrome, and Sports Medicine).

The Royal Free University College Medical School Hospital specializes in vascular disorders (diabetes, DVT, etc.), optimization of IR imaging techniques and Raynaud's Phenomenon.

22.2.6 Germany

University of Leipzig uses IR for open-heart surgery, perfusion and micro-circulation. There are several private clinics and other hospitals that use IR imaging in various applications.

EvoBus-Daimler Chrysler uses IR imaging for screening all their employees for wellness/health assessment (occupational health).

InfraMedic, AG, conducts breast cancer screening of women from 20 to 85 years old for the government under a two-year grant. IR is the sole modality used. Their screening method is called Infrared Regulation Imaging (IRI).

22.2.7 Austria

Ludwig Bolzman Research Institute for Physical Diagnostics has carried out research in IR for many years and it publishes the *Thermology International* (a quarterly journal of IR clinical research and instrumentation). This journal contains papers from many Thermology Societies. A recent issue contains the results of a survey of 2003 international papers dedicated to Thermology [10].

The General Hospital, University of Vienna, does research mainly in angiology (study of blood and lymph vessels) diabetic foot (pedobarography).

22.2.8 Poland

There has been a more recent rapid increase in the use of IR imaging for medicine in Poland since the Polish market for IR cameras was opened up. There are more than 50 cameras being used in the following medical centers: Warsaw University, Technical University of Gdansk, Poznan University, Lodz University, Katowice University, and the Military Clinical Hospital. The research activities are focused on the following areas: Active IR imaging, open-heart surgery, quantitative assessment of skin burns, ophthalmology, dentistry, allergic diseases, neurological disorders, plastic surgery, thermal image database for healthy and pathological cases and multispectral imaging (IR, visual, x-ray, ultrasound).

In 1986 the Eurotherm Committee was created by members of the European Community to promote cooperation in the thermal sciences by gathering scientist and engineers working in the area of Thermology. This organization focuses on quantitative IR thermography and periodically holds conferences and seminars in this field [11].

22.2.9 Italy

Much of the clinical use of IR imaging is done under the public health system, besides private clinics. The ongoing clinical work is in the following areas: dermatology (melanoma), neurology, rheumatology, anesthesiology, reproductive medicine, sports medicine. The University of G. d'Annunzio, Chieti, has an imaging laboratory purely for research on IR applications. It collaborates on these projects with other universities throughout Italy.

There are other places, such as Australia, Norway, South America, Russia, and so on that have ongoing research as well.

22.3 IR Imaging in Breast Cancer

In the United States, breast cancer is a national concern. There are 192,000 cases a year; it is estimated that there are 1 million women with undetected breast cancer; presently, the figure of women affected is

1.8 million; 45,000 women die per year. The cost burden of the U.S. healthcare is estimated at $18 billion per year. The cost for early-stage detection is $12,000 per patient and for late detection it is $345,000 per patient. Hence, early detection would potentially save $12B annually—as well as many lives. As a result, the U.S. Congress created "The Congressionally Directed Medical Research Program for Breast Cancer." Clinical IR has not as yet been supported through this funding. Effort is being directed toward including IR. Since 1982 FDA has approved IR imaging (Thermography) as an adjunct modality to mammography for breast cancer as shown in Table 22.2.

Ideal characteristics for an early breast cancer detection method as defined by the Congressionally Directed Medical Research Programs on Breast Cancer are listed in Table 22.3. IR imaging meets these requirements with the exception of the detection of early lesions at 1000–10,000 cells which has not yet been fully determined.

A program is underway in the United States to develop a prototype web-based database with a collection of approximately 2000 patient thermal signatures to be categorized into three categories: normal, equivocal, suspicious for developing algorithms for screening and early detection of tumor development.

The origin of this program can be traced back to a 1994 multiagency DoD grant sponsored by the Director for Research in the Office of the Director, Defense Research and Engineering, the Defense Advanced Research Projects Agency, and the Army Research Office. This grant funded a study to determine the applicability of advanced military technology to the detection of breast cancer—particularly thermal imaging and automatic target recognition. The study produced two reports, one in 1995 and another in 1998; these studies identified technology, concepts, and ongoing activity that would have direct relevance to a rigorous application of IR. Rigor was the essential ingredient to further progress. The US effort had been dormant since the 1970s because of the limitations imposed by poor sensors, simplistic imaging processing, lack of automatic target recognition, and inadequate computing power. This was complicated by the fact that the virtues of IR had been overstated by a few developers.

TABLE 22.2   Imaging Modalities for Breast Cancer Detection Approved by FDA

Film-screen mammography
Full-field digital mammography
Computer-aided detection
Ultrasound
Magnetic resonance imaging (MRI)
Positron emission tomography (PET)
Thermography
Electrical impedance imaging

Source: Mammography and Beyond, Institute of Medicine, National Academy Press, 2001.

TABLE 22.3   Ideal Characteristics for an Early Breast Cancer Detection Method

Detects early lesion
Available to population (48 million U.S. women age 40–70 y)
High sensitivity/high specificity (in all age groups)
Inexpensive
Noninvasive
Easily trainable and with high quality assurance
Decreases mortality
Infrared imaging meets all the above requirements

In 1999, the director for research in the Office of the Director, Defense Research and Engineering and the deputy assistant secretary of the Army for Installations and Environment; Environmental Safety and Occupational Health formulated a technology transfer program that would facilitate the use of advanced military technology and processes to breast cancer screening. Funds were provided by the Army and the project was funded through the Office of Naval Research (ONR).

A major milestone in the US program was the Tanks to Tumors workshop held in Arlington, VA, Dec. 4–5, 2001. The workshop was co-sponsored by Office of the Director, Defense Research and Engineering, Space and Sensor Technology Directorate; the deputy assistant secretary of the Army for Environment, Safety and Occupational Health; the Defense Advanced Research Projects Agency; and the Army Research Office. The purpose was to explore means for exploiting the technological opportunities in the integration of image processing, web-based database management and development, and IR sensor technology for the early detection of breast cancer. A second objective was to provide guidance to a program. The government speakers noted that significant military advances in thermal imaging, and automatic target recognition coupled with medical understanding of abnormal vascularity (angiogenesis) offer the prospect of automated detection from one to two years earlier than other, more costly and invasive screening methods.

There were compelling reasons for both military and civilian researchers to attend: (1) recognition of breast cancer as a major occupational health issue by key personnel such as Raymond Fatz, deputy assistant secretary of the Army for Installations and Environment; Environmental Safety and Occupational Health; (2) growing use of thermal imaging in military and civilian medicine (especially abroad); (3) maturation of military technology in automatic target recognition (ATR), ATR evaluation, and low-cost thermal imaging; (4) emerging transfer opportunities to and from the military. In particular, ATR assessment technology has developed image data management, dissemination, collaboration, and assessment tools for use by government and industrial developers of ATR software used to find military targets in thermal imagery. Such tools seem naturally suited for adaptation to the creation and use of a national database for IR breast cancer imagery and the evaluation of screening algorithms that would assist physicians in detecting the disease early. Finally, recent IR theories developed by civilian physicians indicate that the abnormal vascularity (angiogenesis) associated with the formation of breast tumors may be detected easily by IR cameras from one to five years before any other technique. Early detection has been shown to be the key to high survival probability.

The workshop involved specialists and leaders from the military R&D, academic, and medical communities. Together they covered a multidisciplinary range of topics: military IR sensor technology, automatic target recognition (ATR), smart image processing, database management, interactive web-based data management, IR imaging for screening of breast cancer, and related medical topics. Three panels of experts considered: (1) Image Processing and Medical Applications; (2) Website and Database; (3) Sensor Technology for Medical Applications. A subject area expert led each. The deliberations of each group were presented in a briefing to the plenary session of the final day. Their outputs were quite general; they still apply to the current program and are discussed below for the benefit of all future US efforts.

22.3.1 Image Processing and Medical Applications

This group focused on the algorithms (ATR approaches) and how to evaluate and use them. It advised that the clinical methods of collection must be able to support the most common ATR approaches, for example, single frame, change detection, multilook, and anomaly detection. They also provided detailed draft guidelines for controlled problem sets for ATR evaluation. Although they thought a multisensor approach would pay dividends, they stressed the need to quantify algorithm performance in a methodical way, starting with approaches that work with single IR images.

22.3.2 Website and Database

This panel concerned itself with the collection and management of an IR image database for breast cancer. It looked particularly at issues of data standards and security. It concluded that the OSD supported Virtual Distributed Laboratory (VDL), created within the OSD ATR Evaluation Program, is a very good model for the medical data repository to include collaborative software, image management software, evaluation concepts, data standards, security, bandwidth, and storage capacity. It also advised that camera calibration concepts and phantom targets be provided to help baseline performance and eliminate unknowns. It noted that privacy regulations would have to be dealt with in order to post the human data but suggested that this would complicate but not impede the formation of the database.

22.3.3 Sensor Technology for Medical Applications

The sensor panel started by pointing out that, if angiogenesis is a reliable early indicator of risk, then thermal imaging is ideally suited to detection at that stage. Current sensor performance is fully adequate. The group discussed calibration issues associated with hardware design and concluded that internal reference is desirable to insure that temperature differences are being measured accurately. However, they questioned the need for absolute temperature measurement; the plenary group offered no counter to this. This group also looked at the economics of thermal imaging, and concluded that recent military developments in uncooled thermal imaging systems at DARPA and the Army Night Vision and Electronic Sensing Division would allow the proliferation of IR cameras costing at most a few thousand dollars each. They cited China's installation of over 60 such cameras. The panel challenged ATR and algorithm developers to look at software methods to help simplify the sensor hardware, for example, frame-to-frame change detection to replace mechanical stabilization.

IR imaging for medical uses is a multidisciplinary technology and must include experts from very different fields if its full potential is to be realized. The Tanks to Tumors workshop is a model for future US efforts. It succeeded in bringing several different communities together—medical, military, academic, industrial, and engineering. These experts worked together to determine how the United States might adopt thermal imaging diagnostic technology in an orderly and demonstrable way for the early detection of breast cancer and other conditions. The panel recommendations will serve to guide the transition of military technology developments in ATR, the VDL, and IR sensors, to the civilian medical community. The result will be a new tool in the war against breast cancer—a major benefit to the military and civilian population. Detailed proceedings of this workshop are available from ACA, Falls Church, VA.

22.4 Guide to Thermal Imaging Systems for Medical Applications

22.4.1 Introduction

The purpose of this section is to provide the physician with an overview of the key features of thermal imaging systems and a brief discussion of the marketplace. It assumes that the reader is somewhat familiar with thermal imaging theory and terminology as well as the fundamentals of digital imaging. It contains a brief, modestly technical guide to buying sensor hardware, and a short list of active websites that can introduce the buyer to the current marketplace. It is intended primarily to aid the newcomer; however, advanced workers may also find some of these websites useful in seeking custom or cutting-edge capabilities in their quest to better understand the thermal phenomenology of breast cancer.

22.4.2 Background

As discussed elsewhere, the last decade has seen a resurgence of interest in thermal imaging for the early detection of breast cancer and other medical applications, both civilian and military. There was a brief period in the 1970s when thermal imaging became the subject of medical interest. That interest waned due to the combination of high prices and modest-to-marginal performance. Dramatic progress has been made in the intervening years; prices have dropped thanks to burgeoning military, domestic, and industrial use; performance has improved significantly; and new technology has emerged from Defense investments. Imaging electronics, digitization, image manipulation software, and automatic detection algorithms have emerged. Cameras can be had for prices that range from about $10,000 on up. These cameras can provide a significant capability for screening and data collection. The camera field is highly competitive; it is possible to rent, lease, or buy cameras from numerous vendors and manufacturers.

22.4.3 Applications and Image Formats

Currently, thermal imaging is being used for research and development into the phenomenology of breast cancer detection, and for screening and cuing in the multimodal diagnosis and tracking of breast cancer in patients. The least stressful and most affordable is the latter. Here, two types of formats can be of general utility: uncalibrated still pictures and simple uncalibrated video. Such formats can be stored and archived for future viewing. Use of such imagery for rigorous research and development is not recommended. Furthermore, there may be legal issues associated with the recording and collection of such imagery unless it is applied merely as a screening aid to the doctor rather than as a primary diagnostic tool. In other words, such imagery would provide the doctor with anecdotal support in future review of a patient's record. In this mode, the thermal imagery has the same diagnostic relevance as a stethoscope or endoscope, neither of which is routinely recorded in the doctor's office. Imagery so obtained would not carry the same diagnostic weight as a mammogram. Still cameras and video imagers of this kind are quite affordable and compact. They can be kept in a drawer or cabinet and be used for thermal viewing of many types of conditions including tumors, fractures, skin anomalies, circulation, and drug affects, to name a few. The marketplace is saturated with imagers under $10,000 that can provide adequate resolution and sensitivity for informal "eyeballing" the thermal features of interest. Virtually any image or video format is adequate for this kind of use.

For medical R&D, in which still imagery is to be archived, shared, and used for the testing of software and medical theories, or to explore phenomenology, it is important to collect calibrated still imagery in lossless archival formats (e.g., the so-called "raw" format that many digital cameras offer). It is thus desirable to purchase or rent a radiometric still camera with uncompressed standard formats or "raw" output that preserves the thermal calibration. This kind of imagery allows the medical center to put its collected thermal imagery into a standard format for distribution to the Virtual Distributed Laboratory and other interested medical centers. There are image manipulation software packages that can transform the imagery if need be. On the other hand, the data can be transmitted in any number of uncompressed formats and transformed by the data collection center. The use of standard formats is critical if medical research centers are to share common databases. There is no obvious need yet for video in R&D for breast cancer, although thermal video is being studied for many medical applications where dynamic phenomena are of interest.

22.4.4 Dynamic Range

The ability of a camera to preserve fine temperature detail in the presence of large scene temperature range is determined by its dynamic range. Dynamic range is determined by the camera's image digitization and formation electronics. Take care to use a camera that allocates an adequate number of bits to the digitization of the images. Most commercially available cameras use 12 bits or more per pixel. This is quite adequate to preserve fine detail in images of the human body. However, when collecting images, make sure there is nothing in the field of view of the camera that is dramatically cooler or hotter than the subject; that is, avoid scene temperature differences of more than roughly 30°C (e.g., lamps, refrigerators, or radiators in the background could cause trouble). This is analogous to trying to use a visible digital camera to capture a picture of a person standing next to headlights—electronic circuits may bloom or sacrifice detail of the scene near the bright lights. Although 12-bit digitization should preserve fine temperature differences at a 30°C delta, large temperature differences generally stress the image formation circuitry, and undesired artifacts may appear. Nevertheless, it is relatively easy to design a collection environment with a modest temperature range. A simple way to do this is to simply fill the camera field of view with the human subject. Experiment with the imaging arrangement before collecting a large body of imagery for archiving.

22.4.5 Resolution and Sensitivity

The two most important parameters for a thermal sensor are its sensitivity and resolution. The sensitivity is measured in degrees Celsius. Modest sensitivity is on the order of a tenth of a degree Celsius. Good sensitivity sensors can detect temperature differences up to 4 times lower or 0.025 degrees. This sensitivity is deemed valuable for medical diagnosis, since local temperature variations caused by tumors and angiogenesis are usually higher than this. The temperature resolution is analogous to the number of colors in a computer display or color photograph. The better the resolution, the smoother the temperature transitions will be. If the subject has sudden temperature gradients, those will be attributable to the subject and not the camera.

The spatial resolution of the sensor is determined primarily by the size of the imaging chip or pixel count. This parameter is exactly analogous to the world of proliferating digital photography. Just as a 4 megapixel digital camera can make sharper photos than a 2 megapixel camera, pixel count is a key element in the design of a medical camera. There are quite economical thermal cameras on the market with 320×240 pixels, and the images from such cameras can be quite adequate for informal screening; imagery may appear to be grainy if magnified unless the viewing area or field of view is reduced. By way of example, if the image is of the full chest area, about 18 inches, then a 320 pixel camera will provide the ability to resolve spatial features of about a 16th of an inch. If only the left breast is imaged, spatial features as low as 1/32 inch can be resolved. On the other hand, a 640×480 camera can cut these feature sizes in half. Good sensitivity and pixel count ensures that the medical images will contain useful thermal and spatial detail. In summary, although 320×240 imagery is quite adequate, larger pixel counts can provide more freedom for casual use, and are essential for R&D in medical centers. Although the military is developing megapixel arrays, they are not commercially available. Larger pixel counts have advantages for consumer digital photography and military applications, but there is no identified, clear need at this time for megapixel arrays in breast cancer detection. Avoid the quest for larger pixel counts unless there is a clear need. Temperature resolution should be a tenth of a degree or better.

22.4.6 Calibration

Another key feature is temperature calibration. Many thermal imaging systems are designed to detect temperature differences, not to map calibrated temperature. A camera that maps the actual surface temperature is a radiographic sensor. A reasonably good job of screening for tumors can be accomplished by only mapping local temperature differences. This application would amount to a third eye for the physician, aiding him in finding asymmetries and temperature anomalies—hot or cold spots. For example, checking circulation with thermal imaging amounts to looking for cold spots relative to the normally warm torso. However, if the physician intends to share his imagery with other doctors, or use the imagery for research, it is advisable to use a calibrated camera so that the meaning of the thermal differences can be quantified and separated from display settings and digital compression artifacts. For example, viewing the same image on two different computer displays may result in different assessments. But, if the imagery is calibrated so that each color or brightness is associated with a specific temperature, then doctors can be sure that they are viewing relevant imagery and accurate temperatures, not image artifacts.

It is critical that the calibration be stable and accurate enough to match the temperature sensitivity of the camera. Here caution is advised. Many radiometric cameras on the market are designed for industrial applications where large temperature differences are expected and the temperature of the object is well over 100°C; for example, the temperature difference may be 5°C at 600°C. In breast cancer, the temperature differences of interest are about a tenth of a degree at about 37°C. Therefore, the calibration method must be relevant for those parameters. Since the dynamic range of the breast cancer application is very small, the calibration method is simplified. More important are the temporal stability, temperature resolution, and accuracy of the calibration. Useful calibration parameters are: of 0.1°C resolution at 37°C, stability of 0.1°C per hour (drift), and accuracy of ±0.3°C. This means that the camera can measure a temperature difference of 0.1°C with an accuracy of ±0.3°C at body temperature. For example, suppose the breast is at 36.5°C; the camera might read 36.7°C.

Two methods of calibration are available—internal and external. External calibration devices are available from numerous sources. They are traceable to NIST and meet the above requirements. Prices are under $3000 for compact, portable devices. The drawback with external calibration is that it involves a second piece of equipment and more complex procedure for use. The thermal camera must be calibrated just prior to use and calibration imagery recorded, or the calibration source must be placed in the image while data are collected. The latter method is more reliable but it complicates the collection geometry.

Internal calibration is preferable because it simplifies the entire data collection process. However, radiometric still cameras with the above specifications are more expensive than uncalibrated cameras by $3000–$5000.

22.4.7 Single Band Imagers

Today there are thermal imaging sensors with suitable performance parameters. There are two distinct spectral bands that provide adequate thermal sensitivity for medical use: the medium wave IR band (MWIR) covers the electromagnetic spectrum from 3 to 5 μm in wavelength, approximately; the long-wave infrared band (LWIR) covers the wavelength spectrum from about 8 to 12 μm. There are advocates for both bands, and neither band offers a clear advantage over the other for medical applications, although the LWIR is rapidly becoming the most economical sensor technology. Some experimenters believe that there is merit to using both bands.

MWIR cameras are widely available and generally have more pixels, hence higher resolution for the same price. Phenomenology in this band has been quite effective in detecting small tumors and temperature asymmetries. MWIR sensors must be cooled to cryogenic temperatures as low as 77 K. Thermoelectric coolers are used for some MWIR sensors; they operate at 175–220 K depending on the design of the imaging chip. MWIR sensors not only respond to emitted radiation from thermal sources but they also sense radiation from broadband visible sources such as the sun. Images in this band can contain structure caused by reflected light rather than emitted radiation. Some care must be taken to minimize reflected light from broadband sources including incandescent light bulbs and sunlight. Unwanted light can cause shadows, reflections, and bright spots in the imagery. Care should be taken to avoid direct illumination of the subject by wideband artificial sources and sunlight. It is advisable to experiment with lighting geometries and sources before collecting data for the record. Moisturizing creams, sweat, and other skin surface coatings should also be avoided.

The cost of LWIR cameras has dropped dramatically since the advent of uncooled thermal imaging arrays. This is a dramatic difference between the current state of the art and what was available in the 1970s. Now, LWIR cameras are being proliferated and can be competitive in price and performance to the thermoelectrically cooled MWIR. Uncooled thermal cameras are compact and have good resolution and sensitivity. Cameras with 320×240 pixels can be purchased for well under $10,000. The trend in uncooled IR cameras is toward larger format arrays with smaller pixel size. Sensors with 640×480 pixels, individual pixel size of 25 μm and sensitivity of less than 50 mk, are on the market. These larger format arrays have thermal sensitivity equal to or greater than the previous generation of smaller format arrays, indicative of advances in the pixel design and manufacturing technology. Sensors in this band are far less likely to be affected by shadows, lighting, and reflections. Nevertheless, it is advisable to experiment with viewing geometry, ambient lighting, and skin condition before collecting data for the record and for dissemination.

Although large format arrays are becoming available, there is a cost advantage in smaller format arrays, either 320×240 or 160×120. The smaller format arrays integrated with signal processing algorithms can produce excellent images for short-term applications encountered in medical imaging. Also, in medical applications, where the targets are static, and data can be collected over several frames, frame integration and image enhancement software can provide excellent imaging, with moderate investment in camera equipment.

22.4.8 Emerging and Future Camera Technology

There are emerging developments that may soon provide for a richer set of observable phenomena in the thermography for breast cancer. Some researchers are already simultaneously collecting imagery in both the MWIR and LWIR bands. This is normally accomplished using two cameras at the same time. Developers of automatic screening algorithms are exploring schemes that compare the images in the two bands and emphasize the common elements of both to get greater confidence in detecting tumors. More sophisticated software (based on neural networks) learns what is important in both bands. Uncooled detector arrays have been demonstrated that operate in both bands simultaneously. It is likely that larger or well-endowed medical centers can order custom imagers with this capability this year.

Spectroscopic (hyperspectral) imaging in the thermal bands is also an important research topic. Investigators are looking for phenomenology that manifests itself in fine spectral detail. Since flesh is a thermally absorptive and scattering medium, it may be possible to detect unique signatures that help detect tumors. Interested parties should ask vendors if such cameras are available for lease or purchase.

In addition, research is underway to integrate tunable spectral filters with the imaging sensor. Since the filters are integrated with the sensor, the overall camera size and weight will be similar to conventional cameras. The spectral tuning range can be flexible, and depending upon filter design, tuning for either the 3–5 or 8–11 μm bands is feasible. A narrow spectral bandwidth, approximately 0.1 μm, will provide a comprehensive set of spectral data for in-depth analysis. Dual band imagery and multispectral data arguably provide physicians with a richer set of observables.

22.4.9 Summary Specifications

Table 22.4 summarizes the key parameters and their nominal values to use in shopping for a camera.

22.4.9.1 How to Begin

Those who are new to thermal phenomenology should carefully study the material in this handbook. Medical centers, researchers, and physicians seeking to purchase cameras and enter the field may wish to contact the authors or leading investigators mentioned in this handbook for advice before looking for sensor hardware. The participants in the Tanks to Tumors workshop and the MedATR program may already have the answers. If possible, compare advice from two or more of these experts before moving on; the experts do not agree on everything. They are currently using sensors and software suitable for building the VDL database. They may also be aware of public domain image screening

TABLE 22.4 Summary of Key Camera Parameters

	Application: Recording	Application: Informal
Format	Digital stills	Video or stills
Compression	None	As provided by mfr
Digitization (dynamic range)	12 bits or more	12 bits nominal
Pixels (array size)	320 × 240 up to 640 × 480	320 × 240
Sensitivity	0.04°C, 0.1°C max	0.1°C
Calibration accuracy	±0.3°C	Not required
Calibration range	Room and body temperature	Not required
Calibration resolution	0.1°C	Not required
Spectral band	MWIR or LWIR	MWIR or LWIR

software. Once advice has been collected, the potential buyer should begin shopping at the one or more of the websites listed in this section. Do not rely on the website alone. Most vendors provide contact information so that the purchaser may discuss imaging needs with a consultant. Take advantage of these advisory services to shop around and survey the field. Researchers may also wish to contact government and university experts before deciding on a camera. Finally, many of the vendors below offer custom sensor design services. Some vendors may be willing to lease or loan equipment for evaluation. High-end, leading-edge researchers may need to contact component developers at companies such as Raytheon, DRS, BAE, or SOFRADIR to see if the state of the art supports their specific needs.

22.4.9.2 Supplier Websites

The reader is advised that all references to brand names or specific manufacturers do not imply an endorsement of the vendor, producer, or its products. Likewise, the list is not a complete survey; we apologize for any omissions. Since the last printing, FLIR Systems Inc. acquired Indigo Systems and L-3 acquired the Raytheon thermal imaging business.

http://www.thermal-eye.com/
http://medicalir.com/
http://www.infrared-camera-rentals.com/
http://www.electrophysics.com/Browse/Brw_AllProductLineCategory.asp
http://www.cantronic.com/ir860.html
http://www.nationalinfrared.com/Medical_Imaging.php
http://www.flirthermography.com/cameras/all_cameras.asp
http://www.mikroninst.com/
http://www.baesystems.com/ProductsServices/bae_prod_s2_mim500.html
http://www.flir.com/US/
http://x26.com/articles.html
http://www.infraredsolutions.com/
http://www.isgfire.com/
http://www.infrared.com/
http://www.sofradir.com/
http://www.drs.com/Products/RSTA/MX2A.aspx

22.5 Summary, Conclusions, and Recommendations

Today, medical IR is being backed by more clinical research worldwide where state-of-the-art equipment is being used. Focus must be placed on the quantification of clinical data, standardization, effective training with high-quality assurance, collaborations, and more publications in leading peer-reviewed medical journals.

For an effective integration of twenty-first century technologies for IR imaging we need to focus on the following areas:

- IR camera systems designed for medical diagnostics
- Advanced image processing
- Image analysis techniques
- High-speed computers
- Computer-aided detection (CAD)
- Knowledge-based databases
- Telemedicine

Other areas of importance are

- Effective clinical use
- Protocol-based image acquisition
- Image interpretation
- System operation and calibration
- Training
- Continued research in the pathophysiological nature of thermal signatures
- Quantification of clinical data

In conclusion, this noninvasive, nonionizing imaging modality can provide added value to the present multi-imaging clinical setting. A thermal image measures metabolic activity in the tissue and thus can noninvasively detect abnormalities very early. It is well known that early detection leads to enhanced survivability and great reduction in healthcare costs. With these becoming exorbitant, this would be of great value. Besides its usefulness at this stage, a second critical benefit is that it has the capability to noninvasively monitor the efficacy of therapies [12].

References

1. Diakides, N.A. (Guest Editor): Special issue on medical infrared imaging, *IEEE/Engineering in Medicine and Biology*, 17(4), Jul/Aug 1998.
2. Diakides, N.A. (Guest Editor): Special issue on medical infrared imaging, *IEEE/Engineering in Medicine and Biology*, 19(3), May/Jun 2000.
3. Diakides, N.A. (Guest Editor): Special issue on medical infrared imaging, *IEEE/Engineering in Medicine and Biology*, 21(6), Nov/Dec 2002.
4. Paul, J.L., Lupo, J.C., From tanks to tumors: Applications of infrared imaging and automatic target recognition image processing for early detection of breast cancer, *Special Issue on Medical Infrared Imaging, IEEE/Engineering in Medicine and Biology*, 21(6), 34–35, Nov/Dec 2002.
5. Diakides, N.A., Medical applications of IR focal plane arrays, Final Progress Report, U.S. Army Research Office, Contract DAAH04–94-C-0020, Mar 1998.
6. Diakides, N.A., Application of army IR technology to medical IR imaging, Technical Report, U.S. Army Research Office Contract DAAH04-96-C-0086 (TCN 97–143), Aug 1999.
7. Diakides, N.A., Exploitation of infrared imaging for medicine, Final Progress Report, U.S. Army Research Office, Contract DAAG55-98-0035, Jan 2001.
8. Diakides, N.A., Medical IR imaging and image processing, Final Report U.S. Army Research Office, Contract DAAH04-96-C-0086 (TNC 01041), Oct 2003.
9. Anbar, M., *Quantitative Dynamic Telethermometry in Medical Diagnosis and Management*, CRC Press, Boca Raton, FL, 1994.
10. Ammer, K. (Ed. In Chief), *Journal of Thermology, Intl.*, 14(1), Jan 2004.

11. Balageas, D., Busse, G., Carlomagno, C., Wiecek, B. (Eds.), *Proceedings of Quantitative Infrared Thermography 4*, Technical University of Lodz, Poland, 1998.
12. Hassan, M. et al., Quantitative assessment of tumor vasculature and response to therapy in Kaposi's sarcoma using functional noninvasive imaging, *Technology in Cancer Research and Treatment*, 3(5), 451–457, Oct 2004.

23

Historical Development of Thermometry and Thermal Imaging in Medicine

Francis J. Ring
University of Glamorgan

Bryan F. Jones
University of Glamorgan

Fever was the most frequently occurring condition in early medical observation. From the early days of Hippocrates, when it is said that wet mud was used on the skin to observe fast drying over a tumorous swelling, physicians have recognized the importance of a raised temperature. For centuries, this remained a subjective skill, and the concept of measuring temperature was not developed until the sixteenth century. Galileo made his famous thermoscope from a glass tube, which functioned as an unsealed thermometer. It was affected by atmospheric pressure as a result.

In modern terms we now describe heat transfer by three main modes. The first is conduction, requiring contact between the object and the sensor to enable the flow of thermal energy. The second mode of heat transfer is convection where the flow of a hot mass transfers thermal energy. The third is radiation. The latter two led to remote detection methods.

Thermometry developed slowly from Galileo's experiments. There were Florentine and Venetian glassblowers in Italy who made sealed glass containers of various shapes, which were tied onto the body surface. The temperature of an object was assessed by the rising or falling of small beads or seeds within the fluid inside the container. Huygens, Roemer, and Fahrenheit all proposed the need for a calibrated scale in the late seventeenth and early eighteenth century. Celsius did propose a centigrade scale based on ice and boiling water. He strangely suggested that boiling water should be zero, and melting ice 100 on his scale. It was the Danish biologist Linnaeus in 1750 who proposed the reversal of this scale, as it is known today. Although International Standards have given the term Celsius to the 0 to 100 scale today, strictly speaking it would be historically accurate to refer to degrees Linnaeus or centigrade [1].

The clinical thermometer, which has been universally used in medicine for over 130 years, was developed by Dr. Carl Wunderlich in 1868. This is essentially a maximum thermometer with a limited scale around the normal internal body temperature of 37°C or 98.4°F. Wunderlich's treatise on body temperature in health and disease is a masterpiece of painstaking work over many years. He charted the progress of all his patients daily, and sometimes two or three times during the day. His thesis was written in German for Leipzig University and was also translated into English in the late nineteenth century [2]. The significance of body temperature lies in the fact that humans are homeotherms who are capable of maintaining a constant temperature that is different from that of the surroundings. This is essential to the preservation of a relatively constant environment within the body known as homeostasis. Changes in temperature of more than a few degrees either way is a clear indicator of a bodily dysfunction; temperature variations outside this range may disrupt the essential chemical processes in the body.

Today, there has been a move away from glass thermometers in many countries, giving rise to more disposable thermocouple systems for routine clinical use.

Liquid crystal sensors for temperature became available in usable form in the 1960s. Originally the crystalline substances were painted on the skin that had previously been coated with black paint. Three of four colors became visible if the paint was at the critical temperature range for the subject. Micro-encapsulation of these substances, that are primarily cholesteric esters, resulted in plastic sheet detectors. Later these sheets were mounted on a soft latex base to mold to the skin under air pressure using a cushion with a rigid clear window. Polaroid photography was then used to record the color pattern while the sensor remained in contact. The system was reusable and inexpensive. However, sensitivity declined over 1–2 years from the date of manufacture, and many different pictures were required to obtain a subjective pattern of skin temperature [3].

Convection currents of heat emitted by the human body have been imaged by a technique called Schlieren photography. The change in refractive index with density in the warm air around the body is made visible by special illumination. This method has been used to monitor heat loss in experimental subjects, especially in the design of protective clothing for people working in extreme physical environments.

Heat transfer by radiation is of great value in medicine. The human body surface requires variable degrees of heat exchange with the environment as part of the normal thermo-regulatory process. Most of this heat transfer occurs in the infrared, which can be imaged by electronic thermal imaging [4]. Infrared radiation was discovered in 1800 when Sir William Herschel performed his famous experiment to measure heat beyond the visible spectrum (see Figure 23.1). Nearly 200 years before, Italian observers

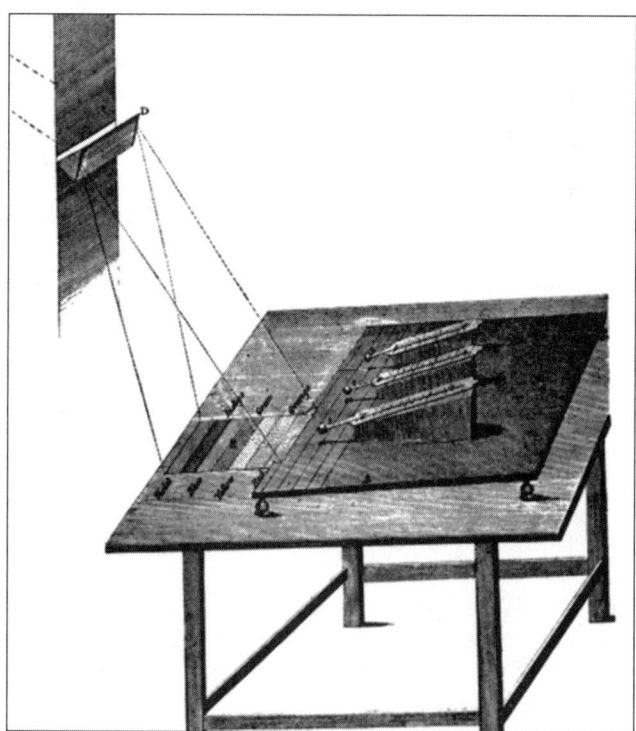

FIGURE 23.1 Herschel's experiment to examine the presence of heat in the spectrum, found beyond the visible red.

had noted the presence of reflected heat. John Della Porta in 1698 observed that when a candle was lit and placed before a large silver bowl in church, that he could sense the heat on his face. When he altered the positions of the candle, bowl, and his face, the sensation of heat was lost.

William Herschel, in a series of careful experiments, showed that not only was there a "dark heat" present, but that heat itself behaved like light, it could be reflected and refracted under the right conditions. William's only son, John Herschel, repeated some experiments after his father's death, and successfully made an image using solar radiation. This he called a "thermogram," a term still in use today to describe an image made by thermal radiation. John Herschel's thermogram was made by focusing solar radiation with a lens onto to a suspension of carbon particles in alcohol. This process is known as evaporography [5].

A major development came in the early 1940s with the first electronic sensor for infrared radiation (see Figure 23.2). Rudimentary night vision systems were produced toward the end of World War II for use by snipers. The electrons from near-infrared cathodes were directed onto visible phosphors which converted the infrared radiation into visible light. Sniperscope devices, based on this principle, were provided for soldiers in the Pacific in 1945, but found little use.

At about the same time, another device was made from indium antimonide; this was mounted at the base of a small Dewar vessel to allow cooling with liquid nitrogen. A cumbersome device such as this, which required a constant supply of liquid nitrogen, was clearly impractical for battlefield use but could be used with only minor inconvenience in a hospital. The first medical images taken with a British prototype system, the "Pyroscan" (see Figure 23.3) were made at The Middlesex Hospital in London and The Royal National Hospital for Rheumatic Diseases in Bath between 1959 and 1961. By modern standards, these thermograms were very crude.

In the meantime, the cascade image tube, that had been pioneered during World War II in Germany, had been developed by RCA into a multialkali photocathode tube whose performance exceeded expectations. These strides in technology were motivated by military needs in Vietnam; they were classified and, therefore, unavailable to clinicians. However, a mark 2 Pyroscan was made for medical use in 1962,

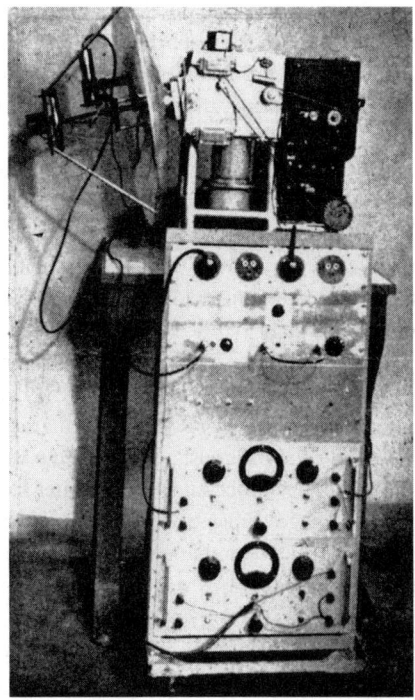

FIGURE 23.2 First English IR prototype camera.

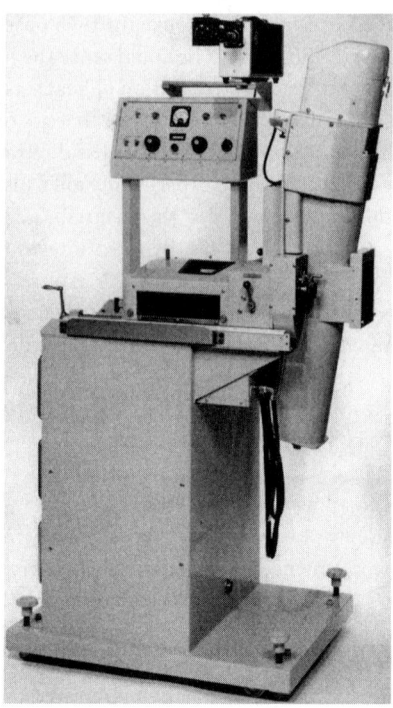

FIGURE 23.3 1960s development from the prototype in 1942. Pyroscan made for medical trials.

with improved images. The mechanical scanning was slow and each image needed from 2 to 5 min to record. The final picture was written line by line on electro-sensitive paper. In the 1970s, the U.S. Military sponsored the development of a multielement detector array that was to form the basis of a real-time framing imager. This led to the targeting and navigation system known as Forward Looking InfraRed (FLIR) systems which had the added advantage of being able to detect warm objects through smoke and fog.

During this time the potential for thermal imaging in medicine was being explored in an increasing number of centers. Earlier work by the American physiologist J. Hardy had shown that the human skin, regardless of color, is a highly efficient radiator with an emissivity of 0.98 which is close to that of a perfect black body. Even so, the normal temperature of skin in the region of 20–30°C generated low intensities of infrared radiation at about 10 μm wavelength [6]. The detection of such low intensities at these wavelengths presented a considerable challenge to the technology of the day. Cancer detection was a high priority subject and hopes that this new technique would be a tool for screening breast cancer provided the motivation to develop detectors. Many centers across Europe, the United States, and Japan became involved. In the United Kingdom, a British surgeon, K. Lloyd Williams showed that many tumors are hot and the hotter the tumor, the worse the prognosis. By this time, the images were displayed on a cathode-ray screen in black and white. Image processing by computer had not arrived, so much discussion was given to schemes to score the images subjectively, and to look for hot spots and asymmetry of temperature in the breast. This was confounded by changes in the breast through the menstrual cycle in younger women. The use of false color thermograms was only possible by photography at this time. A series of bright isotherms were manually ranged across the temperature span of the image, each being exposed through a different color filter, and superimposed on a single frame of film.

Improvements in infrared technology were forging ahead at the behest of the U.S. Military during the 1970s. At Fort Belvoir, some of the first monolithic laser diode arrays were designed and produced with a capability of generating 500 W pulses at 15 kHz at room temperature. These lasers were able to image objects at distances of 3 km. Attention then turned to solid state, gas, and tunable lasers which were used in a wide range of applications.

By the mid-1970s, computer technology made a widespread impact with the introduction of smaller mini and microcomputers at affordable prices. The first "personal" computer systems had arrived. In Bath, a special system for nuclear medicine made in Sweden was adapted for thermal imaging. A color screen was provided to display the digitized image. The processor was a PDP8, and the program was loaded every day from paper-tape. With computerization many problems began to be resolved. The images were archived in digital form, standard regions of interest could be selected, and temperature measurements obtained from the images. Manufacturers of thermal imaging equipment slowly adapted to the call for quantification and some sold thermal radiation calibration sources to their customers to aid the standardization of technique. Workshops that had started in the late 1960s became a regular feature, and the European Thermographic Association was formed with a major conference in Amsterdam in 1974. Apart from a range of physiological and medical applications groups were formed to formulate guidelines for good practice. This included the requirements for patient preparation, conditions for thermal imaging and criteria for the use of thermal imaging in medicine and pharmacology [7,8]. At the IEEE EMBS conference in Amsterdam some 20 years later in 1996, Dr. N. Diakides facilitated the production of a CD-ROM of the early, seminal papers on infrared imaging in medicine that had been published in *ACTA Thermographica* and the *Journal of Thermology*. This CD was sponsored by the U.S. Office of Technology Applications, Ballistic Missile Defence Organisation and the U.S. National Technology Transfer Center Washington Operations and is available from the authors at the Medical Imaging Research Group at the University of Glamorgan, UK [9]. The archive of papers may also be searched online at the Medical Imaging Group's website [9].

A thermal index was devised in Bath to provide clinicians with a simplified measure of inflammation [10]. A normal range of values was established for ankles, elbows, hands, and knees, with raised values obtained in osteoarthritic joints and higher values still in rheumatoid arthritis. A series of clinical trials with nonsteroid, anti-inflammatory, oral drugs, and steroid analogues for joint injection was published using the index to document the course of treatment [11].

Improvements in thermal imaging cameras have had a major impact, both on image quality and speed of image capture. Early single-element detectors were dependent on optical mechanical scanning. Both spatial and thermal image resolutions were inversely dependent on scanning speed. The Bofors and some American imagers scanned at 1–4 frames/s. AGA cameras were faster at 16 frames/s, and used interlacing to smooth the image. Multielement arrays were developed in the United Kingdom and were employed in cameras made by EMI and Rank. Alignment of the elements was critical, and a poorly aligned array produced characteristic banding in the image. Professor Tom Elliott FRS solved this problem when he designed and produced the first significant detector for faster high-resolution images that subsequently became known as the Signal Processing In The Element (Sprite) detector. Rank Taylor Hobson used the Sprite in the high-resolution system called Talytherm. This camera also had a high specification Infrared zoom lens, with a macro attachment. Superb images of sweat pore function, eyes with contact lenses, and skin pathology were recorded with this system.

With the end of the cold war, the greatly improved military technology was declassified and its use for medical applications was encouraged. As a result, the first focal plane array detectors came from the multielement arrays, with increasing numbers of pixel/elements, yielding high resolution at video frame rates. Uncooled bolometer arrays have also been shown to be adequate for many medical applications. Without the need for electronic cooling systems these cameras are almost maintenance free. Good software with enhancement and analysis is now expected in thermal imaging. Many commercial systems use general imaging software, which is primarily designed for industrial users of the technique. A few dedicated medical software packages have been produced, which can even enhance the images from the older cameras. CTHERM is one such package that is a robust and almost universally usable program for medical thermography [9]. As standardization of image capture and analysis becomes more widely accepted, the ability to manage the images and, if necessary, to transmit them over an intranet or Internet for communication becomes paramount. Future developments will enable the operator of thermal imaging to use reference images and reference data as a diagnostic aid. This, however, depends on the level of standardization that can be provided by the manufacturers, and by the operators themselves in the performance of their technique [12].

Modern thermal imaging is already digital and quantifiable, and ready for the integration into anticipated hospital and clinical computer networks.

References

1. Ring, E.F.J., *The History of Thermal Imaging in the Thermal Image in Medicine and Biology*, eds. Ammer, K. and Ring, E.F.J., pp. 13–20. Uhlen Verlag, Vienna, 1995.
2. Wunderlich, C.A., *On the Temperature in Diseases, a Manual of Medical Thermometry*. Translated from the second German edition by Bathurst Woodman, W., The New Sydenham Society, London, 1871.
3. Flesch, U., Thermographic techniques with liquid crystals in medicine. In *Recent Advances in Medical Thermology*, eds. Ring, E.F.J. and Phillips, B., pp. 283–299. Plenum Press, New York, 1984.
4. Houdas, Y. and Ring, E.F.J., *Human Body Temperature, Its Measurement and Regulation*. Plenum Press, New York, 1982.
5. Ring, E.F.J., The discovery of infrared radiation in 1800. *Imaging Science Journal*, 48, 1–8, 2000.
6. Jones, B.F., A reappraisal of infrared thermal image analysis in medicine. *IEEE Transactions on Medical Imaging*, 17, 1019–1027, 1998.
7. Engel, J.M., Cosh, J.A., Ring, E.F.J. et al., Thermography in locomotor diseases: Recommended procedure. *European Journal of Rheumatology and Inflammation*, 2, 299–306, 1979.
8. Ring, E.F.J., Engel, J.M., and Page-Thomas, D.P., Thermological methods in clinical pharmacology. *International Journal of Clinical Pharmacology*, 22, 20–24, 1984.
9. CTHERM website www.medimaging.org.
10. Collins, A.J., Ring, E.J.F., Cash, J.A., and Brown, P.A., Quantification of thermography in arthritis using multi-isothermal analysis: I. The thermographic index. *Annals of the Rheumatic Diseases*, 33, 113–115, 1974.
11. Bacon, P.A., Ring, E.F.J., and Collins, A.J., Thermography in the assessment of antirheumatic agents. In *Rheumatoid Arthritis*, eds. J.L. Gordon and B.L. Hazleman, pp. 105–110. Elsevier/North-Holland Biochemical Press, Amsterdam, 1977.
12. Ring, E.F.J. and Ammer, K., The technique of infrared imaging in medicine. *Thermology International*, 10, 7–14, 2000.

24

Infrared Detectors and Detector Arrays

Paul R. Norton

U.S. Army CERDEC Night Vision and Electronic Sensors Directorate

Stuart B. Horn

U.S. Army CERDEC Night Vision and Electronic Sensors Directorate

Joseph G. Pellegrino

U.S. Army CERDEC Night Vision and Electronic Sensors Directorate

Philip Perconti

U.S. Army CERDEC Night Vision and Electronic Sensors Directorate

There are two general classes of detectors: *photon* (or quantum) and *thermal* detectors [1,2]. Photon detectors convert absorbed photon energy into released electrons (from their bound states to conduction states). The material bandgap describes the energy necessary to transition a charge carrier from the valence band to the conduction band. The change in charge carrier state changes the electrical properties of the material. These electrical property variations are measured to determine the amount of incident optical power. Thermal detectors absorb energy over a broad band of wavelengths. The energy absorbed by a detector causes the temperature of the material to increase. Thermal detectors have at least one inherent electrical property that changes with temperature. This temperature-related property is measured electrically to determine the power on the detector. Commercial infrared imaging systems suitable for medical applications use both types of detectors. We begin by describing the physical mechanism employed by these two detector types.

24.1 Photon Detectors

Infrared radiation consists of a flux of photons, the quantum-mechanical elements of all electromagnetic radiation. The energy of the photon is given by

$$E_{ph} = h\nu = hc/\lambda = 1.986 \times 10^{-19}/\lambda \text{ J}/\mu\text{m} \tag{24.1}$$

where h is the Planck's constant, c is the speed of light, and λ is the wavelength of the infrared photon in micrometers (μm).

Photon detectors respond by elevating a bound electron in a material to a free or conductive state. Two types of photon detectors are produced for the commercial market:

- Photoconductive
- Photovoltaic

24.1.1 Photoconductive Detectors

The mechanism of photoconductive detectors is based upon the excitation of bound electrons to a mobile state where they can move freely through the material. The increase in the number of conductive electrons, n, created by the photon flux, Φ_0, allows more current to flow when the detective element is used in a bias circuit having an electric field E. The photoconductive detector element having dimensions of length L, width W, and thickness t is represented in Figure 24.1.

Figure 24.2 illustrates how the current–voltage characteristics of a photoconductor change with incident photon flux (Chapter 25).

The response of a photoconductive detector can be written as

$$R = \frac{\eta q R E \tau (\mu_n + \mu_p)}{E_{ph}L}(V/W) \tag{24.2}$$

where R is the response in volts per watt, η is the quantum efficiency in electrons per photon, q is the charge of an electron, R is the resistance of the detector element, τ is the lifetime of a photoexcited electron, and μ_n and μ_p are the mobilities of the electrons and holes in the material in volts per square centimeter per second.

Noise in photoconductors is the square root averaged sum of terms from three sources:

- Johnson noise
- Thermal generation–recombination
- Photon generation–recombination

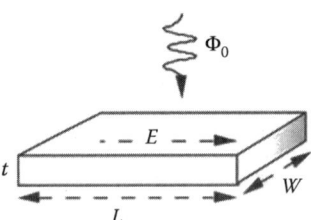

FIGURE 24.1   Photoconductive detector geometry.

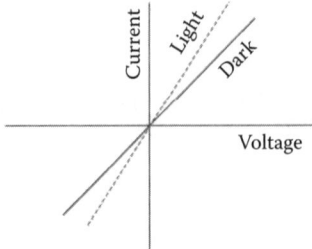

FIGURE 24.2   Current–voltage characteristics of a photoconductive detector.

Expressions for the total noise and each of the noise terms are given in Equations 24.3 through 24.6:

$$V_{\text{noise}} = \sqrt{V_{\text{Johnson}}^2 + V_{\text{ph g-r}}^2 + V_{\text{th g-r}}^2} \tag{24.3}$$

$$V_{\text{Johnson}} = \sqrt{4kTR} \tag{24.4}$$

$$V_{\text{ph g-r}} = \frac{\sqrt{\eta\phi(WL)}\,2qRE\tau(\mu_n + \mu_p)}{L} \tag{24.5}$$

$$V_{\text{th g-r}} = \sqrt{\frac{np}{n+p}\tau\left(\frac{Wt}{L}\right)}\,2qRE(\mu_n + \mu_p) \tag{24.6}$$

The figure of merit for infrared detectors is called D^*. The units of D^* are cm $(\text{Hz})^{1/2}$/W, but are most commonly referred to as Jones. D^* is the detector's signal-to-noise ratio (SNR), normalized to an area of 1 cm², to a noise bandwidth of 1 Hz, and to a signal level of 1 W at the peak of the detectors response. The equation for D^* is

$$D_{\text{peak}}^* = \frac{R}{V_{\text{noise}}}\sqrt{WL}\ (\text{Jones}) \tag{24.7}$$

where W and L are defined in Figure 24.1.

A special condition of D^* for a photoconductor is noted when the noise is dominated by the photon noise term. This is a condition in which the D^* is maximum.

$$D_{\text{blip}}^* = \frac{\lambda}{2hc}\sqrt{\frac{\eta}{E_{\text{ph}}}} \tag{24.8}$$

where "blip" denotes background-limited photodetector.

24.1.2 Photovoltaic Detectors

The mechanism of photovoltaic detectors is based on the collection of photoexcited carriers by a diode junction. Photovoltaic detectors are the most commonly used photon detectors for imaging arrays in current production. An example of the structure of detectors in such an array is illustrated in Figure 24.3

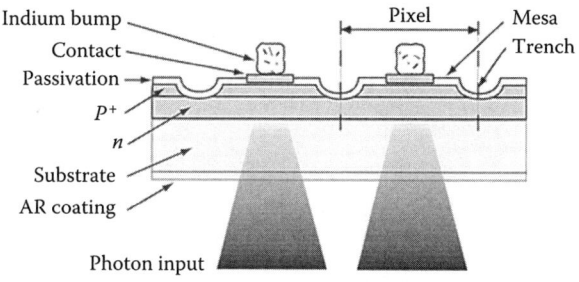

FIGURE 24.3 Photovoltaic detector structure example for mesa diodes.

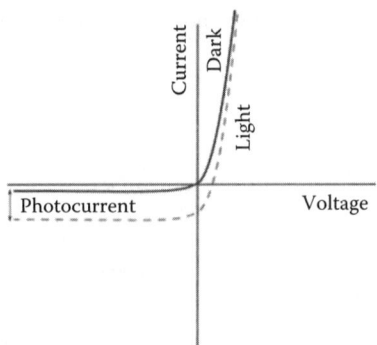

FIGURE 24.4 Current–voltage characteristics of a photovoltaic detector.

for a mesa photodiode. Photons are incident from the optically transparent detector substrate side and are absorbed in the *n*-type material layer. Absorbed photons create a pair of carriers, an electron and a hole. The hole diffuses to the *p*-type side of the junction creating a photocurrent. A contact on the *p*-type side of the junction is connected to an indium bump that mates to an amplifier in a readout circuit where the signal is stored and conveyed to a display during each display frame. A common contact is made to the *n*-type layer at the edge of the detector array. Adjacent diodes are isolated electrically from each other by a mesa etch cutting the *p*-type layer into islands.

Figure 24.4 illustrates how the current–voltage characteristics of a photodiode change with incident photon flux (Chapter 25).

The current of the photodiode can be expressed as

$$I = I_0(e^{qV/kT} - 1) - I_{\text{photo}} \tag{24.9}$$

where I_0 is reverse-bias leakage current and I_{photo} is the photoinduced current. The photocurrent is given by

$$I = I_0(e^{qV/kT} - 1) - I_{\text{photo}} \tag{24.10}$$

where Φ_0 is the photon flux in photons/cm^2/s and A is the detector area.

Detector noise in a photodiode includes three terms: Johnson noise, thermal diffusion generation and recombination noise, and photon generation and recombination. The Johnson noise term is written in terms of the detector resistance $dI/dV = R_0$ at zero bias as

$$i_{\text{Johnson}} = \sqrt{4kT/R_0} \tag{24.11}$$

where k is the Boltzmann's constant and T is the detector temperature. The thermal diffusion current is given by

$$i_{\text{diffusion noise}} = q\sqrt{2I_s\left[\exp\left(\frac{eV}{kT}\right) - 1\right]} \tag{24.12}$$

where the saturation current, I_s, is given by

$$I_s = qn_i^2 \left[\frac{1}{N_a} \sqrt{\frac{D_n}{\tau_{n_0}}} + \frac{1}{N_d} \sqrt{\frac{D_p}{\tau_{p_0}}} \right]$$ (24.13)

where N_a and N_d are the concentration of p- and n-type dopants on either side of the diode junction, τ_{n0} and τ_{p0} are the carrier lifetimes, and D_n and D_p are the diffusion constants on either side of the junction, respectively.

The photon generation–recombination current noise is given by

$$i_{\text{photon noise}} = q\sqrt{2\eta\Phi_0}$$ (24.14)

When the junction is at zero bias, the photodiode D^* is given by

$$D_\lambda^* = \frac{\lambda}{hc}\eta e \frac{1}{\left[(4kT/R_0 A) + 2e^2\eta \right]}$$ (24.15)

In the special case of a photodiode that is operated without sufficient cooling, the maximum D^* may be limited by the dark current or leakage current of the junction. The expression for D^* in this case, written in terms of the junction-resistance area product, $R_0 A$, is given by

$$D_\lambda^* = \frac{\lambda}{hc}\eta e \sqrt{\frac{R_0 A}{4kT}}$$ (24.16)

Figure 24.5 illustrates how D^* is limited by the $R_0 A$ product for the case of dark-current-limited detector conditions.

For the ideal case where the noise is dominated by the photon flux in the background scene, the peak D^* is given by

$$D_\lambda^* = \frac{\lambda}{hc}\sqrt{\frac{\eta}{2E_{\text{ph}}}}$$ (24.17)

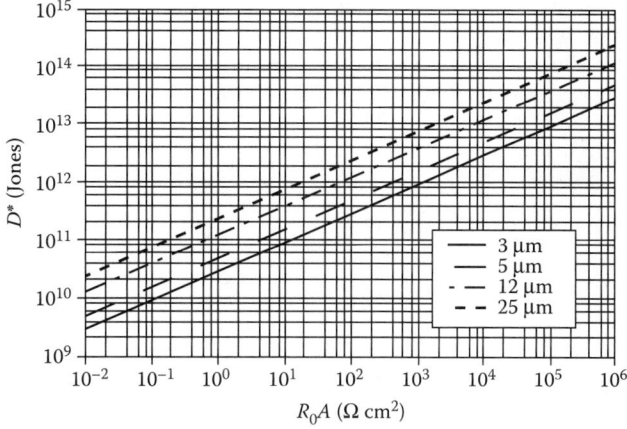

FIGURE 24.5 D^* as a function of the detector resistance–area product, $R_0 A$. This condition applies when detector performance is limited by dark current.

Comparing this limit with that for a photoconductive detector in Equation 24.8, we see that the background-limited D^* for a photodiode is higher by a factor of square root of 2 ($\sqrt{2}$).

24.2 Thermal Detectors

Thermal detectors operate by converting the incoming photon flux to heat [3]. The heat input causes the thermal detector's temperature to rise and this change in temperature is sensed by a bolometer. A bolometer element operates by changing its resistance as its temperature is changed. A bias circuit across the bolometer can be used to convert the changing current to a signal output.

The coefficient α is used to compare the sensitivity of different bolometer materials and is given by

$$\alpha = \frac{1}{R_d}\frac{dR}{dT} \tag{24.18}$$

where R_d is the resistance of the bolometer element, and dR/dT is the change in resistance per unit change in temperature. Typical values of α are 2–3%.

Theoretically, the bolometer structure can be represented as illustrated in Figure 24.6. The rise in temperature due to a heat flux ϕ_e is given by

$$\Delta T = \frac{\eta P_0}{G(1 + \omega^2\tau^2)^{1/2}} \tag{24.19}$$

where P_0 is the radiant power of the signal in watts, G is the thermal conductance (K/W), h is the percentage of flux absorbed, and ω is the angular frequency of the signal. The bolometer time constant, τ, is determined by

$$\tau = \frac{C}{G} \tag{24.20}$$

where C is the heat capacity of the detector element.

The sensitivity or D^* of a thermal detector is limited by variations in the detector temperature caused by fluctuations in the absorption and radiation of heat between the detector element and the background. Sensitive thermal detectors must minimize competing mechanisms for heat loss by the element, namely, convection and conduction.

Convection by air is eliminated by isolating the detector in a vacuum. If the conductive heat losses were less than those due to radiation, then the limiting D^* would be given by

$$D^*(T, f) = 2.8 \times 10^{16}\sqrt{\frac{\varepsilon}{T_2^5 + T_1^5}}\ \text{Jones} \tag{24.21}$$

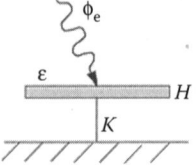

FIGURE 24.6 Abstract bolometer detector structure, where C is the thermal capacitance, G is the thermal conductance, and o is the emissivity of the surface. ϕ_e represents the energy flux in W/cm².

where T_1 is the detector temperature, T_2 the background temperature, and o the value of the detector's emissivity and equally its absorption. For the usual case of both the detector and background temperature at normal ambient, 300 K, the limiting D^* is 1.8×10^{10} Jones.

Bolometer operation is constrained by the requirement that the response time of the detector be compatible with the frame rate of the imaging system. Most bolometer cameras operate at a 30 Hz frame rate—33 ms frame. Response times of the bolometer are usually designed to be on the order of 10 ms. This gives the element a fast-enough response to follow scenes with rapidly varying temperatures without objectionable image smearing.

24.3 Detector Materials

The most popular commercial cameras for thermal imaging today use the following detector materials [4]:

- InSb for 5 μm medium-wavelength infrared (MWIR) imaging
- $Hg_{1-x}Cd_xTe$ alloys for 5 and 10 μm long-wavelength infrared (LWIR) imaging
- Quantum well detectors for 5 and 10 μm imaging
- Uncooled bolometers for 10 μm imaging

We will now review a few of the basic properties of these detector types.

Photovoltaic InSb remains a popular detector for the MWIR spectral band operating at a temperature of 80 K [5,6]. The detector's spectral response at 80 K is shown in Figure 24.7. The spectral response cutoff is about 5.5 μm at 80 K, a good match to the MWIR spectral transmission of the atmosphere. As the operating temperature of InSb is raised, the spectral response extends to longer wavelengths and the dark current increases accordingly. It is thus not normally used above about 100 K. At 80 K, the R_0A product of InSb detectors is typically in the range of 10^5–10^6 Ω cm^2—see Equation 24.16 and Figure 24.5 for reference.

Crystals of InSb are grown in bulk boules up to 3 in. in diameter. InSb materials is highly uniform and combined with a planar-implanted process in which the device geometry is precisely controlled, the resulting detector array responsivity is good to excellent. Devices are usually made with a *p/n* diode polarity using diffusion or ion implantation. Staring arrays of backside illuminated, direct hybrid InSb detectors in 256 # 256, 240 # 320, 480 # 640, 512 # 640, and 1024 # 1024 formats are available from a number of vendors.

HgCdTe detectors are commercially available to cover the spectral range from 1 to 12 μm [7–13]. Figure 24.8 illustrates representative spectral response from photovoltaic devices, the most commonly used type. Crystals of HgCdTe today are mostly grown in thin epitaxial layers on infrared-transparent CdZnTe crystals. Short-wavelength infrared (SWIR) and MWIR material can also be grown on Si substrates with CdZnTe buffer layers. Growth of the epitaxial layers is by liquid-phase melts, molecular

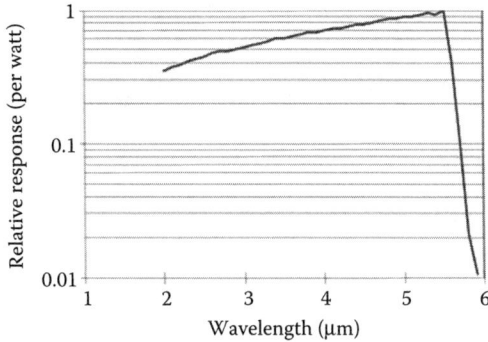

FIGURE 24.7 Spectral response per watt of an InSb detector at 80 K.

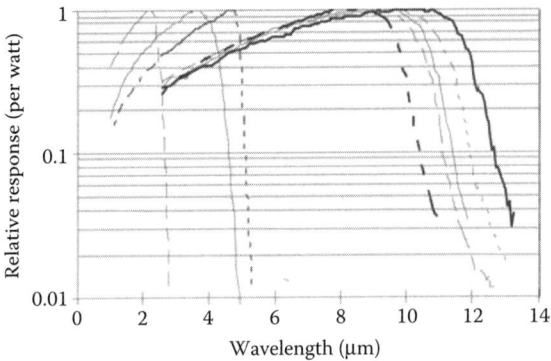

FIGURE 24.8 Representative spectral response curves for a variety of HgCdTe alloy detectors. Spectral cutoff can be varied over the SWIR, MWIR, and LWIR regions.

beams, or by chemical vapor deposition. Substrate dimensions of CdZnTe crystals are in the 25–50 cm^2 range and Si wafers up to 5–6 in. (12.5–15 cm) in diameter have been used for this purpose. The device structure for a typical HgCdTe photodiode is shown in Figure 24.3.

At 80 K, the leakage current of HgCdTe is small enough to provide both MWIR and LWIR detectors that can be photon-noise dominated. Figure 24.9 shows the R_0A product of representative diodes for wavelengths ranging from 4 to 12 μm.

The versatility of HgCdTe detector material is directly related to being able to grow a broad range of alloy compositions in order to optimize the response at a particular wavelength. Alloys are usually adjusted to provide response in the 1–3 μm SWIR, 3–5 μm MWIR, or the 8–12 μm LWIR spectral regions. Short-wavelength detectors can operate uncooled, or with thermoelectric coolers that have no moving parts. Medium- and long-wavelength detectors are generally operated at 80 K using a cryogenic cooler engine. HgCdTe detectors in 256 # 256, 240 # 320, 480 # 640, and 512 # 640 formats are available from a number of vendors.

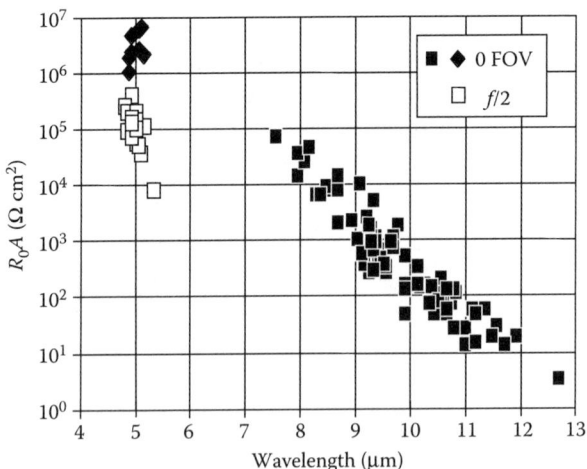

FIGURE 24.9 Values of R_0A product as a function of wavelength for HgCdTe photodiodes. Note that the R_0A product varies slightly with illumination—0° field-of-view compared with $f/2$—especially for shorter-wavelength devices.

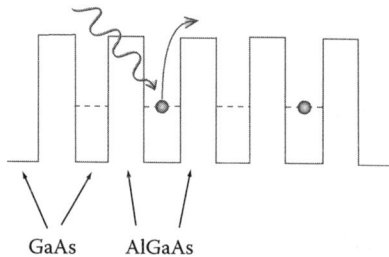

FIGURE 24.10 Quantum wells generate bound states for electrons in the conduction band. The conduction bands for a QWIP structure are shown consisting of $Al_xGa_{1-x}As$ barriers and GaAs wells. For a given pair of materials having a fixed conduction band offset, the binding energy of an electron in the well can be adjusted by varying the width of the well. With an applied bias, photoexcited electrons from the GaAs wells are transported and detected as photocurrent.

Quantum well infrared photodetectors (QWIPs) consist of alternating layers of semiconductor material with larger and narrower bandgaps [14–20]. This series of alternating semiconductor layers is deposited one layer upon another using an ultrahigh vacuum technique such as molecular beam epitaxy (MBE). Alternating large- and narrow-bandgap materials give rise to quantum wells that provide bound and quasi-bound states for electrons or holes [1–5].

Many simple QWIP structures have used GaAs as the narrow-bandgap quantum well material and $Al_xGa_{1-x}As$ as the wide bandgap barrier layers as shown in Figure 24.10. The properties of the QWIP are related to the structural design and can be specified by the well width, barrier height, and doping density. In turn, these parameters can be tuned by controlling the cell temperatures of the gallium, aluminum, and arsenic cells as well as the doping cell temperature. The quantum well width (thickness) is governed by the time interval for which the Ga and As cell shutters are left opened. The barrier height is regulated by the composition of the $Al_xGa_{1-x}As$ layers, which are determined by the relative temperature of the Al and Ga cells. QWIP detectors rely on the absorption of incident radiation within the quantum well and typically the well material is doped n-type at an approximate level of 5×10^{17}.

The QWIP detectors require that an electric field component of the incident radiation be perpendicular to the layer planes of the device. Imaging arrays use diffraction gratings as shown in Figure 24.11. In particular, the latter approach is of practical importance in order to realize two-dimensional detector arrays. The QWIP focal plane array is a reticulated structure formed by conventional photolithographic techniques. Part of the processing involves placing a two-dimensional metallic grating over the focal plane pixels. The grating metal is typically angled at 45° patterns to reflect incident light obliquely so as to couple the perpendicular component of the electric field into the quantum wells thus producing the photoexcitation. The substrate material (GaAs) is backside thinned and a chemical/mechanical polish is used to produce a mirrorlike finish on the backside. The front side of the pixels with indium bumps are

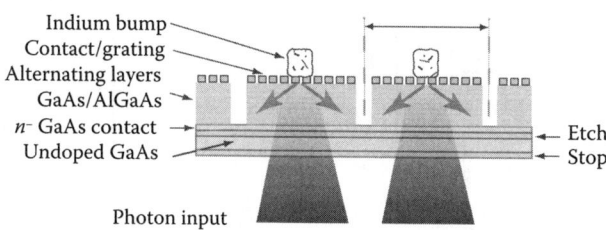

FIGURE 24.11 Backside illuminated QWIP structure with a top side diffraction grating/contact metal. Normally incident light is coupled horizontally into the quantum wells by scattering off a diffraction grating located at the top of the focal plane array.

flip-chip bonded to a readout IC. Light travels through the back side and is unabsorbed during its first pass through the epilayers; upon scattering with a horizontal propagation component from the grating, some of it is then absorbed by the quantum wells, photoexciting carriers. An electric field is produced perpendicular to the layers by applying a bias voltage at doped contact layers. The structure then behaves as a photoconductor.

The QWIP detectors require cooling to about 60 K for LWIR operation in order to adequately reduce the dark current. They also have comparatively low quantum efficiency, generally less than 10%. They thus require longer signal integration times than InSb or HgCdTe devices. However, the abundance of radiation in the LWIR band in particular allows QWIP detectors to still achieve excellent performance in infrared cameras.

The maturity of the GaAs-technology makes QWIPs particularly suited for large commercial focal plane arrays with high spatial resolution. Excellent lateral homogeneity is achieved, thus giving rise to a small fixed-pattern noise. QWIPs have an extremely small $1/f$ noise compared to interband detectors (like HgCdTe or InSb), which is particularly useful if long integration times or image accumulation are required. For these reasons, QWIP is the detector technology of choice for many applications where somewhat smaller quantum efficiencies and lower operation temperatures, compared to interband devices, are tolerable. QWIPs are finding useful applications in surveillance, night vision, quality control, inspection, environmental sciences, and medicine.

Quantum well infrared detectors are available in the 5 and 10 μm spectral region. The spectral response of QWIP detectors can be tuned to a wide range of values by adjusting the width and depth of quantum wells formed in alternating layers of GaAs and GaAlAs. An example of the spectral response from a variety of such structures is shown in Figure 24.12. QWIP spectral response is generally limited to fairly narrow spectral bandwidth—approximately 10–20% of the peak response wavelength. QWIP detectors have higher dark currents than InSb or HgCdTe devices and generally must be cooled to about 60 K for LWIR operation.

The quantum efficiencies of InSb, HgCdTe, and QWIP photon detectors are compared in Figure 24.13. With antireflection coating, InSb and HgCdTe are able to convert about 90% of the incoming photon flux to electrons. The QWIP quantum efficiencies are significantly lower, but work at improving them continues to occupy the attention of research teams.

We conclude this section with a description of Type-II superlattice detectors [21–26]. Although Type-II superlattice detectors are not yet used in arrays for in commercial camera system, the technology is briefly reviewed here because of its potential future importance. This material system mimics an intrinsic detector material such as HgCdTe, but is "bandgap engineered." Type-II superlattice structures

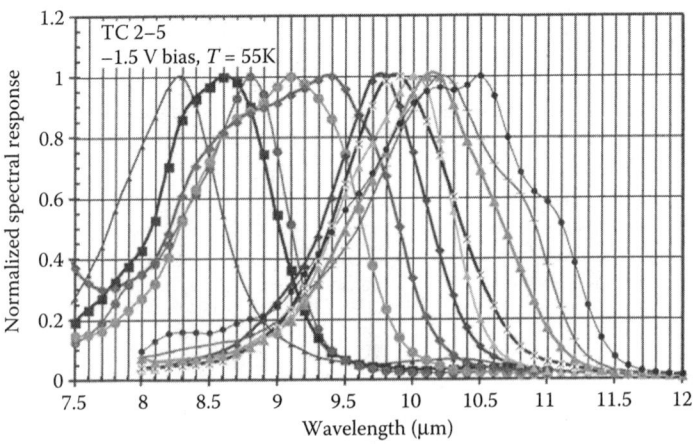

FIGURE 24.12 Representative spectral response of QWIP detectors.

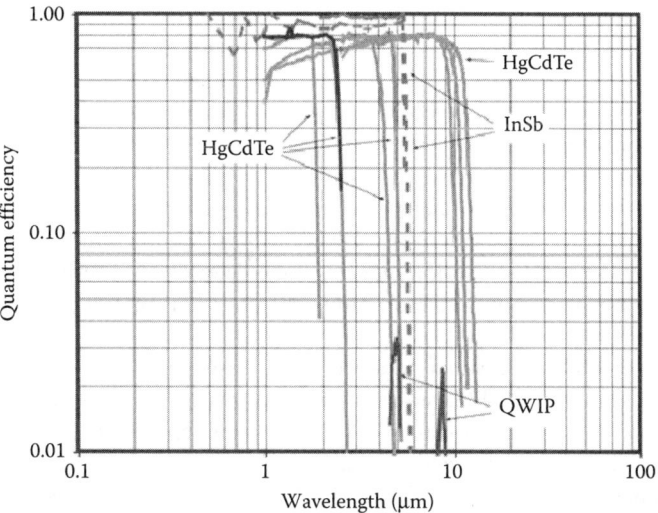

FIGURE 24.13 Comparison of the quantum efficiencies of commercial infrared photon detectors. This figure represents devices that have been antireflection coated.

are fabricated from multilayer stacks of alternating layers of two different semiconductor materials. Figure 24.14 illustrates the structure. The conduction band minimum is in one layer and the valence band minimum is in the adjacent layer (as opposed to both minima being in the same layer as in a Type-I superlattice).

The idea of using Type-II superlattices for LWIR detectors was originally proposed in 1977. Recent work on the MBE growth of Type-II systems by [7] has led to the exploitation of these materials for IR detectors. Short-period superlattices of, for example, strain-balanced InAs/(Ga,In)Sb lead to the

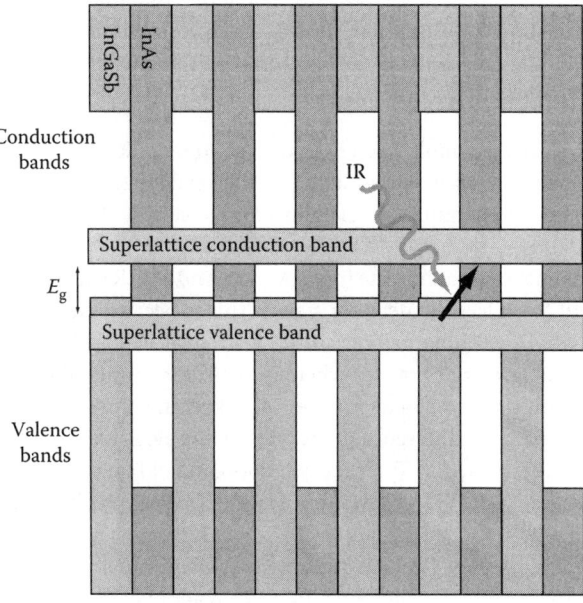

FIGURE 24.14 Band diagram of a short-period InAs/(In,Ga)Sb superlattice showing an infrared transition from the heavy hole (hh) miniband to the electron (e) miniband.

formation of conduction and valence minibands. In these band states heavy holes are largely confined to the (Ga,In)Sb layers and electrons are primarily confined to the InAs layers. However, because of the relatively low electron mass in InAs, the electron wave functions extend considerably beyond the interfaces and have significant overlap with heavy-hole wave functions. Hence, significant absorption is possible at the minigap energy (which is tunable by changing layer thickness and barrier height).

Cutoff wavelengths from 3 to 20 μm and beyond are potentially possible with this system. Unlike QWIP detectors, the absorption of normally incident flux is permitted by selection rules, obviating the need for grating structures or corrugations that are needed with QWIPs. Finally, Auger transition rates, which place intrinsic limits on the performance of these detectors and severely impact the lifetimes found in bulk, narrow-gap detectors, can be minimized by judicious choices of the structure's geometry and strain profile.

In the future, further advantages may be achievable by using the InAs/Ga(As,Sb) material system where both the InAs and Ga(As,Sb) layers may be lattice matched to InAs substrates. The intrinsic quality obtainable in these structures can be in principle superior to that obtained in InAs/(Ga,In)Sb structures. Since dislocations may be reduced to a minimum in the InAs/Ga(As,Sb) material system, it may be the most suitable Type-II material for making large arrays of photovoltaic detectors.

Development efforts for Type-II superlattice detectors are primarily focused on improving material quality and identifying sources of unwanted leakage currents. The most challenging problem currently is to passivate the exposed sidewalls of the superlattice layers where the pixels are etched in fabrication. Advances in these areas should result in a new class of IR detectors with the potential for high performance at high operating temperatures.

24.4 Detector Readouts

Detectors themselves are isolated arrays of photodiodes, photoconductors, or bolometers. Detectors need a readout to integrate or sample their output and convey the signal in an orderly sequence to a signal processor and display [27].

Almost all readouts are integrated circuits (ICs) made from silicon. They are commonly referred to as readout integrated circuits, or ROICs. Here, we briefly describe the functions and features of these readouts, first for photon detectors and then for thermal detectors.

24.4.1 Readouts for Photon Detectors

Photon detectors are typically assembled as a hybrid structure, as illustrated in Figure 24.15. Each pixel of the detector array is connected to the unit cell of the readout through an indium bump. Indium bumps allow for a soft, low-temperature metal connection to convey the signal from the detector to the readout's input circuit.

Commercial thermal imagers that operate in the MWIR and LWIR spectral regions generally employ a direct injection circuit to collect the detector signal. This is because this circuit is simple and works well with the relatively high photon currents in these spectral bands. The direct injection transistor feeds the signal onto an integrating capacitor where it stored for a time called the integration time. The integration time is typically around 200 μs for the LWIR spectral band and 2 ms for the MWIR band, corresponding to the comparative difference in the photon flux available. The integration time is limited by the size of the integration capacitor. Typical capacitors can hold on the order of 3×10^7 electrons.

For cameras operating in the SWIR band, the lower flux levels typically require a more complicated input amplifier. The most common choice employs a capacitive feedback circuit, providing the ability to have significant gain at the pixel level before storage on an integrating capacitor.

Two readout modes are employed, depending upon the readout design:

- Snapshot
- Rolling frame

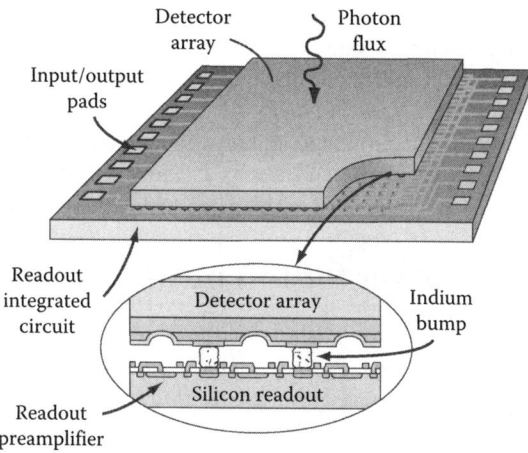

FIGURE 24.15 Hybrid detector array structure consists of a detector array connected to a readout array with indium metal bumps. Detector elements are usually photodiodes or photoconductors, although photocapacitors are sometimes used. Each pixel in the readout contains at least one addressable switch, and more often a preampflifier or buffer together with a charge storage capacitor for integrating the photosignal.

In the snapshot mode, all pixels integrate simultaneously, are stored, and then read out in sequence, followed by resetting the integration capacitors. In the rolling frame mode, the capacitors of each row are reset after each pixel in that row is read. In this case, each pixel integrates in different parts of the image frame. A variant of the rolling frame is an interlaced output. In this case, the even rows are read out in the first frame and the odd rows in the next. This corresponds to how standard U.S. television displays function.

It is common for each column in the readout to have an amplifier to provide some gain to the signal coming from each row as it is read. The column amplifier outputs are then fed to the output amplifiers. Commercial readouts typically have one, two, or four outputs, depending upon the array size and frame rate. Most commercial cameras operate at 30 or 60 Hz.

Another common feature found on some readouts is the ability to operate at higher frame rates on a subset of the full array. This ability is called windowing. It allows data to be collected more quickly on a limited portion of the image.

24.4.2 Thermal Detector Readouts

Bolometer detectors have comparatively lower resistance than photon detectors and relatively slow inherent response times. This condition allows readouts that do not have to integrate the charge during the frame, but only need to sample it for a brief time. This mode is frequently referred to as pulse-biased.

The unit cell of the bolometer contains only a switch that is pulsed on once per frame to allow current to flow from each row in turn to the column amplifiers. Bias is supplied by the row multiplexer. Sample times for each detector are typically on the order of the frame time divided by the number of rows. Many designs employ differential input column amplifiers that are simultaneously fed an input from a dummy or blind bolometer element in order to subtract a large fraction of the current that flows when the element is biased.

The nature of bolometer operation means that the readout mode is rolling frame. Some designs also provide interlaced outputs for input to TV-like displays.

24.4.3 Readout Evolution

Early readouts required multiple bias supply inputs and multiple clock signals for operation. Today, only two clocks and two bias supplies are typically required. The master clock sets the frame rate. The integration clock sets the time that the readout signal is integrated, or that the readout bias pulse is applied. On-chip clock and bias circuits generate the additional clocks and biases required to run the readout. Separate grounds for the analog and digital chip circuitry are usually employed to minimize noise.

Current development efforts are beginning to add on-chip analog-to-digital (A/D) converters to the readout. This feature provides a direct digital output, avoiding significant difficulties in controlling extraneous noise when the sensor is integrated with an imaging or camera system.

24.5 Technical Challenges for Infrared Detectors

Twenty-five years ago, infrared imagining was revolutionized by the introduction of the Probeye Infrared camera. At a modest 8 pounds, Probeye enabled handheld operation, a feature previously unheard of at that time when very large, very expensive IR imaging systems were the rule. Infrared components and technologies have advanced considerably since then. With the introduction of the Indigo Systems Omega camera, one can now acquire a complete infrared camera weighing less than 100 g and occupying 3.5 in.[3]

Many forces are at play enabling this dramatic reduction in camera size. Virtually all of these can be traced to improvements in the silicon IC processing industry. Largely enabled by advancements in photolithography, but additionally aided by improvements in vacuum deposition equipment, device feature sizes have been steadily reduced. It was not too long ago that the minimum device feature size was just pushing to break the 1-μm barrier. Today, foundries are focused on production implementation of 65–90 nm feature sizes.

The motivation behind such significant improvements has been the high-dollar/high-volume commercial electronics business. Silicon foundries have expended billions of dollars in capitalization and R&D aimed at increasing the density and speed of the transistors per unit chip area. Cellular telephones, personal data assistants (PDAs), and laptop computers are all applications demanding smaller size, lower power, and more features—performance—from electronic components. Infrared detector arrays and cameras have taken direct advantage of these advancements.

24.5.1 Uncooled Infrared Detector Challenges

The major challenge for all infrared markets is to reduce the pixel size while increasing the sensitivity. Reduction from a 50-μm pixel to a 25-μm pixel, while maintaining or even reducing noise equivalent temperature difference (NETD), is a major goal that is now being widely demonstrated (see Figure 24.16).

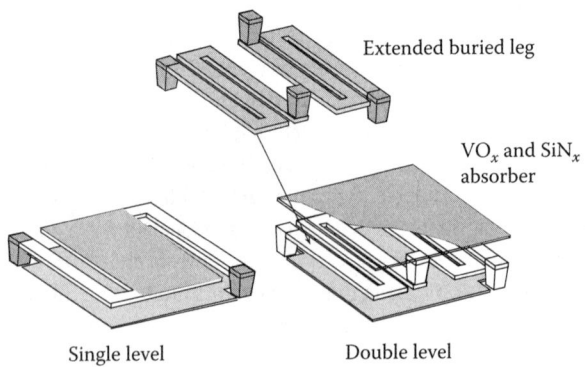

Extended buried leg

VO$_x$ and SiN$_x$ absorber

Single level　　　　　　　Double level

FIGURE 24.16 Uncooled microbolometer pixel structures having noise-equivalent temperature difference (NEΔT) values <50 mK: single level for 2 mil (50 μm) pixels in a 240 × 320 format and double level for 1 mil (25 μm) pixels in a 480 × 640 format. (Courtesy of Raytheon Vision Systems.)

The trends are illustrated by a simple examination of a highly idealized bolometer: the DC response of a detector in which we neglect all noise terms except temperature fluctuation noise, and the thermal conductance value is not detector area dependent (i.e., we are not at or near the radiation conductance limit). Using these assumptions, reducing the pixel area by a factor of four will reduce the SNR by a factor of eight as shown below:

$$\Delta T_{\text{signal|DCresponse}} = \frac{P_{\text{signalDC}}}{G_{\text{th}}} = \frac{\gamma A_{\text{D}} I_{\text{light}}}{G_{\text{th}}} \tag{24.22}$$

where P_{signalDC} is the DC signal from IR radiation (absorbed power) [W], A_{D} is the detector area [m²], I_{light} is the light intensity [W/m²], G_{th} is the thermal conductance [W/K], and γ is a constant that accounts for reflectivity and other factors not relevant to this analysis.

For a detector in the thermal fluctuation limit, the root mean square temperature fluctuation noise is a function of the incident radiation and the thermal conductance of the bolometer bridge.

$$\Delta T_{\text{noise}} \sqrt{\langle \Delta T^2 \rangle} = \sqrt{\frac{kT^2}{C_{\text{th}}}} \tag{24.23}$$

where T is the operating temperature in Kelvin, k is the Boltzmann's constant, and C_{th} is the total heat capacity of the detector in joules per Kelvin [J/K].

The total heat capacity can be written as $C_{\text{th}} = c_{\text{p}} A_{\text{d}} Z_{\text{bridge}}$, where Z_{bridge} is the bolometer bridge thickness in meters and c_{p} is the specific heat of the detector in J/K-m³.

The SNR is then

$$\frac{\Delta T_{\text{signal}}}{\Delta T_{\text{noise}}} = \frac{\gamma A_{\text{D}} I_{\text{light}}}{G_{\text{th}}} \sqrt{\frac{c_{\text{p}} A_{\text{D}} Z_{\text{bridge}}}{kT^2}} = \frac{\gamma A_{\text{D}} I_{\text{light}}}{G_{\text{th}}} A_{\text{D}}^{3/2} \sqrt{\frac{c_{\text{p}} Z_{\text{bridge}}}{kT^2}} \tag{24.24}$$

It can be seen that the SNR goes as the area to the three halves. Therefore, a 4× reduction in detector area reduces the SNR by a factor of eight for this ideal bolometer case. Thermal conductance is assumed constant, that is, the ratio of leg length to thickness remains constant as the detector area is reduced. In practical constructions, reducing the pixel linear dimensions by 2× also reduces the leg length by 2×, thus the thermal conductance increases and aggravates the problem. In order to improve the SNR caused by the 4× loss in area, one may be tempted to reduce the thermal conductance G_{th} by 8×. To accomplish this, the length of the legs must be increased and their thickness reduced. By folding the legs under the detector, as seen in Figure 24.10, one can achieve this result. However, an 8× reduction in thermal conductance would result in a detrimental increase in the thermal time constant.

The thermal time constant is given by $\tau_{\text{thermal}} = C_{\text{th}}/G_{\text{th}}$. The heat capacity is reduced by 4× because of the area loss. If G_{th} is reduced by a factor of 8×, then $\tau_{\text{thermal}} = 2C_{\text{th}}/G_{\text{th}}$ is increased by a factor of two. This image smear associated with this increased time constant would prove problematic for practical military applications.

In order to maintain the same time constant, the total heat capacity must be reduced accordingly. Making the detector thinner may achieve this result except that it also increases the temperature fluctuation noise. From this simple example, one can readily see the inherent relationship between SNR and the thermal time constant.

We would like to maintain both an equivalent SNR and thermal time constant as the detector cell size is decreased. This can be achieved by maintaining the relationships between the thermal conductance, detector area, and bridge thickness as shown in the following.

The thermal time constant is given by

$$\tau_{\text{thermal}} = \frac{C_{\text{th}}}{G_{\text{th}}} = \frac{c_p A_D Z_{\text{bridge}}}{G_{\text{th}}} \tag{24.25}$$

Equating the thermal time constant of the large and small pixels and doing the same with the SNR leads to the following relationships, where the primed variables are the parameters required for the new detector cell:

$$\tau_{\text{thermal}} = \frac{c_p A_D Z_{\text{bridge}}}{G_{\text{th}}} = \frac{c_p A_D' Z_{\text{bridge}}'}{G_{\text{th}}'} \tag{24.26}$$

$$\frac{\Delta T_{\text{signal}}}{\Delta T_{\text{noise}}} = \frac{\gamma A_D I_{\text{light}}}{G_{\text{th}}} \sqrt{\frac{c_p A_D Z_{\text{bridge}}}{kT^2}} = \frac{\gamma A_D' I_{\text{light}}}{G_{\text{th}}'} \sqrt{\frac{c_p A_D' Z_{\text{bridge}}'}{kT^2}} \tag{24.27}$$

Rearranging τ_{thermal} to find the ratio $G_{\text{th}}/G_{\text{th}}'$ and substituting into the SNR, we obtain

$$\frac{Z_{\text{bridge}}'}{Z_{\text{bridge}}} = \frac{A_D'}{A_D}, \quad \text{and it follows that } \frac{G_{\text{th}}'}{G_{\text{th}}} = \left(\frac{Z_{\text{bridge}}'}{Z_{\text{bridge}}} \right)^2 \tag{24.28}$$

So, it becomes evident that a 4× reduction in pixel cell area requires a 16×, and not an 8×, reduction in thermal conductance to maintain equivalent SNR and thermal time constant. This gives some insight into the problems of designing small pixel bolometers for high sensitivity. It should be noted that in current implementations, the state-of-the-art sensitivity is about 10× from the thermal limits.

24.5.2 Electronics Challenges

Specific technology improvements spawned by the commercial electronics business that have enabled size reductions in IR camera signal processing electronics include

- Faster digital signal processors (DSPs) with internal memory 1 MB
- Higher-density field-programmable gate arrays (FPGAs) (>200 K gates and with an embedded processor core)
- Higher-density static (synchronous?) random access memory >4 MB
- Low-power, 14-bit differential A/D converters

Another enabler, also attributable to the silicon industry, is reduction in the required core voltage of these devices (see Figure 24.17). Five years ago, the input voltage for virtually all-electronic components was 5 V. Today, one can buy a DSP with a core voltage as low as 1.2 V. Power consumption of the device is proportional to the square of the voltage. So a reduction from 5- to 1.2-V core represents more than an order of magnitude power reduction.

The input voltage ranges for most components (e.g., FPGAs and memories) are following the same trends. These reductions are not only a boon for reduced power consumption, but also these lower power devices typically come in much smaller footprints. IC packaging advancements have kept up with the higher-density, lower-power devices. One can now obtain a device with almost twice the number of I/Os in 25% of the required area (see Figure 24.18).

All of these lower-power, smaller-footprint components exist by virtue of the significant demand created by the commercial electronics industry. These trends will continue. Moore's law (logic density

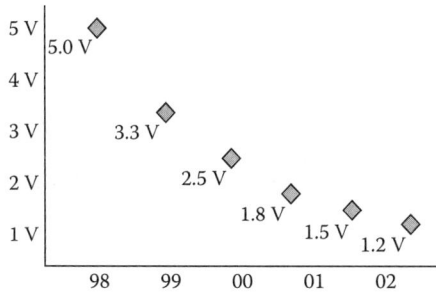

FIGURE 24.17 IC device core voltage versus time.

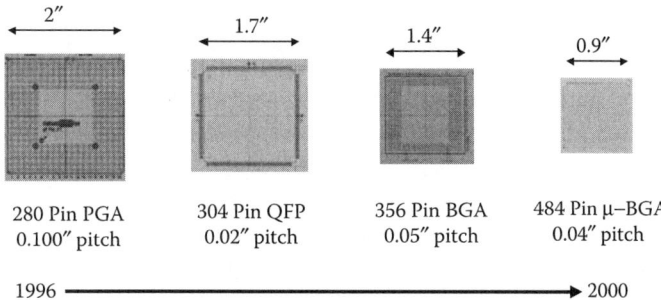

FIGURE 24.18 Advancements in component packaging miniaturization together with increasing pin count that enables reduced camera volume.

in bits/in.² will double every 18 months) nicely describes the degree by which we can expect further advancements.

24.5.3 Detector Readout Challenges

The realization of tighter design rules positively affects reduction in camera size in yet another way. Multiplexers, or ROICs, directly benefit from the increased density. Now, without enlarging the size of the ROIC die, more functions can be contained in the device. On-ROIC A/D conversion eliminates the need for a dedicated, discrete A/D converter. On-ROIC clock and bias generation reduces the number of vacuum dewar feedthroughs to yield a smaller package as well as reducing the complexity and size of the camera power supply. Putting the nonuniformity correction circuitry on the ROIC reduces the magnitude of the detector output signal swing and minimizes the required input dynamic range of the A/D converter. All of these increases in ROIC functionality come with the increased density of the silicon fabrication process.

24.5.4 Optics Challenges

Another continuing advancement that has helped reduced the size of IR cameras is the progress made at increasing the performance of the uncooled detectors themselves. The gains made at increasing the sensitivity of the detectors has directly translated to reduction in the size of the optics. With a sensitivity goal of 100 mK, an *F*/1 optic has traditionally been required to collect enough energy. Given the recent sensitivity improvements in detectors, achievement of 100 mK can be attained with an *F*/2 optic. This reduction in required aperture size greatly reduces the camera size and weight. These improvements

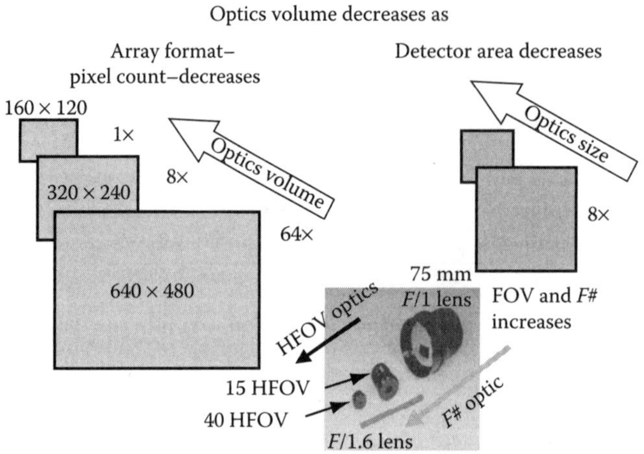

FIGURE 24.19 Trade-off between optics size and volume and *f/#*, array format, and pixel size.

in detector sensitivity can also be directly traceable to improvements in the silicon industry. The same photolithography and vacuum deposition equipments used to fabricate commercial ICs are used to make bolometers. The finer geometry line widths translate directly to increased thermal isolation and increased fill factor, both of which are factors in increased responsivity.

Reduction in optics' size was based on a sequence of NEDT performance improvements in uncooled VO_x microbolometer detectors so that faster optics $F/1.4$ to $F/2$ could be utilized in the camera and still maintain a moderate performance level. As indicated by Equations 24.29 through 24.33, the size of the optics is based on the required field-of-view (FOV), number of detectors (format of the detector array), area of the detector, and *F#* of the optics (see Figure 24.19). The volume of the optics is considered to be approximately a cylinder with a volume of $\pi r^2 L$. In Equations 24.29 through 24.33, FL is the optics focal length equivalent to L, D_o is the optics diameter and $D_o/2$ is equivalent to r, A_{det} is the area of the detector, *F#* is the *f*-number of the optics, and HFOV is the horizontal FOV.

$$\text{FL} = \frac{\#\,\text{horizontal detectors}}{\tan(\text{HFOV}/2)} = \frac{\sqrt{A_{det}}}{2} \tag{24.29}$$

$$D_o = \frac{\#\,\text{horizontal detectors}}{\tan(\text{HFOV}/2)} = \frac{\sqrt{A_{det}}}{2F\#} \tag{24.30}$$

$$F\# = \frac{\text{FL}}{D_o} \tag{24.31}$$

$$\text{Volume}_{\text{optics}} = \pi\left[\frac{D_o}{2}\right]^2 = \text{FL}$$

$$= \pi\left[\frac{(\#\,\text{horizontal detectors}/(\tan(\text{HFOV}/2))) = (\sqrt{A_{det}}/2F\#)}{2}\right]^2 = \text{FL} \tag{24.32}$$

$$\text{Volume}_{\text{optics}} = \pi\left[\frac{(\#\,\text{horizontal detectors}/(\tan(\text{HFOV}/2))) = \sqrt{A_{det}}}{32F\#^2}\right]^3 \tag{24.33}$$

Uncooled cameras have utilized the above enhancements and are now only a few ounces in weight and require only about 1 W of input power.

24.5.5 Challenges for Third-Generation Cooled Imagers

Third-generation cooled imagers are being developed to greatly extend the range at which targets can be detected and identified [28–30]. The U.S. Army rules of engagement now require identification prior to attack. Since the deployment of first- and second-generation sensors, there has been a gradual proliferation of thermal imaging technology worldwide. Third-generation sensors are intended to ensure that the U.S. Army forces maintain a technological advantage in night operations over any opposing force.

Thermal imaging equipment is used to first detect an object, and then to identify it. In the detection mode, the optical system provides a wide FOV (WFOV—*f*/2.5) to maintain robust situational awareness [31]. For detection, LWIR provides superior range under most Army fighting conditions. MWIR offers higher spatial resolution sensing, and a significant advantage for long-range identification when used with telephoto optics (NFOV—*f*/6).

24.5.5.1 Cost Challenges: Chip Size

Cost is a direct function of the chip size since the number of detector and readout die per wafer is inversely proportional to the chip area. Chip size in turn is set by the array format and pixel size. Third-generation imager formats are anticipated to be in a high-definition 16×9 layout, compatible with future display standards, and reflecting the soldier's preference for a wide FOV. An example of such a format is 1280×720 pixels. For a 30-μm pixel, this format yields a die size greater than 1.5×0.85 in. (22×38 mm). This will yield only a few die per wafer, and will also require the development of a new generation of dewar-cooler assemblies to accommodate these large dimensions. A pixel size of 20 μm results in a cost saving of more than 2×, and allows the use of existing dewar designs.

24.5.5.1.1 Two-Color Pixel Designs

Pixel size is the most important factor for achieving affordable third-generation systems. Two types of two-color pixels have been demonstrated. Simultaneous two-color pixels have two indium–bump connections per pixel to allow readout of both color bands at the same time. Figure 24.20 shows an example of a simultaneous two-color pixel structure. The sequential two-color approach requires only one indium bump per pixel, but requires the readout circuit to alternate bias polarities multiple times during each frame. An example of this structure is illustrated in Figure 24.21. Both approaches leave very little area available for the indium bump(s) as the pixel size is made smaller. Advanced etching technology is being developed in order to meet the challenge of shrinking the pixel size to 20 μm.

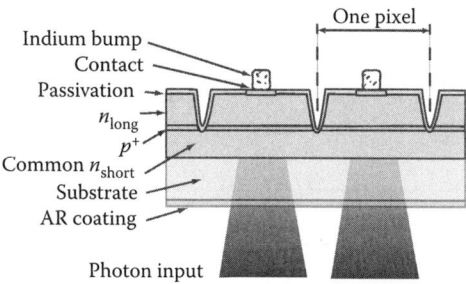
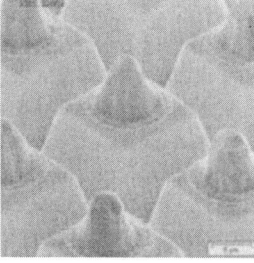

FIGURE 24.20 Illustration of a simultaneous two-color pixel structure—cross section and SEM. Simultaneous two-color FPAs have two indium bumps per pixel. A 50-μm simultaneous two-color pixel is shown.

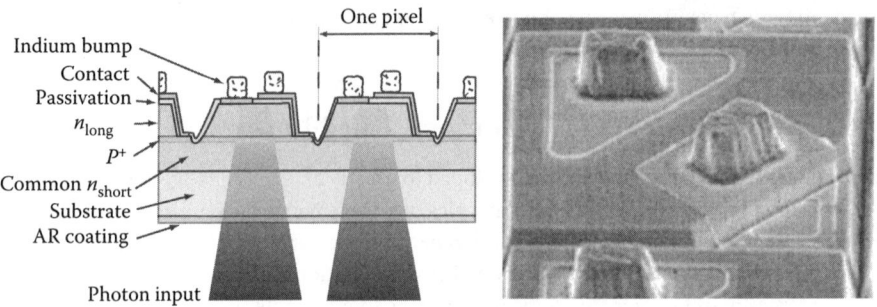

FIGURE 24.21 Illustration of a sequential two-color pixel structure—cross section and SEM. Sequential two-color FPAs have only one indium bump per pixel, helping to reduce pixel size. A 20-μm sequential two-color pixel is shown.

24.5.5.2 Sensor Format and Packaging Issues

The sensor format was selected to provide a wide FOV and high spatial resolution. Target detection in many Army battlefield situations is most favorable in LWIR. Searching for targets is more efficient in a wider FOV, in this case, $f/2.5$. Target identification relies on having 12 or more pixels across the target to adequately distinguish its shape and features. Higher magnification, $f/6$ optics combined with MWIR optical resolution enhances this task.

Consideration was also given to compatibility with future standards for display formats. Army soldiers are generally more concerned with the width of the display than the height, so the emerging 16:9 width to height format that is planned for high-definition TV was chosen.

A major consideration in selecting a format was the packaging requirements. Infrared sensors must be packaged in a vacuum enclosure and mated with a mechanical cooler for operation. Overall array size was therefore limited to approximately 1 in. so that it would fit in an existing standard advanced dewar assembly (SADA) dewar design. Figure 24.22 illustrates the pixel size/format/FOV trade within the design size constraints of the SADA dewar.

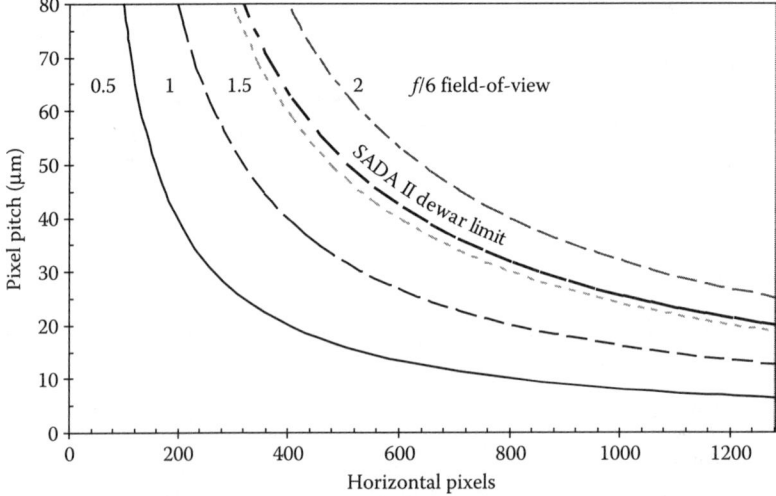

FIGURE 24.22 Maximum array horizontal format is determined by the pixel size and the chip size limit that will fit in an existing SADA dewar design for production commonality. For a 20-μm pixel and a 1.6° FOV, the horizontal pixel count limit is 1280. A costly development program would be necessary to develop a new, larger dewar.

24.5.5.3 Temperature Cycling Fatigue

Modern cooled infrared focal plane arrays are hybrid structures comprising a detector array mated to a silicon readout array with indium bumps (see Figure 24.15).

Very large focal plane arrays may exceed the limits of hybrid reliability engineered into these structures. The problem stems from the differential rates of expansion between HgCdTe and Si, which results in large stress as a device is cooled from 300 K ambient to an operating temperature in the range of 77–200 K. Hybrids currently use mechanical constraints to force the contraction of the two components to closely match each other. This approach may have limits—when the stress reaches a point where the chip fractures.

Two new approaches exist that can extend the maximum array size considerably. One is the use of silicon as the substrate for growing the HgCdTe detector layer using MBE. This approach has shown excellent results for MWIR detectors, but not yet for LWIR devices. Further improvement in this approach would be needed to use it for third-generation MWIR/LWIR two-color arrays.

A second approach that has proven successful for InSb hybrids is thinning the detector structure. HgCdTe hybrids currently retain their thick, 500 μm, CdZnTe epitaxial substrate in the hybridized structure. InSb hybrids must remove the substrate because it is not transparent, leaving only a 10-μm-thick detector layer. The thinness of this layer allows it to readily expand and contract with the readout. InSb hybrids with detector arrays over 2 in. (5 cm) on a side have been successfully demonstrated to be reliable.

Hybrid reliability issues will be monitored as a third-generation sensor manufacturing technology and is developed to determine whether new approaches are needed.

In addition to cost issues, significant performance issues must also be addressed for third-generation imagers. These are now discussed in the following section.

24.5.5.4 Performance Challenges

24.5.5.4.1 Dynamic Range and Sensitivity Constraints

A goal of third-generation imagers is to achieve a significant improvement in detection and ID range over second-generation systems. Range improvement comes from higher pixel count, and to a lesser extent from improved sensitivity. Figure 24.23 shows relative ID and detection range versus pixel size in the MWIR and LWIR, respectively. Sensitivity (D^* and integration time) have been held constant, and the format was varied to keep the FOV constant.

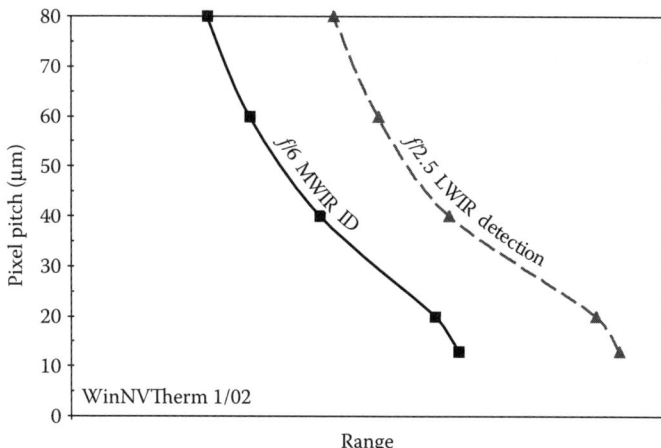

FIGURE 24.23 Range improves as the pixel size is reduced until a limit in optical blur is reached. In the examples above, the blur circle for the MWIR and LWIR cases are comparable since the *f*/number has been adjusted accordingly. D^* and integration time have been held constant in this example.

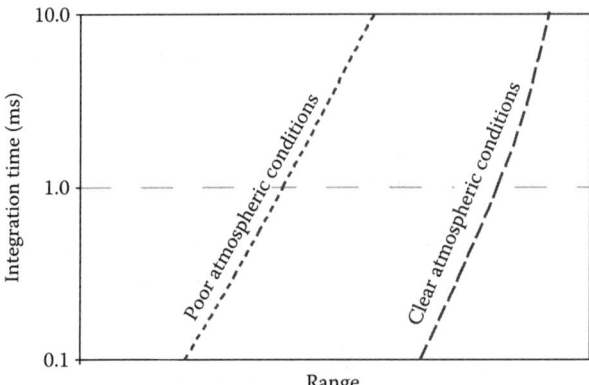

FIGURE 24.24 Range in a clear atmosphere improves only modestly with increased sensitivity. The case modeled here has a 20-μm pixel, a fixed D', and variable integration time. The 100× range of integration time corresponds to a 10× range in SNR. Improvement is more dramatic in the case of lower-atmospheric transmission that results in a reduced target signal.

Sensitivity has less effect than pixel size for clear atmospheric conditions, as illustrated by the clear atmosphere curve in Figure 24.24. Note that here the sensitivity is varied by an order of magnitude, corresponding to two orders of magnitude increase in integration time. Only a modest increase in range is seen for this dramatic change in SNR. In degraded atmospheric conditions, however, improved sensitivity plays a larger role because the signal is weaker. This is illustrated in Figure 24.24 by the curve showing range under conditions of reduced atmospheric transmission.

Dynamic range of the imager output must be considered from the perspective of the quantum efficiency and the effective charge storage capacity in the pixel unit cell of the readout. Quantum efficiency and charge storage capacity determine the integration time for a particular flux rate. As increasing number of quanta are averaged, the SNR improves as the square root of the count. Higher-accuracy A/D converters are therefore required to cope with the increased dynamic range between the noise and signal levels. Figure 24.25 illustrates the interaction of these specifications.

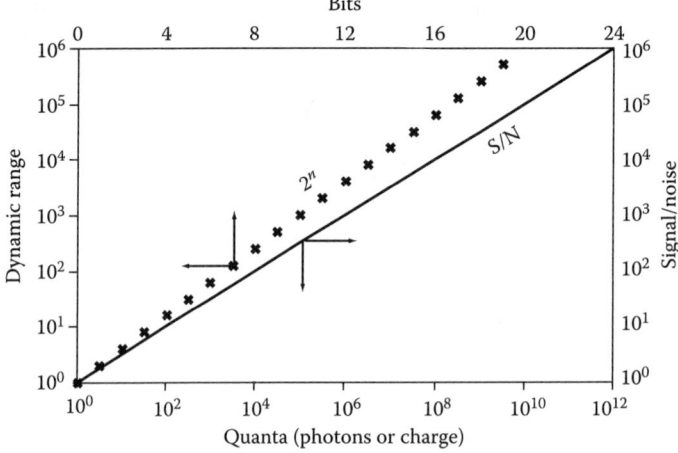

FIGURE 24.25 Dynamic range (2^n) corresponding to the number of digital bits (n) is plotted as a discrete point corresponding to each bit and referenced to the left and top scales. SNR, corresponding to the number of quanta collected (either photons or charge) is illustrated by the solid line in reference to the bottom- and right-hand scales.

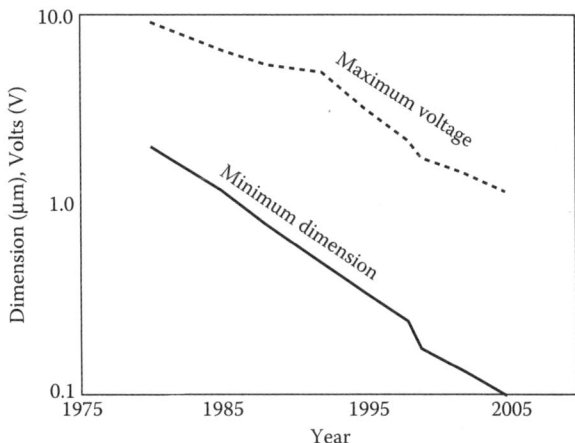

FIGURE 24.26 Trends for design rule minimum dimensions and maximum bias voltage of silicon foundry requirements.

System interface considerations lead to some interesting challenges and dilemmas. Imaging systems typically specify a noise floor from the readout on the order of 300 μV. This is because system users do not want to encounter sensor signal levels below the system noise level. With readouts built at commercial silicon foundries now having submicrometer design rules, the maximum bias voltage applied to the readout is limited to a few volts—this trend has been downward from 5 V in the past decade as design rules have shrunk, as illustrated in Figure 24.26. Output swing voltages can only be a fraction of the maximum applied voltage, on the order of 3 V or less.

This means that the dynamic range limit of a readout is about 10,000—80 db in power—or less. Present readouts almost approach this constraining factor with 70–75 db achieved in good designs. In order to significantly improve sensitivity, the noise floor will have to be reduced.

If sufficiently low readout noise could be achieved, and the readout could digitize on chip to a level of 15–16 bits, the data could come off digitally and the system noise floor would not be an issue. Such developments may allow incremental improvement in third-generation imagers in the future. Figure 24.27 illustrates an example of an on-chip A/D converter that has demonstrated 12 bits on chip.

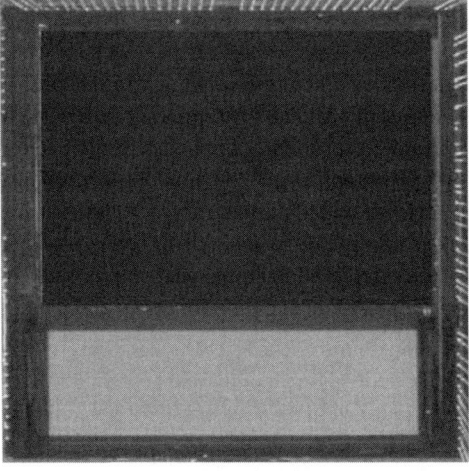

FIGURE 24.27 Focal planes with on-chip A/D converters have been demonstrated. This example shows a 900 × 120 TDI scanning format array. (Photo supplied by Lester Kozlowski of Rockwell Scientific, Camarillo, CA.)

A final issue here concerns the ability to provide high charge storage density within the small pixel dimensions envisioned for third-generation imagers. This may be difficult with standard CMOS capacitors. Reduced oxide thickness of submicrometer design rules does give larger capacitance per unit area, but the reduced bias voltage largely cancels any improvement in charge storage density. Promising technology in the form of ferroelectric capacitors may provide much greater charge storage densities than the oxide-on-silicon capacitors now used. Such technology is not yet incorporated into standard CMOS foundries. Stacked hybrid structures[*] [32] may be needed as at least an interim solution to incorporate the desired charge storage density in detector–readout–capacitor structures.

24.5.5.4.2 High Frame Rate Operation

Frame rates of 30–60 fps are adequate for visual display. In third-generation systems, we plan to deploy high frame rate capabilities to provide more data throughput for advanced signal processing functions such as automatic target recognition (ATR), and missile and projectile tracking. An additional benefit is the opportunity to collect a higher percentage of available signal. Higher frame rates pose two significant issues. First, output drive power is proportional to the frame rate and at rates of 480 Hz or higher; this could be the most significant source of power dissipation on the readout. Increased power consumption on chip will also require more power consumption by the cryogenic cooler. These considerations lead us to conclude that high frame rate capabilities need to be limited to a small but arbitrarily positioned window of 64×64 pixels, for which a high frame rate of 480 Hz can be supported. This allows for ATR functions to be exercised on possible target locations within the full FOV.

24.5.5.4.3 Higher Operating Temperature

Current tactical infrared imagers operate at 77 K with few exceptions—notably MWIR HgCdTe, which can use solid-state thermoelectric (TE) cooling. Power can be saved, and cooler efficiency and cooler lifetime improved if focal planes operate at temperatures above 77 K.

Increasing the operating temperature results in a major reduction of input cryogenic cooler power. As can be seen from Figure 24.28, the coefficient of performance (COP) increases by a factor of 2.4 from 2.5% to 6% as the operating temperature is raised from 80 to 120 K with a 320 K heat sink. If the operating temperature can be increased to 150 K, the COP increases fourfold. This can have a major impact on input power, weight, and size.

Research is underway on an artificial narrow-bandgap intrinsic-like material—strained-layer superlattices of InGaAsSb—which have the potential to increase operating temperatures to even higher

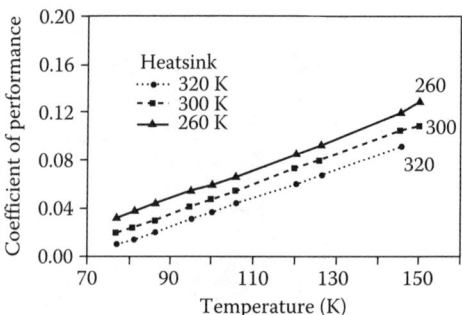

FIGURE 24.28 Javelin cooler coefficient of performance versus temperature.

---

[*] It should be noted that the third-generation imager will operate as an on-the-move wide-area step-scanner with automated ATR versus second-generation systems that rely on manual target searching. This allows the overall narrower field of view for the third-generation imager.

levels [33]. Results from this research may be more than a decade away, but the potential benefits are significant in terms of reduced cooler operating power and maintenance.

The above discussion illustrates some of the challenges facing the development of third-generation cooled imagers. In addition to these are the required advances in signal processing and display technologies to translate the focal plane enhancements into outputs for the user. These advances can be anticipated to not only help to increase the range at which targets can be identified but also to increase the rate of detection and identification through the use of two-color cues. Image fusion of the two colors in some cases is anticipated to help find camouflaged targets in clutter. Improved sensitivity and two-color response is further anticipated to minimize the loss of target contrast now encountered because of diurnal crossover. Future two-color imagers together with novel signal processing methods may further enhance the ability to detect land mines and find obscured targets.

24.6 Summary

Infrared sensors have made major performance strides in the last few years, especially in the uncooled sensors area. Cost, weight, and size of the uncooled have dramatically been reduced, allowing a greater proliferation into the commercial market. Uncooled sensors will find greater use in the medical community as a result. High-performance cooled sensors have also been dramatically improved, including the development of multicolor arrays. The high-performance sensors will find new medical applications because of the color discrimination and sensitivity attributes now available.

References

1. D.G. Crowe, P.R. Norton, T. Limperis, and J. Mudar, Detectors, in *Electro-Optical Components*, W.D. Rogatto, Ed., Vol. 3, ERIM, Ann Arbor, MI; J.S. Accetta and D.L. Schumaker, Executive Eds., *Infrared and Electro-Optical Systems Handbook*, SPIE, Bellingham, WA, 1993, revised 1996, Chapter 4, pp. 175–283.
2. P.R. Norton, Detector focal plane array technology, in *Encyclopedia of Optical Engineering*, R.G. Driggers, Ed., Vol. 1, Marcel Dekker, New York, 2003, pp. 320–348.
3. P.W. Kruse, and D.D. Skatrud, Uncooled infrared imaging arrays and systems, in *Semiconductors and Semimetals*, R.K. Willardson and E.R. Weber, Eds., Academic Press, New York, 1997.
4. P. Norton, Infrared image sensors, *Opt. Eng.*, 30, 1649–1663, 1991.
5. T. Ashley, I.M. Baker, T.M. Burke, D.T. Dutton, J.A. Haigh, L.G. Hipwood, R. Jefferies, A.D. Johnson, P. Knowles, and J.C. Little, *Proc. SPIE*, 4028, 398–403, 2000.
6. P.J. Love, K.J. Ando, R.E. Bornfreund, E. Corrales, R.E. Mills, J.R. Cripe, N.A. Lum, J.P. Rosbeck, and M.S. Smith, Large-format infrared arrays for future space and ground-based astronomy applications, *Proceedings of SPIE; Infrared Spaceborne Remote Sensing IX*, Vol. 4486–38; pp. 373–384, 29 July–3 August, 2001; San Diego, USA.
7. The photoconductive and photovoltaic detector technology of HgCdTe is summarized in the following references: D. Long and J.L. Schmidt, Mercury-cadmium telluride and closely related alloys, in *Semiconductors and Semimetals* 5, R.K. Willardson and A.C. Beer, Eds., Academic Press, New York, pp. 175–255, 1970; R.A. Reynolds, C.G. Roberts, R.A. Chapman, and H.B. Bebb, Photoconductivity processes in 0.09 eV bandgap HgCdTe, in *Proceedings of the 3rd International Conference on Photoconductivity*, E.M. Pell, Ed., Pergamon Press, New York, pp. 217, 1971; P.W. Kruse, D. Long, and O.N. Tufte, Photoeffects and material parameters in HgCdTe alloys, in *Proceedings of the 3rd International Conference on Photoconductivity*, E.M. Pell, Ed., Pergamon Press, New York, pp. 233, 1971; R.M. Broudy and V.J. Mazurczyk (HgCd) Te photoconductive detectors, in *Semiconductors and Semimetals*, 18, R.K. Willardson and A.C. Beer, Eds., Chapter 5, Academic Press, New York, pp. 157–199, 1981; M.B. Reine, A.K. Sood, and T.J. Tredwell, Photovoltaic infrared detectors, in *Semiconductors and Semimetals*, 18, R.K. Willardson and A.C. Beer, Eds., Chapter 6, pp. 201–311;

D. Long, Photovoltaic and photoconductive infrared detectors, in *Topics in Applied Physics* 19, *Optical and Infrared Detectors*, R.J. Keyes, Ed., Springer-Verlag, Heidelberg, pp. 101–147, 1970; C.T. Elliot, infrared detectors, in *Handbook on Semiconductors* 4, C. Hilsum, Ed., Chapter 6B, North Holland, New York, pp. 727–798, 1981.

8. P. Norton, Status of infrared detectors, *Proc. SPIE*, 2274, 82–92, 1994.

9. I.M., Baker, Photovoltaic IR detectors, in *Narrow-Gap II–VI Compounds for Optoelectronic and Electromagnetic Applications*, P. Capper, Ed., Chapman and Hall, London, pp. 450–473, 1997.

10. P. Norton, Status of infrared detectors, *Proc. SPIE*, 3379, 102–114, 1998.

11. M. Kinch, HDVIP® FPA technology at DRS, *Proc. SPIE*, 4369, 566–578, 1999.

12. M.B. Reine., Semiconductor fundamentals—Materials: Fundamental properties of mercury cadmium telluride, in *Encyclopedia of Modern Optics*, Academic Press, London, 2004.

13. A. Rogalski., HgCdTe infrared detector material: History, status and outlook, *Rep. Prog. Phys.*, 68, 2267–2336, 2005.

14. S.D. Guanapala, B.F. Levine, and N. Chand, *J. Appl. Phys.*, 70, 305, 1991.

15. B.F. Levine, *J. Appl. Phys.*, 47, R1–R81, 1993.

16. K.K. Choi., *The Physics of Quantum Well Infrared Photodetectors*, World Scientific, River Edge, New Jersey, 1997.

17. S.D. Gunapala, J.K. Liu, J.S. Park, M. Sundaram, C.A. Shott, T. Hoelter, T.-L. Lin, S.T. Massie, P.D. Maker, R.E. Muller, and G. Sarusi, 9 μm Cutoff 256 × 256 GaAs/AlGaAs quantum well infrared photodetector hand-held camera, *IEEE Trans. Elect. Dev.*, 45, 1890, 1998.

18. S.D. Gunapala, S.V. Bandara, J.K. Liu, W. Hong, M. Sundaram, P.D. Maker, R.E. Muller, C.A. Shott, and R. Carralejo, Long-wavelength 640 × 480 GaAs/AlGaAs quantum well infrared photodetector snap-shot camera, *IEEE Trans. Elect. Dev.*, 44, 51–57, 1997.

19. M.Z. Tidrow et al., Device physics and focal plane applications of QWIP and MCT, *Opto-Elect. Rev.*, 7, 283–296, 1999.

20. S.D. Gunapala and S.V. Bandara, Quantum well infrared photodetector (QWIP) focal plane arrays, in *Semiconductors and Semimetals*, R.K. Willardson and E.R. Weber, Eds., 62, Academic Press, New York, 1999.

21. G.A. Sai-Halasz, R. Tsu, and L. Esaki, *Appl. Phys. Lett.*, 30, 651, 1977.

22. D.L. Smith and C. Mailhiot, Proposal for strained type II superlattice infrared detectors, *J. Appl. Phys.*, 62, 2545–2548, 1987.

23. S.R. Kurtz, L.R. Dawson, T.E. Zipperian, and S.R. Lee, Demonstration of an InAsSb strained-layer superlattice photodiode, *Appl. Phys. Lett.*, 52, 1581–1583, 1988.

24. R.H. Miles, D.H. Chow, J.N. Schulman, and T.C. McGill, Infrared optical characterization of InAs/GaInSb superlattices, *Appl. Phys. Lett.*, 57, 801–803, 1990.

25. F. Fuchs, U. Weimar, W. Pletschen, J. Schmitz, E. Ahlswede, M. Walther, J. Wagner, and P. Koidl, *J. Appl. Phys. Lett.*, 71, 3251, 1997.

26. Gail J. Brown, Type-II InAs/GaInSb superlattices for infrared detection: An overview, *Proc. SPIE*, 5783, 65–77, 2005.

27. J.L. Vampola, Readout electronics for infrared sensors, in *Electro-Optical Components*, Chapter 5, Vol. 3, W.D. Rogatto, Ed., *Infrared and Electro-Optical Systems Handbook*, J.S. Accetta and D.L. Schumaker, Executive Eds., ERIM, Ann Arbor, MI and SPIE, Bellingham, WA, pp. 285–342, 1993, revised 1996.

28. D. Reago, and S. Horn, J. Campbell, and R. Vollmerhausen, Third generation imaging sensor system concepts, *SPIE*, 3701, 108–117, 1999.

29. P. Norton, J. Campbell III, S. Horn, and D. Reago, Third-generation infrared imagers, *Proc. SPIE*, 4130, 226–236, 2000.

30. S. Horn, P. Norton, T. Cincotta, A. Stoltz, D. Benson, P. Perconti, and J. Campbell, Challenges for third-generation cooled imagers, *Proc. SPIE*, 5074, 44–51, 2003.

31. S. Horn, D. Lohrman, P. Norton, K. McCormack, and A. Hutchinson, Reaching for the sensitivity limits of uncooled and minimally cooled thermal and photon infrared detectors, *Proc. SPIE*, 5783, 401–411, 2005.

32. W. Cabanskia, K. Eberhardta, W. Rodea, J. Wendlera, J. Zieglera, J. Fleißnerb, F. Fuchsb, R. Rehmb, J. Schmitzb, H. Schneiderb, and M. Walther, 3rd gen focal plane array IR detection modules and applications, *Proc. SPIE*, 5406, 184–192, 2004.

33. S. Horn, P. Norton, K. Carson, R. Eden, and R. Clement, Vertically-integrated sensor arrays—VISA, *Proc. SPIE*, 5406, 332–340, 2004.

34. R. Balcerak and S. Horn, Progress in the development of vertically-integrated sensor arrays, *Proc. SPIE*, 5783, 384–391, 2005.

25

Infrared Camera
Characterization

Joseph G. Pellegrino
*U.S. Army CERDEC Night
Vision and Electronic
Sensors Directorate*

Jason Zeibel
*U.S. Army CERDEC Night
Vision and Electronic
Sensors Directorate*

Ronald G. Driggers
*U.S. Army CERDEC Night
Vision and Electronic
Sensors Directorate*

Philip Perconti
*U.S. Army CERDEC Night
Vision and Electronic
Sensors Directorate*

Many different types of infrared (IR) detector technology are now commercially available and the physics of their operation has been described in an earlier chapter. IR imagers are classified by different characteristics such as scan type, detector material, cooling requirements, and detector physics. Prior to the 1990s, thermal imaging cameras typically contained a relatively small number of IR photosensitive detectors. These imagers were known as *cooled scanning systems* because they required cooling to cryogenic temperatures and a mechanical scan mirror to construct a two-dimensional (2D) image of the scene. Large 2D arrays of IR detectors, or staring arrays, have enabled the development of *cooled staring systems* that maintain the sensitivity over a wide range of scene–flux conditions, spectral bandwidths, and frame rates. Staring arrays consisting of small bolometric detector elements, or microbolometers, have enabled the development of *uncooled staring systems* that are compact, lightweight, and of low power (see Figure 25.1).

The sensitivity, or thermal resolution, of uncooled microbolometer focal plane arrays (FPA) has improved drastically over the past decade, resulting in IR video cameras that can resolve temperature differences under nominal imaging conditions as small as 20 millidegrees Kelvin using $f/1.0$ optics. Advancements in the manufacturing processes used by the commercial silicon industry have been instrumental in this progress. Uncooled microbolometer structures are typically fabricated on top of the silicon-integrated circuitry (IC) designed to readout the changes in resistance for each pixel in the array. The silicon-based IC serves as an electrical and mechanical interface for the IR microbolometer.

The primary measures of IR sensor performance are sensitivity and resolution. When measurements of the end-to-end or human-in-the-loop (HITL) performance are required, the visual acuity of an observer through a sensor is included. The sensitivity and resolution are both related to the hardware and software that comprises the system, while the HITL includes both the sensor and the observer. Sensitivity is determined through radiometric analysis of the scene environment and the quantum electronic properties of the detectors. Resolution is determined by an analysis of the physical and optical properties, the detector array geometry, and other degrading components of the system in the same manner as complex electronic circuit/signal analysis. The sensitivity of cooled and uncooled staring

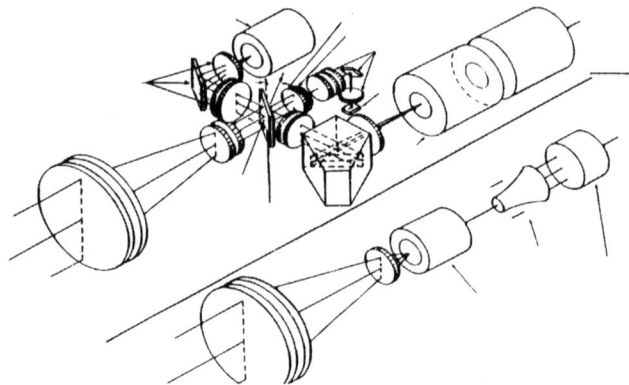

FIGURE 25.1   Scanning and staring system designs.

IR video cameras has improved by more than a factor of 10 compared to scanning systems that were commercially available in the 1980s and the early 1990s [1,2].

Sensitivity describes how the sensor performs with respect to the input signal level. It relates noise characteristics, responsivity of the detector, light gathering of the optics, and the dynamic range of the sensor. Radiometry describes the amount of light leaving the object and background and the amount which is collected by the detector. Optical design and detector characteristics are of considerable importance in sensor-sensitivity analysis. In IR systems, noise-equivalent temperature difference (NETD) is often a first-order description of the system sensitivity. The three-dimensional (3D) noise model [1] describes more detailed representations of the sensitivity parameters. The sensitivity of the scanned long-wave infrared (LWIR) cameras operating at video frame rates is typically limited by very short detector integration times on the order of tens or hundreds of microseconds. The sensitivity of staring IR systems with high quantum efficiency detectors is often limited by the charge integration capacity, or well capacity, of the readout integrated circuit (ROIC). The detector integration time of staring IR cameras can be tailored to optimize the sensitivity for a given application and may range from microseconds to tens of milliseconds.

The second type of measure is resolution. Resolution is the ability of the sensor to image small targets and to resolve fine detail in large targets. Modulation transfer function (MTF) is the most widely used resolution descriptor in IR systems. Alternatively, it may be specified by a number of descriptive metrics such as the optical Rayleigh criterion or the instantaneous field-of-view of the detector. These metrics are component-level descriptions and the system MTF is an all-encompassing function that describes the system resolution. Sensitivity and resolution can be competing system characteristics and they are the most important issues in initial studies for a design. For example, given a fixed sensor aperture diameter, an increase in focal length can provide an increase in resolution, but may decrease sensitivity [2]. A more detailed consideration of the optical design parameters is included in the next chapter.

Quite often metrics such as NETD and MTF, are considered as separable. However, in an actual sensor, sensitivity and resolution performances are interrelated. As a result, the minimum resolvable temperature difference (MRT or MRTD) has become a primary performance metric for IR systems.

This chapter addresses the parameters that characterize a camera's performance. A website advertising IR camera would in general contain a specification sheet that contains some variation of the terms that follow. A goal of this section is to give the reader working knowledge of of these terms so that it will enable them better to obtain the correct camera for their application:

- 3D noise
- NETD
- Dynamic range

- MTF
- MRT and Minimum detectable temperature (MDT)
- Spatial resolution
- Pixel size

25.1 Dimensional Noise

The 3D noise model is essential for describing the sensitivity of an optical sensor system. Modern imaging sensors incorporate complex focal plane architectures and sophisticated postdetector processing and electronics. These advanced technical characteristics create the potential for the generation of complex noise patterns in the output imagery of the system. These noise patterns are deleterious and therefore need to be analyzed to better understand their effects upon performance. Unlike classical systems where "well-behaved" detector noise predominates, current sensor systems have the ability to generate a wide variety of noise types, each with distinctive characteristics temporally, as well as along the vertical and horizontal image directions. Earlier methods for noise measurements at the detector preamplifier port that ignored other system noise sources are no longer satisfactory. System components following the stage that include processing may generate additional noise and even dominate total system noise.

Efforts by the Night Vision and Electronic Sensor Directorate to measure the second-generation IR sensors uncovered the need for a more comprehensive method to characterize noise parameters. It was observed that the noise patterns produced by these systems exhibited a high degree of directionality. The data set is 3D with the temporal dimension representing the frame sequencing and the two spatial dimensions representing the vertical and horizontal directions within the image (see Figure 25.2).

To acquire this data cube, the field of view of a camera to be measured is flooded with a uniform temperature reference. A set number n (typically around 100) of successive frames of video data are then collected. Each frame of the data consists of the measured response (in Volts) to the uniform temperature source from each individual detector in the 2D FPA. When many successive frames of data are "stacked" together, a uniform source-data-cube is constructed. The measured response may be either analog (RS-170) or digital (RS-422, Camera Link, Hot Link, etc.) in nature depending on the camera interface being studied.

To recover the overall temporal noise, first the temporal noise is calculated for each detector in the array. A standard deviation of the n measured voltage responses for each detector is calculated. For an h by v array, there are separate hv values where each value is the standard deviation of n-voltage measurements. The median temporal noise among these hv values is stated as the overall temporal noise in Volts.

Following the calculation of temporal noise, the uniform source-data-cube is reduced along each axis according to the 3D noise procedure. There are seven noise terms as part of the 3D noise definition. Three components measure the average noise present along each axis (horizontal, vertical, and

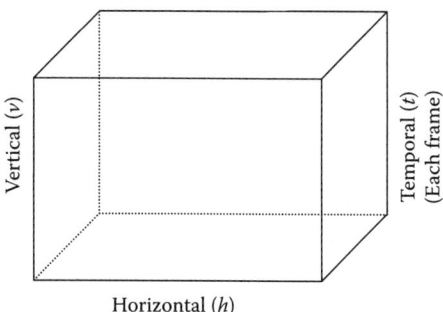

FIGURE 25.2 An example of a uniform source-data-cube for 3D noise measurements. The first step in the calculation of 3D noise parameters is the acquisition of a uniform source-data-cube.

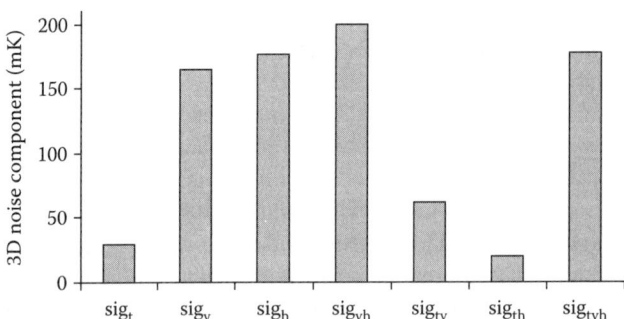

FIGURE 25.3 The 3D noise values for a typical data cube. The spatial nonuniformity can be seen in the elevated values of the spatial 3D noise components σ_h, σ_v, and σ_{vh}. The white noise present in the system (σ_{tvh}) is roughly the same magnitude as the spatial 3D noise components.

temporal) of the data cube (σ_h, σ_v, and σ_t). Three terms measure the noise common to any given pair of the axes in the data cube (σ_{tv}, σ_{th}, and σ_{vh}). The final term measures the uncorrelated random noise (σ_{tvh}). To calculate the spatial noise for the camera, each of the 3D noise components that are independent of time (σ_v, σ_h, and σ_{vh}) are added in quadrature. The result is quoted as the spatial noise of the camera in Volts.

To represent a data cube in a 2D format, the cube is averaged along one of the axes. For example, if a data cube is averaged along the temporal axis, then a time-averaged array is created. This format is useful for purely visualizing spatial noise effects as three of the components are calculated after temporal averaging (σ_h, σ_v, and σ_{vh}). These are the time-independent components of 3D noise. The data cube can also be averaged along both the spatial dimensions. The full 3D noise calculation for a typical data cube is shown in Figure 25.3.

Figure 25.4 shows an example of a data cube that has been temporally averaged. In this case, many spatial noise features are present. Column noise is clearly visible in Figure 25.4; however, the dominant spatial noise component appears to be the "salt and pepper" fixed pattern noise. The seven 3D noise components are shown in Figure 25.5. σ_{vh} is clearly the dominant noise term, as it is expected due to the high fixed pattern noise. The column noise σ_h and the row noise σ_v are also dominant. In this example,

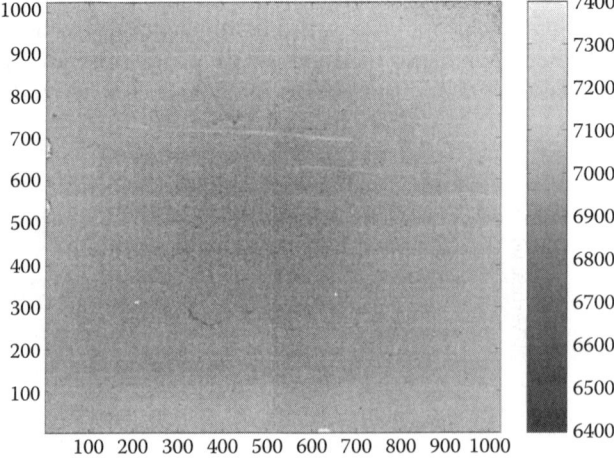

FIGURE 25.4 An example of a camera system with high spatial noise components and very low temporal noise components.

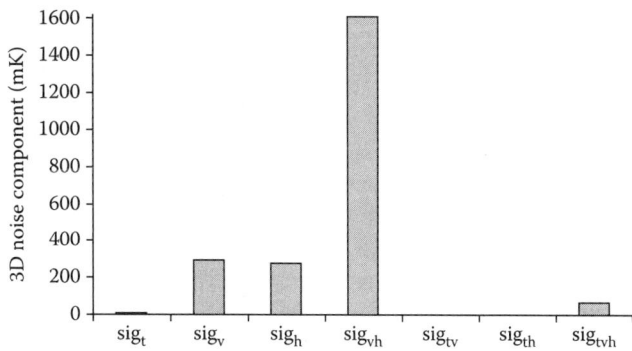

FIGURE 25.5 The 3D noise components for the data cube used to generate the dominant noise as it is expected due to the high fixed pattern noise. Note that the amount of row and column noise is significantly smaller than the fixed pattern noise. All the 3D noise values with a temporal component are significantly smaller than the purely spatial values.

the overall bulls-eye variation in the average frame dominates the σ_v and σ_h terms. Vertical stripes present in the figure add to σ_v, but this effect is negligible in comparison, leading to similar values for σ_v and σ_h. In this example, the temporal components of the 3D noise are two orders of magnitude lower than σ_{vh}. If this data cube were to be plotted as individual frames, we would see that the successive frames would hardly change and the dominant spatial noise would be present (and constant) in each frame.

25.2 Noise-Equivalent Temperature Difference

In general, imager sensitivity is a measure of the smallest signal that is detectable by a sensor. For IR imaging systems, NETD is a measure of sensitivity. Sensitivity is determined using the principles of radiometry and the characteristics of the detector. The system intensity transfer function (SITF) can be used to estimate the NETD. NEDT is the system noise rms voltage over the noise differential output. It is the smallest measurable signal produced by a large target (extended source), in other words, the minimum measurable signal.

The equation below describes NETD as a function of noise voltage and the SITF. The measured NETD values are determined from a line of video-stripped image of a test target, as depicted in Figure 25.10. A square test target is placed before a blackbody source. The delta T is the difference between the blackbody temperature and the mask. This target is then placed at the focal point of an off-axis parabolic mirror. The mirror serves the purpose of a long optical path length to the target and yet relieves the tester from the concerns over atmospheric losses to the difference in temperature The image of the target is shown in Figure 25.6. The SITF slope for the scan line in Figure 25.6 is the $\Delta\Sigma/\Delta T$, where $\Delta\Sigma$ is the signal measured for a given ΔT. The N_{rms} is the background signal on the same line.

$$\text{NETD} = \frac{N_{rms}[\text{volts}]}{\text{SITF\_Slope}[\text{volts / K}]}$$

After calculating both the temporal and spatial noise, a signal transfer function (SiTF) is measured. The field of view of the camera is again flooded with a uniform temperature source. The temperature of the source is varied over the dynamic range of the camera's output while the response of the mean array voltage is recorded. The slope of the resulting curve yields the SiTF responsivity in volts per degree Kelvin change in the scene temperature. Once both the SiTF curve and the temporal and spatial noise in volts are known, the NETD can be calculated. This is accomplished by dividing the temporal and spatial

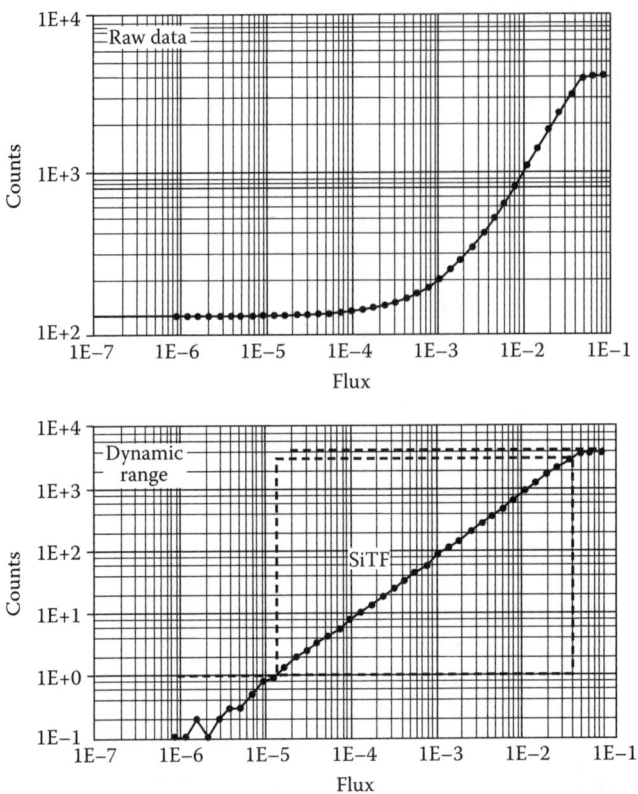

FIGURE 25.6 Dynamic range and system transfer function.

noise in volts by the responsivity in volts per degree Kelvin. The resulting NETD values represent the minimum discernable change in scene temperature for both spatial and temporal observation.

The SiTF of an electro-optical (EO) or IR system is determined by the signal response once the dark offset signal has been subtracted. After subtracting the offset signal due to nonflux effects, the SiTF plots the counts output relative to the input photon flux. The SiTF is typically represented in response units of voltage, signal electrons, digital counts, and so on versus units of the source: blackbody temperature, flux, photons, and so on. If the system behaves linearly within the dynamic range then the slope of the SiTF is constant. The dynamic range of the system, which may be defined by various criteria, is determined by the minimum (i.e., signal-to-noise ratio = 1) and maximum levels of operation.

25.3 Dynamic Range

The responsivity function also provides information on the dynamic range and linearity. The camera dynamic range is the maximum measurable input signal divided by the minimum measurable signal. The NEDT is assumed to be the minimum measurable signal. For AC systems, the maximum output depends on the target size and therefore the target size must be specified if the dynamic range is a specification. Depending upon the application, the maximum input value may be defined by one of the several methods. One method for specifying the dynamic range of a system involves having the ΔV_{sys} signal reach some specified level, say 90% of the saturation level as shown in Figure 25.7. Another method to assess the maximum input value is based on the signal's deviation from linearity. The range of data points that fall within a specified band is designated as the dynamic range. A third approach involves specifying the minimum SiTF of the system.

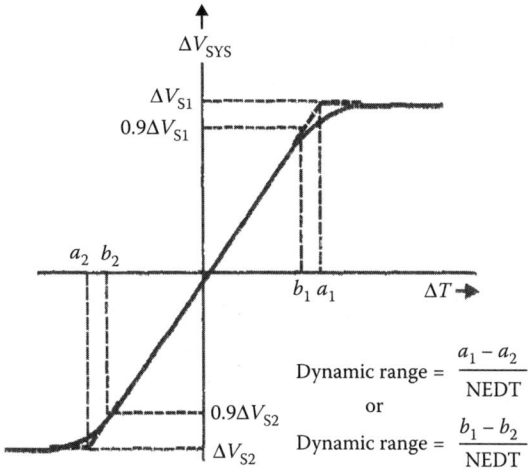

FIGURE 25.7 Dynamic range defined by linearity.

For most systems, the detector output signal is adjusted both in gain and offset system so that the dynamic range of the A/D converter is maximized. Figure 25.8 shows a generic detector system that contains an 8-bit A/D converter. The converter can handle an input signal between 0 and 1 V and an output between 0 and 255 counts. By selecting the gain and offset system, any detector voltage range can be mapped into the digital output. Figure 25.9 shows three different system gains and offsets. When the

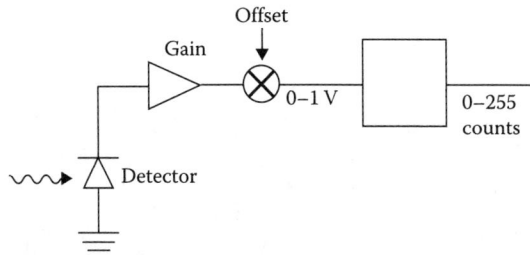

FIGURE 25.8 A system with an 8-bit A/D converter.

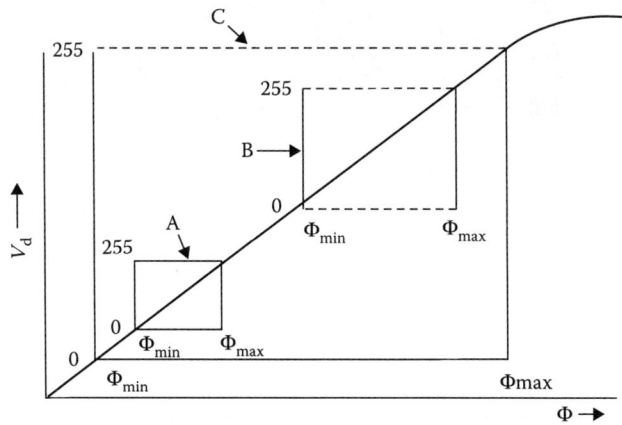

FIGURE 25.9 Different gains and voltage offsets that affect the input-to-output transition.

source flux level is less than Φ_{min}, the source will not be seen (i.e., it will appear as 0 counts). When the flux level is greater than Φ_{max}, the source will appear as 255 counts, and the system is said to be saturated. The gain parameters, Φ_{min} and Φ_{max} are redefined for each gain and offset level setting.

Output A below occurs with the maximum gain. Point B occurs with moderate gain and C with minimum gain. For the various gains, the detector output gets mapped into the full dynamic range of the A/D converter.

25.4 Modulation Transfer Function

The MTF of an optical system measures a system's ability to faithfully image a given object. Consider for example the bar pattern shown in Figure 25.10, with the cross section of each bar being a sine wave. Since the image of a sine wave light distribution is always a sine wave, although the aberrations may be bad, the image is always a sine wave. Therefore, the image will have a sine wave distribution with its intensity shown in Figure 25.10.

When the bars are coarsely spaced, the optical system has no difficulty in faithfully reproducing them. However, when the bars are more tightly spaced, the contrast,

$$\text{Contrast} = \frac{\text{bright} - \text{dark}}{\text{bright} + \text{dark}}$$

begins to fall off as shown in panel c. If the dark lines have an intensity = 0, the contrast = 1, and if the bright and dark lines are equally intense, contrast = 0. The contrast is equal to the MTF at a specified spatial frequency. Furthermore, it is evident that the MTF is a function of spatial frequency and position within the field.

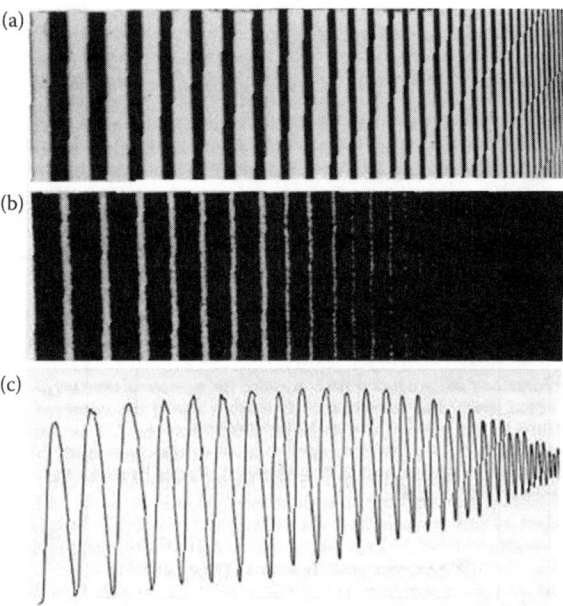

FIGURE 25.10 This figure shows the falloff in MTF as the spatial frequency increases. Panel (a) is a sinusoidal test pattern, panel (b) is the optical system's (negative) response, and panel (c) shows the contrast as a function of spatial frequency.

25.5 Minimum Resolvable Temperature

Whenever a camera is turned on, the observer subconsciously makes a judgment about the image quality. The IR community uses the MRT and the MDT as standard measures of image quality. The MRT and MDT depend upon the IR imaging system's resolution and sensitivity. MRT is a measure of the ability to resolve detail and it is inversely related to the MTF, whereas the MDT is a measure to detect something. The MRT and MDT deal with an observer's ability to perceive low-contrast targets which are embedded in noise.

MRT and MDT are not absolute values rather they are temperature differentials relative to a given background. They are sometimes referred to as the MRTD and the MDTD.

The theoretical MRT is

$$\text{MRT}(f_x) = \frac{k \cdot (\text{NEDT})}{\text{MTF}_{\text{perceived}}(f_x)} \cdot \sqrt{\{\beta_1 + \cdots + \beta_n\}}$$

where $\text{MTF}_{\text{perceived}} = \text{MTF}_{\text{SYS}} \text{MTF}_{\text{MONITOR}} \text{MTF}_{\text{EYE}}$. The $\text{MTF}_{\text{system}}$ is defined by the product $\text{MTF}_{\text{sensor}}$ $\text{MTF}_{\text{optics}} \text{MTF}_{\text{electronics}}$. Each β_i in the equation is an eye filter that is used to interpret the various components of noise. As certain noise sources increase, the MRT also increases. MRT has the same ambient temperature dependence as the NEDT; as the ambient temperature increases, MRT decreases. Because the MTF decreases as the spatial frequency increases, the MRT increases with the increasing spatial frequency. The overall system response depends on both sensitivity and resolution. The MRT parameter is bounded by sensitivity and resolution. Figure 25.10 shows that different systems may have different MRTs. System A has a better sensitivity because it has a lower MRT at low spatial frequencies. At midrange spatial frequencies, the systems are approximately equivalent and it can be said that they provide equivalent performance. At higher frequencies, System B has better resolution and can display finer detail than system A. In general, neither sensitivity, resolution, nor any other single parameter can be used to compare systems and many quantities must be specified for a complete system-to-system comparison.

25.6 Spatial Resolution

The term resolution applies to two different concepts with regard to the vision systems. Spatial resolution refers to the image size in pixels—for a given scene, more pixels means higher resolution. The spatial resolution is a fixed characteristic of the camera and cannot be increased by the frame grabber of postprocessing techniques. For example, the zooming techniques, merely interpolate between pixels to expand an image without adding any new information to what the camera provided. However, it is easy to decrease the resolution, by simply ignoring part of the data. The National Instruments frame grabbers provide a "scaling" feature that instructs the frame grabber to sample the image to return a 1/2, 1/4, 1/8, and so on, scaled image. This is convenient when system bandwidth is limited and you do not require any precision measurements of the image.

The other use of the term "resolution" is commonly found in data acquisition applications and refers to the number of quantization levels used in A/D conversions. In this sense, higher resolution means that you would have improved the capability of analyzing low-contrast images. This resolution is specified by the A/D converter; the frame grabber determines the resolution for analog signals whereas the camera determines digital signals (the frame grabber must have the capability of supporting whatever resolution the camera provides).

25.6.1 Pixel Size

Camera pixel size consists of tiny dots that make up a digital image. So let us say that a camera is capable of taking images at 640×480 pixels. A little math shows us that such an image would contain

3,07,200 pixels or 0.3 megapixels. Now let us say the camera takes 1024×768 images. This gives us 0.8 megapixels. Larger the number of megapixels, the more the image detail . Each pixel can be one of 16.7 million colors.

The detector pixel size refers to the size of the individual sensor elements that make up the detector part of the camera. If we had two charge-coupled device (CCDs) detectors with equal quantum efficiency (QEs), one has 9 µm pixels and the other has 18 µm pixels (i.e., the pixels on CCD#2 are twice the linear size of those on CCD #1) and we put both of these CCDs into cameras that operate identically, then the image taken with CCD#1 will require 4× exposure of the image taken with CCD#2. This seeming discrepancy is due to its entirety to the area of the pixels in the two CCDs and could be compared to the effectiveness of the rain-gathering gauges with different rain collection areas: A rain gauge with a 2-in. diameter throat will collect 4× as much rain water as a rain gauge with a 1-in. diameter throat.

References

1. J. D'Agostino and C. Webb, 3-D analysis framework and measurement methodology for imaging system noise. *Proc. SPIE*, 1488, 110–121, 1991.
2. R.G. Driggers, P. Cox, and T. Edwards, *Introduction to Infrared and Electro-Optical Systems*, Artech House, Boston, MA, 1998, p. 8.

26

Infrared Camera and Optics for Medical Applications

Michael W. Grenn
U.S. Army CERDEC Night Vision and Electronic Sensors Directorate

Jay Vizgaitis
U.S. Army CERDEC Night Vision and Electronic Sensors Directorate

Joseph G. Pellegrino
U.S. Army CERDEC Night Vision and Electronic Sensors Directorate

Philip Perconti
U.S. Army CERDEC Night Vision and Electronic Sensors Directorate

The infrared radiation emitted by an object above 0 K is passively detected by infrared imaging cameras without any contact with the object and is nonionizing. The characteristics of the infrared radiation emitted by an object are described by Planck's blackbody law in terms of spectral radiant emittance.

$$M_\lambda = \varepsilon(\lambda)\frac{c_1}{\lambda^5(e^{c_2/\lambda T} - 1)}\ \text{W/cm}^2\,\mu\text{m}$$

where c_1 and c_2 are constants of 3.7418×10^4 W $\mu\text{m}^4/\text{cm}^2$ and 1.4388×10^4 W μm K. The wavelength, λ, is provided in micrometers and $o(\lambda)$ is the emissivity of the surface. A blackbody source is defined as an object with an emissivity of 1.0, so that it is a perfect emitter. Source emissions of blackbodies at nominal terrestrial temperatures are shown in Figure 26.1. The radiant exitance of a blackbody at a 310 K, corresponding to a nominal core body temperature of 98.6°F, peaks at approximately 9.5 μm in the long-wave infrared (LWIR). The selection of an infrared camera for a specific application requires consideration of many factors including sensitivity, resolution, uniformity, stability, calibratability, user controllability, reliability, object of interest phenomenology, video interface, packaging, and power consumption.

Planck's equation describes the spectral shape of the source as a function of wavelength. It is readily apparent that the peak shifts to shorter wavelengths as the temperature of the object of interest increases. If the temperature of a blackbody approaches that of the sun, or 5900 K, the peak of the

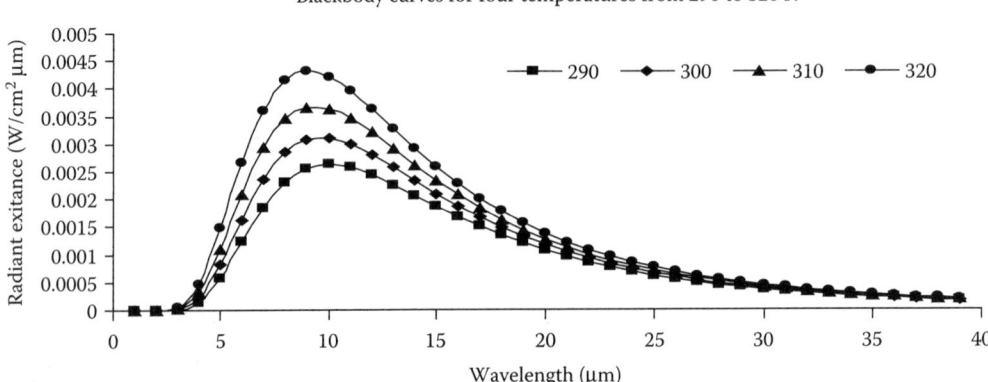

FIGURE 26.1 Planck's blackbody radiation curves.

spectral shape would shift to 0.55 μm or green light. This peak wavelength is described by Wien's displacement law

$$\lambda_{max} = 2898/T \ \mu m$$

Figure 26.2 shows the radiant energy peak as a function of temperature in the LWIR. It is important to note that the difference between the blackbody curves is the "signal" in the infrared bands. For an infrared sensor, if the background temperature is 300 K and the object of interest temperature is 302 K, the signal is the 2 K difference in flux between these curves. Signals in the infrared ride on very large amounts of background flux. This is not the case in the visible. For example, consider the case of a white object on a black background. The black background is generating no signal, while the white object is generating a maximum signal assuming the sensor gain is properly adjusted. The dynamic range may be fully utilized in a visible sensor. For the case of an IR sensor, a portion of the dynamic range is used by the large background flux radiated by everything in the scene. This flux is never a small value; hence sensitivity and dynamic range requirements are much more difficult to satisfy in IR sensors than in visible sensors.

A typical infrared imaging scenario consists of two major components, the object of interest and the background. In an IR scene, the majority of the energy is emitted from the constituents of the scene. This emitted energy is transmitted through the atmosphere to the sensor. As it propagates through the atmosphere it is degraded by absorption and scattering. Obscuration by intervening objects and additional energy emitted by the path also affect the target energy. This effect may be very small in short-range imaging applications under controlled conditions. All these contributors, which are not the object of interest, essentially reduce one's ability to discriminate the object. The signal is further degraded by the optics of the sensor. The energy is then sampled by the detector array and converted to electrical signals. Various electronics amplify and condition this signal before it is presented to either a display for human interpretation or an algorithm like an automatic target recognizer for machine interpretation. A linear systems approach to modeling allows the components' transfer functions to be treated separately as contributors to the overall system performance. This approach allows for straightforward modifications to a performance model for changes in the sensor or environment when performing tradeoff analyses.

The photon flux levels (photons per square centimeter per second) on Earth is 1.5×10^7 in the daytime and around 1×10^{10} at night in the visible. In the MWIR, the daytime and nighttime flux levels are 4×10^{15} and 2×10^{15}, respectively, where the flux is a combination of emitted and solar-reflected flux. In the LWIR, the flux is primarily emitted where both day and night yield a 2×10^{17} level. At first look, it

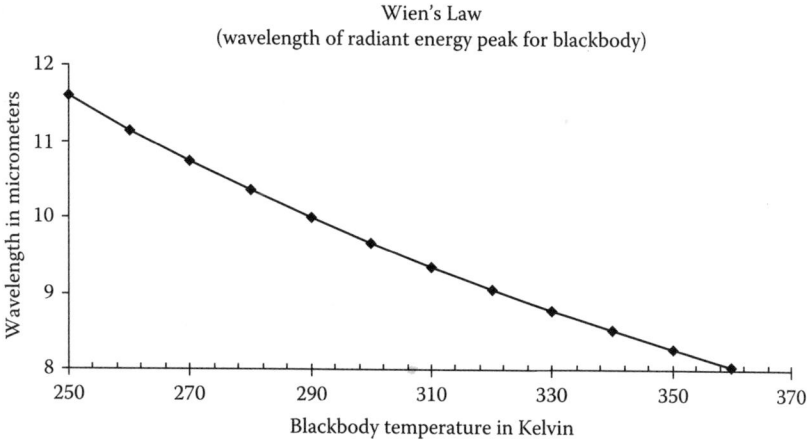

FIGURE 26.2   Location of peak of blackbody radiation, Wien's law.

appears that the LWIR flux characteristics are as good as a daytime visible system, however, there are two other factors limiting performance. First, the energy bandgaps of infrared sensitive devices are much smaller than in the visible, resulting in significantly higher detector dark current. The detectors are typically cooled to reduce this effect. Second, the reflected light in the visible is modulated with target and background reflectivities that typically range from 7% to 20%.

In the infrared, where all terrestrial objects emit, a two-degree equivalent blackbody difference in photon flux between object and background is considered high contrast. The flux difference between two blackbodies of 302 K compared to 300 K can be calculated in a manner similar to that shown in Figure 26.1. The flux difference is the signal that provides an image, hence the difference in signal compared to the ambient background flux should be noted. In the LWIR, the signal is 3% of the mean flux and in the MWIR it is 6% of the mean flux. This means that there is a large flux pedestal associated with imaging in the infrared.

There are two major challenges accompanying the large background pedestal in the infrared. First, the performance of a typical infrared detector is limited by the background photon noise and this noise term is determined by the mean of the pedestal. This value may be relatively large compared to the small signal differences. Second, the charge storage capacity of the silicon input circuit mated to each infrared detector in a staring array limits the amount of integrated charge per frame, typically around 10^7 charge carriers. An LWIR system in a hot desert background would generate 10^{10} charge carriers in a 33 ms integration time. The optical *f*-number, spectral bandwidth, and integration time of the detector are typically tailored to reach half well for a given imaging scenario for dynamic range purposes. This well capacity-limited condition results in a sensitivity, or noise equivalent temperature difference (NETD) of 10–30 times below the photon-limited condition. Figure 26.3 shows calculations of NETD as a function of background temperature for MWIR- and LWIR-staring detectors dominated by the photon noise of the incident IR radiation. At 310 K, the NETD of high-quantum efficiency MWIR and LWIR focal plane arrays (FPAs) is nearly the same, or about 3 millidegrees K, when the detectors are permitted to integrate charge up to the frame time, or in this case about 33 ms. The calculations show the sensitivity limits from the background photon shot noise only and do not include the contribution of detector and system temporal and spatial noise terms. The effects of residual spatial noise on NETD are described later in the chapter. The well capacity assumed here is 10^9 charge carriers to demonstrate sensitivity that could be achieved under large well conditions. The MWIR device is photon limited over the temperature range and begins to reach the well capacity limit near 340 K. The 24 μm pitch 9.5 μm cutoff LWIR device is well capacity limited over the entire temperature range. The 18 μm pitch 9.5 μm cutoff LWIR device becomes photon limited around 250 K. Various on-chip signal processing techniques, such as

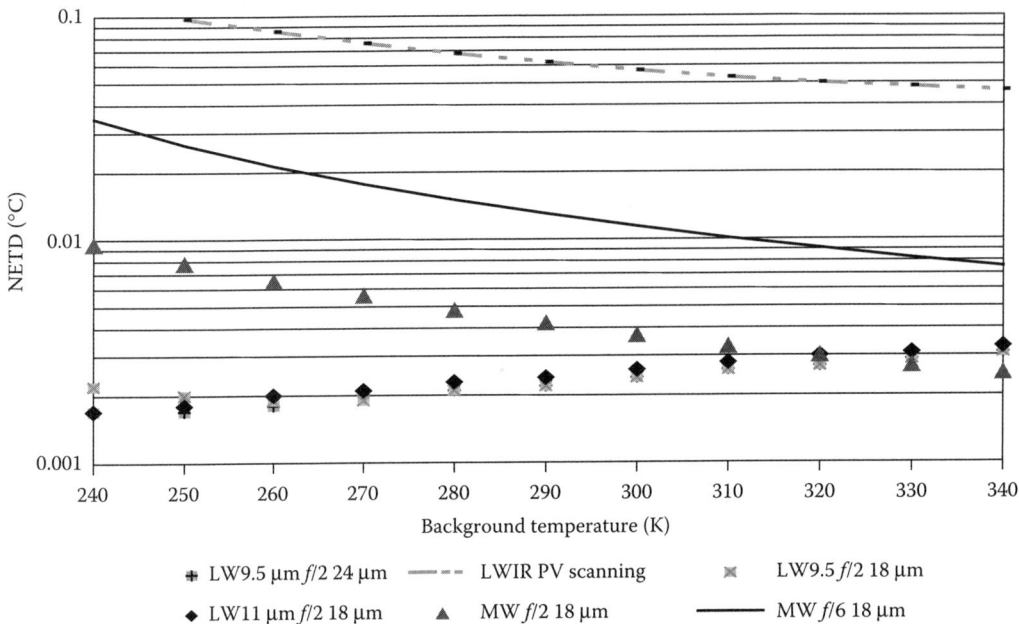

FIGURE 26.3 Background-limited NETD for high quantum efficiency MWIR and LWIR detectors.

charge skimming and charge partitioning, have been investigated to increase the charge capacity of these devices. In addition, as the minimum feature sizes of the input circuitry decreases, more real estate in the unit cell can be allocated to charge storage.

Another major difference between infrared and visible systems is the size of the detector and diffraction blur. Typical sizes for MWIR and LWIR detectors, or pixels, range from 20 to 50 μm. Visible detectors less than 6 μm are commercially available today. The diffraction blur for the LWIR is more than ten times larger than the visible blur and MWIR blur is eight times larger than visible blur. Therefore, the image blur due to diffraction and detector size is much larger in an infrared system than a visible system. It is very common for infrared staring arrays to be sampling limited where the sample spacing is larger than the diffraction blur and the detector size. Dither and microscanning are frequently used to enhance performance. A more detailed discussion of the optical considerations of infrared sensors is provided later in the chapter.

Finally, infrared staring arrays consisting of cooled photon detectors or uncooled thermal detectors may have responsivities that vary dramatically from pixel to pixel. It is common practice to correct for the resulting nonuniformity using a combination of factory preset tables and user inputs. The nonuniformity can cause fixed pattern noise in the image that can limit the performance of the system even more than temporal noise and these effects are demonstrated in the next section.

26.1 Infrared Sensor Calibration

Significant advancement in the manufacturing of high-quality FPAs operating in the short wave infrared (SWIR), MWIR, and LWIR has enabled industry to offer a wide range of affordable camera products to the consumer. Commercial applications of infrared camera technology are often driven by the value of the information it provides and price points set by the marketplace. The emergence of uncooled microbolometer FPA cameras with sensitivity less than 0.030°C at standard video rates has opened many new applications of the technology. In addition to the dramatic improvement in sensitivity over the past several years, uncooled microbolometer FPA cameras are characteristically compact, lightweight, and low power. Uncooled cameras are commercially available from a variety of domestic and foreign vendors including Agema, BAE Systems, CANTRONIC Systems, Inc., DRS and DRS Nytech, FLIR Systems, Inc., Indigo Systems, Inc., Electrophysics Corp., Inc., Infrared Components Corp., IR Solutions, Inc., and Raytheon, Thermoteknix Systems Ltd., ompact, low power. The linearity, stability, and repeatability of the system intensity transfer function (SiTF) may be measured to determine the suitability of an infrared camera for accurate determination of the apparent temperature of an object of interest. LWIR cameras are typically preferred for imaging applications that require absolute or relative measurements of object irradiance or radiance because emitted energy dominates the total signal in the LWIR. In the MWIR, extreme care is required to ensure the radiometric accuracy of data. Thermal references may be used in the scene to provide a known temperature reference point or points to compensate for detector-to-detector variations in response and improve measurement accuracy. Thermal references may take many forms and often include temperature-controlled extended area sources or uniformly coated metal plates with contact temperature sensors. Depending on the stability of the sensor, reference frames may be required in intervals from minutes to hours depending on the environmental conditions and the factory presets. Many sensors require an initial turn-on period to stabilize before accurate radiometric data can be collected. An example of a windows-based graphical user interface (GUI) developed at NVESD for an uncooled imaging system for medical studies is shown in Figure 26.4. The system allows the user to operate in a calibrated mode and display apparent temperature in regions of interest or at any specified pixel location including the pixel defined by the cursor. Single frames and multiple frames at specified time intervals may be selected for storage. Stability of commercially available uncooled cameras is provided earlier.

The LTC 500 thermal imager had been selected as a sensor to be used in a medical imaging application. Our primary goal was to obtain from the imagery calibrated temperature values within an accuracy of approximately a tenth of a degree Celsius. The main impediments to this goal consisted of several sources of spatial nonuniformity in the imagery produced by this sensor, primarily the spatial variation of radiance across the detector FPA due to self heating and radiation of the internal camera components, and to a lesser extent the variation of detector characteristics within the FPA. Fortunately, the sensor provides a calibration capability to mitigate the effects of the spatial nonuniformities.

We modeled the sensor FPA as a 2D array of detectors, each having a gain G and offset K, both of which are assumed to vary from detector to detector. In addition we assumed an internally generated radiance Y for each detector due to the self-heating of the internal sensor components (also varying from

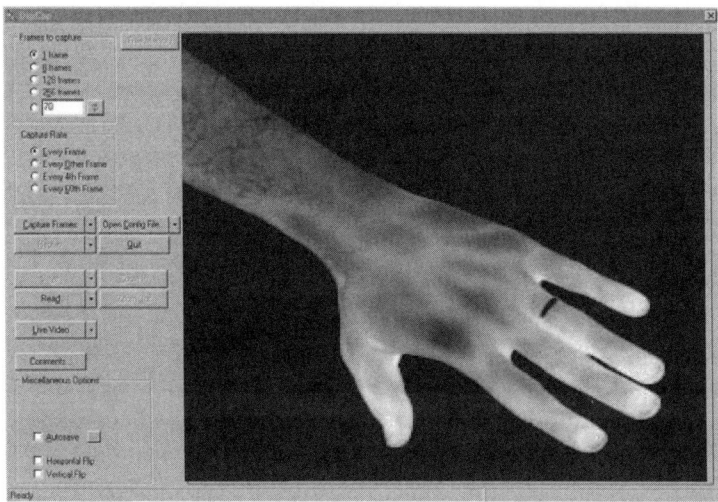

FIGURE 26.4 Windows-based GUI developed at NVESD for an uncooled medical imaging system.

detector to detector, as well as slowly with time). Lastly, there is an internally programmable offset C for each detector which the sensor controls as part of its calibration function. Therefore, given a radiance X incident on some detector of the FPA from the external scene, the output Z for that detector is given by

$$Z = GX + GY + K + C$$

26.2 Gain Detector

Individual detector gains were calculated by making two measurements. First, the sensor was allowed to run for several hours in order for the internal temperatures to stabilize. A uniform blackbody source at temperature T_1 (20°C) was used to fill the field of view (FOV) of the sensor and an output image Z_1 was collected. Next the blackbody temperature was set to T_2 (40°C) and a second output image Z_2 was collected. Since the measurement interval was small (<1–2 min) we assume the Y values remain constant, we have (for each detector):

$$Z_1 = GX_1 + GY + K + C$$
$$Z_2 = GX_2 + GY + K + C$$

where X_1 and X_2 refer to the external scene radiance corresponding to temperatures T_1 and T_2 incident on the detector and were calculated by integrating Planck's blackbody function over the 8–12 μm spectral band of the sensor. Taking the difference, we have (for each detector):

$$G = \frac{Z_2 - Z_1}{X_2 - X_1}$$

where the numbers here refer to measurements at different temperatures and, again, the value G (as well as Z and X) are assumed to vary from detector to detector (detector subscripts were omitted for clarity).

26.2.1 Nonuniformity Calibration

The LTC 500 provides the capability for nonuniformity calibration that allows the user to remove nonuniformities across the FPA assuming they do not change too rapidly with time. The procedure involves placing a uniform blackbody source across the FOV of the sensor and pressing the calibrate button. At this point, the sensor internally adjusts the value of a programmable offset for each detector so that the output Z of each detector is equal to a constant that we will denote Z_{CAL} (which the sensor sets to the midpoint of the digital pixel range, i.e., 16384).

Let D_1 and D_2 be two detectors selected from the 2D FPA, the outputs Z_1, Z_2 are then given by

$$Z_1 = G_1 X_1 + G_1 Y_1 + K_1 + C_1$$
$$Z_2 = G_2 X_2 + G_2 Y_2 + K_2 + C_2$$

where now the numbers refer to different detectors, and as before G is gain, X is the incident radiance from the external scene, Y is the internal self-heating radiance on the detectors, K is a possible offset variation from detector to detector, and C represents the programmable calibration offset for each detector. If we fill the FOV with a uniform blackbody at some temperature (T_{CAL}) producing a uniform radiance X_{CAL} on the FPA and activate the calibration function, we have

$$Z_1 = Z_{CAL} = G_1 X_{CAL} + G_1 Y_1 + K_1 + C_1$$
$$Z_2 = Z_{CAL} = G_2 X_{CAL} + G_2 Y_2 + K_2 + C_2$$

so

$$C_1 = Z_{CAL} - G_1 X_{CAL} - G_1 Y_1 - K_1$$
$$C_2 = Z_{CAL} - G_2 X_{CAL} - G_2 Y_2 - K_2$$

where X_{CAL} is calculated by spectrally integrating Planck's function from 8 to 12 μm at $T = T_{CAL}$. C_1 and C_2 will now retain these values until the sensor is either recalibrated or powered down. Now, for some arbitrary externally supplied radiance X_1, X_2 on the FPA we have

$$Z_1 = G_1 X_1 + G_1 Y_1 + K_1 + C_1$$
$$Z_1 = G_1 X_1 + G_1 Y_1 + K_1 + Z_{CAL} - G_1 X_{CAL} - G_1 Y_1 - K_1$$
$$Z_1 = G_1 X_1 + Z_{CAL} - G_1 X_{CAL}$$
$$Z_1 = G_1 (X_1 - X_{CAL}) + Z_{CAL}$$

and, similarly

$$Z_2 = G_2 (X_2 - X_{CAL}) + Z_{CAL}$$

therefore, the output of each detector depends only on the individual detector gain (which we know) and the external radiance incident on the detector. The spatially varying components (Y and K) have been removed.

Rearranging to solve for radiance input X as a function of the output intensity Z we have

$$X = \frac{(Z - Z_{CAL})}{G} + X_{CAL}$$

Given a precomputed lookup table RAD2TEMP of T, X pairs we can take the radiance value X and look up the corresponding temperature T for any pixel in the image. Hence we have computed temperature T_C as a function of radiance X on any detector:

$$T_C = \text{RAD2TEMP}[X]$$

26.3 Operational Considerations

Upon testing the system in a scenario that more accurately reflected the operational usage anticipated (i.e., with up to 10 ft between the sensor and the measured object), we encountered an unexpected discrepancy between the computed temperature values and the actual values as reported by the blackbody temperature display. We decided to assume that actual temperature values would vary linearly with the values computed by the above method. Therefore, we added a second step to the calibration procedure that requires the user to collect an image at a higher temperature than the calibration temperature T_{CAL}. Also, this second measurement would be made at a sensor to blackbody distance of approximately 10 ft. So now, we have two computed temperatures and two actual corresponding temperatures. Then we compute a slope and y-intercept describing the (assumed) linear relationship between the computed and actual temperatures.

$$T_A = M T_C + B$$

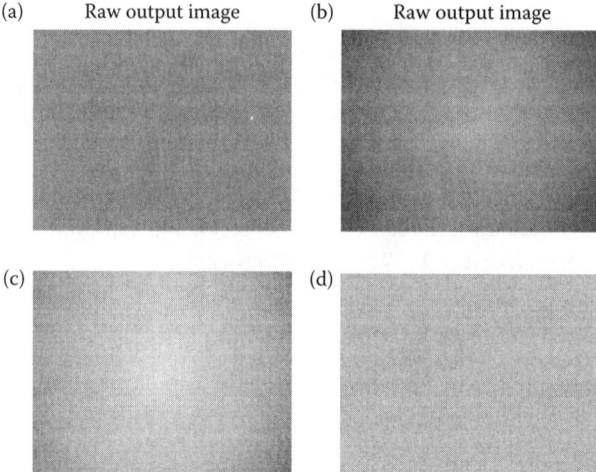

(a) Raw output image (b) Raw output image

(c) (d)

FIGURE 26.5 Gain calculation. (a) *Low temperature*: uniform 30°C black body source, calibrated at 30°, $\mu = 16381$, $\sigma = 1.9$ (raw counts). (b) *High temperature*: uniform 40°C black body source, calibrated at 30°, $\mu = 16842$, $\sigma = 11.3$ (raw counts). (c) *Processed using uniform gain*: uniform 35°C black body source, calibrated at 30°, $\mu = 34.74$, $\sigma = 0.12$ (°C). (d) *Processed using computed gain*: uniform 35°C black body source, calibrated at 30°, $\mu = 34.74$, $\sigma = 0.04$ (°C).

where

$$M = \frac{T_{A_2} - T_{A_1}}{T_{C_2} - T_{C_1}}$$

and

$$B = T_{A_1} - MT_{C_1}$$

where T_A is the adjusted temperature, T_C is the computed temperature from the previously described methodology. M and B are recomputed during each nonuniformity calibration.

From a camera perspective, the SiTF in digital counts for a $DC = A + BeT^4$.

$$T = \left(\frac{DN - A}{B\varepsilon} \right)^{1/4}$$

By adding this second step to the calibration process, we were able to improve the accuracy of the computed temperature to within a tenth of a degree for the test data set (Figure 26.5).

26.4 Infrared Optical Considerations

This section focuses mainly on the MWIR and LWIR since optics in the near infrared (NIR) and SWIR and very similar to that of the visible. This area assumes a basic knowledge of optics, and applies that knowledge to the application of infrared systems.

26.4.1 Resolution

Designing an IR optical system is first initiated by developing a set of requirements that are needed. These requirements will be used to determine the focal plane parameters and desired spectral band.

These parameters in turn drive the first-order design, evolving into the focal length, entrance pupil diameter, FOV, and *f*/number.

If we start with the user inputs of target distance, size, cycle criteria (or pixel criteria), and spectral band, we can begin designing our sensor. First, we calculate the minimum resolution angle (α, in radians). This parameter is also known as the instantaneous field of view (IFOV), and can be calculated by

$$\alpha = \frac{\text{Size}_{tar}}{(\text{Range})(2 \times \text{Cycles})}$$

or

$$\alpha = \frac{\text{Size}_{tar}}{(\text{Range})(\text{Pixels})}$$

On the basis of the wavelength, we can determine the minimum entrance pupil diameter that is necessary to distinguish between the two blur spots.

$$\text{EPD} = \frac{1.22\lambda}{\alpha}$$

Knowing the detector size and pixel pitch we can then determine the minimum focal length based on our IFOV that is required to meet our resolution requirements. Longer focal lengths will provide better spatial resolution.

$$\text{EFL} = \frac{\text{Pitch}}{\alpha}$$

Once we know our focal length, we can determine our FOV based on the height of the detector and the focal length. The vertical and horizontal fields of view are calculated separately based on their respective dimensions.

$$\theta = 2\tan\left[\frac{0.5h}{\text{EFL}}\right]$$

where *h* is the full detector height (or width). Depending on the system requirements, the size of the FPA may want to be scaled to match the desired FOV. Arrays with more pixels provide for greater resolution for a given FOV. However, smaller arrays cost less. Scaling an optical system to match the FOV for a different array format results in the scaling of the focal length, and thus the resolution.

The *f*/number is then calculated as the ratio of the focal length to the entrance pupil diameter.

$$f/\text{number} = \frac{\text{EFL}}{\text{EPD}}$$

The *f*/number of the system can be further optimized based on two parameters: the sensitivity and the blur circle. The minimum *f*/number is already set based on the calculated minimum entrance pupil diameter and focal length. The *f*/number can be adjusted to improve sensitivity by trying to optimize the blur circle to match the diagonal dimension of the detector pixel. This method provides a way to maximize the amount of energy on the pixel while minimizing aliasing.

$$f/\text{number} = \frac{\text{Pixel}_{diagonal}}{2.44\lambda}$$

A faster *f*/number is good in many ways as it can improve the resolution by reducing the blur spot and increasing the optics cutoff frequency. It also allows more signals to the detector and gives a boost in the signal to noise ratio. A fast *f*/number is absolutely necessary for uncooled systems because they have to overcome the noise introduced from operation at warmer temperatures. Faster *f*/numbers also help in environments with poor thermal contrast. However, a faster *f*/number also means that the optics will be larger, and the optical designs will be more difficult. Faster *f*/numbers introduce more aberrations into each lens making all aberrations more difficult to correct, and a diffraction limited system harder to achieve. A cost increase may also occur due to larger optics and tighter tolerances. A tradeoff has to occur to find the optimal *f*/number for the system. The table below shows the tradeoffs between optics diameter, focal length, resolution, and FOV.

26.5 Spectral Requirement

The spatial resolution is heavily dependent on the wavelength of light and the *f*/number. Diffraction limits the minimum blur size based on these two parameters.

$$d_{\text{spot}} = 2.44\lambda(f/\text{number})$$

The table given below compares the blur sizes for various wavelengths and *f*/numbers:

f/Number	Spot Size (µm)			
	$\lambda = 0.6$	$\lambda = 2$	$\lambda = 4$	$\lambda = 10$
1	1.5	4.9	9.8	24.4
2.5	3.7	12.2	24.4	61.0
4	5.9	19.5	39.0	97.6
5.5	8.1	26.8	53.7	134.2
7	10.2	34.2	68.3	170.8

First-Order Parameters Resolution 7.510

	f/Number	Focal Length	Field of View	Entrance Pupil Diameter
Impact resolution	A faster *f*/number results in a smaller optics blur due to diffraction. The result is an improved diffraction limit, and thus better spatial resolution. However, two things can adversely impact this improvement. Aberrations increase with faster *f*/number, potentially moving a system out of being diffraction limited, in which case the faster *f*/number can potentially hurt you. Also, a fixed	Increasing the focal length will increase spatial resolution. However, the amount of improvement may be limited by the size of the allowed aperture, as having to go to a slower *f*/number can reduce some of the gains. Longer focal lengths also result in narrower FOVs, which can	Narrower FOVs are the direct result of longer focal lengths. Longer focal lengths result in improved spatial resolution. The FOV can also vary by changing the size of the FPA. If all other parameters are maintained, and the FPA size is increased merely through the addition of more pixels, then the FOV increases without impacting resolution. If the number of pixels stay the same, but the pixel size is increased, then	The entrance pupil diameter (EPD) can impact the resolution in three ways. Increasing the EPD while maintaining focal length improves resolution by utilizing a faster *f*/number. Increasing the EPD while maintaining a constant *f*/number results in a longer focal length, and thus increase spatial resolution. Maintaining a

	f/Number	Focal Length	Field of View	Entrance Pupil Diameter
	front aperture system will have to reduce its focal length to accommodate the faster *f*/number, thus reducing spatial resolution through a change in focal length	be limited by stabilization issues	resolution is decreased. If pixel size is constant, number of pixels is increased, and focal length is scaled to maintain a constant FOV, then the resolution scales with the focal length	constant EPD while increasing focal length results in an improved spatial resolution due to the focal length, but a reduced resolution due to diffraction. The point where there is no longer significant improvement is dependent on the pixel size

26.5.1 Depth of Field

It is often desired to image targets that are located at different distances in object space. Two targets that are separated by a distance will both appear to be equally in focus if they fall within the depth of field (DOF) of the optics. A target that is closer to the optics than the DOF will appear defocused. In order to bring the out-of-focus target back in focus, it is required to refocus the optics so that the image plane shifts back to the location of the detector. Far targets focus shorter than near targets. If it is assumed that the optics are focused for an infinite target distance, the near DOF, known as the hyperfocal distance (HFD), can be-1pt found by

$$\text{HFD} = \frac{D^2}{2\lambda}$$

where D is the entrance pupil diameter, and λ is the wavelength in the same units as the diameter. This approximation can be made in the infrared because we can assume that we are utilizing a diffraction-limited system.

This formula is dependent only on the aperture diameter and wavelength. It is easily seen that shorter wavelengths and larger apertures have larger HFDs. This relationship is based on the Rayleigh limit which states that as long as the wavefront error is within a 1/4 wavelength of a true spherical surface, it is essentially diffraction limited. The depth of field can then be improved by focusing the optics to be optimally focused at the HFD. The optics are then in focus from that point to infinity based on the 1/4 wave criteria, but also for a 1/4 wave near that target distance. The full DOF of the system then becomes half the HFD to infinity. This is-1pt approximated by

$$\text{DOF} = \frac{D^2}{4\lambda}$$

If the region of interest is not within these bounds, it is possible to approximate the near and far focus points for a given object-1pt distance with

$$Z_{\text{near}} = \frac{\text{HFD} \times Z_0}{\text{HFD} + (Z_0 - f)}$$

$$Z_{\text{far}} = \frac{\text{HFD} \times Z_0}{\text{HFD} - (Z_0 - f)}$$

where X is the object distance that the objects are focused for and f is the focal length of the optics.

Work has been done with digital image-processing techniques to improve the DOF by applying a method known as Wavefront Coding, developed by Cathey and Dowksi at the University of Colorado.

This effectiveness of this technique has been well documented and demonstrated for the visible spectral band. Efforts are underway to demonstrate the effectiveness with LWIR uncooled cameras.

26.6 Selecting Optical Materials

The list of optical materials that transmit in the MWIR and LWIR spectrum is very short compared to that found in the visible spectrum. There are 21 crystalline materials and a handful chalcogenide glasses that transmit radiation at these wavelengths. Of the 21 crystalline materials, only 6 are practical to use in the LWIR, and 9 are usable in the MWIR. The remaining possess poor characteristics such as being hygroscopic, toxic to the touch, and so on, making them impractical for use in a real system. The list grows shorter for multispectral applications as only four transmit in the visible, MWIR, and LWIR. The chalcogenide glasses are an amorphous conglomerate of two or three infrared transmitting materials. Table 26.1 lists practical infrared materials along with a chart of their spectral bands. Transmission losses due to absorption can be calculated from the absorption coefficient of the material at the specified wavelength.

$$T_{abs} = e^{-at}$$

Transmission range for common IR materials

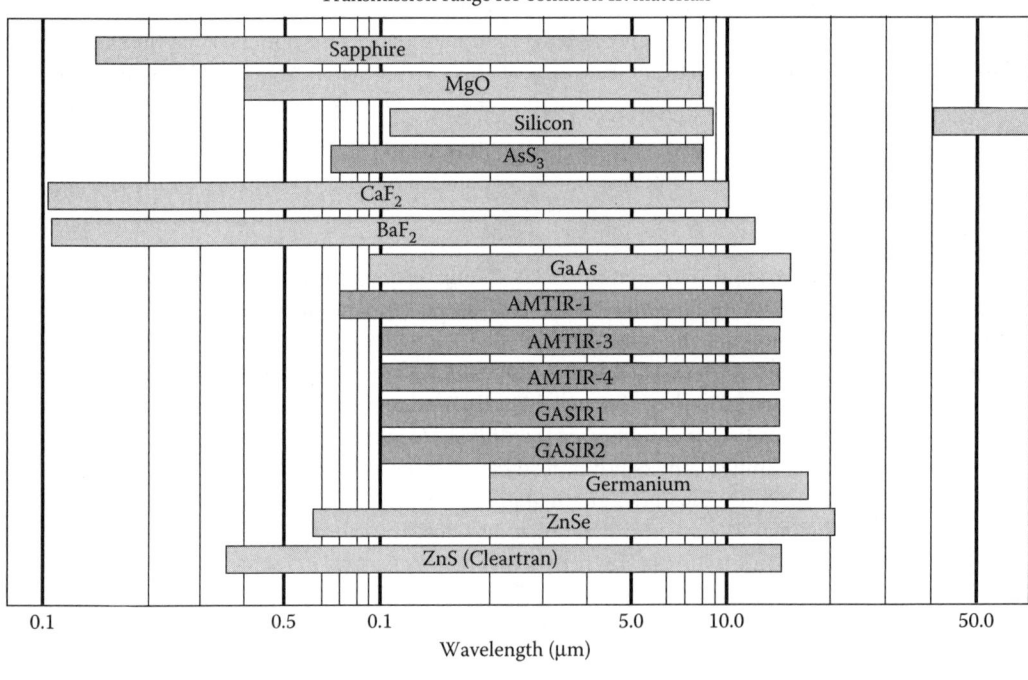

26.6.1 Special Considerations

In the LWIR, germanium is by far the best material to use for color correction and simplicity of design due to its high index of refraction and low dispersion. It is possible to design entire systems with germanium, but there are some caveats to this choice. Temperature plays havoc on germanium in two ways. It has a very high dn/dT (0.000396 K^{-1}), defocusing a lens that changes temperature of only a few degrees. It also has an absorption property in the LWIR for temperatures greater than 57°C. As the optic temperature rises above this point, the absorption coefficient increases, reducing the transmission. The high cost of germanium can also be a factor. It is not always good choice for a low-cost sensor, as

TABLE 26.1 Infrared Optical Materials

Material	Refractive Index 4 μm	= 10 μ	dμ/dT (K⁻¹)	Spectral Range (μm)
Germanium	4.0243	4.0032	0.000396	2.0–17.0
Gallium arsenide	3.3069	3.2778	0.000148	0.9–16.0
ZnSe	2.4331	2.4065	0.000060	0.55–20.0
ZnS (cleartran)	2.2523	2.2008	0.000054	0.37–14.0
AMTIR-1	2.2514	2.4976	0.000072	0.7–14.0
AMTIR-3	2.6200	2.6002	0.000091	1.0–14.0
AMTIR-4	2.6487	2.6353	−0.000030	1.0–14.0
GASIR 1	2.5100	2.4944	0.000055	1.0–14.0
GASIR 2	2.6038	2.5841	0.000058	1.0–14.0
Silicon	3.4255	N/A	0.000160	1.2–9.0
Sapphire	1.6753	N/A	0.000013	0.17–5.5
BaF₂	1.4580	1.4014	−0.000015	0.15–12.5
CaF₂	1.4097	1.3002	−0.000011	0.13–10.0
As₂S₃	2.4112	2.3816	−0.0000086	0.65–8.0
MgO	1.6679	N/A	0.000011	0.4–8.0

the lens may end up costing more than the FPA. A good thermal match to compensate for the dn/dT of germanium is AMTIR-4. Its negative dn/dT provides for an excellent compensator for the germanium. It is possible to design a two lens germanium/AMTIR-4 lens system that does not require refocusing for over a 60°C temperature range.

The low-cost optics are silicon, ZnS, and the chalcogenide glasses. Silicon is only usable in the MWIR, and although the material is very inexpensive, its hardness can make it very difficult to diamond turn, and thus expensive. Although it does not diamond turn well, it does grind and polish easily, providing a very inexpensive solution when complex surfaces such as aspheres and diffractives are not used. ZnS is relatively inexpensive to germanium and ZnSe, but is relatively expensive to silicon and the chalcogenide glasses. The chalcogenide glasses are by far the least expensive to make and manufacture making them an excellent solution for low-cost system design. There are three types of the chalcogenide glasses that are moldable. AMTIR-4, a product of Amorphous Materials, Inc., has a lower melting point that the other chalcogenides making it the easiest to mold. Another material GASIR1 and GASIR2, products of Umicore, have also been demonstrated as being moldable. They have similar optical properties to that of AMTIR-1 and AMTIR-3.

26.6.2 Coatings

The high indices of refraction of most infrared materials lead to large fresnel losses, and thus require AR coatings. The transmission for a plane uncoated surface is shown below. In air, $n_1 = 1$.

$$T = 1 - \left(\frac{n_1 - n_2}{n_1 + n_2} \right)^2$$

The total reflectance off both sides of an uncoated plate is the multiplication of the two surfaces. This is in turn multiplied by the transmission of the material due to absorption. An example is given below:

Example

Uncoated zinc selenide flat, $n = 2.4$ in air, $t = 1.5$ cm thickness, absorption = 0.0005.
Total transmission through both sides = (0.83)(0.999)(0.83) = 0.688.

Standard AR coatings are readily available for all of the materials previously listed. Generally, better than 99% can be expected for an AR-coated lens for either the MWIR or LWIR. If dual band operation is required, expect this performance to drop to 96%, and for the price to go up. The multispectral coatings are more difficult to design, and result in having many more layers. Infrared beamsplitter coatings can be difficult and expensive to manufacture. Care should be taken in specifying both the transmission and reflection properties of the beamsplitter. Specifications that are too stringent often lead to huge costs and schedule delays. Also, it is very important to note that the choice of which wavelength passes through and which wavelength is reflected can make a significant impact on the performance of a beamsplitter. In general, transmitting the longer wavelength and reflecting the shorter wavelength will boost performance and reduce cost.

26.6.3 Reflective Optics

Reflective optics can be a very useful and effective design too in the infrared. Reflective optics have no chromatic aberrations, and allow for diffraction-limited solutions for very wide spectral bands. However, the use of reflective optics is somewhat limited to narrow FOVs and have difficulty with fast *f*/numbers. In addition, the type of reflective system can impact the performance fairly significantly for longer wavelengths. The most common type of design is the Cassegrain, which has two mirrors that are aligned on the same optical axis. The secondary mirror acts as an obscuration to the primary, which results in a degraded MTF due to diffraction around the obscuration. This effect is not apparent in most wavebands because the MTF loss occurs after the Nyquist frequency of the detector. However, this is not the case for the LWIR where the MTF drop occurs before Nyquist. To overcome this effect, most reflective systems used in the LWIR are off-axis reflective optics. These optics will provide diffraction-limited MTF as long as the *f*/numbers do not get too fast, and the FOVs do not get too large. The off-axis nature makes these reflective systems hard to align, and expensive to manufacture.

Acknowledgments

The authors thank John O'Neill, Jason Zeibel, Tim Mikulski, and Kent McCormack for the data; EO-IR Measurements, Inc. for developing the graphical user interface for the medical infrared imaging camera; and Leonard Bonnell, Vipera Systems, Inc., for the development of the infrared endoscope.

References

1. J. D'Agostino and C. Webb, 3-D analysis framework and measurement methodology for imaging system noise. *Proc. SPIE*, 1488, 110–121 (1991).
2. R.G. Driggers, P. Cox, and T. Edwards, *Introduction to Infrared and Electro-Optical Systems*. Artech House, Boston, MA, p. 8 (1998).
3. G.C. Holst, *Electro-Optical Imaging System Performance*. JCD Publishing, Winter Park, FL, p. 347 (1995).
4. M.W. Grenn, Recent advances in portable infrared imaging cameras. *Proc. IEEE–EMBS*, Amsterdam (1996).
5. M.W. Grenn, Performance of portable staring infrared cameras. *Proc. IEEE/EMBS* Oct. 30–Nov. 2, Chicago, IL, USA (1997).

Further Information

Holst, G.C. *Electro-Optical Imaging System Performance*. JCD Publishing, Winter Park, FL, p. 432 (1995).
Johnson, J. Analysis of image forming systems. *Proc. IIS*, 249–273 (1958).

Ratches, J.A. *NVL Static Performance Model for Thermal Viewing Systems*, USA Electronics Command Report ECOM 7043, AD-A011212 (1973).

Schade, O.H. Electro-optical characteristics of television systems. *RCA Review*, IX(1–4) (1948).

Sendall, R. and Lloyd, J.M. Improved specifications for infrared imaging systems. *Proc. IRIS*, 14, 109–129 (1970).

Vollmerhausen, R.H. and Driggers, R.G. NVTHERM: Next generation night vision thermal model. *Proc. IRIS Passive Sensors*, 1 (1999).

27

Physiology of Thermal Signals

David D. Pascoe
Auburn University

James B. Mercer
University of Tromsø

Louis de Weerd
University Hospital of North Norway

27.1 Overview

William Herschel first recognized heat emitted in the infrared (IR) wave spectrum in the 1800s. Medical IR, popularly known as IR-thermography has utilized this heat signature since the 1960s to measure and map skin temperatures. Our understanding of the regulation of skin blood flow, heat transfers through the tissue layers, and skin temperatures has radically changed during these past 40 years, allowing us to better interpret and evaluate these thermographic measurements. During this same period of time, improved camera sensitivity coupled with advances in focal plan array technology and new developments in computerized systems with assisted image analysis have improved the quality of the noncontact, noninvasive thermal map or thermogram [1–3]. In a recent electronic literature search in Medline using the keywords "thermography" and "thermogram" more than 5000 hits were found [4]. In 2003 alone, there were 494 medical references, 188 basic science, 148 applied science (14 combined with Laser Doppler and 28 combined with ultrasound research), and 47 in biology including veterinary medicine [5]. Further databases and references for medical thermography since 1987 are available [6].

This review will highlight some of the literature and applications of thermography in medical and physiological settings. More specifically, IR thermography and the structure and functions of skin thermal microcirculation can provide a better understanding of (1) thermoregulation and skin thermal patterns (e.g., comfort zone, influences of heat, cold, and exercise stressors, etc.), (2) assess skin blood perfusion (e.g., skin grafts), (3) observe and diagnose vascular pathologies that manifest thermal disturbances in the cutaneous circulation, (4) evaluate thermal therapies, and (5) monitor patient/subject/athlete's recovery as evidenced by the resumption of normal thermal patterns during the rehabilitation process for some musculoskeletal injuries.

At the outset, it needs to be stressed that an IR image is a visual map of the skin surface temperature that can provide accurate thermal measurement but cannot quantify measurements of blood flow to the skin tissue. It is also important to stress that recorded skin temperatures may represent heat transferred from within the core through various tissue layers to the skin that may be the result of conductive or radiant heat provided from an external thermal stressor. To interpret thermographic images and thermal measurement, a basic understanding of physiological mechanisms of skin blood flow and factors that influence heat transfers to the skin must be considered to evaluate this dynamic process. With this understanding, objective data from IR-thermography can add valuable information and complement other methodologies in the scientific inquiry and medical practices.

27.2 Skin Thermal Properties in Response to Stress

The thermal properties of the skin surface can change dramatically to maintain our core temperature within a narrowly defined survival range (cardiac arrest at 25°C to cell denaturation at 45°C) [7]. This remarkable task is accomplished despite a large variability in temperatures both from the hostile environment and internal production of heat from metabolism. Further perturbations to core and skin temperature may result from thermal stressors associated with injury, fever, hormonal milieu, and disease. The skin responds to these thermal challenges by regulating skin perfusion.

During heat exposure or intense exercise, skin blood flow can be increased to provide greater heat dissipating capacity. The thermal properties of the skin combined with increased cutaneous circulation operate as a very efficient radiator of heat (emitted radiant heat of 0.98 compared to a blackbody source of 1.0) [8]. Evaporative cooling of sweat on the skin surface further enhances this heat dissipating process. Under hyperthermic conditions, the skin masterfully combines anatomical structure and physiological function to protect and defend the organism from potentially lethal thermal stressors by regulating heat transfers between core, skin, and environment. When exposed to a cold environment, the skin surface nearly eliminates blood flow and becomes an excellent insulator. Under these hypothermic conditions, our skin functions to conserve our body's core temperature. It accomplishes this by reducing convective heat transfers, minimizing heat losses from the core and lessening the possibility of excessive cooling from the environment.

The ability of the skin to substantially increase blood flow, far in excess of the tissue's metabolic needs, alludes to the tissue's role and potential in heat transfer mechanisms. The nutritive needs of skin tissue has been estimated at 0.2 mL/min per cubic centimeter of skin [9], which is considerably lower than the maximal rate of 24 mL/min per cubic centimeter of skin (estimated from total forearm circulatory measurement during heat stress) [10]. If one were to approximate skin tissue as 8% of the forearm, then skin blood would equate to 250–300 mL/100 mL of skin per minute [11]. Applying this flow rate to an estimated skin surface of 1.8 m^2 (average individual), suggests that approximately 8 L of blood flow could be diverted to the skin to dissipate heat at rate of 1750 W to the environment [12,13]. This increased blood flow required for heat transfers from active muscle tissue and skin blood flow for thermoregulation is made available through the redistribution of blood flow (splanchnic circulatory beds, renal tissues) and increases in cardiac output [14]. The increased cardiac output has been suggested to account for two-thirds of the increased blood flow needs, while redistribution provides the remaining one-third [15]. Several good reviews are available regarding cutaneous blood flow, cardiovascular function, and thermal stress [14–19].

27.3 Regulation of Skin Blood Flow for Heat Transfers

In the 1870s, Goltz, Ostromov, and others injected atropine and pilocaprine into the skin to help elucidate the sympathetic neural innervation of the skin tissue for temperature, pressure, pain, and the activation of the sweat glands [20]. The reflex neural regulation of skin blood flow relies on both sympathetic vasoconstrictor and vasodilator controls to modulate internal heat temperature transfers to the skin. The vasoconstrictor system is responsible for eliminating nearly all of the blood flow to the skin during exposure to cold. When exposed to thermal neutral conditions, the vasoconstrictor system maintains the vasomotor tone of the skin vasculature from which small changes in skin blood flow can elicit large changes in heat dissipation. Under these conditions, the core temperature is maintained; mean skin temperature is stable, but dependent upon the extraneous influences of radiant heat, humidity, forced convective airflow, and clothing. A naked individual in a closed room with ambient air temperature between 27°C and 28°C can retain thermal equilibrium without shivering or sweating [21]. Slightly dressed individuals are comfortable in a neutral environment with temperatures between 20°C and 25°C. This thermoneutral zone provides the basis for the clinical testing standards for room temperatures being set at 18–25°C during IR thermographic studies. Controlling room test conditions is important when measuring skin temperature responses as changes in ambient temperatures can alter the fraction of flow shared between the musculature and skin [19]. Under the influence of whole-body hyperthermic conditions, removal of the vasomotor vasoconstrictor tone can account for 10–20% of cutaneous vasodilation, while the vasodilator system provides the remaining skin blood flow regulation [10]. Alterations in the threshold (onset of vascular response and sweating) and sensitivity (level of response) in vasodilation blood flow control can be related to an individual's level of heat acclimation [22], exercise training [22], circadian rhythm [23,24], and women's reproductive hormonal status [10]. Recent literature suggests that some observed shifts in the reflex control are the result of female reproductive hormones. Both estrogen and progesterone have been linked to menopausal hot flashes [10].

Skin blood flow research has identified differences in reflex sympathetic nerve activation for various skin surface regions. In 1956, Gaskell demonstrated that sympathetic neural activation in the acral regions (digits, lips, ears, cheeks, and palmer surfaces of hands and feet) is controlled by adrenergic vasoconstrictor nerve activity [20]. In contrast, I.C. Roddie in 1957 demonstrated that in nonacral regions, the adrenergic vasoconstrictor activity accounts for less than 25% of the control mechanism [25]. In the nonacral region, the sympathetic nervous system has both adrenergic (vasoconstriction) and nonadrenergic (vasodilator) components. While the vasodilator activity in the nonacral region is well accepted, the vasoconstrictor regulation is not fully understood and awaits the identification of neural cotransmitters that mediate the reductions in blood flow. For a more in-depth discussion of regional sympathetic reflex regulation, see Charkoudian [10] and Johnson and Proppe [13].

A further distinction in blood flow regulation can be found in the existence of arteriovenous anastamoses (AVA) that are principally found in acral tissues but not commonly found in nonacral tissues of the legs, arms, and chest regions [10,26,27]. The AVAs are thick-walled, low-resistance vessels that provide a direct blood flow route from arterioles to the venules. The arterioles and AVA, under sympathetic adrenergic vasoconstrictor control, modulate and substantially control flow rates to the skin vascular plexuses in these areas. When constricted, blood flow into subcutaneous venous plexus is reduced to a very low level (minimal heat loss); while, when dilated, extremely rapid flow of warm blood into the venous plexus is allowed (maximal heat loss). The skin sites where these vessels are found are among those where skin blood flow changes are discernible to the IR-thermographer. While the AVA are most active during heat stress, their thick walls and high-velocity flow rates do not support their significant role in heat transfers to adjoining skin tissue [12].

Localized cooling of the skin surface can cause skin blood flow vasoconstriction induced by the stimulation of the nonadrenergic sympathetic nerves. This localized cooling or challenge can be used as a diagnostic tool by IR thermographers to identify clinically significant alterations in skin blood flow response. Using a cold challenge test, Francis Ring developed a vasoplasticity test for Raynaud's syndrome based on the temperature gradient in the hand following a cold water immersion (20°C for 60 s) [28]. Challenge testing and IR imaging has also been used to evaluate blood flow thermal patterns in patients with carpal tunnel syndrome pre- and post-surgery [29]. Skin blood flow vasodilation in response to local heating is stimulated by the release of sensory nerve neuropeptides or the nonneural stimulation of the cutaneous arteriole by nitric oxide. Thermographic imagers have exploited this localized warming response to provide a skin blood flow challenge [10].

As stated earlier, conditions of thermal stress from heat exposure and increased metabolic heat from exercise necessitate increases in skin blood flow to transfer the heat to the environment. This could have serious blood pressure consequences if it were not for baroreflex modulation of skin blood flow in regulating both sympathetic vasoconstriction and vasodilation [30,31]. With mild heat stress for 1 h (38°C and 46°C, 42% relative humidity), cardiac output was not significantly impacted [32–34]. When exposing the individual to longer duration bouts and higher temperatures, significant changes in cardiac output have been observed. During these hyperthermic bouts, skin blood flow will withdraw vasodilation in nonacral regions in response to situations that displace blood volumes to the legs (lower body negative pressure or upright tilting) [35]. In contrast, under normothermic conditions, skin blood flow will demonstrate a sympathetic vasoconstriction to these same blood volume situations. Thus, it appears that the baroreceptor response can activate either sympathetic pathway. Withdrawing vasodilation under normothermic conditions was not an option in this inactive system [36].

In summary, skin blood flow during whole-body thermal stress is regulated by neural reflex control via sympathetic vasoconstriction and vasodilation. There are structural (AVA) and neural mechanisms (vasoconstriction vs. vasodilation) differences between the acral and nonacral regions. During local thermal stress, stimulation of the sensory afferent nerve, nitric oxide stimulation of cutaneous arteriole, and inhibition of sympathetic vasoconstrictor system regulate changes in local blood flow. During thermal stress and increased heat from exercise metabolism, the skin blood flow can be dramatically increased. This increase in skin blood flow is matched to increased cardiac output and peripheral resistance to maintain blood pressure.

27.4 Heat Transfer Modeling Equations for Microcirculation

The capacity and ability of blood to transfer heat through various tissue layers to the skin can be predicted from models. These models are based on calculations from tissue conductivity, tissue density, tissue specific heat, local tissue temperature, metabolic or externally derived heat sources, and blood velocity. Many current models were derived from the 1948 Pennes model of blood perfusion, often referred to as the "bioheat equation" [9]. The bioheat equation calculates volumetric heat that is equated to the proportional volumetric rate of blood perfusion. The Pennes model assumed that thermal equilibrium occurs in the capillaries and venous temperatures were equal to local tissue temperatures. Both of these assumptions have been challenged in more recent modeling research. The assumption of thermal equilibrium within capillaries was challenged by the work of Chato [37] and Chen and Holmes in 1980 [38]. Based on this vascular modeling for heat transfer, thermal equilibrium occurred in "thermally significant blood vessels" that are approximately 50–75 μm in diameter and located prior to the capillary plexus. These thermally significant blood vessels derive from a tree-like structure of branching vessels that are closely spaced in countercurrent pairs. For a historical perspective of heat transfer bioengineering, see Chato in Reference 37 and for a review of heat transfers and microvascular modeling, see Baish in [39].

This modeling literature provides a conceptual understanding of the thermal response of skin when altered by disease, injury, or external thermal stressors to skin temperatures (environment or application of cold or hot thermal sources, convective airflow, or exercise). From tissue modeling, we know that tissue is only slightly influenced by the deep tissue blood supply but is strongly influenced by the cutaneous circulation. With the use of IR-thermography, the skin temperatures can be accurately quantified and the thermal pattern mapped. However, these temperatures cannot be assumed to represent thermal conditions at the source of the thermal stress. Furthermore, the thermal pattern only provides a visual map of the skin surface in which heat is dissipated throughout the skin's multiple microvascular plexuses.

27.5 Cutaneous Circulation Measurement Techniques

A brief review of some of the techniques and procedures that have been employed to reveal skin tissue structure, rates and variability of perfusion, and factors that provide regulatory control of blood flow are provided. This serves to inform the reader as to how these measurement techniques have molded our understanding of skin structure and function. It is also important to recognize the advantages and disadvantages each technique brings to our experimental investigations. It is the opinion of the authors that IR-thermography can provide complimentary data to information obtained from these other methodologies.

27.5.1 Procedures and Techniques

Visual and microscopic views of skin have provided scientists with a structural layout of skin layers and blood flow. Despite our understanding of the structural organization, we still struggle to understand the regulation and functioning of the skin as influenced by the multitude of external and internal stressors. Since ancient times, documents have recorded visible observations made regarding changes to skin color and temperature that underscore some of the skin's functions. These observations include increased skin color and temperature when someone is hyperthermic, skin flushing when embarrassed, and the appearance of skin reddening when the skin is scratched. In contrast, decreases of skin color and temperature are observed during hypothermia, when blood flow is occluded, or during times of circulatory shock. In addition to observations, testing procedures and techniques have been employed in search of an understanding of skin function. Skin blood flow has provided one of the greatest challenges and has been notoriously difficult to record quantitatively in terms of mL/min per gram of skin tissue.

27.5.2 Dyes and Stains

Stains and dyes have been a useful tool to investigate the structure of various histological tissue preparations. In 1889 Overton used Florescin, a yellow dye that glows in visible light, to visualize the lipid bilayer membrane structure [40]. Florescin is still used today to illuminate the blood vessel in various tissues. In the early 1900s, August Krogh was able to identify perfused capillaries by staining them with writer's ink before the tissue was excised and observed under the microscope. Using a different approach to observe the structure of skin blood flow, Michael Salmon in the 1930s developed a radio-opaque preservative mixture that was injected into fresh cadavers and produced detailed pictures of the arterial blood flow to skin tissue regions which were mapped for the entire skin surface [41]. Scientists have also used Evans Blue Dye to investigate changes in blood volume by calculating the dilution factor of pre- and post-samples. Evans Blue and Pontamine Sky Blue dyes have also been used to investigate skin microvascular permeability and leakage as induced by various stimuli [42]. A more recent staining technique involves the use of an IR absorbing dye, indocyanine green (ICG). The dye ICG fluoresces with invisible IR light when captured by special cameras sensitive to these light wavelengths. Recent publications have suggested that ICG video angiographies provide qualitative and quantitative data from which clinicians may assess tissue blood flow in burn wounds [43,44].

27.5.3 Plethysmography

The rationale for venous occlusion plethysmography (VOP) is that a partially inflated cuff around a limb exceeds the pressure of venous blood flow but does not interfere with arterial blood flow to the limb. This can be effectively accomplished when the cuff is inflated to a pressure just below diastolic arterial pressure. Consequently, portions of the limb distal to the cuff will swell as blood accumulates. The original VOP technology relied on measuring the rate of swelling as indicated by the displacement volume of the water-filled chamber around the limb. Later, gauges were used to record changes in limb circumference as the limb expanded. Either way, the geometric forces allows one to express the changes in terms of a starting volume, thus scales are labeled as mL/min per 100 mL in the illustrations of VOP data. Unfortunately, the 100 mL reference quantity refers to the whole limb (not the quantity of the skin) and the VOP technique provides discontinuous measurement, usually four measurements per minute. Currently, VOP represents the most reliable quantitative measure of skin blood flow. More recently, a modified plethysmography technique has been developed that equates changes in blood flow to the changes in electrical impedance, when a mild current is introduced into the blood flow and recorded by serially placed electrodes along the limb.

27.5.4 Doppler Measurement

The Doppler effect describes the shift in wavelength frequency or pitch that result when sound or light from any portion of the electromagnetic spectrum are influenced by the distance and directional movement of the object. Both ultrasound and laser Doppler techniques rely on this physical principle to make the skin blood flow measurement. A continuous-wave Doppler ultrasound emits a high-frequency sound wave from which reflected or echo sounds can be used to calculate the direction of flow and velocity of moving objects (circulating blood cells). When ultrasound equipment is pulsated, the depth of the circulatory flow vessel can be identified. The blood flow is assessed in Doppler units or volts and can be continuously monitored over a small surface area. Similar measurements can be made with the laser Doppler technique, but neither technique is able to yield quantitative blood flow values except through reference data obtained by VOP.

27.5.5 Clearance Measurement

In the 1930s, scientists relied on the thermal conductance method for determining blood flow in tissues. This methodology was based on measurement of heat dissipation in blood flow downstream from a known heat source (thermocouple). The accuracy of the methodology was assumed through strong correlations made with direct drop counting from isolated sheep spleens. However, these blood flow measurements had problems related to trauma associated with the obstruction and insertion of the thermocouple. During the 1950s and 1960s, injection of small amounts of radioactive isotopes was used in an attempt to better quantify skin blood flow [45]. In order to accurately measure skin blood flow, the isotopes had to be freely diffusible and able to cross the capillary endothelium to enter the blood stream. The blood flow measurement (mL blood flow per 100 g of tissue) obtained through this methodology was not reproducible and subjects were exposed to injected radioactive isotope substances.

27.5.6 Thermal Skin Measurement

Physicians and parents have often relied upon touching a child's forehead to identify a fever or elevated temperature. While this is a crude measure of skin temperature, it has demonstrated practical importance. The development of the thermistor has provided quantifiable measurements of the skin surface. This has been extensively used in research related to thermoregulation and in research in which the skin temperature for a particular physiological perturbation must be quantified. Mean skin temperature formulas have been developed in which various regional temperatures (3–15 sites) are combined or a weighted mean based on the DuBois formula for surface area is calculated from the regions measured. When measuring skin temperatures under the influence of colder environments, skin temperature distribution is heterogeneous, especially in the acral regions [46]. Under these conditions, the various placements of the thermistor will provide different temperature measurement that may not be indicative of the mean skin temperature for that region. In contrast, the skin surface temperature is more homogeneous under warm environmental conditions. To provide an accurate measurement, physiologists investigating mean skin temperatures have modified the number of thermistors required during testing as dictated by environmental temperatures [46]. Thermistor attachment to the skin surface is problematic as it creates a microenvironment between the probe, skin, and adhering tape and exerts a pressure on the site. Furthermore, one site placement of the thermistor cannot represent variable responses under conditions and within regions that demonstrate heterogeneous temperature distributions.

IR thermography provides a thermal map of the skin surface area by measuring the radiant heat that is emitted. Current IR-thermography machines provide accurate skin surface temperatures (<0.05°C) that are noninvasive, noncontact measurements through the use of stable detectors. These systems produce high-speed–high-resolution images from which thermal data can be pictorially and quantitatively stored and analyzed. While IR-radiation begins at wavelengths of 0.7 μm, current IR-thermographic imagers are operating at either the mid-range (3–5 μm) or long range (8–14 μm) wavelengths [1–3]. At these wavelengths the skin's ability to emit the radiant heat is 0.98 on a scale of 1.0 for a perfect radiator, blackbody surface [8]. IR-thermographers sometimes rely on "challenge tests" in which the skin thermal response is evaluated after cold or hot water immersion, convective airflow, or an exercise bout that alters skin blood flow. Under these thermally challenging conditions, the clinical importance of abnormalities of skin blood flow may be more apparent. However, one must also recognize that as the heat is being transferred through the various layers of skin, some of the heat is dissipated into the adjoining tissues. The heat decay as the blood traverses the layers of tissue and its dispersion pattern within the circulatory plexus of the skin may disguise the origin of the tissue producing the abnormal thermal response.

27.5.7 Measurement Techniques and Procedures Summary

Since ancient times, significant progress has been made in the quest to understand the anatomy and physiology of skin blood flow and the thermal heat transfers that are dissipated to the skin surface. Current measurement technologies are unable to quantify skin blood flow per skin tissue area (mL/min per 100 mL skin). At this time, our best estimations of skin blood flow come from VOP. VOP provides discontinuous blood flow measurements based on tissue perfusion of a whole limb extremity. In recent years, laser Doppler blood flow measures have been popular when investigating more localized tissue areas, but this technique must be calibrated through the data obtained by plethysmography. In the quest to understand skin surface heat transfers, noncontact IR-thermography provides researchers with accurate measures of skin temperature for specific locations and thermal maps of regions of interest. Thermographic images provide spatial and temporal changes in skin temperature that are representative of spatial and temporal changes in perfusion. However, the scientist and clinician should be aware of blood–skin heat transfer properties prior to interpreting and evaluating the thermal responses of skin perfusion or investigating pathologies that are thermally transferred to the skin.

27.6 Objective Thermography

The main focus of this section is to present some specific examples to show that IR thermal imaging is a useful, objective tool for medical and physiological-based investigations. Although IR thermal imaging cannot determine quantitative measurements of blood flow, this imaging can quantify skin thermal measurement that can be correlated to qualitative evaluations of skin blood flow. As with any technique, it is imperative for the IR-thermographer to understand the anatomical and dynamic physiological features (e.g., vasomotor activity) of the blood vessels involved in skin circulation in order to interpret skin temperature responses. This is particularly important in situations where skin blood flow and temperature are responding to some external or internal thermal stress (e.g., clinician's cold challenge testing, exercise, environment, etc.) or nonthermal stimuli (e.g., disease, injury, medications, etc.). When properly assessed, skin temperature can provide researchers, scientists, and physicians with valuable information about the blood flow and thermal regulation of organs and tissues (see Examples 27.6.1 through 27.6.7).

27.6.1 Efficiency of Heat Transport in the Skin of the Hand (Example 27.1)

The AVA are specialized vascular structures within acral regions. At normal body temperature, sympathetic vasoconstrictor nerves keep these anastomoses closed. However, when the body becomes overheated, sympathetic discharge is greatly reduced so that the anastomoses dilate allowing large quantities of warm blood to flow into the subcutaneous venous plexus, thereby promoting heat loss from the body (Figure 27.1a). In thermal physiology, hands and feet are well recognized as effective thermal windows. By controlling the amount of blood perfusing through these extremities, the temperature of the skin surface can change over a wide range of temperatures. It is at such peripheral sites that the effect of changes in blood flow, and therefore skin temperature are most clearly discernable.

The following example demonstrates how efficient skin blood flow in the hand is dissipating a large incoming radiant heat load. The radiant heat load was provided by a Hydrosun® type 501 water-filtered infrared-A (wIRA) irradiator. The Hydrosun allows a local regional heating of skin tissue with a higher penetration depth than that of conventional IR therapy. The unique principle of operation involves the use of a hermetically sealed water filter in the radiation path to absorb those IR wavelengths emitted by conventional IR lamps which would otherwise harm the skin (OH-group at 0.94, 1.18, 1.38, and 1.87 μm). The total effective radiation from the Hydrosun lamp was 400 mW/cm^2, which is about three times the intensity of the IR-A radiation from the sun. Throughout the time course of the experiment (Figure 27.1a), sequential digital IR-thermal images were taken every 2 s. With the image analysis software, five points within the radiation field of each image were selected for temperature measurement and used to construct temperature curves shown in Figure 27.1b.

In the experiment (Figure 27.1b) a rubber mat with an emissivity close to 1.0 was irradiated with the Hydrosun wIRA lamp for a period of 25 min at a standard distance of 25 cm. At this distance the circular irradiation field had a diameter of about 16 cm. Since the rubber material has a high emissivity it rapidly absorbs heat from the lamp. As can be seen from the time course of the five temperature curves in Figure 27.2 (five fixed measuring points within the radiation field), the center of the irradiated rubber mat rapidly reached temperatures over 90°C during the first 10 min of irradiation. After the first 10 min of irradiation, the hand of a healthy 54-year-old male subject was abruptly placed on the irradiated rubber mat and kept there for a further 10 min, before being removed. When the hand was placed onto the irradiation field, three of the five fixed temperature-measuring sites now measured skin temperature on the dorsal skin surface. Based on the temperature curves in Figure 27.1b, skin temperature on the surface of the hand directed toward the irradiator never increased higher than 40°C, while the two remaining temperature-measuring points on the rubber mat remained at their original high values. The patient suffered no thermal discomfort from placing his hand on the "hot" rubber mat, even though the temperature of the center of the rubber mat was more than 90°C before the hand was placed on it. This was presumably due to a combination of the low heat capacity of the rubber material combined with a high rate of skin blood flow that is capable of rapidly dissipating heat. The visual data created from the IR-thermal images coupled with the temperature curves which were calculated from sequential IR-thermal images clearly demonstrates the large heat transporting capacity of the skin.

27.6.2 Effect of a Reduced Blood Flow (Example 27.2)

During exposure to cold, heat loss from the extremities is minimized by reducing blood flow (vasoconstriction). In cool environments, this vasomotor tone results in a heterogeneous distribution of skin surface temperatures; while in a warm environment the skin surface becomes more homogeneous (see

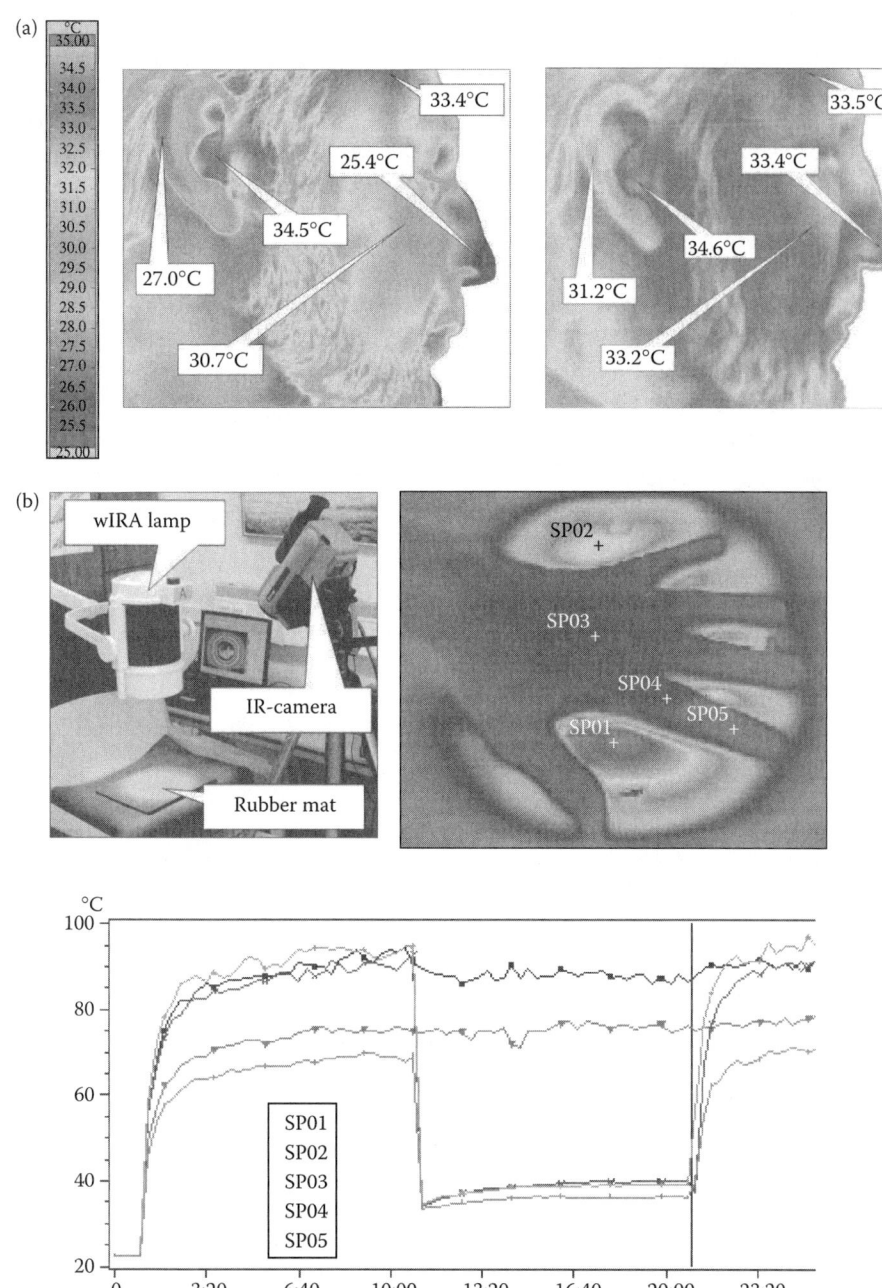

FIGURE 27.1 (a) A thermogram of a healthy 52-year-old male subject in a cold environment (ca. 15°C; left panel) and in a warm environment (ca. 25°C; right panel). In the cold environment arteriovenous anastomoses in the nose and the auricle region of the ears are closed, resulting in low skin temperatures at these sites. Also note reduced blood flow in the cheeks but not on the forehead, where the blood vessels in the skin are unable to vasoconstrict. (b) Efficiency of skin blood flow as a heat transporter. The photograph in the upper left panel shows a rubber mat being heated with a water-filtered IR-A irradiator at high intensity (400 mW/cm²) for a period of 20 min. In the lower panel the time course of surface temperature of the mat at five selected spots as measured by an IR-camera is given. During the last 10 min of the 20-min heating period, the left hand of a healthy 54-year-old male subject was placed on the mat. Note that skin surface temperature of the hand remains below 39°C.

Figure 27.2a). The importance of the integrity of blood flow in a limb as a whole can also be demonstrated at room temperature by totally cutting off the blood supply to the limb with the aid of a pressure cuff. This is demonstrated in the experiment shown in Figure 27.2b. In this experiment, skin surface on the back of the left hand of a 60-year-old healthy male subject was irradiated for a 10-min period with a wIRA lamp (see description in Section 27.6.1). The fingers were not heated. The heating was repeated twice. In the upper panel (Figure 27.2b) intact blood supply is demonstrated. In the lower panel (Figure 27.2b), thermal response to heating of the limb while blood flow was totally restricted using a blood

(a)   30 min equilibration in cool environment (20°C, 30% rh)

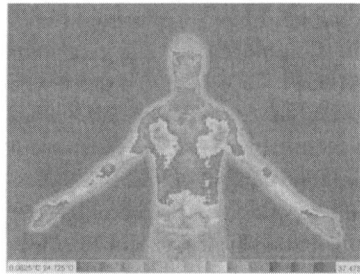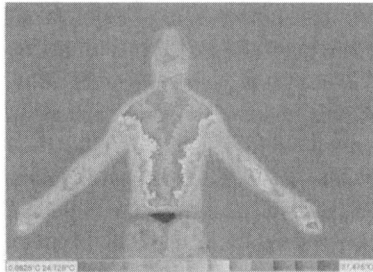

30 min equilibration in warm environment (41°C, 30% rh)

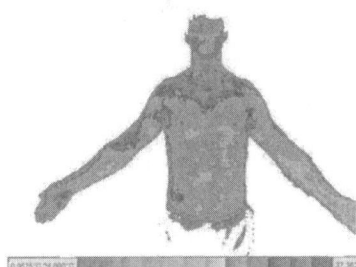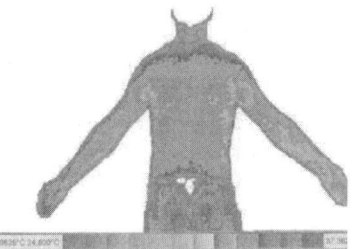

Range of temperature (°C) within regions at two climatic conditions.

	Anterior torso	Posterior torso	Anterior arms	Posterior arms	Palmer hands	Dorsal hands
Cool 20°C	5.0	5.1	6.3	4.5	5.2	4.0
Warm 41°C	3.0	3.2	3.2	3.6	4.0	3.5

FIGURE 27.2   (a) A thermoregulatory response of the torso when exposed to a cool or warm environment. Note the heterogeneous temperature distribution in the cool environment as opposed to the more homogeneous temperature distribution in the warm environment. Different shades of grey represent different temperatures. One might recognize the difficulty related to choosing one point (thermocouple data) as the reference value in a region. (b) Skin heating with and without intact circulation in a 65-year-old healthy male subject. The two panels on the right show the time course of six selected measuring sites (four spot measurements and two area measurements) of skin temperatures as determined by IR-thermography before, during, and after a period in which the skin surface on the back of the left hand was heated with a water-filtered IR-A irradiator at high intensity (400 mW/cm²) in two separate experiments. The results shown in the upper right panel were performed under a situation with a normal intact blood circulation, while the results shown in the lower left panel were made during total occlusion of circulation in the right arm by means of an inflated pressure cuff placed around the upper arm. The time of occlusion is indicated. The IR-thermogram on the left was taken just prior to the end of the heating period in the experiment described in the upper panel. The location of the temperature measurement sites on the hand (four spot measurements [Spot 1 to Spot 4] and the average temperature within a circle [Areas 5 and 6]) are indicated on the thermogram.

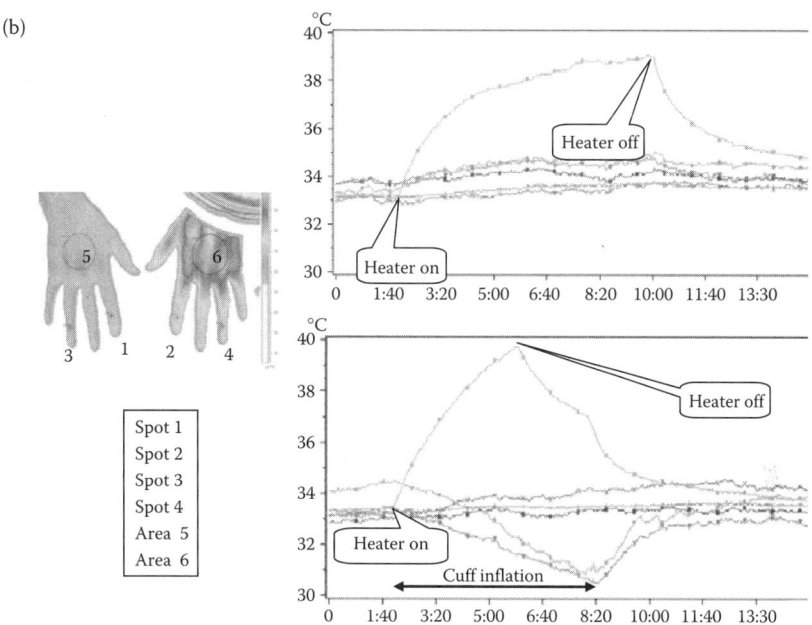

FIGURE 27.2 (Continued.)

pressure cuff is presented. The time course of the temperature curves shown in the upper panel of Figure 27.2b demonstrates a gradual increase in skin temperature, eventually stabilizing just below 39°C. The finger skin temperature on the heated hand only showed a minor increase during the heating period. When the lamp was switched off the accumulated heat was rapidly dissipated and skin temperature of the heated area returned to the preheating level. In the lower panel the experiment was repeated, but as the heater was turned on, a pressure cuff placed around the upper arm was inflated to above systolic pressure to totally cut off blood supply to the arm. As can be seen, the rate of rise of skin temperature over the heated skin area was quite rapid, soon reaching a level deemed to be uncomfortably hot, after which the heater was turned off (at this stage the pressure cuff was still inflated). During the heating period finger skin temperature on the same hand steadily decreased (i.e., the fingers were passively cooling due to lack of circulation). After the heater was turned off the temperature of the back of the left hand also began to decrease indicating a passive cooling. When the pressure cuff was reopened and blood flow to the arm reestablished, the rate of cooling on the back of the hand increased (active cooling) and the skin temperature of the cooled fingers also rapidly returned to normal.

While the same result could have been gained by using other methods to measure skin temperature, such as thermocouples, the visual effect gained by using IR-thermography provides much more information than a single-point measurement. Various points or areas of interest can be investigated during and after the experimental procedures. Modern digital image processing software provides endless possibilities, especially with systems allowing the recording of sequential IR-images. Today modern fire-wire technology permits one to record IR-images at very high frequencies (100 Hz and greater).

27.6.3 Median Nerve Block in the Hand (Example 27.3)

The nervous supply to the hand is via three main nerves: radial, ulnar, and median nerve. The approximate distribution of the sensory innervation by these nerves is shown in Figure 27.3a. With a sudden removal (or disruption) of the sympathetic discharge to one of the main nerves, a maximal vasodilatation of blood vessels in the area supplied by the nerve is observed. Such a vasodilatation will result in a significant increase in skin blood flow to that area and therefore in a rise in skin temperature. The IR-thermogram in Figure 27.3b shows such a response. The subject is a 40-year-old female suffering from excessive sweating in the palms of her hands, a condition known as hyperhidrosis palmaris. Excessive sweating causes cooling of the skin surface. The blue color in Figure 27.3b represents areas of excessive sweating as well as areas of lowest skin temperature. Hyperhidrosis palmaris is treated by subcutaneous injections of botulinum toxin. The skin in the palm of the hand is very sensitive and anesthesia is therefore required. A very effective way to provide adequate anesthesia is the median nerve block. At the level of the wrist, a local anesthetic is injected around the median nerve and blocks the nervous activity in the median nerve. The resulting increase in skin temperature on the palmar side of the left hand after such an injection is clearly seen in Figure 27.3b. One sees that part of the thumb and half of the fourth finger show no increase in temperature, closely matching the predicted area of distribution for this nerve in Figure 27.3a. Although a median nerve block was applied to the right hand, neither vasodilatation nor a change in skin temperature was seen. The botulinum toxin injections on this side were painful. The placement of the anesthetic was therefore incorrect, and as a result, normal nervous activity in the right hand was observed. In Figure 27.3c,d, the thermograms show the hands of a 36-year-old female patient. Her left wrist (middle of the red circle) was punctured with a sharp object, resulting in partial nerve damage. The strong vasodilatory response, due to the nerve damage, results in an increased skin temperature as shown in Figure 27.3d.

The diagnosis of acute nerve damage can be a challenge for a surgeon. In the acute situation, pain makes a proper physical examination often impossible. To evaluate the extent of the nerve injury, cooperation of the patient is necessary and the use of local anesthesia can mask the extent of the injury. IR-thermography proves to be a helpful, noninvasive diagnostic tool by visualizing changes in skin temperature and, indirectly blood flow to the skin, due to the nerve injury.

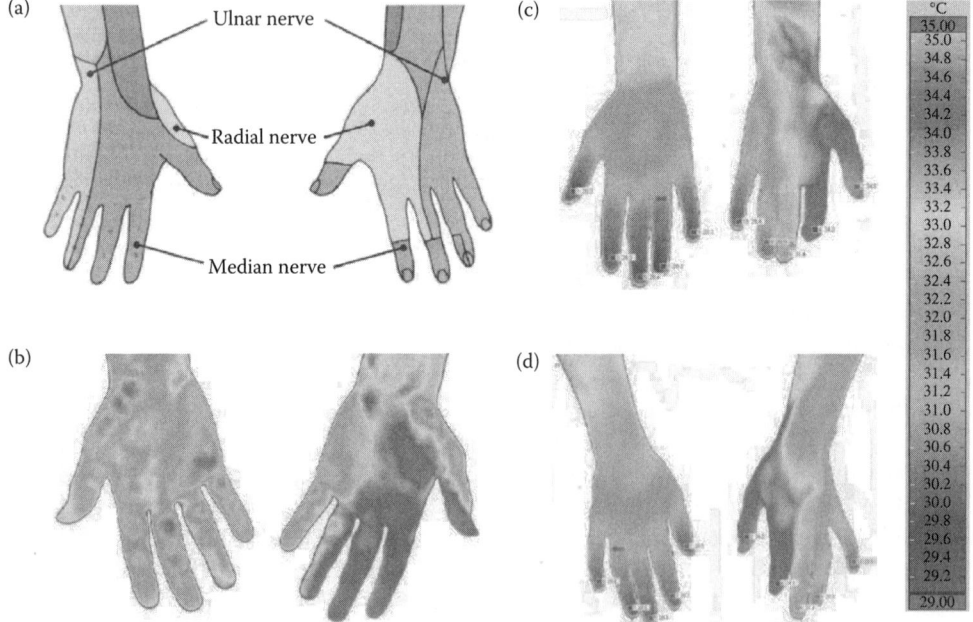

FIGURE 27.3 (a) The distribution of cutaneous nerves to the hand. (b) IR-thermogram of a 40-year-old female patient following a successful nerve block of the left median nerve. (c) and (d) IR-thermograms of the hands of a 36-year-old female patient whose left wrist (middle of the red circle) was punctured with a sharp object resulting in partial nerve damage (motor and sensory loss). The strong vasodilatory response resulting from partially severed nerves can be easily seen.

27.6.4 IR-Thermography and Laser Doppler Mapping of Skin Blood Flow (Example 27.4)

As mentioned in the introduction above, one of the drawbacks of using IR-thermography to indirectly indicate changes in skin blood flow is being able to decide, for example, if an increase in skin temperature is due to a parallel increase in skin blood flow. One way to verify whether observed skin temperature changes are related to changes in skin blood flow is to combine IR-thermography with a more direct measurement technique of skin blood flow. Laser Doppler can ascertain the direction of skin blood flow but these measurements are restricted to small surfaces and blood flow is not quantified but reported as changes in Doppler units or volts [45]. With IR-thermography rapid changes in skin temperature over a large area can be easily measured. Laser-Doppler mapping involves a scanning technique using a lower power laser beam in a raster pattern and requires time to complete a scan (up to minutes depending on the size of the scanned area). During the time it takes to complete a scan it is possible that the skin blood flow has changed in the skin area examined at the start compared to the skin area being examined at the end of each scan. This is most likely to happen in dynamic situations where skin blood flow is rapidly changing. Despite this draw back, the use of IR-thermography and laser Doppler mapping can provide a complimentary investigative view of this dynamic process.

In Figure 27.4, both IR-thermography and scanning laser Doppler mapping have been simultaneously used to examine a healthy 44-year-old female subject. In this experiment the subject was submitted to a 20 min heating of the right side of the abdomen using a water-filtered IR-A irradiation lamp (see Section 27.6.1). During the period of heating, the left side of the abdomen was covered with a drape to prevent this side of the body from being heated. At predetermined intervals prior to, during, and after the heating period both IR-thermal images and laser Doppler mapping images were recorded, the latter with a MoorLDI™ laser Doppler imager (LDI-1), Moor Instruments, England. As can be seen in Figure 27.5, the wIRA heating lamp causes a large increase in skin temperature on the irradiated side of the abdomen. After the end of the heating period, the temperature of the heated area gradually decreases. These changes nicely correspond with the laser Doppler mapping images. A semi quantitative value of blood flow (perfusion units) for each LDI image was also calculated (right panels in Figure 27.5). Each blood flow profile corresponds well with their respective temperature profiles.

27.6.5 Use of Dynamic IR-Thermography to Highlight Perforating Vessels (Example 27.5)

The procedure of dynamic thermography involves promoting changes in skin blood flow by local heating or cooling. In the example shown in Figure 27.5, a mild cooling (2 min period of fan cooling) of the skin overlying the abdominal area of a 36-year-old female patient prior to undergoing breast reconstruction surgery was performed in order to highlight perforating blood vessels [41]. These blood vessels originate in deeper lying tissue and course their way toward the skin surface, although they may not necessarily reach the skin surface. By invoking a local cooling, a temporary vasoconstrictor response is initiated in skin blood vessels. Blood flow in the perforating blood vessels is little affected and following the end of the cooling period they rapidly contribute to the skin rewarming. During the rewarming process the localization of the "hot-spots" caused by these perforating vessels becomes more diffuse as heat from them spreads into neighboring tissue. This technique allows one to more easily identify so-called perforator vessels of the medial and lateral branches of the deep inferior epigastric artery, one or more of which will be selected for reconnection to the internal mammary artery (the usual recipient vessel) during reconstruction of a new breast from this abdominal tissue.

27.6.6 Reperfusion of Transplanted Tissue (Example 27.6)

With the development of microvascular surgery, it has become possible to connect (anastomose) blood vessels with a diameter as small as 0.5 mm to each other. Transplantation of tissue from one place

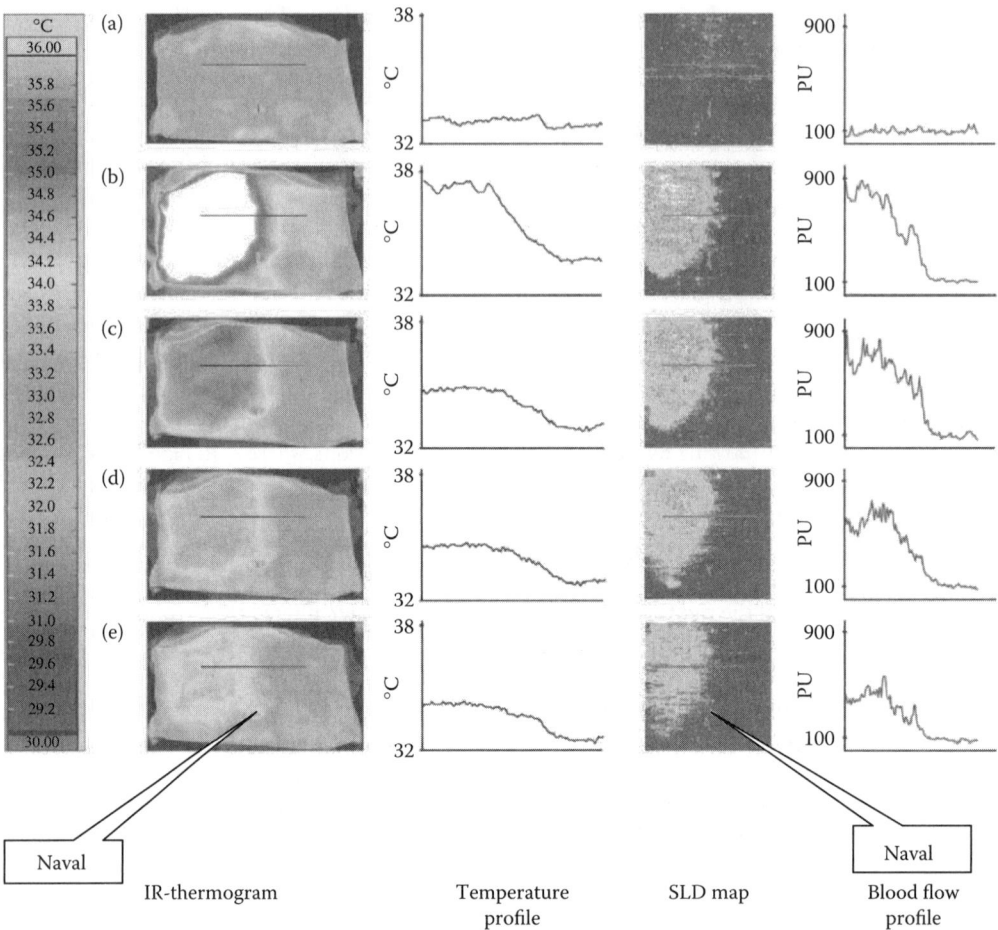

FIGURE 27.4 IR-thermograms, temperature profiles, scanning laser doppler (SLD) scans, and blood flow profiles (perfusion units PU) of the abdominal area of a 44-year-old healthy female subject before (a), immediately after (b), and 5 min (c), 10 min (d), and 20 min (e) after a 20 min heating of the right side of the abdomen with a water-filtered IR-A irradiation lamp. In IR-thermogram (b) the white color indicates skin temperatures greater than 36°C.

to another place in the same patient (autologous transplantation) or from one individual to another (allologous transplantation) has become daily practice in medicine. The technique requires high surgical skills. During the operation, blood supply to the transplant is completely severed and the blood vessels to the transplant are later connected to recipient vessels. These recipient blood vessels will supply blood to the transplant at the new site. Kidney transplantation is a well-known example of allologous transplantation. Here, a patient with a nonfunctional kidney receives a donor kidney to provide normal renal function. Nowadays, autologous tissue transplantation is an integrated part in trauma surgery and cancer surgery. The successful reperfusion of the transplant is obviously essential for its survival. A nonsuccessful operation causes psychological stress for the patient and is indeed an inefficient use of resources stress. IR-thermography provides an ideal noninvasive and rapid method for monitoring the reperfusion status of transplanted tissue.

Autologous breast reconstruction is a critical part of the overall care plan for patients faced with a diagnosis of breast cancer and a plan that includes removal of the breast. The deep inferior epigastric perforator (DIEP) flap is the state of the art in autologous breast reconstruction today. The technique

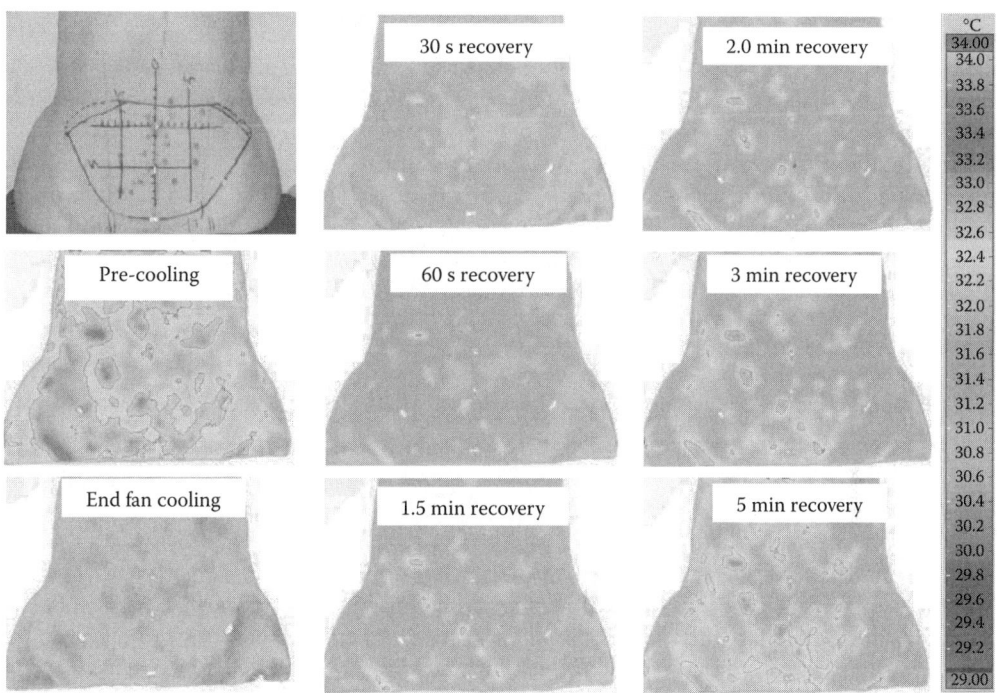

FIGURE 27.5 Abdominal cooling in a 32-year-old female patient prior to breast reconstruction surgery. In this procedure skin and fat tissue from the abdominal area was used to reconstruct a new breast. The localization of suitable perforating vessels for reconnection to the mammary artery is an important part of the surgical procedure. In this sequence of thermograms the patient was first subjected to a mild cooling of the abdominal skin (2 min fan cooling). IR-thermograms of the skin over the entire abdominal area were taken prior to, immediately after, and at various time intervals during the recovery period following the cooling period. To help highlight the perforating vessels, an outline function has been employed in which all skin areas having a temperature greater than 32.5°C are enclosed in solid lines.

uses skin and fatty tissue from the lower abdomen for reconstruction of a new breast (Figure 27.6). The fatty tissue and skin on the lower abdomen are supplied by many blood vessels. By using this tissue as a DIEP flap in autologous breast reconstruction, the blood supply to this tissue is reduced to one single artery and veins, each with a diameter of 1.0–1.5 mm. A critical period during the operative procedure is the connection (anastomosing) of the flap to the recipient vessels. The blood vessels of the DIEP flap are anastomosed to the internal mammary vessels to provide blood supply to the flap. Blood circulation to the newly reconstructed breast is dependent on the viability of the microvascular anastomosis. The series of IR-thermograms shown in Figure 27.6 were taken at various time intervals after reestablishing the blood supply to the flap in a patient undergoing autologous breast reconstruction with a DIEP flap.

During the operation, there is a period (ca. 50 min) with no blood supply to the dissected flap, and as a result, it cools down. The rate and pattern of rewarming of the flap after anastomoses to the recipient vessels provides the surgeon with important information on the blood circulation in the transplanted flap. With a successful and adequate outcome of the anastomosis, the rewarming response was found to be rapid and well distributed (Figure 27.6). A poor rewarming response often made an extra venous anastomosis necessary to improve venous drainage (the most common problem). In such cases, IR-thermography provides an excellent method to quickly verify improvement in the blood flow status in the flap. In addition, in the days following surgery, examination of the skin temperatures using IR-thermography of the newly reconstructed breast was found to be a quick and easy way to monitor its

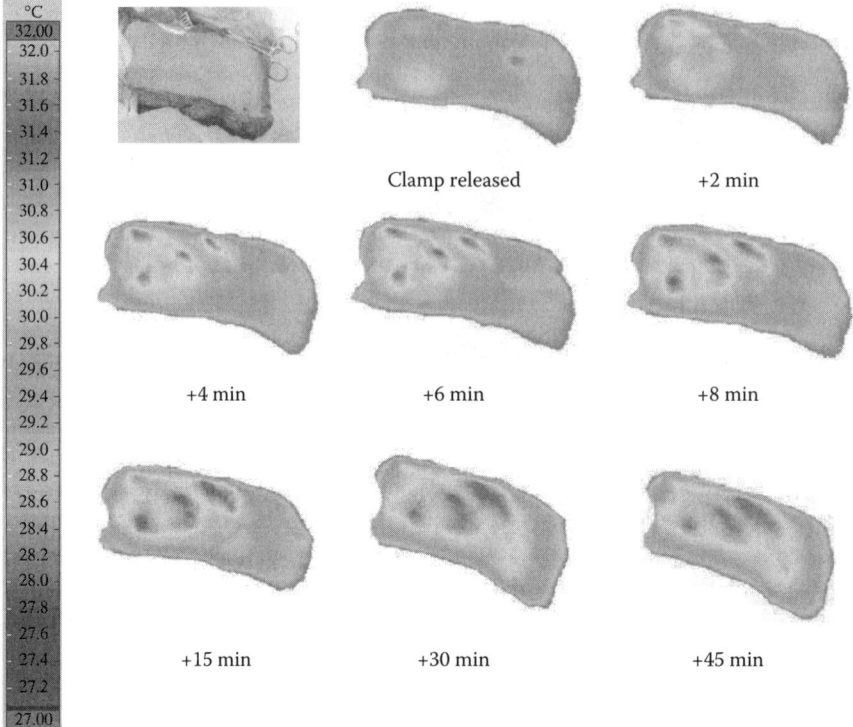

FIGURE 27.6 IR thermal images of an abdominal skin flap during breast reconstruction surgery. The sequence of IR-thermal images demonstrates the return of heat to the excised skin flap following reestablishing its blood supply (anastomizing of a mammary artery and vein to a single branch of the deep inferior epigastric artery and a concomitant vein). Prior to this procedure the excised skin flap had been without a blood supply for about 50 min and consequently cooled down. The photograph in the upper left panel shows the skin flap in position on the chest wall prior to being shaped into a new breast.

blood flow status. The peripheral areas of the new breast can suffer from diminished blood circulation. Improvement in blood circulation could be seen during post surgery.

27.6.7 Sports Medicine Injury (Example 27.7)

Thermal images of an injury sustained by an 18-year-old American football player after a helmet impacted the superior portion of his right shoulder. X-ray and MRI immediately post game showed no structural damage. IR images were taken 12 h post-injury in a controlled environment (22°C, 30% rh, after 20 min equilibration). Upon examination, the athlete was unable to lift his right arm above shoulder level. Note the disruption in the thermal pattern in the right side torso view (T4 spinal region on left side of image) and the very cold temperatures and pattern extending down the left arm. After 3 weeks of rehabilitation, the weakness experienced in the shoulder and arm was resolved. IR imaging confirmed a return to normal symmetrical thermal pattern in the back torso and warmer arm temperatures.

27.6.8 Conclusions

As pointed out in the introduction to this section the main objective of this chapter is to try and persuade those who are not familiar with IR-thermography that this technology can provide objective data, which makes clinical sense. The reader has to be aware that the examples presented above only represent a tiny fraction of the possibilities that this technology provides. It is important to realize that an IR-thermal image of a skin area under examination will more often not provide the examiner with a satisfactory result. It is important to keep in mind that blood flow is a very dynamic event and in many situations useful clinical information can only be obtained by manipulating skin blood flow, for example by local cooling. Thus, the need to have a basic understanding of the physiological mechanisms behind the control of skin blood flow cannot be overemphasized. One also has to realize that this technology should be thought of as an aid to making a clinical diagnosis and in many cases should, if possible, be combined with other complementary techniques. For example, IR-thermography does not have the ability to pinpoint the location of a tumor in the breast. Consequently, IR-thermography's role is in addition to mammography, ultrasound and physical examination, not in lieu of. IR-thermography does not replace mammography and mammography does not replace IR-thermography, the tests complement each other.

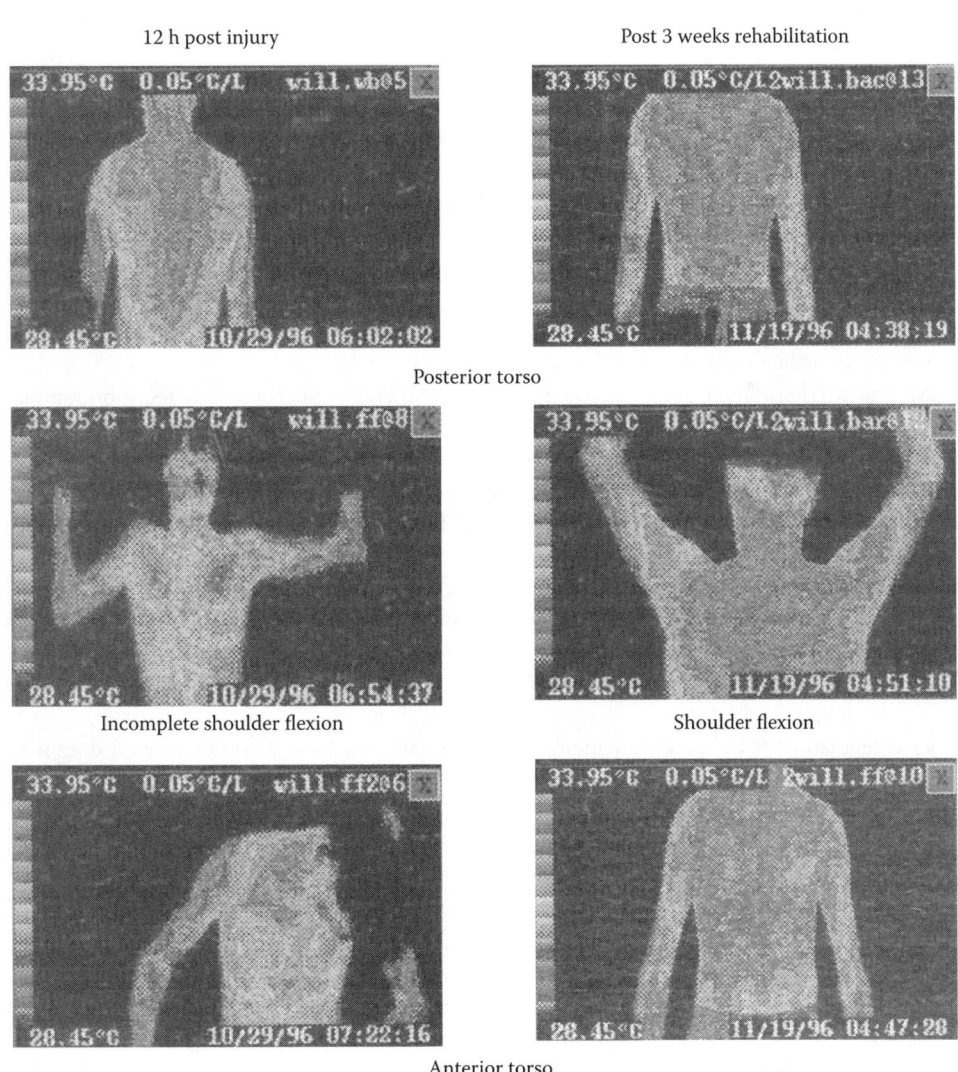

FIGURE 27.7 An American football player who suffered a helmet impact to the right shoulder (left side of image). The athlete was unable to flex his arm above shoulder level. Note the asymmetrical torso pattern in the posterior torso.

Acknowledgments

Examples of IR images from patients and volunteers (Figures 27.1, 27.2b, 27.3 through 27.7) from the Department of Medical Physiology, Faculty of Medicine, University of Tromsø, Norway and the Department of Clinical Physiology, Hillerød Hospital, Hillerød, Denmark. The IR images in these examples were taken using two different IR-cameras: A Nikon Laird S270 cooled camera and a FLIR ThermaCAM® PM695 uncooled bolometer. The respective image analysis software used was ThermaCAM researcher ver. 2.1 and PicWin-IRIS (EBS Systemtechnik GmbH, Munich, Germany). The studies described in Examples 27.1 and 27.2 were carried out at the Department of Clinical Physiology, Hillerød Hospital, Hillerød, Denmark in collaboration with consultant Dr. Stig Pors Nielsen. The assistance of Master student Lise Bøe Setså in the studies described in Examples 27.5 and 27.6 is also acknowledged. Examples of IR images (Figures 27.2a and 27.7) come from the Thermal Lab, Auburn University, Alabama, United States, utilizing a Computerized Thermal Imager 2000. We would like to acknowledge the assistance of John Eric Smith and Estevam Strecker in these projects.

References

1. Jones B.F. and Plassmann P. Digital infrared thermal imaging of human skin. *IEEE Eng. Med. Biol.* 21, 41–48, 2002.
2. Otsuka K., Okada S., Hassan M., and Togawa T. Imaging of skin thermal properties with estimation of ambient radiation temperature. *IEEE Eng. Med. Biol.* 21, 65–71, 2002.
3. Head J.F. and Elliott R.L. Infrared imaging: Making progress in fulfilling its medical promise. *IEEE Eng. Med. Biol.* 21, 80–85, 2002.
4. Park J.Y., Kim S.D., Kim S.H., Lim D.J., and Cho T.H. The role of thermography in clinical practice: Review of the literature. *Thermol. Int.* 13, 77–78, 2003.
5. Ammer K. Thermology 2003—A computer-assisted literature survey with a focus on nonmedical applications of thermal imaging. *Thermol. Int.* 14, 5–36, 2004.
6. Abernathy M. and Abernathy T.B. *International Bibliography of Medical Thermology.* Vol. 2, Washington, DC, American College of Thermology, Georgetown University Medical Center, 1987.
7. Pascoe D.D., Bellinger T.A., and McCluskey B.S. Clothing and exercise II: Influence of clothing during exercise/work in environmental extremes. *Sports Med.* 18, 94–108, 1994.
8. Flesch, U. Physics of skin-surface temperature. In *Thermology Methods.* Engel J.M., Flesch U., and Stüttgen G. (eds), translated by Biederman–Thorson M.A. Federal Republic of Germany Weinheim, pp. 21–37, 1985.
9. Pennes H.H. Analysis of tissue and arterial blood temperatures in resting human forearm. *J. Appl. Physiol.* 1, 93–102, 1948.
10. Charkoudian N. Skin blood flow in adult thermoregulation: How it works, when it does not, and why. *Mayo Clin. Proc.* 78, 603–612, 2003.
11. Greenfield A.D.M. The circulation through the skin. In *Handbook of Physiology—Circulation.* Hamilton W.P. (eds), Washington DC, American Physiological Society, Sec. 3, Vol. 2 (Chapter 39), pp. 1325–1351, 1963.
12. Johnson J.M., Brenglemann G.L., Hales J.R.S., Vanhoutte M., and Wenger C.B. Regulation of the cutaneous circulation. *Fed. Proc.* 45, 2841–2850, 1986.
13. Johnson J.M. and Proppe D.W. Cardiovascular adjustments to heat stress. In *Handbook of Physiology—Environmental Physiology.* Fregly M.J. and Blatteis C.M. (eds), Oxford, Oxford University Press/ American Physiological Society, pp. 215–243, 1996.
14. Rowell L.B. Human cardiovascular adjustments to exercise and thermal stress. *Physiol. Rev.* 54, 75–159, 1974.
15. Rowell L.B. Cardiovascular adjustments in thermal stress. In *Handbook of Physiology. Section 2 Cardiovascular System, Vol. 3 Peripheral Circulation and Organ Flow*, J.T. Shepard and F.M. Abboud (eds), Bethesda, MD: American Physiological Society, pp. 967–1024, 1983.

16. Rowell L.B. *Human Circulation: Regulation during Physiological Stress.* New York: Oxford University Press, 1986.
17. Sawka M.N. and Wenger C.B. Physiological responses to acute exercise–heat stress. In *Human Performance Physiology and Environmental Medicine at Terrestrial Extremes.* Pandolf K.B., Sawka M.N., and Gonzales R.R. (eds), Indianapolis, IN: Benchmark Press, pp. 97–151, 1988.
18. Johnson J.M. Circulation to the skin. In *Textbook of Physiology.* Patton H.D., Fuchs A.F., Hille B., Scher A.M., and Steiner R. (eds), Philadelphia: W.B. Saunders Co., Vol. 2 (Chapter 45), 1989.
19. Johnson J.M. Exercise and the cutaneous circulation. *Exercise Sports Sci. Rev.* 20, 59–97, 1992.
20. Garrison F.H. *Contributions to the History of Medicine.* New York: Hafner Publishing Co., Inc., p. 311, 1966.
21. Kirsh K.A. Physiology of skin-surface temperature. In *Thermology Methods.* Engel J.M., Flesch U., and Stüttgen G. (eds), translated by Biederman–Thorson M.A., Federal Republic of Germany/ Weinheim, pp. 1–9, 1985.
22. Roberts M.P., Wenger C.B., Stölwik J.A.J., and Nadel E.R. Skin blood flow and sweating changes following exercise training and heat acclimation. *J. Appl. Physiol.* 43, 133–137, 1977.
23. Stephenson L.A. and Kolka M.A. Menstrual cycle phase and time of day alter reference signal controlling arm blood flow and sweating. *Am. J. Physiol.* 249, R186–R192, 1985.
24. Aoki K., Stephens D.P., and Johnson J.M. Diurnal variations in cutaneous vasodilator and vasoconstrictor systems during heat stress. *Am. J. Physiol. Regul. Integr. Comp. Physiol.* 281, R591–R595, 2001.
25. Rodie I.C., Shepard J.T., and Whelan R.F. Evidence from venous oxygen saturation that the increase in arm blood flow during body heating is confined to the skin *J. Physiol.* 134, 444–450, 1956.
26. Gaskell P. Are there sympathetic vasodilator nerves in the vessels of the hands? *J. Physiol.* 131, 647–656, 1956.
27. Fox R.H. and Edholm O.G. Nervous control of the cutaneous circulation. *J. Appl. Physiol.* 57, 1688–1695, 1984.
28. Ring E.E.J. Cold stress testing in the hand. In *The Thermal Image in Medicine and Biology.* Ammer K. and Ring E.E.J. (eds), Wein: Uhlen-Verlag, pp. 237–240, 1995.
29. Pascoe D., Purohit R., Shanley L.A., and Herrick R.T. Pre and post operative thermographic evaluations of CTS. In *The Thermal Image in Medicine and Biology.* Ammer K. and Ring E.E.J. (eds), Wein: Uhlen-Verlag, pp. 188–190, 1995.
30. Faithfull N.S., Reinhold P.R., van den Berg A.P., van Roon G.C., Van der Zee J., and Wike-Hooley J.L. Cardiovascular challenges during whole body hyperthermia treatment of advanced malignancy. *Eur. J. Appl. Physiol.* 53, 274–281, 1984.
31. Finberg J.P.M., Katz M., Gazit H., and Berlyne G.M. Plasma rennin activity after acute heat exposure in non-acclimatized and naturally acclimatized man. *J. Appl. Physiol.* 36, 519–523, 1974.
32. Carlsen A., Gustafson A., and Werko L. Hemodynamic influence of warm and dry environment in man with and without rheumatic heart disease. *Acta Med. Scand.* 169, 411–417, 1961.
33. Damato A.N., Lau S.H., Stein E., Haft J.I., Kosowsky B., and Cohen S.J. Cardiovascular response to acute thermal stress (hot dry environment) in unacclimatized normal subjects. *Am. Heart J.* 76, 769–774, 1968.
34. Sancetta S.M., Kramer J., and Husni E. The effects of "dry" heat on the circulation of man. I. General hemodynamics. *Am. Heart J.* 56, 212–221, 1958.
35. Crandall C.G., Johnson J.M., Kosiba W.A., and Kellogg D.L. Jr. Baroreceptor control of the cutaneous active vasodilator system. *J. Appl. Physiol.* 81, 2192–2198, 1996.
36. Kellogg D.L. Jr, Johnson J.M., and Kosiba, W.A. Baroreflex control of the cutaneous active vasodilator system in humans. *Cir. Res.* 66, 1420–1426, 1990.
37. Chato J.C. A view of the history of heat transfer in bioengineering. In *Advances in Heat Transfer.* Cho Y.J. (eds), Boston: Academic Press, Inc./Harcourt Brace Jovanovich Publishers, Vol. 22, pp. 1–19, May 1981.

38. Chen M.M. and Holmes K.R. Microvascular contributions in tissue heat transfer. In *Thermal Characteristics of Tumors: Applications in Detection and Treatment*. Jain R.K. and Guillino P.M. (eds), *Ann. N.Y. Acad. Sci.* 335, 137, 1980.

39. Baish J.W. Microvascular heat transfer. In *The Biomedical Engineering Handbook*. Bronzino J.D. (eds), Boca Raton, FL: CRC Press/IEEE Press, Vol. 2, 98, pp. 1–14, 2000.

40. Hille B. Membranes and ions: Introduction to physiology of excitable cells. In *Textbook of Physiology*. Patton H.D., Fuchs A.F., Hille B., Scher A.M., and Steiner R. (eds), Philadelphia: W.B. Saunders Co., pp. 2–4, 1989.

41. Taylor G.I. and Tempest M.N. (eds), *Michael Salmon: Arteries of the Skin*. London: Churchill Livingstone, 1988.

42. He S. and Walls A.F. Human mast cell trypase: A stimulus of microvascular leakage and mast cell activation. *Eur. J. Pharmacol.* 328, 89–97, 1997.

43. Kalmolz L.P., Haslik A.H., Donner A., Winter W., Meissl G., and Frey M. Indocyanine green video angiographics help identify burns requiring operating. *Burns* 29, 785–791, 2003.

44. Flock S.T. and Jacques S.L. Thermal damage of blood vessels in a rat skin-flap window chamber using indocyanine green and pulsated alexandrite laser: A feasibility study. *Lasers Med. Sci.* 8, 185–196, 1993.

45. Ryan T.J., Jolles B., and Holti G. *Methods in Microcirculation Studies*. London: HK Lewis and Co., Ltd, 1972.

46. Olsen B.W. How many sites are necessary to estimate a mean skin temperature? In *Thermal Physiology*. Hales J.R.S. (eds), New York, Raven Press, pp. 33–38, 1984.

28

Quantitative Active Dynamic Thermal IR-Imaging and Thermal Tomography in Medical Diagnostics

Antoni
Nowakowski
Gdansk University of
Technology

28.1 Introduction

Static infrared (IR) thermal imaging has a number of attractive properties for its practical applications in industry and medicine. The technique is noninvasive and harmless as there is no direct contact of the diagnostic tool to an object under test, the data acquisition is simple and the equipment is transportable and well adapted to mass screening applications. There are also some fundamental limitations concerning this technique. Only processes characterized by changes in temperature distribution on external surfaces directly accessible by an IR-camera can be observed. The absolute value of temperature measurement is usually not very accurate due to generally limited knowledge of the emission coefficient. Many harmful processes are not inducting any changes in surface temperature, for example, in industrial applications material corrosion or cracks are usually not visible in IR thermographs, in medicine in mammography inspection a cyst may mask cancer, and so on. For such cases active dynamic thermal imaging methods with sources of external excitations are helpful. Therefore, the nondestructive evaluation (NDE) of materials using active dynamic thermal IR-imaging is extensively studied; see, for example, proceedings of QIRT [1]. The method is already well developed in some of industrial applications but in medicine this technique is almost unknown.

Active dynamic thermal (ADT) IR-imaging, known in industry either as *infrared-nondestructive testing* (IR-NDT), or as thermographic nondestructive testing (TNDT or just NDT), is under intensive development during at least the past 25 years [1,2]. The concept of material testing by active thermography is based on delivery of external energy to a specimen and observation of the thermal response. In ADT imaging only thermal transients are studied. Such approach allows visualization of material subsurface abnormalities or failures and has already gained high recognition in technical applications [1,2]. In medicine it was applied probably for the first time also around 25 years ago [3,4]. Microwave excitation was applied to evidence breast cancer. Unfortunately, after early experiments the research was suspended, probably due to poor control of microwave energy dissipation. Again some proposals to use ADT in medicine have been published at the end of the last years of the twentieth century [5–7].

The visualization of affected regions needs some extra efforts therefore the role and practical importance of the use of synthetic pictures in ADT for medical applications should be underlined [8–10]. In this case equivalent thermal model parameters are defined and calculated for objective quantitative data visualization and evaluation.

Potential role of medical applications of ADT is clearly visible from experiments on phantoms, and *in vivo* on animals as well as in clinical applications [11,12].

28.1.1 Thermal Tomography

Another concept based on ADT is *thermal tomography* (TT). Vavilow et al. [13–15] dealing with IR-NDTs, proposed this term almost 25 years ago. Even today, the concept is not new this modality may be regarded as being still at the early development stage in technical applications, especially taking into account the limited number of practical applications published up to now. The first proposals to apply the concept of thermal tomography in medicine are just under intensive development in the Department of Biomedical Engineering TUG [16–18]. The main differences comparing TT to simple ADT arise due to necessity of advanced reconstruction procedures applied for determination of internal structure of tested objects.

Tomography is known in medical diagnostics as the most advanced technology for visualization of tested object internal structures. X-rays—CT (computed tomography), NMR—MRI (nuclear magnetic resonance imaging), US—ultrasound imaging, SPECT (single-photon emission computed tomography), PET (positron-emission tomography) are the modalities of already established position in medical diagnostics. There are three additional tomography modalities, still in the phase of intensive research and development—optical tomography (OT), electroimpedance tomography (EIT), and TT. Here we concentrate our notice on ADT and TT. The aim of this chapter is discussion of potential applications of both modalities in medical diagnostics and analysis of existing limitations.

General concept of tomography requires collection of data received in the so-called projections—measurements performed for a specific direction of applied excitation; data from all projections form a scan. Having a model of a tested object the inverse problem is solved showing internal structure of the object. In the oldest tomographic modality—CT—the measurement procedure requires irradiation of a tested object from different directions (projections), all possible projections giving one scan. Then, using a realistic model of a tested object, a reconstruction procedure based on solving the inverse problem allows visualization of external structure of the object. In early systems, a 2D picture of internal organs was shown; nowadays more complex acquisition systems allow visualization of 3D cases. More or less similar procedures are applied in all other tomography modalities, including TT, OT, and EIT. The main advantages of TT, OT, and EIT technologies are: fully safe interaction with tested objects (organisms) and relatively low cost of instrumentation.

The concept and problems of validity in medical diagnostics of ADT imaging as well as of TT are here discussed. In both cases practically the same instrumentation is applied and only the data treatment and object reconstruction differs. Also, the sources of errors influencing quality of measurements and limiting accuracy of reconstruction data are the same. Main limitations are due to the necessity of using proper thermal models of living tissues, which are influenced by physiological processes from one side and are not very accurate due to hardly controlled experiment conditions from the other side.

The main element allowing quantitative evaluation of tested objects is the use of realistic thermal equivalent models. The measurement procedure requires use of heat sources, which should be applied to the object under test (OUT). Thermal response at the surface of OUT to external excitation is recorded using IR-camera. Usually the natural recovery to initial conditions gives reliable data for further analysis. The dynamic response recorded as a series of IR pictures allows reconstruction of properties of the OUT equivalent thermal model. Either thermal properties of the model elements (for defined structure of OUT) or the internal structure (for known material thermal properties) may be determined and recognized. The main problem is correlation of thermal and physiological properties of living tissues, which may strongly differ for *ex vivo* and *in vivo* data. Practical measurement results from phantoms and *in vivo* animal experiments as well as from clinical applications of ADT performed in the Department of Biomedical Engineering Gdansk University of Technology (TUG), Poland and in co-operating clinics of the Medical University of Gdansk are taken into account for illustration of this chapter. The studies in this field are concentrated on applications of burns, skin transplants, cancer visualization, and open-heart surgery, evaluation and diagnostics [19–26].

In the following subchapters all elements of the ADT and TT procedures are described. First, thermal tissue properties are defined. Then basic elements of thermal model construction are described. Following is description of the experiment of active dynamic thermography based on OUT excitation (pulse) and IR recording. Finally the procedures of model identification are described based on phantom and *in vivo* experiments. Some clinical applications illustrate practical value of the described modalities.

28.2 Thermal Properties of Biological Tissues

What is the basic difference between IR-thermography (IRT) and ADT and TT?

In IRT, main information is the absolute value of temperature, T, and distribution of thermal fields, $T(x,y)$. Therefore, regions of high temperature (hot spots) or low temperature (cold spots) are determined giving usually data of important diagnostic value. Unfortunately the accuracy of temperature measurements is limited. It is mainly due to limited accuracy of IR-cameras; due to limited knowledge of the emission coefficient, as individual features of living tissues may be strongly diversified; finally due to hardly controlled conditions of the environment, what may strongly influence temperature distribution at the surface and its absolute values. Additionally surface temperature does not always properly reflect complicated processes, which may exist underneath or in the tissue bulk or which may be masked by fat or other biological structures.

In ADT and TT basic thermal properties of tissues are quantitatively determined; the absolute value of temperature practically is not interesting. Only thermal flows are important. We ask the question—how fast are thermal processes? In ADT, specific equivalent parameters are defined and visualized. In TT directly either spatial distribution of thermal conductivity is of major importance or for known tissue properties the geometry of the structure is determined.

Basic thermal properties (Figures of Merit) of materials and tissues important in ADT and in TT are following:

- k—Thermal conductivity—(W m^{-1} K^{-1}), it describes ability of a material (tissue) to conduct heat in the steady-state conditions

- c_p—Specific heat—($J \; kg^{-1} \; K^{-1}$), describes ability of a material to store the heat energy. It is defined by the amount of heat energy necessary to raise the temperature of a unit mass by 1 K
- ρ—Density of material—($kg \; m^{-3}$)
- ρc_p—Volumetric specific heat—($J \; m^{-3} \; K^{-1}$)
- α—Thermal diffusivity—($m^2 \; s^{-1}$); is defined as

$$\alpha = \frac{k}{\rho \cdot c_p} \qquad (28.1)$$

Volumetric specific heat and thermal conductivity are responsible for thermal transients described by the equation

$$\frac{\partial T}{\partial t} = \alpha \nabla^2 T \qquad (28.2)$$

For one-directional heat flow (what describes the case of infinite plate structures composed of uniform layers and uniformly excited at the surface) this may be rewritten in the form:

$$\frac{\partial T}{\partial t} = \frac{k}{\rho \cdot c_p} \cdot \frac{\partial^2 T}{\partial x^2} \qquad (28.3)$$

Thermal diffusivity describes heat flow and is equivalent to the reciprocal of the time constant τ describing the electrical *RC* circuit:

$$\alpha = \frac{k}{\rho \cdot c_p} \leftrightarrow \frac{1}{\tau} = \frac{1}{RC} \qquad (28.4)$$

Based on this analogy, materials are frequently described by equivalent thermal model composed of thermal resistivity R_{th} and thermal capacity C_{th}, which are responsible for the value of the thermal time constant, τ_{th},

$$\tau_{th} = R_{th} C_{th} \qquad (28.5)$$

Those are the most frequently used equivalent parameters. Determination of such parameters is easy based on measurements of thermal transients and using fitting procedures for determination of the applied model parameters.

Additionally one may define thermal inertia as $k \rho c_p$.

Useful may be also introducing the definition of thermal effusivity β, defined as the root-square of the thermal inertia—($J \; m^{-2} \; K^{-1} \; s^{-1/2}$) or ($W \; s^{1/2} \; m^{-2} \; K^{-1}$).

$$\beta^2 = k \cdot \rho \cdot c_p \qquad (28.6)$$

Importance of IRT and ADT/TT in medical diagnostics is complementary. Regions of abnormal vascularization are detected in IRT as *hot spots* in the cases of intensive metabolic processes or as *cold spots* for regions of affected vascularization or necrosis. The same places may represent higher or lower thermal conductivity, but this is not a rule. Thermal properties of tissues may differ significantly depending on the vascularization, physical structure, water content, and so on. Knowledge of thermal properties and geometry of tested objects may be used in medical diagnostics if correlation of thermal properties and specific physiological features are known. The character of the data allowing objective quantitative description of tissues or organs is the most important.

The main advantage of thermal tissue parameter characterization comparing to absolute temperature measurements is relatively low dependence on external conditions, for example, ambient temperature, what usually is of great importance in IRT. The main disadvantage is still limited knowledge of thermal tissue properties and very complicated structure of biological organs. Although the first results of thermal tissue properties have been published at the end of the nineteenth century, the main data, still broadly cited, were collected around 30 years ago [27–30]. Unfortunately, literature data of thermal tissue properties should be treated as not very reliable, because measurement conditions are not always known [31], *in vivo* and *ex vivo* data are mixed, and so on. Table 28.1 illustrates this problem. Detailed description of measurement methods of biological tissue thermal parameters is given in References 18, 31, and 32.

In Table 28.2 basic thermal tissue properties—mean values of data given by different studies and for different tissues taken *in vitro* at 37°C—are collected [18].

It has to be underlined that thermal tissue properties are temperature dependent (typically around 0.2–1%/°C). In most of ADT and TT measurements this effect may be neglected as being not significant for data interpretation, as possible temperature differences are usually limited. The differences of temperature in *in vivo* experiments may be usually neglected as not important at all. Also there is a strong influence of water content and blood perfusion, see, for example, results of Valvano et al. (1985) in Reference 33. Usually effective thermal conductivity and diffusivity are applied to overcome this problem in modeling of thermal processes. Additionally, in subtle analysis one should remember that some tissues might be anisotropic [18,31].

For mixture of N substances, each characterized by thermal conductivity $k_1,...,k_N$, the effective thermal conductivity is the mean value of the volumetric content of components:

$$k_{tk} = \frac{\sum_{i=1}^{N} k_i \cdot V_i}{\sum_{i=1}^{N} V_i} = \rho_{tk} \sum_{i=1}^{N} k_i \frac{m_i}{m_{tk}} \cdot \frac{1}{\rho_i} \qquad (28.7)$$

TABLE 28.1 Thermal Properties of Muscle Tissue

Muscle	Conditions	Thermal Conductivity (W m^{-1} K^{-1})	Diffusivity (m^2 s^{-1})
Heart	37°C	0.492–0.562	No data
Heart	37°C	0.537	1.47×10^{-7}
Heart	5–20°C	No data	$1.47–1.57 \times 10^{-7}$
Heart (dog)	*In vivo*	0.49	No data
Heart (dog)	37°C	0.536	1.51×10^{-7}
Heart (dog)	21°C	No data	$1.47–1.55 \times 10^{-7}$
Heart (swine)	38°C	0.533	No data
Skeletal	37°C	0.449–0.546	No data
Skeletal (dog)	No data	No data	1.83×10^{-7}
Skeletal (cow)	30°C	No data	1.25×10^{-7}
Skeletal (cow)	24–38°C	0.528	No data
Skeletal (swine)	30°C	No data	1.25×10^{-7}
Skeletal (ship)	21°C	No data	$1.51–1.67 \times 10^{-7}$

Source: From Hryciuk M., PhD dissertation—Investigation of layered biological object structure using thermal excitation (in Polish), *Politechnika Gdanska*, 2003. Shitzer A. and Eberhart R.C., *Heat Transfer in Medicine and Biology*, Plenum Press, New York, London, 1985.

TABLE 28.2 Mean Values of Thermal Tissue Properties Taken *In Vitro*

Parameter	Density	Thermal Conductivity	Specific Heat	Volumetric Specific Heat	Diffusivity	Effusivity
Unit of Measure	(kg m^{-3})	[W/(m K)]	[J/(kg K)]	[J/(m^3 K)]	(m^2 s^{-1})	[J/(m^2 K s$^{1/2}$)]
Symbol	ρ	K	c	ρc ($\times 10^6$)	α ($\times 10^{-7}$)	β
Soft Tissues						
Heart muscle	1060	0.49–0.56	3720	3.94	1.24–1.42	1390–1490
Skeletal muscle	1045	0.45–0.55	3750	3.92	1.15–1.4	1330–1470
Brain	1035	0.50–0.58	3650	3.78	1.32–1.54	1375–1480
Kidney	1050	0.51	3700	3.89	1.31	1410
Liver	1060	0.53	3500	3.71	1.27–1.43	1320–1400
Lung	1050	0.30–0.55	3100	3.26	0.92–1.69	990–1340
Eye	1020	0.59	4200	4.28	1.38	1590
Skin superficial layer	1150	0.27	3600	4.14	0.62	1060
Fat under skin	920	0.22	2600	2.39	0.92	725
Hard Tissues						
Tooth-enamel	3000	0.9	720	2.16	4.17	1400
Tooth-dentine	2200	0.45	1300	2.86	1.57	1130
Cancellous bone	1990	0.4	1330	2.65	1.4–1.89	990–1150
Trabecular bone	1920	0.3	2100	4.03	0.92–1.26	1220–1430
Marrow	1000	0.22	2700	2.70	0.82	770
Fluids						
Blood; 44% HCT	1060	0.49	3600	3.82	1.28	1370
Plasma	1027	0.58	3900	4.01	1.45	1520

Source: From Hryciuk M., PhD dissertation—Investigation of layered biological object structure using thermal excitation (in Polish), *Politechnika Gdanska*, 2003. Shitzer A. and Eberhart R.C., *Heat Transfer in Medicine and Biology*, Plenum Press, New York, London, 1985.

where the index *tk* concerns all tissue, and the index i – *i*th component. Analogically, one may calculate effective specific heat either as the mean value of mass components

$$c_{wtk} = \frac{\sum_{i=1}^{N} c_{wi} \cdot m_i}{\sum_{i=1}^{N} m_i} \qquad (28.8)$$

or as the mean value of volumetric components

$$\rho_{tk} c_{wtk} = \frac{\sum_{i=1}^{N} \rho_i c_{wi} \cdot V_i}{\sum_{i=1}^{N} V_i} \qquad (28.9)$$

Marks and Burton [34] propose for the skin a thermal model, composed of three components—water, fat, and proteins—using the values collected in Table 28.3. Though, it was suggested that more realistic values of thermal conductivity are given by Bowman [18,28].

TABLE 28.3   Thermal Properties for the Equivalent Three-Component Model

Quantity	Density	Thermal Conductivity [W/(mK)]		Specific Heat	Specific Heat (volumetric)
Unit	(kg/m³)	K		[J/(kg K)]	[J/(m³K)]
Symbol	ρ	see Reference 28		c_w	$\rho \cdot c_w\ (\times 10^6)$
Water	1000	0.628	0.6	4200	4.2
Fat	815	0.231	0.22	2300	1.87
Proteins	1540	0.117	0.195	1090	1.68

Source: From Marks R.M. and Bartan S.P., *The Physical Nature of the Skin*, MTP Press, Boston, 1998.

28.3 Thermal Models and Equivalent/Synthetic Parameters

Basic analysis of existing thermal processes in correlation with physiological processes is necessary to understand significance of thermal flows in medical diagnostics. Thermal models are very useful to study such problems. It should be underlined that ADT and TT are based on analysis of thermal models of tested objects. Solution of the so-called direct problem while external excitation (determination of temperature distribution in time and space for assumed boundary conditions and known model parameters) involves simulation of temperature distribution in defined object under test. It allows study on thermal tomography concept, simulation of heat exchange and flows using optimal excitation methods, analysis of theoretical, and practical limitations of proposed methods, and so on.

Direct problems may be properly solved only for realistic thermal models. Having such a model, one can compare the results of experiments and can try to solve the reverse problem. This responds to the question— what is the distribution of thermal properties in the internal structure of a human body? Such knowledge may be directly used in clinical diagnostics if the correlation of thermal and physiological properties is high.

In biologic applications solution of the direct problem is basic to see relationship between excitation and temperature distribution at the surface of a tested object, what is a measurable quantity. This requires solution of the heat flow in 3D space. Equation 28.10, representing the general parabolic heat flow [35] describes this problem mathematically:

$$\operatorname{div}\left(k \cdot \operatorname{grad} T\right) - c_{\mathrm{p}} \rho \frac{\partial T}{\partial t} = -q\left(P, t\right) \tag{28.10}$$

where T is the temperature in K; k the thermal conductivity in W m^{-1} K^{-1}, c_{p} the specific heat in J g^{-1} K^{-1}; ρ the material (tissue) density in g m^{-3}, t the time in seconds, and $q(P,t)$ is the volumetric density of generated or dissipated power in W m^{-3}. For biologic tissues, Pennes [36] defined "the biologic heat flow equation":

$$c_{\mathrm{p}} \rho \frac{\partial T(x, y, z, t)}{\partial t} = k \nabla^2 T(x, y, z, t) + q_{\mathrm{b}} + q_{\mathrm{m}} + q_{\mathrm{ex}} \tag{28.11}$$

where $T(x,y,z,t)$ is the temperature distribution at the moment t, q_{b} (W/m³) the heat power density delivered or dissipated by blood, q_{m} the heat power density delivered by metabolism, and q_{ex} is the heat power density delivered by external sources. Solving of this equation, including all processes influencing tissue temperature, is very complicated and analytically even impossible. Generally there are three approaches in analysis and solving of heat transfers and distribution of temperature.

The first one is analytic, usually very simplified description of an object, typically using the Fourier series method. Analytical solutions of heat flows are known only for very simple structures of well-defined shapes, what usually is not the case acceptable for analysis of biological objects. The simplest solution assumes one-directional flow of energy, as it is for multilayer, infinite structures, thermally uniformly excited. Distribution of temperature, if several sources exist, may be solved assuming the superposition method.

The second option is the use of numerical methods, usually based on the finite element method (FEM); to model more complicated structures. There are several commercial software packages broadly known and used for solving problems of heat flows, usually combining a mechanical part, including generator of a model mesh as well as modules solving specific thermal problems, see, for example, References 37 and 38. Also general mathematical programs, as MATLAB® [39] or Mathematica [40], contain proper tools allowing thermal analysis. FEM methods allow solution of 3D heat flow problems in time. Functional variability of thermal properties and nonlinear parametric description of tested objects may be easily taken into consideration. Again, there are basic limitations concerning the dimension of a problem to be solved (complexity and number of model elements), which should be taken into account from the point of view of the computational costs.

The solution of Equations 28.10 and 28.11 may be given in the explicit form:

$$T_n^{i+1} = \frac{\Delta t}{\rho c_p V_n} \left[\sum_m k_{nm} T_m^i + \left(\frac{\rho c_w V_n}{\Delta t} - \sum_m k_{nm} T_m^i \right) + q_n V_n \right] \tag{28.12}$$

or in the implicit form:

$$T_n^{i+1} - T_n^i = \frac{\Delta t}{\rho c_p V_n} \left[\sum_m k_{nm} \left(T_m^{i+1} - T_n^i \right) + q_n V_n \right] \tag{28.13}$$

where i indicates moment of time, Δt is the time step, n the position in space (node number), V_n the volume of the n node, m indicates neighboring nodes, k_{nm} is thermal conductivity between the nodes n and m, T_n^i the temperature of a node at the beginning of a time step, T_n^{i+1} the temperature of a node at the end of the time step, and q_n is the power density representing generation of heat per unit volume at the nth node. Each node represents a specific part of the modeled structure defined by mass, dimensions, and physical properties. The node is assumed to be thermally uniform and isotropic. Boundary conditions may be assumed discretional, depending on real conditions of experiments to be performed (under analysis). Usually adiabatic or isothermic conditions and a value of excitation power are assumed. The boundary conditions, the value of excitation power as well as individual properties of any node may be modified with time!

In the explicit method the temperature of each node is determined at the end of the time step, taking into account the heat balance based on temperature, heat generation, and thermal properties at the beginning of the time step. Assuming choice of a not proper time step or model geometry may result in lack of stable solution or in poor accuracy of analysis.

In the implicit method, the increase of temperature in each node is calculated from the heat balance resulting from temperatures, heat generation, and thermal properties during the time step. The solution is stable. The duration of a time step may be modified in the adaptation procedure assuming several conditions, for example, maximum rise of temperature in any of the nodes. Increase of iteration steps followed by the need of many possible modifications of parameters during iterations may lead to unacceptable rise in computation time. Still, the mesh geometry may influence accuracy of analysis.

The numerical modeling is preferable in cases where solution of the direct problem may be sufficient, for example, in analysis of methods of investigation, because it allows easy and accurate modifications of important factors influencing measurements. The forward problem may be solved for any configuration of mesh and tissue as well as excitation parameters. Unfortunately, limited knowledge of living tissue properties is reducing possibility of using simulation methods for reliable *in vivo* case analysis.

The third approach is to build simple equivalent models of tested tissues or organs based on such synthetic parameters as thermal resistivity (conductivity) and thermal capacity. This solution, as the simplest one, seems to be the most useful practically. A medical doctor may accept relatively simple, still reliable description, based on synthetic parameters easily determined for such simple models. As an example, thermal structure of the skin may be represented by three equivalent layers described by the $R_{th}(1-3)C_{th}(1-3)$ model. Values of such simple model parameters may be relatively easily determined from experimental data using fitting procedures and well correlated to physical phenomena, for example, depth of burns. This is also probably the easiest method to be applied for solving the inverse problem, and therefore, the best offer for modern computer technology-based diagnostic tools. Also, correlation of model parameters coefficients is not as complicated as in the case of the FEM approach.

28.4 Measurement Procedures

Study of heat transfer enables quantification of thermo-physical material properties such as thermal diffusivity or conductivity and finally detection of subsurface defects. The main drawback of thermal measurement methods is limitation in number of contact sensors distributed within a tested object or application of IR-methods of temperature measurements, allowing observation of the surface temperature distribution only, what in both cases results in limited accuracy of analysis.

The ADT and TT are based on IR technology. The general concept of measurements performed in such applications is shown in Figure 28.1. External thermal excitation source (heating or cooling) is applied to a tested object (TO). First, steady-state temperature distribution on TO surface is registered using the IR-camera. The next step requires thermal excitation application, and registration of temperature transients on the TO surface. The control unit synchronizes the processes of excitation and registration. All data are stored in the data acquisition system (DAS) for further computer analysis.

To allow quantitative evaluation of TO properties, the procedures of both, ADT and TT, are based on determination of thermal models of TO. Typical procedure of model parameter estimation is shown in Figure 28.2. For the measurement structure shown in Figure 28.1 an equivalent model of TO must be assumed (developed and applied in the procedure). In this case usually a simple model, for example, the three layers $R_{th}(1-3)C_{th}(1-3)$, is applied. Thermal excitation (from a physical source as well as simulated for the assumed model), applied simultaneously to TO and to its model, results in thermal transients, registered at the surface of TO by the IR-camera (applied and simulated for the model). For each pixel, the registered temperature course is identified (typically the least-squares approximation—LSA and exponential model for thermal transients are applied). The result (measured thermal course) is compared with the simulated transient and if necessary the thermal model is modified to fit to experimental results.

The registration process is illustrated in Figure 28.3. An example for a pulse excitation and registration of temperature only during the recovery phase (in this case—cooling, after heating excitation) is shown. This is a typical case of practical measurements using optical excitation. Each pixel showing the temperature distribution at the TO surface is represented by an equivalent model, therefore

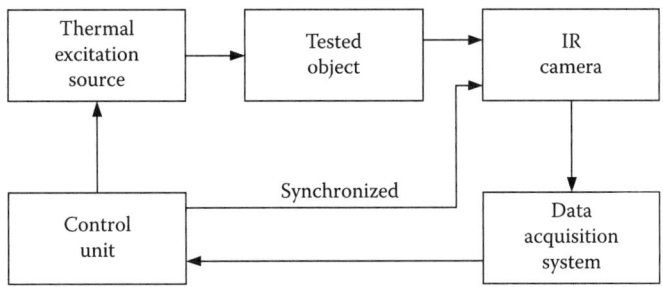

FIGURE 28.1 Schematic diagram of ADT and TT instrumentation.

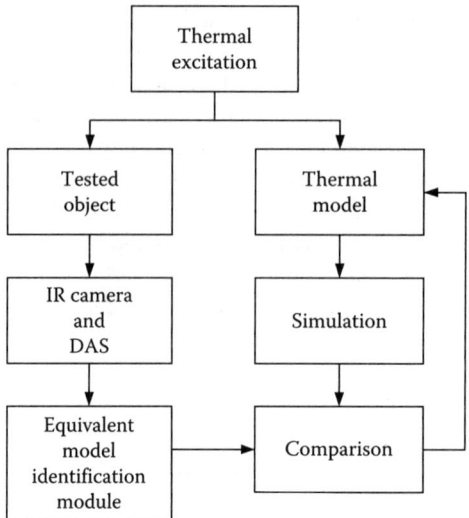

FIGURE 28.2 Model-based identification of a tested structure (object).

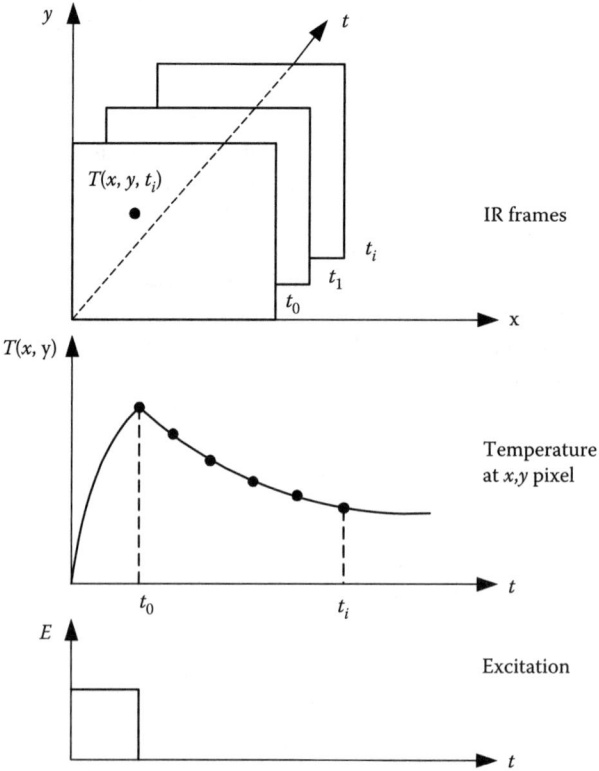

FIGURE 28.3 Registration procedure—after thermal excitation (here heating), a series of IR frames are recorded in controlled moments, starting just at the moment of switching the excitation off; temperature of each pixel is recorded to calculate time constants specific in each pixel.

single excitation and registration of transient temperatures at the position x, y allows identification of the structure *in depth*, resulting in 3D picture of TO.

There are several procedures of NDE of defects by observation of temperature changes of an inspected sample surface using IR-imaging [2]:

1. Continuous heating of a tested object and observation of surface temperature changes during thermal stimulation (step heating, long pulse); the main drawback of the method is limited possibility of quantitative measurements. The information may be similar to classical static thermography with enhancement of specific defects.
2. Sinusoidal heating and synchronized observation of temperature distribution during stimulation (lock-in technique); this is the most accurate NDT–ADT method but not practical in medical applications as the experiment is rather difficult and time consuming. Additionally data analysis is not simple as thermal biofeedback may be influencing values of tissue thermal properties.
3. Pulse excitation (e.g., heating using optical excitation, air fan for cooling, etc.) and observation during the heating and/or the cooling phases. Several procedures are possible, as pulsed ADT, multi-frequency binary sequences (MFBS) technique, pulse phase thermography (PPT), and other. The description in the following text is concentrating on a single pulse excitation, because this experiment is relatively simple, fast and of accuracy acceptable in medical applications. The time of excitation may be set short enough to eliminate biofeedback interactions, which are otherwise difficult in interpretation.

28.5 Measurement Equipment

Typical measurement set is shown in Figure 28.4. The main elements of the set are shown: an IR-camera; a fast data acquisition system; a set of excitation sources with a synchronized driving unit.

The better are the camera properties the higher accuracy measurements are possible, what is a condition for proper reconstruction of thermal properties of TO. Minimal technical requirements for an IR-camera are: repetition rate 30 frames/s; MRTD better than 0.1°C; LW—long wavelengths range preferable; FOV dependent on application—typically in clinical conditions measurements taken from around 1 m distance to a patient are advisable. Still application of a cooled FPA camera with higher

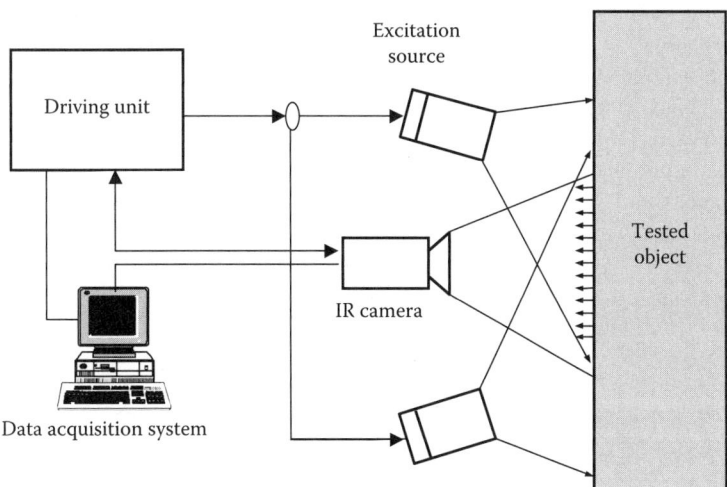

FIGURE 28.4 Measurement set—tested object is exposed to external thermal excitation; the IR-camera, synchronically with excitation records, surface temperature distribution in time.

registration speed and better MRTD would be advisable. SW cameras may be used for other than optical excitations or for analysis of the recovery phase only (time when the excitation is switched off).

Very important is the use of proper excitation sources. Application of optical halogen lamps, laser sources, microwave applicators, even ultrasound generators for heating and air fans or cold sprays for cooling, and some other has been noted [41–44]. As a heating source, an optical or IR lamp, a laser beam, a microwave generator, or an ultrasonic generator can be used. Electromagnetic or mechanical irradiation generated by a source (usually distant) is illuminating a tested object and generating a heating wave proportional to the irradiation energy and to the absorption rate, specific for a tested object material and varying with wavelength of excitation. Microwave irradiation, ultrasonic excitation or electric current flow might generate heat inside a specimen proportional to its dielectric or mechanical properties. For the microwave excitation the main role in the heating process plays the electrical conductivity of a tested object. For the ultrasonic excitation the thermo-elastic effect and mechanical hysteresis are responsible for temperature changes proportional to the applied stress tensor. For the optical irradiation the absorption coefficient is describing the rate of energy converted into heat.

In ADT, the basic information is connected with time-dependent reaction of tested structures therefore it is very important to know the switching properties of the heating or cooling sources, especially the raising and the falling time of generated pulses. Dynamic properties of heating or cooling sources must be taken into account during modeling the different shapes of excitation. Some extra measures should be practically adopted, for example, to avoid the interaction between a lamp, which is self-heated during experiments, and a tested object; sometimes a special shutter is needed to assure proper shape of a heating signal. For microwave excitation the applicator must be directly connected to a tested object therefore a time for mechanical removing of an applicator from the heated object to allow thermographic observation is additionally needed what practically eliminates application of such sources in medical applications.

There are several conclusions regarding application of different sources of thermal excitation:

1. We are dealing with biological objects; therefore, heating should be limited to a safe level, not exceeding 42°C; while cooling temperature of a living tissue should not be lower than 4°C.
2. Thermal excitation should be as uniform as possible; nonuniform excitation results in decrease of accuracy and misinterpretation of measurement data. It is relatively easy to fulfil this condition for optical excitation but very difficult for ultrasonic or microwave methods, even using specially developed applicators.
3. The other important factor is the depth of heat penetration. For different sources of excitation the energy penetration can vary from superficial only absorption to millimeters for some laser beams or even up to a few centimeters for microwave excitation. Ultrasounds are not applicable for biological tissues but of rigid structures only. As an example the data concerning microwave penetration are shown in Table 28.4. High heat penetration may be very interesting for discrimination of deep regions; unfortunately control of microwave energy absorption practically is impossible being dependent on tissue electrical properties. This feature makes use of microwave sources in medical applications very problematic.
4. Temperature interactions should be limited to periods not affected by biological feedback; additionally to assure proper data treatment special care should be devoted to fast switching the

TABLE 28.4 Wavelengths and Penetration Depths of the Microwave Source 2.45 GHz for Typical Tissue with Low and High Water Content

Water Content	λ—In Air (cm)	λ—In Tissue (cm)	σ—Tissue Conductivity (S/m)	Penetration Depth (cm)
High (muscle, skin)	12.2	1.76	2.21	1.70
Low (fat, bones)	12.2	5.21	0.96–2.13	11.2

Source: From Duek A.F., *Physical Properties of Tissue*, Academic Press, London, 1990.

excitation power on and off. For optical sources mechanical shutters are advisable, as electrical switching is effective in the visible range but also other elements as, for example, housing may be heated to a level influencing sensitive IR cameras.

5. Noncontact methods, as optical, seem to be especially appreciated, as aseptic conditions are easy to be secured.
6. Concluding—optical excitation for heating and air fan or cryo-therapy CO_2 devices for cooling seem to be the best options for daily practice in medical diagnostics.

Even ADT is not so sensitive to external conditions as the classical IRT still there are several conditions to be assured. Generally, patients should be prepared for experiments and all "golden standards" valid for classical thermography here should also be applied [46].

28.6 Procedures of Data and Image Processing

Depending on the method of excitation several procedures may be adopted to process the measurement data and then to extract diagnostic information. Here we concentrate only on pulse excitation as it is shown in Figure 28.3. Measurements of transients during the heating and the cooling phases allow further use of procedures developed for pulsed thermography (PT), ADT IR-imaging, pulse phase thermography (PPT), and TT. In all four cases, excitation and registration of thermal transients is performed in the same way using IR-camera. Visualization data differ as it is expressed respectively by thermal contrast images in PT; thermal time constants in ADT and phase shift images in PPT, finally thermal conductivity distribution in TT.

28.6.1 Pulsed Thermography

Pulsed thermography applies calculation of *the maximal thermal contrast index—C(t)* [2].

$$C(t) = \frac{T_d(t) - T_d(0)}{T_s(t) - T_s(0)} \tag{28.14}$$

where T is the temperature, t the time; for $t = 0$ the sample temperature is maximal, d,s are the subscripts indicating the defect and the sample. With given number of temperature images acquired during PT, the thermal contrast image may be expressed also as

$$C(x,y,t) = \frac{T(x,y,t) - T(x_0,y_0,t)}{T(x_0,y_0,t)} \tag{28.15}$$

where x,y is the pixel coordinates and x_0, y_0 the pixel coordinates of the reference point in the chosen defect area.

To calculate contrast images, a defect template or a reference point should be defined. In medical applications, it is almost impossible to indicate such templates therefore to overcome this limitation estimation of the behavior of living tissues in PT conditions is possible. As an example, heat transfer caused by blood flow is different in normal and affected (e.g., cancerous) tissues. During the heating process the affected tissues usually are heated more than the normal tissues, what is caused by reduced thermoregulation. Further image processing (segmentation) allows discrimination of the so-called *hot spots* and *cold spots* images. Another possibility is to define *the normalized differential PT index* (NDPTI) [47]:

$$\text{NDPTI}(x,y,t) = \frac{T(x,y,0) - T(x,y,t)}{T(x,y,0) + T(x,y,t)} \tag{28.16}$$

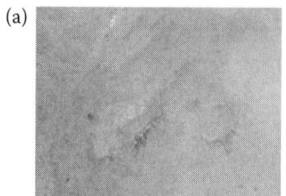
(a)

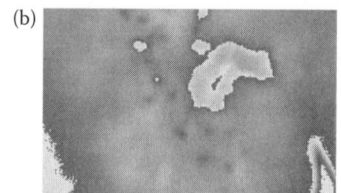
(b)

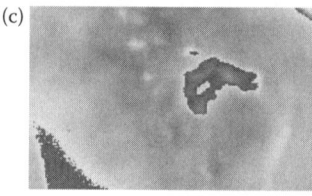
(c)

FIGURE 28.5   Patient with burn wound, first day after the accident—photograph of the burn (a), NDPTI image of the same field (b), and the NDPTI image at the second day (c).

Automatic processing requires definition of thresholds, which can extract only "hot spots" or "cold spots" in the image (i.e., pixels with a value lower than the threshold will compose an image background, while pixels with a value equal or greater than the threshold will compose—"hot spots"). Because popular indexes are constructed to indicate higher probability of detected elements by a higher index value (low values—"cold spots"; high values—"hot spots") it is possible to calculate a negative NDPTI image, too.

$$\text{NPTI}(x,y,t) = 1 - \text{NDPTI}(x,y,t) = \frac{2 * T(x,y,t)}{T(x,y,0) + T(x,y,t)} \tag{28.17}$$

The signal-to-noise ratio (SNR) of this technique is rather small. It can be improved by averaging images, repeating the pulse excitation with time interval long enough for proper cooling.

As an example, Figure 28.5a is a photograph of the burns caused by fire. Figure 28.5b,c shows fields of IIa/b degree burn evidenced at the first and the second day after the accident. The effect of treatment is also very well visible comparing the results of measurements done day by day. In the related example the burn area was small enough to avoid grafting.

28.6.2 Active Dynamic Thermal IR-Imaging

The ADT is based on comparison of measurements with a simple multilayer thermal model described by Equations 28.4 and 28.5 giving a simplified description of parametric images of thermal time constants, whose values are correlated with internal structure of tested objects [11,48]. Recorded in time thermal transients at a given pixel are described by exponential models. Here, the two exponential models are describing the process of natural cooling after switching the heating pulse off.

$$T(t) = T_{\min} + \Delta T_1 e^{-t/\tau_{1c}} + \Delta T_2 e^{-t/\tau_{2c}} \tag{28.18}$$

Model-based identification of a tested structure (object) is performed as it is shown in Figure 28.2. The recorded thermal response is fitted to a model. In many cases the two exponential description is fully sufficient for practical applications. As an example, typical transient in time for a single pixel (e.g., from Figure 28.5) is shown in Figure 28.6, with fitting procedure applied to one and two exponential models.

The two exponential models, as Equation 28.18, are fully sufficient for the data of accuracy available in the performed experiment. Some more pictures and examples of the ADT procedure are shown in the following paragraphs, especially in skin burn evaluation [49,50]. It should be underlined that time constants for the heating phase τ_h and for the cooling phase τ_c usually are different due to different heat flow paths.

28.6.3 Pulse Phase Thermography

The procedure of PPT [2,51] is based on Fourier transform. The sequence of IR images is obtained as in conventional PT experiments, Figure 28.7. Next, for each pixel (x,y) in every of N images the

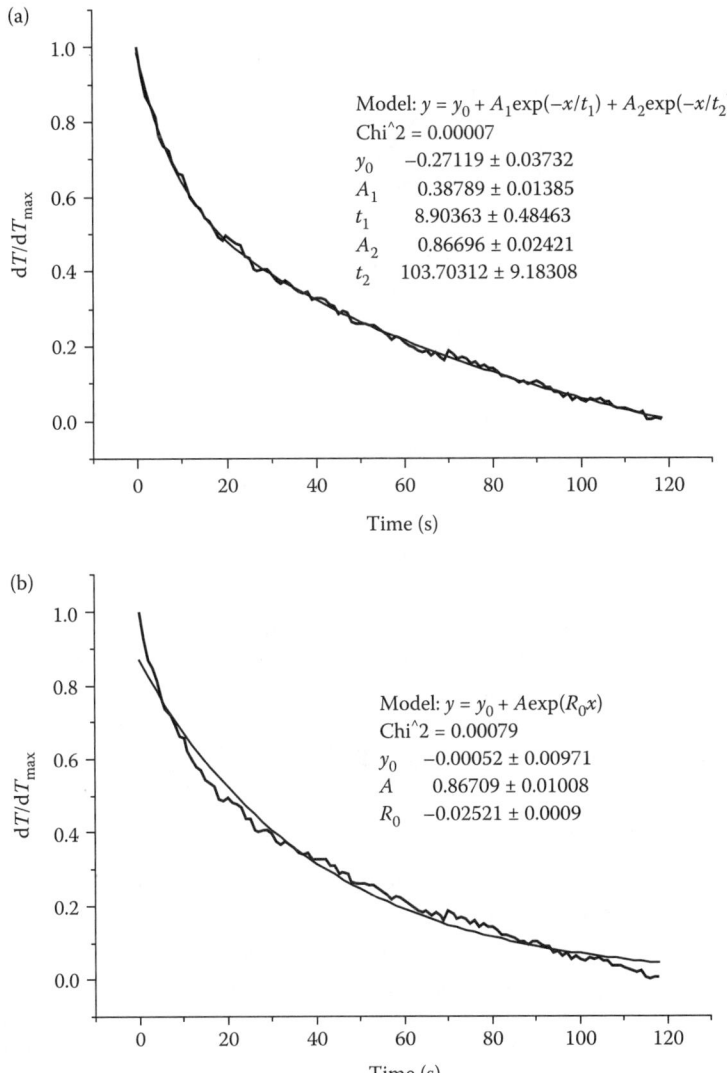

FIGURE 28.6 Fitting of the models to the measurement data—5-parameter model (a) and 3-parameter model (b).

temporal evolution $g_i(t)$ is extracted and then the discrete Fourier transform is performed using the formula:

$$F_i(f) = \frac{1}{N}\sum_{n=0}^{N-1} g_i(t)\exp\left(\frac{-j2\pi f t}{N}\right) = \mathrm{Re}_i(f) + j\mathrm{Im}_i(f)$$

$$\varphi_i(f) = \mathrm{atan}\left(\frac{\mathrm{Im}_i(f)}{\mathrm{Re}_i(f)}\right); \qquad A_i(f) = \sqrt{\mathrm{Re}_i(f)^2 + \mathrm{Im}_i(f)^2}$$

(28.19)

More valuable diagnostic information is given in the phase shift; therefore, this parameter is of major interest.

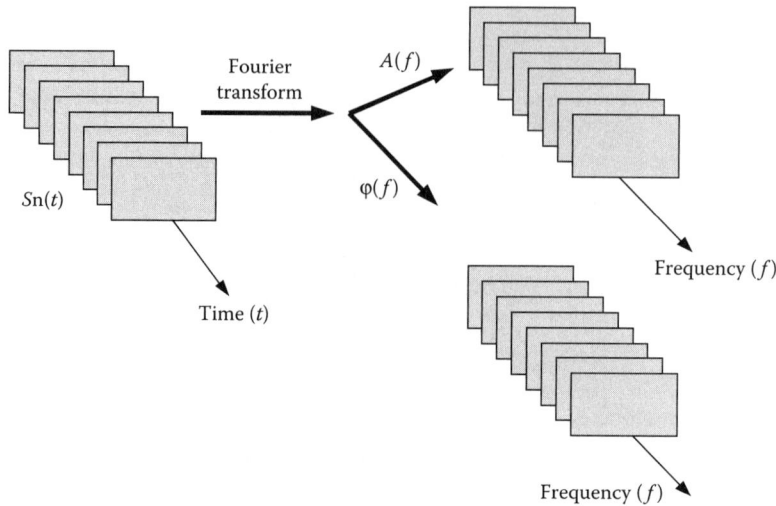

FIGURE 28.7 Procedure of calculation of synthetic pictures in PPT.

Interesting characteristics of PPT are evident since it combines the speed of PT with the features of lock-in approach (the phase and the magnitude image). The condition to get reliable results is application of fast and very high-quality IR-cameras.

As this method was not applied in medicine, yet, we do not show any examples, but extensive discussion of the validity of the procedure may be found in Reference 51.

28.6.4 Thermal Tomography

Thermal tomography should allow tomographic visualization of 3D structures, solving the real inverse problem—find distribution of thermal conductivity inside a tested object. This attempt is fully successful in the case of skin burn evaluation [16–18], giving a powerful tool in hands of medical doctors allowing reliable quantitative evaluation of the burn depth [52–54]. Other applications are under intensive research [55–57].

In TT the first step is determination of thermal properties of a tested object, necessary for development of its thermal equivalent model, to be applied for further data treatment. A typical procedure allowing the model parameters determination is shown in Figure 28.8. The forward problem is solved

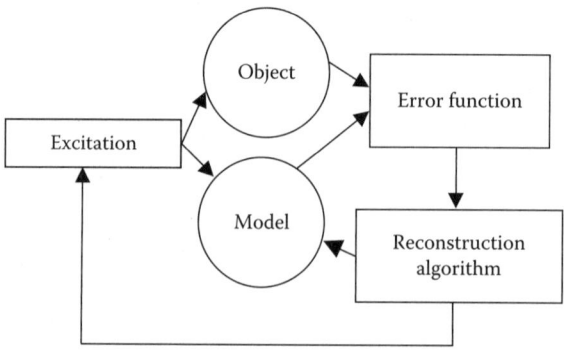

FIGURE 28.8 Determination of model parameters, based on comparison of measurement and simulation data, valid for all kinds of tomography.

and assumed model parameters are modified to satisfy a chosen criterion for model and measurement data comparison. The second step is organization of an active dynamic thermography experiment and registration of thermal transients forced by external excitation.

The next step requires advanced calculations to solve the inverse problem. The information of the correlation of the calculated figure of merit with a specific diagnostic feature is necessary to take a proper diagnostic decision based on the performed measurements. The decision function is directed to determine the internal thermal structure of the tested object based on thermal transients at its surface. In this case, a real inverse problem has to be solved. We perform this procedure using MATLAB scripts [17,18]. As a result the multilayer structure of different thermal properties may be reconstructed. To solve this problem additional assumptions, as number of layers, values of thermal properties or dimensions, are necessary because in general the problem is mathematically ill posed and nonlinear.

The method allows, under some conditions, not only to calculate the thermal effusivity, but also to reconstruct thermal diffusivity distribution in a layered structure. It is done using the nonlinear least-squares optimization algorithm in inversion of the direct problem:

$$\left.\begin{array}{c} T_0(x) \\ T_{exc} \\ \Phi(0,t) \\ k(0) \end{array}\right\} \Rightarrow \alpha(x) \tag{28.20}$$

where $T_0(x)$ is the initial temperature distribution in the object, T_{exc} the temperature of the heater, $\Phi(0,t)$ the heat flux at the surface, and $k(0)$ is the thermal conductivity of the outermost layer. In medical diagnostics of burn depth determination the problem is defined in a discrete form allowing determination of the parameter D, describing the depth of specific thermal properties, for example, depth of the burned tissue (the unknown parameter is local thickness of the tested object $d = D\,\Delta x$):

$$\left.\begin{array}{c} T_m^1, \quad m = 1,\ldots,M \\ \Phi_{exc} \\ T_1^p, \quad p = 1,\ldots,P \\ \left.[k_m,\rho c_m]\right|_{m\le D} = [k_{rub},\rho c_{rub}] \\ \left.[k_m,\rho c_m]\right|_{D<m<M} = [k_{air},\rho c_{air}] \end{array}\right\} \Rightarrow D \tag{28.21}$$

where the upper indexes describe the time domain and lower—the space domain. The inverse problem allows solution for which the direct simulation of temperature distribution is closest to the experiment results. This is by solving the problem, which is set by the goal function $F(D)$:

$$F(D) = \sum_{p=1}^{P} (T_{dir}^p(D) - T_{meas}^p)^2 \xrightarrow{D} \min \tag{28.22}$$

where T_{dir}^p is the surface temperature for simulation performed for assumed value of the parameter D and T_{meas}^p the values measured. In the following examples, the MATLAB *lsqnonlin* function was adopted to solve this problem based on modified interior-reflective Newton method [18]. Description of multilayer structures is also possible and may be defined in the form illustrated in Figure 28.9 [18,54]. One-directional flow of heat energy is assumed.

What should be underlined is that the TT procedure requires advanced calculations and very reliable data, both from measurements as well as for modeling. Comparing with ADT TT is a much more

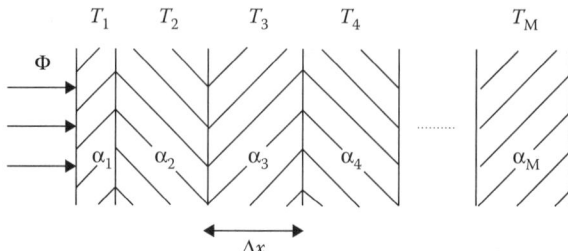

FIGURE 28.9   Spatial discretization of the properties of a multilayer object under test.

demanding method; therefore, it seems that typical for ADT description using thermal time constants at present stage of development seems to be easily accepted by medical staff.

28.7 Experiments and Applications

There are three groups of study performed:

1. On phantoms, for evaluation of technical aspects of instrumentation to be applied for *in vivo* experiments
2. On animals, *in vivo* experiments, for reference data
3. Clinical, for evaluation of the practical meaning of applied procedures

As the ADT as well as TT methods are new in medical diagnostics here we show some results of animal *in vivo* experiments and a few clinical cases. Described applications concern burns diagnostics and evaluation of cardiosurgery interventions. Results of phantom experiments and some other clinical applications were described in other cited publications, for example, References 22, 26, and 43.

28.7.1 Organization of Experiments

The clinical trials are done in *the Department of Plastic Surgery and Burns*, and in *the Department of Cardiac Surgery and Cardiology* of the Medical University of Gdansk. The leading medical personnel had all necessary legal rights for carrying the experiments, approved by the local ethical commission. All clinical experiments were done during normal diagnostic or treatment procedures, as the applied PT, ADT, and TT are noninvasive, aseptic, and safe. The excess of evoked surface temperature rise is around 2–4°C and the observation by the IR-camera is taken from a distance of 1 m. For skin temperature measurements illuminated area usually is kept wet using a thin layer of ointment to satisfy condition of constant evaporation from a tested surface and a constant value of emissivity coefficient. In cardiac surgery experiments with open chest, the surface of the heart is observed where the conditions of emissivity are regarded as constant. The IR-camera is located in a way not disturbing any activity of a surgeon.

The *in vivo* experiments on domestic pigs were performed in *the Department of Animal Physiology, Gdansk University*. The research program received a positive opinion of the institutional board of medical ethics. Housing and care of animals were in accordance with the national regulations concerning experiments on living animals. The choice of animals was intentional. No other animals have skin, blood, or heart properties so close to the human organs than pigs do [45]. Therefore, the experimental data carrying important medical information are of direct relationship to human organ properties.

Our burn experiments were based on the research of Singer et al. [58] and his methodology on standardized burn model. Following his experiment more than 120 paired sets of burns were inflicted on the back skin of 14 young domestic anesthetized pigs using aluminum and copper bars preheated in water

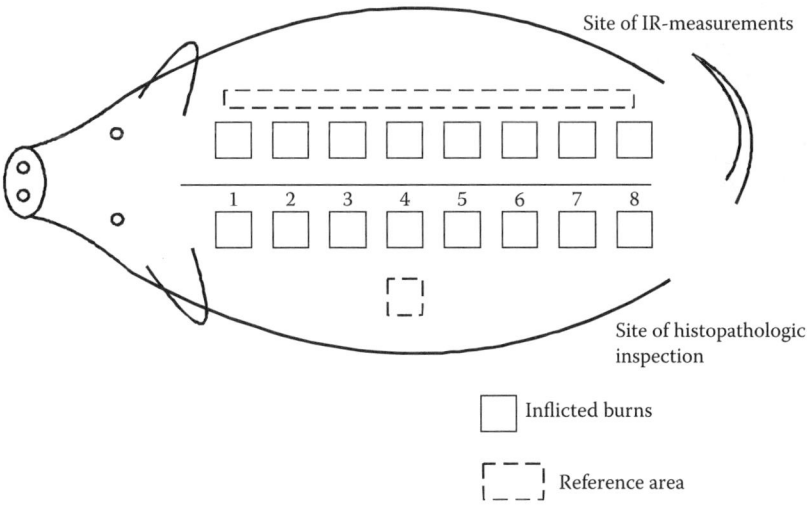

FIGURE 28.10   Location of experimental burns.

in the range from 60°C to 100°C. Typical distribution of burns is shown in Figure 28.10. Each pair was representing different conditions of injury giving a set of controlled burn depths. Additionally, each of measuring points was controlled by full-thickness skin biopsies and followed by histopathologic analysis of burn depth. The results of skin burn degree are in good accordance to the data given by Singer. The pigs were maintained under a surgical plane of anesthesia in conditioned environment of 24°C. The back skin was clipped before creation of burns. The total-body surface area of the burns in each pig was approximately 4%. The animals were observed and treated against pain or discomfort.

After the "burns" experiment was completed, the same pigs were anesthetized, intubated, and used for experimental myocardial infarction by closing the left descending artery. This experiment was lasting 5 h to evidence the nonreciprocal changes of the heart muscle. Full histopathology investigation was performed for objective evaluation of necrosis process.

Basic measurement set-up used in our experiments is composed of instruments shown in Figure 28.4. It consists of the Agema 900 thermographic camera system; IR incandescent lamps of different power or a set of halogen lamps (up to 1000 W) with mechanical shutter or an air-cooling fan as thermal excitation sources; a control unit for driving the system. Additionally a specially designed meter of tissue thermal properties is used to determine the contact reference data necessary for reliable model of the skin or other tissue.

The initial assumptions applied for reconstruction of a tested structure using ADT and TT procedures:

- Tested tissue is a 2- or 3-D medium with two- or three-layer composite structure (e.g., for skin— epidermis, dermis, subcutaneous tissue); (but for simplicity and having limited performance instrumentation even the one-layer model may be useful for diagnostic use in tissue evaluation).
- Tissue properties are independent on its initial temperature.

For skin and under-skin tissues an equivalent three-layer thermal model was developed [11]. For the assumed model its effective parameters have been reconstructed based on the results of transient thermal processes. For known thermal diffusivity and conductivity of specific tissues the local thickness of a two- or three-layer structure may be calculated. In the structural model, each layer should correspond to the anatomy structure of the skin (see Figure 28.11). But in the case of a well-developed burn a two-layer model is sufficient as the skin is totally changed and the new structure is determined by the necrotic layer of burn and modified by injury internal structure of thermal properties drastically different comparing the pre-injury state.

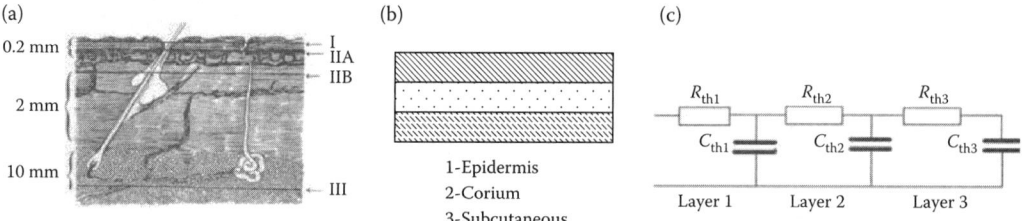

FIGURE 28.11   (a) Anatomy of the skin, (b) three-layer structural model, and (c) equivalent thermo-electric model. (Adapted from Eberhart C. *Heat Transfer in Medicine and Biology, Analysis and Applications*, Vol. 1. Plenum Press, London, 1985.)

28.7.2 Results and Discussion

The related results are divided into groups covering clinical measurements of skin burns and heart surgery and equivalent measurements on pigs. The animal experiments are especially valuable to show importance of the discussed methods. Such experiments assure conditions which may be regarded as reference because fully controlled interventions and objective histopathologic investigations have been performed in this case.

28.7.3 Skin Burns

28.7.3.1 *In Vivo* Experiments on Pigs

The measurements were performed approximately 0.5 h after the burn creation and were repeated after 2 and 5 h and every 24 h during 5 consecutive days after the injury. As the ADT and TT experiments are new in medicine there are several notices concerning methodology of experiments. Especially some biological factors are of high importance. The pigs are growing in extremely fast; therefore, the conditions of measurements are constantly changed. Also the hairs grow anew changing the measurement conditions and cannot be clipped again as the area is affected by injury. This was especially important for direct contact measurements but was not influencing IR measurements. The position of animals in consecutive days was not always the same causing some problems with data interpretation. The results of biopsy and histopathologic observations are used as the reference data of the skin burn thickness. We indicated the same set of parameters as given by Singer, is shown in Figure 28.12 for exemplary burns of one of the pigs. The affected thickness of skin is dependent on the temperature and time of the aluminum and copper bars application. The plots are showing relative thickness of a burn with respect to the thickness of the skin. Such normalization may be important as the skin is of different thickness along the body. All affected points have full histopathologic description. Here only one example is shown for points of the aluminum bar applications of different temperature but constant 30 s time of application.

Some thermographic data of one of pigs taken 5 h after the burn injury are shown in Figure 28.13a [11]. A thermogram while heating is switched off with indicated six measurement areas is shown. Two bottom fields are uninjured reference points, four others are burns made using the aluminum bar—from the left: 100°C/30 s; 100°C/10 s, and 90°C/30 s; 80°C/30 s. The set of halogen lamps was applied for PT and ADT experiment. The result of NDPTI pictures show temperature distribution 100 and 200 ms after the excitation Figure 28.13b,c. The burns are clearly visible and the relative temperature rise is very strongly correlated to the condition of the injury. For the indicated areas the mean value of temperature changes are calculated. This is shown for the first phase of cooling in Figure 28.14. The data might be fitted to thermal models giving ADT specific synthetic pictures of thermal time constants. The quality of the fitting procedure of measurement data to the equivalent model parameters is shown as an example in Figure 28.6a,b for one- and two-layer models.

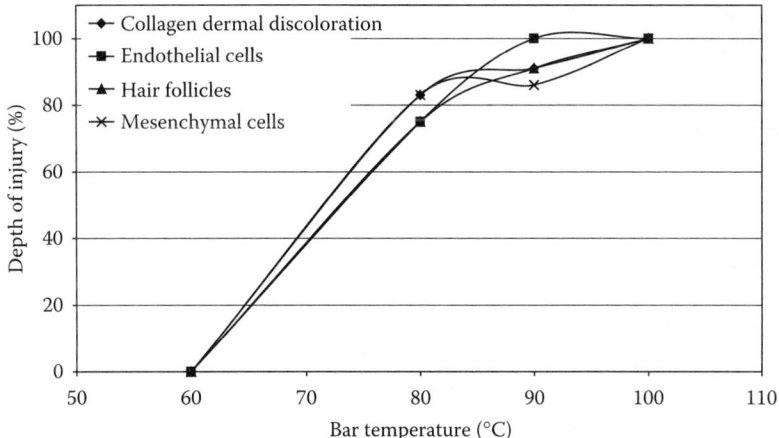

FIGURE 28.12 Relative thickness of the burned skin for several aluminum bar temperatures for time of application equal 30 s—different indicators describing burns are listed (biopsy results).

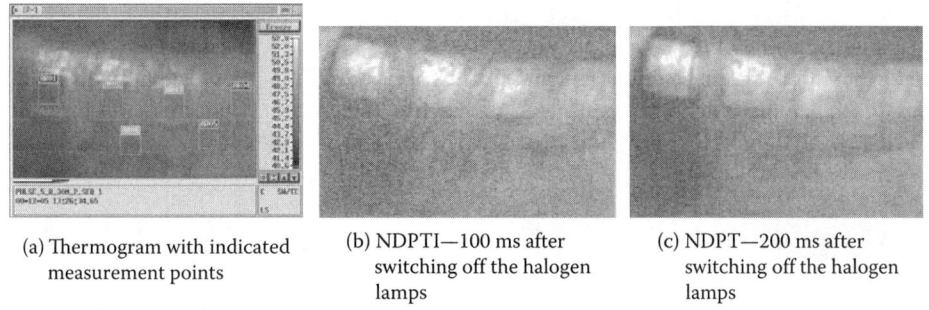

(a) Thermogram with indicated measurement points

(b) NDPTI—100 ms after switching off the halogen lamps

(c) NDPT—200 ms after switching off the halogen lamps

FIGURE 28.13 Classical thermogram (a) and PT normalized differential thermography index pictures of burns (b) and (c).

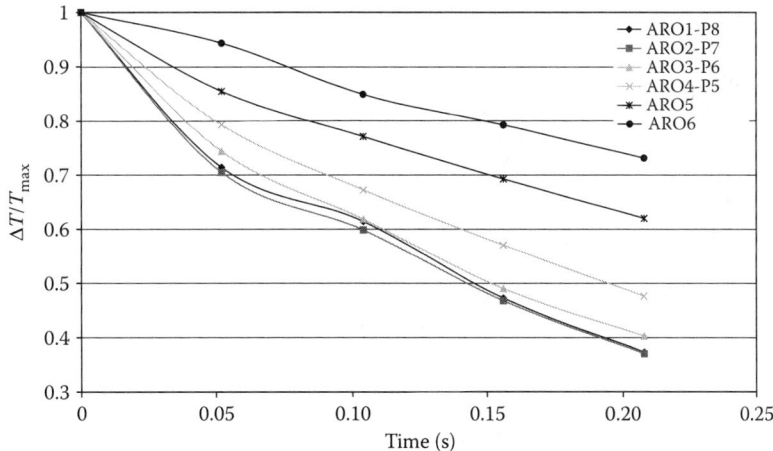

FIGURE 28.14 The normalized averaged temperature changes at the first phase after the excitation is switched off for indicated in Figure 28.13a points.

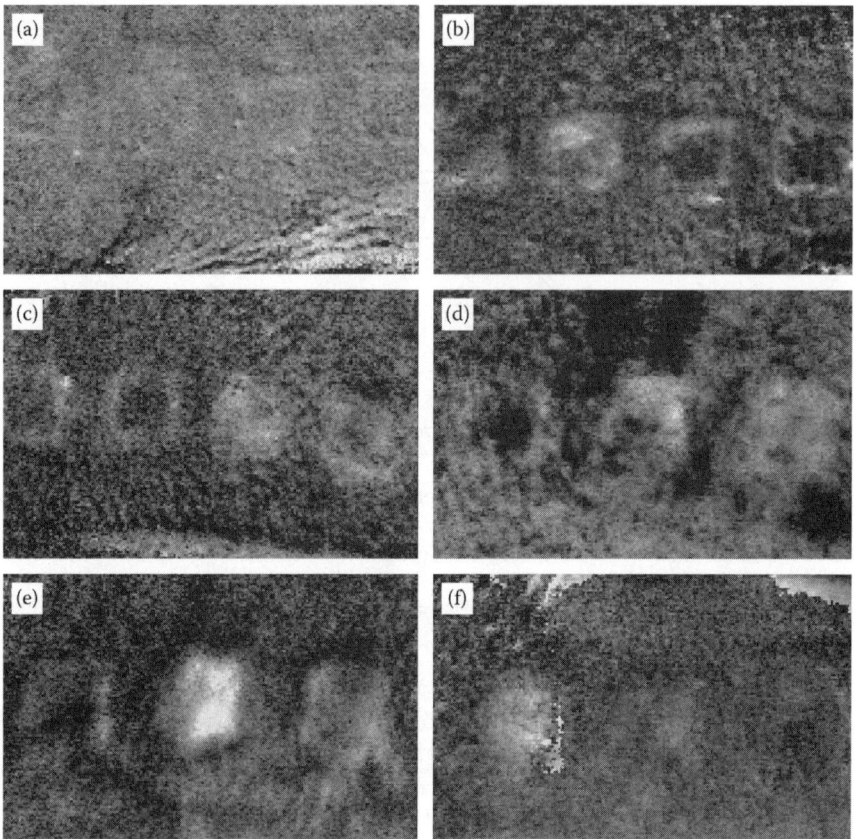

FIGURE 28.15 Thermal time constant representation for the same case as showed in Figures 28.13 and 28.14 in consecutive days, starting from the moment of injury (upper left) and ending on the 5th day (bottom right). The placement of injures seems to be shifted due to different positions of the animal from day-to-day. Specific burn areas are easy recognizable. Additional studies are necessary for making full diagnostic medical recognition of injury, as there are two factors influencing each other—healing process and fast growth of the animal.

There is a possibility to transform each of the pixels into the equivalent model descriptor. In Figure 28.15a–f thermograms taken in consecutive days are transformed according to the formula $A \exp(-R_0 t)$. Distribution of the parameter—the thermal time constant—is shown.

Diagnostic importance of thermal transients is especially clearly visible in Figure 28.16 [18], where different injuries are responding differently to thermal excitation. The line mode of the IR-camera is here applied for fast data registration (>3000 scans/s), allowing reduction of noise.

Based on the same material, the TT procedure and reconstruction of thermal conductivity is also possible [18,54]. Assuming that we know the initial state of the object, the value of excitation flux, thermal response on the surface and spatial distribution of volumetric specific heat within the object it is possible to find the distribution of thermal conductivity:

$$
\left.
\begin{array}{l}
T_m^1, \quad m = 1,\ldots,M \\[4pt]
\Phi_{\text{exc}} \\[4pt]
T_1^p, \quad p = 1,\ldots,P \\[4pt]
\rho c_m, m = 1,\ldots,M
\end{array}
\right\}
\Rightarrow k_m, \quad m = 1,\ldots,M
\tag{28.23}
$$

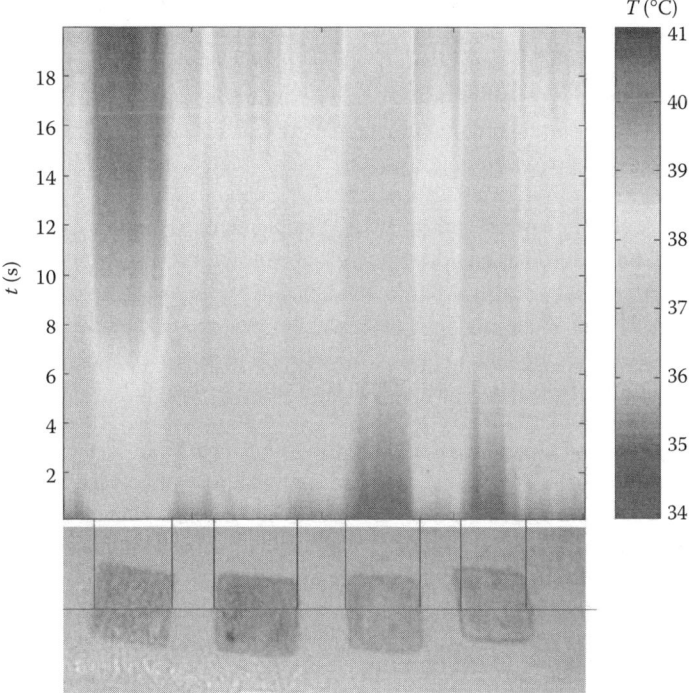

FIGURE 28.16 Thermal transients of burn fields of degree: I, IIa, IIb, IIb.

The inverse problem defined by Equation 28.23 is highly justified due to practical reasons: the volumetric specific heat of biological tissues is much less dependent on water and fat content and other physiological factors than thermal conductivity is (especially effective thermal conductivity, which includes blood perfusion) [45]. Hence, the distribution of $\rho c(x)$ may be regarded with good approximation as known, and irregularities in thermal conductivity distribution should be searched for.

Figure 28.17 presents the results of minimization based on measurements taken during experiments with controlled degree burn fields as it was shown in Figure 28.16. The distribution of specific heat has been assumed identical with the healthy tissue, because of its low dependency on burn [18]. On the reconstructed

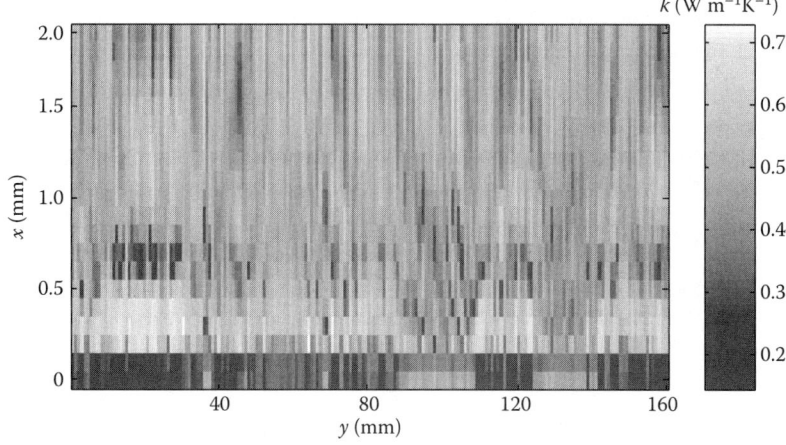

FIGURE 28.17 Results of the reconstruction of thermal conductivity distribution in burn fields.

thermal tomogram, a distinct layered structure of the skin can be seen, as well as the changes in its thermal structure caused by burns. The outermost two slices (0–0.2 mm) represent the epidermis and have thermal conductivity close to 0.3 W m^{-1} K^{-1}, which is almost not affected by burns. Fundamental changes in thermal properties induced by burns may be noticed in the next four slices (0.2–0.5 mm). From the anatomical point of view, this region represents the superficial plexus and adjacent layer of the dermis. As one can expect, for superficial burns we observe increase of k in this region, and decrease of k for severe burns. Based on this observation, quantitative classification criteria can be proposed [18].

For examination of skin burns it seems optimal to implement expression 28.23. It allows obtaining thermal tomography images, which reflect pathologic changes in thermal conductivity distribution up to 2–3 mm.

28.7.3.2 Clinics

We have examined around 100 patients with different skin injuries. Burn injuries were formed in different accidents as a result of flame action directly on skin, hands and faces, and on burning clothes, thorax. The investigations were performed during the first 5 days following an accident. To illustrate the clinical importance of the discussed methods an example of burns caused by an accident is shown in Figure 28.5. The well-determined area of the second-degree burn is evident. The next step—after collecting more clinical data—will be quantitative classification based on data of the burn thickness. Long-lasting effects of treatment and scars formation are still studied and not related here, yet. Already we claim that the value of the thermal time constant taken on the second day after the accident allows quantitative, objective discrimination between IIa and IIb burn [60,61]. More results of skin burns classification using ADT and TT procedures with application of CO_2 external cooling as thermal excitation are in reference [62].

28.7.4 Cardiac Surgery

28.7.4.1 *In Vivo* Experiments on Pigs

Understanding the thermal processes existing during the open chest heart operations is essential for proper surgical interventions, performed for saving the life. Experiments on pigs may be giving answers to several important questions impossible to be responded in clinical situations. This especially may concern sudden heart temperature changes and proper interpretation of the causes.

Clamping the left descending artery and evoking a heart infarct performs the study. Temperature changes have been correlated with the histopathologic observations. The macroscopic thickness of the necrosis was evaluated. This was confirmed by the microscopic data. In Figure 28.18a anatomy of the heart with the clamp is shown. The cross-section line is visible. In the Figure 28.18b the macroscopic cross-section is shown and the evidence of tissue necrosis is by the microscopic histopathology is shown in Figure 28.18c. The widths of the left and right ventricle as well as septum were also measured. The

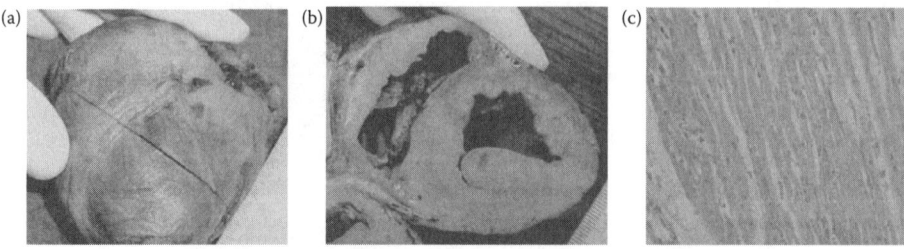

FIGURE 28.18 Pig's heart after heart infarct evoked by the indicated clamp (a), the cross section of the heart with visible area of the stroke (the necrosis of the left ventricle wall—under the finger—is evidenced by darker shadow) (b) and the micro-histopathologic picture showing the cell necrosis (c).

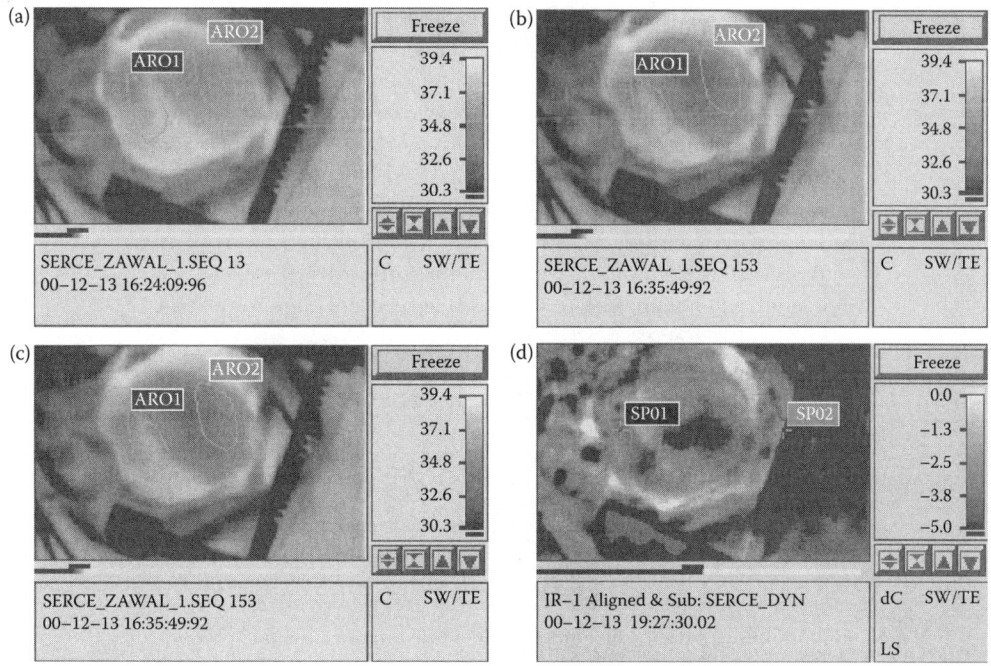

FIGURE 28.19 Thermograms of the heart: before (a) and after the evoked infarct (b). The change of the PT/ADT pictures in time (indicated in the subscript of the thermogram) 0.5 h after the LAD clamping (the tissue is still alive) (c), and 3 h later (the necrosis is evidenced by the change of thermal properties of the tissue) (d).

mass of the necrosis tissue was calculated. The evident correlation between the thickness of the left and right ventricle walls and the thermographic data are found. Thermographic views of this heart are shown in Figure 28.19a,b respectively before and after application of the clamp. The left ventricle wall is cooling faster than the right one as the left ventricle wall thickness is bigger and the heating effect caused by the flowing blood (of the same temperature in both ventricles) is here weaker. The cooling process of the heart caused by stopping the blood flow in LAD is shown in Figure 28.20—the mean temperature changes are indicated in Figure 28.18a, regions AR01 and AR02 are plotted.

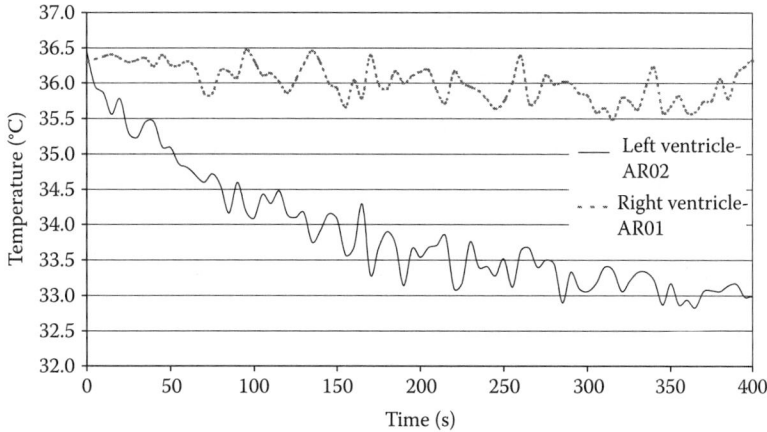

FIGURE 28.20 Temperature changes of the left and right ventricle after the LAD clamping related to Figure 28.19a,b.

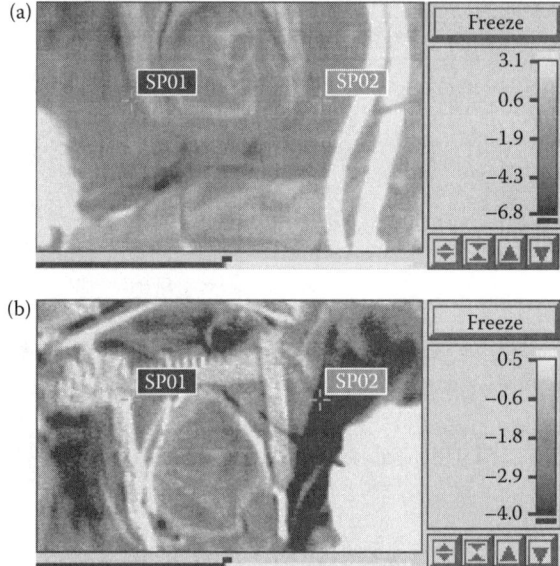

FIGURE 28.21 ADT picture of clinical intervention—before the CABG (a) and after the operation (b). Important is more uniform temperature distribution after the operation proving that intervention was fully successful.

The PT/ADT picture 0.5 h after the clamp was applied (Figure 28.19c) is still showing that thermal properties of the walls are unchanged even the temperature of the left ventricle wall is evidently decreased (Figure 28.19b). Progressing in time the necrosis process is changing thermal tissue properties what is clearly visible after 3 h in Figure 28.19d.

28.7.4.2 Clinics

Operation under extracorporeal circulation is normally a typical clinical situation. Two cases before and after CABG—coronary artery by-pass grafting—are shown for ADT in Figure 28.21a,b respectively. Areas of necrosis and of ischemia as well as volume of the healthy heart muscle were evaluated with respect to coronaroangiographic and radioisotope data showing high correlation. The observations performed before and after CABG show evident recovery of heart functioning. It is evidenced by smaller temperature rise after optical excitation of the heart in the same conditions. ADT shows the level and efficiency of revascularization. The region of heart muscle dysfunction due to heart stroke was possible to be differentiated using both—normal thermography as well as ADT method—what leads to the conclusion that both modalities should be taken into account for diagnostics. The application of thermography for instant evaluation of the quality of the CABG intervention is prompt—the patency of the LIMA—LAD graft is unbeatable by any other method [63], but thermal tissue properties reflecting real state of the tissue is given only by ADT.

Application of all discussed modalities PT, ADT, PPT, and TT during the cardiosurgical interventions gives important indications how to improve surgical procedures.

28.8 Conclusions

The study shows that ADT as well as TT have been successfully used in medical applications giving not only qualitative improvement of diagnostics but in several applications allowing also quantitative evaluation of affected structures.

The importance of active dynamic thermal imaging and thermal tomography applied to burn evaluation and in the inspection of the open chest cardiology interventions was verified. Most probably there are also other attractive fields of medical applications of ADT and TT as, for example, cancer diagnostics [62]. ADT can be applied in medical procedures for monitoring the state of the skin and subdermal tissue structure during burns treatment giving objective, measurable ratings of the treatment procedure. The moment of thermal investigation after an accident is of the highest significance. The most valuable results are obtained during the first and the second days following an accident. The clinical valuable features of the method in skin burns evaluation are the early objective determination of the burn depth—up to two days after an accident and possibility of quantitative evaluation of burn surface and depth as well as objective classification of burn degree. Also, the monitoring role of the method in interoperation of cardiac protection seems to be unbeatable. Changes of tissue vascularization are important for prediction of treatment progress. In all applications, the method is noncontact, noninvasive, clean and nonstressed, allows wide area of investigation and clear and objective documentation of diagnoses and treatment process.

The use of different excitation sources should be limited to those of the best measurement properties. Based on the described experiments most handy are optical sources of irradiation but probably cooling may give even better results in terms of higher signal-to-noise ratio. The operation of such sources is safe, harmless, and easy. The distribution of light may be relatively uniform; the control of irradiated power is also easy.

The work in the field of ADT and TT is still under fast development. Important is extensive IR instrumentation progress giving radical imaging improvement. The problem to be solved is development of a method of noncontact automatic determination of basic properties of thermal parameters of affected tissue what is one of main tasks for the future. Special software is under development for objective and automatic generation of affected tissue depth maps. Important will be to find not only qualitative information but also application of quantitative measures; to describe ratings of the burn wounds or calculate the thickness of affected heart tissues. Still more experiments giving statistically significant knowledge are necessary.

One of important goals is combination of different modalities and application of automatic classification procedures for improved diagnostics. This requires some progress in standardization of IR imaging, which still is not offered in the DICOM standard. For sure, distant consultation of images and automatic data retrieval will be pushing proper work in this field.

Acknowledgments

The author thanks his coworkers and PhD students, who participated in the development of ADT & TT in medicine and who produced the presented data. Most of the reported *in vivo* experiments have been performed with the help of Dr. M. Kaczmarek, Dr. M. Hryciuk, A. Galikowski, and others from the Department of Biomedical Engineering, Gdansk University of Technology. Participation of medical staff: Dr. A. Renkielska and Dr. J. Grudziński (from the Department of Plastic Surgery and Burns), Professor J. Siebert (from the Department of Cardiac Surgery and Cardiology, Medical University of Gdansk) and others are highly appreciated. *In vivo* animal experiments have been performed at the Department of Animal Physiology, Gdansk University with the main assistance of Dr. W. Stojek. Others are listed in the attached bibliography as coauthors of common publications. The work was supported by several grants from KBN (Polish Ministry of Science and Information).

References

1. *Proc. Quantitative InfraRed Thermography:* Chatenay-Malabary-1992, Naples-94, Stuttgart-1996, Lodz-1998, Venice-2000, Reims-2002, Brussels-2004, Dubroynik-2006, Krakow-2008, and Quebec-2010. See also *QIRT Journal*, 2004.
2. Maldague X.P.V. *Theory and Practice of Infrared Technology for Nondestructive Testing*, John Wiley & Sons, Inc., New York, 2001.

3. Van Denhaute E., Ranson W., Cornelis J., Barel A., and Steenhaut O., Contrast enhancement of IR thermographic images by microwave heating in biomedical applications, *Application mikro-und-optolelktronischer Systemelemente*, pp. 71–75, 1985.

4. Steenhaut O., Van Denhaute E., and Cornelis J., Contrast enhancement in IR-thermography by application of microwave irradiation applied to tumor detection, *MECOMBE'86*, pp. 485–488, 1986.

5. Nowakowski A., and Kaczmarek M., Dynamic thermography as a quantitative medical diagnostic tool, *Med. Biol. Eng. Comput. Incorporate Cell. Eng*, 37(Suppl. 1), Part 1, 244–245, 1999.

6. Kaczmarek M., Rumiński J., and Nowakowski A., Measurement of thermal properties of biological tissues—Comparison of different thermal NDT techniques, *Proceedings of the Advanced Infrared Technology and Application*, Venice, 1999, pp. 322–329, 2001.

7. Rumiński J., Kaczmarek M., and Nowakowski A., Data visualization in dynamic thermography, *J. Med. Inform. Technol*, 5, IT29–IT36, 2000.

8. Rumiński J., Nowakowski A., Kaczmarek M., and Hryciuk M., Model-based parametric images in dynamic thermography, *Polish J. Med. Phys. Eng*, 6, 159–164, 2000.

9. Rumiński J., Kaczmarek M., and Nowakowski A., Medical active thermography—A new image reconstruction method, *Lecture Notes in Computer Science*, LNCS 2124, Springer, Berlin, pp. 274–281, 2001.

10. Nowakowski A., Kaczmarek M., and Rumiński J., Synthetic pictures in thermographic diagnostics, *Proceedings of the EMBS-BMES Conference*, CD, Houston, pp. 1131–1132, 2002.

11. Nowakowski A., Kaczmarek M., Rumiński J., Hryciuk M., Renkielska A., Grudziński J., Siebert J. et al., Medical applications of model based dynamic thermography, Thermosense XIII, Orlando, *Proc. SPIE*, 4360, 492–503, 2001.

12. Sakagami T., Kubo S., Naganuma T., Inoue T., Matsuyama K., and Kaneko K., Development of a new diagnosis method for caries in human teeth based on thermal images under pulse heating, Thermosense XIII, Orlando, *Proc. SPIE*, 4360, 511–515, 2001.

13. Vavilov V., and Shirayev V., Thermal Tomograph—USSR Patent no. 1.266.308, 1985.

14. Vavilov V.P., Kourtenkov D., Grinzato E., Bison P., Marinetti S., and Bressan C., Inversion of experimental data and thermal tomography using "Thermo Heat" and "Termidge" Software, *Proc. QIRT '94*, 273–278, 1994.

15. Vavilov V.P., 1D–2D–3D transition conditions in transient IR thermographic NDE, *Seminar 64—Quantitative Infra-Red Thermography—QIRT'2000*, Reims, 74, 2000. http://qirt.gel.ulaval.ca/dynamique/index.php?idD=45.

16. Hryciuk M., Nowakowski A., and Renkielska A., Multi-layer thermal model of healthy and burned skin, *Proc. 2nd European Medical and Biological Engineering Conference*, EMBEC'02, Vol. 3, Pt. 2., pp. 1614–1617, Vienna, 2002.

17. Nowakowski A., Kaczmarek M., and Hryciuk M., Tomografia Termiczna, pp. 615–696, in Chmielewski L., Kulikowski J.L., and Nowakowski A., *Obrazowanie Biomedyczne* (Biomedical Imaging—*in Polish*) Biocybernetyka i Inżynieria Biomedyczna 2000, 8, Akademicka Oficyna Wydawnicza EXIT, Warszawa, 2003.

18. Hryciuk M., Badanie struktury biologicznych obiektów warstwowych z wykorzystaniem pobudzenia cieplnego (PhD Dissertation—Investigation of layered biological object structure using thermal excitation, *in Polish*), *Politechnika Gdanska*, 2003.

19. Kaczmarek M., Nowakowski A., and Renkielska A., Rating burn wounds by dynamic thermography, in D. Balageas, J. Beaudoin, G. Busse, and G. Carlomagno, eds., *Quantitative InfraRed Thermography* 5, pp. 376–381, Reims, 2000. http://qirt.gel.ulaval.ca/dynamique/index.php?idD=45.

20. Kaczmarek M., Nowakowski A., Renkielska A., Grudziński J., and Stojek W., Investigation of skin burns based on active thermography, *Proc. 23rd Annual International Conference IEEE EMBS*, CD-ROM, Istanbul, 2001.

21. Nowakowski A, Kaczmarek M., Wtorek J., Siebert J., Jagielak D., Roszak K., and Topolewicz J., Thermographic and electrical measurements for cardiac surgery inspection, *Proc. of 23rd Annual International Conference IEEE EMBS*, CD-ROM, Istanbul, 2001.

22. Nowakowski A., Kaczmarek M., Hryciuk M., and Rumiński J., *Postépy termografii–aplikacje medyczne,* Wyd. Gdańskie (Advances of Thermography–Medical Applications, *in Polish*), Gdańsk, 2001.
23. Hryciuk M. and Nowakowski A., Multi-layer thermal model of healthy and burned skin, *Proc. 2nd European Medical and Biological Engineering Conference,* EMBEC'02, Vol. 3, Pt. 2., pp. 1614–1617, Vienna, 2002.
24. Hryciuk M., and Nowakowski A., Evaluation of thermal diffusivity variations in multi-layered structures, *Proc. 6 QIRT,* Zagreb, pp. 267–274, 2003.
25. Kaczmarek M. and Nowakowski A., Analysis of transient thermal processes for improved visualization of breast cancer using IR imaging, *Proc. IEEE EMBC,* Cancun, pp. 1113–1116, 2003.
26. Kaczmarek M., Modelowanie właściwości tkanek ż ywych dla potrzeb termografii dynamicznej, PhD dissertation—Modeling of living tissue properties for dynamic thermography, *in Polish,* Politechnika Gdańska, 2003.
27. Chato J.C., A method for the measurement of the thermal properties of biological materials, thermal problems in biotechnology, *ASME Symp,* Philadelphia, Pennsylvania, pp. 16–25, 1968.
28. Bowman H.F., Cravalho E.G., and Woods M., Theory, measurement and application of thermal properties of biomaterials, *Ann. Rev. Biophys. Bioeng,* 4, 43–80, 1975.
29. Chen M.M., Holmes K.R., and Rupinskas V., Pulse-decay method for measuring the thermal conductivity of living tissues, *J. Biomech. Eng,* 103, 253–260, 1981.
30. Balasubramaniam T.A. and Bowman H.F., Thermal conductivity and thermal diffusivity of biomaterials: A simultaneous measurement technique, *J. Biomech. Eng,* 99, 148–154, 1977.
31. Shitzer A. and Eberhart R.C., *Heat Transfer in Medicine and Biology,* Vols. 1, 2, Plenum Press, New York, London, 1985.
32. Balageas D.L., Characterization of living tissues from the measurement of thermal effusivity, *Innov. Tech. Biol. Med,* 12, 145–153, 1991.
33. Valvano J.W., Cochran J.R., and Diller K.R., Thermal conductivity and diffusivity of biomaterials measured with self-heating thermistors, *Int. J. Thermophys,* 6, 301–311, 1985.
34. Marks R.M., and Barton S.P., *The Physical Nature of the Skin,* Boston, MTP Press, 1998.
35. Janna W.S., *Engineering Heat Transfer,* CRC Press, Washington, DC, 2000.
36. Pennes H.H., Analysis of tissue and arterial blood temperatures in the resting human forearm, *J. Appl. Physiol,* 1, 93–122, 1948.
37. IDEAS operating manual.
38. NASTRAN operating manual.
39. MATLAB operating manual.
40. Mathematica operating manual.
41. Salerno A., Dillenz A., Wu D., Rantala J., and Busse G., Progress in ultrasound lock-in thermography, *Proc. QIRT '98,* pp. 154–160, Lodz, 1998.
42. Maldague X., and Marinetti S., Pulse phase thermography, *J. Appl. Phys,* 79(5), 2694–2698, 1996.
43. Nowakowski A., Kaczmarek M., and Dêbicki P., Active thermography with microwave excitation, D. Balageas, J., Beaudoin, G., Busse, G., and Carlomagno, G., eds., *Quantitative InfraRed Thermography,* Vol. 5, pp. 387–392, 2000. http://qirt.gel.ulaval.ca/dynamique/index.php?idD=45.
44. Nowakowski A., Kaczmarek M., Renkielska A., Grudziński J., and Stojek J., Heating or cooling to increase contrast in thermographic diagnostics, *Proc. EMBS-BMES Conference,* CD, Houston, pp. 1137–1138, 2002.
45. Duck A.F., *Physical Properties of Tissue,* Academic Press, London, 1990.
46. Ring E.F.J., Standardization of thermal imaging technique, *Thermology Oesterrich,* 3, 11–13, 1993.
47. Rumiński J., Kaczmarek M., Nowakowski A., Hryciuk M., and Werra W., Differential analysis of medical images in dynamic thermography, *Proc. V National Conference on Application of Mathematics in Biology and Medicine,* Zawoja, pp. 126–131, 1999.
48. Nowakowski A., Kaczmarek M., and Rumiński J., Synthetic pictures in thermographic diagnostics, *Proc. EMBS-BMES Conf,* 2002, CD, pp. 1131–1132, Houston, 2002.

49. Kaczmarek M., Nowakowski A., and Renkielska A., Rating burn wounds by dynamic thermography, D. Balageas, J. Beaudoin, G. Busse, and G. Carlomagno, eds., *Quantitative InfraRed Thermography*, Vol. 5, pp. 376–381, 2000. http://qirt.gel.ulaval.ca/dynamique/index.php?idD=45.

50. Kaczmarek M., Rumiński J., Nowakowski A., Renkielska A., Grudziński J., and Stojek W., In-vivo experiments for evaluation of new diagnostic procedures in medical thermography, *Proceedings of 6th International Conference on Quantitative Infrared thermography, Proc. Quantitative Infrared Thermography 6-QIRT'02*, pp. 260–266, Zagreb, 2003.

51. Ibarra-Castanedo C., and Maldague X., Pulsed phase thermography reviewed, *QIRT J*, 1(1), 47–70, 2004.

52. Hryciuk M., and Nowakowski A., Multilayer thermal model of healthy and burned skin, *Proc. 2nd European Medical and Biological Engineering Conference*, EMBEC'02, Vol. 3, Pt. 2, pp. 1614–1617, Vienna, 2002.

53. Hryciuk M. and Nowakowski A., Evaluation of thermal diffusivity variations in multi-layered structures, *Proceedings of 6th International Conference on Quantitative Infrared thermography, Proc. Quantitative Infrared Thermography 6-QIRT'02*, pp. 267–274, Zagreb, 2003.

54. Hryciuk M. and Nowakowski A., Formulation of inverse problem in thermal tomography for burns diagnostics, *Proc. SPIE*, 5505, 11–18, 2004.

55. Kaczmarek M., Rumiński J., and Nowakowski A., Data processing methods for dynamic medical thermography, *Proceedings of International Federation for Medical and Biological Engineering*, EMBEC'02, pp. 1098–1099, Vienna, 2002.

56. Nowakowski A., Kaczmarek M., Siebert J., Rogowski J., Jagielak D., Roszak K., Topolewicz J., and Stojek W., Role of thermographic inspection in cardiosurgery, *Proc. Int. Federation for Medical and Biological Engineering*, EMBEC'02, pp. 1626–1627, Vienna, 2002.

57. Kaczmarek M. and Nowakowski A., Analysis of transient thermal processes for improved visualization of breast cancer using IR imaging, *25th Annual International Conference of the IEEE Engineering in Medicine and Biology Society* "A New Beginning for Human Health," Cancun, Mexico, CD, 2003.

58. Singer A.J., Berruti L., Thode HC J.R., and McClain S.A., Standardized burn model using a multiparametric histologic analysis of burn depth. *Academic Emergency Medicine*, 7(1), 1–6, 2000.

59. Eberhart C. *Heat Transfer in Medicine and Biology, Analysis and Applications*, Vol. 1. Plenum Press, London, 1985.

60. Renkielska A., Nowakowski A., Kaczmarek M., Ruminski J., Burn depths evaluation based on active dynamic IR thermal imaging—A preliminary study, *Burns*, 32(7), 867–875, 2006.

61. Rumiński J., Kaczmarek M., Renkielska A., Nowakowski A., Thermal parametric imaging in the evaluation of skin burn depth, *IEEE Transactions on Biomedical Engineering*, 54(2), 303–312, 2007.

62. Nowakowski A. et al., Rozwój diagnostyki termicznej metodami detekcji podczerwieni (ilościowa diagnostyka ran oparzeniowych i inne aplikacje), in *Polish*, EXIT, Warszawa, 2009.

63. Kaczmarek M., Nowakowski A., Suchowirski M., Siebert J., Stojek W., Active dynamic thermography in cardiosurgery, *QIRT J.*, 4(1), 107–123, 2007.

29

Dynamic Thermal Assessment

Michael Anbar
*University at Buffalo, State
University of New York*

29.1 Introduction

The purpose of this chapter is not just to summarize studies on dynamic thermal assessment (DTA) [aka *dynamic infrared imaging* (DIRI) or *dynamic thermal imaging* (DTI)] published since 1987, but to present this topic from a general, critical perspective, focusing on studies published since 2000, which have significantly extended the scope of this promising biomedical technique. The latter most interesting achievements have not been reviewed up-to-date in the context of DTI. This chapter is not a tutorial on DTI or DTA, replicating previously published reviews. Interested readers are, therefore, encouraged to consult appropriate review papers pointed out below. Further, since this chapter is likely to be the last first-hand account of the history of DTI, written by the person who conceptualized and initiated this field of endeavor, it will include historical details that were not published before. The nature of this chapter also allows the author to include personal views on some of the topics discussed.

To bring readers up to speed, they must understand the concept of DTA as compared with classical *static thermal imaging*. Whereas the former methodology monitors or quantitatively measures temporal *changes* in temperature over areas of interest, the latter technique involves observation of temperature distribution over such areas. Thermal changes can be *monotonic*—warming or cooling of areas of interest or parts thereof—or they can be *periodic*, manifested as temperature *modulation*. Monitoring of either kind of temperature change over an area can be done just by one kind of technology—using infrared cameras, preferably in the 8–12 μm range, to monitor the blackbody radiation of the areas of interest. Consequently, one can describe this technique as dynamic *infrared* monitoring or *DIRI*.

In brief, whenever we use in this review the terms DTI or DTA, it is implied that the measurement of temperature was done remotely using infrared detection.

Certain clinical applications of DTI have been monitoring monotonic temperature changes—warming of organs following a cold challenge, following surgical reperfusion, or cooling of organs following perfusion with a cold fluid (used occasionally in cardiac surgery). Such slow monotonic warming or cooling processes can be visually monitored in real time. This is one kind of DTI—display of sequential thermal images over a period of time to be observed visually. These sequential observations can also be represented by single images of the *rates* of gradual temperature change, which may be different for different subareas of the region of interest (ROI). The spatial distribution of rates over the ROI can be displayed on color-coded bitmaps.

Physiological processes that affect the temperature of live surfaces (e.g., skin, cornea, or the surface of the brain) are generally *periodic*, resulting in *temperature modulation*. Observing gradual warming of biological surfaces ignores the minute underlying modulations and averages them out. However, those minute modulations, which generally require higher precision of temperature measurement, convey important physiological information. Moreover, those modulations can be monitored when no gross changes in average surface temperature take place. In fact, the use of DTI in this mode, with no prior thermal challenge, is generally far more informative, as it monitors physiology noninvasively under *undisturbed* conditions.

Quantitative assessment of temperature modulation requires accumulation of hundreds or even thousands of sequential thermal images acquired at a significantly higher rate than the frequencies of the physiological or pathophysiological temperature modulation monitored. Presented generally to the end user is the spatial distribution of amplitudes of temperature modulation at discrete frequencies or range of frequencies. This modulation amplitude versus frequency presentation is derived from fast Fourier transformation (FFT) of the observed periodic temperature changes. This spatial distribution can be displayed as color bitmaps of *amplitudes* distribution or of the *microhomogeneity of amplitude* distribution [1], at a given frequency or range of frequencies. These can then be visually spatially correlated with anatomical features over the ROI.

With the exception of real-time continuous DTI, generally used in surgical intraoperative applications, DTI "images" do not represent spatial distribution of infrared radiation flux or of temperature, but are a computerized presentation of periodic temperature *changes*. Furthermore, certain applications of "DIRI" that monitor well-defined anatomical features, requiring no anatomic spatial correlation, do not require display of any images altogether. Thus the term "imaging" in these cases is an utter misnomer.

Notwithstanding semantic finesse, while discussing DTA, we will often use the term "DTI" interchangeably with DTA, because "*thermal* imaging," that is, imaging of thermal phenomena, which are generally *dynamic*, is distinct from classical *static* thermographic "*temperature* imaging."

29.2 Biomedical Dynamic Thermal Assessment

29.2.1 Early History

Dynamic thermal assessment (DTA) was conceptualized in the late 1980s by Michael Anbar [2–5]. Anbar discovered that rapid *changes* in human skin temperature convey valuable physiological and pathophysiological information, information that cannot be derived from static temperature mapping (i.e., measurement of temperature distribution over areas of skin). These ideas crystallized further on the basis of rudimentary experimental studies in the early 1990s [1,6–18].

Since under physiological conditions the temperature of skin depends on blood supply to cutaneous and subcutaneous tissues, blood being the heat exchange fluid, skin temperature manifests a variety of hemodynamic processes. These processes are modulated by pulsatile cardiogenic changes in blood flow as well as by neuronal control of blood flow in the vasculature and microvasculature. Since blood perfusion affects skin temperature differently at different areas of skin, depending on the underlying vascular anatomy, assessment of these processes requires repeated temperature imaging of ROI at frequencies higher than the highest frequency of measurable blood supply modulation. In brief, DTI of ROI can provide new information on the anatomy of the vasculature, on systemic changes in blood flow due to both heart function and neuronal systemic and local control of vascular blood flow and perfusion of the capillary bed.

In addition to useful anatomic and physiologic information, DTI can also be clinically useful. Pathologies that affect any anatomic or physiologic parameters of blood supply can be diagnosed by this technique. For these discoveries Anbar was awarded the President's Award of the American Academy of Thermology for 1990.

The only thermometric technique that can attain the spatial resolution, thermal sensitivity, and speed of data acquisition of skin temperature is infrared imaging with a large ($\Box 256 \times 256$) solid-state detector array in the 8–12 μm range (temperature can be measured also by infrared sensors in the 3–5 μm range—however, at a significantly lower sensitivity and subject to substantial reflectivity artifacts). In the early 1990s, infrared detection technology was still in its infancy (multidetector two-dimensional arrays were still on the drawing board) and thus it could not meet the requirement of a practical dynamic diagnostic technique. Anbar's early experiments were, therefore, rudimentary, far from offering a practical solution to any clinical problem. Medical technology had to wait, therefore, for additional developments in infrared detection and image-processing technologies.

29.2.2 "Quantitative Dynamic Area Telethermometry in Medical Diagnosis and Management": An Imaginative Speculative Treatise

In 1994, Anbar summarized his ideas and preliminary experimental research in this new field in a monograph titled *Quantitative Dynamic Area Telethermometry in Medical Diagnosis and Management* [19]. The term "area telethermometry" was used to distinguish remote, noncontact, infrared thermal imaging from the, now obsolete, contact thermometric imaging methods (e.g., liquid crystals, thermistor arrays). Today, the term "thermal imaging" implies *infrared* imaging. That monograph described the scientific background of this imaging technique, which is uniquely suited for dynamic applications.

The book projected a large variety of clinical applications that would be feasible using DTI.

It describes potential clinical uses of DTA in a variety of neurological disorders that affect circulatory behavior and/or cutaneous perfusion. These include carpal tunnel syndrome and Raynaud's syndrome, complex regional pain syndrome (earlier named "reflex sympathetic dystrophy"), back pain and leg pain due to spinal stenosis or herniation, as well as migraines and other headaches involving vasospasms.

Among other neurological effects that can be monitored by DTI the book describes sympathetic nervous response to mental stress. The latter entails numerous potential clinical applications in psychiatry both as a diagnostic as well as therapeutic tool (using biofeedback). DTI could as well effectively monitor mental stress induced by deception ("lie detection"). Since sympathetic vasoconstriction or vasodilation are much more sensitive manifestations of mental stress than perspiration, Anbar suggested that remote monitoring of subjects by DTI (which also readily measures heart rate) is likely to be a far more effective "lie detector" than the best of polygraphs.

Vascular disorders are the next group of clinical applications of DTI discussed in the book. These include occlusions (including peripheral vascular occlusive disease) and aneurysms, as well as vascular effects of diabetes. Anbar suggested that DTI could distinguish between diabetic neuropathies and diabetic vascular occlusive disease, helping optimize treatment of diabetes mellitus.

Then Anbar's book discusses how DTI can be useful in the differential diagnosis and monitoring of treatment of inflammatory processes, including rheumatic disease, local infections, and burns.

Potential surgical applications of DTI are the next topic discussed in the 1994 book. These include monitoring of reperfusion of transplanted organs (e.g., kidneys) and of the heart following cardioplegia in open heart surgery, reperfusion of skin grafts and skin flaps in plastic surgery, and monitoring reperfusion following reconnection of blood vessels and of intestines or in colostomy. It also suggests the use of DTI in monitoring anesthesia.

Quantitative Dynamic Area Telethermometry suggests the use of DTI to monitor metabolic processes also at the cellular level. Metabolic processes are either endothermic or exothermic. At the cellular level they are periodical, that is, oscillatory, owing to thermal and nonthermal autocatalysis, as well as because of the complex interactive kinetics of diffusion of nutrients, oxygen, and metabolites through cellular membranes and cytoplasm. Anbar suggested to monitor the metabolism of mammalian cells in tissue cultures and thus rapidly detect, using DTI, changes in cellular metabolism (a physiological approach) due to the effect of antimetabolites or toxins, instead of waiting for the effects manifested in replication (essentially an anatomic approach).

Clinical applications of the cellular DTI methodology include rapid evaluation of the effect of chemotherapeutic agents on cells extracted by biopsy from malignant tumors, rapid evaluation of the effect of antigens on such cells, and rapid evaluation of their radiation sensitivity. Another potential clinical application of DTI discussed in the book was rapid determination of the sensitivity of bacteria or fungi to antibiotics, without the needed follow-up *in vitro* of proliferation of such pathogens.

A preliminary study done at the University at Buffalo by the author in collaboration with Dr. Malcolm Slaughter indicates the feasibility of cellular DTI. In a study on the thermal behavior of live retinal neurons *in vitro*, retinas of newts were isolated and their thermal behavior was dynamically observed with the aid of a 1:1 germanium macro lens (AIM, Infrarot Module, Heilbrunn, Germany). The study tried to find out if temperature modulation of the neurons (four neurons per pixel), due to cellular metabolism, observed in the 2–8 Hz range, was altered by pulsed light stimulation. The findings were positive though not sufficiently reproducible because of experimental limitations (mainly spatial resolution at 256×256 pixels). However, this has been the first attempt to monitor *in vitro* cellular metabolism by DTI. Commercially available equipment with 16 times higher spatial resolution could be used today to verify DTI's potential in this field.

Cellular DTI could be extended to detection of viral infection of cells in tissue cultures because the metabolism of affected cells changes dramatically owing to the effect of the virus on their transcriptive apparatus. Cellular DTI could be much faster than radiotracer uptake studies. This might allow rapid detection of viruses and testing the effectiveness of antiviral drugs. Although Anbar discussed in his book the use of DTI for detecting viral infections *in vivo*, due to their effect on macrophages, which locally generate nitric oxide (NO) very much like cancerous cells (see below), he overlooked, at the time, this potentially highly important *in vitro* application of cellular DTI in clinical virology. This is, therefore, a new idea whose time will hopefully come soon.

Among the most exciting of the potential clinical applications of DTI discussed by Anbar were those related to oncology. Neoplastic lesions are generally associated with angiogenesis and subsequent local hypervascularization. This by itself must produce aberration in the local anatomy of perfusion. Moreover, newly formed neoplastic blood vessels are likely to be sparsely innervated, if at all, and therefore their response to neuronal vascular control is likely to be abnormal and therefore detectable by DTI, which monitors neuronal modulation of vascular flow. However, even a more specific feature of neoplastic lesions from the standpoint of potential detection and management of cancer by DTI is their generation of NO.

Back in 1978, Anbar has discovered that humans and other mammals produce and carry measurable amounts of endogenic NO in their blood [20]. The physiologic function of this highly reactive substance was unknown at the time and remained unknown until the late 1980s and early 1990s, when it was shown to be a neurotransmitter that induces vasodilatation [21–23]. Since it had been well documented that neoplastic disease is associated with local hyperthermia of the overlying skin, Anbar showed in 1994 by quantitative analysis that this phenomenon must be associated with local vasodilatation [24]. He then advanced a hypothesis that this manifestation of neoplasms is due to generation of NO by cancerous tissues.

He showed that this abnormality of neoplastic cells gives them a substantial advantage over normal cells by enhancing blood supply to the neoplastic tissue (before it induces angiogenesis) and by enhancing potential metastasis [25]. This hypothesis has been experimentally corroborated independently already in 1994 in different types of cancerous cell lines [26–28].

Since it was known by 1994 that NO is a chemical messenger in regulation of vascular tone, Anbar speculated that NO produced by cancerous lesions will interfere with vasomotor regulation of perfusion. Thus Anbar's hypothesis predicted that not only will cancerous lesions enhance regional vascular perfusion but also that perfusion in the surrounding tissues will not be normally modulated. The corollary of this hypothesis is that DTI might detect the effect of cancer-produced NO on the neuronal modulation of perfusion, and thereby detect cancerous lesions more effectively than by just monitoring local hyperthermia. A recent thermographic study confirmed Anbar's conclusion that breast-cancer-induced hyperthermia is not due to local hypervascularity [29], and it must, therefore, be associated with local vasodilatation.

An important parameter conceptualized by Anbar and described in his monograph is the micro-homogeneity of temperature modulation or spatial thermal homogeneity (STH = 1/SD (standard deviation) of temperature values of spots in a given subarea) [1]. Quantitative DTI can also measure the modulation of local homogeneity of subareas at any given frequency or range of frequencies. The latter parameter measures the level of perfusion of a given subcutaneous region: that is, when the region's perfusion reaches a maximum so does the microhomogeneity.

Finally, another novel concept highlighted by Anbar already in 1994 was the direct *objective* use of digital data in clinical diagnosis. DTI is essentially not an anatomic imaging technique but a physiological one. It produces its findings on the oscillatory behavior of the temperature of biological surfaces in terms of frequencies and their relative amplitudes (following FFT, as demonstrated by Anbar in 1991). DTI expresses pathology or biological abnormalities as frequency–amplitude aberrations, analogously to electrocardiogram (ECG) or electroencephalogram (EEG). When these aberrations are monitored over large areas of skin their spatial distribution can be bitmapped, color coded, and visually evaluated by the human eye. However, these are not images of temperature but images of the distribution of temperature *changes*. This is the only meeting point between DTI and anatomy. Now, in many clinical applications the anatomical information is absolutely unnecessary, because the physiological data contain all the diagnostics information. As these data are digital to begin with, they can be processed further to provide *objective* diagnostic measures of pathology, or of the probability of pathology. DTI can therefore become a forerunner of computerized medicine in the twenty-first century.

In brief, at the risk of repetition, it must be concluded that in spite of its common name, DTI is essentially not an imaging technique. Clinical imaging techniques require always evaluation of images by experts to achieve a diagnosis. DTA is, therefore, more than an imaging technique.

Back in 1994, all these scores of novel-computerized clinical applications were essentially just a glimpse in the eye of the author. At that time, this well-documented, scientific book with hundreds of references was still not far from being good science fiction, because none of the applications envisioned there had been reduced to practice. Like Jules Verne in his time or Arthur Clarke, Anbar recognized the potential of a new technology in an entirely different field. In this case it was infrared imaging, which was likely to rapidly develop so to meet emerging needs of military surveillance and targeting. Anbar foresaw that this technology will meet the sensitivity and speed requirements of clinically useful DTI. Also computational speed and computer memory available in 1994 were insufficient to process DTI data in any practical manner. This did not deter Anbar from projecting that these will be available when infrared technology will meet DTI requirements. Many of these "dreams" were realized within less than a decade.

After publicizing his new ideas on DTA [30,31], and extending the ideas on the mechanism of breast cancer hyperthermia [25,32], Anbar advanced a hypothesis on the role of NO in pathophysiological pain, explaining the mechanism of hyperthermia associated with pain [33,34]. Yet all these plausible speculations awaited experimental verification.

29.2.2.1 Hypothesis on the Effect of Cancer on Perfusion Confirmed

Anbar's hypothesis that NO generated in neoplastic cells affects vascular behavior in the vicinity of solid tumor has been confirmed already in the following 3 years [35–39]. The role of NO in cancer biology has been demonstrated in breast cancer [40–42], cancer of the colon [43–45], squamous cell carcinomas of the head and neck [46–48], brain malignancies [49–52], melanoma [53–55], lung cancer [56–58], cancer of the prostate [59], ovarian cancer [60], cancer of the pancreas [61], chondrosarcoma [62], cancer of the bladder [63,64; see, however, 65], and gastric cancer [66,67]. In brief, the production of NO in malignant tissues has been well established, corroborating Anbar's prediction [24,25], as has been its vasodilatatory effect. (For a more detailed discussion see the introduction in Reference 68.)

What remained to be demonstrated was to what extent can the specific effect of solid tumors on the modulation of tissue perfusion be detected at skin level by DTI, refining the information on the tumor-associated local skin hyperthermia (an effect that has been well known for decades—although its mechanism remained obscure before the NO mechanism has been elucidated) [24].

29.2.3 Considering the Realities

The 1994 publication of Anbar's monograph was a landmark in the history of DTI, but this technique would have been forgotten if not for his research efforts to make his dream come through. In making DTI a practical technique one must consider its scope and limitations.

After discussing the wide scope of DTI's potential applications, we must also consider the limitations of this technique when applied to the live human body. It must be realized that because of the very high absorption coefficient of skin tissue to photons in the 8–10 μm range, blackbody radiation emitted from the skin and detectable by infrared cameras represents the temperature of a layer less than 0.1 mm thick of skin. Since no temperature changes can occur intrinsically within that thin skin layer, any modulation in local skin temperature of the upper layer of skin represents temperature modulation of subcutaneous tissues, including blood vessels, conducted to the skin's surface. The modulation of skin temperature is due to modulation of perfusion of the subcutaneous capillary bed as well as modulation of blood flow through vessels in proximity of the skin. These modulations are driven by two processes—cardiogenic pulses and neurological modulation of the vascular tone (i.e., vasodilatation and vasoconstriction). Locally elevated or lower temperature due to hypermetabolism or hypometabolism of tissues, respectively, or to environmental factors, are not expected to manifest any modulation below 0.001 Hz and will not be detectable by appropriately programmed computerized DTI.

Further, modulation of perfusion of tissues or vasculature situated deep (>10 mm) below the skin is unlikely to be detectable at skin level because of heat dissipation, which results in impedance of the modulated thermal signal. The latter effect will result in blurred modulated images of deep vessels detectable at skin level; the deeper the vessel the more blurred will be its modulated thermal image until it fades into the background. Since the impedance of temperature modulation increases with frequency, only low-frequency modulation of heat sources situated deep under the skin will be detectable at skin level. It can be expected that temperature modulation of heat sources below, say, 10 mm, will not be detectable at all at skin level even if unmodulated skin temperature might be higher in a given area due to a low-lying heat source. The level of detectable modulation depends obviously on the precision of temperature measurement. The higher the precision the more sensitive will be the detection of modulation due to perfusion of deeper structures.

In brief, the higher the frequency of the modulation the more pronounced will be the attenuation of the heat-dissipated signals. Consequently, we expect to detect high-frequency modulation (>1 Hz) only of modulated cutaneous microvasculature or over superficially situated large vessels. However, temperature modulation of large vessels will be predominantly driven by cardiogenic pulses with only minor effects of vasodilatation or vasoconstriction that occur at other frequencies. In any case, temperature modulation at the skin surface is necessarily a biased representation of the modulation of subcutaneous tissue perfusion. While modulation frequencies >2 Hz can occasionally be detectable at skin surface (excluding FFT artifactual harmonics of cardiac pulsation) most useful DTI information is expected in the below the 2 Hz frequency region. These may include low-frequency waves due to reflection and interference of cardiogenic waves and to beats of interference between higher frequency neurogenic vasoconstriction or vasodilatation modulations.

It must be concluded, therefore, that assessment of perfusion dynamics by DTI is rather limited in spite of the relative simplicity of measurement, and more precise information on perfusion dynamics of deeper tissues might be obtained by other technologies, such as laser Doppler flowmetry, Doppler ultrasound, or MRI. Yet all the basic predictions developed by Anbar regarding the diagnostic usefulness of monitoring *modulation* of blood perfusion (described above) are valid irrespective of the monitoring technique. It must also be realized that the limitations on DTI of skin do not apply to DTI of cells in tissue cultures or of microorganisms.

29.3 DTA Experimentation (1997–2001)

29.3.1 Early DTA Experimentation

Modulation of skin temperature due to hemodynamic effects is of the order of 10 mK [69], which requires a precision of temperature measurement better than 2 mK. If the hemodynamic modulation frequencies of interest are 2–10 Hz, a data acquisition rate of at least 100 Hz is required as is a stability of 1 mK over >30 min—the duration of a complete multi-image DTI study [70]. Anbar's attempts from 1992 till mid-1997 to experimentally use different commercial infrared camera systems available at that time to verify basic concepts of quantitative DTA on human subjects have ended with ambiguous results because of the inadequate sensitivity, reproducibility, and speed of those systems. None of those failed experiments were published.

Finally, by the end of 1996 Anbar became aware of the new type of fast and sensitive Ga/As 256 × 256 array quantum-well infrared photodetectors (QWIP) developed by Gunapala et al. [71,72] at the Jet Propulsion Laboratory (JPL) in Pasadena. The availability of a sensitive 256 × 256 focal plane detector array has been a minimal prerequisite for meaningful DTA biomedical applications. At the time, that camera could be transferred to and used in a DOD laboratory only. Consequently, Anbar joined Dr. Kaveh Zamani at the Walter Reed Army Institute of Research (WRAIR) in Washington DC and explored a variety of potential biomedical uses of DTA with this unique camera.

These studies included demonstration of monitoring cardiac pulsatile hemodynamics and measurement of blood flow rate in peripheral vasculature [69,73], and demonstration of DTA use in assessment of cutaneous lesions and neuropathies caused by chemicals and of observation of significant changes in facial perfusion under mental stress [74]. Shortly later, DTI was also applied, though with less advanced equipment, to study joint inflammation and pain, presumably mediated by NO [75–77].

Following the promising preliminary findings at WRAIR, Dr. Gunapala loaned his camera to facilitate preliminary DTI clinical studies at Buffalo. At the Erie County Hospital, in collaboration with Dr. William Flynn of the Department of Surgery, Anbar demonstrated the effective use of DTI in assessment of microsurgical attachment of a severed penis. Then, in collaboration with Dr. Kenneth Eckert, he demonstrated, at the Windsong Clinic of Buffalo, the use of DTA in assessment of hemodynamic behavior of cancerous breasts [78]. These brief preliminary demonstration studies with borrowed equipment confirmed the potential usefulness of DTA in the clinic. The conclusions of these preliminary findings were then summarized in review papers that pointed out the instrumental and software requirements of this technique [70,79–81].

29.3.2 Research at the Millard Fillmore Hospital at Buffalo

By 1999 Anbar received from a company (OmniCorder Technologies Inc., now Advanced Biophotonics Inc., East Setauket, New York) a state-of-the-art commercial fast digital infrared camera with a QWIP 8–9 μm 256 × 256 detector array, operating at a rate of 100 frames/s (AIM, Infrarot Module, Heilbrunn, Germany). That camera incorporated a highly reliable and stable Stirling helium cooler, which is essential for meaningful DTA studies (because of the high temperature dependence of the sensitivity of QWIP detectors). Anbar received this camera, placed at the Millard Fillmore University Hospital in Buffalo, for experimental DTA studies on breast cancer.

The goal of the research project at Buffalo was twofold:

1. Develop algorithms that will *objectively* differentiate between cancerous and cancer-free breasts without the need for human expertise of "reading" bitmaps of DTI modulation amplitudes. In other words, alleviate *imaging* from DTI and make it a genuine DTA-computerized technique. DTI, which is essentially a wholly computerized technique, which produces FFT-generated modulation amplitude spectra for each pixel of the image, lends itself uniquely to the latter end when the whole organ in question, or well-defined regions of it, are treated as an anatomically undifferentiated ROI [68,70,82].

2. Establish the feasibility of using the algorithms developed meeting the first goal to *objectively* detect breast cancer in patients who have had suspicious x-ray mammograms before undergoing exploratory biopsy, that is, to distinguish between true- and false-positive x-ray mammograms; the DTA findings were to be compared with the pathology of calcified biopsied tissue as the "gold standard."

Using algorithms developed by Dr. Lorin Milescu [83,84], Anbar's group studied DTI data of a total of 100 breasts, 64 free of cancer and 36 with biopsy-confirmed breast cancers (three DTI views were taken for each breast), of patients examined at the Millard Fillmore Hospital at Buffalo and at the Department of Radiology, University Hospital and Medical Center at Stony Brook, New York [68,85]. That was the first study to demonstrate the potential use of DTA as an *objective* quantitative diagnostic technique. Because of this and since this may be the last time this study will be reviewed in the general context of DTA, we shall include here certain clarifying details and somewhat newer and more effective computational analysis procedures used in the last phase of this 3-year research effort.

To summarize, the objective of that study was to demonstrate that DTA can effectively differentiate between cancerous breasts (irrespective of the type of the cancer) and breasts free of cancer. Once this objective has been achieved, a follow-on study would have had to use the criteria developed in the first study to test the effectiveness of the new methodology under clinical field conditions. Although the objective of the first study has been fully achieved [68,85], unfortunately, no follow-up clinical study under similar experimental and computational conditions was implemented up-to-date.

29.3.2.1 Methodology of Assessment

The working hypothesis of the Buffalo study was that the skin of cancerous breasts will manifest significantly lower temperature modulation because of higher perfusion, primarily owing to the vasodilatatory effect of NO.

The following DTA methodology was developed to quantify the temperature modulation of the surface of breasts and identify breasts with low modulation.

Following the acquisition of 1200 sequential thermal images at a rate of 100 frames/s, the projected area of the thermal image of the breast was subdivided into square subareas (spots) of 4×4 pixels each, corresponding to approximately 16 mm² of skin. The total area of interest delineated manually on the primary thermal image, comprised of about 1700± spots, depending on the size of the breast. The average temperature of each of those spots was then calculated, and a time series of 1024 temperature values was obtained for each spot. After linear regression eliminated slow (<0.1 mHz) temperature changes, and after correction for spurious modulation of the camera or of the environment (common interference removal), each time series underwent FFT analysis [69,83]. Using the FFT data of 160 intervals, 50 mHz each, in the frequency range 2–10 Hz, the modulation amplitude of each spot at each of these 160 discrete frequencies was obtained. The cardiogenic modulation frequencies (0.5–2 Hz) were excluded, primarily because their assessment would require longer observation times, exacerbating motion artifacts (primarily patient breathing).

For each discrete frequency a subarea (or subareas) of spots with lowest modulation amplitudes (□24 spots in the published study) was (were) identified. Such a subarea was named a *cluster* of low-amplitude spots. These clusters were identified and demarcated as follows: all the spots that represented the area of interest (the whole demarcated breast) were rank ordered by their amplitudes (the spot with the lowest amplitude first, the spot with the second lowest second, up to the spot with the highest amplitude). Spots with low amplitude, owing to one or more "dead" pixels, caused by corresponding inactive detector elements, were excluded from the ranking. The position of the spots with the lowest amplitudes was then registered. If these spots were adjacent to other such spots, a cluster of two or more low-amplitude spots was identified. Then spots with the next to lowest amplitude were identified and those in the proximity of a spot with the lowest amplitude were counted as members of a recognized cluster.

This computerized process was continued until a cluster of low-amplitude spots with a specified size was identified (24 spots in this study, corresponding approximately to 4 cm² (that number could be larger than 24 because the last step could have added more than one sequential spot to the low-amplitude cluster, or more than a single cluster with more than 24 spots was formed in the last step of clustering). The amplitude of the spot with the highest amplitude in the identified cluster was then registered. Then the ratio between the number of spots in the identified low-amplitude cluster (or clusters with ☐24 spots) and all the other spots (nonclustered or less clustered) that, at that frequency, had amplitudes smaller or equal to the spot with the highest amplitude value in the identified low-amplitude cluster was determined. That ratio was defined as "first cluster ratio" (FCR).

Another differentiating parameter used was the "first cluster amplitude ratio" (FCA) = the ratio between the average amplitude of the first cluster and the average of the amplitudes of all the spots over the whole demarcated area of interest (the whole breast). The working hypothesis was that both FCR and FCA in a cancerous breast will be significantly lower than in a cancer-free breast.

As discussed earlier, computerized DTA produced information on modulation of both temperature and STH [1,68]; thus we computed in parallel also FCR and FCA values for STH of the spots.

For each case studied and for each of its three views, the computerized output was a spectrum of FCR and FCA values of both temperature and homogeneity for each of the 160 frequencies analyzed.

This large data matrix was statistically analyzed to find out if these parameters can differentiate between cancerous and cancer-free breasts.

The working hypothesis predicted cancerous breasts to have higher FCR and FCA values, at least at certain frequencies, because local attenuation of modulation by extravascular, cancer-produced NO is expected to result in larger clusters with attenuated temperature amplitudes and greater homogeneity compared with breasts free of cancerous lesions. This hypothesis could be tested by a statistical analysis of the FCR and FCA values obtained for the 100 breasts studied.

29.3.2.2 Statistical Analysis and Findings

Using a macroprocedure, a computer sequentially processed each of the image series (cases) in our database, that is, each of the views of each case. For each view, the researchers obtained as the output four ASCII files that listed the FCR(temp), FCR(STH), FCA(temp), and FCA(STH) values for each of the 160 discrete frequencies analyzed. This output could be displayed as a spreadsheet with 160 columns (frequencies), with each row corresponding to a single case (a single view of a specified breast). The same spreadsheet also contained demographic and clinical data. These spreadsheets were then fed to a statistical program, developed at Buffalo by Dr. Aleksey Naumov, for further analysis. The statistical analysis, described before for other DTA-derived parameters [85], reaches the same conclusion—DTA can highly effectively differentiate between cancerous and cancer-free breasts; sensitivities and diagnostic powers >0.95 were obtained, with STH data providing a somewhat higher significance. It was also found that frontal views of cancerous breasts yield significantly higher sensitivity and specificity values than lateral views of the same breast. A description of the statistical procedures and findings are, however, outside the purview of this review chapter.

29.3.2.3 Limitations

The Buffalo study was limited to assessing only high-frequency modulation >2 Hz because the motion artifacts limited the acquisition time to 12 s. While the discrete structures of the average spectra and the highly significant difference between the averages of the two groups of subjects indicates manifestation of hemodynamic process in the 2–8 Hz region [68,85], it is regrettable that no reliable information could be produced at lower frequencies. (This limitation has been recently removed by sophisticated motion correction algorithms to be published soon, and those algorithms have already been used to process data in a very recent breast cancer study [86]; see below.)

Removal of motion artifacts will evidently revolutionize many of DTI's clinical applications, especially its use in breast cancer detection. It is now possible to study the hemodynamic behavior of the breast or other tissues down to 0.01 Hz. This could open up a new era in the application of DTA to breast cancer detection and evaluation.

29.3.2.4 Physiological Considerations and Their Implications

From the physiological mechanistic standpoint, the positive findings of the Buffalo study pose interesting questions. While it is expected that a hyperperfused breast will appear warmer, as found in classical thermal imaging, how could changes in perfusion modulation kinetics of a tumor situated, say 20 mm below the skin, affect temperature modulation and the homogeneity of temperature distribution at the skin level. It must be concluded, therefore, that the presence of a cancerous lesion inside the breast affects the behavior of the cutaneous capillary bed. Were it only due to the higher heat dissipation of cancerous breasts, DTI would not have had a higher sensitivity, and especially specificity, of breast cancer detection than classical thermography. Moreover, ductal carcinoma *in situ* (DCIS) that is unlikely to affect the heat dissipation of the whole breast would not have been detectable as it was by DTA [68,85]. We must advance the hypothesis that the NO produced in a tumor inside the breast affects *cutaneous* perfusion dynamics measurable by DTI.

Then one must ask whether it is NO that diffuses from the cancerous lesion to the cutaneous capillary bed and, if so, how does it diffuse? Is it carried in the arterial blood supply? This is rather unlikely in view of its short lifetime in the presence of hemoglobin. Does it diffuse through the lymphatic system or in the interstitial space? This again is not very plausible in view of the rate of oxidation of NO in aqueous media.

We venture here the hypothesis that cancerous breasts build up a significant level of NO in their fat wherein the half-life of NO is likely to be quite long. Then the NO diffuses slowly from the fat into the cutaneous capillary bed, affecting its hemodynamic behavior. This hypothesis awaits, evidently, experimental verification. The fact that cancerous breasts were identified irrespective of the size of the tumors by examining temperature modulation over the whole breast, irrespective of the site of the tumor, supports this new hypothesis, presented here for the first time.

The NO–fat hypothesis implies that subcutaneous fat of cancerous breasts retrieved by needle liposuction will have a significant NO content, while fat of cancer-free breasts would be virtually free of NO. This suggests a quasi-invasive preliminary test of breasts that were found suspicious by x-ray mammography. Such a test could be an attractive alternative to exploratory biopsy, which has a significant level of false negatives, in addition to its invasiveness and costs. It is noteworthy that the presence of NO in subcutaneous fat is less dependent on the locale and nature of the cancerous lesion and might be, therefore, a highly sensitive and specific test, actually alleviating the need for DTI for this clinical problem. Furthermore, if this test proved reliable, it could be streamlined to become the first-line diagnostic test to be followed by surgery. If this hypothesis was verified and such a diagnostic test was found effective, it can be considered a conceptual offshoot of the Buffalo DTI study, justifying inclusion of this suggestion in this review paper.

29.3.3 Preliminary DTA Findings on Melanoma and Diabetes

Although the main trust of DTA studies at Buffalo were on breast cancer patients, two other exploratory studies done there warrant being mentioned. Preliminary studies of patients with osteosarcoma and melanoma undergoing chemotherapy gave encouraging results. In the first study, carried out in collaboration with Dr. C. Karakousis of the Department of Surgery, it was found that cancer induced characteristic DTI "signatures" of melanoma disappeared following chemotherapy, suggesting that inoperative metastatic tumors lost their capacity of NO production as a result of chemotherapy, as a result of their metabolic arrest. In other patients DTI was also able to pick up indication of the presence of residual malignant tissue following excision of the primary lesion.

The other preliminary study was done by Dr. C. Carthy in collaboration with Dr. P. Dandona on diabetic patients. These investigators explored the use of DTI in staging of diabetes mellitus by examining the perfusion of the extremities. The preliminary findings, though promising, however, were not conclusive.

29.4 Recent DTA Studies (2000–2005)

29.4.1 Detection of and Treatment of Malignancy

Following the preliminary findings in Buffalo there have been a number of attempts in different clinical research centers to use DTI in oncology. This included detection of malignant lesions as well as follow-up of treatment of cancer.

Janicek et al. [87] studied the response of soft tissue sarcomas to chemotherapy with DTI, in parallel with CT and PET. DTA detected the malignancy in superficially located sarcomas, and the findings were reported to correlate well with assessments by the two other imaging modalities. Janicek et al. [88–90] showed enhanced temperature modulation, probably due to hypervascularization since they monitored in the 0.8–2 Hz range, also in the case of metastatic gastrointestinal stromal tumors; the finding correlated well with those of Doppler ultrasound. Similar results were observed also in the case of malignant lymphomas. The malignant lesions studied by Janicek et al. [91] might have been too deep to exhibit frequencies higher than 2 Hz; thus only the cardiogenic pulsatile modulations were observable. The conclusion of these preliminary clinical studies and suggestions to use DTI in other than breast cancer studies were summarized in 2003.

Lately, a research project was undertaken by Dr. Johan Nilsson at the Karolinska Institute in Stockholm to explore the use of DTI in the detection of metastatic melanoma. In a preliminary series of tests on two patients, melanoma metastases were detectable as spots of enhanced modulation on DTI temperature amplitude bitmaps, both in the cardiogenic frequency range of 0.9–1.7 Hz and in the low vasomotor frequency range of 0.05–0.2 Hz. The DTI detected melanoma metastases, some of which were visible on the skin and palpable, and confirmed *prior* to the DTI study by thin needle aspiration biopsy. Unfortunately, this preliminary study was not extended to include detection of lesions that were not known beforehand, like in the case of the prebiopsy breast cancer study in Buffalo. These preliminary measurements in the <2 Hz modulation frequency range complement Anbar's earlier observations (see above) on the effect of melanoma metastases on localized temperature modulation in the 2–8 Hz range. This far an optimal frequency range for detection of melanoma by DTI has yet to be established.

Following the Buffalo study, there have been just two more DTI studies aimed at breast cancer detection. A major multicenter study by Parisky et al. [92] involved close to a thousand prebiopsy patients. These investigators tried to identify emerging characteristic thermal patterns on thermal images of breasts, in response to external cooling by a stream of cold air. In this study Parisky used hundreds of sequential thermal images. This subset of what has been done in Buffalo 4 years earlier is based on Anbar's hypothesis that vasculature surrounding cancerous lesions is less likely to respond to sympathetic vasoconstriction induced by cold stimuli. The findings corroborated this hypothesis. Unfortunately this extensive study was limited by inferior IR equipment that lacked the sensitivity and speed necessary to monitor temperature modulation. The other limitation of this study was the use of human "experts" in evaluating the computerized images. As was pointed out by Moskowitz [93], the usefulness of this subjective DTI protocol is rather limited.

Another study on breast cancer detection was done by Button et al. [94] at Stony Brook University Hospital. Button used up-to-date equipment and computational procedures in his study of temperature modulation in the cardiogenic frequency range. His findings on a limited number of prebiopsy patients were indicative but nonconclusive, partially because he, like Parisky, used trained human "experts" to evaluate the DTI images.

The latest use of DTI in breast oncology has been in a study by Fanning et al. [86] at the Cleveland Clinic. In their preliminary experiments they assessed the effect of chemotherapeutic agents on established cancerous lesions, on the basis of the assumption that as the viability of the lesion diminishes so will the effect of the NO on temperature modulation. Their preliminary findings were encouraging. However, this use of DTI has limited sensitivity because NO is also produced by phagocytes during the necrosis of the shrinking tumors [33].

In summary, in spite of several encouraging attempts by several groups, the use of DTA in breast oncology still awaits extensive, well-designed clinical trials. A major obstacle to acquisition of reliable DTA data over a wide range of frequencies has been recently removed by motion corrections algorithms. However, this new promising approach to detection of breast cancer has yet to be tested in large-scale clinical studies. Such studies are warranted in view of independent experimental findings that confirmed the vascular effect of cancer-produced NO.

Button et al. [94] have shown in an animal study that the generation of NO by a neoplastic lesion can be detected by DTI. Mice were implanted subcutaneously with human epithelial caner cells. Once these cells established a viable neoplastic lesion 7 days after implantation, the lesion was unambiguously manifested on a DTI bitmap. This manifestation was totally abolished by administration of a conventional NO synthesis inhibitor (LNAME) but reappeared 3 days later, when the effect of the inhibitor abated. This study also demonstrated detection by DTI of the vasodilatatory effect of NO on the vasculature of mice following topical treatment with nitroglycerin.

29.4.2 Use of DTI in the Study of Brain Function and Brain Malignancies

Up to this point we discussed only DTI studies of skin, the huge exposed organ of the body. However, the exposed parenchyma of any other organ could be studied by DTI if its blackbody radiation can be exposed to an IR camera. During open brain surgery for intracranial vascular repair or removal of malignant or benign space-occupying lesions, the outer surface of the brain is exposed, allowing infrared imaging, including DTI.

Alexander Gorbach conceptualized the idea of using infrared imaging to monitor the brain already in 1993 when he was still in Russia [95]. Gorbach persisted with his studies in this field at NIH and has published since 2002 a series of highly impressive studies, starting with animal experimentation [96] and ending with numerous clinical open brain intraoperative investigations. Gorbach's studies covered two major aspects:

1. Monitoring the physiology of neurological functions in different regions of the brain by manifestations of changes in local perfusion and metabolic activity [97,98].
2. Clinical uses of DTI, including real-time follow-up of reperfusion in the course of vascular neurosurgery, and localization of benign or malignant space-occupying lesions by their abnormal vascular structure and perfusion dynamics, allowing then the following up of their surgical removal [96,99,100].

Gorbach has shown that local metabolism even in hypermetabolic brain tissues is just a minor contributor of temperature change following mental stimulation compared with enhanced perfusion of the ROI [97,98]; this confirmed Anbar's conclusion regarding the metabolism versus perfusion in cancerous breasts [24]. Gorbach's findings on regional perfusional changes in response to somatosensory stimulation have been most recently independently confirmed [101].

Unlike Anbar, Gorbach used a 3–5 μm camera with a lower thermal sensitivity and stability, and lower acquisition rate, as well as lower accuracy because of the need for a much greater correction for the reflectivity of the monitored surface. These studies were limited, therefore, to monitoring of changes in brain surface temperature following stimulation or surgical manipulations rather than changes in modulation amplitudes of perfusion. In view of these limitations Gorbach's beautifully designed experiments and their unambiguous conclusions are even more praiseworthy. Moreover, Gorbach did not limit his studies to visual observations of temperature change or of the rate of temperature change (which are generally sufficient for neurosurgeons), but he used computerized data processing, similar to that used by Anbar 4 years earlier [83], to receive off-line *objective* information [97]. Since we believe that this is going to be a major advantage of DTA, the independent use of similar algorithms in processing DTI data is quite gratifying.

In parallel with Gorbach's studies of the brain at NIH, Ecker et al. [102] at the Mayo Clinic in Rochester, MN, carried out a DTI study using up-to-date IR imaging equipment and superior data processing software. The superior equipment used at the Mayo clinic allowed demonstration of the same clinical uses of DTI demonstrated at NIH, that is, visualization of brain reperfusion following vascular operations and localization of brain tumors by their abnormal perfusion patterns and vascular dynamics. The equipment used by Ecker et al. [102] (200 frames/s) and its FFT algorithms allowed detection of pathology with a much higher sensitivity and resolution. This demonstrated again the pronounced advantages of computerized analysis of temporal temperature modulation at high spatial resolution.

Ecker's study, independently corroborated by Gorbach's later findings, unambiguously indicates the use of DTI in neurosurgery. What is preventing today the routine use of this modality are not the cost of the equipment (<$300,000 for a surgical procedure costing >$20,000 each) or its sophistication (it can be fully automated). What is needed is a multicenter clinical study that will demonstrate the added value, in terms of outcomes of open brain surgical procedures, of using DTI as a tool. From the commercial standpoint, such a multimillion dollar study is not attractive because of the relatively limited commercial market for such equipment (brain surgery is not a common medical procedure). Also from the standpoint of public health, problems that call for brain surgery are not very common compared to other public healthcare problems. Therefore, expenditure of millions on this problem might be of low priority. Neurosurgeons will have to wait, therefore, for manufacturers of DTI equipment to build up a sufficiently large market for their products in other clinical fields to be in position to sponsor an outcome-driven clinical study in cranial neurosurgery, so as to open up another, though limited, market for their equipment.

Amazingly, Ecker's paper does not refer at all to Gorbach's closely related work, whereas Gorbach refers only once to Ecker's study. In the closely knit community of neurosurgeons of the top institutions in the United States, including NIH and the Mayo Clinic, people must have been aware of the parallel efforts. It seems that science calls for more collegial information exchange and collaboration. It is perhaps equally surprising that Ecker, who unlike Gorbach was not a pioneer in this field, did not refer also to Anbar's monograph, which summarized in detail the history of uses of IR imaging in neurosurgery up to 1993 and strongly recommends the use of DTI in this clinical field. Chances are that Ecker got the idea of using DTI in his clinic from that book, as he used Anbar's algorithms in his study (which he does refer to). Moreover, Ecker's paper's title starts with the pretentious phrase: "Vision of the Future": Whose vision has this been to begin with? It is quite conceivable that Ecker would never have undertaken his study without having been made aware of Anbar's monograph by the distributor of the IR equipment he used.

This teaches us something about the sociology of science, studied by Anbar many years earlier [103]. Academicians are often more ready to give due credit to developers of new hardware or software, or to producers of new data, rather than to people who conceptualized new ideas. However, new ideas are those that have driven science through the ages. Scientists ought to be recognized and rewarded for their ideas first of all.

To summarize, the clinical use of DTI in neurosurgery is one of the first to have verified Anbar's vision on the potential clinical value of this science-based approach.

29.4.3 Use of DTI Intraoperatively in Other Surgical Procedures

There are numerous potential uses of DTI used in surgery. We discussed in Section 29.3.2 neurosurgical applications separately, because open cranial surgery has yielded substantial new physiological neurological information, in addition to is potential clinical uses. Other surgical applications to be discussed next are primarily of clinical value only.

Different surgical applications were suggested in Anbar's monograph, based predominantly on previous static infrared imaging studies. All surgical applications of DTI are based on intraoperative monitoring of perfusion. Two groups of surgical applications of DTI have been recently reduced to practice in well-documented clinical studies—uses in reconstructive and vascular surgery (which have been first demonstrated by Anbar in 1998; see above) and uses in cardiac and transplant surgery. These uses will be described below.

29.4.3.1 Reconstructive and Vascular Surgery

Intraoperative DTI is potentially an ideal tool for reconstructive and vascular surgery, as it allows to assess perfusion and reperfusion in real time and thus provide the surgeon immediate feedback. Surgeons can thus take corrective action when it is most effective. Zeroing in on and displaying bitmaps of the spatial distribution of cardiogenic frequency modulation in real time enhances significantly the sensitivity of the technique. DTI can also be a highly useful preoperative and postoperative evaluation tool.

In addition, DTI at cardiogenic frequency allows the precise localization of perforator vessels, which perfuse subcutaneous tissue from below, preoperatively, and thus significantly improving the outcome of grafting. The currently used laser Doppler flowmetry has inferior capacity to provide information on the vasculature over large areas of skin. The application of DTI to this important surgical problem, which has been first demonstrated by Binzoni et al. [104] at the University of Geneva, is likely to be adopted by plastic surgeons as a routine preoperative procedure once a broad scale multicenter clinical study demonstrates its usefulness in a controlled outcome study.

While the use of DTI in reconstructive and vascular surgery is self-evident, it is surprising that only two other clinical studies have been published in this field in recent years. In addition to the pioneering study in Geneva, a study on the intraoperative use of DTI in vascular surgery was carried out in Dundee University in Scotland [105]. A study at Tohoku University demonstrated the advantage of long-wave IR cameras in DTI-assisted vascular surgery [106]. Those three demonstration studies are expected to be just a beginning to a highly beneficial array of routine uses of DTI in these surgical specialties.

29.4.3.2 Cardiac and Transplant Surgery

The use of DTI in open heart surgery is an obvious clinical application, as it involves perfusion and reperfusion of a highly vascular organ. It also involves grafting of vessels (discussed in Section 29.4.3.1). Mohr et al. [107] demonstrated this application on a large number of patients and documented improved outcomes when this technique was used [108,109]. Mohr actually extended the use of DTI in cardiac surgery he pioneered in 1989, using later much better equipment. The former study was cited in Anbar's 1994 monograph as a model for surgical uses of DTI. Surprisingly, in spite of these well-documented positive clinical results, no other studies on the use of DRI in cardiac surgery in other clinical centers were published to date.

Another surgical application that depends on assessment of reperfusion is transplant surgery. Gorbach et al. [110] have demonstrated the effectiveness of using DTI in kidney transplant surgery. They showed the rate of reperfusion to be an important predictive parameter of the success of transplantation, especially in the case of allografts from cadavers that have been subjected to extended periods of ischemic cooling. The history of this application of thermal imaging, which dates back to the early 1970s, was reviewed in Anbar's 1994 monograph. Yet only modern DTI equipment enabled a reproducible quantitative noninvasive assessment of perfusion rates, making this an attractive procedure for routine kidney transplant surgery, as well as for other transplant situations. Like in the case of cardiac surgery, there has been so far no other follow-up studies of these pioneering efforts.

It seems that introduction of a new technology into surgical suits requires more than just good clinical demonstration studies. Surgery is a relatively conservative discipline, and changes in protocol take a considerable effort, especially when they involve the installation of substantial instrumentation in the operating room. It is often easier to find an enthusiastic research clinician to test a new technological modality and get academic credit for it, than to convince a hospital administrator to acquire a new instrument for a clinic with the sole benefit of better clinical outcomes. As long as there is no competition that forces a hospital to modernize, modernization is less likely. Moreover, the use of any new technique in the clinic requires appropriate compensation by medical insurance, Medicare in particular. Insurance companies are, obviously, reluctant to approve new technology unless it cuts the cost of hospitalization. In the case of cardiac surgery it can be readily claimed that early detection of failure in vascular grafting or of rejection in the case of transplant surgery will cut hospitalization costs. Yet we see how slow has been the acceptance of routine use of DTI even in these surgical procedures.

29.4.4 Clinical Applications of DTI in Other Fields

The use of infrared imaging to monitor reperfusion of tissues, of the extremities in particular, is as old as classic infrared imaging [19]. DTI in its most rudimentary mode—quantitative assessment of warming rates at different subareas of the ROI—makes this methodology of clinical value. After our review of its uses in surgery (see above), we shall discuss a few recent studies that have used this approach in nonsurgical clinical situation.

Gold et al. [111] have recently used DTI to diagnose upper extremity musculoskeletal disorders, including carpal tunnel syndrome, by following the perfusion dynamics of hands during and after a standardized typing task. The findings were consistent with earlier ones [19], but the more precise DTI assessment allowed meaningful statistical evaluation. It remains to be seen if this technique, which has been known for decades among neurologists, will become more accepted with more precise computerized equipment available today. As was pointed out by Anbar already in 1994, it is conceivable that more precise differential diagnosis could be achieved if temperature modulation was monitored in addition to gross cooling or warm-up rates.

Rewarming of extremities following brief immersion (10 s) in cold water has been used as a diagnostic test also for neurovascular damage resulting from type-2 diabetes mellitus [112]. Since the test performed used classic thermal imaging at 5 min intervals, it can hardly be classified as a DTI procedure. A similar study, though more sophisticated and precise, was carried out more recently on type-1 diabetes patients by Zotter et al. [113] at the University of Graz. In this study differential diagnosis was based on the relative rewarming rates of different toes, adding an anatomic dimension to the test.

Regretfully, up-to-date, no studies have confirmed the value of DTI in differential diagnosis between diabetes-induced vascular occlusions and vascular neuropathies, which should be possible by comparing thermal modulation of the skin of extremities in the cardiogenic and vasomotor frequency ranges, respectively [19]. This could be done without thermal stress, although response to a transient thermal stress could add diagnostic information. Also no attempts have been made so far to use DTI as a management tool to stage diabetes and monitor the effectiveness of treatment.

The same limitations on the acceptance of DTI routinely in surgery, discussed above, apply also to its use in diabetic clinics. Feasibility studies are first needed, and then large-scale clinical tests must prove the added value of the diagnostic technique, before a new technology reaches routine clinical use.

Finally, in the field of peripheral neuronal diseases we will cite a recent quantitative DTI study on complex regional pain syndrome [114]. Huygen et al. [114] at Rotterdam, studied the dynamics of temperature change in the hands of patients following systemic major thermal challenge by a thermosuit. While the DTI temperature imaging was done at 10 min intervals, their computerized diagnostic test allowed *objective* evaluation of patients, as in Anbar's diagnostic test on breast cancer [83]. Moreover, this application of DTA has been among those suggested by Anbar 10 years earlier [19].

Other early DTI studies have had recent follow-ups. Fifteen years after Anbar had first demonstrated the use of DTI in monitoring the temperature of the cornea [11,115], a 2005 review recommends the use of dynamic ocular thermography in ophthalmology [116]. The early use of DTI in pain assessment [33,76] have been recently followed in patients with postoperative neuralgia [117]. The results in this group of patient have shown, however, no correlation between cutaneous blood flow and tactile induced pain, unlike pain in rheumatic inflammation [76], suggesting that the former pain is not due to a local vasoactive process. The latter suggestion has been corroborated by another independent thermographic study [118].

Completing the review of thermal imaging warm-up studies since 1999, one has to mention a study on the warm up of teeth and gingival tissue following a brief cooling period with a stream of cold air, to assess the perfusion and thereby the vitality of teeth [119,120]. This study essentially establishes that all normal teeth in a patient's mouth have a similar warm-up pattern, implying that an affected tooth will show a lower rate of thermal recovery. The competing technology is, however, laser Doppler flowmetry (LDF), which can provide the same information at a lower cost. This study is an example of an unjustified use of DTI. Since the area of interest is quite small and DTI equipment is bulkier and more expensive than LDF, there is no justification for the use of DTI for this specific dental problem. It is not surprising, therefore, that there has been no follow-up to this study. However, DTI has a potential use in dental surgery (e.g., in the management of TMJ pain [75,76]).

29.5 Conclusion

It has been both a gratifying experience and a disappointment for me writing this chapter. I found that the ideas I advanced in the early 1990s, summarized in my 1994 monograph, on the potential advantages of physiology-based DTI as a clinical tool have merit. Many investigators, most of them new users of thermal imaging, have accepted and adopted these notions. At the same time, static, anatomic thermal imaging, which has been around since the early 1970s, has failed to gain acceptance by the medical community. By now it has been universally recognized that thermal imaging manifests physiology and it must, therefore, measure the *dynamics* of physiological processes. A fair number of clinical applications of DTI suggested in my 1994 monograph have been successfully demonstrated since 2000, when appropriate computerized infrared monitoring equipment became commercially available. By now DTI is a recognized domain in medical technology. This has been truly gratifying.

On the other hand, this far none of those applications has reached the stage of routine use in a clinical setting. This may not be as disappointing as it looks, compared with the long time it took to get ultrasonic imaging or even MRI into routine clinical use. In either of these two cases it took time until major medical equipment manufacturers realized the potential of those technologies and marketed them on a large scale. It all boils down to marketing. DTI has not yet reached this stage.

However, it has become more difficult with time to market new medical technologies because of economic constraints. One must prove that the benefits of using a new technology (in terms of better clinical outcomes—patients' survival and quality of life, days of hospitalization, patients' pain and suffering, and so on) outweigh its costs (including the equipment, space, training of personnel, risks, etc.). Moreover, the benefit/cost of the given technology must exceed those of competing technologies. For reasons I pointed out already in 1994 [19], classic clinical thermal imaging has not met these criteria over 30+ years of its existence, in spite of a few successful preliminary attempts. It was left behind, while ultrasound imaging, CT, and MRI have flourished.

Will DTI be more successful? For one, it is based on firmer biomedical grounds (users can understand what they are measuring in physiological terms), it is quantitative and is potentially the most *objective* among all medical-imaging techniques (as described above, computerized DTA can be used without *any* imaging output), and its hardware costs a fraction of that of CT, PET, or MRI. It also exceeds competing technologies—laser Doppler flowmetry and ultrasound Doppler imaging—in its ability to acquire information extremely rapidly on large anatomical areas. Moreover, while DTI can become an invaluable tool in surgery by providing real-time information on facets unavailable to the clinician in any other way, DTA allows completely automated objective diagnosis, as I have demonstrated. DTA heralds therefore a new paradigm in clinical medicine alleviating the need for imaging experts, thus substantially reducing heath care costs. It must be realized that DTA poses a threat to radiologists, the experts who interpret clinical images, and it might be fought by them for obvious reasons. In spite of this, DTI and especially DTA are, with all likelihood, going to become someday a mainstream biomedical technology. This may take more time, possibly not during the lifetime of this reviewer.

The author is comforted by another personal experience. In the late 1950s Anbar pioneered the use of F^{18} in nuclear medicine [121,122], and demonstrated its use in brain tumor localization by coincidence detection of positrons [123–125]. This was long before computers allowed CT to develop. It took more than 30+ years revolutionary developments in computer technology before PET scanners became clinically useful. Hopefully, DTA will have a similar fate.

The author wishes to conclude this review with a personal note.

Note: In his desire to make this review of DTI as inclusive as possible, the author covered all relevant papers that have appeared up to January 2006 in the National Library of Medicine database, in the European *EMbase* (Excerpta Medica). Also covered were *Thermology* (discontinued), *Thermology International* (and its discontinued predecessors *Thermologie Osterreich* and *European Journal of Thermology*), and *Biomedical Thermology* (Japan), which are not covered in full in the international medical databases. The author also consulted Professor K. Ammer and Professor K. Mabuchi, the editors of the two latter current journals. Consequently, publications on DTI outside these resources could have been left out.

References

Note: Review papers are demarcated by an asterisk (*).

1. Anbar M. and Haverly R.F. Local "micro" variance in temperature distribution evaluated by digital thermography. *Biomedical Thermology*, 13, 173–187, 1994. Also in *Advanced Techniques and Clinical Applications in Biomedical Thermology*. Mabuchi K., Mizushina S. and Harrison B. (eds.) Chur, Harwood Academic Publishers, 173–187, 1994.
2. Anbar M. Computerized thermography. The emergence of a new diagnostic imaging modality. *International Journal of Technology Assessment in Health Care*, 3, 613–621, 1987.
3. Montoro J. and Anbar M. New modes of data handling in computerized thermography. *Proceedings of the 10th Annual International Conference of the IEEE Engineering in Medicine and Biology Society*; Harris G. and Walker C. (eds.), Vol. 10, 845–847, 1988.
4. Montoro J., Hershey L.A., and Anbar M. Enhancement of interpretation of thermograms through on-line software. *Thermology*, 3, 121–124, 1989.
5. Montoro J., Lee K.-H., and Anbar M. Study of regulation of skin temperature using dynamic digital thermal imaging. *Proceedings of the 11th Annual International Conference of the IEEE Engineering in Medicine and Biology Society*. Seattle, WA, 1158–1159, 1989.
6. Montoro J., Lee K.-H., Spangler R.A., and Anbar M. Assessment of skin temperature regulation by dynamic digital thermal imaging. *Proceedings of the 34th Annual Meeting of the Biophysical Society. Biophysical Journal*, 57, 280a, 1990.
7. Montoro J., Lee K.-H., and Anbar M. Skin temperature regulation parameters derived from temporal studies of infrared images. *The FASEB Journal*, Abstracts Part I, 4, A698, 1990.
8. Montoro J. and Anbar M. Visualization and analysis of dynamic thermographic changes. *Proceedings of the First Conference on Visualization in Biomedical Computing*, Atlanta, GA, 486–489, 1990.

9. Montoro J., D'Arcy S., and Anbar M. Temporal analysis of thermal images. *Proceedings of the 12th Annual International Conference of the IEEE Engineering in Medicine and Biology Society*, 12, 1578–1579, 1990.

10. Anbar M. Objective assessment of clinical computerized thermal images. *SPIE Proceedings* 1445, 479–484, 1991.

11. Montoro J.C., Haverly R.F., D'Arcy S.J., Gyimesi I.M., Coles W.H., Spangler R.A., and Anbar M. Use of digital infrared imaging to objectively assess thermal abnormalities in the human eye. *Thermology* 3, 242–248, 1991.

12. Anbar M., Montoro J.C., Lee K.-H., and D'Arcy S.J. Manifestation of neurological abnormalities through frequency analysis of skin temperature regulation. *Thermology*, 3, 234–241, 1991.

13. Anbar M., D'Arcy S., and Montoro J. Characteristic frequencies of human skin temperature regulation derived from temporal analysis of infrared images. *The FASEB Journal*, 5, 4303, 1991.

14. Anbar M. and D'Arcy S. Localized regulatory frequencies of human skin temperature derived from the analysis of series of infrared images. *Proceedings of the 4th Annual IEEE Symposium on Computer Based Medical Systems (CBMS '91)*, 184–191, 1991.

15. Anbar M. Recent technological developments in thermology and their impact on clinical applications. *Biomedical Thermology*, 10, 270–276, 1992.

16. Anbar M. Thermoregulatory processes affecting skin temperature derived from time series of infrared images. *Thermologie Osterreich*, 2S, 18, 1992.

17. *Anbar M. Dynamic area telethermometry—a new field in clinical thermology Part I. *Medical Electronics*, 146, 62–73, 1994.

18. *Anbar M. Dynamic area telethermometry—a new field in clinical thermology Part II. *Medical Electronics*, 147, 73–85, 1994.

19. *Anbar M. *Quantitative Dynamic Telethermometry in Medical Diagnosis and Management*. Boca Raton, FL, CRC Press Inc., 1994.

20. Freeman G., Dyer R.L., Juhos L., St. John G.A., and Anbar M. Identification of nitric oxide (NO) in human blood. *Archives of Environmental Health*, 33, 19–23, 1978.

21. Moncada S. The first Robert Furchgott lecture: From endothelium-dependent relaxation to the 811L-arginine: NO pathway. *Blood Vessels*, 27, 208–217, 1990.

22. Luscher T.F. Endothelium-derived nitric oxide: The endogenous nitrovasodilator in the human cardiovascular system. *European Heart Journal*, 12 (Suppl E), 2–11, 1991.

23. Moncada S. and Higgs A. The 811L-arginine-nitric oxide pathway. *New England Journal of Medicine*, 329, 2002–2012, 1993.

24. Anbar M. Hyperthermia of the cancerous breast—analysis of mechanism. *Cancer Letters*, 84, 23–29, 1994.

25. Anbar M. Mechanism of hyperthermia of the cancerous breast. *Biomedical Thermology*, 15, 135–139, 1995.

26. Thomsen L.L., Lawton F.G., Knowles R.G., Beesley J.E., Riveros-Moreno V., and Moncada S. Nitric oxide synthase activity in human gynecological cancer. *Cancer Research*, 54, 1352–1354, 1994.

27. Fujisawa H., Ogura T., Kurashima Y., Yokoyama T., Yamashita J., and Esumi H. Expression of two types of nitric oxide synthase mRNA in human neuroblastoma cell lines. *Journal of Neurochemistry*, 63, 140–145, 1994.

28. Jenkins D.C., Charles I.G., Baylis S.A., Lelchuk R., Radomski M.W., and Moncada S. Human colon cancer cell lines show a diverse pattern of nitric oxide synthase gene expression and nitric oxide generation. *British Journal of Cancer*, 70, 847–849, 1994.

29. Xie W., McCahon P., Jakobsen K., and Parish C. Evaluation of the ability of digital infrared imaging to detect vascular changes in experimental animal tumours. *International Journal of Cancer*, 108, 790–794, 2004.

30. *Anbar M. Quantitative and dynamic telethermometry—a fresh look at clinical thermology. *IEEE Engineering in Medicine and Biology Magazine*, 14, 15–16, 1995.

31. *Anbar M. Dynamic area telethermometry and its clinical applications. *SPIE Proceedings*, 2473, 312–322, 1995.

32. Anbar M. The role of nitric oxide as a synchronizing chemical messenger in the hyperperfusion of the cancerous breast. In *The Biology of Nitric Oxide Part 5*, Moncada S. et al. (eds.), London, Portland Press, pp. 288a–288d, 1996.

33. Anbar M. and Gratt B.M. Role of nitric oxide in the physiopathology of pain. *Journal of Pain and Symptom Management*, 14, 225–254, 1997.

34. Anbar M. Mechanism of the association between local hyperthermia and local pain in joint disorders. *European Journal of Thermology*, 7, 173–188, 1997.

35. Jenkins D.C., Charles I.G., Thomsen L.L., Moss D.W., Holmes L.S., Baylis S.A., Rhodes P., Westmore K., Emson P.C., and Moncada S. Roles of nitric oxide in tumor growth. *Proceedings of the Natural Academy of Science USA*, 92, 4392–4396, 1995.

36. Maeda H., Noguchi Y., Sato K., and Akaike T. Enhanced vascular permeability in solid tumor is mediated by nitric oxide and inhibited by both new nitric oxide scavenger and nitric oxide synthase inhibitor. *Japan Journal of Cancer Research*, 85, 331–334, 1994.

37. Tozer G.M., Prise V.E., and Bell K.M. The influence of nitric oxide on tumour vascular tone. *Acta Oncology*, 34, 373–377, 1995.

38. Tozer G.M., Prise V.E., and Chaplin D.J. Inhibition of nitric oxide synthase induces a selective reduction in tumor blood flow that is reversible with 811L-arginine. *Cancer Research*, 57, 948–955, 1997.

39. Fukumura D. and Jain R.K. Role of nitric oxide in angiogenesis and microcirculation in tumors. *Cancer Metastasis Review*, 17, 77–89, 1998.

40. Thomsen L.L., Miles D.W., Happerfield L., Bobrow L.G., Knowles R.G., and Moncada S. Nitric oxide synthase activity in human breast cancer. *British Journal Cancer*, 72, 41–44, 1995.

41. Zeillinger R., Tantscher E., Schneeberger C., Tschugguel W., Eder S., Sliutz G., and Huber J.C. Simultaneous expression of nitric oxide synthase and estrogen receptor in human breast cancer cell lines. *Breast Cancer Research Treatment*, 40, 205–207, 1996.

42. Duenas-Gonzalez A., Isales C.M., del Mar Abad-Hernandez M., Gonzalez-Sarmiento R., Sangueza O., and Rodriguez-Commes J. Expression of inducible nitric oxide synthase in breast cancer correlates with metastatic disease. *Modern Pathology*, 10, 645–649, 1997.

43. Blachier F., Selamnia M., Robert V., M'Rabet-Touil H., and Duee P.H. Metabolism of 811L-arginine through polyamine and nitric oxide synthase pathways in proliferative or differentiated human colon carcinoma cells. *Biochimica et Biophysica Acta*, 1268, 255–262, 1995.

44. Ambs S., Merriam W.G., Bennett W.P., Felley-Bosco E., Ogunfusika M.O, Oser S.M., Klein S., Shields P.G., Billiar T.R., and Harris C.C. Frequent nitric oxide synthase-2 expression in human colon adenomas: Implication for tumor angiogenesis and colon cancer progression. *Cancer Research*, 58, 334–341, 1998.

45. Kojima M., Morisaki T., Tsukahara Y., Uchiyama A., Matsunari Y., Mibu R., and Tanaka M. Nitric oxide synthase expression and nitric oxide production in human colon carcinoma tissue. *Journal of Surgical Oncology*, 70, 222–229, 1999.

46. Rosbe K.W., Prazma J., Petrusz P., Mims W., Ball S.S., and Weissler M.C. Immunohistochemical characterization of nitric oxide synthase activity in squamous cell carcinoma of the head and neck. *Otolaryngology Head and Neck Surgery*, 113, 541–549, 1995.

47. Gallo O., Masini E., Morbidelli L., Franchi A., Fini-Storchi I., Vergari W.A., and Ziche M. Role of nitric oxide in angiogenesis and tumor progression in head and neck cancer. *Journal of Natural Cancer Institute*, 90, 587–596, 1998.

48. Gavilanes J., Moro M.A., Lizasoain I., Lorenzo P., Perez A., Leza J.C., and Alvarez-Vicent J.J. Nitric oxide synthase activity in human squamous cell carcinoma of the head and neck. *Laryngoscope*, 109, 148–152, 1999.

49. Cobbs C.S., Brenman J.E., Aldape K.D., Bredt D.S., and Israel M.A. Expression of nitric oxide synthase in human central nervous system tumors. *Cancer Research*, 55, 727–730, 1995 and *British Journal of Cancer*, 73, 189–196, 1996.

50. Ellie E., Loiseau H., Lafond F., Arsaut J., and Demotes-Mainard J. Differential expression of inducible nitric oxide synthase mRNA in human brain tumours. *Neuro Report*, 7, 294–296, 1995.

51. Whittle I.R., Collins F., Kelly P.A., Ritchie I., and Ironside J.W. Nitric oxide synthase is expressed in experimental malignant glioma and influences tumour blood flow. *Acta Neurochir (Wien)*, 138, 870–875, 1996.

52. Bakshi A., Nag T.C., Wadhwa S., Mahapatra A.K., and Sarkar C. The expression of nitric oxide synthases in human brain tumours and peritumoral areas. *Journal of Neurology Science*, 155, 196–203, 1998.

53. Joshi M., Strandhoy J., and White W.L. Nitric oxide synthase activity is up-regulated in melanoma cell lines: A potential mechanism for metastases formation. *Melanoma Research*, 6, 121–126, 1996.

54. Joshi M. The importance of 811L-arginine metabolism in melanoma: An hypothesis for the role of nitric oxide and polyamines in tumor angiogenesis. *Free Radical Biology and Medicine*, 22, 573–578, 1997.

55. Ahmad N., Srivastava R.C., Agarwal R., and Mukhtar H. Nitric oxide synthase and skin tumor promotion. *Biochemical and Biophysical Research Communication*, 232, 328–331, 1997.

56. Edwards P., Cendan J.C., Topping D.B., Moldawer L.L., MacKay S., Copeland E.M., and Lind D.S. Tumor cell nitric oxide inhibits cell growth *in vitro*, but stimulates tumorigenesis and experimental lung metastasis *in vivo*. *Journal of Surgical Research*, 63, 49–52, 1996.

57. Liu C.Y., Wang C.H., Chen T.C., Lin H.C., Yu C.T., and Kuo H.P. Increased level of exhaled nitric oxide and up-regulation of inducible nitric oxide synthase in patients with primary lung cancer. *British Journal of Cancer*, 78, 534–541, 1998.

58. Fujimoto H., Ando Y., Yamashita T., Terazaki H., Tanaka Y., Sasaki J., Matsumoto M., Suga M., and Ando M. Nitric oxide synthase activity in human lung cancer. *Japan Journal of Cancer Research*, 88, 1190–1198, 1997.

59. Klotz T., Bloch W., Volberg C., Engelmann U., and Addicks K. Selective expression of inducible nitric oxide synthase in human prostate carcinoma. *Cancer*, 82, 1897–1903, 1998.

60. Thomsen L.L., Sargent J.M., Williamson C.J., and Elgie A.W. Nitric oxide synthase activity in fresh cells from ovarian tumour tissue: Relationship of enzyme activity with clinical parameters of patients with ovarian cancer. *Biochemical Pharmacology*, 56, 1365–1370, 1998.

61. Hajri A., Metzger E., Vallat F., Coffy S., Flatter E., Evrard S., Marescaux J., and Aprahamian M. Role of nitric oxide in pancreatic tumour growth: *In vivo* and *in vitro* studies. *British Journal of Cancer*, 78, 841–849, 1998.

62. Di Cesare P.E., Carlson C.S., Attur M., Kale A.A., Abramson S.B., Della Valle C., Steiner G., and Amin A.R. Up-regulation of inducible nitric oxide synthase and production of nitric oxide by the Swarm rat and human chondrosarcoma. *Journal of Orthopaedic Research*, 16, 667–674, 1998.

63. Swana H.S., Smith S.D., Perrotta P.L., Saito N., Wheeler M.A., and Weiss R.M. Inducible nitric oxide synthase with transitional cell carcinoma of the bladder. *Journal of Urology*, 161, 630–634, 1999.

64. Morcos E., Jansson O.T., Adolfsson J., Kratz G., and Wiklund N.P. Endogenously formed nitric oxide modulates cell growth in bladder cancer cell lines. *Urology*, 53, 1252–1257, 1999.

65. Jansson O.T., Morcos E., Brundin L., Bergerheim U.S., Adolfsson J., and Wiklund N.P. Nitric oxide synthase activity in human renal cell carcinoma. *Journal of Urology*, 160, 556–560, 1998.

66. Eroglu A., Demirci S., Ayyildiz A., Kocaoglu H., Akbulut H., Akgul H., and Elhan H.A. Serum concentrations of vascular endothelial growth factor and nitrite as an estimate of *in vivo* nitric oxide in patients with gastric cancer. *British Journal of Cancer*, 80, 1630–1634, 1999.

67. Goto T., Haruma K., Kitadai Y., Ito M., Yoshihara M., Sumii K., Hayakawa N., and Kajiyama G. Enhanced expression of inducible nitric oxide synthase and nitrotyrosine in gastric mucosa of gastric cancer patients. *Clinical Cancer Research*, 5, 1411–1415, 1999.

68. Anbar M., Naumov A., Milescu L., and Brown C. Objective detection of breast cancer by DAT—an update. *Thermology International*, 11, 11–18, 2001.

69. Anbar M., Grenn M.W., Marino M.T., Milescu L., and Zamani K. Fast dynamic area telethermometry (DAT) of the human forearm with a Ga/As quantum well infrared focal plane array camera. *European Journal of Thermology*, 7, 105–118, 1997.

70. *Anbar M. and Milescu L. Hardware and software requirements of clinical DAT. *SPIE Proceedings*, 3698, 63–74, 1999.

71. Gunapala S.D., Liu J.K., Sundaram M., Bandara S.V., Shott C.A., Hoelter T.R., Maker P.D., and Muller R.E. Long-wavelength 256 × 256 QWIP hand-held camera. *SPIE Proceedings*, 2746, 124–133, 1996.

72. Gunapala S.D., Liu J.K., Park J.S., Sundaram M., Shott C.A., Hoelter T., Lin T.-L., Massie S.T., Maker P.D., Muller R.E., and Sarusi G. 9 μm cutoff 256 × 256 GaAs/AlxGal-xAs quantum well infrared photodetector hand-held camera. *IEEE Transactions of Electron Devices*, 44, 51–57, 1997.

73. Anbar M., Milescu L., Grenn M.W., Zamani K., and Marino M.T. Study of skin hemodynamics with fast dynamic area telethermometry (DAT). *Proceedings of the 19th IEEE EMBS International Conference*, 644–648, 1997.

74. Zamani K., Marino M.T., Bonner M., and Anbar M. Assessment of mental stress as well as neurological effects of chemical warfare agents by dynamic area telethermometry. *Proceedings of the 21th Army Science Conference*, 125–130, 1998.

75. Gratt B.M. and Anbar M. Thermology and facial thermography: Part II. Current and future clinical applications in dentistry. *Journal of Dentomaxillofacial Radiology*, 27, 68–74, 1998.

76. Anbar M. and Gratt B.M. The possible role of nitric oxide in the physiopathology of pain associated with temporomandibular disorders. *Journal of Oral and Maxillofacial Surgery*, 56, 872–882, 1998.

77. Anbar M. and Zamani K. A DAT study of a painful knee—comparison with MRI findings. *Proceedings of the 4th Congress of the International College of Thermology* and *the Annual Meeting of the American Academy of Thermology*, Fort Lauderdale, FL, 25, 1998.

78. Anbar M., Eckhert K.H. Jr., and Milescu L. Preliminary study of women's breasts with dynamic area telethermometry (DAT). *Proceedings of the 4th Congress of the International College of Thermology* and *the Annual Meeting of the American Academy of Thermology*, Fort Lauderdale, FL, 27–28, 1998.

79. *Anbar M. Clinical thermal imaging today—shifting from phenomenological thermography to pathophysiologically based thermal imaging. *IEEE EMBS Magazine*, 17, 25–33, 1998.

80. Anbar M. and Milescu L. Scope and limitations of dynamic area telethermometry (DAT). *Proceedings of the 20th IEEE EMBS International Conference*, Hong Kong, HK, 928–931, 1998.

81. Anbar M., Brown C.A., Milescu L., and Babalola J.A. Clinical applications of DAT using a QWIP FPA camera. *SPIE Proceedings*, Orlando, FL, 3698, 93–104, 1999.

82. Anbar M., Brown C.A., Milescu L., Babalola J.A., and Gentner L. Potential applications of dynamic area telethermometry (DAT) in assessment of cancer in the breasts. *IEEE EMBS Magazine*, 19, 58–62, 2000.

83. Anbar M., Brown C.A., and Milescu L. Objective identification of cancerous breasts by dynamic area telethermometry (DAT). *Thermology International*, 9, 137–143, 1999.

84. Anbar M., Brown C.A., and Milescu L. Objective detection of beast cancer by dynamic area telethermometry. *Proceedings of the 21st Annual International Conference of EMBS*, 1115–1116, 1999.

85. Anbar M., Milescu L., Naumov A., Brown C.A., Button T., Carty C., and AlDulaimi K. Detection of cancerous breasts by dynamic area telethermometry (DAT). *IEEE EMBS Magazine*, 20, 80–91, 2001.

86. Fanning S.R., Short S., Coleman K., Andresen S., Budd G.T., Moore H., Rim A., Crowe J., and Weng D.E. Correlation of dynamic infrared imaging with radiologic and pathologic response for patients treated with primary systemic therapy for locally advanced breast cancer. *American Society of Clinical Oncology (ASCO) Annual Meeting*, Atlanta, GA, 2006.

87. Janicek M.J., Waxman A., Janicek M.R., and Demetri G.D. Assessment of early response to therapy in sarcomas: Dynamic infrared imaging (DIRI), computerized tomography (CT) and F-18 FDG positron emission tomography (PET). *American Society of Clinical Oncology (ASCO) Annual Meeting*, 2001, Abstract #1390.

88. Janicek M.J., van Sonnenberg E., and Demetri G.D. Monitoring of early response to treatment in metastatic gastrointestinal stromal tumor (gist): Model of multimodality approach including f-18 fdg pet, infrared imaging and Doppler ultrasound. *SGR (Society of Gastrointestinal radiologists) Abdominal radiology Conference*, 2001.

89. Janicek M.J., Janicek M.R., Merriam P., Potter A., Silberman S., Dimitrijevic S., Fauci M., and Demetri G.D. Imaging responses to Imatinib mesylate (Gleevec, STI571) in gastrointestinal stromal tumors (GIST): Vascular perfusion patterns with Doppler ultrasound (DUS) and dynamic infrared imaging (DIRI). *American Society of Clinical Oncology (ASCO) Annual Meeting*, 2002, Abstract #333.

90. Janicek M.J., Demetri G.D., Janicek M.R., Shaffer K., and Fauci M.A. Dynamic infrared imaging of newly diagnosed malignant lymphoma compared with Gallium-67 and Fluorine-18 fluorodeoxyglucose (FDG) positron emission tomography. *Cancer Research and Treatment*, 2, 571–578, 2003.

91. Janicek M.J., Demetri G., Janicek M.R., Shaffer K., and Fauci M.A. Dynamic infrared imaging of newly diagnosed malignant lymphoma compared with gallium-67 and fluorine-18 fluorodeoxyglucose (FDG) positron emission tomography. *Technology in Cancer Research and Treatment*, 2, 71–77, 2003.

92. Parisky Y.R., Sardi A., Hamm R., Hughes K., Esserman L., Rust S., and Callahan K. Efficacy of computerized infrared imaging analysis to evaluate mammographically suspicious lesions. *American Journal of Roentgenology*, 180, 263–269, 2003.

93. Moskowitz M. Efficacy of computerized infrared imaging. *American Journal of Roentgenology*, 180, 596, 2003.

94. Button T.M., Li H., Fisher P., Rosenblatt R., Dulaimy K., Li S., O'Hea B., Salvitti M., Geronimo V., Geronimo C., Jambawalikar S., Carvelli P., and Weiss R. Dynamic infrared imaging for the detection of malignancy. *Physics in Medicine and Biology*, 49, 3105–3116, 2004.

95. Gorbach A.M. Infrared imaging of brain function. *Advances in Experimental Medicine and Biology*, 333, 95–123, 1993.

96. Watson J.C., Gorbach A.M., Pluta R.M., Rak R., Heiss J.D., and Oldfield E.H. Real-time detection of vascular occlusion and reperfusion of the brain during surgery by using infrared imaging. *Journal of Neurosurgery*, 96, 918–923, 2002.

97. Gorbach A.M., Heiss J., Kufta C., Sato S., Fedio P., Kammerer W.A., Solomon J., and Oldfield E.H. Intraoperative infrared functional imaging of human brain. *Annals of Neurology*, 54, 297–309, 2003.

98. Gorbach A.M. Local alternated temperature gradients as footprints of cortical functional activation. *Journal of Thermal Biology*, 29, 589–598, 2004.

99. Gorbach A.M., Heiss J.D., Kopylev L., and Oldfield E.H. Intraoperative infrared imaging of brain tumors. *Journal of Neurosurgery*, 101, 960–969, 2004.

100. Gorbach A.M., Ntziachristos V., and Perelman L. Advances in optical imaging of cancer. In *New Techniques in Oncologic Imaging*, Padhani A.M. and Choyke P.L. (eds.), New York, Taylor and Francis, Chapter 18, pp. 351–370, 2005.

101. Trubel H.K., Sacolik L.I., and Hyder F. Regional temperature changes in the brain during somatosomatic stimulation. *Journal Cerebral Blood Flow and Metabolism*, 26, 68–78, 2006.

102. Ecker R.D., Goerss S.J., Meyer F.B., Cohen-Gadol A.A., Britton J.W., and Levine J.A. Vision of the future: Initial experience with intraoperative real-time high-resolution dynamic infrared imaging. *Journal of Neurosurgery*, 97, 1460–1471, 2002.

103. Cohen B.P., Kruse R.J., and Anbar M. The social structure of scientific research teams. *Pacific Sociological Review*, 25, 205–245, 1982.

104. Binzoni T., Leung T., Delpy D.T., Fauci M.A., and Rufenacht D. Mapping human skeletal muscle perforator vessels using a quantum well infrared photodetector (QWIP) might explain the variability of NIRS and LDF measurements. *Physics in Medicine and Biology*, 49, N165–N173, 2004.

105. Campbell P.A., Cresswell A.B., Frank T.G., and Cuschieri A. Real-time thermography during energized vessel sealing and dissection. *Surgical Endoscopy*, 17, 1640–1645, 2003.

106. Nakagawa A., Hirano T., Uenohara H., Utsunomiya H., Suzuki S., Takayama K., Shirane R., and Tominaga T. Use of intraoperative dynamic infrared imaging with detection wavelength of 7–14 μm in the surgical obliteration of spinal arteriovenous fistula: Case report and technical considerations. *Minimally Invasive Neurosurgery*, 47, 136–139, 2004.

107. Mohr F.W. and Falk V. Thermal coronary angiography: A method for assessing graft patency and coronary anatomy in coronary bypass surgery. *Annals of Thoracic Surgery*, 47, 441–449, 1989. Updated in 1997 *Annals of Thoracic Surgery*, 63, 1506–1507.

108. Falk V., Walther T., Philippi A., Autschbach R., Krieger H., Dalichau H., and Mohr F.W. Thermal coronary angiography for intraoperative patency control of arterial and saphenous vein coronary artery bypass grafts: Results in 370 patients. *Journal of Cardiac Surgery*, 10, 147–160, 1995.

109. van Son J.A., Falk V., Walther T., Diegeler A., and Mohr F.W. Thermal coronary angiography for intraoperative testing of coronary patency in congenital heart defects. *Annals of Thoracic Surgery*, 64, 1499–1500, 1997.

110. Gorbach A., Simonton D., Hale D.A., Swanson S.J., and Kirk A.D. Objective, real-time, intraoperative assessment of renal perfusion using infrared imaging. *American Journal of Transplantation*, 3, 988–993, 2003.

111. Gold J.E., Cherniack M., and Buchholz B. Infrared thermography for examination of skin temperature in the dorsal hand of office workers. *European Journal of Applied Physiology*, 93, 245–251, 2004.

112. Fujiwara Y., Inukai T., Aso Y., and Takemura Y. Thermographic measurement of skin temperature recovery time of extremities in patients with type 2 diabetes mellitus. *Experimental and Clinical Endocrinology and Diabetes*, 108, 463–469, 2000.

113. Zotter H., Kerbl R., Gallistl S., Nitsche H., and Borkenstein M. Rewarming index of the lower leg assessed by infrared thermography in adolescents with type 1 diabetes mellitus. *Journal of Pediatric Endocrinology Metabolism*, 16, 1257–1262, 2003.

114. Huygen F.J., Niehof S., Klein J., and Zijlstra F.J. Computer-assisted skin videothermography is a highly sensitive quality tool in the diagnosis and monitoring of complex regional pain syndrome type I. *European Journal of Applied Physiology*, 91, 516–524, 2004.

115. Haverly R.F. and Anbar M. A telethermometric study of the age dependence of corneal temperature. *Biomedical Thermology*, 14, 10–26, 1994.

116. Purslow C. and Wolffsohn J.S. Ocular surface temperature: A review. *Eye Contact Lens*, 31, 117–123, 2005.

117. Besson M., Brook P., Chizh B.A., and Pickering A.E. Tactile allodynia in patients with postherpetic neuralgia: Lack of change in skin blood flow upon dynamic stimulation. *Pain*, 117, 154–191, 2005.

118. Kemppainen P., Forster C., and Handwerker H.O. The importance of stimulus site and intensity in differences of pain-induced vascular reflexes in human orofacial regions. *Pain*, 91, 331–338, 2001.

119. Kells B.E., Kennedy J.G., Biagioni P.A., and Lamey P.J. Computerized infrared thermographic imaging and pulpal blood flow: Part 1. A protocol for thermal imaging of human teeth. *International Endodontic Journal*, 33, 442–447, 2000.

120. Kells B.E., Kennedy J.G., Biagioni P.A., and Lamey P.J. Computerized infrared thermographic imaging and pulpal blood flow: Part 2. Rewarming of healthy human teeth following a controlled cold stimulus. *International Endodontic Journal*, 33, 448–462, 2000.

121. Anbar M., Guttmann S., and Lewitus Z. The accumulation of fluoroborate ions in thyroid glands of rats. *Endocrinology*, 66, 888–890, 1960.

122. Anbar M. Application of fluorine 18 in biological studies with special reference to bone physiology. In *Production and Use of Short Lived Radioisotopes*, Vienna, IAEA, Vol. II, pp. 227–245, 1963.

123. Anbar M., Kosary I., Laor Y., Guttmann S., Lewitus Z., and Askenasy H. The localization of intracranial tumors by positron emitting F18 labelled fluoborate. *Proceedings of the Beilinson Hospital*, 10, 50–52, 1961.

124. Askenasy H., Kosary I., Toledo E., Lewitus Z., and Anbar M. The use of radioisotopes in the detection of brain tumors. *Proceedings of the Beilinson Hospital*, 10, 53–58, 1961.

125. Ashkenazy H.M., Anbar M., Laor Y., Kosary I.Z., and Guttmann S. The localization of intracranial space-occupying lesions by fluoroborate ions labelled with fluorine 18. *American Journal of Roentgenology and Nuclear Medicine*, 88, 350–354, 1962.

30

Thermal Texture Mapping: Whole-Body Infrared Imaging and Its Holistic Interpretation

H. Helen Liu
*Institute of Holistic Health
and Science*

Zhong Qi Liu
*Academy of TTM
Technologies and Bioyear
Medical Instrument*

30.1 Introduction

A live human body emits heat, part of which is radiated as infrared (IR) photons. Heat is one of a few basic features that distinguish a live body from a dead one, because heat is continuously being generated through metabolic, blood flow, and other important biological processes such as thermogenesis processes. Thus, although IR photons represent only a narrow band of the electromagnetic spectrum, information contained in such images is fundamentally associated with the functional status and movement in our body.

In radiological science, functional imaging is a fast evolving field that focuses on imaging and assessing biological functions of the body. Based on the physical and physiological characteristics of IR imaging, it can fit perfectly into this category and attract tremendous medical interests [1,2]. However, despite many appealing features of IR as compared to other imaging modalities, IR has not entered the field of radiology in mainstream medicine so far. This is an unfortunate fact, and many historical, social–political as well as scientific factors can be attributed to it.

In our opinion, there are two major misconceptions about IR that have hindered its development in the past. The first misconception is related to the depth of IR photons that can penetrate through the skin. At present, IR is generally perceived to be useful for imaging skin, blood flow and conditions near superficial depths only, for example, breast imaging, pain management, skin perfusion, and so on. This perception came into dominance because IR photons can only go through a minuscule distance inside tissues. Thus, it has been conventionally believed that heat from sources deep within the body cannot be easily seen from IR images, and thus, IR has very limited role to play in studying internal organs and in the field of radiology.

The second misconception about IR is that it merely reflects the thermal activity of the body. This misconception came into existence because physics has taught us that heat gives off IR photons, and there is a relationship between temperature and intensity of IR photons. Thus, we tend to believe that IR imaging is only about seeing the thermal activity of the body. This has significantly limited the use of the IR, because heat only represents a narrow range of biological functions in the body.

Quite contrary to these conventionally held beliefs, through continuous research and development efforts over the past 15 years, we have found that first of all, surface thermal patterns are strongly associated with internal organ functions and biological processes. More importantly, IR images represent essentially a type of energy maps of the human body within the IR spectral window, in other words, they are intrinsically holographic or reflexiological maps of the human energy structure.

These important findings came into light when we carried out earlier experiments and theoretical analyses, followed by a large number of clinical observations of various diseases and health conditions. On the basis of continuous availability of clinical data and accumulated experience over a decade of work, a new system of acquiring and interpreting the images was developed. In differentiating traditional thermography from this new approach, it received a new name of "thermal texture mapping" or TTM which refers to the way how the images are acquired, analyzed, and interpreted [3–10]. TTM has evolved to be essentially a new tool to evaluate the functional balance and health environment of the body. IR-TTM is in fact a bridge between mainstream medicine and alternative medicine, the merging of two will lead to a new era of holistic medicine.

In parallel to the research efforts, commercial development was undertaken in the 1990s for TTM. Complete hardware and software systems were developed, facilitating the use of TTM in hospital settings as well as in public health. Applications in mainstream medicine and holistic medicine, and other emerging fields are being actively investigated at present. Meanwhile, we would like to point out that the methodology of TTM is still in its developmental stage. We anticipate its continuous and dynamic growth in the coming years as more basic research and clinical investigations are added to the field.

30.2 Early Experiments and Analyses

A live human body must maintain thermal homeostasis within a few degree Celsius to ensure proper functions of its biological integrity. In the meantime, heat exchange is constantly ongoing to reach a steady state of thermal equilibrium within the body and with the environment. It is then apparent that our body, through millions if not billions of years of natural evolution, must be equipped with extraordinary means of maintaining the thermal homeostasis and equilibrium of itself. Various thermal pathways must exist to conduct the heat in an extremely efficient and harmonious manner for our basic survival. In classic context, it is believed that heat transfer in the body is assisted by blood flow and perfusion, respiration and perspiration, direct heat conduction, convection, and radiation. There are likely other means of transferring the heat efficiently, for example, through meridian and other subtle energy systems [11] of which presently science has little knowledge about.

It is then not difficult to realize that the thermal patterns observed on the skin surface must be affected and related to the internal body function and the entire heat exchange process. In fact, this concept has been used in many industrial and military applications in which underground targets are detected through surface thermal patterns. Even in considering the adipose tissue (fat) which does not contain a large amount of blood vessels and is well insulated to protect the body, heat exchange is constantly ongoing, and the thermal patterns on the skin surface must be related intrinsically to the thermal characteristics underneath it. Earlier works have explored this topic and showed promising results that warrant further investigations [12–17].

This work was inspired by earlier observations of diseases known to have thermogenesis properties, such as inflammation and cancer growth that are highly metabolically active [3,7–10]. From conventional thermographs of human subjects with these health conditions, we observed that certain thermal patterns seen on the skin surface could be closely related to local lesions that are thermal active. Our body seems to be rather thermal transparent, allowing internal heat to be transferred efficiently to the skin surface as a means to maintain thermal homeostasis and equilibrium in the body.

30.2.1 *Ex Vivo* Measurements and Modeling

In an attempt to address the question on how surface heat is related to its internal source, we have conducted experiments and analyses using *ex vivo* animal tissues [6]. In the simulation, heat sources with a temperature close to the human body temperature were imbedded inside freshly dissected animal tissue samples. A typical piece of such tissue sample includes shaved skin, subcutaneous fat, connected tissues, and muscular tissues. The experimental setup is shown in Figure 30.1. In this particular case, a piece of adipose tissue was used, with the size being approximately 15 cm × 15 cm × 2 cm. A brass ball was buried in the tissue as a heat source. The diameter of the ball could be changed from 5 mm to a few centimeters. The surface temperature of the tissue was scanned using a commercial IR camera (spectral response in 8–14 μm) at a distance of approximately 1 m. The brass ball was heated for about 2 h to reach steady state of the surface temperature. Figure 30.2 shows the heat distribution measured from the tissue surface.

We found that the heat going through the tissue sample and emitted from the surface showed a bell-shaped thermal distribution. The center of this bell-shaped function is where the imbedded heat source was the closest to the surface. We found that there is a unique relationship between the depth of the heat source and the width of the bell-shaped function. In other words, we found that the area covered by certain isothermal contours was related to the depth of the heat source itself.

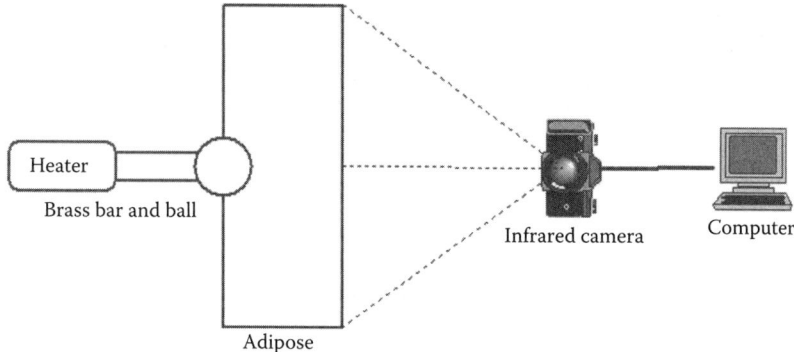

FIGURE 30.1 Illustration of the experimental setup where an internal ball heat source (e.g., brass ball) was imbedded in a piece of adipose tissue. For color figures, see www.holistichealthscience.org.

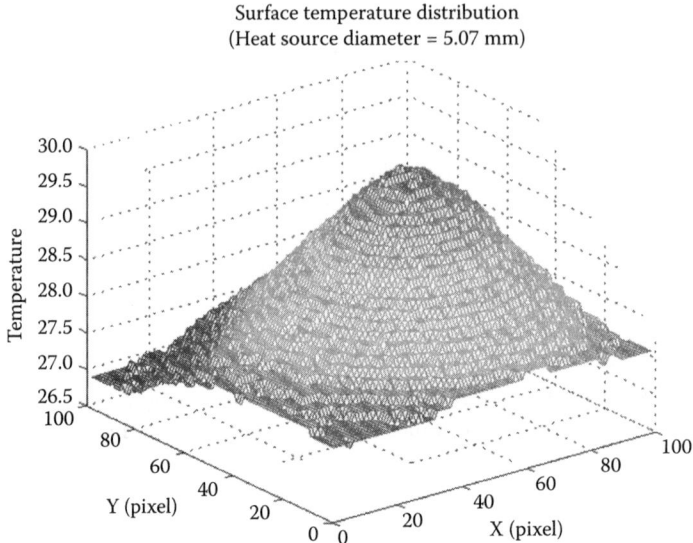

FIGURE 30.2 Illustration of the surface temperature distribution of the internal source of Figure 30.1. For color figures, see www.holistichealthscience.org.

To explore the theoretical basis of this observation, we used the commonly applied bio-heat transfer equation [18],

$$bc\frac{\partial T}{\partial t} = \nabla \cdot (k\nabla T) + Q_b + Q_m \tag{30.1}$$

which describes the energy conservation in a volume of tissue with a constant blood flow rate Q_b and metabolic rate Q_m, and c, b, and k denote the specific heat, the density, and the effective thermal conductivity of the tissue, respectively. If the *ex vivo* tissue sample is in a steady state, Q_b and Q_m equal to zero and the bio-heat transfer equation is reduced to,

$$\nabla \cdot (k\nabla T) = 0 \tag{30.2}$$

To arrive at an analytical solution to Equation 30.2, we consider that the temperature distribution T can be approximated by concentric spheres in a large isotropic phantom, where the center of the spheres coincides with the center of the ball heat source. In spherical coordinates with radius ρ. Equation 30.2 can be expressed as,

$$\frac{d}{d\rho}\left(\rho^2 \frac{dT}{d\rho}\right) = 0 \tag{30.3}$$

If the total heat emanating from the ball heat source is Q, the heat density q of the spot at a distance of ρ from the ball center is

$$q = \frac{Q}{4\pi\rho^2} \tag{30.4}$$

The heat density also can be obtained through the Fourier's Law

$$q = -\frac{dT}{d\rho} \quad (30.5)$$

From Equations 30.4 and 30.5, the temperature field function $T(\rho)$ can be found after taking the integral,

$$T(\rho) = T_1 - \frac{Q}{4\pi}\frac{1}{k}\left(\frac{1}{R} - \frac{1}{\rho}\right) \quad (30.6)$$

where T_1 is the temperature of the heat source and R is the radius of the ball. Next, we assume that at any spot on the boundary, heat density transferring from internal heat source is fully exchanged with the environment, that is,

$$q_{in} = q_{out} \quad (30.7)$$

where

$$q_{in} = \frac{Q}{4\pi\rho^2} = k\frac{T_1 - T_D(r)}{(\rho/R)(\rho - R)} \quad (30.8)$$

$$q_{out} = h_r(T_D(r) - T_0) + h_c(T_D(r) - T_0) = \alpha(T_D(r) - T_0) \quad (30.9)$$

in which h_r, h_c, and α are the radiative, convection, and total heat exchange coefficients used to approximate the boundary heat exchange using the first-order approximation. Finally, the surface temperature distribution can be obtained with an analytical solution,

$$T_D(r) = T_0 + \frac{(T_1 - T_0)}{(\alpha/k)\cdot\left(\sqrt{D^2 + r^2}/R\right)\cdot\left(\sqrt{D^2 + r^2} - R\right) + 1} \quad (30.10)$$

where D is the distance from the surface to the center of the heat source.

The calculated thermal distribution $T_D(r)$ was found to behave in a bell-shaped function, similar to those observed in the *ex vivo* tissue testing.

The effort in deriving the analytical solution to Equation 30.2 helped us understand the characteristics of the surface heat distribution versus the heat source itself in an extremely simplified setting. The results were very encouraging because they showed that in *ex vivo* conditions, surface heat is related to the depth of the source D and its spherical radius R. If the source radius R is relatively small compared to the depth of D, then the surface heat is primarily influenced by the depth of the source. This is an important finding, which identifies that the primary influence of the heat distribution is the depth of the heat source, and it is relatively independent of many other factors associated with the heat-exchange process in the tissue. There were earlier experimental work [14,15] which drew essentially the same conclusion.

30.2.2 Phantom Simulations

To further explore the surface heat distribution under more realistic phantom conditions, we simulated a cylindrical phantom where a spherical heat source was imbedded along the central axis of the phantom at different depths. The phantom consists of layers of tissues including skin, fat, and visceral tissues. We relied on solving Equation 30.1 using a finite-element approach (see more details in Reference 19) to obtain the surface temperature distribution. The effects of various parameters related to the heat source, physiological and environmental factors were studied extensively. Similar works have been done by other investigators using different approaches [20,21].

We found that the relative temperature distribution was essentially affected by radius R and depth D of the heat source only, which is consistent to both the analytical results and the one obtained from the *ex vivo* experiment, even though more layers of tissues and blood flow were included in the simulation. Furthermore, the range of the relative temperature distribution was mainly influenced by the depth D of the source only, relatively independent of other parameters used in the simulation (Figure 30.3).

What these results suggested is that when a source is deeply situated in the tissue, the width of the bell-shaped function is larger, resulting in a more gradual change of the surface heat; the shallower the source, the sharper the change of surface heat, resulting in a greater temperature drop away from the central axis of the cylinder (see Figure 30.3). Therefore, the temperature gradient of the surface heat can indicate the depth of the source. This makes obvious sense as we can see that the heat loss from the source center to any point on the surface has to be governed by the distance between these two points. The depth of the source determines how this distance is increased from the source center to peripheral areas. And the shallower the source, the sharper this distance will be increased away from the center, thereby, the greater the temperature will be reduced. Therefore, by evaluating the temperature gradient of the source surface temperature distribution, one could estimate whether the source is close to the skin surface or deeply situated away from the surface.

In practical terms, the temperature gradient can be displayed by isothermal contours for a given heat source, similar to the idea of using topology maps [6,12,13,19]. For a deeply situated source, its surface isothermal contours appear as densely packed, meaning the distance between the isothermal contours is closer because of a more gradual decrease of temperature from the source center, in contrast to a shallow source; whereas for a source situated near the skin surface, the isothermal contours near the source center will spread out with a greater distance in between.

Figure 30.4 illustrates this concept comparing deep and shallow heat sources. Another technique that we have developed to display the topology of the isothermal contours is called "dynamic slicing technique" shown in Figure 30.5. Here we reduce the displayed temperature level one step at a time,

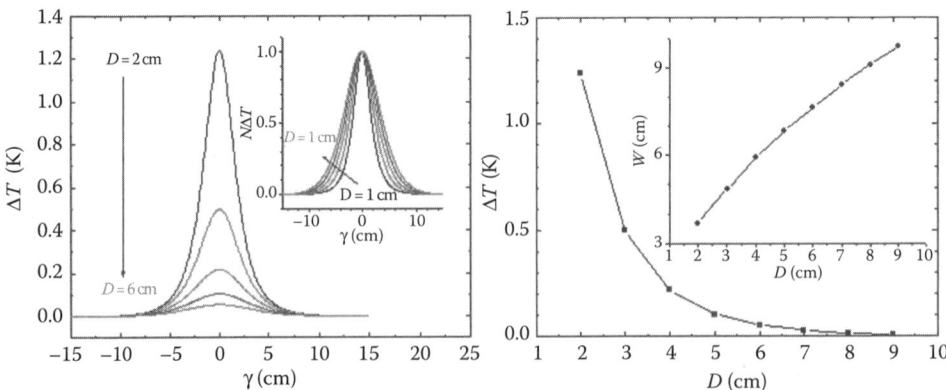

FIGURE 30.3 Left: temperature distributions on the phantom surface of the heat source. Baseline temperature was subtracted to obtain the relative temperature DT(r) and its normalized term NDT(r); r is the radius on the phantom surface away from the center of the source. Right: change of the DT(r=0) and its width W versus the source depth D. For color figures, see www.holistichealthscience.org.

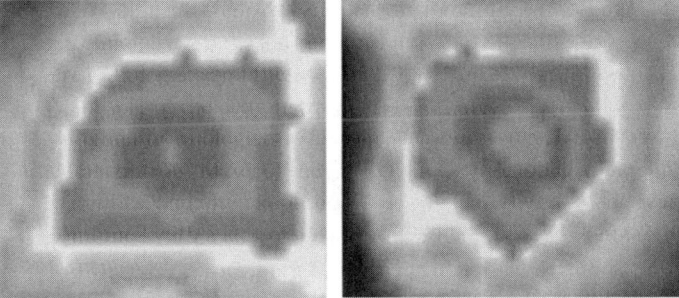

FIGURE 30.4 Illustration of the isothermal contours of the surface temperature distributions of heat sources at different depths. Left: a skin surface source with a greater distance between the isothermal contours. Right: a deep tissue source with closer distance between the isothermal contours. For color figures, see www.holistichealth-science.org.

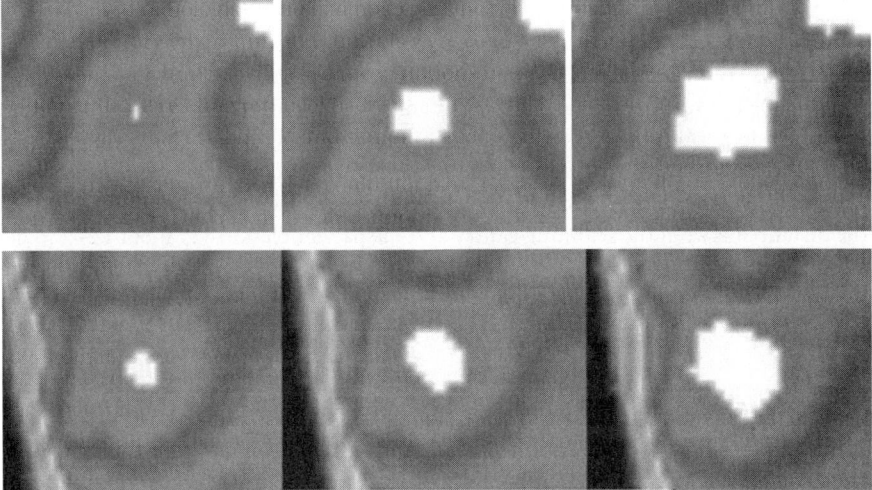

FIGURE 30.5 Illustration of the dynamic slicing technique in displaying the isothermal contours. The white area is the isothermal contour above certain temperature level corresponding to those contours shown in Figure 30.4. The temperature level is dynamically reduced every 0.05°C in a movie mode (three frames of the movie are shown here). Top: a skin surface source with greater changes between the isothermal contours. Bottom: a deep tissue source with gradual changes between the isothermal contours. For color figures, see www.holistichealthscience.org.

for example, every 0.05°C, allowing the surface isothermal contour to appear one level at a time corresponding to the chosen displayed temperature. In visualizing the changes of the isothermal contours dynamically with the displayed temperature, we can compare depths of different heat sources, in a way to differentiate a deep internal source versus skin surface heat source.

30.2.3 Summary of Early Findings

Results of our *ex vivo* experiments and simplified theoretical simulations were quite encouraging, because they pointed to the possibility of identifying deep situated heat sources based on the gradient of their surface temperature distribution. This conclusion was derived based on the condition that the tissue serving as the heat-exchange medium between the source and the surface is relatively homogeneous and isotropic in terms of their thermal properties.

Let us consider a realistic situation where a heat source is imbedded in live tissues, for example, a small tumor growing inside the muscle. The tumor-generated excessive metabolic heat will undergo heat exchange to reach thermal equilibrium with its surrounding tissues and the environment. Under steady-state conditions, heat from the tumor will be eventually distributed to the skin surface, though the surface temperature distribution will also depend on heat transfer processes involving different tissues, for example, blood flow and other thermal pathways. Therefore, whether we could detect deep-tissue heat sources will depend on the temperature contrast between the source and its surrounding tissues, sensitivity of the IR imager itself, and influence of many other physical and physiological factors associated with the heat exchange.

In the next phase of our investigation, we performed a large number of clinical studies and developed corresponding hardware system and software tools in acquiring and processing the image data. Before we present results of these clinical studies, the components of the TTM system and other relevant details are explained here for the purpose of clarification.

30.3 The TTM System

30.3.1 Hardware

To facilitate image acquisition of human subjects in clinical settings, we have developed an IR imaging system in the 1990s. This system consists of a scanner gantry, patient platform, and computer workstations (Figure 30.6). The scanner gantry has an IR camera mounted and a mechanical platform which allows the camera to perform pan, tilt, and vertical movement operations. The patient platform has a base unit where a patient can stand straight on the top and be rotated and scanned from different angles. This hardware system was designed to acquire whole-body images of the patient from any angle and height. The distance between the scanning gantry and the patient platform is about 1.5–2 m depending on the optical property of the camera.

At present, a typical TTM image series consists of 10–20 images with patients performing a sequence of poses. See Figure 30.7 for examples of these poses.

30.3.2 Software

Upon image acquisition, the images are sent to the computer workstation to be reviewed and analyzed. A commercial TTM software package was developed to manage patient database and image processing.

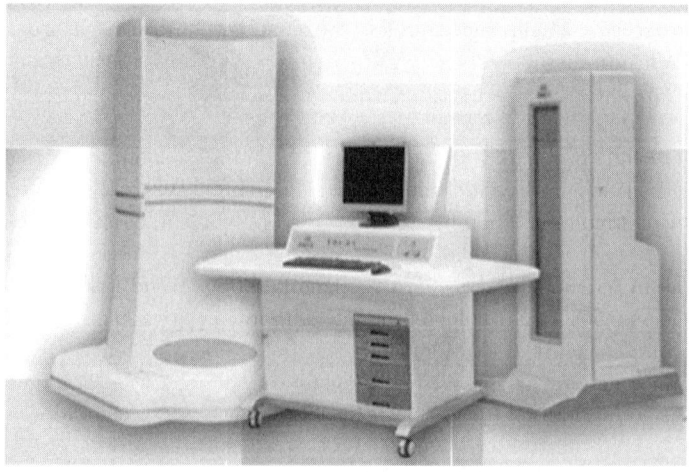

FIGURE 30.6 Illustration of the hardware equipment of a TTM system. For color figures, see www.holisti-chealthscience.org.

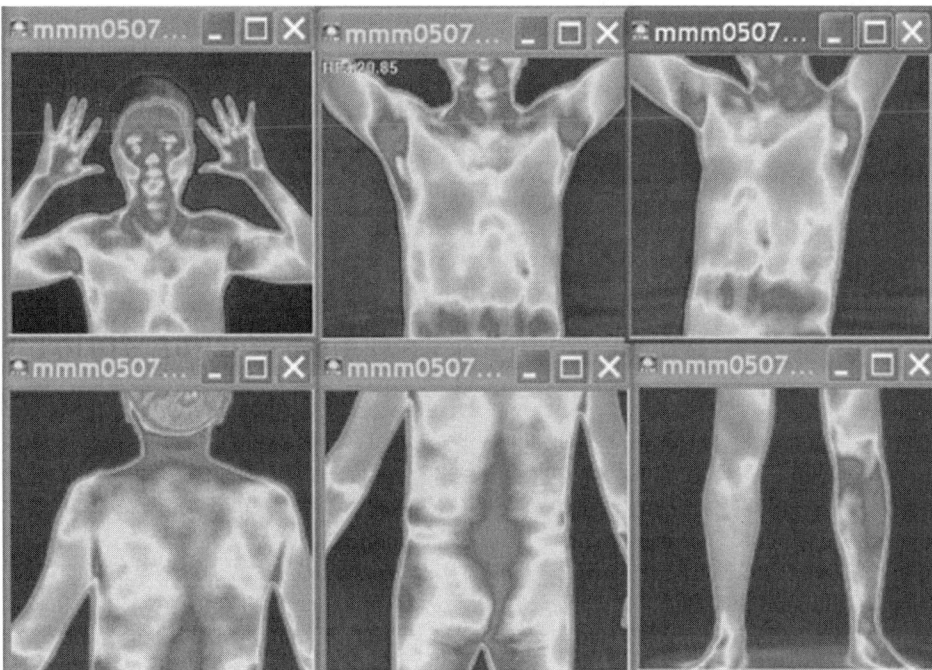

FIGURE 30.7 Typical poses used in a whole-body scan using the TTM system. For color figures, see www.holistichealthscience.org.

The image processing tools allow adjustment of color maps, displayed window and level of the images (brightness and contrast), image fusion and comparison, image measurements, and other associated functions. We also implemented tools to display the isothermal contours of the images along with the dynamic slicing technique. These tools help us visualize and analyze the topology, shape, texture, and anatomical features of the images.

The name "thermal texture mapping" or TTM came from the way that these images are displayed and analyzed. The terminology is still being used today for the purpose of continuity only, though the way we use the images today has evolved with a great degree of difference from the earlier versions. TTM differs from traditional thermography on several aspects. First of all, relative temperature and isothermal contour maps are used in TTM rather than the absolute temperature maps in traditional thermography. It is well known that absolute temperature is influenced by many physical and physiological factors and can vary significantly depending on the processes involved. By using the relative temperature maps and isothermal contours, effects of many of these factors, for example, how the IR signal is converted into temperature, environmental conditions, and camera conditions, and so on, can be minimized.

Second, we emphasize on assessing the topology information of the images in TTM in addition to the conventional temperature maps. The topological and morphological properties of the isothermal contours including shapes, textures, connection between different spots and other anatomical features are used to analyze the thermal distributions and their associated physiological implications.

Furthermore, in TTM software, image tools were implemented allowing image registration and fusion of TTM images with standard anatomical template as well as radiological images (x-ray/CT, MRI, PET, etc.). This feature was particularly effective in combining and comparing information obtained from other radiological modalities. An example of such fused TTM image is given in Figure 30.8. There are other unique features developed in interpreting the images in the TTM system. Details will be given in the next sections.

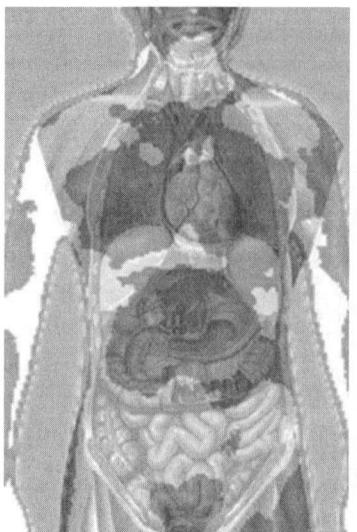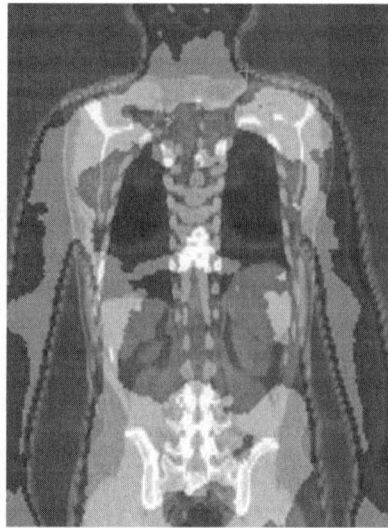

FIGURE 30.8 TTM images are fused with anatomical template (left) and reconstructed CT images of a coronal plane of the studied subject. For color figures, see www.holistichealthscience.org.

30.4 Clinical Observations of Internal Body Heat

30.4.1 Study Procedures

It is known that excessive cell growth, blood flow, or aggregated blood vessels such as those seen in cancer development or inflammation could be associated with a higher metabolic rate and a thermogenesis rate. These types of abnormalities can then serve as internal thermal sources. To investigate surface thermal patterns and how they are affected by the internal heat, we performed multiple studies of commonly seen solitary tumors, hyperplasia, and other tumor types. In addition, diseases associated with local infection and inflammation were observed as well. Interesting studies involved subjects of acquired immune deficiency syndrome (AIDS) and severe acute respiratory syndrome (SARS) which involved infection/inflammation in the lungs [7]. These studies typically included the following procedures.

Patients with one particular type of abnormality, for example, prostate cancer, were recruited with certain predetermined selection criteria (details varied depending on the type of disease and the design of that study). Typically, these patients had clinically confirmed abnormality based on combined radiological studies, clinical tests, and manifested symptoms. Before any surgical procedures and therapeutic intervention, patients were scanned with a TTM system to acquire images of the whole body of the study subject.

When acquiring the images, factors that could possibly influence thermal patterns of the body were minimized, similar to the requirements of conventional thermography procedures. For example, patients were asked to fast for at least 2 h prior to the image scan. Alcohol, use of other stimulants and medications were stopped for at least 8 h before the scan. Skin conditioning such as use of cosmetics and perfume was minimized. Patients were asked to take all clothes off and expose the body in a temperature-controlled room for 10–15 min prior to the scan. Images were then taken for typically about 10–15 min depending on the specific protocol requirements.

We also collected radiological images and other medical reports whenever available, including the lesion's depth, size, clinical stage, and other relevant demographic and clinical data. We used these data in combination with the TTM images to study whether certain thermal signatures were observed near the physical location of the lesion underneath the skin surface. If reconstructed radiological images were available, we also fused such images with TTM images, allowing further examination of the thermal patterns corresponding to the physical location of the lesion identified on the radiological images. These radiological images could come from x-ray/CT, MRI, or PET/CT images available for the studied subjects. Results from representing cases are discussed below.

30.4.2 Case Studies

Figure 30.9 shows a case of liver hemangioma which forms a cluster of entangled blood vessels in the liver. The tumor was approximately 4 cm in size and 5 cm deep inside the liver, diagnosed through an ultrasound exam. This type of tumor serves as an ideal heat source in internal organs because of their simple physiological and anatomical structures. On thermal images, hemangiomas in the liver often appear as distinct hot spots in close proximity to their anatomical locations. Results confirmed our initial finding that under steady-state condition, local heat generated by thermal sources such as a hemangioma will be eventually transferred to skin surface to reach thermal equilibrium. Using the dynamic slicing technique, we can analyze the features of the isothermal contours of the tumor in comparison with other known surface hot spots on the same image. This tumor that is situated inside the liver had isothermal contours that were closely packed in contrast to those of a shallow skin spot. A comparison of the isothermal contours is given in Figure 30.5.

Figure 30.10 shows a stage III stomach cancer case involving the gastrointestinal junction of the stomach and the end of the esophagus. On the thermal map, thermal elevation was seen corresponding to the anatomical location of the lesion and in an agreement with findings from the PET/CT scan. The fact that heat from this deep lesion could be seen on the skin surface was both intriguing and encouraging because of the complexity of the anatomy and in homogeneity of the tissues involved. The heat from the lesion had to go through sections of the stomach, liver, diaphragm, bones of the rib cages, and various connective tissue layers in between to reach the skin surface. However, this complex matrix of tissues surrounding the lesion did not seem to prevent the internal heat from being detected on the skin surface, indicating the capability of heat transfer in the body to reach thermal equilibrium conditions.

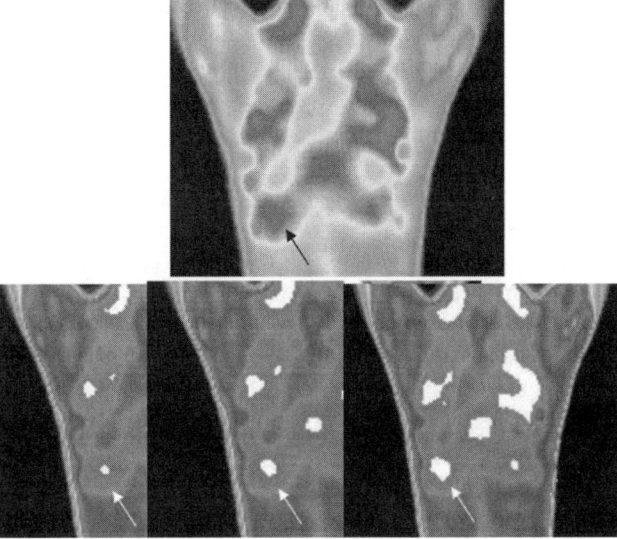

FIGURE 30.9 TTM images of a studied subject with hemangioma of the liver, shown by the arrow. Top: temperature map; bottom: dynamic slicing used in TTM and isothermal contours shown by the white areas. For color figures, see www.holistichealthscience.org.

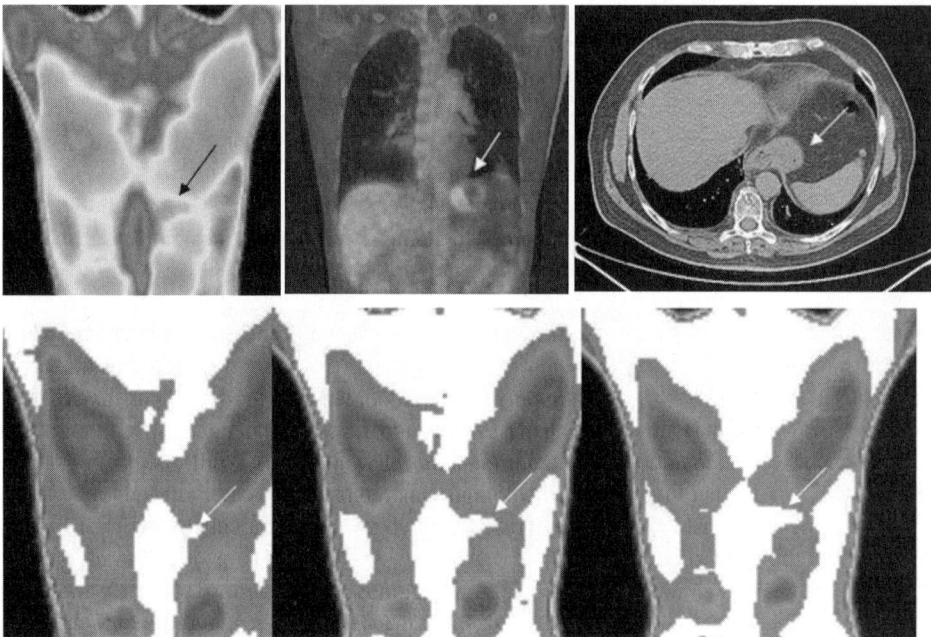

FIGURE 30.10 TTM images of a studied subject with stage III cancer of the stomach, shown by the arrow. Top: temperature map, PET/CT, and a CT axial cut; bottom: dynamic slicing used in TTM and isothermal contours shown by the white areas of the lesion.

Figure 30.11 shows another case of liver cancer, however, with more complex presentations and multiple lesions (stave IV multifocal hepatocellular carcinoma). A cluster of lesions were found from the MRI study near the anterior portion of the liver by the junction of the left and right lobes. TTM images showed that the skin surface near the anatomical location of the liver displayed abnormal hot spots seen from the anterior, right side, and posterior surface of the studied subject. These hot spots were quite irregular, naturally, because of the cancer lesions themselves were at an advanced stage and far more complex than a simple hemoangioma.

30.4.3 Further Discussions

It is known that the angiogenesis process involved in cancer development also helps cancer lesions develop a matrix of blood vessels that supplies metabolic need of the cancer growth. Likely, these vessels are also involved in dissipating the excessive heat from the cancer lesions to their surrounding tissues. At an advanced stage of cancer development, tissue necrosis also occurs because of hypoxia in the core of the lesions. All these factors make the heat-exchange process far more complex than that of an infancy cancer or a simple solid tumor. For such advanced stage cancer cases, we observed several important phenomena that are worth discussing here.

First of all, the topology of the isothermal contours of this type of cancer lesions become far more irregular and complex. The results came as no surprise, because, in addition to the factors of angiogenesis and necrosis, multiple heat sources could be superimposed together, each may have irregular shape and extend to different depths and layers of tissues. Second, the hot-spot locations appearing on the surface thermal maps could deviate from those seen from radiological images, likely caused by the necrosis process and blood flow-related factors as well. Naturally as the cancer lesions grow larger, heat produced by the lesions may be more intense at the edge of the lesions where metabolic rate is greater than the core of the lesions where necrosis could occur. Blood vessels could also carry the heat to surrounding

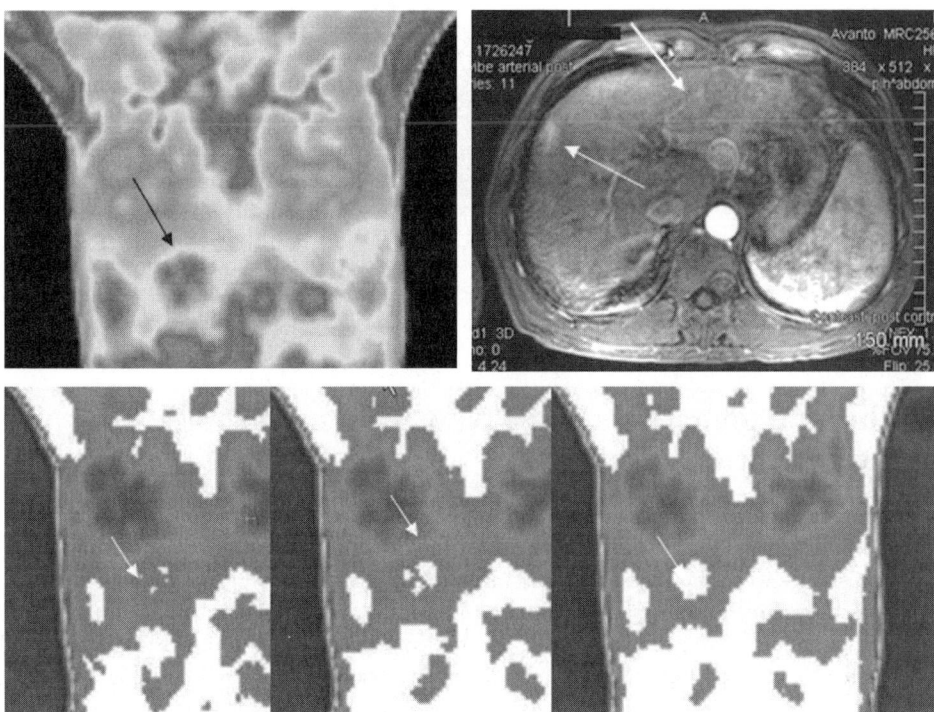

FIGURE 30.11 TTM images of a studied subject with stage IV cancer of the liver, shown by the arrows. Top: temperature map, an MRI axial cut; bottom: dynamic slicing used in TTM and isothermal contours shown by the white areas of the lesions. For color figures, see www.holistichealthscience.org.

tissues and skin surface at locations away from the cancer lesions themselves, making their thermal patterns appear differently than those observed on anatomical images. Third, because of reduced metabolic and thermogenesis rate near the core of the lesions, advanced cancer lesions may not show significant thermal contrast, making it more difficult to distinguish near their corresponding anatomical locations.

Another more interesting and important observation we found is that heat generated by cancer lesions could also be carried elsewhere far away from the source itself through thermal pathways where thermal exchange happens at a greater rate, in other words, pathways that are least thermal resistance. For example, heat transfer through muscular tissue is greater than adipose tissue and bones, and is greater along the muscular fiber orientation than transverse from it. Examples will be given in the next section. There are likely other thermal pathways, for example, involving blood or lymphatic circulation, meridian systems and network of subtle energy [22–24], that can carry the heat away from the source. For stomach and esophageal cancers, for example, we found hot spots that we refer to as "thermal acupoints" that are located near the throat, abdomen and back far away from the stomach itself (Figure 30.12). These acupoints appear as distinct circular or other regularly shaped structures, with locations consistent across different studied subjects. The exact mechanism and physiological basis of these acupoints are unknown, but they seem to indicate a template of such structures in correspondence to the local stress such as cancer growth of the area.

To account for these complex processes and their effects on isothermal contours, we had to extend our original method used for simple solid heat sources in tissues. By reviewing images from many clinical cases on various diseases and health conditions, we found interesting features of thermal patterns or thermal signatures that are associated with disease development and the ways of heat exchange in our body, for example, thermal acupoints as just mentioned.

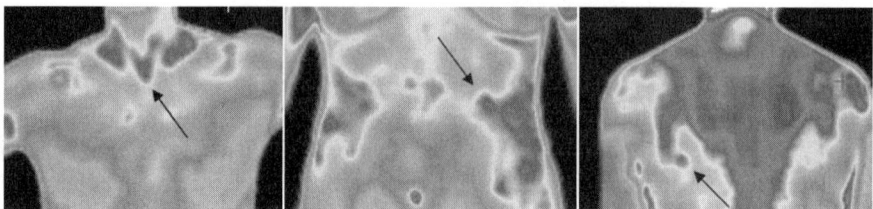

FIGURE 30.12 Thermal acupoints that are associated with stomach disorders. Left: acupoint near the supercla-vicular notch of the same subject of Figure 30.10. Mid and right: acupoints near the left middle abdomen and left back of another subject. For color figures, see www.holistichealthscience.org.

30.5 Thermal Signatures and a New System of Image Interpretation

It has been long recognized that cancer, autoimmune disorders, and many other serious conditions are systematic diseases that affect the whole body. Thus, disease development not only affects the local area, but may also involve whole-body response and impacts the functionality of the entire system. At pres-ent, radiological imaging is often confined to study a limited area of the body because these modalities such as ultrasound, CT and MRI are mainly used for the purpose of examining local anatomy and tis-sues only rather than functional aspects of the whole body. On the other hand, IR images intrinsically reflect function status of the body. Being noninvasive and simple to operate, IR can be used to scan the whole body. This feature allows us to investigate thermal signatures of diseases, their developmental processes, the overall health environment and body response to such local conditions. Some of the rep-resentative cases are presented here to illustrate our findings.

30.5.1 Case Studies

Figure 30.13 shows a case of prostate hyperplasia involving enlargement of the prostate. The ther-mal image of the front pelvic area indicates the increase of heat dissipated near the local area of the prostate. The back view shows hot spots by both sides of the buttock area, which is a typical feature observed from thermal patterns of prostate hyperplasia and prostate cancer. Likely, sacrum and coccyx of the pelvic girdle are quite thermal insulating, preventing the heat of the prostate from coming to the posterior skin surface directly. Thermal pathways through blood flow and muscular conduction could carry the heat more efficiently farther away from the prostate to the outer edges of the pelvic area.

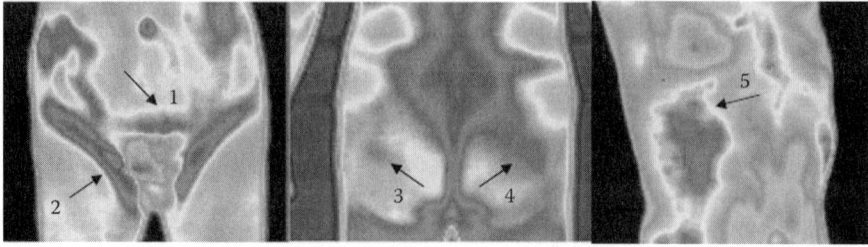

FIGURE 30.13 TTM images of a studied subject with prostate hyperplasia shown by arrow #1. Abnormal thermal activities were also observed at the pelvic lymph node area (arrow #2, back of the buttock (arrow #3, #4), and in the liver area (arrow #5). For color figures, see www.holistichealthscience.org.

In addition to heat associated with local prostate, we also observed the elevation of thermal activities accompanied by thermal asymmetry of the pelvic lymph node area. Thermal asymmetry refers to the temperature difference between the left and right side of the pelvic nodal region seen from the images. This thermal signature may be associated with increased metabolic activity and blood flow of the pelvic nodes which are involved in the process of cancer development.

Furthermore, we also observed that subjects with prostate disorder had accompanying symptoms of abnormal thermal signatures of the liver area as well, indicating certain association between the liver and prostate functions. It is unknown whether such an association is a simple correlation (both occur simultaneously) or it has a causal effect (one causes the other to occur). But this finding has suggested the importance of observing liver function and its effect on the development of prostate cancer or vice versa. To the best of our knowledge, this phenomenon has not been documented in the current clinical research, but it indicates that using whole-body IR can reveal important relationship and interconnection among functions of different organs. One interesting clinical question to be explored is whether treatment of the prostate cancer by local therapy will impact the liver function, and how these two organs are related.

Figure 30.14 shows another clinical case involving cancer of the apex of the right lung. Although PET and CT images showed highlighted regions near this anatomical location only, abnormal thermal activities were seen on the mid right chest and upper left chest, along with right supraclavicular lymph node and right mediastinum lymph node areas. As mentioned earlier, at an advanced stage of disease development, thermal patterns of local diseases can become rather complex, and thermal elevation is no longer constrained to local areas. Local–regional lymph nodes and other abnormal thermal patterns may be involved, indicating the involvement and response of the entire region or even the whole-body under the stress condition. Figure 30.15 shows a case with nasopharynx cancer. Apparent change of

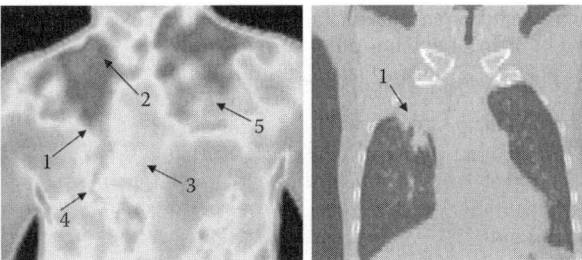

FIGURE 30.14 Images of a studied subject with cancer of the lung shown by arrow #1 on TTM image (left) and chest CT (right). Abnormal thermal activities were also observed near the right supraclavicular and mediastinum lymph node areas (arrow #2, #3, respectively), and mid right chest and upper left chest areas (arrow #4, #5, respectively). For color figures, see www.holistichealthscience.org.

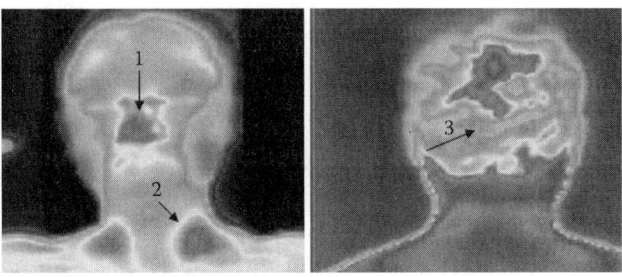

FIGURE 30.15 Images of a studied subject with nasopharynx cancer near the nose cavities (arrow #1). Abnormal thermal activities were also observed near the left neck area and supraclavicular lymph node (arrow #2) and from the back of the head (arrow #3). For color figures, see www.holistichealthscience.org.

thermal pattern in the nasal cavity area can be observed. In addition, thermal elevation was seen by the left neck area and supraclavicular node. Abnormal thermal activity was also observed on the back of head corresponding to the posterior side of the cancer lesion.

30.5.2 Features of Whole-Body Thermal Signatures

Results from imaging the commonly occurring cancer types and systematic diseases showed that these cases are associated with several important thermal signatures accompanying the thermal activities of local conditions. First of all, local and regional lymph nodes near the cancer lesions have elevated and abnormal thermal activities, shown by the cases above. This observation is in good agreement with standard clinical findings on the role of lymphatic-activated immuno-response in disease development. For example, in addition to thermal patterns observed in conventional thermography studies, breast cancer cases may also have abnormal thermal activities near the axillary nodes, maxillary nodes, and thermal asymmetry of both underarm areas.

Second, in cancer, autoimmune, and other systematic disorders, thermal highlight was seen from the endocrine organs that possibly involve thyroids, pancreas, ovaries, or prostate. Again, in breast cancer cases, for example, abnormal thermal patterns, either hot spots or cold spots of the thyroids, and highlighted area of the ovaries and uterus were often seen. This finding is also consistent with current clinical observation that breast cancer itself may be associated with abnormal hormonal status, and functions of the endocrine and reproductive organs.

Next, certain thermal signatures were seen along the spine areas of the back and other "feature spots" corresponding to the diseases. The mechanism of these thermal features is unknown and may be related to other subtle thermal pathways discussed earlier. The spine is where the central nerve system passes through. This is also an area rich with sympathetic and parasympathetic nerves, as well as acupoints that are associated with important functions of the internal organs in the entire torso. For example, patients with cardiac diseases were found to have the back of the spine highlighted near vertebrae of C7 to T2, in an agreement with the sympathetic nerves and acupoints associated with the heart function.

Furthermore, we have found that irregularity of the thermal patterns is associated with a high mental stress level and in patients with cancer and other systematic diseases. This thermal irregularity has a unique feature that we name as a "leopard spot" pattern of the whole body, which is highly distinguishable on thermal images (Figure 30.16). This pattern was identified initially from subjects who reported themselves to experience a high level of mental stress from their work environment or family relationship. This thermal pattern can be mitigated or smoothed out after studied subjects performed relaxation exercises (e.g., musical therapy or meditation exercises) to reduce mental stress.

Thermal signatures for certain psychological burden and illness are currently under study, for example, depression and bipolar disorder. Abnormal thermal patterns have been observed on the back of the

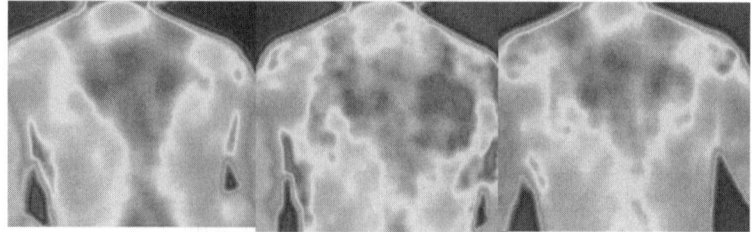

FIGURE 30.16 The effect of stress and its mitigation shown by TTM images. Left: morning condition with low mental stress; middle: evening condition with high mental stress; right: 1 h after the evening scan of the middle panel with 30 min of relaxation meditation. For color figures, see www.holistichealthscience.org.

head, suggesting disorders of brain activities and associated thermogenesis from the area. The results are encouraging because they suggested that IR can serve as an imaging tool to study emotional and mental disorders and their important effects on disease development and physical health. This topic has been quickly recognized in mainstream medicine recently and will continue to attract a surge of scientific interests in medical research [25].

30.5.3 A New System of Image Interpretation

In summary, clinical observations have shown that systematic diseases such as cancer have unique thermal signatures that are not only confined to the local area, but are also presented in the whole body. Using these thermal signatures may aid in the screening and diagnosis processes of these diseases and studying functional relationship among different organs and physiological systems. Based on the characteristics of the thermal signatures, we have developed a new system of image interpretation using the whole-body images in combination with the TTM technique discussed above.

In general, this new system of holistic image interpretation involves the following steps:

1. Assess overall topological features of the whole body, patterns and locations of areas with either thermal elevation or depression;
2. Assess thermal symmetry of the whole body from three axes—front vs. back, left vs. right, and head to feet; (Thermal asymmetry and thermal depression will be discussed further in the next section.)
3. Assess the presence of mental stress and other psychological burden by their thermal signatures;
4. Assess thermal activities of important endocrine organs including the thyroids, pancreas, ovary, and prostate;
5. Assess thermal activities of the regional lymph nodes, and further compare thermal symmetry if the nodal areas are located on either sides of the body (e.g., head-neck, supraclavicular, axillary, and pelvic nodes on both sides of the body);
6. Assess thermal patterns of the central spine area of the back and appearance of specific thermal acupoints associated with certain diseases;
7. Assess local hot spots and surrounding areas by using the TTM technique, measuring the relative temperatures of the suspected hot spots or cold areas, examining thermal topological features and their relationship with other parts of the body;
8. Perform additional stress tests if necessary to examine thermal pattern changes of suspected areas before and after the stress, for example, in taking certain drugs or contrast enhancing agents for suspected diseases (more details will be given in the next section).

We can appreciate that in this new system of holistic image interpretation, eight metrics are used to assess thermal patterns of the whole body and its overall health conditions that we refer to as the "health environment" of an individual. The first six steps have to do with thermal signatures of the functional balance and harmony of the body, and the last two steps are associated with the local suspected areas only.

We believe that the strength of whole-body IR with the use of this set of metrics would enable a comprehensive assessment of the health environment of a person and the status of one's overall wellbeing. In the current medical practice, this information is missing yet extremely important in health evaluation, and none of other radiological imaging test or lab tests can provide such critical information at this point. This is the unique advantage of the whole-body IR and the TTM system, which can serve as an effective tool for wellness focused medicine.

We also want to emphasize that the health environment is a key concept in maintaining the wellbeing of a person and in risk assessment of diseases and health conditions. If the overall health environment is out of order, systematic diseases such as cancer, cardiovascular diseases, autoimmune diseases, and many other types of disorders could arise as a result of such imbalance of the body functions. For example, if the first six metrics are problematic, it is simply a matter of what specific types of diseases will arise subsequently and where the disorder will appear first or to be diagnosed. The focus of the TTM-based health evaluation is always on the overall conditions and environment of the whole-body system rather than appearance of specific diseases.

In other words, if we ignore the overall health environment of a person, and simply focus all attention on diagnosing and treating local disease by itself, then we would lose the overall big picture of the whole body and getting lost in specific details. This is precisely the difference between wellness focused medicine or holistic medicine, versus disease focused medicine or allopathic medicine. In the later case, one may be working hard in removing specific types of symptoms and disorders without appreciating the overall balance of the system. Often such an approach will result in recurrence of the same issues or trigger other more serious conditions as a result of aggressive local treatment if the overall health environment is not restored. We believe that tools such as TTM will help us gain a deeper appreciation of this principle and adopt more holistic approaches in medical practices.

30.6 Other Important Applications of the TTM System

So far, we have been mainly focused on discussing the applications of TTM in studying internal heat sources and their thermal signatures. However, the concept of TTM is not limited to this scope, it can also be applied to study thermal patterns of many other types of diseases and conditions. Clinical studies are being conducted, for example, in the areas of cardiovascular diseases, autoimmune disorders, metabolic disorders, epidemic and infection diseases, and even in mental health. Some of the important cases are shown here to illustrate the use of the TTM concept in these fields.

30.6.1 Thermal Imbalance and Its Associated Disorders

Figure 30.17 shows representative images of subjects who had cardiac ischemia caused by coronary artery diseases and those who had chronic fatty liver, high cholesterol, and high blood pressure syndromes. These examples are shown here to illustrate that certain health conditions can also be manifested as thermal deficiency from excessive coldness of an area on the body. In other words, thermal imbalance in the form of either excessive heat or coldness likely indicates certain disorders or health conditions of the area. In subjects with coronary artery diseases, lack of blood flow to the heart causes reduced perfusion, thus compromised metabolic activity of the cardiac tissues. Asymmetry thermal patterns with coldness in the left chest area seen either from the front or back

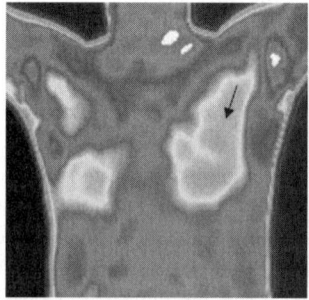 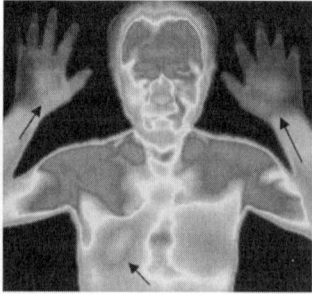

FIGURE 30.17 Left: thermal deficiency in the left chest area (shown by the arrow) associated with a subject with coronary artery disease and cardiac ischemia. Right: thermal deficiency in the right chest area and of the palms and the smaller fingers (shown by the arrows) in a subject who had chronic fatty liver and high cholesterol. High blood pressure experienced by this subject shown as thermal elevation in the head and upper shoulder area. For color figures, see www.holistichealthscience.org.

body surface have been found in such subjects, who have a risk of heart attack, stroke, and other cardiovascular diseases.

Subjects with fatty liver and liver cirrhosis were found to have coldness in the area slightly above the liver on the right side of the chest. These subjects who had accompanying chronic history of high cholesterol also manifest a cold finger symptom (shown in Figure 30.17) in which temperature drops remarkably across from the five fingers likely associated with reduced blood flow and disorder of microcirculation in the smaller fingers. High blood pressure could be experienced by such subjects as well which shows a thermal signature of excessive heat in the entire head or in the forehead area with heat radiating from the neck and upper shoulder. Seen from the whole-body image, thermal imbalance shown as temperature drop from the head to feet direction has been found in these subjects with high blood pressure, consistent with the feelings of head being heavy or hot in the manifestation of the clinical symptoms. Thermal asymmetry has also been observed in patients with recent history of transient ischemia attack or stroke in the brain. The left and right sides of the body showed thermal difference consistent with the loss of function in one side of the body typically experienced by such subjects. In general, healthy normal subjects showed thermal symmetry along three axes of the body: front to back, left to right, and head to feet. Asymmetric temperature distributions could indicate imbalance of energy and functions along either axes of the body.

As emphasized earlier, the advantage of whole-body IR is that it helps us study and explore the inter-connection among different health conditions and underlying relationship weaving through different symptoms that appear to be isolated and uncorrelated. In reality, many of these events are correlated or have causal effects that need to be addressed as a whole rather than being treated as isolated occurrence. For example, we mentioned about the findings in our prostate cancer study that liver and prostate functions were found to be closely related. In studying cardiovascular diseases and metabolic disorders, we also found similar inter-connection among liver conditions, high cholesterol and high blood pressure, and their combined effects on the health of the heart. Kidney function also plays an important role in this group of conditions. Abnormal thermal signatures in the kidney, either as thermal deficiency shown by excessive coldness or local hot spots have been seen in such patient population as well.

30.6.2 Temporal and Functional Changes of the Body

IR imaging and information contained in such images have unique temporal or frequency properties that are very different from those of anatomical images. In the later case, images of the body essentially capture specific physical properties and structures of the body. For example, x-ray CT reflects the medium density, and MRI is about proton density and other related factors. Such anatomical images are static and will not change quickly over time (except in the case that imaging contrast agent is injected in the blood or in the tissue artificially). IR images on the other hand, reflect the metabolic, blood flow, and other activities which occur in a much faster fashion. Such changes could happen in a matter of few minutes to a few hours. Therefore, IR images are more dynamic and fluid compared to anatomical images; this is an intrinsic property of IR that one has to bear in mind in using this modality. In a way, we can observe the body being live and moving in an interactive way in responding to its internal undulations and environmental stimulants.

Results from our clinical observations showed that within the scope of the IR itself, changes of image intensity follow different temporal patterns as well. First of all, fast changes can come from the need to respond to environment (room temperature, air flow, clothing, etc.), body movement, and even mental changes such as mood and emotional swings. Such changes can happen in a matter of a few minutes assisted by hormonal, blood circulation, and metabolic responses of the body. For example, a person's blood pressure could rise in a few minutes in responding to a burst of anger, and heat from the head will increase correspondingly. The next category is normal physiological functions and cycles that are constantly ongoing in the body, for example, digestion, resting, sleeping, menstrual cycle, and so on. Such changes happen in the scale of hours, days, and weeks depending on the specific physiological functions. More significant changes accompanying disease progression or other physiological or psychological factors can last for months or even years.

In general, we found that the body tends to preserve a steady state of equilibrium and thermal pattern of itself. Thus, although small scales of changes are constantly ongoing in the body, there is a stable whole-body thermal pattern that is being maintained for individual people. Each person carries a set of unique thermal signature that can last for months to years. In a good analogy, temperature of different locations on the Earth is constantly changing, but over a scale of decades to centuries, there is an overall stable pattern that is being preserved for the Earth's thermal stability.

Understanding the temporal properties of IR is extremely important in clinical studies, because this feature governs how the images should be acquired, analyzed, and interpreted. For example, precise quantitative measurement of certain temperatures associated with a disease will be both difficult and meaningless when we intend to use IR for disease diagnosis because of the constant changes of the body and person-to-person variations. Rather, we have to look for and capture the essential topographic features of the thermal patterns or thermal signatures qualitatively of a disease. This is what we want to emphasize in TTM image interpretation.

IR is also an effective tool in observing body changes in response to certain diseases, stress, or stimulant conditions [3,4,26–28]. In our experiments, we found that drugs that are taken orally can start to change the body as fast as 10–20 min. The effects are most apparent in the window of about 30–40 min, and stabilize in about 45–60 min. Details of this time sequence depend greatly on the pharmacokinetics of individual drugs and sensitivity of the person. After 1 h, the changes can be brought by other biophysical factors and normal physiological cycle of the body. Therefore, it is important to minimize other environmental, physiological, and psychological factors when IR is used in studying the drug effect and therapy response.

Figure 30.18 shows the changes of the body of a studied subject who underwent cancer chemotherapy and upon oral intake of a dose of herbal supplement to reduce side effects of the chemotherapy. The changes of the body over 2 months before and after the chemotherapy are also shown, illustrating the apparent difference in body functions consistent with lab test results and clinical symptoms of the studied subject. Obviously, the ability of the whole-body IR in observing body response will be very important in drug development and comparing efficacy of different therapies. The principle of the dynamic responding test has also been used in identifying properties of suspected abnormalities under certain stress conditions. For example, cold stress test has been used in thermography to differentiate benign versus malignant lesions in breast cancer [26,27]. It is also possible to use contrast-enhancing agents or drugs to stimulate response of the lesions and observe its temporal course, from which certain physiological characteristics can be derived [29]. This approach has been commonly used in radiological imaging and is included in our metrics of system interpretation of IR.

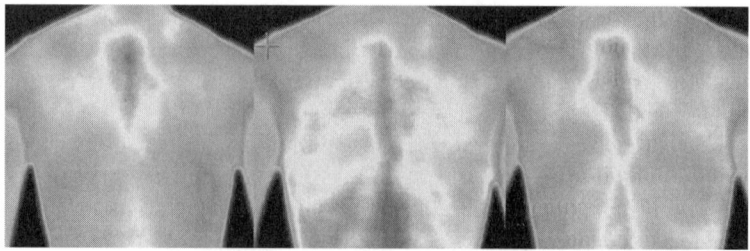

FIGURE 30.18 Thermal pattern changes of a studied subject undergoing cancer chemotherapy. Left: prior to chemotherapy; middle: post chemotherapy 2 months after the first scan; right: 1 h after the scan of the middle panel and with oral intake of a dose of herbal supplement to mitigate side effects of chemotherapy. For color figures, see www.holistichealthscience.org.

30.6.3 Energy Mapping and Subtle Energy Pathways

In fact, whole-body IR is not limited to only study drug or therapy response. We can also use this tool to understand the effects of many other types of stimulants, stress, or change of body energy level on the body thermal patterns. For example, Figure 30.16 shows changes of the body throughout one day, in the morning when the subject reported to be relatively relaxed after a full-night resting, in the evening when the subject reported to experience a high level of fatigue and mental stress after a full-day work, and the effect of taking 30 min relaxation meditation of the subject. We can appreciate the dynamic changes of the body and how it responds to different environmental and mental inputs. In other words, what we can see from the whole-body IR is a dynamic and live body system at work, which constantly undergoes changes and interactions within itself and with its environment.

What forces are driving the life and movement of this dynamic and live system at work? This seems to be an eternal question for us since the beginning of human life, and it is the same question that inspires us in the research of IR and TTM. We can find answers of this question in many branches of science, philosophy, religions and spiritual studies. Indeed, current medical science has started to embrace the holistic view of the body, mind, and spirit connection, and the power of emotional and mental health on our physical body.

Conventionally, IR images have been believed to represent "thermal" activities of the body. This is because in the history of physics, scientists found that heat sources radiate electromagnetic spectrum in the window of the IR photons, and a relationship was thus developed in converting IR energy to temperature according to the theory of black-body radiation. Thus in classic scientific context, we tend to believe that intensity in the IR images is related to heat of the body, and such heat is mainly caused by metabolic activities and blood flow related phenomena.

Although we have been using the word of "thermal" in compliance with conventional terminology so far, our recent work revealed that the IR images of the body reflect essentially the energy system of the human body within the IR window. This is a more accurate and broader description of intrinsic nature of the IR images, in contrast to the conventional belief and a narrow definition that IR images merely reflect "thermal" activities of the body.

Even though IR images occupies only a narrow window on the electromagnetic spectrum, we want to clarify that IR image itself is a "holographic" or "reflexiologic" map of the energy structure of the body. This IR energy map of the body is intrinsically associated with other types of energy that the current science has little knowledge about. This source of energy has been called "subtle energy" in recent years in describing its invisibility and subtleness that are different from other more familiar forms of energy such as electromagnetic energy [11]. In ancient texts, this energy has also been referred to as "Qi" in Chinese medicine and "Prana" in Indian ayurvedic medicine.

Because all energy has continuous spectra and can change freely from one form to the other as a fundamental nature of the energy, it is then not difficult to realize that IR images have to be connected with this subtle form of energy as well. This insight have opened up exciting new areas of research in IR because imaging studies on subtle energy has been extremely limited so far, and they could bring fundamental breakthroughs in medical research and in understanding other subtle forces at work for human health. Thus, in clinical studies of TTM, we have extended its application in holistic medicine, in particular, energy medicine that primarily deals with this form of subtle energy.

Figure 30.19 illustrates examples of a study on meridian system and heat conduction in the body. The images were obtained by heating an acupoint on the shoulder (GB 21 of the gall bladder meridian) with a traditional moxibustion technique and observing the passage of heat along this meridian. Previous publications have shown conflicting results of thermal conduction along the meridian system, which motivated us to pursue further studies on this topic [22–24,30–33].

Results of our experiments showed that not all meridian channels and acupoints are thermal sensitive and conductive. Rather, there are specific acupoints that are highly active and involved in the heat exchange process. When moxibustion is applied to these acupoints, studied subjects experienced

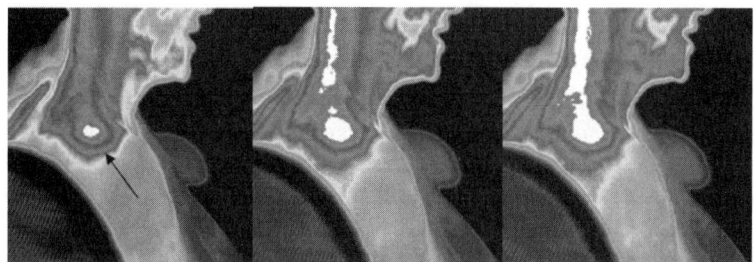

FIGURE 30.19 Thermal pattern changes of a studied subject after applying moxibustion treatment at an acupoint on the shoulder (GB21 of the gall bladder meridian, shown by the arrow). Thermal increase was seen along the side of the neck along this meridian after 5, 10, and 15 min (left, middle, and right panels, respectively) after the treatment and was in agreement with the same feeling of warming up of the neck experienced by the subject. For color figures, see www.holistichealthscience.org.

warming up of certain areas, either along the same meridian channel or at other locations. This finding is consistent with clinical observations that certain diseases are associated with thermal acupoints at distinct locations. Perhaps one of the functions of these acupoints is to provide additional thermal pathways allowing internal heat to be transferred to the body surface.

Therefore, in addition to the regular heat transfer mechanisms including blood flow and conduction, there may be other subtle channels that help the body maintain thermal equilibrium and homeostasis. IR-TTM is a new scientific tool for alternative medicine in studying subtle energy and how it influences our body in intricate ways. Thus, TTM can serve essentially as a bridge between the mainstream and alternative medicine. The merging of the two medical fields will lead to quantum leaps in medicine, revolutionizing the way we look at human health and its improvement.

30.7 Summary

In this chapter, we presented the basic idea of how internal heat source is related to its surface thermal distribution under extremely simplified *ex vivo* conditions. This idea was explored in live human bodies through clinical observations of different types of diseases and conditions. Though the depth of tissue that IR photons can go through is very limited, heat from internal organs can be expressed on the body surface through different mechanisms. The technique of thermal texture mapping or TTM was developed initially to visualize and analyze thermal gradient of heat sources and whether such sources are surface based or deeply situated inside tissues. For live bodies, surface thermal distribution becomes very complex, and the technique of thermal gradient analysis has to be extended in real situations. In this case, topology of the thermal distributions, including shapes, textures, anatomical locations and other morphological features have to be used in understanding the nature of the heat sources.

Results of clinical observations suggested that systematic diseases and health conditions such as cancer and autoimmune disorders are associated with certain whole-body thermal signatures that can be used to assess the presence and risk of such disorders. These thermal signatures were obtained from the atlas of whole-body IR images, and they suggested the association or inter-connection of different parts of the body in responding to certain stress conditions. Development of serious conditions such as cancer not only involves abnormal thermal patterns of the local region, but also presents as unique thermal signatures of the whole body including thermal asymmetry, deficiency, and irregularity. These findings motivated us to develop a new system for image interpretation, which emphasizes on combining information of the whole-body images in a holistic and integrative way. This is an essential extension of the TTM technique in image interpretation and evaluation of the health environment of the whole body.

The concept and methodology of TTM has also been tested in other applications including the study of drug or therapy response, holistic medicine, and epidemic diseases in public health. Findings of these studies showed that IR with TTM is an effective tool in observing functions of the body, its dynamic changes, overall balance and associations of different subcomponents. This modality also helps us explore advanced topics such as meridian channels, subtle energy, and their manifestation on the IR images.

On the basis of our experience from available clinical observations, we want to emphasize in the end that IR images are essentially energy maps of the body within the IR spectral window. Our body energy system is live and dynamic, as our mind and body are constantly undergoing changes and movement inside and outside. In addition, there are other sources or channels of subtle energy that are continuously influencing the intensity of such energy maps. It is important to realize that the information contained in IR images goes far beyond the heat emitted from the metabolic activities and blood flow in the body, which is what we have believed so far in the context of traditional thermography.

The beauty of IR is that it provides us a new angle of seeing the body as a whole, and inter-connected system, live and moving. And the secret of maintaining its health is about the intricate balance inside this system and harmonious interactions with its environment. This new perspective is drastically different from the traditional reductionist view of treating the body as made up of separated mechanical parts that are static and isolated, as how the present anatomical and disease-driven paradigms are dominating in medicine and radiological imaging. The adoption of the new holistic view will fundamentally revolutionize medicine and healthcare, allowing setting up new scientific directions and medical practices in congruence with the operating principles of the nature. We expect that IR will serve an even more important role in the new era of integrative and holistic medicine in the coming years.

References

1. Diakides, N.A. and J.D. Bronzino, Editors, *Medical Infrared Imaging*. CRC Press, Taylor & Francis Group, USA, 2008.
2. Fujimasa, I., T. Chinzei, and I. Saito, Converting far infrared image information to other physiological data. *IEEE Engineering in Medicine and Biology Magazine*, 2000. **19**(3): 71–6.
3. Li, Q., Y.E. Yuan, and W.D. Han, Experimental animal model in breast cancer development using thermal texture maps. *Chinese Journal of Medical Imaging and Technologies*, 2006. **22**(6): 819–20.
4. Li, X., X. Huang, and X. Li, Effects and mechanisms of *Herba dendrobii* on rats with stomach-heat syndrome. *Zhongguo Zhong Yao Za Zhi*, 2010. **35**(6): 750–4.
5. Liu, Z.Q. and C. Wang, *Method and Apparatus for Thermal Radiation Imaging*. Technical Report 6,023,637, United States Patent., 2000.
6. Shang, Z. and G. Jiang, Fundamental theoretic research of thermal texture maps I—Simulation and analysis of the relation between the depth of inner heat source and surface temperature distribution in isotropy tissue. *Conf Proc IEEE Eng Med Biol Soc*, 2004. **7**: 5271–3.
7. Wang, W. et al., Clinical study on using thermal texture maps in SARS diagnosis. *Conf Proc IEEE Eng Med Biol Soc*, 2004. **7**: 5258–64.
8. Yuan, C., C. Wang, and S.T. Song, Thermal texture mapping in breast cancer. *Chinese Journay of Medical Imaging and Technologies*, 2006. **16**(1): 7–10.
9. Yuan, Y. et al., Image analysis of breast tumors using thermal texture mapping (TTM). *Conf Proc IEEE Eng Med Biol Soc*, 2005. **1**: 697–9.
10. Yuan, Y.E., C. Wang, and R. Yuan, Image analysis of thermal texture maps on breast cancer. *Chinese Journal of Medical Imaging and Technologies*, 2004. **20**(12): 1803–05.
11. Dale, C., *The Subtle Body: An Encyclopedia of Your Energetic Anatomy*. Sounds True, Incorporated; 2009.
12. Chunfang, G., L. Kaiyang, and Z. Shaoping, A novel approach of analyzing the relation between the inner heat source and the surface temperature distribution in thermal texture maps. *Conf Proc IEEE Eng Med Biol Soc*, 2005. **1**: 623–6.
13. Deng, Z.S. and J. Liu, Mathematical modeling of temperature mapping over skin surface and its implementation in thermal disease diagnostics. *Comput Biol Med*, 2004. **34**(6): 495–21.

14. Draper, J.W. and J.W. Boag, Skin temperature distributions over veins and tumours. *Phys Med Biol*, 1971. **16**(4): 645–54.

15. Draper, J.W. and J.W. Boag, The calculation of skin temperature distributions in thermography. *Phys Med Biol*, 1971. **16**(2): 201–11.

16. Gustafsson, S.E., S.K. Nilsson, and L.M. Torell, Analytical calculation of the skin temperature distribution due to subcutaneous heat production in a spherical heat source. *Phys Med Biol*, 1975. **20**(2): 219–24.

17. Weinbaum, S., L.M. Jiji, and D.E. Lemons, Theory and experiment for the effect of vascular microstructure on surface tissue heat transfer—Part I: Anatomical foundation and model conceptualization. *J Biomech Eng*, 1984. **106**(4): 321–30.

18. Pennes, H.H., Analysis of tissue and arterial blood temperatures in the resting human forearm. *J Appl Physiol*, 1948. **1**(2): 93–122.

19. Wu, Z. et al., A basic step toward understanding skin surface temperature distributions caused by internal heat sources. *Phys Med Biol*, 2007. **52**(17): 5379–92.

20. Chan, C.L., Boundary element method analysis for the bioheat transfer equation. *J Biomech Eng*, 1992. **114**(3): 358–65.

21. Mital, M. and E.P. Scott, Thermal detection of embedded tumors using infrared imaging. *J Biomech Eng*, 2007. **129**(1): 33–9.

22. Wang, P., X. Hu, and B. Wu, Displaying of the infrared radiant track along meridians on the back of human body. *Zhen Ci Yan Jiu*, 1993. **18**(2): 90–3, 89.

23. Xu, J.S. et al. Comparison of the thermal conductivity of the related tissues along the meridian and the non-meridian. *Zhongguo Zhen Jiu*, 2005. **25**(7): 477–82.

24. Yang, H.Q. et al., Appearance of human meridian-like structure and acupoints and its time correlation by infrared thermal imaging. *Am J Chin Med*, 2007. **35**(2): 231–40.

25. *Advances in Mind – Body Medicine*. InnoVision Communications, USA.

26. Amalu, W.C., Nondestructive testing of the human breast: The validity of dynamic stress testing in medical infrared breast imaging. *Conf Proc IEEE Eng Med Biol Soc*, 2004. **2**: 1174–7.

27. Hu, L. et al., Effect of forced convection on the skin thermal expression of breast cancer. *J Biomech Eng*, 2004. **126**(2): 204–11.

28. Hassan, M., V. Chernomordik, and A. Vogel, *Infrared Imaging for Functional Monitoring of Disease Processes*. Medical Infrared Imaging; Edited by Diakides and Bronzino; CRC Press, USA, 2008.

29. Gescheit, I.M. et al., Minimal-invasive thermal imaging of a malignant tumor: A simple model and algorithm. *Med Phys*, 2010. **37**(1): 211–16.

30. Hu, X., B. Wu, and P. Wang, Displaying of meridian courses travelling over human body surface under natural conditions. *Zhen Ci Yan Jiu*, 1993. **18**(2): 83–9.

31. Litscher, G., Infrared thermography fails to visualize stimulation-induced meridian-like structures. *Biomed Eng Online*, 2005. **4**(1): 38.

32. Lo, S.Y., Meridians in acupuncture and infrared imaging. *Med Hypotheses*, 2002. **58**(1): 72–6.

33. Zhang, D. et al., Research on the acupuncture principles and meridian phenomena by means of infrared thermography. *Zhen Ci Yan Jiu*, 1990. **15**(4): 319–23.

31

Infrared Imaging of the Breast: A Review

William C. Amalu
Pacific Chiropractic and Research Center

William B. Hobbins
Women's Breast Health Center

Jonathan F. Head
Elliot-Elliot-Head Breast Cancer Research and Treatment Center

Robert L. Elliot
Elliot-Elliot-Head Breast Cancer Research and Treatment Center

31.1 Introduction

The use of infrared imaging in healthcare is not a recent phenomenon. However, its utilization in breast cancer screening is seeing renewed interest. This attention is fueled by research that clearly demonstrates the value of this procedure and the tremendous impact it has on the mortality of breast cancer.

Since the late 1950s, extensive research has been performed on the use of infrared imaging in breast cancer screening. Over 800 papers can be found in the indexed medical literature. In this database, well over 300,000 women have participated as study subjects. The numbers of participants in many studies are very large and range from 10,000 to 85,000 women. Some of these studies have followed patients for up to 12 years in order to investigate and establish the technology's unique ability as a risk marker.

With strict standardized interpretation protocols having been established for over 15 years, infrared imaging of the breast has obtained an average sensitivity and specificity of 90%. As a future risk indicator for breast cancer, a persistent abnormal thermogram carries a 22 times higher risk and is 10 times more significant than a first-order family history of the disease. Studies clearly show that an abnormal infrared image is the single most important risk marker for the existence of or future development of breast cancer.

The first recorded use of thermobiological diagnostics can be found in the writings of Hippocrates around 480 BC [1]. A mud slurry spread over the patient was observed for areas that would dry first and was thought to indicate underlying organ pathology. Since this time, continued research and clinical observations proved that certain temperatures related to the human body were indeed indicative of normal and abnormal physiologic processes.

In the 1950s, military research into infrared monitoring systems for nighttime troop movements ushered in a new era in thermal diagnostics. Once declassified in the mid-1950s, infrared imaging technology was made available for medical purposes. The first diagnostic use of infrared imaging came in 1956 when Lawson discovered that the skin temperature over a cancer in the breast was higher than that of normal tissue [2–4]. He also showed that the venous blood draining the cancer is often warmer than its arterial supply.

The Department of Health Education and Welfare released a position paper in 1972 in which the director, Thomas Tiernery, wrote, "The medical consultants indicate that thermography, in its present state of development, is beyond the experimental state as a diagnostic procedure in the following 4 areas: (1) Pathology of the female breast …" (1972 HEW position paper). On January 29, 1982, the Food and Drug Administration published its approval and classification of thermography as an adjunctive diagnostic screening procedure for the detection of breast cancer. Since the late 1970s, numerous medical centers and independent clinics have used thermography for a variety of diagnostic purposes.

Since Lawson's groundbreaking research, infrared imaging has been used for over 40 years as an adjunctive screening procedure in the evaluation of the breast. In this time, significant advances have been made in infrared detection systems and the application of sophisticated computerized image processing.

31.2 Fundamentals and Standards in Infrared Breast Imaging

Clinical infrared imaging is a procedure that detects, records, and produces an image of a patient's skin surface temperatures or thermal patterns. The image produced resembles the likeness of the anatomic area under study. The procedure uses equipment that can provide both qualitative and quantitative representations of these temperature patterns.

Infrared imaging does not entail the use of ionizing radiation, venous access, or other invasive procedures; therefore, the examination poses no harm to the patient. Classified as a functional imaging technology, infrared imaging of the breast provides information on the normal and abnormal physiologic functioning of the sensory and sympathetic nervous systems, vascular system, and local inflammatory processes.

31.2.1 Physics

All objects with a temperature above absolute zero (–273 K) emit infrared radiation from their surface. The Stefan–Boltzmann Law defines the relation between radiated energy and temperature by stating that the total radiation emitted by an object is directly proportional to the object's area and emissivity and the fourth power of its absolute temperature. Since the emissivity of human skin is extremely high (within 1% of that of a blackbody), measurements of infrared radiation emitted by the skin can be converted directly into accurate temperature values. This makes infrared imaging an ideal procedure to evaluate surface temperatures of the body.

31.2.2 Equipment Considerations

Infrared rays are found in the electromagnetic spectrum within the wavelengths of 0.75 μm to 1 mm. Human skin emits infrared radiation mainly in the 2–20 μm wavelength range, with an average peak at 9–10 μm [5]. With the application of Planck's equation and Wein's Law, it is found that approximately 90% of the emitted infrared radiation in humans is in the longer wavelengths (6–14 μm).

There are many important technical aspects to consider when choosing an appropriate clinical infrared imaging system. (The majority of which is outside the scope of this chapter.) However, minimum equipment standards have been established from research studies, applied infrared physics, and human anatomic and physiologic parameters [6,7]. Absolute, spatial, and temperature resolution along with thermal stability and adequate computerized image processing are just a few of the critical specifications to be taken into account. Real-time image capture is a basic requirement in modern clinical imaging systems. Absolute resolution, or the number of distinct infrared detectors dedicated to forming the image (resolvable elements per line in a scanning system), must be adequate enough to produce a quality image. The ability of the system to resolve discrete areas on the surface of the skin is defined as spatial resolution. Standards for clinical systems require that the spatial resolution of the camera should be able to resolve 1 mm² at the surface of the skin when the patient is placed at 40 cm from the detector (2.5 mrad). The temperature resolution, or thermal sensitivity, of the camera should be 0.1°C. This level of temperature discernment is necessary to maintain adequate objective temperature measurements when performing quantitative analyses. Although these specifications are extremely important, the most fundamental consideration in the selection of clinical infrared imaging equipment is the wavelength sensitivity of the infrared detector. The decision on which area in the infrared spectrum to select a detector from depends on the object one wants to investigate and the environmental conditions in which the detection is taking place. Considering that the object in question is the human body, Planck's equation leads us to select a detector in the 6–14 μm region. Assessment of skin temperature by infrared measurement in the 3–5 μm region is less reliable due to the emissivity of human skin being farther from that of a blackbody in that region [8,9]. The environment under which the examination takes place is well controlled, but not free from possible sources of detection errors. Imaging room environmental artifacts such as reflectance can cause errors when shorter wavelength detectors (under 7 μm) are used [10]. Consequently, the optimum infrared detector to use in imaging the breast, and the body as a whole, would have sensitivity in the longer wavelengths spanning the 9–10 μm range [7–14].

The problems encountered with first-generation infrared camera systems, such as incorrect detector sensitivity (shorter wavelengths), thermal drift, calibration, analog interface, and so forth have been solved for almost two decades. Modern clinical infrared imaging systems exceed the minimum specification standards mentioned earlier. However, no studies have been published demonstrating the need for a change in the standards. Modern computerized infrared imaging systems have the ability to discern minute variations in thermal emissions while producing extremely high-resolution images that can undergo digital manipulation by sophisticated computerized analytical processing.

31.2.3 Laboratory and Patient Preparation Protocols

In order to produce diagnostic quality infrared images, certain laboratory and patient preparation protocols must be strictly adhered to. Infrared imaging must be performed in a controlled environment. The primary reason for this is the nature of human physiology. Changes from a different external (noncontrolled room) environment, clothing, and so forth produce thermal artifacts. In order to properly prepare the patient for imaging, the patient should be instructed to refrain from sun exposure, stimulation or treatment of the breasts, cosmetics, lotions, antiperspirants, deodorants, exercise, and bathing before the examination.

The imaging room must be temperature- and humidity controlled and maintained between 18°C and 23°C, and kept to within 1°C of change during the examination. This temperature range ensures that the patient is not placed in an environment in which their physiology is stressed into a state of shivering or perspiring. The room should also be free from drafts and infrared sources of heat (i.e., sunlight and incandescent lighting). In keeping with a physiologically neutral temperature environment, the floor should be carpeted or the patient must wear shoes in order to prevent increased physiologic stress.

Lastly, the patient must undergo 15 min of waist-up nude acclimation in order to reach a condition in which the body is at thermal equilibrium with the environment. At this point, further changes in the surface temperatures of the body occur very slowly and uniformly; thus, not affecting changes in homologous anatomic regions. Thermal artifacts from clothing or the outside environment are also removed at this time. The last 5 min of this acclimation period is usually spent with the patient placing their hands on top of their head in order to facilitate an improved anatomic presentation of the breasts for imaging. Depending on the patient's individual anatomy, certain positioning maneuvers may need to be implemented such that all of the pertinent surfaces of the breasts may be imaged. In summary, adherence to proper patient and laboratory protocols is absolutely necessary to produce a physiologically neutral image free from artifact and ready for interpretation.

31.2.4 Imaging

The actual process of imaging is undertaken with the intent to adequately detect the infrared emissions from the pertinent surface areas of the breasts. As with mammography, a minimum series of images is needed in order to facilitate adequate coverage. The series includes the bilateral frontal breast along with the right and left oblique views (a right and left single breast close-up view may also be included). The bilateral frontal view acts as a scout image to give a baseline impression of both breasts. The oblique views (~45° to the detector) expose the lateral and medial quadrants of the breasts for analysis. The optional close-up views maximize the use of the detector allowing for the highest thermal and spatial resolution image of each breast. This series of images takes into consideration the infrared analyses of curved surfaces and adequately provides for an accurate analysis of all the pertinent surface areas of the breasts (see Figures 31.1 through 31.5).

Positioning of the patient prior to imaging facilitates acclimation of the surface areas and ease of imaging. Placing the patient in a seated or standing posture during the acclimation period is ideal to facilitate these needs. In the seated position, the patient places their arms on the arm rests away from the body to allow for proper acclimation. When positioning the patient in front of the camera, the use of a rotating chair or having the patient stand makes for uncomplicated positioning for the necessary views.

Because of differing anatomy from patient to patient, special views may be necessary to adequately detect the infrared emissions from the pertinent surface areas of the breasts. The most common problem encountered is inadequate viewing of the inferior quadrants due to nipple ptosis. This is easily remedied by adding "lift views." Once the baseline images are taken, the patient is asked to gently "lift" each breast from the superior most aspect of the Tail of Spence exposing the inferior quadrants for detection. Additional images are then taken in this position in order to maintain the surface areas covered in the standard views.

31.2.5 Special Tests

In the past, an optional set of views may have been added to the baseline images. Additional views would be taken after the patient placed their hands in ice cold water as a thermoregulatory challenge. It was hoped that this dynamic methodology would increase the sensitivity and specificity of the thermographic procedure.

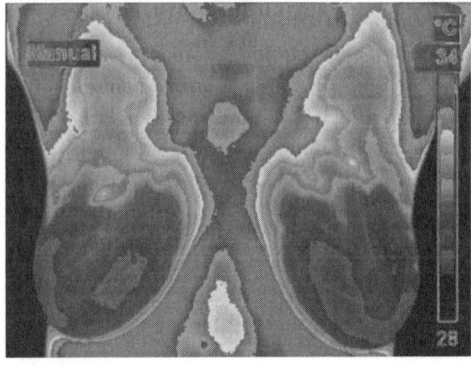

FIGURE 31.1   Bilateral frontal.

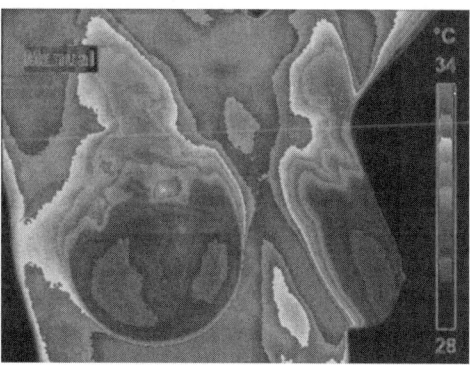

FIGURE 31.2   Right oblique.

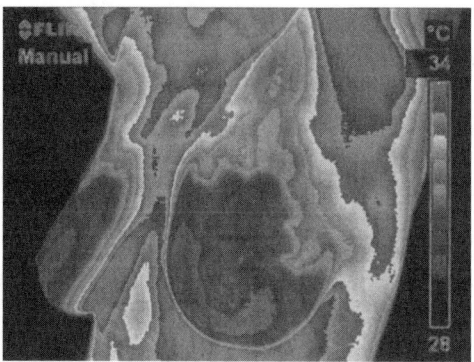

FIGURE 31.3   Left oblique.

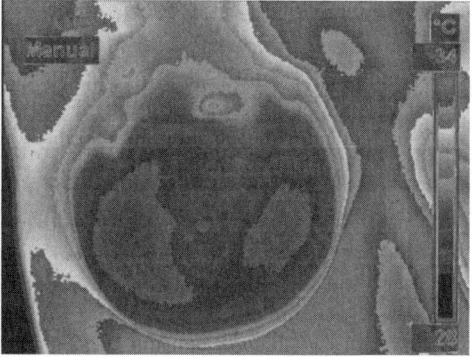

FIGURE 31.4   Right close-up.

In order to understand the hopes placed on this test, one needs to understand the underlying physiologic mechanisms of the procedure. The most common and accepted method of applied thermoregulatory challenge involves ice water immersion of the hands or feet (previous studies investigating the use of fans or alcohol spray noted concerns over the creation of thermal artifacts along with the methods causing a limited superficial effect). The mechanism is purely neurovascular and involves a primitive survival reflex initiated from peripheral neural receptors and conveyed to the central nervous system.

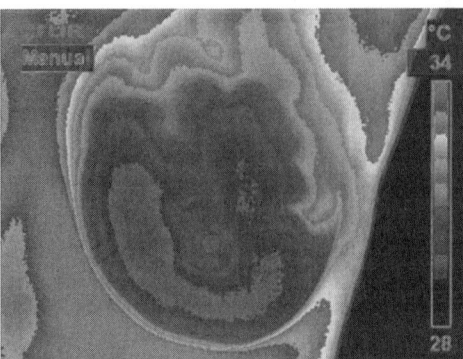

FIGURE 31.5   Left close-up.

To protect the body from hypothermia, the reflex invokes a sympathetically mediated blood vessel constriction in the periphery in an attempt to maintain the normal core temperature set point. This stress test is intended to increase the sensitivity of the thermogram by attempting to identify nonresponding blood vessels such as those involved in angiogenesis associated with neoplasm. Blood vessels produced by cancerous tumors are simple endothelial tubes devoid of a muscular layer and the neural regulation afforded to embryologic vessels. As such, these new vessels would fail to constrict in response to a sympathetic stimulus. In the normal breast, test results would produce an image of relative cooling with attenuation of vascular diameter. A breast harboring a malignancy would theoretically remain unchanged in temperature or demonstrate hyperthermia with vascular dilatation. However, to date it has not been found that the stress test offers any advantage over the baseline images [15].

For well over a decade, the largest infrared breast imaging centers worldwide, along with the leading experts and researchers in the field of infrared breast imaging, have discontinued the use of the cold challenge. Yet, in a 2004 detailed review of the literature combined with an investigational study, Amalu explored the validity of the thermoregulatory challenge test [15]. Results from 23 patients with histologically confirmed breast cancers along with 500 noncancerous patients were presented demonstrating positive and negative responses to the challenge. From the combined literature review and study analysis it was found that the test did not alter the clinical decision-making process for following up suspicious thermograms, nor did it enhance the detection of occult cancers found in normal thermograms. In summary, it was found that there was no evidence to support the use of the cold challenge. The study noted insufficient evidence to warrant its use as a mandated test with all women undergoing infrared breast imaging. It also warned that it would be incorrect to consider a breast thermogram substandard, inaccurate, or incomplete if a thermoregulatory challenge was not included. In conclusion, Amalu stated that "Until further studies are performed and ample evidence can be presented to the contrary, a review of the available data indicates that infrared imaging of the breast can be performed excluding the cold challenge without any known loss of sensitivity or specificity in the detection of breast cancers."

31.2.6 Image Interpretation

Early methods of interpretation of infrared breast images was based solely on qualitative (subjective) criteria. The images were read for variations in vascular patterning with no regard to temperature variations between the breasts (Tricore method) [16]. This led to wide variations in the outcomes of studies preformed with inexperienced interpreters. Research throughout the 1970s proved that when both qualitative and quantitative data were incorporated in the interpretations, an increase in sensitivity and specificity was realized. In the early 1980s, a standardized method of thermovascular analysis was proposed. The interpretation was composed of 20 discrete vascular and temperature attributes

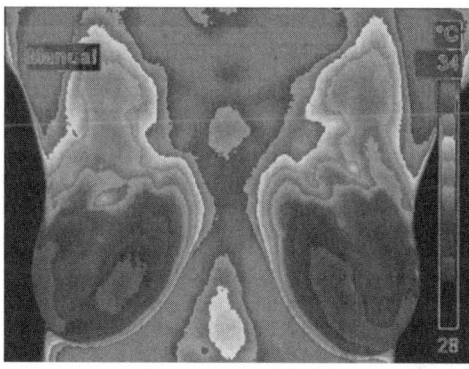

FIGURE 31.6   TH1 (normal uniform nonvascular).

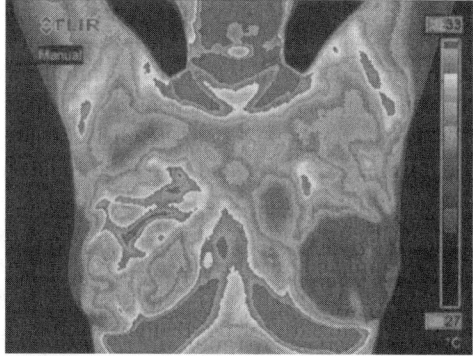

FIGURE 31.7   Right TH5 (severely abnormal).

in the breast [17,18]. This method of analysis was based on previous research and large-scale studies comprising tens of thousands of patients. Using this methodology, thermograms would be graded into one of 5 TH (thermobiological) classifications. Based on the combined vascular patterning and temperatures across the two breasts, the images would be graded as TH1 (normal uniform nonvascular), TH2 (normal uniform vascular), TH3 (equivocal), TH4 (abnormal), or TH5 (severely abnormal) (see Figures 31.6 and 31.7). The use of this standardized interpretation method significantly increased infrared imaging's sensitivity, specificity, positive and negative predictive value, and inter-/intraexaminer interpretation reliability. Continued patient observations and research over the past two decades has caused changes in some of the thermovascular values; thus keeping the interpretation system up-to-date. Variations in this methodology have also been adopted with great success. However, it is recognized that, as with any other imaging procedure, specialized training and experience produces the highest level of screening success.

31.2.7 Correlation between Pathology and Infrared Imaging

The empirical evidence that an underlying breast cancer alters regional skin surface temperatures was investigated early on. In 1963, Lawson and Chughtai, two McGill University surgeons, published an elegant intraoperative study demonstrating that the increase in regional skin surface temperature associated with breast cancer was related to venous convection [19]. This early quantitative experiment added credence to previous research suggesting that infrared findings were linked to increased vascularity.

Infrared imaging of the breast may also have critical prognostic significance since it may correlate with a variety of pathologic prognostic features such as tumor size, tumor grade, lymph node status, and markers of tumor growth [20]. Continued research is underway investigating the pathologic basis for these infrared findings. One possibility is increased blood flow due to vascular proliferation (assessed by quantifying the microvascular density [MVD]) as a result of tumor-associated angiogenesis. Although in one study [21], the MVD did not correlate with abnormal infrared findings. However, the imaging method used in that study consisted of contact plate technology (liquid crystal thermography [LCT]), which is not capable of modern computerized analysis. Consequently, LCT does not possess the discrimination and digital processing necessary to begin to correlate histological and discrete vascular changes [22].

In 1993, Head and Elliott reported that improved images from second-generation infrared systems allowed more objective and quantitative analysis [20], and indicated that growth-rate-related prognostic indicators were strongly associated with the infrared image interpretation.

In a 1994 detailed review of the potential of infrared imaging [23], Anbar suggested that the previous empirical observation that small tumors were capable of producing notable infrared changes could be due to enhanced perfusion over a substantial area of the breast surface via regional tumor induced nitric oxide (NO) vasodilatation. NO is synthesized by nitric oxide synthase (NOS), found both as a constitutive form of NOS, especially in endothelial cells, and as an inducible form of NOS, especially in macrophages [24]. NOS has been demonstrated in breast carcinoma [25] using tissue immunohistochemistry, and is associated with a high tumor grade.

Nitric oxide is a molecule with potent vasodilating properties. It is a simple highly reactive free radical that readily oxidizes to form nitrite or nitrate ions. It diffuses easily through both hydrophilic and hydrophobic media. Thus, once produced, NO diffuses throughout the surrounding tissues, inside and outside the vascular system, and induces a variety of biochemical changes depending on the specific receptors involved. NO exerts its influence by binding to receptor sites in the endothelium of arteries or arterioles. This causes inhibition of sympathetic vasoconstriction. The end result is NO induced vasodilatation, which in turn may produce an asymmetrical thermovascular infrared image.

The largest body of evidence surrounding the physiologic mechanism by which infrared imaging detects precancerous and malignant states of the breast lies in the recruitment of existing blood vessels and the formation of new ones (angiogenesis). The process of angiogenesis begins with the release of angiogenesis factors (AF) from precancerous or cancerous cells. In the early stages of tumor growth, the majority of neoplasms exhibit a lower cellular metabolic demand. As such, the release of AF causes the existing vessels to resist constriction in order to maintain a steady supply of nutrients to the growing mass. As the tumor increases in size, the need for nutrients becomes greater. AF begins to exert its influence by opening the dormant vessels in the breast. Once this blood supply becomes too little to maintain the growth of the neoplasm, AF causes the formation of new blood vessels. These new vessels are simple endothelial tubes connecting the tumor to existing nearby arteries and arterioles. This augmented blood supply produces the increase in heat and vascular asymmetry seen in infrared images.

The concept of angiogenesis, as an integral part of early breast cancer, was emphasized in 1996 by Guidi and Schnitt. Their observations suggested that it is an early event in the development of breast cancer and may occur before tumor cells acquire the ability to invade the surrounding stroma and even before there is morphologic evidence of an *in situ* carcinoma [26]. In 1996, in his highly reviewed textbook entitled *Atlas of Mammography—New Early Signs in Breast Cancer*, Gamagami studied angiogenesis by infrared imaging and reported that hypervascularity and hyperthermia could be shown in 86% of nonpalpable breast cancers. He also noted that in 15% of these cases infrared imaging helped to detect cancers that were not visible on mammography [27].

The greatest evidence supporting the underlying principle by which infrared imaging detects precancerous growths and cancerous tumors surrounds the well-documented recruitment of existing vascularity and angiogenesis that is necessary to maintain the increased metabolism of malignant cellular growth and multiplication. The biomedical engineering evidence of infrared imaging's value, both in model *in vitro* and clinically *in vivo* studies of various tissue growths, normal and neoplastic, has been established [28–34].

31.3 Role of Infrared Imaging in the Detection of Cancer

To determine the value of infrared imaging, two viewpoints must be considered: first, the sensitivity of thermograms taken preoperatively in patients with known breast carcinoma; and second, the incidence of normal and abnormal thermograms in asymptomatic populations (specificity) and the presence or absence of malignancy in each of these groups.

In 1965, Gershon-Cohen, a radiologist and researcher from the Albert Einstein Medical Center, introduced infrared imaging to the United States [35]. Using a Barnes thermograph, he reported on 4000 cases with a sensitivity of 94% and a false-positive rate of 6%. This data was included in a review of the then current status of infrared imaging published in 1968 in *California—A Cancer Journal for Physicians* [36].

In prospective studies, Hoffman first reported on thermography in a gynecologic practice. He detected 23 carcinomas in 1924 patients (a detection rate of 12.5 per 1000), with an 8.4% false-negative (91.6% sensitivity) and a 7.4% false-positive (92.6% specificity) rate [37].

Stark and Way screened 4621 asymptomatic women, 35% of whom were under 35 years of age, and detected 24 cancers (detection rate of 7.6 per 1000), with a sensitivity and specificity of 98.3% and 93.5%, respectively [38].

In a study comprising 25,000 patients screened and 1878 histologically proven breast cancers, Amalric and Spitalier reported on their results with infrared imaging. From this group, a false-negative and false-positive rate of 9% (91% sensitivity and specificity) was found [39].

In a mobile unit examination of rural Wisconsin, Hobbins screened 37,506 women using thermography. He reported the detection of 5.7 cancers per 1000 women screened with a 12% false-negative and 14% false-positive rate. His findings also corroborated with others that thermography is the sole early initial signal in 10% of breast cancers [17,40].

Reporting his Radiology division's experience with 10,000 thermographic studies done concomitantly with mammography over a 3-year period, Isard reiterated a number of important concepts including the remarkable thermal and vascular stability of the infrared image from year to year in the otherwise healthy patient and the importance of recognizing any significant change [41]. In his experience, combining these modalities increased the sensitivity rate of detection by approximately 10%; thus, underlining the complementarity of these procedures since each one did not always suspect the same lesion. It was Isard's conclusion that, had there been a preliminary selection of his group of 4393 asymptomatic patients by infrared imaging, mammographic examination would have been restricted to the 1028 patients with abnormal infrared imaging, or 23% of this cohort. This would have resulted in a cancer detection rate of 24.1 per 1000 combined infrared and mammographic examinations as contrasted to the expected 7 per 1000 by mammographic screening alone. He concluded that since infrared imaging is an innocuous examination, it could be utilized to focus attention upon asymptomatic women who should be examined more intensely. Isard emphasized that, like mammography and other breast imaging techniques, infrared imaging does not diagnose cancer, but merely indicates the presence of an abnormality.

Spitalier and associates screened 61,000 women using thermography over a 10-year period. The false-negative and false-positive rate was found to be 11% (89% sensitivity and specificity). Thermography also detected 91% of the nonpalpable cancers (Grade T0: tumors less than 1 cm in size). The authors noted that of all the patients with cancer, thermography alone was the first alarm in 60% of the cases [42].

Two small-scale studies by Moskowitz (150 patients) [43] and Treatt (515 patients) [44] reported on the sensitivity and reliability of infrared imaging. Both used unknown experts to review the images of breast cancer patients. While Moskowitz excluded unreadable images, data from Threatt's study indicated that less than 30% of the images produced were considered good, the rest being substandard. Both of these studies produced poor results; however, this could be expected considering the lack of adherence to accepted imaging methods and protocols. The greatest error in these studies is found in the methods used to analyze the images. The type of image analysis consisted of the sole use of abnormal vascular pattern recognition. At the time these studies were performed, the accepted method of infrared image interpretation consisted of a combined vascular pattern and quantitative analysis of temperature variations across the breasts. Consequently, the data obtained from these studies is highly questionable. Their findings were also inconsistent with numerous previous large-scale multicenter trials. The authors suggested that for infrared imaging to be truly effective as a screening tool, there needed to be a more objective means of interpretation and proposed that this would be facilitated by computerized evaluation. This statement is interesting considering that recognized quantitative and qualitative reading protocols (including computer analysis) were being used at the time.

In a unique study comprising 39,802 women screened over a 3-year period, Haberman and associates used thermography and physical examination to determine if mammography was recommended. They reported an 85% sensitivity and 70% specificity for thermography. Haberman cautioned that the findings of thermographic specificity could not be extrapolated from this study as it was well-documented that long-term observation (8–10 years or more) is necessary to determine a true false-positive rate. The authors noted that 30% of the cancers found would not have been detected if it were not for thermography [45].

Gros and Gautherie reported on a large-scale study comprising 85,000 patients screened. Culmination of the data resulted in a 90% sensitivity and 88% specificity for thermography [46–49].

In a large-scale multicenter review of nearly 70,000 women screened, Jones reported a false-negative and false-positive rate of 13% (87% sensitivity) and 15% (85% sensitivity), respectively for thermography [50].

In a study performed in 1986, Usuki reported on the relation of thermographic findings in breast cancer diagnosis. He noted an 88% sensitivity for thermography in the detection of breast cancers [51].

Parisky and associates published a study from a multicenter 4-year clinical trial using infrared imaging to evaluate mammographically suspicious lesions. Data from a blinded subject set was obtained in 769 women with 875 biopsied lesions resulting in 187 malignant and 688 benign findings. The index of suspicion resulted in a 97% sensitivity in the detection of breast cancers [52].

In a study comparing clinical examination, mammography, and thermography in the diagnosis of breast cancer, three groups of patients were used: 4716 patients with confirmed carcinoma, 3305 patients with histologically diagnosed benign breast disease, and 8757 general patients (16,778 total participants). This paper also compared clinical examination and mammography to other well-known studies in the literature including the National Cancer Institute (NCI) sponsored Breast Cancer Detection and Demonstration Projects (BCDDPs). In this study, clinical examination had an average sensitivity of 75% in detecting all tumors and 50% in cancers less than 2 cm in size. This rate is exceptionally good when compared to many other studies at between 35% and 66% sensitivity. Mammography was found to have an average of 80% sensitivity and 73% specificity. Thermography had an average sensitivity of 88% (85% in tumors less than 1 cm in size) and a specificity of 85%. An abnormal thermogram was found to have a 94% predictive value. From the findings in this study, the authors suggested that "none of the techniques available for screening for breast carcinoma and evaluating patients with breast-related symptoms is sufficiently accurate to be used alone. For the best results, a multimodal approach should be used" [53].

In a series of 4000 confirmed breast cancers, Thomassin and associates observed 130 subclinical carcinomas ranging in diameter of 3–5 mm. Both mammography and thermography were used alone and in combination. Of the 130 cancers, 10% were detected by mammography, 50% by thermography, and 40% by both techniques. Thus, there was a thermal alarm in 90% of the patients and the only sign in 50% of the cases [54].

In a study performed at Cornell University, a prospective clinical trial comprising 92 patients investigated digital infrared imaging for breast cancer screening. Based on prior mammograms or ultrasound, all 92 patients were recommended for biopsy. Of the 94 biopsies performed 60 were malignant and 34 were benign. Digital infrared imaging identified 58 of 60 malignancies for a sensitivity of 97%. The study summary noted that "Digital infrared thermal imaging is a valuable adjunct to mammography and ultrasound, especially in women with dense breast parenchyma" [55].

Wang and associates conducted a study on 276 women with a comparison made between findings on infrared imaging and mammographic BI-RADS categories. In all, 174 malignant lesions (22 DCIS and

152 invasive carcinomas) were discovered among BI-RADS categories 3 through 5. When compared to the BI-RADS scale, the sensitivities for infrared imaging were highest in the 4–5 categories. For BI-RADS category 3 lesions, infrared imaging correctly identified the only one cancerous lesion. An 82% overall sensitivity was found for infrared imaging across the BI-RADS categories 3–5. A sensitivity of 92% was noted for infrared imaging when compared to the BI-RADS 4 and 5 categories [56].

In a study utilizing a new computerized analysis methodology, 100 women scheduled for biopsy underwent infrared imaging. In total, 106 biopsies were performed with 65 malignant and 41 benign lesions noted. With the use of the computer analysis alone a sensitivity of 78% and specificity of 75% was realized. When combined with mammography, the sensitivity was increased to 89% in women under the age of 50. The study concluded that the combined sensitivity of infrared imaging and mammography in women under 50 was encouraging, suggesting a potential way forward for a dual imaging approach in this younger age group [57].

In a simple review of over 15 large-scale studies from 1967 to 1998, infrared imaging of the breast has showed an average sensitivity and specificity of 90%. With continued technological advances in infrared imaging in the past decade, some studies are showing even higher sensitivity and specificity values. However, until further large-scale studies are performed, these findings remain in question.

31.4 Infrared Imaging as a Risk Indicator

As early as 1976, at the *Third International Symposium on Detection and Prevention of Cancer* held in New York, thermal imaging was established by consensus as the highest risk marker for the possibility of the presence of an undetected breast cancer. It had also been shown to predict such a subsequent occurrence [58–60]. The Wisconsin Breast Cancer Detection Foundation presented a summary of its findings in this area, which has remained undisputed [60]. This, combined with other reports, has confirmed that an abnormal infrared image is the highest risk indicator for the future development of breast cancer and is 10 times as significant as a first-order family history of the disease [61].

In a study of 10,000 women screened, Gautherie found that, when applied to asymptomatic women, thermography was very useful in assessing the risk of cancer by dividing patients into low- and high-risk categories. This was based on an objective evaluation of each patient's thermograms using an improved reading protocol that incorporated 20 thermopathological factors [62].

A screening of 61,000 women using thermography was performed by Spitalier over a 10-year period. The authors concluded that "in patients having no clinical or radiographic suspicion of malignancy, a persistently abnormal breast thermogram represents the highest known risk factor for the future development of breast cancer" [42].

From a patient base of 58,000 women screened with thermography, Gros and associates followed 1527 patients with initially healthy breasts and abnormal thermograms for 12 years. Of this group, 44% developed malignancies within 5 years. The study concluded that "an abnormal thermogram is the single most important marker of high-risk category for the future development of breast cancer" [49].

Spitalier and associates followed 1416 patients with isolated abnormal breast thermograms. It was found that a persistently abnormal thermogram, as an isolated phenomenon, is associated with an actuarial breast cancer, a risk of 26% at 5 years. Within this study, 165 patients with nonpalpable cancers were observed. In 53% of these patients, thermography was the only test which was positive at the time of initial evaluation. It was concluded that:

1. A persistently abnormal thermogram, even in the absence of any other sign of malignancy, is associated with a high risk of developing cancer.
2. This isolated abnormality also carries with it a high risk of developing interval cancer, and as such the patient should be examined more frequently than the customary 12 months.
3. Most patients diagnosed as having minimal breast cancer have abnormal thermograms as the first warning sign [63,64].

In a study by Gautherie and associates, the effectiveness of thermography in terms of survival benefit was discussed. The authors analyzed the survival rates of 106 patients in whom the diagnosis of breast cancer was established as a result of the follow-up of thermographic abnormalities found on the initial examination when the breasts were apparently healthy (negative physical and mammographic findings). The control group consisted of 372 breast cancer patients. The patients in both groups were subjected to identical treatment and followed for 5 years. A 61% increase in survival was noted in the patients who were followed-up due to initial thermographic abnormalities. The authors summarized the study by stating that "the findings clearly establish that the early identification of women at high risk of breast cancer based on the objective thermal assessment of breast health results in a dramatic survival benefit" [65,66].

Infrared imaging provides a reflection of functional tumor-induced angiogenesis and metabolic activity rather than structurally based parameters (i.e., tumor size, architectural distortion, and microcalcifications). Recent advances in cancer research have determined that the biological activity of a neoplasm is far more significant an indicator of aggressiveness than the size of the tumor. As a direct reflection of the biological activity in the breast, infrared imaging has been found to provide a significant biological risk marker for cancer.

31.5 Infrared Imaging as a Prognostic Indicator

Studies exploring the biology of cancers have shown that the amount of thermovascular activity in the breast is directly proportional to the aggressiveness of the tumor. As such, infrared imaging provides the clinician with an invaluable tool in prognosis and treatment monitoring.

In a study of 209 breast cancers, Dilhuydy and associates found a positive correlation between the degree of infrared abnormalities and the existence of positive axillary lymph nodes. It was reported that the amount of thermovascular activity seen in the breast was directly related to the prognosis. The study concluded that infrared imaging provides a highly significant factor in prognosis and that it should be included in the pretherapeutic assessment of a breast cancer [67].

Amalric and Spitalier reported on 25,000 patients screened and 1878 histologically proven breast cancers investigated with infrared imaging. The study noted that the amount of infrared activity in the breast was directly proportional to the survival of the patient. The "hot" cancers showed a significantly poorer prognosis with a 24% survival rate at 3 years. A much better prognosis with an 80% survival rate at 3 years was seen in the more biologically inactive or "cooler" cancers. The study also noted a positive association between the amount of thermal activity in the breast and the presence of positive axillary nodes [68].

Reporting on a study of breast cancer doubling times and infrared imaging, Fournier noted significant changes in the thermovascular appearance of the images. The shorter the tumor doubling time, the more thermographic pathological signs were evident. It was concluded that infrared imaging served as a warning signal for the faster-growing breast cancers [69].

A retrospective analysis of 100 normal patients, 100 living cancer patients, and 126 deceased cancer patients was published by Head. Infrared imaging was found to be abnormal in 28% of the normal patients, compared to 65% of the living cancer patients and 88% of the deceased cancer patients. Known prognostic indicators related to tumor growth rate were compared to the results of the infrared images. The concentration of tumor ferritin, the proportion of cells in DNA synthesis and proliferating, and the expression of the proliferation-associated tumor antigen Ki-67 were all found to be associated with an abnormal infrared image. It was concluded that "the strong relationships of thermographic results with these three growth rate-related prognostic indicators suggest that breast cancer patients with abnormal thermograms have faster-growing tumors that are more likely to have metastasized and to recur with a shorter disease-free interval" [20].

In a paper by Gros and Gautherie, the use of infrared imaging in the prognosis of treated breast cancers was investigated. The authors considered infrared imaging to be absolutely necessary for assessing pretherapeutic prognosis or carrying out the follow-up of breast cancers treated by exclusive radio-therapy. They noted that before treatment, infrared imaging yields evidence of the cancer growth rate (aggressiveness) and contributes to the therapeutic choice. It also indicates the success of radio-sterilization or the suspicion of a possible recurrence or radio-resistance. The authors also noted a weaker 5-year survival with infrared images that showed an increase in thermal signals [70].

In a study by Keyserlingk, 20 women with core-biopsy proven locally advanced breast cancer underwent infrared imaging before and after chemohormonotherapy. All 20 patients were found to have abnormal thermovascular signs prior to treatment. Upon completion of the final round of chemotherapy, each patient underwent curative-intent surgery. Prior to surgery, all 20 patients showed improvement in their initial infrared scores. The amount of improvement in the infrared images was found to be directly related to the decrease in tumor size. A complete normalization of prechemotherapy infrared scores was seen in five patients. In these patients, there was no histological evidence of cancer remaining in the breast. In summary, the authors stated that "Further research will determine whether lingering infrared detected angiogenesis following treatment reflects tumor aggressiveness and ultimately prognosis, as well as early tumor resistance, thus providing an additional early signal for the need of a therapeutic adjustment" [71].

31.6 Breast Cancer Detection and Demonstration Project

The BCDDP is the most frequently quoted reason for the decreased interest in infrared imaging. The BCDDP was a large-scale study performed from 1973 through 1979, which collected data from many centers around the United States. Three methods of breast cancer detection were studied: physical examination, mammography, and infrared imaging.

Just before the onset of the BCDDP, two important papers appeared in the literature. In 1972, Gerald D. Dodd of the University of Texas Department of Diagnostic Radiology presented an update on infrared imaging in breast cancer diagnosis at the *Seventh National Cancer Conference* sponsored by the National Cancer Society and the NCI [72]. In his presentation, he suggested that infrared imaging would be best employed as a screening agent for mammography. He proposed that in any general survey of the female population aged 40 and over, 15–20% of these subjects would have positive infrared imaging and would require mammograms. Of these, approximately 5% would be recommended for biopsy. He concluded that infrared imaging would serve to eliminate 80–85% of the potential mammograms. Dodd also reiterated that the procedure was not competitive with mammography and, reporting the Texas Medical School's experience with infrared imaging, noted that it was capable of detecting approximately 85% of all breast cancers. Dodd's ideas would later help to fuel the premise and attitudes incorporated into the BCDDP.

Three years later, J.D. Wallace presented to another Cancer Conference, sponsored by the American College of Radiology, the American Cancer Society and the Cancer Control Program of the NCI, an update on infrared imaging of the breast [73]. The author's analysis suggested that the incidence of breast cancer detection per 1000 patients screened could increase from 2.72 when using mammography to 19 when using infrared imaging. He then underlined that infrared imaging poses no radiation burden on the patient, requires no physical contact, and, being an innocuous technique, could concentrate the sought population by a significant factor selecting those patients that required further investigation. He concluded that "the resulting infrared image contains only a small amount of information as compared to the mammogram, so that the reading of the infrared image is a substantially simpler task."

Unfortunately, this rather simplistic and cavalier attitude toward the generation and interpretation of infrared images was prevalent when it was hastily added and then prematurely dismissed from the BCDDP, which was just getting underway. Exaggerated expectations led to the ill-founded premise that infrared imaging might replace mammography rather than complement it. A detailed review of the Report of the Working Group of the BCDDP, published in 1979, is essential to understand the subsequent evolution of infrared imaging [74].

The work scope of this project was issued by the NCI on March 26, 1973 with six objectives, the second being to determine if a negative infrared image was sufficient to preclude the use of clinical examination and mammography in the detection of breast cancer. The Working Group, reporting on results of the first 4 years of this project, gave a short history regarding infrared imaging in breast cancer detection. They wrote that, as of the 1960s, there was intense interest in determining the suitability of infrared imaging for large-scale applications, and mass screening was one possibility. The need for technological improvement was recognized and the authors stated that efforts had been made to refine the technique. One of the important objectives behind these efforts had been to achieve a sufficiently high sensitivity and specificity for infrared imaging in order to make it useful as a prescreening device in selecting patients for referral for mammographic examination. It was thought that, if successful, the incorporation of this technology would result in a relatively small proportion of women having mammography (a technique that had caused concern at that time because of the carcinogenic effects of radiation). The Working Group indicated that the sensitivity and specificity of infrared imaging readings, with clinical data emanating from interinstitutional studies, were close to the corresponding results for physical examination and mammography. They noted that these three modalities selected different subgroups of breast cancers, and for this reason further evaluation of infrared imaging as a screening device in a controlled clinical trial was recommended.

31.6.1 Poor Study Design

While the Working Group describes in detail the importance of quality control of mammography, the entire protocol for infrared imaging was summarized in one paragraph and simply indicated that infrared imaging was conducted by a BCDDP-trained technician. The detailed extensive results from this report, consisting of over 50 tables, included only one that referred to infrared imaging showing that it had detected only 41% of the breast cancers during the first screening while the residual were either normal or unknown. There is no breakdown as far as these two latter groups were concerned. Since 28% of the first screening and 32% of the second screening were picked up by mammography alone, infrared imaging was dropped from any further evaluation and consideration. The report stated that it was impossible to determine whether abnormal infrared images could be predictive of interval cancers (cancers developing between screenings) since they did not collect these data.

By the same token, the Working Group was unable to conclude, with their limited experience, whether the findings were related to the then available technology of infrared imaging or with its application. They did, however, conclude that the decision to dismiss infrared imaging should not be taken as a determination of the future of this technique, rather that the procedure continued to be of interest because it does not entail the risk of radiation exposure. In the Working Group's final recommendation, they state that "infrared imaging does not appear to be suitable as a substitute for mammography for routine screening in the BCDDP." The report admitted that several individual programs of the BCDDP had results that were more favorable than what was reported for the BCDDP as a whole. They encouraged investment in the development and testing of infrared imaging under carefully controlled study conditions and suggested that high priority be given to these studies. They noted that a few suitable sites appeared to be available within the BCDDP participants and proposed that developmental studies should be solicited from sites with sufficient experience.

31.6.2 Untrained Personnel and Protocol Violations

JoAnn Haberman, who was a participant in this project [75], provided further insight into the relatively simplistic regard assigned to infrared imaging during this program. The author reiterated that expertise in mammography was an absolute requirement for the awarding of a contract to establish a screening center. However, the situation was just the opposite with regard to infrared imaging—no experience was required at all. When the 27 demonstration project centers opened their doors, only five had any preexisting expertise in infrared imaging. Of the remaining screening centers, there was no experience at all in this technology. Finally, more than 18 months after the project had begun, the NCI-established centers where radiologists and their technicians could obtain sufficient training in infrared imaging. Unfortunately, only 11 of the demonstration project directors considered this training of sufficient importance to send their technologists to learn proper infrared technique. The imaging sites also disregarded environmental controls. Many of the project sites were mobile imaging vans that had poor heating and cooling capabilities, and often kept their doors open in the front and rear to permit an easy flow of patients. This, combined with a lack of adherence to protocols and preimaging patient acclimation, lead to unreadable images.

In summary, with regard to infrared imaging, the BCDDP was plagued with problems and seriously flawed in five critical areas:

1. The study was initiated with an incorrect premise that infrared imaging might replace mammography. A functional imaging procedure that detects metabolic thermovascular aberrations cannot replace a test that looks for specific areas of structural changes in the breast.
2. Completely untrained technicians were used to perform the scans.
3. The study used radiologists who had no experience or knowledge in reading infrared images.
4. Proper laboratory environmental controls were completely ignored. In fact, many of the research sites were mobile trailers with extreme variations in internal temperatures.
5. No standardized reading protocol had yet been established for infrared imaging. It was not until the early 1980s that established and standardized reading protocols were adopted.

Considering these facts, the BCDDP could not have properly evaluated infrared imaging. Since the termination of the BCDDP, a considerable amount of published research has demonstrated the true value of this technology.

31.7 Mammography and Infrared Imaging

From a scientific standpoint, mammography and infrared imaging are completely different screening tests. As a structural imaging procedure, mammography cannot be compared to a functional imaging technology such as infrared imaging. While mammography attempts to detect architectural tissue shadows, infrared imaging observes for changes in the subtle metabolic milieu of the breast. Even though mammography and infrared imaging examine completely different aspects of the breast, research has been performed that allows for a statistical comparison of the two technologies. Since a review of the research on infrared imaging has been covered, data on the current state of mammography is presented.

In a study by Rosenberg, 183,134 screening mammograms were reviewed for changes in sensitivity due to age, breast density, ethnicity, and estrogen replacement therapy. Out of these screening mammograms 807 cancers were discovered at screening. The results showed that the sensitivity for mammography was 54% in women younger than 40 years, 77% in women aged 40–49, 78% in women aged 50–64, and 81% in women older than 64 years. Sensitivity was 68% in women with dense breasts and 74% in estrogen replacement therapy users [76].

Investigating the cumulative risk of a false-positive result in mammographic screening, Elmore and associates performed a 10-year retrospective study of 2400 women aged 40–69 years of age. A total of 9762 mammograms were investigated. It was found that a woman had an estimated 49.1% cumulative risk of having a false-positive result after ten mammograms. Even though no breast cancer was present, over one-third of the women screened were required to have additional evaluations [77].

In a review of the literature, Head investigated the sensitivity, specificity, positive predictive value, and negative predictive values for mammography and infrared imaging. The average reported performance for mammography was 86% sensitivity, 79% specificity, 28% positive predictive value, and 92% negative predictive value. For infrared imaging the averaged performance was: 86% sensitivity, 89% specificity, 23% positive predictive value, and 99.4% negative predictive value [78].

Pisano, along with a large investigational group, provided a detailed report on the Digital Mammographic Imaging Screening Trial (DMIST). The study investigated the diagnostic performance of digital versus film mammography in breast cancer screening. Both digital and film mammograms were taken on 42,760 asymptomatic women presenting for screening mammography. Data were gathered from 33 sites in the United States and Canada. Digital mammography was found to be more accurate in women under age 50 and in women whose breasts were radiographically dense. The sensitivity for both film and digital mammography was found to be 69% [79].

Keyserlingk and associates published a retrospective study reviewing the relative ability of clinical examinations, mammography, and infrared imaging to detect 100 new cases of ductal carcinoma *in situ*, stage I and II breast cancers. Results from the study found that the sensitivity for clinical examination alone was 61%, mammography alone was 66%, and infrared imaging alone was 83%. When suspicious and equivocal mammograms were combined the sensitivity was increased to 85%. A sensitivity of 95% was found when suspicious and equivocal mammograms were combined with abnormal infrared images. However, when clinical examination, mammography, and infrared images were combined a sensitivity of 98% was reached [80].

From a review of the cumulative literature database, it can be found that the average sensitivity and specificity for mammography is, at best, 80% and 79%, respectively, for women over the age of 50 [81–83]. A significant decrease in sensitivity and specificity is seen in women below this age. This same research also shows that mammography routinely misses interval cancers (cancers that form between screening exams) [80] that may be detected by infrared imaging. Taking into consideration all the available data, mammography leaves much to be desired as the current gold standard for breast cancer screening. As a stand alone screening procedure, it is suggested that mammography may not be the best choice. In the same light, infrared imaging should also not be used alone as a screening test. The two technologies are of a complementary nature. Neither used alone are sufficient, but when combined each builds on the deficiencies of the other. In reviewing the literature it seems evident that a multimodal approach to breast cancer screening would serve women best. A combination of clinical examination, mammography, and infrared imaging would provide the greatest potential for breast conservation and survival.

31.8 Current Status of Breast Cancer Detection

Current first-line breast cancer detection strategy still depends essentially on clinical examination and mammography. The limitations of the former, with its reported sensitivity rate often below 65% [80,84] is well-recognized, and even the proposed value of self-breast examination is being contested [85]. While mammography is accepted as the most cost-effective imaging modality, its contribution continues to be challenged with persistent false-negative rates ranging up to 30% [76,79,86,87]; with decreasing sensitivity in younger patients and those on estrogen replacement therapy [76,87,88]. In addition, there is recent data suggesting that denser and lesser informative mammography images are precisely those associated with an increased cancer risk [89,90]. Echoing some of the shortcomings of the BCDDP concerning their study design and infrared imaging, Moskowitz indicated that mammography is also not a procedure to be performed by the inexperienced technician or radiologist [91].

With the current emphasis on earlier detection, there is now renewed interest in the parallel development of complementary imaging techniques that can also exploit the precocious metabolic, immunological, and vascular changes associated with early tumor growth. While promising, techniques such as scintimammography [92], Doppler ultrasound [93], and magnetic resonance imaging (MRI) [94], are associated with a number of disadvantages that include exam duration, limited accessibility, need of intravenous access, patient discomfort, restricted imaging area, difficult interpretation, and limited availability of the technology. Like ultrasound, they are more suited to be used as second-line options to pursue the already abnormal screening evaluations. While practical, this stepwise approach currently results in the nonrecognition, and thus delayed utilization of second-line technology in approximately 10% of established breast cancers [91]. This is consistent with a study published by Keyserlingk et al. [80].

As an addition to the breast health screening process, infrared imaging has a significant role to play. Owing to infrared imaging's unique ability to image the metabolic aspects of the breast, extremely early warning signals (8–10 years before any other detection method) have been observed in long-term studies. It is for this reason that an abnormal infrared image is the single most important marker of high risk for the existence of or future development of breast cancer. This, combined with the proven sensitivity, specificity, and prognostic value of the technology, places infrared imaging as one of the major front-line methods of breast cancer screening.

31.9 Future Advancements in Infrared Imaging

Modern high-resolution uncooled focal plane array cameras coupled with high-speed computers running sophisticated image analysis software are commonplace in today's top infrared imaging centers. However, research in this field continues to produce technological advancements in image acquisition and digital processing.

Research is currently under way investigating the possible subtle alterations in the blood supply to the breast during the earliest stages of malignancy. Evidence suggests that there may be a normal vasomotor oscillation frequency in the arterial structures of the human body. It is theorized that there may be disturbances in this normal oscillatory rate when a malignancy is forming. Research using infrared detection systems capturing 200 frames per second with a sensitivity of 0.009 of a degree centigrade may be able to monitor alterations in this vasomotor frequency band.

Another unique methodology is investigating the possibility of using infrared emission data to extrapolate depth and location of a metabolic heat source within the body. In the case of cancer, the increased tissue metabolism resulting from rapid cellular multiplication and growth generates heat. With this new approach in infrared detection, it is theorized that an analysis based on an analogy to electrical circuit theory—termed the thermal-electric analog—may possibly be used to determine the depth and location of the heat source.

The most promising of all the advances in medical infrared imaging are the adaptations being used from military developments in the technology. Hardware advances in narrow-band filtering hold promise in providing multispectral and hyperspectral images. One of the most intriguing applications of multispectral/hyperspectral imaging may include real-time intraoperative cytology. Investigations are also underway utilizing smart processing, also known as artificial intelligence. This comes in the form of postimage processing of the raw data from the infrared sensor array. Some of the leading-edge processing currently under study includes automated target recognition (ATR), artificial neural networks (ANN), and a host of other proprietary algorithms. The uses of ATR and similar algorithms are dependent on a reliable normative database. The images are processed based on what the system has learned as normal and compares the new image to that database. Unlike ATR, ANN uses data summation to produce pattern recognition. This is extremely important when it comes to the complex thermovascular patterns seen in infrared breast imaging. Ultimately, these advancements should lead to a substantial increase in both objectivity and accuracy as an analytical aid to the human interface.

In another and possibly critical role, infrared imaging of the breast may hold a significant potential in breast cancer prevention. Due to the ability of infrared imaging's detection of changes in the dermal circulation, any exogenous pharmacological intervention or endogenous release of biochemicals that have the propensity to alter vascular profusion may be detected. This is especially true of chemicals that are target specific for the tissues of the breast. Being a primary target tissue for the hormone estrogen, the hormone's effect in the breast is anabolic to the ductal cells. As such, the outcome is one of increased cellular metabolism. This increase in cellular activity necessitates the need for nutrients above and beyond the norm. In order to facilitate this need, an increase in blood supply must occur. This translates to an infrared image demonstrating a uniform increase in vascular patterning. The importance of this observation lies in one of the primary risk factors for breast cancer—lifetime exposure to estrogen. If infrared imaging has the ability to warn of increased thermovascular activity secondary to levels of estrogen in the breast, action can be taken to lower this activity and ultimately the patient's risk for future breast cancer. Treatments can be monitored for positive effects by incorporating infrared imaging as a method of observing these effects. Studies have shown this effect and the positive outcome of pharmacological intervention. Many patients with this condition also demonstrate signs and symptoms that include breast pain, tenderness, cysts, and benign lumps. In many patients, a reversal or reduction in these signs and symptoms are also noted when treatment is initiated [95–97]. Infrared imaging's ability to detect increased thermovascular activity secondary to levels of estrogen in the breast, and to monitor the effects of treatment targeted at the breast, may play a significant role in breast cancer prevention.

New breast cancer treatments are also exploring methods of targeting the angiogenic process. Owing to a tumor's dependence on a constant blood supply to maintain growth, antiangiogenesis therapy is becoming one of the most promising therapeutic strategies and has been found to be pivotal in the new paradigm for consideration of breast cancer development and treatment [98]. The future may see infrared imaging and antiangiogenesis therapy combined as the state-of-the-art in the biological assessment and treatment of breast cancer.

These and other new methodologies in medical infrared imaging are being investigated and may prove to be significant advancements.

31.10 Conclusion

The large patient populations and long survey periods in many of the above clinical studies yields a high significance to the various statistical data obtained. This is especially true for the contribution of infrared imaging to early cancer diagnosis, as an invaluable marker of high-risk populations, and in therapeutic decision making.

Currently available high-resolution digital infrared imaging technology benefits greatly from enhanced image production, computerized image processing and analysis, and standardized image interpretation protocols. Over 40 years of research and 800 indexed papers encompassing well over 300,000 women participants has demonstrated infrared imaging's abilities in the early detection of breast cancer. Infrared imaging has distinguished itself as the earliest detection technology for breast cancer. It may be able to signal an alarm that a cancer may be forming 8–10 years before any other procedure can detect it. In seven out of ten cases, infrared imaging will detect signs of a cancer before it is seen on a mammogram. Clinical trials have also shown that infrared imaging significantly augments the long-term survival rates of its recipients by as much as 61%. And when used as part of a multimodal approach (clinical examination, mammography, and infrared imaging), 95% of all early stage cancers will be detected. Ongoing research into the thermal characteristics of breast pathologies will continue to investigate the relationships between neoangiogenesis, chemical mediators, and the neoplastic process.

It is unfortunate, but many clinicians still hesitate to consider infrared imaging as a useful tool in spite of the considerable research database, steady improvements in both infrared technology and image analysis, and continued efforts on the part of the infrared imaging societies. This attitude may be due in part to the average clinician's unfamiliarity with the physical and biological basis of infrared imaging. The other methods of cancer investigations refer directly to topics of medical teaching. For instance, radiography and ultrasonography refer to structural anatomy. Infrared imaging, however, is based on thermodynamics and thermokinetics, which are unfamiliar to most clinicians; though man is experiencing heat production and exchange in every situation he undergoes or creates.

Considering the contribution that infrared imaging has demonstrated thus far in the field of early breast cancer detection, all possibilities should be considered for promoting further technical, biological, and clinical research along with the incorporation of the technology into common clinical use.

References

1. Adams, F., *The Genuine Works of Hippocrates*. Williams & Wilkins, Baltimore, 1939.
2. Lawson, R. N., Implications of surface temperatures in the diagnosis of breast cancer. *Can. Med. Assoc. J.,* 75, 309, 1956.
3. Lawson, R. N., Thermography—A new tool in the investigation of breast lesions. *Can. Serv. Med.,* 13, 517, 1957.
4. Lawson, R. N., A new infrared imaging device. *Can. Med. Assoc. J.* 79, 402, 1958.
5. Archer, F., Gros, C., Classification thermographique des cancers mammaries. *Bull. Cancer,* 58, 351, 1971.
6. Amalu, W. et al., Standards and protocols in clinical thermographic imaging. International Academy of Clinical Thermology, September 2002.
7. Kurbitz, G., Design criteria for radiometric thermal-imaging devices, in *Thermological Methods*, VCH mbH, 94–100, 1985.
8. Houdas, Y., Ring E.F.J., Models of thermoregulation, in *Human Temperature: Its Measurement and Regulation*, Plenum Press, New York, 136–141.
9. Flesch, U., Physics of skin-surface temperature, in *Thermological Methods*, VCH mbH, 21–33, 1985.
10. Anbar M., *Quantitative Dynamic Telethermometry in Medical Diagnosis and Management*, CRC Press, FL, 106, 1994.
11. Anbar, M., Potential artifacts in infrared thermographic measurements. *Thermology,* 3, 273, 1991.
12. Friedrich, K. (Optic research laboratory, Carl Zeiss—West Germany), Assessment criteria for infrared thermography systems. *Acta Thermographica,* 5, 68–72.
13. Engel, J. M., Thermography in locomotor diseases. *Acta Thermographica,* 5, 11–13.
14. Cuthbertson, G. M., The development of IR imaging in the United Kingdom, in *The Thermal Image in Medicine and Biology*. Uhlen-Verlag, Wien, 21–32, 1995.
15. Amalu, W., Nondestructive testing of the human breast: The validity of dynamic stress testing in medical infrared breast imaging. *Proceedings of the 26th Annual International Conference of the IEEE EMBS,* 1174–1177, 2004.
16. Gautherie, M., Kotewicz, A., Gueblez, P., Accurate and objective evaluation of breast thermograms: Basic principles and new advances with special reference to an improved computer-assisted scoring system: in *Thermal assessment of Breast Health*, MTP Press Limited, 72–97, 1983.
17. Hobbins, W. B., Abnormal thermogram—Significance in breast cancer. *Interamer. J. Rad.,* 12, 337, 1987.
18. Gautherie, M., New protocol for the evaluation of breast thermograms, in *Thermological Methods*, VCH mbH, 227–235, 1985.
19. Lawson, R. N., Chughtai, M. S., Breast cancer and body temperatures. *Can. Med. Assoc. J,* 88, 68, 1963.
20. Head, J. F., Wang, F., Elliott, R. L., Breast thermography is a noninvasive prognostic procedure that predicts tumor growth rate in breast cancer patients. *Ann N Y Acad. Sci,* 698, 153, 1993.
21. Sterns, E. E., Zee, B., Sen Gupta, J., Saunders, F. W., Thermography: Its relation to pathologic characteristics, vascularity, proliferative rate and survival of patients with invasive ductal carcinoma of the breast. *Cancer,* 77, 1324, 1996.
22. Head, J. F., Elliott, R. L., Breast thermography. *Cancer,* 79, 186, 1995.
23. Anbar M., in *Quantitative Dynamic Telethermometry in Medical Diagnosis and Management*. CRC Press, Boca Raton, FL, pp. 84–94, 1994.
24. Rodenberg, D. A., Chaet, M. S., Bass, R. C. et al. Nitric oxide: An overview. *Am. J Surg.* 170, 292, 1995.
25. Thomsen, L. L., Miles, D. W., Happerfield, L. et al. Nitric oxide synthase activity in human breast cancer. *Br. J. Cancer,* 72(1), 41, 1995.
26. Guidi, A. J., Schnitt, S. J., Angiogenesis in pre-invasive lesions of the breast. *The Breast J.,* 2, 364, 1996.
27. Gamagami, P., Indirect signs of breast cancer: Angiogenesis study, in *Atlas of Mammography*, Blackwell Science, Cambridge, MA, 231–226, 1996.

28. Love, T., Thermography as an indicator of blood perfusion. *Proc NY Acad Sci J*, 335, 429, 1980.
29. Chato, J., Measurement of thermal properties of growing tumors. *Proc NY Acad Sci*, 335, 67, 1980.
30. Draper, J., Skin temperature distribution over veins and tumors. *Phys. Med. Biol.*, 16(4), 645, 1971.
31. Jain, R., Gullino, P., Thermal characteristics of tumors: Applications in detection and treatment. *Ann. NY Acad. Sci.*, 335, 1, 1980.
32. Gautherie, M., Thermopathology of breast cancer; measurement and analysis of *in-vivo* temperature and blood flow. *Ann. NY Acad. Sci.*, 365, 383, 1980.
33. Gautherie, M., Thermobiological assessment of benign and malignant breast diseases. *Am. J Obstet. Gynecol.*, 147(8), 861, 1983.
34. Gamigami, P., *Atlas of Mammography: New Early Signs in Breast Cancer*. Blackwell Science, 1996.
35. Gershen-Cohen, J., Haberman, J., Brueschke, E., Medical thermography: A summary of current status. *Radiol. Clin. North Am.*, 3, 403, 1965.
36. Haberman, J., The present status of mammary thermography. *Ca—A Cancer J. Clin.*, 18, 314, 1968.
37. Hoffman, R., Thermography in the detection of breast malignancy. *Am. J Obstet. Gynecol.*, 98, 681, 1967.
38. Stark, A., Way, S., The screening of well women for the early detection of breast cancer using clinical examination with thermography and mammography. *Cancer*, 33, 1671, 1974.
39. Amalric, D. et al., Value and interest of dynamic telethermography in detection of breast cancer. *Acta Thermogr.*, 1, 89–96.
40. Hobbins, W., Mass breast cancer screening. *Proceedings, Third International Symposium on Detection and Prevention of Breast Cancer*, New York City, NY, 637, 1976.
41. Isard, H. J., Becker, W., Shilo, R. et al., Breast thermography after four years and 10,000 studies. *Am. J Roentgenol.*, 115, 811, 1972.
42. Spitalier, H., Giraud, D. et al., Does infrared thermography truly have a role in present-day breast cancer management? *Biomedical Thermology*, Alan R. Liss, New York, NY, 269–278, 1982.
43. Moskowitz, M., Milbrath, J., Gartside, P. et al., Lack of efficacy of thermography as a screening tool for minimal and stage I breast cancer. *N Engl. J Med.*, 295, 249, 1976.
44. Threatt, B., Norbeck, J.M., Ullman, N.S. et al., Thermography and breast cancer: An analysis of a blind reading. *Ann. N Y Acad Sci*, 335, 501, 1980.
45. Haberman, J., Francis, J., Love, T., Screening a rural population for breast cancer using thermography and physical examination techniques. *Ann. NY Acad. Sci.*, 335, 492, 1980.
46. Sciarra, J., Breast cancer: Strategies for early detection, in *Thermal Assessment of Breast Health (Proceedings of the International Conference on Thermal Assessment of Breast Health)*. MTP Press LTD, 117–129, 1983.
47. Gautherie, M., Thermobiological assessment of benign and malignant breast diseases. *Am. J Obstet. Gynecol.*, 147(8), 861, 1983.
48. Louis, K., Walter, J., Gautherie, M., Long-term assessment of breast cancer risk by thermal imaging, in *Biomedical Thermology*. Alan R. Liss Inc., 279–301, 1982.
49. Gros, C., Gautherie, M., Breast thermography and cancer risk prediction. *Cancer*, 45, 51, 1980.
50. Jones, C. H., Thermography of the female breast, in *Diagnosis of Breast Disease*, C.A. Parsons (Ed.), University Park Press, Baltimore, 214–234, 1983.
51. Useki, H., Evaluation of the thermographic diagnosis of breast disease: Relation of thermographic findings and pathologic findings of cancer growth. *Nippon Gan Chiryo Gakkai Shi*, 23, 2687, 1988.
52. Parisky, Y. R., Sardi, A. et al., Efficacy of computerized infrared imaging analysis to evaluate mammographically suspicious lesions. *AJR*, 180, 263, 2003.
53. Nyirjesy, I., Ayme, Y. et al., Clinical evaluation, mammography, and thermography in the diagnosis of breast carcinoma. *Thermology*, 1, 170, 1986.
54. Thomassin, L., Giraud, D. et al., Detection of subclinical breast cancers by infrared thermography, in *Recent Advances in Medical Thermology (Proceedings of the Third International Congress of Thermology)*, Plenum Press, New York, NY., 575–579, 1984.
55. Arora, N., Martins, D., Ruggerio, D. et al., Effectiveness of a noninvasive digital infrared thermal imaging system in the detection of breast cancer. *Am. J Surg.*, 196(4), 523–526, 2008.

56. Wang et al., Evaluation of the diagnostic performance of infrared imaging of the breast: A preliminary study. *Biomedical Engineering*, 9, 3, 2010.

57. Wishart, G. C., Lampiri, M., Boswell, M. et al., The accuracy of digital infrared imaging for breast cancer detection in women undergoing breast biopsy. *Eur. J Surg. Oncol.*, 36(6), 535–540, 2010.

58. Amalric, R., Gautherie, M., Hobbins, W., Stark, A., The future of women with an isolated abnormal infrared thermogram. *La Nouvelle Presse Med*, 10(38), 3153, 1981.

59. Gautherie, M., Gros, C., *Contribution of Infrared Thermography to Early Diagnosis, Pretherapeutic Prognosis, and Post-Irradiation Follow-up of Breast Carcinomas*. Laboratory of Electroradiology, Faculty of Medicine, Louis Pasteur University, Strasbourg, France, 1976.

60. Hobbins, W., Significance of an "isolated" abnormal thermogram. *La Nouvelle Presse Medicale*, 10, 3155, 1981.

61. Hobbins, W., Thermography, highest risk marker in breast cancer. *Proceedings of the Gynecological Society for the Study of Breast Disease,* 267–282, 1977.

62. Gauthrie, M., Improved system for the objective evaluation of breast thermograms, in *Biomedical Thermology*. Alan R. Liss, Inc., New York, NY, 897–905, 1982.

63. Amalric, R., Giraud, D. et al., Combined diagnosis of small breast cancer. *Acta Thermographica*, 1984.

64. Spitalier, J., Amalric, D. et al., The importance of infrared thermography in the early suspicion and detection of minimal breast cancer, *in Thermal Assessment of Breast Health*, MTP Press Ltd., 173–179, 1983.

65. Gautherie, M. et al., Thermobiological assessment of benign and malignant breast diseases. *Am. J Obstet. Gynecol.*, 147(8), 861, 1983.

66. Jay, E., Karpman, H., Computerized breast thermography, in *Thermal Assessment of Breast Health*, MTP Press Ltd., 98–109, 1983.

67. Dilhuydy, M. H. et al., The importance of thermography in the prognostic evaluation of breast cancers. *Acta Thermogr.*, 130–136.

68. Amalric, D. et al., Value and interest of dynamic telethermography in detection of breast cancer. *Acta Thermogr.*, 89–96.

69. Fournier, V. D., Kubli, F. et al., Infrared thermography and breast cancer doubling time. *Acta Thermogr.*, 107–111.

70. Gros, D., Gautherie, M., Warter, F., Thermographic prognosis of treated breast cancers. *Acta Thermogr.*, 11–14.

71. Keyserlingk, J. R., Ahlgren P. D. et al., Preliminary evaluation of high resolution functional infrared imaging to monitor pre-operative chemohormonotherapy-induced changes in neo-angiogenesis in patients with locally advanced breast cancer. Ville Marie Oncology Center/St. Mary's Hospital, Montreal, Canada. In submission for publication, 2003.

72. Dodd, G. D., Thermography in breast cancer diagnosis, in *Abstracts for the Seventh National Cancer Conference Proceedings*. Lippincott, Philadelphia, Los Angeles, CA, 267, 1972.

73. Wallace, J. D., Thermographic examination of the breast: An assessment of its present capabilities, in *Early Breast Cancer: Detection and Treatment,* Gallagher, H.S. (Ed.). American College of Radiology, Wiley, New York, 13–19, 1975.

74. Report of the Working Group to Review the National Cancer Institute Breast Cancer Detection Demonstration Projects. *J. Natl. Cancer Inst.*, 62, 641, 1979.

75. Haberman, J., An overview of breast thermography in the United States, in *Medical Thermography*, M. Abernathy, S. Uematsu (Eds), American Academy of Thermology, Washington, 218–223, 1986.

76. Rosenberg, R. D., Hunt, W. C. et al., Effects of age, breast density, ethnicity, and estrogen replacement therapy on screening mammographic sensitivity and cancer stage at diagnosis: Review of 183,134 screening mammograms in Albuquerque, New Mexico. *Radiology*, 209(2), 511, 1998.

77. Elmore, J. et al, Ten-year risk of false positive screening mammograms and clinical breast examinations. *N. Engl. J Med.*, 338, 1089, 1998.

78. Head, J. F., Lipari, C. A., Elliot, R. L., Comparison of mammography, and breast infrared imaging: Sensitivity, specificity, false negatives, false positives, positive predictive value and negative predictive value. *IEEE*, 1999.

79. Pisano, E. D., Gatsonis, C. et al., Diagnostic performance of digital versus film mammography for breast-cancer screening. *N. Engl. J Med.*, 353, 2005.

80. Keyserlingk, J. R., Ahlgren, P. D. et al., Infrared imaging of the breast; initial reappraisal using high-resolution digital technology in 100 successive cases of stage 1 and 2 breast cancer. *Breast J.*, 4, #4, 1998.

81. Schell, M. J., Bird, R. D., Desrochers, D. A., Reassessment of breast cancers missed during routine screening mammography. *Am. J Roentgenol.*, 177, 535, 2001.

82. Poplack, S. P., Tosteson, A. N., Grove, M. et al., The practice of mammography in 53,803 women from the New Hampshire mammography network. *Radiology*, 217, 832, 2000.

83. Pullon, S., McLeod, D., The early detection and diagnosis of breast cancer: A literature review. General Practice Department, Wellington School of Medicine, December 1996.

84. Sickles, E. A., Mammographic features of "early" breast cancer. *Am. J Roentgenol.*, 143, 461, 1984.

85. Thomas, D. B., Gao, D. L., Self, S. G. et al., Randomized trial of breast self-examination in Shanghai: Methodology and preliminary results. *J. Natl. Cancer Inst.*, 5, 355, 1997.

86. Moskowitz, M., Screening for breast cancer. How effective are our tests? *CA Cancer J. Clin.*, 33, 26, 1983.

87. Elmore, J. G., Wells, C. F., Carol, M. P. et al., Variability in radiologists interpretation of mammograms. *NEJM*, 331(22), 1493, 1994.

88. Gilliland, F. D., Joste, N., Stauber, P. M. et al., Biologic characteristics of interval and screen-detected breast cancers. *J. Natl. Cancer Inst.*, 92, 743, 2000.

89. Laya, M. B., Effect on estrogen replacement therapy on the specificity and sensitivity of screening mammography. *J. Natl. Cancer Inst.*, 88, 643, 1996.

90. Boyd, N. F., Byng, J. W., Jong, R. A. et al., Quantitative classification of mammographic densities and breast cancer risk. *J. Natl. Cancer Inst.*, 87, 670, 1995.

91. Moskowitz, M., Breast imaging, in *Cancer of the Breast*, Donegan, W. L., Spratt, J.S. (Eds), Saunders, New York, 206–239, 1995.

92. Khalkhali, I., Cutrone, J. A. et al., Scintimammography: The complementary role of Tc-99m sestamibi prone breast imaging for the diagnosis of breast carcinoma. *Radiology*, 196, 421, 1995.

93. Kedar, R. P., Cosgrove, D. O. et al., Breast carcinoma: Measurement of tumor response in primary medical therapy with color doppler flow imaging. *Radiology*, 190, 825, 1994.

94. Weinreb, J. C., Newstead, G., MR imaging of the breast. *Radiology*, 196, 593, 1995.

95. Verzini, L., Romani, L., Talia, B., (Radiology department university of Modena (Italy)). Thermographic variations in the breast during the menstrual cycle. *Acta Thermographica*, 143–149, 1980s.

96. Huber, C., Pons, J., Pateau, A., (Gynecology and department of radiology Cretei hospital (Paris) France). Breast fibrocystic disease and thermography. *Acta Thermographica*, 48–50, 1980s.

97. Borten, M., Ransil, B. et al. (Department of obstetrics and gynecology, Beth Israel Hospital, Harvard Medical School). Regional differences in breast surface temperature by liquid crystal thermography. *Thermology*, 1, 216–220, 1986.

98. Love, S. M., Barsky, S. H., Breast cancer: An interactive paradigm. *Breast J.*, 3, 171, 1996.

32

Functional Infrared Imaging of the Breast: Historical Perspectives, Current Application, and Future Considerations

John R. Keyserlingk
Ville Marie Medical and Women's Health Center

P.D. Ahlgren
Ville Marie Medical and Women's Health Center

E. Yu
Ville Marie Medical and Women's Health Center

Normand Belliveau
Ville Marie Medical and Women's Health Center

Mariam Yassa
Ville Marie Medical and Women's Health Center

There is a general consensus that earlier detection of breast cancer should result in improved survival. For the last two decades, first-line breast imaging has relied primarily on mammography. Despite better equipment and regulation, particularly with the recent introduction of digital mammography, variability in interpretation and tissue density can affect mammography accuracy. To promote earlier diagnosis, a number of adjuvant functional imaging techniques have recently been introduced, including Doppler ultrasound and gadolinium-enhanced magnetic resonance imaging (MRI) that can detect cancer-induced regional neovascularity. While valuable modalities, problems relating to complexity, accessibility, cost, and in most cases the need for intravenous access make them unsuitable as components of a first-line imaging strategy.

In order to reassess the potential contribution of infrared (IR) imaging as a first-line component of a multi-imaging strategy, using currently available technology, we will first review the history of its introduction and early clinical application, including the results of the Breast Cancer Demonstration Projects (BCDDP). We will then review the Ville Marie Multidisciplinary Breast Center's more recent experience with currently available high-resolution computerized IR technology to assess IR imaging both as a complement to clinical exam and mammography in the early detection of breast cancer and also as a tool to monitor the effects of preoperative chemohormonotherapy in advanced breast cancer. Our goal is to show that high-resolution IR imaging provides additional safe, practical, cost-effective, and objective information in both of these instances when produced by strict protocol and interpreted by sufficiently trained breast physicians. Finally, we will comment on its further evolution.

32.1 Historical Perspectives

32.1.1 Pre-Breast Cancer Detection Demonstration Projects Era

In 1961, in the *Lancet*, Williams and Handley [1] using a rudimentary handheld thermopile, reported that 54 of 57 of their breast cancer patients were detectable by IR imaging, and "among these were cases in which the clinical diagnosis was in much doubt." The authors reported that the majority of these cancers had a temperature increase of 1–2°C, and that the IR imaging permitted excellent discrimination between benign and malignant processes. Their protocol at the Middlesex Hospital consisted of having the patient strip to the waist and be exposed to the ambient temperature for 15 min.

The authors demonstrated a precocious understanding of the significance of IR imaging by introducing the concept that increased cooling to 18°C further enhanced the temperature discrepancy between cancer and the normal breast. In a follow-up article the subsequent year, Handley [2] demonstrated a close correlation between the increased thermal pattern and increased recurrence rate. While only 4 of 35 cancer patients with a 1–2°C discrepancy recurred, five of the six patients with over 3°C rise developed recurrent cancer, suggesting already that the prognosis could be gauged by the amount of rise of temperature in the overlying skin.

In 1963, Lawson and Chughtai [3], two McGill University surgeons, published an elegant intraoperative study demonstrating that the increase in regional temperature associated with breast cancer was related to venous convection. This quantitative experiment added credence to Handley's suggestion that IR findings were related to both increased venous flow and increased metabolism.

In 1965, Gershon-Cohen [4], a radiologist and researcher from the Albert Einstein Medical Center, introduced IR imaging to the United States. Using a Barnes thermograph that required 15 min to produce a single IR image, he reported 4000 cases with a remarkable true-positive rate of 94% and a false-positive rate of 6%. These data were included in a review of the then current status of infrared imaging published in 1968 in *CA—A Cancer Journal for Physicians* [5]. The author, JoAnn Haberman, a radiologist from Temple University School of Medicine, reported the local experience with IR imaging, which produced a true-positive rate of 84% compared with a concomitant true-positive rate of 80% for mammography. In addition, she compiled 16,409 IR imaging cases from the literature between 1964 and 1968 revealing an overall true-positive rate of 87% and a false-positive rate of 13%.

A similar contemporary review compiled by Jones, consisting of nearly 70,000 cases, revealed an identical true-positive rate of 85% and an identical false-positive rate of 13%. Furthermore, Jones [6] reported on over 20,000 IR imagings from the Royal Marsden Hospital between 1967 and 1972, and noted that approximately 70% of Stage I and Stage II cancers and up to 90% of Stage III and Stage IV cancers had abnormal IR features. These reports resulted in an unbridled enthusiasm for IR imaging as a front-line detection modality for breast cancer.

Sensing a potential misuse of this promising but unregulated imaging modality, Isard made some sobering comments in 1972 [7] in a publication of the *American Journal of Roentengology*, where he emphasized that, like other imaging techniques, IR imaging does not diagnose cancer but merely indicates the presence of an abnormality. Reporting his Radiology division's experience with 10,000 IR studies done concomitantly with mammography between 1967 and 1970, he reiterated a number of important concepts, including the remarkable stability of the IR image from year to year in the otherwise healthy patient, and the importance of recognizing any significant change. Infrared imaging detected 60% of occult cancers in his experience, versus 80% with mammography. The combination of both these modalities increased the sensitivity by approximately 10%, thus underlining the complementarity of both of these processes, since each one did not always suspect the same lesion.

It was Isard's conclusion that, had there been a preliminary selection of his group of 4393 asymptomatic patients by IR imaging, mammography examination would have been restricted to the 1028 patients with abnormal IR imaging (23% of this cohort). This would have resulted in a cancer detection rate of 24.1 per 1000 mammographic examinations, as contrasted to the expected 7 per 1000 by mammographic screening. He concluded that since IR imaging is an innocuous examination, it could be utilized to focus attention upon asymptomatic women who should be examined more intensely.

In 1972, Gerald D. Dodd [8] of the Department of Diagnostic Radiology of the University of Texas presented an update on IR imaging in breast cancer diagnosis at the Seventh National Cancer Conference sponsored by the National Cancer Society and the National Cancer Institute (NCI). He also suggested that IR imaging would be best employed as a screening agent for mammography and proposed that in any general survey of the female population age 40 and over, 15–20% would have positive IR imaging and would require mammograms. Of these, approximately 5% would be recommended for biopsy. He concluded that IR imaging would serve to eliminate 80–85% of the potential mammograms. Reporting the Texas Medical School's experience with IR imaging, he reiterated that IR was capable of detecting approximately 85% of all breast cancers. The false-positive rate of 15–20% did not concern the author, who stated that these were false-positives only in the sense that there was no corroborative evidence of breast cancer at the time of the examination and that they could serve to identify a high-risk population.

Feig et al. [9] reported the respective abilities of clinical exam, mammography, and IR imaging to detect breast cancer in 16,000 self-selected women. While only 39% of the initial series of overall established cancer patients had an abnormal IR imaging, this increased to 75% in his later cohort, reflecting an improved methodology. Of particular interest was the ability of IR imaging to detect 54% of the smallest tumors, four times that of clinical examination. This potential important finding was not elaborated, but it could reflect IR's ability to detect vascular changes that are sometimes more apparent at the initiation of tumor genesis. The authors suggested that the potential of IR imaging to select high-risk groups for follow-up screening merited further investigation.

Wallace [10] presented an update on IR imaging of the breast to another contemporary Cancer Conference sponsored by the American College of Radiology, the American Cancer Society, and the Cancer Control Programme of the NCI. The analysis suggested that the incidence of breast cancer detection per 1000 screenees could increase from 2.72 when using mammography to 19 when using IR imaging. He then underlined that IR imaging poses no radiation burden on the patient, requires no physical contact, and, being an innocuous technique, could concentrate the sought population by a significant factor, selecting those patients that required further investigation. He concluded that "the resulting IR image contains only a small amount of information as compared to the mammogram, so that the reading of the IR image is a substantially simpler task."

Unfortunately, this rather simplistic and cavalier attitude toward the acquisition and interpretation of IR imaging was widely prevalent when it was hastily added to the BCDDP, which was just getting underway. Rather than assess, in a controlled manner, its potential as a complementary first-line detection modality, it was hastily introduced into the BCDDP as a potential replacement for mammography and clinical exam.

32.1.2 Breast Cancer Detection Demonstration Projects Era

A detailed review of the Report of the Working Group of the BCDDP is essential to understand the subsequent evolution of IR imaging [11]. The scope of this project was issued by the NCI on March 26, 1973, with six objectives, the second being to determine if a negative IR imaging was sufficient to preclude the use of clinical examination and mammography in the detection of breast cancer. The Working Group, reporting on results of the first 4 years of this project, gave a short history regarding IR imaging in breast cancer detection. They reported that as of the 1960s, there was intense interest in determining the suitability of IR imaging for large-scale applications, and mass screening was one possibility. The need for technological improvement was recognized and the authors stated that efforts had been made to refine the technique. One of the important objectives behind these efforts had been to achieve a sufficiently high sensitivity and specificity for IR imaging under screening conditions to make it useful as a prescreening device in selecting patients who would then be referred for mammographic examination. It was thought that if successful, this technology would result in a relatively small proportion of women having mammography, a technique that caused concern because of the carcinogenic effects of radiation. The Working Group indicated that the sensitivity and specificity of IR imaging readings from clinical data emanating from interinstitutional studies were close to the corresponding results for physical examination and for mammography. While they noted that these three modalities selected different subgroups of breast cancers, further evaluation of IR imaging as a potential stand-alone screening device in a controlled clinical trial was recommended.

The authors of the BCDDP Working Group generated a detailed review of mammography and efforts to improve its quality control in image quality and reduction in radiation. They recalled that in the 1960s, the Cancer Control Board of the U.S. Public Health Service had financed a national mammography training program for radiologists and their technologists. Weekly courses in mammography were taught at approximately 10 institutions throughout the country with material supplied by the American College of Radiology. In 1975, shortly after the beginning of this project, the NCI had already funded seven institutions in the United States in a 3-year effort aimed at reorienting radiologists and their technologists in more advanced mammographic techniques and interpretation for the detection of early breast cancer.

In the interim, the American College of Radiology and many interested mammographers and technologists had presented local postgraduate refresher courses and workshops on mammography. Every year for the previous 16 years, the American College of Radiology had supported, planned, and coordinated week-long conferences and workshops aimed at optimizing mammography to promote the earlier detection and treatment of breast cancer. It was recognized that the well-known primary and secondary mammographic signs of a malignant condition, such as ill-defined mass, skin thickening, skin retraction, marked fibrosis and architectural distortion, obliteration of the retromammary space, and enlarged visible axillary lymph nodes, could detect an established breast cancer. However, the authors emphasized that more subtle radiographic signs that occur in minimal, clinically occult, and early cancers, such as localized punctate calcifications, focal areas of duct prominence, and minor architectural distortion, could lead to an earlier diagnosis even when the carcinoma was not infiltrating, which was a rare finding when previous mammographic techniques were used.

The authors reiterated that the reproduction of early mammography signs required a constant high-quality technique for fine image detail, careful comparison of the two breasts during interpretation, and the search for areas of bilateral, parenchymal asymmetry that could reflect underlying cancer. The BCDDP Working Group report stated that mammographies were conducted by trained technicians and that, while some projects utilized radiological technicians for the initial interpretation, most used either a radiologist or a combination of technician and radiologist. Quality control for mammography consisted of reviews by the project radiologists and site visits by consultants to identify problems in procedures and the quality of the films.

On the other hand, the entire protocol for IR imaging within this study was summarized in one paragraph, and it indicated that IR imaging was conducted by a BCDDP-trained technician. Initial interpretation was made mostly by technicians; some projects used technicians plus radiologists and a few used radiologists and/or physicians with other specialties for all readings. Quality control relied on review of procedures and interpretations by the project physicians. Positive physical exams and mammographies were reported in various degrees of certainty about malignancy or as suspicious-benign; IR imaging was reported simply as normal or abnormal. While the protocol for the BCDDP required that the three clinical components of this study (physical examination, IR imaging, and mammography) be conducted separately, and initial findings and recommendations be reported independently, it was not possible for the Working Group to assess the extent to which this protocol was adhered to or to evaluate the quality of the examinations.

The detailed extensive results from this Working Group report consisted of over 50 tables. There was, however, only one table that referred to IR imaging, showing that it had detected 41% of the breast cancers during the first screening, while the residuals were either normal or unknown. There is no breakdown as far as these two latter groups were concerned. Since 28% of the first screening and 32% of the second screening were picked up by mammography alone, IR imaging was dropped from any further evaluation and consideration. The report stated that it was impossible to determine whether abnormal IR imaging could be predictive of interval (developing between screenings) cancers, since these data were not collected.

By the same token, the Working Group was unable to conclude, with their limited experience, whether the findings were related to the then existing technology of IR imaging or with its application. They did, however, indicate that the decision to dismiss IR imaging should not be taken as a determination of the future of this technique, rather that the procedure continued to be of interest because it does not entail the risk of radiation exposure. In the Working Group's final recommendation, they state that "infrared imaging does not appear to be suitable as a substitute for mammography for routine screening in the BCDDP" but could not comment on its role as a complementary modality. The report admitted that several individual programs of the BCDDP had results that were more favorable than for the BCDDP as a whole. They also insisted that high priority be given to development and testing of IR imaging under carefully controlled study conditions. They noted that a few suitable sites appeared to be available among the BCDDP and proposed that developmental studies should be solicited from the sites with sufficient experience.

Further insight into the inadequate quality control assigned to IR imaging during this program was provided by Haberman, a participant in that project [12]. The author reiterated that, while proven expertise in mammography was an absolute requirement for the awarding of a contract to establish a Screening Center, the situation was just the opposite as regards IR imaging. As no experience was required, when the 27 demonstration projects opened their doors, only five of the centers had preexisting expertise in IR imaging. Of the remaining screening centers, there was no experience at all in this technology. Finally, more than 18 months after the BCDDP project had begun operating, the NCI, recognizing this problem, established centers where radiologists and their technicians could obtain further training in IR imaging. Unfortunately, only 11 of the demonstration project directors considered this training of sufficient importance to send their technologists. In some centers, it was reported that there was no effort to cool the patient prior to examination. In other centers, there was complete lack of standardization, and a casual attitude prevailed with reference to interpretation of results. While quality control of this imaging technology could be considered lacking, it was nevertheless subjected to the same stringent statistical analysis as was mammography and clinical breast examination.

32.1.3 Post-Breast Cancer Detection Demonstration Projects Era

Two small-scale studies carried out in the 1970s by Moskowitz [13] and Threatt [14] reported on the sensitivity and reliability of IR imaging. Both used "experts" to review the images of breast cancer patients. While Moskowitz excluded unreadable images, data from Threatt's study indicated that less than 30% of the images produced were considered good, with the rest being substandard. Both these studies produced poor results, inconsistent with numerous previous multicenter trials, particularly that of Stark [15] who, 16 years earlier, reported an 81% detection rate for preclinical cancers.

Threatt noted that IR imaging demonstrated an increasing accuracy as cancers increased in size or aggressiveness, as did the other testing modalities (i.e., physical examination and mammography). The author also suggested that computerized pattern recognition would help solve the reproducibility problems sometimes associated with this technology and that further investigation was warranted. Moskowitz also suggested that for IR imaging to be truly effective as a screening tool, there needed to be more objective means of interpretation. He proposed that this would be much facilitated by computerized evaluation. In a frequently cited article, Sterns and Cardis [16] reviewed their group's limited experience with IR in 1982. While there were only 11 cancer cases in this trial, they were concerned about a sensitivity of 60% and a false-positive rate of IR of 12%. While there was no mention of training, they concluded, based on a surprisingly low false-positive rate of clinical exam of only 1.4%, that IR could not be recommended for breast diagnosis or as an indication for mammography.

Thirteen years later, reviewing the then status of breast imaging, Moskowitz [17] challenged the findings of the recent Canadian National Breast Screening Study (NBSS) that questioned the value of mammography, much in the same way that the Working Group of the BCDDP questioned IR imaging 20 years previously. Using arguments that could have qualified the disappointing results of the IR imaging used in the BCDDP study, the author explained the poor results of mammography in the NBSS on the basis of inadequate technical quality. He concluded that only 68% of the women received satisfactory breast imaging.

In addition to the usual causes of poor technical quality, failure to use the medial lateral oblique view resulted in exclusion of the tail of Spence and of much of the upper outer quadrant in many of the subjects screened. There was also a low interobserver agreement in the reading of mammographies, which resulted in a potential diagnostic delay. His review stated that of all noncontrast, nondigital radiological procedures, mammography required the greatest attention to meticulous detail for the training of technologists, selection of the film, contrast monitoring of processing, choosing of equipment, and positioning of the patient. For mammography to be of value, it required dedicated equipment, a dedicated room, dedicated film, and the need to be performed and interpreted by dedicated people. Echoing some of the criticisms that could be pertinent to the BCDDP's use of IR imaging, he indicated that mammography is not a procedure to be performed by the untutored. In rejecting any lack of quality control of IR imaging during the BCDDP studies by stating that "most of the investigators in the BCDDP did undergo a period of training," the author once again suggested that the potential of IR imaging would only increase if there was better standardization of technology and better-designed clinical trials.

Despite its initial promise, this challenge was not taken up by the medical community, who systematically lost interest in this technique, primarily due to the nebulous BCDDP experience. Nevertheless, during the 1980s, a number of isolated reports continued to appear, most emphasizing the risk factors associated with abnormal IR imaging. In *Cancer* in 1980, Gautherie and Gros [18] reported their experience with a group of 1245 women who had a mildly abnormal infrared image along with either normal or benign disease by conventional means, including physical exam, mammography, ultrasonography, and fine needle aspiration or biopsy. They noted that within 5 years, more than one-third of this group had histologically confirmed cancers. They concluded that IR imaging is useful not only as a predictor of breast cancer risk but also to identify the more rapidly growing neoplasms.

The following year, Amalric et al. [19], expanded on this concept by reporting that 10–15% of patients undergoing IR imaging will be found to be mildly abnormal when the remainder of the examination is essentially unremarkable. They noted that among these "false-positive" cases, up to 38% will eventually develop breast cancer when followed closely. In 1981, Mariel [20] carried out a study in France on 655 patients and noted an 82% sensitivity. Two years later, Isard [21] discussed the unique characteristics and respective roles of IR imaging and ultrasonography and concluded that, when used in conjunction with mammography in a multi-imaging strategy, their potential advantages included enhanced diagnostic accuracy, reduction of unnecessary surgery, and improved prognostic ability. The author emphasized that neither of these techniques should be used as a sole screening modality for breast cancer in asymptomatic women, but rather as a complementary modality to mammography.

In 1984, Nyirjesy [22] reported in *Obstetrics and Gynecology* a 76% sensitivity for IR imaging of 8767 patients. The same year, Bothmann [23] reported a sensitivity of 68% from a study carried out in Germany on 2702 patients. In 1986, Useki [24] published the results of a Japanese study indicating an 88% sensitivity.

Despite newly available IR technology, due in large part to military research and development, as well as compelling statistics of over 70,000 documented cases showing the contribution of functional IR imaging in a hitherto structurally based strategy to detect breast cancer, few North American centers have shown an interest, and fewer still have published their experience. This is surprising in view of the current consensus regarding the importance of vascular-related events associated with tumor initiation and growth that finally provide a plausible explanation for the IR findings associated with the early development of smaller tumors. The questionable results of the BCDDP and a few small-scale studies are still being referred to by a dwindling authorship that even mention the existence of this imaging modality. This has resulted in a generation of imagers that have neither knowledge of nor training in IR imaging. However, there are a few isolated centers that have continued to develop an expertise in this modality and have published their results.

In 1993, Head et al. [25] reported that improved images of the second generation of IR systems allowed more objective and quantitative visual analysis. They also reported that growth-rate-related prognostic indicators were strongly associated with the IR results [26]. In 1996, Gamagami [27] studied angiogenesis by IR imaging and reported that hypervascularity and hyperthermia could be shown in 86% of nonpalpable breast cancers. He also noted that in 15% of these cases, this technique helped to detect cancers that were not visible on mammography.

The concept of angiogenesis, suggested by Gamagami as an integral part of early breast cancer, was reiterated in 1996 by Guidi and Schnitt [28], whose observations suggested that angiogenesis is an early event in the development of breast cancer. They noted that it may occur before tumor cells acquire the ability to invade the surrounding stroma and even before there is morphologic evidence of an *in situ* carcinoma.

In contemporary publications, Anbar [29,30], using an elegant biochemical and immunological cascade, suggested that the empirical observation that small tumors capable of producing notable IR changes could be due to enhanced perfusion over a substantial area of breast surface via tumor-induced nitric oxide vasodilatation. He introduced the importance of dynamic area telethermometry to validate IRs full potential.

Parisky and his colleagues working out of six radiology centers [31] published an interesting report in *Radiology* in 2003 relating to the efficacy of computerized infrared imaging analysis of mammographi-cally suspicious lesions. They reported a 97% sensitivity, a 14% specificity, and a 95% negative predic-tive value when IR was used to help determine the risk factors relating to mammographically noted abnormal lesions in 875 patients undergoing biopsy. They concluded that infrared imaging offers a safe, noninvasive procedure that would be valuable as an adjunct to mammography, determining whether a lesion is benign or malignant.

32.2 Ville Marie Multidisciplinary Breast Center Experience with High-Resolution Digital Infrared Imaging to Detect and Monitor Breast Cancer

32.2.1 Infrared Imaging as Part of a First-Line Multi-Imaging Strategy to Promote Early Detection of Breast Cancer

There is still a general consensus that the crucial strategy for the first-line detection of breast cancer depends essentially on clinical examination and mammography. Limitation of the former, with its reported sensitivity rate below 65% is well recognized [32], and even the proposed value of breast self-examination is now being contested [33]. With the current emphasis on earlier detection, there is an increasing reliance on better imaging. Mammography is still considered our most reliable and cost-effective imaging modality [17]. However, variable interreader interpretation [34] and tissue density, now proposed as a risk factor itself [35] and seen in both younger patients and those on hormonal replacement

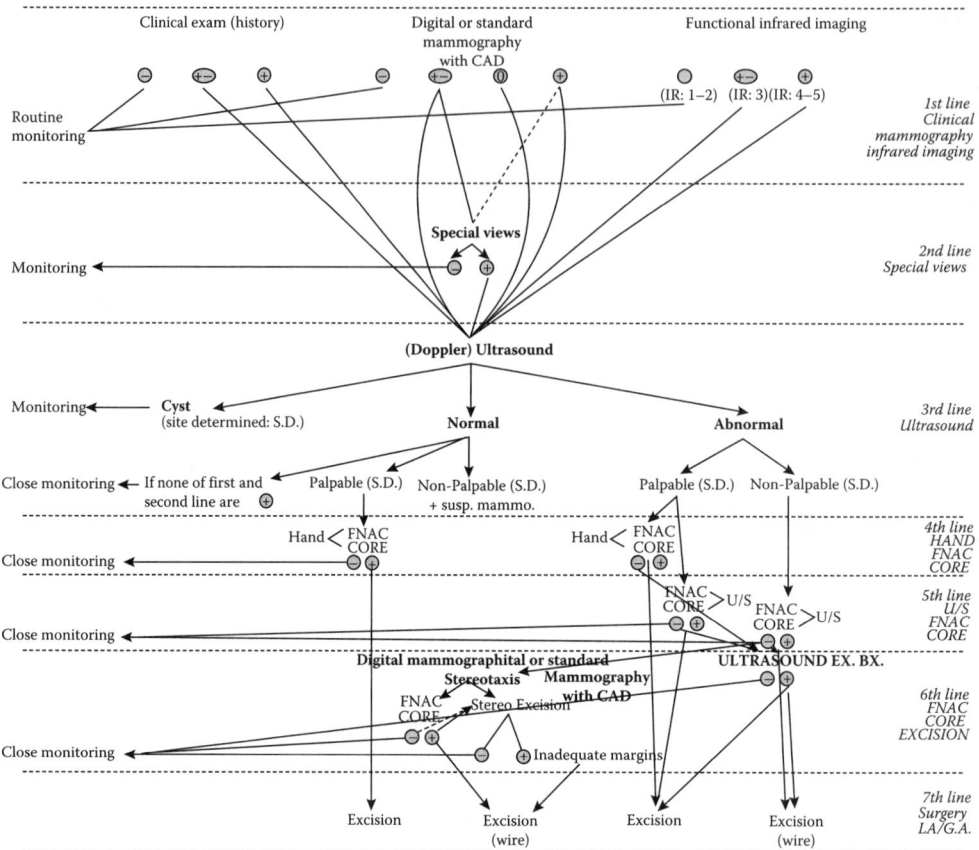

FIGURE 32.1   Ville Marie Breast Center: clinical and multi-imaging breast cancer detection strategy.

[36], prompted us to reassess currently available IR technology spearheaded by military research and development, as a first-line component of a multi-imaging breast cancer detection strategy (Figure 32.1).

This modality is capable of quantifying minute temperature variations and qualifying abnormal vascular patterns, probably associated with regional angiogenesis, neovascularization (Figure 32.2), and nitric oxide-induced regional vasodilatation [29], frequently associated with tumor initiation and progression, and potentially an early predictor of tumor growth rate [26,28]. We evaluated a new fully integrated high-resolution computerized IR imaging station to complement mammography units. To validate its reported ability to help detect early tumor-related regional metabolic and vascular changes [27], we limited our initial review to a series of 100 successive cases of breast cancer who filled the following three criteria: (a) minimal evaluation included a clinical exam, mammography, and IR imaging; (b) definitive surgical management constituted the preliminary therapeutic modality carried out at one of our affiliated institutions; and (c) the final staging consisted of noninvasive cancer ($n = 4$), Stage I ($n = 42$), or Stage II ($n = 54$) invasive breast cancer.

While 94% of these patients were referred to our Multidisciplinary Breast Center for the first time, 65% from family physicians and 29% from specialists, the remaining 6% had their diagnosis of breast cancer at a follow-up visit. Age at diagnosis ranged from 31 to 84 years, with a mean age of 53. The mean histologic tumor size was 2.5 cm. Lymphatic, vascular, or neural invasion was noted in 18% of patients, and concomitant noninvasive cancer was present, along with the invasive component, in 64%. One-third of the 89 patients had axillary lymph node dissection, one-third had involved nodes, and 38% of the tumors were histologic Grade III.

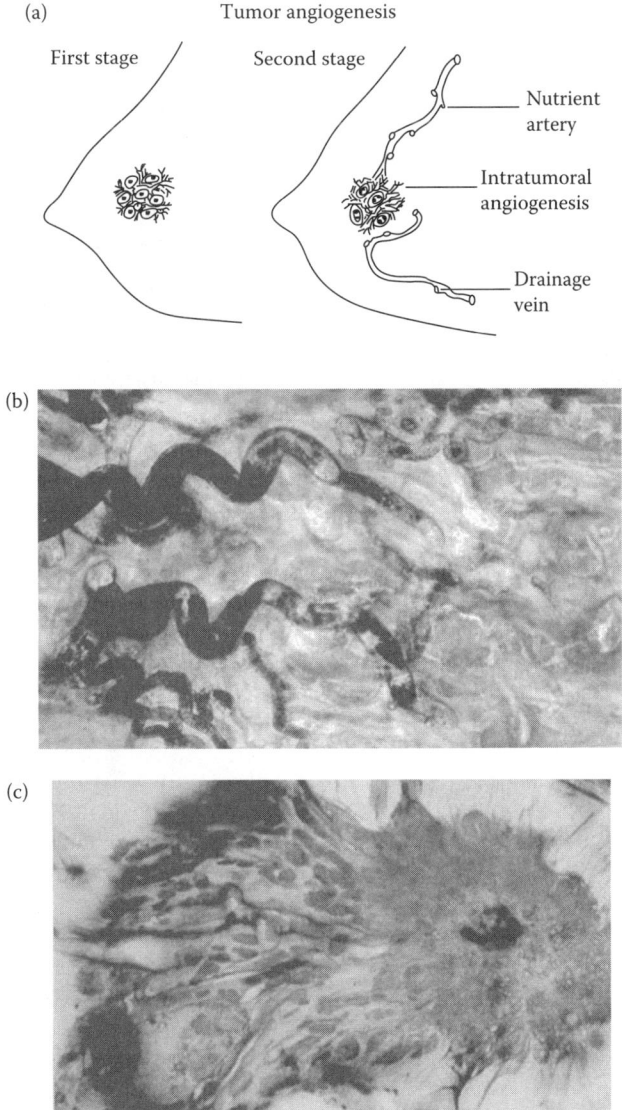

FIGURE 32.2 (a) Tumor angiogenesis. (b) High nuclear-grade ductal carcinoma *in situ* with numerous blood vessels (angiogenesis) (Tabar). (c) Invasive ductal carcinoma with central necrosis and angiogenesis (Tabar).

While most of these patients underwent standard four-view mammography, with additional views when indicated, using a GE DMR apparatus at our center, in 17 cases we relied on recent and adequate quality outside films. Mammograms were interpreted by our examining physician and radiologist, both having access to the clinical findings. Lesions were considered suspicious if either of them noted findings indicative of carcinoma. The remainder were considered either contributory but equivocal or nonspecific. A nonspecific mammography required concordance with our examining physician, radiologist, and the authors.

Our integrated IR station at that time consisted of a scanning-mirror optical system containing a mercury–cadmium–telleride detector (Bales Scientific, CA) with a spatial resolution of 600 optical lines, a central processing unit providing multitasking capabilities, and a high-resolution color monitor

TABLE 32.1   Ville Marie Infrared (IR) Grading Scale

Abnormal signs

1. Significant vascular asymmetry[a]
2. Vascular anarchy consisting of unusual tortuous or serpiginous vessels that form clusters, loops, abnormal arborization, or aberrant patterns
3. A 1°C focal increase in temperature (ΔT) when compared to the contralateral site and when associated with the area of clinical abnormality[a]
4. A 2°C focal ΔT versus the contralateral site[a]
5. A 3°C focal ΔT versus the rest of the ipsilateral breast when not present on the contralateral site[a]
6. Global breast ΔT of 1.5°C versus the contralateral breast[a]

Infrared scale

IR1 = Absence of any vascular pattern to mild vascular symmetry
IR2 = Significant but symmetrical vascular pattern to moderate vascular asymmetry, particularly if stable
IR3 = One abnormal sign
IR4 = Two abnormal signs
IR5 = Three abnormal signs

[a] Unless stable on serial imaging or due to known noncancer causes (e.g., abscess or recent benign surgery).
   Infrared imaging takes place in a draft-free, thermally controlled room maintained between 18°C and 20°C, after a 5 min equilibration period during which the patient is disrobed with her hands locked over her head. Patients are asked to refrain from alcohol, coffee, smoking, exercise, deodorant, and lotions 3 h prior to testing.

capable of displaying 1024×768 resolution points and up to 110 colors or shades of gray per image. IR imaging took place in a draft-free thermally controlled room, maintained at between 18°C and 20°C, after a 5 min equilibration period during which the patient sat disrobed with her hands locked over her head. We requested that the patients refrain from alcohol, coffee, smoking, exercise, deodorant, and lotions 3 h prior to testing.

Four images (an anterior, an undersurface, and two lateral views) were generated simultaneously on the video screen. The examining physician would digitally adjust them to minimize noise and enhance the detection of more subtle abnormalities prior to exact on-screen computerized temperature reading and IR grading. Images were then electronically stored on retrievable laser discs. Our original Ville Marie grading scale relies on pertinent clinical information, comparing IR images of both breasts with previous images. An abnormal IR image required the presence of at least one abnormal sign (Table 32.1). To assess the false-positive rate, we reviewed, using similar criteria, our last 100 consecutive patients who underwent an open breast biopsy that produced a benign histology. We used the Carefile Data Analysis Program to evaluate the detection rate of variable combinations of clinical exam, mammography, and IR imaging.

Of this series, 61% presented with a suspicious palpable abnormality, while the remainder had either an equivocal (34%) or a nonspecific clinical exam (5%). Similarly, mammography was considered suspicious for cancer in 66%, while 19% were contributory but equivocal, and 15% were considered nonspecific. Infrared imaging revealed minor variations (IR-1 or IR-2) in 17% of our patients while the remaining 83% had at least one (34%), two (37%), or three (12%) abnormal IR signs. Of the 39 patients with either a nonspecific or equivocal clinical exam, 31 had at least one abnormal IR sign, with this modality providing pertinent indication of a potential abnormality in 14 of these patients who, in addition, had an equivocal or nonspecific mammography.

Among the 15 patients with a nonspecific mammography, there were 10 patients (mean age of 48; 5 years younger than the full sample) who had an abnormal IR image. This abnormal finding constituted a particularly important indicator in six of these patients who also had only equivocal clinical findings. While 61% of our series presented with a suspicious clinical exam, the additional information provided by the 66 suspicious mammographies resulted in an 83% detection rate. The combination of only suspicious mammograms and abnormal IR imaging increased the sensitivity to 93%, with a further increase to 98% when suspicious clinical exams were also considered (Figure 32.3).

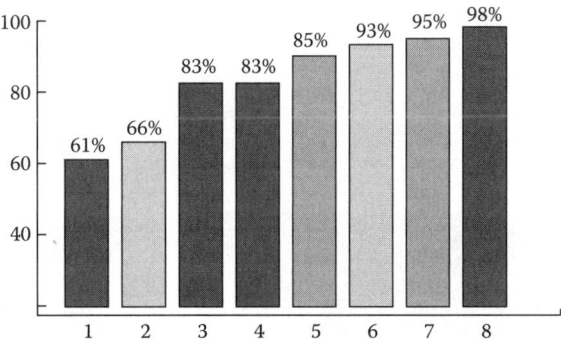

FIGURE 32.3 Relative contribution of clinical exam, mammography, and IR imaging to detect breast cancer in the Ville Marie Breast Center series. In this series, adding infrared imaging to both suspicious and equivocal mammographies increased the detection rate. (1) Suspicious clinical exam; (2) suspicious mammography; (3) suspicious clinical exam or suspicious mammography; (4) abnormal infrared imaging; (5) suspicious or equivocal mammography; (6) abnormal infrared imaging or suspicious mammography; (7) abnormal infrared imaging or equivocal or suspicious mammography; and (8) abnormal infrared imaging or suspicious mammography or suspicious clinical exam.

The mean histologically measured tumor size for those cases undetected by mammography was 1.66 cm while those undetected by IR imaging averaged 1.28 cm. In a concurrent series of 100 consecutive eligible patients who had an open biopsy that produced benign histology, 19% had an abnormal IR image while 30% had an abnormal preoperative mammography that was the only indication for surgery in 16 cases.

The 83% sensitivity of IR imaging in this series is higher than the 70% rate for similar Stage I and II patients tested from the Royal Marsden Hospital two decades earlier [6]. Although our results might reflect an increased index of suspicion associated with a referred population, this factor should apply equally to both clinical exam and mammography, maintaining the validity of our evaluation. Additional factors could include our standard protocol, our physicians' prior experience with IR imaging, their involvement in both image production and interpretation, as well as their access to much improved image acquisition and precision (Figure 32.4).

While most previous IR cameras had 8-bit (one part in 256) resolution, current cameras are capable of one part in 4096 resolution, providing enough dynamic range to capture all images with 0.05°C discrimination without the need for range switching. With the advancement of video display and enhanced gray and colors, multiple high-resolution views can be compared simultaneously on the same monitor. Faster computers now allow processing functions such as image subtraction and digital filtering techniques for image enhancement. New algorithms provide soft tissue imaging by characterizing dynamic heat-flow patterns. These and other innovations have made vast improvements in the medical IR technology available today.

The detection rate in a series where half the tumors were under 2 cm, would suggest that tumor-induced thermal patterns detected by currently available IR technology are more dependent on early vascular and metabolic changes. These changes possibly are induced by regional nitric oxide diffusion and ferritin interaction, rather than strictly on tumor size [29]. This hypothesis agrees with the concept that angiogenesis may precede any morphological changes [28]. Although both initial clinical exam and mammography are crucial in signaling the need for further investigation, equivocal and nonspecific findings can still result in a combined delayed detection rate of 10% [17].

When eliminating the dubious contribution of our 34 equivocal clinical exams and 19 equivocal mammograms, which is disconcerting to both physician and patient, the alternative information provided by IR imaging increased the index of concern of the remaining suspicious mammograms by 27% and the combination of suspicious clinical exams or suspicious mammograms by 15% (Figure 32.3).

An imaging-only strategy, consisting of both suspicious and equivocal mammography and abnormal IR imaging, also detected 95% of these tumors, even without the input of the clinical exam. Infrared imaging's most tangible contribution in this series was to signal an abnormality in a younger cohort of breast cancer patients who had noncontributory mammograms and also nonspecific clinical exams who conceivably would not have been passed on for second-line evaluation.

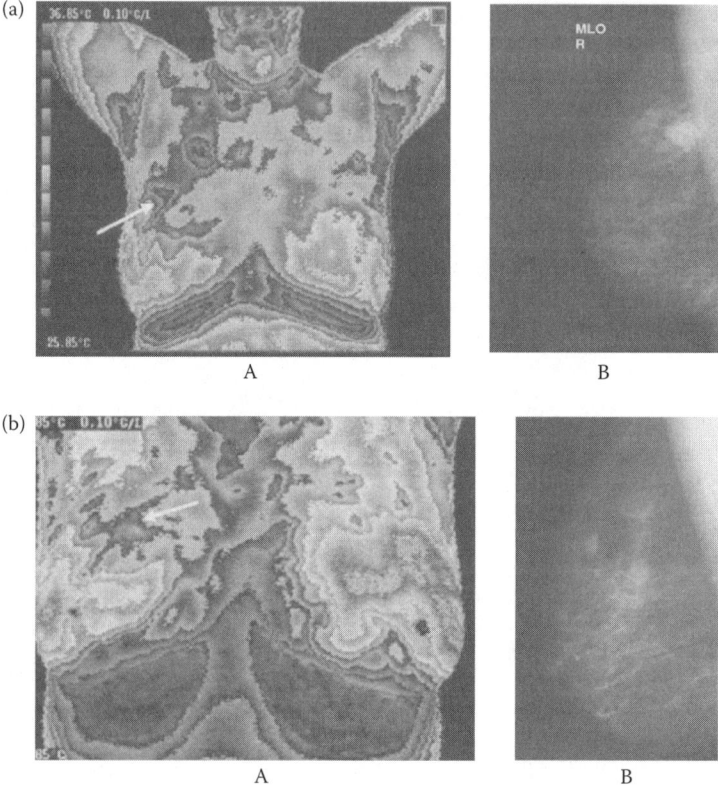

FIGURE 32.4 (a) A 46-year-old patient: Lump in the upper central area of the right breast. *Infrared imaging* (A): significant vascular asymmetry (SVA) in the upper central area of the right breast (IR-3). *Mammography* (B): corresponding speculated opacity. *Surgical histology*: 2 cm infiltrating ductal carcinoma with negative sentinel nodes. (b) A 44-year-old patient. *Infrared imaging* (A): revealed a significant vascular asymmetry in the upper central and inner quadrants of the right breast with a ΔT of 1.8°C (IR-4.8). *Corresponding mammography* (B): reveals a spiculated lesion in the upper central portion of the right breast. *Surgical histology*: 0.7 cm infiltrating ductal carcinoma. Patient underwent adjuvant brachytherapy. (c) A 52-year-old patient presented with a mild fullness in the lower outer quadrant of the right breast. *Infrared imaging* (A): left breast (B): right breast reveals extensive significant vascular asymmetry with a ΔT of 1.35°C (IR-5.3). A 2 cm cancer was found in the lower outer area of the right breast. (d) A 37-year-old patient. *Infrared image* (A): significant vascular asymmetry in the upper inner quadrant of the left breast with a ΔT of 1.75°C (IR-4) (mod IR-4.75). *Mammography* (B): corresponding spiculated lesion. *Ultrasound* (C): 6 mm lesion. *Surgical histology*: 0.7 cm infiltrating ductal carcinoma. (e) An 82-year-old patient. *Infrared imaging anterior view*: significant vascular asymmetry and a ΔT of 1.90°C (IR-4) in the left subareolar area. *Corresponding mammography*: (not included) asymmetrical density in the left areolar area. *Surgical histology*: left subareolar 1 cm infiltrating ductal carcinoma. (f) A 34-year-old patient with a palpable fullness in the supra-areolar area of the right breast. *Infrared imaging* (A): extensive significant vascular asymmetry and a ΔT of 1.3°C in the right supra-areolar area (IR-4) (mod IR-5.3). *Mammography* (B): scattered and clustered central microcalcifications. *Surgical histology*: after total right mastectomy and TRAM flap: multifocal DCIS and infiltrating ductal CA centered over a 3 cm area of the supra-areolar area.

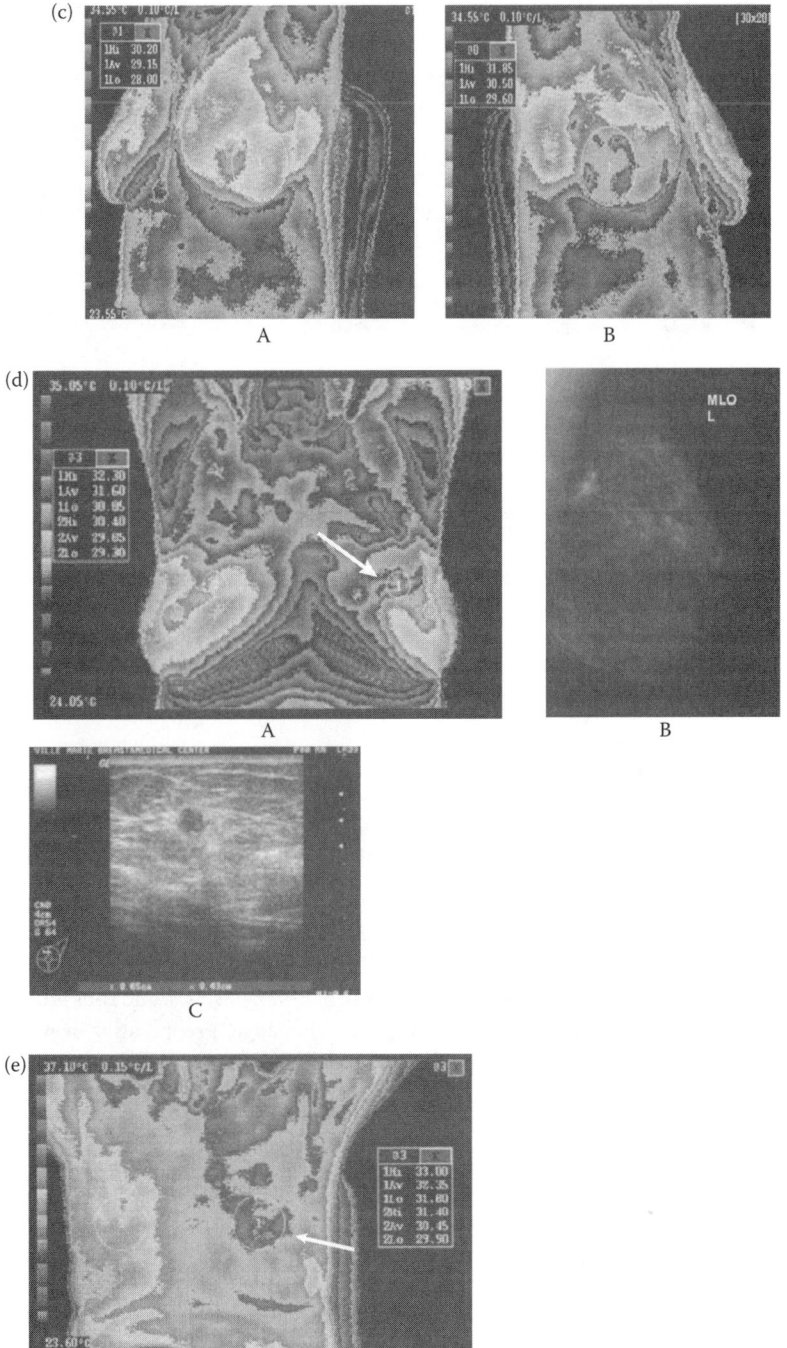

FIGURE 32.4 (Continued.)

While 17% of these tumors were undetected by IR imaging, due to either insufficient production or detection of metabolic or vascular changes, the 19% false-positive rate in histologically proven benign conditions, in part a reflection of our current grading system, suggests sufficient specificity for this modality to be used in an adjuvant setting.

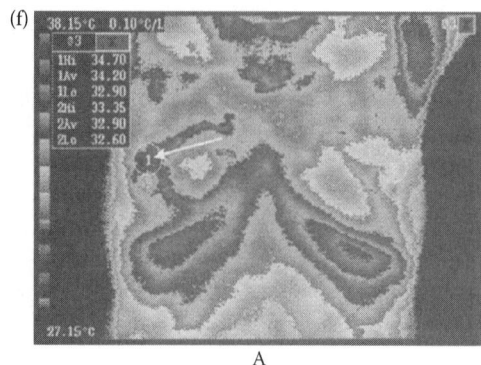
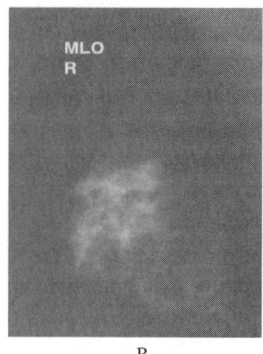

A   B

FIGURE 32.4   (Continued.)

Our validation of prior data would also suggest that IR imaging, based more on process than structural changes and not requiring contact, compression, radiation, or venous access, can provide pertinent and practical complementary information to both clinical exam and mammography, our current first-line detection modalities. Quality-controlled abnormal IR imaging heightened our index of suspicion in cases where clinical or mammographic findings were equivocal or nonspecific, thus signaling further investigation rather than observation or close monitoring (Figure 32.5) and to minimize the possibility of further delay (Figure 32.6).

32.2.2 Preliminary Evaluation of Digital High-Resolution Functional Infrared Imaging to Monitor Preoperative Chemohormonotherapy-Induced Changes in Neoangiogenesis in Patients with Advanced Breast Cancer

Approximately 10% of our current breast cancer patients present with sufficient tumor load to be classified as having locally advanced breast cancer (LABC). This heterogeneous subset of patients, usually diagnosed with either stage T3 or T4 lesions without evidence of metastasis, and thus judged as potential surgical candidates, constitutes a formidable therapeutic challenge. Preoperative or neoadjuvant chemotherapy (PCT), hormonotherapy, or both, preferably delivered within a clinical trial, is the current favored treatment strategy.

Preoperative chemotherapy offers a number of advantages, including ensuring improved drug access to the primary tumor site by avoiding surgical scarring, the possibility of complete or partial tumor reduction that could downsize the extent of surgery and also the ability to better plan breast reconstruction when the initial tumor load suggests the need for a possible total mastectomy. In addition, there is sufficient data to suggest that the absence of any residual tumor cells in the surgical pathology specimen following PTC confers the best prognosis, while those patients achieving at least a partial clinical response as measured by at least a 50% reduction in the tumor's largest diameter often can aspire to a better survival than nonresponders [37]. While current clinical parameters do not always reflect actual PCT-induced tumor changes, there is sufficient correlation to make measuring the early clinical response to PTC an important element in assessing the efficacy of any chosen regimen. Unfortunately, the currently available conventional monitoring tools, such as palpation combined with structural/anatomic imaging such as mammography and ultrasound, have a limited ability to precisely measure the initial tumor load, and even less to reflect the effect of PCT [34].

These relatively rudimentary tools are dependent on often-imprecise anatomical and structural parameters. A more effective selection of often quite aggressive therapeutic agents and ideal duration of

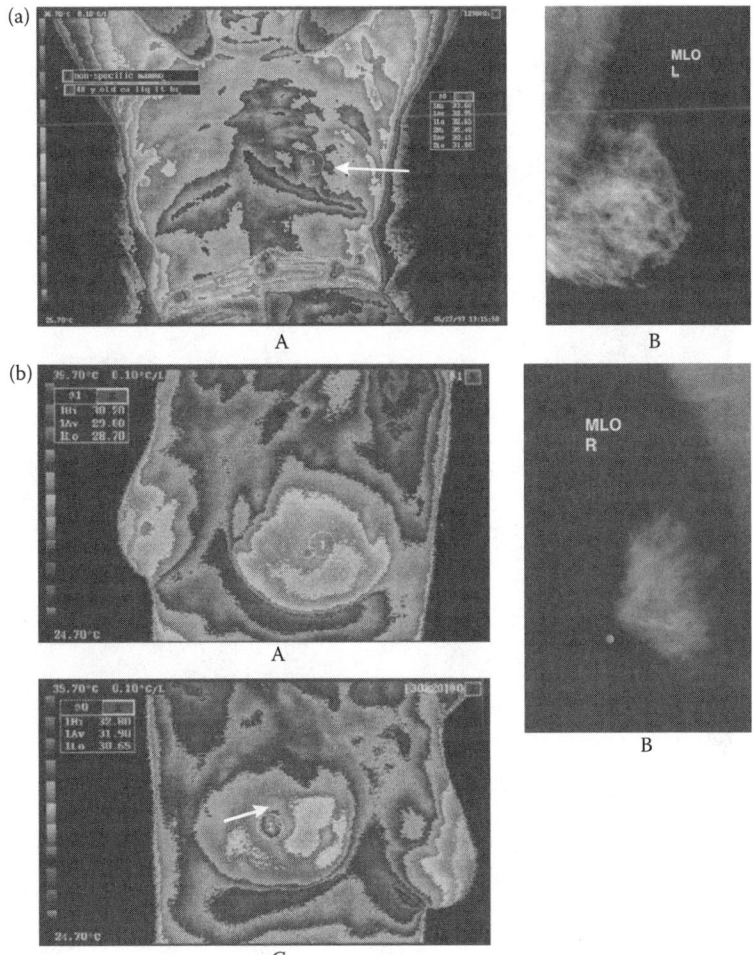

FIGURE 32.5 (a) A 48-year-old patient. *Infrared imaging* (A): significant vascular asymmetry and a ΔT of 0.8°C (IR-3) in the lower inner quadrant of the left breast. *Corresponding mammography* (B): a nonspecific density. *Surgical histology*: 1.6 cm left lower inner quadrant infiltrating ductal carcinoma. (b) A 40-year-old patient. *Infrared imaging* (A): left breast, (B) right breast: focal hot spot in the right subareolar area on a background of increased vascular activity with a ΔT of 1.1°C (IR-4). *Corresponding mammography* (C): reveals dense tissue bilaterally. *Surgical histology*: reveals a 1 cm right infiltrating ductal carcinoma and positive lymph nodes. (c) A 51-year-old patient. *Infrared imaging* (A): significant vascular asymmetry and a ΔT of 2.2°C (IR-5) in the upper central area of the left breast. *Corresponding mammography* (B): mild scattered densities. *Surgical histology*: 2.5 cm infiltrating ductal carcinoma in the upper central area of the left breast. (d) A 44-year-old patient. *Infrared imaging* (A): significant vascular asymmetry and a ΔT of 1.58°C (IR-4) in the upper inner quadrant of the left breast. *Corresponding mammography* (B): a nonspecific corresponding density. *Surgical histology*: a 0.9 cm left upper inner quadrant infiltrating ductal carcinoma. (e) A 45-year-old patient with a nodule in central area of left breast. *Infrared imaging* (A): extensive significant vascular asymmetry (SVA) in the central inner area of the left breast with a ΔT of 0.75°C (IR-3) (mod IR-4.75). *Mammography* (B): noncontributory. *Surgical histology*: 1.5 cm infiltrating ductal carcinoma with necrosis in the central inner area and 3+ axillary nodes. (f) A 51-year-old patient. *Infrared imaging* (A): extensive significant vascular asymmetry and a ΔT of 2.2° (IR-5) (mod IR-6.2) in the upper central area of the left breast. *Corresponding mammography* (B): scattered densities. *Surgical histology*: 2.5 cm infiltrating ductal carcinoma in the upper central area of the left breast. (g) A 74-year-old patient. *Infrared imaging* (A): significant vascular asymmetry in the upper central portion of the right breast with a ΔT of 2.8°C (IR-5) (Mod VM IR: 6.8). *Corresponding mammography* (B): bilateral extensive density. *Surgical histology*: 1 cm right central quadrant infiltrating ductal carcinoma.

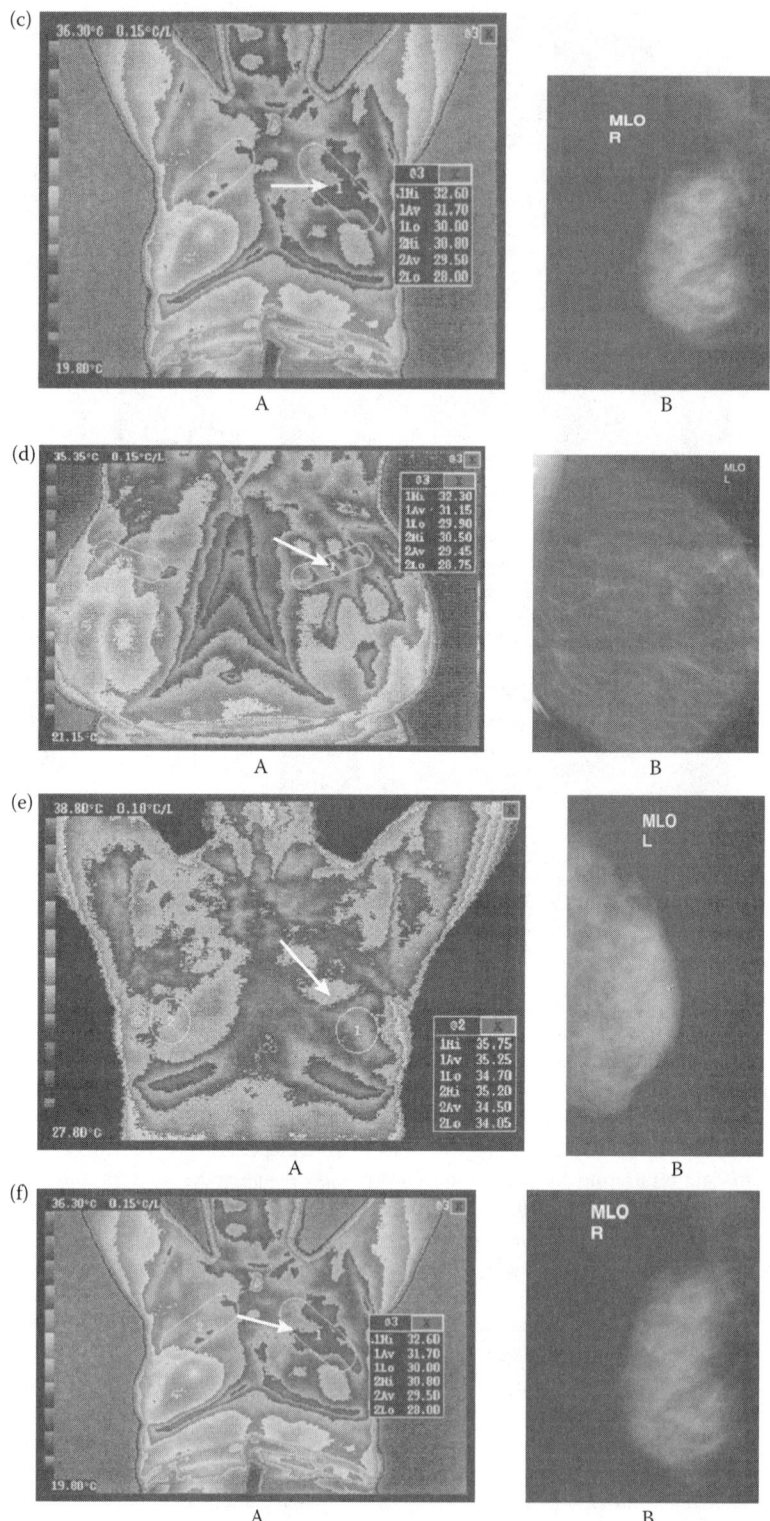

FIGURE 32.5   (Continued.)

(g)

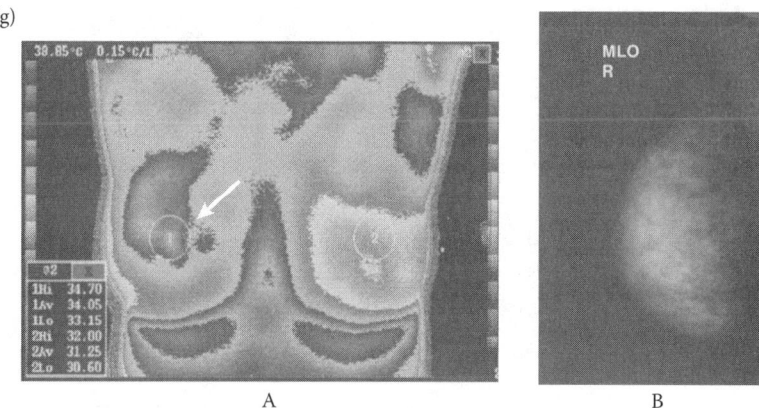

A   B

FIGURE 32.5 (Continued.)

their use could be enhanced by the introduction of a convenient, safe, and accessible modality that could provide an alternative and serial measurement of their therapeutic efficacy.

There is thus currently a flurry of interest to assess the potential of different functional imaging modalities that could possibly monitor tumor changes looking at metabolic and vascular features to fill the void. Detecting early metabolic changes associated early tumor initiation and growth using positron emission tomography [38,39], MRI, and Sestamibi scanning are all potential candidates to help monitor PCT-related effects. Unfortunately, they are all hampered by limited access for serial use, duration of the exam, costs, and the need of intravenous access. High-resolution digital infrared imaging, on the other hand, a convenient functional imaging modality free of these inconveniences and not requiring radiation, nuclear material, contact, or compression, can be used repeatedly without safety issues. There are ample data indicating its ability to effectively and reliably detect, in a multi-imaging strategy, neoangiogenesis related to early tumor growth [40]. The premise of our review is that this same phenomenon should even be more obvious when using IR as a monitoring tool in patients with tumors associated with extensive vascular activity as seen in LABC.

To evaluate the ability of our high-resolution digital IR imaging station and a modified Ville Marie scoring system to monitor the functional impact of PCT, 20 successive patients with LABC underwent prospective IR imaging, both prior to and after completion of PCT, usually lasting between 3 and 6 months, which was then followed by curative-intent surgery [41]. Ages ranged between 32 and 82 with a mean of 55. Half of the patients were under 50. Patients presented with T2, T3, or inflammatory carcinoma were all free of any distant disease, thus remaining post-PCT surgical candidates. IR was done at the initial clinical evaluation and prior to core biopsy, often ultrasound guided to ensure optimal specimen harvesting, which was used to document invasive carcinoma. Both sets of IR images were acquired according to our published protocol [38] using the same integrated infrared station described in our previous section.

We used a modification of the original Ville Marie IR scale (Table 32.2) where IR-1 reflects the absence of any significant vascular pattern to minimal vascular symmetry; IR-2 encompasses symmetrical to moderately asymmetrical vascular patterns, including focal clinically related significant vascular asymmetry (SVA); IR-3 implies a regional SVA while an extensive SVA, occupying more than a third of the involved breast, constitutes an IR-4. Mean temperature difference (ΔT) in degrees centigrade between the area of focal, regional, or extensive SVA and the corresponding area of the noninvolved breast is then added, resulting in the final IR score.

Conventional clinical response to PCT was done by measuring the maximum tumor diameter in centimeters, both before beginning and after completion of PCT.

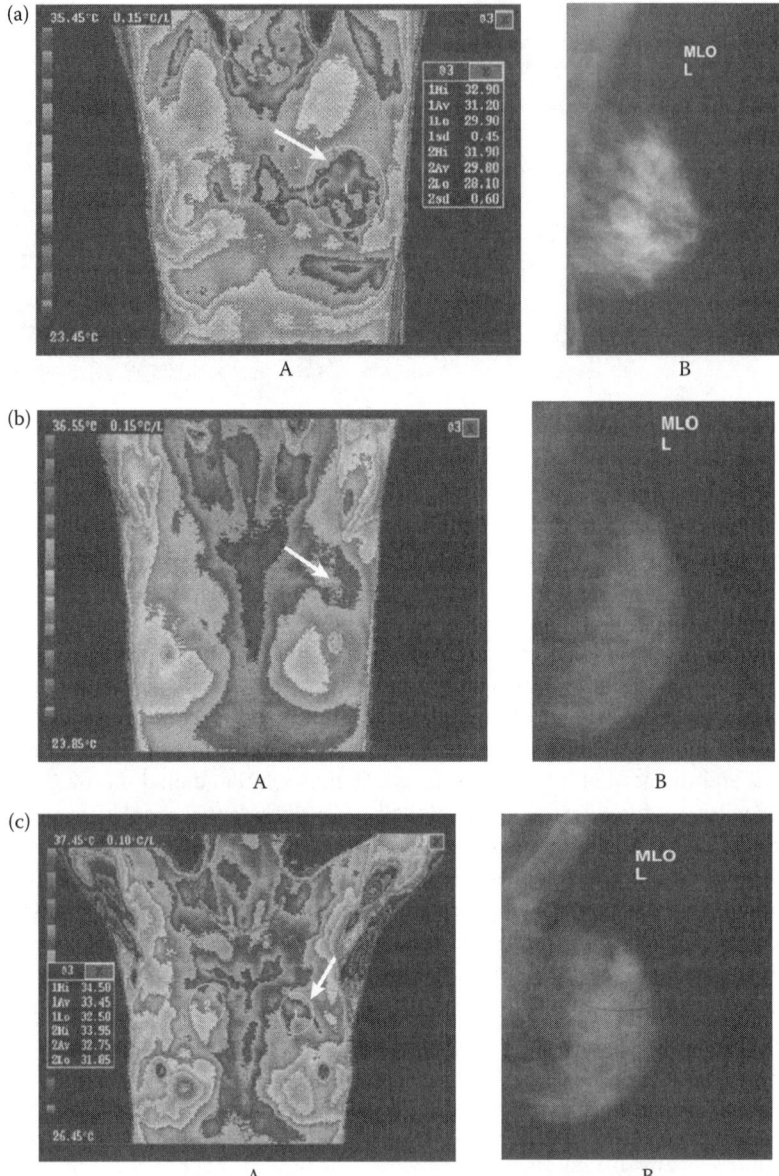

FIGURE 32.6 (a) A 66-year-old patient. Initially seen 2 years prior to diagnosis of left breast cancer for probable fibrocystic disorder (FCD) and scattered cysts, mostly on the left side. *Initial infrared imaging* (A): extensive significant vascular asymmetry left breast and a near global ΔT of 1.4°C (IR-4) (Mod IR: 5.4). *Initial mammography* (B): scattered opacities and ultrasound and cytologies were consistent with FCD. Two years later a 1.7 cm cancer was found in the central portion of the left breast. (b) A 49-year-old patient. *Infrared imaging* 1997 (A): significant vascular asymmetry in the upper central aspect of the left breast (IR-3) *Corresponding mammography* 1997 (B): dense tissue (contd. 6B2). (c) Patient presents 2 years later with a lump in the upper central portion of the left breast. *Corresponding infrared imaging* (A): still reveals significant vascular asymmetry and a ΔT of 0.7°C (IR-3) (Mod VM IR: 3.7). *Corresponding mammography* (B): now reveals an opacity in the upper aspect of the left breast. *Surgical histology*: 1 cm infiltrating ductal carcinoma.

TABLE 32.2 Modified Ville Marie Infrared Scoring Scale

IR-1	Absence of any vascular pattern to mild vascular symmetry
IR-2	Symmetrical vascular pattern to moderate vascular asymmetry, particularly if stable or due to known noncancer causes (e.g., infection, abscess, recent or prior surgery, or anatomical asymmetry). Local clinically related vascular assymetry
IR-3	Regional significant vascular asymmetry (SVA)
IR-4	Extensive SVA, involving at least one-third of the breast area

Add the temperature difference (ΔT) in degrees centigrade between the involved area and the corresponding area of the noninvolved contralateral breast to calculate the final IR score.

Induction PCT in 10 patients, 8 on a clinical trial (NSABP B-27 or B-57) consisted of four cycles of adriamycin (A) 60 mg/m² and cyclophosphamide (C) 600 mg/m², with or without additional taxotere (T) 100 mg/m², or six cycles of AT every 21 days. Eight other patients received AC with additional 5 FU (1000 mg/m²) and methotrexate (300 mg/m²). Tamoxifen, given to select patients along with the chemotherapy, was used as sole induction therapy in two elderly patients.

Values in both clinical size and IR scoring both before and after chemotherapy were compared using a paired *t*-test.

32.2.3 Results

All 20 patients in this series with LABC presented with an abnormal IR image (IR ≥ 3). The preinduction PCT mean IR score was 5.5 (range: 4.4–6.9). Infrared imaging revealed a decrease in the IR score in all 20 patients following PCT, ranging from 1 to 5 with a mean of 3.1 ($p < .05$). This decrease following PCT reflected the change in the clinical maximum tumor dimension, which decreased from a mean of 5.2 cm prior to PCT to 2.2 cm ($p < .05$) following PCT in the two-thirds of our series who presented with a measurable tumor. Four of the complete pathological responders in this series saw their IR score revert to normal (<3) following PCT (Figure 32.7) while a fifth had a post-PCT IR score of 3.6. An additional seven patients had a final post-PCT IR score that reflected the final tumor size as measured at surgery (Figure 32.8).

LABC is considered an aggressive process that is typically associated with extensive neoangiogenesis required to sustain rapid and continued tumor growth [27]. Functional IR imaging provided a vivid real-time visual reflection of this invasive process in all our patients. The dramatic IR findings associated with LABC, often occupying more than a third of the breast, are further emphasized by the comparative absence of any significant vascular findings in the uninvolved breast. These images thus provided a new parameter and baseline to complement the traditional structurally based imaging, particularly for the seven patients with clinically nonmeasurable LABC.

The significant reduction in the mean IR score following PCT is primarily an indication of its effect on neoangiogenesis. While this reduction can sometimes correspond to tumor size, as it did in half of this series, IR's main contribution concerns functional parameters that can both precede and linger after structural tumor-induced changes occur. Because IR-detected regional angiogenesis responded slightly slower to PCT than did the anatomical parameters in nine patients, it underscores the fundamental difference between functional imaging such as IR and structural-dependent parameters such as clinical tumor dimensions currently used to assess PCT response. IR has the advantage of not being dependent on a minimal tumor size but rather on the tumor's very early necessity to develop an extensive network to survive and proliferate. This would be the basis of IR's ability to sometimes detect tumor growth earlier than can structurally based modalities. The slight discrepancy between the resolving IR score and the anatomical findings in nine of our patients could suggest that this extensive vascular network, most evident in LABC, requires more time to dismantle in some patients. It could reflect the variable volume of angiogenesis, the inability of PCT to affect

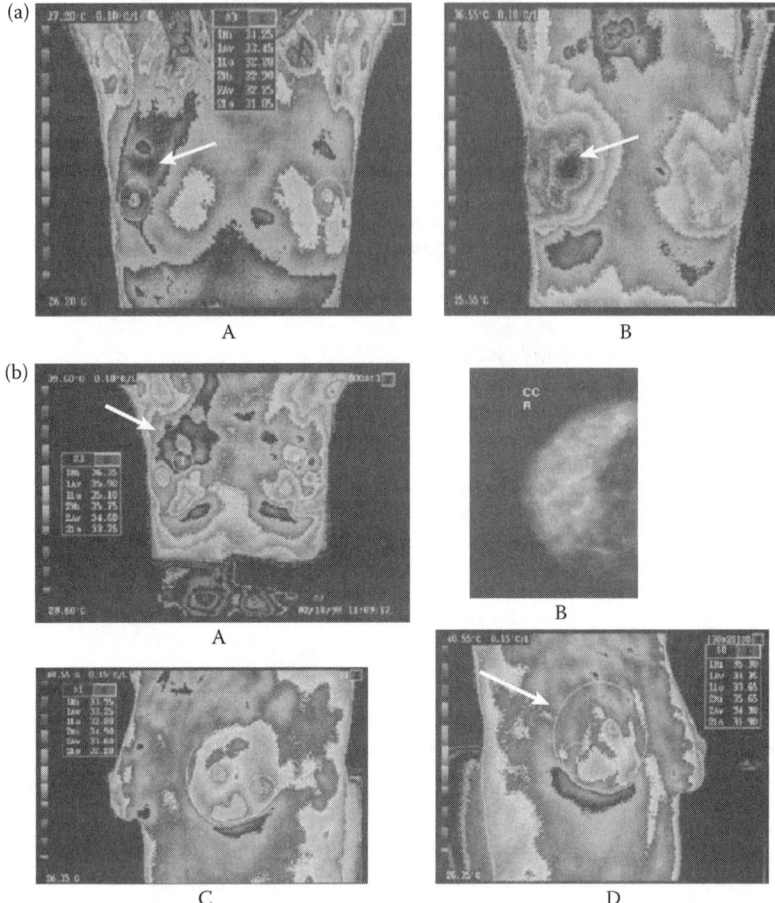

FIGURE 32.7 (a) A 52-year-old patient. *Infrared imaging* (A): extensive vascular asymmetry (SVA) in the right breast with a ΔT of 1.2°C (IR-5.2). The patient was started on preoperative chemotherapy (PCT). *Post-PCT infrared imaging* (B): resolution of previously noted SVA (IR-2). *Surgical histology*: no residual carcinoma in the resected right breast specimen. (b) A 32-year-old patient. *Infrared imaging* (A): extensive significant vascular asymmetry and tortuous vascular pattern and a ΔT of 1.3°C (IR-5.3) in the right breast. *Corresponding mammography* (B): scattered densities. Patient was started on preoperative chemotherapy (PCT). *Post-PCT infrared image* (C—left breast; D—right breast): Notable resolution of SVA, with a whole breast ΔT of 0.7°C (IR-2). *Surgical histology*: no residual right carcinoma and chemotherapy induced changes. (c) A 47-year-old patient. *Infrared imaging* (A): extensive significant vascular asymmetry in the inner half of the left breast with a ΔT of 2°C (IR-6.0). The patient was started on preoperative chemotherapy (PCT). *Post-PCT infrared imaging* (B): no residual asymmetry (IR-1). *Surgical histology*: no viable residual carcinoma, with chemotherapy-induced dense fibrosis surrounding nonviable tumor cells. (d) A 56-year-old patient. *Prechemotherapy infrared imaging* (A): significant vascular asymmetry overlying the central portion of the left breast with a ΔT of 1.35°C (IR-4.35). The patient was given preoperative chemotherapy (PCT). *Post-PCT infrared* (B): mild bilateral vascular symmetry (IR-). *Surgical histology*: no residual tumor. (e) A 54-year-old patient. *Infrared image* (A): extensive significant vascular asymmetry right breast with an rT of 2.8°C (IR-6.8). Received preoperative chemotherapy (PCT). *Post-PCT infrared* (B): mild local residual vascular asymmetry with an rT of 1.65°C (IR-3.65). *Surgical pathology*: no residual viable carcinoma.

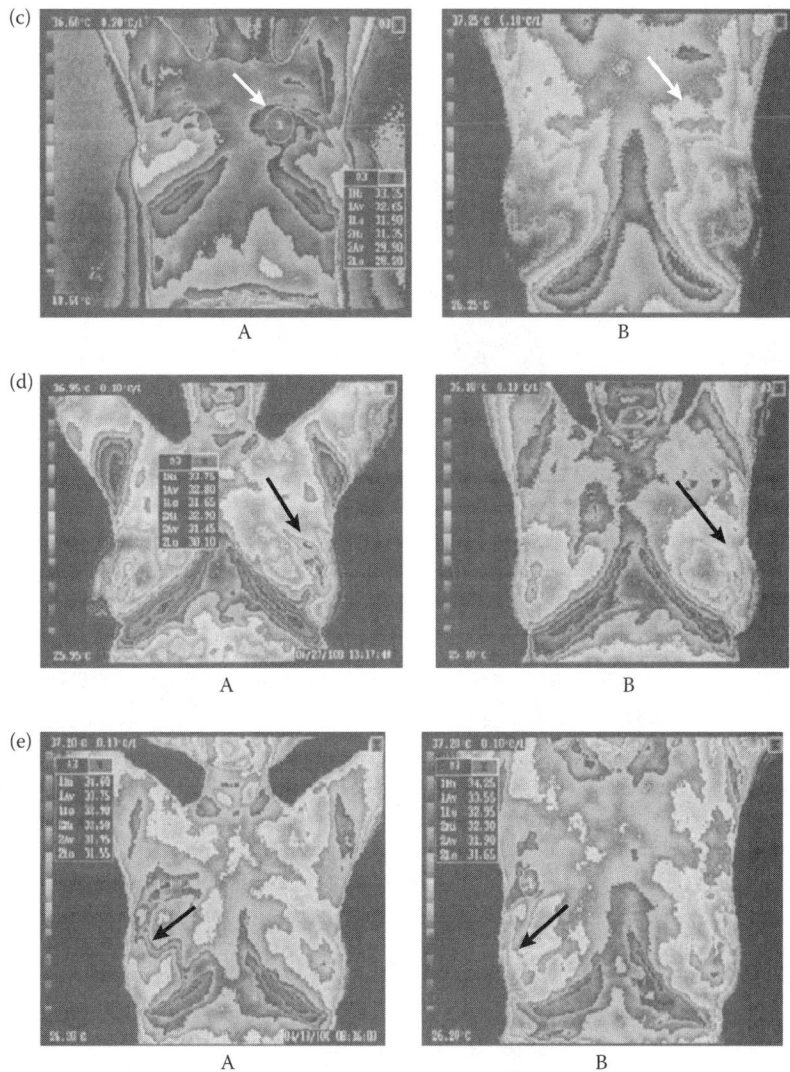

FIGURE 32.7 (Continued.)

it, and thus possibly constitute a prognostic factor. This feature could also result from a deficiency in our proposed scoring scale.

Further study and follow-up are needed to better evaluate whether the sequential utilization of this practical imaging modality can provide additional pertinent information regarding the efficacy of our current and new therapeutic strategies, particularly in view of the increasing number with antiangiogenesis properties, and whether lingering IR-reflected neoangiogenesis following PCT ultimately reflects on prognosis.

32.3 Future Considerations Concerning Infrared Imaging

Mammography, our current standard first-line imaging modality only reflects an abnormality that could then prompt the alert clinician to intervene rather than to observe. This decision is crucial since

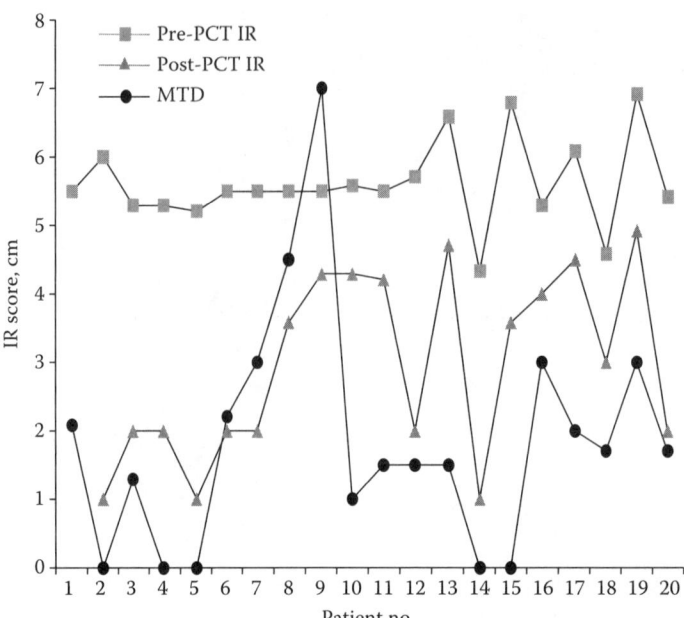

FIGURE 32.8   Pre- and post-PCT IR score and histological maximum tumor dimension (MTD).

it is at this first level that sensitivity and specificity are most vulnerable. There is a clear consensus that we have not yet developed the ideal breast cancer imaging technique and this is reflected in the flurry of new modalities that have recently appeared. While progress in imaging and better training have resulted in the gradual decrease in the average size of breast tumors over the previous decade, the continued search for improved imaging must continue to further reduce the false-negative rate and promote earlier detection.

Digital mammography is already recognized as a major imaging facilitator with the capability to do tomosynthesis and subtraction, along with state-of-the-art 3D and 4D ultrasound. However, there is now new emphasis on developing functional imaging that can exploit early vascular and metabolic changes associated with tumor initiation that often predate morphological changes that most of our current structural imaging modalities still depend on; thus, the enthusiasm in the development of Sestamibi scanning, Doppler ultrasound, and MRI of the breast [42,43]. Unfortunately, as promising as these modalities are, they are often too cumbersome, costly, inaccessible, or require intravenous access to be used as first-line detection modalities alongside clinical exam and mammography.

On the other hand, integrating IR imaging, a safe and practical modality into the first-line strategy, can increase the sensitivity at this crucial stage by also providing an early warning signal of an abnormality that in some cases is not evident in the other components. Combining IR imaging and mammography in an "IR-Assisted Mammography Strategy" is particularly appealing in the current era of increased emphasis on detection by imaging with less reliance on palpation as tumor size further decreases.

Intercenter standardization of a protocol concerning patient preparation, temperature-controlled environment, digital image production, enhanced grading, and archiving, as well as data collection and sharing are all important factors that are beginning to be addressed. New technology could permit real-time image acquisition that could be submitted to computerized assisted image reading which will further enhance the physician's ability to detect subtle abnormalities.

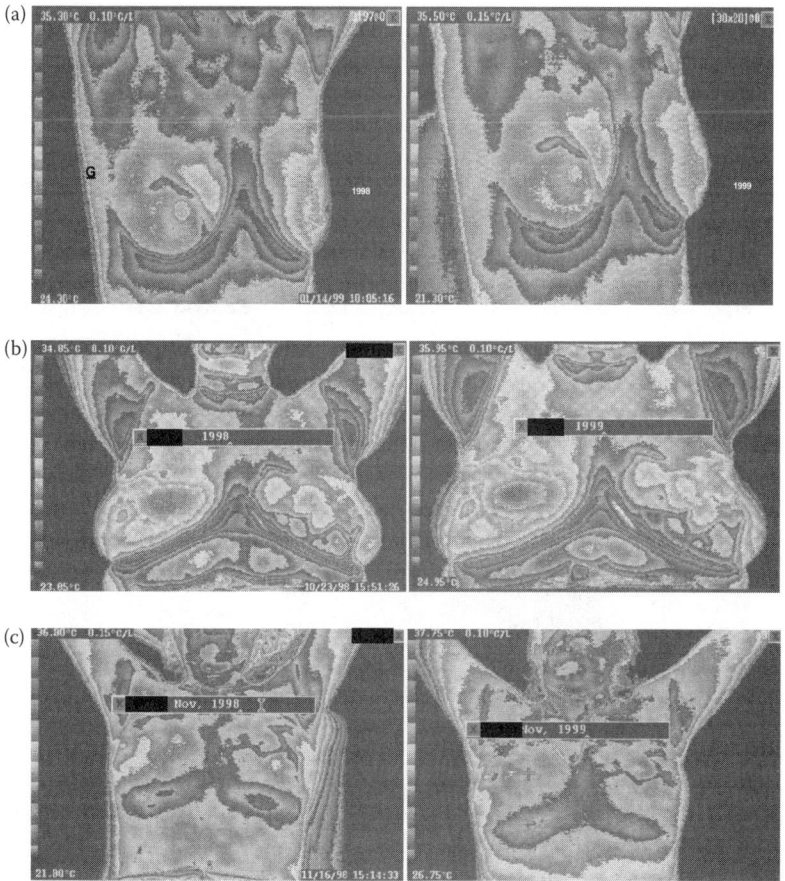

FIGURE 32.9 (a) A stable vascular distribution in the lower inner quadrant of the left breast over a 12-month period. *Infrared imaging* of the breast usually remains remarkably stable in the absence of any ongoing developing significant pathology. It is important in grading these images to determine if the findings are to be considered evolving and important or stable and possibly relating to the patient's vascular anatomy. (b) An identical vascular distribution of the left breast over a 12-month period. (c) A stable vascular distribution in both breasts over a 12-month period.

Physician training is an essential quality control component for this imaging modality to contribute its full potential. A thorough knowledge of all aspects of benign and malignant breast pathology and concomitant access to prior IR imaging that should normally remain stable (Figure 32.9) are all contributory features. This modality needs to benefit from the same quality control previously applied to mammography and should not, at this time, be used as stand-alone. It should benefit from the same interaction between clinical knowledge and other imaging tools as is the case in current breast cancer detection in the clinical environment. This is especially important since there are no current IR regulations, as it poses no health threat and does not use radiation, and could thus fall victim to untrained personnel who could misuse it on unsuspecting patients as was previously the case.

Its future promise, however, resides primarily in its ability to qualify and quantify vascular and metabolic changes related to early tumor genesis. The proposals that a higher temperature difference (ΔT) and increased vascular asymmetry are prognostic factors of tumor aggressivity need to be validated

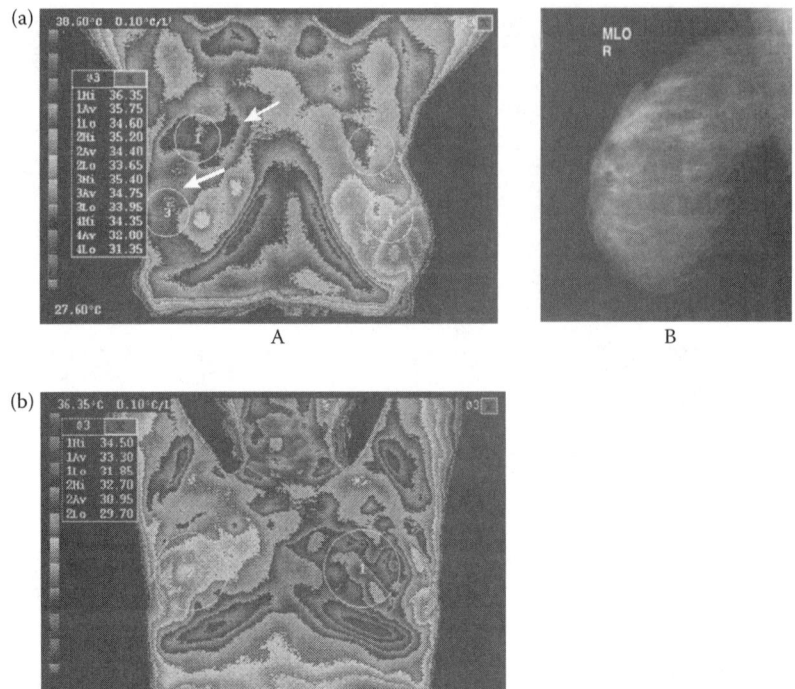

FIGURE 32.10   (a) A 50-year-old patient. *Infrared imaging* (A): significant vascular asymmetry and a ΔT of 3.4°C (IR-5) in the right breast. *Corresponding mammography* (B): increased density and microcalcifications in the right breast. Surgical histology: extensive right multifocal infiltrating ductal carcinoma requiring a total mastectomy. (b) A 50-year-old patient. *Infrared imaging*: significant vascular asymmetry with a near global ΔT of 2.35°C in the left breast (IR-5). *Mammography* (not available) diffuse density. *Surgical histology*: left multifocal infiltrating ductal carcinoma requiring a total mastectomy.

by further research (Figure 32.10). The same applies to the probability that the reduction of IR changes seen with preoperative chemohormonotherapy reflect reduction in neoangiogenesis and thus treatment efficacy. These remain, at the very least, extremely interesting and promising areas for future research, particularly in view of the current interest in new angiogenesis-related therapeutic strategies. Its contribution to monitoring postoperative patients (Figure 32.11) which is problematic with both mammography and ultrasound [44] and its ability to recognize recurrent cancer (Figure 32.12) are other areas for further clinical trials. Adequate physician training and strict attention to image acquisition are essential to avoid false-negative interpretation (Figure 32.13).

As is the case for all current imaging modalities, the fact that this modality does not detect all tumors should not detract from its contribution as a functional adjuvant addition to our current first-line imaging strategy that is still based essentially on mammography alone, a structural modality that has reached its full potential. There are already sufficient data regarding IR's sensitivity and specificity that has been more recently validated and ongoing data collection will be important to justify its continued use in the ever-evolving breast imaging field. Infrared imaging may become an alternative to a more costly and invasive imaging modality, and possibly integrated as an informative first-line tool. In the meantime, to ignore its contribution to the very complex process of promoting earlier breast cancer detection could be questioned. A good first-line imaging modality must be safe, convenient, and able to help detect primarily the more aggressive tumors where early intervention can have a greater impact on survival.

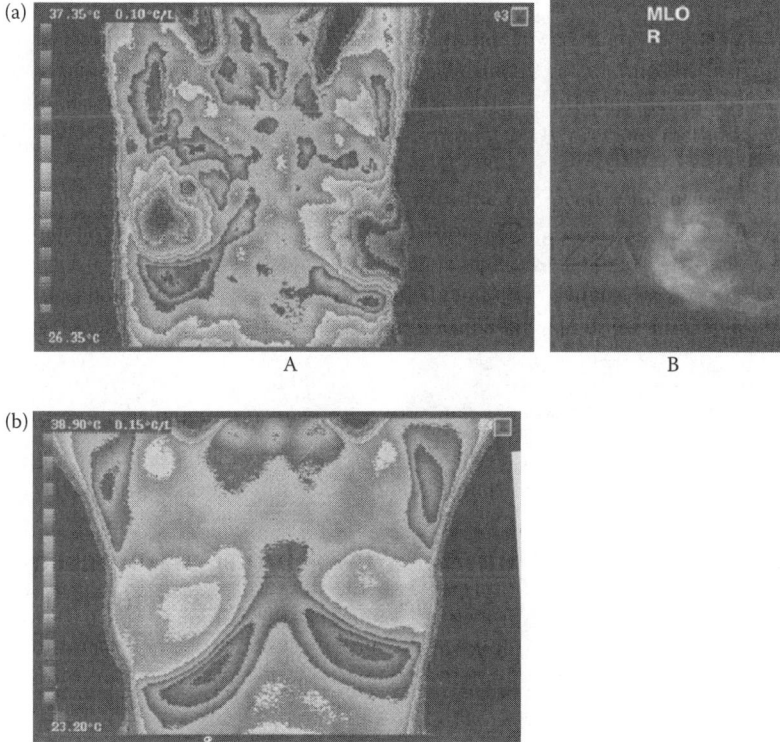

FIGURE 32.11 (a) Four years post-right partial mastectomy, the patient is recurrence free. Current *infrared imaging* (A): shows no activity and *mammography* (B): shows scar tissue. (b) *Infrared imaging*: 5 years following a left partial mastectomy and radiotherapy for carcinoma revealing slight asymmetry of volume, but no abnormal vascular abnormality and resolution of radiation-induced changes. The patient is disease free.

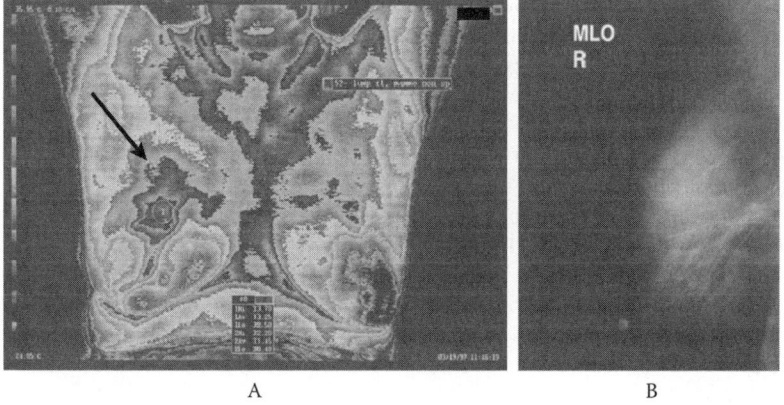

FIGURE 32.12 A 52-year-old patient, 5 years following right partial mastectomy, radiation, and chemotherapy for right breast cancer. Recent follow-up *infrared imaging* (A) now reveals significant vascular asymmetry (SVA) in the right breast with a ΔT of 1.5°C in the area of the previous surgery (IR-4). *Corresponding mammography* (B): density and scar tissue versus possible recurrence. *Surgical histology*: 4 cm, recurrent right carcinoma in the area of the previous resection.

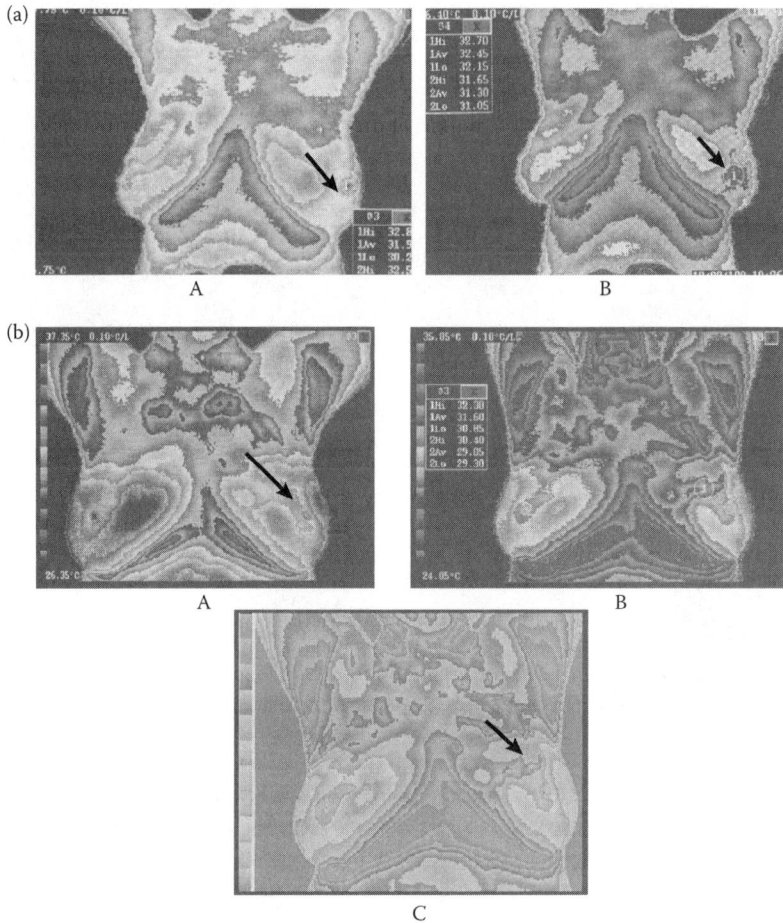

FIGURE 32.13 (a) A 45-year-old patient with small nodular process just inferior and medial to the left nipple areolar complex. *Infrared imaging* (A), without digital enhancement, was carried out and circles were placed on the nipple area rather than just below and medial to it. The nonenhanced IR image was thus initially misinterpreted as normal with a ΔT of 0.25°C. The same image was recalled and *repeated* (B), now with appropriate digital enhancement and once again, documented the presence of increased vascular activity just inferior and medial to the left nipple areolar complex with a ΔT of 1.15°C (IR-4.15). A 1.5 cm cancer was found just below the left nipple. (b) A 37-year-old patient with lump in the upper inner quadrant of the left breast. Mammography confirms spiculated mass. *Infrared imaging* (A): reported as "normal." Infrared imaging was repeated after appropriate *digital adjustment* (B): now reveals obvious significant vascular asymmetry in the same area and a ΔT of 1.75°C (Ir-4) (mod IR-4.75). Using a different IR camera on the *same patient* (C) confirms same finding. *Surgical histology*: 1.5 cm infiltrating ductal CA.

References

1. Lloyd-Williams K. and Handley R.S. Infra-red thermometry in the diagnosis of breast disease. *Lancet* 2, 1371–1381, 1961.
2. Handley R.S. The temperature of breast tumors as a possible guide to prognosis. *Acta Unio. Int. Contra. Cancrum.* 18, 822, 1962.
3. Lawson R.N. and Chughtai M.S. Breast cancer and body temperatures. *Can. Med. Assoc. J.* 88, 68–70, 1963.

4. Gershen-Cohen J., Haberman J., and Brueschke E.E. Medical thermography: A summary of current status. *Radiol. Clin. North. Am.* 3, 403–431, 1965.
5. Haberman J. The present status of mammary thermography. *Ca—Can. J. Clin.* 18, 314–321, 1968.
6. Jones C.H. Thermography of the female breast. In Parsons C.A. (ed.), *Diagnosis of Breast Disease*, University Park Press, Baltimore, pp. 214–234, 1983.
7. Isard H.J., Becker W. et al. Breast thermography after four years and 10,000 studies. *Am. J. Roentgenol.* 115, 811–821, 1972.
8. Dodd G.D. Thermography in breast cancer diagnosis. In *Proceedings of the 7th National Cancer Conference.* Los Angeles, CA, September 27–29, Lippincott, Philadelphia, Toronto, p. 267, 1972.
9. Feig S.A., Shaber G.S. et al. Thermography, mammography, and clinical examination in breast cancer screening. *Radiology* 122, 123–127, 1977.
10. Wallace J.D. Thermographic examination of the breast: An assessment of its present capabilities. In Gallagher H.S. (ed.), *Early Breast Cancer: Detection and Treatment.* American College of Radiology, Wiley, New York, pp. 13–19, 1975.
11. Report of the Working Group to Review the National Cancer Institute Breast Cancer Detection Demonstration Projects. *J. Natl. Cancer Inst.* 62, 641–709, 1979.
12. Haberman J. An overview of breast thermography in the United States. In Abernathy M. and Uematsu S. (eds), *Medical Thermography.* American Academy of Thermology, Washington, pp. 218–223, 1986.
13. Moskowitz M., Milbrath J. et al. Lack of efficacy of thermography as a screening tool for minimal and stage I breast cancer. *N. Engl. J. Med.* 295, 249–252, 1976.
14. Threatt B., Norbeck J.M. et al. Thermography and breast cancer: An analysis of a blind reading. *Ann. N.Y. Acad. Sci.* 335, 501–519, 1980.
15. Stark A. The use of thermovision in the detection of early breast cancer. *Cancer* 33, 1664–1670, 1964.
16. Sterns E. and Cardis C. Thermography in breast diagnosis. *Cancer* 50, 323–325, 1982.
17. Moskowitz M. Breast imaging. In Donegan W.L. and Spratt J.S. (eds), *Cancer of the Breast.* Saunders, New York, pp. 206–239, 1995.
18. Gautherie M. and Gros C.M. Breast thermography and cancer risk prediction. *Cancer* 45, 51–56, 1980.
19. Amalric R., Gautherie M. et al. Avenir des femmes à thermogramme infra-rouge mammaire anormal isolé. *La. Nouvelle. Presse Médicale* 38, 3153–3155, 1981.
20. Mariel L., Sarrazin D. et al. The value of mammary thermography. A report on 655 cases. *Sem. Hop.* 57, 699–701, 1981.
21. Isard H.J. Other imaging techniques. *Cancer* 53, 658–664, 1984.
22. Nyirjesy I. and Billingsley F.S. Detection of breast carcinoma in a gynecological practice. *Obstet. Gynecol.* 64, 747–751, 1984.
23. Bothmann G.A. and Kubli F. Plate thermography in the assessment of changes in the female breast. 2. Clinical and thermographic results. *Fortschr. Med.* 102, 390–393, 1984.
24. Useki H. Evaluation of the thermographic diagnosis of breast disease: Relation of thermographic findings and pathologic findings of cancer growth. *Nippon. Gan. Chiryo. Gakkai. Shi.* 23, 2687–2695, 1988.
25. Head J.F., Wang F., and Elliott R.L. Breast thermography is a noninvasive prognostic procedure that predicts tumor growth rate in breast cancer patients. *Ann. N.Y. Acad. Sci.* 698, 153–158, 1993.
26. Head J.F. and Elliott R.L. Breast thermography. *Cancer* 79, 186–188, 1995.
27. Gamagami P. Indirect signs of breast cancer: Angiogenesis study. In *Atlas of Mammography.* Blackwell Science, Cambridge, MA, pp. 231–26, 1996.
28. Guidi A.J. and Schnitt S.J. Angiogenesis in preinvasive lesions of the breast. *Breast J.* 2, 364–369, 1996.
29. Anbar M. Hyperthermia of the cancerous breast: Analysis of mechanism. *Cancer Lett.* 84, 23–29, 1994.

30. Anbar M. Breast cancer. In *Quantitative Dynamic Telethermometry in Medical Diagnosis and Management*. CRC Press, Ann Arbor, MI, pp. 84–94, 1994.

31. Parisky H.R., Sard A. et al. Efficacy of computerized infrared imaging analysis to evaluate mammographically suspicious lesions. *Am. J. Radiol.* 180, 263–272, 2003.

32. Sickles E.A. Mammographic features of "early" breast cancer. *Am. J. Roentgenol.* 143, 461, 1984.

33. Thomas D.B., Gao D.L. et al. Randomized trial of breast self-examination in Shanghai: Methodology and preliminary results. *J. Natl. Cancer Inst.* 5, 355–365, 1997.

34. Elmore J.G., Wells C.F. et al. Variability in radiologists interpretation of mammograms. *N. Engl. J. Med.* 331, 99–104, 1993.

35. Boyd N.F., Byng J.W. et al. Quantitative classification of mammographic densities and breast cancer risk. *J. Natl. Cancer Inst.* 87, 670–675, 1995.

36. Laya M.B. Effect on estrogen replacement therapy on the specificity and sensibility of screening mammography. *J. Natl. Cancer Inst.* 88, 643–649, 1996.

37. Singletary S.E., McNeese M.D., and Hortobagyi G.N. Feasibility of breast-conservation surgery after induction chemotherapy for locally advanced breast carcinoma. *Cancer* 69, 2849–2852, 1992.

38. Jansson T., Westlin J.E. et al. Position emission tomography studies in patients with locally advanced and/or metastatic breast cancer: A method for early therapy evaluation? *J. Clin. Oncol.* 13, 1470–1477, 1995.

39. Hendry J. Combined positron emission tomography and computerized tomography. Whole body imaging superior to MRI in most tumor staging. *JAMA* 290, 3199–3206, 2003.

40. Keyserlingk J.R., Ahlgren P.D., Yu E., and Belliveau N. Infrared imaging of the breast: Initial reappraisal using high-resolution digital technology in 100 successive cases of stage I and II breast cancer. *Breast J.* 4, 245–251, 1998.

41. Keyserlingk J.R., Yassa, M., Ahlgren, P., and Belliveau N. Tozzi. Ville Marie Oncology Center and St. Mary's Hospital, Montreal, Canada D. *Preliminary Evaluation of Digital Functional Infrared Imaging to Reflect Preoperative Chemohormonotherapy-Induced Changes in Neoangiogenesis in Patients with Locally Advanced Breast Cancer*. European Oncology Society, Milan, Italy, September 2001.

42. Berg W. Tumor type and breast profile determine value of mammography, ultrasound and MR. *Radiology* 233, 830–849, 2004.

43. Oestreicher N. Breast exam and mammography. *Am. J. Radiol.* 151, 87–96, 2004.

44. Mendelson, Berg et al. Ultrasound in the operated breast. Presented at the *RSNA*. Chicago, November 2005.

33

MammoVision (Infrared Breast Thermography) Compared to X-Ray Mammography and Ultrasonography: 114 Cases Evaluated

Reinhold Berz
German Society of Thermography and Regulation Medicine (DGTR)

Claus Schulte-Uebbing
German Society of Thermography and Regulation Medicine (DGTR)

33.1 Introduction

Breast cancer is the leading deadly cancer in women at least in the developed countries. X-ray mammography (MG) is called the gold standard for detecting breast cancer, but the method has some limitations: For many women MG may be painful, and the ionizing radiation could cause malignancy. More importantly: Cancerous lumps must have a diameter of at least 5 mm (often much more) to be detected by MG. Many breast cancers at this stage are 5–10 years old. Earlier detection is requested, but seems to be not easy to do by the established methods. MRI could be a better way, but there is a lack of experience, and it is costly. Ultrasonography (USG) can be helpful, too, but is recognized as a complementary examination.

33.1.1 Breast Metabolism and Heat Signs

There is a well known relationship between breast cancer and breast heat signs. Especially aggressive and fast growing breast cancers have an exaggerated metabolism causing a high blood supply. Intraoperative studies have demonstrated that breast cancer leads to an increased venous flow and to heat convection [1]. Usually the healthy breast is, depending on its size, colder than the surrounding chest and abdominal areas without thermographically visible signs of vessels or hot spots. Both breasts should have an average temperature differing not more than 0.5°C (thermal symmetry, Figure 33.1).

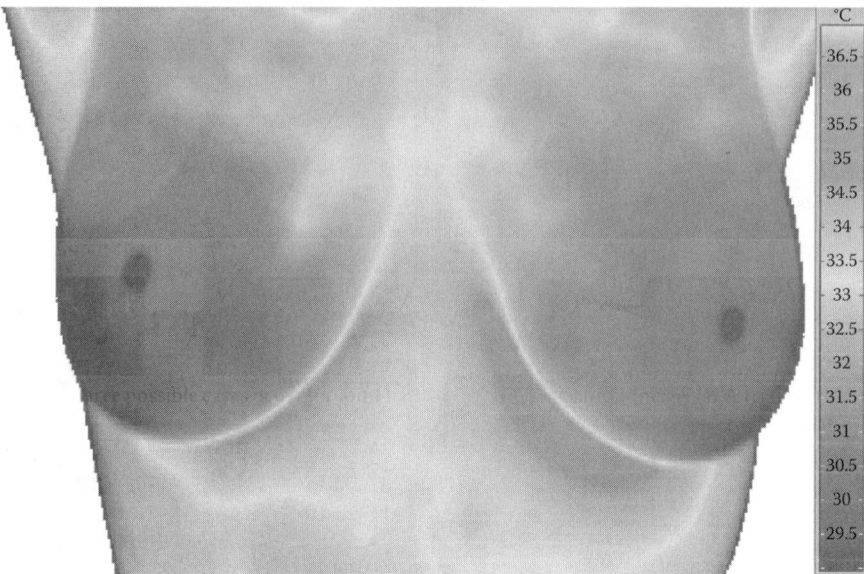

FIGURE 33.1 Normal MammoVision result of a 29-year-old healthy woman: symmetrically cool, no visible vessels, no hot spots, nipple and areola cold, contour without bulge or edge sign.

33.1.2 Infrared Thermography

The heat patterns of the breasts can be recorded with infrared detecting devices (infrared cameras), that have been in use for medical purposes since 1956 [2–5]. Since the late 1990s, due to the technological progress and sensor development infrared imaging devices since the late 1990s are much more suitable for medical measurements [6]. According to PLANCK's law, the infrared radiation of the human skin of 30°C (303 K) peaks at a wavelength of about 10 μm, and so called long wave infrared cameras (LWIR) are suitable to record and measure the heat pattern of the breast (Figure 33.2). Comparable to the US FDA approval, in Europe medical temperature measurement devices have to comply with the Medical Devices Directive, Council Directive 93/42/EEC [7]. This approval regards the whole

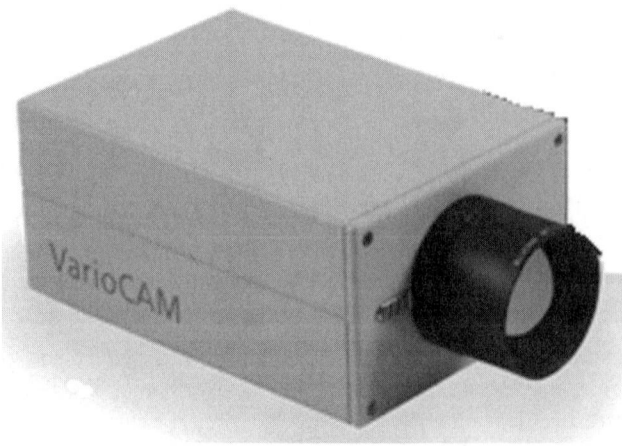

FIGURE 33.2 Medically approved infrared camera Jenoptik (formerly Carl Zeiss Jena) VarioCam Head.

equipment: IR camera, cable connections, power supply, computer and other hardware, software and examination rack.

33.2 MammoVision Methodology of Regulation Thermography

There are different approaches to conduct infrared thermography of the female breast. To solve the problem of lacking standardization, in Europe the method of Regulation Thermography, with decades of applications, was chosen. This approach is based on the idea that the response to a stimulus (like in other medical examinations, for example, ECG or EEG) enhances the diagnostic value and acuteness. Regulation Thermography or IRI (Infrared Regulation Imaging) applies a cool air stress exposure to the patient (disrobed at room temperature of 19–21°C) and measures the thermal pattern immediately after disrobing (comfort temperature) and a second time after adapting to the cold ambient (down regulated skin temperature after 10 min) [8–15]. This method has shown to be appropriate for female breast imaging [16]. For other applications different cold stress tests are common [17–20]. The thermal down regulation leads to a skin temperature decrease of about 1.0°C within the breast areas (Figure 33.3).

Very important is the appropriate preparation of the patient, the adaptation to the examination room (patient dressed) of 30 min, the ambient conditions of the examination room (19–21°C, humidity between 30 and 50%, shielding of the patient from sources of heat or cold (Figure 33.4).

33.2.1 MammoVision Equipment

MammoVision requires a complete medically approved temperature measurement system: infrared camera, cable connections, power supply, computer and other hardware, software and examination rack. The IR camera used for this study was a German made Jenoptik (formerly Carl Zeiss Jena) VarioCam

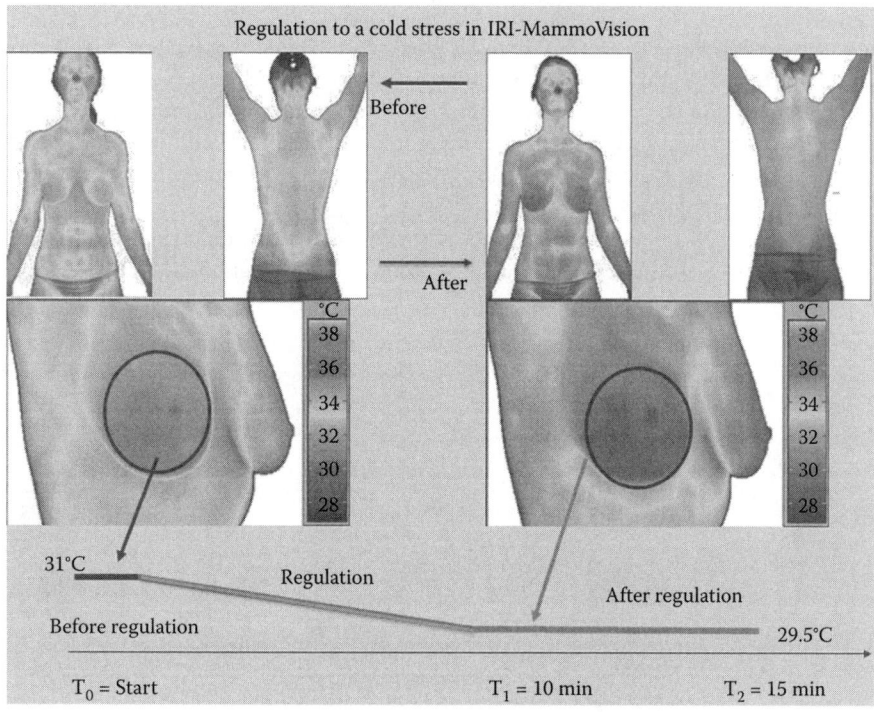

FIGURE 33.3   Principles of IRI (Infrared Regulation Imaging) and MammoVision.

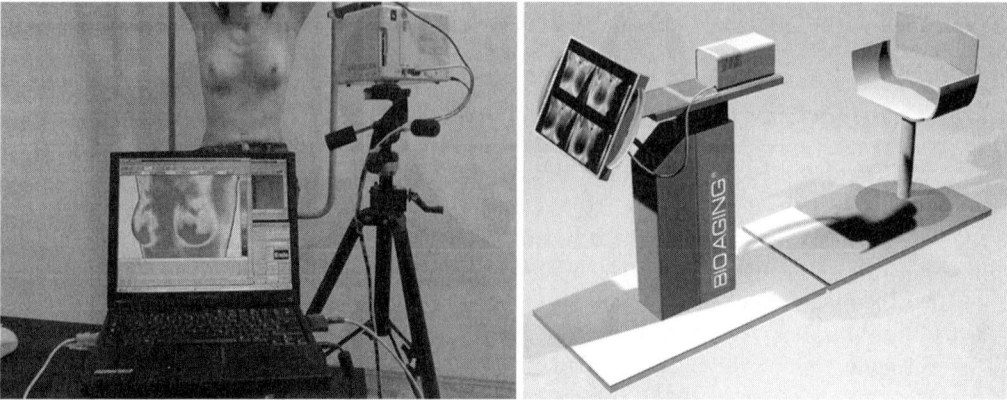

FIGURE 33.4 Early prototype of MammoVision (2000, left) and recent MammoVision device (bioaging Stuttgart, Germany, right).

Head with a spatial resolution of 320×240 sensors, detector pitch 35×35 µm, sensitivity 60 mK and better, accuracy $\pm 0.4°C$, stability over time 20 min after onset better than $\pm 0.5°C$, lens aperture $f = 1/1.0$, focal length $f = 25$ mm. An additional digital camera (webcam) takes a colour picture in parallel for the documentation of scarves or other visible breast abnormalities.

Core of the MammoVision system is the medically approved software EXAM for administration, examination, measurement and imaging control, data storage and, most importantly, data evaluation, and generating a medical report [21].

33.2.2 MammoVision Evaluation Guideline

The MammoVision examination needs 10 images: 5 before and 5 after thermal down regulation due to the cooling. The patented equipment and procedure [22] ensures that the views are more or less identical, which is important for the evaluation (Figure 33.5). After recording the measurement and images, the evaluation process starts: A patented evaluation procedure including a grid system marks the breast areas that will be mathematically evaluated. This grid should cover the same breast areas of the images taken before and after regulation (Figure 33.6).

The next step demands a detailed description of the vascular situation (a grayscale image is more suitable than a colour masked one, Figure 33.7). MammoVision evaluation criteria include the lateral

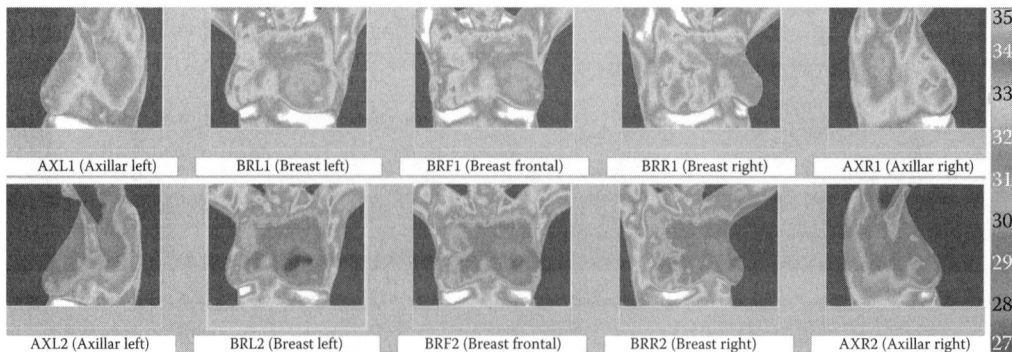

FIGURE 33.5 Measurement views of MammoVision: upper row before cold stimulus, lower row after cold stimulus and cooling down.

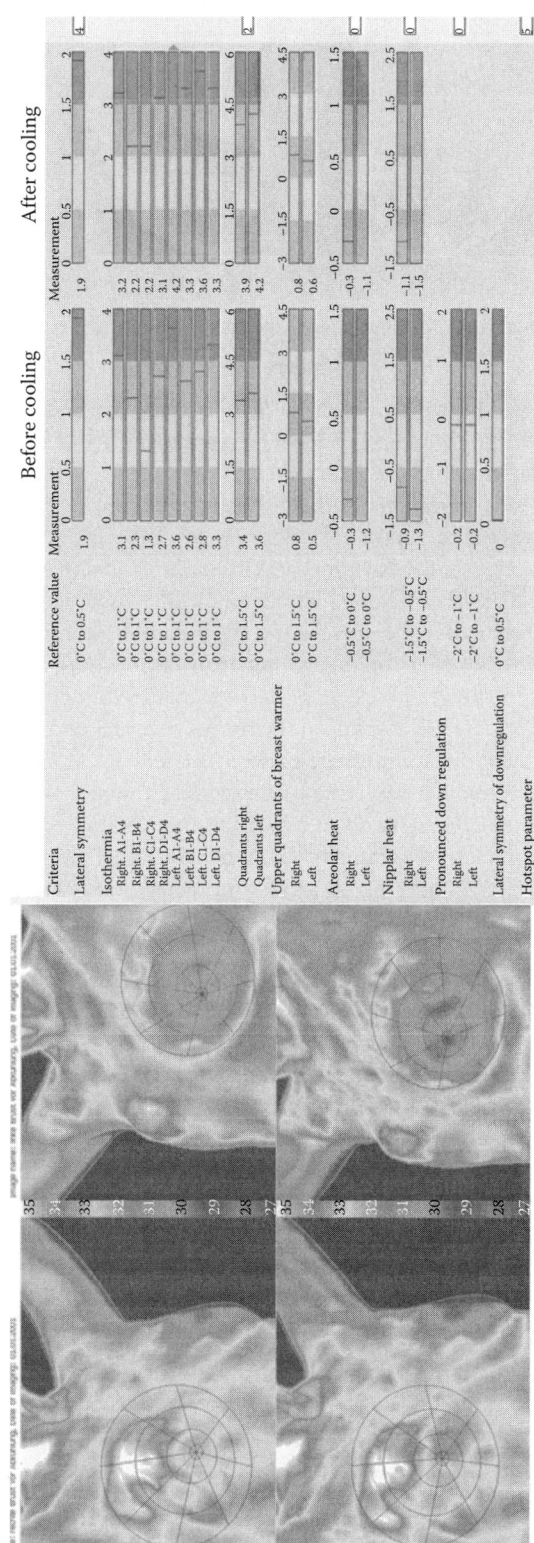

Criteria	Reference value	Before cooling Measurement	After cooling Measurement
Lateral symmetry	0°C to 0.5°C	1.9	1.9
Isothermia			
Right. A1-A4	0°C to 1°C	3.1	3.2
Right. B1-B4	0°C to 1°C	2.3	2.2
Right. C1-C4	0°C to 1°C	1.3	2.2
Right. D1-D4	0°C to 1°C	2.7	3.1
Left. A1-A4	0°C to 1°C	3.6	4.2
Left. B1-B4	0°C to 1°C	2.6	3.3
Left. C1-C4	0°C to 1°C	2.8	3.6
Left. D1-D4	0°C to 1°C	3.3	3.3
Quadrants right	0°C to 1.5°C	3.4	3.9
Quadrants left	0°C to 1.5°C	3.6	4.2
Upper quadrants of breast warmer			
Right	0°C to 1.5°C	0.8	0.8
Left	0°C to 1.5°C	0.5	0.6
Areolar heat			
Right	−0.5°C to 0°C	−0.3	−0.3
Left	−0.5°C to 0°C	−1.2	−1.1
Nipplar heat			
Right	−1.5°C to −0.5°C	−0.9	−1.1
Left	−1.5°C to −0.5°C	−1.3	−1.5
Pronounced down regulation			
Right	−2°C to −1°C	−0.2	
Left	−2°C to −1°C	−0.2	
Lateral symmetry of downregulation	0°C to 0.5°C	0	
Hotspot parameter			

FIGURE 33.6 Positioning of the evaluation grid in MammoVision (left): upper row before, lower row after cold stimulus and cooling (woman with hot cancer in the right breast); MammoVision results in an evaluation graph (right).

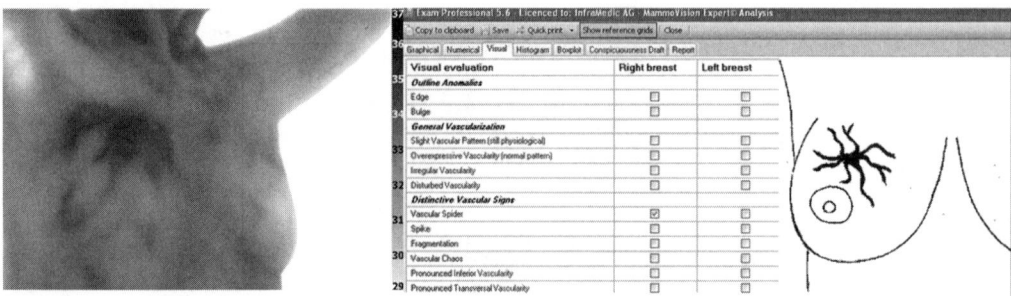

FIGURE 33.7 Grayscale masked MammoVision image for vascular description (left); MammoVision vascular description form (right).

symmetry of the breasts, the isothermia (homogeneous tempered breast areas with a small span of temperatures), areolar or nipplar heat, the extent of down regulation and the hotspot parameter [23]. The shapes of the breasts and vascular signs have to be assessed.

According to the assessment criteria [24,25] the results have been classified into 5 BIRAS groups (**B**reast **I**nfra**R**ed **A**ssessment **S**ystem):

BIRAS I: Inconspicuous; average lateral symmetry 0.5°C or better; isothermia/homogeneous areas with temperatures in a range of 1.5°C or less; no thermographically visible vascularity or few small vessels with homogeneous vessel characteristics including comparison with contra lateral breast; vascularity thermographically disappearing after cooling; no hot areas or hot spots, nipples and areola colder than the average of the breast, no bulge or edge signs, down regulation after cooling −0.5°C or more;

BIRAS II: Slightly conspicuous; fairly lateral symmetry between 0.5 and 1.0°C; fairly isothermia/homogeneous areas with temperatures in a range between 1.5 and 3.0°C; more impressive, but still physiological vessel characteristics, that can remain after cooling; nipples and areola colder than the average of the breast, no bulge or edge signs, down regulation after cooling −0.5°C or more;

BIRAS III: Conspicuous; often lateral asymmetry of more than 1.0°C; thermal pattern of the breasts more inhomogeneous, isothermia/homogeneous areas with temperatures more than 3.0°C differing; intensive and/or slightly abnormal vascular signs; slight edge or bulk signs; warm areas or warm spots; warm areola; most signs decreasing after cooling;

BIRAS IV: Very conspicuous; obvious lateral asymmetry of more than 1.5°C; pronounced unmodified hot spots and hot areas; very inhomogeneous, isothermia/homogeneous areas with temperatures more than 4.5°C differing; hot spikes; clear edge or bulk signs; areola and/or nipple hot; often one breast unilaterally affected, the other without or with less symptoms and signs; most signs resistive to cooling.

BIRAS V: Significantly conspicuous; like BIRAS IV, impressive lateral asymmetry of more than 2.0°C; cancer-related vascular signs (hot spiders, circular vessels, vascular chaos; very abnormal vascularity); paradoxical heating of spots or areas instead of cooling down regulation.

33.3 Patients Examined

114 women were enrolled in the study at the breast center Prof. Schulte-Uebbing, Munich, who were asked and agreed to participate. All women have had an x-ray mammogram (MG) in a radiological institute within the same time period as the MammoVision had been performed, from January 2006 to June 2007. The reasons for the MG examinations differed: either for screening purposes, or a lump had been detected, or other symptoms were recorded. The age of the patients ranged between 29 and 69 years, with an average of 48.5 years. Based on the MG BI-RADS classification the patients formed 5 groups, because MG is called the gold standard for breast cancer diagnosis. Group BI-RADS I $n = 41$; group BI-RADS II $n = 45$; group BI-RADS III $n = 15$; group BI-RADS IV $n = 8$; group BI-RADS V $n = 5$; totally 114 women.

Most of the patients had additional ultrasonography (USG), some had MRI, in some women biopsies were examined.

33.4 Results

33.4.1 Illustrations of BIRAS Classified Results

The illustrations show women with typical signs and classifications before and after cooling, focused on the symptomatic breast. Figure 33.8 shows a woman with a typical BIRAS I result, completely inconspicuous, symmetrical and homogeneous thermal breast pattern without thermographically visible vascularity.

Figure 33.9 represents a typical BIRAS II finding: still symmetrical, but with a broader range of temperatures within each breast (isothermia/homogeneity slightly affected), nipple cold, areola slightly warm, but cooling down after down regulation, warm vascular pattern above the breast that is sufficiently cooling down.

Figure 33.10 is a good example for a BIRAS III result: especially the very warm periareolar areas on both breasts are suspicious and should give reason for further examinations; even after down regulation, the warm areolar region is visible.

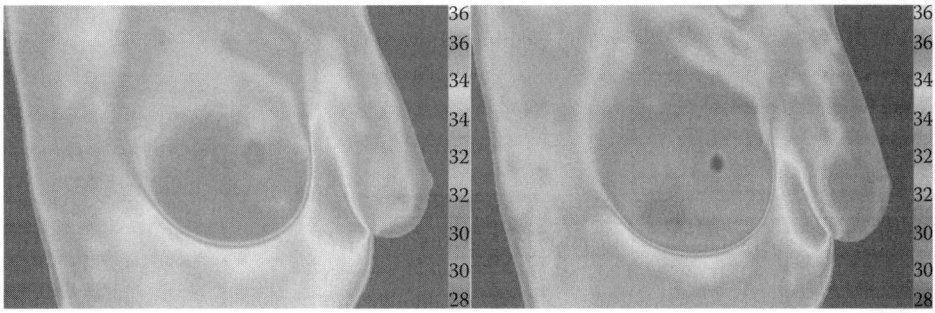

FIGURE 33.8 BIRAS I example; 29-year-old woman, left picture before cold stimulus, right picture after cold stimulus and cooling down; no clinical signs of breast disorder; in MammoVision very homogeneous, symmetrical thermal patterns, no vessels visible.

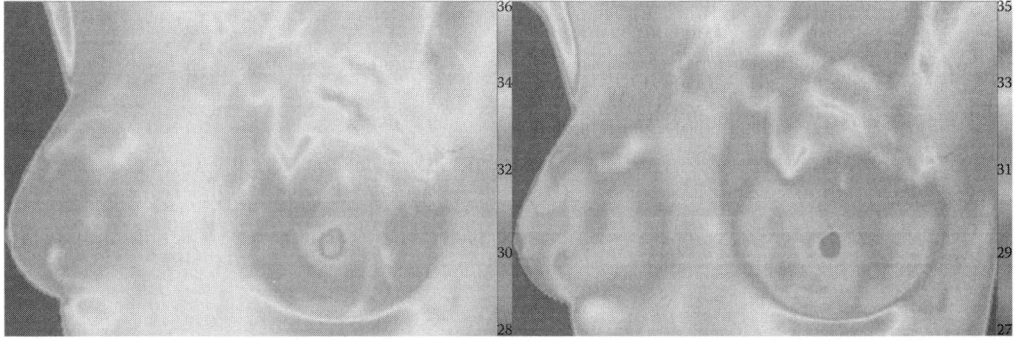

FIGURE 33.9 BIRAS II example; 42-year-old woman, left picture before cold stimulus, right picture after cold stimulus and cooling down; mastopathia, no other breast disease; MammoVision: symmetrical thermal pattern, areola and nipple cool, sufficient thermal down cold stimulus, small vessels that mostly disappear to be visible after cooling.

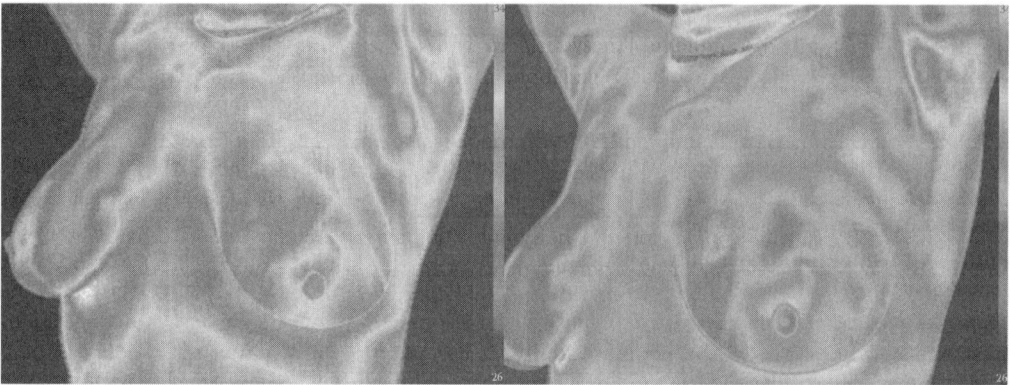

FIGURE 33.10 BIRAS III example; 43-year-old woman, left picture before cold stimulus, right picture after cold stimulus and cooling down; mastopathia, palpable nodules. MammoVision: suspicious result, areolar heat both sides, intensive down cold stimulus.

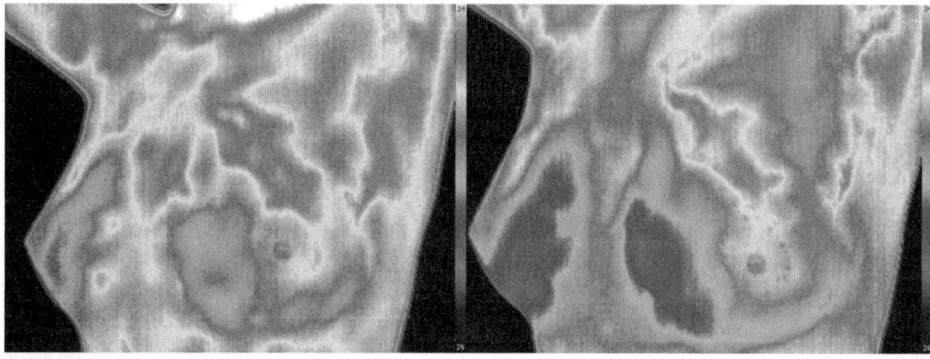

FIGURE 33.11 BIRAS IV example; 55 year old woman, left picture before cold stimulus, right picture after cold stimulus and cooling down; palpable lump in the left breast, questionable palpable axillary lymph nodes; MammoVision: very suspicious, highly asymmetrical, insufficient down cold stimulus, inflammatorious area above left areola; persisting heat even after cooling; biopsy: invasive ductal carcinoma pT2 pN1, G3, ER +, PR +, HER −.

The woman presented in Figure 33.11 shows a highly suspicious result. The thermal symmetry is lost, and the left breast seems clearly affected with heat signs. Impressively the areolar heat increases instead of cooling after thermal down regulation. In the upper quadrants there are classified hot spot/hot areas signs, like an inflammation. This woman had a biopsy, and the result was an invasive ductal carcinoma (pT2 pN1, G3, ER +, PR +, HER −).

Figure 33.12 shows a rare sign of malignancy in the right breast. The whole right breast is over heated compared to the left side; especially the vascular pattern is highly suspicious due to the circular vessel with aspects of a thermal vascular spider. Vascular abnormalities like this are highly conspicuous that there is already breast cancer. In this case it was an invasive ductal carcinoma; pT2 pN1, G3, ER +, PR +, HER +.

33.4.2 Statistical Results

All patients of the BI-RADS IV and V groups (highly suspicious to have breast cancer) have had clearly pathological signs in the MammoVision examination. The same holds true, with one exception, for the women of the BI-RADS III group. But in the BI-RADS I and II groups (not suspicious to

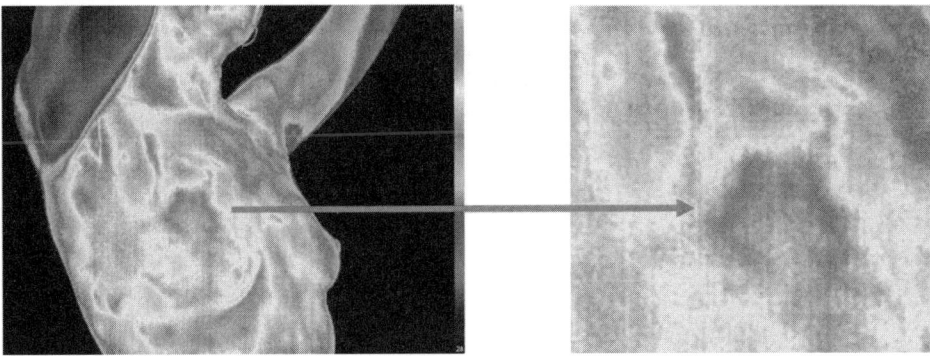

FIGURE 33.12 BIRAS V example; MammoVision very suspicious: extreme asymmetry, right breast heated intensively, absolute pathological vessel (circular structure with vascular spider aspects); biopsy: invasive ductal carcinoma; pT2 pN1, G3, ER +, PR +, HER +.

have breast cancer) there were remarkable differences between the MG classification and many of the MammoVision results. Especially in group BI-RADS II, half of the patients had slightly to very conspicuous thermal signs.

For a more detailed evaluation each BI-RADS group (I to V) was separately compared with the differentiated MammoVision results (BIRAS I to V) as presented in Figure 33.13. It can be stated that in the x-ray MG BI-RADS I group the MammoVision findings mostly are classified as non conspicuous. In 9 of 41 women there were BIRAS II results to be found.

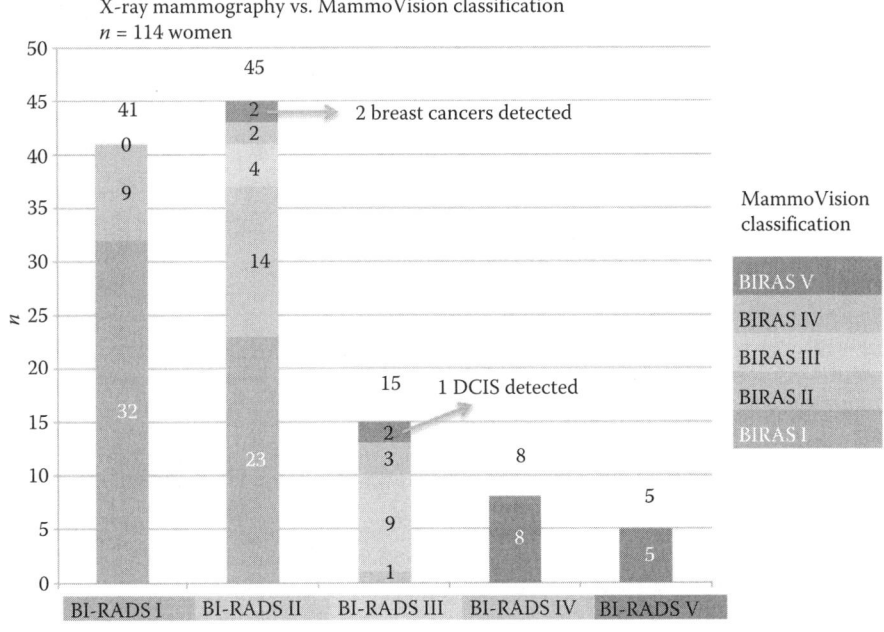

FIGURE 33.13 Comparison of x-ray mammography classification (BI-RADS I to V) versus MammoVision classification (BIRAS I to V).

The MG BI/RADS III group looked very inhomogeneous regarding the MammoVision results. About 50% of the women hat inconspicuous MammoVision findings, 30% slightly suspicious results, but 8 of 45 women showed more conspicuous results, two of them classified as BIRAS IV and two as BIRAS V. They were therefore consequently examined by USG and MRI. Three of them had a biopsy, and in two of these women cancer was found.

Also in the BI-RADS III group, MammoVision gave the reason for additional USG, MG and MRI examinations. Two women underwent biopsy, one of them had DCIS.

33.5 Conclusion

The results of this study should be regarded as preliminary. The number of women included is too small to obtain statistically valid conclusions.

In the past only few studies have stressed the issue of comparing x-ray MG to infrared thermography [26–29]. One problem of comparing infrared thermography to x-ray MG is the amount of false positive and false negative results of MG. Even in this limited 114 women study, x-ray MG failed to detect 2 cases of invasive breast cancer and one case of DCIS, whereas the MammoVision results gave reason for further examinations and at last for confirmation of these three cases of malignancy. Infrared thermography of the breast should therefore be compared to MRI (which actually is proving to be more accurate than MG) or to biopsy results. But MRI is expensive and rarely applied, and biopsy is invasive and only done in highly suspicious cases.

Regarding the future applications of breast thermography, this study wanted to contribute and to pinpoint the increased possibilities given by last generation high accuracy and reliable thermal measurement equipment. Further comparison and outcome research for infrared thermography of the breast is urgently needed.

References

1. Lawson, R.N. and Chughtai, M.S., Breast cancer and body temperatures. *Can Med Assoc J* 88, 68–70, 1963.
2. Lawson, R.N., Implications of surface temperature in the diagnosis of breast lesions. *Canad Med Assoc J* 75, 309, 1956.
3. Lloyd Williams, K., Thermography in breast cancer. *Br J Radiol* 5, 75, 1969.
4. Lloyd Williams, K., Lloyd Williams, F., and Handley, R.S., Infrared thermometry in the diagnosis of breast diseases. *Lancet* 2, 1378, 1971.
5. Lewis, J.D., Milbrath, J.R., Shaffer, K.A., and Das Gupta, T.K., Implications of suspicious findings in breast cancer screening. *Arch Surg* 110, 903–907, 1975.
6. Berz, R. and Sauer, H., The medical use of infrared-thermography history and recent applications. In: Deutsche Gesellschaft für Zerstörungsfreie Prüfung e.V. (Ed): Thermografie-Kolloquium 2007. DGZfP-Berichtsband BB 107-CD. Berlin 2007.
7. Council Directive 92/42/EEC of 14 January 1993 on Medical Devices, 1993.
8. Schwamm, E., Thermoregulation und Thermodiagnostik. In Rost, A. (Ed), Thermographie und Thermoregulationsdiagnostik. Uelzen, 96–107, 1980.
9. Heim, G., Thermographie im Zeitablauf unter verschiedenen Belastungsformen. In Rost, A. (Ed), Thermographie und Thermoregulationsdiagnostik. MLV, Uelzen 64–73, 1980.
10. Berz, R., Das Wärmebild und die Reaktion auf Abkühlung bei jungen gesunden Probanden. *Ärztezeitschrift f Naturheilverfahren* 26, 237–243, 1985.
11. Berz, R., Regulation thermography—a survey. In: Baleagas, D., Busse, G., Carlomagno, C.M., Wiecek, B. (Eds), *Medical InfraRed Thermography MIRT'98*. Technical University of Lodz, Poland, 1998.

12. Berz, R., *About Regulation Thermography—A Sensitive Tool for Early Diagnose and Therapy Control.* Proceedings of the Focus Symposium on Health, Healing and Medicine, V 01 V. University of Windsor, Canada 1999.

13. Berz, R., Infrared Regulation Imaging (IRI)—a different approach to health, wellness, and to prevention. ThermoMed 16, 49–58, 2000.

14. Berz, R., Introducing Regulation into Infrared Imaging: ReguVision and MammoVision. In: Institute of Electronics, Technical University of Lodz (Ed): Proceedings of the 4th National Conference "Termografia i Termometria w Podczerwieni" TTP 2000. Lodz, Poland, 206–212, 2000.

15. Berz, R., MammoVision—a new approach to diagnosis and prevention of breast cancer. In: Benkö, I., Kovaczicz, I., and Lovak, I. (Eds.): 12th Inter-national Conference on Thermal Engineering and Thermogrammetry (THERMO), June 2001, Budapest. Mate, Hungary, 265–272, 2001.

16. Berz, R. and Sauer, H., Comparing effects of thermal regulation tests (cool air stimulus vs. cold water stress test) on infrared imaging of the female breast. In: *Institute of Physics and Engineering in Medicine* Ed), Clinical temperature measurement and thermography. York, UK, 36–41, 2007.

17. Ring, E.F.J., Aarts, N.J.M., Black, C.M., and Boesiger, P., Raynaud's phenomenon assessment by thermography. *Thermology* 3, 69–73, 1988.

18. Ring, E.F.J., Cold stress test for the hands. In Ammer, K. and Ring, E.F.J. (Eds), *The Thermal Image in Medicine and Biology*. Uhlen, Vienna, 237–240, 1995.

19. Pascoe, D.D., Purohit, R.C., Shanley, L.A., and Herrick, R.T., Pre- and post-operative evaluation of carpal tunnel syndrome. In Ammer, K. and Ring, E.F.J. (Eds), *The Thermal Image in Medicine and Biology*. Uhlen, Vienna, 188–190, 1995.

20. Berz R. and Bucher W., Procedure for the evaluation of thermograhically images of a female or male breast (Verfahren zur Auswertung von Wärmebildern einer weiblichen oder männlichen Brust), German Patent Nr. 101 50 918, Munich, 2003.

21. Medical Device Certification GmbH Stuttgart (Germany), CE-0483, 2007.

22. Berz R., Equipment for measuring the temperature pattern at the body surface of a person (Vorrichtung zur Bestimmung der Temperaturverteilung an der Körperoberfläche einer Person), German Patent Nr. 199 56 346, Munich, 2004.

23. Boesiger, P. and Stucki, D., Quantitative auswertung und interpretation von infrarotthermogrammen der weiblichen Brust. In Lauth, G. and Eulenburg, R. (Eds), *Thermographie der weiblichen Brust*. VCH, Weinheim, 185–219, 1986.

24. Schulte-Uebbing, C., Breast Cancer and Heavy Metals, New Aspects for Diagnosis and Therapy, Oncology Meeting, Bad Aibling, Germany, February 2008.

25. Schulte-Uebbing, C., Mammovision—ein komplementäres Mamma—Diagnostik—Verfahren, zaenmagazin 2, 13–19, 2010.

26. Parisky, Y.R., Sardi, A., Hamm, R., Hughes, K., Esserman, L., Rust, S., and Callahan, K., Efficacy of computerized infrared imaging analysis to evaluate mammographically suspicious lesions. *Am J Roentgenol* 180, 263–269, 2003.

27. Ng, E.Y.K., Ung, L.N., Ng, F.C., and Sim, L.S.J., Statistical analysis of healthy and malignant breast thermography. *J Med Eng Tech*, 25, 253–263, 2001.

28. Qi, H., Liu, Z.Q., and Wang, C., Breast cancer identification through shape analysis in thermal texture maps. Annual International Conference of the IEEE Engineering in Medicine and Biology Proceedings, 2, 1129–1130, 2002.

29. Qi, H., Kuruganti, P.T., and Snyder, W.E., Detecting breast cancer from thermal infrared images by asymmetry analysis. In: Diakides, N.A., Bronzino, J.D. (Eds), *Medical Infrared Imaging*. CRC Press, Boca Raton, 11-1–11-13, 2008.

34

Detecting Breast Cancer from Thermal Infrared Images by Asymmetry Analysis

Hairong Qi
University of Tennessee

Phani Teja
Kuruganti
*Oak Ridge National
Laboratory*

Wesley E. Snyder
*North Carolina State
University*

One of the popular methods for breast cancer detection is to make comparisons between contralateral images. When the images are relatively symmetrical, small asymmetries may indicate a suspicious region. In thermal infrared (IR) imaging, asymmetry analysis normally needs human intervention because of the difficulties in automatic segmentation. In order to provide a more objective diagnostic result, we describe an automatic approach to asymmetry analysis in thermograms. It includes automatic segmentation and supervised pattern classification. Experiments have been conducted based on images provided by Elliott Mastology Center (Inframetrics 600M camera) and Bioyear, Inc. (Microbolometer uncooled camera).

34.1 Introduction

The application of IR imaging in breast cancer study starts as early as 1961 when Williams and Handley first published their results in the *Lancet* [1]. However, the premature use of the technology and its poorly controlled introduction into breast cancer detection in the 1970s have led to its early demise [2]. IR-based diagnosis was criticized as generating a higher false-positive rate than mammography, and thus was not recommended as a standard modality for breast cancer detection. Therefore, despite its deployment in many areas of industry and military, IR usage in medicine has declined [3]. Three decades later, several papers and studies have been published to reappraise the use of IR in medicine [2,3] for the following three reasons: (1) we have greatly improved IR technology. New generations of IR cameras have been developed with much enhanced accuracy; (2) we have much better capabilities in image processing. Advanced techniques including image enhancement, restoration, and segmentation have been effectively used in processing IR images; and (3) we have a deeper understanding of the patho-physiology of heat generation.

The main objective of this work is to evaluate the viability of IR imaging as a noninvasive imaging modality for early detection of breast cancer so that it can be performed both on the symptomatic and the asymptomatic patient and can thus be used as a complement to traditional mammography. This report summarizes how the identification of the asymmetry can be automated using image segmentation, feature extraction, and pattern recognition techniques. We investigate different features that contribute the most toward the detection of asymmetry. This kind of approach helps reduce the false-positive rate of the diagnosis and increase chances of disease cure and survival.

34.1.1 Measuring the Temperature of Human Body

Temperature is a long-established indicator of health. The Greek physician, Hippocrates, wrote in 400 B.C. "In whatever part of the body excess of heat or cold is felt, the disease is there to be discovered" [4]. The ancient Greeks immersed the body in wet mud and the area that dried more quickly, indicating a warmer region, was considered the diseased tissue. The use of hands to measure the heat emanating from the body remained well into the sixteenth and the seventeenth centuries. It was not until Galileo, who made a thermoscope from a glass tube, that some form of temperature-sensing device was developed, but it did not have a scale. It is Fahrenheit and later Celsius who have fixed the temperature scale and proposed the present-day clinical thermometer. The use of liquid crystals is another method of displaying skin temperature. Cholesteric esters can have the property of changing colors with temperature and this was established by Lehmann in 1877. It was involved in use of elaborative panels that encapsulated the crystals and were applied to the surface of the skin, but due to large area of contact, they affected the temperature of the skin. All the methods discussed above are contact based.

Major advances over the past 30 years have been with IR thermal imaging. The astronomer, Sir William Herschel, in Bath, England discovered the existence of IR radiation by trying to measure the heat of the separate colors of the rainbow spectrum cast on a table in the darkened room. He found that the highest temperature was found beyond the red end of the spectrum. He reported this to the Royal society as Dark Heat in 1800, which eventually has been turned the IR portion of the spectrum. IR radiation occupies the region between visible and microwaves. All objects in the universe emit radiations in the IR region of the spectra as a function of their temperature. As an object gets hotter, it gives off more intense IR radiation, and it radiates at a shorter wavelength [3]. At moderate temperatures (above 200°F), the intensity of the radiation gets high enough that the human body can detect that radiation as heat. At sufficiently high temperatures (above 1200°F), the intensity gets high enough and the wavelength gets short enough that the radiation crosses over the threshold to the red end of the visible light spectrum. The human eye cannot detect IR rays, but they can be detected by using the thermal IR cameras and detectors.

34.1.2 Metabolic Activity of Human Body and Cancer Cells

Metabolic process in a cell can be briefly defined as the sum total of all the enzymatic reactions occurring in the cell. It can be further elaborated as a highly coordinated, purposeful activity in which many sets of interrelated multienzyme systems participate, exchanging both matter and energy between the cell and its environment. Metabolism has four specific functions: (1) to obtain chemical energy from the fuel molecules; (2) to convert exogenous nutrients into the building blocks or precursor of macromolecular cell components; (3) to assemble such building blocks into proteins, nucleic acids, lipids, and other cell components; and (4) to form and degrade biomolecules required in specialized functions of the cell.

Metabolism can be divided into two major phases, catabolism and anabolism. Catabolism is the degradative phase of metabolism in which relatively large and complex nutrient molecules (carbohydrates, lipids, and proteins) are degraded to yield smaller, simpler molecules such as lactic acid, acetic acid, CO_2, ammonia, or urea. Catabolism is accompanied by conservation of some of the energy of the nutrient in the form of phosphate bond energy of adenosine triphosphate (ATP). Conversely, anabolism is the building up phase of metabolism, the enzymatic biosynthesis of such molecular components of cells as the nucleic acids, proteins, lipids, and carbohydrates from their simple building block precursors. Biosynthesis of organic molecules from simple precursors requires input of chemical energy, which is furnished by ATP generated during catabolism. Each of these pathways is promoted by a sequence of specific enzymes catalyzing consecutive reactions. The energy produced by the metabolic pathways is utilized by the cell for its division. Cells undergo mitotic cell division, a process in which a single cell divides into many cells and forms tissues, leading further into the development and growth of the multicellular organs. When cells divide, each resultant part is a complete relatively small cell. Immediately after division the newly formed cells grow rapidly soon reaching the size of the original cell. In humans, growth occurs through mitotic cell division with subsequent enlargement and differentiation of the reproduced cells into organs. Cancer cells also grow similarly but lose the ability to differentiate into organs. So, a cancer may be defined as an actively dividing undifferentiated mass of cells called the "tumor."

Cancer cells result from permanent genetic change in a normal cell triggered by some external physical agents such as chemical agents, x-rays, UV rays, and so on. They tend to grow aggressively and do not obey normal pattern of tissue formation. Cancer cells have a distinctive type of metabolism. Although they possess all the enzymes required for most of the central pathways of metabolism, cancer cells of nearly all types show an anomaly in the glucose degradation pathway (namely, glycolysis). The rate of oxygen consumption is somewhat below the values given by normal cells. However, the malignant cells tend to utilize anywhere from 5 to 10 times as much glucose as normal tissue and convert most of it into lactate instead of pyruvate (lactate is a low energy compound whereas pyruvate is a high-energy compound). The net effect is that in addition to the generation of ATP in mitochondria from respiration, there is a very large formation of ATP in extra mitochondrial compartment from glycolysis. The most important effect of this metabolic imbalance in cancer cells is the utilization of a large amount of blood glucose and release of large amounts of lactate into blood. The lactate so formed is recycled in the liver to produce blood glucose again. Since the formation of blood glucose by the liver requires six molecules of ATP whereas breakdown of glucose to lactate produces only two ATP molecules, the cancer cells are looked upon as metabolic parasites dependent on the liver for a substantial part of their energy. Large masses of cancer cells thus can be a considerable metabolic drain on the host organism. In addition to this, the high metabolic rate of cancer cells causes an increase in local temperature as compared to normal cells. Local metabolic activity ceases when blood supply is stopped since glycolysis is an oxygen-dependent pathway and oxygen is transported to the tissues by the hemoglobin present in the blood; thus, blood supply to these cells is important for them to proliferate. The growth of a solid tumor is limited by the blood supply. If it were not invaded by capillaries a tumor would be dependent on the diffusion of nutrients from its surroundings and could not enlarge beyond a diameter of a few millimeters. Thus, in order to grow further the tumor cells stimulate the blood vessels to form a capillary network that invades the tumor mass. This phenomenon is popularly called "angiogenesis," which is a process of vascularization of a tissue involving the development of new capillary blood vessels.

Vascularization is a growth of blood vessels into a tissue with the result that the oxygen and nutrient supply is improved. Vascularization of tumors is usually a prelude to more rapid growth and often to metastasis (advanced stage of cancer). Vascularization seems to be triggered by angiogenesis factors that stimulate endothelial cell proliferation and migration. In the context of this chapter the high metabolic rate in the cancer cells and the high density of packaging makes them a key source of heat concentration (since the heat dissipation is low) thus enabling thermal IR imaging as a viable technique to visualize the abnormality.

34.1.3 Early Detection of Breast Cancer

There is a crucial need for early breast cancer detection. Research has shown that if detected earlier (tumor size <10 mm), the breast cancer patient has an 85% chance of cure as opposed to 10% if the cancer is detected late [5].

Different kinds of diagnostic imaging techniques exist in the field of breast cancer detection. The most popularly used method presently is x-ray mammography. The drawback of this technique is that it is invasive and experts believe that electromagnetic radiation can also be a triggering factor for cancerous growth. Because of this, periodic inspection might have a negative effect on the patient's health. Research shows that the mammogram sensitivity is higher for older women (age group 60–69 years) at 85% compared with younger women (<50 years) at 64% [5]. A new study in a British medical journal (the *Lancet* [6]) has asserted that there is no reliable evidence that screening with mammography for breast cancer reduces mortality. They show that screening actually leads to more aggressive treatment, increasing the number of mastectomies by about 20%, and the number of mastectomies and tumorectomies by about 30%.

In contrast to this, IR imaging uses a noninvasive imaging technique as the diagnostic tool. The main source of IR rays is heat emitted from different bodies whose temperature is above absolute zero. Thus a thermogram of a patient provides the heat distribution in the body. The cancerous cells, due to high metabolic rates and angiogenesis, are at a higher temperature than the normal cells around it. Thus the cancer cells can be imaged as hotspots in the IR images. The thermogram provides more dynamic information of the tumor since the tumor can be small in size but can be fast growing making it appear as a high-temperature spot in the thermogram [7,8]. However, this is not the case in mammography, in which unless the tumor is beyond certain size, it cannot be imaged as x-rays essentially pass through it unaffected. This qualifies IR imaging as an effective diagnostic tool for early detection of breast cancer. Keyserlingk et al. [2] reported that the average tumor size undetected by thermal imaging is 1.28 and 1.66 cm by mammography. It is also reported that thermography can provide results that can be correct even 8–10 years before mammography can detect a mass in the patient's body [9,10].

34.2 Asymmetric Analysis in Breast Cancer Detection

Radiologists routinely make comparisons between contralateral images. When the images are relatively symmetrical, small asymmetries may indicate a suspicious region. This is the underlying philosophy in the use of asymmetry analysis for mass detection in breast cancer study [11]. Unfortunately, due to various reasons such as fatigue, carelessness, or simply because of the limitation of human visual system, these small asymmetries might not be easy to detect. Therefore, it is important to design an automatic approach to eliminate human factors.

There have been a few papers addressing techniques for asymmetry analysis of mammograms [11–16]. Head et al. [17,18] recently analyzed the asymmetric abnormalities in IR images. In their approach, the thermograms are segmented first by an operator. Then breast quadrants are derived automatically based on unique point of reference, that is, the chin, the lowest, rightmost, and leftmost points of the breast.

This chapter describes an automatic approach to asymmetry analysis in thermograms. It includes automatic segmentation and pattern classification. Hough transform is used to extract the four feature curves that can uniquely segment the left and right breasts. The feature curves include the left and the right body boundary curves, and the two parabolic curves indicating the lower boundaries of the breasts. Upon segmentation, different pattern recognition techniques are applied to identify the asymmetry.

Both segmentation and classification results are shown on images provided by Elliott Mastology Center (Inframetrics 600M camera) and Bioyear, Inc. (Microbolometer uncooled camera).

34.2.1 Automatic Segmentation

There are several ways to perform segmentation, including *threshold-based* techniques, *edge-based* techniques, and *region-based* techniques. Threshold-based techniques assign pixels above (or below) a specified threshold to be in the same region. Edge-based techniques assume that the boundary formed by adjacent regions (or segments) has high edge strength. Through edge detection, we can identify the boundary that surrounds a region. Region-based methods start with elemental regions and split or merge them [19].

34.2.1.1 Edge Image Generation

In this research work, we choose to use the edge-based segmentation technique as we have identified four dominant curves in the edge image, which we call "feature curves," including the left and right body boundaries, and the two lower boundaries of the breasts (Figure 34.3) or the two shadow boundaries that are below the breasts (Figure 34.2) whichever is stronger.

Edges are areas in the image where the brightness changes suddenly. One way to find edges is to calculate the amplitude of the first derivative (Equation 34.1) that generates the so-called gradient magnitude image where $\partial f / \partial x$ is the derivative of the image f along the x direction, and $\partial f / \partial y$ is the derivative along the y direction (the x and y directions are orthogonal to each other) and to threshold the amplitude image.

$$\text{Gradient magnitude} = \sqrt{\left(\frac{\partial f}{\partial x}\right)^2 + \left(\frac{\partial f}{\partial y}\right)^2} \tag{34.1}$$

Another way is to calculate the second derivative and to locate the zero-crossing points, as the second derivative at edge pixels would appear as a point where the derivatives of its left and right pixels change signs.

Although effective, both derivative images are very sensitive to noise. In order to eliminate or reduce the effect of noise, a Gaussian smoothing low-pass filter is applied before taking the derivatives. The smoothing process, on the other hand, also results in thicker edges. The Canny edge detector [20] solves this problem by taking two extra steps, the *nonmaximum suppression* (NMS) step and the *hysteresis thresholding* step, in order to locate the true edge pixels (only one pixel wide along the gradient direction).

For each edge pixel in the gradient magnitude image, the NMS step looks one pixel in the direction of the gradient, and another pixel in the reverse direction. If the magnitude of the current pixel is not the maximum of the three, then this pixel is not a true edge pixel. NMS helps locate the true edge pixels properly. However, the new edges still suffer from extra edge points problem due to noise and missing edge points.

The hysteresis thresholding improves the quality of edge image by using a dual-threshold approach, in which two thresholds, τ_1 and τ_2 (τ_2 is significantly larger than τ_1), are applied on the NMS-processed edge image to produce two binary edge images, denoted as T_1 and T_2, respectively. Since T_1 was created using a lower threshold, it will contain more extra edge pixels than T_2. Edge pixels in T_2 are therefore considered to be parts of true edges. When some discontinuities in edges occur in the T_2 image, the pixels at the same location of the T_1 image is looked up that could be continuations of the edge. If such pixels are found, they are included in the true edge image. This process continues until the continuation of pixels in T_1 connects with an edge pixel in T_2 or no connected T_1 points are found. (See Figures 34.2 and 34.3 for examples of the edge image derived from Canny edge detector.)

34.2.1.2 Hough Transform for Edge Linking

From Figures 34.2 and 34.3, we find that the edge images still cannot be used directly for segmentation as the edge detector picks up all the intensity changes, which would complicate the segmentation. On the other hand, many edges show gaps among edge pixels that would result in segments that are not closed. We have identified four feature boundaries that could enclose the breast. The body boundaries are easy to detect. Difficulties lie in the detection of the lower boundaries of the breasts or the shadow. We observe that the breast boundaries are generally parabolic in shape. Therefore, the Hough transform [21] is used to detect the parabola.

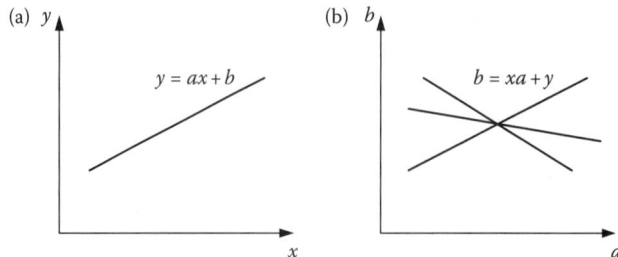

FIGURE 34.1 Illustration of the Hough transform. (a) The original image domain and (b) the parametric domain.

The Hough transform is one type of parametric transforms, in which the object in an image is expressed as a mathematical function of some parameters and the object can be represented in another transformation domain by these parameters. Take a straight edge in an image as an example, in the original image representation domain (or the x–y domain), we can use $y = ax + b$ to describe this edge with a slope of a and an intercept of b, as shown in Figure 34.1a. In order to derive the two parameters, a and b, we can convert the problem to a parametric domain (or the a–b domain) from the original x–y space, and treat x and y as parameters. We find that for each point (x, y) on the edge, there are infinite number of possible corresponding (a, b)s and they form a line in the a–b space, $b = xa + y$. We can imagine that for all the points on the edge, if each of which corresponds to a straight line in the a–b space, then in theory, these lines must intersect at one and only one point (Figure 34.1b), which indicates the true slope and intercept of the edge.

Similarly, the problem of deriving the parameters that describe the parabola can be formulated in a three-dimensional (3D) parametric space of x_0–y_0–p as there are three unknown parameters:

$$y - y_0 = p(x - x_0)^2 \tag{34.2}$$

Each point on the parabola in the x–y space corresponds to a parabola in the x_0–y_0–p space. All the points on the parabola in the x–y space intersect at one point in the x_0–y_0–p space. In order to locate this intersection point in the parametric space, the idea of *accumulator array* is used in which the number of times that a certain pixel in the parametric space is "hit" by a transformed curve (line, parabola, etc.) is treated as the intensity of the pixel. Therefore, the value of the parameters can be derived based on the coordinates of the brightest pixel in the parametric space. The readers are referred to Reference 19 for details on how to implement this accumulator array.

The coordinates of the two brightest spot in the parametric space are used to describe the parabolic functions that form the lower boundaries of the breasts, as shown in Figures 34.2 and 34.3.

34.2.1.3 Segmentation Based on Feature Boundaries

Segmentation is based on three key points, the two armpits (P_L, P_R) derived from the left and right body boundaries by picking up the point where the largest curvature occurs and the intersection (O) of the two parabolic curves derived from the lower boundaries of the breasts/shadow of the breasts. The vertical line that goes through point O and is perpendicular to line $P_L P_R$ is the one used to separate the left and right breasts.

34.2.1.4 Experimental Results

The first set of testing images are obtained using the Inframetrics 600M camera, with a thermal sensitivity of 0.05 K. The images are collected at Elliott Mastology Center. Results from two testing images (*lr, nb*) are shown in Figure 34.2 that includes the intermediate results from edge detection, feature curve extraction, and segmentation. From the figure, we can see that Hough transform can derive the parabola at the accurate location.

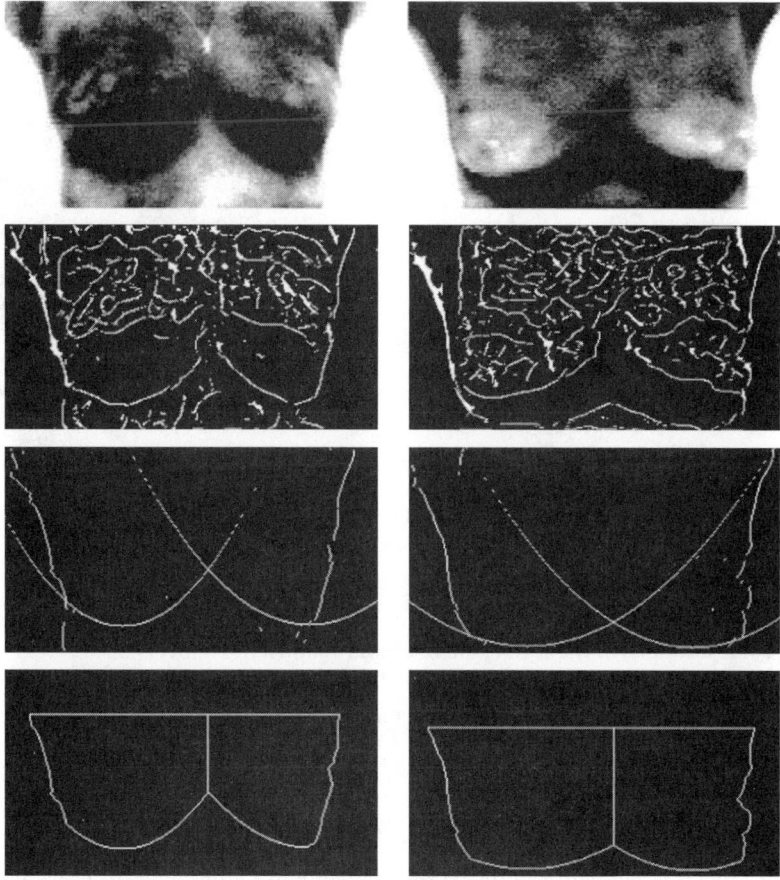

FIGURE 34.2 Segmentation results of two images. Left: results from *lr*. Right: results from *nb*. From top to bottom: original image, edge image, four feature curves, and segments. (Copyright 2005 IEEE.)

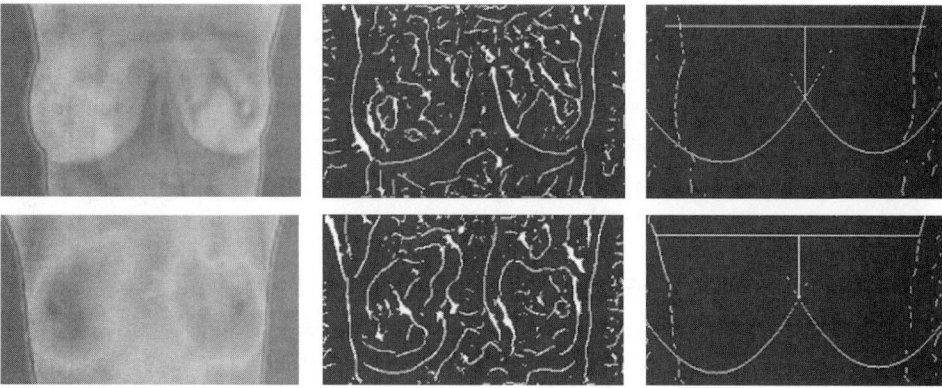

FIGURE 34.3 Hough transform-based image segmentation. Top: image of a patient with cancer. Bottom: image of a patient without cancer. From left to right: the original TIR image, the edge image using Canny edge detector, and the segmentation based on Hough transform. (Copyright 2005 IEEE.)

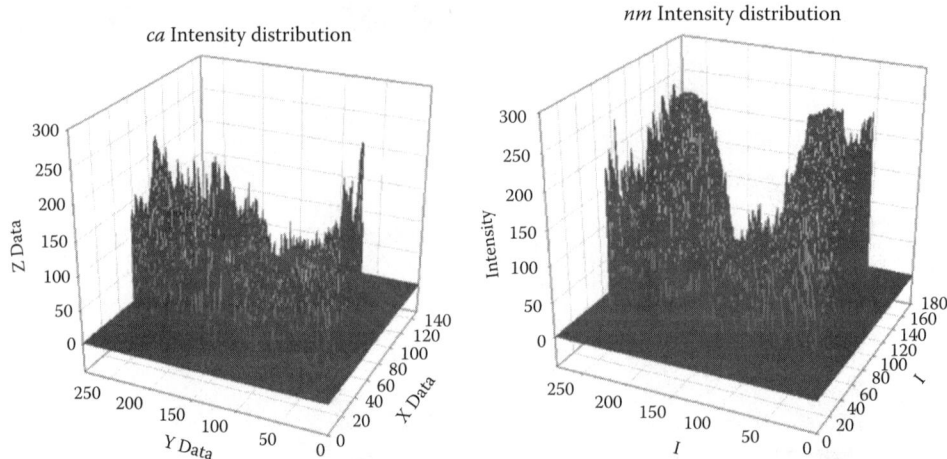

FIGURE 34.4 The left figure show the intensity distribution of a cancerous image and the right figure shows the same for a noncancerous image. The cancerous image is more asymmetrical than the noncancerous one.

Another set of images are obtained using Microbolometer uncooled camera, with a thermal sensitivity of 0.05 K. Some examples of the segmented images are shown in Figure 34.3.

Figure 34.4 shows the 3D histogram of the thermal distribution described in the intensity component of the cancerous (*ca*) and noncancerous (*nm*) images. From the graphs, we observe that the *ca* image is more asymmetrical than the *nm* image.

34.2.2 Asymmetry Identification by Unsupervised Learning

Pixel values in a thermogram represent the thermal radiation resulting from the heat emanating from the human body. Different tissues, organs, and vessels have different amount of radiation. Therefore, by observing the heat pattern, or in other words, the pattern of the pixel value, we should be able to discover the abnormalities if there are any.

Usually, in pattern classification algorithms, a set of training data are given to derive the decision rule. All the samples in the training set have been correctly classified. The decision rule is then applied to the testing data set where samples have not been classified yet. This classification technique is also called supervised learning. In unsupervised learning, however, data sets are not divided into training sets or testing sets. No *a priori* knowledge is known about which class each sample belongs to.

In asymmetry analysis, none of the pixels in the segment knows its class in advance, thus there will be no training set or testing set. Therefore, this is an unsupervised learning problem. We use *k*-means algorithm to do the initial clustering. *k*-Means algorithm is described as follows:

1. Begin with an arbitrary set of cluster centers and assign samples to nearest clusters
2. Compute the sample mean of each cluster
3. Reassign each sample to the cluster with the nearest mean
4. If the classification of all samples has not changed, then stop, else go to step 2

After each sample is relabeled to a certain cluster, the cluster mean can then be calculated. The segmented image can also be displayed in labeled format. From the difference of mean distribution, we can tell if there is any asymmetric abnormalities.

Figure 34.5 provides the histogram of pixel value from each segment that generated in Figure 34.2 with 10-bin setup. We can tell just from the shape of the histogram that *lr* is more asymmetric than *nb*. However, the histogram only reveals global information. Figure 34.6 displays the classification results for

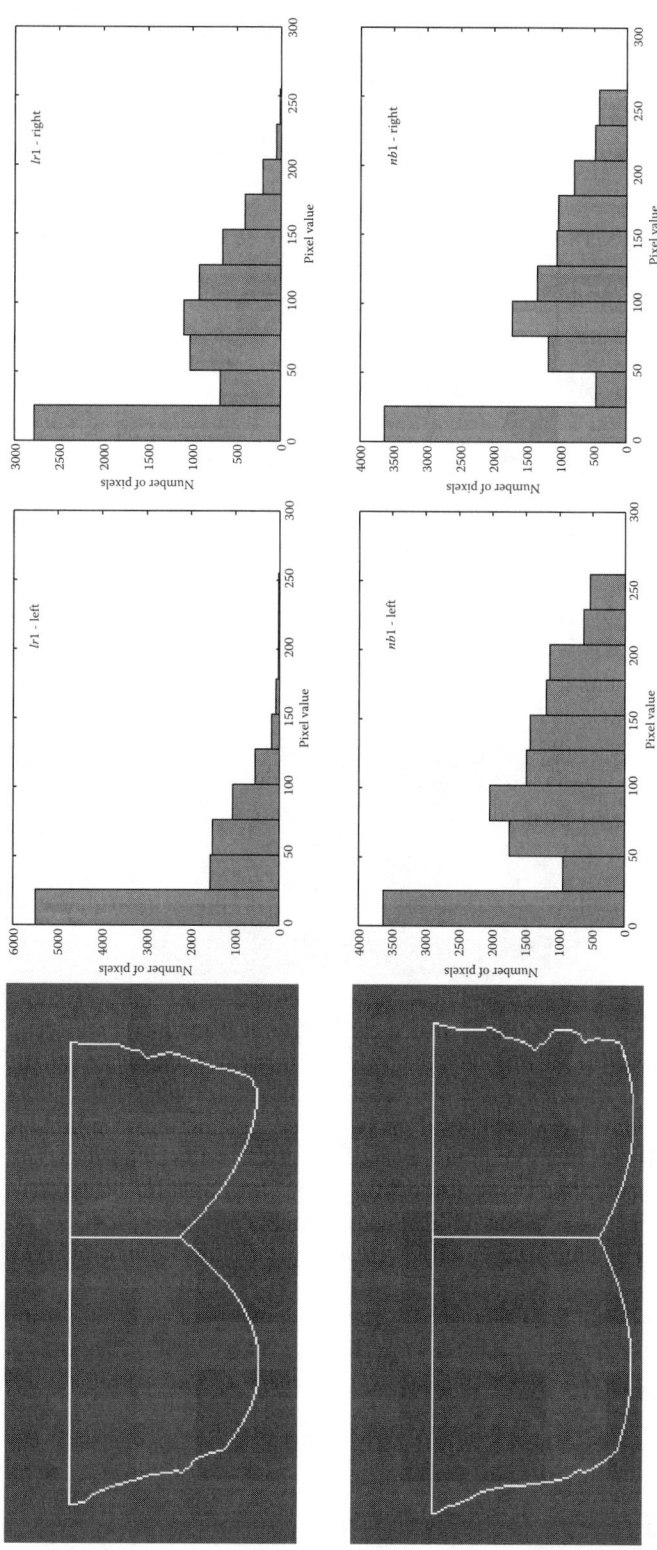

FIGURE 34.5 Histogram of the left and right segments. Top: results from *lr*. Bottom: results from *nb*. From left to right: the segments, histogram of the left segment, histogram of the right segment. (Copyright 2005 IEEE.)

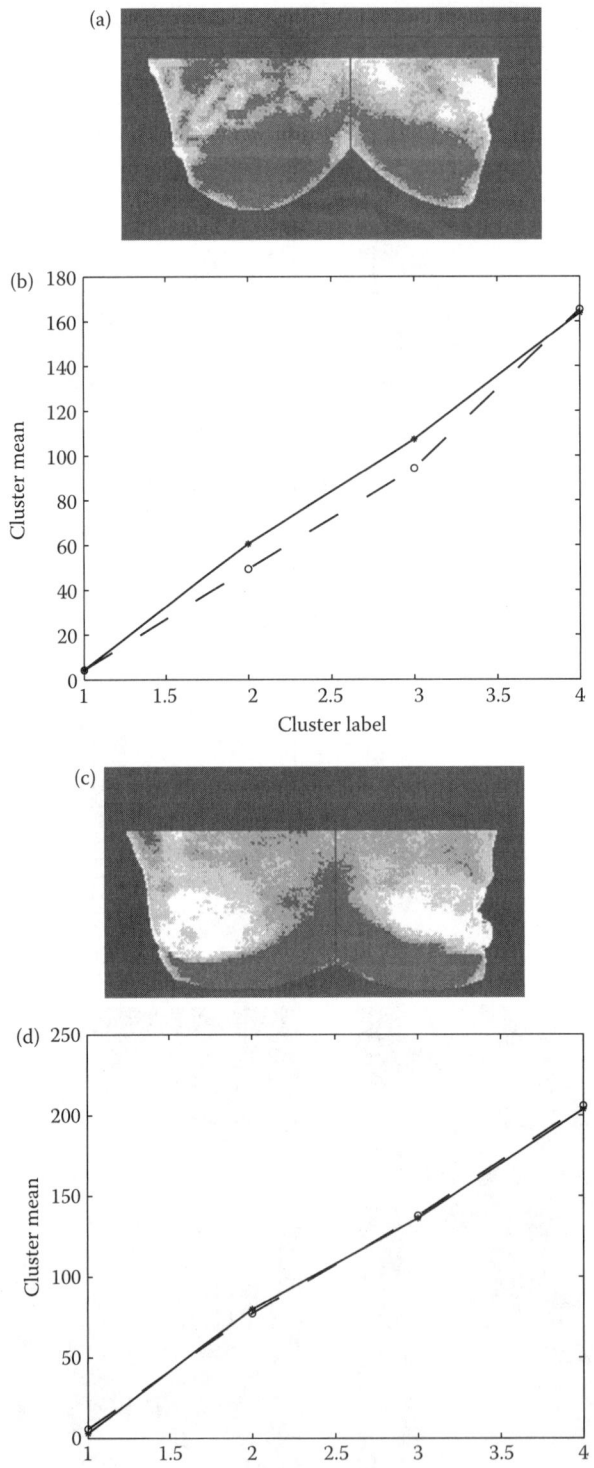

FIGURE 34.6 Labeled image and the profile of mean for each cluster. (a) Results from *lr*, (b) labeled image, (c) results from *nb*, and (d) average pixel value profile of each cluster. (Copyright 2005 IEEE.)

each segment in its labeled format. Here, we choose to use four clusters. The figure also shows the mean difference of each cluster in each segmented image. From Figure 34.6, we can clearly see the much bigger difference shown in the mean distribution or image *lr*, which can also be observed from the labeled image.

34.2.3 Asymmetry Identification Using Supervised Learning Based on Feature Extraction

Feature extraction is performed on the segmented images. The aim of this research is to identify the effectiveness of the features in contributing toward the asymmetry analysis.

As discussed earlier, TIR imaging is a functional imaging technique representing thermal information as a function of intensity. The TIR image is a pseudo-colored image with different colors assigned to different temperature ranges.

The distribution of different intensities can now be quantified by calculating some high-order statistics as feature elements. We design the following features to form the feature space:

- *Moments of the intensity image*: The intensity component of the image directly corresponds to the thermal energy distribution in the respective areas. The histogram describing the intensity distributions essentially describes the texture of the image. The moments of the histogram give statistical information about the texture of the image. Figure 34.5 shows the intensity distribution of images of a cancerous patient and noncancerous patient. The four moments, mean, variance, skewness, and kurtosis are taken as

$$\text{Mean } \mu = \frac{1}{N} \sum_{j=1}^{N} p_j \tag{34.3}$$

$$\text{Variance } \sigma^2 = \frac{1}{N-1} \sum_{j=1}^{N} (p_j - \mu)^2 \tag{34.4}$$

$$\text{Skewness} = \frac{1}{N} \sum_{j=1}^{N} \left[\frac{p_j - \mu}{\sigma} \right]^3 \tag{34.5}$$

$$\text{Kurtosis} = \frac{1}{N} \sum_{j=1}^{N} \left(\frac{p_j - \mu}{\sigma} \right)^4 \tag{34.6}$$

where p_j is the probability density of the *j*th bin in the histogram, and *N* is the total number of bins.

- *The peak pixel intensity of the correlated image*: The correlated image between the left and right (reflected) breasts is also a good indication of asymmetry. We use the peak intensity of the correlated image as a feature element since the higher the correlation value, the more symmetric the two breast segments.
- *Entropy*: Entropy measures the uncertainty of the information contained in the segmented images. The more equal the intensity distribution, the less information. Therefore, the segment with hot spots should have a lower entropy.

$$\text{Entropy } H(X) = -\sum_{j=1}^{N} p_j \log p_j \tag{34.7}$$

TABLE 34.1   Moments of the Histogram

	Cancerous		Noncancerous	
Moments	Left	Right	Left	Right
Mean	0.0010	0.0008	0.0012	0.0010
Variance (10^{-6})	2.0808	1.1487	3.3771	2.7640
Skewness (10^{-6})	2.6821	1.1507	4.8489	4.5321
Kurtosis (10^{-8})	1.0481	0.3459	2.1655	2.3641

- *Joint Entropy*: The higher the joint entropy between the left and right breast segments, the more symmetric they are supposedly to be, and the less possible of the existence of tumor.

$$\text{Joint Entropy } H(X,Y) = \sum_{i=1}^{N_X} \sum_{j=1}^{N_Y} p_{ij} \log(p_{ij}) \tag{34.8}$$

where p_{ij} is the joint probability density, N_X and N_Y are the number of bins of the intensity histogram of images X and Y, respectively.

From the set of features derived from the testing images, the existence of asymmetry is decided by calculating the ratio of the feature from the left segment to the feature from the right segment. The closer the value to 1, the more correlated the features or the less asymmetric the segments. Classic pattern classification techniques like the maximum posterior probability and the kNN classification [22] can be used for the automatic classification of the images. Table 34.1 describes the typical moments for the cancerous and noncancerous images.

The typical values of the cancerous images and noncancerous images are tabulated in Table 34.2. The asymmetry can be clearly stated with a close observation of the given feature values. We used six normal patient thermograms and 18 cancer patient thermograms. With a larger database, a training feature set can be derived and supervised learning algorithms such as discriminant function or kNN classification can be implemented for a fast, effective, and automated classification.

Figure 34.7 evaluates the effectiveness of the features used. The first data point along the *x*-axis indicates *entropy*, the second to the fifth points indicate the four statistical moments (*means, variance, skewness,* and *kurtosis*). The *y*-axis shows the *closeness* metric we defined as

$$\text{Bilateral ratio closeness to } 1 = \left| \frac{\text{feature value from left segment}}{\text{feature value from right segment}} - 1 \right| \tag{34.9}$$

From the figure, we observe that the high-order statistics are the most effective features to measure the asymmetry, while low-order statistics (*mean*) and *entropy* do not assist asymmetry detection.

TABLE 34.2   Entropy and Correlation Values

Feature	Cancerous	Noncancerous
Correlation	$\times 10^8$	2.35719×10^8
Joint entropy	9.0100	17.5136
Entropy		
Left	1.52956	1.70684
Right	1.3033	1.4428

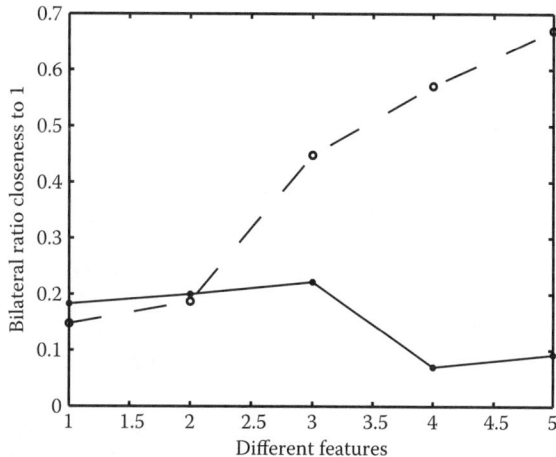

FIGURE 34.7 Performance evaluation of different feature elements. Solid line: noncancerous image; dashed line: cancerous image. The five data points along the *x*-axis indicate (from left to right): entropy, mean, variance, skewness, and kurtosis. (Copyright 2005 IEEE.)

34.3 Conclusions

This chapter develops a computer-aided approach for automating asymmetry analysis of thermograms. This kind of approach will help the diagnostics as a useful second opinion. The use of TIR images for breast cancer detection and the advantages of thermograms over traditional mammograms are studied. From the experimental results, it can be observed that the Hough transform can be effectively used for breast segmentation. We propose two pattern classification algorithms, the unsupervised learning using k-means and the supervised learning using kNN based on feature extraction. Experimental results show that feature extraction is a valuable approach to extract the signatures of asymmetry, especially the joint entropy. With a larger database, supervised pattern classification techniques can be used to attain more accurate classification. These kind of diagnostic aids, especially in a disease such as breast cancer where the reason for the occurrence is not totally known, will reduce the false-positive diagnosis rate and increase the survival rate among the patients since the early diagnosis of the disease is more curable than in a later stage.

References

1. Llyod-Williams, K. and Handley, R.S., Infrared thermometry in the diagnosis of breast disease. *Lancet*, 2, 1378–1381, 1961.
2. Keyserlingk, J.R., Ahlgren, P.D., Yu, E., Belliveau, N., and Yassa, M., Functional infrared imaging of the breast. *IEEE Engineering in Medicine and Biology*, 19, 30–41, 2000.
3. Jones B.F., A reappraisal of the use of infrared thermal image analysis in medicine. *IEEE Transactions on Medical Imaging*, 17, 1019–1027, 1998.
4. Thermology, http://www.thermology.com/history.htm
5. Ng, E.Y.K. and Sudarshan, N.M., Numerical computation as a tool to aid thermographic interpretation. *Journal of Medical Engineering and Technology*, 25, 53–60, 2001.
6. Oslen, O. and Gotzsche, P.C., Cochrane review on screening for breast cancer with mammography. *Lancet*, 9290, 1340–1342, 2001.
7. Hay, G.A., *Medical Image: Formation, Perception and Measurement*. The Institute of Physics, John Wiley & Sons, New York, NY, 1976.

8. Watmough, D.J., The role of thermographic imaging in breast screening, discussion by C.R. Hill. In *Medical Images: Formation, Perception and Measurement, 7th L H Gray Conference: Medical Images*, pp. 142–158, 1976.

9. Gautheire, M., *Atlas of breast thermography with specific guidelines for examination and interpretation.* Milan, Italy, PAPUSA, 1989.

10. Ng, E.Y.K., Ung, L.N., Ng, F.C., and Sim, L.S.J., Statistical analysis of healthy and malignant breast thermography. *Journal of Medical Engineering and Technology*, 25, 253–263, 2001.

11. Good, W.F., Zheng, B., Chang, Y. et al., Generalized procrustean image deformation for subtraction of mammograms. In *Proceedings of SPIE Medical Imaging—Image Processing*, Vol. 3661, pp. 1562–1573, San Diego, CA, SPIE, 1999.

12. Shen, L., Shen, Y.P., Rangayyan, R.M., and Desautels J., Measures of asymmetry in mammograms based upon shape spectrum. In *Proceedings of the Annual Conference on EMB*, Vol. 15, pp. 48–49, San Diego, CA, 1993.

13. Yin, F.F., Giger, M.L., Doi, K. et al., Computerized detection of masses in digital mammograms: Analysis of bilateral subtraction images. *Medical Physics*, 18, 955–963, 1991.

14. Yin, F.F., Giger, M.L., Doi, K. et al., Computerized detection of masses in digital mammograms: Automated alignment of breast images and its effect on bilateral-subtraction technique. *Medical Physics*, 21, 445–452, 1994.

15. Yin, F.F., Giger, Vyborny C.J. et al., Comparison of bilateral-subtraction and single-image processing techniques in the computerized detection of mammographic masses. *Investigative Radiology*, 6, 473–481, 1993.

16. Zheng, B., Chang, Y.H., and Gur, D., Computerized detection of masses from digitized mammograms: Comparison of single-image segmentation and bilateral image subtraction. *Academic Radiology*, 2, 1056–1061, 1995.

17. Head J.F., Lipari, C.C., and Elliott R.L., Computerized image analysis of digitized infrared images of the breasts from a scanning infrared imaging system. In *Proceedings of the 1998 Conference on Infrared Technology and Applications XXIV, Part I*, Vol. 3436, pp. 290–294, San Diego, CA, SPIE, 1998.

18. Lipari C.A. and Head J.F., Advanced infrared image processing for breast cancer risk assessment. In *Proceedings for 19th International Conference of IEEE/EMBS*, pp. 673–676, Chicago, IL, Oct. 30–Nov. 2. IEEE, 1997.

19. Snyder, W.E. and Qi, H., *Machine Vision*, Cambridge University Press, New York, 2004.

20. Canny, J., A computational approach to edge detection. *IEEE Transactions on Pattern Analysis and Machine Intelligence*, 6, 679–698, 1995.

21. Jafri M.Z. and Deravi, F., Efficient algorithm for the detection of parabolic curves. In *Vision Geometry III*, Vol. 2356, pp. 53–62, SPIE, 1998.

22. Duda, R.O., Hart, P.E., and Strok, D.G., *Pattern Classification*, 2nd ed. John Wiley & Sons, New York, NY, 2001.

35

Application of Nonparametric Windows in Estimating the Mutual Information between Bilateral Breasts in Thermograms

M. Etehadtavakol
Isfahan University of Medical Science

E.Y.K. Ng
Nanyang Technological University

Caro Lucas
University of Tehran

S. Sadri
Isfahan University of Technology

Isfahan University of Medical Science

N. Gheissari
Isfahan University of Technology

Isfahan University of Medical Science

35.1 Preamble

All things in the universe radiate infrared radiation as a function of their temperature [1]. The surface temperature of the human body is influenced by the level of blood perfusion which directs the infrared radiation from the skin. The variations in temperature can be captured by a sensitive infrared (IR) camera [2]. Cancerous cells send signals to the surrounding normal host tissue by which certain genes in the host tissue can make some proteins that can develop new blood vessels [3]. The cells are shown as hot spots in the thermal images.

Since symmetry is usually a sign of healthy subjects [4], an asymmetrical temperature distribution between the right breast and the left breast could be a sign of abnormality [5–10]. Studies have shown that some factors such as environmental stresses and genetic mutations would affect individuals and consequently the homeostatic mechanisms that preserve the symmetry of paired structures such as the breast tend to demote [11]. There are also studies concerning the relationships between asymmetry and hormonal concentrations. Estrogen is extremely essential in the development and growth of the breast. An individual's ability to tolerate disruptive hormonal variations can affect the symmetrical breast development [12]. Consequently, an increase in the unstable asymmetry of paired structures could be a sign of poor health.

The mutual information (MI) is a similarity measure that can be used to indicate the temperature distribution similarity between the two breast IR images. In order to estimate it, the joint PDF of the two IR breast images and the marginal PDF of each breast IR image are required.

Nonparametric (NP) windows are signal densities and distribution estimators that are based on the Shannon–Whittaker–Nyquist theory of sampled signals. It estimates signal statistics by directly calculating each piecewise section of the signal. Interpolation and smoothing are performed in the signal domain rather than in the probability domain. The advantages of NP windows make the technique attractive to estimate MI. NP windows are applied to estimate the joint distribution and consequently the joint intensity histogram of image pairs.

35.2 Mutual Information

Information has a broad concept. When any probability distribution entropy is defined, it has many properties that agree with the notion of measuring information [13].

The MI can be defined as the relative entropy between the joint distribution and the product distribution.

$$MI(x, y) = \sum_{x \in X} \sum_{y \in Y} p(x, y) \log \frac{p(x, y)}{p(x)p(y)} \tag{35.1}$$

MI is a nonlinear measure and it can be used to measure both linear and nonlinear correlations [14]. Independent component analysis [15,16], registration of remote sensing [17], and medical images [18] are some of its applications.

In this chapter, the similarity between the two breast images is measured by calculating the MI which is a similarity measure of intensity between the two regions.

When a tumor is initiated, its growth can be described by a separate mathematical function or a stochastic process model. The tumor growth function starting from a single cell may be described by a simple logistic cell kinetic function predicting the volume of cells viable in the tumor as a logistic function. For example, a gamma-distributed mixture of exponential tumor growth functions [19]. As a result, the variations of the right and the left breasts' IR images are due to the cancerous cells that are comparatively nonlinear. Consequently, the MI technique for the detection of the asymmetry between the two breasts becomes very useful.

Estimation of MI can be difficult which has been a common problem in many MI applications and this estimation sometimes is unreliable, noisy, and even biased.

Parametric and NP approaches are the two basic approaches for the estimation of MI. In NP approaches, the form of the function is not given and the estimation techniques include nearest neighbor, histogram-based, adaptive partitioning, spline, and kernel density [20].

In parametric estimation, it is assumed that the data belong to a given density function and the form of the density function is given. In this study, the accuracy of the estimated MI is important and it is estimated from the joint intensity histogram of the image pair.

The joint intensity histogram can be described as a two-dimensional (2D) histogram of combinational intensity pairs, I1, I2, where I1 and I2 denote the intensity level (0–255) of image 1 and image 2, respectively. Traditionally, histograms are built-up by using each intensity sample to populate the histogram bin. The limitation of the quantization of intensity and the number of intensity samples available to populate the histogram is a disadvantage of this method. For example, the number of bins are limited with too few samples and consequently an under populated histogram is resulted, so that usable MI values are not achievable from such a histogram.

To avoid under-populated histograms, several algorithms have been proposed [21–25]. For this achievement, the number of bins in the histogram and also an appropriate kernel size are needed. Practically, there are some limitations for estimating the joint histogram.

By proposing NP windows, Kadir and Brady solved this problem [26,27]. NP is a technique which is established by the Shannon–Whittaker–Nyquist theory of the sampled signal. For a given interpolation model, signal density and distribution are estimated by directly calculating the distribution of each piecewise section of a signal. In this technique, interpolation or smoothing is accomplished in the signal domain and not in the probability domain which is contrary to the previous methods. The benefits of NP windows make it appropriate for the estimation of MI [28].

By using the joint PDF of the two breast images with their respective intensities i_1 and i_2, the MI between the two breast images can be obtained as Equation 35.2

$$MI = \sum_{i_1}\sum_{i_2} p_{f_1 f_2}(i_1,i_2) \log \frac{p_{f_1 f_2}(i_1,i_2)}{p_{f_1}(i_1)p_{f_2}(i_2)} \qquad (35.2)$$

$p_{f_1 f_2}$ denotes the joint PDF of f_1 and f_2. The marginal PDFs are $p_{f_1} = \sum_{i_2} p_{f_1 f_2}$ and $p_{f_2} = \sum_{i_1} p_{f_1 f_2}$. The finite bin size of the histogram from which $p_{f_1 f_2}$ is calculated can be indicated by discrete variables i_1 and i_2. Bin size is inversely proportional to the number of bins in the histogram.

35.3 Nonparametric Windows to Estimate the Joint Histogram for a Pair of Images

In this study, two interpolation methods are investigated; bilinear interpolation and half-bilinear interpolation.

35.3.1 Bilinear Interpolation

Bilinear interpolation can be regarded as the intuitive generalization of the one-dimensional linearly interpolated signal to the two-dimensional form. The linear interpolation is accomplished in one direction first and then again in the other direction. Suppose, the value of the unknown function f at the point $m = (x,y)$ is derived, the values of f at the four points are assumed to be $f_1, f_2, f_3,$ and f_4.

The following equations are obtained by doing the linear interpolation in the X direction as shown in Figure 35.1.

$$f(R_1) = \frac{x_1 - x}{x_1 - x_2} f_1 + \frac{x_2 - x}{x_2 - x_1} f_2 \qquad (35.3)$$

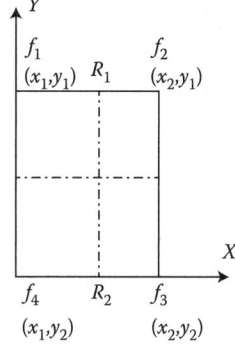

FIGURE 35.1 f at the four points (x_1,y_1), (x_2,y_2), (x_3,y_3), and (x_4,y_4) are $f_1, f_2, f_3,$ and f_4, respectively and are known values. The desired point for interpolation is $m = (x,y)$.

$$f(R_2) = \frac{x_1 - x}{x_1 - x_2} f_4 + \frac{x_2 - x}{x_2 - x_1} f_3 \tag{35.4}$$

Then, interpolating in the Y direction we obtain Equation 35.5

$$f(m) = \frac{y_1 - y}{y_1 - y_2} f(R_1) + \frac{y_2 - y}{y_1 - y_2} f(R_2) \tag{35.5}$$

$$f(m) = \frac{y_1 - y}{y_1 - y_2}\left(\frac{x_1 - x}{x_1 - x_2} f_1 + \frac{x_2 - x}{x_2 - x_1} f_2\right)$$
$$+ \frac{y_2 - y}{y_1 - y_2}\left(\frac{x_1 - x}{x_1 - x_2} f_4 + \frac{x_2 - x}{x_2 - x_1} f_3\right) \tag{35.6}$$

A coordinate system in which the four points are (0,0), (0,1), (1,0), and (1,1) may be chosen, then the interpolant can be obtained as

$$f(p) = axy + bx + cy + d \tag{35.7}$$

For a pair of two-dimensional images and by applying the bilinear interpolation, we obtain Equations 35.8 and 35.9.

$$f_1 = a_1 x_1 x_2 + b_1 x_1 + c_1 x_2 + d_1 \tag{35.8}$$

$$f_2 = a_2 x_1 x_2 + b_2 x_1 + c_2 x_2 + d_2 \tag{35.9}$$

The probability of f can be developed by using the transformation formula. It depends on the absolute value of the gradient x with respect to f (Jacobian) [29]

$$p_f(f) = \left|\frac{\partial x}{\partial f}\right| p_x(x(f)) \tag{35.10}$$

The joint probability is derived as Equation 35.11 for this case.

$$p_f(f_1, f_2) = \left|\det(J_{x \circ f})\right| p_x(x(X)) \tag{35.11}$$

The Jacobian is also acquired as Equation 35.12

$$\left|\det J_{xof}\right| = [(b_2 c_1 - b_1 c_2 + a_2(d_1 - f_1) - a_1(d_2 - f_2))^2$$
$$- 4(a_2 c_1 - a_1 c_2)(b_2(d_1 - f_1) - b_1(d_2 - f_2))]^{-\frac{1}{2}} \tag{35.12}$$

A polygon bounded by four edges is the valid region for this PDF. The total probability over a particular bin covered by the polygon is achieved by integrating Equation 35.12 directly to determine the histogram.

Integration of $|\det(J_{x\circ f})|$ is almost unworkable as it is shown in Equation 35.13. However, if the half-bilinear interpolation which is illustrated in the following section is applied, an estimation of the histogram would be possible.

$$\rho = k_1\sqrt{\phi(f_1,2)} + \phi(f_1)(k_2 + \log[\phi(f_1) + k_3\sqrt{\phi(f_1,2)}]) + k_4\log[\phi(f_1)]$$
$$+ k_5\sqrt{\phi(f_1,2)}] + k_6\log\left[\frac{\phi(f_1) + k_7\sqrt{\phi(f_1,2)}}{\phi(f_1)}\right]$$

(35.13)

35.3.2 Half-Bilinear Interpolation

Suppose the value of the unknown function f at the point $m = (x,y)$ is derived assuming that $f_1, f_2,$ and f_3 are known and are the values of f at the three points (x_1,y_1), (x_2,y_2), and (x_3,y_3), respectively are indicated in Figure 35.2.

A_1, A_2, and A_3 are areas of triangle f_2pf_3, triangle f_1pf_3, and triangle f_1pf_2, respectively, are defined in Equations 35.14 through 35.16.

$$A_1 = \frac{1}{2}\det\begin{bmatrix} x & x_2 & x_3 \\ y & y_2 & y_3 \\ 1 & 1 & 1 \end{bmatrix}$$

(35.14)

$$A_2 = \frac{1}{2}\det\begin{bmatrix} x & x_1 & x_3 \\ y & y_1 & y_3 \\ 1 & 1 & 1 \end{bmatrix}$$

(35.15)

$$A_3 = \frac{1}{2}\det\begin{bmatrix} x & x_1 & x_2 \\ y & y_1 & y_2 \\ 1 & 1 & 1 \end{bmatrix}$$

(35.16)

$$A = \frac{1}{2}\det\begin{bmatrix} x_1 & x_2 & x_3 \\ y_1 & y_2 & y_3 \\ 1 & 1 & 1 \end{bmatrix}$$

(35.17)

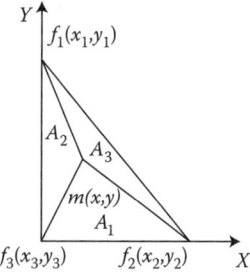

FIGURE 35.2 f at the three points (x_1,y_1), (x_2,y_2), and (x_3,y_3) are $f_1, f_2,$ and f_3, respectively which are known values. The desired point for interpolation is $m = (x,y)$.

$$f(m) = \frac{A_1}{A} f_1 + \frac{A_2}{A} f_2 + \frac{A_3}{A} f_3 \tag{35.18}$$

$$f(m) = ax + by + c \tag{35.19}$$

If the cross-term of Equation 35.7 is removed from the bilinear interpolant, Equation 35.19 would be obtained. Only three basis samples (α, β, γ) are required because there are only three coefficients in Equation 35.20 which must be computed. Their relation yields

$$\begin{pmatrix} a \\ b \\ c \end{pmatrix} = \begin{pmatrix} -1 & 1 & 0 \\ 0 & -1 & 1 \\ 1 & 0 & 0 \end{pmatrix} \begin{pmatrix} \alpha \\ \beta \\ \gamma \end{pmatrix} \tag{35.20}$$

The interpolated intensity $f(x_1, x_2)$ for an image is depicted in Figure 35.3, where dark indicates low intensity and light indicates high intensity.

Suppose we have two images instead of one image. For the images, the image lattice may be separated to neighbors of regular 45° right-angled nonoverlapping triangles.

Assuming that the basis samples lay on the triangle ($\alpha \beta \gamma$) where β is 90° angle. If for a pair of images the half-bilinear interpolation is applied, the following functions would be derived:

$$f_1 = a_1 x_1 + b_1 x_2 + c_1 \tag{35.21}$$

$$f_2 = a_2 x_1 + b_2 x_2 + c_2 \tag{35.22}$$

The inverse functions are obtained as Equations 35.23 and 35.24

$$x = \frac{c_1 b_2 - b_1 c_2 - b_2 f_1 + b_1 f_2}{b_1 a_2 - a_1 b_2} \tag{35.23}$$

$$y = \frac{c_1 a_2 - a_1 c_2 - a_2 f_1 + a_1 f_2}{-b_1 a_2 + a_1 b_2} \tag{35.24}$$

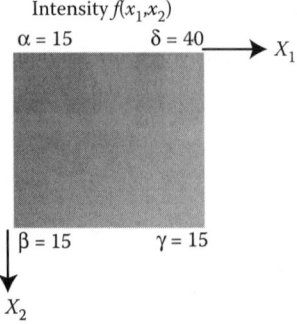

FIGURE 35.3 An example of interpolated image ($f(x_1, x_2)$) light shade indicates high intensity and dark shade indicates low intensity.

and then the Jacobian is given as Equation 35.25

$$\det(J_{x \circ f}) = \begin{vmatrix} \dfrac{\partial x_1}{\partial f_1} & \dfrac{\partial x_1}{\partial f_2} \\[2ex] \dfrac{\partial x_2}{\partial f_1} & \dfrac{\partial x_2}{\partial f_2} \end{vmatrix} = \dfrac{1}{|a_1 b_2 - b_1 a_2|} \tag{35.25}$$

According to the standard probability theory, the joint probability distribution of a pair of two-dimensional signals with transformation yields

$$p_f(f_1, f_2) = \left| \det(J_{x \circ f}) \right| p_x(x(X)) \tag{35.26}$$

and it demonstrates that the absolute determinant of the Jacobian for a pair of basis sample triplets is constant. In addition, the area of the triangle given by (α_1, α_2), (β_1, β_2), and (γ_1, γ_2) is described as Equation 35.27.

$$\frac{1}{2}\left[(\beta_1 - \alpha_1)(\gamma_2 - \beta_2) - (\gamma_1 - \beta_1)(\beta_2 - \alpha_2)\right] = \frac{1}{2}(a_1 b_2 - b_1 a_2) \tag{35.27}$$

Multiplying this area by the probability within the triangle accompanies to 1/2. It is an unsurprised value, because only half a pixel has been calculated.

Suppose we have a cell of four basis samples $(\alpha_1, \beta_1, \gamma_1, \delta_1)$ and $(\alpha_2, \beta_2, \gamma_2, \delta_2)$. By each neighborhood (a single pair of triangles), the PDF contribution is constant and bounded within a triangle. Accordingly, the vertex coordinating in the joint PDF are the intensity values in the two images.

First, the individual contribution of each neighborhood is weighted to normalize it and then the results are aggregated to determine the overall PDF. The smaller triangle possesses a higher weighting and the probability over each triangle aggregates to 1/2. They are depicted in Figure 35.4.

Two special cases may occur geometrically: the triangle yields a line and the triangle yields a point. The three possible cases are demonstrated in Figure 35.5.

Since the probability value within the regions of integration is always constant. Hence, the integral corresponds to calculating three cases: an area for triangles and a length for lines, and a value for points. It takes the value of one for points. Assuming that the vertices of one of the triangles are shown in Figure 35.6a.

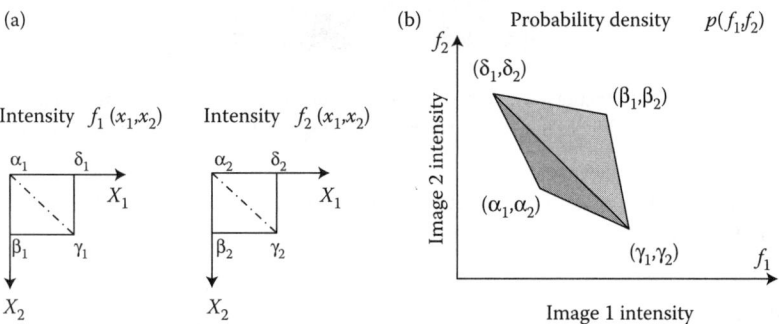

FIGURE 35.4 (a) Two images with $f_1(x_1, x_2)$ and $f_2(x_1, x_2)$ intensities. (b) Triangles of uniform probability in the joint PDF of intensity, for each triangle, the probability must integrate to one, the smaller triangle possesses a higher weight, and the vertices of the two triangles are matching the intensity values in part (a).

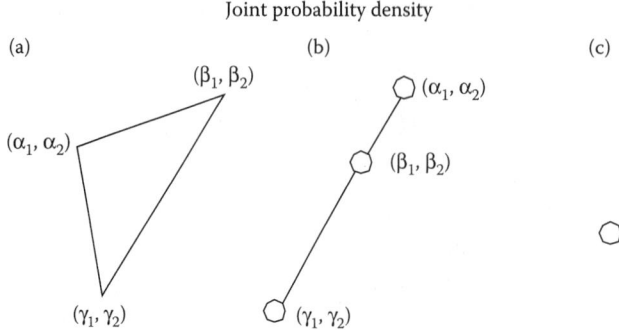

FIGURE 35.5 Three possible cases occur for joint half-bilinear interpolation image. (a) A triangle, (b) a line and (c) a point.

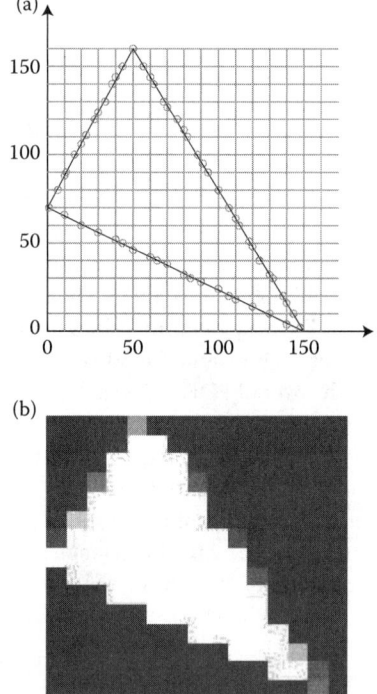

FIGURE 35.6 (a) Example of a triangle with circles indicating the intersection of the triangle sides and bin boundaries. (b) The proportional coverage of the triangle over each histogram bin is obtained and cumulatively added.

We suggest an algorithm in order to calculate the proportional coverage of the triangle over each histogram bin. It consists of the following steps:

Step 1. The intersections of the sides of the triangles with bin boundaries (they are depicted by circles) are found.

Step 2. The inside region from the outside region of the triangle is separated (zero code for inside region and one for outside region).

Step 3. Regions with code one come into the polygon shape in different bins and the vertices for each bin are found.

Step 4. Vertices are ordered in counter clockwise.

Step 5. For each bin the area of the polygon is calculated.

Step 6. The area of the polygon for each bin is divided by the area of the triangle.

In the above example, the result is shown in Figure 35.6b.

The histogram is an image whose bins are individual pixels and the probability in each bin is the image intensity.

35.4 Experimental Results

In the following experiments, we applied the MI algorithm on 60 breast-simulated images which are in six groups. For instance, image *a* is the real image of a patient's right breast which is accessible by the Sunstate Thermal Imaging Center in Australia [30]. Simulated images *b* through *f* are retained as follows: mirroring image *a*, image *b* is achieved. Images *c* through *f* are retained by sequential color changes to the preceding images. By pseudo-color algorithms, the main output images of IR cameras which are gray-scale images are transformed to RGB images. The map of the heat profile is experimentally evident by inspecting the real color images, so that it is possible to detect low-temperature parts from the high-temperature parts. Fittingly, in our simulated images, we have tried to simulate the color changes in one breast in comparison with the other one just for the hotter parts. In consonance with natural phenomena, the changes between the sequential images are kept small. In each step, the MI between the pairs of real image *a* and image *b* through *f* is calculated. In this way we study the power of MI technique for monitoring sequential images of a patient. One image from each group is depicted in Figure 35.7 and their matching, calculated, and normalized MI values are presented in Table 35.1.

As it is shown in Table 35.1, the more similar the IR image of the right breast to the IR image of the left breast, the closer will be the normalized MI value which is equal to 1. Means and standard deviations for each group of simulated images are shown in Table 35.2. The standard deviation and the mean of the MI between the pairs of real image *a* and image *b* through *f* are provided bold in Table 35.2. The mean of abnormal and also normal cases are provided bold in Table 35.3.

Estimated normalized MI value of an investigated patient, as an additional feature, may be then fed into a trained classification system such as support vector machine to achieve more reliable and more authentic results to identify malignant anomalies in breast thermograms. Furthermore, the regions of interest can be different matching quadrants of each breast.

35.5 The Algorithm for Real Case Issue

In the recommended protocols for the measurement of the human body temperature [31–34], all the instrumental setup, environmental control, patients' preparation, and data-collecting procedures performed should follow the recommended guidelines [31–33], relevant standards, and protocols in clinical thermographic imaging [34]. This practice is to minimize as much as possible those potential background uncertainties which may affect the false-positive prediction.

In practice, most of the real IR breast images which are accommodated under the standard protocol of IR screening contrasting our simulated images do not have symmetry boundaries. This phenomenon can be studied in real images that are used in this study. These real images are provided by Sunstate Thermal Imaging Center in Australia [30].

Therefore, a registration for two breasts is required for real images. Applying shape contexts, an approach was proposed by Belongie and Malik [35]. In this study, the algorithm follows the below-mentioned steps:

1. Correspondences between the points on the boundaries on the two breasts are solved.
2. The correspondences are used to estimate an aligning transform (mapping function). The procedures have been shown in Figures 35.8 and 35.9.

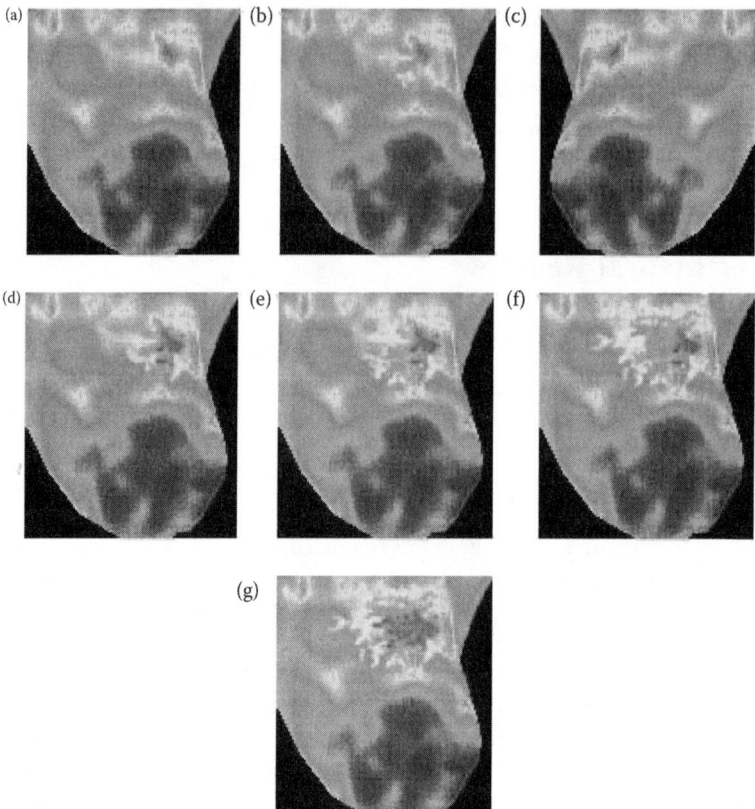

FIGURE 35.7 One image from each group. (a) Real right breast, (b) simulated left breast, (c) simulated left breast with small changes with respect to b, (d) simulated left breast with small changes with respect to c, (e) simulated left breast with small changes with respect to d, (f) simulated left breast with small changes with respect to e, (g) simulated left breast with small changes with respect to f.

TABLE 35.1 Normalized Mutual Information Values Corresponding to the Images of Figure 35.7

A,f	A,e	A,d	A,c	A,b	A,g	Images
0.9475	0.9585	0.9615	0.9833	1	0.9189	Normalized mutual information

TABLE 35.2 Means and Standard Deviations for Six Groups of Simulated Images

A,f		A,e		A,d		A,c		A,b		A,g		Images
SD	Mean	SD	Mean	SD	SD	SD	SD	SD	Mean	SD	Mean	Normalized mutual information
0.0838	0.9351	0.0701	0.9531	0.0681	0.0539	0.0574	0.0539	0.0539	1	0.0539	0.9183	

TABLE 35.3 Means and Standard Deviations for Normal and Abnormal Simulated Images along with *P*-Value

Normal Mean ± SD	Abnormal Mean ± SD	*P*-Value
0.9829 ± 0.0139	**0.9355** ± 0.0153	0.0294

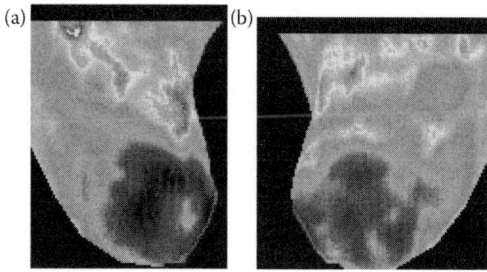

FIGURE 35.8   Original images (a) left breast, (b) right breast.

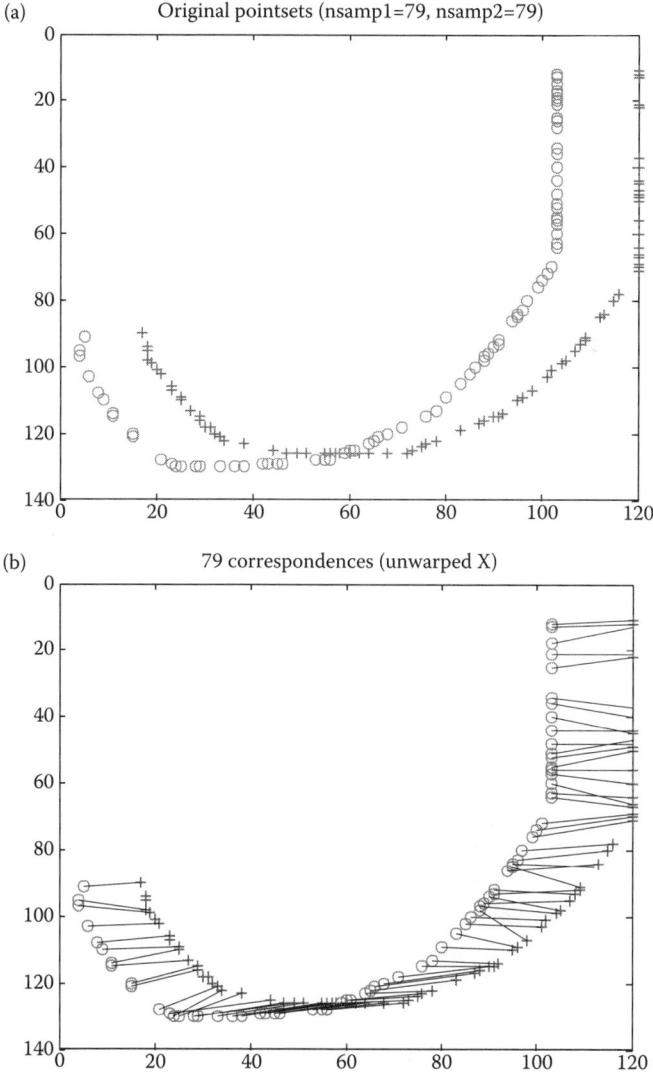

FIGURE 35.9   (a) Boundary samples of right breast (+), boundary samples of left breast (o), (b) unwarped boundaries, (c) warped boundaries, (d) boundaries of the two breasts after employing the mapping function.

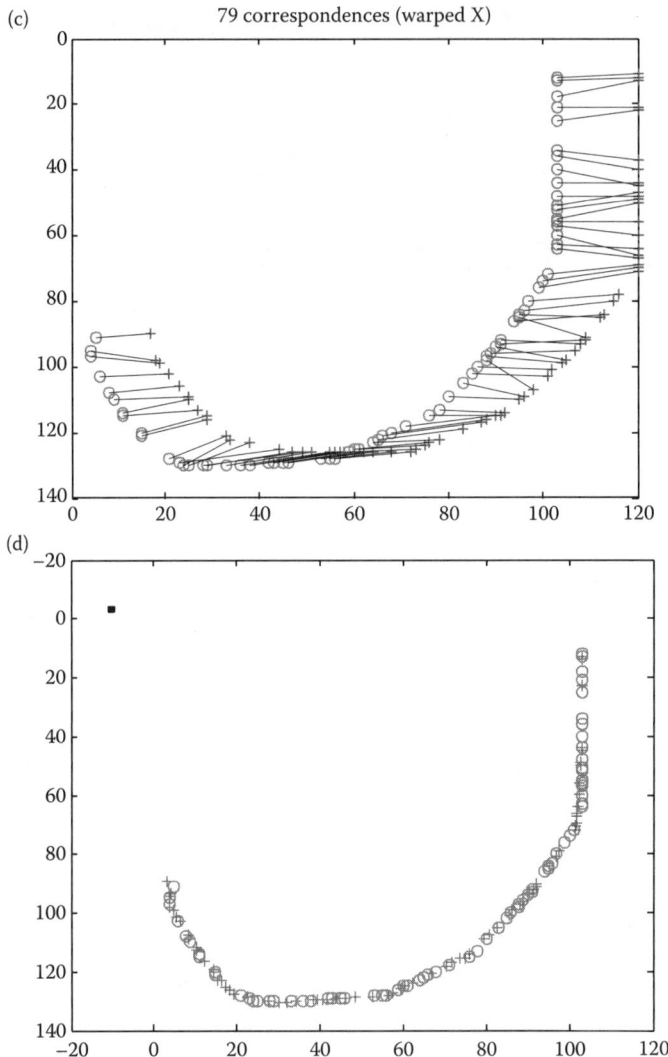

FIGURE 35.9   (Continued.)

3. Calculated mapping function of boundary points is used to map the interior points of the breasts. In digital images, the discrete picture elements, or pixels, are restricted to lie on a sampling grid, taken to be in an integer lattice. The output grid does not generally coincide with the integer lattice. Rather, the positions of the grid points may take on any of the continuous values that are allocated by the mapping function.

   Consequently, an interpolation must be presented to fit a continuous surface through the input data samples. The continuous surface may then be sampled at noninteger positions of the output grid. The accuracy of the interpolation has a significant influence on the quality of the output image.

4. Cubic spline for interpolation is used to determine the R, G, B amounts of the output grid appropriately.

The algorithm is implemented for 15 normal and nine abnormal cases. Results are shown in Table 35.4.

TABLE 35.4 Means and Standard Deviations for Normal and Abnormal Real Cases

Normalized Mutual Information	Normal	Abnormal
Mean	0.9601	0.9249
Standard deviation	0.0167	0.0354

35.6 Conclusion

Symmetry of the two breasts is usually a sign of a healthy breast. Collation between contra-lateral breast images is one of the impressive methods in breast cancer detection. Unhealthy breasts have asymmetric temperature distribution.

The MI is a measure that grasps linear and nonlinear dependencies, without demanding the specification of any kind of model of dependence. Hence, it is appropriate for our investigation. We applied NP windows to estimate the MI.

Although NP windows is a computationally expensive technique, it does not demand parameters such as prior selection of a kernel. It obtains accurate histograms since it coordinates an interpolation model which enhances the resolution to a highly oversampled image.

For our determination, we used 60 simulated breast thermal images. Experimental results indicate that the more similar the thermal image of the left breast to the thermal image of the right breast, the closer will be the normalized MI value equal to 1. Hence, we are capable of capturing very small dissimilarities between the two breasts. Future work could be focusing on the different regions of interest such as the different matching quadrants of each breast.

References

1. R. Siegel, J. R. Howell, *Thermal Radiation Heat Transfer*, Hemisphere, Washington, DC, 1992.
2. J. M. Barreiro, F. M. Sanchez, V. Maojo, F. Sanz, *Biological and Medical Data Analysis, 5th International Symposium*, Barcelona, Spain, Springer, November 18–19, 2004.
3. Y. Singh, Tumor angiogenesis: Clinical implications, *Nepal Journal of Neuroscience*, 1(1): 61–63, 2004.
4. S. Uematsu, Symmetry of skin temperature comparing one side of the body to the other, *International Journal of Thermology*, 1(1): 4–7, 1985.
5. H. Qi, P. T. Kuruganti, W. E. Snyder, Detecting breast cancer from thermal infrared images by asymmetry analysis, *Biomedical Engineering Handbook*, CRC Press, Boca Raton, FL, Chapter 27, pp. 1–14, 2006.
6. N. Diakides, J. D. Bronzino, *Medical Infrared Imaging*, CRC Press, Taylor & Francis Group, Boca Raton, FL, 2008.
7. T. Z. Tan, C. Quek, G. S. Ng, E. Y. K. Ng, A novel cognitive interpretation of breast cancer thermography with complementary learning fuzzy neural memory structure, *Expert Syst. Appl.*, 33(3): 652–666, 2007.
8. M. Frize, C. H. Herry, R. Roberge, Processing of thermal images to detect breast cancer: Comparison with previous work, *IEEE EMBS/BMES Conference*, Houston, Texas, Vol. 2, pp. 1159–1160, 2002.
9. T. Jakubowska, B. Wiecek, M. Wysocki, C. Drews Peszynski, Thermal signatures for breast cancer screening comparative study, In *Proceedings of the 25th Annual International Conference of the IEEE EMBS Conference*, Cancun, Mexico, Vol. 2, pp.1117–1120, 2003.
10. G. Schaefer, M. Zavisek, T. Nakashima, Thermography based breast cancer analysis using statistical features and fuzzy classification, *Pattern Recognition*, 42(6): 1133–1137, 2009.
11. N. H. Eltonsy, A. S. Elmaghraby, G. D. Tourassi, Bilateral breast volume asymmetry in screening mammograms as a potential marker of breast cancer: Preliminary experience, *Image Processing, IEEE International Conference in Image Processing*, San Antonio, Texas, Vol. 5, pp. 5–8, 2007.
12. D. Scutt, G. A. Lancaster, J. T. Manning, Breast asymmetry and predisposition to breast cancer, *Breast Cancer Research*, doi: 10.1186/bcr1388, 8 R14, 2006.

13. T. M. Cover, J. A. Thomas, *Elements of Information Theory*, John Wiley & Sons, Inc., New York, 1991.
14. F. Rossi, A. Lendasse, D. François, V. Wertz, M. Verleysen, Mutual information for the selection of relevant variables in spectrometric nonlinear modeling, *Chemometrics and Intelligent Laboratory Systems*, 80, 215–226, 2006.
15. K. C. Chiu, Z. Y. Liu, L. Xu, A statistical approach to testing mutual independence of ICA recovered sources, *4th International Symposium on Independent Component Analysis and Blind Signal Separation*, Nara, Japan, April 2003.
16. G. A. Darbellay, The mutual information as a measure of statistical dependence, *IEEE International Symposium on Information Theory*, Ulm, Germany, 405pp., 1997.
17. H. M. Chen, P. Varshney, M. K. Arora, A study of joint histogram estimation methods to register multi sensor remote sensing images using mutual information, *IEEE Geoscience and Remote Sensing Symposium*, Toulouse, France, Vol. 6, pp. 4035–4037, July 2003.
18. P. W. Josien, J. B. Pluim, A. Maintz, M. A. Viergever, Mutual information based registration of medical images: A survey, *IEEE Transactions on Medical Imaging*, 22(8): 986–1004, 2003.
19. K. G. Manton, I. Akushevick, J. Kravchenko, *Cancer Mortality and Morbidity Patterns in the US Population*, Statistics for Biology and Health, Springer, New York, 2009.
20. J. W. Williams, Y. Li, *Estimation of Mutual Information: A Survey*, Springer-Verlag, Berlin Vol. 5589/2009, pp. 389–396, 2009.
21. E. Parzen, On estimation of a probability density function and mode, *Annals of Mathematical Statistics*, 33(3): 1065–1076, 1962.
22. P. Thevenaz, M. Unser, Optimization of mutual information for multi-resolution image registration, *IEEE Transactions on Image Processing*, 9(12): 2083–2099, 2000.
23. F. Maes, A. Collignon, D. Vandermeulen, G. Marchal, P. Suetens, Multimodality image registration by maximization of mutual information, *IEEE Transactions on Medical Imaging*, 16(2): 187–198, 1997.
24. H. Chen, P. Varshney, Mutual information-based CT-MR brain image registration using generalised partial volume joint histogram estimation, *IEEE Transactions on Medical Imaging*, 22(9): 1111–1119, 2003.
25. E. D'Agostino, F. Maes, D. Vandermeulen, P. Suetens, An information theoretic approach for non-rigid image registration using voxel class probabilities, *Medical Image Analysis*, 10, 413–430, 2006.
26. T. Kadir, M. Brady, Estimating statistics in arbitrary regions of interest, *Proceedings of the 16th British Machine Vision Conference*, Oxford, Vol. 2, pp. 589–598, Sept. 2005.
27. T. Kadir, M. Brady, Nonparametric estimation of probability distributions from sampled signals, *Technical Report OUEL No: 2283/05*, Robotics Research Laboratory, Oxford University, July 2005.
28. N. Dowson, T. Kadir, R. Bowden, Estimating the joint statistics of images using nonparametric windows with application to registration using mutual information, *IEEE Transactions on Pattern Analysis and Machine Intelligence*, 30(10): 1841–1857, 2008.
29. A. Papoulis, S. U. Pillai, *Probability, Random Variables and Stochastic Processes*, McGraw-Hill, New York, 4th Edition, 2002.
30. STImaging: *http://www.stimaging.com.au/page2.html* (last accessed March 2010).
31. E. F. J. Ring, Progress in the measurement of human body temperature, *Engineering in Medicine & Biology Magazine*, 17: 19–24, 1998.
32. E. Y. K. Ng, A review of thermography as promising non-invasive detection modality for breast tumour. *International Journal of Thermal Sciences*, 48(5): 849–855, 2009.
33. E. F. J. Ring, H. McEvoy, A. Jung, J. Zuber, G. Machin, New standards for devices used for the measurement of human body temperature. *Journal of Medical Engineering & Technology*, 34(4): 249–253, 2010.
34. *Thermography Guidelines: Standards and Protocols in Clinical Thermographic Imaging*, Sept. 2002, http://www.iact-org.org/professionals/thermog-guidelines.html, also: http://www.blatmanpain-clinic.com/blat_cancerscreening.htm
35. S. Belongie, J. Malik, J. Puzicha, Shape matching and object recognition using shape contexts, *IEEE Transactions on Pattern Analysis and Machine Intelligence*, 24(24): 509–522, 2002.

Boguslaw Wiecek
Technical University of Lodz

Maria Wiecek
Technical University of Lodz

Robert Strakowski
Technical University of Lodz

M. Strzelecki
Technical University of Lodz

T. Jakubowska
Technical University of Lodz

M. Wysocki
Technical University of Lodz

C. Drews-Peszynski
Technical University of Lodz

Breast Cancer Screening Based on Thermal Image Classification

Thermal imaging can be a useful technique for early detection of many diseases, for example, skin lesions, breast cancers, benign and malignant skin tumors, and so on. Thermal image features (indexes, signatures) and image classification can be one of the possible approaches for fast, noninvasive, contactless screening. There are many different methods that describe image features. A large group of methods is based on statistical parameters [4,9,10]. Parameters such as mean value, standard deviation, skewness, kurtosis, and so on can be used to compare and differentiate thermal images. We consider both the first and the second-order statistical parameters [3,4,7,10,15–17]. The first-order ones use histograms of the thermal image to compute signatures (see Figure 36.1), while the second-order statistical parameters are defined for the so-called co-occurrence matrix of the image [4,7,10].

In the medical applications, one of the basic features of a thermal image is its axis symmetry of temperature patterns. The human body and its thermal pattern are symmetric in most of the physiological cases, while they are usually asymmetric in the pathological conditions. However, sometimes a significant asymmetry can indicate the physiologic abnormality as well. Thermal asymmetry may correspond to pathology, including cancer, fibrocystic diseases, an infection (see Figure 36.2) or a vascular disease or it might indicate an anatomical variant [1,2,11,12,16]. This makes the difficulty to achieve the high efficiency of the image classifications and screening and it is the main reason that the researchers are still looking for the new effective methods of image processing for medical applications.

The next group of methods is based on image transformations, such as linear and nonlinear filtering, Fourier or wavelet analysis. All these methods allow regenerating an image (data) in another domain, and in consequence, the thermal signatures are defined based on new kind of data corresponding to frequency, time delay, scale in wavelet transform, and so on. Well-known Karhunen–Loeve transform can be implemented in the form of principle component analysis (PCA). PCA is a technique that is usually used for reducing the dimensionality and decorrelating of multivariate data preserving most of the variance [3,6,9,14].

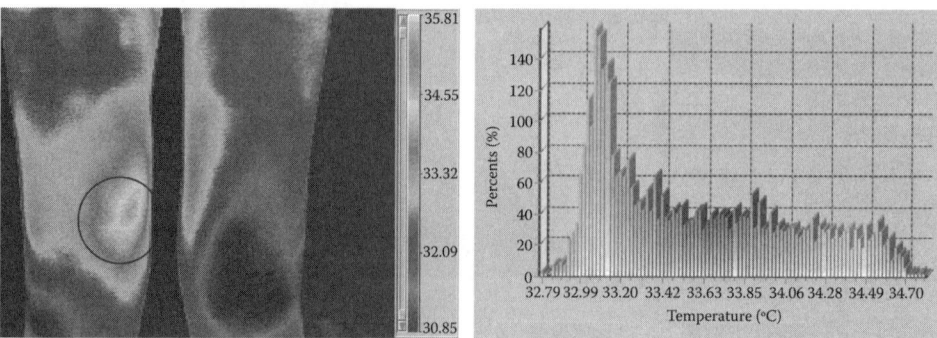

FIGURE 36.1 Thermal image and its histogram.

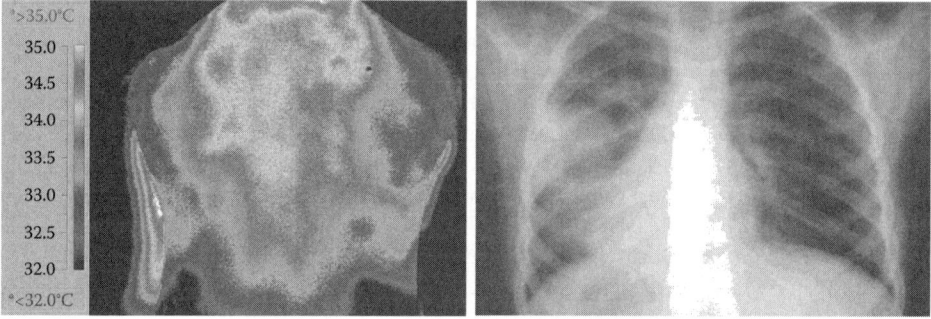

FIGURE 36.2 Thermal and x-ray images of pneumonia with asymmetric distribution of temperature.

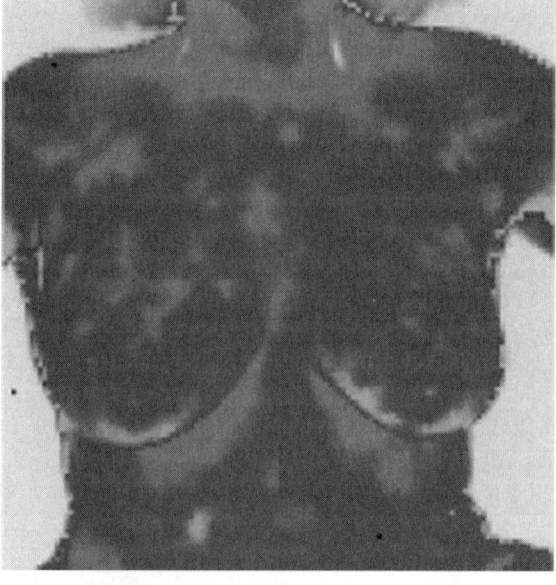

FIGURE 36.3 Thermal image of the healthy breast.

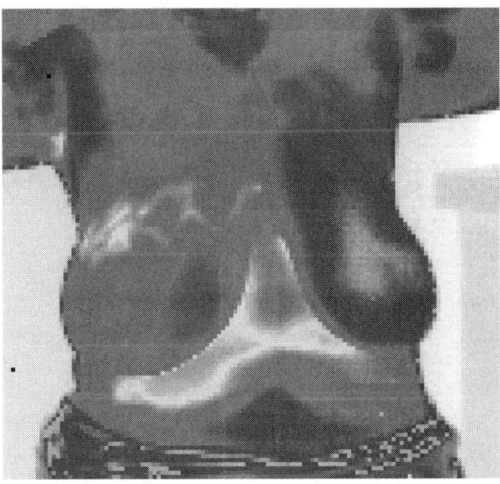

FIGURE 36.4 Thermal image of the breast with malignant tumor (left side of the image).

Thermal image classification is a powerful tool for many medical diagnostic protocols, including breast cancer screening [15–17]. Figures 36.3 and 36.4 show thermal images of a healthy breast and that with malignant tumor, respectively. Among the variety of different image features, statistical thermal signatures (first and second order) have been already effectively used for classification of images represented by raw data [15–17]. In another approach, the features obtained from the wavelet transformation can also be used for successful classification [8,16,17].

It is possible to define many features for an image, and obviously, the selection and reduction of them are needed. Two approaches may be applied, based on Fischer coefficient as well as by using minimization of classification error probability (POE) and average correlation coefficients (ACC) between chosen features [2,10,17]. It can reduce the number of features to a few ones. Features preprocessing which generates new parameters after linear or nonlinear transformations can be the next step in the procedure. It allows getting less correlated and lower order data. Two approaches are used, that is, PCA and linear discriminant analysis (LDA) [6,10]. Finally, classification can be performed using different methods, for example, artificial neural network (ANN) or nearest-neighbor classification (NNC) [16,17].

36.1 Histogram-Based First-Order Statistical Thermal Signatures

An image is assumed to be a rectangular matrix of discretized data (pixels) pix[*m,n*], where *m* = 0, 1, ..., *M*, *n* = 0,1, ... *N*. Each pixel takes a value from the range $i \in <0, L-1>$. The histogram describes the frequency of existence of pixels of the same intensity in whole image or in the region of interest (ROI). Formally, the histogram represents the distribution of the probability function of existence of the given image intensity and it is expressed using Kronecker delta function as

$$H(i) = \sum_{n}^{N-1}\sum_{m}^{M-1} \delta(p[m,x],i) \quad \text{for } i = 0,1,...,L-1, \tag{36.1}$$

where

$$\delta(p[m,n],i) = \begin{cases} 1 & \text{for } p[m,n] = i \\ 0 & \text{for } p[m,n] \neq i \end{cases} \tag{36.2}$$

Histogram is used for defining first-order statistical features of the image, such as mean value μ_H, variance σ_H, skewness, kurtosis, energy, and entropy. The definitions of these parameters are given below.

$$\mu_H = \sum_{i=0}^{L-1} i p(i)$$

$$\sigma_H = \sum_{i=0}^{L-1} (i - \mu_H)^2 p(i)$$

$$\text{skewness} = \frac{\sum_{i=0}^{L-1} (i - \mu_H)^3 p(i)}{\sigma_H^3}$$

$$\text{kurtosis} = \frac{\sum_{i=0}^{L-1} (i - \mu_H)^4 p(i)}{\sigma_H^4} - 3 \qquad (36.3)$$

$$\text{energy} = \sum_{i=0}^{L-1} p^2(i)$$

$$\text{entropy} = -\sum_{i=0}^{L-1} \log_2(p(i)) p(i)$$

Histogram describes the global information of an image (see Figure 36.1). By processing the histogram, one can obtain very useful image improvement, such as contrast enhancement or intensity adjustment [3,9]. First-order statistical parameters can be employed to separate physiological and pathological cases using infrared (IR) imaging. The preliminary results for breast cancer screening are presented in the following subchapters.

In the first clinical trial, 32 healthy patients and 10 patients with malignant tumors were analyzed using thermography. There were four images registered for every patient that represented each breast in direct (frontal) and lateral direction to the camera. Histograms were created for these images and on the basis of statistical parameters, the following features were calculated: mean temperature, standard deviation, variance, skewness, and kurtosis. Afterward, differences of parameter values for left and right breast were calculated. The degree of symmetry on the basis of these differences was then estimated (see Figures 36.5 and 36.6).

The mean temperature in the healthy group was estimated at the level 30.2 ± 1.8°C in the direct position and 29.7 ± 1.9°C in the lateral one. The mean temperature was higher in eight cases out of 10 in malignant tumor group. Moreover, six cases out of 32 in the healthy group with mean temperatures exceeded normal level. Therefore, we have found that it is necessary to analyze symmetry between left and right breast. Comparison of mean temperature was insufficient to separate physiological and pathological images.

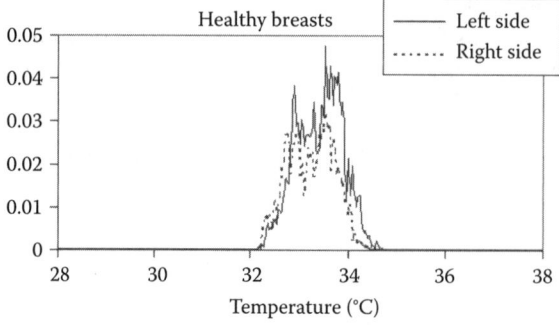

FIGURE 36.5 Histograms of thermal image for healthy breasts, see Figure 36.3.

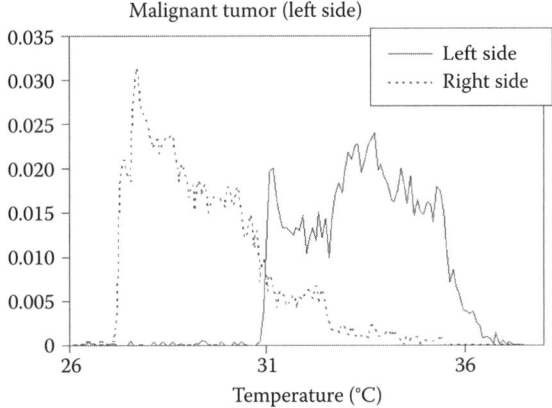

FIGURE 36.6 Histograms of thermal images for breasts presented in Figure 36.4 (malignant tumor on the left side).

Among analyzed parameters, skewness was the most promising for successful classification of thermal images. Absolute differences of skewness for left and right side was equal to $0.4 \pm 0.3°C$ in frontal position and $0.6 \pm 0.4°C$ in lateral one for the healthy group. These differences were higher for images in lateral position for all cases in the pathological group in comparison to the healthy patients' images.

The images in Figures 36.3 and 36.4 confirm the evidence of asymmetry between left and right side for healthy and malignant tumor cases.

Analyzing the first-order statistical parameter, let us conclude that it is quite hard to use them for the image classification and detecting tumors with high efficiency. Only mean temperature and skewness allow separating and classifying thermal images of breasts with and without malignant tumors. Frontal and lateral positions were used during this investigation, but no significant difference of the obtained result was noticed.

It is concluded that the first-order parameters do not give the satisfactory results, and due to some physiological changes of the breast, we could observe that these parameters do not allow separating patients with and without tumors. That was the main reason, that the second-order statistical parameters were used for further investigations.

36.2 Second-Order Statistical Parameters

More advanced statistical information on thermal images can be derived from the second-order parameters. They are defined using the so-called co-occurrence matrix [2,10,16,17]. Such a matrix represents the joint probability of two pixels having ith and jth intensity (temperature) at the different distances d, in the different directions. Co-occurrence matrix gives more information on intensity distribution over the whole image, and in this sense, it can effectively be used to separate and classify thermal images.

Let us assume that each pixel has eight neighbors lying in four directions: horizontal, vertical, diagonal, and antidiagonal. One can consider only the nearest neighbors, so the distance $d = 1$ (see Figure 36.7). As an example let us take an image 4×4 with four intensity levels given as (see Figure 36.8).

For horizontal direction, the co-occurrence matrix for the data presented in Figure 36.8 takes a form:

$$m_{\text{horizontal}} = \begin{bmatrix} 2 & 1 & 0 & 0 \\ 1 & 4 & 2 & 2 \\ 0 & 2 & 4 & 2 \\ 0 & 2 & 2 & 0 \end{bmatrix} \tag{36.4}$$

The co-occurrence matrix is always square and diagonal with the dimension equal to the number of intensity levels L in the image. After normalization we get the matrix of the probabilities $p(i,j)$.

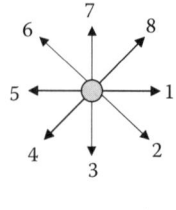

6	7	8
5	*	1
4	3	2

FIGURE 36.7 Eight neighboring pixels in four direct horizontal, vertical, diagonal, and antidiagonal.

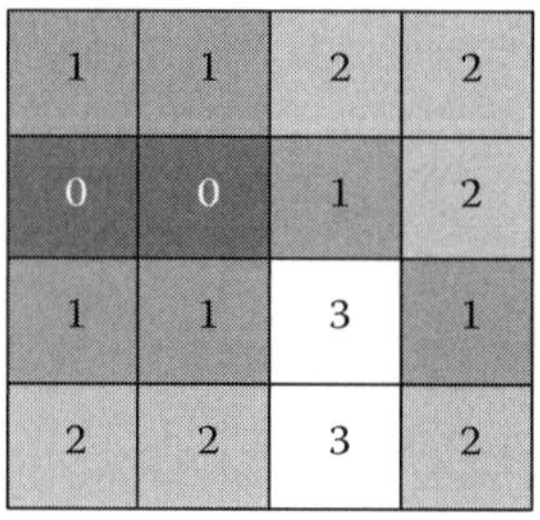

1	1	2	2
0	0	1	2
1	1	3	1
2	2	3	2

FIGURE 36.8 Example of 4×4 image with four discrete intensity levels.

Normalization is done by dividing all elements by the number of possible couple pixels for a given direction of analysis. For horizontal, vertical, and diagonal directions this numbers are equal to $2N(M–1)$, $2M(N–1)$, and $2(M–1)(N–1)$, respectively.

Second-order parameters are presented by Equations 36.5 and 36.6. As an example of comparing thermal images, mean values and standard deviations (μ_x, μ_y, σ_x, σ_y) for the elements of co-occurrence matrixes were calculated for horizontal and vertical directions, respectively. The quantitative results are presented in Figures 36.9 and 36.10.

Second-order statistical parameters can effectively be used to discriminate the physiological and pathological cases, for example, breast cancers. Most of them successfully discriminate healthy and malignant tumor cases. The protocol of the investigation assumes the symmetry analysis in the following way. At first, a polygon-shape ROI were chosen for analysis of the part of the skin corresponding to the breast. Then, the co-occurrence matrixes were calculated for left and right breasts to evaluate

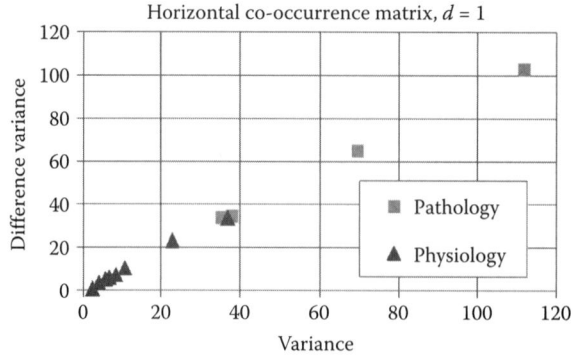

FIGURE 36.9 Difference variance versus variance obtained from co-occurrence matrix for horizontal direction.

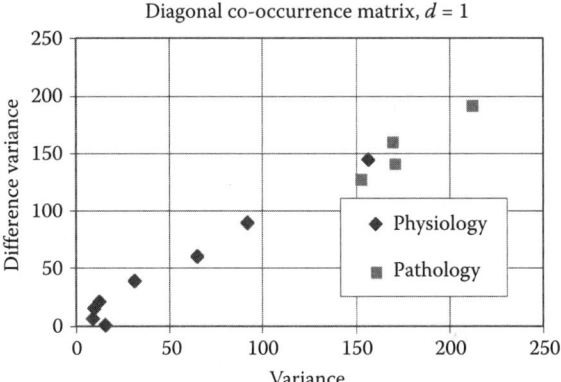

FIGURE 36.10 Difference variance versus variance obtained from co-occurrence matrix for diagonal direction.

second-order statistical parameters for different directions. Only the neighbor pixels are considered in these investigations ($d = 1$). Finally, the differences of the values of these parameters for left and right sides were used for the image classification. Figures 36.9 and 36.10 illustrate that the differences of second-order parameters for left and right sides are typically greater for pathological cases. Taking only two second-order parameters, that is, difference variance and variance allow separating successfully almost all healthy and malignant tumor cases.

$$\text{Variance} = \sum_{i=0}^{L-1} \sum_{j=0}^{L-1} (i-j)^2 \, p(i,j)$$

$$\text{Angular second moment} = \sum_{i=0}^{L-1} \sum_{j=0}^{L-1} p(i,j)^2$$

$$\text{Contrast} = \sum_{n=0}^{L-1} n^2 \sum_{\substack{i=0 \\ |i-j|=n}}^{L-1} \sum_{j=0}^{L-1} p(i,j)$$

$$\text{Correlation} = \frac{\sum_{i=0}^{L-1} \sum_{j=0}^{L-1} (ij) p(i,j) - \mu_x \mu_y}{\sigma_x \sigma_y}$$

$$\text{Sum of squares} = \sum_{i=0}^{L-1} \sum_{j=0}^{L-1} (i - \mu_x)^2 p(i,j)$$

$$\text{Inverse difference moment} = \sum_{i=0}^{L-1} \sum_{j=0}^{L-1} \frac{p(i,j)}{1 + (i-j)^2}$$

$$\text{Sum average} = \sum_{i=0}^{2(L-1)} i p_{x+y}(i)$$

$$\text{where } p_{x+y}(l) = \sum_{i=0}^{L-1} \sum_{j=0}^{L-1} p(i,j), \text{ for } |i+j| = l, l = 0,1,...,2(L-1)$$

$$\text{Sum variance} = \sum_{i=0}^{2(L-1)} (i - \text{Sum average})^2 p_{x+y}(i)$$

$$\text{Sum entropy} = -\sum_{i=0}^{2(L-1)} p_{x+y}(i) \log_2 \left[p_{x+y}(i) \right]$$

$$\text{Entropy} = -\sum_{i=0}^{L-1} \sum_{j=0}^{L-1} p(i,j) \log_2 \left[p(i,j) \right]$$

$$\text{Difference variance} = Var(p_{x-y})$$

$$\text{where } p_{x-y}(l) = \sum_{i=0}^{L-1} \sum_{j=0}^{L-1} p(i,j), \text{for} \left| i-j \right| = l, l = 0,1,...,L-1$$

$$\text{Difference entropy} = -\sum_{i=0}^{L-1} p_{x-y}(i) \log_2 \left[p_{x-y}(i) \right]$$

$$\text{Energy} = \sum_{i=0}^{L-1} \sum_{j=0}^{L-1} p^2(i,j) \tag{36.5}$$

where

$$p_{x-y}(l) = \sum_{i=0}^{L-1} \sum_{j=0}^{L-1} p(i,j), \text{ for} \left| i-j \right| = l, l = 0,1,...,L-1 \tag{36.6}$$

36.3 D-Wavelet Transformation

Among many known 2-dimensional (2D) transformations, wavelet method becomes more and more useful tool for image processing [8,15–17]. Wavelets allow performing time–frequency analysis, similar to the so-called short-time Fourier and more general Gabor transforms. Practically, it works as 1D low (L) and high (H) pass filtering for an image represented by its rows and columns alternatively (see Figure 36.11). After each step of filtering, decimation is applied to reduce the size of the result image. Four images (LL_1, LH_1, HL_1, HH_1) are the results of such a processing, as shown in Figure 36.12. Next, LL_1 image becomes an input data for the next level of processing, where exactly the same procedure is repeated. Theoretically, it can be performed many times until the result images have 1×1 dimensions. In practice, the algorithm stops maximally after 3–4 steps (levels).

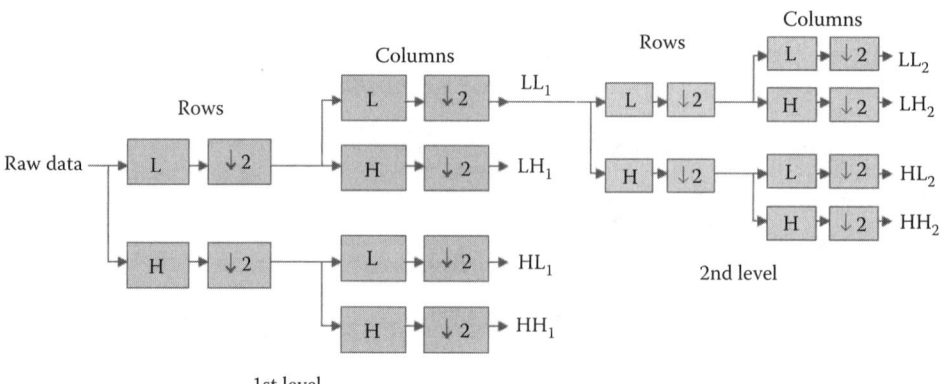

FIGURE 36.11   2D wavelet transform concept.

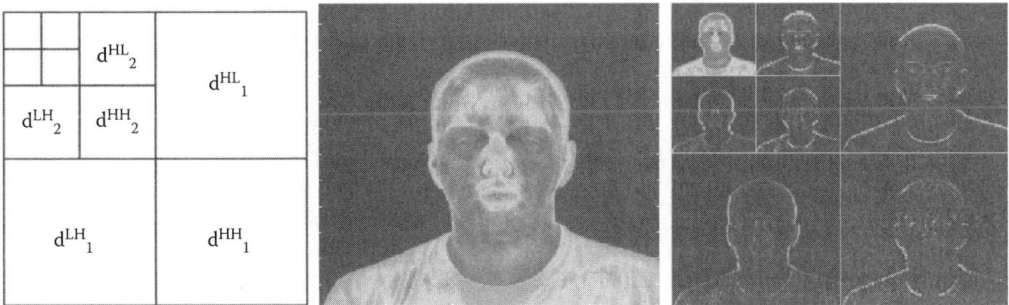

FIGURE 36.12 Typical result of 2D wavelet filtering, images' map, original and filtered images.

On each level, four images are available for further processing. These images are now used to calculate image features of the IR image. The technique of representing an image by the set of features is well known and frequently used in medical imaging. The features are then used in the classification process.

Tumors typically have better perfusion. They should have higher temperature, but in many cases, the network of blood vessels are much better developed and it has a special structural pattern. In such cases, the second-order parameters seem to be more effective to separate and classify healthy and pathological thermal images.

There are tens of thermal signatures that can be easily calculated. One of the problems in choosing the right thermal parameters is their dependency on the noise and size of the image taken for the investigations. Noise strongly depends on the type of the camera used in measurements [15]. This issue seems to be important as we have today two main thermovision camera types on the market—microbolometer, uncooled and photon, cooled ones. Obviously, uncooled, cost-effective cameras have the thermal resolution significantly lower, reaching the level 40–50 mK in contrast to 15–20 mK for cooled ones. The practical question can be posed, if there is a way to compensate the lower performance of the equipment by choosing the thermal signature less dependent on noise. In addition, because of the need of standardization of thermal images [7,15], it is necessary to estimate the right distance between the camera and the subject. Definitely, the closer the patient, the more accurate is the thermal imaging, but due to practical reason, it is very difficult to keep the constant distance in time, during massive screening. For this reason the sensitivity of the parameters as a function of distance and size of the subject should be as low as possible.

In order to find thermal parameters less dependent on the level of additive noise and the size of ROI, the preliminary research has been performed. The first- and second-order statistical parameters were considered. In addition, 2D wavelet transform was applied to calculate both histogram and co-occurrence matrix-based thermal signatures. A hypothesis was assumed that wavelet transform based on filtering (see Figures 36.11 and 36.12), should reduce the noise influence. Additionally, the considered parameter should allow differentiating the pathological and physiological cases in the acceptable range of noise and size variation.

As an example, the investigations of 10 patients with recognized breast tumors, as well as 30 healthy patients are presented. All healthy and pathological cases were confirmed by other diagnostic methods, such as mammography, USG, and/or biopsy. We have used thermographic camera to take two images for each breast: frontal and lateral ones. Each patient was relaxing before the experiment for 15 min in a room where temperature was stabilized at 20°C. Figure 36.13 presents the pathological case. Left breast has evidently higher temperature and the temperature distribution is very asymmetric.

In order to verify the noise and image size influence on the chosen features, the numerical procedure using 2D wavelet transformation was implemented. The wavelet transformation with biorthogonal filters was used. In order to differentiate healthy and pathological cases in breast investigation,

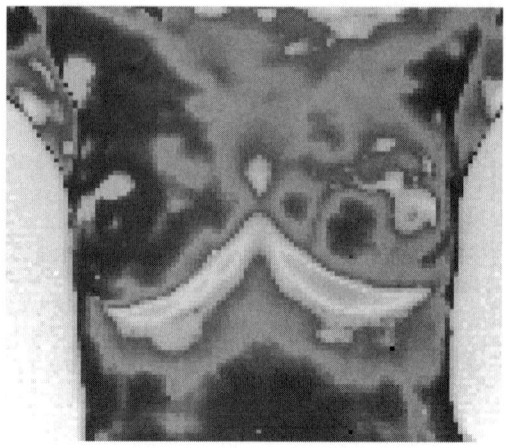

FIGURE 36.13 Example of thermal image showing the tumor (left breast).

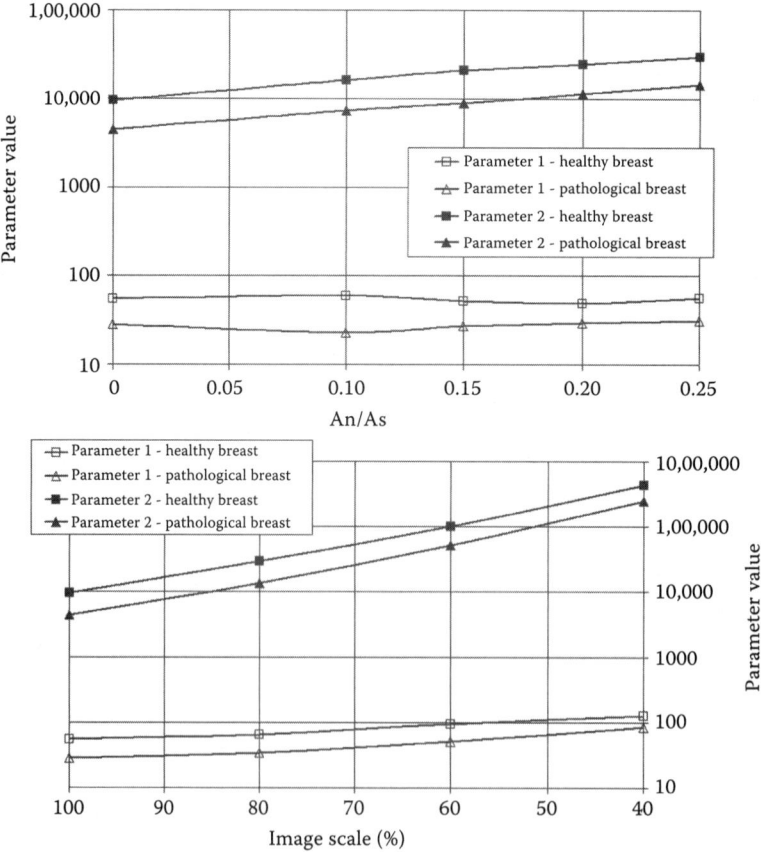

FIGURE 36.14 Second-order contrast (parameter 1) and correlation (parameter 2) chosen for breast investigation, parameter values versus noise level (top), and image scale (bottom).

second-order contrast and correlation were selected (see Figure 36.14). The chosen parameters depend on noise and size, but can still be used for classification in the wide range of noise and size variation. For example, decreasing the size of the thermal image to 40% of the original one and adding 25% noise to the image, change the parameter values both for healthy and pathological cases, but preserves possibility of the tumor detection (see Figure 36.14).

The investigations confirmed the expectation that among many different thermal signatures, the parameters calculated after 2D wavelet transformation using second-order statistical parameters are very promising for the screening purposes. Definitely, this investigation proved the necessity of selecting the best parameters. Different criteria have to be considered for such a selection. The proper discriminating healthy and pathological images have to be the main criterion. This investigation proved that such an approach can be a powerful tool for the medical diagnosis, and can be implemented as an automatic or semiautomatic software procedure.

36.4 ANN Classification

Thermal image classification can be a powerful tool for many medical diagnostic protocols such as breast cancer screening [15–17]. The classification process begins with image features calculation (see Figure 36.15). Because it is possible to define hundreds of different features for an image, obviously selection and reduction are needed. Many approaches are known for feature selection. One can use Fischer coefficient or POE together with ACC. These methods allow selecting the most effective and discriminative features [2,9,10]. Features' preprocessing which generates new parameters after linear or nonlinear transformation can be the next step in the overall procedure. It allows getting less correlated data and data of the lower order. Two approaches are used, PCA (Principal Component Analysis) and LDA [2,10]. Finally, classification can be performed using different ANNs, with or without additional hidden layers, and with different number of neurons. Alternatively, NNC can also be effective for thermal image classification.

ANN is typically used for classification. The selected image features are used as inputs. It means that the number of input nodes is equal to number of features. Number of neurons in the first hidden layer can be equal, lower or higher than the number of features in the classification, as illustrated in Figure 36.16. ANN can have user-defined next hidden layers which allow additional nonlinear processing of the input features. As ANN is the nonlinear system, such technique allows the additional decorrelating and data reduction.

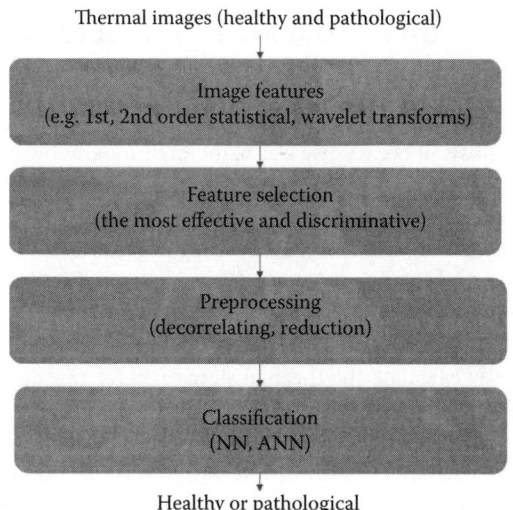

FIGURE 36.15 A typical image classification procedure.

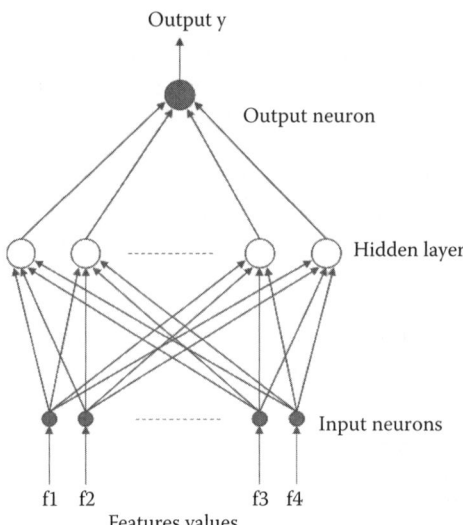

FIGURE 36.16 A typical one-directional ANN structure for thermal image classification.

Decorrelation of data, if possible, is always recommended for classification. Features of thermal images are more or less correlated with each other. It is because the change of certain thermal image content simultaneously changes the values of different features. Decorrelated set of features, describing different properties of thermal images are the best for classification. It can be achieved by preprocessing using PCA or Nonlinear Discriminant Analysis (NDA) [5,6,14].

It is well known that a proper training of ANN is the very important step in the entire protocol. It is a multivariable optimization problem, typically based on back-propagation technique. In the general case it can lead to wrong solutions if there is no single minimum of an error function. Therefore, one needs sufficient data size during training phase, and sometimes it is better or necessary to repeat training of ANN with different initial values of the neuron weight coefficients.

36.5 Software for Medical Diagnosis and Screening

To verify the research assumptions, novel software was created in MATLAB® environment (see Figures 36.18 and 36.19). In Laser Diagnostic and Therapy Center, at Technical University of Lodz, the laboratory for parallel diagnosis of breast diseases using mammography, ultrasonography, and thermography was created a few years ago and now is continuously using for medical treatment. In the same place and at the same time, a patient can be diagnosed using thermography, digital mammography, and ultrasonography. In our laboratory, a screening program has just been started, so we hope to collect enough images for ANN learning process. The software which is discussed in this chapter is suitable for features' calculations and image classification either for x-ray, acoustic or thermal images.

As shown in Figure 36.8, thermal camera operator can capture thermal image, define ROI, generate the histogram, and finally calculate the thermal signatures for raw data (first and second order). Having the left and right breast images, it is possible to evaluate the asymmetry of temperature patterns in the chosen ROI. In addition, the group of methods based on image transformations is implemented in the software. It is linear and nonlinear filtering, and Fourier or wavelet analysis (see Figure 36.18). Finally, classification can be performed using different ANN, with or without additional hidden layers, and with different number of neurons. NN method can also be used, as an alternative images' classification.

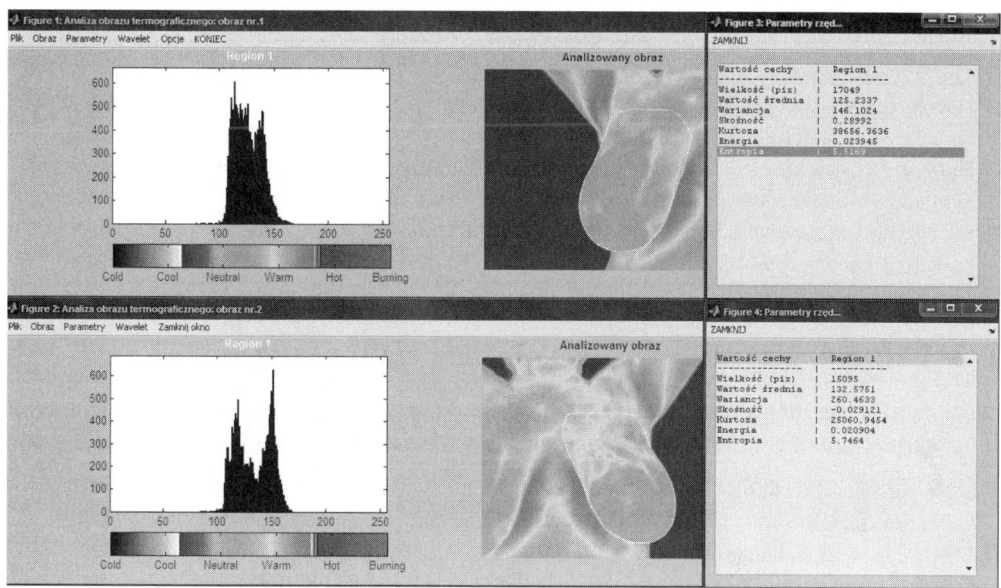

FIGURE 36.17 Application window with selected region and displayed the first-order features values.

In this research, both first- and second-order thermal features for left and right breasts were calculated (see Figures 36.17 and 36.18). Table 36.1 shows the values of chosen exemplary parameters for two breasts of the same patient, one is healthy and the second one is from the risky group. They can easily differentiate the thermal patterns on both images. These features were selected manually, just to confirm their usefulness in the thermal image classification. In practice, the automatic objective method can be used for features selection.

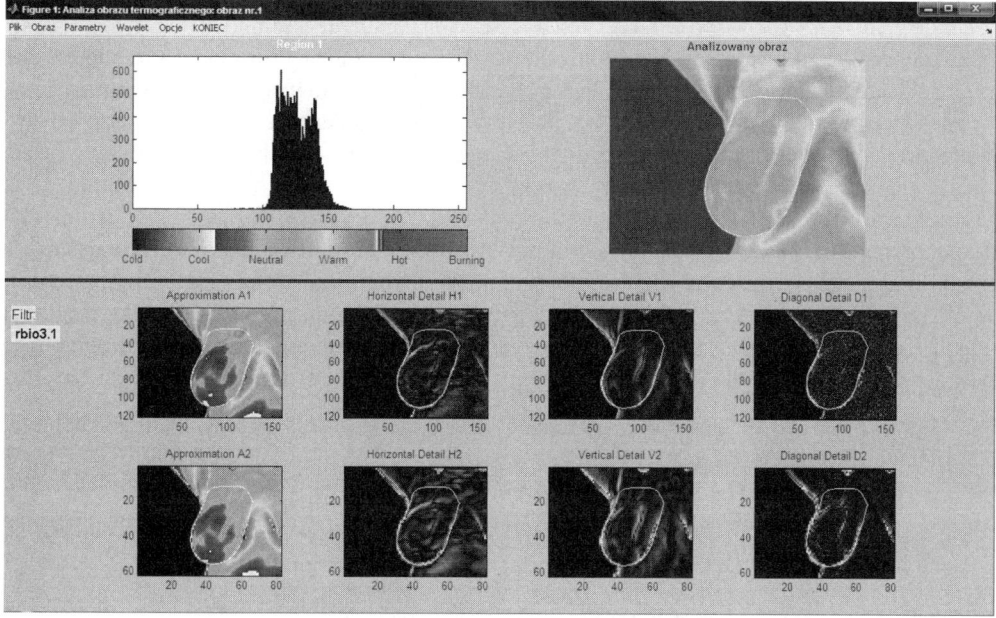

FIGURE 36.18 Results after wavelet transform for first and second filtering steps.

TABLE 36.1   Exemplary Parameter Values Differentiating Left and Right Breasts Shown in Figure 36.17

Parameters	Left Breast	Right Breast
First order, skewness for raw image	−0.029	0.29
Second order in vertical direction, correlation for raw image	107	1.24
First-order skewness after wavelets, LL1 image	0.0255	0.252
First-order variance after wavelets, LH2 image	452	223
Second order in diagonal direction, variance after wavelets, LH2 image	3060	599
Second order in antidiagonal direction, variance after wavelets, LH2 image	223	79.9

36.6 Clinical Results of Breast Cancer Screening

The preliminary screening investigations using thermal image processing has been made during the routine mammography inspection. The mammography investigations gave the results divided in five-stage scale.

1. No pathological change
2. Benign change
3. Possible benign change
4. Suspicious pathological change
5. Pathological change

The investigations have been carried out in the Laser Diagnostics and Therapy Centre at the Technical University of Lodz. During the medical diagnostics, 240 images were taken, two frontal and two lateral ones for 60 patients. Based on the mammography investigation, each breast image was classified into one of five groups. The same classification was made for the patients. There were patients with two healthy breasts without any pathological change classified to group no. 1. In addition, we had found patients with one breast which was selected to one of four groups other than the groups mentioned above. In this way, the small database of thermal images and patients was created (see Table 36.2). The images of patient breasts from group nos. 3 and 4 were recognized as suspicious. No patients with pathological change were found during this investigation.

Four different tests were performed. Each test was based on the simple assumption that having N images in each trail, $N-1$ images were used for training the neural network and one separated for testing. Then the one directional neural network with the hidden layer was trained using all images except the one separated. Finally, the separated image was used for the classification test. In order to minimize the statistical error, this process was repeated several times with different images for testing, and the average result was taken.

Test no. 1

The first test was carried out for 15 images of breasts classified into the 3rd and 4th risk group. The next 15 images were selected to the group without any change. The training data consisted of 29 sets of selected parameters. Frontal thermal images were taken into account only. The results are presented in Table 36.3. Selection using Fisher coefficient reduces the set of features into six ones as below.

- Contrast—Second-order statistical parameter after Haar wavelet, matrix HL-2, horizontal direction with distance $d = 1$.

TABLE 36.2   Number of Patients for Five Risk Groups during the Screening Investigations

No. of group	1	2	3	4	5
No. of patients	25	20	10	5	0
No. of images	170	40	20	10	0

TABLE 36.3   Classification Results for Frontal Thermal Images

No.	Risk Group	% of Correctly Classified	No. of Correctly Classified	No. of Classification Trials
1	3	27.3	3	11
2	3	81.8	9	11
3	3	72.7	8	11
4	3	72.7	8	11
5	3	63.6	7	11
6	3	90.9	10	11
7	3	81.8	9	11
8	3	63.6	7	11
9	3	54.5	6	11
10	3	72.7	8	11
11	4	72.7	8	11
12	4	27.2	3	11
13	4	27.2	3	11
14	4	18.2	2	11
15	4	72.7	8	11
16	1	18.2	2	11
17	1	0	0	11
18	1	18.2	2	11
19	1	100	11	11
20	1	36.4	4	11
21	1	36.4	4	11
22	1	18.2	2	11
23	1	72.7	8	11
24	1	63.6	7	11
25	1	72.7	8	11
26	1	54.5	6	11
27	1	81.8	9	11
28	1	72.7	8	11
29	1	100	11	11
30	1	63.6	7	11

- Sum variance—Second-order statistical parameter after Haar wavelet, matrix HL-2, antidiagonal direction (135°) with distance $d = 1$.
- Difference entropy—Second-order statistical parameter after Haar wavelet, matrix HL-1, diagonal direction (45°) with distance $d = 2$.
- Skewness—First-order statistical parameter after Haar wavelet, matrix LH-1.
- Kurtosis skewness—First-order statistical parameter after reverse biorthogonal 3.1 wavelet, matrix LL-2.
- Difference variance—First-order statistical parameter, diagonal direction (45°) with distance $d = 2$.

Test no. 2

Test no. 2 was made for the same group of patients as test no. 1. The lateral thermal images were analyzed (see Table 36.4 and Figure 36.19). Another six features were chosen using the Fisher criterion.

- Sum entropy—Second-order statistical parameter after Haar wavelet, matrix HL-1, diagonal direction (45°) with distance $d = 3$.
- Difference entropy—Second-order statistical parameter after Haar wavelet, matrix HL-1, antidiagonal direction (135°) with distance $d = 3$.

TABLE 36.4 Classification Results for Lateral Thermal Images

No.	Risk Group	% of Correctly Classified	No. of Correctly Classified	No. of Classification Trials
1	3	63.6	7	11
2	3	45.5	5	11
3	3	36.4	4	11
4	3	81.8	9	11
5	3	81.8	9	11
6	3	54.5	6	11
7	3	63.6	7	11
8	3	81.8	9	11
9	3	27.2	3	11
10	3	9.1	1	11
11	4	81.8	9	11
12	4	54.5	6	11
13	4	45.4	5	11
14	4	81.8	9	11
15	4	90.9	10	11
16	1	18.1	2	11
17	1	9.1	1	11
18	1	45.4	5	11
19	1	0	0	11
20	1	45.4	5	11
21	1	9.1	1	11
22	1	63.6	7	11
23	1	54.5	6	11
24	1	45.4	5	11
25	1	27.2	3	11
26	1	18.1	2	11
27	1	54.5	6	11
28	1	45.4	5	11
29	1	36.3	4	11
30	1	27.2	3	11

- Entropy—First-order statistical parameter after Haar wavelet, matrix HL-1.
- Difference entropy—First-order statistical parameter, horizontal direction with distance $d = 1$.
- Short run emphasis inverse moments—Run length matrix-based parameters [10,17].
- Kurtosis for gradient-based parameters [10,17].

Test no. 3

Test no. 3 was carried out for 40 patients. Twenty-five women were healthy (with both breasts belonging to group no. 1), and 15 with changes from 3rd and 4th risk group (only one breast belonged to group no. 3 or 4). Simulation in this case took into account the difference of chosen parameters for both patients' breasts seen in front (see Table 36.5). The following six features were used in the calculations.

- Contrast—Second-order statistical parameter after Haar wavelet, matrix LH-1, diagonal direction (45°) with distance $d = 1$.
- Difference variance—Second-order statistical parameter after Haar wavelet, matrix HL-2, horizontal direction with distance $d = 1$.
- Sum of squares—Second-order statistical parameter after Haar wavelet, matrix LH-2, diagonal direction (45°) with distance $d = 1$.

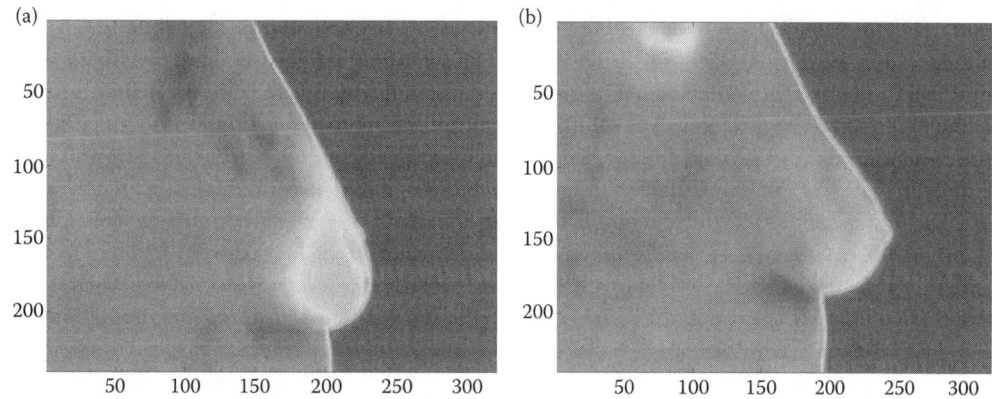

FIGURE 36.19 Exemplary side thermal images of breasts (a) with, (b) without pathological change.

- Difference entropy—Second-order statistical parameter after reverse biorthogonal 3.1 wavelet, matrix LH-1, vertical direction with distance $d = 2$.
- Sum average—Second-order statistical parameter after reverse biorthogonal 3.1 wavelet, matrix LH-1, antidiagonal direction (135°) with distance $d = 1$.
- Variance—First-order statistical parameter after reverse biorthogonal 3.1 wavelet, matrix LH-2.

Test no. 4

The test no. 4 was made for the same group of patients as test no. 3. Simulation in this case took into account the difference of chosen parameters for both breasts seen from the lateral side (see Table 36.6). The same (as in test no. 3) six features were used in the calculations.

- Contrast—Second-order statistical parameter after Haar wavelet, matrix LH-1, diagonal direction (45°) with distance $d = 1$.
- Difference variance—Second-order statistical parameter after Haar wavelet, matrix HL-2, horizontal direction with distance $d = 1$.
- Sum of squares—Second-order statistical parameter after Haar wavelet, matrix LH-2, diagonal direction (45°) with distance $d = 1$.
- Difference entropy—Second-order statistical parameter after reverse biorthogonal 3.1 wavelet, matrix LH-1, vertical direction with distance $d = 2$.
- Sum average—Second-order statistical parameter after reverse biorthogonal 3.1 wavelet, matrix LH-1, anti-diagonal direction (135°) with distance $d = 1$.
- Variance—First-order statistical parameter after reverse biorthogonal 3.1 wavelet, matrix LH-2.

Table 36.7 presents the summarized results of the classification. The efficiency of detection is higher for pathological changes than for healthy cases. The lateral thermal imaging of breasts allows getting the better results. The best detection of pathological changes was for test no. 4, that is, for features calculated as the difference of chosen parameters for healthy and suspicious breasts seen from the lateral direction. Detectivity for pathological changes was at 70%, while 57% for healthy cases. One can notice that it is a good result for low number of images available for training neural network and classification.

36.7 Conclusions

This chapter presents the preliminary results of the feature analysis for thermal images for different medical applications, mainly used in breast oncology. Thermography as the additional and adjacent method can be very helpful for early screening it helps to detect and even recognize the tumors. At first, we consider first- and second-order statistical parameters. Although we do not have many pathological

TABLE 36.5   Classification Results for Frontal Thermal Images for the Parameter Difference between Pathological and Healthy Breast

No.	Risk Group	% of Correctly Classified	No. of Correctly Classified	No. of Classification Trials
1	3	57.1	4	7
2	3	28.6	2	7
3	3	85.7	6	7
4	3	57.1	4	7
5	3	42.9	3	7
6	3	85.7	6	7
7	3	85.7	6	7
8	3	42.9	3	7
9	3	71.4	5	7
10	3	100	7	7
11	4	100	7	7
12	4	85.7	6	7
13	4	85.7	6	7
14	4	28.6	2	7
15	4	0	0	7
16	1	85.7	6	7
17	1	85.7	6	7
18	1	71.4	5	7
19	1	57.1	4	7
20	1	71.4	5	7
21	1	71.4	5	7
22	1	42.9	3	7
23	1	57.1	4	7
24	1	42.9	3	7
25	1	71.4	5	7
26	1	42.9	3	7
27	1	28.6	2	7
28	1	57.1	4	7
29	1	28.6	2	7
30	1	0	0	7
31	1	71.4	5	7
32	1	0	0	7
33	1	85.7	6	7
34	1	57.1	4	7
35	1	85.7	6	7
36	1	57.1	4	7
37	1	71.4	5	7
38	1	14.3	1	7
39	1	71.4	5	7
40	1	0	0	7

cases for investigations yet, the first results are very promising. The second-order parameters are more sensitive to the overall structure of an image. Lately, the study has been extended by choosing second-order parameters for multivariate data classification. The presented approach includes the PCA analysis to reduce the dimensionality of the problem and by selecting the eigen vectors it is possible to generate data which represents the tumors more evidently.

Breast cancer screening is a challenge today for medical engineering. Breast temperature depends not only because of some pathological changes, but it also varies in normal physiological situations, even

TABLE 36.6 Classification Results for Lateral Thermal Images for the Parameter Difference between Pathological and Healthy Breast

No.	Risk Group	% of Correctly Classified	No. of Correctly Classified	No. of Classification Trials
1	3	57.14	4	7
2	3	28.57	2	7
3	3	85.71	6	7
4	3	57.14	4	7
5	3	42.86	3	7
6	3	85.71	6	7
7	3	85.71	6	7
8	3	42.86	3	7
9	3	71.43	5	7
10	3	100	7	7
11	4	100	7	7
12	4	85.71	6	7
13	4	85.71	6	7
14	4	28.57	2	7
15	4	100	7	7
16	1	85.71	6	7
17	1	85.71	6	7
18	1	71.43	5	7
19	1	57.14	4	7
20	1	71.43	5	7
21	1	71.43	5	7
22	1	42.86	3	7
23	1	57.14	4	7
24	1	42.86	3	7
25	1	71.43	5	7
26	1	42.86	3	7
27	1	28.57	2	7
28	1	57.14	4	7
29	1	28.57	2	7
30	1	0	0	7
31	1	71.43	5	7
32	1	0	0	7
33	1	85.71	6	7
34	1	57.14	4	7
35	1	85.71	6	7
36	1	57.14	4	7
37	1	71.43	5	7
38	1	14.29	1	7
39	1	71.43	5	7
40	1	100	7	7

it is a consequence of emotional state of a patient. It was a main reason that we are looking for more advanced methods of thermal image processing that could give satisfactory results.

One of the possible alternatives for such processing in ANN Classification based on multidimensional feature domain, with use of image transformations, for example, wavelet analysis. The preliminary investigations were quite successful, and can be improved by increasing the number of samples taken for processing.

Future research will concentrate around selection of features and adjusting wavelet transformation parameters to get the best classification. We assume that the more satisfactory results can be obtained

TABLE 36.7   Summary of the Classification Tests

	True Positive (%)	False Negative (%)	True Negative (%)	False Positive (%)
Test 1	60	40	54	46
Test 2	60	40	33	67
Test 3	64	36	53	47
Test 4	70	30	57	43

by using features based on asymmetry between left and right side of a patient. It could help for one-side cancerous lesion classification, what is the most typical pathological case and frequently happens today.

References

1. W.C. Amalu, W.B. Hobbins, F.J. Head Elliot, Infrared imaging of the breast—An overview, *Medical Devices and Systems*, Ed. J.D. Bronzino, Boca Raton, FL, CRC Press, 2006, Section III, Chapters 25-1 to 25-21.
2. M. Bennett Breast cancer screening using high-resolution digital thermography, *Total Health*, 22(6) 44, 1985.
3. R. Causton, *A Biologist's Advanced Mathematics*, London, Allen and Unwin, 1987.
4. P. Cichy, Texture analysis of digital images–doctoral thesis, *Technical University of Lodz, Institute of Electronics*, Lodz, 2000, in Polish.
5. P. Debiec, M. Strzelecki, A. Materka, Evaluation of texture generation methods based on CNN and GMRF image texture models, *Proceedings of International Conference on Signals and Electronic Systems*, October 17–20, 2000, Ustron, pp. 187–192.
6. I. T. Jolliffe, *Principal Component Analysis*, New York, Springer-Verlag, 1986.
7. T. Jakubowska, B. Wiecek, M. Wysocki, C. Drews-Peszynski, Thermal signatures for breast cancer screening comparative study, *Proc. IEEE EMBS Conf.*, Cancun, Mexico, Sept. 17–21, 2003.
8. M. Kociolek, A. Materka, M. Strzelecki, P. Szczypinski, Discrete wavelet transform-derived features for digital image texture analysis, *Proceedings of International Conference on Signals and Electronic Systems ICSES'2001*, Lodz, 18–21 Sept. 2001, pp. 111–116.
9. B.F.J. Manly, *Multivariate Statistical Method: A Primer*. London, Chapman & Hall, 1994.
10. A. Materka, M. Strzelecki, R. Lerski, L. Schad, Evaluation of texture features of test objects for magnetic resonance imaging, *Infotech Oulu Workshop on Texture Analysis in Machine Vision*, Oulu, Finland, June 1999.
11. E.Y.K. Ng, L.N. Ung, F.C. Ng, L.S.J. Sim, Statistical analysis of healthy and malignant breast thermography, *Journal of Medical Engineering and Technology*, 25(6), 253–263, 2001.
12. E.Y-K. Ng, A review of thermography as promising non-invasive detection modality for breast tumour, *International Journal of Thermal Sciences*, 2008, DOI: 10.1016/j.ijthermalsci.2008.06.015.
13. E.Y-K. Ng, and N.M. Sudharsan, Numerical modelling in conjunction with thermography as an adjunct tool for breast tumour detection, *BMC Cancer, Medline Journal* 4(17), 1–26, 2004.
14. J. Schürman, *Pattern Classification*, John Wiley & Sons, 1996.
15. B. Wiecek, S. Zwolenik, Thermal wave method—Limits and potentialities of active thermography in biology and medicine, *2nd Joint EMBS-BMES Conference, 24th Annual International Conference of the IEEE Engineering in Medicine and Biology Society*, BMES-EMS 2002, Houston, Oct. 23–26, 2002.
16. B. Wiecek, M. Strzelecki, T. Jakubowska, M. Wysocki, C. Drews-Peszynski, Advanced thermal image processing, *Handbook of Medical Devices and Systems*, Ed. Joseph D. Bronzino, Boca Raton, FL, CRC Press, 2006, Chapters 28-1–28-13.
17. M. Wiecek, R. Strakowski, T. Jakubowska, B. Wiecek, Software for classification of thermal imaging for medical applications, *9th International Conference on Quantitative InfraRed Thermography QIRT2008, Inżynieria Biomedyczna*, Vol. 14, nr 2/2008, str. 143.

37

Fuzzy C Means Segmentation and Fractal Analysis of the Benign and Malignant Breast Thermograms

M. Etehadtavakol
Isfahan University of Medical Science

E.Y.K. Ng
School of Mechanical and Aerospace Engineering

Nanyang Technological University

Caro Lucas
University of Tehran

S. Sadri
Isfahan University of Technology

Isfahan University of Medical Science

37.1 Preamble

Breast cancer is one of the main problems in women's health today. Early detection of breast cancer plays a significant role in lowering the mortality rate. Cancer threats could be halted by identifying and removing malignant tumors in the early stages before they metastasize and spread to adjacent regions. Breast thermography [1] is a potential early detection method which is fast, nonradiating, noninvasive, low cost, passive, painless, and risk free with no contact with the body [2–4]. It is effective for women with all sizes of breast as well as with all ages, for women with breast with dense tissue, and for nursing or pregnant women [5,6].

In 1956, Lawson declared that the skin temperature of breast with cancer was hotter than the normal one. Hence, he proposed that in the infrared (IR) images, the cancer tissues can be differentiated as hot spots [7]. The cancerous tissue emits with angiogenesis and it has an inflammation temperature pattern different from the healthy one. In IR pseudocolor images, different colors indicate different rates of temperature. Color segmentation of IR thermal images can be very useful in detecting the tumor regions.

Cancer is often designated as a chaotic, poorly regulated growth [8]. Cancerous cells and tumors have irregular shapes, and traditional Euclidean geometry based on smooth shapes such as line, plane, cylinder, and sphere are not able to delineate them. When the focus is on irregularities of tumor growth, fractal geometry is thus useful. Fractal geometry can be a more powerful means of quantifying the spatial complexity of real objects [9].

37.2 Color Segmentation

37.2.1 K Means Clustering

The K means algorithm that has been used in many pattern recognition problems was suggested in the 1960s [10]. It is one of the most straightforward unsupervised learning techniques for clustering.

It divides N data points to K disjoint subsets S_j where $j = 1,2,\ldots,K$.

It works with the minimization of the objective function which is expressed as

$$J = \sum_{j=1}^{K} \sum_{n \in S_j} \left\| x_n - \mu_j \right\|^2 \tag{37.1}$$

where x_n is a vector for the nth data point in S_j and μ_j is the geometric centroid of data points. The algorithm consists of two steps: the number of cluster k must be chosen, and then the K means clustering to the image must be implied.

37.2.2 Mean Shift Clustering

Mean shift clustering (MS) was proposed by Fukunaga and Hosteler in 1975 [11]. The mean shift algorithm is a nonparametric clustering technique which does not require prior knowledge of the number of clusters, and does not constrain the shape of the clusters [12–15]. Assuming x_i ($i = 1,\ldots,n$) be a set of feature vectors in a d-dimensional feature space. The density at any point x can be estimated by the Parzen window kernel density estimator $K(x)$ with window size h as described below.

$$f_{h,K}(x) = \frac{c_{k,d}}{nh^d} \sum_{i=1}^{n} k\left(\left\| \frac{x - x_i}{h} \right\|^2 \right) \tag{37.2}$$

The normalization constant $c_{k,d}$ assures that $K(x)$ integrates to one. Three different kernel estimators are Epanechnikov, Uniform, and Normal. They are introduced in Equations 37.3, 37.4, and 37.5, respectively.

$$K(x) = \begin{bmatrix} c(1 - \|x\|^2) & \text{for} \|x\| \leq 1 \\ 0 & \text{otherwise} \end{bmatrix} \tag{37.3}$$

$$K(x) = \begin{bmatrix} c & \text{for} \|x\| \leq 1 \\ 0 & \text{otherwise} \end{bmatrix} \tag{37.4}$$

$$K(x) = c.\exp\left(-\frac{1}{2}\|x\|^2\right) \tag{37.5}$$

Taking the gradient of Equation 37.2 leads to

$$0 = \nabla f_{h,K}(x) = \frac{2c_{k,d}}{nh^{(d+2)}} \sum_{i=1}^{n} (x - x_i) g\left(\left\|\frac{x - x_i}{h}\right\|^2\right) \tag{37.6}$$

$$= \frac{2c_{k,d}}{nh^{(d+2)}} \left[\sum_{i=1}^{n} g\left(\left\|\frac{x - x_i}{h}\right\|^2\right)\left(\frac{\sum_{i=1}^{n} x_i g\left(\left\|\frac{x - x_i}{h}\right\|^2\right)}{\sum_{i=1}^{n} g\left(\left\|\frac{x - x_i}{h}\right\|^2\right)} - x\right)\right] \tag{37.7}$$

where $g(s) = -K'(s)$. Equation 37.7 is a product of two terms. The first term is proportional to the density estimate at x, and the second term is the mean shift vector as expressed below as

$$m_h(x) = \frac{\sum_{i=1}^{n} x_i g\left(\left\|\frac{x - x_i}{h}\right\|^2\right)}{\sum_{i=1}^{n} g\left(\left\|\frac{x - x_i}{h}\right\|^2\right)} - x \tag{37.8}$$

It is observed that the mean shift vector always points toward the direction of the maximum increase in the density. If we start from a point X^t in feature space, we move with the mean shift vector to the point X^t+1. The mean shift procedure is obtained by successive

1. Computation of the mean shift vector $m_h(X^t)$
2. Translation of the window $X^t+1 = X^t + m_h(X^t)$

It is important to note that the number of clusters is not a parameter, but rather an output of the clustering algorithm. The only parameter of the mean shift clustering is the window size parameter h and its influence on the obtained results is significant.

37.2.3 Fuzzy C Means Clustering

Fuzzy C means (FCM) was first suggested by Bezdek et al. [16]. A value between 0 and 1, called the partition matrix, is given by the algorithm. It means the degree of membership between each data and centers of clusters is determined by minimizing the objective function as shown below

$$J_m(U,C) = \sum_{i=1}^{c} \sum_{k=1}^{n} u_{ik}^m \|X_k - C_i\|^2 \tag{37.9}$$

where $X_1, X_2, \ldots, X_n$ are n data sample vectors and m is any real number greater than one. $U \equiv [u_{ik}]$ is a $c \times n$ matrix, where u_{ik} is the ith membership value of the kth input sample X_k such that $\sum_{i=1}^{c} u_{ik} = 1$ and $C \equiv \{C_1, C_2, \ldots, C_c\}$ are cluster centers.

The fuzziness of the membership function is controlled by $m \in [1, \infty)$ which is an exponent weight factor. The similarity between any input sample and its corresponding cluster center is expressed by $\|*\|$.

The objective function of Equation 37.10 is optimized with updating of the membership u_{ik}, and cluster center C_i

$$u_{ik} = \cfrac{1}{\displaystyle\sum_{j=1}^{C} \left\{ \cfrac{\|X_k - C_i\|}{\|X_k - C_j\|} \right\}^{\frac{2}{m-1}}}$$ (37.10)

$$C_i = \cfrac{\displaystyle\sum_{k=1}^{n} u_{ik}^m . X_k}{\displaystyle\sum_{k=1}^{n} u_{ik}^m}$$ (37.11)

The standard FCM involves the following steps:

1. The number of clusters C is chosen.
2. The exponent weight m is chosen.
3. The membership u_{ik} is initialized.
4. The cluster center C_i (Equation 37.11) is calculated.
5. The membership u_{ik} (Equation 37.10) is updated for $i = 1,2,...,c$ and $k = 1,2,...,n$.
6. Steps 4 and 5 are repeated until the distortion is less than a specified value.

In color segmentation of IR images by FCM clustering, the colors are compared in a relative sense and grouped in clusters which are not with crisp boundaries. Moreover, data points can belong to more than one cluster. That is, pixels can belong to many clusters with different degrees of membership. The constraint of $\sum_{i=1}^{c} u_{ik} = 1$ for $1 \leq k \leq n$ points out that the sum of the membership values for all clusters of a data vector equals one. Hence, the trivial solution $U = 0$ is prevented and reasonable results with no empty cluster are provided.

It is worth noting that the data points in this implementation for segmentation of the IR image are pixels of the corresponding color space CIELAB (L*a*b*).

37.3 Results for Color Segmentation

We studied 15 breast thermograms available from the Ann Arbor thermography center [17], thermal imaging lab in the San Fransisco Bay Area [18], American College of Clinical Thermology [19], Thermography of Iowa [20], and Sunstate Thermal Imaging Center in Australia [21].

All cases studied are implemented using K means, mean shift, and C means algorithms. In some trials, empty clusters appeared when applying the K means algorithm, and if the algorithm is repeated several times, the results for different trials may be different showing that K means clustering is not stable. Figure 37.1b shows the trial in which two clusters are empty for a cancer case of Figure 37.1a. Figure 37.2b shows the trial in which three clusters are empty for a normal case of Figure 37.2a.

Mean shift clustering is very sensitive to the window size parameter h. Results of implementation of the mean shift clustering with $h = 12$ and $h = 15$ are presented in Figure 37.2c and d, respectively. In this implementation, 11 empty clusters and four empty clusters are found with $h = 12$ and $h = 15$, respectively.

As we expected, by implementing the FCM algorithm for both cases, as shown in Figures 37.1d and 37.2e, however, no empty cluster appeared. Hence, by using this segmentation technique for breast IR images, we are able to find the first and the second hottest regions for each case where some useful features could be extracted.

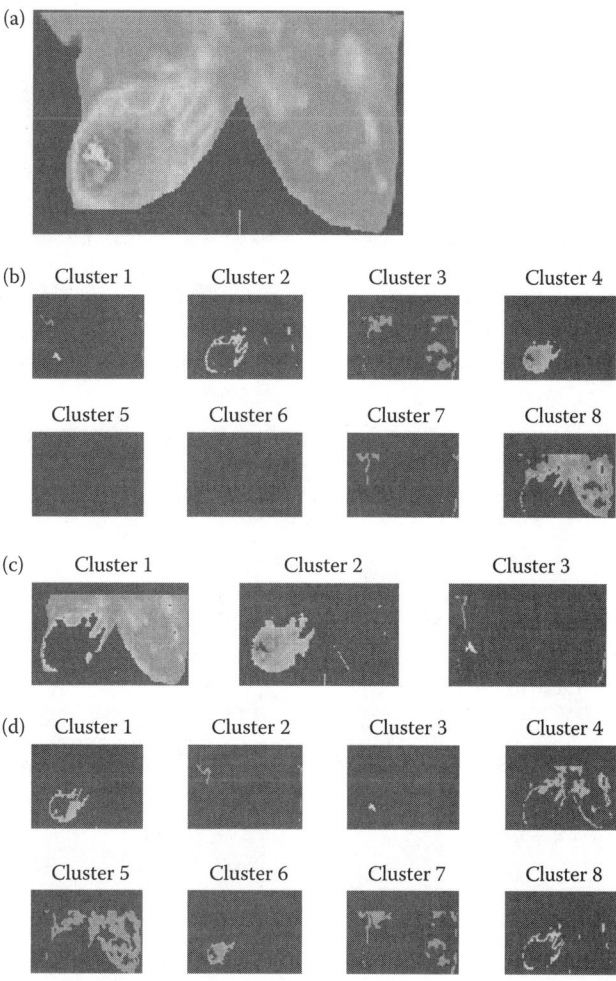

FIGURE 37.1 Inflammatory cancer case. (a) Original image (inflammatory cancer case). (b) Color segmentation by K means; two empty clusters (inflammatory cancer case). (c) Color segmentation by mean shift with $h = 35$. (d) Color segmentation by fuzzy C means.

In our work, despite the fact that different images are taken from different thermography with different color palettes and different numbers of clusters, the FCM approach is however capable of identifying the first and the second hottest regions by comparing their colors with the color palette spectrum which has been applied. With segmentation of thermal images, the hottest cluster can be recognized. We are capable of extracting some useful information from the suspicious regions by comparing the hottest region color with the spectrum of color palette used.

Next, we will examine and have a better understanding of those factors that are affecting the breast surface temperature.

37.4 Factors That Determine Breast Temperature

37.4.1 Angiogenesis

There have been a number of studies on the angiogenesis of tumors. The vascular construction of tumors is experienced to be remarkably different from that of normal tissues [22].

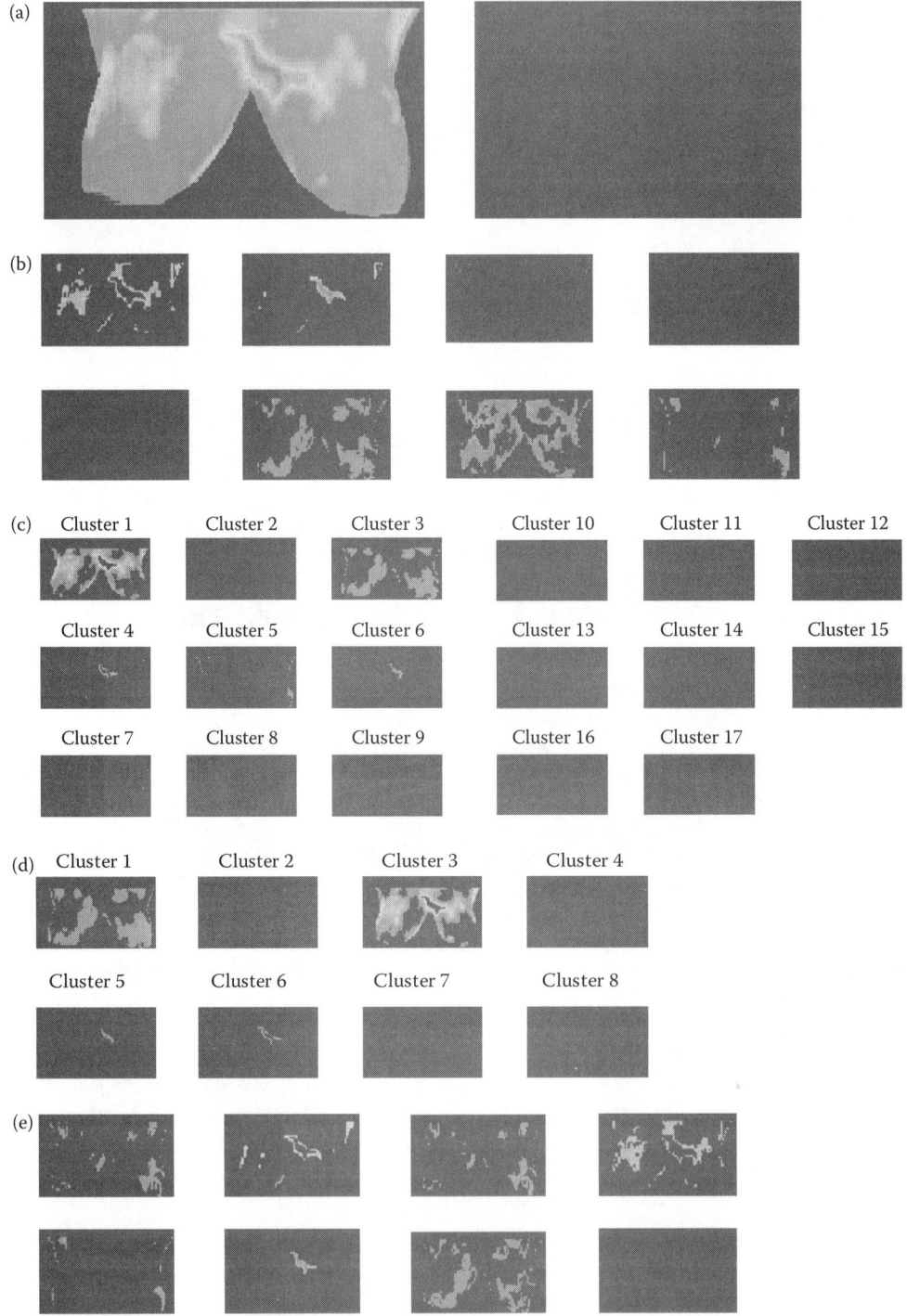

FIGURE 37.2 Normal case. (a) Original image (normal case). (b) Color segmentation by K means (three empty clusters). (c) Color segmentation by mean shift with $h = 12$ (11 empty clusters). (d) Color segmentation by mean shift with $h = 15$ (4 empty clusters). (e) Color segmentation by fuzzy C means.

In normal vascular networks, tree-like branching patterns or nearly constant intravascular distances are persistent features, while no such features exist in disorganized tumor vascular networks. One normal situation where angiogenesis occurs is wound repairing where the fundamental process of the development and growth of new blood vessels from the preexisting vasculature is extremely regulated. A developing child in the mother's womb where the vast network of arteries, veins, and capillaries are created is another example of normal angiogenesis [23]. Some studies have been directed with regard to angiogenesis in breast thermography. Gamagami discovered hypervascularity and hyperthermia in 1996 in 86% of non-palpable breast cancers with thermograms [24]. He also observed that in 15% of those cases, thermography helped to catch cancers that were not visible through mammography. Guido and Schnitt [25] described that angiogenesis is an early event in the development of breast cancer that might occur before tumor cells achieved the ability to invade the surrounding stoma and even before there was any morphologic evidence of a ductal carcinoma *in situ* (DCIS). Correspondingly, angiogenesis has been discovered as a critical event in tumor growth. Alarcon et al. investigated the influences of blood flow and red blood cell heterogeneity on tumor growth and angiogenesis with a mathematical model [26]. Another model of tumor angiogenesis taking into consideration the biochemical processes was proposed by Smiley and Levine [27].

37.4.2 High-Metabolic-Rate Angiogenesis

Tumor angiogenesis relates the proliferation of a network of blood vessels which supply nutrients and oxygen into tumor cells and remove waste products from them [28]. Molecules that send signals to surrounding normal host tissue are released by cancerous tumor cells. Certain genes (oncogenes) in the host tissue could be activated and make the proteins raise the growth of new blood vessels by these signals.

The local interaction between cells and the vascular system is modeled by Scalerandi et al. [29].

37.4.3 Local Vasodilatation

Anbar observed that notable IR changes in small tumor were produced by enhanced perfusion over a substantial area of breast surface via tumor-induced nitric oxide vasodilatation [30,31].

Nitroxide distribution is different between the tumor and normal tissues. This fact may reflect the differences in vasculatures of microenvironment associated with tumors. Also, in tumors of different sizes, the nitroxide distribution differs substantially [32].

37.5 Applications of Fractal Analysis in Biomedical Images and Fractal Dimension

In biomedical areas, fractal analysis has been widely used. Lee et al. compared several shape factors, including fractal dimension (FD) on the irregularity of the borders of melanocytic lesions [33]. Zheng and Chan proposed a model to employ fractals to detect abnormal regions in mammograms [34]. Guo et al. [35] computed FD in mammograms to identify the abnormality of breast masses by employing a support vector machine [35]. FD was also computed by Caldwell et al. [36] and Byng et al. [37] using the box counting method (BCM) to characterize the breast tissue. Gazit et al. used the fractal concept to analyze the vessel networks that surround a tumor and the hemodynamics within these vessel structures [38]. Grizzi et al. introduced the surface FD that was able to explain the geometric complexity of cancerous vascular networks [39]. They indicated that the number of vessels and their patterns of distribution have a significant impact on the surface FD. Investigations were further carried out by applying FD for classification of tumors in magnetic resonance images of brain [40,41], images related to colonic cancer [42], and ultrasonic images of liver [43]. Rangayyan and Nguyen applied fractal analysis for the classification of breast masses by using only their contours [44].

Fractal analysis plays an important role in discriminating malignant tumors from benign tumors in mammograms [45]. The edge sharpness of malignant mass as well as the benign mass has been studied in several investigations. It has been shown that malignant masses are rough and have complicated boundaries while benign masses are usually round and smooth with well-defined boundaries [46,47]. We can evaluate geometrical complexity by quantifying the irregularities of the boundary.

37.6 Fractal Dimension

A fractal is a nonregular geometric shape that can be split into parts which possess self-similarity or have the same degree of irregularity on all scales [48–53]. FD is a statistical quantity that denotes how completely a fractal would fill the space in different scales or magnification in a fractal geometry. The concept of fractal was introduced by Mandelbrot to denote an object whose Hausdorff dimension is greater than its topological dimension [48].

The relation between D, the self-similarity dimension, and a, the number of self-similar pieces at reduction factor $(1/S)$ is defined by the following power law:

$$a \propto \frac{1}{S^D} \tag{37.12}$$

D is expressed as

$$D = \frac{\log(a)}{\log\left(\frac{1}{S}\right)} \tag{37.13}$$

That is, D is estimated by the slope of the straight line approximation for a plot of log (a) versus log ($1/S$). Analytical and box counting methods are among several approaches for estimating FD. By using an analytical rule which is based upon a recursive mathematical relation, we can generate fractals. To explain BCM, we may partition the image into square boxes of equal sizes and then count the number of boxes which contain a part of the image. The process is repeated with partitioning the images into smaller and smaller size of boxes. To compute the FD of pattern, we may use the plot of log of the number of boxes counted versus the log of the magnification index for each stage of partitioning. The slope of the best-fitting line to the aforementioned plot is the FD of pattern.

Supposing a grid of boxes is laid over the curve as shown in Figure 37.3. The number of grid boxes that contain a part of the curve (viz. the boxes having intersections with the curve, shaded in gray) is calculated. In Figure 37.3, the number of these boxes is 10 out of 25 boxes, hence, $a = 10$, $1/S = 25$. This is kept on for increased numbers of squares, and the FD is estimated by the gradient of the logarithm of the number of squares occupied by the edge contour, viz. log(a), over the logarithm of the number of squares, log(1/S).

Ten contour shapes of different irregularities are shown in Figure 37.4. Their FDs are determined by BCM and results are included in Table 37.1. We may consider that the more complicated the shape boundary is, the larger the value of FD would be.

FD can be a potentially valuable tool for explaining the pathological architecture of breast tumors and providing insights into the mechanisms of tumor growth as it is demonstrated above. In this study, we examine whether the vascular networks in thermal images own a fractal nature and if so, what would be the FD values in different stages of abnormality.

37.7 Processing Steps and Results for Fractal Analysis

If we share the IR images with others or use them for research, it is more convenient by using a calibrated standard IR camera; then, we can ensure that relevant IR images and accurate temperatures can be viewed since each color is associated with a specific temperature. Although only mapping the local temperature differences are enough to accomplish the imaging for tumors, an accurate and stable calibration

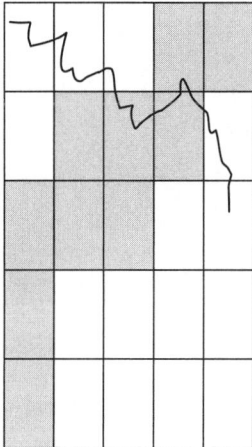

FIGURE 37.3 Box counting method.

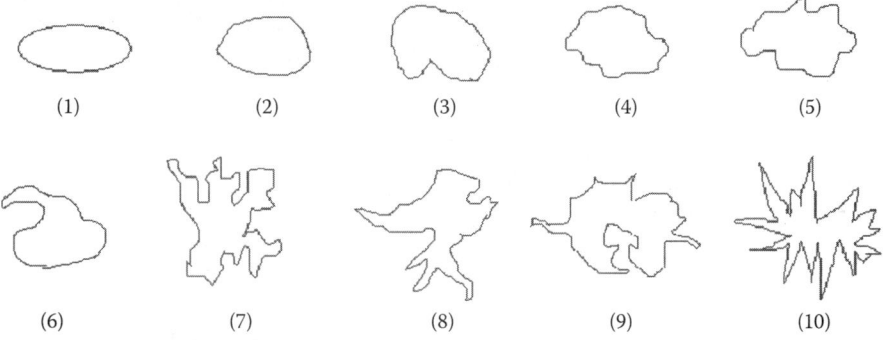

FIGURE 37.4 Sample contours of different irregularities.

TABLE 37.1 Calculated FDs for 10 Different Contour Shapes

Contours	1	2	3	4	5	6	7	8	9	10
FD	1.0711	1.1573	1.2162	1.2204	1.2750	1.2962	1.4076	1.4194	1.4370	1.4464

in order to satisfy the temperature sensitivity of the camera is significant. For the breast cancer case, the calibration method must be carried out such that the temperature difference is about one tenth of 37°C [3]. There are also other crucial factors so as to make thermal images in a standard form. The environmental conditions of thermal imaging such as humidity, ambient temperature, and illumination are essential to be controlled. Also, preparation of the patient in certain conditions is necessary.

Although the images we used are from sources which are varied in their resolutions and generally did not follow a unified protocol, our fractal analysis could demonstrate significant difference between the benign and malignant cases.

In this work, the right breast was separated from the left breast automatically. Canny edge detector and the morphological bridging operations for obtaining closed contour regions were used to extract left and right body boundaries. The two lower boundaries of the breasts were extracted as follows: for a data set, nine landmark points for two breasts were localized in a training procedure. The points with maximum curvature of two breasts correspond to the first and the last points. Then, for a new case, the

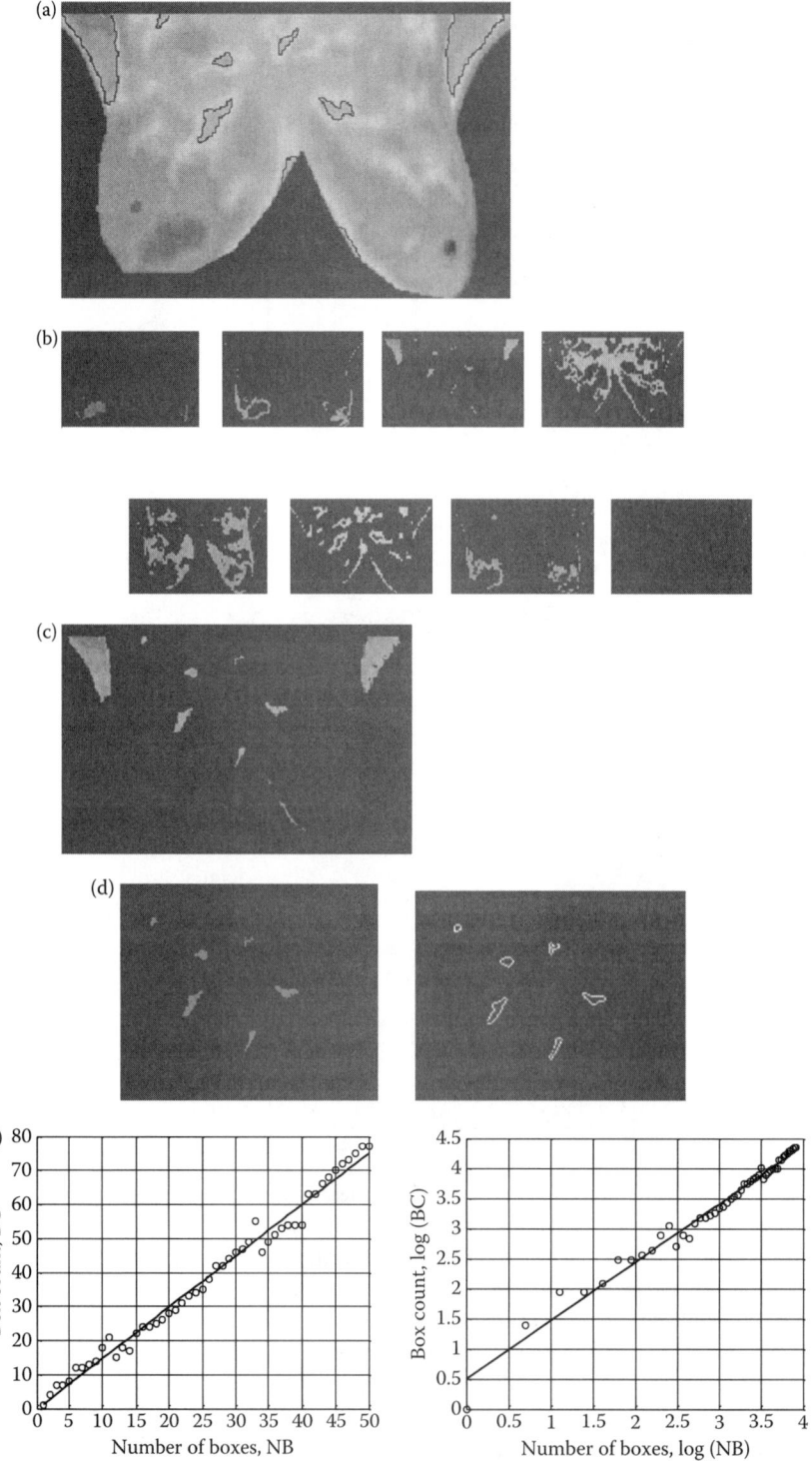

FIGURE 37.5 (a) Benign case 1 (B1). (b) Segmentation of (a) by fuzzy C mean. (c) The first hottest regions of B1. (d) B1: (1) The first hottest regions after removing the axilla and close sternal boundaries. (2) Boundaries of part (1). (e) B1: (1) Box count (BC) versus number of boxes (NB). (2) log(BC) versus log (NB).

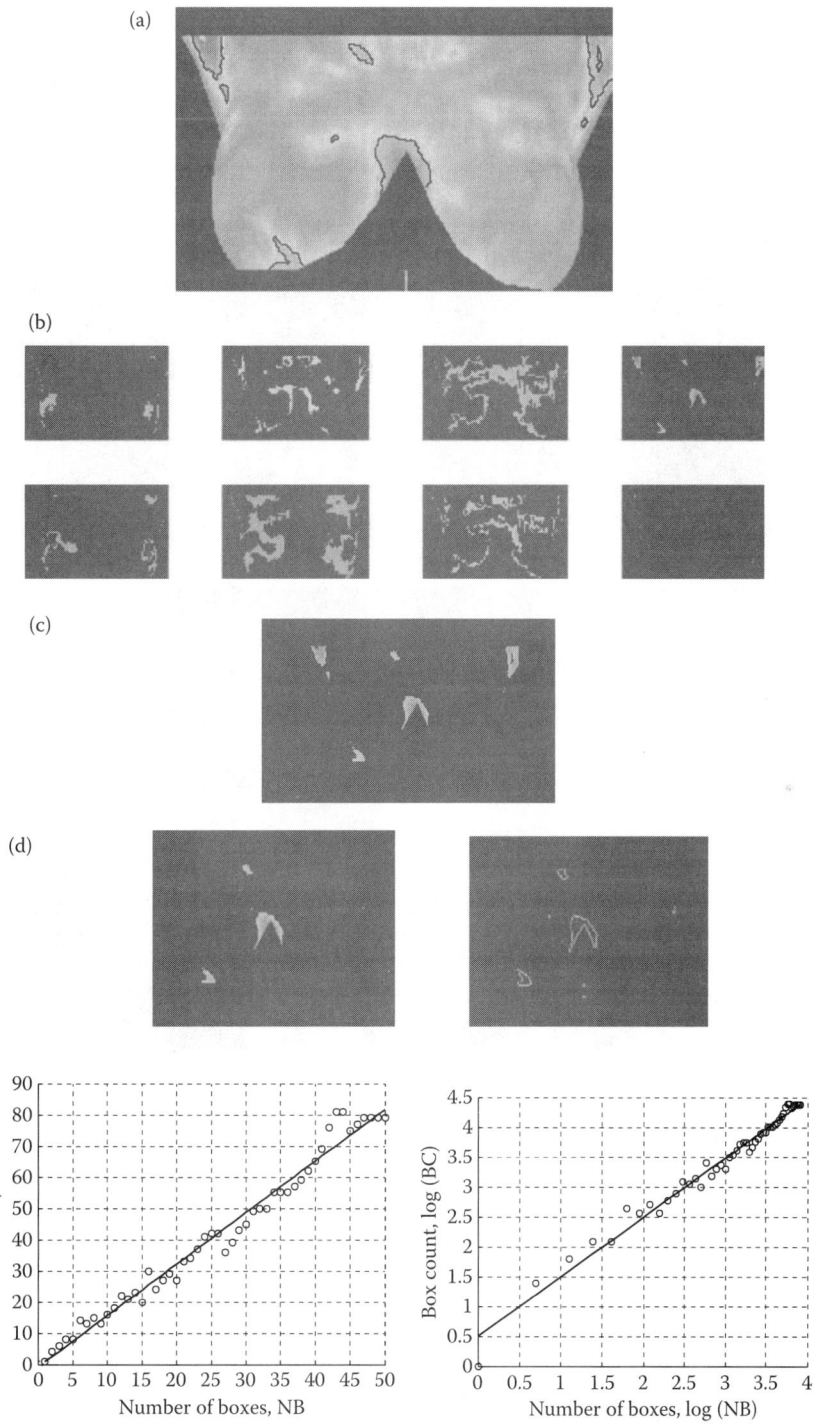

FIGURE 37.6 (a) Benign case 2 (B2). (b) Segmentation of (a) by fuzzy C mean. (c) The first hottest regions of B2. (d) B2: (1) The first hottest regions after removing the axilla boundaries. (2) Boundaries of part (1). (e) B2: (1) Box count (BC) versus number of boxes (NB). (2) log(BC) versus log (NB).

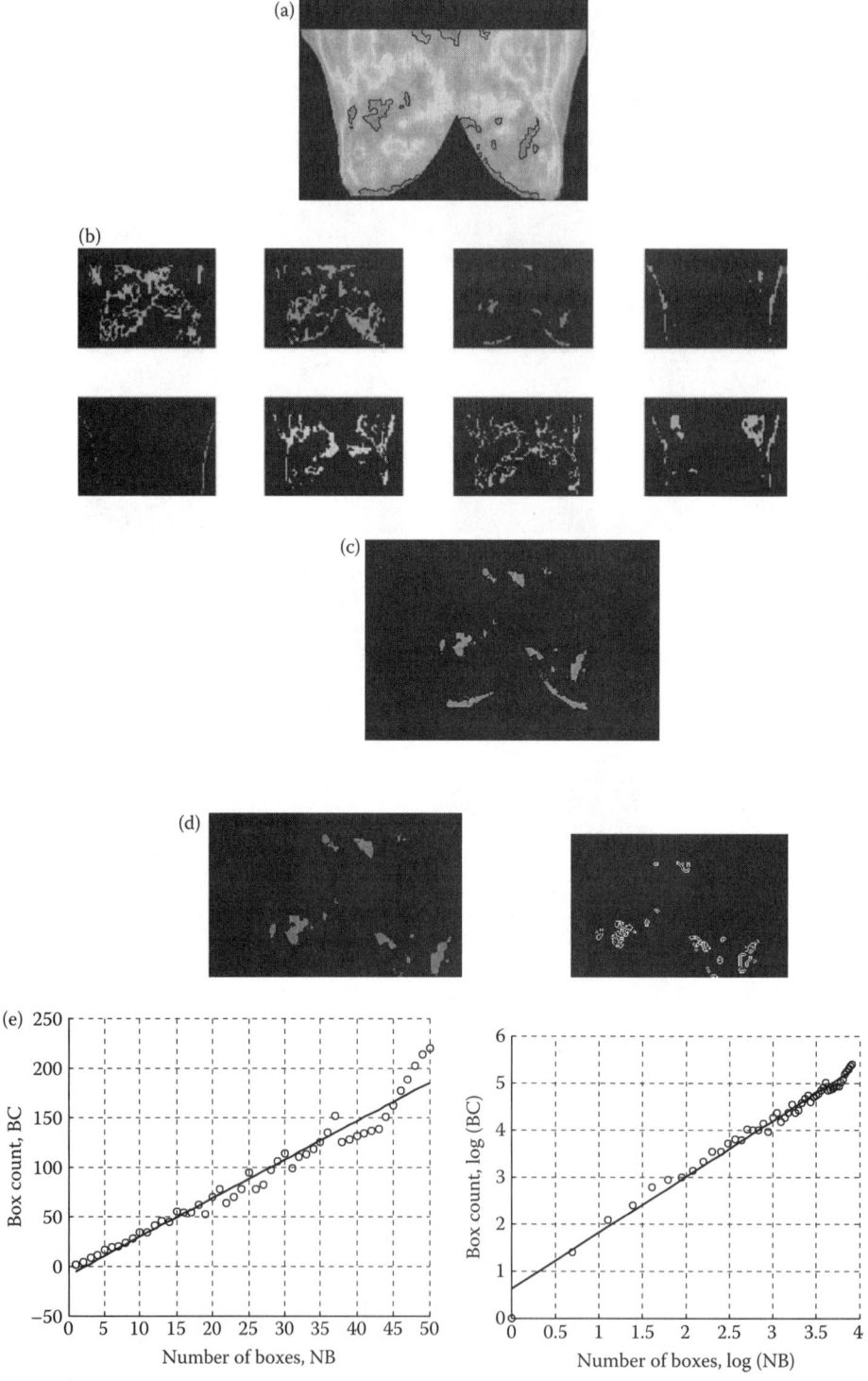

FIGURE 37.7 (a) Benign case 3 (B3). (b) Segmentation of (a) by fuzzy C mean. (c) The first hottest regions of B3. (d) B3: (1) The first hottest regions after removing close sternal boundaries. (2) Boundaries of part (1). (e) B3: (1) Box count (BC) versus number of boxes (NB). (2) log(BC) versus log (NB).

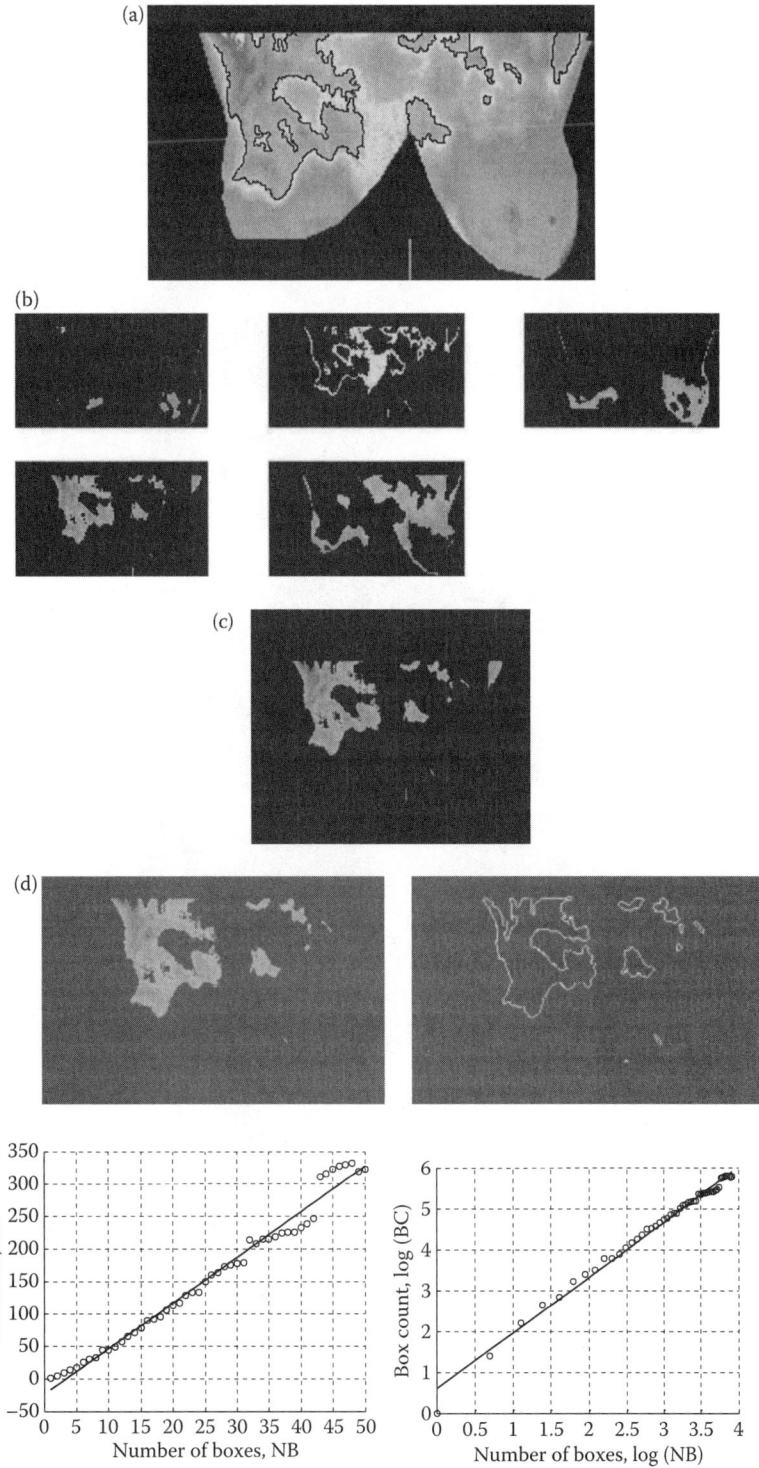

FIGURE 37.8 (a) Malignant case 1 (M1). (b) Segmentation of (a) by fuzzy C mean. (c) The first hottest regions of M1. (d) M1: (1) The first hottest regions after removing the axilla boundaries. (2) Boundaries of part (1). (e) M1: (1) Box count (BC) versus number of boxes (NB). (2) log(BC) versus log (NB).

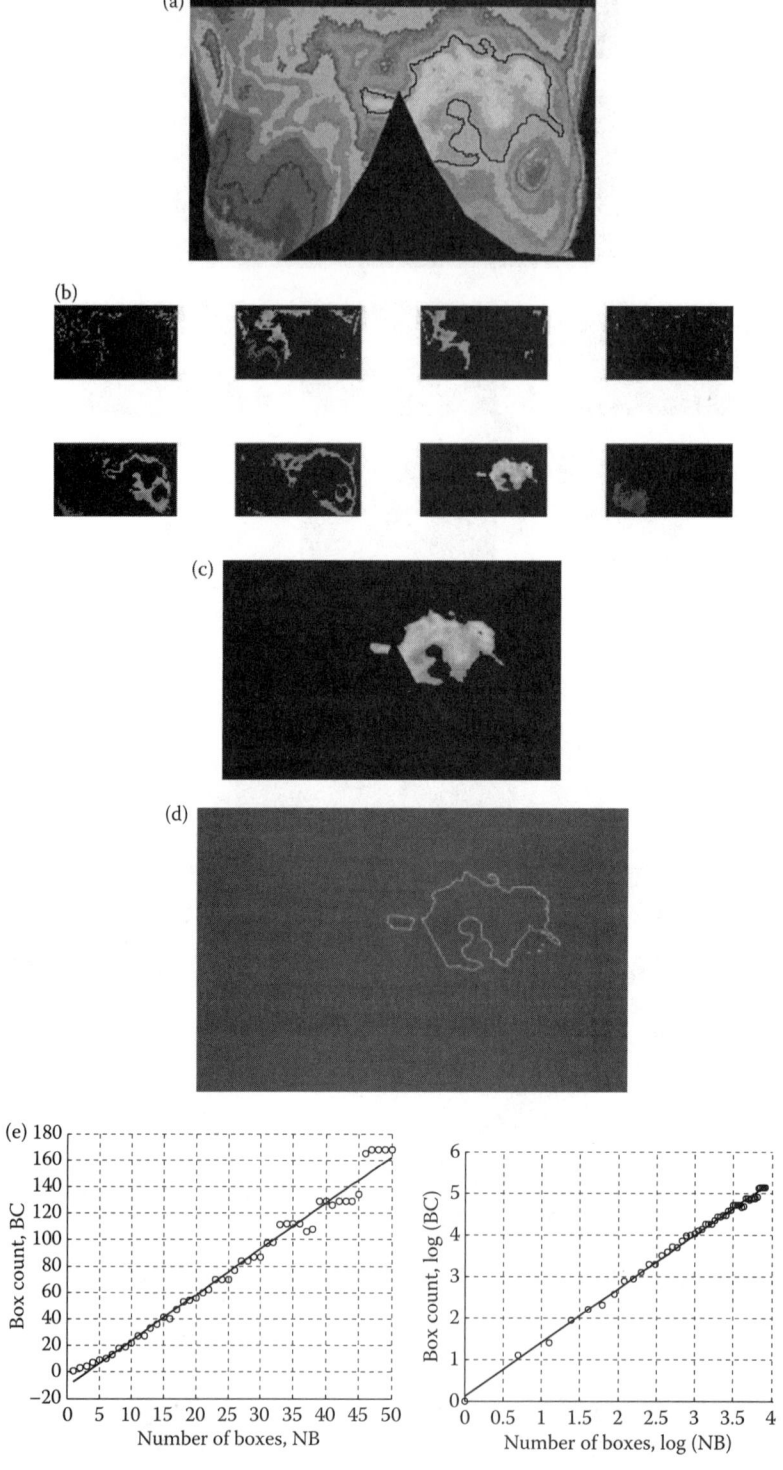

FIGURE 37.9 (a) Malignant case 2 (M2). (b) Segmentation of (a) by fuzzy C mean. (c) The first hottest regions of M2. (d) Boundaries of the first hottest regions of M2. (e) M2: (1) Box count (BC) versus number of boxes (NB). (2) log(BC) versus log (NB).

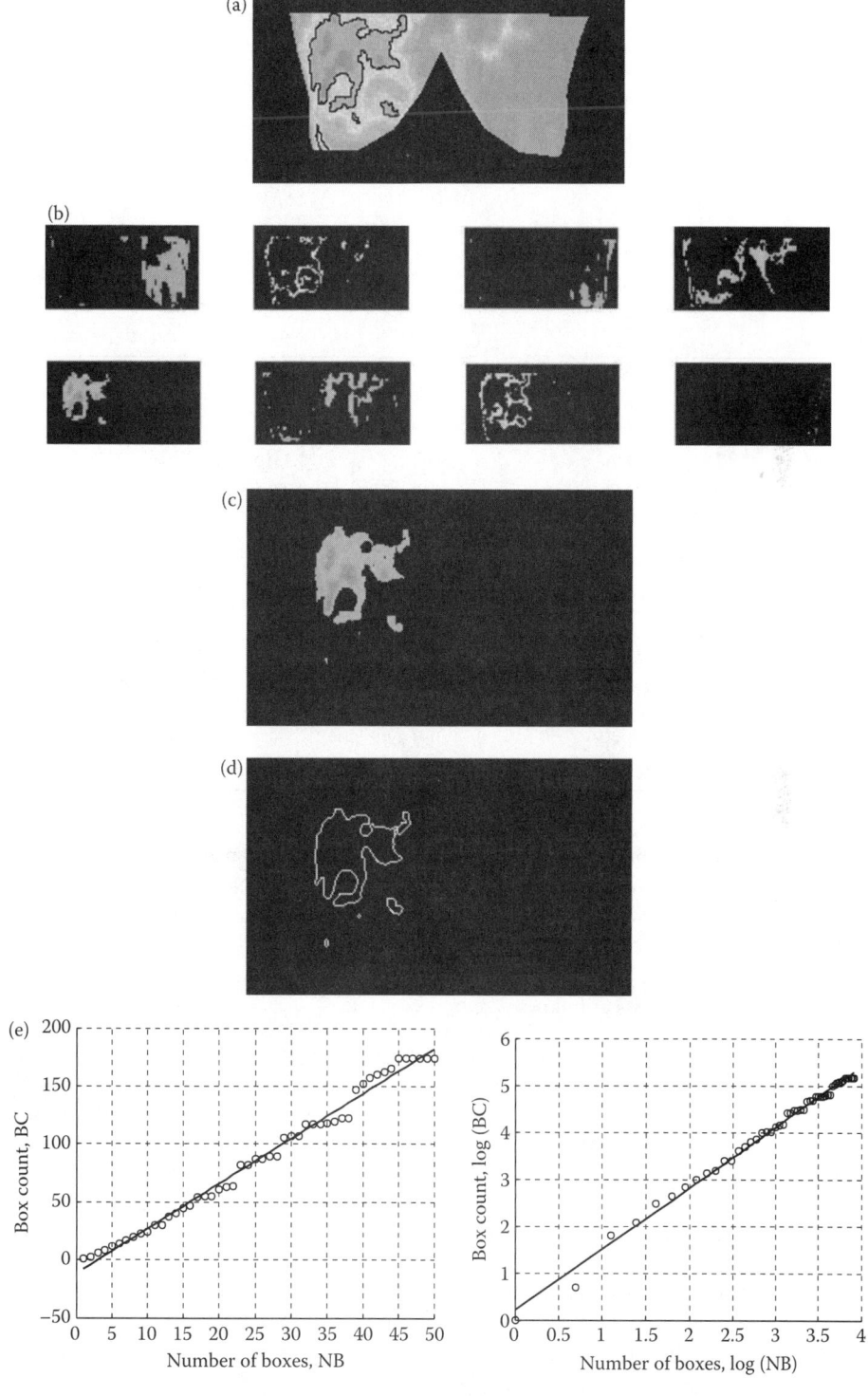

FIGURE 37.10 (a) Malignant case 3 (M3). (b) Segmentation of (a) by fuzzy C mean. (c) The first hottest regions of M3. (d) Boundaries of the first hottest regions of M3. (e) M3: (1) Box count (BC) versus number of boxes (NB). (2) log(BC) versus log (NB).

TABLE 37.2 Calculated FDs for Eight Benign and Seven Malignant Cases by BCM

B1	0.9675
B2	0.9911
B3	1.1321
B4	1.1060
B5	1.0382
B6	0.9781
B7	1.1218
B8	1.0081
M1	1.3538
M2	1.2992
M3	1.3479
M4	1.2787
M5	1.4001
M6	1.3310
M7	1.2884

B: benign, M: malignant.

TABLE 37.3 Mean and Standard Deviation of Calculated FDs for Eight Benign and Seven Malignant Cases

	Benign	Malignant
Mean	1.0429	1.3284
Standard deviation	0.2600	0.2074
Accuracy rate (%)	91.9	93.1

two points with maximum curvature of breasts were determined and geometrically transformed to the first and the last points of the averaged set points of the training results. Next, to fit two curves between the points with maximum curvature of each breast and the fifth point of it, a linear interpolation was employed. It performed faultlessly for 90% of all the cases at hand.

The proposed algorithm for detecting malignancy or benignity of breast tumors is then applied to both the left and the right breasts as follows:

1. The breast IR images are segmented by FCM algorithm. The number of clusters depends on the number of the camera palette colors.
2. The first hottest regions which have the color matching to the maximal temperature are diagnosed. The axilla and close sternal boundaries are removed and are not considered.
3. The FD of step (2) is estimated by BCMs as follows:
   - The image of the first hottest regions is made in binary.
   - The edges are detected.
   - A grid of boxes is set up.
   - The number of occupied boxes is counted.
   - The boxes sizes are changed and the previous step is repeated.
   - The slope of the best-fitting line to the plot of the log of the number of box count versus the log of the number of boxes is calculated.

It is notable that the breast IR images are normalized before using the BCM.

Three typical benign cases of breast thermograms are shown in Figures 37.5a, 37.6a, and 37.7a, respectively. Their images are color segmented by using the FCM algorithm and are illustrated respectively in Figures 37.5b, 37.6b, and 37.7b. The first hottest regions of thermal images are shown in Figures 37.5c, 37.6c, and 37.7c, with the axilla and close sternal boundaries removed in Figures 37.5d1, 37.6d1, and 37.7d1, and their corresponding boundaries are presented in Figures 37.5d2, 37.6d2, and 37.7d2. Plot of the number of box count (BC) versus the number of boxes (NB) and plot of the log(BC) versus log(NB) are depicted in Figures 37.5e, 37.6e, and 37.7e, respectively. For the three typical malignant cases, similar information is presented in Figures 37.8, 37.9, and 37.10, respectively.

The FDs for eight benign and seven malignant cases were estimated as tabulated in Table 37.2, and the mean and standard deviation of estimated FDs are presented in Table 37.3. The FD results for benign cases are not significantly different from 1, the topological dimension of a line, while those for malignant cases are however significantly greater.

37.8 Conclusion

Although there is no conclusive evidence that pseudocolor coding of gray images provides more information to the observer, the fact shows that carefully designed pseudocolor image coding does give lesion detection performance that equals gray scale and improves the performance of other tasks such as recognition and interpretation of a lesion. For color segmentation of IR breast images, we used the following three techniques.

Mean shift algorithm is very sensitive to the window size parameter h. Hence, in this investigation, we are frequently confronted with empty clusters, and choosing an appropriate h was not an easy task. K means algorithm minimizes the sum of within-cluster results mathematically and when clusters are compact and well separated, it provides accurate results. However, in many situations, K means clustering is not suitable where clusters are not disjoint and a sample pattern or a pixel in an image may belong to different clusters. It is very important for K means to have good initial cluster centers. Poor initial centers may cause empty clusters. There are some algorithms developed recently to improve the initial centers. In FCM clustering, pixels may belong to many clusters with different degrees of membership. In this study, due to the fuzzy nature of the thermal images, FCM technique gives more accurate results to segmentation of the IR images.

We also analyzed thermal images of breast using FD to identify the possible difference between malignant and benign patterns. The present numerical experimental results verify the theoretical concepts and show a significant difference in FD between malignant and benign cases, with the FDs for benign cases close to 1, while those for malignant cases significantly greater. This suggests that fractal analysis may potentially improve the reliability of thermography in breast tumor detection. Fractal dimension is very sensitive to the algorithm that segments images. The fuzzy nature of IR breast images helps the FCM segmentation and provides more accurate results than the others with no empty cluster.

For future work with a vast library of IR images at hand, validation of FCM to extract pathologically relevant structures can be demonstrated through comparing the regions segmented by FCM with the regions found by other modalities such as mammograms. Likewise, other popular descriptors, including principal components, area/perimeter, and so on, can be applied to characterize the regularity of the shape so as to compare with the FD. Lastly, one may try a better clustering algorithm such as Kohonen map and compare with K means.

References

1. Jones, B.F., A reappraisal of the use of infrared thermal image analysis in medicine. *IEEE Transactions on Medical Imaging.* 17:6,1019–1027, 1998, doi:10.1109/42.746635.
2. Ng, E.Y.K., A review of thermography as promising non-invasive detection modality for breast tumour. *International Journal of Thermal Sciences.* 48:5,849–855, 2009, doi:10.1016/j.ijthermalsci.2008.06.015.

3. Diakides, N., and Bronzino, J.D., *Medical Infrared Imaging*. New York: CRC, Taylor & Francis, 3rd edition, 2008.

4. Ng, E.Y.K., and Kee, E.C., Integrative computer-aided diagnostic with breast thermogram, *Journal of Mechanics in Medicine and Biology*, 7(1):1–10, 2007.

5. www.earlycancerdetection.com/breast_thermo.html (last accessed August 2010).

6. Foster, K.R., Thermographic detection of breast cancer, *IEEE Engineering in Medicine and Biology Magazine*, 17:610–614, 1998, doi:10.1109/51.734241.

7. Lawson, R.N., Implications of surface temperature in the diagnosis of breast cancer, *Canadian Medical Association Journal*, 75:4309–4310, 1956.

8. Ahmed, E., Fractals and chaos in cancer models, *International Journal of Theoretical Physics*, 32(2):353–355, 2004.

9. Baish, J.W., and Jain, R.K., *Fractals and Cancer, American Association for Cancer Research, Cancer Research*, 60, 3683–3688, 2000.

10. Zhou, X., Zhang, C., and Li, S. A perceptive uniform pseudo-color coding method of SAR images, Radar, CIE. *468 International Conference*, Shanghai, China, October 2006, IEEE, pp. 1–4.

11. Li, H., and Burgess, A.E., Evaluation of signal detection performance with pseudo-color display and lumpy backgrounds. In: Kundel H.L. (Ed.), *SPIE, Medical Imaging: Image Perception*, Vol 3036, Newport Beach, CA, USA, pp. 143–149, 1997.

12. Connolly, C., and Fliess, T., A study of efficiency and accuracy in the transformation from RGB to CIELAB color space, *IEEE Transactions on Image Processing*, 6(7):1046–1048, 1997.

13. Cheng, Y., Mean shift, mode seeking, and clustering, *IEEE Transactions on Pattern Analysis and Machine Intelligence*, 17(8):790–799, 1995.

14. Kybic, J., Mean shift segmentation, Winter Semester Course 2007, http://cmp.felk.cvut.cz/cmp/courses/33DZOzima2007/slidy/meanShiftSeg.pdf.

15. Mayer, A. and Greenspan, H., Segmentation of brain MRI by adaptive mean shift, *3rd IEEE International Symposium on Biomedical Imaging: Macro to Nano*, Arlington, VA, pp. 319–322, 2006.

16. Bezdek, J.C., Keller, J., Krisnapuram, R., and Pal, N.R. *Fuzzy Models and Algorithms for Pattern Recognition and Image Processing*, Norwell, MA: Kluwer, 1999.

17. AAT: http://aathermography.com (last accessed July 2010).

18. MII: http://www.breastthermography.com/case_studies.htm (last accessed July 2010).

19. ACCT: www.thermologyonline.org/Breast/breast_thermography_what.htm (last accessed July 2010).

20. http://www.thermographyofiowa.com/casestudies.htm (last accessed July 2010).

21. STImaging: http://www.stimaging.com.au/page2.html (last accessed July 2010).

22. Gazit, Y., Baish J.W., Safabakhsh, N., Leuning M., Baxter, L.T., and Jaim, R.K., Fractal characteristics of tumor vascular architecture during tumor growth and regression, *Microcirculation*, 4(4):395–402, 1997.

23. NCI: www.cancer.gov/cancertopics/UnderstandingCancer/angiogenesis (last accessed July 2009).

24. Gamagami, P. (Ed.), Indirect signs of breast cancer: Angiogenesis study, In: *Atlas of Mammography*, Cambridge, MA: Blackwell Science, pp. 231–236, 1996.

25. Guidi, A.J., and Schnitt, S.J., Angiogenesis in preinvasive lesions the breast, *The Breast Journal*, 2(4):364–369, 1996.

26. Alarcon, T., Byrne, H.M., and Maini, P.K., A cellular automaton model for tumour growth in inhomogeneous environment, *Journal of Theoretical Biology*, 225(2):257–274, 2003.

27. Smiley, M.W., and Levine, H.A., Numerical simulation of capillary formation during the onset of tumor angiogenesis, *Proceedings of the 4th International Conference on Dynamical System and Differential Equations*, Wilmington, NC, USA, 817–826, 2000.

28. Singh, Y., Tumor angiogenesis: Clinical implications, *Nepal Journal of Neuroscience*, 1(2):61–63, 2004.

29. Pisano, E.D., *Breast Imaging, Vol. 13 Breast Disease*, 130 pp, ISBN: 978-1-58603-168-8, VA, USA: IOS Press, 2002.

30. Scalerandi, M., Pescarmona, G.P., Delsanto, P.P., and Capogrosso Sansone B., Local interaction simulation approach for the response of the vascular system to metabolic changes of cell behavior, *Physical Review. E, Statistical, Nonlinear and Soft Matter Physics*, 63(1 Pt 1):011901, 2001.

31. Anbar, M., Hyperthermia of the cancerous breast: Analysis of mechanism, *Cancer Letters*, 84(1):23–29, 1994.

32. Anbar, M. (Ed.), Breast cancer. In: *Quantitative Dynamic Telethermometry in Medical Diagnosis and Management*, Ann Arbor, MI: CRC Press, pp. 84–94, 1994.

33. Lee, T.K., McLean, D.I., and Atkins, M.S., Irregularity index, a new border irregularity measure for cutaneous melanocytic lesions, *Medical Image Analysis*, 7(1):47–64, 2003.

34. Zheng, L., and Chan A.K., An artificial intelligent algorithm for tumor detection in screening mammogram, *IEEE Transactions on Medical Imaging*, 20(7):559–567, 2001.

35. Guo, Q., Ruiz, V., Shao, J., and Guo, F., A novel approach to mass abnormality detection in mammographic images, *Proceedings of the IASTED International Conference on Biomedical Engineering*, Innsbruck, Austria, pp. 180–185, 2005.

36. Caldwell, C.B., Stapleton, S.J., Holdsworth, D.W., Jong, R.A., Weiser, W.J., Cooke, G., and Yaffe, M.J., Characterization of mammographic parenchymal pattern by fractal dimension, *Physics in Medicine and Biology*, 35(2):235–247, 1990.

37. Byng, J.W., Boyd, N.F., Fishell, E., Jong, R.A., and Yaffe, M.J., Automated analysis of mammographic densities, *Physics in Medicine and Biology*, 41:909–923, 1996.

38. Gazit, Y., Berk, D.A., Leunig, M., Baxter, L.T., and Jain, R.K., Scale-invariant behavior and vascular network formation in normal and tumor tissue, *Physical Review Letters*, 75(12):2428–2431, 1995.

39. Grizzi, F., Russo, C., Colombo, P., Franceschini, B., Frezza, E., Cobos, E., and Chiriva-Internati, M., Quantitative evaluation and modeling of two-dimensional neovascular network complexity: The surface fractal dimension, *BMC Cancer*, 5(14), DOI: 10.1186/1471-2407-5-14, 2005.

40. Liu, J.Z., Zhang, L.D., and Yue, G.H., Fractal dimension in human cerebellum measured by magnetic resonance imaging, *Biophysical Journal*, 85(6):4041–4046, 2003.

41. Kuczynski, K., and Mikotajczak, P., *Magnetic Resonance Image Classification Using Fractal Analysis, Information Technologies in Biomedicine*, Berlin: Springer, 2008.

42. Esgiar, A.N., and Chakravorty, P.K., Fractal based classification of colon cancer tissue images, *IEEE, 9th International Symposium on Signal Processing and Its Application*, Sharjah, United Arab Emirates, February 1–4, 2007.

43. Lee, W.L., Chen, Y.C., and Chen, Y. Ch., Unsupervised segmentation of ultrasonic liver images by multiresolution fractal feature vector, *Information Science*, 175(3):177–195, 2005.

44. Rangayyan, R.M., and Nguyen, T.M., Fractal analysis of contours of breast masses in mammograms, *Journal of Digital Imaging*, 20(3):223–237, 2007.

45. Mastsubara, T., Fujita, H., Kasai, S., Goto, M., Tani, Y., Hara, T., and Endo, T., Development of new schemes for detection and analysis of mammographic masses, *Proceedings of the 1997 IASTED International Conference on Intelligent Information Systems (IIS97)*, Grand Bahamas Island, Bahamas, December 1997, pp. 63–66.

46. Homer, M.J., *Mammographic Interpretation, A Practical Approach*, Boston, MA: McGraw-Hill, 2nd edition, 1997.

47. Reston, V.A., *American College of Radiology, Illustrated Breast Imaging Reporting and Data System (BI-RADSTM)*, 3rd edition, Reston, VA: American College of Radiology, 1998.

48. Peitgen, H.O. Jurgens, H., and Saupe, D., *Chaos and Fractal, New Frontiers of Science*, New York, NY: Springer, 2004.

49. Liu, S.H., Formation and anomalous properties of fractals, *IEEE Engineering in Medicine and Biology Magazine*, 11(2):28–39, 1992.

50. Deering, W., and West, B.J., Fractal physiology, *IEEE Engineering in Medicine and Biology Magazine*, 11(2):40–46, 1992.

51. Schepers, H.E., Van Beek, J.H.G.M., and Bassingthwaighte, J.B., Four methods to estimate the fractal dimension from self affine signals, *IEEE Engineering in Medicine and Biology Magazine*, 11(2):57–64, 1922.

52. Fortin, C.S., Kumaresan, R., Ohley, W.J., and Hoefer, S., Fractal dimension in the analysis of medical images, *IEEE Engineering in Medicine and Biology Magazine*, 11(2):65–71, 1992.

53. Goldberger, A.L., Rigney, D.R., and West, B.J., Chaos and fractals in human physiology, *Scientific American*, 262(2):42–49, 1990.

38

The Role of Thermal Monitoring in Cardiosurgery Interventions

Antoni Nowakowski
Gdansk University of Technology

Mariusz Kaczmarek
Gdansk University of Technology

Jan Rogowski
Gdansk University of Medicine

38.1 Introduction

Applications of nondestructive testing based on IR-thermal imaging (NDT TI) are of a very high importance in industry. Classical quantitative IR-thermal imaging (QIRT) and active dynamic thermography (ADT) belong to this field of technology. During the last 25 years, one may observe a very rapid development of solutions such as lock-in, pulsed phase (PPT), ADT, and thermal tomography (TT) in a variety of different applications and just recently also in medical diagnostics [1]. This is due to increased availability of mature technology based on uncooled FPA (focal plane array) IR-detectors, significant decrease of equipment prices, as well as implementation of advanced digital image analysis methods. Therefore, it is not surprising that IR-thermal imaging was also implemented as a useful tool in surgery and cardiosurgery inspection. Probably the first published case of such an application was the use of a thermal camera in the Department of Cardiac Surgery, Heartcenter, University of Leipzig [2–4]. We are involved in the practical use of IR-thermal imaging in cardiosurgery for more than 12 years [5,6], also implementing ADT and TT procedures unknown in medical applications.

In this chapter, the results of a research project devoted to the analysis of the value of IR-thermal imaging in monitoring the quality of cardiosurgery interventions are presented. The research was performed at the Department of Biomedical Engineering, Gdansk University of Technology in cooperation with the Department of Cardiosurgery, Gdansk University of Medicine. *In vivo* experiments on animals have been performed at the Department of Animal Physiology, Gdansk University. The aim of the project was to show which procedures may be directly applied in clinics and which one in specific fields of research. To better understand physiology, apart from thermal studies, active and passive electrical properties of the tested tissues have also been studied. In the following text, basic problems related to practical applications of QIRT in the evaluation of cardiosurgery procedures quality are discussed. The results of the research have already been published, for example, Reference 7.

It should be underlined that medical applications of QIRT in comparison to technical NDT TI applications are much more difficult as heat transfers in living tissues are far more complicated compared to technical applications of nondestructive testing based on IR-thermal imaging. Additionally, in cardiosurgery, the basic problem is nonlinear and the strongly stochastic nature of the beating heart mechanical action which is changing all the dimensions in the tested field. Also, the natural biofeedback reactions of living organisms and tissues should be avoided to get a clear interpretation of measurement results.

One important feature of the application of ADT in medicine should be underlined—analysis of a given problem requires high skills in the modeling of a tested case as all processes of diagnostics use objective model-based evaluation of measurement data. There are also other problems, which have to be taken into account to perform reliable analysis of measurement data, such as elimination of displacement errors, choice of proper measurement conditions, and so on. The following text contains a discussion of problems present in QIRT and ADT IR-thermal analysis of living objects—here, the beating heart.

38.2 Measurement Set-Up

The general concept (block diagram of the measurement set) of measurements performed in QIRT and ADT adapted to cardiosurgery is shown in Figure 38.1. The basic components applied as individual instruments are exchangeable. IR-thermal camera is applied for measurements of temperature distribution at the surface of the heart muscle. To avoid problems with the interpretation of series of thermal images of the beating heart (problems of the heart motion), the registration of images may be synchronized with the heart action using the QRS detector. Versatile acquisition of electrical and thermal data may be set using automatic procedures run in the applied computer-driven system. The electrical instruments allow measurements of cardiac potential and collection of electrical impedance spectroscopy data. Additionally, the thermal excitation source may be applied to perform ADT experiments.

First, the steady-state temperature distribution on the tested surface is recorded using an IR camera. Next, in ADT, an external thermal excitation is applied to force thermal transients at the tested surface. Recording of the temperature allows the calculation of thermal parameters, such as thermal

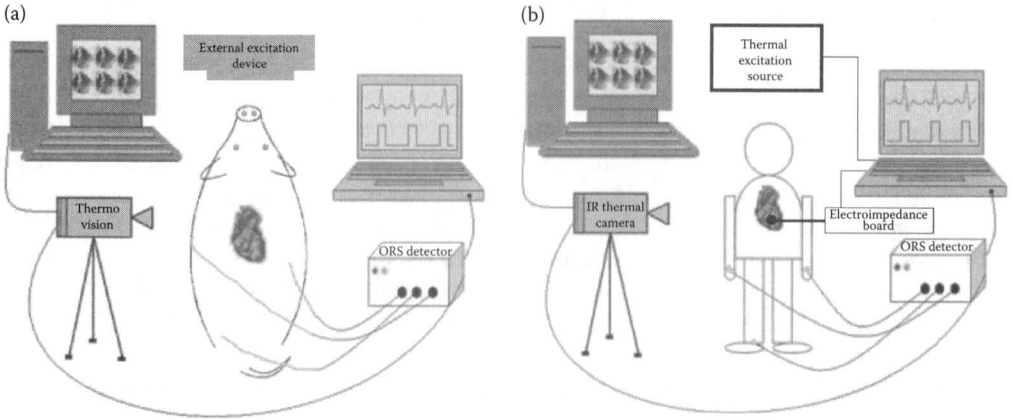

FIGURE 38.1 Measurement set-up for QIRT, ADT, and electrical experiments in cardiosurgery applications: (a) animal experiment, (b) in clinics.

time constants, dependent on the state of the tested structure. We apply external pulse excitation lasting several seconds, up to 1 min, using several solutions, as an apparatus for cryotherapy for cooling or optical excitation for heating. The IR camera is used for capturing series of thermal images, allowing measurements of temperature transients on the tested surface.

The IR camera synchronized with an excitation source (in the experiments described here, this was a set of halogen lamps or an air cooling system, but we are now mainly using CO_2 cryotherapy instrumentation for cooling) allows the surface temperature of the object under examination to be recorded at a speed of 30 frames/s for the AGEMA 900 SW 0.1°C resolution system; similar conditions are used for the uncooled Flir A320G system and 60 frames/s for the SC 3000 QWIP FPA LW 0.02°C system. Changes in tested surface temperature are caused by an external source and are dependent on the internal state of the heart muscle. More detailed description of the instrumentation and procedures applied in thermal monitoring are discussed in Reference 1, where the concept of nondestructive testing using thermal instrumentation is generally described. Our approaches are also presented in several former publications, for example, References 6–8.

To show that the application of the IR camera and an external excitation source is not disturbing the work of doctors, a view of the ADT experiment with halogen lamp excitation is presented in Figure 38.2a, animal experiments, and Figure 38.2b, at the clinic. There is plenty of space for a surgeon to perform interventions as the optical path must be free only at the moment of ADT measurements, while for the rest of the time the image may be disturbed as even a glimpse of the surgeon is sufficient for control of the situation. Additionally, a typical high-resolution RGB camera may be applied for continuous observation of surgical interventions. A prototype system developed in our project with all elements allowing QIRT and ADT experiments is shown in Figure 38.3.

A typical procedure of thermal image capture after cooling is shown in Figure 38.4. Moments of measurements are dotted. Usually, image registration should be synchronized with the heart action to obtain a stable position of the heart in thermal images.

Visual and IR images may be matched, as it is shown in Figure 38.5. Such a procedure may be important for the precise localization of the heart muscle position in thermal images. Also, external markers may be applied for the stabilization of images in time.

Single excitation and registration of transient temperatures at the position x–y allows the identification of the structure "in depth" on the basis of the equivalent thermal model. For all pixels, reconstruction of shallow 3D images of the tested object is possible. In the ADT case, the temperature of each pixel

(a) 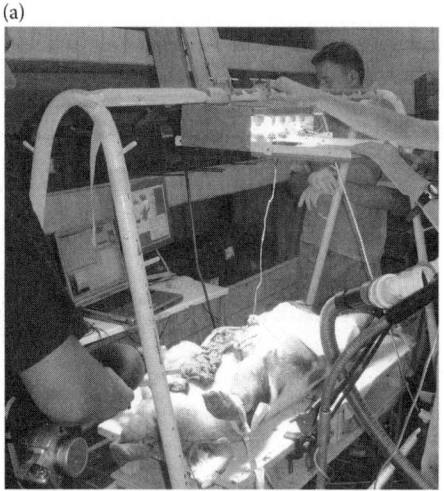 (b)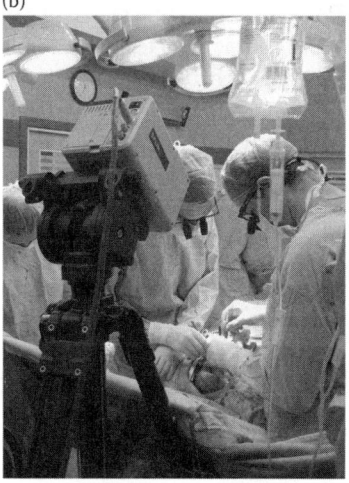

FIGURE 38.2 Placement of an IR-camera during cardiosurgery. (a) Agema THV 900, (b) FLIR SC3000.

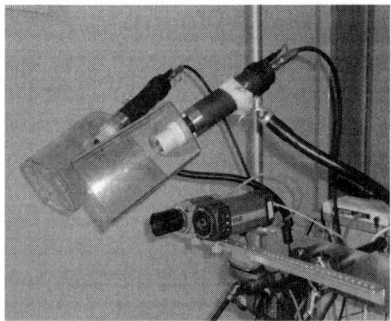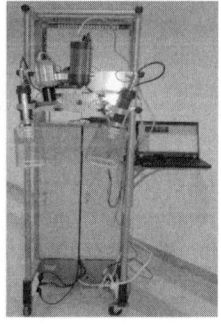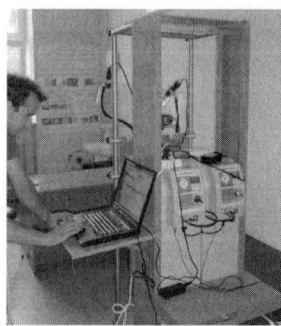

FIGURE 38.3 The experimental set—view from three perspectives. IR and RGB cameras are visible as well as cooling heads of the CO_2 cryotherapy system.

is recorded to calculate thermal time constants specific at each pixel. The parametric image of the time constants then enables the tested surface to be visualized, owing the high degree of correlation with the depth of the affected tissue.

38.3 Instrumentation: Software Problems

There are at least three levels of the software necessary to perform data acquisition and analysis of collected data, leading to diagnostic conclusions in QIRT and ADT. The first one combines specific software for the execution of all necessary actions of the system, as starting measurements, synchronization of excitation sources and recording cameras, and so on. If several imaging modalities are applied, visible and IR, then it is important that synchronization is performed between different cameras.

The second level of the software combines all elements of communication interfaces, including user-friendly manipulation of the system (GUI). In a typical solution, such a software is written in C++ and is specific for the technology applied.

Still, and within the third level of the software, there are different practical problems requiring additional software tools, for example, to eliminate natural movements of a living object or synchronization of images during cardiosurgery interventions, when the beating heart is changing its volume, position, and shape in a nonlinear way. This leads to the question how to analyze thermal transients and apply procedures of automatic understanding of image content, when in the following moments, each detector of the FPA sees not the same region of a tested object and additionally, the temperature at each pixel is also changing in time. Two factors are influencing the measurements based on series of images: first, displacement of a patient, and second, change of the thermal content in the following images. To solve the problems, some actions are needed to eliminate unwanted factors responsible for errors induced in sequences of thermal images collected in time. The first obvious action must be matching (stabilization) of following images to see the same area of a tested object/region, to allow further thermal analysis of series of thermal images. This task is not always easy, especially when the object is moving its position and shape in time. This is a typical case of the heart during open-chest cardiosurgical interventions. Dynamic changes of the heart in time combine not only change of the position but also the angle of observation, volume, and temperature at the surface of the heart, limiting the possibility of using ADT for proper diagnostics of the state of the heart muscle. We asked if there are any possibilities to monitor cardiosurgery interventions to assure a high quality of such operations based on quantitative evaluation of the content of the following images. Unfortunately, the heart during one cycle of action is strongly changing not only its position but also its volume. Practically, all visible elements at its surface are changing positions and are stressed and expanded in a nonlinear way. In effect, the application of simple affine transformations, typically sufficient in studies of other applications, is in this case not effective. What algorithms would be sufficient to make such transformations that will force the structure of

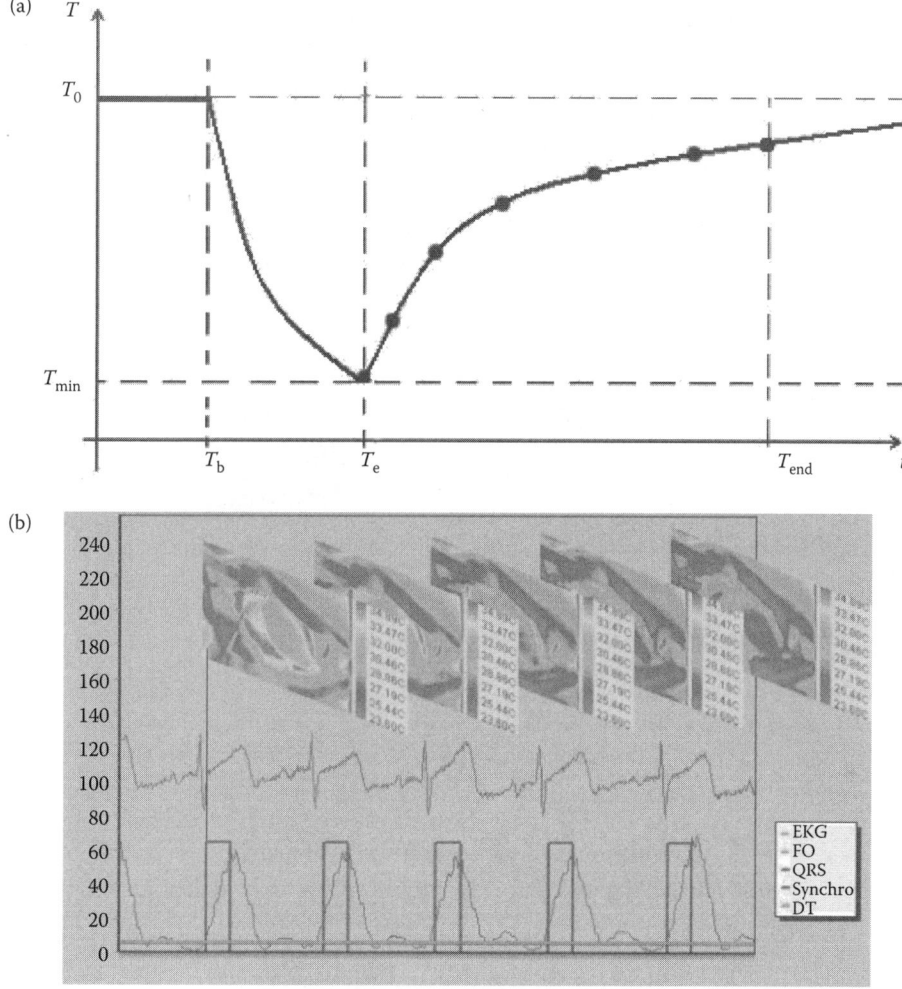

FIGURE 38.4 Measurement procedure requires registration of temperature transients at any pixel x,y in time. The example (a) shows the trace of temperature at x,y—cooling excitation; $t_{b/e}$—moments at which the cooling source is switched *on* (beginning) and *off* (end of excitation), respectively, t_{end}—time of termination of the recording; dots are indicating moments of thermal image capture; (b) shows that thermal images are measured synchronically with the heart rate, according to QRS.

images to unchanged positions? This means the elimination of all artifacts of position, angle of observation, and dimensions of the heart muscle in such a way that those pixels representing specific regions of the heart surface always stay in the same position, independently of the evolution of the tested structure in time. Unfortunately, solving such problems is not trivial and there are no software packages available that support this task. We tried several algorithms of image stabilization and matching but the problem is still generally unsolved. For objective evaluation of different correction algorithms, we prepared software "phantoms" of easy modified distortions, based on real images of the beating heart [9]. For the objective comparison of images after transformations, the following figures of merit are applied: correlation of images (CORR) (Equation 38.1)—which is the best in terms of a clear description of image differences (the value 1 means full identity); root mean square (RMS) (Equation 38.2)—0 means the identity; and the normalized mean square error (NMSE) (Equation 38.3)—the smaller the value the better the fitting of images:

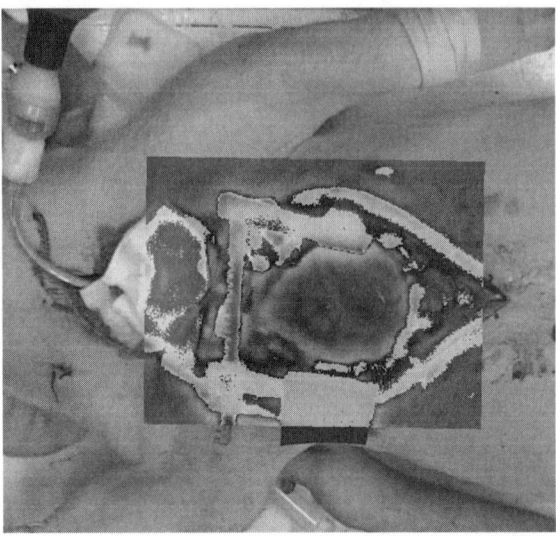

FIGURE 38.5   Matching of visible and IR images may help in recognition of the region of interest.

$$\text{CORR} = \frac{\sum_{x=0}^{X}\sum_{y=0}^{Y}[F(x,y) - \bar{F}][G(x,y) - \bar{G}]}{\sqrt{\sum_{x=0}^{X}\sum_{y=0}^{Y}[F(x,y) - \bar{F}]^2[G(x,y) - \bar{G}]^2}} \tag{38.1}$$

$$\text{RMS} = \frac{1}{N}\sum_{x=0}^{X}\sum_{y=0}^{Y}\sqrt{[F(x,y) - G(x,y)]^2} \tag{38.2}$$

$$\text{NMSE} = \frac{\sum_{x=0}^{X}\sum_{y=0}^{Y}[F(x,y) - G(x,y)]^2}{\sum_{x=0}^{X}\sum_{y=0}^{Y}[F(x,y)]^2} \tag{38.3}$$

where $F(x,y)$ is the pixel value at the point (x,y) in the unchanged image, $G(x,y)$ is the pixel value at the point (x,y) in the deformed image, N is the number of the gray-scale levels, and $\bar{F}$ is the mean value of the image intensity.

To show the simulation methodology, a thermal image of the heart during open-chest cardiosurgery animal experiment is shown in Figure 38.6. The region of interest (ROI), here showing the position of the tested heart, is calculated and indicated as the bright polygon (Figure 38.6a). This area is cut off and a new polygon of assumed parameters is inserted, representing the required mechanical and thermal changes (Figure 38.6b). In this case, the arrows show the direction of shrinking forces and the mechanical deformation is clearly visible in the deformed grid. The next step is the application of a reconstruction algorithm. One has to apply an algorithm generating the anti-deformed grid, as it is shown in Figure 38.6c. Unfortunately, usually the reconstruction is not perfect due to the loss of some data caused by, for example, numerical errors. Additionally, a specific pattern of thermal fields may be applied. Also, this pattern is suffering transformation errors, resulting in the limitation of visualization accuracy. In this way, a series of images in time may be simulated, giving data for further analysis of reconstruction algorithms or thermal tomography procedures to be applied.

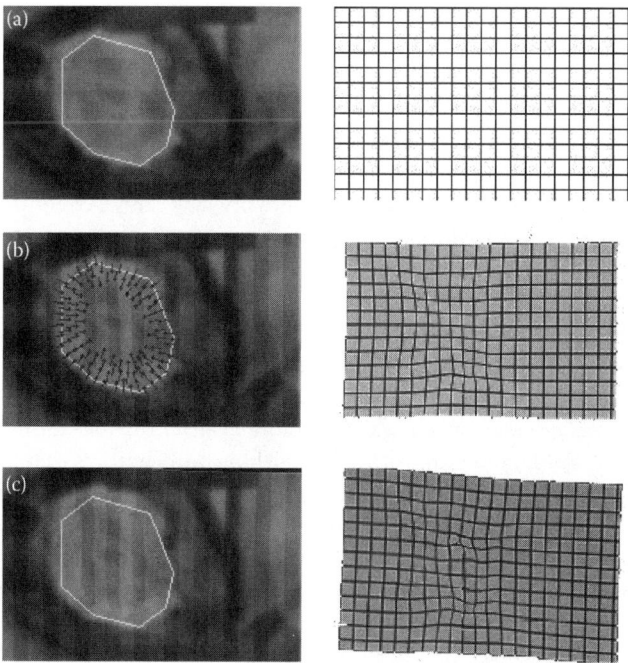

FIGURE 38.6 (a) Original thermal image of a heart and regular geometry transformation grid; (b) the same image after forward transformation (directions of the inserted geometry distortions are indicated by arrows and the grid is respectively deformed); additionally, pattern showing modulation of external temperature is visible; (c) application of the reverse algorithm represented by the geometry of the modified (anti-deformed) grid.

One should note that the segmentation of the heart from thermal images is not an easy task as the differences of temperature between the heart tissues and surrounding tissues may be not high enough to differentiate tissues or organs. Also, during the collection of the series of images, the temperature field in different parts of the ROI is usually changed, which makes the problem even more complicated. To enhance and facilitate the segmentation procedure, an additional RGB camera may be applied and a fusion of the visible and IR images may significantly improve this step of the analysis. Generally, using different approaches, one may regard the segmentation to be successful if the correlation of the indicated ROI and the real ROI exceeds the value 0.96. It means that, for the heart, the probability that a chosen pixel represents the proper part of the heart equals 96%. This work is still continuing.

38.4 Experiments and Measurements

The following text is divided into two parts, the first devoted to animal experiments, to answer several research questions, and the second to clinical applications, to show the practical value of the technology. In both cases, to meet the high accuracy of the experiments, all reference environmental and procedural conditions required for static thermography examination have been secured. The experiments have been conducted in an air-conditioned environment, the temperature and humidity being, respectively, typically 20°C and 60% in the operation theatre and 22–23°C and 45–55% in the animal quarters.

38.4.1 Animal Experiments: Methods and Materials

Pigs were taken as the experimental animals due to their closeness to the human physiological and anatomical structure of the heart muscle and circulatory system. Studies based on *in vivo* animal experiments were performed according to all legal regulations and permission by the Gdansk Ethics Commission for Experimentation on Animals.

Optimized solutions of instrumentation have been analyzed during the experiments, such as evoked heart stroke, coronary artery by-pass grafting CABG, off pump OP CABG procedures, and others. One of the important problems was to compare thermal and electrical measurements, as the response of the heart muscle to electrical stimulation may be nonlinear. We expect that such a measurement may hold important diagnostic information as the level of nonlinearity may carry extra information of the heart tissue properties. The question was—is there a correlation between thermal and electrical tissue properties? Here, the results presented in References 10, 11 are summarized.

The experiments were conducted on several young domestic pigs, each weighing approximately 25 kg. Anesthesia and analgesia were obtained by the administration of ketamine (im), pentobarbital (iv), and fentanyl (iv) at doses of 20, 30–50, and 0.5–0.1 mg/kg, respectively. The animal chest was open by sternotomy; the pericardium was stitched off to have full access to the heart muscle as it is shown in Figure 38.7. The intubation procedure was applied to keep the animal alive. To evoke the heart muscle ischemia, the left descending artery (LAD) was clamped, totally blocking the delivery of the blood (see Figure 38.8).

The short-term effects of ischemia preconditioning and blood arrest in the left ventricle were studied in a swine model of beating heart coronary artery revascularization using ADT instrumentation and image processing. The open-chest experiments with full accessibility to the heart were performed to test typical surgical procedures.

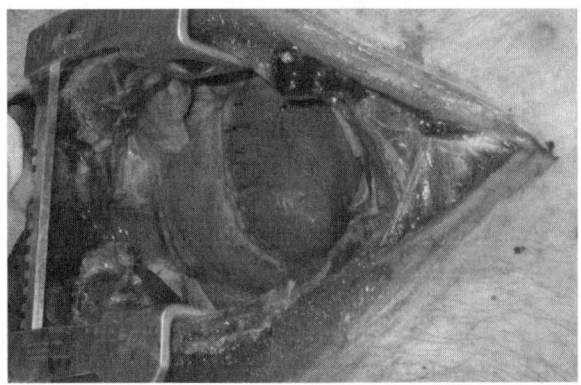

FIGURE 38.7   Exposition of a pig heart before clamping LAD.

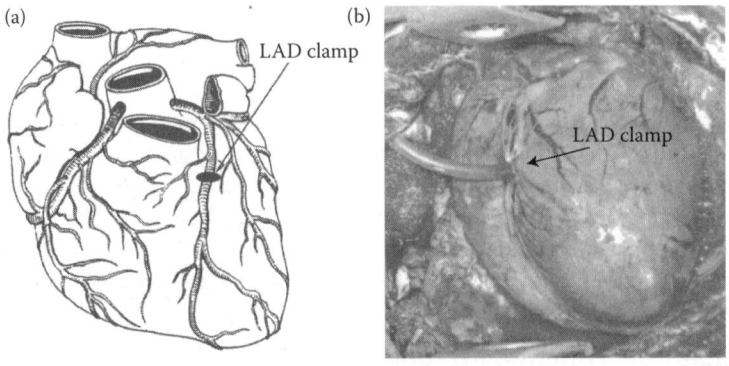

FIGURE 38.8   (a) Diagram of the heart muscle circulatory system [12]; (b) the heart photo with indicated site of clamped LAD.

Permanent clamping of the LAD procedure was damaging the heart muscle in the same way as the heart infarct, resulting in a strong modification of tissue structure and changes of thermal and electrical properties of the heart muscle in time. The heart fibrillation and following death of the animal was observed typically 35–70 min following permanent clamping of LAD. The thermal state of the heart was monitored using an IR thermal camera and simple recording of radiation emitted by the observed surface of the heart. Additionally, the thermal properties of the heart muscle were calculated from ADT experiments based on external thermal excitation.

One of the several protocols applied in the research experiments is the protocol presented in Figure 38.9. The ischemia episodes and thermal investigation are marked on the time chart. The camera indicates the registration of static thermography and ADT—the active dynamic thermography procedure with cooling excitations. The two ischemic preconditioning episodes lasting 2 min each was followed by the permanent clamping of LAD. Seven measuring sessions were performed during the total period of experiment. Several similar experiments have been performed to obtain reliable conclusions.

Ischemic preconditioning (IP), defined as a rapid adaptation response to a brief ischemic episode, was tested as a protecting procedure following the high-risk cardiosurgery. Evidence of ischemic preconditioning has been shown in a large number of previous studies developed in animal and human procedures, for example, References 13–15. IP has been found to increase myocardial tolerance for blood arrest, to reduce the rate of anaerobic glycolysis, and to reduce the area of necrosis during prolonged ischemia. On the other hand, this technique has also been found to fail, and since there is no reliable and clinically suitable method for intrasurgery monitoring of efficacy, the IP is performed "blindly." To our knowledge, presented here (after the paper [10]) are the first ADT parametric images of the myocardium recorded just after removing occlusion from LAD during the preconditioning procedure. One of the goals of this study was to understand ischemic preconditioning in protecting the heart muscle and its role in therapeutic procedures. We asked if one may see the effect of preconditioning on ADT images.

The ADT experiment was performed using a cooling device, generating an air stream with a temperature of 5°C, and the timing was 30 s of the stimulus and 90 s of the recording temperature at the recovery phase (self-rewarming). As an example of measurements performed using the acquisition system, which is shown in Figure 38.1a and according to the experimental protocol shown in Figure 38.9, typical results are presented in Tables 38.1 and 38.2 and in Figures 38.10 through 38.12. The chosen ROIs represent the left (AR01, AR02) and the right ventricle (AR03) surfaces. The AR01 is located above the clamp site and the AR02 below the site of clamping the LAD.

The two exponential thermal model for the calculation of parametric images is applied. The results for τ_1 and τ_2 at ROI for the self-rewarming phase are presented in Tables 38.1 and 38.2.

Strong changes of tissue properties are visible for both time constants. The physical factors responsible for decrease or increase in time of the value of time constants are not fully recognized. Several

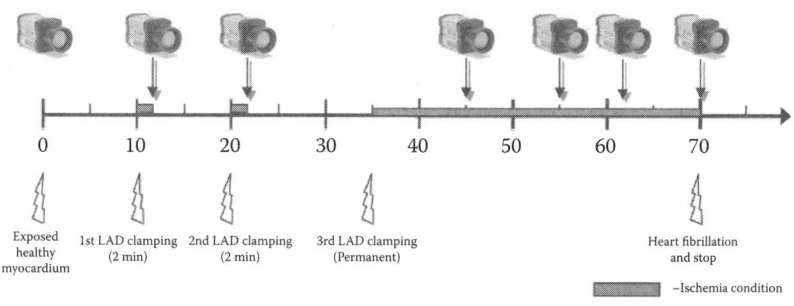

Time of experiment (min)

FIGURE 38.9 Experiment schedule with indicated surgery incidents and measurements points; static thermography and ADT as well as electrical impedance measurements.

TABLE 38.1 Time Constants τ_1 (s) for the Schedule Shown in Figure 38.9

	ROI		
Time (min)	AR01	AR02	AR03
0	2.059 ± 0.226	2.672 ± 0.441	3.709 ± 0.309
12	1.130 ± 0.174	0.797 ± 0.081	0.806 ± 0.145
24	0.426 ± 0.107	0.187 ± 0.057	1.705 ± 0.231
45	2.352 ± 1.526	3.114 ± 0.276	2.007 ± 0.489
55	2.166 ± 0.556	3.441 ± 0.319	3.856 ± 0.427
62	2.035 ± 0.299	2.976 ± 0.325	0.664 ± 0.112
70	4.220 ± 0.229	4.926 ± 0.235	0.618 ± 0.071

TABLE 38.2 Time Constants τ_2 (s) for the Schedule Shown in Figure 38.9

	ROI		
Time (min)	AR01	AR02	AR03
0	23.876 ± 0.969	14.971 ± 1.168	19.660 ± 1.800
12	19.473 ± 0.568	15.276 ± 0.323	10.449 ± 0.331
24	17.449 ± 0.770	11.709 ± 0.388	10.684 ± 0.770
45	26.273 ± 4.090	39.601 ± 2.373	13.552 ± 2.007
55	32.364 ± 4.053	45.636 ± 2.353	14.463 ± 2.637
62	42.052 ± 5.097	47.051 ± 3.956	8.418 ± 0.281
70	35.253 ± 2.017	48.586 ± 3.751	21.122 ± 0.245

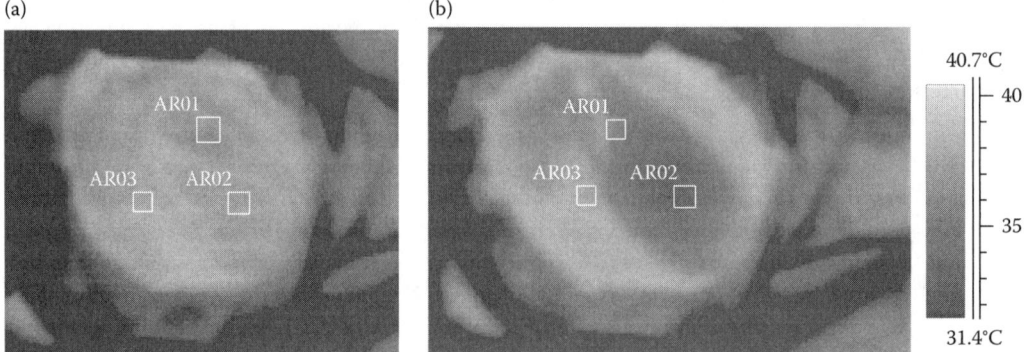

FIGURE 38.10 Thermograms of the myocardium with marked regions of interest AR0x; (a) for normal condition, (b) after clamping of LAD.

factors, mainly the changes in vascularization and changes in cell structures in the affected regions, what can be confirmed by histopathology examination, may be regarded as important. Influence of red blood cells or/and content of water extravasated within the interstitial space, drying of the myocardium surface, and some other phenomena may be taken into account too.

We found that ischemic preconditioning usually is followed by coronary flow increase as the autonomic reaction to blood delivery decrease. It is manifested by decreasing values of the time constants τ_1 and τ_2 for all ROI for measurements collected in the 24th minute, compared to measurements performed at the 0 minute, according to the experiment schedule. This observation is similar to that described in References 16, 17 for ultrasonic imaging.

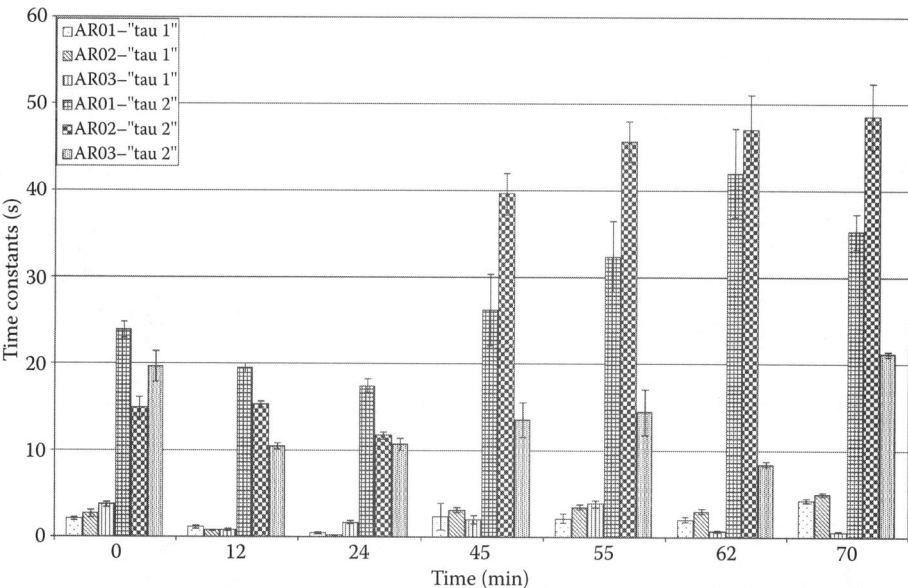

FIGURE 38.11 Estimated time constants (τ_1 and τ_2) for regions of interest AR0x; measurements according to the schedule shown in Figure 38.9.

Measurements acquired after the permanent clamping of LAD show that calculated time constants are getting longer during the blood arrest episode for the left ventricle area—about 4 times longer than for IP condition, while for the right ventricle the time constants stay almost the same or are even decreased. Parametric images of the time constant based on the sequence of thermograms recorded during the self-rewarming transient thermal processes show exactly the area of limited or increased blood perfusion (Figure 38.12).

For the measurements acquired just after the second preconditioning episode, the temperature and the time constant images are relatively uniform with visible big blood arteries (LAD and diagonal branches). In the 20 min following the permanent clamping of LAD, the static temperature image shows that the left ventricle of the heart is of lower temperature than the right ventricle. This temperature is also lower compared to the measurement taken just after the second preconditioning episode. But this lower temperature is almost the same as for the measurements taken in the 10 and the 27 min following the permanent clamping of LAD! We conclude that the static temperature of the left ventricle during blood arrest is significantly lower than for the right ventricle, but after few minutes following clamping of LAD temperature, it reaches the stabilized level. So, the static temperature could not be a discriminating parameter for monitoring the myocardium perfusion quality. The time constant image (Figure 38.12d) shows the area of limited blood flow region characterized by longer time constants. However, there is still a serious lack of information concerning thermal and physiological processes during and after ischemic preconditioning episodes and during progressed heart infarct. Furthermore, the cardioprotective effect (increase of perfusion) of ischemic preconditioning is evident. In our further work, we want to correlate thermal imaging data with bioimpedance measurements of the myocardium.

These preliminary findings show that the proposed methodology is able to determine the changes of blood flow intensity in the myocardium.

Apart from ADT, the thermal behavior of the heart muscle using classical QIRT measurements is very interesting, as illustrated in Figure 38.13. In contrast to ADT, where structural thermal tissue properties are measured, a very important functional information is evidenced here. On the other hand,

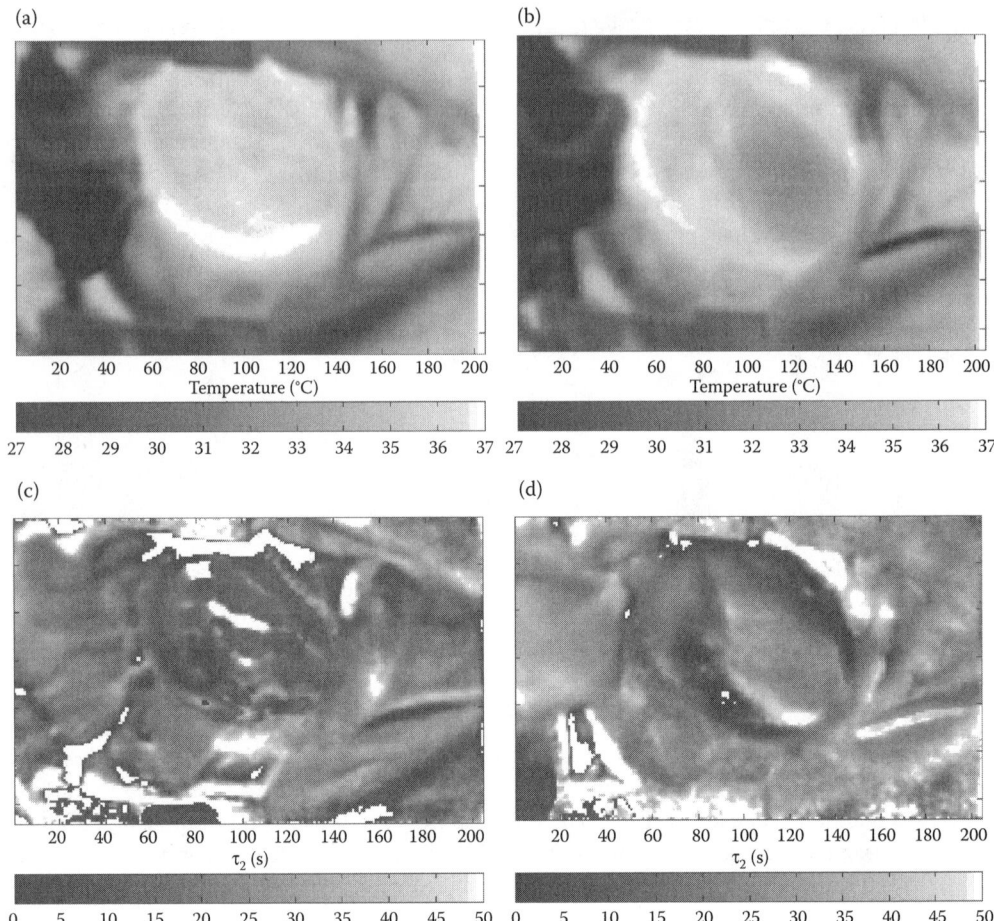

FIGURE 38.12   (a) and (b) Static thermograms; (c) and (d) estimated time constants τ_2 images for measurements taken in 24 min (the first column) and 55 min (the second column) of the experiment schedule presented in Figure 38.9.

there is a strong correlation between both modalities. The analysis of thermal images also allows the understanding of ADT experiment, what is evidenced in Figure 38.14. Series of thermal images show rapid change of vascularization and functionality of the affected tissue after clamping the LAD.

Based on images shown in Figures 38.13 and 38.14, one may calculate ADT parametric images, as shown in Figure 38.15. The content of such images relates to the change of thermal tissue properties in consequence of the time passing after clamping LAD and physiological changes caused by ischemia. There is still a problem of calibration of such images which requires more experience.

Another example of a research problem solved based on thermal investigations is the question of the quality of OP CABG. A special mechanical heart stabilizer (holder) is applied to hold the place where a by-pass graft should be inserted. This region of the heart should be stable in space and time, allowing normal action of the heart during OP CABG. We asked a question that if by using such a mechanical holder, additional control of the tissue electrical properties would be possible by the application of electrodes inserted to the holder. Another question was the quality of such intervention, the time duration of the operation to be safe for a patient, and so on. A prototype of a holder with inserted electrodes for electrical impedance measurements is shown in Figure 38.16a. The four-pole configuration of electrodes is typically applied as shown in Figure 38.16b. Current electrodes are placed at the outer

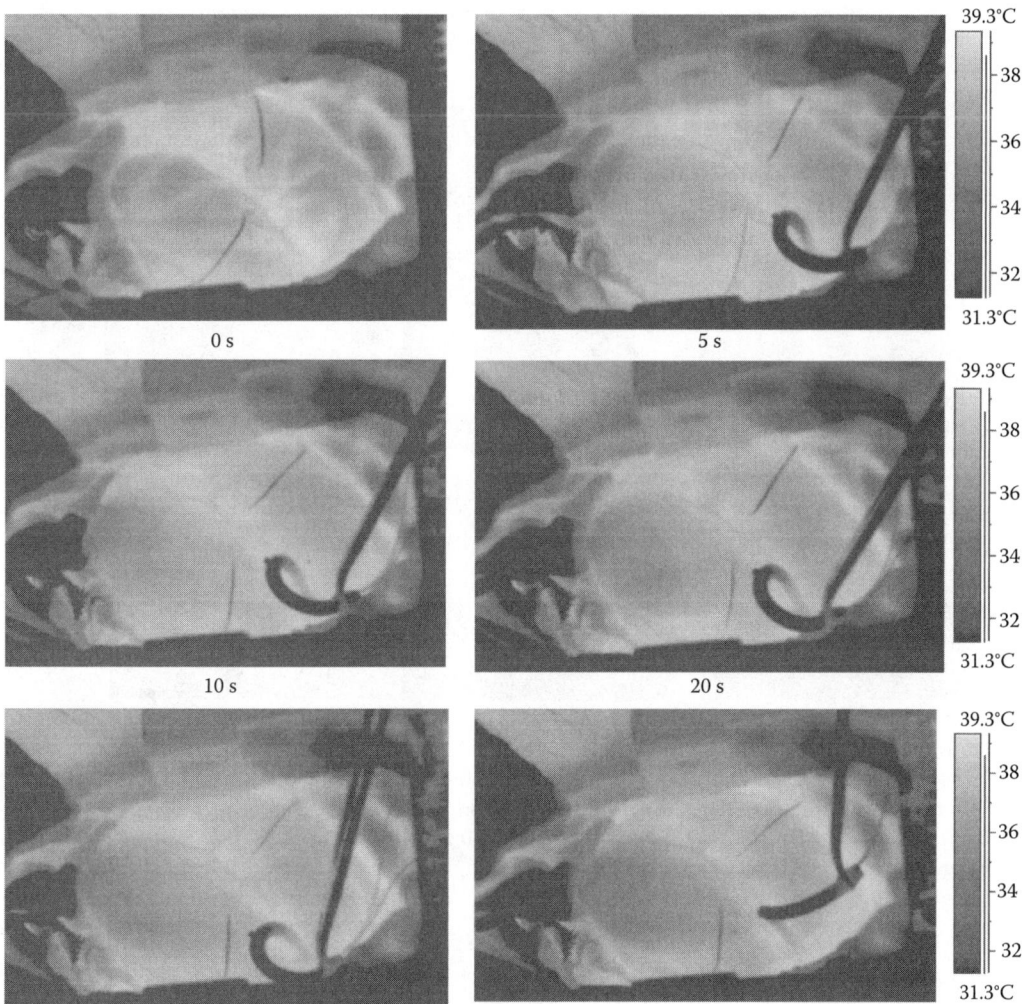

FIGURE 38.13 The static thermograms of the pig heart taken at the indicated times after clamping LAD taken by a camera synchronized with the heart rate. Temperature at the affected region is slowly decreasing; affected vascularization after clamping LAD is evident.

part of the sucking arms. In our experimental arrangement, several voltage electrodes are applied, also allowing measurements of electrical field distribution. The applied Solartron Impedance Analyzer 1260 allows spectral measurements of electrical impedance in a broad range of frequencies. Placing a set of electrodes to the suckers of the stabilizer allows continuous measurements of electrical signals, at all times of the use of the stabilizer, also assuring a very good electrical contact of the electrodes to the heart muscle. Unfortunately, the use of the stabilizer may affect the heart muscle, as illustrated in Figure 38.17. Still, this effect belongs to a procedure claimed to be "minimally invasive."

The important confirmation of the correlation of thermal and electrical tissue properties is illustrated in Figure 38.18, showing change of electrical impedance in time after clamping LAD and showing the devastating influence of ischemia. This experiment is in a perfect agreement with the changes of parametric ADT images in time after forming ischemia and is confirmed by IR-thermal observation. Both functional and structural electrical and thermal properties of the heart muscle are affected by ischemia. This is not only due to limited vascularization but also due to visible changes in cell structures in the affected regions. An example of thermal monitoring of clinical OPCABG is shown in the following section.

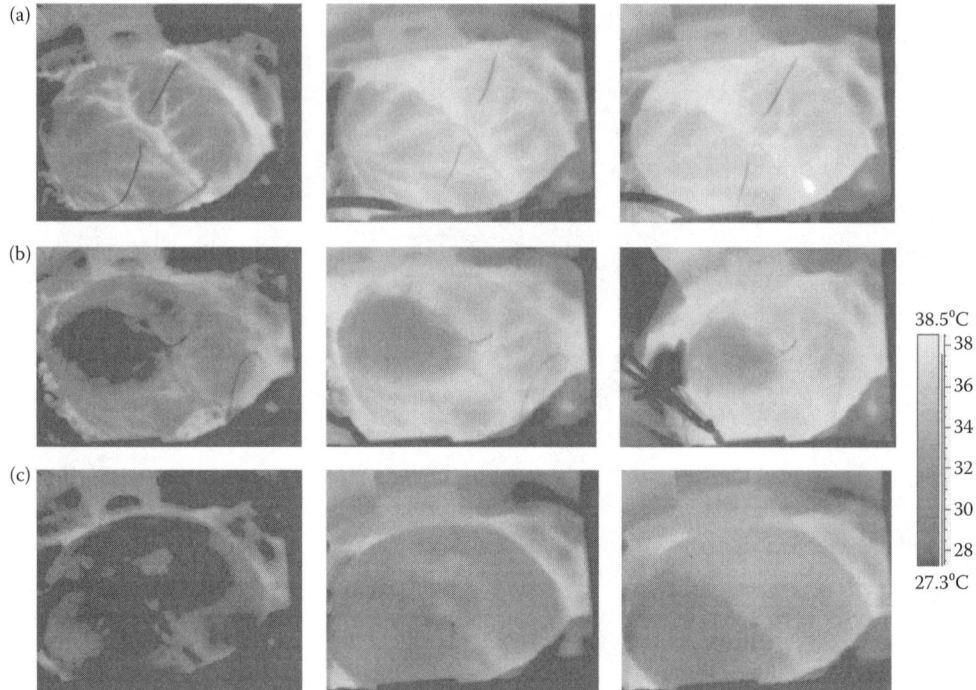

FIGURE 38.14 ADT experiment on the heart during induced heart infarct for different phases of the blood arrest. Thermograms at different moments after stopping cold excitation using CO_2; first column—end of cold excitation, second column—20 s following stopping of cold excitation, third column—90 s following stopping of cold excitation, rows: (a) examination of a healthy heart (before clamping LAD according to Figure 38.9); (b) 40 min after stopping blood flow in LAD; (c) 80 min after blood arrest.

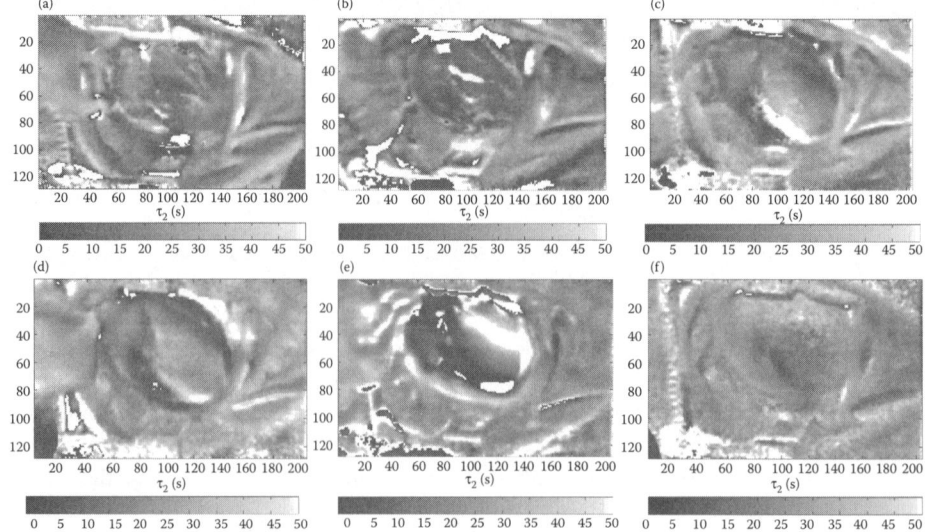

FIGURE 38.15 Images of thermal time constant τ_2 calculated for the phase of rewarming, after excitation using the cryo-instrument generating cold air of temperature 5°C during 30 s; (a) the healthy heart; (b) the heart muscle after the preconditioning lasting 2 min; (c) 10 min after clamping LAD; (d) 20 min after clamping LAD; (e) after 27 min; (f) just after the stop of the heart beating (30 min after clamping LAD).

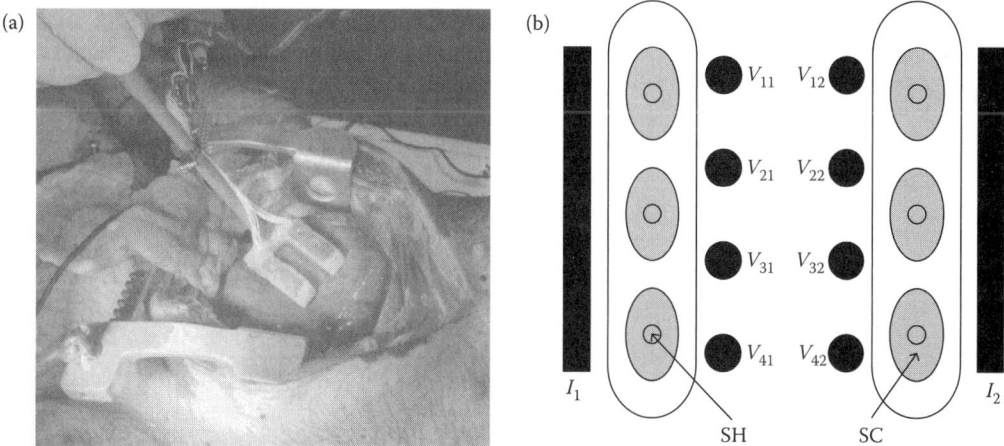

FIGURE 38.16 (a) Mechanical stabilizer with electroimpedance electrodes applied to the heart muscle; (b) the schematic diagram (bottom view) of the probe combined with sucking holder; I and V stand for current and voltage electrodes while SH and SC mark sucking holes and cups, respectively.

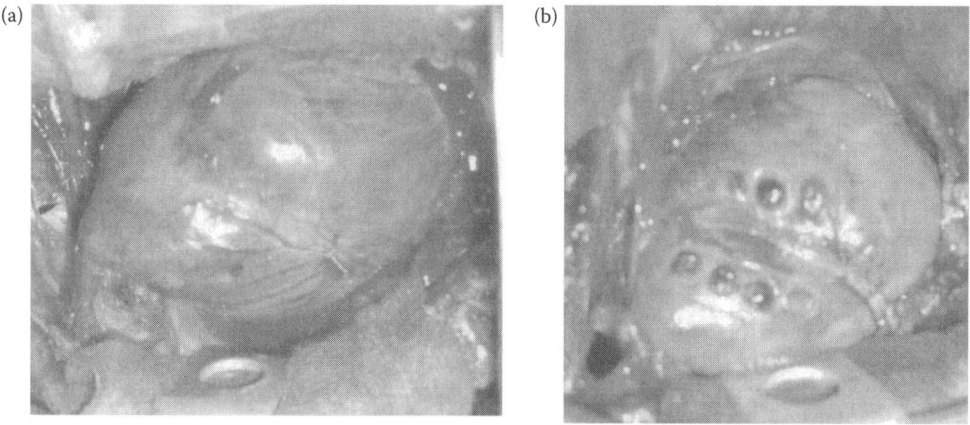

FIGURE 38.17 (a) The pig heart before application of the stabilizer; (b) after intervention—the hematoma visible at the positions of the sucking chambers.

38.4.2 Clinical Applications

Several examples of clinical thermal measurements are already shown in Reference 1. Here, we will summarize the final results of the research based on comparison of the value of applied monitoring tools and also illustrated by a few practical cases in clinics using absolute temperature and temperature courses during surgical interventions, including the ADT method.

38.5 Thermal Monitoring of Surgical Procedures during CABG

Although CABG interventions are today regarded as very invasive and are replaced by OP CABG, the thermal monitoring of several procedures typical in CABG still seems to be important. In all cases, when blood circulation is totally blocked even for a while, such a state is dangerous as there is a deficit of oxygen and metabolites necessary for the survival of the affected tissue. To minimize the negative effects

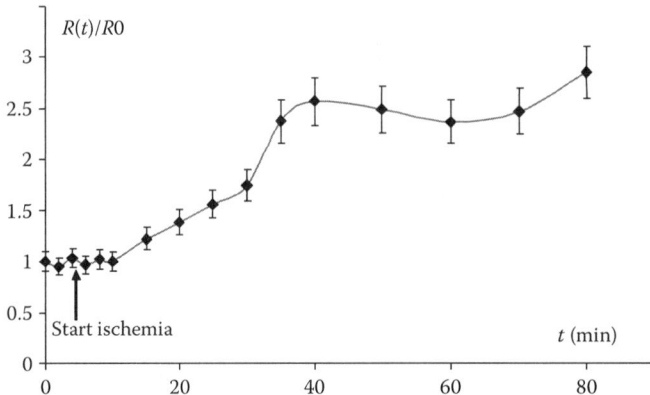

FIGURE 38.18 Resistivity measured at 5 kHz for the set of electrodes in Figure 38.16 (I_1, I_2, V_{21}, and V_{22}) and the mechanical stabilizer placed close to the center of the affected vascularization region of the heart muscle.

of anoxemia, deep hypothermia of the heart muscle is necessary. The heart muscle should be cooled to a temperature of 10–14°C, which allows for a safe surgical intervention lasting up to 120–180 min. Deep cooling is possible by the application of liquid cardioplegia solution at a temperature of 4°C to blood vessels, aorta, and/or descending artery. There are different strategies to perform cardioplegia, called antegrade and retrograde cardioplegia. Examples of effective procedures are shown in Figures 38.19 and 38.20 where images taken in time evidence progressive cooling of the heart muscle.

Thermal monitoring allows precise control of the state of the heart muscle. Typically, during cardiosurgery intervention, the temperature rises slowly, which may be dangerous, causing fibrillation of the heart muscle. Even though the aorta is blocked (clammed), there exists some inflow of blood via arteries, which heats the heart muscle slowly—this is shown in Figure 38.21.

The first thermogram is taken at the moment of stopping cardioplegia. The following images are taken after 3 and 13 s. Control of the temperature allows for a reduction of the fibrillation risk and intraoperation heart stroke.

Additionally, thermal images may be useful in finding coronary arteries to be grafted. Usually, such arteries are covered by a layer of fat which leads to problems in the precise localization using the traditional approach (palpation). After cardioplegia, those arteries are clearly visible at thermograms.

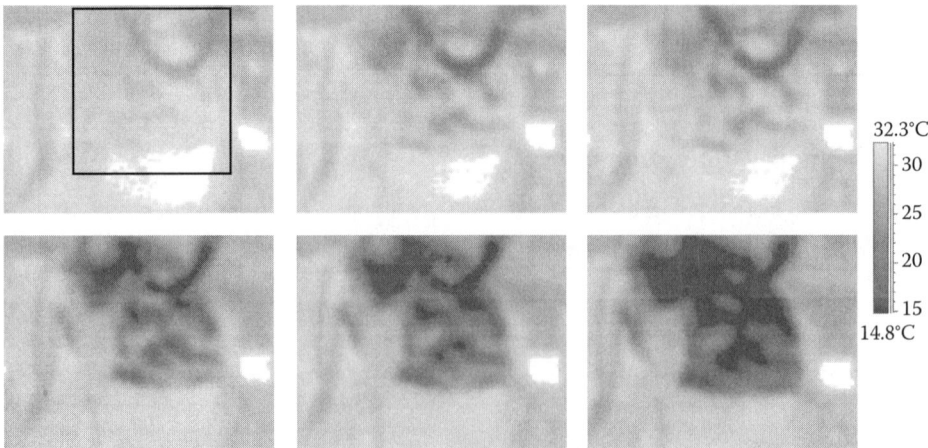

FIGURE 38.19 Series of thermograms during antegrade cardioplegia taken every 10 s; one can see a progressive decrease of the heart muscle temperature; position indicated by the rectangle.

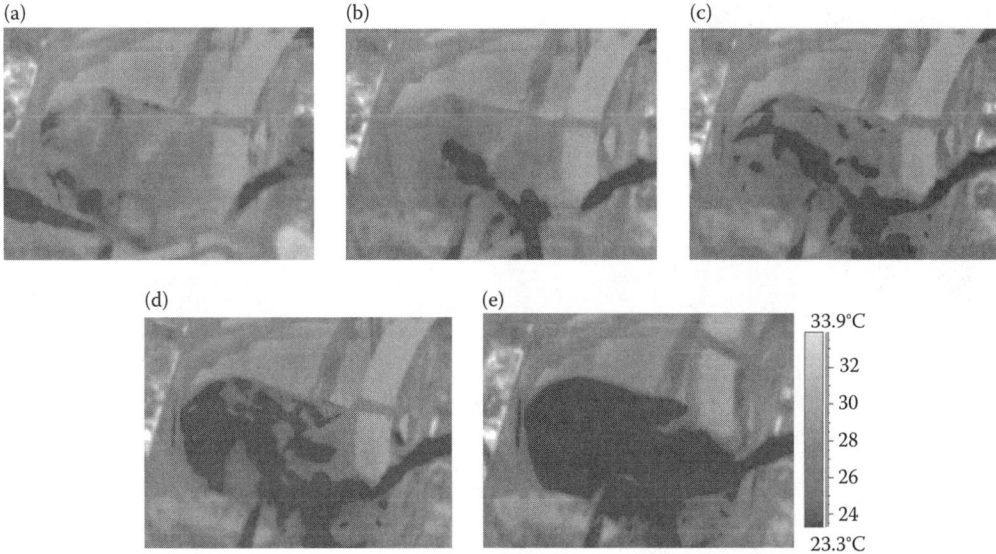

FIGURE 38.20 Series of thermograms during cardioplegia (retro/ante); (a) application of 500 mL of cardioplegia liquid retrograde; (b) continuation using antegrade cardioplegia at 10 s after beginning of antegrade, (c) 25 s, (d) 45 s, (e) 75 s.

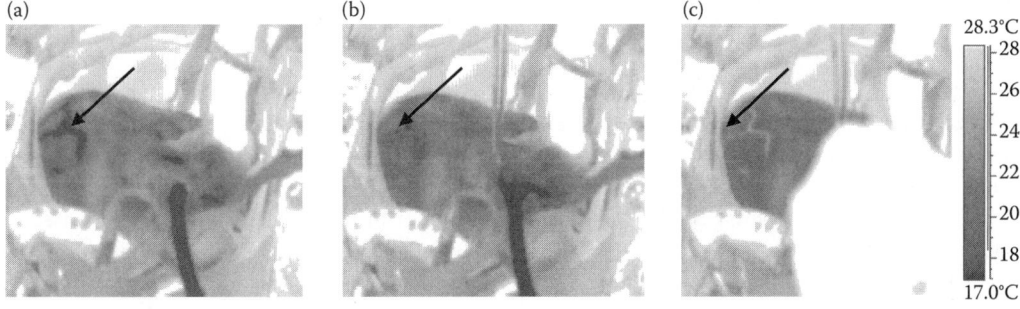

FIGURE 38.21 (a) Thermogram after stopping cardioplegia and respectively (b) after 3 s and (c) after 13 s; the arrow shows LAD.

The next very important surgical procedure is the evaluation of the quality of an inserted graft. Here, one may use thermography just to see the temperature distribution on the myocardium; after a successful CABG operation, it should be a uniform thermal image. On the other hand, all grafts are clearly visible. Especially, the moment of blood circulation recovery is important as one may see an instant rise of temperature on thermal images in all of the important places. Based on thermal images, it is even possible to evaluate the rate of the blood flow, assuming the simplest exponential model of temperature changes:

$$T(t) = T_0 - \Delta T \cdot (1 - e^{-\frac{t}{\tau}}) \tag{38.4}$$

where $T(t)$ is the temperature at the heart surface, ΔT is the increase of temperature due to the inflowing blood, T_0 is the temperature of the myocardium, τ is the time constant—a factor related to the value of free flow-out of blood from LIMA (left internal mammary artery), and t is the time. Two cases of such analysis are presented in Figure 38.22 for correct and failed cases of grafts inserted during CABG

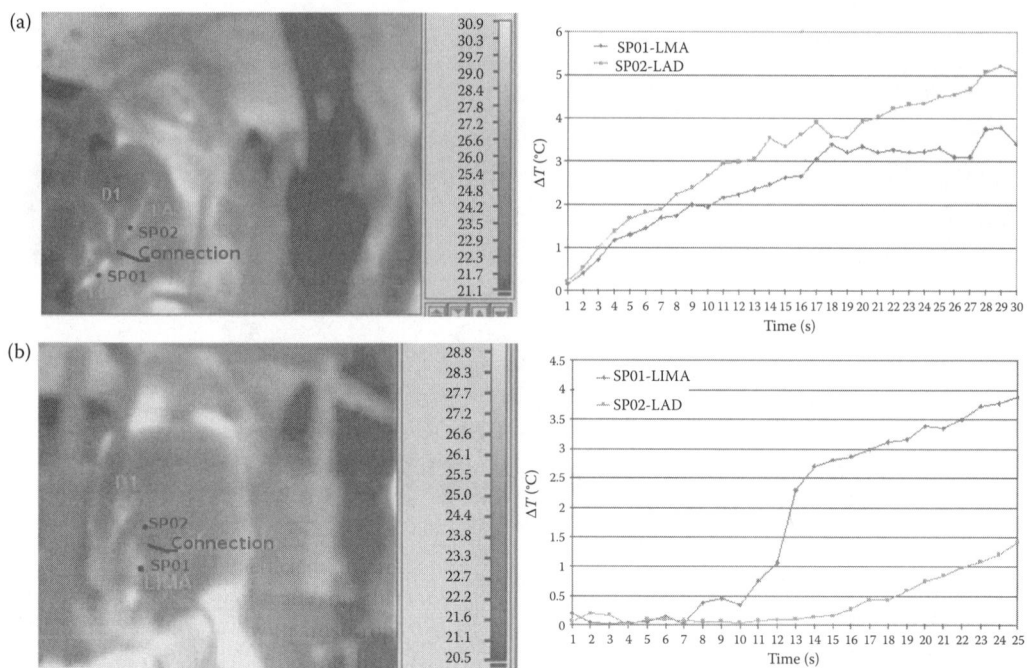

FIGURE 38.22 Quantitative analysis of the graft LIMA-LAD; (a) correct case with temperatures rising in time at the points SP01 and SP02; (b) nonfunctioning graft at SP02—lack or affected rise of temperature in LAD.

interventions. Thermal images and traces of temperature in time after opening the blood circulation in specific points of interest are presented. A noncorrect flow (Figure 38.22b) is manifested by lack of temperature rise below the place of the graft insertion.

Also, ADT parametric images allow for clear evaluation of the graft quality. This is illustrated in Figure 38.23 for two cases: the correct one, the left column, and the graft requiring reoperation, the right column. The time constants at the regions where blood is supplied properly are of the value of 20 s, while in ischemic parts, the time constants are very long. The images show (a) temperature distribution at 20 s after unclamping the graft, (b) temperature difference at this moment, and (c) time constants distribution. At the parametric images, it is clearly visible which fragments of myocardium are characterized by big changes of temperature and those being at almost steady state (the uniform area). For the left column, one may see the branch of LAD with diagonal vessels. For the right case, the only region of increased temperature is in pectoral artery till the LAD joint; the rest is cold. Similarly, in ΔT images, the increase of temperature is around 4°C.

38.6 Thermal Monitoring of Surgical Procedures during OP CABG

OP CABG is regarded as a minimally invasive procedure, even if it is a drastic intervention inside the body of a patient. The practical use of a mechanical stabilizer holding the heart muscle in the place of graft insertion is shown in Figure 38.24a. Practically, it allows maintaining the heart action during the intervention, without applying the procedure of external blood circulation. Especially important is the state of the myocardium, its temperature, in the vicinity of the holder. The decrease of temperature below 28°C may be dangerous, leading to fibrillation. We suggested some changes in the new construction of a heart stabilizer just to decrease the thermal conductivity of the construction, to decrease heat out-flow, and to increase the time of possible surgical intervention.

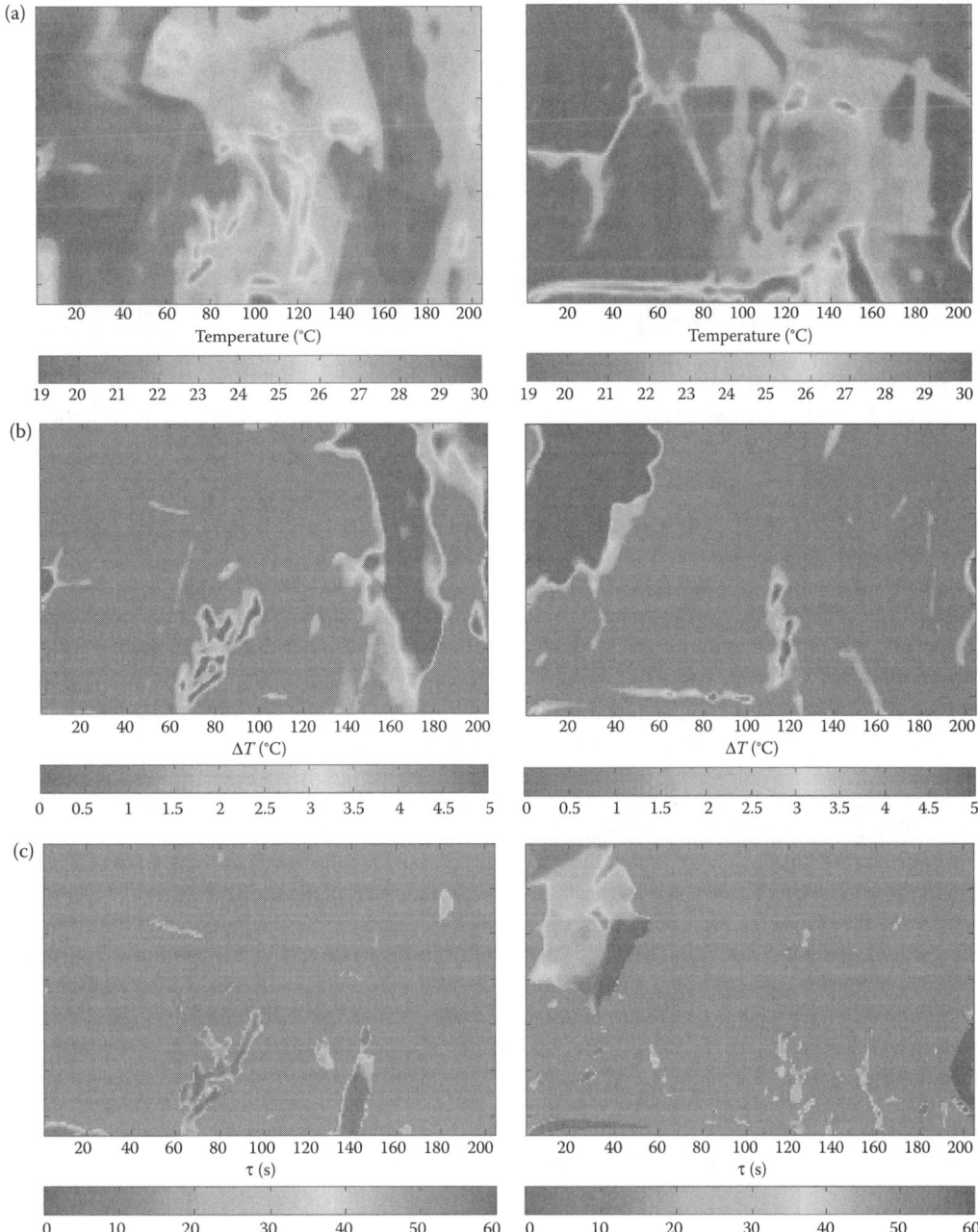

FIGURE 38.23 Correct (left column) and requiring reoperation (right column) LIMA-LAD grafts; (a) thermal images at 20 s after unclamping the graft; (b) recorded rise of temperature; (c) time constants according to Equation 38.4.

Another important problem is finding the optimal position where the graft should be inserted. On thermograms, it is usually clearly visible in the place where the artery is blocked, as is shown in Figure 38.24b (see arrow). The next procedure is the evaluation of the quality of the graft. A properly inserted graft responds to the unclamping procedure by a rapid increase in the temperature of the myocardium below the joint as illustrated in Figure 38.24c.

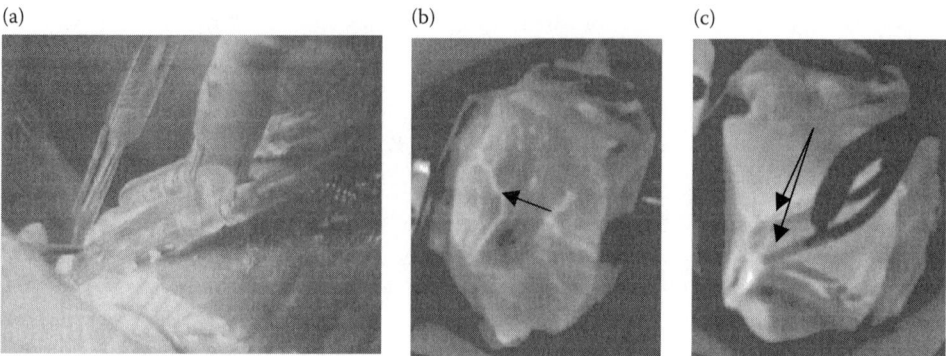

FIGURE 38.24 OP CABG intervention: (a) view of the mechanical heart stabilizer, (b) thermogram showing blockade at the LAD (see arrow), (c) myocardium under LAD with the stabilizer arms sucked to hold it in a stable position (see arrows).

38.7 ADT Monitoring of the Heart Muscle Perfusion and Other Applications

The final effect of different cardiosurgical procedures is properly distributed vascularization of myocardium and effective mechanical heart action. Thermography allows for the evaluation of the global state of the heart muscle. A positive result of any of the interventions may be therefore evidenced by using the described technologies. As an example, the case of CABG intervention is shown in Figure 38.25, based on QIRT measurements. Similarly, ADT images might also be applied, but data treatment is in this case much more advanced. One may see an important change of the temperature distribution which after CABG is much more uniform and the mean value of temperature is higher, which shows that blood supply and flow is regular in all parts of the treated heart.

Another possibility of using classical thermography concerns studies such as the analysis of specific surgery procedures. In Figure 38.26, a thermogram shows the vascularization of an arm after physical exercise. This measurement was performed in studies of extracting the hand radial artery for a by-pass. The same patient, after the extraction and using his artery for a successful by-pass operation within the next 3 months, was under the same examination, and only a slight decrease of temperature, not exceeding 0.5°C, has been noticed. The result is very positive in terms of full recovery of vascularization in the hand. This study on 50 patients showed reasonable use of this artery in cardiosurgery by-pass operations.

38.8 Summary and Conclusions

IR-thermal measurements are noncontact and fully aseptic. Temperature is a functional parameter allowing for nonspecific evaluation of complex physiological processes existing in the tested organ. Observation of thermal fields at the surface of tested organs allows for fast and quantitative evaluation of complex physiological processes. It is similar in ADT measurements but this is a structural parameter showing thermal properties of a tested tissue, thermal conductivity, and thermal capacity. In both cases, thermal visualization allows for an elegant, quantitative illustration of tested processes, as cardiosurgery interventions. ADT allows for precise planning of surgical interventions without the need for big safety margins. Both modalities are complementing each other, allowing better understanding of the state of a tested organ. This also allows for fast and objective monitoring of cardiosurgical interventions, quantitative evidence of the results of such interventions, as well as for objective observation of treatment progress.

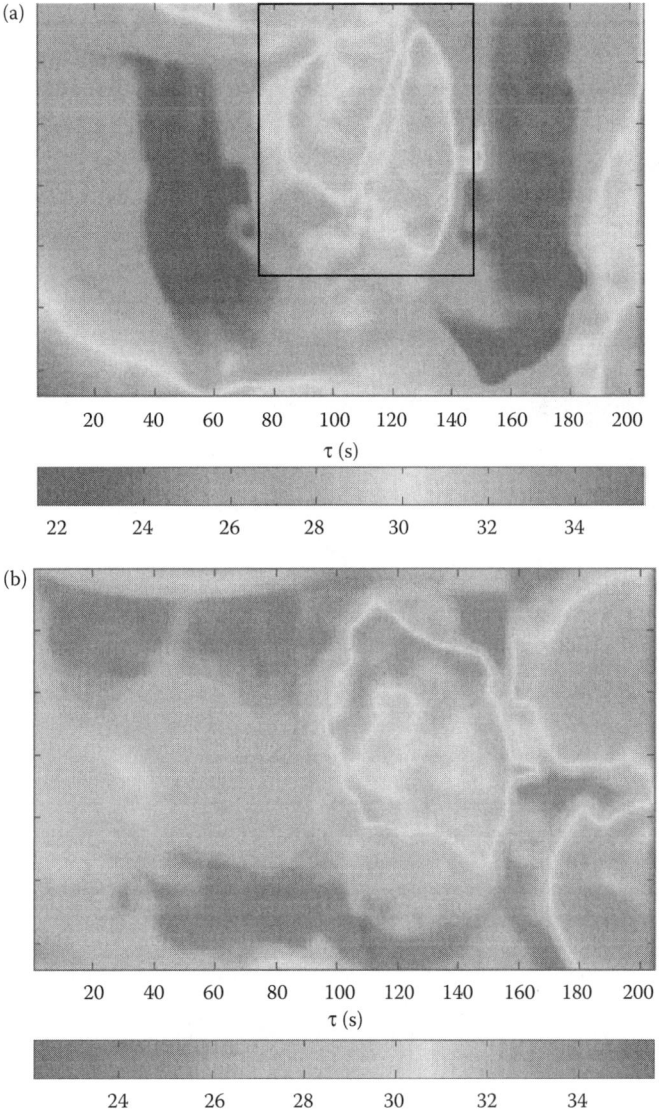

FIGURE 38.25 Perfusion of myocardium (a) before and (b) after CABG; the heart region is indicated by a rectangle.

We have shown an important role of both modalities in research and also in clinics. The boundary conditions are still very important in the interpretation of thermal and ADT parameters; therefore, this should be the main condition for assuring a high quality of such measurements. Especially, proper segmentation of thermal images would be impossible without assuring standard conditions of measurements, which should also be regarded as the highest possible knowledge of boundary conditions.

Absolute temperature may be an important parameter in the monitoring of the state of a patient before, during, and after surgical interventions. Unfortunately, there are no defined standards—clear boundaries of the values of temperature for specific interventions and treatment procedures. This means that further investigations are necessary for filling the existing gap in such knowledge. This notice concerns both experiments on animals and clinical practice.

Temperature allows monitoring of vascularization in each phase of cardiosurgery interventions. This is a perfect method for the evaluation of the quality of the inserted graft, of the efficiency of cardioplegia,

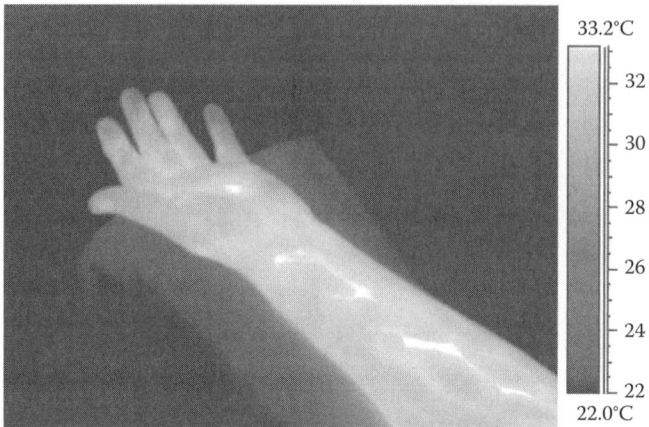

FIGURE 38.26   Vascularization of a hand after mechanical exercise before extracting the radial artery for a bypass. This is a reference image for further analysis of hand function recovery after reconvalescence lasting typically 3 months.

and of the quality of many surgical procedures in clinical practice. Such monitoring is prompt, easy, and objective, especially if dynamic processes are investigated. It allows for noncontact observations of the blood circulation, especially after the elimination of any blockades.

Temperature measurements allow for easy discrimination of the regions of affected circulation and also of hyperemia or inflammation, and any increased or decreased metabolism.

ADT identification of regions of affected thermal properties may be used for the evaluation of tissues and organs for transplants, and so on. These parameters are also important in the evaluation of the state of blood deficit or progress of tissue necrosis. This is an important factor in cardiosurgery interventions as repairing of the heart is nowadays more important than transplantations. Very important are observations of changes of tissue parameters in time. Necrosis is evidenced within around 30 min after blood arrest!

Visualization of temperature distribution at the surface of the heart muscle is less invasive than electroimpedance measurements, being a fully noncontact procedure. The only condition for measurements in this case is visual accessibility to the tested region, what is not always possible, as thermal inspection should not disturb surgical interventions.

The set of ADT parametric images gives rather structural information of the tested tissue. Properties of tissues are dependent on the blood flow and the physical structure which is devastated after long-lasting processes of ischemia. Blood arrest has a damaging influence on the structure of cells which may be easily evidenced by histopathology. Therefore, the ADT images are differentiating tissues already affected but are not sensitive to short deficits in blood flow. Analysis of the ADT measurement results leads to the conclusion that special care must be taken to secure proper measurement conditions.

Information gathered in both modalities is of different character. Thermography shows regions of increased or decreased temperature, usually caused by a change of vascularization due to different clinical reasons—increased metabolism, necrosis, ischemia, and so on. The minimal requirement for instrumentation is the use of a thermal camera of a resolution of at least 0.1°C and a lens with FOV adequate for the chosen application.

IR thermography instrumentation and application of dedicated data processing for the analysis of thermal transients after external excitations allow to obtain objective, quantitative thermal data of tested tissues; therefore, it has a potential value as an intraoperative monitoring and predictive tool, especially in beating heart myocardial revascularization procedures, where, during the grafting process, the heart muscle is forced to work in ischemic conditions and there is a high possibility that the revascularization procedure can fail or be incomplete. Generally, this approach allows validation of ADT in medical applications such as diagnostics of the heart transplants but also open-heart surgery evaluation.

ADT allows the determination of the thermal properties of a tested region. It employs the external thermal excitation source with the aim of analysis of thermal transients to determine thermal conductivity and thermal capacity, represented by thermal time constants, being the product of both parameters.

The choice of SW or LW IR-camera is of secondary importance, as modern cameras in both ranges of radiation are of similar thermal resolution and speed of operation. We prefer LW spectral region because it is easier to avoid interaction while optical excitation is applied.

Acknowledgments

The authors acknowledge contributions of all coworkers from the Department of Biomedical Engineering, Gdansk University of Technology, and from the Department of Cardiosurgery and other departments of the Gdansk Medical University, especially professor J. Siebert and doctors J. Topolewicz, B. Trzeciak, Ł. Jaworski, K. Roszak, and S. Beta as well as engineering staff: M. Suchowirski, M. Bajorek, A. Galikowski and K. Kudlak. *In vivo* animal experiments have been performed at the Department of Animal Physiology, Gdansk University with the main assistance of Dr. W. Stojek. Coworkers are listed in the attached bibliography as coauthors of common publications. This is to underline that most of the illustrations presented here are taken from the cited own publications. The work was supported by several grants from KBN and recently by the development grant R13 027 01 from the Polish Ministry of Science and Higher Education.

References

1. Nowakowski A., Quantitative active dynamic thermal IR-imaging and thermal tomography in medical diagnostics, *The Biomedical Engineering Handbook, Third Edition, Medical Devices and Systems*, ed. J. B. Bronzino, CRC Press, Taylor & Francis, Boca Raton, FL, III Infrared Imaging, 22, pp. 22-1–22-30, 2006.
2. Mohr F. W. et al., IMA-graft patency control by thermal coronary angiography during coronary bypass surgery, *Eur. J. Cardio-Thorac. Surg.*, 5, 534–541, 1986.
3. Mohr F. W. et al., Intraoperative assessment of internal mammary artery bypass graft patency by thermal coronary angiography, *Cardiovasc-Surg.*, 2(6), 703–710, 1994.
4. Falk V., Walther T., Diegeler A., Rauch T., Kitzinger H., Mohr F.W., Thermal-coronary-angiography (TCA) for intraoperative evaluation of graft patency in coronary artery bypass surgery, *Eutotherm. Seminar 50 Proc. QIRT*, 96, 348–353, 1996.
5. Kaczmarek M., Nowakowski A., Siebert J., Rogowski J., Intraoperative thermal coronary angiography—Correlation between internal mammary artery (IMA) free flow and thermographic measurement during coronary grafting, *Seminar 60—Quantitative InfraRed Thermography—QIRT'98, Proc.*, 1, 250–258, 1998.
6. Kaczmarek M., Nowakowski A., Siebert J., Rogowski J., Infrared thermography—Applications in heart surgery, *Proc. SPIE*, 3730, 184–188, 1999.
7. Nowakowski A., ed., Analiza technik diagnostycznych i terapeutycznych w celu oceny procedur kardiochirurgicznych (in Polish) [Analysis of diagnostic and therapeutic methods in terms of evaluation of cardiosurgery procedures], AOW EXIT, Warsaw, 2008.
8. Nowakowski A, Kaczmarek M., Dynamic thermography as a quantitative medical diagnostic tool, *Medical and Biological Engineering and Computing Incorporate Cellular Engineering*, 37(Suppl. 1, Part 1), 244–245, 1999.
9. Suchowirski M., Nowakowski A., Problems in analysis of thermal images sequences for medical diagnostics, EMBEC 2008, *4th European Conference of the International Federation for Medical and Biological Engineering*, Antwerp, Belgium, 23–27 November, abstracts, 355, 2008.

10. Kaczmarek M., Nowakowski A., Stojek W., Topolewicz J., Siebert J., Rogowski J., Thermal monitoring of the myocardium under blood arrest—Preliminary study, *Proceedings of the 29th IEEE EMBS Annual International Conference*, Lyon, CD, 254–257, 2007.

11. Nowakowski A., Kaczmarek M., Wtorek J., Stojek W., Rogowski J., Siebert J., Electrical and thermal monitoring during cardiosurgery interventions, *IFMBE Proceedings*, 17, 150–153, 2007.

12. Sokołowska-Pituchowa J., Ed., in Polish: Anatomia człowieka [Human anatomy], p. 249, Warszawa, PZWL, 1992.

13. Murry C.E., Jennings R.B., Reimer K.A., Preconditioning with ischemia: A delay of lethal cell injury in ischemic myocardium, *Circulation*, 74(5), 1124–1136, 1986.

14. Flameng W.J., Role of myocardial protection for coronary bypass grafting on the beating heart, *Ann. Thorac. Surg.*, 63, 18–22, 1997.

15. Yellon D.M., Baxter G.F., Garcia-Dorado D., Heusch G., Sumeray M., Ischaemic preconditioning: Present position and future directions, *Cardiovasc. Res.*, 37(1), 21–33, 1998.

16. Hao X., Bruce Ch., Pislaru C., Greenleaf J., Characterization of reperfused infarcted myocardium from high-frequency intracardiac ultrasound imaging using homodyned K-distribution, *IEEE Transactions on Ultrasonics, Ferroelectrics, and Frequency Control*, 49(11), 1530–1542, 2002.

17. Hossaek J., Li Y., Yang Z., French B., Assessment of transient myocardial perfusion defects in intact mice using a microbubble contrast destruction/refill approach, *IEEE International Ultrasonics, Ferroelectrics and Frequency Control, Joint 50th Anniversary Conference*, 9–12, 2004.

39

Physiology-Based Face Recognition in the Thermal Infrared Spectrum

Pradeep Buddharaju
University of Houston

Ioannis Pavlidis
University of Houston

39.1 Introduction

Biometrics has received a lot of attention during the past few years from both the academic and business communities. It has emerged as a preferred alternative to traditional forms of identification, like card IDs, which are not embedded into one's physical characteristics. Research into several biometric modalities, including face, fingerprint, iris, and retina recognition, has produced varying degrees of success [1]. Face recognition stands as the most appealing modality, since it is the natural mode of identification among humans and is totally unobtrusive. At the same time, however, it is one of the most challenging modalities [2]. Research into face recognition has been biased toward the visible spectrum for a variety of reasons. Among those is the availability and low cost of visible band cameras and the undeniable fact that face recognition is one of the primary activities of the human visual system. Machine recognition of human faces, however, has proven more problematic than the seemingly effortless face recognition performed by humans. The major culprit is light variability, which is prevalent in the visible spectrum owing to the reflective nature of incident light in this band. Secondary problems are associated with the difficulty of detecting facial disguises [3].

As a solution to the aforementioned problems, researchers have started investigating the use of thermal infrared (IR) for face recognition purposes [4–6]. However, many of these research efforts in thermal face recognition use the thermal IR band only as a way to see in the dark or reduce the deleterious effect of light variability [7,8]. Methodologically, they do not differ very much from face recognition algorithms in the visible band, which can be classified as appearance- [9,10] and feature-based approaches [11,12]. Recently, attempts have been made to fuse the visible and IR modalities to increase the performance of face recognition [13–16].

In this chapter, we present a novel approach to the problem of thermal facial recognition that realizes the full potential of the thermal IR band. It consists of a statistical face segmentation and a physiological feature extraction algorithm tailored to thermal phenomenology. The use of vein structure for human identification has been studied during the recent years using traits such as hand vein patterns [17,18] and finger vein patterns [19,20]. Prokoski and Riedel [21] anticipated the possibility of extracting the vascular network from thermal facial images and using it as a feature space for face recognition. However, they did not present an algorithmic approach for achieving this. To the best of our knowledge, this is the first attempt to develop a face recognition system using physiological information on the face. An early stage of this research was reported briefly in the *Proceedings of the 2005 IEEE Conference on Advanced Video and Signal Based Surveillance* [22]. Our goal is to promote a different way of thinking in the area of face recognition in thermal IR, which can be approached in a distinct manner when compared with other modalities.

Figure 39.1 shows the architecture of the proposed system. The goal of face recognition is to match a query face image against a database of facial images to establish the identity of an individual. Our system operates in the following two phases to achieve this goal:

1. *Off-line phase*: The thermal facial images are captured by an IR camera. For each subject to be stored in the database, we record five different poses. A two-step segmentation algorithm is applied on each pose image to extract the vascular network from the face. Thermal minutia points (TMPs) are detected on the branching points of the vascular network and are stored in the database (see Figure 39.1).

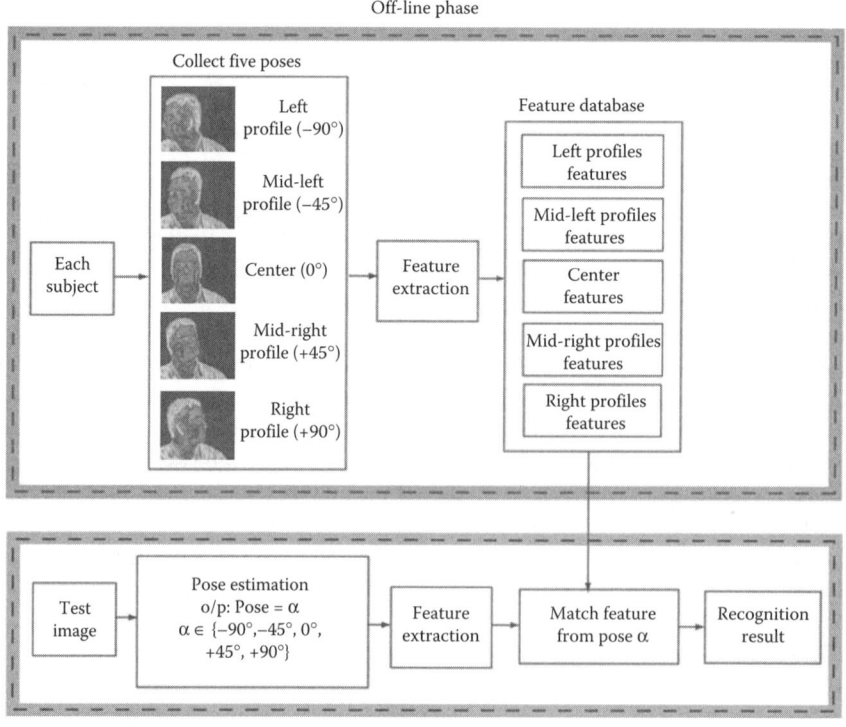

FIGURE 39.1   Architecture of our face recognition system.

   2. *On-line phase*: Given a query image, TMPs of its vascular network are extracted and are matched against those of the corresponding pose images stored in the database (see Figure 39.1).

In the following sections, we will describe our face recognition system in detail. In Section 39.2, we present the feature extraction algorithm. In Section 39.3, we discuss our approach for vascular network matching. In Section 39.4, we present the experimental results and attempt a critical evaluation. We conclude this chapter in Section 39.5.

39.2 Feature Extraction

A thermal IR camera with good sensitivity provides the ability to directly image superficial blood vessels on the human face [23]. The pattern of the underlying blood vessels (see Figure 39.2) is characteristic to each individual, and the extraction of this vascular network can provide the basis for a feature vector. Figure 39.3 outlines the architecture of our feature extraction algorithm.

39.2.1 Face Segmentation

Owing to its physiology, a human face consists of "hot" parts that correspond to tissue areas that are rich in vasculature and "cold" parts that correspond to tissue areas with sparse vasculature. This casts the human face as a bimodal temperature distribution entity, which can be modeled using a mixture of two normal distributions. Similarly, the background can be described by a bimodal temperature distribution with walls being the "cold" objects and the upper part of the subject's body dressed in cloths being the "hot" object. Figure 39.4b shows the temperature distributions of the facial skin and the background from a typical IR facial image. We approach the problem of delineating facial tissue from background using a Bayesian framework [22,24] since we have *a priori* knowledge of the bimodal nature of the scene.

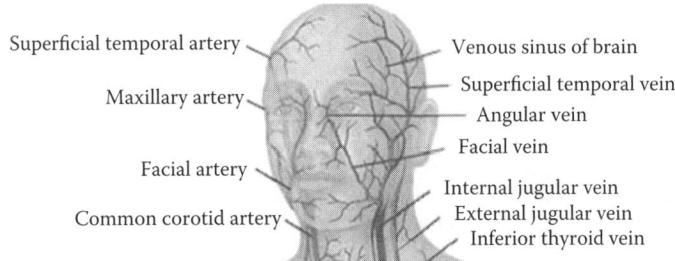

FIGURE 39.2   Superficial blood vessels on the face.

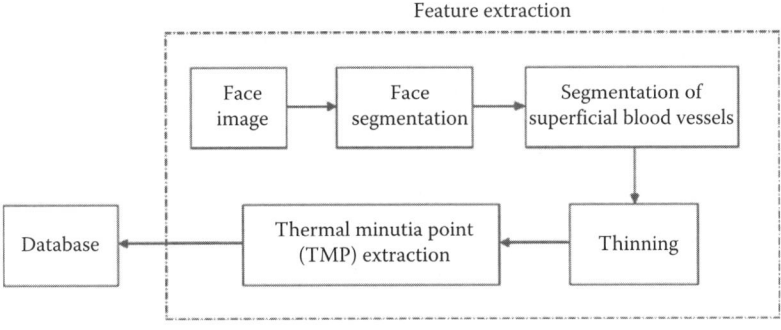

FIGURE 39.3   Architecture of feature extraction algorithm.

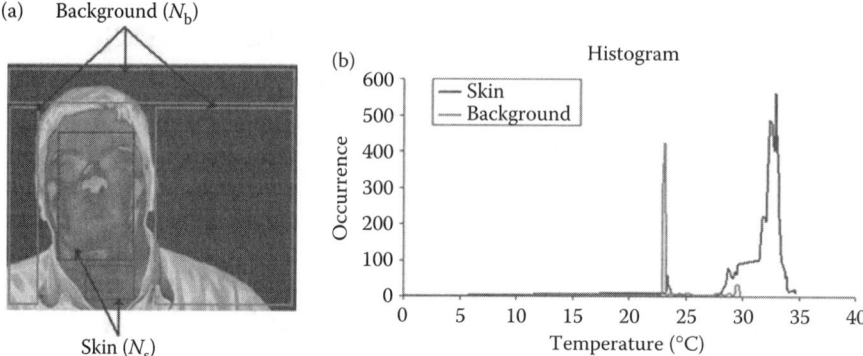

FIGURE 39.4 Skin and background: (a) selection of samples for EM algorithm and (b) corresponding bimodal temperature distributions.

We call θ the parameter of interest, which takes two possible values (skin s or background b) with some probability. For each pixel x in the image at time t, we draw our inference of whether it represents skin (i.e., $\theta = s$) or background (i.e., $\theta = b$) based on the posterior distribution $p^{(t)}(\theta|x_t)$ given by

$$p^{(t)}(\theta \mid x_t) = \begin{cases} p^{(t)}(s \mid x_t), & \text{when } \theta = s \\ p^{(t)}(b \mid x_t) = 1 - p^{(t)}(s \mid x_t), & \text{when } \theta = b \end{cases} \tag{39.1}$$

We develop the statistics only for skin, and then the statistics for the background can easily be inferred from Equation 39.1.

According to the Bayes' theorem

$$p^{(t)}(s|x_t) = \frac{\pi^{(t)}(s)f(x_t|s)}{\pi^{(t)}(s)f(x_t|s) + \pi^{(t)}(b)f(x_t|b)} \tag{39.2}$$

Here, $\pi^{(t)}(s)$ is the prior skin distribution and $f(x_t|s)$ is the likelihood for pixel x representing skin at time t. In the first frame ($t = 1$), the prior distributions for skin and background are considered equiprobable:

$$\pi^{(1)}(s) = \frac{1}{2} = \pi^{(1)}(b) \tag{39.3}$$

For $t > 1$, the prior skin distribution $\pi^{(t)}(s)$ at time t is equal to the posterior skin distribution at time $t - 1$:

$$\pi^{(t)}(s) = p^{(t-1)}(s \mid x_{t-1}) \tag{39.4}$$

The likelihood $f(x_t|s)$ of pixel x representing skin at time $t = 1$ is given by

$$f(x_t \mid s) = \sum_{i=1}^{2} w_{s_i}^{(t)} N(\mu_{s_i}^{(t)}, \sigma_{s_i}^{2(t)}) \tag{39.5}$$

where the mixture parameters w_{s_i} (weight), μ_{s_i} (mean), $\sigma_{s_i}^2$ (variance) : $i = 1,2$, and $w_{s_2} = 1 - w_{s_1}$ of the bimodal skin distribution can be initialized and updated using the Expectation-Maximization (EM) algorithm. For that, we select N representative facial frames (off-line) from a variety of subjects that we call the training set. Then, we manually segment, for each of the N frames, skin (and background) areas, which yields N_s skin (and N_b background) pixels as shown in Figure 39.4a.

To estimate the mixture parameters for the skin, we initially provide the EM algorithm with some crude estimates of the parameters of interest: $w_{s_0}, \mu_{s_0}, \sigma_{s_0}^2$. Then, we apply the following loop for $k = 0,1,\ldots$:

$$z_{ij}^{(k)} = \frac{w_{s_i}^{(k)}(\sigma_{s_i}^{(k)})^{-1}\exp-\left\{\frac{1}{2(\sigma_{s_i}^{(k)})^2}(x_j - \mu_{s_i}^{(k)})^2\right\}}{\sum_{t=1}^{2} w_{s_t}^{(k)}(\sigma_{s_t}^{(k)})^{-1}\exp\left\{-\frac{1}{2(\sigma_{s_t}^{(k)})^2}(x_j - \mu_{s_t}^{(k)})^2\right\}}$$

$$w_{s_i}^{(k+1)} = \frac{\sum_{j=1}^{N_s} z_{ij}^{(k)}}{N_s}$$

$$\mu_{s_i}^{(k+1)} = \frac{\sum_{j=1}^{N_s} z_{ij}^{(k)} x_j}{N_s w_{s_i}^{(k+1)}}$$

$$(\sigma_{s_i}^{(k+1)})^2 = \frac{\sum_{j=1}^{N_s} z_{ij}^{(k)}(x_j - \mu_{s_i}^{(k+1)})^2}{N_s w_{s_i}^{(k+1)}}$$

where $i = 1,2$ and $j = 1,\ldots,N_s$. Then, we set $k = k + 1$ and repeat the loop. The condition for terminating the loop is

$$| w_{s_i}^{(k+1)} - w_{s_i}^{(k)} | < \varepsilon, \quad i = 1,2 \tag{39.6}$$

We apply a similar EM process for determining the initial parameters of the background distributions. Once a data point x_t becomes available, we decide that it represents skin if the posterior distribution for the skin, $p^{(t)}(s|x_t) > 0.5$ and that it represents background if the posterior distribution for the background, $p^{(t)}(b|x_t) > 0.5$. Figure 39.5b depicts the visualization of Bayesian segmentation on the subject shown in Figure 39.5a. Part of the subject's nose has been erroneously classified as background and a couple of cloth patches from the subject's shirt have been erroneously marked as facial skin. This is due to occasional overlapping between portions of the skin and background distributions. The isolated nature of these mislabeled patches makes them easily correctable through postprocessing. We apply our three-step postprocessing algorithm on the binary segmented image. Using foreground (and

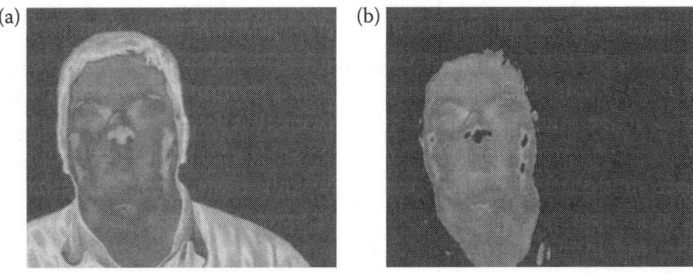

(a)   (b)

FIGURE 39.5 Segmentation of facial skin region: (a) original thermal facial image and (b) result of Bayesian segmentation.

background) correction, we find the mislabeled pixels in the foreground (and background) and remove them. Following is the algorithm for achieving this:

1. Label all the regions in the foreground and background using a simple floodfill or connected component labeling algorithm [25]. Let the foreground regions be $R_f(i)$, $i = 1,...,N_f$, where N_f represents the number of foreground regions, and let the background regions be $R_b(j)$, $j = 1,...,N_b$, where N_b represents the number of background regions.
2. Compute the number of pixels in each of the foreground and background regions. Find the maximum foreground (R_f^{max}) and background (R_b^{max}) areas:

$$R_f^{max} = \max\{R_f(i), i = 1,...,N_f\}$$
$$R_b^{max} = \max\{R_b(i), i = 1,...,N_b\}$$

3. Change all foreground regions that satisfy the condition $R_f(i) < R_f^{max}/4$ to background. Similarly, change all background regions that satisfy the condition $R_b(i) < R_b^{max}/4$ to foreground. We found experimentally that outliers tend to have an area smaller than one-fourth of the maximum area, and hence can be corrected with the above conditions. Figure 39.6 shows the result of our post-processing algorithm.

39.2.2 Segmentation of Superficial Blood Vessels

Once a face is delineated from the rest of the scene, the segmentation of superficial blood vessels from the facial tissue is carried out in the following two steps [23,24]:

1. The image is processed to reduce noise and enhance edges.
2. Morphological operations are applied to localize the superficial vasculature.

In thermal imagery of human tissue, the major blood vessels have weak sigmoid edges, which can be handled effectively using anisotropic diffusion. The anisotropic diffusion filter is formulated as a process that enhances object boundaries by performing intraregion as opposed to interregion smoothing. The mathematical equation for the process is

$$\frac{\partial I(\bar{x},t)}{\partial t} = \nabla(c(\bar{x},t)\nabla I(\bar{x},t)) \tag{39.7}$$

In our case, $I(\bar{x},t)$ is the thermal IR image, $\bar{x}$ refers to the spatial dimensions, and t to time. $c(\bar{x},t)$ is called the diffusion function. The discrete version of the anisotropic diffusion filter of Equation 39.7 is as follows:

$$\begin{aligned} I_{t+1}(x,y) = I_t &+ \frac{1}{4} * [c_{N,t}(x,y)\nabla I_{N,t}(x,y) + c_{S,t}(x,y)\nabla I_{S,t}(x,y) \\ &+ c_{E,t}(x,y)\nabla I_{E,t}(x,y) + c_{W,t}(x,y)\nabla I_{W,t}(x,y)] \end{aligned} \tag{39.8}$$

The four diffusion coefficients and four gradients in Equation 39.8 correspond to four directions (i.e., north, south, east, and west) with respect to the location (x,y). Each diffusion coefficient and the corresponding gradient are calculated in the same manner. For example, the coefficient along the north direction is calculated as follows:

$$c_{N,t}(x,y) = \exp\left(\frac{-\nabla I_{N,t}^2(x,y)}{k^2}\right) \tag{39.9}$$

where $I_{N,t} = I_t(x,y+1) - I_t(x,y)$.

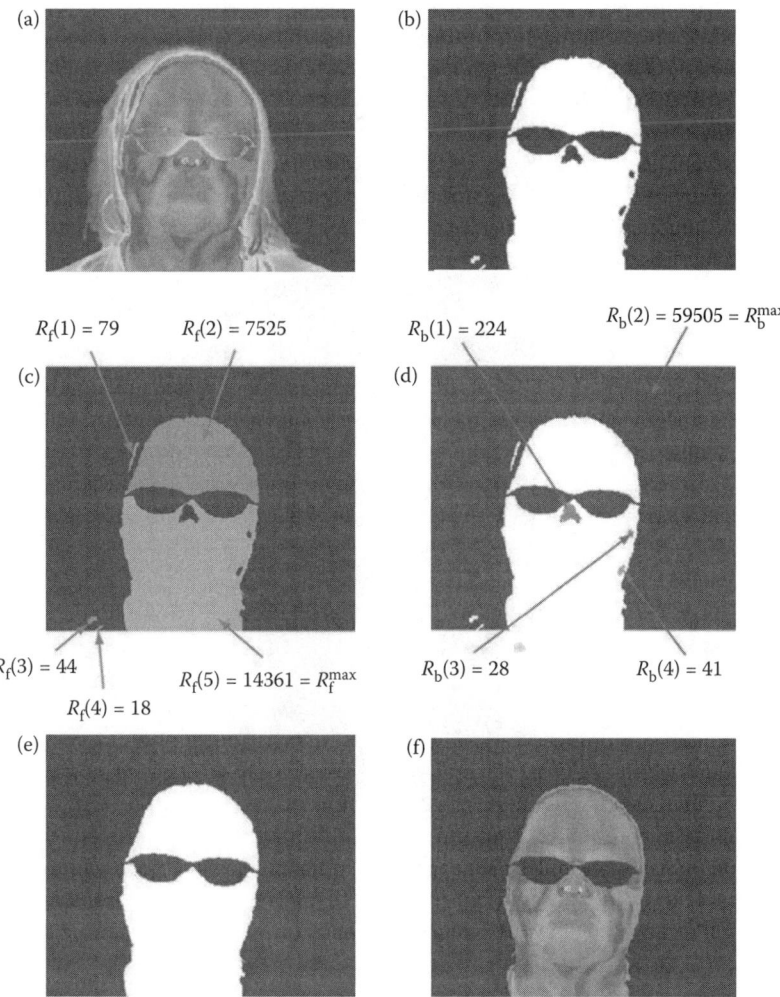

FIGURE 39.6 Segmentation of facial skin region: (a) original thermal facial image; (b) binary segmented image; (c) foreground regions each represented in different color; (d) background regions each represented in different color; (e) binary mask after foreground and background corrections; and (f) final segmentation result after postprocessing.

Image morphology is then applied on the diffused image to extract the blood vessels that are at a relatively low contrast compared with that of the surrounding tissue. We employ for this purpose a top-hat segmentation method, which is a combination of erosion and dilation operations. Top-hat segmentation takes two forms. The first form is the white top-hat segmentation that enhances the bright objects in the image, while the second one is the black top-hat segmentation that enhances dark objects. In our case, we are interested in the white top-hat segmentation because it helps with enhancing the bright ("hot") ridge-like structures corresponding to the blood vessels. In this method the original image is first opened and then this opened image is subtracted from the original image as shown below:

$$I_{\text{open}} = (I \ominus S) \oplus S$$
$$I_{\text{top}} = I - I_{\text{open}}$$

(39.10)

(a)

(b)

(c)

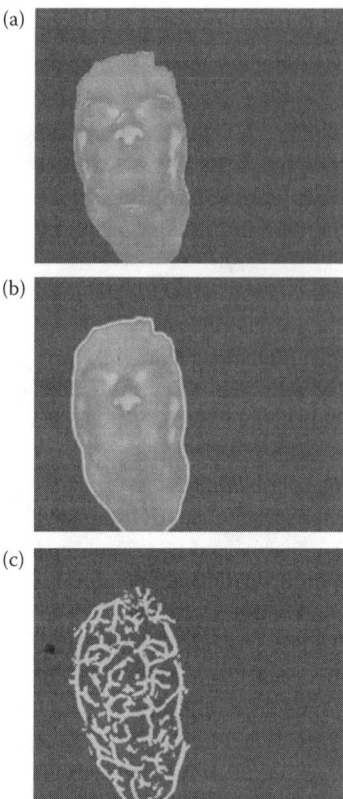

FIGURE 39.7   Vascular network extraction: (a) original segmented image; (b) anisotropically diffused image; and (c) blood vessels extracted using white top-hat segmentation.

where I, I_{open}, and I_{top} are the original, opened, and white top-hat segmented images, respectively, S is the structuring element, and $\ominus$, $\oplus$ are morphological erosion and dilation operations, respectively. Figure 39.7a depicts the result of applying anisotropic diffusion to the segmented facial tissue shown in Figure 39.4b, and Figure 39.7b shows the corresponding blood vessels extracted using white top-hat segmentation.

39.2.3 Extraction of TMPs

The extracted blood vessels exhibit different contour shapes between subjects. We call the branching points of the blood vessels TMPs. TMPs can be extracted from the blood vessel network in ways similar to those used for fingerprint minutia extraction. A number of methods have been proposed [26] for robust and efficient extraction of minutia from fingerprint images. Most of these approaches describe each minutia point by at least three attributes, including its type, its location in the fingerprint image, and the local vessel orientation. We adopt a similar approach for extracting TMPs from vascular networks, which is outlined in the following steps:

1. The local orientation of the vascular network is estimated.
2. The vascular network is skeletonized.
3. The TMPs are extracted from the thinned vascular network.
4. The spurious TMPs are removed.

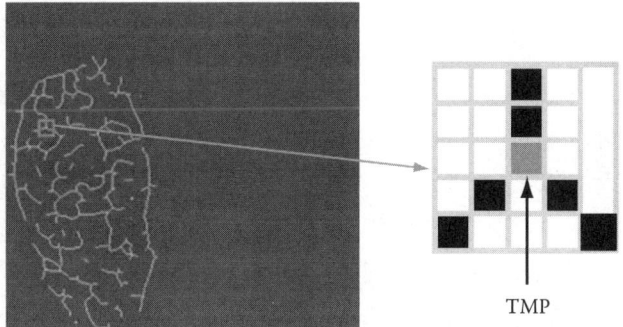

FIGURE 39.8 TMP extracted from the thinned vascular network.

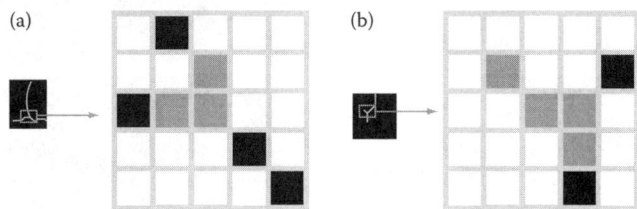

FIGURE 39.9 Spurious TMPs: (a) clustered TMPs and (b) spike formed due to a trivially short branch.

Local orientation $\psi(x,y)$ is the angle formed at (x,y) between the blood vessel and the horizontal axis. Estimating the orientation field at each pixel provides the basis for capturing the overall pattern of the vascular network. We use the approach proposed in Reference 27 for computing the orientation image because it provides pixel-wise accuracy.

Next, the vascular network is thinned to one-pixel thickness [28]. Each pixel in the thinned map contains a value of 1 if it is on the vessel and 0 if it is not. Considering eight-neighborhood $(N_0, N_1, \ldots, N_7)$ around each pixel, a pixel (x,y) represents a TMP if $(\sum_{i=0}^{7} N_i) > 2$ (see Figure 39.8).

It is desirable that the TMP extraction algorithm does not leave any spurious TMPs since this will adversely affect the matching performance. Removal of clustered TMPs (see Figure 39.9a) and spikes (see Figure 39.9b) helps to reduce the number of spurious TMPs in the thinned vascular network.

The vascular network of a typical facial image contains around 50–80 genuine TMPs whose location (x,y) and orientation (ψ) are stored in the database. Figure 39.10 shows the results of each stage of the feature extraction algorithm on a thermal facial image.

39.3 Matching

Each subject's record in the database consists of five different poses to account for pose variation during the testing phase. Since facial images from the same person look quite different across multiple views, it is very important that the search space includes facial images with pose similar to the pose of the test image. Given a test image, we first estimate its pose. Then, the task is simply to match the TMP network extracted from the test image against the TMP database corresponding to the estimated pose.

39.3.1 Estimation of Facial Pose

To the best of our knowledge, it is the first time that the issue of pose estimation in thermal facial imagery is addressed. However, as it is the case with face recognition in general, a number of efforts have been

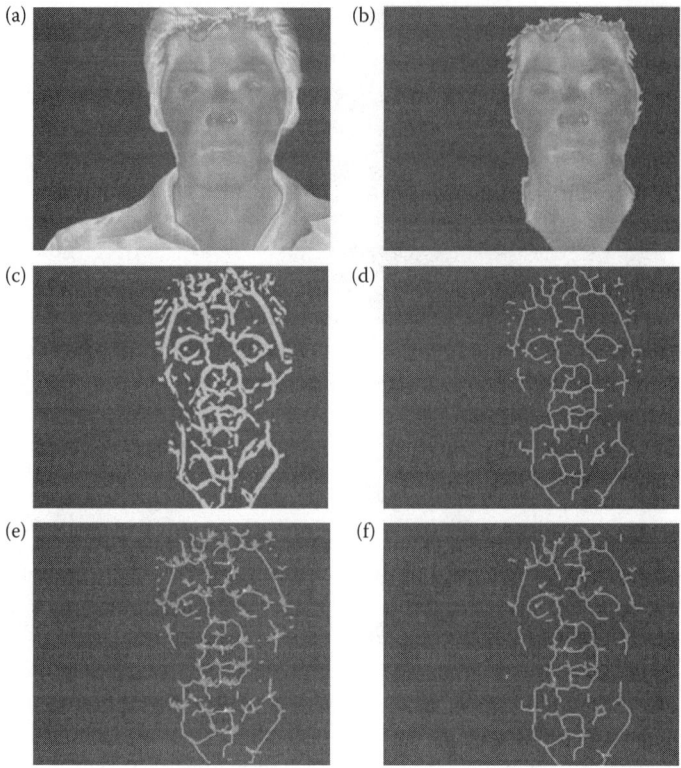

FIGURE 39.10 Visualization of the various stages of the vascular feature extraction algorithm: (a) a typical thermal facial image; (b) facial tissue delineated from the background; (c) network of vascular contours extracted from the thermal facial image; (d) skeletonized vessel map; (e) extracted TMPs from branching points; and (f) cleaned TMP set.

made to address the issue of facial pose estimation in visible band imagery [29,30]. We capitalize upon the algorithm proposed in Reference 29 for estimating head pose across multiple views. We apply principal component analysis (PCA) on the thermal facial images in the training set to reduce the dimensionality of the training examples. Figure 39.11 illustrates sample face images in the database across multiple views. Then, we train the support vector machine (SVM) classifier with the PCA vectors of face samples. Given a test image, SVM can classify it against one of the five poses (center, mid-left profile, left profile, mid-right profile, and right profile) under consideration.

39.3.2 Matching of TMPs

Numerous methods have been proposed for matching fingerprint minutiae, most of which try to simulate the way forensic experts compare fingerprints [26]. Popular techniques are alignment-based point pattern matching, local structure matching, and global structure matching. Local minutiae matching algorithms are fast, simple, and more tolerant to distortions. Global minutiae matching algorithms feature high distinctiveness. A few hybrid approaches [31,32] have been proposed where the advantages of both local and global methods are exploited. We use such a method [31] to perform TMP matching.

For each TMP $M(x_i,y_i,\psi_i)$ that is extracted from the vascular network, we consider its N nearest-neighbor TMPs $M(x_n,y_n,\psi_n)$, $n = 1,\ldots,N$. Then, the TMP $M(x_i,y_i,\psi_i)$ can be defined by a new feature vector:

$$L_M = \{\{d_1,\varphi_1,\vartheta_1\},\{d_2,\varphi_2,\vartheta_2\},\ldots,\{d_N,\varphi_N,\vartheta_N\},\Psi_i\} \tag{39.11}$$

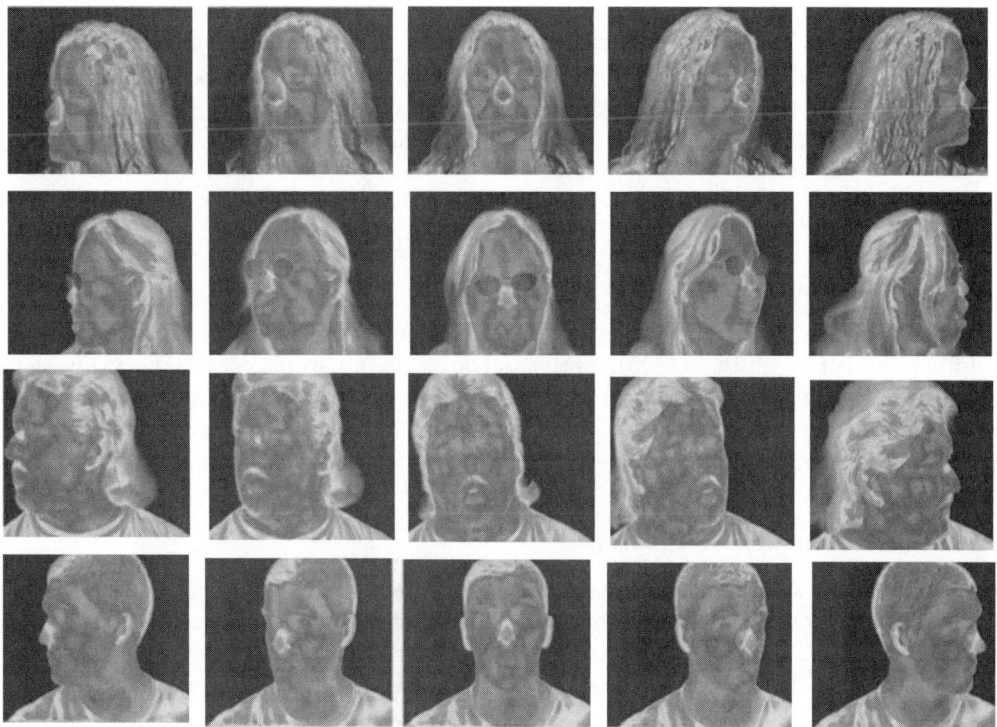

FIGURE 39.11 Samples from our training set featuring five different poses per subject. From left to right the views depicted are left profile, mid-left profile, center, mid-right profile, and right profile.

where

$$d_n = \sqrt{(x_n - x_i)^2 + (y_n - y_i)^2}$$
$$\varphi_n = \text{diff}(\Psi_n, \Psi_i), \quad n = 1, 2, \dots, N$$
$$\vartheta_n = \text{diff}\left(\arctan\left(\frac{y_n - y_i}{x_n - x_i}\right), \Psi_i\right)$$

(39.12)

The function diff () calculates the difference of two angles and scales the result within the range [0, 2π) [32]. Given a test image $\mathbf{I}_t$, the feature vector of each of its TMP is compared with the feature vector of each TMP of a database image. Two TMPs M and M' are marked to be a matched pair if the absolute difference between corresponding features is less than specific threshold values {$\delta_d, \delta_\varphi, \delta_\vartheta, \delta_\psi$}. The threshold values should be chosen in such a way that they accommodate linear deformations and translations. The final matching score between the test image and a database image is given by

$$\text{Score} = \frac{\text{NUM}_{\text{match}}}{\max(\text{NUM}_{\text{test}}, \text{NUM}_{\text{database}})}$$

(39.13)

where $\text{NUM}_{\text{match}}$ represents the number of matched TMP pairs, and NUM_{test} and $\text{NUM}_{\text{database}}$ represent the number of TMPs in test and database images, respectively. If the highest matching score between the test and database images is greater than a specific threshold, the corresponding database image is classified as a match. If not, the test image is classified to be not in the database.

39.4 Experimental Results

We collected a large database of thermal facial images in our laboratory from volunteers representing different sex, race, and age groups. The images were captured using a high-quality mid-wave IR Phoenix camera produced by Indigo Systems. The following are the specifications of the camera:

Detector: InSb 640 × 512 element FPA
Spectral range: 3.0–5.0 μm
NETD (sensitivity): 0.01°C
Focal length: 50 mm

We used a subset of the dataset for evaluating the performance of the proposed face recognition algorithm. The dataset consists of 7590 thermal facial images from 138 different subjects (55 images per subject) with varying pose and facial expressions. Five images from each subject (each image representing one of the five training poses) were used for training, TMPs of which were extracted and stored in the database. The remaining 50 images per subject at arbitrary poses were used for testing.

39.4.1 Low Permanence Problem

A major challenge associated with thermal face recognition is the recognition performance over time [33]. Facial thermograms may change depending on the physical condition and environmental conditions. This makes the task of acquiring similar features for the same person over time difficult. A few approaches that use direct temperature data for recognition reported degraded performance over time [10]. However, our approach attempts to solve this problem by using facial anatomical information as feature space, which is unique to each person and at the same time is invariable to physical and environmental conditions as shown in Figure 39.12. The vascular network extracted from the same person with a time gap of about 6 months exhibits a similar pattern.

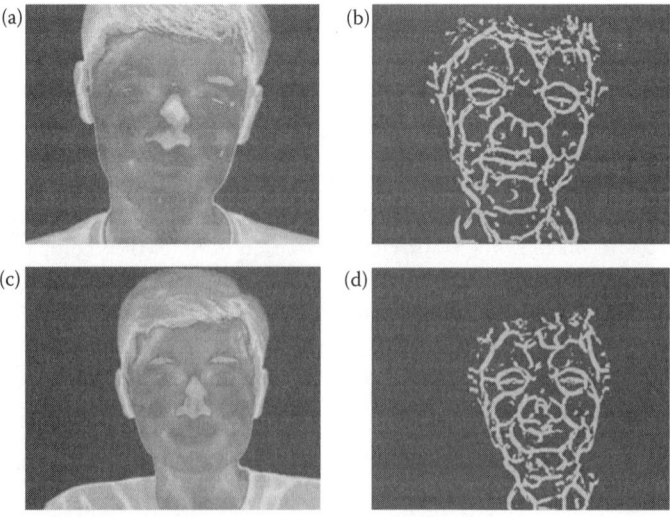

FIGURE 39.12 (a) Thermal facial image of a subject acquired on October 17, 2003; (b) corresponding vascular network; (c) thermal facial image of the same subject acquired on April 29, 2004; and (d) corresponding vascular network.

39.4.2 Frontal Pose and Arbitrary Pose Experiments

Many face recognition algorithms that perform well on the frontal image dataset often have problems when tested on images with arbitrary poses [2]. Our face recognition algorithm overcomes this problem by using multiple pose images for training, which allows pose invariance in the test image. We found experimentally that the five poses we used for training our face recognition algorithm are sufficient to accommodate all yaw rotations (including tilt rotations to a certain extent) without confusing our matching algorithm significantly. As shown in Figure 39.13, when an image that is close to the mid-left profile is queried, pose estimation picked the corresponding mid-left profile image from the training dataset for matching. The small variation in pose that still exists between the query and database images might cause minor position and angle differences in corresponding TMPs extracted from those images. This can be compensated by choosing appropriate values for thresholds $\{\delta_d, \delta_\varphi, \delta_\theta, \delta_\psi\}$, discussed in Section 39.3.2.

We conducted two sets of experiments in order to evaluate the performance of our face recognition system. The first experiment is the frontal pose experiment where the test set contains images with poses between mid-left and mid-right profiles. This test set is matched against only frontal images of the training database. This is the typical experimental procedure used for testing most of the current face recognition algorithms. The second experiment is the arbitrary pose experiment where test set contains all possible poses between left and right profiles. This test set is matched against the entire training set containing five pose images per subject. Figures 39.14 and 39.15 show comparative results of these two experiments. We noticed that the arbitrary pose experiment showed better results when compared to the frontal pose experiment in both cases.

Figure 39.14 shows the cumulative math characteristic (CMC) curves of the two experiments, and Figure 39.15 shows the receiver operating characteristic (ROC) curves based on various threshold values for the matching score discussed in Section 39.3.2. The results demonstrate the promise as well as some problems with our proposed approach. Specifically, CMC shows that rank 1 recognition is over 86% and rank 5 recognition is over 96%. This performance puts a brand new approach very close to the performance of mature visible band recognition methods. In contrast, ROC reveals a weakness of the current method, as it requires false acceptance rate over 20% to reach positive acceptance rate above the 86% range. To address this problem, we believe we need to estimate and eliminate the incorrect TMPs and nonlinear deformations in the extracted vascular network.

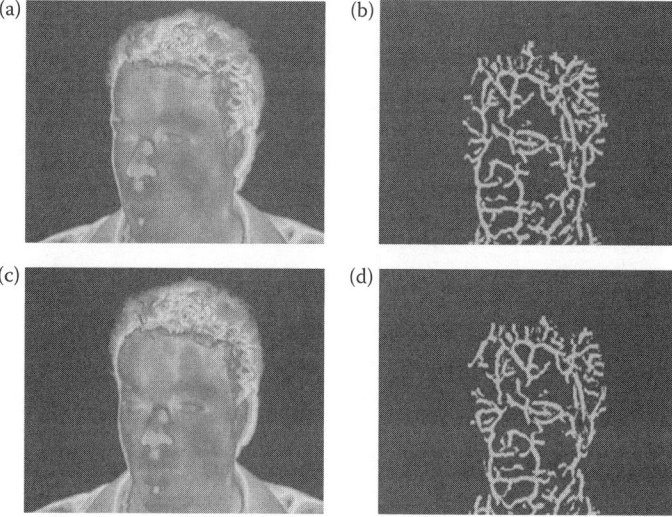

FIGURE 39.13 (a) Test image and (b) corresponding vascular network. (c) Mid-left profile image picked from training database by pose estimation and (d) corresponding vascular network.

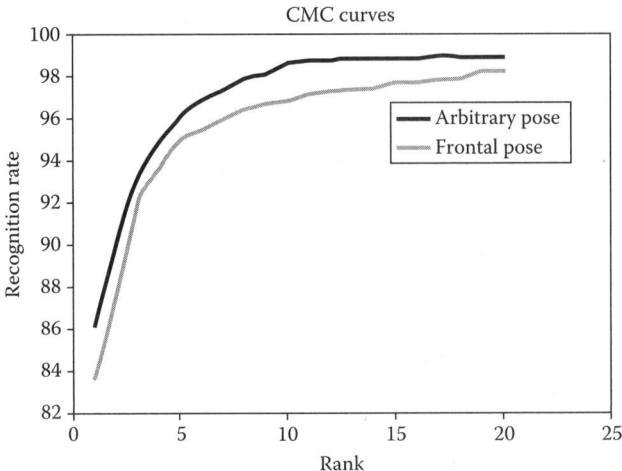

FIGURE 39.14   CMC curves of our method for the frontal and arbitrary pose experiments.

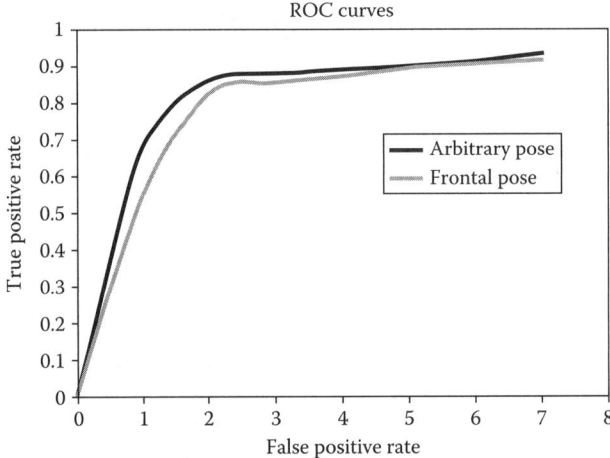

FIGURE 39.15   ROC curves of our method for the frontal and arbitrary pose experiments.

39.5 Conclusions and Future Work

We have outlined a novel approach to the problem of face recognition in thermal IR—one of the fastest-growing biometrics. The cornerstone of the approach is the use of unique and time-invariant physiological information as feature space. We collect five different poses for each subject to be stored in the training database. We have shown that these five poses are capable of accommodating all yaw rotations in the test image. The facial tissue is first separated from the background using a Bayesian segmentation method. The vascular network on the surface of the skin is then extracted based on a white top-hat segmentation preceded by anisotropic diffusion. TMPs are extracted from the vascular network and are used as features for matching the test to database images. The experimental results demonstrate that our approach is very promising.

The method, although young, performed well in a nontrivial database. Our ongoing work is directed toward improving the sophistication of the method regarding nonlinear deformations of the vascular network and testing it comparatively in larger databases.

References

1. Jain, A., Bolle, R., and Pankanti, S., *Biometrics: Personal Identification in Networked Society*, 1st edn., Kluwer Academic Publishers, Norwell, MA, USA, 1999.
2. Zhao, W., Chellappa, R., Phillips, P.J., and Rosenfeld, A., Face recognition: A literature survey, *ACM Computing Surveys (CSUR)*, 35, 399, 2003.
3. Pavlidis, I. and Symosek, P., The imaging issue in an automatic face/disguise detection system. In *Proceedings of IEEE Workshop on Computer Vision Beyond the Visible Spectrum: Methods and Applications*, Hilton Head Island, SC, USA, 2000, p. 15.
4. Prokoski, F., History, current status, and future of infrared identification. In *Proceedings of IEEE Workshop on Computer Vision Beyond the Visible Spectrum: Methods and Applications*, Hilton Head Island, SC, USA, 2000, p. 5.
5. Socolinsky, D.A. and Selinger, A., A comparative analysis of face recognition performance with visible and thermal infrared imagery. In *Proceedings of 16th International Conference on Pattern Recognition*, 4, Quebec, Canada, 2002, p. 217.
6. Wilder, J., Phillips, P.J., Jiang, C., and Wiener, S., Comparison of visible and infrared imagery for face recognition. In *Proceedings of the Second International Conference on Automatic Face and Gesture Recognition*, Killington, VT, 1996, p. 182.
7. Socolinsky, D.A., Wolff, L.B., Neuheisel, J.D., and Eveland, C.K., Illumination invariant face recognition using thermal infrared imagery. In *Proceedings of the IEEE Computer Society Conference on Computer Vision and Pattern Recognition (CVPR 2001)*, 1, Kauai, H1, USA, 2001, p. 527.
8. Selinger, A. and Socolinsky, D.A., Face recognition in the dark. In *Proceedings of the Joint IEEE Workshop on Object Tracking and Classification Beyond the Visible Spectrum*, Washington, DC, 2004.
9. Cutler, R., Face recognition using infrared images and eigenfaces, cs.umd.edu/rgc/face/face.htm, 1996.
10. Chen, X., Flynn, P.J., and Bowyer, K.W., PCA-based face recognition in infrared imagery: Baseline and comparative studies. In *Proceedings of the IEEE International Workshop on Analysis and Modeling of Faces and Gestures*, Nice, France, 2003, p. 127.
11. Srivastava, A. and Liu, X., Statistical hypothesis pruning for recognizing faces from infrared images, *Journal of Image and Vision Computing*, 21, 651, 2003.
12. Buddharaju, P., Pavlidis, I., and Kakadiaris, I., Face recognition in the thermal infrared spectrum. In *Proceedings of the Joint IEEE Workshop on Object Tracking and Classification Beyond the Visible Spectrum*, Washington, DC, 2004.
13. Heo, J., Kong, S.G., Abidi, B.R., and Abidi, M.A., Fusion of visual and thermal signatures with eyeglass removal for robust face recognition. In *Proceedings of the Joint IEEE Workshop on Object Tracking and Classification Beyond the Visible Spectrum*, Washington, DC, 2004.
14. Gyaourova, A., Bebis, G., and Pavlidis, I., Fusion of infrared and visible images for face recognition. In *Proceedings of the eighth European Conference on Computer Vision*, Prague, Czech Republic, 2004.
15. Socolinsky, D.A. and Selinger, A., Thermal face recognition in an operational scenario. In *Proceedings of the IEEE Computer Society Conference on Computer Vision and Pattern Recognition*, 2, Washington DC, 2004, p. 1012.
16. Wang, J.G., Sung, E., and Venkateswarlu, R., Registration of infrared and visible-spectrum imagery for face recognition. In *Proceedings of the Sixth IEEE International Conference on Automatic Face and Gesture Recognition*, Seoul, Korea, 2004, p. 638.
17. Lin, C.L. and Fan, K.C., Biometric verification using thermal images of palm-dorsa vein patterns, *IEEE Transactions on Circuits and Systems for Video Technology*, 14, 199, 2004.
18. Im, S.K., Choi, H.S., and Kim, S.W., A direction-based vascular pattern extraction algorithm for hand vascular pattern verification, *ETRI Journal*, 25, 101, 2003.
19. Shimooka, T. and Shimizu, K., Artificial immune system for personal identification with finger vein pattern. In *Proceedings of the Eighth International Conference on Knowledge-Based Intelligent*

Information and Engineering Systems, Lecture Notes in Computer Science, Wellington, New Zealand, 3214, 2004, p. 511.

20. Miura, N., Nagasaka, A., and Miyatake, T., Feature extraction of finger vein patterns based on iterative line tracking and its application to personal identification, *Systems and Computers in Japan*, 35, 61, 2004.

21. Prokoski, F.J. and Riedel, R., *BIOMETRICS: Personal Identification in Networked Society*, Infrared Identification of Faces and Body Parts, Kluwer Academic Publishers, Norwell, MA, USA, 1998, Chapter 9.

22. Buddharaju, P., Pavlidis, I.T., and Tsiamyrtzis, P., Physiology-based face recognition. In *Proceedings of the IEEE Advanced Video and Signal based Surveillance*, IEEE Conference on Advanced Video and Signal Based Surveillance (AVSS 2005), Como, Italy, 2005.

23. Manohar, C., Extraction of superficial vasculature in thermal imaging, Master's thesis, University of Houston, Houston, TX, 2004.

24. Pavlidis, I., Tsiamyrtzis, P., Manohar, C., and Buddharaju, P., *Biomedical Engineering Handbook*, Biometrics: Face Recognition in Thermal Infrared, CRC Press, Boca Raton, FL, 2006, Chapter 22.

25. Di Stefano, L. and Bulgarelli, A., Simple and efficient connected components labeling algorithm. In *Proceedings of the International Conference on Image Analysis and Processing*, Venice, Italy, 1999, p. 322.

26. Maltoni, D., Maio, D., Jain, A.K., and Prabhakar, S., *Handbook of Fingerprint Recognition*, Springer-Verlag, NY, USA, 2003.

27. Oliveira, M.A. and Leite, N.J., Reconnection of fingerprint ridges based on morphological operators and multiscale directional information, In *The Brazilian Symposium on Computer Graphics and Image Processing*, Curitiba, PR, Brazil, 2004, p. 122.

28. Jang, B.K. and Chin, R.T., One-pass parallel thinning: Analysis, properties, and quantitative evaluation, *IEEE Transactions on Pattern Analysis and Machine Intelligence*, 14, 1129, 1992.

29. Yang, Z., Ai, H., Wu, B., Lao, S., and Cai, L., Face pose estimation and its application in video shot selection. In *Proceedings of the 17th International Conference on Pattern Recognition*, 1, Cambridge, UK, 2004, p. 322.

30. Li, Y., Gong, S., Sherrah, J., and Liddell, H., Support vector machine based multi-view face detection and recognition, *Image and Vision Computing*, 22, 413, 2004.

31. Yang, S. and Verbauwhede, I.M., A secure fingerprint matching technique. In *Proceedings of the 2003 ACM SIGMM Workshop on Biometrics Methods and Applications*, Berkley, CA, 2003, p. 89.

32. Jiang, X. and Yau, W.Y., Fingerprint minutiae matching based on the local and global structures. In *Proceedings of the 15th International Conference on Pattern Recognition*, 2, Barcelona, Catalonia, Spain, 2000, p. 1038.

33. Socolinsky, D.A. and Selinger, A., Thermal face recognition over time. In *Proceedings of the 17th International Conference on Pattern Recognition*, 4, Cambridge, UK, 2004, p. 23.

40

Noninvasive Infrared Imaging for Functional Monitoring of Disease Processes

Moinuddin Hassan
*U.S. Food and Drug
Administration (FDA)*

Jana Kainerstorfer
*National Institutes of
Health*

Victor
Chernomordik
*National Institutes of
Health*

Abby Vogel
*Georgia Institute of
Technology*

Israel Gannot
Tel Aviv University

Richard F. Little
*National Institutes of
Health*

Robert Yarchoan
*National Institutes of
Health*

Amir H.
Gandjbakhche
*National Institutes of
Health*

Noninvasive imaging techniques are emerging into the forefront of medical diagnostics and treatment monitoring. Both near- and mid-infrared imaging techniques have provided invaluable information in the clinical setting. Most *in vivo* biomedical applications of functional imaging use light in the near-infrared spectrum. The main advantage of the interaction of near-infrared light with tissue is increased penetration: light with wavelengths between 700 and 1100 nm passes through skin and other tissues better than visible light.

In the infrared thermal waveband, information about blood circulation, local metabolism, sweat gland malfunction, inflammation, and healing can be extracted. Originally used to detect breast carcinoma, IR imaging was subsequently reported to have clinical utility in a multitude of neuromusculoskeletal, vascular, and rheomatolgy disorders. There is an especially strong interest in developing optical technologies that have the capability of performing *in situ* tissue diagnosis without the need for sample excision and processing. At present, excisional biopsy followed by histology is considered to be the "gold standard" for the diagnosis of early neoplastic changes and carcinoma. In some cases, cytology, rather than excisional biopsy, is performed. These techniques are powerful diagnostic tools because they provide high-resolution spatial and morphological information of the cellular and subcellular structures of tissues. The use of staining and processing can enhance visual contrast and specificity of histopathology. Both these diagnostic procedures, however, require physical removal of specimens followed by tissue processing in a laboratory. The current status of modern infrared imaging is that of a first-line supplement to both clinical exams and current imaging methods. Using infrared imaging to detect breast pathology is based on the principle that both metabolic and vascular activity in the tissue surrounding a new and developing tumor is usually higher than in normal tissue. Early cancer growth is dependent on increasing blood circulation by creating new blood vessels (angiogenesis). This process results in regional variations that can often be detected by infrared imaging.

The spectroscopic power of light, along with the revolution in molecular characterization of disease processes have given rise to new methods and instrumentation for the early or noninvasive diagnosis of various medical conditions, including arteriosclerosis, heart arrhythmia, cancer, and many other diseases. Near-infrared imaging has been used to functionally monitor diseases processes, including cancer and lymph node detection and optical biopsies. Spectroscopic imaging modalities have been shown to improve the diagnosis of tumors and add new knowledge about the physiological properties of the tumor and surrounding tissues. Particular emphasis should be placed on identifying markers that predict the risk of precancerous lesions progressing to invasive cancers, thereby providing new opportunities for cancer prevention. This might be accomplished through the use of markers as contrast agents for imaging using conventional techniques or through refinements of newer technologies such as magnetic resonance imaging (MRI) or positron emission tomography (PET) scanning.

Infrared imaging techniques have the potential for performing *in vivo* diagnosis on tissue without the need for sample excision and processing. Another advantage of diagnosis through infrared imaging is that the resulting information can be available in real time. In addition, since removal of tissue is not required for diagnosis, a more complete examination of the organ of interest can be achieved than with excisional biopsy or cytology.

Section 40.1 discusses near-infrared imaging and its applications in imaging biological tissues. Mid-infrared thermal imaging techniques, calibration, and a current clinical trial of Kaposi's sarcoma (KS) are described in Section 40.2.

40.1 Near-Infrared Quantitative Imaging of Deep Tissue Structure

In vivo optical imaging has traditionally been limited to superficial tissue surfaces, directly or endoscopically accessible. These methods are based on geometric optics. Most tissues scatter light so strongly, however, that for geometric optics-based equipment to work, special techniques are needed to remove multiply scattered light (such as pinholes in confocal imaging or interferometry in optical coherence microscopies). Even with these special designs, high-resolution optical imaging fails at depths of more than 1 mm below the tissue surface.

Collimated visible or infrared (IR) light impinging upon thick tissue is scattered many times in a distance of ~1 mm, so the analysis of light–tissue interactions requires theories based on the diffusive nature of light propagation. In contrast to x-ray and PET, a complex underlying theoretical picture is needed to describe photon paths as a function of scattering and absorption properties of the tissue.

Approximately two decade ago, a new field called "photon migration" was born that seeks to characterize the statistical physics of photon motion through turbid tissues. The goal is to image macroscopic structures in 3D at greater depths within tissues and to provide reliable pathlength estimation for noninvasive spectral analysis of tissue changes. Although geometrical optics fails to describe light propagation under these conditions, the statistical physics of strong, multiply scattered light provides powerful approaches to macroscopic imaging and subsurface detection and characterization. Techniques using visible and near-infrared light offer a variety of functional imaging modalities, in addition to density imaging, while avoiding ionizing radiation hazards.

In Section 40.1.1, the optical properties of biological tissue are discussed. Section 40.1.2 is devoted to different measurement methods. Theoretical models for spectroscopy and imaging are discussed in Section 40.1.3. In Sections 40.1.4 and 40.1.5, two studies on breast imaging and the use of exogenous fluorescent markers are presented as examples of near-infrared spectroscopy. Finally, the future direction of the field is discussed in Section 40.1.6.

40.1.1 Optical Properties of Biological Tissue

The difficulty of tissue optics is to define optical coefficients of tissue physiology and quantify their changes to differentiate structures and functional status *in vivo*. Light–tissue interactions dictate the way that these parameters are defined. The two main approaches are the wave and particle descriptions of light propagation. Wave propagation uses Maxwell's equations and therefore quantifies the spatially varying permittivity as a measurable quantity. For simplistic and historic reasons, the particle interpretation of light has been used more often (see Section 40.1.3). In photon transport theory, one considers the behavior of discrete photons as they move through the tissue. This motion is characterized by absorption and scattering, and when interfaces (e.g., layers) are involved, refraction. The absorption coefficient, μ_a (mm^{-1}), represents the inverse mean pathlength of a photon before absorption. The distance in a medium where intensity is attenuated by a factor of 1/e (Beer–Lambert law) is considered to be $1/\mu_a$. Absorption in tissue is strongly wavelength dependent and is due to chromophores including water. Among the chromophores in tissue, the dominant component is the hemoglobin in blood. In Figure 40.1, hemoglobin absorption is divided into oxygenated and deoxygenated hemoglobin. As seen in this figure, in the visible range (600–700 nm), the blood absorption is relatively high compared to absorption in the near-infrared. By contrast, water absorption is low in the visible and NIR regions and increases rapidly above approximately 950 nm. Thus, for greatest penetration of light in tissue, wavelengths in the 650–950 nm spectra are used most often. This region of the light spectrum is called the "therapeutic window." One should note that different spectra of chromophores allow one to separate the contribution of varying functional species in tissue (e.g., quantification of oxy- and deoxyhemoglobin to study tissue oxygenation). Similarly, scattering is characterized by a coefficient, μ_s, which is the inverse mean free path of photons between scattering events. The average size of the scattered photons in tissue, proportional to the wavelength of light, places the scattering in the Mie region. In the Mie region, a scattering event does not result in isotropic scattering angles [1,2]. Instead, the scattering in tissue is biased in the forward direction.

For example, by studying the development of neonatal skin, Saidi et al. were able to show that the principal sources of anisotropic scattering in muscle are collagen fibers [3]. The fibers were determined to have a mean diameter of 2.2 μm. In addition to the Mie scattering from the fibers, there is isotropic Rayleigh scattering due to the presence of much smaller scatterers such as organelles in cells.

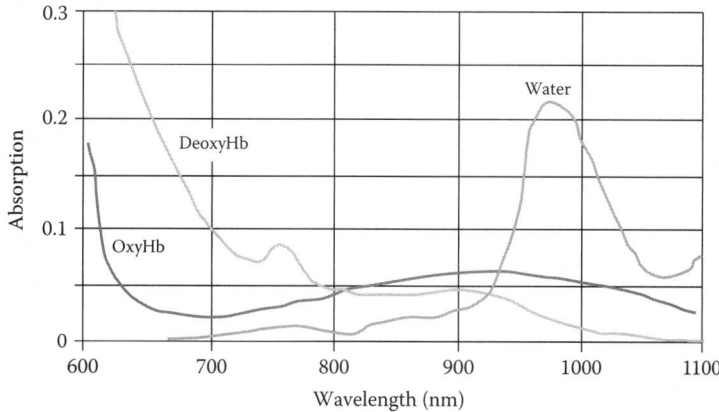

FIGURE 40.1 Absorption spectra of the three major components of tissue in the NIR region: oxy- and deoxyhemoglobin, and water.

Anisotropic scattering is quantified in a coefficient, the mean cosine of the scattering angle g:

$$g \equiv \langle \cos(\theta) \rangle \equiv \frac{\int\limits_{0}^{\pi} p(\theta) \cos(\theta) \sin(\theta) d\theta}{\int\limits_{0}^{\pi} p(\theta) \sin(\theta) d\theta} \tag{40.1}$$

where, $p(\theta)$ is the probability of a particular scattering angle. For isotropic scattering, $g = 0$. For complete forward scattering, $g = 1$, and for complete back scattering, $g = -1$. In tissue, g is typically 0.7–0.98 [3–5].

Likewise, different tissue types have differing scattering properties that are wavelength dependent. The scattering coefficients of many soft tissues have been measured at a variety of optical wavelengths, and are within the range of 10–100 mm^{-1}. Compared to absorption, however, scattering changes, as a function of wavelength, are more gradual and have smaller extremes. Abnormal tissues such as tumors, fibro-adenomas, and cysts all have scattering properties that are different from normal tissue [6,7]. Thus, the scattering coefficient of an inclusion may also be an important clue to disease diagnosis.

Theories of photon migration are often based on isotropic scattering. Therefore, one must find the appropriate scaling relationships that will allow for an isotropic scattering model. For the case of diffusion-like models (e.g., [8]), it has been shown that one may use an isotropic scattering model with a corrected scattering coefficient, μ_s', and obtain equivalent results, where

$$\mu_s' = \mu_s(1 - g) \tag{40.2}$$

The corrected scattering coefficient is smaller than the actual scattering that corresponds to a greater distance between isotropic scattering events than would occur with anisotropic scattering. For this reason, μ_s' is typically called the transport-corrected scattering coefficient.

There are instances when the spectroscopic signatures will not be sufficient to detect disease. This can occur when the specific disease results in only very small changes to the tissue's scattering and absorption properties, or when the scattering and absorption properties are not unique to the disease. Although it is not clear what the limits of detectability are in relation to diseased tissue properties, it is clear that there will be cases for which optical techniques based on elastic absorption are inadequate. In such cases, another source of optical contrast, such as fluorescence, will be required to detect and localize the disease. The presence of fluorescent molecules in tissue can provide useful contrast mechanisms. Concentration of these endogenous fluorophores in the body can be related to functional and metabolic activities, and therefore to the disease processes. For example, the concentrations of fluorescent molecules such as collagen and NADH have been used to differentiate between normal and abnormal tissue [9].

Advances in the molecular biology of disease processes, new immunohistopathological techniques, and the development of fluorescently labeled cell surface markers have led to a revolution in specific molecular diagnosis of disease by histopathology, as well as in research on molecular origins of disease processes (e.g., using fluorescence microscopy in cell biology). As a result, an exceptional level of specificity is now possible due to the advances in the design of exogenous markers. Molecules can now be tailor-made to bind only to specific receptor sites in the body. These receptor sites may be antibodies or other biologically interesting molecules. Fluorophores may be bound to these engineered molecules and injected into the body, where they will preferentially concentrate at specific sites of interest [10,11].

Furthermore, fluorophore may be used as a probe to measure environmental conditions in a particular locality by capitalizing on changes in fluorophore lifetime [12,13]. Each fluorophore has a characteristic lifetime that quantifies the probability of a specific time delay between fluorophore excitation and emission. In practice, this lifetime may be modified by specific environmental factors such as temperature, pH, and concentrations of substances such as oxygen. In these cases, it is possible to quantify local concentrations of specific substances or specific environmental conditions by measuring the lifetime of fluorophores at the site. Whereas conventional fluorescence imaging is very sensitive to nonuniform fluorophore transport and distribution (e.g., blood does not transport molecules equally to all parts of the body), fluorescence lifetime imaging is insensitive to transport nonuniformity as long as a detectable quantity of fluorophores is present in the site of interest. Throughout the following sections, experimental techniques and differing models used to quantify these sources of optical contrast are presented.

40.1.2 Measurable Quantities and Experimental Techniques

Three classes of measurable quantities prove to be of interest to transform results of remote sensing measurements in tissue into useful physical information. The first is the spatial distribution of light or the intensity profile generated by photons reemitted through a surface and measured as a function of the radial distance from the source and the detector when the medium is continually irradiated by a point source (e.g., a laser). This type of measurement is called continuous wave (CW). The intensity, nominally, does not vary in time. The second class is the temporal response to a very short pulse (~ps) of photons impinging on the surface of the tissue. This technique is called time-resolved and the temporal response is known as the time-of-flight (TOF). The third class is the frequency-domain technique in which an intensity-modulated laser beam illuminates the tissue. In this case, the measured outputs are the AC modulation amplitude and the phase shift of the detected signal. These techniques can be implemented in geometries with different arrangements of source(s) and detector(s): (a) In reflection mode, source(s) and detector(s) are placed at the same side of the tissue. (b) In transmission mode, source(s) and detector(s) are located on opposite sides of the tissue. In the latter, the source(s) and detector(s) can move in tandem while scanning the tissue surface and detectors with lateral offsets can also be used. (c) Tomographic sampling often uses multiple sources and detectors placed around the circumference of the target tissue.

For CW measurements, the instrumentation is simple and requires only a set of light sources and detectors. In this technique, the only measurable quantity is the intensity of light, and, due to multiple scattering, strong pathlength dispersion occurs, which results in a loss of localization and resolution. Hence, this technique is widely used for spectroscopic measurements of bulk tissue properties in which the tissue is considered to be homogeneous [14,15]. However, CW techniques for imaging abnormal targets that use only the coherent portion of light, and thereby reject photons with long pathlengths, have also been investigated. Using the transillumination geometry, collimated detection is used to isolate nonscattered photons [16–18]. Spatial filtering has been proposed which employs a lens to produce the Fourier spectrum of the spatial distribution of light from which the high-order frequencies are removed. The resulting image is formed using only the photons with angles close to normal [19]. Polarization discrimination has been used to select those photons which undergo few scattering events and therefore preserve a fraction of their initial polarization state, as opposed to those photons which experience multiple scattering resulting in complete randomization of their initial polarization state [20]. Several investigators have used heterodyne detection which involves measuring the beat frequency generated by the spatial and temporal combination of a light beam and a frequency modulated reference beam. Constructive interference occurs only for the coherent portion of the light [20–22]. However, the potential of direct imaging using CW techniques in very thick tissue (e.g., breast) has not been established. On the other hand, use of models of photon migration implemented in inverse method based on backprojection techniques has shown promising results. For example, Phillips Medical has used 256 optical fibers placed at the periphery of a white conical-shaped vessel. The area of interest, in this case the breast, is suspended in the vessel, and surrounded by a matching fluid. Three CW laser diodes sequentially illuminate the breast using one fiber. The detection is done simultaneously by 255 fibers.

It is now clear that CW imaging cannot provide direct images with clinically acceptable resolution in thick tissue. Attempts are underway to devise inverse algorithms to separate the effects of scattering and absorption and therefore use this technique for quantitative spectroscopy as proposed by Phillips [23]. However, until now, clinical application of CW techniques in imaging has been limited by the mixture of scattering and absorption of light in the detected signal. To overcome this problem, time-dependent measurement techniques have been investigated.

Time-domain techniques involve the temporal resolution of photons traveling inside the tissue. The basic idea is that photons with smaller pathlengths are those that arrive earlier to the detector. In order to discriminate between unscattered or less scattered light and the majority of the photons, which experience a large number of multiple scattering, sub-nanosecond resolutions are needed. This short time gating of an imaging system requires the use of a variety of techniques involving ultra-fast phenomena and/or fast detection systems. Ultra-fast shuttering is performed using the Kerr effect. The birefringence in the Kerr cell, placed between two crossed polarizers, is induced using very short pulses. Transmitted light through the Kerr cell is recorded, and temporal resolution of a few picoseconds is achieved [19]. When an impulse of light (~picoseconds or hundreds of femtoseconds) is launched at the tissue surface, the whole temporal distribution of photon intensity can be recorded by a streak camera. The streak camera can achieve temporal resolution on the order of few picoseconds up to several nanoseconds detection time. This detection system has been widely used to assess the performance of breast imaging and neonatal brain activity [24,25]. The time of flight recorded by the streak camera is the convolution of the pulsed laser source (in practice with a finite width) and the actual temporal point spread function (TPSF) of the diffuse photons. Instead of using very short pulse lasers (e.g., Ti-Sapphire lasers), the advent of pulse diode lasers with relatively larger pulse width (100–400 ps) have reduce the cost of time-domain imaging much lower. However, deconvolutions of the incoming pulse and the detected TPSF have been a greater issue. Along with diode laser sources, several groups have also used time-correlated single photon counting with photomultipliers for recording the TPSF [26,27]. Fast time gating is also obtained by using stimulated Raman scattering. This phenomenon is a nonlinear Raman interaction in some materials such as hydrogen gas involving the amplification of photons with Stokes shift by a higher energy pump beam. The system operates by amplifying only the earliest-arriving photons [28]. Less widely used techniques such as second-harmonic generation [29], parametric amplification [30], and a variety of others have been proposed for time domain (see an excellent review in [31]).

For frequency-domain measurements, the requirement is to measure the DC amplitude, the AC amplitude, and the phase shift of the photon density wave. For this purpose, a CW light source is modulated with a given frequency (~100 MHz). Lock-in amplifiers and/or phase-sensitive CCD camera have been used to record the amplitude and phase [32,33]. Multiple sources at different wavelengths can be modulated with a single frequency or multiple frequencies [6,34]. In the latter case, a network analyzer is used to produce modulation swept from several hundreds of MHz to up to 1 GHz.

40.1.3 Models of Photon Migration in Tissue

Photon migration theories in a biomedical optics have been borrowed from other fields such as astrophysics, atmospheric science, and specifically from nuclear reactor engineering [35,36]. The common properties of these physical media and biological tissues are their characterization by elements of randomness in both space and time. Because of many difficulties surrounding the development of a theory based on a detailed picture of the microscopic processes involved in the interaction of light and matter, investigations are often based on statistical theories. These can take a variety of forms, ranging from quite detailed multiple-scattering theories [36] to transport theory [37]. However, the most widely used theory is the time-dependent diffusion approximation to the transport equation:

$$\vec{\nabla} \cdot (D\vec{\nabla}\Phi(\vec{r},t)) - \mu_a \Phi(\vec{r},t) = \frac{1}{c}\frac{\partial \Phi(\vec{r},t)}{\partial t} - S(\vec{r},t) \tag{40.3}$$

where $\vec{r}$ and t are spatial and temporal variables, c is the speed of light in tissue, and D is the diffusion coefficient related to the absorption and scattering coefficients as follows:

$$D = \frac{1}{3[\mu_a + \mu_s']} \tag{40.4}$$

The quantity $\Phi(\vec{r},t)$ is called the fluence, defined as the power incident on an infinitesimal volume element divided by its area. Note that the equation does not incorporate any angular dependence, therefore assuming an isotropic scattering. However, for the use of the diffusion theory for anisotropic scattering, the diffusion coefficient is expressed in terms of the transport-corrected scattering coefficient. $S(\vec{r},t)$ is the source term. The gradient of fluence, $J(\vec{r},t)$, at the tissue surface is the measured flux of photons by the detector:

$$J(\vec{r},t) = -D\vec{\nabla}\Phi(\vec{r},t) \tag{40.5}$$

For CW measurements, the time dependence of the flux vanishes, and the source term can be seen as the power impinging in its area. For time-resolved measurement, the source term is a Dirac delta function describing a very short photon impulse. Equation 40.3 has been solved analytically for different types of measurements such as reflection and transmission mode assuming that the optical properties remain invariant through the tissue. To incorporate the finite boundaries, the method of images has been used. In the simplest case, the boundary has been assumed to be perfectly absorbing which does not take into account the difference between indices of refraction at the tissue–air interface. For semi-infinite and transillumination geometries, a set of theoretical expressions has been obtained for time-resolved measurements [38].

The diffusion approximation equation in the frequency domain is the Fourier transformation of the time domain with respect to time. Fourier transformation applied to the time-dependent diffusion equation leads to a new equation:

$$\vec{\nabla} \cdot (D\vec{\nabla}\Phi(\vec{r},\omega)) - \left[\mu_a + \frac{i\omega}{c}\right]\Phi(\vec{r},\omega) + S(\vec{r},\omega) = 0 \tag{40.6}$$

Here, the time variable is replaced by the frequency ω. This frequency is the modulation angular frequency of the source. In this model, the fluence can be seen as a complex number describing the amplitude and phase of the photon density wave, dumped with a DC component:

$$\Phi(\vec{r},\omega) = \Phi_{AC}(\vec{r},\omega) + \Phi_{DC}(\vec{r},0) = I_{AC}\exp(i\theta) + \Phi_{DC}(\vec{r},0) \tag{40.7}$$

In the right-hand side of Equation 40.7, the quantity θ is the phase shift of the diffusing wave. For a nonabsorbing medium, its wavelength is

$$\lambda = 2\pi\sqrt{\frac{2c}{3\mu_s'\omega}} \tag{40.8}$$

Likewise in the time domain, Equation 40.3 has an analytical solution for the case where the tissue is considered homogeneous. The analytical solution permits one to deduce the optical properties in a spectroscopic setting.

For imaging where the goal is to distinguish between structures in tissue, the diffusion coefficient and the absorption coefficient in Equations 40.3 and 40.6 become spatial-dependent and be replaced by $D(r)$ and $\mu_a(r)$. For the cases where an abnormal region is embedded in otherwise homogeneous tissue, perturbation methods based on Born approximation or Rytov approximation have been used (see excellent review in [39]). However, for the cases where the goal is to reconstruct the spectroscopic signatures inside the tissue, no analytical solution exists. For these cases, inverse algorithms are devised to map the spatially varying optical properties. Numerical methods such as finite-element or finite-difference methods have been used to reconstruct images of breast, brain, and muscle [40–42]. Furthermore, in those cases where structural heterogeneity exists, *a priori* information from other image modalities can be useful such as MRI. An example is given in Figure 40.2. Combining MRI and NIR imaging, rat cranium functional imaging during changes in inhaled oxygen concentration was studied [43]. Figure 40.2a and b corresponds to the MRI image and the corresponding constructed finite-element mesh. Figure 40.2c and d corresponds to the oxygen map of the brain with and without incorporation of MRI geometry and constraints.

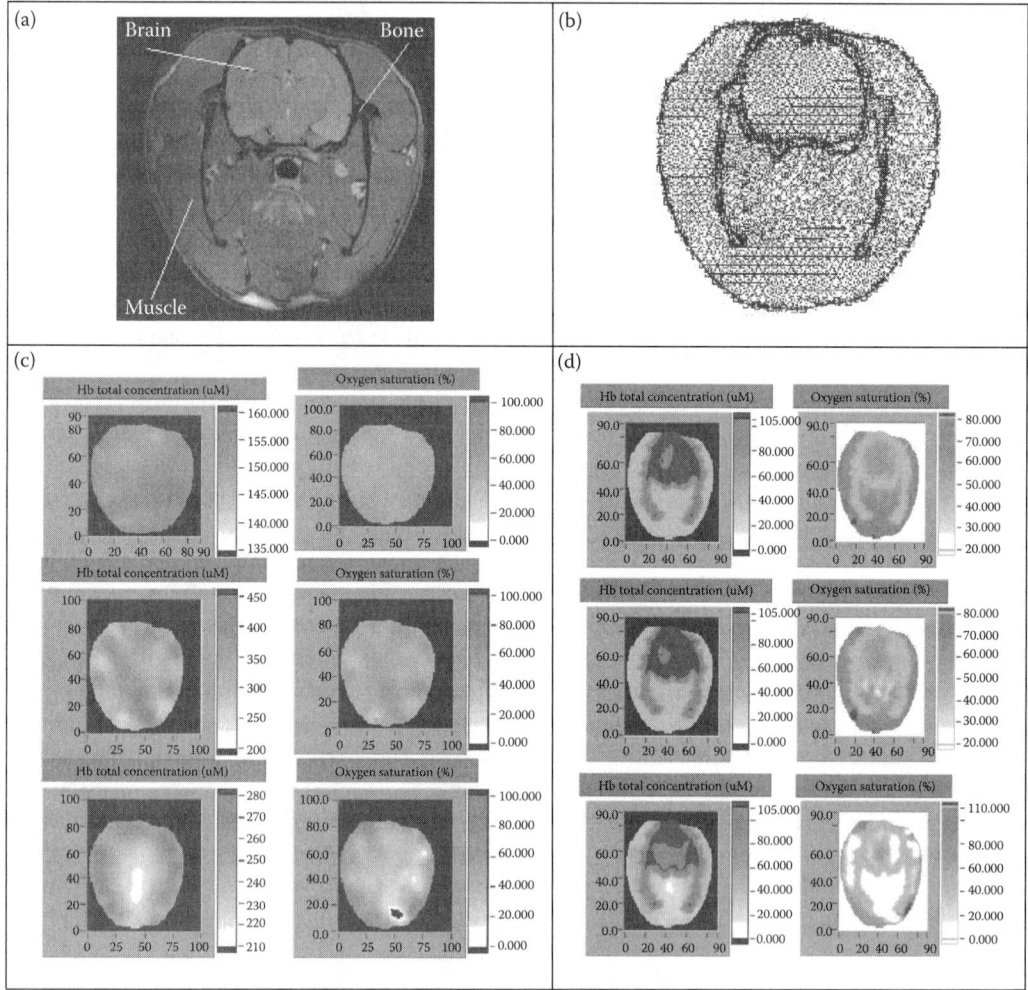

FIGURE 40.2 Functional imaging of rat cranium during changes in inhaled oxygen concentration. (a) MRI image; (b) creation of the mesh to distinguish different compartments in the brain; (c) map of hemoglobin concentration and oxygen saturation of the rat brain without structural constraints from MRI; (d) same as (c) with structural constraints, including tissue heterogeneity. In (c) and (d), the rows from top correspond to 13%, 8%, and 0% (after death) oxygen inhaled. (Courtesy of Dartmouth College.)

The use of MRI images has improved dramatically the resolution of the oxygen map. The use of optical functional imaging in conjunction with other imaging modalities has opened new possibilities in imaging and treating diseases at the bedside.

The second theoretical framework used in tissue optics is the random walk theory (RWT) on a lattice developed at the National Institutes of Health [44,45] and historically precedes the use of the diffusion approximation theory. It has been shown that RWT may be used to derive an analytical solution for the distribution of photon pathlengths in turbid media such as tissue [44]. RWT models the diffusion-like motion of photons in turbid media in a probabilistic manner. Using RWT, an expression may be derived for the probability of a photon arriving at any point and time given a specific starting point and time.

Tissue may be modeled as a 3D cubic lattice containing a finite inclusion, or region of interest, as shown in Figure 40.3. The medium has an absorbing boundary corresponding to the tissue surface, and the lattice spacing is proportional to the mean photon scattering distance, $1/\mu_s'$. The behavior of photons in the RWT model is described by three dimensionless parameters, ρ, n, and μ, which are respectively the radial distance, the number of steps, and the probability of absorption per lattice step. In the RWT model, photons may move to one of the six nearest-neighboring lattice points, each with probability 1/6. If the number of steps, n, taken by a photon traveling between two points on the lattice is known, then the length of the photon's path is also known.

RWT is useful in predicting the probability distribution of photon pathlengths over distances of at least five mean-photon scattering distances. The derivation of these probability distributions is described in review papers [44,45]. For simplicity in this derivation, the tissue–air interface is considered to be perfectly absorbing; a photon arriving at this interface is counted as arriving at a detector on the tissue surface. The derivation uses the central limit theorem and a Gaussian distribution around lattice points to obtain a closed-form solution that is independent of the lattice structure.

The dimensionless RWT parameters, ρ, n, and μ, described above, may be transformed to actual parameters, in part, by using time, t, the speed of light in tissue, c, and distance traveled, r, as follows:

$$\rho \to \frac{r\mu_s'}{\sqrt{2}}, n \to \mu_s'ct, \mu \to \frac{\mu_a}{\mu_s'} \tag{40.9}$$

As stated previously, scattering in tissue is highly anisotropic. Therefore, one must find the appropriate scaling relationships that will allow the use of an isotropic scattering model such as RWT. Like diffusion theory, for RWT [46], it has been shown that one may use an isotropic scattering model with

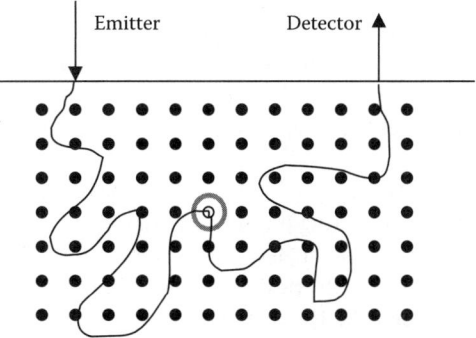

FIGURE 40.3 2D random walk lattice showing representative photon paths from an emitter to a specific site and then to a detector.

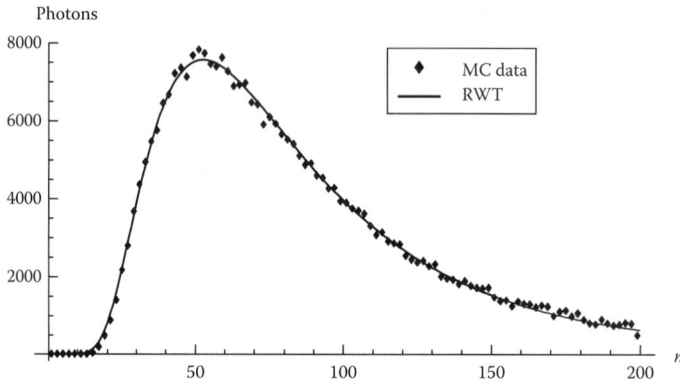

FIGURE 40.4 RWT prediction and Monte Carlo simulation results for transillumination of a 15-mm-thick slab with scattering 1/mm and 109 photons.

a corrected scattering coefficient, μ_s', and obtain equivalent results. The corrected scattering coefficient is smaller than the actual scattering that corresponds to a greater distance between isotropic scattering events than would occur with anisotropic scattering. RWT has been used to show how one would transition from the use of μ_s to μ_s' as the distance under consideration increases [47].

As an example, for a homogeneous slab into which a photon has been inserted, the probability P of a photon arriving at a point ρ after n steps is [48]

$$P(n,\rho) = \frac{\sqrt{3}}{2}\left[\frac{1}{2\pi(n-2)}\right]^{\frac{3}{2}} e^{\frac{-3\rho^2}{2(n-2)}} \sum_{k=-\infty}^{\infty}\left[e^{\frac{-3\left[(2k+1)L-2\right]^2}{2(n-2)}} - e^{\frac{-3\left[(2k+1)L\right]^2}{2(n-2)}}\right]e^{-n\mu} \quad (40.10)$$

where L is the thickness of the slab. The method of images has been used to take into account the two boundaries of the slab. Plotting Equation 40.10 yields a photon arrival curve as shown in Figure 40.4; Monte Carlo simulation data are overlaid. In the next two sections, the use of RWT for imaging will be presented.

40.1.4 RWT Applied to Quantitative Spectroscopy of the Breast

One important and yet extremely challenging area to apply diffuse optical imaging of deep tissues is the human breast (see the review article of Hawrysz and Sevick-Muraca [49]. It is clear that any new imaging or spectroscopic modalities that can improve the diagnosis of breast tumors or can add new knowledge about the physiological properties of the breast and surrounding tissues will have a great significance in medicine.

Conventional transillumination using CW light was used for breast screening several decades ago [50]. However, because of the high scattering properties of tissue, this method resulted in poor resolution. In the late 1980s, time-resolved imaging techniques were proposed to enhance spatial resolution by detecting photons with very short TOF within the tissue. In this technique, a very short pulse, of picosecond duration, impinges upon the tissue. Photons experience dispersion in their pathlengths, resulting in temporal dispersion in their TOF.

To evaluate the performance of time-resolved transillumination techniques, RWT on a lattice was used. The analysis of breast transillumination was based on the calculation of the point spread function (PSF) of time-resolved photons as they visit differing sites at different planes inside a finite slab. The PSF

[51] is defined as the probability that a photon inserted into the tissue visits a given site, is detected at the nth step (i.e., a given time), and has the following rather complicated analytical expression:

$$W_n(\mathbf{s},\mathbf{r},\mathbf{r}_0) = \sum_{l=0}^{n} p_l(\mathbf{r},\mathbf{s}) p_{n-l}(\mathbf{s},\mathbf{r}_0) = \frac{9}{16\pi^{5/2} n^{3/2}} \sum_{k=-\infty}^{\infty} \sum_{m=-\infty}^{\infty} \{F_n[\alpha_+(k),\beta_+(m,\rho)]$$
$$+ F_n[\alpha_-(k),\beta_-(m,\rho)] - F_n[\alpha_+(k),\beta_-(m,\rho)] - F_n[\alpha_-(k),\beta_+(m,\rho)]\} \tag{40.11}$$

$$F_n(a,b) = \left(\frac{1}{a} + \frac{1}{b}\right) \exp\left[-\frac{(a+b)^2}{n}\right] \tag{40.12}$$

$$\alpha_\pm(k) = \left\{\frac{3}{2}\left[s_1^2 + (s_3 + 2kN \pm 1)^2\right]\right\}^{1/2} \tag{40.13}$$

$$\beta_\pm(k,\rho) = \left\{\frac{3}{2}\left[(\rho - s_1)^2 + (N - s_3 + 2kN \pm 1)^2\right]\right\}^{1/2} \tag{40.14}$$

where $N = (L\mu_s'/\sqrt{2}) + 1$ is the dimensionless RWT thickness of the slabs and $\bar{s}(s_1,s_2,s_3)$ are the dimensionless coordinates (see Equation 40.9). Evaluation of time-resolved imaging showed that strong scattering properties of tissues prevent direct imaging of abnormalities [52]. Hence, devising theoretical constructs to separate the effects of the scattering from the absorption was proposed, thus allowing one to map the optical coefficients as spectroscopic signatures of an abnormal tissue embedded in thick, otherwise normal tissue. In this method, accurate quantification of the size and optical properties of the target becomes a critical requirement for the use of optical imaging at the bedside. RWT on a lattice has been used to analyze the time-dependent contrast observed in time-resolved transillumination experiments and deduce the size and optical properties of the target and the surrounding tissue from these contrasts. For the theoretical construction of contrast functions, two quantities are needed. First, the set of functions [51] defined previously. Second, the set of functions [53] defined as the probability that a photon is detected at the nth step (i.e., time) in a homogeneous medium (Equation 40.10) [48].

To relate the contrast of the light intensity to the optical properties and location of abnormal targets in the tissue, one can take advantage of some features of the theoretical framework. One feature is that the early time response is most dependent on scattering perturbations, whereas the late time behavior is most dependent on absorptive perturbations, thus allowing one to separate the influence of scattering and absorption perturbations on the observed image contrast. Increased scattering in the abnormal target is modeled as a time delay. Moreover, it was shown that the scattering contrast is proportional to the time-derivative of the PSF, dW_n/dn, divided by P_n [53]. The second interesting feature in RWT methodology assumes that the contrast from scattering inside the inclusion is proportional to the cross section of the target (in the z direction) [51,53], instead of depending on its volume as modeled in the perturbation analysis [54].

Several research groups intend to implement their theoretical expressions into general inverse algorithms for optical tomography, that is, to reconstruct three-dimensional maps of spatial distributions of tissue optical characteristics [49], and thereby quantify optical characteristics, positions, and sizes of abnormalities. Unlike these approaches, the method is a multistep analysis of the collected data. From images observed at differing flight times, construct the time-dependent contrast functions, fit theoretical expressions, and compute the optical properties of the background, and those of the abnormality along with its size. The outline of the data analysis is given in Reference 55.

By utilizing the method for different wavelengths, one can obtain diagnostic information (e.g., estimates of blood oxygenation of the tumor) for corresponding absorption coefficients that no other imaging modality can provide directly. Several research groups have already successfully used multiwavelength measurements using frequency-domain techniques, to calculate physiological parameters (oxygenation, lipid, water) of breast tumors (diagnosed with other modalities) and normal tissue [56].

Researchers at Physikalich.-Techniche-Bundesanstalt (PTB) of Berlin have designed a clinically practical optical imaging system, capable of implementing time-resolved *in vivo* measurements on the human breast [27]. The breast is slightly compressed between two plates. A scan of the whole breast takes but a few minutes and can be done in mediolateral and craniocaudal geometries. The first goal is to quantify the optical parameters at several wavelengths and thereby estimate blood oxygen saturation of the tumor and surrounding tissue under the usual assumption that the chromophores contributing to absorption are oxy- and deoxyhemoglobin and water. As an example, two sets of data, obtained at two wavelengths ($\lambda = 670$ and 785 nm), for a patient (84 year old) with invasive ductal carcinoma, were analyzed. Though the images exhibit poor resolution, the tumor can be easily seen in the optical image shown in Figure 40.5a. In this figure, the image is obtained from reciprocal values of the total integrals of the distributions of TOFs of photons, normalized to a selected "bulk" area. The tumor center is located at $x = -5, y = 0.25$ mm.

The best spatial resolution is observed, as expected, for shorter time-delays allowing one to determine the position of the tumor center on the 2-D image (transverse coordinates) with accuracy ~2.5 mm. After preliminary data processing that includes filtering and deconvolution of the raw time-resolved data, we created linear contrast scans passing through the tumor center and analyzed these scans, using the algorithm. It is striking that one observes similar linear dependence of the contrast amplitude on the derivative of PSF ($\lambda = 670$ nm), as expected in the model (see Figure 40.5b). The slope of this linear dependence was used to estimate the amplitude of the scattering perturbation [55].

Dimensions and values of optical characteristics of the tumor and surrounding tissues were then reconstructed for both wavelengths. Results show that the tumor had larger absorption and scattering than the background. Estimated parameters are presented in Table 40.1.

Both absorption and scattering coefficients of the tumor and background all proved to be larger at the red wavelength (670 nm). Comparison of the absorption in the red and near-infrared range is used to estimate blood oxygen saturation of the tumor and background tissue. Preliminary results of the analysis gave evidence that the tumor tissue is in a slightly deoxygenated state with higher blood volume, compared to surrounding tissue.

The spectroscopic power of optical imaging, along with the ability to quantify physiological parameters of human breast have opened a new opportunity for assessing metabolic and physiological activities of human breast during treatment.

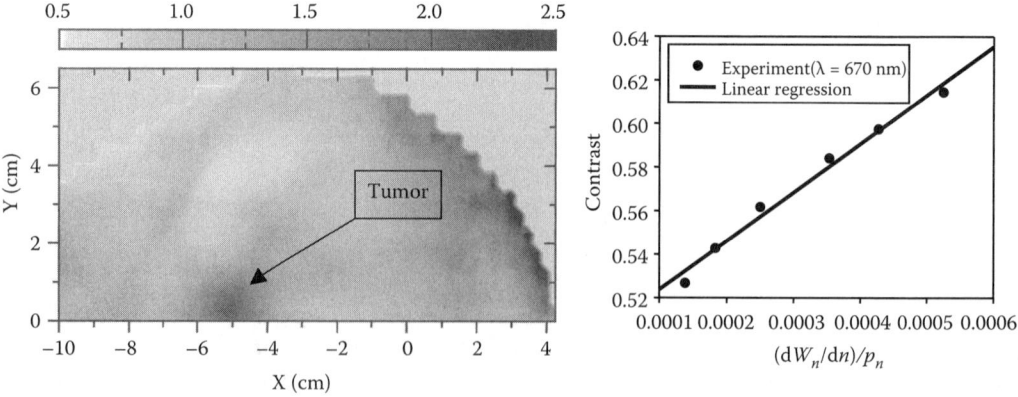

FIGURE 40.5 (a) 2-D optical image of the breast with the tumor. (Courtesy of Physikalich.-Techniche-Bundesanstalt, Berlin.) (b) Contrast obtained from linear scan through the tumor plotted versus the derivative of PSF. From the linear regression, the scattering coefficient of the tumor is deduced.

TABLE 40.1   Optical Parameters of Tumor and Background Breast Tissue

Unknown Coefficients	Reconstructed Values, $\lambda = 670$ nm	Reconstructed Values, $\lambda = 785$ nm
Absorption (background)	0.0029 mm^{-1}	0.0024 mm^{-1}
Scattering (background)	1.20 mm^{-1}	1.10 mm^{-1}
Absorption (Tumor)	0.0071 mm^{-1}	0.0042 mm^{-1}
Scattering (Tumor)	1.76 mm^{-1}	1.6 mm^{-1}

40.1.5 Quantitative Fluorescence Imaging and Spectroscopy

As mentioned in Section 40.1.1, advances in the molecular biology of disease processes, new immuno-histopathological techniques, and the development of specific fluorescently labeled cell surface markers have led a revolution in research on the molecular origins of disease processes. On the other hand, reliable, sensitive, and specific, noninvasive techniques are needed for *in vivo* determinations of abnormalities within the tissue. If successfully developed, noninvasive "optical biopsies" may replace conventional surgical biopsies and provide the advantages of smaller sampling errors, reduction in cost and time for diagnosis, resulting in easier integration of diagnosis and therapy by following the progression of disease or its regression in response to therapy. Clinically practical fluorescence imaging techniques must meet several requirements. First, the pathology under investigation must lie above a depth where the attenuation of the signal results in a poor signal-to-noise ratio and resolvability. Second, the specificity of the marker must be high enough that one can clearly distinguish between normal and abnormal lesions. Finally, one must have a robust image reconstruction algorithm which enables one to quantify the fluorophore concentration at a given depth.

The choices of projects in this area of research are dictated by the importance of the problem, and the impact of the solution on healthcare. Below, the rationale of two projects is described in Section on Analytical and Functional Biophotonics (SAFB), at the National Institutes of Health is pursuing.

Sjøgren's syndrome (SS) has been chosen as an appropriate test case for developing a noninvasive optical biopsy based on 3D localization of exogenous specific fluorescent labels. SS is an autoimmune disease affecting minor salivary glands which are near (0.5–3.0 mm below) the oral mucosal surface [57]. Therefore, the target pathology is relatively accessible to noninvasive optical imaging. The hydraulic conductivity of the oral mucosa is relatively high, which, along with the relatively superficial location of the minor salivary glands, makes topical application and significant labeling of diseased glands with large fluorescent molecules easy to accomplish. Fluorescent ligands (e.g., fluorescent antibodies specific to CD4$^+$ T cell-activated lymphocytes infiltrating the salivary glands) are expected to bind specifically to the atypical cells in the tissue, providing high contrast and a quantitative relationship to their concentration (and therefore to the stage of the disease process). The major symptoms (dry eyes and dry mouth due to decreased tear and saliva secretion) are the result of progressive immune-mediated dysfunction of the lacrimal and salivary glands. Currently, diagnosis is made by excisional biopsies of the minor salivary glands in the lower lip. This exam, though considered the best criterion for diagnosis, involves a surgical procedure under local anesthesia followed by postoperative discomfort (swelling, pain) and frequently a temporary loss of sensation at the lower lip biopsy site. Additionally, biopsy is inherently subject to sampling errors and the preparation of histopathological slides is time consuming, complicated, expensive, and requires the skills of several professionals (dentist, pathologist, and laboratory technician). Thus, there is a clear need for a noninvasive diagnostic procedure which reflects the underlying gland pathology and has good specificity. A quantitative noninvasive assay would also allow repetition of the test to monitor disease progression and the effect of treatment. However, the quantification of fluorophore concentration within the tissue from surface images requires determining the intensities of different fluorophore sources, as a function of depth and transverse distance and predicting the 3-D distribution of fluorophores within the tissue from a series of images [58].

The second project involves the lymphatic imaging-sentinel node detection. The stage of cancer at initial diagnosis often defines prognosis and determines treatment options. As part of the staging procedure of melanoma and breast cancer, multiple lymph nodes are surgically removed from the primary lymphatic draining site and examined histologically for the presence of malignant cells. Because it is not obvious which nodes to remove at the time of resection of the primary tumor, standard practice involves dissection of as many lymph nodes as feasible. Since such extensive removal of lymphatic tissue frequently results in compromised lymphatic drainage in the examined axilla, alternatives have been sought to define the stage at the time of primary resection. A recent advance in lymph node interrogation has been the localization and removal of the "sentinel" node. Although there are multiple lymphatic channels available for trafficking from the primary tumor, the assumption was made that the anatomic location of the primary tumor in a given individual drains into lymphatic channels in an orderly and reproducible fashion. If that is in fact the case, then there is a pattern by which lymphatic drainage occurs. Thus, it would be expected that malignant cells from a primary tumor site would course from the nearest and possibly most superficial node into deeper and more distant lymphatic channels to ultimately arrive in the thoracic duct, whereupon malignant cells would gain access to venous circulation. The sentinel node is defined as the first drainage node in a network of nodes that drain the primary cancer. Considerable evidence has accrued validating the clinical utility of staging breast cancer by locating and removing the sentinel node at the time of resection of the primary tumor. Currently, the primary tumor is injected with a radionucleotide one day prior to removal of the primary tumor. Then, just before surgery, it is injected with visible dye. The surgeon localizes crudely the location of the sentinel node using a hand-held radionucleotide detector, followed by a search for visible concentrations of the injected dye. The method requires expensive equipment and also presents the patient and hospital personnel with the risk of exposure to ionizing radiation. As an alternative to the radionucleotide, we are investigating the use of IR-dependent fluorescent detection methods to determine the location of sentinel node(s).

For *in vivo* fluorescent imaging, a complicating factor is the strong attenuation of light as it passes through tissue. This attenuation deteriorates the signal-to-noise ratio of detected photons. Fortunately, the development of fluorescent dyes (such as porphyrin and cyanine) that excite and reemit in the "biological window" at near-infrared (NIR) wavelengths, where scattering and absorption coefficients are relatively low, have provided new possibilities for deep fluorescence imaging in tissue. The theoretical complication occurs at depths greater than 1 mm where photons in most tissues enter a diffusion-like state with a large dispersion in their pathlengths. Indeed, the fluorescent intensity of light detected from deep tissue structures depends not only on the location, size, concentration, and intrinsic characteristics (e.g., lifetime, quantum efficiency) of the fluorophores but also on the scattering and absorption coefficients of the tissue at both the excitation and emission wavelengths. Hence, in order to extract intrinsic characteristics of fluorophores within tissue, it is necessary to describe the statistics of photon pathlengths which depend on all these differing parameters.

Obviously, the modeling of fluorescent light propagation depends on the kinds of experiments that one plans to perform. For example, for frequency-domain measurements, Patterson and Pogue [59] used the diffusion approximation of the transport equation to express their results in terms of a product of two Green's function propagators multiplied by a term that describes the probability of emission of a fluorescent photon at the site. One Green's function describes the migration of an incident photon to the fluorophore, and the other describes migration of the emitted photon to the detector. In this representation, the amount of light emitted at the site of the fluorophore is directly proportional to the total amount of light impinging on the fluorophore, with no account for the variability in the number of visits by a photon before an exciting transformation. Since a transformation on an early visit to the site precludes a transformation on all later visits, this results in an overestimation of the number of photons which have a fluorescence transformation at a particular site. This overestimation is important when fluorescent absorption properties are spatially inhomogeneous and largest at later arrival times. RWT has been used to allow for this spatial inhomogeneity by introducing the multiple-passage probabilities concept, thus rendering the model more physically plausible [60]. Another incentive to devise a general theory of diffuse fluorescence photon migration is the capability to quantify local changes in fluorescence lifetime. By selecting fluorophore probes with known lifetime dependence on specific environmental variables, lifetime imaging enables one to localize and quantify such metabolic parameters as temperature and pH, as well as changes in local molecular concentrations *in vivo*.

In the probabilistic RWT model, the description of a photon path may be divided into three parts: the path from the photon source to a localized, fluorescing target; the interaction of the photon with the fluorophore; and finally, the path of the fluorescently emitted photon to a detector. Each part of the photon path may be described by a probability: first, the probability that an incident photon will arrive at the fluorophore site; second, the probability that the photon has a reactive encounter with the fluorophore and the corresponding photon transit delay, which is dependent on the lifetime of the fluorophore and the probability of the fluorophore emitting a photon; and third, the probability that the photon emitted by the fluorophore travels from the reaction site to the detector. Each of these three sequences is governed by a stochastic process. The mathematical description of the three processes is extremely complicated. The complete solution for the probability of fluorescence photon arrival at the detector is [61]

$$\hat{\gamma}(r,s,r_0) = \frac{\eta \; \Phi \hat{p}'_\xi(r|s) \; \hat{p}_\xi(s|r_0)}{\langle \Delta n \rangle (1-\eta)[\exp(\xi)-1] + \left\{ \eta \langle \Delta n \rangle [\exp(\xi)-1] + 1 \right\} \left\{ 1 + \left[(1/8)(3/\pi)^{3/2} \sum_{j=1}^{\infty} (\exp(-2j\xi)/j^{3/2}) \right] \right\}}$$

(40.15)

where η is the probability of fluorescent absorption of an excitation wavelength photon, Φ is the quantum efficiency of the fluorophore which is the probability that an excited fluorophore will emit a photon at the emission wavelength, $\langle \Delta n \rangle$ is the mean number of steps the photon would have taken had the photon not been exciting the fluorophore (which corresponds to the fluorophore lifetime in random walk parameters), and ξ is a transform variable corresponding to the discrete analog of the Laplace transform and may be considered analogous to frequency. The probability of a photon going from the excitation source to the fluorophore site is $\hat{p}_\xi(s|r_0)$, and the probability of a fluorescent photon going from the fluorophore site to the detector is $\hat{p}'_\xi(r|s)$; the prime indicates that the wavelength of the photon has changed and therefore the optical properties of the tissue may be different. In practice, this solution is difficult to work with, so some simplifying assumptions are desired. With some simplification the result in the frequency domain is

$$\hat{\gamma}(r,s,r_0) = \eta \Phi \left\{ \hat{p}'_\xi(r|s) \; \hat{p}_\xi(s|r_0) - \xi \langle \Delta n \rangle \hat{p}'_\xi(r|s) \hat{p}_\xi(s|r_0) \right\}.$$

(40.16)

The inverse Laplace transform of this equation gives the diffuse fluorescent intensity in the time domain, and the integral of the latter over time leads to CW measurements. The accuracy of such cumbersome equations is tested in well-defined phantoms and fluorophores embedded in *ex vivo* tissue. In Figure 40.6, a line scan of fluorescent intensity collected from 500 μm^3 fluorescent dye (Molecular Probe, far red microspheres: 690 nm excitation; 720 nm emission), embedded in 10.4 mm porcine tissue with a lot of heterogeneity (e.g., fat), are presented. The dashed line is the corresponding RWT fit. The inverse algorithm written in C++ was able to construct the depth of the fluorophore with 100% accuracy. Knowing the heterogeneity of the tissue (seen in the intensity profile), this method presents huge potential to interrogate tissue structures deeply embedded in tissue for which specific fluorescent labeling such as antibodies for cell surfaces exists.

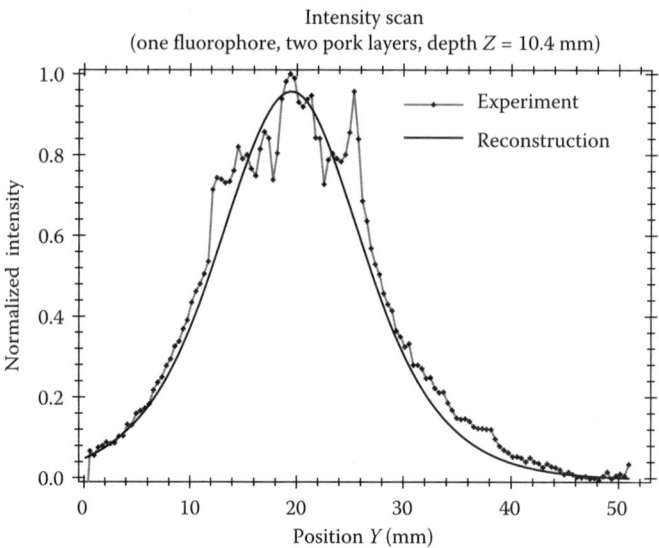

Intensity scan
(one fluorophore, two pork layers, depth Z = 10.4 mm)

FIGURE 40.6   Intensity scan of a fluorophore 10.4 mm below the tissue surface.

40.1.6 Future Directions

A clinically useful optical imaging device requires multidisciplinary and multistep approaches. At the desk, one devises quantitative theories, and develop methodologies applicable to *in vivo* quantitative tissue spectroscopy and tomographic imaging in different imaging geometries (i.e., transmission or reflection), different types of measurements (e.g., steady-state or time-resolved). Effects of different optical sources of contrast such as endogenous or exogenous fluorescent labels, variations in absorption (e.g., hemoglobin or chromophore concentration) and scattering should be incorporated in the model. At the bench, one designs and conducts experiments on tissue-like phantoms and runs computer simulations to validate the theoretical findings. If successful, one tries to bring the imaging or spectroscopic device to the bedside. For this task, one must foster strong collaborations with physicians who can help to identify physiological sites where optical techniques may be clinically practical and can offer new diagnostic knowledge and/or less morbidity over existing methods. An important intermediate step is the use of animal models for pre-clinical studies. Overall, this is a complicated path. However, the spectroscopic power of light, along with the revolution in molecular characterization of disease processes has created a huge potential for *in vivo* optical imaging and spectroscopy. Maybe the twenty-first century will be the second *"siecle des lumieres."*

40.2 Monitoring of Disease Processes: Clinical Study

40.2.1 Thermal Imaging

The relationship between a change in body temperature and health status has been of interest to physicians since Hippocrates stated "should one part of the body be hotter or colder than the rest, then disease is present in that part." Thermography provides a visual display of the surface temperature of the skin. Skin temperature recorded by an infrared scanner is the resultant balance of thermal transport within the tissues and transport to the environment. In medical applications, thermal images of human skin contain a large amount of clinical information that can help to detect numerous patho-logical conditions ranging from cancer to emotional disorders. For the clinical assessment of cancer, physicians need to determine the activity of the tumor and location, extent, and response to therapy. All of these factors make it possible for tumors to be examined using thermography. Advantages to using this method are that it is completely nonionizing, safe, and can be repeated as often as required without exposing the patient to risk. Unfortunately, the skin temperature distribution is misinterpreted in many cases, because any high skin temperature does not always indicate a tumor. Therefore, thermography requires thorough investigation to interpret the temperature distribution patterns as well as additional research to clarify various diseases based on skin temperature.

Before applying the thermal technique in the clinical setting, it is important to consider how to avoid misinterpretation of the results. Before the examination, the body should attain thermal equilibrium with its environment. A patient should be unclothed for at least 20 min in a controlled environment at a temperature of approximately 22°C. Under such clinical conditions, thermograms will show only average temperature patterns over an interval of time. The evaluation of surface temperature by infrared techniques requires wavelength and emissive properties of the surface (emissivity) to be examined over the range of wavelengths to which the detector is sensitive. In addition, a thermal camera should be calibrated with a known temperature reference source to standardize clinical data.

An accurate technique for measuring emissivity is presented in Section 40.2.1. In Section 40.2.2, a procedure for temperature calibration of an infrared detector is discussed. The clinical application of thermography with KS is detailed in Section 40.2.3.

40.2.1.1 Emissivity Corrected Temperature

Emissivity is described as a radiative property of the skin. It is a measure of how well a body can radiate energy compared to a black body. Knowledge of emissivity is important when measuring skin temperature with an infrared detector system at different ambient radiation temperatures. Currently, different spectral band infrared detector systems are used in clinical studies such as 3–5 and 8–14 μm. It is well known that the emissivity of the skin varies according to the spectral range. The skin emits infrared radiation mainly between 2 and 20 μm with maximum emission at a wavelength around 10 μm [62]. Jones [63] showed with an InSb detector that only 2% of the radiation emitted from a thermal black body at 30°C was within the 3–5 μm spectral range; the wider spectral response of HgCdTe detector (8–14 μm) corresponded to 40–50% of this black body radiation.

Many investigators have reported on the values for emissivity of skin *in vivo*, measured in different spectral bands with different techniques. Hardy [64] and Stekettee [65] showed that the spectral emissivity of skin was independent of wavelength (λ) when λ > 2 μm. These results contradicted those obtained by Elam et al. [66]. Watmough and Oliver [67] pointed out that emissivity lies within 0.98 to 1 and was not less than 0.95 for a wavelength range of 2–5 μm. Patil and Williams [68] reported that the average emissivity of normal breast skin was 0.99 ± 0.045, 0.972 ± 0.041, and 0.975 ± 0.043 within the ranges 4–6, 6–18, and 4–18 μm, respectively. Steketee [65] indicated that the average emissivity value of skin was 0.98 ± 0.01 within the range 3–14 μm. It is important to know the precise value of emissivity because an emissivity difference of 0.945 to 0.98 may cause an error of skin temperature of 0.6°C [64].

There is considerable diversity in the reported values of skin emissivity even in the same spectral band. The inconsistencies among reported values could be due to unreliable and inadequate theories and techniques employed for measuring skin emissivity. Togawa [69] proposed a technique in which the emissivity was calculated by measuring the temperature upon a transient stepwise change in ambient radiation temperature [69,70] surrounding an object surface as shown in Figure 40.7.

The average emissivity of skin for the 12 normal subjects measured by a radiometer and infrared camera are presented in Table 40.2. The emissivity values were found to be significantly different between the 3–5 and 8–14 μm spectral bands ($P < 0.001$). An example of a set of images obtained during measurement using an infrared camera (3–5 μm bands) on the forearm of a healthy male subject is shown in Figure 40.8.

An accurate value of emissivity is important because an incorrect value of emissivity can lead to a temperature error in radiometric thermometry especially when the ambient radiation temperature varies widely. The extent to which skin emissivity depends on the spectral range of the infrared

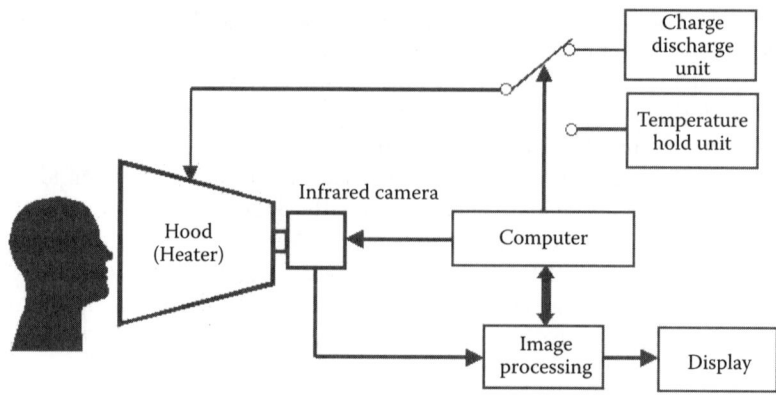

FIGURE 40.7   Schematic diagram of the emissivity measurement system. (From M. Hassan and T. Togawa, *Physiol. Meas.*, 22, 187–200, 2001.)

TABLE 40.2   Average Normal Forearm Skin of 12 Subjects

Emissivity Values	
Infrared camera (3–5 μm)	0.958 ± 0.002
Radiometer (8–14 μm)	0.973 ± 0.0003

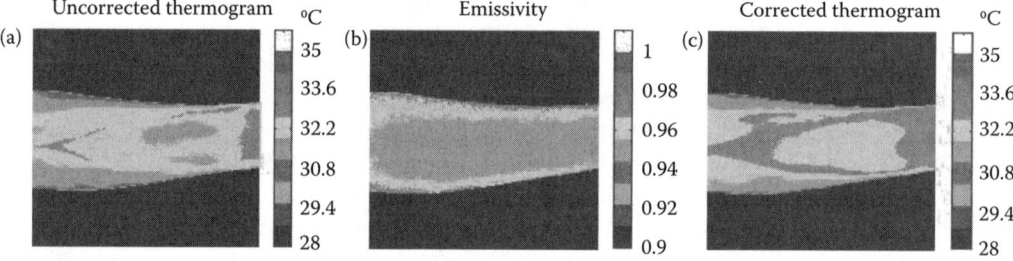

FIGURE 40.8   An example of images obtained from the forearm of a normal healthy male subject. (a) Original thermogram; (b) emissivity image; and (c) thermogram corrected by emissivity.

detectors is demonstrated in Table 40.2, which shows emissivity values measured at 0.958 ± 0.002 and 0.973 ± 0.003 by an infrared detector with spectral bands of 3–5 and 8–14 μm, respectively. These results can give skin temperatures that differ by 0.2°C at a room temperature of 22°C. Therefore, it is necessary to consider the wavelength dependence of emissivity, when high precision temperature measurements are required.

Emissivity not only depends on the wavelength but is also influenced by surface quality, moisture on the skin surface, and so on. In the infrared region of 3–50 μm, the emissivity of most nonmetallic substances is higher for a rough surface than a smooth one [71]. The presence of water also increases the value of emissivity [72]. These influences may account for the variation in results.

40.2.1.2 Temperature Calibration

In infrared thermography, any radiator is suitable as a temperature reference if its emissivity is known and constant within a given range of wavelengths. Currently, many different commercial blackbody calibrators are available to be used as temperature reference sources. A practical and simple blackbody

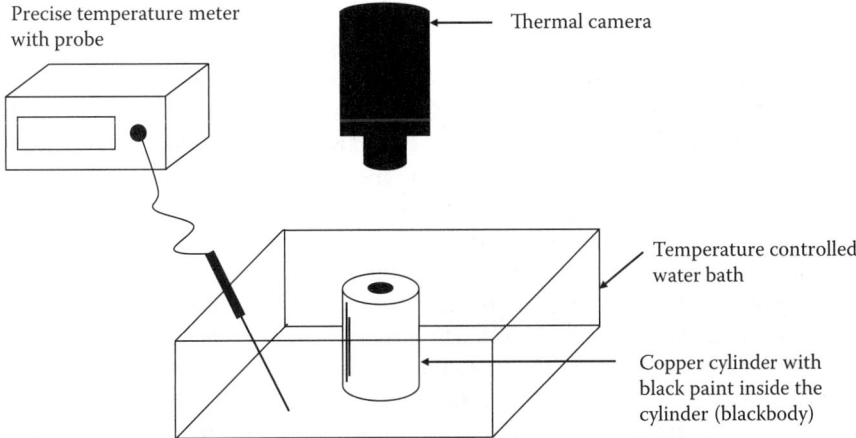

FIGURE 40.9 Schematic diagram of temperature calibration system.

radiator with a known temperature and measurement system is illustrated in Figure 40.9. The system consists of a hollow copper cylinder, a temperature-controlled water bath and a precise temperature meter with probe. The height of the cylinder is 15 cm and the diameter is 7.5 cm. The cylinder is closed except for a hole in the center of the upper end which is 2 cm in diameter. To make the blackbody radiator, the inner surface of the cylinder is coated with black paint (3M Velvet Coating no. 2010) with emissivity of 0.93. Before the calibration, 3/4 of the cylinder is placed vertically in the water and the thermal camera is placed on the top of the cylinder in a vertical direction with a distance of focus length between the surface of the hole and the camera. The water temperature ranges from 18°C to 45°C by 2°C increments. This range was selected since human temperature generally varies from 22°C to 42°C in clinical studies. After setting the water temperature, the thermal camera measures the surface temperature of the hole while the temperature meter with probe measures the water temperature. The temperature of the camera is calibrated according to the temperature reading of the temperature meter.

40.2.2 Near-Infrared Multispectral Imaging

Near-infrared multispectral imaging is most closely related to visual assessment. At National Institutes of Health (NIH) in collaboration with the Lawrence Livermore National Laboratory, a portable spectral imaging system was designed. The system captures images with a high-resolution CCD camera at six near-infrared wavelengths (700, 750, 800, 850, 900, and 1000 nm). Based on differences in absorption coefficients, tissue differences can be assessed. A white light held approximately 45 cm from tissue illuminates the surface uniformly. Using optical filters, images are obtained at the six wavelengths and the intensity images are used in a mathematical optical model of skin containing two layers: an epidermis and much thicker, highly scattering dermis. Each layer contains major chromophores that determine absorption in the corresponding layer and the layers together determine the total reflectance of the skin. Local variations in melanin, oxygenated hemoglobin (HbO_2), and blood volume can be reconstructed through a multivariate analysis.

For the mathematical optical skin model, the effect of the thin epidermis layer on the intensity of the diffusely reflected light is determined by the effective attenuation of light, A_{epi}:

$$A_{epi}(\lambda) = e^{-\mu_{a(epi)}(\lambda)t}$$

where $\mu_{a(epi)}(\lambda)$ is the epidermis absorption coefficient (mm^{-1}), λ is the wavelength (nm), and t is the thickness of the epidermis (mm). The epidermis absorption coefficient is determined by the percentage of melanin, the absorption coefficient of melanin, and the absorption coefficient of normal tissue. Researchers have used different equations to calculate the melanin [73,74] and baseline skin [73–76] absorption coefficients. This model uses the equations of Meglinski and Matcher [77] and Jacques [73] for the melanin and baseline skin absorption coefficients, respectively. The influence of the much thicker, highly scattering dermis layer on the skin reflectance should be estimated by a stochastic model of photon migration, for example, RWT. Fitting the known random walk expression for diffuse reflectivity of the turbid slab [45] yields a formula that depends on the reduced scattering coefficient and dermis absorption coefficient. The dermis absorption coefficient is based on the volume of blood in the tissue and hemoglobin oxygenation, that is, relative fractions of HbO_2 and deoxygenated hemoglobin (Hb). At wavelengths greater than 850 nm, the contribution of water and lipids should be taken into account. The absorption coefficient of blood was calculated by the volume fraction of HbO_2 times the absorption coefficient of HbO_2 plus the volume fraction of Hb times the absorption coefficient of Hb. In the dermis, large cylindrical collagen fibers are responsible for Mie scattering, while smaller-scale collagen fibers and other microstructures are responsible for Rayleigh scattering [73]. The reduced scattering coefficient was calculated by combining Mie and Rayleigh components [78].

Each multispectral image was corrected for the light intensity by calibration of the light source, and camera. Then, each was divided by a weight factor to bring the intensity of the images into the physiologically acceptable range. A best-fit procedure was used to reconstruct for HbO_2 fraction, and blood volume fraction. Melanin concentrations as well as the epidermis thickness were assumed to be constant. The epidermis thickness was assumed to be 60 μm [78] and the melanin content was based on [79].

Thus, near-infrared diffuse multispectral imaging of the skin combined with an analytical, numerical, or stochastic skin model can provide this information by producing spatial maps of skin chromophore concentrations [80–82]. The disadvantage of finding these parameters by fitting the data to an analytical skin model lies in the computationally expensive data postprocessing. This makes immediate conclusions difficult or even impossible if the image size is large, whereas in clinical routines it is often desired to assess the metabolic state of a tumor in real time. An alternative to image reconstruction has been proposed, which can provide real-time blood volume and blood oxygenation maps, which is based on principal component analysis (PCA). PCA [83] linearly transforms the data into an orthogonal coordinate system whose axes correspond to the principal components in the data, that is, the first principal component accounts for as much variance in the data as possible and, successively, further components capture the remaining variance. Through an eigenanalysis, the principal components are determined as eigenvectors of the dataset's covariance matrix and the corresponding eigenvalues refer to the variance that is captured within each eigenvector. It has been shown that, when applied to multispectral images in the near-infrared range (700 nm–850 nm), the first eigenvector corresponds to blood volume and the second to blood oxygenation [84].

40.2.2.1 Validation of Multispectral Images

In order to validate the use of multispectral imaging for assessing fractional blood volume and blood oxygenation, images from healthy volunteers were acquired. A pressure cuff was used to occlude the upper right arm with 180 mm Hg pressure. This amount of pressure was chosen to achieve arterial occlusion and the pressure lasted for 5 min. Multispectral images were taken every 30 s before occlusion, during occlusion, and for 5 min afterwards, resulting in 21 time points in total [80,84,85]. Occlusion experiments were chosen as the behavior of blood volume and blood oxygenation over time is well known. Blood volume remains constant, blood oxygenation undergoes ischemia during, and reactive hyperemia after occlusion [80,86–88].

Figure 40.10 shows 2D reconstruction maps of fractional blood volume and blood oxygenation concentrations over time for one representative healthy volunteer's lower forearm over time. The first row shows the baseline before occlusion, and row 2 and 3 show the results during and after occlusion,

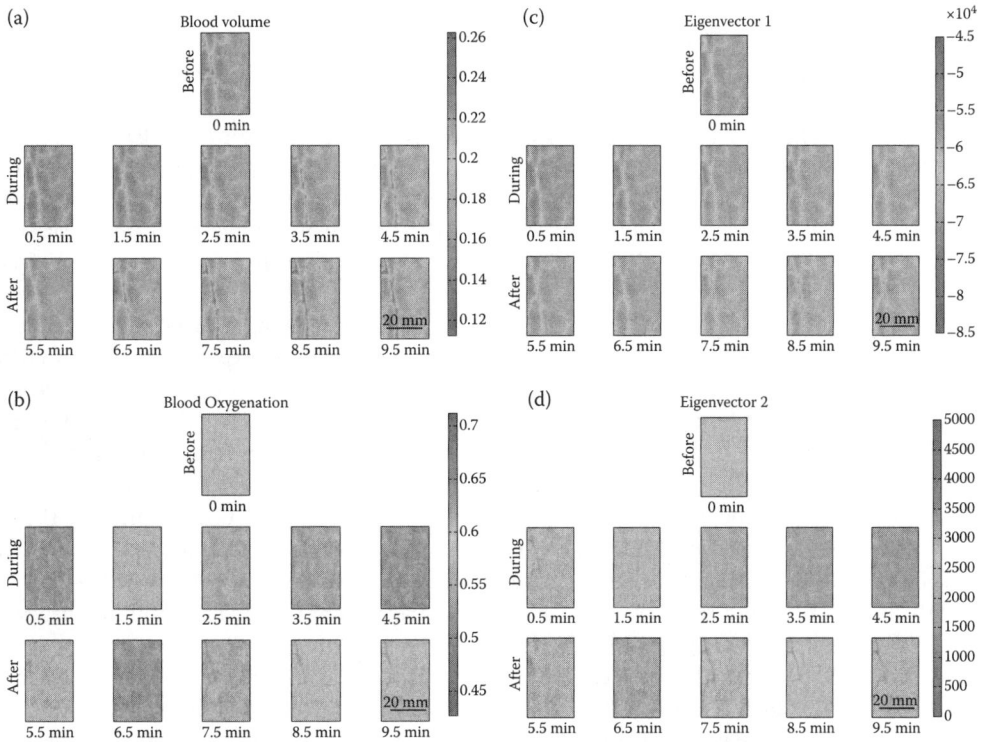

FIGURE 40.10 Typical multispectral results from a healthy volunteer's forearm. Reconstructed fractional blood volume (a) and blood oxygenation (b) over time. Principal component analysis results with eigenvector 1 (c) and eigenvector 2 (d). (From J. Kainerstorfer, M. Ehler, F. Amyot et al., *J. Biomed. Opt.*, 15, 046007, 2010. With permission.)

respectively. Veins contain more blood than the surrounding tissue and are clearly separable in the reconstruction maps by increased blood volume. The overall tissue oxygenation follows the typical expected trend of ischemia during occlusion (drop of oxygenation compared to baseline) and reactive hyperemia after occlusion (overshoot compared to baseline).

The corresponding PCA results show the same spatial distribution, as well as temporal behavior, validating PCA as an alternative tool for chromophore assessment.

40.2.3 Clinical Study: Kaposi's Sarcoma

The oncology community is testing a number of novel targeted approaches such as antiangiogenic, antivascular, immuno-, and gene therapies for use against a variety of cancers. To monitor such therapies, it is desirable to establish techniques to assess tumor vasculature and changes with therapy [89]. Currently, several imaging techniques such as dynamic contrast-enhanced MRI [90–92], PET [93–95], computed tomography (CT) [96–99], color Doppler ultrasound (US) [100,101], and fluorescence imaging [102,103] have been used in angiogenesis-related research. With regard to monitoring vasculature, it is desirable to develop and assess noninvasive and quantitative techniques that can not only monitor structural changes, but can also assess the functional characteristics or the metabolic status of the tumor. There are currently no standard noninvasive techniques to assess parameters of angiogenesis in lesions of interest and to monitor changes in these parameters with therapy. For antiangiogenic therapies, factors associated with blood flow are of particular interest.

KS is a highly vascular tumor that occurs frequently among people infected with acquired immu-nodeficiency syndrome (AIDS). During the first decade of the AIDS epidemic, 15–20% of AIDS patients developed this type of tumor [104]. Patients with KS often display skin and oral lesions and KS frequently involves lymph nodes and visceral organs [105]. KS is an angio-proliferative disease characterized by angiogenesis, endothelial spindle-cell growth (KS cell growth), inflammatory-cell infiltration, and edema [106]. A gamma herpesvirus called KS-associated herpesvirus (KSHV) or human herpesvirus type 8 (HHV-8) is an essential factor in the pathogenesis of KS [107]. Cutaneous KS lesions are easily accessible for noninvasive techniques that involve imaging of tumor vascula-ture, and they may thus represent a tumor model in which to assess certain parameters of angiogen-esis [108,109].

Two potential noninvasive imaging techniques, infrared thermal imaging (thermography) and laser Doppler imaging (LDI), have been used to monitor patients undergoing an experimental anti-KS ther-apy [110,111]. Thermography graphically depicts temperature gradients over a given body surface area at a given time. It is used to study biological thermoregulatory abnormalities that directly or indirectly influence skin temperature [112–116]. However, skin temperature is only an indirect measure of skin blood flow, and the superficial thermal signature of skin is also related to local metabolism. Thus, this approach is best used in conjunction with other techniques. LDI can more directly measure the net blood velocity of small blood vessels in tissue, which generally increases as blood supply increases dur-ing angiogenesis [117,118]. Thermal patterns were recorded using an infrared camera with a uniform sensitivity in the wavelength range of 8–12 μm and LDI images were acquired by scanning the lesion area of the KS patients at two wavelengths, 690 nm and 780 nm.

An example of the images obtained from a typical KS lesion using different modalities is shown in Figure 40.11 [111]. As can be seen in the thermal image, the temperature of the lesion was approximately 2°C higher than that of the normal tissue adjacent to the lesion. Interestingly, in a number of lesions, the area of increased temperature extended beyond the lesion edges as assessed by visual inspection or palpation. This may reflect relatively deep involvement of the tumor in areas underlying normal skin. However, the thermal signature of the skin not only reflects superficial vascularity but also deep tissue metabolic activity. In the LDI image of the same lesion, there was increased blood flow in the area of the lesion as compared to the surrounding tissue, with a maximum increase of over 600 AU (arbitrary units). Unlike the thermal image, the increased blood velocity extended only slightly beyond the area of this visible lesion, possibly because the tumor process leading to the increased temperature was too deep to be detected by LDI. Both these techniques were used successfully to visualize KS lesions, and although each measure an independent parameter (temperature or blood velocity), there was a strong correlation in a group of 16 patients studied by both techniques (Figure 40.12). However, there were

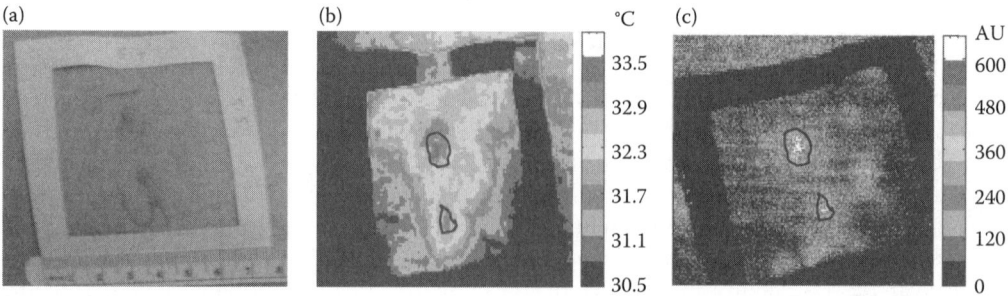

FIGURE 40.11 Typical multimodality images obtained from a patient with KS lesion. The numbers "1" and "5" in the visual image were written on the skin to identify the lesions for tumor measurement. The solid line in the ther-mal and LDI demarks the border of the visible KS lesion. Shown is a representative patient from the study reported in Reference 111. (a) Photo; (b) Thermal image; and (c) Laser Doppler image.

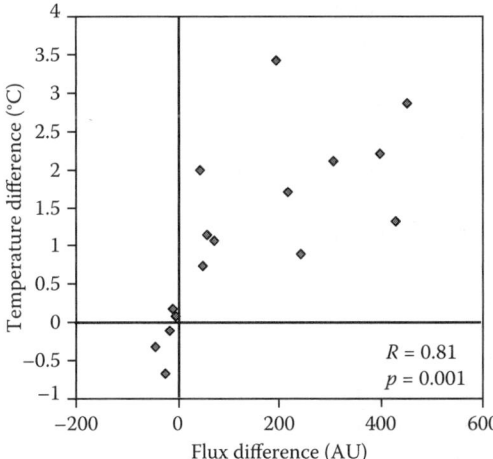

FIGURE 40.12 Relationship between the difference in temperature and flux assessed by LDI of the lesion and surrounding area of the lesion of each subject. A positive correlation was observed between these two methods ($R = 0.8$, $p < 0.001$). (From M. Hassan, R. F. Little, A. Vogel et al., *TCRT*, 3, 451–457, 2004. With permission.)

some differences in individual lesions since LDI measured blood flow distribution in the superficial layer of the skin of the lesion, whereas the thermal signature provided a combined response of superficial vascularity and metabolic activities of deep tissue.

In patients treated with an anti-KS therapy, there was a substantial decrease in temperature and blood velocity during the initial 18-week treatment period as shown in Figure 40.13 [111]. The changes in

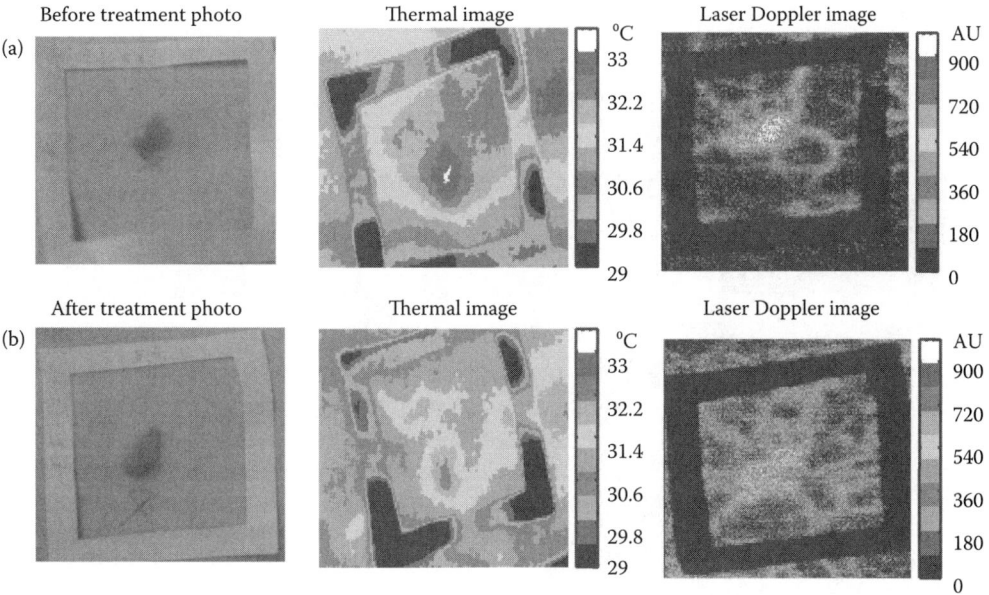

FIGURE 40.13 Typical example of lesion obtained from a subject with KS (a) before and (b) after the treatment. Improvement after the treatment can be assessed by the thermal or LDI images after 18 weeks. Shown is a patient from the clinical trial reported in Reference 111.

these two parameters were generally greater than those assessed by either measurement of tumor size or palpation. In fact, there was no statistically significant decrease in tumor size overall. These results suggest that thermography and LDI may be relatively more sensitive in assessing the response of therapy in KS than conventional approaches. Assessing responses to KS therapy is now generally performed by visual measuring and palpating the numerous lesions and using rather complex response criteria. However, the current tools are rather cumbersome and often subject to observer variation, complicating the assessment of new therapies. The techniques described earlier, possibly combined with other techniques to assess vasculature and vessel function, have the potential of being more quantitative, sensitive, and reproducible than established techniques.

Diffuse multispectral imaging for noncontact and noninvasive monitoring changes in concentrations of blood volume and oxygenated and deoxygenated hemoglobin has also been been used in this clinical study to assess the pathogenesis of the status and changes of KS lesions during therapy. Such an approach can be used to provide early markers for tumor responses and to learn about the pathophysiology of the disease and its changes in response to treatment.

An example of multimodality images obtained from a KS patient before any anti-KS therapy is shown in Figure 40.14. Relatively high contrast of oxygenated hemoglobin and tissue blood volume are observed in the tumor region, which is expected for a metabolically active tumor. The normal tissue blood volume fraction is approximately 5%. This follows previous research that the volume fraction of blood in tissue is 0.2–5% [119]. Another example of multispectral images of a KS patient over the course of treatment is seen in Figure 40.15 in combination of PCA results [120]. Results of oxygenation and blood volume showed an increase and decrease, respectively, inside the lesion over the course of the treatment. Results indicated remission of the disease already at week 14, even though the lesion on the surface did not clinically decrease in size. Pathologic complete remission of disease was confirmed by the clinic in week 48.

The novel imaging modality could potentially be used as predictive tools for the outcome, and therefore also used for individualization of therapeutic strategies.

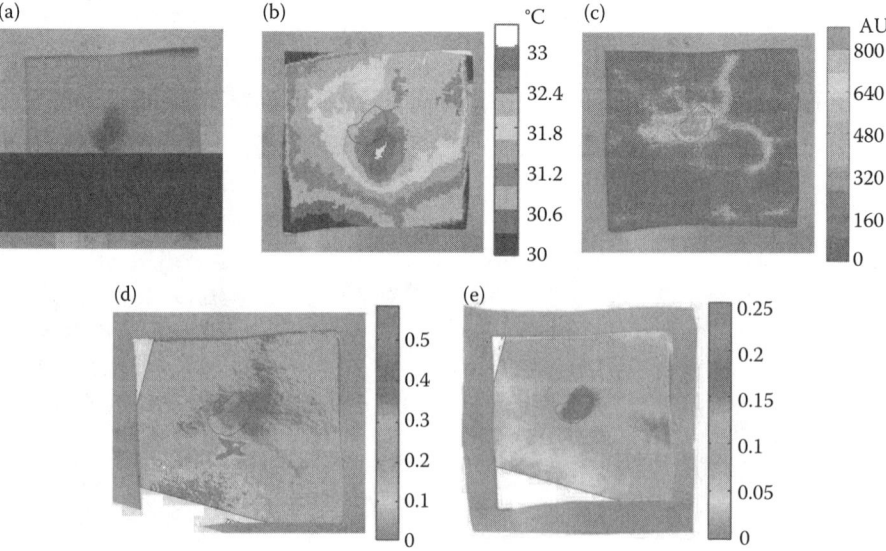

FIGURE 40.14 Set of comparative images of a KS patient. (a) Visual, (b) thermal, (c) laser Doppler, (d) HbO$_2$ fraction, and (e) tissue blood volume fraction images are provided. (From A. Vogel, M. Hassan, F. Amyot et al., *Biomedical Optics 2006, Technical Digest*, p. SG2, 2006.)

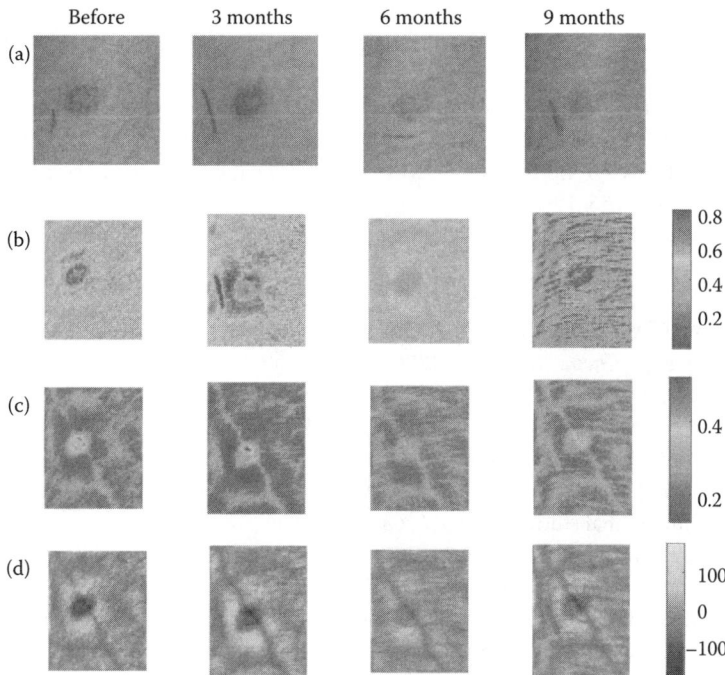

FIGURE 40.15 Digital images of KS lesion over time. Left to right: week 0, 14, 26, and 38 (a); blood oxygenation over time (b); blood volume over time (c); projection along the first principal component (d). (From Kainerstorfer, J. M., F. Amyot, M. Hassan et al., *Biomedical Optics, OSA Technical Digest*, p. BME6, 2010. With permission.)

Acknowledgments

Special thanks go to Dr. Herbert Rinneberg (Physikalich.-Techniche-Bundesanstalt, Berlin) and Dr. Brian Pogue (Dartmouth College) for providing optical images. The authors also wish to express their thanks to Dr. Tatsuo Togawa, a former professor of the Institutes of Biomaterials and Bioengineering, Tokyo Medical and Dental University, Tokyo, Japan for his valuable suggestions and allowing emissivity measurements to be performed in his lab. The authors also thank Stavros Demos at the Lawrence Livermore National Laboratory for helping to design and construct the multispectral imaging system used in the KS clinical trials. This research is supported by the Intramural Research Program of the Eunice Kennedy Shriver National Institute of Child Health and Human Development and the National Cancer Institute, National Institutes of Health.

References

1. M. Born and E. Wolf, *Principles in Optics*, 7th ed. Cambridge: Cambridge University Press, 1999.
2. A. T. Young, Rayleigh scattering, *Phys. Today*, 35, 42–48, 1982.
3. I. S. Saidi, S. L. Jacques, and F. K. Tittel, Mie and Rayleigh modeling of visible-light scattering in neonatal skin, *Appl. Opt.*, 34, 7410, 1995.
4. M. J. C. Van Gemert, S. L. Jacques, H. J. C. M. Sterenberg, and W. M. Star, Skin optics, *IEEE Trans.*, 36, 1146, 1989.
5. R. Marchesini, A. Bertoni, S. Andreola, E. Melloni, and A. Sicherolli, Extinction and absorption coefficients and scattering phase functions of human tissues *in vitro*, *Appl. Opt.*, 28, 2318, 1989.

6. J. Fishkin, O. Coquoz, E. Anderson, M. Brenner, and B. Tromberg, Frequency-domain photon migration measurements of normal and malignant tissue optical properties in a human subject, *Appl. Opt.*, 36, 10, 1997.

7. T. L. Troy, D. L. Page, and E. M. Sevick-Muraca, Optical properties or normal and diseased breast tissues: prognosis for optical mammography, *J. Biomed. Opt.*, 1, 342, 1996.

8. A. H. Gandjbakhche, R. F. Bonner, and R. Nossal, Scaling relationships for anisotropic random walks, *J. Statistical Phys.*, 69, 35, 1992.

9. G. A. Wagnieres, W. M. Star, and W. B. C, *In vivo* fluorescence spectroscopy and imaging for oncological applications, *Photochem. Photobiol.*, 68, 603, 1998.

10. R. Weissleder, A clearer vision for *in vivo* imaging, *Nat. Biotechnol.*, 19, 316, 2001.

11. V. F. Kamalov, I. A. Struganova, and K. Yoshihara, Temperature dependent radiative lifetime of J-aggregates, *J. Phys. Chem.*, 100, 8640, 1996.

12. S. Mordon, J. M. Devoisselle, and V. Maunoury, *In vivo* pH measurement and imaging of a pH-sensitive fluorescent probe (5–6 carboxyfluorescein): Instrumental and experimental studies, *Photochem. Photobiol.*, 60, 274, 1994.

13. C. L. Hutchinson, J. R. Lakowicz, and E. M. Sevick-Muraca, Fluorescence lifetime-based sensing in tissues: A computational study, *Biophys. J.*, 68, 1574, 1995.

14. F. F. Jobsis, Noninvasive infrared monitoring of cerebral and myocardial oxygen sufficiency and circulatory parameters, *Science*, 198, 1264, 1977.

15. T. J. Farrell, M. S. Patterson, and B. Wilson, A diffusion theory model of spatially resolved, steady-state diffuse reflectance for the noninvasive determination of tissue optical properties *in vivo*, *Med. Phys.*, 9, 879, 1992.

16. P. C. Jackson, P. H. Stevens, J. H. Smith, D. Kear, H. Key, and P. N. T. Wells, Imaging mammalian tissues and organs using laser collimated transillumination, *J. Biomed. Eng.*, 6, 70, 1987.

17. G. Jarry, S. Ghesquiere, J. M. Maarek, F. Fraysse, S. Debray, M.-H. Bui, and D. Laurent, Imaging Mammalian tissues and organs using laser collimated transillumination, *J. Biomed. Eng.*, 6, 70, 1984.

18. M. Kaneko, M. Hatakeyama, P. He et al., Construction of a laser transmission photo-scanner: Preclinical investigation, *Radiat. Med.*, 7, 129, 1989.

19. L. Wang, P. P. Ho, C. Liu, G. Zhang, and R. R. Alfano, Ballistic 2-D imaging through scattering walls using an ultrafast optical Kerr gate, *Science*, 253, 769, 1991.

20. A. Schmitt, R. Corey, and P. Saulnier, Imaging through random media by use of low-coherence optical heterodyning, *Opt. Lett.*, 20, 404, 1995.

21. H. Inaba, M. Toida, and T. Ichmua, Optical computer-assisted tomography realized by coherent detection imaging incorporating laser heterodyne method for biomedical applications, *SPIE Proc.*, 399, 108, 1990.

22. H. Inaba, Coherent detection imaging for medical laser tomography, *Medical Optical Tomography: Functional Imaging and Monitoring*, ed. Muller, G., SPIE Optical Engineering Press, Bellingham, WA, p. 317, 1993.

23. S. B. Colak, D. G. Papaioannou, G. W. T'Hoooft, M. B. van der Mark, H. Schomberg, J. C. J. Paasschens, J. B. M. Melissen, and N. A. A. J. van Austen, Tomographic image reconstruction from optical projections in light diffusing media, *Appl. Opt.*, 36, 180, 1997.

24. J. C. Hebden, D. J. Hall, M. Firbank, and D. T. Delpry, Time-resolved optical imaging of a solid tissue-equivalent phantom, *Appl. Opt.*, 34, 8038, 1995.

25. J. C. Hebden, Evaluating the spatial resolution performance of a time-resolved optical imaging system, *Med. Phys.*, 19, 1081, 1992.

26. R. Cubeddu, A. Pifferi, P. Taroni, A. Torriceli, and G. Valentini, Time-resolved imaging on a realistic tissue phantom: μ_s' and μ_a images versus time-integrated images, *Appl. Opt.*, 35, 4533, 1996.

27. D. Grosenick, H. Wabnitz, H. Rinneberg, K. T. Moesta, and P. Schleg, Development of a time-domain optical mammograph and first in-vivo application, *Appl. Opt.*, 38, 2927, 1999.

28. M. Bashkansky, C. Adler, and J. Reinties, Coherently amplified Raman polarization gate for imaging through scattering media, *Opt. Lett.*, 19, 350, 1994.

29. K. M. Yoo, Q. Xing, and R. R. Alfano, Imaging objects hidden in highly scattering media using femtosecond second-harmonic-generation cross-correlation time gating, *Opt. Lett.*, 16, 1019, 1991.

30. G. W. Faris and M. Banks, Upconverting time gate for imaging through highly scattering media, *Opt. Lett.*, 19, 1813, 1994.

31. J. C. Hebden, S. R. Arridge, and D. T. Delpry, Optical imaging in medicine I: Experimental techniques, *Phys. Med. Biol.*, 42, 825, 1997.

32. J. R. Lakowitz and K. Brendt, Frequency domain measurements of photon migration in tissues, *Chem. Phys. Lett.*, 166, 246, 1990.

33. M. A. Franceschini, K. T. Moesta, S. Fantini, G. Gaida, E. Gratton, H. Jess, W. W. Mantulin et al., Frequency-domain techniques enhance optical mammography: Initial clinical results, *Proc. Natl. Acad. Sci.*, *Med. Sci.*, 94, 6468, 1997.

34. B. Tromberg, O. Coquoz, J. B. Fishkin, T. Pham, E. Anderson, J. Butler, M. Cahn et al., Non-invasive measurements of breast tissue optical properties using frequency-domain photon migration, *Philos. Trans. R. Soc. London Ser.*, B352, 661, 1997.

35. J. J. Duderstadt and L. J. Hamilton, *Nuclear Reactor Analysis*. New York: Wiley, 1976.

36. K. M. Case and P. F. Zweifel, *Linear Transport Theory*. Reading: Addison Wesley, 1967.

37. A. Ishimaru, *Wave Propagation and Scattering in Random Media*. New York: Academic Press, 1978.

38. M. S. Patterson, B. Chance, and B. Wilson, Time resolved reflectance and transmittance for the non-invasive measurement of tissue optical properties, *Appl. Opt.*, 28, 2331, 1989.

39. S. R. Arridge and J. C. Hebden, Optical imaging in medicine: II. Modelling and reconstruction, *Phys. Med. Biol.*, 42, 841, 1997.

40. S. R. Nioka, M. Miwa, S. Orel, M. Schnall, M. Haida, S. Zhao, and B. Chance, Optical imaging of human breast cancer, *Adv. Exp. Med. Biol.*, 361, 171, 1994.

41. S. Fantini, S. A. Walker, M. A. Franceschini, M. Kaschke, P. M. Schlag, and K. T. Moesta, Assessment of the size, position, and optical properties of breast tumors *in vivo* by noninvasive optical methods, *Appl. Opt.*, 37, 1982, 1998.

42. M. Maris, E. Gratton, J. Maier, W. Mantulin, and B. Chance, Functional near-infrared imaging of deoxygenated haemoglobin during exercise of the finger extensor muscles using the frequency-domain techniques, *Bioimaging*, 2, 174, 1994.

43. B. W. Pogue and K. D. Paulsen, High-resolution near-infrared tomographic imaging simulations of the rat cranium by use of *a priori* magnetic resonance imaging structural information, *Opt. Lett.*, 23, 1716, 1998.

44. R. F. Bonner, R. Nossal, S. Havlin, and G. H. Weiss, Model for photon migration in turbid biological media, *J. Opt. Soc. Am. A*, 4, 423, 1987.

45. A. H. Gandjbakhche and G. H. Weiss, Random walk and diffusion-like models of photon migration in turbid media, *Progress in Optics*, ed. Wolf, E. Elsevier Science B.V., North Holland, Amsterdam, vol. XXXIV, p. 333, 1995.

46. A. H. Gandjbakhche, R. Nossal, and R. F. Bonner, Scaling relationships for theories of anisotropic random walks applied to tissue optics, *Appl. Opt.*, 32, 504, 1993.

47. V. Chernomordik, R. Nossal, and A. H. Gandjbakhche, Point spread functions of photons in time-resolved transillumination experiments using simple scaling arguments, *Med. Phys.*, 23, 1857, 1996.

48. A. H. Gandjbakhche, G. H. Weiss, R. F. Bonner, and R. Nossal, Photon path-length distributions for transmission through optically turbid slabs, *Phys. Rev. E*, 48, 810, 1993.

49. D. J. Hawrysz and E. M. Sevick-Muraca, Developments toward diagnostic breast cancer imaging using near-infrared optical measurements and fluorescent contract agents, *Neoplasia*, 2, 388, 2000.

50. M. Cutler, Transillumination as an aid in the diagnosis of breast lesions, *Surg. Gynecol. Obstet.*, 48, 721, 1929.

51. A. H. Gandjbakhche, V. Chernomordik, J. C. Hebden, and R. Nossal, Time-dependent contract functions for quantitative imaging in time-resolved transillumination experiments, *Appl. Opt.*, 37, 1973, 1998.

52. A. H. Gandjbakhche, R. Nossal, and R. F. Bonner, Resolution limits for optical transillumination of abnormalities deeply embedded in tissues, *Med. Phys.*, 21, 185, 1994.

53. V. Chernomordik, D. Hattery, A. Pifferi, P. Taroni, A. Torricelli, G. Valentini, R. Cubeddu et al., A random walk methodology for quantification of the optical characteristics of abnormalities embedded within tissue-like phantoms, *Opt. Lett.*, 25, 951, 2000.

54. M. Morin, S. Verreault, A. Mailloux, S. Frechette, Y. Chatingny, Y. Painchaud, and P. Beaudry, Inclusion characterization in a scattering slab with time-resolved transmittance measurements: Perturbation analysis, *Appl. Opt.*, 39, 2840–2852, 2000.

55. V. Chernomordik, D. W. Hattery, D. Grosenick, H. Wabnitz, H. Rinneberg, K. T. Moesta, P. M. Schlag et al., Quantification of optical properties of a breast tumor using random walk theory, *J. Biomed. Opt.*, 7, 80–7, 2002.

56. A. P. Gibson, J. C. Hebden, and S. R. Arridge, Recent advances in diffuse optical imaging, *Phys. Med. Biol.*, 50, R1–43, 2005.

57. R. I. e. Fox, Treatment of the patient with Sjogren syndrome, *Rheumatic Dis. Clinic N. Am.*, 18, 699–709, 1992.

58. V. Chernomordik, D. Hattery, I. Gannot, and A. H. Gandjbakhche, Inverse method 3D reconstruction of localized in-vivo fluorescence. Application to Sjogren syndrome, *IEEE J. Sel. Topics Quant. Elec.*, 5, 930, 1999.

59. M. S. Patterson and B. W. Pogue, Mathematical model for time-resolved and frequency-domain fluorescence spectroscopy in biological tissue, *Appl. Opt.*, 33, 1963, 1994.

60. A. H. Gandjbakhche, R. F. Bonner, R. Nossal, and G. H. Weiss, Effects on multiple passage probabilities on fluorescence signals from biological media, *Appl. Opt.*, 36, 4613, 1997.

61. D. Hattery, V. Chernomordik, M. Loew, I. Gannot, and A. H. Gandjbakhche, Analytical solutions for time-resolved fluorescence lifetime imaging in a turbid medium such as tissue, *JOSA(A)*, 18, 1523, 2001.

62. E. Samuel, Thermography—some clinical applications, *Biomed. Eng.*, 4, 15–9, 1969.

63. C. H. Jones, Physical aspects of thermography in relation to clinical techniques, *Bibl. Radiol.*, 1–8, 1975.

64. J. Hardy, The radiation power of human skin in the infrared, *Am. J. Physiol.*, 127, 454–462, 1939.

65. J. Steketee, Spectral emissivity of skin and pericardium, *Phys. Med. Biol.*, 18, 686–94, 1973.

66. R. Elam, D. Goodwin, and K. Willams, Optical properties of human epidermics, *Nature*, 198, 1001–1002, 1963.

67. D. J. Watmough and R. Oliver, Emissivity of human skin in the waveband between 2 micron and 6 micron, *Nature*, 219, 622–624, 1968.

68. K. D. Patil and K. L. William, Spectral study of human radiation. Non-ionizing Radiation, *Nonionizing Radiat.*, 1, 39–44, 1969.

69. T. Togawa, Non-contact skin emissivity: Measurement from reflectance using step change in ambient radiation temperature, *Clin. Phys. Physiol. Meas.*, 10, 39–48, 1989.

70. M. Hassan and T. Togawa, Observation of skin thermal inertia distribution during reactive hyperaemia using a single-hood measurement system, *Physiol. Meas.*, 22, 187–200, 2001.

71. W. H. McAdams, *Heat Transmission*, New York: McGraw Hill, p. 472, 1954.

72. H. T. Hammel, J. D. Hardy, and D. Murgatroyd, Spectral transmittance and reflectance of excised human skin, *J. Appl. Physiol.*, 9, 257–64, 1956.

73. S. L. Jacques, Skin Optics, http://omlc.ogi.edu/news/jan98/skinoptics.html, 1998.

74. R. Zhang, W. Verkruysse, B. Choi, J. A. Viator, B. Jung, L. O. Svaasand, G. Aguilar et al., Determination of human skin optical properties from spectrophotometric measurements based on optimization by genetic algorithms, *J. Biomed. Opt.*, 10, 024030, 2005.

75. L. F. A. Douven and G. W. Lucassen, Retrieval of optical properties of skin from measurement and modeling the diffuse reflectance, *Proc. SPIE*, 3914, 312–323, 2000.

76. I. O. Svaasand, L. T. Norvang, E. J. Fiskerstrand, E. K. S. Stopps, M. W. Berns, and J. S. Nelson, Tissue parameters determining the visual appearance of normal skin and port-wine stains, *Laser Med. Sci.*, 10, 55–65, 1995.

77. I. V. Meglinski and S. J. Matcher, Quantitative assessment of skin layers absorption and skin reflectance spectra simulation in the visible and near-infrared spectral regions, *Physiol. Meas.*, 23, 741–53, 2002.

78. I. Nishidate, Y. Aizu, and H. Mishina, Estimation of absorbing components in a local layer embedded in the turbid media on the basis of visible and near-infrared (VIS-NIR) reflectance spectra, *Opt. Rev.*, 10, 427–435, 2003.

79. S. L. Jacques, Origins of tissue optical properties in the UVA, visible, and NIR regions, *OSA TOPS on Advances in Optical Imaging and Photon Migration*, eds, R.R. Alfano and James G. Fujimoto, vol. 2, Optical Society of America, Washington, DC, pp. 364–371, 1996.

80. J. Kainerstorfer, F. Amyot, S. G. Demos, M. Hassan, V. Chernomordik, C. K. Hitzenberger, A. H. Gandjbakhche et al., Quantitative assessment of ischemia and reactive hyperemia of the dermal layers using multi—Spectral imaging on the human arm, *Progr. Biomed. Opt. Imaging—Proc. SPIE*, 7369, 2009.

81. A. Vogel, V. V. Chernomordik, J. D. Riley, M. Hassan, F. Amyot, B. Dasgeb, S. G. Demos et al., Using noninvasive multispectral imaging to quantitatively assess tissue vasculature, *J. Biomed. Opt.*, 12, 051604, 2007.

82. A. Vogel, B. Dasgeb, M. Hassan, F. Amyot, V. Chernomordik, Y. Tao, S. G. Demos et al., Using quantitative imaging techniques to assess vascularity in AIDS-related Kaposi's sarcoma, *Conf. Proc. IEEE Eng. Med. Biol. Soc.*, 1, 232–5, 2006.

83. K. Pearson, On lines and planes of closest fit to systems of points in space, *Philos. Mag.*, 2, 559–572, 1901.

84. J. Kainerstorfer, M. Ehler, F. Amyot, M. Hassan, S. G. Demos, V. Chernomordik, C. K. Hitzenberger, A. H. Gandjbakhche, and J. D. Riley, Principal component model of multi spectral data for near real time skin chromophore mapping, *J. Biomed. Opt.*, 15, 046007, 2010.

85. J. Kainerstorfer, F. Amyot, M. Ehler, M. Hassan, S. G. Demos, V. Chernomordik, C. K. Hitzenberger et al., Direct curvature correction for non-contact imaging modalities—applied to multi-spectral imaging, *J. Biomed. Opt.*, 15, 2010.

86. S. H. Tseng, P. Bargo, A. Durkin, and N. Kollias, Chromophore concentrations, absorption and scattering properties of human skin *in-vivo*, *Opt. Express*, 17, 14599–617, 2009.

87. D. J. Cuccia, F. Bevilacqua, A. J. Durkin, F. R. Ayers, and B. J. Tromberg, Quantitation and mapping of tissue optical properties using modulated imaging, *J. Biomed. Opt.*, 14, 024012, 2009.

88. U. Merschbrock, J. Hoffmann, L. Caspary, J. Huber, U. Schmickaly, and D. W. Lubbers, Fast wavelength scanning reflectance spectrophotometer for noninvasive determination of hemoglobin oxygenation in human skin, *Int. J. Microcirc. Clin. Exp.*, 14, 274–81, 1994.

89. D. M. McDonald and P. L. Choyke, Imaging of angiogenesis: From microscope to clinic, *Nat. Med.*, 9, 713–25, 2003.

90. J. S. Taylor, P. S. Tofts, R. Port, J. L. Evelhoch, M. Knopp, W. E. Reddick, V. M. Runge et al., MR imaging of tumor microcirculation: Promise for the new millennium, *J. Magn. Reson. Imaging*, 10, 903–907, 1999.

91. K. L. Verstraete, Y. De Deene, H. Roels, A. Dierick, D. Uyttendaele, and M. Kunnen, Benign and malignant musculoskeletal lesions: Dynamic contrast-enhanced MR imaging—parametric "first-pass" images depict tissue vascularization and perfusion, *Radiology*, 192, 835–43., 1994.

92. L. D. Buadu, J. Murakami, S. Murayama, N. Hashiguchi, S. Sakai, K. Masuda, S. Toyoshima et al., Breast lesions: Correlation of contrast medium enhancement patterns on MR images with histopathologic findings and tumor angiogenesis, *Radiology*, 200, 639–49, 1996.

93. A. Fredriksson and S. Stone-Elander, PET screening of anticancer drugs. A faster route to drug/target evaluations *in vivo*, *Methods Mol. Med.*, 85, 279–94, 2003.

94. G. Jerusalem, R. Hustinx, Y. Beguin, and G. Fillet, The value of positron emission tomography (PET) imaging in disease staging and therapy assessment, *Ann. Oncol.*, 13, 227–34., 2002.

95. H. C. Steinert, M. Hauser, F. Allemann, H. Engel, T. Berthold, G. K. von Schulthess, and W. Weder, Non-small cell lung cancer: Nodal staging with FDG PET versus CT with correlative lymph node mapping and sampling, *Radiology*, 202, 441–446, 1997.

96. S. D. Rockoff, The evolving role of computerized tomography in radiation oncology, *Cancer*, 39, 694–6, 1977.

97. K. D. Hopper, K. Singapuri, and A. Finkel, Body CT and oncologic imaging, *Radiology*, 215, 27–40., 2000.

98. K. A. Miles, M. Hayball, and A. K. Dixon, Colour perfusion imaging: A new application of computed tomography, *Lancet*, 337, 643–645, 1991.

99. K. A. Miles, C. Charnsangavej, F. T. Lee, E. K. Fishman, K. Horton, and T. Y. Lee, Application of CT in the investigation of angiogenesis in oncology, *Acad. Radiol.*, 7, 840–50, 2000.

100. N. Ferrara, Role of vascular endothelial growth factor in physiologic and pathologic angiogenesis: Therapeutic implications, *Semin. Oncol.*, 29, 10–4, 2002.

101. D. E. Goertz, D. A. Christopher, J. L. Yu, R. S. Kerbel, P. N. Burns, and F. S. Foster, High-frequency color flow imaging of the microcirculation, *Ultrasound Med. Biol.*, 26, 63–71, 2000.

102. E. M. Gill, G. M. Palmer, and N. Ramanujam, Steady-state fluorescence imaging of neoplasia, *Methods Enzymol.*, 361, 452–81, 2003.

103. K. Svanberg, I. Wang, S. Colleen, I. Idvall, C. Ingvar, R. Rydell, D. Jocham et al., Clinical multi-colour fluorescence imaging of malignant tumours—initial experience, *Acta Radiol.*, 39, 2–9, 1998.

104. V. Beral, T. A. Peterman, R. L. Berkelman, and H. W. Jaffe, Kaposi's sarcoma among persons with AIDS: A sexually transmitted infection?, *Lancet*, 335, 123–8, 1990.

105. B. A. Biggs, S. M. Crowe, C. R. Lucas, M. Ralston, I. L. Thompson, and K. J. Hardy, AIDS related Kaposi's sarcoma presenting as ulcerative colitis and complicated by toxic megacolon, *Gut*, 28, 1302–1306, 1987.

106. E. Cornali, C. Zietz, R. Benelli, W. Weninger, L. Masiello, G. Breier, E. Tschachler et al., Vascular endothelial growth factor regulates angiogenesis and vascular permeability in Kaposi's sarcoma, *Am. J. Pathol.*, 149, 1851–69, 1996.

107. Y. Chang, E. Cesarman, M. S. Pessin, F. Lee, J. Culpepper, D. M. Knowles, and P. S. Moore, Identification of herpesvirus-like DNA sequences in AIDS-associated Kaposi's sarcoma, *Science*, 266, 1865–1869, 1994.

108. R. Yarchoan, Therapy for Kaposi's sarcoma: Recent advances and experimental approaches, *J. Acquir. Immune Defic. Syndr.*, 21(Suppl 1), S66–S73, 1999.

109. R. F. Little, K. M. Wyvill, J. M. Pluda, L. Welles, V. Marshall, W. D. Figg, F. M. Newcomb et al., Activity of thalidomide in AIDS-related Kaposi's sarcoma, *J. Clin. Oncol.*, 18, 2593–602, 2000.

110. M. Hassan, D. Hattery, V. Chernomordik, K. Aleman, K. Wyvill, F. Merced, R. F. Little et al., Non-invasive multi-modality technique to study angiogenesis associated with Kaposi's sarcoma, *Proc. EMBS BMES*, 1139–1140, 2002.

111. M. Hassan, R. F. Little, A. Vogel, K. Aleman, K. Wyvill, R. Yarchoan, and A. Gandjbakhche, Quantitative assessment of tumor vasculature and response to therapy in Kaposi's sarcoma using functional non-invasive imaging, *TCRT*, 3, 451–457, 2004.

112. C. Maxwell-Cade, Principles and practice of clinical thermography, *Radiography*, 34, 23–34, 1968.

113. J. F. Head and R. L. Elliott, Infrared imaging: making progress in fulfilling its medical promise, *IEEE Eng. Med. Biol. Mag.*, 21, 80–85, 2002.

114. S. Bornmyr and H. Svensson, Thermography and laser-Doppler flowmetry for monitoring changes in finger skin blood flow upon cigarette smoking, *Clin. Physiol.*, 11, 135–41, 1991.

115. K. Usuki, T. Kanekura, K. Aradono, and T. Kanzaki, Effects of nicotine on peripheral cutaneous blood flow and skin temperature, *J. Dermatol. Sci.*, 16, 173–81, 1998.

116. M. Anbar, Clinical thermal imaging today, *IEEE Eng. Med. Biol. Mag.*, 17, 25–33, 1998.
117. J. Sorensen, M. Bengtsson, E. L. Malmqvist, G. Nilsson, and F. Sjoberg, Laser Doppler perfusion imager (LDPI)—for the assessment of skin blood flow changes following sympathetic blocks, *Acta Anaesthesiol. Scand.*, 40, 1145–1148, 1996.
118. A. Rivard, J. E. Fabre, M. Silver, D. Chen, T. Murohara, M. Kearney, M. Magner et al., Age-dependent impairment of angiogenesis, *Circulation*, 99, 111–20, 1999.
119. A. Vogel, M. Hassan, F. Amyot, V. Chernomordik, S. Demos, R. Little, R. Yarchoan et al., Using multi-modality imaging techniques to assess vascularity in AIDS-related Kaposi's sarcoma, *Biomedical Optics 2006, Technical Digest*, p. SG2, 2006.
120. Kainerstorfer, J. M., F. Amyot, M. Hassan, M. Ehler, R. Yarchoan, K. M. Wyvill, T. Uldrick et al., Reconstruction-free imaging of Kaposi's Sarcoma using multi-spectral data, *Biomedical Optics, OSA Technical Digest*, p. BME6, 2010.

41

Biomedical Applications of Functional Infrared Imaging

Arcangelo Merla
University of Chieti-Pescara

Gian Luca Romani
University of Chieti-Pescara

41.1 Introduction

Infrared imaging provides quantitative representation of the surface thermal distribution of the human body. The skin temperature distribution of the human body depends on the complex relationships defining the heat exchange processes between skin tissue, inner tissue, local vasculature, and metabolic activity. All of these processes are mediated and regulated by the sympathetic and parasympathetic activity to maintain the thermal homeostasis. The presence of a disease can affect the heat balance or exchange processes, resulting in an increase or in a decrease of the skin temperature and altered dynamics of the local control of the skin temperature. Therefore, the characteristic parameters modeling the activity of the skin thermoregulatory system can be used as diagnostic parameters. The functional infrared (fIR) imaging is the study for diagnostic purposes, based on the modeling of the bio-heat exchange processes, of the functional properties and alterations of the human thermoregulatory system. In this chapter, we present some of the clinical applications in order to show the potentialities of the technique.

41.2 Diagnosis of Varicocele and Follow-Up of Treatment

Varicocele is a widely spread male disease consisting of a dilatation of the pampiniform venous plexus and of the internal spermatic vein. Consequences of such a dilatation are an increase of the scrotal temperature and a possible impairment of the potential fertility [22,31].

In normal men, testicular temperature is 3–4°C lower than core body temperature [22]. Two thermoregulatory processes maintain this lower temperature: heat exchange with the environment through the scrotal skin and heat clearance by blood flow through the pampiniform plexus. Venous stasis due to the varicocele may increase the temperature of the affected testicle or pampiniform plexus. Thus, an abnormal temperature difference between the two hemiscrota may suggest the presence of varicocele [15,31] (see Figure 41.1).

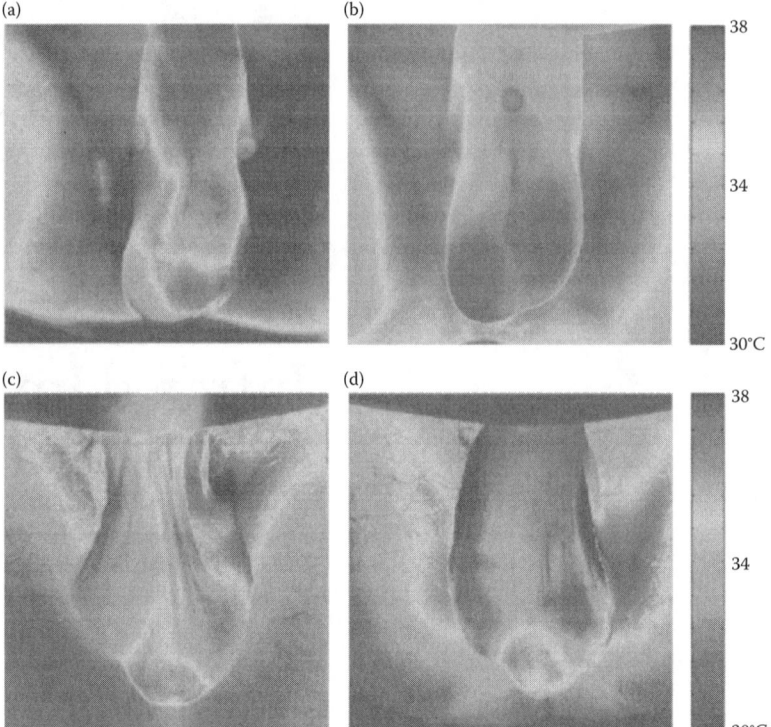

FIGURE 41.1   (a) Second-grade right varicocele. The temperature distribution all over the scrotum clearly highlights significant differences between affected and unaffected testicles. (b) The same scrotum after varicocelectomy. The surgical treatment reduced the increased temperature on the affected hemiscrotum and restored the symmetry in the scrotal temperature distribution. (c) Third-grade left varicocele. (d) The same scrotum after varicocelectomy. The treatment was unsuccessful in repairing the venous reflux, as documented by the persisting asymmetric scrotal distribution.

Telethermography can reveal abnormal temperature differences between the two testicles and altered testicular thermal recovery after an induced cold stress. Affected testicles return to prestress equilibrium temperatures faster than do normal testicles [15].

fIR imaging has been used to determine whether altered scrotal thermoregulation is related to subclinical varicocele [19]. In a study conducted in 2001, Merla and Romani enrolled 60 volunteers, 18–27 years of age (average age, 21 ± 2 years), with no symptoms or clinical history of varicocele. After clinical examination, echo color Doppler imaging (the gold standard) and functional infrared imaging were performed. fIR imaging evaluation consisted of obtaining scrotal images, measuring the basal temperature at the level of the pampiniform plexus (T_p) and the testicles (T_t), and determining thermal recovery of the scrotum after cold thermal stress.

The temperature curve of the hemiscrotum during rewarming showed an exponential pattern and was, therefore, fitted to an exponential curve. The time constant τ of the best exponential fit depends on the thermal properties of the scrotum and its blood perfusion [15,17]. Therefore, τ provides a quantitative parameter assessing how much the scrotal thermoregulation is affected by varicocele. Cooling was achieved by applying a dry patch to the scrotum that was 10°C colder than the basal scrotal temperature. The fIR measurements were performed accordingly with usual standardization procedures [14]. The basal prestress temperature and the recovery time constant τ_p at the level of the pampiniform plexus and of the testicles (τ_t) were evaluated on each hemiscrotum. A basal testicular temperature greater than 32°C and basal pampiniform plexus temperature greater than 34°C were considered warning thresholds. Temperature differences among testicles (ΔT_t) or pampiniform plexus ΔT_p temperature greater than 1.0°C were also considered warning values, as were $\Delta \tau_t$ and $\Delta \tau_t$ values longer than 1.5 min.

The fIR imaging evaluation classified properly the stages of disease, as confirmed by the echo color Doppler imaging and clinical examination in a blinded manner.

In 38 subjects, no warning basal temperatures or differences in rewarming temperatures were observed. These subjects were considered to be normal according to infrared functional imaging. Clinical examination and echo color Doppler imaging confirmed the absence of varicocele ($p < 0.01$, one-way ANOVA test).

In 22 subjects, one or more values were greater than the warning threshold for basal temperatures or differences in rewarming temperatures. Values for ΔT_p and the $\Delta \tau_p$ were higher than the warning thresholds in 8 of the 22 subjects, who were classified as having grade 1 varicocele. Five subjects had ΔT_t and $\Delta \tau_t$ values higher than the threshold. In nine subjects, three or more infrared functional imaging values were greater than the warning threshold values. The fIR imaging classification was grade 3 varicocele. Clinical examination and echo color Doppler imaging closely confirmed the fIR imaging evaluation of the stage of the varicocele. fIR imaging yielded no false-positive or false-negative results. All participants with positive results on infrared functional imaging also had positive results on clinical examination and echo color Doppler imaging. The sensitivity and specificity of fIR test were 100% and 93%, respectively.

An abnormal change in the temperature of the testicles and pampiniform plexus may indicate varicocele, but the study demonstrated that impaired thermoregulation is associated with varicocele-induced alteration of blood flow. Time to recovery of prestress temperature in the testicles and pampiniform plexus appears to assist in the classification of the disease. fIR imaging accurately detected 22 asymptomatic varicocele.

The control of the scrotum temperature should improve after varicocelectomy as a complementary effect of the reduction of the blood reflux. Moreover, follow-up of the changes in scrotum thermoregulation after varicocelectomy may provide early indications on possible relapses of the disease.

To answer the above questions, Merla et al. [13] used fIR imaging to study changes in the scrotum thermoregulation of 20 patients (average age, 27 ± 5 years) that were judged eligible for varicocelectomy on the basis of the combined results of the clinical examination, Echo color Doppler imaging, and spermiogram. No bilateral varicoceles were included in the study.

Patients underwent to clinical examination, echo color Doppler imaging and instrument varicocele grading, and infrared functional evaluation before varicocelectomy and every 2 weeks thereafter, up to the 24th week. Fourteen out of the 20 patients suffered from grade 2 left varicocele. All of them were characterized by basal temperatures and recovery time after cold stress according to Reference 13. Varicoceles were surgically treated via interruption of the internal spermatic vein using modified Palomo's technique. fIR imaging documented the changes in the thermoregulatory control of the scrotum after the treatment as follows: 13 out of the 14 grade 2 varicocele patients exhibited normal basal T_t, T_p on the varicocele side of the scrotum, and normal temperature differences ΔT_t and ΔT_p starting from the 4th week after varicocelectomy. Their $\Delta \tau_t$ and $\Delta \tau_p$ values returned to the normal range from the 4th to the 6th week. Four out of the six grade 3 varicocele patients exhibited normal basal T_t, T_p on the varicocele side of the scrotum, and normal temperature differences ΔT_t and ΔT_p starting from the 6th week after varicocelectomy. Their $\Delta \tau_t$ and $\Delta \tau_p$ values returned to normal range from the 6th to the 8th week. The other three patients did not return to normal values of the above specified parameters. In particular, $\Delta \tau_t$ and $\Delta \tau_p$ remained much longer than the threshold warning values [13] up to the last control (Figure 41.1). Echo color Doppler imaging and clinical examination assessed relapses of the disease.

The study proved that the surgical treatment of the varicocele induces modification in the thermoregulatory properties of the scrotum, reducing the basal temperature of the affected testicle and pampiniform plexus, and slowing down its recovery time after thermal stress. Among the 17 with no relapse, 4 exhibited return to normal T_t, T_p, ΔT_t, and ΔT_p for the latero-anterior side of the scrotum, while the posterior side of the scrotum remained hyperthermal or characterize by ΔT_t and ΔT_p higher than the threshold warning value.

This fact suggested that the surgical treatment via interruption of the internal spermatic vein using Palomo's technique may not be the most suitable method for those varicoceles. The time requested by the scrotum to restore normal temperature distribution and control seems to be positively correlated to the volume and duration of the blood reflux lasting: the greater the blood reflux, the longer the time.

The study demonstrated that IR imaging may provide an early indication on the possible relapsing of the disease and may be used as a suitable complementary follow-up tool.

41.3 Raynaud's Phenomenon and Scleroderma

Raynaud's phenomenon (RP) is defined as a painful vasoconstriction—that may follow cold or emotional stress—of small arteries and arterioles of extremities, like fingers and toes. RP can be primary (PRP) or secondary (SSc) to scleroderma. The latter is usually associated with a connective tissues disease.

RP precedes the systemic autoimmune disorders development, particularly scleroderma, by many years and it can evolve into secondary RP. The evaluation of vascular disease is crucial in order to distinguish between PRP and SSc. In PRP, episodic ischemia in response to cold exposure or to emotional stimuli is usually completely reversible: absence of tissue damage is the typical feature [1], but mild structural changes are also demonstrated [30]. In contrast, scleroderma RP shows irreversible tissue damage and severe structural changes in the finger vascular organization [25].

None of the physiological measurement techniques currently in use, except infrared imaging, are completely satisfactory in focusing primary or secondary RP [10]. The main limit of such techniques (nail fold capillary microscopy, cutaneous laser Doppler flowmetry, and plethysmography) is the fact that they can proceed just into a partial investigation, usually assessing only one finger once. The measurement of skin temperature is an indirect method to estimate change in skin thermal properties and blood flow.

Thermography protocols [4,6,7,9,10,12,23,26,29] usually include cold patch testing to evaluate the capability of the patient hands to rewarm. The pattern of the rewarming curves is usually used to depict the underlying structural diseases. Analysis of rewarming curves has been used in several studies to differentiate healthy subjects from PRP or SSc Raynaud's patients. Parameters usually considered so far are the lag time preceding the onset of rewarming or to reach a preset final temperature; the rate of the rewarming and the maximum temperature of recovery; and the degree of temperature variation between different areas of the hands.

Merla et al. [18] proposed to model the natural response of the fingertips to exposure to a cold environment to get a diagnostic parameter derived by the physiology of such a response. The thermal recovery following a cold stress is driven by thermal exchange with the environment, transport by the incoming blood flow, conduction from adjacent tissue layers, and metabolic processes. The finger temperature is determined by the net balance of the energy input/output. The more significant contributions come from the input power due to blood perfusion and the power lost to the environment [18]:

$$\frac{dQ}{dt} = -\frac{dQ_{env}}{dt} + \frac{dQ_{ctr}}{dt} \tag{41.1}$$

Normal finger recovery after a cold stress is reported in Figure 41.2.

In absence of thermoregulatory control, fingers exchange heat only with the environment: in this case, their temperature T_{exp} follows an exponential pattern with time constant τ given by

$$\tau = \frac{\rho \cdot c \cdot V}{h \cdot A} \tag{41.2}$$

where ρ is the mass density, c the specific heat, V the finger volume, h the combined heat transfer coefficient between the finger and the environment, and A the finger surface area. Thanks to the

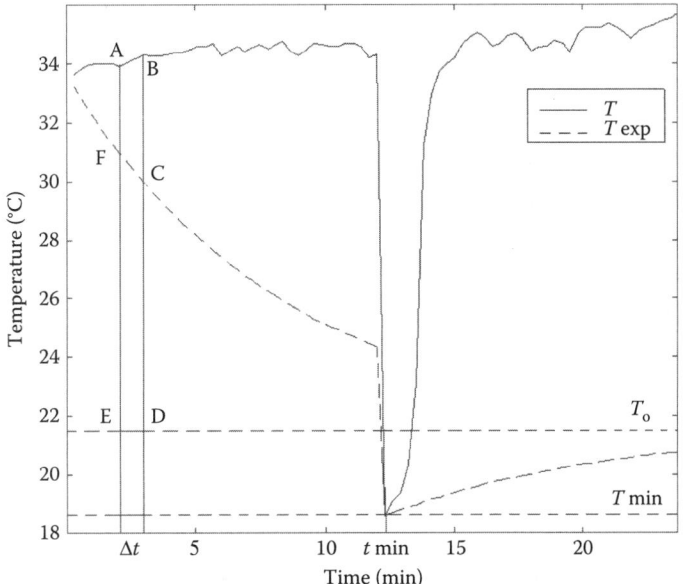

FIGURE 41.2 Experimental rewarming curves after cold stress in normal subjects. The continuous curve represents the recorded temperature finger. The outlined curve represents the exponential temperature pattern exhibited by the finger in the absence of thermoregulatory control. In this case, the only heat source for the finger is the environment. (From Merla, A. et al., Infrared functional imaging applied to Raynaud's phenomenon, *IEEE Eng. Med. Biol. Mag.*, 21, 73, 2002, by permission of the editor.)

thermoregulatory control, the finger maintains its temperature T greater than T_{exp}. For a Δt time, the area of the trapezoid $ABCF$ times $h\,A$ in Figure 41.2 computes the heat provided by the thermoregulatory system, namely ΔQ_{ctrl}. This amount summed to ΔQ_{env} yields Q, the global amount of heat stored in the finger.

Then, the area of the trapezoid $ABDE$ is proportional to the amount Q of heat stored in the finger during a Δt interval. Therefore, Q can be computed integrating the area surrounded by the temperature curve T and the constant straight line T_0:

$$Q = -h \cdot A \cdot \int_{t_1}^{t_2} \left(T_0 - T(\varsigma)\right) \mathrm{d}\varsigma \tag{41.3}$$

where the minus sign takes into account that the heat stored by the finger is counted as positive. Q is intrinsically related to the finger thermal capacity, according to the expression

$$\Delta Q = \rho \cdot c \cdot V \cdot \Delta T \tag{41.4}$$

Under the hypothesis of constant T_0, the numerical integration in (Equation 41.3) can be used to characterize the rewarming exhibited by a healthy or a suffering finger.

The Q parameter has been used in References 16, 18 to discriminate and classify PRP, SSc, and healthy subjects on a set of 40 (20 PRP, 20 SSc) and 18 healthy volunteers. For each subject, the response to a mild cold challenge of hands in water was assessed by fIR imaging. Rewarming curves were recorded for each of the five fingers of both hands; the temperature integral Q was calculated along the 20 min following the cold stress. Ten subjects, randomly selected within the 18 normal ones, repeated two times

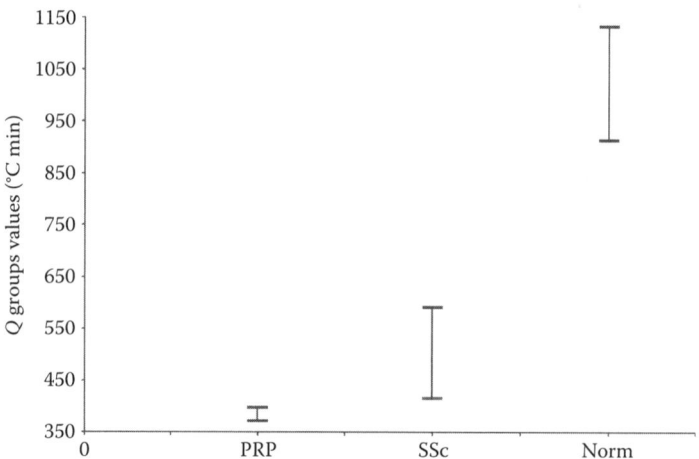

FIGURE 41.3 One-way ANOVA test applied to the Q parameter calculated for each group (PRP, SSc, and healthy). The Q parameter clearly discriminates the three groups. (From Merla, A. et al., Infrared functional imaging applied to Raynaud's phenomenon, *IEEE Eng. Med. Biol. Mag.*, 21, 73, 2002, by permission of the editor.)

and in different days the test to evaluate the repeatability of the fIR imaging findings. The repeatability test confirmed that fIR imaging and Q computation is robust tool to characterize the thermal recovery of the fingers.

The grand average Q values provided by the first measurement was 1060.0 ± 130.5°C min, while for the second assessment it was 1012 ± 135.1°C min ($p > 0.05$, one-way ANOVA test). The grand average Q values for PRP, SSc, and healthy subjects groups are in shown in Figure 41.3, whereas single values obtained for each finger of all of the subjects are reported in Figure 41.4.

The results in References 16, 18 highlight that the PRP group features low intraindividual and inter-individual variability whereas the SSc group displays a large variability between healthy and unhealthy fingers. Q values for SSc finger are generally greater than PRP ones.

The temperature integral at different finger regions yields very similar results for all fingers of the PRP group, suggesting common thermal and blood flow (BF) properties. SSc patients showed different thermoregulatory responses in the different segments of the finger. This feature is probably due to the local modification in the tissue induced by the scleroderma. Scleroderma patients also featured a significantly different behavior across the five fingers depending on the disease involvement.

In normal and PRP groups, all fingers show a homogeneous behavior and PRP fingers always exhibit a poorer recovery than normal ones. Additionally, in both groups, the rewarming always starts from the finger distal area differently from what happens in SSc patients. The sensitivity of the method in order to distinguish patients from normal is 100%. The specificity in distinguishing SSc from PRP is 95%.

Q clearly highlights the difference between PRP, SSc, and between and normal subjects. It provides useful information about the abnormalities of their thermoregulatory finger properties.

The PRP patients exhibited common features in terms of rewarming. Such behavior can be explained in terms of an equally low and constant BF in all fingers and to differences in the amount of heat exchanged with the environment [25].

Conversely, no common behavior was found for the SSc patients, since their disease determines—for each finger—very different thermal and blood perfusion properties. Scleroderma seems to increase the tissue thermal capacity with a reduced ability to exchange. As calculated from the rewarming curves, the Q parameter seems to be particularly effective to describe the thermal recovery capabilities of the finger. The method clearly highlighted the difference between PRP and SSc patients and provides useful information about the abnormalities of their thermal and thermoregulatory finger properties.

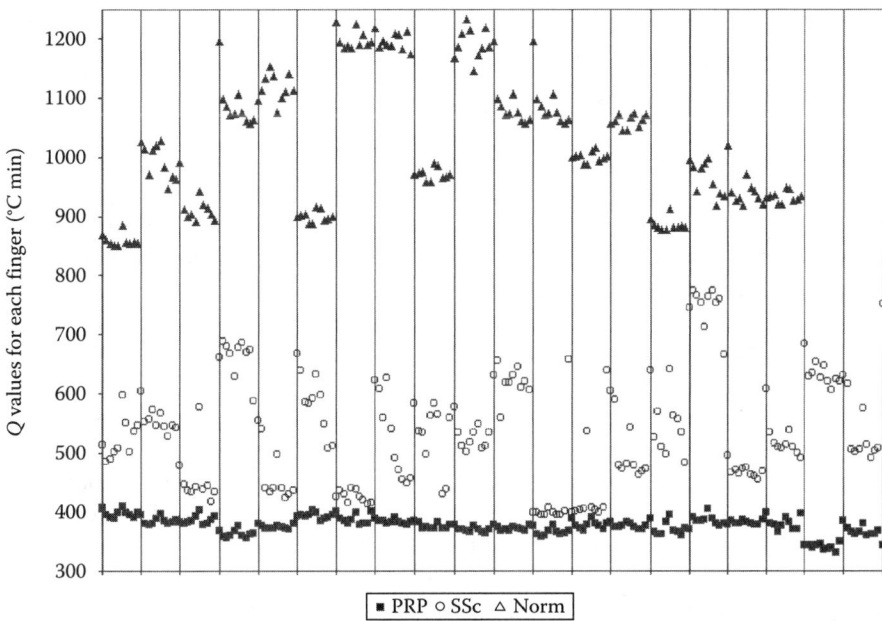

FIGURE 41.4 *Q* values calculated for each finger of each subject. Vertical grid lines are placed to discriminate the 10 fingers. PRP fingers are characterized by a strong intra- and interindividual homogeneity. Greater mean *Q* values and greater intra- and interindividual variations characterize the SSc fingers. (From Merla, A. et al., Infrared functional imaging applied to Raynaud's phenomenon, *IEEE Eng. Med. Biol. Mag.*, 21, 73, 2002, by permission of the editor.)

In consideration of the generally accepted theory that the different recovery curves of the patients is a reflection of the slow deterioration of the microcirculation, so that over time in the same patients it is possible to observe changes in the thermal recovery curves, the method described above could be used to monitor the clinical evolution of the disease. In addition, pharmacological treatment effects could be advantageously followed up.

The contribution that functional IR imaging may provide to the clinicians also regards other body regions potentially affected by scleroderma, especially in the systemic sclerosis form [20]. Men with systemic sclerosis (SSc) present an increased risk of developing erectile dysfunction (ED). In a recent study, Merla et al. [20] evaluated the extent of penile vascular damage in sclerodermic patients using Duplex ultrasonography.

The aim of that study was to investigate whether there exist penile thermal differences among sclerodermic patients and healthy controls. For this reason 10 men with systemic sclerosis under current treatment for their disease and 10 healthy controls were enrolled; penile thermal properties were assessed functional IR. Erectile function was evaluated using the sexual health inventory for men (SHIM) questionnaire [27]. The SHIM results confirmed the presence of ED in sclerodermic patients. Baseline penile temperature in patients (32.1 ± 1.4°C) was lower than in controls (34.1 ± 0.9°C). Recovery from cooling test was seen to be faster in healthy controls than in patients, both in terms of recovery amplitude (patients 3.75 ± 2.09°C, controls 9.80 ± 2.77°C) and amplitude to time constant ratio (patients 1.21 ± 0.64°C/min, controls 1.96 ± 0.48°C/min).

The results indicated that penile thermal abnormalities occur in almost all sclerodermic patients. Noncontact thermal imaging not only identifies thermal alterations but also clearly distinguishes between SSc patients and healthy controls and therefore could represent a valuable instrument in identifying early ED in systemic sclerosis patients.

41.4 Comparison of Functional IR and Laser Doppler Imaging in Assessment of Cutaneous Perfusion in Healthy Controls and Scleroderma Patients

In recent years, laser Doppler imaging (LDI) has been widely used to quantify microvascular flow and to provide a flux map showing possible microcirculatory defects [2,3,5,11,28]. It is based on the laser Doppler technique that measures blood flow in very small blood vessels of the microvascular network, such as low-speed flows associated with nutritional blood flow in capillaries close to the skin surface and in the underlying arterioles and venules involved in skin temperature regulation. LDI also permits the noninvasive assessment of modifications in cutaneous blood flow (CBF). In fact, although the flow signals are generated by the movement of blood cells (the blood cell flux), it has been demonstrated that relative changes in CBF can be monitored as well [2].

The term commonly used to describe blood flow measured by the laser Doppler technique is "flux": a quantity proportional to the product of the average speed of the blood cells and their numerical concentration (often referred to as blood volume). This is expressed in arbitrary "perfusion units." Standardization of LDI instrument measurements in perfusion units can be achieved by measuring a flux due to the Brownian motion of polystyrene microspheres in water [3].

Temperature measurement is widely used as an indirect assessment of cutaneous circulation. Spatial distribution and time-course of the cutaneous temperature (T_c) can be effectively obtained by means of thermal infrared imaging (IR), that can be then used for the indirect assessment of possible impairments of cutaneous microvasculature or tissues [16,17].

Few studies quantitatively compare CBF and T_c. Bornmyr et al. [2] studied the interrelation between changes in skin temperature (measured by means of contact probes) and changes in blood flow (measured by laser Doppler techniques) in healthy volunteers' feet. The main findings indicated an exponential interrelation between laser Doppler flowmetry and temperature readings, and that relative changes in LDI and temperatures showed a weak linear relationship. Clark et al. [5] compared IR thermography and LDI in the assessment of digital blood flow in subjects with RP. They found a poor correlation between the outcomes obtained with the two techniques and they concluded that one technique cannot substitute the other.

However, CBF is just one of the factors concurring in determining the actual T_c values, as the latter also depend on the tissue metabolism, heat exchange with surrounding tissue and environment, and local thermophysical properties. Therefore, a direct relationship between CBF and T_c may not be observable, especially in the presence of tissue pathologies.

Bio-heat transfer models permit the calculation of CBF from high-resolution IR image series (9). A major advantage for computing CBF from thermal imagery is that CBF images can be obtained at approximately the same frame rate as thermal imaging (up to 100 complete 524×524 pixels images per second using the most advanced commercially available thermal cameras), thus overcoming one of the main limits for LDI, that is low time resolution. In any case, quantitative comparison between LDI-measured CBF values and CBF values obtained from thermal imagery has not been previously evaluated.

In a recent study Merla et al. [21] compared CBF obtained from thermal imagery and CBF measured with LDI in order to verify whether combined LDI and thermal imaging provide useful and effective diagnostic information concerning tissue and/or microvascular impairment. Therefore, the comparison was extended to both healthy subjects and patients suffering from systemic sclerosis.

The model adopted derives from previous works of Fujimasa [8] and Pavlidis [24]. At thermal equilibrium (i.e., stationary state), the heat balance equation for cutaneous tissue can be expressed as

$$Q_r + Q_e + Q_f = Q_c + Q_m + Q_b \tag{41.5}$$

where Q_r is the heat radiated from the skin to air; Q_e is the basic evaporated heat; Q_f is the heat loss via convection to the neighboring air; Q_c is the heat conducted by subcutaneous tissue; Q_m is the heat generated by tissue metabolism; and Q_b is the heat gain/loss via convection attributable to blood flow of subcutaneous blood vessels.

According to Pavlidis and Levine [24], cutaneous temperature change (ΔT_c) over a short time period (Δt) is expressed by the following equation:

$$C\Delta T_c \cong (\Delta Q_c + \Delta Q_b) \tag{41.6}$$

where C is the heat capacity of the cutaneous tissue and the terms ΔQ_b and ΔQ_c are defined as

$$\Delta Q_b = \alpha C_b \cdot S \cdot [\omega_{c2}(T_b - T_{c2}) - \omega_{c1}(T_b - T_{c1})] \tag{41.7}$$

and

$$\Delta Q_c = (K_c/3d) \cdot [(T_b - T_{c2}) - (T_b - T_{c1})] \tag{41.8}$$

where α is the countercurrent heat exchange coefficient in normal condition; C_b is the heat capacity of blood; S is the thickness of the skin; ω_{ci}, with $i = 1,2$ is the cutaneous blood flow rate at times t_1 and t_2; T_b is the blood temperature in the core; T_{ci}, with $i = 1,2$ is the cutaneous temperature at times t_1 and t_2; K_c is the thermal conductivity of the skin; and d is the depth of the core temperature point from the cutaneous surface.

Equation 41.6 can be then solved using numerical methods to compute the time derivative of the blood flow rate ω_c according to the following equation:

$$d\omega_c/dt = [\psi/(T_b T_c)^2]dT_c/dt \tag{41.9}$$

where Ψ is a constant acting like a scale factor and it is given by

$$\psi = C - (K_c/3d) \tag{41.10}$$

The expression for $d\omega_c/dt$ can be integrated numerically twice over time to obtain an estimate for ω_c (i.e., the blood flow rate) and then the cutaneous blood flow V_c (i.e., the LDI flux equivalent):

$$V_c = V_c(\psi(C,K_c,d),c_1,c_2) \tag{41.11}$$

where c_1 and c_2 are numerical integration constants.

Given a series of thermal digital images of a region of interest, the above-described algorithm can be repeated for each pixel (x,y) of each raw thermal image of the series. Therefore, it is possible to transform raw thermal image series in blood flow image series. CBF-like images from raw thermal data (namely, IR-CBF) can thus be obtained. Such images can then be quantitatively compared to the CBF-LDI images.

Both methods, LDI and thermal imaging based, report CBF in arbitrary units. Therefore, an unknown scale factor between CBF values from LDI and thermal imaging must be introduced.

Each full hand LDI recording lasted 3 min and produced one $n \times n$ (with $n = 64$) pixels CBF image (henceforth named LDI-CBF image). In the same time period, $n + 1$ (=65) 256 × 256 pixels IR images were recorded. From this set of 65 IR images, we computed $n = 64$ IR-CBF images, as the CBF computation required a frame-by-frame time derivative. This meant that during the time interval required to obtain one full IR-CBF image, the LDI imager scanned just one row out of the $n = 64$ forming the full LDI-CBF image. Therefore, it is necessary to fuse in a single image the series of the n CBF images, opportunely resampled over time, for a meaningful comparison of IR-CBF and LDI-CBF images.

For this reason, each IR-CBF image was resampled in a $n \times n$ grid creating a new "fused" IR-CBF image where the i-th row was copied from the i-th row of the i-th image of the IR-CBF images series,

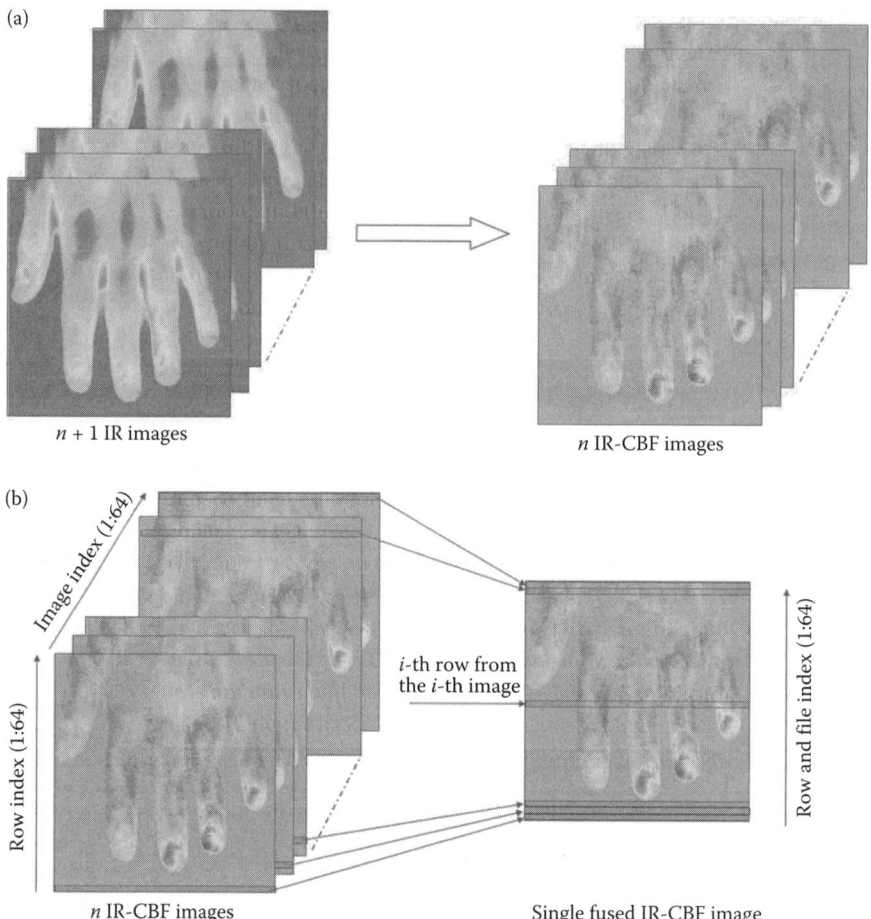

FIGURE 41.5 From the thermal IR images series to the IR-CBF image. (a) The series of $n + 1$ IR images is converted into a series of n IR-CBF images by applying the proposed bio-heat model. (b) The series of n IR-CBF images is then condensed in a single IR-CBF image. Each i-th row of the IR-CBF image is obtained by pasting the i-th row ($i = 1:64$) of the i-th image ($i = 1:64$) of the IR-CBF image series. In this way, each row out of the 64 rows of the final and single IR-CBF image is synchronous with the corresponding row out of the 64 ones in the LDI-IR image.

with I ranging from 1 to n (Figure 41.5). Therefore, each row of the final IR-CBF image and of the LDI-CBF image resulted synchronized over time and a meaningful quantitative comparison between the same regions of interest could be possible.

In order to quantitatively compare the CBF estimated by the two methods, after having performed skin segmentation, the mean CBF value for each LDI and IR-CBF image, namely V_{LDI} and V_{IR}, respectively, were computed. Correlation between V_{LDI} and V_{IR} values was assessed through Pearson product moment correlation.

Figure 41.5 shows the IR-CBF image obtained from a series of thermal images for a healthy subject. Figure 41.6 shows an example of IR-CBF and LDI-CBF images reporting, in arbitrary units, the map of the cutaneous perfusion for a representative subject. Figure 41.7 shows the scatter plots of the mean values of the cutaneous perfusion obtained with the two methods for the two groups. While a linear correlation between perfusion values obtained through the two methods was found for the healthy group ($V_{IR} = \alpha \cdot V_{LDI} + \beta$, $R = 0.85$, $\alpha = 0.35$, and $\beta = 0.06$), a correlation among V_{LDI} and V_{IR} values for

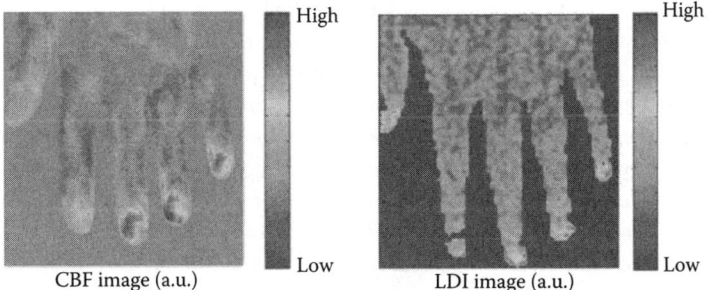

CBF image (a.u.) LDI image (a.u.)

FIGURE 41.6 CBF images (in arbitrary units) obtained with the proposed method (upper panel, IR-CBF) and recorded with LDI imager (lower panel). Color bar reports false-color visualization of the perfusion distribution. The overall distributions appear to be consistent, both images similarly showing the same high-perfusion and low-perfusion regions.

the SSc group was not observed. The lacking of correlation indicates that the bio-heat transfer exchanges among microvasculature and cutaneous tissues are altered in presence of SSc. Therefore, normal bio-heat transfer models do not apply for SSc.

According to Equation 41.11, actual V_{IR} values depended on local skin thermal conductivity K, depth of core temperature point from cutaneous surface d, and tissue heat capacity C. Such parameters are lumped together in the Ψ value (see Equation 41.10) that played the role of a scale factor with respect to the unknown absolute perfusion value.

Absolute perfusion values from thermal imaging can be obtained only by adopting realistic models of heat exchanges at cutaneous and subcutaneous levels, and taking into account the specific microvasculature geometry. This would also require an *in vivo* estimation of the heat capacity of blood and tissues and the quantification of countercurrent heat exchanges between arterioles, veins, and capillaries.

With reference to the comparison of the two methods, it must to be pointed out that both methods assume that all of the relevant thermophysical features for estimating perfusion values did not change

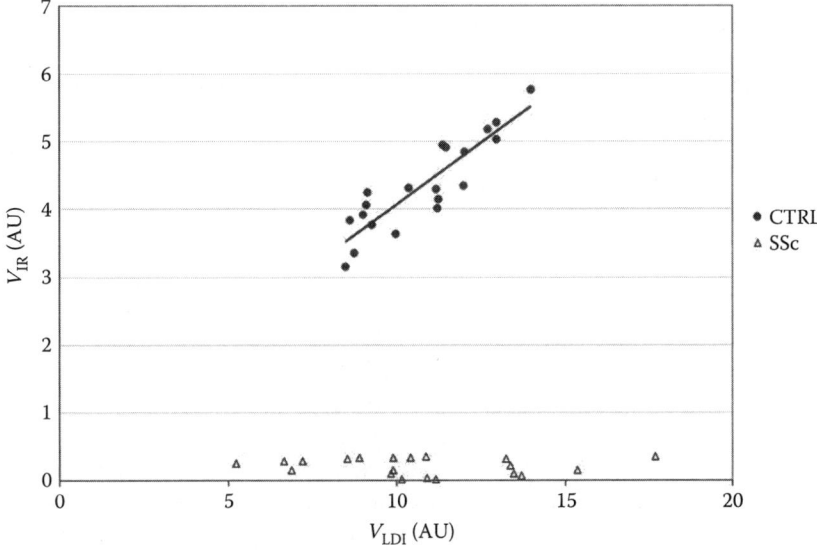

FIGURE 41.7 V_{IR} versus V_{LDI} scatter plot with regression line. Measures are reported in arbitrary units. V_{IR} and V_{LDI} are linearly correlated ($V_{IR} = 0.35V_{LDI} + 0.06$; $R = 0.85$) for the healthy group, but not for the SSc.

among individuals. Such an assumption was correct for the healthy controls group, but it may not have been in the presence of ailments involving cutaneous tissue or cutaneous microvasculature, as is the case of scleroderma. In fact, V_{IR} and V_{LDI} values correlated positively for the healthy controls group. Therefore, in spite of the fact that *in vivo* values of the bio-heat parameters remains unknown, the bio-heat transfer model itself and the assumptions made for computing CBF from thermal IR data appeared to be well-sounded. The proportionality constant α between V_{IR} and V_{LDI} values depends on the normalization factors and the actual choice for the parameters involved in the bio-heat model. Such a constant could be regarded as a conversion factor between the output of the two methods.

The parameter β indicated that zero V_{LDI} readings did not correspond to zero V_{IR} value. Therefore, β could be regarded as a tuning factor of the bio-heat model parameters to achieve the perfect agreement between the readings of the two methods. Also, it could represent the parametric error associated to the bio-heat model.

Interestingly, the bio-heat model failed when applied to the SSc group. This fact suggests that the model parameters, that had been calibrated for normal conditions, does not apply in the presence of a pathology, as the thermophysical properties of the tissue and microvasculature are altered by the morphofunctional changes induced by the disease itself. In fact, SSc determines a global skin tissue rearrangement, which is characterized by decreased capillary density, interstitial edema, especially in the early stage of inflammation, and extracellular matrix deposition. These modifications may lead to local or global thermophysical parameters changes as, for example, an increase of the local tissue thermal capacity due to the local blood flow decrease and to a concomitant increase of water content of the interstitial tissue.

The thermal imaging-based method provided faster and better time-resolved imaging of cutaneous perfusion than standard laser Doppler techniques as thermal cameras can provide up to 100 full 524×524 pixels images per second, thus allowing real-time monitoring of tissue perfusion rate.

The results reported hereby suggest that combined bio-heat models and thermal imaging data may provide accurate and fast assessment of the cutaneous tissue perfusion rate and flow. Also, they suggest that combined LDI and thermal imaging may allow an effective discrimination between healthy versus impaired cutaneous tissue thermal properties and cutaneous vasculature, thus providing a potential effective imaging-based tool for a variety of biomedical and clinical applications, ranging from diagnostics to the follow-up of treatments.

41.5 Discussion and Conclusion

fIR imaging is a biomedical imaging technique that relies on high-resolution infrared imaging and on the modeling of the heat exchange and control processes at the skin layer. fIR imaging is aimed to provide quantitative diagnostic parameters through the functional investigation of the thermoregulatory processes. It is also aimed to provide further information about the studied disease to the physicians, like explanation of the possible physics reasons of some thermal behaviors and their relationships with the physiology of the involved processes. One of the great advantages of fIR imaging is the fact that is not invasive and it is a touchless imaging technique. fIR is not a static imaging investigation technique. Therefore, data for fIR imaging need to be processed adequately for movement. Adequate bio-heat modeling is also required. The medical fields for possible applications of fIR imaging are numerous, ranging from those described in this chapter, to psychometrics, cutaneous blood flow modeling, peripheral nervous system activity, and some angiopathies. The applications described in this chapter show that fIR imaging provides highly effective diagnostic parameters. The method is highly sensitive, but also highly specific in discriminating different conditions of the same disease. For the studies reported hereby, fIR imaging is sensitive and specific as the corresponding golden standard techniques, at least. In some cases, fIR represents a useful follow-up tool (like in varicocelectomy to promptly assess possible relapses) or even an elective diagnostic tool, as in the RP. More advantages from this technique may come from advancement and development in bio-heat transfer processes modeling.

References

1. Allen, E.V. and Brown, G.E., Raynaud's disease: A critical review of minimal requisites for diagnosis, *Am. J. Med. Sci.*, 183,187, 1932.

2. Bornmyr, S., Svensson, H., Lilja, B., Sundkvist, G. Skin temperature changes and changes in skin blood flow monitored with laser Doppler flowmetry and imaging: A methodological study in normal humans. *Clin. Physiol.*, 17, 71–81, 1997.

3. Briers, J.D. Laser Doppler, speckle and related techniques for blood perfusion mapping and imaging. *Physiol. Meas.*, 22, R35–R66, 2001.

4. Clarks, S. et al., The distal-dorsal difference as a possible predictor of secondary Raynaud's phenomenon, *J. Rheumatol.*, 26, 1125, 1999.

5. Clark, S. et al., Laser Doppler imaging—A new technique for quantifying microcirculatory flow in patients with primary Raynaud's phenomenon and systemic sclerosis. *Microvasc. Res.*, 57, 284–291, 1999.

6. Clark S. et al., Comparison of thermography and laser Doppler imaging in the assessment of Raynaud's phenomenon. *Microvasc. Res.*, 66, 73–76, 2003.

7. Del Bianco et al., Raynaud's phenomenon (primary or secondary to systemic sclerosis). The usefulness of laser-Doppler flowmetry in the diagnosis. *Int. Angiol.*, 20, 307–313, 2001.

8. Fujimasa, I., Chinzei, T., Saito, I. Converting far infrared image information to other physiological data. *IEEE Eng. Med. Biol. Mag.*, 19, 71–76, 2000.

9. Guiducci, S., Giacomelli, R., Cerinic, M.M., Vascular complications of scleroderma. *Autoimmun. Rev.*, 6, 520–23, 2007.

10. Herrick, A.L. and Clark, S., Quantifying digital vascular disease in patients with primary Raynaud's phenomenon and systemic sclerosis, *Ann. Rheum. Dis.*, 57, 70, 1998.

11. Herron, G.S., Romero, L. Vascular abnormalities in scleroderma. *Semin. Cutan. Med. Surg.*, 17(1), 12–17, 1998.

12. Javanetti, S. et al., Thermography and nailfold capillaroscopy as noninvasive measures of circulation in children with Raynaud's phenomenon. *J. Rheumatol.*, 25, 997, 1998.

13. Merla, A., Ledda, A., Di Donato, L., Romani, G.L., Assessment of the effects of the varicocelectomy on the thermoregulatory control of the scrotum. *Fertil. Steril.*, 81, 471, 2004.

14. Merla, A. and Romani, G. L. Functional infrared imaging in clinical applications, in *The Biomedical Engineering Handbook*, ed., J.D. Bronzino, CRC Press, Boca Raton, FL, 32.1–32.13, 2006.

15. Merla, A. et al., Dynamic digital telethermography: A novel approach to the diagnosis of varicocele, *Med. Biol. Eng. Comp.*, 37, 1080, 1999.

16. Merla, A. et al., Infrared functional imaging applied to Raynaud's phenomenon. *IEEE Eng. Med. Biol. Mag.*, 21, 73, 2002.

17. Merla, A. et al., Quantifying the relevance and stage of disease with the Tau image technique. *IEEE Eng. Med. Biol. Mag.*, 21, 86, 2002.

18. Merla, A. et al., Raynaud's phenomenon: Infrared functional imaging applied to diagnosis and drugs effects. *Int. J. Immun. Pharm.*, 15, 41, 2002.

19. Merla, A. et al., Use of infrared functional imaging to detect impaired thermoregulatory control in men with asymptomatic varicocele. *Fertil. Steril.*, 78, 199, 2002.

20. Merla, A. et al., Penile cutaneous temperature in systemic sclerosis: A thermal imaging study. *Int. J. Immunopathol. Pharmacol.*, 20(1):139–44, 2007.

21. Merla, A. et al., Comparison of thermal infrared and laser Doppler imaging in the assessment of cutaneous tissue perfusion in scleroderma patients and healthy controls. *Int. J. Immunopathol. Pharmacol.*, 21(3), 679–86, 2008.

22. Mieusset, R. and Bujan, L., Testicular heating and its possible contributions to male infertility: A review. *Int. J. Andr.*, 18,169, 1995.

23. O'Reilly, D. et al., Measurement of cold challenge response in primary Raynaud's phenomenon and Raynaud's phenomenon associated with systemic sclerosis. *Ann. Rheum. Dis.*, 51, 1193, 1992.
24. Pavlidis, I. and Levine, J. Thermal image analysis for polygraph testing. *IEEE Eng. Med. Biol. Mag.*, 21, 56–64, 2002.
25. Prescott et al., Sequential dermal microvascular and perivascular changes in the development of scleroderma, *J. Pathol.*, 166, 255, 1992.
26. Ring, E.F.J., Cold stress test for the hands. in *The Thermal Image in Medicine and Biology*, Ammer, K. and Ring, E. F. G., ed., Uhlen Verlag, Wien, 1995.
27. Rosen, R.C. et al., The International Index of Erectile Function (IIEF): A multidimensional scale for assessment of erectile dysfunction. *Urology*, 49, 822, 1997.
28. Salsano, F. et al., Significant changes of peripheral perfusion and plasma adrenomedullin levels in *N*-acetylcysteine long term treatment of patients with sclerodermic Raynauds phenomenon. *Int. J. Immunopathol. Pharmacol.*, 18, 761–70, 2005.
29. Schuhfried, O. et al., Thermographic parameters in the diagnosis of secondary Raynaud's phenomenon, *Arch. Phys. Med. Rehabil.*, 81, 495, 2000.
30. Subcommittee for Scleroderma Criteria of the American Rheumatism Association Diagnostic and Therapeutic Criteria Committee, Preliminary criteria for the classification of systemic sclerosis (scleroderma). *Arthritis Rheum.*, 23, 581, 1980.
31. Tucker, A., Infrared thermographic assessment of the human scrotum. *Fertil. Steril.*, 74, 802, 2000.

42

Modeling Infrared Imaging Data for the Assessment of Functional Impairment in Thermoregulatory Processes

Alessandro Mariotti
G. d'Annunzio University

Arcangelo Merla
University of Chieti-Pescara

42.1 Introduction

Infrared imaging permits the study of cutaneous thermoregulation through its capability of accurate recording of the cutaneous temperature dynamics. Such a dynamics depends on the complex heat exchange processes between cutaneous tissue, inner tissue, local vasculature, and metabolic activity, all of these processes being mediated and regulated by the sympathetic and parasympathetic activity. The main function of such processes is to preserve the homeostasis. The presence of a disease alters this heat exchange processes, with respect to the corresponding healthy condition, resulting in an increase or in a decrease of the cutaneous temperature and in an alteration of local thermoregulation. The characteristic parameters modeling the activity of the cutaneous thermoregulatory system can be used as diagnostic parameters, thus increasing the diagnostic specificity of the technique.

While fine *in vivo* modeling of the heat exchange processes is indeed extremely complex, the mathematical theory of the control system offers easy-to-manage tools for modeling feedback processes, which are the basis of homeostatic controls. These tools are often used in bioengineering to model biological functions as in the devices for automatic glucose control or pace maker. Very few studies combining thermal imaging data and automatic system control theory are available. In this chapter, we provide examples of such an approach for two important pathologies: Raynaud's phenomenon and varicocele.

42.2 Modeling and Assessment of Thermoregulatory Impairment in Raynaud's Phenomenon and Scleroderma

Raynaud's phenomenon (RP) is a paroxysmal vasospastic disorder of small arteries, precapillary arteries, and cutaneous arteriovenous shunts of the extremities. RP is typically induced by cold exposure and emotional stress [3]. The main clinical signature of RP is cutaneous triphasic color changes: well-demarcated pallor due to a sudden vasospasm, cyanotic phase secondary to local hemoglobin desaturation, and then red flush caused by reactive hyperemia. RP usually involves fingers and toes, even though tongue, nose, ears, and nipples may also be involved. The presence of the initial ischemic phase is mandatory for diagnosis, whereas the reactive hyperemic phase may not occur.

RP can be classified as *primary* (PRP), with no identifiable underlying pathological disorder, and *secondary*, usually associated with a connective tissue disease, use of certain drugs, or exposition to toxic agents [16]. Secondary RP is frequently associated with systemic sclerosis. In this case, RP typically may precede the onset of other symptoms and signs of disease by several years [2]. While PRP is generally characterized by an abnormal vasospastic response in the absence of specific structural abnormalities, RP secondary to systemic sclerosis is characterized by a peculiar rearrangement of the microvascular structures [20,38].

It has been estimated that 12.6% of patients suffering from primary RP develop a secondary disease. In particular, 5–20% of subjects suffering from secondary RP will develop either limited or diffuse systemic sclerosis [45]. On the other hand, all of the systemic sclerosis subjects (SSc) will experience episodes of RP. This indicates the importance of early and proper differential diagnosis.

IR imaging is a noninvasive technique which provides a map of the superficial temperature of a given body by measuring emitted infrared energy [24,28]. Several IR imaging studies have been performed to differentiate primary from secondary RP, often in combination with the monitoring of the finger thermoregulatory response to a controlled cold challenge [6,8,15,17,24,31].

Cutaneous circulation is a major effector of finger thermoregulation [18]. Exposure to cold stress elicits generalized cutaneous vasoconstriction, which may be extremely pronounced at the fingertip surface. Cutaneous vasoconstriction is a response mediated by a sympathetic control process triggered partly by stimulation of the cutaneous cold receptors in the cooled area, and partly by cooled blood returning to the general circulation, which stimulates the temperature-regulating center in the anterior hypothalamus [39,42]. Homeostasis is basically maintained by a negative feedback loop, similar to a thermostat [34], which regulates the energy exchange with the environment at the cutaneous level through metabolic and hemodynamic processes that determine finger temperature at any given time [37]. Employing control system theory, the homeostatic process can be seen as a feedback-controlled system. This kind of system considers a reference signal (i.e., prestress finger temperature) to produce the desired output (i.e., the actual finger temperature). A cold challenge induces a finger temperature (plant-controlled output) change from the basal value (reference value). The difference between the plant-controlled output and the reference value (i.e., output error) prompts the thermoregulatory reaction in order to restore the basal value. In other words, the thermoregulatory reaction steers the output error to zero. The temperature–time evolution can be recorded by means of thermal IR imaging [24]. Examples of temperature versus time curves obtained from experimental recovery data in HCS, SSc, and PRP are reported in Figure 42.1. According to the control system theory, differences in the temperature recovery curves depend on the efficacy of the finger thermoregulatory system, which in turn can be represented by the actual values of a given set of functional modeling parameters.

The finger thermoregulatory response after the cold stress challenge is not instantaneous. The time delay from the onset of the rewarming process and the end of the cold challenge is often referred to as lag time (LT). LT in healthy controls (HCS) is usually around 4–5 min long [43], while it may vary largely in PRP and SSc (Figure 42.1). LT may depend on both physics and physiological factors such as environmental temperature, basal finger temperature, vascular smooth muscle tone,

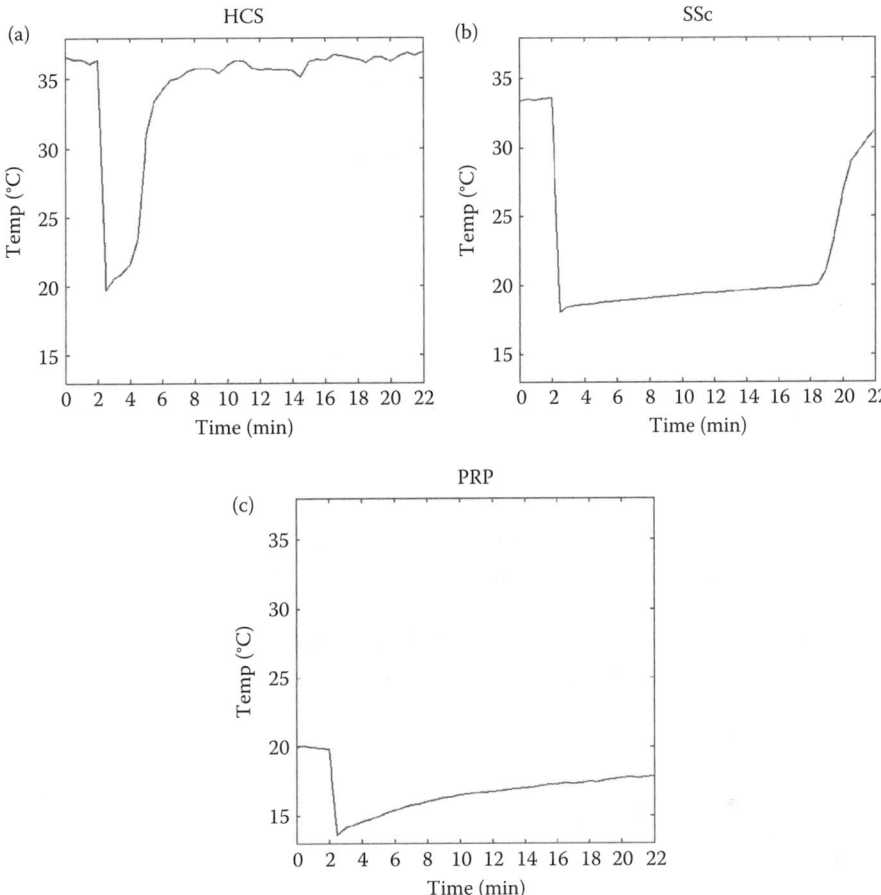

FIGURE 42.1   Temperature versus time curves obtained from thermal imaging data during cold stress test in (a) HCS, (b) SSc, and (c) PRP. (From Mariotti, A., G. Grossi, P. Amerio et al. *Ann. Biomed. Eng.* 37(12):2631–2639, 2009.)

cold-receptor efficacy, and autonomic activity. The cold challenge test activates specific responses of the thermoregulatory system, which operate at both local (i.e., peripheral) and systemic (i.e., central) levels attempting to restore the basal temperature [5]. These two levels of the thermoregulatory system can be modeled through two hierarchical control units: a higher-level unit (supervisor), and a feedback lower-level executor driven by the supervisor [1,11,46]. The supervisor sets the reference signal on the basis of the basal prestress temperature and the onset time. The overall performance of the thermoregulatory system depends on the activity of both the supervisor and the executor. Besides the contribution of the thermoregulatory system, the finger temperature (i.e., system output) is also influenced by the thermal exchange between the finger and the surrounding environment. This thermal exchange depends on the temperature difference, which constitutes the external input to the thermoregulatory system [5,37].

Figure 42.2a shows the overall architecture of the system. The only observable output is the finger cutaneous temperature $y(t)$, obtained through thermal IR imaging. Even though no information about internal variables is available, the theory of automatic system control allows to both quantitatively and qualitatively describe the control action, on the basis of the assumption of an input/output feedback control [32]. The system is characterized by an external input (room temperature) and a

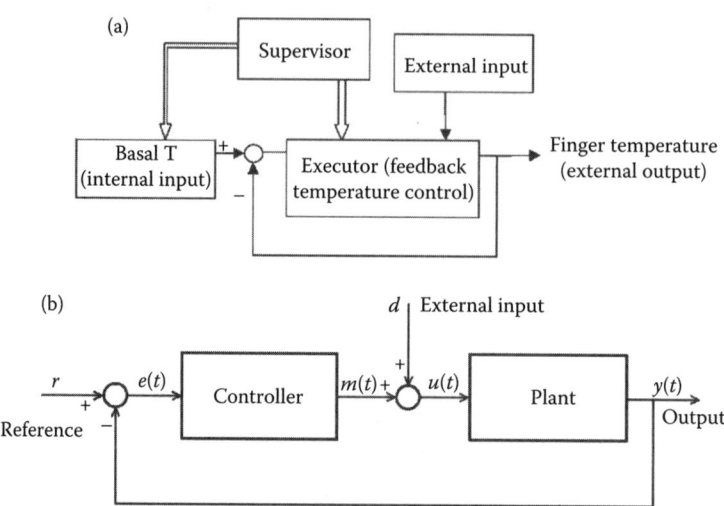

FIGURE 42.2 (a) Logical architecture of the thermoregulatory system. (b) Block diagram of executor unit. (From Mariotti, A., G. Grossi, P. Amerio et al. *Ann. Biomed. Eng.* 37(12):2631–2639, 2009.)

steady-state regime reference signal (basal finger cutaneous temperature). The reference signal can be measured by IR imaging before the exposure to the cold stress, and averaged over time to provide a constant reference value *r*. In particular, the dynamics of the thermal recovery after cold stress (Figure 42.1) classifies the system as a second-order time-invariant feedback system [35]. In particular, the feedback lower-level unit is composed of a controller and a plant block in sequence (Figure 42.2b), both assumed to be time-invariant systems described by first-order transfer functions. The theory provides the differential equation to model the plant output $y(t)$ (i.e., the finger temperature) in the time domain:

$$\dot{y}(t) = -a \cdot y(t) + b \cdot u(t) \tag{42.1}$$

where *u* is the plant input, and *a* and *b* are constant coefficients.

The cold stress stimulation directly affects the system output, lowering the cutaneous temperature. The poststress temperature $y(0)$ (i.e., the temperature measured immediately after the cessation of the cold stress) constitutes the initial condition for the response of the control system. The plant input $u(t)$ is then the sum of the feedback controller output $m(t)$ plus the additional external input *d* as shown in Figure 42.2b:

$$u(t) = m(t) + d \tag{42.2}$$

Input *d* represents passive heat exchange with the environment. Therefore, it depends on room temperature and $y(t)$. In other words, input *d* can be seen as the uncontrolled effect of environmental conditions on the finger temperature.

The feedback controller block generates the signal $m(t)$ stimulated by the difference between the system output and the reference signal *r*, namely, *output error e(t)*:

$$e(t) = r - y(t) \tag{42.3}$$

The feedback controller acts on the plant by the signal $m(t)$ to steer the *output error* to zero.

Common approaches for modeling homeostatic processes are based on an integral-type feedback controller system, which nullifies stepwise variation of the error signal [46]. The differential equation that describes the controller behavior in the time domain is

$$\dot{m}(t) = k \cdot e(t) \tag{42.4}$$

where k is a proportionality constant.

The supervisor unit activates this controller by means of logic signals (on/off transition). When the supervisor unit logical output is "on," the feedback is closed on the integral-type controller and then the active temperature recovery can start. Otherwise, when the supervisor unit logical output is "off" (during the LT), the controller is disabled to restore the initial condition, while the external input d is independent of this switching logic.

The evolution of the plant can be described more easily in the Laplace domain. The Laplace transform (L-transform) of Equation 42.1 is given by

$$Y(s) = \frac{1}{(s+a)} \cdot y(0) + \frac{b}{(s+a)} \cdot U(s) \tag{42.5}$$

where s is the Laplace variable, and $Y(s)$ and $U(s)$ are the output and input L-transforms, respectively. The ratio between plant input and output defines the plant transfer function $P(s)$, which is computed assuming null $y(0)$ [22]:

$$P(s) = \frac{Y(s)}{U(s)} = \frac{b}{(s+a)} \tag{42.6}$$

where b is the plant gain coefficient and $s = -a$ is its pole, that is, the negative reciprocal of the plant time constant.

According to Equation 42.4, the transfer function of the integral-type controller $G(s)$ is given by

$$G(s) = \frac{k}{s} \tag{42.7}$$

where k is the controller gain.

As described above and as depicted in Figure 42.3, the overall model works in open loop for $t < $ LT

$$Y(s) = P(s) \cdot d \tag{42.8}$$

and in closed loop for $t > $ LT:

$$Y(s) = \frac{G(s) \cdot P(s)}{1 + G(s) \cdot P(s)} \cdot r + \frac{P(s)}{1 + G(s) \cdot P(s)} \cdot d \tag{42.9}$$

Therefore, the model (Figure 42.3) is unequivocally described by $-a$, k, d, and LT, which can be estimated based on measurements of r and $y(t)$.

In particular, the reciprocal of the plant time constant a represents the speed of the response of the thermal process to external and internal stimuli. A low a value is indicative of a very slow recovery process. The controller gain k refers to the control action and determines the efficiency of the feedback control system in achieving the steady state, restoring the reference basal conditions. This parameter

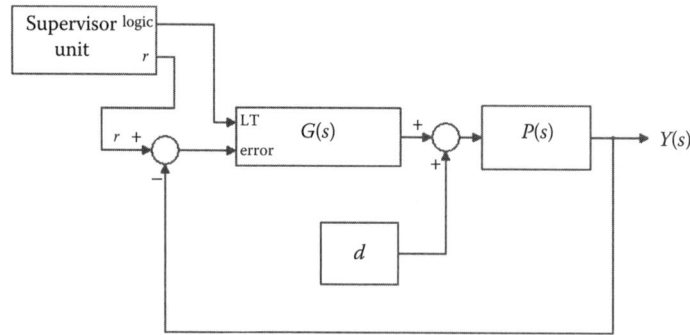

FIGURE 42.3 Thermoregulatory model block diagram for the finger. (From Mariotti, A., G. Grossi, P. Amerio et al. *Ann. Biomed. Eng.* 37(12):2631–2639, 2009.)

quantifies the power of an active and internal vasodilation process. The disturbance input d is related to the response induced by an external input, namely thermal exchange of the system with the environment. d, which is one of the fitted parameters, represents passive heat exchange with the environment, and, therefore, depends on room temperature and $y(t)$. LT is the time interval between the end of the cold stress and the onset of internal rewarming process. During this time, the thermal variations are mostly attributable to the passive heat exchange with the environment. Once LT is finished, there is the onset of the rewarming process and the controller starts to restore the reference basal conditions r.

The model was tested in a previous experimental study by Mariotti et al. [23], which can be referred to for detailed information. Fourteen SSc, 14 patients affected by PRP, and 16 HCS participated in this study. SSc and PRP patients were classified according to the criteria established in 2001 by the American College of Rheumatology [20,21,47].

For each subject, the functional response to a mild cold challenge of hands in water was assessed by functional IR imaging [23,24]. Thermal IR imaging was performed by means of a digital thermal camera (FLIR SC3000, FlirSystems, Sweden), with a Focal Plane Array of 320×240 QWIP detectors, capable of collecting the thermal radiation in the 8–9 μm band, with a 0.02 s time resolution, and 0.02 K temperature sensitivity. Cutaneous emissivity was estimated as $\varepsilon \approx 0.98$. The thermal camera response was blackbody-calibrated to null noise effects related to the sensor drift/shift dynamics and optical artifacts. Thermal images of the dorsum of each subject's hands were recorded. Recording was performed for 25 min, acquiring images every 30 s, and recording five thermal images before the cold stress to obtain the baseline of finger temperature. The thermal camera was placed 1.5 m away from the dorsum. Each image series was corrected for motion artifacts by means of a contour alignment algorithm. The cold stress was achieved by immersing the hands (protected from getting wet by thin, disposable latex gloves) for 3 min in a 3-L water bath maintained at 10°C. After removal of the gloves, the hands were placed in the same position as before the cold stress. Rewarming curves were obtained for each of the five fingertips of both hands, by averaging the temperature of the pixels within the nail-bed region.

For data and graphic analysis, a self-implemented software was used under a MATLAB® platform (www.themathworks.com). The control model was implemented using the Matlab Simulink Graphical User Interface®. The model parameters (a, k, d, and LT) were computed and optimized through the Matlab Simulink Parameter Estimation Toolbox®, by using a nonlinear least square algorithm, while r and $y(t)$ were directly measured by fIRI. Thermoregulation model responses were simulated by the variable-step ODE45 (Dormand-Price) solver. The distributions of the averaged parameters for each class of subjects were tested for normality by visual inspection of the frequency distribution and Shapiro–Wilk test, and then compared through a Student's t-test (STATISTICA, www.statsoft.it). The level of statistical significance was fixed at 0.01.

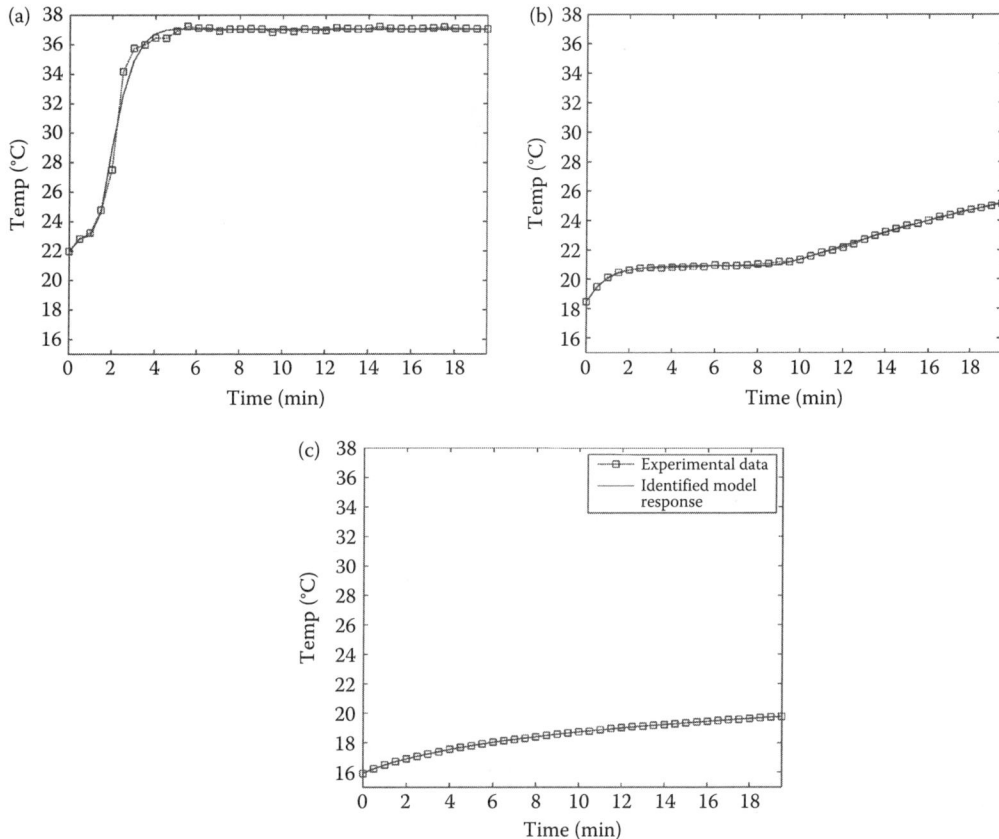

FIGURE 42.4 Comparison between experimental data and identified model response, for (a) HCS, (b) SSc, and (c) PRP. (From Mariotti, A., G. Grossi, P. Amerio et al. *Ann. Biomed. Eng.* 37(12):2631–2639, 2009.)

Figure 42.4 shows an example of the comparison between the identified response and the experimental temperature curves for three representative subjects randomly chosen, from HCS, SSc, and PRP groups. Mean and confidence interval for each parameter are reported in Figure 42.5. The mean values of k and a resulted statistically different in the three groups. The PRP group presented the lowest a and k values, with the lowest interindividual variability. The HCS group was instead characterized by the highest values for both parameters, with the largest interindividual variability for only the k parameter. SSc presented intermediate average values for both parameters and the highest variability with respect to the mean a value. d appeared to clearly discriminate PRP from SSc and HCS. The PRP group presented the highest average for d while the SSc and HCS groups showed lower values, without statistically significant intergroup differences. The LT parameter distinguished SSc from the other two groups, with the highest value. HCS and PRP presented very similar LT values. Mean values of r appeared to replicate the same behavior as the a parameter.

HCS parameters indicate that healthy thermoregulatory systems are fast and efficient in reestablishing the reference basal conditions. High a and k values are suggestive of fast and efficient control over vasomotor and metabolic processes. This observation is in agreement with the fact that the steady-state basal temperature, r, is the highest. HCS d values indicate that the system is driven less by heat exchange with the surrounding environment and dominated more by active temperature control through the controller unit. HCS LT values are the smallest, indicating a prompt reaction of the

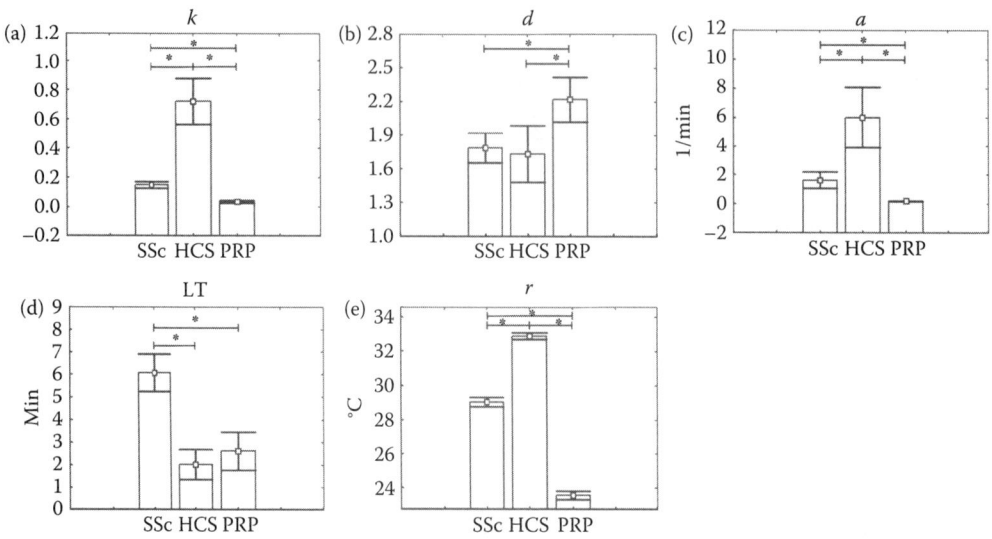

FIGURE 42.5 Comparison of model parameters among groups (Whisker Box plot) Mean and 95% confidence interval are reported for each parameter (a–e). The asterisks on the horizontal bars specify the groups with significant statistical difference. (From Mariotti, A., G. Grossi, P. Amerio et al. *Ann. Biomed. Eng.* 37(12):2631–2639, 2009.)

thermoregulatory process to the thermal stimuli. LT values in SSc indicated that the onset of the active control was strongly delayed in comparison to both HCS and PRP. SSc rewarming processes are slower than HCS, with the controllers less effective in achieving the steady state. In fact, for several fingers in several cases, SSc were not able to restore the reference basal conditions within the poststress monitoring time. The variability of *a* and *k* values in SSc was high even within the fingers of the same hand, which may be linked to variable structural and functional vascular changes at different stages of scleroderma in each finger. Systemic sclerosis is a generalized connective tissue disease, which is pathologically characterized by microvascular injury and immune activation, resulting in increased synthesis of extracellular matrix components, including collagen, fibronectin, and proteoglycans, cutaneously and viscerally. Interstitial fibrosis and occlusive microvascular damage induce a progressive decrease of capillary density [7]. These structural alterations lead to a reduction in cutaneous blood flow with increased periods of stasis. The estimated LT values for the PRP group were similar to HCS, indicating a proper onset of active recovery. The efficiency of the controller, however, was extremely weak, almost negligible. In fact, PRP fingers had the slowest and weakest recovery, as indicated by *a* and *k* values. All PRP fingers exhibited a very similar rewarming pattern, never able to restore the reference basal conditions during the monitoring time. PRP *d* values were the highest with low controller gain levels indicating that heat exchange with the environment dominated the thermal recovery process. This observation is in agreement with previous fIR imaging studies which reported homogeneous digital thermal behavior for PRP fingers in response to cold stress [24], which may be related to the hypothesis that in PRP subjects an excessive vasoconstrictor tone and a weak systemic vasodilation process, both centrally mediated, do not allow an active thermal recovery [15].

Experimental result from Mariotti et al. [23] and those reported in the literature prove that SSc, HCS, and PRP exhibit different thermoregulatory responses to the standardized external stimuli, administered in strictly controlled environmental conditions. These different responses appear to be due to pathological functional and morphological alterations at the local or central level. The goal of this chapter was to identify a feedback thermoregulatory model to describe and to distinguish the functional differences in the recoveries, at both central and peripheral levels. In fact, the parameters so far identified to define each model describe how the system acts at the two different levels, in terms of process speed, efficiency of control action, and heat exchanges mechanisms, in order to restore the prestress basal conditions. Several advantages may be derived from this approach. The estimated model parameter values for each subject can aid in estimating the level of functional impairment expressed in the different forms of the disease. Thus, it is possible to more effectively monitor both the evolution of the disease and the efficacy of the treatment and its follow-up. The application of this control system theory model to SSc and primary RP diagnosis would also help to treat the causes of different conditions appropriately. In future studies, the proposed approach could be applied to distinguish additional expressions or causes of secondary RP such as limited or diffused scleroderma, lupus, or other prompting factors of the syndrome.

42.3 Scrotal Thermoregulatory Model Assessing Functional Impairment in Varicocele

In healthy men, testicular temperature is 3–4°C lower than the core body temperature. Two main thermoregulatory processes control testicular temperature: heat exchange with the environment through the scrotum skin and heat clearance by blood flow through the pampiniform plexus. Varicocele is defined as the pathological dilatation of the pampiniform plexus and scrotal veins with venous blood reflux. It is present in 15% of the adult male population, in 35% of men with primary infertility, and in 80% of men with secondary infertility [36]. Varicocele usually affects the left hemiscrotum because of valve insufficiency and right-angled mouth of the left testicular vein into the left renal vein. The venous reflux into the testicular vein and the pampiniform plexus results in venous hyperemia leading to hyperthermia and hypoxia of testicular tissue, which may cause infertility [12,29]. The assessment of the vascular impairment is generally performed by means of echo color Doppler, while scrotal hyperthermia is usually evaluated through the measurement of the scrotal cutaneous temperature by means of thermal infrared (IR) imaging [24,26,27,30,41,46]. It has been demonstrated that alteration of the scrotal blood flow secondary to varicocele impairs scrotal thermoregulation. Patients suffering from varicocele present higher scrotal cutaneous temperature and shorter time constant to recover from mild controlled cold stress of the scrotum [26] (Figure 42.6).

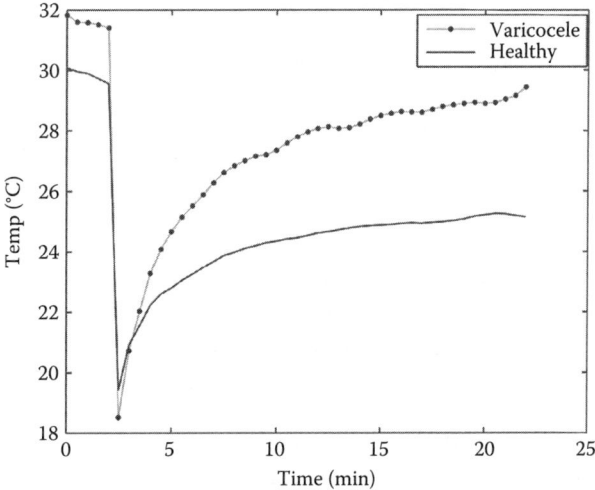

FIGURE 42.6 Cutaneous temperature versus time curves obtained from thermal imaging of the scrotum during cold stress test.

Scrotal thermoregulation serves to liberate the large amount of heat produced during spermatogenesis. A number of supporting mechanisms like thin skin with abundant vascularization, numerous sweat glands, and absence of subcutaneous fat facilitates heat exchange and contributes to maintaining the testicular temperature below body temperature [44].

Venous stasis associated with varicocele increases the cutaneous temperature of the affected testicle or pampiniform plexus [26]. Exposure to cold stress elicits cutaneous vasoconstriction, accompanied by increased skin rugosity to reduce the surface area involved in the heat exchange with the environment [39]. After the cessation of cold exposure, homeostatic processes restore basal prestress conditions, mostly through vasodilatation, favoring heat exchange with deeper layers [24]. In the presence of varicocele, affected testicles return to prestress equilibrium temperature faster than normal testicles [26]. Homeostasis is basically maintained by a negative feedback loop, similar to a thermostat [33] which regulates the energy exchange with the environment at the cutaneous level through metabolic and hemodynamic processes that determine the cutaneous temperature at any given time [37].

Experimental evidence shows that thermoregulatory response after the cold stress challenge is instantaneous. Thus, it can be assumed that the regulatory processes are activated instantaneously and simultaneously just after the cold stress, determining the actual value of the cutaneous temperature through a lumped action. From the control system theory, the basic functional components of homeostasis can be thought as arranged in a feedback loop: a controlled plant (scrotum thermal processes) whose output (cutaneous scrotum temperature) is constrained to follow a given set-point (reference basal value) through an internal feedback loop (homeostatic mechanism). The cutaneous basal temperature can be considered the reference value and assumed to be almost constant. To study the system dynamics and to evoke thermoregulatory processes that produce recovery patterns, the system has to be stimulated by a proper functional input. Namely, a cold challenge induces a scrotum cutaneous temperature (plant-controlled output) change from the basal value (reference value). In other words, the cold stress induces a variation from basal value of the controlled output. In feedback systems, the output signal is compared with the reference value generating an error signal, which stimulates the thermoregulatory control reaction in order to restore the basal value. In other words, the thermoregulatory reaction steers the error to zero.

Time evolution of scrotal temperature can be recorded by means of thermal IR imaging. Examples of temperature versus time curves obtained from experimental recovery data are reported in Figure 42.6. The temperature recovery curves can be interpreted, according to the control system theory, as the feedback system response to a perturbation of operative conditions. Differences in recovery curves depend on the capability of the control system to recover and to calibrate heat generation, thus determining internal and cutaneous temperature up to possible functional impairment associated with the presence of varicocele.

Varicocele can affect just one or both hemiscrota [29] and the only affected hemiscrotum (generally the left) presents marked alteration of thermoregulatory control [26]. In this chapter, we characterize differences in model parameters between healthy and left affected hemiscrota.

As mentioned, experimental evidence showed that scrotum thermoregulatory response after the cold stress challenge is instantaneous. Different from other body regions, the recovery patterns did not show a time delay from the onset of the rewarming process and the end of the cold challenge, often referred to as lag time (LT) [43]. The rewarming pattern after a cold challenge test was preliminarily modeled as an exponential function [25]. The cold challenge test activates specific responses of the thermoregulatory system, which operate at both local (i.e., peripheral) and systemic (i.e., central) levels, attempting to restore basal temperature [10]. These two levels are here modeled through two hierarchical control units: a high-level unit (supervisor) driving a feedback low-level executor [23]. The supervisor sets the reference signal on the basis of the basal prestress temperature. Albeit the overall performance of the thermoregulatory system is also affected by the surrounding environment, the speed of rewarming and the hemiscrotum temperature at the end of recovery allows the neglect of the thermal exchange with the environment with respect to thermoregulatory system contribution.

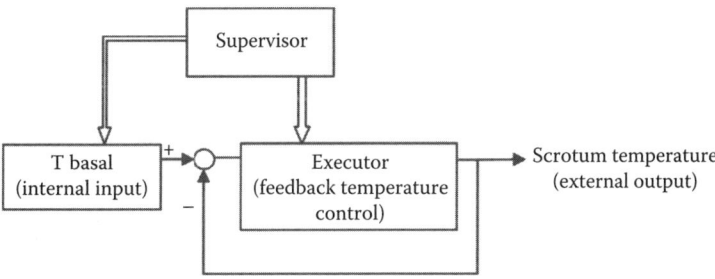

FIGURE 42.7 Logical architecture of the thermoregulatory system for the scrotum.

The model adopted is very similar to the one formulated for the finger thermoregulation and described in the previous section. Figure 42.7 shows the overall architecture of the system. The only measurable output is the scrotum (i.e., hemiscrotum) cutaneous temperature $y(t)$, obtained through thermal IR imaging. The steady-state regime reference signal (basal cutaneous temperature of hemiscrotum) has been measured before the exposure to the cold stress, and time-averaged to provide a constant reference value r. The system is a second-order time-invariant feedback system [35], with the feedback lower-level unit composed of a cascaded controller and plant blocks (Figure 42.8a), both assumed to be time-invariant systems described by first-order transfer functions.

As for the previous model, the plant evolution can be described more easily in the Laplace domain. The transfer function of the controller $G(s)$ is given by

$$G(s) = \frac{k}{s} + h \tag{42.10}$$

where k is the integral controller gain, h is the gain of the proportional-type controller, and s is the Laplace variable. The model (Figure 42.9) is unequivocally described by the triple a, k, h, which can be estimated by measurements of r and $y(t)$.

The controller gain k refers to the control action and determines the efficiency of the feedback control system in achieving the steady state, restoring the reference basal conditions. This parameter quantifies the power of an active and systemic vasodilation process. h is the gain of the proportional-type controller and represents a measure of the efficiency of the thermal exchange between the cutaneous layer and

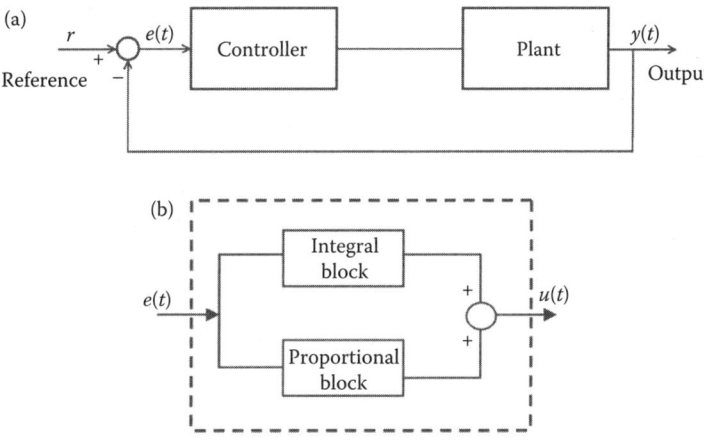

FIGURE 42.8 (a) Block diagram of executor unit. (b) Controller structure.

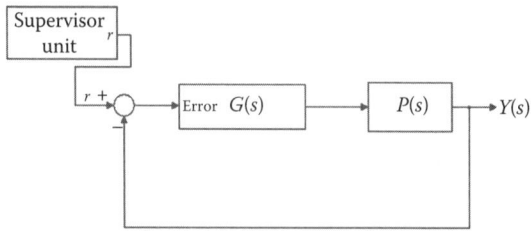

FIGURE 42.9   Thermoregulatory model block diagram for the scrotum.

the inner structures. a, the reciprocal of the plant time constant, represents the speed of the response of the thermal process to external and internal stimuli. A low a value is indicative of a slow recovery process.

The model was tested in 90 young patients (average age: 20 ± 4 years) suffering from left varicocele, and 40 healthy controls (average age: 21 ± 3 years) participated in this study. Only pure left varicoceles were included in this study to avoid possible confounding due to right or bilateral varicocele.

After clinical examination, participants underwent echo color Doppler imaging (ATL 5000 echo color Doppler imaging system, Philips Medical System, Eindhoven, The Netherlands) which is so far considered the gold standard for varicocele diagnosis.

For each subject, the functional response to a mild cold challenge of scrotum was assessed by thermal infrared imaging. All participants were asked to refrain from physical activities and intake of vasoactive substances for 2 h prior to the measurements. Participants were seated comfortably in an environment-controlled room. Before undergoing measurements, the subjects observed a 20-min acclimatization period to the recording room, which was set at standardized temperature (23°C), humidity (50–60%), and without direct ventilation. Thermal infrared imaging was performed by means of a digital thermal camera (FLIR SC3000, FlirSystems, Sweden), with a Focal Plane Array of 320×240 QWIP detectors, capable of collecting the thermal radiation in the 8–9 µm band, with a 0.02 s time resolution, and 0.02 K temperature sensitivity. Cutaneous emissivity was estimated as $\varepsilon \approx 0.98$. The thermal camera response was blackbody-calibrated to null noise effects related to the sensor drift/shift dynamics and optical artifacts. Thermal images of the scrotum of each subject were recorded for 25 min, acquiring images every 30 s. Five thermal images were recorded before the cold stress to obtain the baseline of scrotum temperature. Each image series was corrected for motion artifacts by means of a contour alignment algorithm. The cold stress was achieved by applying a dry patch to the scrotum maintained at 10°C. Rewarming curves were obtained separately for each of the two hemiscrota, by averaging the temperature of the pixels within the cutaneous projection of the testis.

For data and graphic analysis, a self-implemented software was used under MATLAB platform (www.themathworks.com). The control model was implemented using the Matlab Simulink Graphical User Interface. The model parameters (a, k, and h) were computed and optimized through the Matlab Simulink Parameter Estimation Toolbox, by using a nonlinear least square algorithm, while r and $y(t)$ were measured directly by thermal infrared imaging. Thermoregulatory model responses were simulated by the variable-step ODE45 (Dormand-Price) solver. The statistical analysis was performed to compare differences in model parameters and cutaneous temperature between healthy individuals and those affected by varicocele hemiscrota. All parameters for each group were compared through Wilcoxon–Mann–Whitney test [14].

The comparison between the identified response and the experimental temperature curves for two representative cases randomly chosen from varicocele and healthy control groups is shown in Figure 42.10. The mean and confidence interval of each parameter for each hemiscrota are reported in Figure 42.11. None of the parameters were statistically different between hemiscrota in healthy subjects. The mean values of k are not statistically different among hemiscrota, in both healthy and left

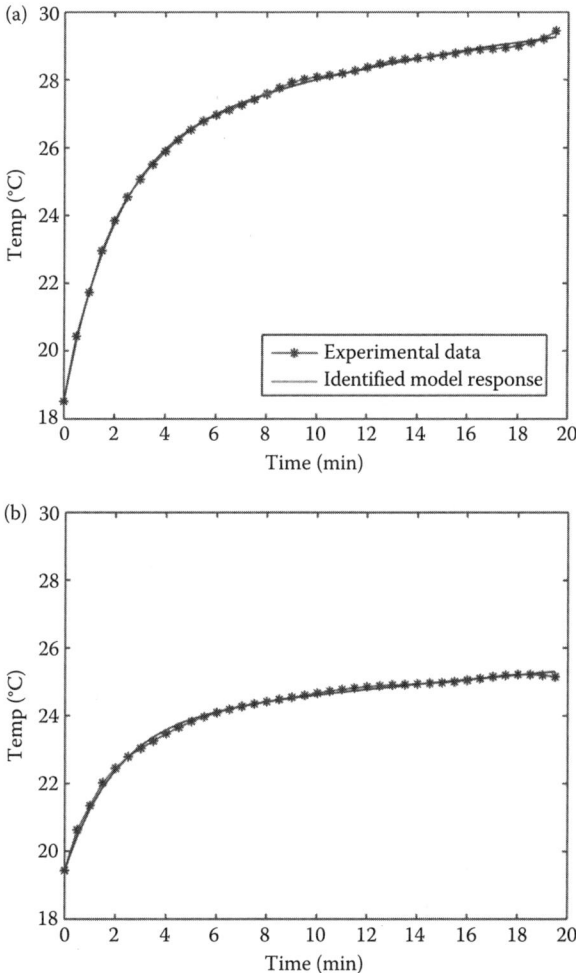

FIGURE 42.10 Comparison between experimental data and identified model response for (a) left varicocele and (b) healthy control.

varicocele groups, and between groups. h and a resulted significantly different between groups for left hemiscrotum ($p < 0.001$; $p < 0.01$, respectively). r resulted significantly different between groups for both left ($p < 0.001$) and right hemiscrotum ($p < 0.01$).

The first important issue that comes from these results is that the presence of left varicocele induced a faster rewarming of the affected hemiscrotum with respect to the homolateral healthy control. In fact the group average a value is lower for the left varicocele group with respect to the healthy side, thus indicating that the presence of this pathology accelerated the return to the basal homeostatic thermoregulatory conditions. This result is concordant with previous published results [26,29].

Basal conditions for left varicocele corresponded to higher cutaneous temperature of the left hemiscrotum with respect to the healthy left hemiscrotum, as proved by higher r values. This result was in agreement with previously reported indications [26,29]. Moreover, the left hemiscrotum affected by varicocele presents higher h values while no difference appears to characterize the average value of the k parameter. Overall, these results suggest that the accelerated recovery of the left hemiscrotum in the presence of varicocele was mostly due to the increased rate, with respect to normal conditions, of heat exchange from inner scrotal structures (veins and testes) with the skin. In fact, the active processes of

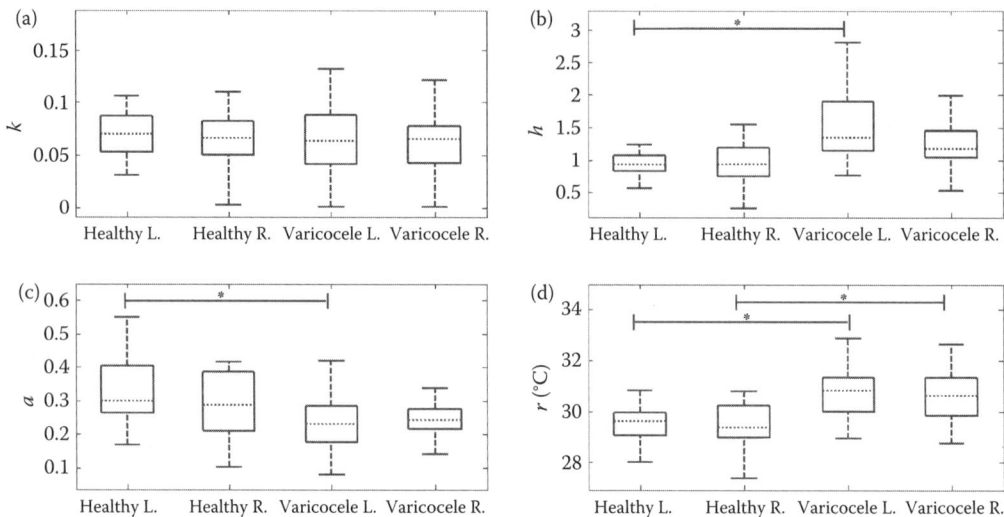

FIGURE 42.11 Comparison of model parameters among groups (Whisker Box plot). Median, first and third quartile, minimum and maximum are reported for each parameter (a–d). The asterisks on the horizontal bars specify the groups with statistically significant differences.

thermoregulatory vasodilatation induced by the cold exposure similarly acted in either the presence or the absence of varicocele, as proven by the average values of k, not significantly different between the two groups. This finding suggested that the true altered process in scrotal cutaneous hyperthermia secondary to varicocele did not depend on an increased effectiveness of the active thermoregulatory control, but was attributable to larger thermal exchange, probably by convection, between inner structures and the skin. In other words, it appeared that the increased blood reflux in the spermatic vein may have induced a diffused reflux in the testicular vessel network [19,40].

Average values for modeling parameters in healthy controls did not present statistically significant differences between right and left hemiscrota. This fact indicated and confirmed that in the absence of increased reflux secondary to varicocele, there were no thermoregulatory differences between healthy hemiscrota.

Interestingly, and not previously reported, right hemiscrotum in the presence of left varicocele presented higher basal temperature (i.e., r values) than healthy right hemiscrotum, thus suggesting that left hyperthermic hemiscrota induced a warming effect on the contralateral site. Differences in other functional parameters did not have a statistically significant relevance. Therefore, it seemed that such thermal interaction between hemiscrota in the presence of left varicocele may have been due to the proximity of the hemiscrota or intrascrotal vascular shunts and were not related to systemic vascular control [9,13].

The goal of this study was to identify a thermoregulatory feedback model to describe and to distinguish the functional differences in the recoveries, at both central and peripheral levels. In fact, the parameters so far identified to define each model described how the system acts at the two different levels, in terms of process speed, efficiency of control action, and heat exchanges mechanisms, in order to restore the prestress basal conditions. Several advantages may be derived from this approach. The estimated model parameter values for each subject can aid in estimating the level of functional impairment expressed in the different stages of the disease. Thus, it is possible to more effectively monitor both the evolution of the disease and the efficacy of the treatment and its follow-up. The application of this model to scrotal hyperthermia secondary to varicocele would also help to understand at which specific functional level is the possible spermatogenesis damage determined. The study proved that for scrotal hyperthermia, even pure left varicocele appeared to behave like a bilateral disease, thus providing further elements to understand the functional impairment.

42.4 Discussion and Conclusions

The goal of this chapter was to show that control system theory applied to cutaneous thermal data obtained from thermal imaging may provide a powerful tool to identify a thermoregulatory feedback model. Such an approach is particularly relevant as the cutaneous thermoregulation is based on feedback mechanisms. The model parameters describe and distinguish the functional differences in the recoveries, at both central and peripheral levels. In fact, the parameters so far identified to define each model described how the system acts at the two different levels, in terms of process speed, efficiency of control action, and heat exchanges mechanisms, in order to restore the prestress basal conditions. Several advantages may be derived from this approach. The estimated model parameter values for each subject can aid in estimating the level of functional impairment expressed in the different stages of the disease. Thus, it is possible to more effectively monitor both the evolution of the disease and the efficacy of the treatment and follow-up. The application of this model would also help to understand at which specific functional stage of the regulatory process is the possible functional impairment determined. Functional infrared imaging can take great advantage from this approach, in a variety of clinical applications expressed through abnormalities and deviation from normal thermoregulatory behavior.

References

1. Agresti, A. *Categorical Data Analysis* (2nd edition). Hoboken, NJ: Wiley InterScience, pp. 165–166, 2002.
2. Belch, J. Raynaud's phenomenon. Its relevance to scleroderma. *Ann. Rheum. Dis.* 50:839–845, 2005.
3. Block, J.A., and W. Sequeira. Raynaud's phenomenon. *Lancet.* 357:2042–2048, 2001.
4. Chakravarthy, N., K. Tsakalis, S. Sabesan, and L. Iasemidis. Homeostasis of brain dynamics in epilepsy: A feedback control system perspective seizure. *Ann. Biomed. Eng.* 37(3):565–585, 2009.
5. Charkoudian, N. Skin blood flow in adult human thermoregulation: How it works, when it does not, and why. *Mayo Clin. Proc.* 78:603–612, 2003.
6. Clark, S., F. Campbell, T. Moore, M.I.V. Jayson, T.A. King, and A.L. Herrick. Laser Doppler imaging. A new technique for quantifying microcirculatory flow in patients with primary Raynaud's phenomenon and systemic sclerosis. *Microvasc. Res.* 57:284–291, 1999.
7. Cutolo, M., C. Pizzorni, and A. Sulli. Capillaroscopy. *Best Pract. Res. Clin. Rheum.* 3:437–452, 2005.
8. Di Carlo, A. Thermography and the possibilities for its applications in clinical and experimental dermatology. *Clin. Dermatol.* 13:329–336, 1995.
9. Elbendary, M., and A. Elbadry. Right subclinical varicocele: How to manage in infertile patients with clinical left varicocele? *Fertil. Steril.* 92(6):2050–2053, 2009.
10. Fette, A., and J.M. Austria. Homeostatic control mechanism. *J. Pediatr. Surg.* 35(8):1222–1225, 2002.
11. Forssel, U., and L. Ljung Closed loop identification revisited. *Automatica.* 35:1215–1241, 1999.
12. Gat, Y., G. Bachar, Z. Zukerman, A. Belenky, and M. Gorenish. Physical examination may miss the diagnosis of bilateral varicocele: A comparative study of 4 diagnostic modalities. *J. Urol.* 172(4):1414–1417, 2004.
13. Gat, Y., G. Bachar, Z. Zukerman, A. Belenky, and M. Gornish. Varicocele: A bilateral disease. *Fertil. Steril.* 81(2):424–429, 2004.
14. Glantz, S. *Primer of BioStatistics* (6th edition.). New York: McGraw-Hill, pp. 353–358, 2005.
15. Hahn, M., C. Hahn, M. Jünger, A. Steins, D. Zuder, T. Klyscz, A. Büchtemann, G. Rassner, and V. Blazek. Local cold exposure test with a new arterial photoplethysmography sensor in healthy controls and patients with secondary Raynaud's phenomenon. *Microvasc. Res.* 57:187–198, 1999.
16. Herrick, A.L. Pathogenesis of Raynaud's phenomenon. *Rheumatology.* 44:587–596, 2005.
17. Herrick, A.L., and S. Clark. Quantifying digital vascular disease in patients with primary Raynaud's phenomenon and systemic sclerosis. *Ann. Rheum. Dis.* 57:70–78, 1998.

18. Kellog, D.L. A physiological systems approach to human and mammalian thermoregulation. *J. Appl. Physiol.* 100:1709–1718, 2006.

19. Kessler, A., S. Meirsdorf, M. Graif, P. Gottlieb, and S. Strauss. Intratesticular varicocele: Gray scale and color Doppler sonographic appearance. *J. Ultrasound Med.* 24(12):1711–1716, 2005.

20. Kuryliszin-Moskal, A., P.A. Klimiuk, and S. Sierakowski. Soluble adhesion molecules (sVCAM-1, sE-selectin), vascular endothelial growth factor (VEGF) and endothelin-1 in patient with systemic sclerosis: Relationship to organ systemic involvement. *Clin. Rheumatol.* 24:111–116, 2005.

21. LeRoy E.C., and T.A. Medsger. Criteria for the classification of early systemic sclerosis. *J. Rheumatol.* 28:1573–1576, 2001.

22. Ljung, L. *System Identification.* Upper Saddle River: Prentice Hall PTR, pp. 511–512, 2007.

23. Mariotti, A., G. Grossi, P. Amerio, G. Orlando, P.A. Mattei, A. Tulli, G.L. Romani, and A. Merla. Finger thermoregulatory model assessing functional impairment in Raynaud's phenomenon. *Ann. Biomed. Eng.* 37(12):2631–2639, 2009.

24. Merla, A., L. Di Donato, S. Di Luzio, G. Farina, S. Pisarri, M. Proietti, F. Salsano, and G.L. Romani. Infrared functional imaging applied to Raynaud's phenomenon. *IEEE Eng. Med. Biol. Mag.* 6:73–79, 2002.

25. Merla, A., L. Di Donato, S. Di Luzio, and G.L. Romani. Quantifying the relevance and stage of disease with the Tau image technique. *IEEE Eng. Med. Biol. Mag.* 21(6):86–91, 2002.

26. Merla, A., A. Ledda, L. Di Donato, S. Di Luzio, and G.L. Romani. Use of infrared functional imaging to detect impaired thermoregulatory control in men with asymptomatic varicocele. *Fertil. Steril.* 18(1):199–200, 2002.

27. Merla, A., A. Ledda, L. Di Donato, and G.L. Romani. Assessment of the effects of varicocelectomy on the thermoregulatory control of the scrotum. *Fertil. Steril.* 81(2):471–472, 2004.

28. Merla, A., G.L. Romani, S. Di Luzio, L. Di Donato, G. Farina, M. Proietti, S. Pisarri, and S. Salsano. Raynaud's phenomenon: Infrared functional imaging applied to diagnosis and drug effect. *Int. J. Immunopathol. Pharmacol.* 15:41–52, 2002.

29. Mieusset, R., and L. Bujan. Testicular heating and its possible contributions to male infertility: A review. *Int. J. Androl.* 14(8):169–184, 1995.

30. Nogueira, F., L. Barroso, E. Miranda, J.D. Castro, and F.M. Filho. Infrared digital telethermography: A new method for early detection of varicocele. *Fertil. Steril.* 92(1):361–362, 2009.

31. O'Reilly, D., L. Taylor, K. El-Hadivi, and M.I. Jayson. Measurement of cold challenge response in primary Raynaud's phenomenon and Raynaud's phenomenon associated with systemic sclerosis. *Ann. Rheum. Dis.* 11:1193–1196, 1992.

32. Oussar, Y., and G. Dreyfus. How to be a gray Box: Dynamic semi-physical modelling. *Neural Networks.* 14:1161–1172, 2001.

33. Ren, T., and D. Thieffry. Dynamical behaviour of biological regulatory networks-I. Biological role of feedback loops and practical use of the concept of the loop-characteristic state. *Bull. Math. Biol.* 57:274–276, 1995.

34. Renè, T., and D. Thieffry. Dynamical behaviour of biological regulatory networks- I. Biological role of feedback loops and practical use of the concept of the loop-characteristic state. *Bull. Math. Biol.* 57:247–276, 1995.

35. Rollins, D., N. Bhabdar, and S. Hulting. System identification of the human thermoregulatory system using continuous-time block-oriented predictive modelling. *Chem. Eng. Sci.* 61:1516–1527, 2006.

36. Romeo, C., and G. Santoro. Varicocele and infertility: Why a prevention? *J. Endocrinol. Invest.* 32(6):559–561, 2009.

37. Sanial, D.C., and N.K. Maji. Thermoregulation through cutaneous under variable atmospheric and physiological conditions. *J. Theor. Biol.* 208:451–456, 2001.

38. Sato, S., M. Hasegawa, K. Takehara, and T.F. Tedder. Altered B lymphocyte function induces systemic autoimmunity in systemic sclerosis. *Mol. Immunol.* 42:821–831, 2005.

39. Sawasaki, N., S. Iwase, and T. Mano. Effect of cutaneous sympathetic response to local or systemic cold exposure on thermoregulatory functions in humans. *Auton. Neurosci.* 87:274–281, 2001.

40. Shafik, A. Advances in male contraception. *Arch. Androl.* 45(3):155–167, 2000.

41. Shiraishi, K., K. Naito, and H. Takihara. Indication of varicocelectomy in the era of assisted reproductive technology: Prediction of treatment out come by noninvasive diagnostic methods. *Arch. Androl.* 49(6):475–478, 2003.

42. Shitzer, A., On the thermal efficiency of cold-stressed finger. *Ann. NY Acad. Sci.* 858:74–87, 1998.

43. Shitzer, A., A. Stroscheine, R.R. Gonzalez, and K.B. Pandolf. Lumped parameter tissue temperature-blood perfusion model of a cold stressed finger. *J. Appl. Physiol.* 80:1829–1834, 1996.

44. Skandhan, K., and A. Rajahariprasad. The process of spermatogenesis liberates significant heat and the scrotum has a role in body thermoregulation. *Med. Hypotheses.* 68:303–307, 2007.

45. Suter, L.G., J.M. Murabito, D.T. Felson, and L. Fraenkel. The incidence and natural history of Raynaud's phenomenon in the community. *Arthritis Rheum.* 52(4):1259–1263, 2005.

46. Waterhouse, J. Homeostatic control mechanism. *Anaesth. Intensive Care.* 5:236–240, 2004.

47. Lonzetti, L.S., F. Joyal, J.P. Raynauld, A. Roussin, J.R. Goulet, E. Rich, D. Choquette, Y. Raymond, and J.L. Senécal. Updating the American College of Rheumatology preliminary criteria for systemic sclerosis: Addition of severe nailfold capillaroscopic abnormalities markedly increases sensitivity for limited scleroderma. *Arthritis Rheum.* 44:735–736, 2001.

43

Infrared Thermal Imaging Standards for Human Fever Detection

Francis J. Ring
University of Glamorgan

E.Y.K. Ng
School of Mechanical and Aerospace Engineering

Nanyang Technological University

43.1 Introduction

Infrared (IR) thermal imaging provides an efficient means of recording the surface temperatures of the human body. It is a noncontact radiometric technique that has improved considerably since its early trials in medicine in the late 1950s.[1]

In recent years concerns about the spread and containment of infectious diseases, especially among the travelling public has brought this technology into use as a means of detecting high fever in passengers. The Severe Acute Respiratory Syndrome (SARS) outbreak around 2003 saw the introduction on IR imaging cameras in Chinese airports.[2,3] While there were a small percentage of passengers who were stopped because they had elevated facial temperatures, the policy of locating these cameras high above a crowd of passers by, is now recognized as being not fully efficient. Passengers wearing hats and face masks, for example, may have a large area of their face covered and escape recognition.

The Singapore Standards Organisation SPRING examined the use of these cameras in 2003 and published two excellent guides to the most suitable devices and how they should be calibrated and deployed.[4,5] Subsequently the International Standards Organisation (ISO) was invited to consider these documents and review their potential application in the international community.

As a result an international writing group worked on the contents of these reports, to update and widen the details and references to the supporting information. It also was able to link sections and definitions of the new documents to existing standards, which provided valuable, cross referencing.

Following the form of the SPRING documents, the ISO produced two new documents, the first to describe the essential performance specification of suitable imaging systems for fever detection in humans, and the second on the effective deployment, installation, maintenance, and staff training required to obtain optimum performance in the field. Full details of these documents should be obtained by all who are directly concerned with the specification manufacture and sales of these devices.[6,7] Equally, the detail of the correct deployment of the fever screening installations is found in the full ISO documentation. This chapter aims to merely highlight some of those details, and some of which could have a useful bearing on the clinical application of IR imaging.

43.2 Definitions

The standard documents contain full details of definitions used throughout, and it is not intended to reproduce all in this chapter. Many of the terms and definitions are those that are found across the same technical area, but additional terms have been added for this specific application.

Examples of these additional terms are:

Calibration Source 201.3.202
IR radiation blackbody reference source of known and traceable temperature and emissivity

Detector 201.3.203
IR thermal sensor or array of sensors able to detect IR thermal energy radiating from the surface of the face or other object

External Temperature Reference Source 201.3.205
Part of the screening thermograph that is used to ensure accurate operation between calibration using IR radiation source of known temperature and emissivity. Note: the external temperature reference source is normally imaged in each thermogram or prior to each thermogram.

Face 201.3.206
Anterior cranial face of the patient being measured.

Screening Thermograph 201.3.209 and 201.7.3.101
Medical electrical equipment or ME system (201.3.209) that:
Detects IR radiation emitted from the face from which a thermogram is obtained from the target.
Detects IR radiation emitted from an external temperature radiation source;
Displays a radiometric image;
Obtains a temperature reading from the target and
Compares that temperature reading to the threshold temperature to determine if the patient is febrile
The technical description (201.7.3.101) shall include:

A. A reference to ISO/TR13154 Medical electrical equipment—deployment, implementation, and operational guidelines for identifying febrile humans using a screening thermograph (the guidance document for the application of screening thermographs)
B. A recommendation that the relative humidity in the area of screening should be maintained below 50% and temperature below 24°C to achieve the intended use and an explanation of the effects of elevated humidity and ambient temperature on the temperature reading caused by sweating.

Note 1: The measurements provided by a screening thermograph in intended use can be influenced when the patient is sweating. Sweating thresholds can vary, according to the patient's fitness level, environment of residence, length of adaptation, and the relative humidity.

C. An explanation of the effects due to environmental IR sources such as sunlight, nearby electrical sources and lighting, and instructions on how these should be minimized.

Note 2: The responsible organization needs to be aware of the type of lighting used in the screening area. Lighting such as incandescent, halogen, quart tungsten halogen, and other type of lamps that produce significant interference (heat) should be avoided.

Note 3: The area chosen for screening should have a nonreflective background and minimal reflected IR radiation from the surroundings.

D. An explanation of the effects due to airflow, and instructions that this should be minimized.

Note 4: Drafts from air conditioning ducts can cause forced cooling or heating of the face and should be baffled or diffused to prevent airflow from blowing directly onto the patient.

Skin Temperature 201.3.210

Skin surface temperature as measured from the workable target plane of a screening thermograph, with an appropriate adjustment for skin emissivity.

Note: the emissivity of dry human skin is accepted to be 0.98

Target Plane 201.3.213

Infocus plane perpendicular to the line of sight of a screening thermograph.

43.3 Discussion

From the above it is clear that the standard requires more from the manufacturer than a simple IR camera and temperature reference source. The minimal acceptable performance of the camera is clearly defined, and the accuracy and stability required are based on the expectation that the device will operate continuously throughout a full day. The recommendation is that an un-cooled detector system is used since there is a shortened life expectancy of a cooling system that can be expensive to replace or renew.

The manufacturer needs to be fully aware of the specification details and ensure that the end user (described as the responsible organization) is alerted to the ISO document that specifies optimal conditions for installation and management of the screening set up. There is evidence to indicate that some manufacturers seem to be unaware of this standard, and certainly failing to pass on the kind of information shown in the above extract. However, clinical users of IR thermal imaging will be already familiar with most of these criteria, that play an important role is achieving consistent and reliable thermograms used in medicine. It is interesting that the ISO document chooses to refer to the human target for

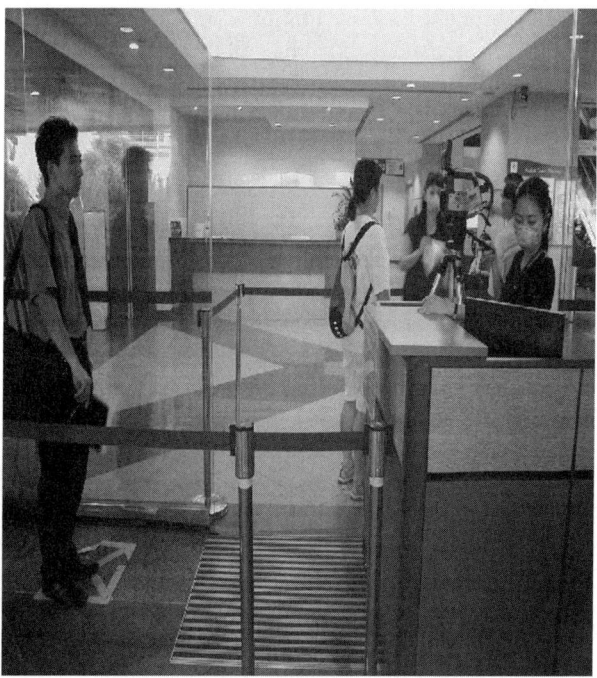

FIGURE 43.1 Setup for a typical IR camera system at a medical center entrance.

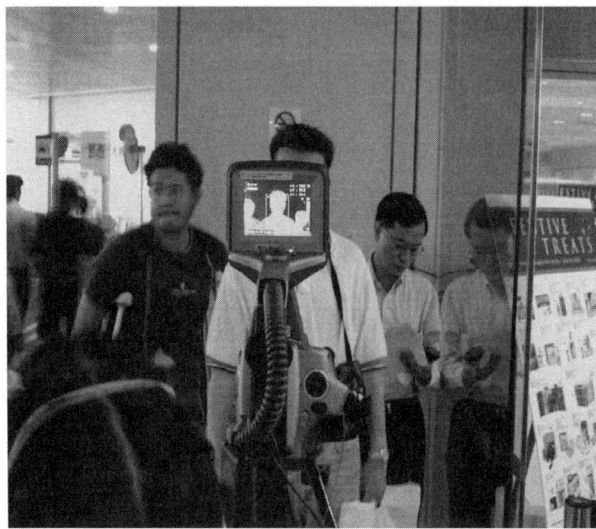

FIGURE 43.2   Operator's viewpoint (with subject standstill within a designated box for a few seconds).

screening as the patient on the grounds that this technique is designed to indicate a person who is likely to have a fever, and on subsequent medical examination will have that diagnosis accepted or rejected. It is also the reason why the screening thermograph is described as "medical equipment."

In this latter case, this is a new departure from other screening systems used in security screening in airports. Detection of metal objects and drugs are now routine operations for airport passengers.

However, thermal imaging brought into use in a pandemic fever, can be used in other buildings and organizations. Schools, factories, and civil public buildings can equally use this technique. In the Guidance document on deployment, there are two situations described. A high volume transit, where screening can be carried out at maximum speed using automatic software to alert the operator of temperature found in excess of 38°C, from whence the passenger is diverted to a medical check that will include a questionnaire and a thermometry test. However, in a smaller application less-expensive installations can be used where the operator may be required to position the camera, and read the result from the screen image. Figures 43.1 and 43.2 show a typical set-up for the IR system at an entrance to a hospital and an operator's viewpoint.

One critical part of the specification for use in both documents is the positioning and location of the site for temperature measurement.

The forehead, lateral temporal artery locations have both been used, but are less reliable as a site for indicating fever. The inner canthus of the eye, has been shown to be reliable. It is fed from the internal carotid artery, and is less influenced by ambient and physiological stress, than other areas of the face. For this reason the standard specifies that all spectacles must be removed, and hats, and facemasks, if they interfere with a clear reading from the eye region. It is also clear that at a distance from the camera lens it will be impossible to obtain sufficient pixels and temperature readings to read the temperature with certainty. Oblique angles between camera and patient are also inaccurate. It is therefore necessary to stop the passenger for a few seconds (Figures 43.1 and 43.2), to ensure that the camera is in line with the eyes before the image is registered.[8] It is anticipated that only positive findings leading to a thermogram being stored with its appropriate identity including passport details. Only time will reveal if this is adequate given the possible litigation should a febrile passenger be missed in screening, and go on to infect a large number of fellow travellers.

References

1. Ring, E.F.J., Progress in the measurement of human body temperature. *Engineering in Medicine & Biology Magazine*, 17, 1998, 19–24.
2. Bitar, D., Goubar, A., and Desenclos, J.C., International travels and fever screening during epidemics: A literature review on the effectiveness and potential use of non-contact infrared thermometers. *Euro Surveill*, 14(6), 2009, 1–5.
3. Ng, E.Y.K. and Rajendra Acharya, U., A review of remote-sensing infrared thermography for indoor mass blind fever screening in containing an epidemic. *Engineering in Medicine and Biology*, 28(1), 2009, 76–83.
4. Thermal Imagers for human temperature screening Part 1: Requirements and test methods. *Technical Reference TR15:* part 1:2003 SPRING Singapore.
5. Thermal imagers for human temperature screening Part 2: Implementation and Guidelines. *Technical Reference TR15:* part 2:2004 SPRING Singapore.
6. Particular requirements for the basic safety and essential performance of screening thermographs for human febrile temperature screening. *ISO TC121/SC3-IEC SC62D*, 2008.
7. Medical Electrical Equipment—Deployment, implementation and operational guidelines for identifying febrile humans using a screening thermograph. *ISO/TR 13154; ISO/TR 80600*, 2009.
8. Ring, E.F.J., McEvoy, H., Jung, A., Zuber, J., and Machin, G., New standards for devices used for the measurement of human body temperature. *Journal of Medical Engineering & Technology*, 34(4), 2010, 249–253.

44

Francis J. Ring
University of Glamorgan

A. Jung
Military Institute of Medicine

B. Kalicki
Military Institute of Medicine

J. Zuber
Military Institute of Medicine

A. Rustecka
Military Institute of Medicine

R. Vardasca
Polytechnic Institute of Leiria

Infrared Thermal Imaging for Fever Detection in Children

44.1 Introduction

Over recent years, pandemic influenza virus infections have caused concerns about an ever-increasing mobility of populations, especially in air travel. Limiting exposure to fellow travellers who may be suffering from a febrile high temperature has been employed with some success. Pandemic influenza virus is a virulent human form that causes global outbreak, or pandemic, of serious illness. Because there is little natural immunity, the disease can spread easily from person to person. There have been pandemic outbreaks in the United States in 1918, 1958, and 1968 with varying degrees of morbidity and virulence. Children under 18 years have tended to have the highest rates of illness, though not of severe disease and death.[1]

Infrared thermal imaging has in recent years become more accessible and affordable as a means of remote sensing for human body temperature. Historically, a clinical fever has been checked with a clinical thermometer, and these devices have been slowly replaced by infrared radiometers mainly for inner ear temperature measurement. However, the number of scientific reports and papers confirming the reliability of the infrared methods are limited. Furthermore, there is a need for critical technique, which has not always been well defined in these publications.[2]

Some use of infrared imaging for fever screening has been made since 2006 in international airports, most of which have not used optimal technique. For this reason, the International Standards Organisation produced two documents in 2008 and 2009 (ISO TC121/SC3-IEC SC62D)[3,4] (see Chapter 43 by Ring and Ng).

One important issue that is most important to a correct technique is the positioning of both camera and subject. Typical screening installations use cameras mounted at an angle to survey passing groups of passengers. The best site for temperature measurement is the inner corner (or canthus) of the eye.

This requires the camera to be mounted close up and on level with the eyes, thus providing a cluster of image pixels in the region of interest. The study described here has employed a good specification radiometric camera at a correct position, to ensure a minimum of 9 pixels in each eye canthus.

44.2 Method

Cohorts of children at the Pediatric Clinic in Warsaw were checked for fever by three different methods. The routine department procedure was carried out by a nurse using a clinical thermometer under the armpit (axilla), and left there for a full 5 min.

They then entered a room for thermal imaging maintained at 22–23°C where they were seated before the FLIR infrared camera SC640. The image of the face was set to occupy at least 75% of the image, and regions around the inner canthi (i.c.) were measured for temperature. A second area of interest over the forehead was also recorded, as some claims have been made that forehead temperature would be an adequate target for fever. Both inner ear measurements (tympanic membrane) with a clinical radiometer were then recorded and documented, with the child's demographic data.

44.3 Results

A total of 402 children were examined between 2006 and 2011. The majority of children attending the hospital were not febrile, they were compared with those known to have a clinically defined fever, and examined prior to medication. Of this group 350 (85%) were found to be free from fever, and 52 (15%) cases of definite fever were recorded. There were 192 male and 210 female individuals.

All subjects had infrared thermograms and axilla recordings, not all subjects were measured by the ear tympanic membrane thermometer, due to equipment failure.

The age distribution is shown in Table 44.1.

44.3.1 Temperature Data

The data were analyzed for any differences between male and female individuals, no statistical differences were found for sex dependency. Similarly for age dependency, again no statistical differences were found. In the control subjects (afebrile) left eye vs right eye data were compared and found to be not significant. As a result both readings were combined and the mean temperature of both eyes was used for each subject (Table 44.2). While temperatures of 38°C and above are considered to be found in children over 5 years and adults in fever, 37.5°C and above is considered to be a fever level in under 5-year olds. In this study we have categorized all temperatures over 37.6°C as fever. In most cases they are higher than 38°C (Table 44.3).

To examine the possible relationship between the different measurement sites and methods, Pearson's correlation tests were performed on the temperature data. See Tables 44.4a and 44.4b.

This shows the existence of a linear relationship between the measurements among sites in the cases of fever. This is highest when comparing the inner canthus eye measurements by thermography and axilla temperature measured by the clinical contact thermometer. The forehead temperatures and ear measurements correlate less well with statistical significance ($p < 0.1$).

TABLE 44.1 Age Distribution of Subjects

<3 years	50
3–6	128
7–12	136
13–16	82
>16	6

TABLE 44.2   Temperature Data: Nonfever Group

Afebrile	Mean (°C)	Std. Dev.	Number
Eyes i.c.	36.48	0.49	354
Forehead	36.44	0.65	326
Axilla	36.34	0.59	347
Ear	36.12	0.71	178

TABLE 44.3   Temperature Data: Fever Group (49% Male, 51% Female)

Febrile	Mean (°C)	Std. Dev.	Number
Eyes i.c.	38.9	0.84	52
Forehead	34.7	0.86	52
Axilla	38.9	0.68	52
Ear	37.4	1.41	24

TABLE 44.4A   Afebrile

Pair	Pearson's Correlation	p-Value
Eyes i.c./axilla	0.507	0.0006
Forehead/axilla	0.432	0.000
Ear/axilla	0.420	0.014

TABLE 44.4B   Febrile (Fever) Cases

Pair	Pearson's Correlation	p-Value
Eyes i.c./axilla	0.587	0.000
Forehead/axilla	0.432	0.022
Ear/axilla	0.276	0.267

In the analysis of these data it was found that in febrile children the eye temperature measurements and the thermometric axilla temperatures are closer that those measured from the forehead (thermographic) or ear (tympanic membrane radiometer). The eye and axilla measurements also showed more internal consistency than the others (reliability coefficient alpha of 0.724).

44.4 Discussion

This study has been performed on children in Warsaw, Poland according to the recommended technique described in the new ISO standards of 2008/2009. The advantage of performing the study in a hospital environment is that the diagnosis was known prior to the study measurements, but was not conveyed to those undertaking the study until after the data had been examined. There were no cases of clinical fever that were undetected by the study.

It had been questioned if another source of mild infection such as sinusitis could confuse the data and cause a false-positive result. Such cases have been documented by the pediatric department and there was known to be a clear difference between sinusitis and generalized fever. In the case of sinusitis, there is often a bilateral increase in heat affecting the face, and rarely affecting the i.c. temperatures.

The clinical fever cases in this study showed excellent symmetry, so that a close correlation was always found between the left and the right eye, in both the febrile and afebrile patients. Those with sinusitis or dental infection showed a characteristic localized and asymmetric temperature increase.

The examination room was thermally stable, and air conditioning could be used prior to a clinical session if required. However, unlike the normal protocols recommended for clinical tests using infrared imaging, the patients were not required to rest and stabilize prior to the test. This would not be practical in a traveller screening situation, and the promise that the i.c. of the eye should be the most stable site for measurement was borne out by this study. The forehead on the other hand, also measured from the thermogram using a rectangular region of interest occupying some 60% of the exposed area, did not show such consistency. It was sometimes necessary to use a disposable paper hat to contain long hair prior to the imaging procedure.

For the most efficient positioning of the subject before the camera a stool was used, which limited the range of height adjustment required for the camera stand. This was a counterbalanced single pillar stand as used in photographic studios, because, the ISO has specifically warned of the potential for error in reproducible positions, when using a pan and tilt head tripod as the infrared camera mount.

This study has also endorsed the methodology recommended in the ISO document for fever screening where a close-up stationary image is recorded of the subject's face. With the current infrared cameras, even using the best available, the system error could be as high as 0.4°C which is a large proportion of the actual difference in temperatures found between afebrile and febrile cases. It is therefore clear that a camera mounted over a meter from the subject, and possibly also at an oblique angle will fail to have sufficient pixels in the relatively small target area of the i.c. of an eye. Increasing the number of pixels over the measurement site is not only good but essential practice in this application.

Fever screening in a global pandemic has yet to be taken seriously, but it is clear that there can be legal repercussions from false-positive measurements due to bad technique or inadequate technology.

In this study also we decided to include very young children over the age of 6 months. At this age a parent facing the camera held them, and because the distance between subject and camera lens was short, there was no difficulty in filling the screen with the child's face. It was also not a problem if the child was asleep, but only in the case of persistent crying, producing tears, the temperature readings were aborted. In a few cases, they were resumed after the child had been pacified, and a bright colored object moved above the lens of the camera was sufficient to make the child look in the right direction.

In this study, the commercial software proved entirely adequate for the analysis of two regions of the face. However, some recent studies have proposed software that will automatically track the human face and obtain measurements with minimal intervention by the operator. This approach will lead the way to rapid screening in the future.[5,6]

44.5 Conclusion

The use of an infrared radiometric camera can be a reliable tool for the detection of fever in children. The technique recommended by the ISO in document TR 13154:2009 ISO/TR80600 is endorsed by the results of this study. There was a significant difference between the temperatures measured in afebrile patients and those with known fever, with the thermal imaging of the eye region being the most rapid noncontact site for measurement.

Acknowledgments

We are extremely grateful for the complete support of FLIR Infrared Systems, Warsaw, for the regular support of Mr. Pawel Rutkowski, and the loan of the Infrared camera. We also thank the staff and patients of the Military Institute of Medicine, Warsaw for their willing participation in this study.

References

1. *Pandemic Influenza: Preparedness, Response & Recovery. Guide for Critical Infrastructure and Key Resources.* Homeland Security. Sept. 19th, 2006, USA.
2. Dodd S.R., Lancaster G.A., Craig J.V., Smyth R.L., Williamson P.R. In a systematic review, infrared ear thermometry for fever diagnosis in children finds poor sensitivity. *J. Clin. Epidemiol.* 59(4), 354–57, 2006.
3. ISO TC121/SC3-IEC SC62D Particular requirements for the basic safety and essential performance of screening thermographs for human febrile temperature screening, 2008.
4. ISO/TR 13154:2009 *ISO/TR 8-600: Medical Electrical Equipment—Deployment, Implementation and Operational Guidelines for Identifying Febrile Humans Using a Screening Thermograph.*
5. Strakowska M., Strzelecki M., Wiecek B. Automatic measurement of human body temperature in the eye canthi using a thermovison camera. *Thermology International* 21(2), 57–58, 2011.
6. Bajwa U.I., Taj I.A., Bhatti Z.E. A comprehensive comparative performance analysis of Laplacian faces and Eigen faces for face recognition. *The Imaging Science Journal* 59, 32–40, 2011.

45

Thermal Imager as Fever Identification Tool for Infectious Diseases Outbreak

E.Y.K. Ng
School of Mechanical and Aerospace Engineering

Nanyang Technological University

45.1 Introduction

Thermography is a noninvasive diagnostic method that is economic, quick, and does not inflict any pain on the subject. It is a relatively straightforward method of imaging that detects the variation of temperature on the surface of the human skin. Thermography is widely used in the medical arena [1–29]. This includes the detection of an elevated body temperature [6–29], which is the focus of this chapter. Thermograms alone will not be sufficient for the medical practitioner to make a diagnosis. Analytical tools such as bio-statistical methods and artificial neural network (ANN) such as radical basis function network (RBFN) is utilized to analyze the thermograms. Neural network is a pattern recognition program that has the ability to predict the outcome based on the various inputs fed into the program. For an elevated body temperature thermography, the program will predict if the subject is febrile or nonfebrile. Figures 45.1 and 45.2 reveal two typical examples of normal and febrile thermograms.

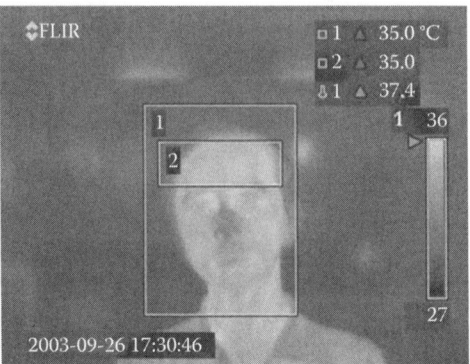

FIGURE 45.1   Nonfebrile thermogram (aural temperature = 36.9°C).

In the late 2009, the World Health Organization (WHO) is urging the world to brace for a second wave of the H1N1 pandemic as the heavily populated Northern Hemisphere edges toward the cooler season when flu thrives. There had been second and third waves in previous pandemics. Thus, one has to be prepared for whatever surprises this capricious new virus would deliver in the coming years. More than 6000 people have died since H1N1 was uncovered in Mexico nearly 7 months ago (April to mid-October 2009). Twenty-two million Americans were infected by the H1N1 during the earlier period of which 4000 were killed after a new counting method yielded an estimate six times higher than the last one. The virus is more infectious than seasonal flu and more durable through the warmer months. It is mystified at the "most worrying" characteristic of this virus. Nearly 40% of the most severe or fatal cases occur in people who are in perfect health.

Fever has been regarded as an important symptom of pandemic influenza though a recent research reveals that one in five of the H1N1 or swine flu pandemic will not be detected, some have mild or no fever, and their general symptoms make them hard to identify and still pass on the virus. It was reported lately that only half had high fever of 37.8°C or more which is one of the symptoms the United States uses to identify H1N1 cases. If we use this cut-off, then 46% of the confirmed cases would not have been picked up. Cough was the most common symptom; affecting four in five patients, although only half had sore throats. For most H1N1, the fever receded a day after they started taking Tamiflu. Thus, the doctors do not know whether the virus is alive or dead and hence they are uncertain if the person is still infectious. However, an improvement in the accuracy of using noncontact infrared (IR) system to detect feverish subjects is useful for other flu pandemics such as SARS and H5N1.

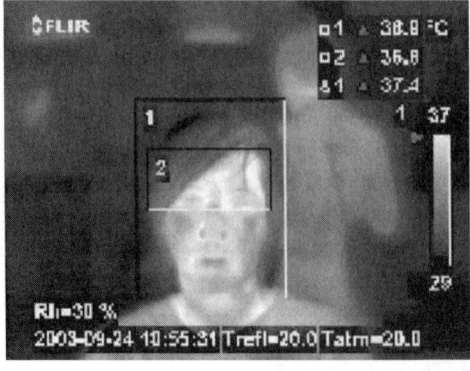

FIGURE 45.2   Febrile thermogram (aural temperature = 38.4°C).

There are many well-documented articles including comprehensive review papers in renowned journals [7,11,12,16,18,21,22,24,26–28] as well as the recent International Standard Organization (ISO) procedures and standards (ISO/TR 13154 and IEC 80601-2-59) as published recently [29–30] that are closely related to the present topic. These standards are related to "Deployment, implementation, and operational guidelines for identifying febrile humans using a screening thermograph" and "Particular requirements for the basic safety and essential performance of screening thermographs for human febrile temperature screening."

45.2 Methodology

45.2.1 Data Acquisition

The blind mass data were collected (502 without duplicate measurements, confirmed later as 86 febrile and 416 healthy cases with ear thermometer) from the designated SARS hospital (A & E Department, Tan Tock Seng Hospital [TTSH]) and the Civil Defense Force Academy [SCDF] in Singapore (in-door screening with ambient temperature of 25 ± 2°C, humidity ≈60%) in which thermal imagers are used as a first-line tool for the blind screening of hyperthermia. The subjects are considered febrile if his/her mean ear temperature is ≥37.7°C for adults (37.9°C for children) using Braun Thermoscan IRT 3520+. Results are drawn for the two important pieces of information: the best and yet a practical region on the face to screen and guidance on optimal preset threshold temperature for the same handheld radiometric IR ThermaCAM S60 FLIR system [31]. The focal length from the subject to the scanner was fixed at 2 m and the duration of time patients scanned was 3 s. Figure 45.3 illustrates an example of temperature profiles from a temperature operation using thermal imager with temperature reading. Visitors were directed to line up in a single file with the aid of barricades. Stand in position, remove spectacles, and look at the imager so that his/her face fills at least 1/3 vertical height of the display screen (Figures 45.4 and 45.5). The detector was a focal plane array, an uncooled microbolometer of 320 × 240 pixels with a thermal sensitivity of 0.06°C at 30°C, a spectral range of 7.5–13 μm, and its measurement accuracy at ±2% of the real-time reading [31]. The average temperature of the skin surface was measured from the field-of-view of the thermal imager with an appropriate adjustment for skin emissivity. Human skin emissivity may vary from site to site ranging from 0.94 to 0.99 (0.98 was used here). Figures 45.6 and 45.7 present an example of the processed thermal images of both frontal and side (left) profiles from

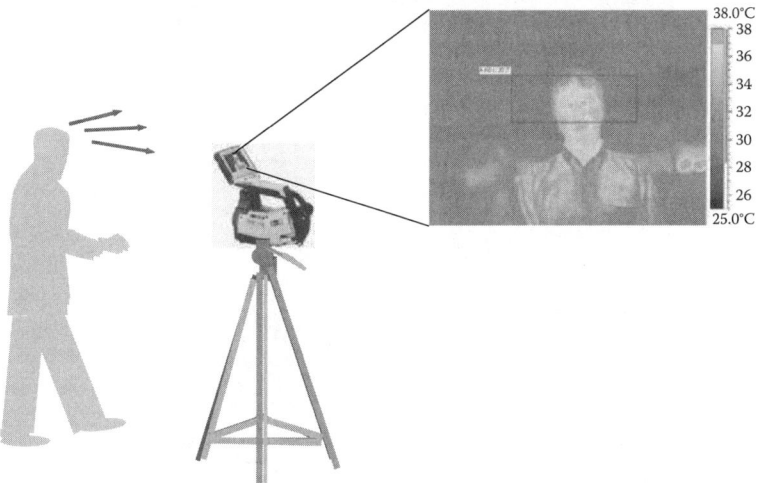

FIGURE 45.3 A typical thermal imager with direct threshold temperature setting. (Adapted from Zugo. www.zugophotonics.com/)

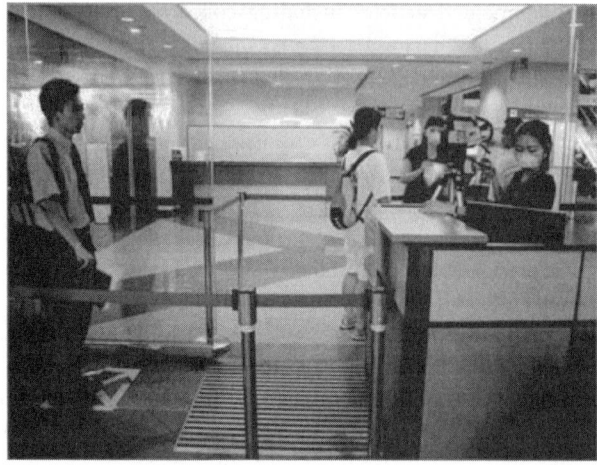

FIGURE 45.4 A yellow square marked on the ground for visitors to stand in.

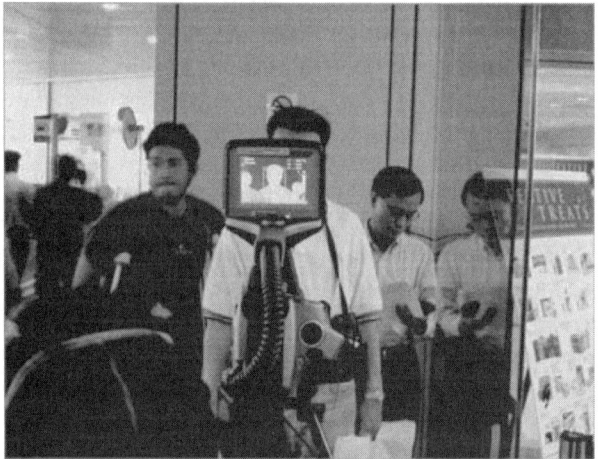

FIGURE 45.5 Face fills at least one-third vertical height for the field of view.

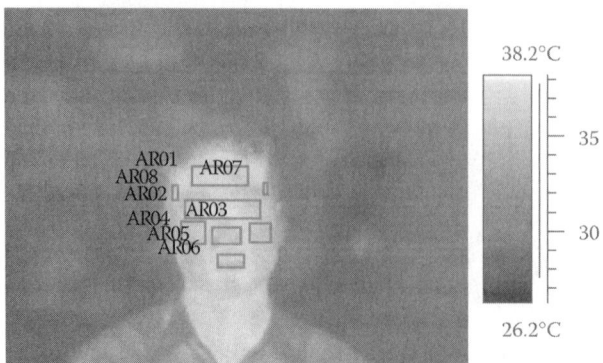

FIGURE 45.6 Processed thermal images of the frontal profile.

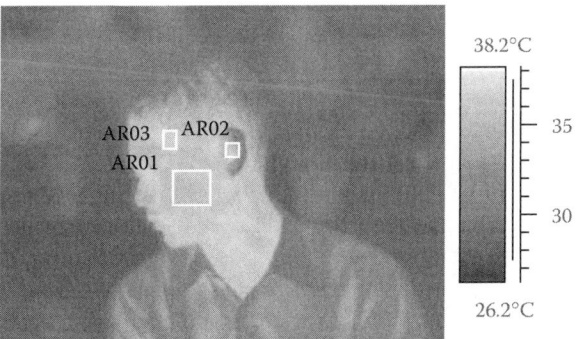

FIGURE 45.7   Processed thermal images of the side profile.

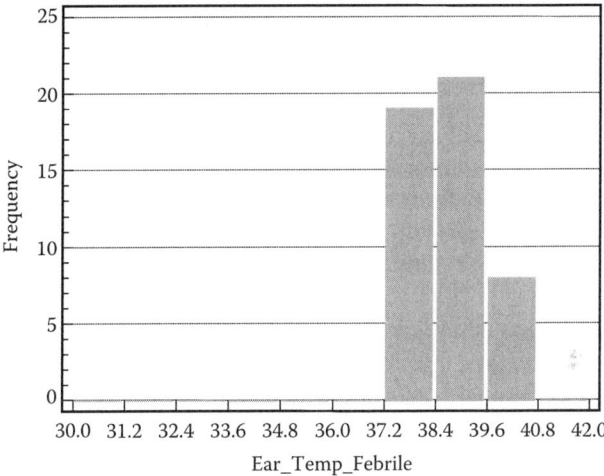

FIGURE 45.8   Distribution of ear temperature for febrile cases.

the same subject. The following spots were logged and analyzed from the subjects with frontal and side profiles: forehead, eye region, average cheeks, nose, mouth (closed), average temple, side face, ears, and side temple (the last three are for the side profile).

Reproducibility of both the instrument and physiological assumptions was established by comparing paired left–right readings of the temples and cheeks [32,33]. Comparing the ear's core temperature of febrile and nonfebrile data (Figures 45.8 through 45.11), it is noted that the mode of the nonfebrile data falls between 36.0°C and 37.2°C. For febrile, it spread over a larger region, from 37.2°C to 39.6°C.

45.2.2 Artificial Neural Networks

ANN are a group of techniques for numerical learning [34]. They are made up of many nonlinear computational elements called neurons. These neurons, also known as network nodes (NN), are linked to one another. Through this weighted interconnection, they formed the main architect of the NN. To draw an analogy, ANN is similar to the neurological system in humans and animals, which are made up of real NN. One important point to note is that ANN is much less complex than the biological NN (BNN). As a result, it is not realistic to expect ANN to emulate BNN, which is responsible for the behavior of humans and animals. However, ANN has the capability to assist us in some tasks. This includes nonlinear estimation, classification, clustering, and content-addressable memory.

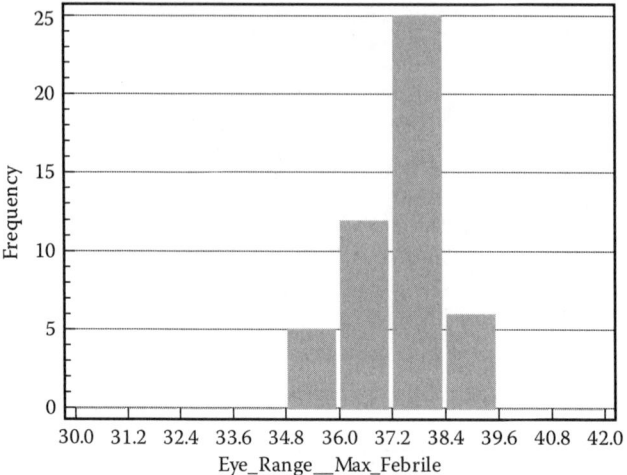

FIGURE 45.9 Distribution of maximum temperature at eye range for febrile cases.

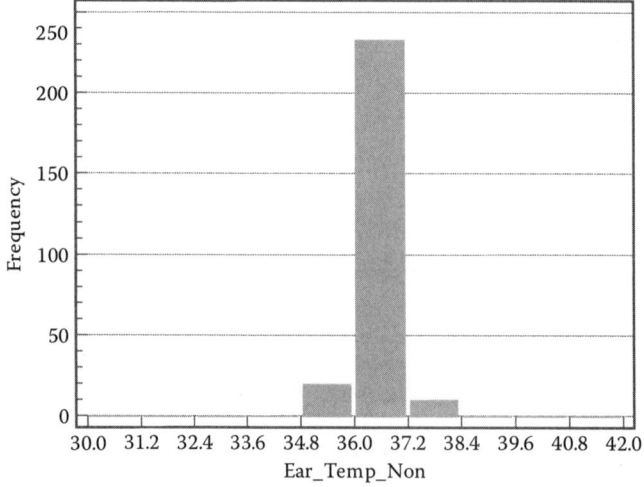

FIGURE 45.10 Distribution of ear temperature for nonfebrile cases.

Two or more inputs are connected to a node in an ANN [34]. Each of them has a weighted linkage attached to it (Figure 45.12). Based on the input values, a node has the ability to perform simple calculation. Both inputs and outputs are real numbers or integers between −1 and 1. All the input data have to be normalized before being fed into the program. The output from one individual node can either be inputted into another node or be a part of the NN's overall output. Each node performs its calculation and function independently from the rest of the nodes. The only association between the nodes is that the output from a node might be the input for another node. This type of architect is also known as a parallel structure, which allows for the exploration of numerous hypotheses. In addition, this parallel architect also permits the NN to make full use of the conventional personal computers.

The main advantage of ANN is that the tolerance of failure of an individual node or neuron is relatively high. This includes the weighted interconnection, because it might be erroneous too. The weights can be obtained by utilizing a trained algorithm, through iteration, and adjustments. The eventual transfer function is obtained with regard to the desired output.

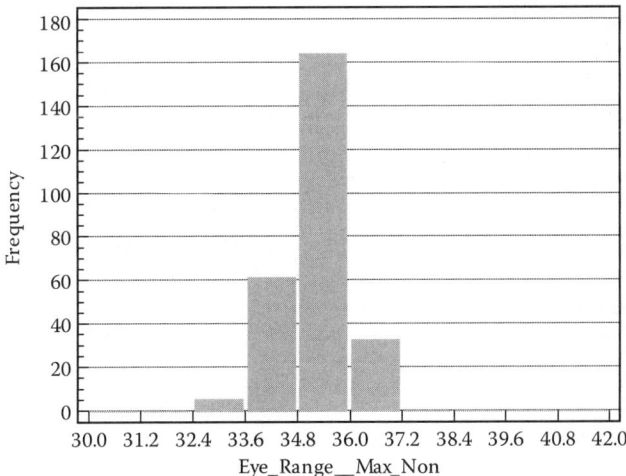

FIGURE 45.11   Distribution of maximum temperature at eye region for nonfebrile cases.

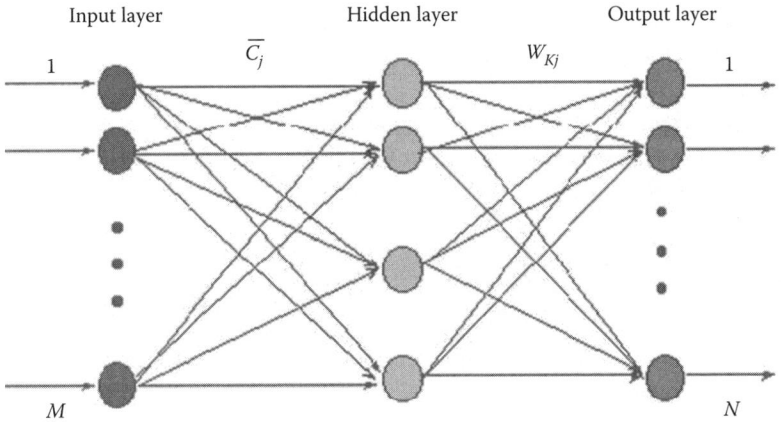

FIGURE 45.12   RBFN architect. (Adapted from Battelle: http://www.battelle.org/pipetechnology/ (assessed 10 June 2009); Receiver operating characteristics (ROC): http://www.medcalc.be/ (accessed 17 July 2010).)

When a set of inconsistent or incomplete data is given, ANN is able to give an approximate answer rather than a wrong answer. The performance of the NN will undergo a gradual degradation should there be any failures from individual nodes in the network. This is very useful in the medical arena as many a times, it is difficult to run a comprehensive test. The disadvantage of using ANN is that it does not have the capability to predict and forecast accurately beyond the range of previously trained data. In other words, the predicted outcome is based on the available set of data.

45.2.3 Radial Basis Function Network

Radial basis function network is a kind of feed-forward and unsupervised learning paradigm. A simple RBFN consists of three separate layers—input layer, hidden layer, and output layer as shown in Figure 45.12. The first part of the training cycle involves the clustering of input vectors. Mathematically, the clustering is done using Dynamic K-Means algorithm [35]. At the end of the clustering process, the radius of the Gaussian functions at the middle of the clusters will be equivalent to the distance between the two nearest cluster centers [34].

During the training, the RBFN is required to fulfill two tasks. First, it is to determine the middle of each hypersphere (circle in 2-D and hypersphere in *n*-dimensional pattern space) and second, to obtain its radius. For the first task, it is done by allocating the weights of the processing elements. This can be done by using an unsupervised clustering algorithm. It is important to note that the output neuron in the prototypical layer of a RBFN is in a function of the Euclidean distance. This distance measures from the input vector to the weighted vector. The unsupervised learning phase in the hidden layer of RBFN is followed by another different supervised learning phase. This is the stage where the output neurons are trained to associate each individual cluster with their own distinct shapes and sizes. RBFN is selected for the current work since its training speed is faster than the Back-Propagation network, able to detect data that are not within the norm, and make a better decision during classification problems.

The input and output neurons of RBFN and perceptron are alike [34]. The major difference lies in the hidden neuron. In most cases, it is governed by the Gaussian function. This is different from other processing neurons that produce an output based on the weighted sum of the inputs. On the contrary, the input neurons of the RBFN are not involved in the processing of information. Their sole function is to input the given data to the receiving nodes. Using a linear transfer function, these receiving nodes will decide the weights to be allocated to each subsequent processing element. They are governed by the transfer functions:

$$y_i = f_r(r_i), \quad r_i = \sqrt{\sum_{j=1}^{n}(x_j - w_{ij})^2}$$

where x_j is the input vector, W_{ij} represents the amount of weights allocated to the inputs of the neuron i. f_r is a symmetrical function known as the radial basis function or the Gaussian function, which is the preferred choice of most researchers.

$$f_r(r_i) = \exp\left(\frac{-r_i^2}{2\sigma_i^2}\right)$$

where σ_i is the standard deviation of the Gaussian distribution. Every neuron at each hidden layer will have its own unique σ_i value.

45.2.4 Bio-Statistical Methods

45.2.4.1 Regression Analysis

Regression (least-squares) analysis is a statistical technique used to determine the unique curve or a line that "best fits" all the data points (Figure 45.13). The underlying principle is to minimize the square of the distance of each data point to the line itself. In the regression analysis, there are two variables—namely, dependent and independent. The former is the variable to be estimated or predicted.

The most important result obtained in the analysis is the *R*-squared, or the coefficient of determination. *R*-squared is an indication of how tightly or sparsely clustered the data points are and it is a value that lies between 0 and 1. Thus, it is a measure of the correlation between the two variables. Correlation is the predictability of the change in the dependent variable given a change in the independent variable.

Parabolic regression refers to using a parabolic curve to fit the data points. It is a simple yet effective way to obtain the correlation between the two variables. However, a few assumptions are made in using the learn rule (LR). First, a parabolic relationship is assumed between the two variables, which might not always be the case. Second, the dependent variable is assumed to be normally distributed with the same variance with its corresponding value of the independent variable. Mathematically, the parabolic regression (PR) model is given by $Y = Ax^2 + Bx + C$ (Figure 45.14). PR usually offers a more realistic and better correlation between the two variables compared with LR.

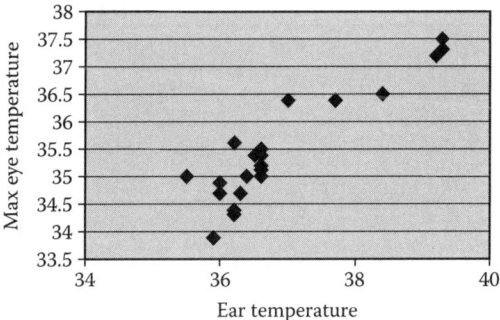

FIGURE 45.13 A typical scattered plot.

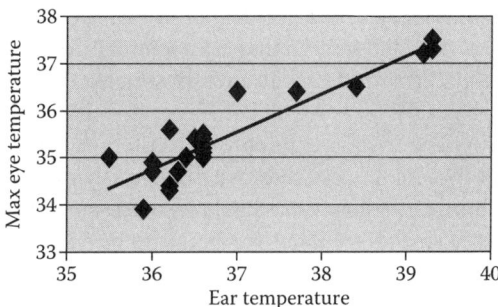

FIGURE 45.14 A regression line being fitted.

45.2.4.2 Receiver Operating Characteristics Curve

Receiver operating characteristics (ROC) curves are used to assess the diagnostic performance of a medical test to discriminate unhealthy cases from healthy cases [36]. Very often, in a medical test, the perfect separation between unhealthy and healthy cases is not possible if we were to discriminate them based on a threshold value. To illustrate this phenomenon, let us call the threshold value γ.

Figure 45.15 suggests that at the threshold value γ, the majority of those without the disease will be correctly diagnosed as healthy (TN). Similarly, the majority of those with the disease will be correctly diagnosed as unhealthy (TP). However, there will also be one group of diseased patients wrongly diagnosed as healthy (FN) and one group of healthy patients wrongly diagnosed as unhealthy (FP). Table 45.1 summarizes all the possibilities—TN, TP, FN, and FP and their respective algebraic representation.

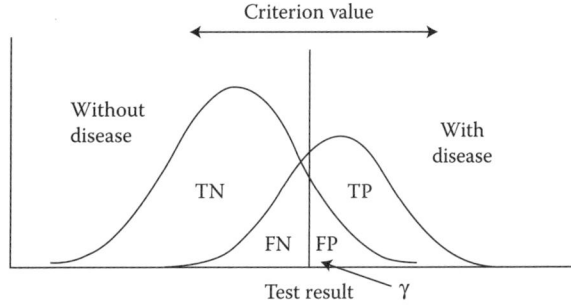

FIGURE 45.15 Discrimination curve.

TABLE 45.1 Basic Mathematical Formulae for ROC Analysis

Test	Disease	Number	Disease	Number	Total
Result	Present	*n*	Absent	*m*	
Positive	True positive	*a*	False positive	*c*	*a* + *c*
Negative	False negative	*b*	True negative	*d*	*b* + *d*
Total		*a* + *b*		*c* + *d*	

TABLE 45.2 Important Terminology for ROC Analysis

Sensitivity	$a/(a + b)$
Specificity	$d/(c + d)$
Positive predictive value	Sensitivity/(1 – specificity)
Negative predictive value	(1 – sensitivity)/specificity

With that, four important criterions can be defined—sensitivity,* specificity,† positive predictive value (PPV),‡ and negative predictive value (NPV)§ and they are commonly used in the ROC analysis to assess the credibility of the test. The mathematical formulas are summarized in Table 45.2.

In the ROC curves analysis result (Figure 45.16), both sensitivity and specificity will be displayed for all criterions. This will allow the user to choose the optimum criterion, which ought to have a high value for both sensitivity and specificity. The value of sensitivity is inversely proportional to that of specificity. This can be easily illustrated by the threshold value γ. A low γ will ensure that those with the disease will be detected. But this will also cause those without the disease to be classified as diseased. On the other hand, a high γ will allow to correctly categorize the healthy group but will miss out on the diseased group.

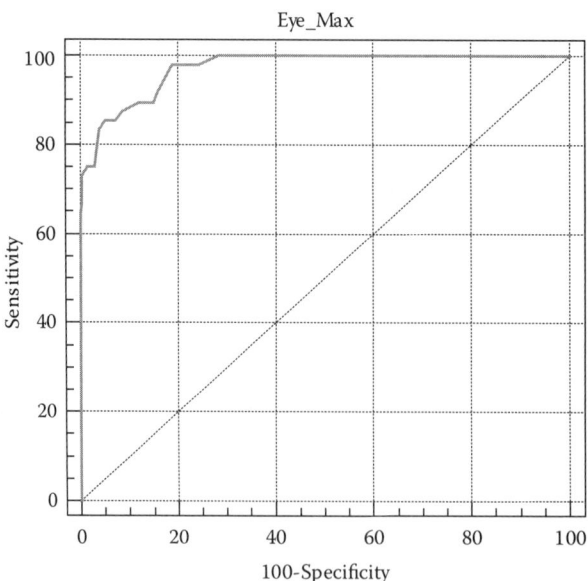

FIGURE 45.16 A typical ROC curve. (Adapted from Hopgood, A. Intelligent systems for engineers and scientists. Library of Congress Catalogingin-Publication Data, 2000.)

---

* Sensitivity—The probability that test is positive in the unhealthy population.
† Specificity—The probability that the test is negative in the healthy population.
‡ PPV—Given a positive forecast, the probability that it is correct.
§ NPV—Given a negative forecast, the probability that it is correct.

An example of the ROC curves is presented in Figure 45.16. The vertical axis shows the sensitivity while the horizontal axis shows the (100—specificity). Once again, this reinforces the fact that there is a trade-off between sensitivity and specificity.

The area under the ROC curve is an important information obtained in the analysis. The value lies between 0.5 and 1. A value of 0.5 implies that the test cannot discriminate the unhealthy from the healthy group, whereas a value of 1 implies that the test can distinguish the two groups perfectly.

45.3 Designed-Integrated Approach

45.3.1 Case 1: Advanced-Integrated Technique (Parabolic Regression + Artificial Neural Network Radial Basis Function Network + Receiver Operating Characteristics) for Febrile and Nonfebrile Cases

The proposed approach is a multipronged approach that comprises of PR, RBFN, and ROC analysis. It is a novel, integrative, and powerful technique that can be used to analyze complicated and large numerical data.

45.3.1.1 Step 1: Parabolic Regression

PR reflects the correlation between the variables and the actual health status (febrile or nonfebrile) of the subject, which is decided by the means of a thermometer placed in the ear. The output is either 1 or 0, corresponding to febrile and nonfebrile cases, respectively. The two input variables with the best correlation are chosen. The rational behind using PR over LR is it offers a more accurate and realistic approach in providing the correlation coefficient (LR results are also tabulated here for comparison purposes). Table 45.3 summarizes the temperature data from the thermograms [27].

45.3.1.2 Step 2: ANN Radial Basis Function Network

On the basis of the various inputs fed into the network, RBFN is trained to produce the desired outcome, which are either positive (1) for febrile cases, or negative (0) for nonfebrile cases. When this is done, the RBFN algorithm will possess the ability to predict the outcome when there are new input variables.

45.3.1.3 Step 3: ROC Analysis

Next, ROC is used to evaluate the accuracy, sensitivity, and specificity of the outcome of RBFN test files (i.e., Is RBFN well built or not?).

Table 45.4 and Figure 45.17 reveal the software needed for the entire process, including the steps prior to the advanced integrated technique.

45.3.2 Case 2: Conventional Bio-Statistical Technique (LR + ROC) for Febrile and Nonfebrile Cases

The conventional bio-statistical technique comprises of LR and ROC to analyze the data collected from the thermal imager [22]. Similar to the previous approach, regression is used to select the variable and the strongest correlation with the outcome (health status of the patient). Subsequently, ROC is applied to obtain the optimal preset temperature based on the chosen variables. The temperature is dependent on

TABLE 45.3   Temperature Data of Forehead and Near Eye Regions

Forehead Region	Near Eye Region
Minimum temperature	Minimum temperature
Maximum temperature	Maximum temperature
Average temperature	Average temperature

TABLE 45.4   Software Used for Advanced Integrated Technique for Febrile and Nonfebrile Thermograms

Purpose	Software
Views thermograms from thermal imager and extracts temperature data	Image J
Normalizes raw temperature data and performs statistical analysis (e.g., mean, median, and standard deviation)	MS Excel Statistical Toolbox
Determines the correlation of each variable with the output (health status)	MedCal
Training and testing of data, building an algorithm for the data	NeuralWorks Pro II
To evaluate the effectiveness of the computed method	MedCal

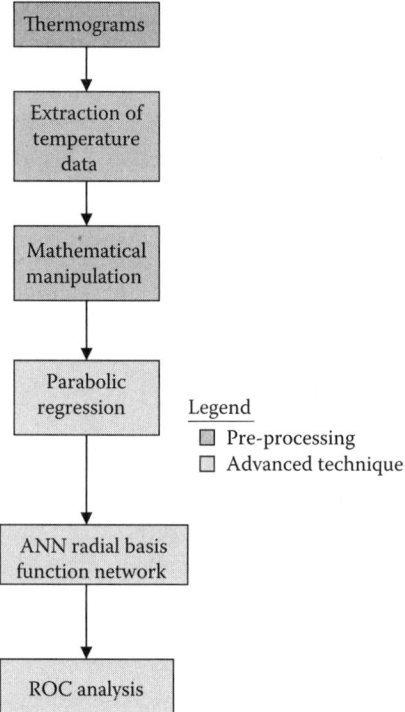

FIGURE 45.17   Flow chart for advanced integrated technique.

the values of sensitivity and specificity from the ROC analysis results. The chosen threshold temperature must have high values of sensitivity and specificity. Also, the area under the ROC curve is to be high to determine whether or not a subject should be considered as febrile (diseased) or nonfebrile (healthy). Table 45.5 and Figure 45.18 show the procedure of the conventional technique used during the SARS-2003 outbreak [22–24,27–28].

45.4 Results and Discussion

45.4.1 Case 1: Advanced Integrated Technique (PR + ANNRBFN + ROC) for Febrile and Nonfebrile Cases

Table 45.6 tabulates the results for PR and LR results are also included for comparison purposes. The PR coefficient of determination is always higher than that of LR. Thus, using simple LR with the present nonlinear data set are not always the best possible ways to "fit the data," as it is frequently used.

TABLE 45.5 Software Used for Conventional Approach

Purpose	Software
Views thermograms from thermal imager and extracts temperature data	Image J
Normalizes raw temperature data	MS Excel statistical toolbox
Performs statistical analysis (e.g., mean, median, and standard deviation)	
Determines correlation of each variable on the output (health status)	MedCal
Determines the optimal preset temperature and evaluates the effectiveness on the basis of sensitivity and specificity	MedCal

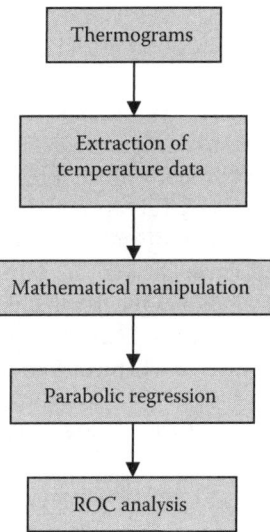

FIGURE 45.18 Flow chart for conventional approach.

When a parabolic curve is used to generate the correlation coefficient, the *maximum temperature of the near eye* and *the maximum temperature of the forehead regions* still remain to be the best correlated spots on the frontal face with regard to the core temperature. Hence, temperature data from these two regions are selected as input variables for the training of ANN. Although, using the parabolic function gives the better correlation coefficient, the outcome of the NN remains the same even if LR is used.

TABLE 45.6 Summarized Results for Step 1 for Advanced Integrated Technique

	Coefficient of Determination	
Independent Variable	Linear	Parabolic
Maximum temperature at eye range	0.5507	0.6315
Minimum temperature at eye range	0.0672	0.1114
Standard deviation at eye range	0.0303	0.0588
Total average at eye range	0.4489	0.5721
Maximum temperature at forehead range	0.4973	0.6362
Minimum temperature at forehead range	0.1169	0.1798
Standard deviation at forehead range	0.0053	0.0053
Total average at forehead range	0.3759	0.5379

TABLE 45.7 Selected Results for RBFN SLP of Advanced Integrated Technique

Learn Rule	Transfer Rule	Score (%)
Delta rule	Sigmoid	96
Delta rule	DNNA	96
Norm-cum-delta	Linear	96
Norm-cum-delta	TanH	96
Norm-cum-delta	Sigmoid	96
Norm-cum-delta	Sine	96
Ext DBD	Linear	96

Table 45.7 gives the selected results for RBFN SLP with a various combination of learn rule and transfer rate. The results for the selected combination of learn rule and transfer rule (with various *options* tested) for RBFN SLP are included in Table 45.8.

Various combinations of learn rule, transfer rule, and *options* were tested. With the inclusion of *options* (e.g., Connect Prior, Connect Bias), more NNs with an accuracy of 96% can be generated. The RBFN is credible and has the ability to differentiate the febrile from the nonfebrile cases to a very large extent. There are always four input data which the model always predicts wrongly and accounts for the 4% error. This is due to the inconsistencies between the patient's facial temperature (deduced from the thermograms) and his core temperature. For example, the Max Temp in the near eye region and Max Temp in the forehead region are very high and it indicates the fact that the person is having fever. Hence, ANN predicts that the person is having fever. However, the core temperature taken by the thermometer suggests that the person is not having fever. Thus, ANN's prediction is wrong. This is certainly not the ANN's

TABLE 45.8 Selected Results for RBFN SLP (with *Options* for Advanced Integrated Technique)

Learn Rule	Transfer Rule	Option	Score (%)
Delta rule	Sigmoid	Connect Prior	96
Delta rule	Sigmoid	Connect Bias	96
Delta rule	Sigmoid	MinMax Table	96
Delta rule	DNNA	Connect Prior	96
Delta rule	DNNA	Linear O/P	96
Delta rule	DNNA	Softmax O/P	96
Delta rule	DNNA	Connect Bias	96
Delta rule	DNNA	MinMax Table	96
Norm-cum-delta	TanH	Connect Prior	96
Norm-cum-delta	TanH	Linear O/P	96
Norm-cum-delta	TanH	Connect Bias	96
Norm-cum-delta	TanH	MinMax Table	96
Norm-cum-delta	Sigmoid	Connect Prior	96
Norm-cum-delta	Sigmoid	Linear O/P	96
Norm-cum-delta	Sigmoid	Connect Bias	96
Norm-cum-delta	Sigmoid	MinMax Table	96
Norm-cum-delta	Sine	Connect Prior	96
Norm-cum-delta	Sine	Linear O/P	96
Norm-cum-delta	Sine	Connect Bias	96
Norm-cum-delta	Sine	MinMax Table	96
Ext DBD	Linear	Connect Prior	96
Ext DBD	Linear	Linear O/P	96
Ext DBD	Linear	Connect Bias	96
Ext DBD	Linear	MinMax Table	96

TABLE 45.9   ROC Results for RBFN SLP with Various Combination of Learn Rule and Transfer Rule

No.	Learn Rule	Transfer Rule	Score (%)	Area Under Curve	Sensitivity	Specificity
1	Delta rule	Sigmoid	96	0.972	100	84.1
2	Delta rule	DNNA	96	0.971	91.7	94.3
3	Norm-cum-delta	Sigmoid	96	0.975	100	88.6

TABLE 45.10   ROC Results for RBFN SLP with Selected Combination of Learn Rule and Transfer Rule (with Various *Options* Tested)

No.	Learn Rule	Transfer Rule	Option	Score (%)	Area Under Curve	Sensitivity	Specificity
1	Delta rule	Sigmoid	Connect prior	96	0.972	100	84.1
2	Delta rule	Sigmoid	MinMax table	96	0.974	91.7	94.3
3	Delta rule	DNNA	Connect prior	96	0.971	91.7	94.3
4	Delta rule	DNNA	Linear O/P	96	0.971	91.7	94.3
5	Delta rule	DNNA	Softmax O/P	96	0.971	91.7	94.3
6	Delta rule	DNNA	Connect bias	96	0.970	91.7	94.3
7	Norm-cum-delta	TanH	Connect bias	96	0.973	91.7	94.3
8	Norm-cum-delta	TanH	MinMax table	96	0.978	100	87.5
9	Norm-cum-delta	Sigmoid	Connect prior	96	0.975	100	88.6
10	Norm-cum-delta	Sigmoid	Linear O/P	96	0.975	100	88.6
11	Norm-cum-delta	Sigmoid	Connect bias	96	0.970	100	85.2
12	Norm-cum-delta	Sigmoid	MinMax table	96	0.981	100	94.3
13	Norm-cum-delta	Sine	Connect bias	96	0.975	91.7	94.3
14	Norm-cum-delta	Sine	MinMax table	96	0.975	91.7	94.3
15	Ext DBD	Linear	Connect bias	96	0.980	100	93.2
16	Ext DBD	Linear	MinMax table	96	0.984	100	94.3

fault because in these cases, the person's facial temperature has a poor correlation with his core temperature. Without these exceptional cases, ANN should achieve a higher accuracy rate. Tables 45.9 and 45.10 (with various *options* tested) summarize the selected results (of ROC area >0.970) for ROC analysis.

The ROC area under the curve for all the RBFNs shown in Tables 45.9 and 45.10 is larger than 0.97. These RBFNs also have high sensitivities (>90%) and high specificities (>80%). This suggests that the RBFN is well-built and the overall diagnostic performance is reliable, and can be used for mass screening of febrile subjects. The best performing RBFN is a single-layered perceptron with Ext DBD as the learn rule, linear function as the transfer rule, and MinMax table as the selected option. The area under the ROC curve is 0.984 and its sensitivity and specificity are 100% and 94.3%, respectively.

45.4.2 Case 2: Conventional Bio-Statistical Technique (LR + ROC) for Febrile and Nonfebrile Cases

The LR analysis shows that the particular area on the skin surface that will produce the most consistent results with regard to the core temperature (taken using ear scanner) is the maximum temperature in the eye region with a coefficient correlation of 0.5507 (Table 45.11). The least correlated independent variable with the core temperature is the standard deviation for the forehead and eye regions (0.0053 and 0.0303), and the minimum temperature in the eye region (0.0672). Figure 45.19 shows the ROC plot in which the false positives are weighted similarly as false negatives. Table 45.12 summarizes the sensitivity and specificity for various preset scanner temperature.

TABLE 45.11   Summarized Results of LR for Conventional Approach

Independent Variable	Coefficient of Determination (linear)
Maximum temperature at eye range	0.5507
Minimum temperature at eye range	0.0672
Standard deviation at eye range	0.0303
Total average at eye range	0.4489
Maximum temperature at forehead range	0.4973
Minimum temperature at forehead range	0.1169
Standard deviation at forehead range	0.0053
Total average at forehead range	0.3759

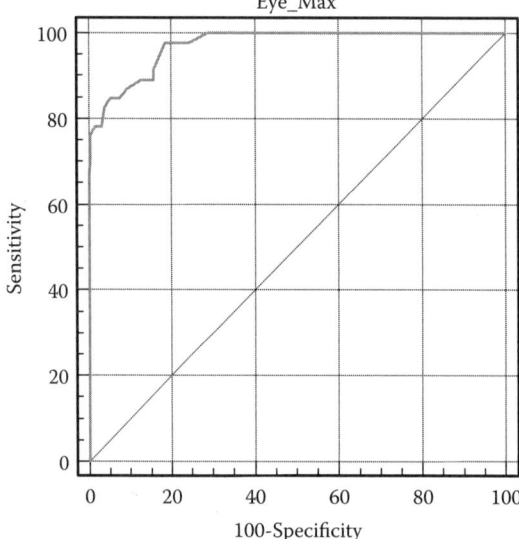

FIGURE 45.19   ROC curve for conventional technique (area of ROC = 0.972). (Adapted from Ng, E.Y.-K., Kaw, G.J.L, Chang, W.M., *Microvascular Research*, 68(2), 2004, 104–109; Ng, E.Y.-K., Chong, C., Kaw, G.J.L., *Journal of Mechanics in Medicine and Biology*, 5(1), 2005, 165–190; Ng, E.Y.-K., *Medical Physics*, 32(1), 2005, 93–97.)

ROC curve analysis for the maximum eye region shows that the optimal preset (cut-off) temperature is 36.3°C. If a subject's maximum temperature in the eye region exceeds 36.3°C, it implies that one is having fever. At this cut-off temperature, the sensitivity and specificity are 85.4% and 95.0%, respectively, with an accuracy rate of 93%.

45.4.3 Comparison between the Advanced Integrated Technique and Conventional Bio-Statistical Technique

The advanced technique achieves 96% of the accuracy rate whereas the conventional bio-statistical technique has 93% accuracy rate. Hence, there is a greater promise in using the advanced integrated technique for the thermogram analysis. In the conventional technique, after the "Max Temp in the Eye region" is found to have the strongest correlation with the output, the rest of the variables (e.g., Max Temp in the forehead region, Min Temp in the forehead region, Min Temp in the eye region, mode, median, etc.) are discarded. This implies that they will no longer be used in ANN. But in the advanced technique, it is possible and a common practice to use more than one input variable (besides Max Temp in the eye region). For this study Max Temp in the forehead region is used as the second input variable

TABLE 45.12 Selected Results of ROC Analysis for Conventional Bio-Statistical Technique [22–24]

Criterion	Sensitivity	Specificity
36.1	85.4	92.7
36.2	85.4	93.9
36.3[a]	85.4	95.0
36.4	83.3	96.2
36.5	75	96.9

[a] Selected criterion for preset temperature: 36.3°C.

for ANN training and testing. These are the two variables with the strongest correlation with the output. Further studies could be carried out to check if third, fourth, fifth, … input variables would further improve the effectiveness of the advanced technique.

45.5 Conclusion and Future Work

The chapter focuses on the numerical analyses of the data, to the detriment of performing a scientifically rigorous test of the hypotheses that febrile patients can be detected using simple thermograms. Through the use of ANN and bio-statistical methods, progress is made in thermography application with regard to achieving a higher level of consistency. This is made possible with the introduction of the novel advanced integrated technique in thermogram analysis.

The advanced technique has a high level of accuracy rate in prediction on the basis of the temperature data extracted from the thermograms. It improves the correlation and may prove more efficacious for mass fever screening. For elevated body temperature thermography, the advanced technique enables us to have in place a reliable system for the mass screening of fever cases. The proposed approach (PR + ANN + ROC) has surpassed the conventional bio-statistical approach (LR + ROC), which was used for analytical purposes during the SARS-2003 pandemic. In other words, the advanced technique enables us to possibly differentiate the febrile from nonfebrile cases in a short time . This is important with regard to the SARS outbreak in 2003 and the potentially lethal Avian flu or malaria. Recently Indonesia has reported the world's first laboratory-confirmed cluster of human-to-human transmission of bird flu, although scientists are as yet unsure of the significance for the multiple mutations in the H5N1 virus. In the event of such a virus being pandemic, we will be better prepared to set up thermography units in public places to mass screen populations for epidemic outbreaks.

In brief, thermography application is like an unpolished gemstone, waiting for us to unlash its full potential. The future development of an integrative fever screening system may incorporate the effectiveness of Laser Doppler Flowmeter (for heart rate), microwave radar (for respiration rate), and thermography (for skin temperature) to eliminate setbacks or noises that are prevalent in each individual device. All the medical images/data obtainable from these screening devices can then be supplied into the self-developed software that is built on the basis of ANN. With sufficient data collected from the affected patients, the software can be trained to carry out the automatic feature definition and image classification objectively.

Acknowledgments

To pay a tribute to the late Dr. Nicholas Diakides, this chapter is a revised version of Chapter 37, *Biomedical Engineering Handbook, Infrared Imaging Spin-off Edition*, ISBN-0-8493-9027-3, CRC Press.

References

1. Ring, E.F.J., Progress in the measurement of human body temperature, *Engineering in Medicine and Biology Magazine*, 17, 1998, 19–24.

2. Merla, A., Donato, L.D., Luzio, S.D., Farina, G., Pisarri, S., Proietti, M., Salsano, F., Romani, G.L., Infrared functional imaging applied to Raynaud's phenomenon, *IEEE Engineering in Medicine and Biology Magazine*, 21(6), 2002, 73–79.

3. Ng, E.Y.-K., Chen, Y., Segmentation of breast thermogram: Improved boundary detection with modified snake algorithm, *Journal of Mechanics in Medicine and Biology*, 6(2), 2006, 123–136.

4. Ng, E.Y.-K., A review of thermography as promising non-invasive detection modality for breast tumour, *International Journal of Thermal Sciences*, 48(5), 2009, 849–855.

5. Tan, J.H., Ng, E.Y.-K., Acharya R.U., Chee, C., Infrared thermography on ocular surface temperature: A review, *Infrared Physics and Technology*, 52(4), 2009, 97–108.

6. Pang, C., Gu, D.L., Some problems about detecting the suspected cases of SARS according to the local skin temperatures on face, *Space Medical and Medical Engineering*, 16(3), 2003, 231–234.

7. Chan, L.S., Cheung, G.T.Y., Lauder, I.J., Kumana, C.R., Screening for fever by remote-sensing infrared thermographic camera, *Journal of Travel Medicine*, 11, 2004, 273–278.

8. Peacock, G.R., Human radiation thermometry and screening for elevated body temperature in humans, *Thermosense XXVI, Proceedings of SPIE*, Vol. 5405, 2004, pp. 48–53, Orlando, USA.

9. Wu, M., Stop outbreak of SARS with infrared cameras, *Thermosense XXVI, Proceedings of SPIE*, Vol. 5405, 2004, pp. 98–105, Orlando, USA.

10. Samaan, G., Patel, M., Spencer, J., Roberts, L., Border screening for SARS in Australia: What has been learnt? *The Medical Journal of Australia*, 180(5), 2004, 220–223.

11. Hay, A.D., Peters, T.J., Wilson, A., Fahey, T., The use of infrared thermometry for the detection of fever, *The British Journal of General Practice*, 54, 2004, 448–450.

12. Liu, C.C., Chang, R.E., Chang, W.C., Limitations of forehead infrared body temperature detection for fever screening for SARS, *Infection Control and Hospital Epidemiology*, 25(12), 2004, 1109–1111.

13. Itoi, M., Yanai, Y., Abe, S., Is the using of thermography useful for the active surveillance of infectious disease at quarantine spot? *Journal of Japanese Quarantine Medicine*, 6, 2004, 125–132.

14. Health Canada. Thermal image scanners to detect fever in airline passengers, Vancouver and Toronto, 2003. *Canada Communicable Disease Report*, 30, (19), 2004, 165–167.

15. Ng, D.K., Chan, C.H., Lee, R.S., Leung, L.C., Non-contact infrared thermometry temperature measurement for screening fever in children, *Annals of Tropical Paediatrics*, 25(4), 2005, 267–275.

16. Shu, P.Y., Chien, L.J., Chang, S.F., Su, C.L., Kuo, Y.C., Liao, T.L., Fever screening at airports and imported dengue, *Emerging Infectious Diseases*, 11(3), 2005, 460–462.

17. Chiu, W.T., Lin, P.W., Chiou, H.Y., Lee, W.S., Lee, C.N., Yang, Y.Y., Lee, H.M., Hsieh, M.S., Hu, C.J., Ho, Y.S., Deng, W.P., Hsu, C.Y., Infrared thermography to mass-screen suspected SARS patients with fever, *Asia-Pacific Journal of Public Health*, 17(1), 2005, 26–28.

18. St John, R.K., King, A., de Jong, D., Bodie-Collins, M., Squires, S.G., Tam, T.W., Border screening for SARS, *Emerging Infectious Diseases*, 11(1), 2005, 6–10.

19. Wong, J.J., Wong, C.Y., Non-contact infrared thermal imagers for mass fever screening: State of the art or myth? *Hong Kong Medical Journal*, 12(3), 2006, 242–244.

20. Matsui, T., Suzuki, S., Ujikawa, K., Usui, T., Gotoh, S., Sugamata, M., Abe, S., The development of a non-contact screening system for rapid medical inspection at a quarantine depot using a laser Doppler blood-flow meter, microwave radar and infrared thermography, *Journal of Medical Engineering and Technology*, 33(6), 2009, 481–487.

21. Bitar, D., Goubar, A., Desenclos, J.C., International travels and fever screening during epidemics: A literature review on the effectiveness and potential use of non-contact infrared thermometers, *Eurosurveillance*, 14(6), 2009, 1–5.

22. Ng, E.Y.-K., Kaw, G.J.L, Chang, W.M., Analysis of IR thermal imager for mass blind fever screening, *Microvascular Research*, 68(2), 2004, 104–109.

23. Ng, E.Y.-K., Chong, C., Kaw, G.J.L., Classification of human facial and aural temperature using neural networks and IR fever scanner: A responsible second look, *Journal of Mechanics in Medicine and Biology*, 5(1), 2005, 165–190.

24. Ng, E.Y.-K., Is thermal scanner losing its bite in mass screening of fever due to SARS?, *Medical Physics*, 32(1), 2005, 93–97.

25. Ng, E.Y.-K., Chong, C., ANN based mapping of febrile subjects in mass thermogram screening: Facts and myths, *International Journal of Medical Engineering and Technology*, 30(5), 2006, 330–337.

26. Ng, E.Y.-K., Rajendra Acharya, U., A review of remote-sensing infrared thermography for indoor mass blind fever screening in containing an epidemic, *IEEE Engineering in Medicine and Biology*, 28(1), 2009, 76–83.

27. Ng, E.Y.-K., Kaw, G.J.L., IR scanners as fever monitoring devices: Physics, physiology and clinical accuracy, in *Biomedical Engineering Handbook*, CRC Press, Boca Raton, FL, N. Diakides, ed., pp. 24-1 to 24-20. (Mar. 2006).

28. Ng, E.Y.-K., Wiryani, M., Wong, B.S., Study of facial skin and aural temperature using IR with and w/o TRS, *IEEE Engineering in Medicine and Biology Magazine*, 25(3), 2006, 68–74.

29. ISO TC121/SC3-IEC SC62D:2008 Particular requirements for the basic safety and essential performance of screening thermographs for human febrile temperature screening.

30. ISO/TR 13154:2009 ISO/TR 80600: Medical electrical equipment:Deployment, implementation and operational guidelines for identifying febrile humans using a screening thermograph.

31. FLIR Systems: http://www.flir.com (accessed 17th July 2010).

32. Togawa, T., Body temperature measurement, *Clinical Physics Physiology Measure*, 6, 1985, 83–108.

33. Kaderavek, F., Clinical thermometry (Czech), *Casopis Lekaru Ceskych*, 111, 1972, 1135–1138.

34. Hopgood, A. Intelligent systems for engineers and scientists. Library of Congress Cataloging-in-Publication Data, 2000.

35. Battelle: http://www.battelle.org/pipetechnology/ (assessed 10 June 2009).

36. Receiver operating characteristics (ROC): http://www.medcalc.be/ (accessed 17 July 2010).

46

Thermal Imaging in Diseases of the Skeletal and Neuromuscular Systems

Francis J. Ring
University of Glamorgan

Kurt Ammer
*Ludwig Boltzmann
Research Institute for
Physical Diagnostics*

University of Glamorgan

46.1 Introduction

Clinical medicine has made considerable advances over the last century. The introduction of imaging modalities has widened the ability of physicians to locate and understand the extent and activity of a disease. Conventional radiography has dramatically improved, beyond the mere demonstration of bone and calcified tissue. Computed tomography ultrasound, positron emission tomography, and magnetic resonance imaging are now available for medical diagnostics.

Infrared imaging has also added to this range of imaging procedures. It is often misunderstood, or not been used, due to lack of knowledge of thermal physiology and the relationship between temperature and disease.

In rheumatology, disease assessment remains complex. There are a number of indices used, which testify to the absence of any single parameter for routine investigation. Most indices used are subjective. Objective assessments are of special value, but may be more limited due to their invasive nature. Infrared imaging is noninvasive, and with modern technology has proved to be reliable and useful in rheumatology.

From early times, physicians have used the cardinal signs of inflammation, that is, pain, swelling, heat, redness, and loss of function. When a joint is acutely inflamed, the increase in heat can be readily detected by touch. However, subtle changes in joint surface temperature occur and increase and decrease in temperature can have a direct expression of reduction or exacerbation of inflammation.

46.2 Inflammation

Inflammation is a complex phenomenon, which may be triggered by various forms of tissue injury. A series of cellular and chemical changes take place that are initially destructive to the surrounding tissue. Under normal circumstances, the process terminates when healing takes place, and scar tissue may then be formed.

A classical series of events take place in the affected tissues. First, a brief arteriolar constriction occurs, followed by a prolonged dilatation of arterioles, capillaries, and venules. The initial increased blood flow caused by the blood vessel dilation becomes sluggish and leucocytes gather at the vascular endothelium. Increased permeability to plasma proteins causes exudates to form, which is slowly absorbed by the lymphatic system. Fibrinogen, left from the reabsorption, partly polymerizes to fibrin. The increased permeability in inflammation is attributed to the action of a number of mediators, including histamines, kinins, and prostaglandins. The final process is manifest as swelling caused by the exudates, redness, and increased heat in the affected area resulting from the vasodilation, and increased blood flow. Loss of function and pain accompany these visible signs.

Increase in temperature and local vascularity can be demonstrated by some radionuclide procedures. In most cases, the isotope is administered intravenously and the resulting uptake is imaged or counted with a gamma camera. Superficial increases in blood flow can also be shown by laser Doppler imaging, although the response time may be slow. Thermal imaging, based on infrared emission from the skin is both fast and noninvasive.

This means that it is a technique that is suitable for repeated assessment, and especially useful in clinical trials of treatment whether by drugs, physical therapy, or surgery.

Intra-articular injection, particularly to administer corticosteroids came into use in the middle of the last century. Horvath and Hollander in 1949 [1] used intra-articular thermocouples to monitor the reduction in joint inflammation and synovitis following treatment. This method of assessment while useful to provide objective evidence of anti-inflammatory treatment was not universally used for obvious ethical reasons.

The availability of noncontact temperature measurement for infrared radiometry was a logical progression. Studies in a number of centers were made throughout the 1960s to establish the best analogs of corticosteroids and their effective dose. Work by Collins and Cosh in 1970 [2] and Ring and Collins in 1970 [3] showed that the surface temperature of an arthritic joint was related to the intra-articular joint, and to other biochemical markers of inflammation obtained from the exudates. In a series of experiments with different analogs of prednisolone (all corticosteroids), the temperature measured by thermal imaging in groups of patients can be used to determine the duration and degree of reduction in inflammation [4,5].

At this time, a thermal challenge test for inflamed knees was being used in Bath, UK, based on the application of a standard ice pack to the joint. This form of treatment is still used, and results in a marked decrease of joint temperature, although the effect may be transient.

The speed of temperature recovery after an ice pack of 1 kg of crushed ice to the knee for 10 min was shown to be directly related to the synovial blood flow and inflammatory state of the joint. The mean temperature of the anterior surface of the knee joint could be measured either by infrared radiometry or by quantitative thermal imaging [6].

A number of new nonsteroid anti-inflammatory agents were introduced into rheumatology in the 1970s and 1980s. Infrared imaging was shown to be a powerful tool for the clinical testing of these drugs, using temperature changes in the affected joints as an objective marker. The technique had been successfully used on animal models of inflammation, and effectively showed that optimal dose–response curves could be obtained from temperature changes at the experimental animal joints. The process with human patients suffering from acute rheumatoid arthritis was adapted to include a washout period for previous medication. This should be capable of relieving pain but no direct anti-inflammatory action per se. The compound used by all the pharmaceutical companies was paracetamol. It was shown by

Bacon et al. [7] that small joints such as fingers and metacarpal joints increased in temperature quite rapidly while paracetamol treatment was given, even if pain was still suppressed. Larger joints, such as knees and ankles required more than 1 week of active anti-inflammatory treatment to register the same effect. Nevertheless, the commonly accepted protocol was to switch to the new test anti-inflammatory treatment after 1 week of washout with the analgesic therapy. In every case, if the dose was ineffective, the joint temperature was not reduced. At an effective dose, a fall in temperature was observed, first in the small joints, then later in the larger joints. Statistical studies were able to show an objective decrease in joint temperature by infrared imaging as a result of a new and successful treatment. Not all the new compounds found their way into routine medicine; a few were withdrawn as a result of undesirable side effects. The model of infrared imaging to measure the effects of a new treatment for arthritis was accepted by all the pharmaceutical companies involved and the results were published in the standard peer-reviewed medical journals. More recently, attention has been focused on a range of new biological agents for reducing inflammation. These are also being tested in trials that incorporate quantitative thermal imaging.

To facilitate the use and understanding of joint temperature changes, Ring and Collins [3] and Collins et al. [8] devised a system for quantitation. This was based on the distribution of isotherms from a standard region of interest. The thermal index was calculated as the mean temperature difference from a reference temperature. The latter was determined from a large study of 600 normal subjects where the average temperature threshold for ankles, knees, hands, elbows, and shoulder were calculated. Many of the clinical trials involved the monitoring of hands, elbows, knees, and ankle joints. Normal index figure obtained from controls under the conditions described was from 1 to 2.5 on this scale. In inflammatory arthritis, this figure was increased to 4–5, while in osteoarthritic joints, the increase in temperature was usually less, 3–4. In gout and infection, higher values around 6–7 on this scale were recorded.

However, to determine normal values of finger joints is a very difficult task. This difficulty arises partly from the fact that cold fingers are not necessarily a pathological finding. Tender joints showed higher temperatures than nontender joints, but a wide overlap of readings from nonsymptomatic and symptomatic joints was observed [9]. Evaluation of finger temperatures from the reference database of normal thermograms [10] of the human body might ultimately solve the problem of being able to establish a normal range for finger joint temperatures in the near future.

46.3 Paget's Disease of Bone

The early descriptions of Osteitis Deformans by Czerny [11] and Paget [12] refer to "chronic inflammation of bone." An increased skin temperature over an active site of this disease has been a frequent observation and that the increase may be around 4°C. Others have shown an increase in peripheral blood flow in almost all areas examined. Increased periosteal vascularity has been found during the active stages of the disease. The vascular bed is thought to act as an arterio-venous shunt, which may lead to high output cardiac failure. A number of studies, initially to monitor the effects of calcitonin, and later bisphosphonate therapy, have been made at Bath. As with the clinical trials previously mentioned, a rigorous technique is required to obtain meaningful scientific data. It was shown that the fall in temperature during calcitonin treatment was also indicated more slowly, by a fall in alkaline phosphatase, the common biochemical marker. Relapse and the need for retreatment was clearly indicated by thermal imaging. Changes in the thermal index often preceded the onset of pain and other symptoms by 2–3 weeks. It was also shown that the level of increased temperature over the bone was related to the degree of bone pain. Those patients who had maximal temperatures recorded at the affected bone experienced severe bone pain. Moderate pain was found in those with raised temperature, and no pain in those patients with normal temperatures. The most dramatic temperature changes were observed at the tibia, where the bone is very close to the skin surface. In a mathematical model, Ring and Davies [13] showed that the increased temperature measured over the tibia was primarily derived from osseous blood flow and not from metabolic heat. This disease is often categorized as a metabolic bone disease.

46.4 Soft Tissue Rheumatism

46.4.1 Muscle Spasm and Injury

Muscle work is the most important source for metabolic heat. Therefore, contracting muscles contribute to the temperature distribution at the body's surface of athletes [14,15]. Pathological conditions such as muscle spasms or myofascial trigger points may become visible at regions of increased temperature [16]. An anatomic study from Israel proposes in the case of the levator scapulae muscle that the frequently seen hot spot on thermograms of the tender tendon insertion on the medial angle of the scapula might be caused by an inflamed bursae and not by a taut band of muscle fibers [17].

Acute muscle injuries may also be recognized by areas of increased temperature [18] due to inflammation in the early state of trauma. However, long-lasting injuries and also scars appear at hypothermic areas caused by reduced muscle contraction and therefore reduced heat production. Similar areas of decreased temperature have been found adjacent to peripheral joints with reduced range of motion due to inflammation or pain [19]. Reduced skin temperatures have been related to osteoarthritis of the hip [20] or to frozen shoulders [21,22]. The impact of muscle weakness on hypothermia in patients suffering from paresis was discussed elsewhere [23].

46.4.2 Sprains and Strains

Ligamentous injuries of the ankle [24] and meniscal tears of the knee [25] can be diagnosed by infrared thermal imaging. Stress fractures of bone may become visible in thermal images prior to typical changes in x-rays [26]. Thermography provides the same diagnostic prediction as bone scans in this condition.

46.4.3 Enthesopathies

Muscle overuse or repetitive strain may lead to painful tendon insertions or where tendons are shielded by tendon sheaths or adjacent to bursae, to painful swellings. Tendovaginitis in the hand was successfully diagnosed by skin temperature measurement [27]. The acute bursitis at the tip of the elbow can be detected through an intensive hot spot adjacent to the olecranon [28]. Figure 46.1 shows an acute tendonitis of the Achilles tendon in a patient suffering from inflammatory spondylarthropathy.

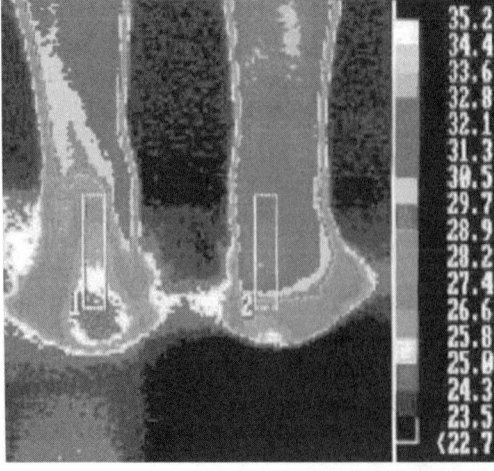

FIGURE 46.1 Acute tendonitis of the right Achilles tendon in a patient suffering from inflammatory spondylarthropathy.

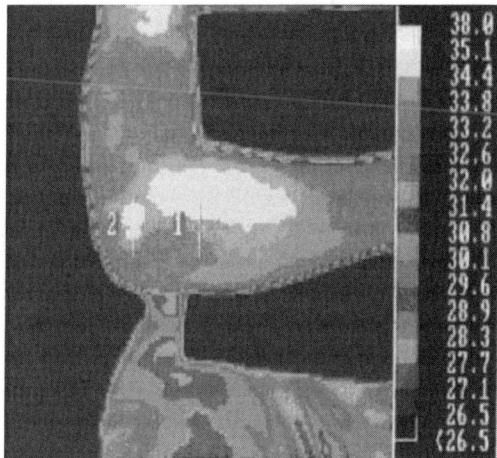

FIGURE 46.2 Tennis elbow with a typical hot spot in the region of tendon insertion.

46.4.3.1 Tennis Elbow

Painful muscle insertion of the extensor muscles at the elbow is associated with hot areas on a thermogram [29]. Thermal imaging can detect persistent tendon insertion problems of the elbow region in a similar way as isotope bone scanning [30]. Hot spots at the elbow have also been described as having a high association with a low threshold for pain on pressure [31]. Such hot areas have been successfully used as outcome measure for monitoring treatment [32,33]. In patients suffering from fibromyalgia, bilateral hot spots at the elbows is a common finding [34]. Figure 46.2 is the image of a patient suffering from tennis elbow with a typical hot spot in the region of tendon insertion.

46.4.3.2 Golfer Elbow

Pain due to altered tendon insertions of flexor muscles on the medial side of the elbow is usually named Golfer elbow. Although nearly identical in pathogenesis as the tennis elbow, temperature symptoms in this condition were rarely found [35].

46.4.3.3 Periarthropathia of Shoulder

The term "periarthropathia" includes a number of combined alterations of the periarticular tissue of the humero-scapular joint. The most frequent problems are pathologies at the insertion of the supraspinous and infraspinous muscles, often combined with impingement symptoms in the subacromial space. Long-lasting insertion alteration can lead to typical changes seen on radiographs or ultrasound images, but unfortunately there are no typical temperature changes caused by the disease [22,36]. However, persistent loss in range of motion will result in hypothermia of the shoulder region [21,22,36,37]. Figure 46.3 gives an example of an area of decreased temperature over the left shoulder region in patient with restricted range of motion.

46.4.4 Fibromyalgia

The terms "tender points" (important for the diagnosis of fibromyalgia) and "trigger points" (main feature of the myofascial pain syndrome) must not be confused. Tender points and trigger points may give a similar image on the thermogram. If this is true, patients suffering from fibromyalgia may present with a high number of hot spots in typical regions of the body. A study from Italy could not find different patterns of heat distribution in patients suffering from fibromyalgia and patients with osteoarthritis of the spine [38]. However, they reported a correspondence of nonspecific hyperthermic patterns with painful

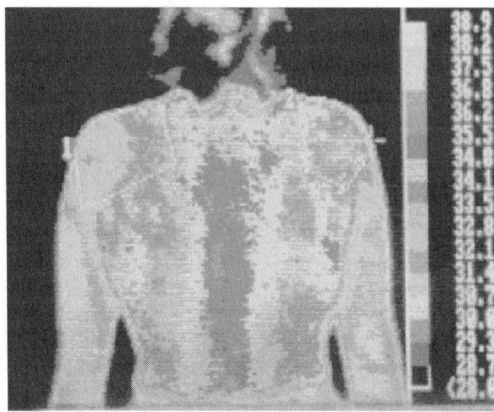

FIGURE 46.3   Decreased temperature in patient with a frozen shoulder on the left-hand side.

muscle areas in both groups of patients. Our thermographic investigations in fibromyalgia revealed a diagnostic accuracy of 60% of hot spots for tender points [34]. The number of hot spot was greatest in fibromyalgia patients and the smallest in healthy subjects. More than 7 hot spots seem to be predictive for tenderness of more than 11 out of 18 specific sites [39]. Based on the count of hot spots, 74.2% of 252 subjects (161 fibromyalgia, 71 with widespread pain but less than 11 tender sites out of 18, and 20 healthy controls) have been correctly diagnosed. However, the intra- and interobserver reproducibility of hot spot count is rather poor [40]. Software-assisted identification of hot or cold spots based on the angular distribution around a thermal irregularity [41] might overcome that problem of poor repeatability.

46.5 Peripheral Nerves

46.5.1 Nerve Entrapment

Nerve entrapment syndromes are compression neuropathies at specific sites in the human body. These sites are narrow anatomic passages where nerves are situated. The nerves are particularly prone to extrinsic or intrinsic pressure. This can result in paresthesias such as tingling or numb feelings, pain, and ultimately in muscular weakness and atrophy.

Uematsu [42] has shown in patients with partial and full lesion of peripheral nerves that both conditions can be differentiated by their temperature reaction to the injury. The innervated area of partially lesioned nerve appears hypothermic, caused by the activation of sympathetic nerve fibers. Fully dissected nerves result in a total loss of sympathetic vascular control and therefore in hyperthermic skin areas.

The spinal nerves, the brachial nerve plexus, and the median nerve at the carpal tunnel are the most frequently affected nerves with compression neuropathy.

46.5.1.1 Radiculopathy

A slipped nucleus of an intervertebral disk may compress the adjacent spinal nerve or better the sensory and motor fibers of the dorsal root of the spinal nerve. This may or must not result in symptoms of compression neuropathy in the body area innervated by these fibers.

The diagnostic value of infrared thermal imaging in radiculopathies is still under debate. A review by Hoffman et al. [43] from 1991 concluded that thermal imaging should be used only for research and not in clinical routine. This statement was based on the evaluation of 28 papers selected from a total of 81 references.

The study of McCulloch et al. [44], planned and conducted at a high level of methodology, found thermography not valid. However, the applied method of recording and interpretation of thermal images was not sufficient. The chosen room temperature of 20–22°C might have been too low for the identification of hypothermic areas. Evaluation of thermal images was based on the criterion that at least 25% of a dermatome present with hypothermia of 1°C compared to the contralateral side. This way of interpretation might be feasible for contact thermography, but does not meet the requirements of quantitative infrared imaging.

The paper of Takahashi et al. [45] showed that the temperature deficit identified by infrared imaging is an additional sign in patients with radiculopathy. Hypothermic areas did not correlate with sensory dermatomes and only slightly with the underlying muscles of the hypothermic area. The diagnostic sensitivity (22.9–36.1%) and the positive predictive value (25.2–37.0%) were low both for muscular symptoms such as tenderness or weakness and for spontaneous pain and sensory loss. In contrast, high specificity (78.8–81.7%), high negative predictive values (68.5–86.2%), and a high diagnostic accuracy were obtained.

Only the papers by Kim and Cho [46] and Zhang et al. [47] found thermography of high value for the diagnosis of both lumbosacral and cervical radiculopathies. However, these studies have several methodological flaws. Although a high number of patients were reported, healthy control subjects were not mentioned in the study on lumbosacral radiculopathy. The clinical symptoms are not described and the reliability of the used thermographic diagnostic criteria remains questionable.

46.5.1.2 Thoracic Outlet Syndrome

Similar to fibromyalgia, the disease entity of the thoracic outlet syndrome (TOS) is under continuous debate [48]. Consensus exists, that various subforms related to the severity of symptoms must be differentiated. Recording thermal images during diagnostic body positions can reproducibly provoke typical temperature asymmetries in the hands of patients with suspected TOS [49,50]. Temperature readings from thermal images from patients passing that test can be reproduced by the same and by different readers with high precision [51]. The original protocol included a maneuver in which the fist was opened and closed 30 times before an image of the hand was recorded. As this test did not increase the temperature difference between index and little finger, the fist maneuver was removed from the protocol [52]. Thermal imaging can be regarded as the only technique that can objectively confirm the subjective symptoms of mild TOS. It was successfully used as outcome measure for the evaluation of treatment for this pain syndrome [53]. However, in a patient with several causes for the symptoms paresthesias and coldness of the ulnar fingers, thermography could show only a marked cooling of the little finger, but could not identify all reasons for that temperature deficit [54]. It was also difficult to differentiate between subjects whether they suffer from TOS or carpal tunnel syndrome (CTS). Only 66.3% of patients were correctly allocated to three diagnostic groups, while none of the CTSs have been identified [55].

46.5.1.3 Carpal Tunnel Syndrome

Entrapment of the median nerve at the carpal tunnel is the most common compression neuropathy. A study conducted in Sweden revealed a prevalence of 14.4%; for pain, numbness, and tingling in the median nerve distribution in the hands. Prevalence of clinically diagnosed CTS was 3.8% and 4.9% for pathological results of nerve conduction of the median nerve. Clinically and electrophysiologically confirmed CTS showed a prevalence of 2.7% [56].

The typical distribution of symptoms leads to the clinical suspect of CTS [57], which must be confirmed by nerve conduction studies. The typical electroneurographic measurements in patients with CTS show a high intra- and interrater reproducibility [58]. The course of nerve conduction measures for a period of 13 years in patients with and without decompression surgery was investigated and it was shown that most of the operated patients presented with less pathological conduction studies within 12 months after operation [59]. Only 2 of 61 patients who underwent a simple nerve decompression by division of the carpal ligament as therapy for CTS had pathological findings in nerve conduction studies 2–3 years after surgery [60].

However, nerve conduction studies are unpleasant for the patient and alternative diagnostic procedures are welcome. Liquid crystal thermography was originally used for the assessment of patients with suspected CTS [61–64]. So et al. [65] used infrared imaging for the evaluation of entrapment syndromes of the median and ulnar nerves. Based on their definition of abnormal temperature difference to the contralateral side, they found thermography without any value for assisting diagnosis and inferior to electrodiagnostic testing. Tchou reported infrared thermography of high diagnostic sensitivity and specificity in patients with unilateral CTS. He has defined various regions of interest representing mainly the innervation area of the median nerve. Abnormality was defined if more than 25% of the measured area displayed a temperature increase of at least 1°C when compared with the asymptomatic hand [66].

Ammer has compared nerve conduction studies with thermal images in patients with suspected CTS. Maximum specificity for both nerve conduction and clinical symptoms was obtained for the temperature difference between the third and fourth finger at a threshold of 1°C. The best sensitivity of 69% was found if the temperature of the tip of the middle finger was by 1.2°C less than the temperature of the metacarpus [67].

Hobbins [68] combined the thermal pattern with the time course of nerve injuries. He suggested the occurrence of a hypothermic dermatome in the early phase of nerve entrapment and hyperthermic dermatomes in the late phase of nerve compression. Ammer et al. [69] investigated how many patients with a distal latency of the median nerve greater than 6 ms present with a hyperthermic pattern. They reported a slight increase of the frequency of hyperthermic patterns in patients with severe CTS, indicating that the entrapment of the median nerve is followed by a loss of the autonomic function in these patients.

Ammer and Melnizky [70] has also correlated the temperature of the index finger with the temperature of the sensory distribution of the median nerve on the dorsum of the hand and found nearly identical readings for both areas. A similar relationship was obtained for the ulnar nerve. The author concluded from these data that the temperature of the index or the little finger is highly representative for the temperature of the sensory area of the median or ulnar nerve, respectively.

Many studies on CTS have used a cold challenge to enhance the thermal contrast between affected fingers. A slow recovery rate after cold exposure is diagnostic for Raynaud's phenomenon [71]. The coincidence of CTS and Raynaud's phenomenon was reported in the literature [72,73].

46.5.1.4 Other Entrapment Syndromes

No clear thermal pattern was reported for the entrapment of the ulnar nerve [65]. A pilot study for the comparison of hands from patients with TOS or entrapment of the ulnar nerve at the elbow found only one out of seven patients with ulnar entrapment who presented with temperature asymmetry of the affected extremity [74]. All patients with TOS who performed provocation test during image recording showed at least in one thermogram an asymmetric temperature pattern.

46.5.2 Peripheral Nerve Paresis

Paresis is an impairment of the motor function of the nervous system. Loss of function of the sensory fibers may be associated with motor deficit, but sensory impairment is not included in the term "paresis." Therefore, most of the temperature signs in paresis are related to impaired motor function.

46.5.2.1 Brachial Plexus Paresis

Injury of the brachial plexus is a severe consequence of traffic accidents and motor cyclers are most frequently affected. The loss of motor activity in the affected extremity results in paralysis, muscle atrophy, and decreased skin temperature. Nearly 0.5% to 0.9% of newborns acquire brachial plexus paresis during delivery [75]. Early recovery of the skin temperature in babies with plexus paresis precede the recovery of motor function as shown in a study from Japan [76].

46.5.2.2 Facial Nerve

The seventh cranial nerve supplies the mimic muscles of the face and an acquired deficit is often named Bell's palsy. This paresis has normally a good prognosis for full recovery. Thermal imaging was used as outcome measure in acupuncture trials for facial paresis [77,78]. Ammer et al. [79] found slight asymmetries in patients with facial paresis, in which hyperthermia of the affected side occurred more frequently than hypothermia. However, patients with apparent herpes zoster causing facial palsy presented with higher temperature differences to the contralateral side than patients with nonherpetic facial paresis [80].

46.5.2.3 Peroneal Nerve

The peroneal nerve may be affected by metabolic neuropathy in patients with metabolic disease or by compression neuropathy due to intensive pressure applied at the site of fibula head. This can result in "foot drop," an impairment in which the patient cannot raise his forefoot. The thermal image is characterized by decreased temperatures on the anterior lower leg, which might become more visible after the patient has performed some exercises [81].

46.6 Complex Regional Pain Syndrome

A temperature difference between the affected and the nonaffected limb equal or greater than 1°C is one of the diagnostic criteria of the complex regional pain syndrome (CRPS) [82]. Ammer conducted a study in patients after radius fracture treated conservatively with a plaster cast [83]. Within 2 h after plaster removal and 1 week later, thermal images were recorded. After the second thermogram, an x-ray image of both hands was taken. The mean temperature difference between the affected and unaffected hand was 0.6 after plaster removal and 0.63 1 week later. In 21 out of 41 radiographs, slight bone changes suspected of algodystropy have been found. Figure 46.4 summarizes the results with respect to the outcome of x-ray images. Figure 46.5 shows the time course of an individual patient.

It was also shown that the temperature difference decrease during successful therapeutic intervention and temperature effect was paralleled by reduction of pain and swelling and resolution of radiologic changes [84].

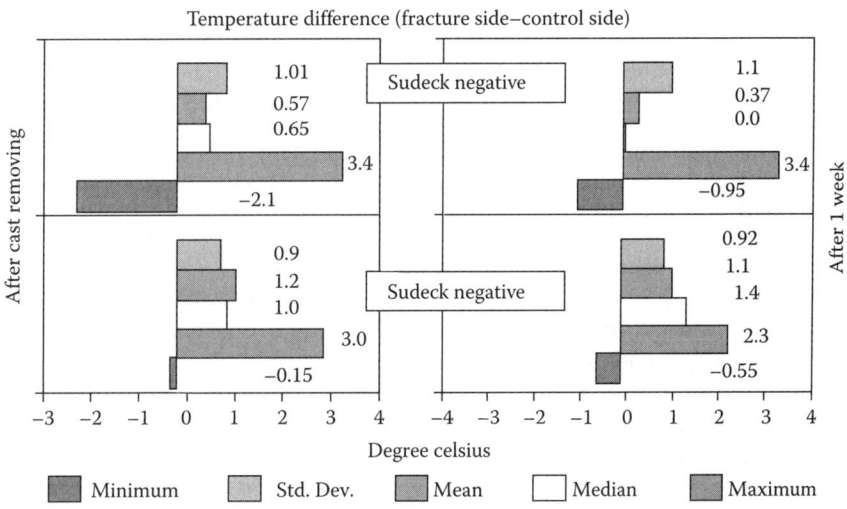

FIGURE 46.4 Diagram of temperatures obtained in patients with positive or negative x-ray images. (From Ammer, K. *Thermol. Österr.*, 1, 4, 1991. With permission.)

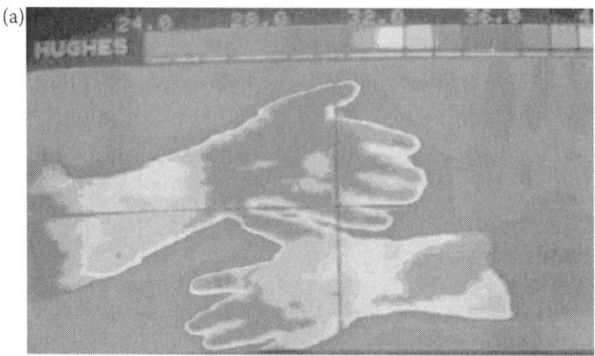

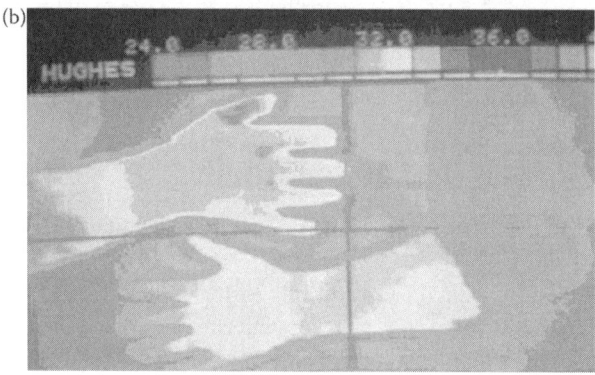

FIGURE 46.5   Early CRPS after radius fracture. (a) Two hours after cast removal; (b) 1 week later.

Disturbance of vascular adaptation mechanism and delayed response to temperature stimuli was obtained in patients suffering from CRPS [85,86]. These alterations have been interpreted as being caused by abnormalities of the autonomic nerve system. It was suggested to use a cold challenge on the contralateral side of the injured limb for prediction and early diagnosis of CRPS. Gulevich et al. [87] confirmed the high diagnostic sensitivity and specificity of cold challenge for the CRPS. Wasner et al. [88] achieved similar results by whole-body cooling or whole-body warming. Most recently, a Dutch study found that the asymmetry factor, which was based on histograms of temperatures from the affected and nonaffected hand, had the highest diagnostic power for CRPS, while the difference of mean temperatures did not discriminate between disease and health [89].

46.7 Thermal Imaging Technique

The parameters for a reliable technique have been described in the past. Reference 90 is a report published in 1978 by a European working group on thermography in locomotor diseases. This paper discusses aspects of standardization, including the need for adequate temperature control of the examination room and the importance of standard views used for image capture. More recently, Ring and Ammer [91] described an outline of necessary considerations for good thermal imaging technique in clinical medicine. This outline has been subsequently expanded to encompass a revised set of standard views, and associated regions of interest for analysis. The latter is especially important for standardization, since the normal approach used is to select a region of interest subjectively. This means that without a defined set of reference points, it is difficult for the investigator to reproduce the same region of interest on subsequent occasions. It is also even more difficult for another investigator to achieve the same, leading to unacceptable variables in the derived data. The aspects for standardization of the technique and the standard views and regions of interest recently defined are the product of a multicentered Anglo-Polish study that is pursuing the concept of a database of normal reference thermograms. The protocol can be found on a British University Research Group's website from University of Glamorgan [10].

46.7.1 Room Temperature

Room temperature is an important issue when investigating this group of diseases. Inflammatory conditions such as arthritis are better revealed in a room temperature of 20°C, for the extremities, and may need to be at 18°C for examining the trunk. This presumes that the relative humidity will not exceed 45%, and a very low airspeed is required. At no time during preparatory cooling or during the examination should the patient be placed in a position where they can feel a draught from moving air. However, in other clinical conditions where an effect from neuromuscular changes is being examined, a higher room temperature is needed to avoid forced vasoconstriction. This is usually performed at 22–24°C ambient. At higher temperatures, the subject may begin to sweat, and below 17°C, shivering may be induced. Both of these thermoregulatory responses by the human body are undesirable for routine thermal imaging.

46.7.2 Clinical Examination

In this group of diseases, it can be particularly important that the patient receives a clinical examination in association with thermal imaging. Observations on medication, range of movement, experience of pain related to movement, or positioning may have a significant effect on the interpretation of the thermal images. Documentation of all such clinical findings should be kept on record with the images for future reference.

References

1. Horvath, S.M. and Hollander, J.L. Intra-articular temperature as a measure of joint reaction. *J. Clin. Invest.*, 13, 615, 1949.
2. Collins, A.J. and Cosh, J.A. Temperature and biochemical studies of joint inflammation. *Ann. Rheum. Dis.*, 29, 386, 1970.
3. Ring, E.F.J. and Collins, A.J. Quantitative thermography. *Rheumatol. Phys. Med.*, 10, 337, 1970.
4. Esselinckx, W. et al. Thermographic assessment of three intra-articular prednisolone analogues given in rheumatoid arthritis. *Br. J. Clin. Pharm.*, 5, 447, 1978.
5. Bird, H.A., Ring, E.F.J., and Bacon, P.A. A thermographic and clinical comparison of three intra-articular steroid preparations in rheumatoid arthritis. *Ann. Rheum. Dis.*, 38, 36, 1979.
6. Collins, A.J. and Ring, E.F.J. Measurement of inflammation in man and animals. *Br. J. Pharm.*, 44, 145, 1972.
7. Bacon, P.A., Ring, E.F.J., and Collins, A.J. Thermography in the assessment of anti rheumatic agents, in *Rheumatoid Arthritis*. Gordon, J.L. and Hazleman, B.L., Eds., Elsevier/North Holland Biomedical Press, Amsterdam, 1977, p. 105.
8. Collins, A.J. et al. Quantitation of thermography in arthritis using multi-isothermal analysis. I. The thermographic index. *Ann. Rheum. Dis.*, 33, 113, 1974.
9. Ammer, K., Engelbert, B., and Kern, E. The determination of normal temperature values of finger joints. *Thermol. Int.*, 12, 23, 2002.
10. Website address, Standard protocol for image capture and analysis, www.medimaging.org.
11. Czerny, V. Eine fokale Malazie des Unterschenkels. *Wien. Med. Wochenschr.*, 23, 895, 1873.
12. Paget, J. On a form of chronic inflammation of bones. *Med. Chir. Transact.*, 60, 37, 1877.
13. Ring, E.F.J. and Davies, J. Thermal monitoring of Paget's disease of bone. *Thermology*, 3, 167, 1990.
14. Tauchmannova, H., Gabrhel, J., and Cibak, M. Thermographic findings in different sports, their value in the prevention of soft tissue injuries. *Thermol. Österr.* 3, 91–95, 1993.

15. Smith, B.L, Bandler, M.K., and Goodman, P.H. Dominant forearm hyperthermia, a study of fifteen athletes. *Thermology*, 2, 25–28, 1986.

16. Fischer, A.A. and Chang, C.H. Temperature and pressure threshold measurements in trigger points. *Thermology*, 1, 212, 1986.

17. Menachem, A., Kaplan, O., and Dekel, S. Levator scapulae syndrome: An anatomic–clinical study. *Bull. Hosp. Jt. Dis.*, 53, 21, 1993.

18. Schmitt, M. and Guillot, Y. Thermography and muscle injuries in sports medicine, in *Recent Advances in Medical Thermography*. Ring, E.F.J. and Philips, J., Eds., Plenum Press, London, 1984, p. 439.

19. Ammer, K. Low muscular activity of the lower leg in patients with a painful ankle. *Thermol. Österr.*, 5, 103, 1995.

20. Kanie, R. Thermographic evaluation of osteoarthritis of the hip. *Biomed. Thermol.*, 15, 72, 1995.

21. Vecchio, P.C. et al. Thermography of frozen shoulder and rotator cuff tendinitis. *Clin. Rheumatol.*, 11, 382, 1992.

22. Ammer, K. et al. Thermography of the painful shoulder. *Eur. J. Thermol.*, 8, 93, 1998.

23. Hobbins, W.B. and Ammer, K. Controversy: Why is a paretic limb cold, high activity of the sympathetic nerve system or weakness of the muscles? *Thermol. Österr.*, 6, 42, 1996.

24. Ring, E.F.J. and Ammer, K. Thermal imaging in sports medicine. *Sports Med. Today*, 1, 108, 1998.

25. Gabrhel, J. and Tauchmannova, H. Wärmebilder der Kniegelenke bei jugendlichen Sportlern. *Thermol. Österr.*, 5, 92, 1995.

26. Devereaux, M.D. et al. The diagnosis of stress fractures in athletes. *JAMA*, 252, 531, 1984.

27. Graber, J. Tendosynovitis detection in the hand. *Verh. Dtsch. Ges. Rheumatol.*, 6, 57, 1980.

28. Mayr, H. Thermografische Befunde bei Schmerzen am Ellbogen. *Thermol. Österr.*, 7, 5–10, 1997.

29. Binder, A.I. et al. Thermography of tennis elbow, in *Recent Advances in Medical Thermography*. Ring, E.F.J. and Philips, J., Eds., Plenum Press, London, 1984, p. 513.

30. Thomas, D. and Savage, J.P. Persistent tennis elbow: evaluation by infrared thermography and nuclear medicine isotope scanning. *Thermology*, 3, 132; 1989.

31. Ammer, K. Thermal evaluation of tennis elbow, in *The Thermal Image in Medicine and Biology*. Ammer, K. and Ring, E.F.J., Eds., Uhlen Verlag, Wien, 1995, p. 214.

32. Devereaux, M.D., Hazleman, B.L., and Thomas, P.P. Chronic lateral humeral epicondylitis—A double-blind controlled assessment of pulsed electromagnetic field therapy. *Clin. Exp. Rheumatol.*, 3, 333, 1985.

33. Ammer, K. et al. Thermographische und algometrische Kontrolle der physikalischen Therapie bei Patienten mit Epicondylopathia humeri radialis. *ThermoMed*, 11, 55–67, 1995.

34. Ammer, K., Schartelmüller, T., and Melnizky, P. Thermography in fibromyalgia. *Biomed. Thermol.* 15, 77, 1995.

35. Ammer, K. Only lateral, but not medial epicondylitis can be detected by thermography. *Thermol. Österr.*, 6, 105, 1996.

36. Hirano, T. et al. Clinical study of shoulder surface temperature in patients with periarthritis scapulohumeralis (abstract). *Biomed. Thermol.*, 11, 303, 1991.

37. Jeracitano, D. et al. Abnormal temperature control suggesting sympathetic dysfunction in the shoulder skin of patients with frozen shoulder. *Br. J. Rheumatol.*, 31, 539, 1992.

38. Biasi, G. et al. The role computerized telethermography in the diagnosis of fibromyalgia syndrome. *Minerva Medica*, 85, 451, 1994.

39. Ammer, K. Thermographic diagnosis of fibromyalgia. *Ann. Rheum. Dis. XIV European League Against Rheumatism Congress, Abstracts*, 135, 1999.

40. Ammer, K., Engelbert, B., and Kern, E. Reproducibility of the hot spot count in patients with fibromyalgia, an intra- and inter-observer comparison. *Thermol. Int.*, 11, 143, 2001.

41. Anbar, M. Recent technological developments in thermology and their impact on clinical applications. *Biomed. Thermol.*, 10, 270, 1990.

42. Uematsu, S. Thermographic imaging of cutaneous sensory segment in patients with peripheral nerve injury. *J. Neurosurg.*, 62, 716–720, 1985.

43. Hoffman, R.M., Kent, D.L., and. Deyo, R.A. Diagnostic accuracy and clinical utility of thermography for lumbar radiculopathy. A meta-analysis. *Spine*, 16, 623, 1991.

44. McCulloch, J. et al. Thermography as a diagnostic aid in sciatica. *J. Spinal Disord.*, 6, 427, 1993.

45. Takahashi, Y., Takahashi, K., and Moriya, H. Thermal deficit in lumbar radiculopathy. *Spine*, 19, 2443, 1994.

46. Kim, Y.S. and Cho, Y.E. Pre- and postoperative thermographic imaging of lumbar disk herniations. *Biomed. Thermol.*, 13, 265, 1993.

47. Zhang, H.Y., Kim, Y.S., and Cho, Y.E. Thermatomal changes in cervical disc herniations. *Yonsei Med. J.*, 40, 401, 1999.

48. Cuetter, A.C. and Bartoszek, D.M. The thoracic outlet syndrome: controversies, overdiagnosism overtreatment and recommendations for management. *Muscle Nerve*, 12, 419, 1989.

49. Schartelmüller, T. and Ammer, K. Thoracic outlet syndrome, in *The Thermal Image in Medicine and Biology*. Ammer, K. and Ring, E.F.J., Eds., Uhlen Verlag, Wien, 1995, p. 201.

50. Schartelmüller, T. and Ammer, K. Infrared thermography for the diagnosis of thoracic outlet syndrome. *Thermol. Österr.*, 6, 130, 1996.

51. Melnizky, P., Schartelmüller, T., and Ammer, K. Prüfung der intra-und interindividuellen Verläßlichkeit der Auswertung von Infrarot-Thermogrammen. *Eur. J. Thermol.*, 7, 224, 1997.

52. Ammer, K. Thermographie der Finger nach mechanischem Provokationstest. *ThermoMed*, 17/18, 9, 2003.

53. Schartelmüller, T., Melnizky, P., and Engelbert, B. Infrarotthermographie zur Evaluierung des Erfolges physikalischer Therapie bei Patenten mit klinischem Verdacht auf Thoracic Outlet Syndrome. *Thermol. Int.*, 9, 20, 1999.

54. Schartelmüller, T. and Ammer, K. Zervikaler Diskusprolaps, Thoracic Outlet Syndrom oder periphere arterielle Verschlußkrankheit-ein Fallbericht. *Eur. J. Thermol.*, 7, 146, 1997.

55. Ammer, K. Diagnosis of nerve entrapment syndromes by thermal imaging, in *Proceedings of the First Joint BMES/EMBS Conference. Serving Humanity, Advancing Technology*, October 13–16, 1999, Atlanta, GA, USA, p. 1117.

56. Atroshi, I. et al. Prevalence of carpal tunnel syndrome in a general population. *JAMA*, 282, 153, 1999.

57. Ammer, K., Mayr, H., and Thür, H. Self-administered diagram for diagnosing carpal tunnel syndrome. *Eur. J. Phys. Med. Rehab.*, 3, 43, 1993.

58. Melnizky, P., Ammer, K., and Schartelmüller, T. Intra- und interindividuelle Verläßlichkeit der elektroneurographischen Untersuchung des Nervus medianus. *Österr. Z. Phys. Med. Rehab.*, 7, S83, 1996.

59. Schartelmüller, T., Ammer, K., and Melnizky, P. Natürliche und postoperative Entwicklung elektroneurographischer Untersuchungsergebnisse des N. medianus von Patienten mit Carpaltunnelsyndrom (CTS). *Österr. Z. Phys. Med.*, 7, 183, 1997.

60. Rosen, H.R. et al. Is surgical division of the carpal ligament sufficient in the treatment of carpal tunnel syndrome? *Chirurg*, 61, 130, 1990.

61. Herrick, R.T. et al. Thermography as a diagnostic tool for carpal tunnel syndrome, in *Medical Thermology*, Abernathy, M. and Uematsu, S., Eds., American Academy of Thermology, Washington, DC, 1986, p. 124.

62. Herrick, R.T. and Herrick, S.K., Thermography in the detection of carpal tunnel syndrome and other compressive neuropathies. *J. Hand Surg.*, 12A, 943–949, 1987.

63. Gateless, D., Gilroy, J., and Nefey, P. Thermographic evaluation of carpal tunnel syndrome during pregnancy. *Thermology*, 3, 21, 1988.

64. Meyers, S. et al. Liquid crystal thermography, quantitative studies of abnormalities in carpal tunnel syndrome. *Neurology*, 39, 1465, 1989.

65. So, Y.T., Olney, R.K., and Aminoff, M.J. Evaluation of thermography in the diagnosis of selected entrapment neuropathies. *Neurology*, 39, 1, 1989.

66. Tchou, S. and Costich, J.F. Thermographic study of acute unilateral carpal tunnel syndromes. *Thermology*, 3, 249–252, 1991.

67. Ammer, K. Thermographische Diagnose von peripheren Nervenkompressionssyndromen. *ThermoMed*, 7, 15, 1991.

68. Hobbins, W.B. Autonomic vasomotor skin changes in pain states: Significant or insignificant? *Thermol. Österr.*, 5, 5, 1995.

69. Ammer, K. et al. The thermal image of patients suffering from carpal tunnel syndrome with a distal latency higher than 6.0 msec. *Thermol. Int.*, 9, 15, 1999.

70. Ammer, K. and Melnizky, P. Determination of regions of interest on thermal images of the hands of patients suffering from carpal tunnel syndrome. *Thermol. Int.*, 9, 56, 1999.

71. Ammer, K. Thermographic diagnosis of Raynaud's phenomenon. *Skin Res. Technol.*, 2, 182, 1996.

72. Neundörfer, B., Dietrich, B., and Braun, B. Raynaud–Phänomen beim Carpaltunnelsyndrom. *Wien. Klin. Wochenschr.*, 89, 131–133, 1977.

73. Grassi, W. et al. Clinical diagnosis found in patients with Raynaud's phenomenon: A multicentre study. *Rheumatol. Int.*, 18, 17, 1998.

74. Mayr, H. and Ammer, K. Thermographische Diagnose von Nervenkompressionssyndromen der oberen Extremität mit Ausnahme des Karpaltunnelsyndroms (abstract). *Thermol. Österr.*, 4, 82, 1994.

75. Mumenthaler, M. and Schliack, H. *Läsionen periphere Nerven*. Georg Thieme Verlag, Stuttgart-New York, Auflage, 1982, p. 4.

76. Ikegawa, S. et al. Use of thermography in the diagnosis of obstetric palsy (abstract). *Thermol. Österr.*, 7, 31, 1997.

77. Zhang, D. et al. Preliminary observation of imaging of facial temperature along meridians. *Chen Tzu Yen Chiu*, 17, 71, 1992.

78. Zhang, D. et al. Clinical observations on acupuncture treatment of peripheral facial paralysis aided by infra-red thermography—A preliminary report. *J. Tradit. Chin. Med.*, 11, 139, 1991.

79. Ammer, K., Melnizky, P. and Schartelmüller, T. Thermographie bei Fazialisparese. *ThermoMed*, 13, 6–11, 1997.

80. Schartelmüller, T., Melnizky, P., and Ammer, K. Gesichtsthermographie, Vergleich von Patienten mit Fazialisparese und akutem Herpes zoster ophthalmicus. *Eur. J. Thermol.*, 8, 65, 1998.

81. Melnizky, P., Ammer, K., and Schartelmüller, T. Thermographische Überprüfung der Heilgymnastik bei Patienten mit Peroneusparese. *Thermol. Österr.*, 5, 97, 1995.

82. Wilson, P.R. et al. Diagnostic algorithm for complex regional pain syndromes, in *Reflex Sympathetic Dystrophy, A Re-appraisal*. Jänig, W. and Stanton-Hicks, M., Eds., IASP Press, Seattle, 1996, p. 93.

83. Ammer, K. Thermographie nach gipsfixierter Radiusfraktur. *Thermol. Österr.*, 1, 4, 1991.

84. Ammer, K. Thermographische Therapieüberwachung bei M.Sudeck. *ThermoMed*, 7, 112–115, 1991.

85. Cooke, E.D. et al. Reflex sympathetic dystrophy (algoneurodystrophy): Temperature studies in the upper limb. *Br. J. Rheumatol.*, 8, 399, 1989.

86. Herrick, A. et al. Abnormal thermoregulatory responses in patients with reflex sympathetic dystrophy syndrome. *J. Rheumatol.*, 21, 1319, 1994.

87. Gulevich, S.J. et al. Stress infrared telethermography is useful in the diagnosis of complex regional pain syndrome, type I (formerly reflex sympathetic dystrophy). *Clin. J. Pain*, 13, 50, 1997.

88. Wasner, G., Schattschneider, J., and Baron, R. Skin temperature side differences—A diagnostic tool for CRPS? *Pain*, 98, 19, 2002.

89. Huygen, F.J.P.M. et al. Computer-assisted skin videothermography is a highly sensitive quality tool in the diagnosis and monitoring of complex regional pain syndrome type I. *Eur. J. Appl. Physiol.*, 91, 516, 2004.

90. Engel, J.M. et al. Thermography in locomotor diseases, recommended procedure. Anglo-dutch thermographic society group report. *Eur. J. Rheumatol. Inflam.*, 2, 299–306, 1979.

91. Ring, E.F.J. and Ammer, K. The technique of infra red imaging in medicine. *Thermol. Int.*, 10, 7, 2000.

47

Functional Infrared Imaging in the Evaluation of Complex Regional Pain Syndrome, Type I: Current Pathophysiological Concepts, Methodology, Case Studies, and Clinical Implications

Timothy D. Conwell
Colorado Infrared Imaging Center

James Giordano
Potomac Institute for Policy Studies
George Mason University
University of Oxford

47.1 Introduction

47.1.1 Overview, History, and Contemporary Issues

Complex Regional Pain Syndrome, Type I (CRPS I) is a potentially disabling neuropathic condition characterized by regional pain that is often disproportionate to or occurs in the absence of an identifiable inciting event. This poorly understood disease is the result of a multifactorial interplay between altered somatosensory, motor, autonomic, and inflammatory systems. Peripheral and central sensitization is a common feature in CRPS. The condition is associated with hyperalgesia, allodynia, spontaneous pain, abnormal skin color, changes in skin temperature, abnormal sudomotor activity, edema, active and passive movement disorders, and trophic changes of nails and hair. CRPS I usually begins after minor or major trauma to soft tissue (e.g., strain, sprain, or surgery). Although rare, it can also occur following fracture, visceral trauma, or central nervous system insult (e.g., cerebrovascular accident; CVA). Although similar—if not identical—in presentation, a related syndrome, Type II (CRPS II), occurs following direct insult or injury to peripheral nerve. A complete address of CRPS II is beyond the scope of this chapter (see [1], for review). Sandroni et al. [2] report that CRPS I occurs more frequently than CRPS II (i.e., CRPS I incidence of 5.5/100,000 person years at risk vs. CRPS II incidence of 0.8/100,000 person years at risk), is more prevalent (21/100,000 vs. 4/100,000), and occurs more in females than males with reported ratios of 2:1 or greater [3].

Diagnosis of CRPS I is based upon patient history and evaluation of presenting clinical signs and symptoms. Diagnosis can be complicated by the facts that (1) the severity of the symptoms is characteristically far greater than that of the instigating insult; (2) there is a tendency of the symptoms to spread proximally and in some cases to the contralateral limb, trunk, and face; and (3) although somewhat more rare, all four extremities may be involved [4,5]. In light of these diagnostic issues, a consensus workshop was convened in Orlando in 1993 to posit evaluative criteria and develop a more effective nomenclature for these disorders. From this work, the term "CRPS" was first introduced [7]. Subsequently, The International Association for the Study of Pain (IASP) modified their taxonomy of pain to include these disorders, thus formalizing the use of CRPS I to identify and describe distinct syndromes [6–8]. During the same time period (i.e., circa early 1990s), Veldman et al. developed similar criteria for CRPS [9]. Previously, CRPS I and II were known as reflex sympathetic dystrophy (RSD) and causalgia, respectively, although both syndromes were rather arbitrarily referred to as algodystrophy, Sudeck's atrophy, sympathalgia, and sympathetically maintained pain (SMP). However, it should be noted that SMP remains in use as a diagnostic category for any pain syndrome that involves, and/or is perpetuated by autonomic hyperreactivity, and is identifiable by positive response to sympatholytic intervention.

The IASP diagnostic criteria for CRPS I is based upon nonstandardized signs and symptoms [10–13]. Rigorous discriminant function analyses (DFA) applied to these criteria have revealed problems in reliability and external validity. Results of validation studies have shown that there is significant potential for overdiagnosis due to low specificity [14–16], low interobserver reliability [17,18], and considerable variability in the recognition of relevant clinical signs. Consequently, the maximum potential benefits of the IASP criteria have been unsuccessful. As a result, an international consensus group revised the IASP criteria for CRPS [19]. The schema, known as the "Budapest Criteria" revealed a diagnostic sensitivity of 99%, with an improved specificity of 68%, thereby significantly enhancing the poor specificity (41%) obtained when utilizing the original IASP criteria [20]. Yet, other researchers have expressed a need for more regionally based CRPS diagnostic criteria that differ from the "Budapest Criteria" [21].

Such disparities in diagnostic criteria promote inherent difficulties in the clinical management of CRPS I. Lack of coherence in detection, discernment, and diagnostic acumen arises from a tendency to rely on sympathetic blockade as a diagnostic measure. Reiteratively, it is important to note that while some CRPS I patients will be responsive to sympatholytics (e.g., systemically administered adrenergic antagonists; interventional sympathetic blockade), such SMP does not occur in all CRPS I, and therefore is not an exclusory criterion. Also, given the heterogeneity of signs, symptoms, and overall presentations, there is a level of suspicion among non-subspecialists regarding the validity of CRPS I as a diagnosis. Taken together, these lead to a tendency for either frank undertreatment or excessive utilization of therapeutic interventions that incur significant cost, time, and even health burdens for the patient. Thus, it can be seen that diagnosis is the foundation upon which effective and sound treatment is built. Clearly, more reliable diagnostic tests are needed to advance both our understanding and treatment of CRPS I.

47.1.2 Ethics and Imperatives for Evidence-Based Use of Functional Infrared Imaging in Research and Practice

It is important to emphasize that detection alone is not diagnosis. In formulating any diagnosis, the clinician must utilize distinct domains and types of knowledge to apprehend the objective and subjective features of a disorder as expressed in a particular patient. While this is important in the diagnosis of any malady, it is particularly critical to diagnosing (and treating) pain syndromes. By its nature, pain is subjective, and thus the clinician must utilize patient narrative and history, together with any/all objective findings to formulate a clinical impression [22]. The "goal" of this initial step of pain medicine is to detect what and how a disorder presents in a particular patient, differentiate these signs and symptoms from other possible disorders, discern the contextual basis of these features, and establish a diagnosis, literally a "...seeing or a knowledge into the problem." This provides the basis for the scope, nature, and extent of subsequent care, and allows for more accurate prognosis (knowledge of what could occur). It is clear that this process—often referred to as the nosological method—is not simply one of applied science, but takes on considerable ethical weight as it names the disorder (and by extension categorizes the patient), frames the patient within a larger community of others, and creates a foundation for the development and implementation of prudent care [23]. The diversity and individuality of signs and symptoms of CRPS I complicates this process. The ethical obligation to treat pain [23] compels research to determine those techniques and technologies that facilitate diagnoses and treatments that are safe and effective, and sustains the utilization of these approaches in clinical practice [24–26].

By classical definition, medicine is dedicated to providing patient care that is technically correct and ethically sound, enacted within the clinical encounter [27]. Research facilitates these ends by affording knowledge that (1) enables the clinician to evaluate the relative value(s), benefits, burdens, and risks of particular diagnostic and therapeutic approaches, so as to ultimately resolve clinical equipoise, and (2) empowers patients to be informed participants in clinical decisions relevant to care, thereby lessening their inherent vulnerability and decreasing the inequalities of knowledge, power, and capacity [25]. The ethical obligations of research and practice are reciprocal: findings from research inform practice, and evaluation of outcomes gained by employing various techniques in practice contributes to a progressive revision and expansion of evidentiary knowledge to instigate and guide further study [26,28]. Thus, we argue that the investigational and clinical use of functional infrared (fIR) imaging is both pragmatically valid and ethically imperative.

47.1.3 Detection, Discernment, and Diagnosis: Bases for Effective Treatment

fIR effectively detects the thermal signature of vasomotor disturbances that are an important factor in establishing a diagnosis of CRPS I. Early detection of CRPS I is essential for successful treatment, yet detection of early-stage CRPS I is difficult because the signs and symptoms mimic other pathologies. Several studies have supported the utility of infrared imaging (thermography) in early detection of CRPS [29–33]. Most studies have utilized quantitative, homologous side-to-side temperature differences as the sole criterion in establishing the diagnosis. These temperature differences have ranged from 0.5°C [29], 0.6°C [34,35], 1°C [32,36–38], 1.5°C [39], and 2°C [33].

Bruehl et al. [34] evaluated thermal asymmetries in patients with CRPS I following equilibration in a 20°C examining room for 20 min, and demonstrated a sensitivity of 60% and specificity of 67% utilizing an asymmetry cutoff of 0.6°C in side-to-side computer-generated temperature differences. Gulevich et al. [38] demonstrated a 93% sensitivity and 89% specificity when three of the following four infrared image categories were present: (1) quantitative homologous side-to-side computer-generated temperature differences of greater than 1.0°C in the region of interest (ROI); (2) the presence of abnormal, disrupted transverse distal thermal gradient lines visualized in the symptomatic extremity; (3) the presence of a "thermal marker" of the symptomatic extremity visualized in the isotherm view; and (4) abnormal warming of the symptomatic extremity secondary to functional cold-water autonomic stress testing of an asymptomatic limb. These contingencies are addressed elsewhere in this chapter (see Section 47.3). Similarly, Wasner et al. [40] showed a sensitivity of 76% and specificity of 93% when patients underwent controlled alteration of sympathetic activity by using thermoregulatory whole-body cooling followed by computer-generated side-to-side temperature differences of homologous body regions. Conwell et al. [41] showed a sensitivity of 72% and specificity of 94%, with a positive predictive value 82% and negative predictive value 90%, when using cold-water autonomic functional stress testing as compared with the modified IASP criteria for CRPS. The use of quantitative temperature differences alone lacks diagnostic specificity because numerous pathologies may present with skin temperature asymmetry. For example, differences in skin temperature occur in focal inflammation and vascular disease. Moreover, thermal asymmetry can result from somatoautonomic vasoconstriction secondary to acute trauma [42], limb immobilization [43], fracture [44], antidromic vasodilatation from small fiber distal neuropathy, and neuropathic pain with sympathetic activity. Infrared imaging (thermography) does not merely measure limb temperature; the infrared thermogram yields a temperature map (IR signature) of an extremity through which a highly trained and experienced examiner can differentiate the IR signatures (thermal patterns) of CRPS I from trauma, inflammation, and vascular disease. The quantitative assessment of the IR signature (vasomotor changes) is instrumental, if not mandatory, for establishing an accurate diagnosis of CRPS I and II [45–47]. Furthermore, the infrared thermographic study is significantly enhanced when the IR data are interfaced with software that enables the examiner to obtain three IR indices [38]: (1) computer-generated side-to-side temperature differences, (2) statistical evaluation of the integrity (i.e., normality vs. abnormality) of distal thermal gradient IR signatures, and (3) responses to cold-water autonomic functional stress testing [41].

An understanding of the capabilities and limitations of fIR technology is critical to establishing its significance in detecting physiological changes that are relevant and meaningful to the diagnosis of CRPS I. Thus, this chapter will present (1) a brief overview of the pathophysiology of CRPS I, with particular emphasis upon those autonomically mediated vasomotor effects that evoke clinically relevant changes in the radiant heat signature; (2) current fIR methodology that has been shown to be capable of effectively detecting such changes; (3) discussion of the current procedures and protocol methods for performing fIR studies of presumed CRPS I (and differentiating this from other pain syndromes); and (4) selected cases of acute trauma, neurogenic inflammation without sympathetic activity, small-caliber fiber distal neuropathy, and acute and chronic CRPS I, to illustrate clinical applications of this technology.

47.2 Pathophysiology of CRPS I

47.2.1 Sympathetic Neural Involvement

Any discussion of CRPS I, II, SMP, and other dysautonomias must address the role of autonomic dysfunction. Ordinarily, sympathetic efferents and sensory afferents are not conjoined [48,49]. However, functional and perhaps structural interactions between nociceptive C-fiber afferents and sympathetic efferent fibers in both the periphery and within the dorsal root ganglion have been elucidated in both animal models of sympathetically mediated pain [50] and in humans with CRPS I [51,52]. This interaction involves the *de novo* expression of alpha-2 adrenoceptors on C-fiber processes, resulting in an increased sensitivity to adrenergic stimulation [52,53]. It remains unclear whether structural synaptogenesis is involved in the periphery or the dorsal root, but clearly the functional properties of C-fiber afferents change, with alteration in excitation threshold(s), after-response duration and frequencies, and perhaps expansion of receptive fields [39,54]. However, while sympathetic contribution to C-fiber activity may be influential and can contribute to the loss of thermoregulatory function (via sensitized alpha-adrenoceptor responses to norepinephrine) that evokes C-fiber-mediated pain and a concomitant axon reflex vasodilatation [55–58], such sympathetically mediated mechanisms are not uniform in all instances of CRPS I, and sympathetic dysregulation does not account for the entire constellation of neurological features of the disorder. Using microneurography to evaluate possible electrophysiological interactions by simultaneously recording single identified sympathetic efferent fibers and C nociceptors while provoking sympathetic neuronal discharges in cutaneous nerves, Campero et al. assessed potential effects of sympathetic activity upon 35 polymodal nociceptors and 19 mechano-insensitive nociceptors in patients with CRPS I and II. These studies failed to reveal activation of nociceptors related to sympathetic discharge, thereby suggesting that sympathetic–nociceptor interactions are the exception [59].

47.2.2 Neurogenic Inflammatory and Central Neural Interactions

Irrespective of sympathetic effects, a neurogenic inflammatory response appears to be perpetuated in CRPS I [60,61,63], thereby supporting the century-old work of Sudeck et al. [62]. This inflammatory response is initiated, at least in part, by substance-P, and involves a nitric oxide-mediated peripheral vasodilatation [64], with enhanced extravasation of serotonin (5-hydroxytryptamine; 5-HT) [65,66], as well a variety of peptides [67] that restimulate C-fiber afferents and elevate local concentrations of proinflammatory cytokines [68–70]. The continued activation of C-fiber afferents, second-order neurons of the spinothalamic tract (STT), and higher supraspinal loci in the neuraxis can evoke functional and perhaps structural changes in the CNS that (1) suppress endogenous pain modulatory mechanisms, (2) decrease pain thresholds, and (3) increase the duration and intensity of pain sensation and perception [24,71]. Such changes have been demonstrated in CRPS I, and may be responsible for "top-down" effects upon the sympathetic system that initiate and/or maintain increased activation of pronociceptive mechanisms [72,73], alter peripheral vaso- and sudomotor control, and may affect the structural integrity of the innervated tissues (e.g., skin, hair, nails, and bone).

47.2.3 Putative Genetic Factors

These plastic changes occur over a variable time course, and it is almost impossible to predict the rapidity of these effects. Thus, there is considerable temporal and individual variation in the presentation of CRPS I. It is not known whether this variability reflects some genetic and/or phenotypic diathesis, a circumstantial effect relative to the provocative insult, or a combination of both. Genetically, particular histocompatibilty complexes have been linked to (certain forms of) CRPS I; Van De Beek and colleagues [74] have shown that spontaneous-onset CRPS I is associated with a newly identified HLA I complex, and increased HLA-DQ1 and HLA-DR13 have been found in CRPS I patients [75,76]. To date, however, it is unclear whether the presence of these histocompatibility complexes are predictive, precipitative, or simply a copresentation (or even epi-phenomenon) of CRPS I. Still, these findings suggest that with further research, HLA testing may become a valuable contribution to the diagnosis of CRPS I. But while genetic testing may be useful to predict or correlate a predisposition to CRPS I, the strength of these findings remains dependent upon other objective measures that detect pathologic changes in support of patients' subjective reports (of pain, sensory and autonomic dysfunction, etc.) and thus reveal the disorder in its pattern of expression. It is in this light that we argue for the utility of fIR as a critical component in the evaluation of CRPS I.

47.3 Methodology: fIR Imaging

47.3.1 Description

Functional infrared thermography (fIR) is a nonionizing, pain-free physiological assessment procedure that has no known adverse biological side effects, is completely safe for (1) women who may become or are pregnant, (2) patients with intractable pain, and (3) patients who cannot tolerate painful invasive procedures. Functional IR imaging is not recommended for patients with casts, bandages, or other technical factors (i.e., patients bound to a wheelchair) that preclude the ability to expose skin to temperature equilibration and imaging.

47.3.2 Brief Historical Context

Measuring human skin temperature as a means of medical assessment began in antiquity with practitioners and scholars who recognized that body temperature is altered during infection and disease. As early as 400 BCE, Hippocrates applied thin layers of moistened clay to various body regions and measured drying times in order to show differences in body temperature, believing that ". . .in whatever part of the body heat or cold is seated, there is disease" [77]. Some 2000 years later, Galileo Galilee invented the "thermoscope" to detect human body temperature. In the early eighteenth century, Gabriel Fahrenheit invented the mercury thermometer, a device that is strikingly similar to its contemporary counterpart. However, it was not until 1870 that the thermometer was used in medicine. In 1800, William Herschel discovered the infrared spectrum [78], and this ultimately provided the impetus for studies on thermal heat that culminated in the development of imaging of radiant emissions some 200 years later. The incipient use of infrared technology provided a rudimentary depiction of biological heat signatures, and it was not until the mid-1960s that these methods were directly employed as a potentially viable evaluative tool in medicine. In the early 1980s, highly sensitive infrared cameras were interfaced with computer software specifically designed for medical applications. The development of sophisticated computerized electronic infrared detectors that are coupled to the state-of-the-art analytic software has overcome many of the technical and practical limitations of infrared thermography, that now allows accurate real-time, side-to-side homologous temperature differences of the extremities, as well as additional sophisticated computer-enhanced thermal images.

47.3.3 Medical Infrared Equipment

Medical infrared thermographic equipment is able to image and record the radiant infrared emission from skin surface radiation. Optimal detection must be capable of measuring human skin temperature with a thermal energy within the 7.5–13.5 Mm IR waveband. The infrared radiant emission is focused through 25–50 mm lens and detected by an indium antimonide (InSb) focal plane array, third-generation microbolometer (or better) with a 320×240 resolution (or better) and 12–16 bit dynamic range. The thermal resolution should be 60 mK NETD (noise equivalent temperature difference) or less. The IR emission is converted into an electronic signal that is processed by a computer and displayed on a color monitor in real time. Current infrared equipment can detect temperature differences as small as 0.02°C, with high thermal sensitivity and resolution. This high-resolution infrared image is able to detect the subtle temperature differences that are required to evaluate patients with mild sensory and autonomic neuropathies. Advances in medical infrared cameras (focal plane array microbolometer detectors) and sophisticated medical software allows for very accurate computer-generated side-to-side homologous temperature differences of the regions of interest to provide objective discrimination of thermal emissions. The thermal sensitivity range utilized by most clinicians with modern high-resolution IR equipment ranges from 0.2°C to 1.0°C. The thermal range is set according to the anatomic region being studied, as well as the discriminate information relative to the pathology studies. In addition, advanced software is capable of enhancing the thermal image to evaluate autonomic vasomotor tone and maintenance of the sympathetic vasoconstrictor reflex during cold-water autonomic functional stress testing.

47.3.4 Infrared Laboratory Environment

The infrared laboratory environment must be controlled to ensure obtaining accurate readings of the thermal emission that are free of artifact. The laboratory must be maintained at a constant temperature of $20 \pm 1°C$, and may require a 2–4°C reduction in temperature during the hot summer months in order to achieve the necessary ANS arousal (i.e., body cooling) prior to imaging. It is imperative that the subjects' autonomic thermoregulatory function is not affected by the ambient environment. Thus, the laboratory must be free of any ultraviolet rays that may cause aberrant heating of the surface skin temperature, and should be lit with fluorescent light bulbs. Similarly, all windows should be covered to eliminate solar radiation. The laboratory must maintain low humidity to ensure protection from diffuse cooling, and must be as draft-free as possible to prevent cold air blowing on the patient. The laboratory must be carpeted to prevent an inadvertent cooling artifact of the plantar surface of the feet.

47.3.5 Patient Selection: Indication

Patients that are presumed or suspected to have CRPS I and/or II are commonly selected for fIR studies, as are those patients with signs and symptoms of conditions that mimic CRPS I [79,80]. Some of these latter conditions include small fiber distal mononeuropathies, acute trauma, localized inflammation, vascular pathology, peripheral neuropathy, and vasospastic disorders. Follow-up fIR studies may be helpful in determining the effectiveness of sympathetic blockade, sympathectomy, and/or spinal cord stimulator placement. Follow-up fIR studies may also be indicated when evaluating patients' response to treatment, or evaluating progression of the underlying disease state.

47.3.6 Patient Preprocedure Protocol

Patients undergoing fIR testing must follow very specific preprocedure protocols [79,80]. These include discontinuing the use of nicotine and caffeine products 4 h before testing; discontinuing physical therapy and TENS unit the day before testing, and the avoidance of skin lotions, deodorants, moisturizers, liniments, topical OTC medications, skin powders, and makeup the day of testing. Patients are advised not to wear any tight-fitting clothing on the day of the test, and to discontinue the use of braces, bandaging, or neoprene wraps for 24 h before evaluation. Also, patients must not have any form of invasive diagnostic procedures for 24 h before testing. Patients may be required to discontinue certain opioid and nonopioid analgesics, and sympatholytic medications up to 24 h before testing, as these may impact the sympathetic function and alter surface skin temperature. All interventional (sympathetic, Bier, and neurolytic) blocks must be discontinued for a minimum of 3 days before testing.

47.3.7 Patient Protocol

Prior to initiating IR imaging, the patient is required to equilibrate body temperature in a $20 \pm 1°C$ environment for a minimum of 15 min in order to stimulate the thermoregulatory autonomic response. The equilibration time may be prolonged in patients who are carrying a heat load from a warm outside environment or who may have a high basal metabolic rate (BMR). A patient assessment should be performed before equilibration. This includes assessing the ability to tolerate the procedure, evaluation of any contraindications, taking an appropriate medical history, and conducting a physical examination. In addition, mental status, pain levels, symptoms/signs of allodynia, hyperalgesia, hyperpathia, vasomotor or sudomotor findings, and risk of vasomotor instability should be assessed. Documentation of the patient's current medications and therapies, results of any previous thermographic or vascular studies, and results of any previous sympathetic or vascular interventions should also be acquired [79,80].

Before beginning equilibration, the patient is asked to disrobe and put on a loose-fitting cotton gown that covers the breasts and genitalia. The patient is required to stand during the equilibration period and is asked not to scratch, rub, or touch any area of the skin that is going to be imaged. During the equilibration period, the technician should ensure that the patient has followed all preprocedure protocols [79,80].

47.3.8 Study Protocol for fIR Pain Studies

Upper body fIR pain study (qualitative and quantitative images are of the same views):
Capture IR images of

1. Posterior cervical region
2. Posterior thoracic region that includes posterior arms
3. Anterior thoracic region that includes anterior arms
4. Anterior forearms and palmar hands (preferably in one image)
5. Posterior forearms and dorsal hands (preferably in one image)
6. Radial forearms and hands (preferably in one image)
7. Ulnar forearms and hands (preferably in one image)

Evaluate the following three (3) IR signature indices required for an interpretive impression for presumptive CRPS of the upper extremities:

Index 1: Quantitative side-to-side homologous computer-generated temperature measurements of

1. Anterior forearms and palmar hands (preferably in one image)
2. Posterior forearms and dorsal hands (preferably in one image)
3. Radial and ulnar forearms also

Index 2: Black–white distal thermal gradient IR signatures

1. Palmar hands (preferably in one image)
2. Dorsal hands (preferably in one image)

Index 3: Cold-water autonomic functional stress test IR signatures

1. Distal posterior forearms and dorsal hands (one image)

Lower body fIR pain study (qualitative and quantitative images are of the same views):
Capture IR images of

1. Posterior lumbar and buttock region
2. Posterior thighs and legs (preferably in one image)
3. Anterior thighs and legs (preferably in one image)
4. Left lateral thigh and leg with medial right thigh and leg (one image)
5. Right lateral thigh and leg with medial left thigh and leg (one image)
6. Dorsal feet (preferably in one image)
7. Plantar feet (preferably in one image)

Evaluate the following IR signature indices required for an interpretive impression for presumptive CRPS of the lower extremities:

Index 1: Quantitative side-to-side homologous computer-generated temperature measurements of

1. Anterior legs (preferably in one image)
2. Posterior legs (preferably in one image)
3. Dorsal feet (preferably in one image)
4. Plantar feet (preferably in one image)

Index 2: Black–white distal thermal gradient imaging of

1. Dorsal feet (preferably in one image)
2. Plantar feet (preferably in one image)

Index 3: Cold-water autonomic functional stress testing of

1. Distal anterior legs and dorsal feet (one image)

47.3.9 Methods for Obtaining Three Specific fIR Indices Required for an Interpretive Impression for Patients with Presumptive CRPS

Index 1: Qualitative/quantitative side-to-side homologous computer-generated temperature views. Both the quantitative and qualitative images are obtained by capturing baseline color qualitative thermal images 0–50°C, with 0.05° accuracy. The user can display the 12-bit data in color or gray scale with software-installed color maps. The images are displayed with an 85–100-color palette and 0.15°C thermal window. Once the qualitative thermal images are captured, the technician outlines the region of interest using the polygon drawing tool that is embedded in the medical software. In an upper body pain study, the technician draws a polygon around the anterior forearms, posterior forearms, palmar hands, and dorsal hands. In a lower body pain study, the technician draws a polygon around the anterior legs, posterior legs, dorsal feet, and plantar feet. The computer software calculates average temperature(s) within each polygon, allowing calculation of side-to-side homologous temperature differences. A side-to-side homologous temperature difference >1.0°C is generally considered indicative of an autonomic abnormality secondary to an underlying pathology. This 1.0°C temperature difference may range from 0.5°C to 1.5°C depending on the laboratory bias.

Index 2: Black–white distal thermal gradient IR signatures. The black–white distal transverse thermal gradient signature views are obtained by imaging the palmar and dorsal surfaces of the hand in an upper body pain study and the dorsal and plantar surfaces of the feet in a lower body pain study. The images are viewed in the black–white mode with a 10-color palette and 0.05°C thermal window.

Index 3: Cold-water autonomic functional stress test IR signatures. Cold-water autonomic functional stress testing is best performed by utilizing real-time dynamic subtraction imaging that is available on most medical IR software programs. Real-time image subtraction is achieved by choosing a starting reference image, then choosing to view only the differences from the reference-to-the-current image. If the individual pixel temperature rises, the difference will be shown in color; if the temperature drops, the image will be displayed in shades of gray. At any time during the imaging process the user can choose to view the reference, delta, or current image. All thermal data have a dynamic range of 12 bits, enabling the user to view 0.05° difference in a 0–50°C temperature range. This testing is performed by imaging the symptomatic and contralateral asymptomatic distal extremity for 5 min while an asymptomatic limb is placed in a 12–16°C cold-water bath. The immersion of a noninvolved limb activates autonomic thermoregulatory function. If autonomic function is intact, there is vasoconstriction in all four extremities due to the central vasoconstrictor reflex. If the autonomic vasoconstrictor reflex is inhibited or there is autonomic failure, then an axon vasodilatation reflex will occur. This reflex will be visualized by a warming of the symptomatic distal extremity, and on occasion the bilateral asymptomatic distal extremity, during the 5-min cold-water autonomic functional stress test.

Conwell et al. [41] have described cold-water autonomic functional stress testing and the sensitivity, specificity, and predictive value in comparing stress test results with modified IASP criteria for CRPS. This IR index, in and of itself, reveals a 72% sensitivity, 94% specificity, positive predictive value 82%, negative predictive value 90%, and kappa statistical analysis of 0.69 (95% confidence interval: 0.55 and 0.83). The authors posited that cold-water autonomic functional stress testing may be helpful in identifying those patients with a sympathetically mediated component that have a high probability to positively respond to sympatholytic intervention(s). Those patients who have an empirically normal cold-water stress test response characteristically do not respond to sympathetic nerve blocks, and are considered to have the sympathetically independent pain (SIP) form of CRPS I.

47.4 Case Studies

47.4.1 Integrating Pathophysiology of CRPS I to Findings from fIR Case Studies

Functional infrared imaging detects the thermal signature produced by changes in cutaneous blood flow regulated by central thermal and respiratory control that affects vasoconstrictor and sudomotor reflexes. This vaso- and sudomotor activity is predominantly, but not exclusively, dependent upon hypothalamic mechanisms. Sympathetic preganglionic neurons project to the paravertebral ganglia and synapse upon postganglionic neurons innervating target organs and cells. Postganglionic sympathetic neurons release norepinephrine (NE) and neuropeptide Y (NPY) to regulate cutaneous blood flow. Studies suggest that the thermoregulatory dysfunction in CRPS I is due to central inhibition of the cutaneous sympathetic vasoconstrictor reflex [81].

In addition to inhibition of efferent sympathetic neurons, afferent neurons also regulate cutaneous blood flow. Sensitization of cutaneous, small-caliber C fibers evokes orthodromic release of the tachykinin substance-P (SubsP) within the dorsal horn to engage the nociceptive neuraxis, and may also cause antidromic release of SubsP, as well as calcitonin gene-related peptide (CGRP) to (1) elicit peripheral vasodilatation, causing extravasation of other pronociceptive and proinflammatory mediators (e.g., serotonin [5-HT], bradykinin, vasoactive intestinal peptide [VIP]), and (2) perpetuate a neurogenic inflammatory response [24,61–65,68,82–85]. This cutaneous vasodilatation may be involved in the clinically observed vasomotor changes in patients with acute CRPS I, and is easily demonstrated with fIR imaging by visualizing the infrared hyperthermic radiation. Wasner et al. revealed that vascular hyperthermic abnormalities seen in acute CRPS I (and visualized via IR signature(s)) are the result of complete inhibition of sympathetic nerve activity, rather than antidromic vasodilatation secondary to activation of nociceptive afferents [86].

47.4.2 Interpretation of fIR Signatures

Gulevich et al. [38] demonstrated 93% sensitivity and 89% specificity with fIR in diagnosing cases presumed to be CRPS I. These results were obtained by evaluating three separate and distinct IR indices:

1. Computer-generated side-to-side quantitative homologous temperature differences of the symptomatic and asymptomatic distal extremities obtained after the patient equilibrated in a controlled temperature environment of ≤20°C for 15 min (see Section 47.3).
2. Black-and-white distal transverse thermal gradient IR signatures evaluated for maintenance or presence of well-defined transverse gradient lines, which represents normal vasomotor presentation or disruption of the transverse gradient lines, which represent normal vasomotor presentation or disruption of the tranverse gradient lines that represent an abnormal vasomotor presentation. The distal thermal gradient patterns are visualized in the hands or feet, paying particular attention to fingers and toes.
3. Responses to cold-water autonomic functional stress testing [38,41,87,88] of the symptomatic and asymptomatic distal extremity to evaluate for autonomic function with concomitant maintenance of the vasoconstrictor reflex. When autonomic function is intact, there is evidentiary cooling of the distal symptomatic extremity due to maintenance of the vasoconstrictor reflex. With autonomic dysfunction, there is warming of the distal symptomatic extremity [38,41]. This warming may be due to inhibition/failure of the vasoconstrictor reflex [38,41,89–92] or adrenergic

sensitization of nociceptors (viz., upregulation and/or hyperaffinity of alpha adrenergic receptors [93]) producing an axon reflex-mediated vasodilatation. This axon reflex-mediated vasodilatation is not suppressed by sympathetic activity due to central inhibition of sympathetic efferent fibers.

47.4.3 Normal fIR Signatures

In an asymptomatic (i.e., healthy, normal control) patient population, the three fIR image indices are entirely normal as demonstrated by (1) symmetrical thermal emission; (2) normal well-defined transverse thermal gradient lines; and (3) normal response (i.e., cooling) to cold-water autonomic functional stress testing [38] (Table 47.1).

IR findings:

- Bilateral thermal symmetry in region of interest (ROI)
- Normal, well-defined and uniform, transverse distal thermal gradient lines
- Cooling of the symptomatic distal extremity during cold-water autonomic functional stress testing

IR indices description:

1. *Quantitative thermal emission (computer-generated side-to-side temperature) image finding*: Uematsu et al. [94] in a pioneering normative study demonstrated that in a normal healthy asymptomatic patient population, the quantitative computer-generated side-to-side temperature differences of homologous body parts is in the range of 0.17–0.45°C, with a human surface temperature symmetry averaging 0.24 ± 0.073°C between homologous sides [95]. The mean standard deviation for repetitive readings over time of computer-generated side-to-side temperature differences of homologous body parts was 30.8 ± 0.032°C [96]. Uematsu's data have been confirmed by numerous authors [38,97,98].
2. *Distal thermal gradient image pattern findings*: In normal, healthy asymptomatic patients, the distal transverse thermal gradient lines visualized in the distal extremities, particularly in the fingers and toes, are well maintained [38]. Normal distal thermal gradient patterns in the fingers and toes are represented by distinct uniform transverse lines that are closely aligned, forming an alternating black–white–black linear pattern. Normal distal thermal gradient IR signatures may be a result of the normal rhythmic cycling of cutaneous blood flow that is seen in healthy asymptomatic individuals [99].

TABLE 47.1 Normal Study

Normal Study	fIR Index 1: ROI delta T°	fIR Index 2: Distal Thermal Gradient IR Signatures	fIR Index 3: Cold-Water Autonomic Functional Stress Test
IR Signature:	IR Signature:	IR Signature:	IR Signature:
1. Quantitative and qualitative thermal symmetry in the ROI	1. ROI symmetrical IR signature <1.0°C	1. Maintained distal gradient IR signature	1. Normal cooling of the symptomatic and asymptomatic distal extremity
			Putative mechanism:
			1. Normal ANS function with maintenance of the vasoconstrictor reflex
Upper body fIR study			
IR Signatures			
Lower body fIR study			
IR Signatures			

3. *Cold-water autonomic functional stress test findings:* In normal, healthy asymptomatic patients with intact autonomic function, there is cooling of the distal extremities when a noninvolved extremity is placed in a ≤15°C cold-water bath [38,41] or when subjected to whole-body cooling by perfusion of circulating water into a thermal suit [40,100]. Additional studies have shown that following the arousal stimuli and the cold pressor test, the vasoconstrictor response is observed in asymptomatic patients and is diminished or absent in patients with CRPS I [89–92].

47.4.4 Abnormal fIR Studies

47.4.4.1 Mimics of CRPS I

In symptomatic patients, numerous conditions *mimic* the modified IASP CRPS criteria, and these make differentiation difficult by the nonexpert clinician. Instead, we argue that the following three fIR image indices, with their specific thermal signatures, provides significant aid in differentiating CRPS I from other pain syndromes.

47.4.5 Acute Trauma (Post-Traumatic Injury): fIR Signatures

Following acute trauma, patients without strong clinical signs of sympathetic dysfunction or acute nerve injury may present with symptoms similar to CRPS I (Table 47.2). This patient population shows clinically relevant hypothermia in the symptomatic extremity that is likely due to maintenance of the vasoconstrictor reflex secondary to a peripheral pain generator [101].

Image findings:

- Unilateral hypothermic vascular disturbances in ROI
- Normal well-defined transverse distal thermal gradient lines
- Cooling of the symptomatic distal extremity during cold-water autonomic functional stress testing due to normal autonomic function with maintenance of the vasoconstrictor reflex

TABLE 47.2 Acute Trauma

Acute Trauma	fIR Index 1: ROI delta T°	fIR Index 2: Distal Thermal Gradient IR Signatures	fIR Index 3: Cold-Water Autonomic Functional Stress Test
IR Signature:	IR Signature:	IR Signature:	IR Signature:
1. Quantitative and qualitative thermal asymmetry in the ROI	1. ROI hypothermic IR signature >1.0°C	1. Maintained distal gradient IR signatures	1. Normal cooling of the symptomatic and asymptomatic distal extremity
Putative mechanism:			Putative mechanism:
1. Increased sympathetic vasomotor tone secondary to a peripheral pain generator			1. Normal ANS function with maintenance of the vasoconstrictor reflex
2. No evidence of neurogenic inflammation–antidromic vasodilatation			
Upper body fIR study			
IR Signatures			
Lower body fIR study			
IR Signatures			

Image indices description:

1. *Quantitative thermal emission (computer-generated side-to-side temperature) findings*: In cases of acute trauma with an intact autonomic function, skin temperature cooling is a common finding of the affected symptomatic extremity when compared to the unaffected, contralateral extremity. Cooling in the symptomatic extremity is due to a somatoautonomic reflex secondary to a peripheral pain generator, with a resultant increase in sympathetic vasoconstrictor activity. This normal somatoautonomic reflex vasoconstriction is due to excitation of sensory receptors and/ or irritation of a sensory nerve that elicits increased sympathetic tone, resulting in skin cooling. This vasoconstriction is predominantly visualized in the territory in which the afferent stimulus originates [102].

2. *Distal thermal gradient lined patterns*: In post-traumatic states, the distal thermal gradient lines are well maintained. This is believed to be due to maintenance of normal sympathetic vasomotor tone.

3. *Cold-water autonomic functional stress test findings*: In post-traumatic states, autonomic function is intact and elicits cooling of the symptomatic extremity during cold-water autonomic functional stress testing. Several researchers believe that maintenance of the sympathetic vasoconstrictor reflex may be a feature that allows differentiation between normal, post-traumatic states, and CRPS I [41,85,92,103,104].

47.4.6 C-Fiber (Small-Caliber Nociceptive Afferent Excitation) Mononeuropathy: fIR Signatures

Excitation of peripheral sensory C-fiber nociceptive afferents produces both orthodromic and antidromic release of vasodilator substances from the involved nerve terminals (Table 47.3). The vasodilatatory substances include SubsP and CGRP. The (antidromic) vasodilatatory effects induce a rise in surface temperature and increase in the resultant radiant heat signature. This hyperthermia is independent of sympathetic activity, and is localized to the skin territory innervated by the particular C-fiber [83,105,106].

TABLE 47.3   C-Fiber (Small-Caliber Nociceptive Afferent Excitation) Mononeuropathy

Small-Caliber Fiber Distal Sensory Mononeuropathy (ABC Syndrome)	fIR Index 1: ROI delta T°	fIR Index 2: Distal Thermal Gradient IR Signatures	fIR Index 3: Cold-Water Autonomic Functional Stress Test
IR Signature:	IR Signature:	IR Signature:	IR Signature:
1. Vasodilatation (visualized hyperthermic emission) localized in specific skin territory of the involved nerve	1. ROI hyperthermic IR signature >1.0°C localized to the specific skin territory of the involved nerve	1. Disrupted distal gradient IR signature localized to the skin territory of the sensitized peripheral nerve	1. Normal cooling of the symptomatic and asymptomatic distal limb
Putative mechanism:			Putative mechanism:
1. Antidromic vasodilatation unrelated to sympathetic activity			1. Normal ANS function that overrides the antidromic vasodilatation with maintenance of the vasoconstrictor reflex
Upper body fIR study			
IR Signatures			

Image findings:

- Unilateral hyperthermic vascular disturbances isolated to a specific nerve territory
- Disrupted transverse distal thermal gradient lines isolated to a specific nerve territory
- Normal cooling of the symptomatic distal extremity during cold-water autonomic functional stress testing due to normal autonomic function that suppresses vasodilatation induced by antidromic release of pro-inflammatory substances

Image indices description:

1. *Quantitative thermal emission (computer-generated side-to-side temperature) findings*: In these cases there is skin temperature warming (hyperthermia) localized to the skin territory of the involved nerve that is independent of sympathetic activity. There is normal thermal symmetry of the asymptomatic extremity.
2. *Distal thermal gradient lined patterns*: The distal thermal gradient lines are disrupted solely in the skin territory of the involved nerve with loss of the normal transverse lines.
3. *Cold-water autonomic functional stress test findings*: Normal cooling of the symptomatic extremity is observed during cold-water autonomic functional stress testing because the observed vasodilatation is independent of sympathetic activity in this pathology. Therefore, the normal cooling is most likely due to intact autonomic function with maintenance of the vasoconstrictor reflex that suppresses vasodilatation [41,90,94,96–98,107].

47.4.7 Acute CRPS I fIR Signatures

47.4.7.1 Abnormal fIR Signatures Visualized Solely in Symptomatic Limb

The following fIR images were taken from case studies of patients who met both the IASP and Gulevich et al. [34] criteria for CRPS I, which, when taken together, demonstrated a 93% sensitivity and 89% specificity in diagnosing patients with presumed CRPS I (Table 47.4). These fIR cases show hyperthermia of the symptomatic distal extremity visualized by computer-generated side-to-side homologous temperature differences >1.0°C. These cases also show evidence of inhibition of the vasoconstrictor reflex as revealed by abnormal hyperthermic response to cold-water autonomic functional stress testing [41]. This fIR thermal presentation appears to be consistent with the hypothesized central inhibition of sympathetic activity that occurs in acute-stage CRPS I, producing decreased release of NE at the terminal sites, and resulting in vasodilatation and increased cutaneous blood flow [82]. This central sympathetic inhibition results in abnormal warming during cold-water autonomic functional stress testing.

Image findings:

- Unilateral hyperthermic vascular disturbances in ROI
- Disrupted transverse distal thermal gradient lines in ROI
- Abnormal warming of the distal symptomatic extremity (generally seen in the fingers or toes of the involved extremity) during cold-water autonomic functional stress testing

Image indices description:

1. *Quantitative thermal emission (computer-generated side-to-side temperature) findings*: In the acute phase of CRPS I, the affected distal extremity shows abnormal vasodilatation with subsequent skin warming as compared to the contralateral asymptomatic extremity [81,92,108–111]. This vasodilatation is due, in part, to central inhibition of sympathetic activity and a decreased release of NE and NPY at terminal sites of sympathetic neurons [112–114]. Decreased NE activity at the terminal sites results in an increased cutaneous blood flow, which produces the clinical picture of

TABLE 47.4 Acute CRPS I

Acute CRPS I	fIR Index 1: ROI delta T°	fIR Index 2: Distal Thermal Gradient IR Signatures	fIR Index 3: Cold-Water Autonomic Functional Stress Test
IR Signature:	IR Signature:	IR Signature:	IR Signature:
1. Vasodilatation (visualized hyperthermic emission) with global, nondermatomal skin warming in the affected distal extremity	1. ROI hyperthermic IR signature >1.0°C	1. Disrupted distal gradient IR signature in a global, nondermatomal distribution in the symptomatic distal extremity and rarely may be visualized in the asymptomatic contralateral distal extremity	1. Abnormal warming of symptomatic distal extremity with occasional warming of the contralateral side
Putative mechanism:			Putative mechanism:
1. Neurogenic inflammation–afferent axon reflex vasodilatation 2. Central sympathetic inhibition			1. Abnormal ANS function with impairment of the sympathetic vasoconstrictor reflex or sympathetic failure 2. Intense axon reflex vasodilatation secondary to C-fiber sensitivity to circulating NE
Upper body fIR study IR Signatures **Lower body fIR study** IR Signatures			

a warm, discolored extremity. Inhibition of neuronally mediated vasoconstrictor reflexes is not believed to be due to major damage to the peripheral nerve (as in CRPS II), but rather due to a central inhibition of the thermoregulatory function [40,108,111].

2. *Distal thermal gradient line patterns*: In symptomatic patients with thermoregulatory dysfunction, the distal transverse thermal gradient lines visualized in the distal extremities (particularly in the fingers and toes) are disrupted [38]. The disrupted lines are represented by irregular black–white–black gradient lines that are highly irregular without evidence of the normal transverse well-maintained pattern alignment. The disrupted irregular patterns are felt to represent aberrations produced by abnormal sympathetic vasomotor tone.

3. *Cold-water autonomic functional stress test patterns*: In the acute phase of CRPS I, the affected extremity abnormally warms during cold-water autonomic functional stress testing [38,41]. It is hypothesized that this abnormal warming is due to inhibition or complete failure of the vasoconstrictor reflex and concomitant axon reflex-mediated vasodilatation. The axon reflex vasodilatation prevails due to the absence or inhibition of vasoconstrictor reflexes that would normally suppress vasodilatation. This has been illustrated by a case presentation of a patient who developed complete failure of the tonic vasoconstrictor response to cooling within 2 weeks of CRPS I onset [108]. This has been further supported by literature showing diminished sympathetic vasoconstrictor reflexes in the affected limb during the early-acute phases of CRPS I [110,111]. This abnormal warming may be due to adrenergic sensitization of nociceptors [93].

47.4.8 Acute CRPS I fIR Signatures: Bilateral Presentation

47.4.8.1 Abnormal fIR Signatures Visualized in Both Symptomatic and Asymptomatic Limbs

There are reports in the literature of subclinical *contralateral* sympathetic involvement in CRPS I [89,90,99] that are associated with axon reflex vasodilatation (hyperthermia) in both the distal symptomatic and asymptomatic limbs [115]. The following fIR images are taken from case studies of patients who met IASP CRPS I criteria and the criteria of Gulevich et al. [38], which demonstrated 93% sensitivity and 89% specificity in diagnosing patients with presumed CRPS I who demonstrated bilateral vasomotor findings (Table 47.5). These fIR cases show hyperthermia of both the symptomatic and asymptomatic distal extremity, evidenced by computer-generated side-to-side homologous temperature differences of a >1°C hyperthermia of the symptomatic distal extremity. These studies also show evidence of inhibition of the vasoconstrictor reflex subserved by an abnormal axon reflex vasodilatation during cold-water autonomic functional stress testing [41]. The hypothermia is likely due to supersensitivity to circulating catecholamines evoking vasoconstriction [116]. These findings tend to support the notion that CRPS I may also involve central mediation via an increased activation of brainstem or hypothalamic–pituitary–adrenal mechanisms.

Image findings:

- Bilateral distal hyperthermic vascular disturbances with the symptomatic distal extremity (ROI) demonstrating a >1.0°C hyperthermic difference with the contralateral asymptomatic limb
- Bilateral disrupted transverse distal thermal gradient lines in ROI
- Bilateral abnormal warming of the distal extremities (generally seen in the fingers or toes) during cold-water autonomic functional stress testing.

TABLE 47.5   Acute CRPS I (Bilateral Thermal Findings)

Acute CRPS I Bilateral Thermal Findings	fIR Index 1: ROI delta T°	fIR Index 2: Distal Thermal Gradient IR Signatures	fIR Index 3: Cold-Water Autonomic Functional Stress Test
IR Signature:	IR Signature:	IR Signature:	IR Signature:
1. Vasodilatation (visualized hyperthermic emission) with global, nondermatomal skin warming in the affected distal extremity	1. ROI hyperthermic IR signature >1.0°C	1. Bilateral disrupted distal thermal gradient IR signature (seen in the fingers or toes) visualized in a global nondermatomal distribution in the effected distal extremity and asymptomatic contralateral distal limb	1. Abnormal warming of symptomatic and asymptomatic distal extremity
Putative mechanism:			Putative mechanism:
1. Central sympathetic inhibition 2. Neurogenic inflammation–afferent axon reflex vasodilatation			1. Abnormal ANS function with bilateral impairment of the sympathetic vasoconstrictor reflex or sympathetic failure 2. Bilateral axon reflex vasodilatation secondary to C-fiber sensitivity to circulating NE
Upper body fIR study			
IR signatures			

47.4.9 Chronic CRPS I fIR Signatures

The following fIR images are taken from case studies of patients who met the IASP criteria for chronic CRPS I as well as the Gulevich et al. [38] criteria (Table 47.6). These fIR studies show hypothermia of the symptomatic distal extremity visualized by computer-generated side-to-side homologous temperature differences >1.0°C. These case studies also show evidence of inhibition of the vasoconstrictor reflex associated with an axon reflex vasodilatation that is readily visualized in the symptomatic distal extremity, and occasionally the asymptomatic distal extremity during the cold-water autonomic functional stress testing [41].

Image findings:

- Unilateral hypothermic vascular disturbances with the ROI being >1.0°C colder than the contralateral asymptomatic limb
- Unilateral or bilateral disrupted transverse distal thermal gradient lines
- Unilateral or bilateral (warming) abnormal response to cold-water autonomic functional stress testing

Image indices description:

1. *Quantitative thermal emission (computer-generated side-to-side temperature) findings*: In the chronic phase of CRPS I, the affected distal extremity shows abnormal vasoconstriction with subsequent skin cooling of the involved distal limb as compared to the contralateral asymptomatic limb [37,38,40,116,117]. This vasoconstriction is felt to be due to supersensitivity to circulating catecholamines [118]. Numerous mechanisms are responsible for this adrenergic supersensitivity, including, but not limited to, diminished neurotransmitter reuptake, enzyme degradation, increased alpha adrenoceptor binding affinity, and/or density of receptor sites, increased expression of sodium channels and/or sodium–potassium pump inefficiency [119].

TABLE 47.6   Chronic CRPS I

Chronic CRPS I	fIR Index 1: ROI delta T°	fIR Index 2: Distal Thermal Gradient IR Signatures	fIR Index 3: Cold-Water Autonomic Functional Stress Test
IR Signature:	IR Signature:	IR Signature:	IR Signature:
1. Vasoconstriction (visualized hypothermic emission) with skin cooling in the affected distal extremity	1. ROI hypothermic IR signature >1.0°C	1. Bilateral disrupted distal thermal gradient IR signature (seen in the fingers or toes) visualized in a global nondermatomal distribution in the effected distal extremity and asymptomatic contralateral distal limb	1. Abnormal warming of the symptomatic distal extremity with occasional warming of the contralateral asymptomatic extremity
Putative mechanism:			Putative mechanism:
1. Supersensitivity to circulating catecholamines–adrenergic supersensitivity			1. Abnormal ANS function with bilateral impairment of the sympathetic vasoconstrictor reflex or sympathetic failure
2. Minimal or absent sympathetic inhibition			2. Bilateral axon reflex vasodilatation secondary to C-fiber sensitivity to circulating NE
Upper body fIR study			
IR signatures			

2. *Distal thermal gradient line patterns*: The distal transverse thermal gradient lines in chronic CRPS I are disrupted with a loss of the normal well-defined transverse gradient lines [38]. It is hypothesized that this disruption is the result of vasomotor disturbances evoked by circulating catecholamines.
3. *Cold-water autonomic functional stress test findings*: In the chronic phase of CRPS I, the affected extremity, and occasionally the contralateral unaffected extremity, shows abnormal warming during cold-water autonomic functional stress testing [38,41]. It is hypothesized that this abnormal warming is due to inhibition or complete loss of the vasoconstrictor reflex resulting in an axon reflex-induced vasodilatation.

47.4.10 Clinical Implications and Potential

These findings support our contention that fIR, when coupled to advanced computational software, can effectively detect thermal signatures that reflect particular vaso- and sudomotor disturbances that are important in establishing a differential diagnosis of CRPS I. Obviously, it is important to restate that these objective features cannot be taken in isolation, and thus we do not advocate that fIR be considered or utilized as a stand-alone diagnostic modality. However, it is equally important to recognize that the inherent ambiguities in the presentation of CRPS I (and a persistent reticence to acknowledge the validity of a diagnosis of CRPS I based upon lesser objective findings) fortify the utility of this technology as a part of the diagnostic workup. Functional IR testing, when administered and evaluated by a competently trained professional, can provide reliable data that can contribute to both the diagnosis of a particular patient and a progressive database that can be utilized to develop an objective standard for clinical discernment and diagnoses.

Extant concerns and refutations of the plausibility of IR thermography reflected inadequacies of older technology, and were valid criticisms of the lack of specificity, inappropriate and/or inapt use by untrained personnel, and the entrepreneurial overuse of IR as a "diagnostic" test. However, these biases are no longer applicable as the enjoinment of current technology (based upon declassified military instrumentation) and advanced statistical software has rendered all prior iterations of thermographic detection almost obsolete and established a new benchmark for technical efficiency and accuracy.

This technology will only improve, and thus it is important to both study fIR further to develop new avenues for clinical use and employ these methods in the detection of CRPS I and other diagnostically difficult syndromes.

Dedication

This chapter is dedicated to the memory of Nicholas A. Diakides, D.Sc. Dr. Diakides was a pioneer in the development of knowledge-based databases of standardized IR signatures validated by pathology which was instrumental in setting the groundwork for numerous advances in medical IR imaging. The scientific contribution, by this exceptional human being, to the understanding and potential benefit of medical IR imaging will most certainly play a role in improving the health and well-being of future generations.

Acknowledgments

Contributions to this work were supported in part by Colorado Infrared Imaging Center, Denver Colorado. The fIR case studies were obtained from the center's patient files.

TC gratefully acknowledges Drs. Nicholas Diakides (deceased), William Hobbins, Stephen Gulevich, L. Barton Goldman, Floyd Ring, Richard Stieg, and Neil Rosenberg (deceased) for their support and encouragement over many years.

Contributions to this work were also supported in part by the Institute for Biotechnology Futures, The William H. and Sara Crane Schaeffer Endowment, and Nour Foundation (JG). JG gratefully acknowledges Kim Abramson for assistance on this chapter.

We express our sincere thanks to Maurice Bales, founder and president, Bales Scientific, for his valuable and lifelong dedication to medical infrared imaging. The fIR images in this chapter were captured by a Bales Scientific advanced image acquisition Tip-50 infrared camera interfaced with sophisticated medical computerized analytic system imaging software.

References

1. Hendler, N., Complex regional pain syndrome types I and II, in *Weiner's Pain Management: A Practical Guide for Clinicians*. 7th ed., Boswell, M.V. and Cole, B.E., Eds., CRC Press, Boca Raton, FL, 2005.

2. Sandroni, P. et al., Complex regional pain syndrome type I: Incidence and prevalence in Olmsted County—A population based study, *Pain*, 103, 199, 2003.

3. Allen, G., Galer, B.S., and Schwartz, L., Epidemiology of complex regional pain syndrome: A retrospective chart review of 134 patients, *Pain*, 80, 539, 1999.

4. Harden, R.N., Baron, R., and Janig, W., *Complex Regional Pain Syndrome, Progress in Pain Research and Management*, IASP Press, Seattle, Vol. 22, 2001.

5. Janig, W. and Levine, J.D., Autonomic-endocrine-immune interactions in acute and chronic pain, in *Wall and Melzack's Textbook of Pain*, 5th ed., McMahon, S.P. and Koltzenburg, M., Eds., Churchill Livingston, Edinburgh, 2005.

6. Merskey, H. and Bogduk, N. *Classification of Chronic Pain: Descriptions of Chronic Pain Syndrome and Definitions of Pain Terms*, 2nd ed., IASP Press, Seattle, 1994.

7. Stanton-Hicks, M. et al., Reflex sympathetic dystrophy: Changing concepts and taxonomy, *Pain*, 63, 127, 1995.

8. Janig, W. and Stanton-Hicks, M., Eds. *Reflex Sympathetic Dystrophy: A Reappraisal, Progress and Pain Research and Management*, IASP Press, Seattle, Vol. 6, 1996.

9. Veldman, P.H. et al., Signs and symptoms of reflex sympathetic dystrophy: Prospective study of 829 patients. *Lancet*, 342, 1012, 1993.

10. Bonica, J.J., *The Management of Pain*, Lea and Febiger, Philadelphia, PA, 1953.

11. Kozin, F. et al., Reflex sympathetic dystrophy (RSDS), III: Scintigraphic studies, further evidence for the therapeutic efficacy of systemic corticosteroids and proposed diagnostic criteria, *Am. J. Med.*, 70, 23, 1981.

12. Blumberg, H., A new clinical approach for diagnosing reflex sympathetic dystrophy, in *Proceedings of the VI World Congress on Pain*, Bond, M.R., Charlton, J.E., and Woolf, C.J., Eds., Elsevier, New York, p. 399, 1991.

13. Gibbons, J.J. and Wilson, P.R., RSD score: Criteria for the diagnosis of reflex sympathetic dystrophy and causalgia, *Clin. J. Pain*, 8, 260, 1992.

14. Harden, R.N. and Bruehl, S.P., Diagnostic criteria: The statistical deviation of the four criteria factors, in *CRPS: Current Diagnosis and Therapy*, Wilson, P.R., Stanton Hicks, M., and Harden, R.N., Eds., IASP Press, Seattle, Vol. 32, 2005.

15. Galer, B.S., Bruehl, S., and Harden, R.N., IASP diagnostic criteria for complex regional pain syndrome: A preliminary comparable validation study, *Clin. J. Pain*, 14, 48, 1998.

16. Bruehl, S. et al., External validation of IASP diagnostic criteria for complex regional pain syndrome and proposed research diagnostic criteria, *Pain*, 81, 147, 1999.

17. Van de Beek, W.J. et al., Diagnostic criteria used in studies of reflex sympathetic dystrophy, *Neurology*, 8, 522, 2002.

18. Van den Vusse, A.C. et al., Interobserver reliability of the diagnosis in patients with CRPS, *Eur. J. Pain*, 7, 259, 2003.

19. Harden, R.N. et al., Proposed new diagnostic criteria for complex regional pain syndrome, *Pain Med.*, 8(4), 326, 2007.

20. Harden, R.N. et al., Validation of proposed diagnostic criteria (the "Budapest Criteria") for Complex Regional Pain Syndrome, *Pain*, 150(2), 268, 2010.

21. Sumitani, M. et al., Development of comprehensive diagnostic criteria for complex regional pain syndrome in the Japanese population, *Pain*, 150(2), 243, 2010.

22. Giordano, J., *Pain: Mind, Meaning and Medicine*. Glen Falls, PA: PPM Books, 2009.

23. Giordano, J., Prolegomenon: Engaging philosophy, ethics and policy in, and for pain medicine, in *Pain Medicine: Philosophy, Ethics, and Policy*. Giordano J. and Boswell M.V., Eds., Linton Atlantic Books, Oxon, 2009, pp. 13–20.

24. Giordano, J., The neuroscience of pain and analgesia, in *Weiner's Pain Management: A Practical Guide for Clinicians* 7th ed., Boswell, M.V. and Cole, B.E., Eds., CRC Press, Boca Raton, FL, 2005.

25. Giordano, J., Moral agency in pain medicine: Philosophy, practice and virtue, *Pain Phys.*, 9, 71, 2006.

26. Giordano, J., Good as gold? The randomized controlled trial—Pragmatic and ethical issues in pain research, *Am. J. Pain Manage.*, 16, 68, 2006.

27. Pellegrino, E.D., The healing relationship: The architectonics of clinical medicine, in *The Clinical Encounter: The Moral Fabric of the Patient-Physician Relationship*, Philosophy and Medicine Series 4, Shelp, E.E., Ed. Dordrecht, D., Reidel, 1983.

28. Giordano, J., Pain research: Can paradigmatic revision bridge the needs of medicine, scientific philosophy and ethics? *Pain Phys.*, 7, 459, 2004.

29. Karstetter, K.W. and Sherman, R.A., Use of thermography in initial detection of early reflex sympathetic dystrophy, *J. Am. Podiatr. Med. Assoc.*, 81, 198, 1991.

30. Perelman, R.B., Adler, D., and Humphries, M., Reflex sympathetic dystrophy: Electronic thermography as an aid in diagnosis, *Orthop. Rev.*, 16, 561, 1987.

31. Lightman, H.I. et al., Thermography in childhood reflex sympathetic dystrophy, *J. Pediatr.*, 111, 551, 1987.

32. Lewis, R., Racz, G., and Fabian, G., Therapeutic approaches to reflex sympathetic dystrophy of the upper extremity, *Clin. Issues Reg. Anesth.*, 1, 1, 1985.

33. Uematsu, S. et al., Thermography and electromyography in the differential diagnosis of chronic pain syndromes and reflex sympathetic dystrophy, *Electromyogr. Clin. Neurophysiol.*, 21, 165, 1981.

34. Bruehl, S. et al., Validation of thermography in the diagnosis of reflex sympathetic dystrophy, *Clin. J. Pain.*, 12, 316, 1996.

35. Cooke, E.D. et al., Reflex sympathetic dystrophy (algoneurodystrophy): Temperature studies in the upper limb, *Br. J. Rheumatol.*, 28, 399, 1989.

36. McLeod, J.G. and Tuck, R.R., Disorders of the autonomic nervous system, *Ann. Neurol.*, 21, 419, 1987.

37. Low, P.A. et al., Laboratory findings in reflex sympathetic dystrophy: A preliminary report, *Clin. J. Pain.*, 10, 235, 1994.

38. Gulevich, S.J. et al., Stress infrared telethermography is useful in the diagnosis of complex regional pain syndrome, type 1 (formally reflex sympathetic dystrophy), *Clin. J. Pain.*, 13, 50, 1997.

39. Birklein, F. et al., Neurological findings in complex regional pain syndrome-analysis of 145 cases, *Acta Neurol. Scand.*, 101, 262, 2000.

40. Wasner, G., Schattschneider, J., and Baron, R., Skin temperature side differences: A diagnostic tool for CRPS? *Pain*, 98, 19, 2002.

41. Conwell, T.D. et al., Sensitivity, specificity and predictive value of infrared cold water autonomic functional stress testing as compared with modified IASP criteria for CRPS, *Thermol. Int.*, 20-2, 60, 2010.

42. Schurmann, M. et al., Imaging in early posttraumatic complex regional pain syndrome: A comparison of diagnostic methods, *Clin. J. Pain.*, 23(5), 449, 2007.

43. Terkelsen, A.J. et al., Experimental forearm immobilization in humans induces cold and mechanical hyperalgesia, *Anesthesiology*, 109(2), 297, 2008.

44. Niehof, S.P. et al., Using skin surface temperature to differentiate between complex regional pain syndrome type I patients after a fracture and control patients with various complaints after a fracture, *Anesth. Analg.*, 106(1), 270, 2008.

45. Rommel, O., Habler, H.J., and Schurmann, M., Laboratory tests for complex regional pain syndrome, in *CRPS: Current Diagnosis and Therapy*, Wilson, P.R., Stanton-Hicks, M., Harden, R.N., Eds., IASP Press, Seattle, Vol. 32, 2005.

46. Hooshmand, H., *Chronic Pain: Reflex Sympathetic Dystrophy Prevention and Management*, CRC Press, Boca Raton, FL, 1993.

47. Stanton-Hicks, M., Janig, W., and Boas, R.A., *Reflex Sympathetic Dystrophy*, Kluwer Academic Publications, Norwell, MA, 1990.

48. Baron, R. and Maier C., Reflex sympathetic dystrophy: Skin blood flow, sympathetic vasoconstrictor reflexes and pain before and after surgical sympathectomy, *Pain*, 67, 317, 1996.

49. Wasner, G. et al., No effect of sympathetic sudomotor activity on capsaicin-evoked ongoing pain and hyperalgesia, *Pain*, 84, 331, 2000.

50. McLachlan, E.M. et al., Peripheral nerve injury triggers noradrenergic sprouting within the dorsal root ganglia, *Nature*, 363, 543, 1993.

51. Ali, Z. et al., Intradermal injection of norepinephrine evokes pain in patients with sympathetically maintained pain, *Pain*, 88, 161, 2000.

52. Baron, R. et al., Relation between sympathetic vasoconstrictor activity and pain and hyperalgesia in complex regional pain syndromes: A case control study, *Lancet*, 359, 1655, 2002.

53. Shi, T.S. et al., Distribution and regulation of alpha(2)—Adrenoceptors in rat dorsal root ganglia, *Pain*, 84, 319, 2000.

54. Sieweke, N. et al., Patterns of hyperalgesia in complex regional pain syndrome, *Pain*, 80, 171, 1999.

55. Janig, W. and Habler, H.J., Organization of the autonomic nervous system: Structure and function, in *Handbook of Clinical Neurology*, Appenzeller, O., Ed., Elsevier, Amsterdam, Vol. 74, p. 1, 1999.

56. Janig, W. and Habler, H.J., Neurophysiological analysis of target-related sympathetic pathways from animal to human: Similarities and differences, *Acta Physiol. Scand.*, 177, 255, 2003.

57. Janig, W. and MacLachlan, E.M., Neurobiology of the autonomic nervous system, in *Autonomic Failure: A Textbook of Clinical Disorders of the Autonomic Nervous System*, 4th ed., Mathias, C.J. and Bannister, R., Eds., Oxford University Press, Oxford, p. 3, 1999.

58. Janig, W., The autonomic nervous system and its coordination by the brain, in *Handbook of Affective Sciences, Part II*, Davidson, R.J., Scherer, K.R., Goldsmith, H.H., Eds., Oxford University Press, Oxford, p. 135, 2003.

59. Campero, M., Bostock, H., Baumann, T.K., and Ochoa, J. L., A search for activation of C nociceptors by sympathetic fibers in complex regional pain syndrome, *Clin. Neurophysiol.*, 121(7), 1072, 2010.

60. Oyen, W.J. et al., Reflex sympathetic dystrophy of the hand: An excessive inflammatory response? *Pain*, 55, 151, 1993.

61. Weber, M. et al., Facilitated neurogenic inflammation in complex regional pain syndrome, *Pain*, 91, 251, 2001.

62. Sudeck, P., Über die acute (trophoneurotische) Knochenatrophie nach Entzündugen und Traumen der Extremitüten, *Deutsche Medizinische Wochenschrift*, 28, 336, 1902.

63. Bove, G.M., Focal nerve inflammation induces neuronal signs consistent with symptoms of early complex regional pain syndromes, *Exp. Neurol.*, 219, 223, 2010.

64. Hartrick, C.T., Increased production of nitric oxide stimulated by interferon-gamma from peripheral blood monocytes in patients with complex regional pain syndrome, *Neurosci. Lett.*, 323, 75, 2002.

65. Giordano, J. and Dyche, J., Differential analgesic action of serotonin 5-HT3 receptor antagonists in three pain tests, *Neuropharmacology*, 28, 431, 1989.

66. Giordano, J. and Schultea, T., Serotonin 5-HT3 receptor mediation of pain and anti-nociception, *Pain Phys.*, 7, 141, 2003.

67. Kozin, F. et al., The reflex sympathetic dystrophy syndrome: I. Clinical and histologic studies: Evidence for bilaterality, response to corticosteroids and articular involvement, *Am J. Med.*, 60, 321, 1976.

68. Sufka, K., Schomberg, F., and Giordano, J., Receptor mediation of 5-HT-induced inflammation and nociception in rats, *Pharmacol. Biochem. Behav.*, 41, 53, 1992.

69. Giordano, J. and Sacks, S., Topical ondansetron attenuates capsaicin-induced inflammation and pain, *Eur. J. Pharmacol.*, 354, 13, 1998.

70. Huygen, F.J. et al., Evidence for local inflammation in complex regional pain syndrome type 1, *Mediators Inflamm.*, 11, 47, 2002.

71. Giordano, J., Neurobiology of nociceptive and anti-nociceptive systems, *Pain Phys.*, 8, 277, 2005.

72. Apkarian, A.V. et al., Prefrontal cortical hyperactivity in patients with sympathetically mediated chronic pain, *Neurosci. Lett.*, 311, 193, 2001.

73. Juttonen, K. et al., Altered central sensorimotor processing in patients with complex regional pain syndrome, *Pain*, 98, 315, 2002.

74. Van de Beek, W.J. et al., Susceptibility loci for complex regional pain syndrome, *Pain*, 103, 93, 2003.

75. Kemler, M.A. et al., HLA-DQ1 associated with reflex sympathetic dystrophy, *Neurology*, 53, 1350–1351, 1999.

76. Van Hilten, J.J., Van de Beek, W.J., and Roep, B.O., Multifocal or generalized tonic dystonia of complex regional pain syndrome: A distinct clinical entity associated with HLA-DR13, *Ann. Neurol.*, 48, 113–116, 2000.

77. Galenus, C. (Galen), *Hippocrates Writings*, Franklin Library, Franklin Center, PA, 1979.

78. Clark, R.P., Human skin temperature and its relevance in physiology and clinical assessment, in *Recent Advances in Medical Thermology*, Ring, E.F.J. and Phillips, B., Eds. Plenum Press, New York, 5, 1984.

79. American Chiropractic College of Infrared Imaging a College of the Council on Diagnostic Imaging, *Technical Protocols for High Resolution Infrared Imaging*, American Chiropractic Association, 1999.

80. Schwartz, R.G., Chair, Practice guidelines committee, Guidelines for neuromusculoskeletal thermography, American Academy of Thermology, *Thermology International*, 16, 5, 2006.

81. Wasner, G. et al., Vascular abnormalities in reflex sympathetic dystrophy (CRPS I): Mechanisms and diagnostic value, *Brain*, 124, 587, 2001.

82. Giordano, J. and Gerstmann, H., Patterns of serotonin- and 2-methylserotonin-induced pain may reflect 5-HT3 receptor sensitization, *Eur. J. Pharmacol.*, 483, 267, 2004.

83. Ochoa, J.L. et al., Intrafascicular nerve stimulation elicits regional skin warming that matches the projected field of evoked pain, in *Fine Afferent Nerve Fibers and Pain*, Schmidt, R.F., Schaible, H.G., Vahle-Hinz, C., Eds., VCH Verlagsgesellschaft, Weinheim, Germany, 1987.

84. Holzer, P., Peptidergic sensory neurons in the control of vascular functions: Mechanisms and significance in the cutaneous and splanchnic vascular beds, *Rev. Physiol. Biochem. Pharmacol.*, 121, 49, 1992.

85. Birklein, F., Kunzel, W., and Sieweke, N., Despite clinical similarities there are significant differences between acute limb trauma and complex regional pain syndrome I (CRPS I), *Pain*, 93, 165, 2001.

86. Wasner, G. et al., Vascular abnormalities in acute reflex sympathetic dystrophy (CRPS I): Complete inhibition of sympathetic nerve activity with recovery, *Arch Neurol.*, 56(5), 613, 1999.

87. Hobbins, W.B., Differential diagnosis of painful conditions and thermography, in *Contemporary Issues in Chronic Pain Management*, Norwell, M.A., Ed., Kluwer Academic Publishers, Paris 251, 1991.

88. Edwards, B.E. and Hobbins, W.B., Pain management and thermography, in *Practical Management of Pain*, 2nd ed., Raj, P.P., Mosby-Year Book, St. Louis, p. 168, 1992.

89. Rosen, L. et al., Skin microvascular circulation in the symptomatic dystrophy is evaluated by video-photometric capillaroscopy and laser Doppler fluxmetry, *Eur. J. Clin. Invest.*, 18, 305, 1998.

90. Kurvers, H.J. et al., The spinal component to skin blood flow abnormalities in reflex sympathetic dystrophy, *Arch. Neurol.*, 53, 50, 1996.

91. Schurmann, M., Grab, G., and Furst, H., A standardized bedside test for assessment of peripheral sympathetic nervous function using laser Doppler flowmetry, *Microvasc. Res.*, 52, 157, 1996.

92. Schurmann, M. et al., Assessment of peripheral sympathetic nervous function for diagnosing early post-traumatic complex regional pain syndrome type 1, *Pain*, 80, 149, 1999.

93. Campbell, J.N., Maier, R.A., and Raja, S.N., Is nociceptor activation by alpha-1 adrenoceptors the culprit in sympathetically maintained pain? *APS J.*, 1, 3, 1992.

94. Uematsu, S., Thermographic imaging of the sensory dermatomes, *Soc. Neurosci.*, abstract, 9, 324, 1983.

95. Uematsu, S., Thermographic imaging of cutaneous sensory segments in patients with peripheral nerve injury, *J. Neurosurg.*, 62, 716, 1985.

96. Uematsu, S. et al., Quantification of thermal asymmetry, Part 1: Normal values and reproducibility, *J. Neurosurg.*, 69, 552, 1988.

97. Feldman, F. and Nickoloff, E.L., Normal thermographic standards for the cervical spine and upper extremities, *Skeletal Radiol.*, 12, 235, 1984.

98. Goodman, P.A., Computer-assisted thermography, *Proceedings of the 14th annual meeting of the American Academy of Thermology*, abstract, 36, 1985.

99. Bej, M.D. and Schwartzman, R.J., Abnormalities of cutaneous blood flow regulation in patients with reflex sympathetic dystrophy as measured by laser doppler fluxmetry, *Arch. Neurol.*, 48, 912, 1991.

100. Bini, G. et al., Thermography and rhythm-generating mechanisms governing the sudomotor and vasoconstrictor outflow in human cutaneous nerves, *J. Physiol.*, (London), 206, 537, 1980.

101. Ochoa, J.L. et al., Interactions between sympathetic vasoconstrictor outflow and C-nociceptors-induced antidromic vasodilatation, *Pain*, 54, 191, 1993.

102. Bennett, G.J. and Ochoa, L.J., Thermographic observations on rats with experimental neuropathic pain, *Pain*, 45, 61, 1991.

103. Schurmann, M. et al., Peripheral sympathetic function as a predictor of complex regional pain syndrome type I (CRPS I) in patients with radial fracture, *Autonom. Neurosci.*, 86, 127, 2000.

104. Rosenbaum, R.B. and Ochoa, J.L., Thermography, in *Carpal Tunnel Syndrome and Other Disorders of the Median Nerve*, Rosenbaum, R.B. and Ochoa, J.L., Eds., Butterworth-Heindmann, Boston, p. 185, 1993.

105. Cline, M.A., Ochoa, J.L., and Torebjork, H.E., Chronic hyperalgesia and skin warming caused by sensitized C nociceptors, *Brain*, 112, 621, 1989.

106. Ochoa, J.L., The newly recognize painful ABC syndrome: Thermographic aspects, *Thermology*, 2, 65, 1986.

107. Ochoa, J.L. et al., Antidromic vasodilatation overridden by somatosympathetic reflexes in man-intraneural stimulation and thermography (abstract), *Soc. Neurosci.*, 16, 1280, 1990.

108. Wasner, G. et al., Vascular abnormalities in acute reflex sympathetic dystrophy (CRPS I): Complete inhibition of sympathetic nerve activity with recovery, *Arch. Neurol.*, 56, 613, 1999.

109. Hornyak, M.E. et al., Sympathetic activity influences the vascular axon reflex in the skin, *Acta Physiol. Scand.*, 139, 77, 1990.

110. Kurvers, H.J. et al., Reflex sympathetic dystrophy: Evolution of microcirculatory disturbances in time, *Pain*, 60, 333, 1995.

111. Birklein, F. et al., Sympathetic vasoconstrictor reflex pattern in patients with complex regional pain syndrome, *Pain*, 75, 93, 1998.

112. Drummond, P.D., Finch, P.M., and Smythe, G.A., Reflex sympathetic dystrophy: The significance of differing plasma catecholamine concentrations in affected and unaffected limbs, *Brain*, 114, 2025, 1991.

113. Drummond, P.A. et al., Plasma neuropeptide Y in the symptomatic limb of patients with causalgia pain, *Clin. J. Pain*, 12, 222, 1996.

114. Harden, R.N. et al., Norepinephrine and epinephrine levels in affected versus unaffected limbs in sympathetically maintained pain, *Clin. J. Pain,* 10, 324, 1994.

115. Leis, S. et al., Facilitated neurogenic inflammation in unaffected limbs of patients with complex regional pain syndrome, *Neurosci. Lett.,* 359, 163, 2004.

116. Baron, R. and Maier, C., Reflex sympathetic dystrophy: Skin blood flow, sympathetic vasoconstrictor reflexes and pain before and after surgical sympathectomy, *Pain,* 67, 317, 1996.

117. Birklein, F. et al., Pattern of autonomic dysfunction in time course of complex regional pain syndrome, *Clin. Auto. Res.,* 8, 79, 1998.

118. Cannon, W.B. and Rosenblueth, A., *The Supersensitivity of Denervation Structures: A Law of Denervation,* Macmillan, New York, 1949.

119. Fleming, W.W. and Westphal, D.P., Adaptive supersensitivity, in *Catecholamines I, Handbook of Experimental Pharmacology,* Trendelenburg, U. and Weiner, N., Eds., New York, Springer, Vol. 9, p. 509, 1988.

48

Thermal Imaging in Surgery

Paul Campbell
Ninewells Hospital

Roderick Thomas
Swansea Institute of Technology

48.1 Overview

Advances in miniaturization and microelectronics, coupled with enhanced computing technologies, have combined to see modern infrared imaging systems develop rapidly over the past decade. As a result, the instrumentation has considerably improved, not only in terms of its inherent resolution (spatial and temporal) and detector sensitivity (values ca. 25 mK are typical) but also in terms of its portability: the considerable reduction in bulk has resulted in light, camcorder (or smaller)-sized devices. Importantly, cost has also been reduced so that entry to the field is no longer prohibitive. This attractive combination of factors has led to an ever-increasing range of applicability across the medical spectrum. Whereas the mainstay application for medical thermography over the past 40 years has been with rheumatological and associated conditions, usually for the detection and diagnosis of peripheral vascular diseases such as Raynaud's phenomenon, the latest generations of thermal imaging systems have seen active service within new surgical realms such as orthopedics, coronary by-pass operations, and also in urology. The focus of this chapter relates not to a specific area of surgery per se, but rather to a generic and pervasive aspect of all modern surgical approaches: the use of *energized* instrumentation during surgery. In particular, we will concern ourselves with the use of thermal imaging to accurately monitor temperature within the tissue locale surrounding an energy-activated instrument. The rationale behind this is that it facilitates optimization of operation-specific protocols that may either relate to thermally based therapies or else to reduce the extent of collateral damage that may be introduced when inappropriate power levels, or excessive pulse durations, are implemented during surgical procedures.

48.2 Energized Systems

Energy-based instrumentation can considerably expedite fundamental procedures such as vessel sealing and dissection. The instrumentation is most often based around ultrasonic, laser, or radio-frequency (RF)-current-based technologies. Heating tissue into distinct temperature regimes is required in order to achieve the desired effect (e.g., vessel sealing, cauterization, or cutting). In the context of electrical current heating, the resultant effect of the current on tissue is dominated by two factors: the temperature attained by the tissue and the duration of the heating phase, as encapsulated in the following equation:

$$T - T_0 = \frac{1}{\sigma \rho c} J^2 \delta t \tag{48.1}$$

where T and T_0 are the final and initial temperatures (in degrees Kelvin [K]) respectively, σ is the electrical conductivity (in S/m), ρ is the tissue density, c is the tissue specific heat capacity (J kg^{-1} K^{-1}), J is the current density (A/m^2), and δt is the duration of heat application. The resultant high temperatures are not limited solely to the tissue regions in which the electrical current flow is concentrated. Heat will flow away from hotter regions in a time-dependent fashion given by the Fourier equation

$$Q(r,t) = -k\nabla T(r,t) \tag{48.2}$$

where Q is the heat flux vector, the proportionality constant k is a scalar quantity of the material known as the thermal conductivity, and $\nabla T(r,t)$ is the temperature gradient vector. The overall spatio-temporal evolution of the temperature field is embodied within the differential equation of heat flow (alternatively known as the diffusion equation)

$$\frac{1}{\alpha}\frac{\partial T(r,t)}{\partial t} = \nabla^2 T(r,t) \tag{48.3}$$

where α is the thermal diffusivity of the medium defined in terms of the physical constants, k, ρ, and c as

$$\alpha = k/\rho c \tag{48.4}$$

and the temperature T is a function of both the three dimensions of space (r) and the time t. In other words, high temperatures are not limited to the region specifically targeted by the surgeon, and this is often the source of an added surgical complication caused by collateral or proximity injury. Electrosurgical damage, for example, is the most common cause of iatrogenic bowel injury during laparoscopic surgery and 60% of mishaps are missed, that is, the injury is not recognized during surgery and declares itself with peritonitis several days after surgery or even after discharge from the hospital. This level of morbidity can have serious consequences, in terms of the expense incurred by readmission to hospital or even the death of the patient. By undertaking *in vivo* thermal imaging during energized dissection, it becomes possible to determine, in real time, the optimal power conditions for the successful accomplishment of specific tasks, and with minimal collateral damage. As an adjunct imaging modality, thermal imaging may also improve surgical practice by facilitating easier identification and localization of tissues such as arteries, especially by less experienced surgeons. Further, as tumors are more highly vascularized than normal tissue, thermal imaging may facilitate their localization and staging, that is, the identification of the tumor's stage in its growth cycle. Figure 48.1 shows a typical set-up for implementation of thermography during surgery.

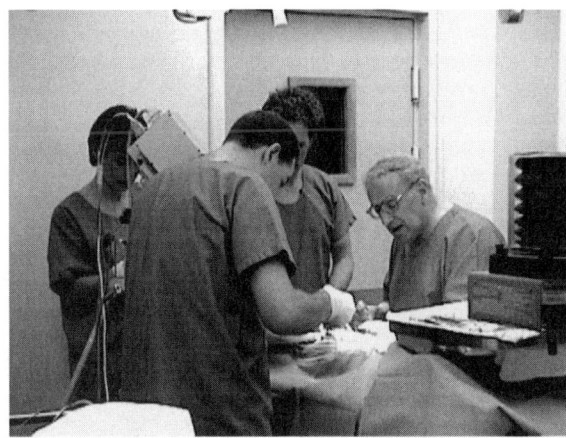

FIGURE 48.1 Typical set-up for a thermal imaging in surgery. The camera is tripod mounted toward the foot of the operating table and aimed at the surgical access site (camera visible over the left shoulder of the nearest surgeon).

48.3 Thermal Imaging Systems

As skin is a close approximation to an ideal black body (the emissivity, o, of skin is 0.98, whereas that of an ideal black body is o = 1), then we can feel reasonably confident in applying the relevant physics directly to the situation of thermography in surgery. One important consideration must be the waveband of detector chosen for thermal observations of the human body. It is known from the thermal physics of black bodies, that the wavelength at which the maximum emissive power occurs, λ_{max} (i.e., the peak in the Planck curve), is related to the body's temperature T through Wien's law:

$$\lambda_{max}T = 0.002898 \tag{48.5}$$

Thus, for bodies at 310 K (normal human body temperature), the peak output is around 10 μm, and the majority of the emitted thermal radiation is limited to the range from 2 to 20 μm. The optimal detectors for passive thermal imaging of normal skin should thus have best sensitivity around the 10 μm range, and this is indeed the case with many of the leading thermal imagers manufactured today, which often rely on GaAs quantum well infrared photodetectors (QWIPs) with a typical waveband of 8–9 μm. A useful alternative to these longwave detectors involves the use of indium–antimonide (InSb)-based detectors to detect radiation in the mid-wave infrared (3–5 μm). Both these materials have the benefit of enhanced temperature sensitivity (ca. 0.025 K), and are both wholly appropriate even for quantitative imaging of hotter surfaces, such as may occur in energized surgical instrumentation.

48.4 Calibration

While the latest generation of thermal imaging systems are usually robust instruments exhibiting low drift over extended periods, it is sensible to recalibrate the systems at regular intervals in order to preserve the integrity of captured data. For some camera manufacturers, recalibration can be undertaken under a service agreement and this usually requires shipping of the instrument from the host laboratory. However, for other systems, recalibration must be undertaken in-house, and on such occasions, a black body source (BBS) is required.

Most BBS are constructed in the form of a cavity at a known temperature, with an aperture to the cavity that acts as the black body, effectively absorbing all incident radiation upon it. The cavity temperature

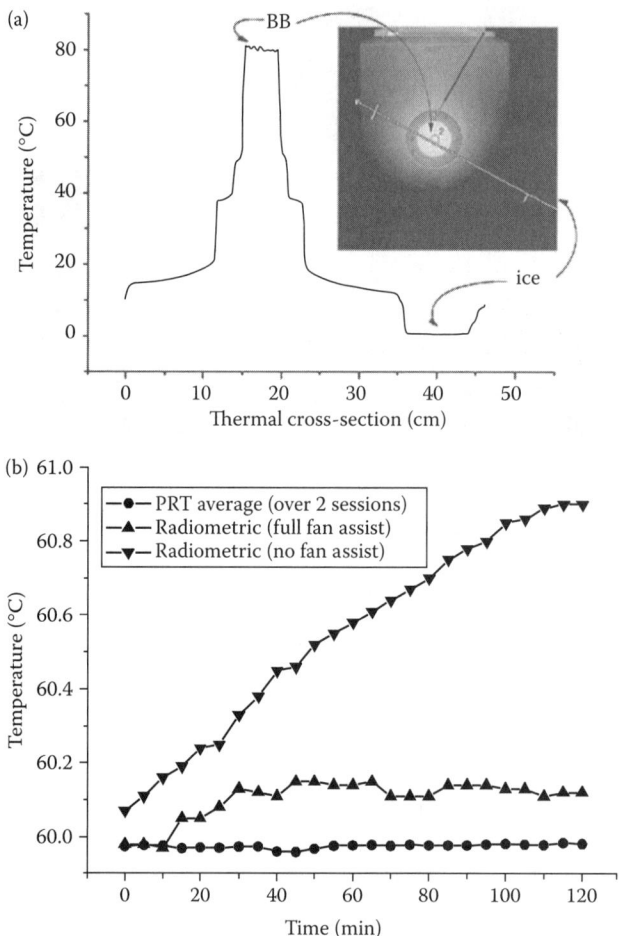

FIGURE 48.2 Thermal cross-section (profile) through the black body calibration source together with equilibrated crushed ice, which acts as a convenient secondary temperature gauge *in situ*. (Insert [left] thermal view with linear region of interest highlighted, and [right] optical view of the black body cavity and beaker of [equilibrated] crushed ice to the lower right.) (b) Radiometric detector drift during start up under two different ambient conditions. The detector readout is centered on the black body cavity source shown in (a), which was itself maintained at a target temperature of 59.97°C throughout the measurements (solid circles). Without fan-assisted cooling of the camera exterior, the measured temperature drifted by 0.8°C over 2 h, hence the importance of calibration under typical operating conditions. With fan-assisted cooling, the camera "settles" within around 30 min of switching on. (Camera: Raytheon Galileo [Raytheon Systems].)

must be measured using a high-accuracy thermometric device, such as a platinum resistance thermometer (PRT), with performance characteristics traceable to a thermometry standard. Figure 48.2b shows one such system, as developed by the UK National Physical Laboratory at Teddington, and whose architecture relies on a heat-pipe design. The calibration procedure requires measurement of the aperture temperature at a range of temperature set-points that are simultaneously monitored by the PRT (e.g., at intervals of 5° between temperature range of 293 and 353 K). Direct comparison of the radiometric temperature measured by the thermal camera with the standard temperature monitored via the PRT allows a calibration table to be generated across the temperature range of interest. During each measurement, sufficient time must be allowed in order to let the programmed temperature set-point equilibrate, otherwise inaccuracies will result. Further, the calibration procedure should ideally be undertaken under similar ambient conditions to those under which usual imaging is undertaken. This may include aspects such as laminar, or even fan-assisted, flow around the camera body which will affect the heat transfer rate from the camera to the ambient and in turn may affect the performance of the detector (Figure 48.2b).

48.5 Thermal Imaging during Energized Surgery

Fully remote-controlled cameras may be ideally suited to overhead bracket mountings above the operating table so that a bird's eye view over the surgical site is afforded. However, without a robotized arm to fully control pitch and location, the view may be restrictive. Tripod mounting, as illustrated in Figure 48.1, and with a steep look-down angle from a distance of about 1 m to the target offers the most versatile viewing without compromising the surgeon's freedom of movement. However, this type of set-up demands that a camera operator be on hand continually in order to move the imaging system to those positions offering best viewing for the type of energized procedure being undertaken.

48.5.1 RF Electrosurgery

As mentioned earlier, the most common energized surgical instrumentation employ a physical system reliant on (high-frequency) electrical current, an ultrasonic mechanism, or else incident laser energy in order to induce tissue heating. Thermal imaging has been used to follow all three of these procedures. There are often similarities in approach between the alternative modalities. For example, vessel sealing often involves placement of elongated forcep-style electrodes across a target vessel followed by ratcheted compression, and then a pulse of either RF current or alternatively ultrasonic activation of the forceps is applied through the compressed tissue region. The latest generations of energized instrumentation may have active feedback control over the pulse to facilitate optimal sealing with minimal thermal spread (e.g., the Valleylab *Ligasure* instrument); however, under certain circumstances, such as with calcified tissue or in excessively liquid environments, the performance may be less predictable.

Figure 48.3 illustrates how thermal spread may be monitored during the instrument activation period of one such "intelligent" feedback device using RF current. The initial power level for each application is determined through a fast precursor voltage scan that determines the natural impedance of the compressed tissue. Then, by monitoring the temperature dependence of impedance (of the compressed tissue) during current activation, the microprocessor-controlled feedback loop automatically maintains an appropriate power level until a target impedance is reached, indicating that the seal is complete. This process typically takes between 1 and 6 s, depending on the nature of the target tissue. The termination of the pulse is indicated by an audible tone burst from the power supply box. The performance of the system has been evaluated in preliminary studies involving gastric, colonic, and small bowel resection [1]; hemorraoidectomy [2]; prostatectomy [3]; and cholecystectomy [4].

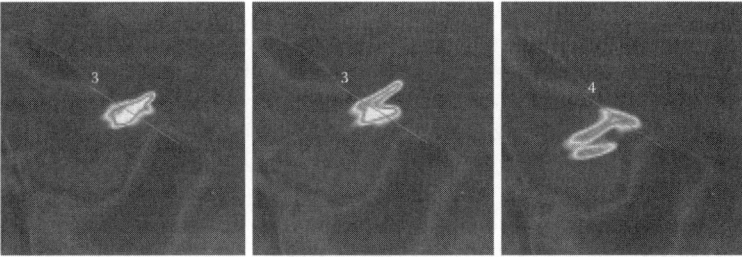

FIGURE 48.3 Thermographic sequence taken with the Dundee thermal imaging system and showing (1) energized forceps attached to bowel (white correlates with temperature), (2) detachment of the forceps revealing hot tissue beneath, and (3) remnant hot spot extending across the tissue and displaying collateral thermal damage covering 4.5 mm on either side of the instrument jaws.

Perhaps most strikingly, the facility for real-time thermographic monitoring, as illustrated in Figure 48.3, affords the surgeon immediate appreciation of the instrument temperature, providing a visual cue that automatically alerts to the potential for iatrogenic injury should a hot instrument come into close contact with vital structures. By the same token, the *in situ* thermal image also indicates when the tip of the instrument has cooled to ambient temperature. It should be noted that the amount by which the activated head's temperature rises is largely a function of device dimensions, materials, and the power levels applied together with the pulse duration.

48.5.2 Analysis of Collateral Damage

While thermograms typical of Figure 48.3 offer a visually instructive account of the thermal scene and its temporal evolution, a quantitative analysis of the sequence is more readily achieved through the identification of a linear region of interest (LROI), as illustrated by the line bisecting the device head in Figure 48.4a. The data constituted by the LROI is effectively a snapshot thermal profile across those pixels lying on this designated line (Figure 48.4b). A graph can then be constructed to encapsulate the time-dependent evolution of the LROI. This is displayed as a 3D surface (a function of spatial co-ordinate along the LROI, time, and temperature) upon which color-mapped contours are evoked to represent the different temperature domains across the LROI (Figure 48.4c). In order to facilitate measurement of the thermal spread, the 3D surface, as represented in matrix form, can then be interrogated with a mathematical programming package, or alternatively inspected manually, a process that is most easily undertaken after projecting the data to the 2D coordinate–time plane, as illustrated in Figure 48.4d. The critical temperature beyond which tangible heat damage can occur to tissue is assumed to be 45°C [5]. Thermal spread is then calculated by measuring the maximum distance between the 45°C contours on the planar projection, then subtracting the electrode "footprint" diameter from this to get the total spread. Simply dividing this result by two gives the thermal spread on either side of the device electrodes.

The advanced technology used in some of the latest generations of vessel sealing instrumentation can lead to a much reduced thermal spread, compared with the earlier technologies. For example, with the Ligasure LS1100 instrument, the heated peripheral region is spatially confined to less than 2 mm, even when used on thicker vessels/structures. A more advanced version of the device (LS1200 [*Precise*]) consistently produces even lower thermal spreads, typically around 1 mm (Figure 48.4). This performance is far superior to other commercially available energized devices.

For example, Kinoshita and coworkers [6] have observed (using infrared imaging) that the typical lateral spread of heat into adjacent tissue is sufficient to cause a temperature of over 60°C at radial distances of up to 10 mm from the active electrode when an ultrasonic scalpel is used. Further, when standard bipolar electrocoagulation instrumentation is used, the spread can be as large as 22 mm. Clearly, the potential for severe collateral and iatrogenic injury is high with such systems unless power levels are tailored to the specific procedure in hand and real-time thermal imaging evidently represents a powerful adjunct technology to aid this undertaking.

While the applications mentioned thus far relate to "open" surgical procedures requiring a surgical incision to access the site of interest, thermal imaging can also be applied as a route to protocol optimization for other less invasive procedures. Perhaps the most important surgical application in this regime involves laser therapy for various skin diseases/conditions. Application of the technique in this area is discussed below.

48.6 Laser Applications in Dermatology

48.6.1 Overview

Infrared thermographic monitoring (ITM) has been successfully used in medicine for a number of years and much of this has been documented by Professor Francis Ring (http://www.medimaging.org/),

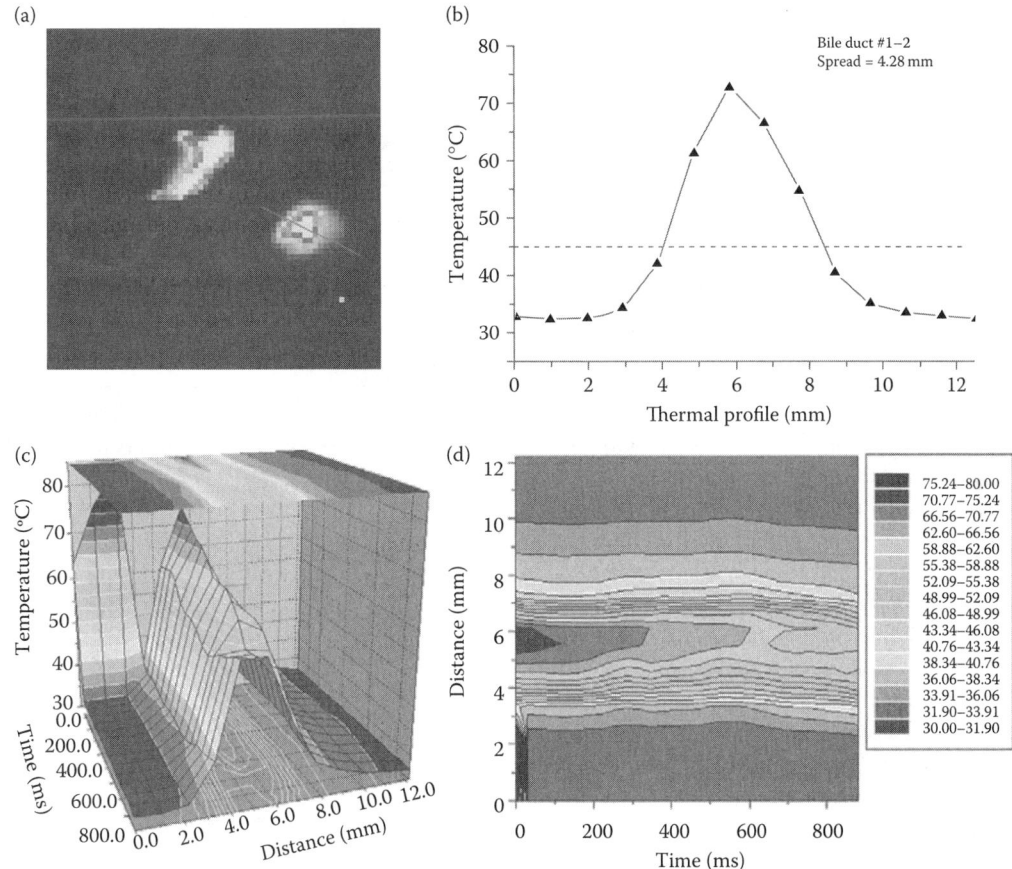

FIGURE 48.4 (a) Mid-infrared thermogram taken at the instant an energized forceps (Ligasure LS1200 *"Precise"*) is removed from the surgical scene after having conducted a seal on the bile duct. The hot tips of the forceps are clearly evident in the infrared view (just left of center), as is the remnant hot spot where the seal has occurred on the vessel. By generating a linear region of interest (LROI) through the hot spot, as indicated by the highlighted line in the figure, it is possible to monitor the evolution of the hot spot's temperature in a quantitative fashion. (b) Thermal profile corresponding to the LROI shown in (a). (c) By tracking the temporal evolution of the LROI, it is possible to generate a 3D plot of the thermal profile by simply stacking the individual profiles at each acquisition frame. In this instance, the cooling behavior of the hot spot is clearly identified. Manual estimation of the thermal spread is most easily achieved by resorting to the 2D contour plot of the thermal profile's temporal evolution, as shown in (d). In this instance, the maximal spread of the 45°C contours is measured as 4.28 mm. By subtracting the forcep "footprint" (2.5 mm for the device shown) and dividing the result by 2, we arrive at the thermal spread for the device. The average thermal spread (for six bile-duct sealing events) was 0.89 ± 0.35 mm.

who has established a database and archive within the Department of Computing at the University of Glamorgan, UK, spanning over 30 years of ITM applications. Examples include monitoring abnormalities such as malignancies, inflammation, and infection that cause localized increases in skin temperature, which show as hot spots or as asymmetrical patterns in an infrared thermogram.

A recent medical example that has benefited by the intervention of ITM is the treatment by laser of certain dermatological disorders. Advancements in laser technology have resulted in new portable laser therapies, examples of which include the removal of vascular lesions (in particular port-wine stains [PWS]), and also cosmetic enhancement approaches such as hair (depilation) and wrinkle removal.

TABLE 48.1 Characteristics of Laser Therapy during and after Treatment

General Indicators	Dye Laser Vascular Lesions	Ruby Laser Depilation
During treatment	Varying output parameters	Varying output parameters
	Portable	Portable
	Manual and scanned	Manual and scanned
	Selective destruction of target chromophore (hemoglobin)	Selective destruction of target chromophore (melanin)
After treatment (desired effect)	Slight bruising (purpura)	Skin returns to normal coloring (no bruising)
	Skin retains its elasticity	Skin retains surface markings
	Skin initially needs to be protected from UV and scratching	Skin retains its ability to tan after exposure to ultraviolet light
	Hair follicles are removed	Hair removed

In these laser applications, it is a common requirement to deliver laser energy uniformly without overlapping of the beam spot to a subdermal target region, such as a blood vessel, but with the minimum of collateral damage to the tissue locale. Temperature rise at the skin surface, and with this the threshold to burning/scarring is of critical importance for obvious reasons. Until recently, this type of therapy had not yet benefited significantly from thermographic evaluation. However, with the introduction of the latest generation thermal imaging systems, exhibiting the essential qualities of portability, high resolution, and high sensitivity, significant inroads to laser therapy are beginning to be made.

Historically, lasers have been used in dermatology for some 40 years [7]. In recent years, there have been a number of significant developments, particularly regarding the improved treatment of various skin disorders, most notably the removal of vascular lesions using dye lasers [8–12] and depilation using ruby lasers [13–15]. Some of the general indicators as to why lasers are the preferred treatment of choice are summarized in Table 48.1.

48.7 Laser–Tissue Interactions

The mechanisms involved in the interaction between light and tissue depend on the characteristics of the impinging light and the targeted human tissue [16]. To appreciate these mechanisms the optical properties of tissue must be known. It is necessary to determine the tissue reflectance, absorption, and scattering properties as a function of wavelength. A simplified model of laser light interaction with the skin is illustrated in Figure 48.5.

Recent work has shown that laser radiation can penetrate through the epidermis and basal structure to be preferentially absorbed within the blood layers located in the lower dermis and subcutis. The process is termed selective photothermolysis, and is the specific absorption of laser light by a target

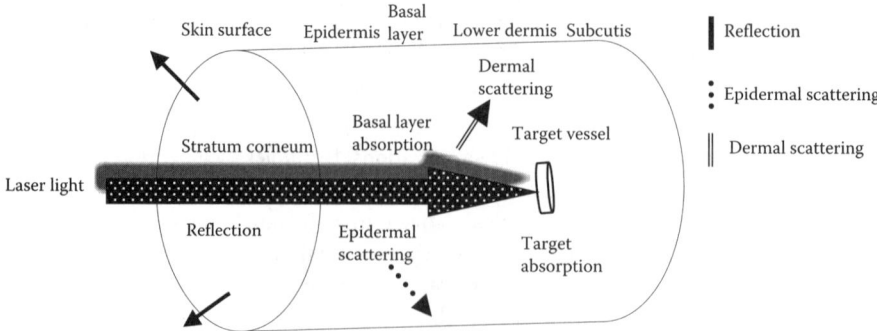

FIGURE 48.5 Passage of laser light within skin layers.

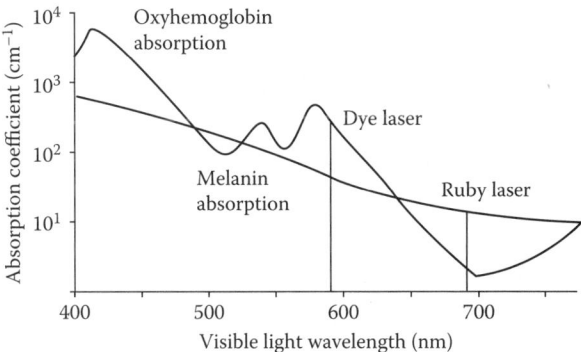

FIGURE 48.6 Spectral absorption curves for human blood and melanin.

TABLE 48.2 Interaction Effects of Laser Light and Tissue

Effect	Interaction
Photothermal	
Photohyperthermia	Reversible damage of normal tissue (37–42°C)
Photothermolysis Photocoagulation	Loosening of membranes (odema), tissue welding (45–60°C)
Photocarbonization	Thermal-dynamic effects, micro-scale overheating
Photovaporization	Coagulation, necrosis (60–100°C)
	Drying out, vaporization of water, carbonization (100–300°C)
	Pyrolysis, vaporization of solid tissue matrix (>300°C)
Photochemical	Photodynamic therapy, black light therapy
Photochemotherapy Photoinduction	Biostimulation
Photoionization Photoablation	Fast thermal explosion, optical breakdown, mechanical shockwave

tissue in order to eliminate that target without damaging surrounding tissue. For example, in the treatment of PWS, a dye laser of wavelength 585 nm has been widely used [17] where the profusion of small blood vessels that comprise the PWS are preferentially targeted at this wavelength. The spectral absorption characteristics of light through human skin have been well established [18] and are replicated in Figure 48.6 for the two dominant factors: melanin and oxyhemoglobin.

There are three types of laser–tissue interaction, namely photothermal, photochemical, and protoionization (Table 48.2), and the use of lasers on tissue results in a number of differing interactions, including photodisruption, photoablation, vaporization, and coagulation, as summarized in Figure 48.7.

The application of appropriate laser technology to medical problems depends on a number of laser operating parameters, including matching the optimum laser wavelength for the desired treatment. Some typical applications and the desired wavelengths for usage are highlighted in Table 48.3.

48.8 Optimizing Laser Therapies

There are a number of challenges in optimizing laser therapy, mainly related to the laser parameters of wavelength, energy density, and spot size. Combined with these are difficulties associated with poor positioning of hand-held laser application that may result in uneven treatment (overlapping spots and/or uneven coverage [stippling] of spots), excessive treatment times, and pain. Therefore, for enhanced

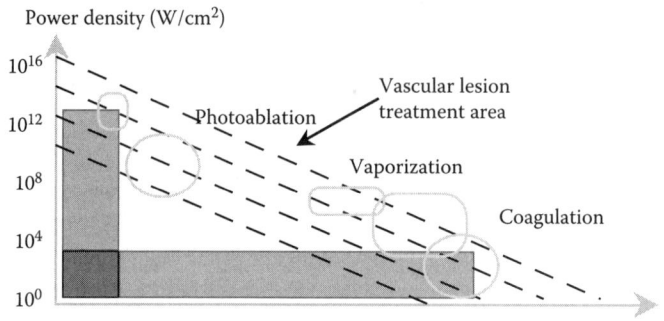

FIGURE 48.7 Physiological characteristics of laser therapy. (From Thomas, R.A. et al. 2002. *Thermosense XXIV, Proceedings of SPIE*, April 1–4, Orlando, USA. With permission.)

TABLE 48.3 Laser Application in Dermatology

Laser	Wavelength (nm)	Treatment
Flashlamp short-pulsed dye	510	Pigmented lesions, for example, freckles, tattoos
Flashlamp long-pulsed dye	585	PWS in children, warts, hypertrophic scars
Ruby single-pulse or Q-switched	694	Depilation of hair
Alexandrite Q-switched	755	Multicolored tattoos, viral warts, depilation
Diode variable	805	Multicolored tattoos, viral warts
Neodymium yitrium aluminum (Nd-YAG) Q-switched	1064	Pigmented lesions; adult port-wine stains, black/blue tattoos
Carbon dioxide continuous pulsed	10600	Tissue destruction, warts, tumors

efficacy, an improved understanding of the thermal effects of laser–tissue interaction benefits therapeutic approaches. Here, variables for consideration include

1. Thermal effects of varying spot size
2. Improved control of hand-held laser minimizing overlapping and stippling
3. Establishment of minimum gaps
4. Validation of laser computer scanning

Evaluation (Figure 48.8) was designed to elucidate whether or not measurements of the surface temperature of the skin are reproducible when illuminated by nominally identical laser pulses. In this case, a 585 nm dye laser and a 694 nm ruby laser were used to place a number of pulses manually on tissue. The energy emitted by the laser is highly repeatable. Care must be taken to ensure that both the laser and

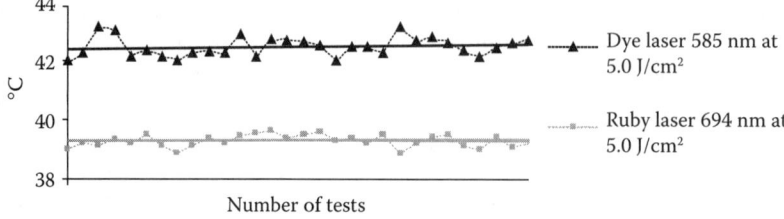

FIGURE 48.8 Repeatability of initial maximum skin temperatures (°C) of two lasers with similar energy density but different wavelengths.

radiometer positions are kept constant and that the anatomical location used for the test had uniform tissue pigmentation.

Figure 48.8 shows the maximum temperature for each of 20 shots fired on the forearm of a representative Caucasian male with type 2 skin*. Maximum temperature varies between 48.90°C and 48.10°C representing a variance of 1°C (±0.45°C). This level of reproducibility is pleasing since it shows that, despite the complex scenario, the radiometer is capable of repeatedly and accurately measuring surface tissue temperatures. In practice, the radiometer may be used to inform the operator when any accumulated temperature has subsided, allowing further treatment without exceeding some damage threshold.

Energy density is also an important laser parameter and can be varied to match the demands of the application. It is normal in the discipline to measure energy density (fluence) in J/cm^2. In treating vascular lesions, most utilize an energy density for therapy of 5–10 J/cm^2 [19]. The laser operator needs to be sure that the energy density is uniform and does not contain hot spots that may take the temperature above the damage threshold inadvertently. Preliminary characterization of the spot with thermal imaging can then aid with fine tuning of the laser and reduce the possibility of excessive energy density and with that the possibility of collateral damage.

48.9 Thermographic Results of Laser Positioning

During laser therapy, the skin is treated with a number of spots, applied manually depending on the anatomical location and required treatment. It has been found that spot size directly affects the efficacy of treatment. The wider the spot size the higher the surface temperature [20]. The type and severity of lesion also determine the treatment required. Its color severity (dark to light) and its position on skin (raised to level). Therefore, the necessary treatment may require a number of passes of the laser over the skin. It is therefore essential as part of the treatment that there is a physical separation between individual spots so that

1. The area is not overtreated with overlapping spots that could otherwise result in local heating effects from adjacent spots resulting in skin damage.
2. The area is not undertreated leaving stippled skin.
3. The skin has cooled sufficiently before second or subsequent passes of the laser.

Figure 48.9 shows two laser shots placed next to each other some 4 mm apart. The time between the shots is 1 s. There are no excessive temperatures evident and no apparent temperature build-up in the

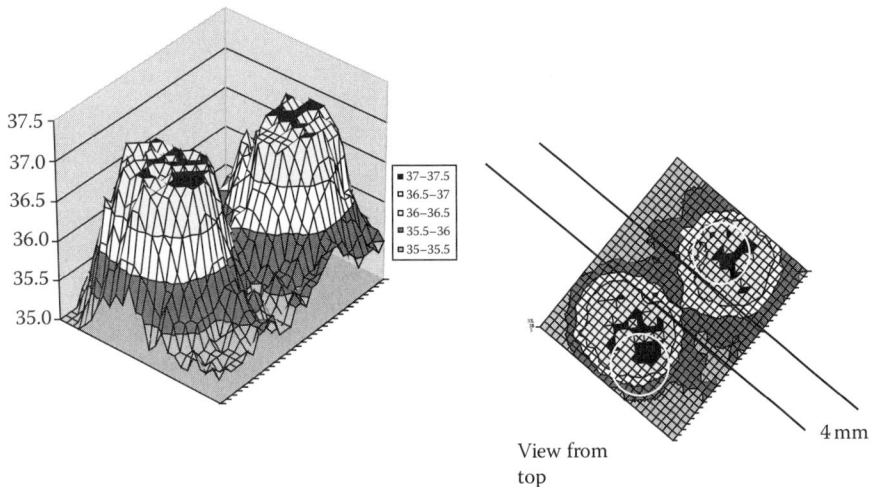

FIGURE 48.9 Two-dye laser spots with a minimum of 4 mm separation (585 nm at 4.5 J/cm^2, 5 mm spot).

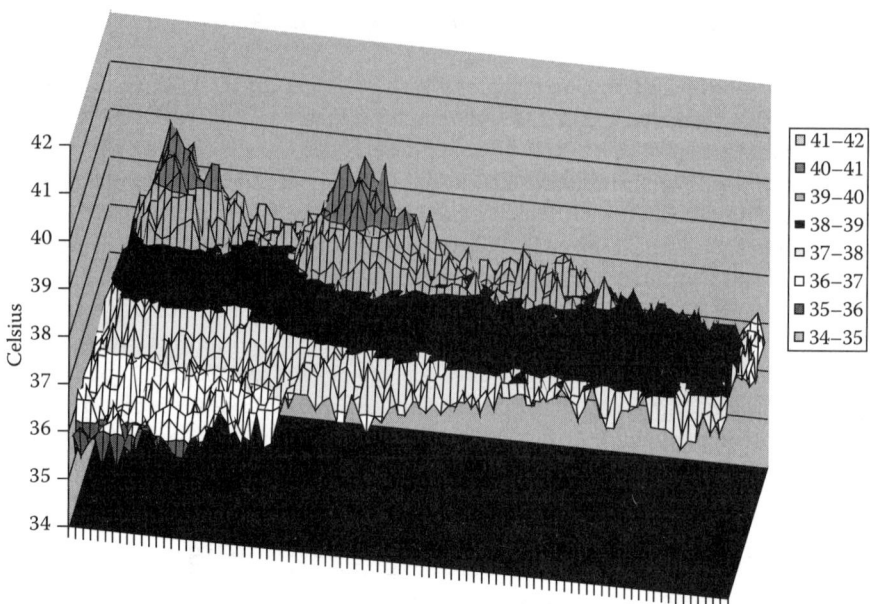

FIGURE 48.10   Three-dye laser spots, 2 s apart with a 5 mm separation (585 nm at 5 J/cm^2, 5 mm spot).

gap. This result, which concurs with Lanigan [21], suggests a minimum physical separation of 5 mm between all individual spot sizes.

The intention is to optimize the situation leading to a uniform therapeutic and aesthetic result without either striping or thermal build-up. This is achieved by initially determining the skin color (Chromotest) for optimum energy settings, followed by a patch test and subsequent treatment. Increasing the number of spots to 3 with the 4 mm separation reveals a continuing trend, as shown in Figure 48.10. The gap between the first two shots is now beginning to merge in the 2 s period that has lapsed. The gap between shots 2 and 3 remains clear and distinct and there are clearly visible thermal bands across the skin surface between 38–39°C and 39–40°C. These experimental results supply valuable information to support the development of both free-hand treatment and computer-controlled techniques.

48.10 Computerized Laser Scanning

Having established the parameters relating to laser spot positioning, the possibility of achieving reproducible laser coverage of a lesion by automatic scanning becomes a reality. This has potential advantages, which include

  1. Accurate positioning of the spot with the correct spacing from the adjacent spots
  2. Accurate timing allowing the placement at a certain location at the appropriate lapsed time

There are some disadvantages that include the need for additional equipment and regulatory approvals for certain market sectors.

A computerized scanning system has been developed [13] that illuminates the tissue in a predefined pattern. Sequential pulses are not placed adjacent to an immediately preceding pulse thereby ensuring the minimum of thermal build-up. Clement et al. [13] carried out a trial, illustrating treatment coverage using a hand-held system compared to a controlled computer scanning system. Two adjacent areas (lower arm) were selected and shaved. A marked hexagonal area was subjected to 19 shots using a hand-held system, and an adjacent area of skin was treated with a scanner whose computer control

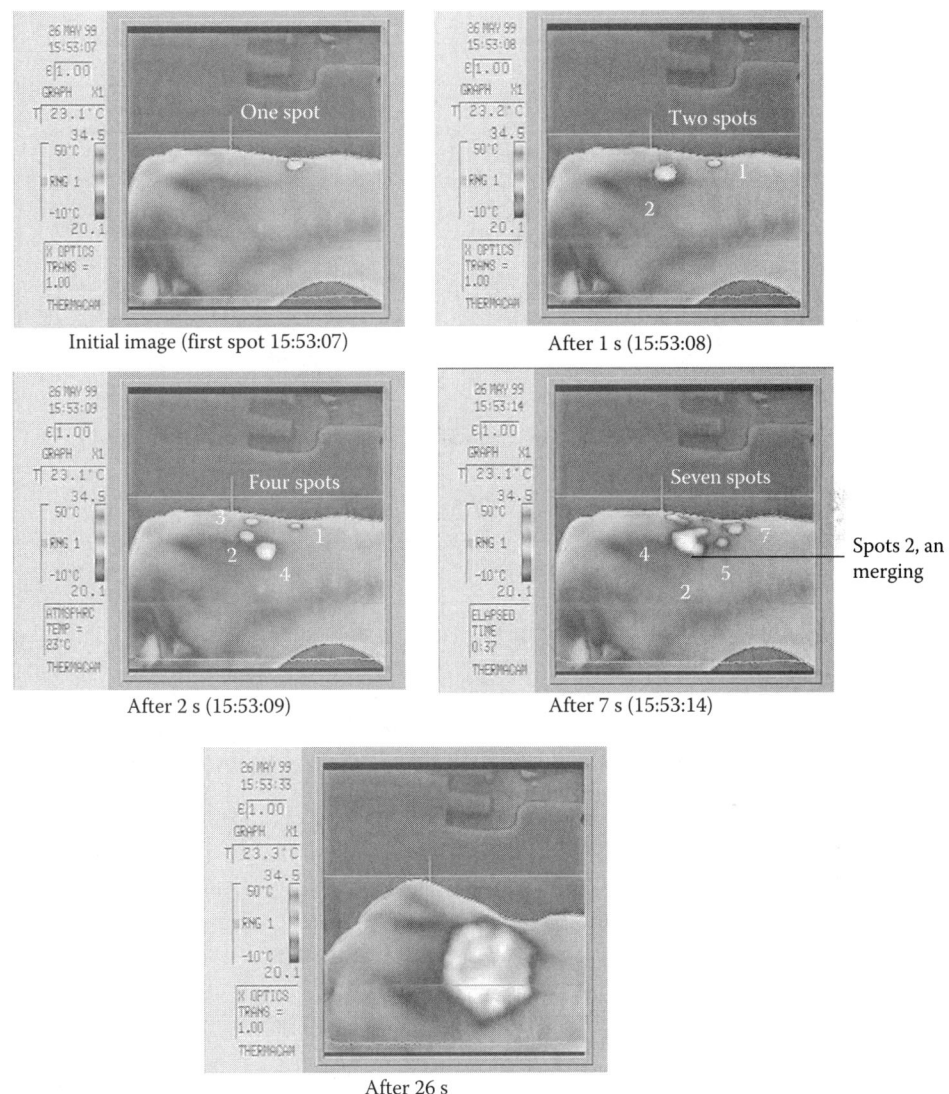

FIGURE 48.11 Sample sequences during computer laser scanning.

is designed to uniformly fill the area with exactly 19 shots. Such tests were repeated and the analyzed statistics showed that, on average, only 60% of area is covered by laser spots. The use of thermography allowed the validation and optimization of this automated system in a way that was impossible without thermal imaging technology. The following sequence of thermal images, Figure 48.11, captures the various stages of laser scanning of the hand using a dye laser at 5.7 J/cm². Thermography confirms that the spot temperature from individual laser beams will merge and that both the positioning of spots and the time duration between spots dictate the efficacy of treatment.

48.10.1 Case Study 1: Port-Wine Stain

Vascular nevi are common and are present at birth or develop soon after. Superficial lesions are due to capillary networks in the upper or mid dermis, but larger angiomas can be located in the lower dermis

TABLE 48.4 Vasculature Treatment Types

Treatment Type	Process	Possible Concerns
Camouflage	Applying skin colored pigments to the surface of the skin. Enhancement to this technique is to tattoo skin colored inks into the upper layer of the lesion	Only a temporary measure and is very time consuming. Efficacy dependent on flatter lesions
Cryosurgery	Involves applying supercooled liquid nitrogen to the lesion to destroy abnormal vasculature	May require several treatments
Excision	Common place where the lesion is endangering vital body functions	Not considered appropriate for purely cosmetic reasons. Complex operation resulting in a scar. Therefore, only applicable to the proliferating hemangioma lesion
Radiation therapy	Bombarding the lesion with radiation to destroy vasculature	Induced number of skin cancer in a small number of cases
Drug therapy	Widely used administering steroids	Risk of secondary complications affecting bodily organs

and subcutis. An example of vascular nevi is the PWS often present at birth, which is an irregular red or purple macule which often affects one side of the face. Problems can arise if the nevus is located close to the eye, and in some cases where a PWS involves the trigeminal nerve's ophthalmic division may have an associated intracranial vascular malformation known as Sturge Weber syndrome. The treatment of vascular nevi can be carried out in a number of ways, often dependent on the nature, type, and anatomical and severity of lesion location, as highlighted in Table 48.4.

A laser wavelength of 585 nm is preferentially absorbed by hemoglobin within the blood, but there is partial absorption in the melanin-rich basal layer in the epidermis. The objective is to thermally damage the blood vessel, by elevating its temperature, while ensuring that the skin surface temperature is kept low. For a typical blood vessel, the temperature–time graph appears similar to Figure 48.12. This suggests that it is possible to selectively destroy the PWS blood vessels, by

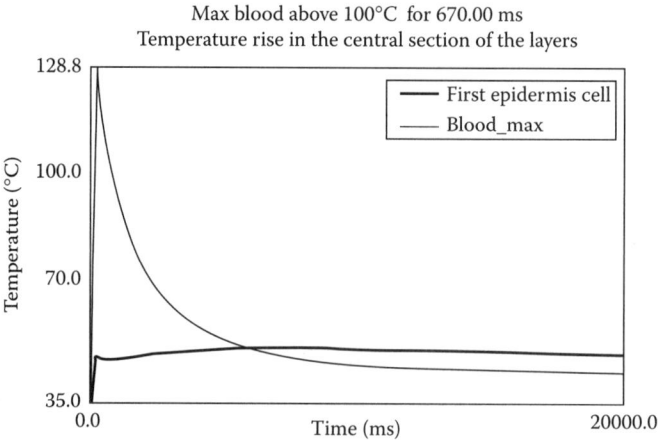

FIGURE 48.12 Typical temperatures for PWS problem, indicating thermal disruption of blood vessel, while skin surface temperature remains low.

elevating them to a temperature in excess of 100°C, causing disruption to the small blood vessels, while maintaining a safe skin surface temperature. This has been proven empirically via thermographic imaging with a laser pulsing protocol that was devised and optimized on the strength of Monte-Carlo-based models [22] of the heat dissipation processes [23]. The two-dimensional Cartesian thermal transport equation is

$$\nabla T^2 + \frac{Q(x,y)}{k} = \frac{1}{\alpha}\frac{\partial T}{\partial t} \tag{48.6}$$

where temperature T has both an implied spatial and temporal dependence, and the volumetric source term, $Q(x,y)$, is obtained from the solution of the Monte-Carlo radiation transport problem [24].

48.10.2 Case Study 2: Laser Depilation

The 694 nm wavelength laser radiation is preferentially absorbed by melanin, which occurs in the basal layer and particularly in the hair follicle base, which is the intended target using an oblique angle of laser beam (see Figure 48.13). A Monte-Carlo analysis was performed in a similar manner to *Case Study 1* above, where the target region in the dermis is the melanin-rich base of the hair follicle. Figure 48.14a and b shows the temperature–time profiles for 10 and 20 J cm² laser fluence [25]. These calculations suggest that it is possible to thermally damage the melanin-rich follicle base while restricting the skin surface temperature to values that cause no superficial damage. Preliminary clinical trials indicated that there is indeed a beneficial effect, but the choice of laser parameters still required optimizing.

Thermographic analysis has proved to be indispensable in this work. Detailed thermometric analysis is shown in Figure 48.15a. Analysis of this data shows that in this case, the surface temperature is raised to about 50°C. The thermogram also clearly shows the selective absorption in the melanin-dense hair. The temperature of the hair is raised to over 207°C. This thermogram illustrates direct evidence for selective wavelength absorption leading to cell necrosis. Further clinical trials have indicated a maximum fluence of 15 J cm² for type III Caucasian skin. Figure 48.15b illustrates a typical thermographic image obtained during the real-time monitoring.

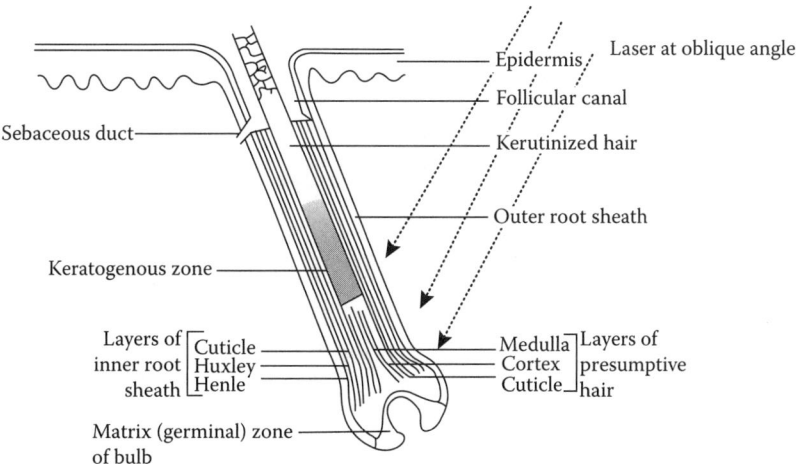

FIGURE 48.13 Oblique laser illumination of hair follicle.

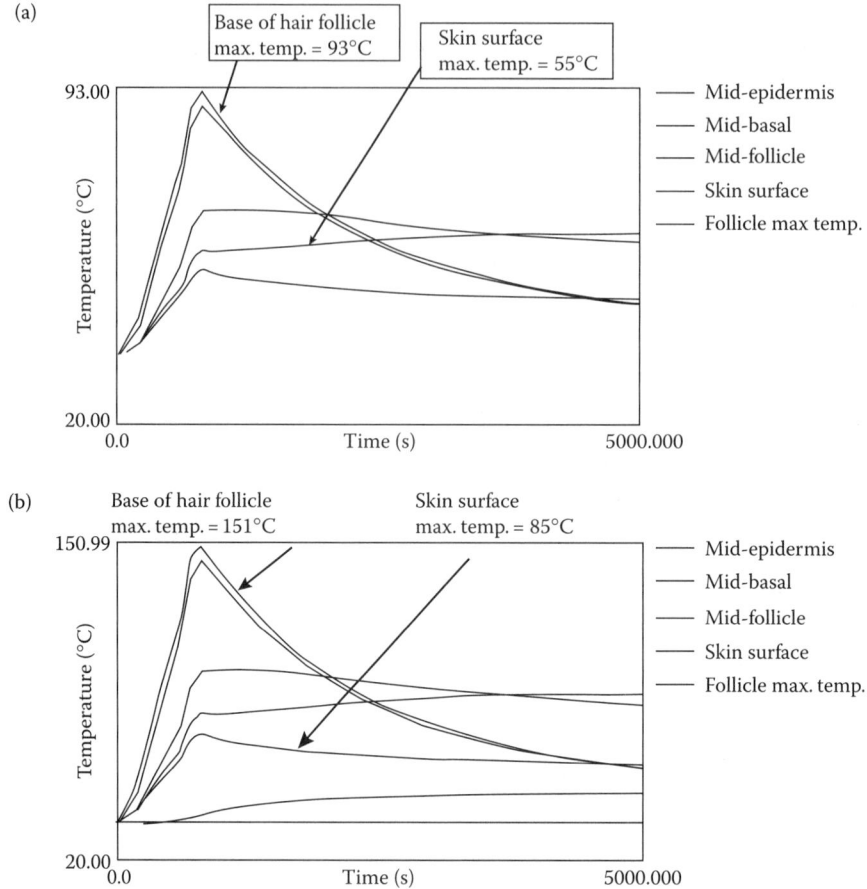

FIGURE 48.14   (a) Temperature–time profiles at 10 J cm² ruby (694 nm), 800 μs laser pulse on Caucasian skin type III. (b) Temperature–time profiles for 20 J cm² ruby (694 nm), 800 μs laser pulse on Caucasian skin type III.

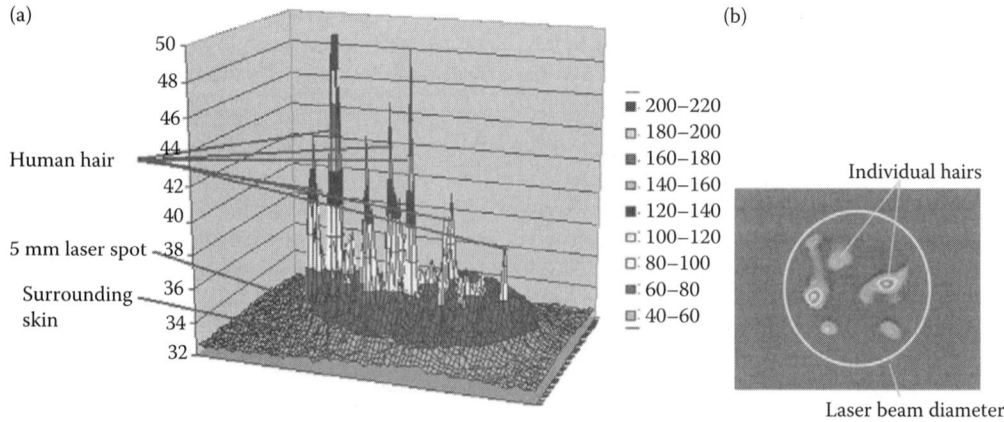

FIGURE 48.15   (a) Postprocessed results of 5 mm. (b) Simplified thermogram diameter 694 nm 20 J cm² 800 μs ruby pulse of ruby laser pulse, with 5 mm spot at 20 J cm².

48.11 Conclusions

The establishment, development, and consequential success of medical infrared thermographic (MIT) intervention with laser therapy is primarily based on the understanding of the following:

1. Problem/condition to be monitored
2. Set-up and correct operation of infrared system (appropriate and validated training)
3. Appropriate conditions during the monitoring process
4. Evaluation of activity and development of standards and protocol

With reference to (1) above, that is, the condition to be monitored, there needs to be a good knowledge as to the physiological aspects of the desired medical process; in laser therapy an understanding as to the mechanisms involved in laser–tissue interaction. A good reference source of current practice can be found in the *Handbook of Optical Biomedical Diagnostics*, published by The International Society for Optical Engineering (SPIE).

In this application, fast data capture (>50 Hz), good image quality (256 × 256 pixels), temperature sensitivity, and repeatability were considered important and an Inframetrics SC1000 Focal Plane Array Radiometer (3.4–5 μm, CMOS PtSi Cooled Detector) with a real-time data acquisition system (Dynamite) was used. There are currently very fast systems available with data acquisition speeds in terms of hundreds of Hertz with detectors that provide excellent image quality. In (2), the critical aspect is training [26]. Currently, infrared equipment manufacturers design systems with multiple applications in mind. This has resulted in many aspects of good practice and quality standards. This is one of the reasons why industrial infrared thermography is so successful. This has not necessarily been the case in medicine. However, it is worth noting that there are a number of good infrared training organizations throughout the world, particularly in the United States. The advantages of adopting training organizations such as these is that they have experience of training with reference to a very wide range and type of infrared thermographic systems, in a number of different applications. This will help in the identification of the optimum infrared technology. In (3), consideration as to the conditions surrounding the patient and the room environment are important for optimum results. In the United Kingdom, for example, Professor Francis Ring, University of Glamorgan, has led the way in the development and standardizations of clinical infrared practice [27]. Finally, (4) the evaluation of such practice is crucial if lessons are to be learnt and protocol and standards are to emerge.

Infrared thermal imaging provides an important tool for optimizing energized surgical interventions and facilitates validation of theoretical models of evolving temperature fields.

References

1. Heniford, B.T., Matthews, B.D., Sing, R.F., Backus, C., Pratt, P., and Greene, F.L. 2001 Initial results with an electrothermal bipolar vessel sealer. *Surg. Endosc.* 15: 799–801.
2. Palazzo, F.F., Francis, D.L., and Clifton, M.A. 2002 Randomised clinical trial of ligasure versus open haemorrhoidectomy. *Br. J. Surg.* 89: 154–157.
3. Sengupta, S. and Webb, D.R. 2001 Use of a computer controlled bipolar diathermy system in radical prostatectomies and other open urological surgery. *ANZ J. Surg.* 71: 538–540.
4. Schulze, S., Krztiansen, V.B., Fischer-Hansen, B., and Rosenberg, J. 2002 Sealing of the cystic duct with bipolar electrocoagulation. *Surg. Endosc.* 16: 342–344.
5. Reidenbach, H.D. and Buess, G. 1992. Anciliary technology: Electrocautery, thermoregulation and laser. In Cuschieri, A., Buess, G., and Perrisat, L. Eds., *Operative Manual of Endoscopic Surgery.* Springer-Verlag, Berlin, pp. 44–60.
6. Kinoshita, T., Kanehira, E., Omura, K., Kawakami, K., and Watanabe, Y. 1999 Experimental study on heat production by a 23.5 kHz ultrasonically activated device for endoscopic surgery. *Surg. Endosc.* 13: 621–625.

7. Wheeland, R.G. 1995 Clinical uses of lasers in dermatology. *Lasers Surg. Med.* 16:2–23.

8. Barlow, R.J., Walker, N.P.J., and Markey, A.C. 1996 Treatment of proliferative haemangiomas with 585 nm pulsed dye laser. *Br. J. Dermatol.* 134: 700–704.

9. Garden, J.M., Polla, L.L., and Tan, O.T. 1988 Treatment of port wine stains by pulsed dye laser—Analysis of pulse duration and long term therapy. *Arch. Dermatol.* 124: 889–896.

10. Glassberg, E., Lask, G., Rabinowitz, L.G., and Tunnessen, W.W. 1989 Capillary haemangiomas: Case study of a novel laser treatment and a review of therapeutic options. *J. Dermatol. Surg. Oncol.* 15: 1214–1223.

11. Kiernan, M.N. 1997 An analysis of the optimal laser parameters necessary for the treatment of vascular lesions, PhD thesis, The University of West of England.

12. Motley, R.J., Katugampola, G., and Lanigan, S.W. 1996 Microvascular abnormalities in port wine stains and response to 585 nm pulsed dye laser treatment. *Br. J. Dermatol.* 135(Suppl. 47): 13–14.

13. Clement, R.M., Kiernan, M.N., Thomas, R.A., Donne, K.E., and Bjerring, P.J. 1999 The use of thermal imaging to optimise automated laser irradiation of tissue. *Skin Research and Technology.* Vol. 5, No. 2, *th Congress of the International Society for Skin Imaging*, July 4–6, 1999, Royal Society London.

14. Gault, D., Clement, R.M., Trow, R.B., and Kiernan, M.N. 1998 Removing unwanted hairs by laser. *Face* 6: 129–130.

15. Grossman et al. 1997 Damage to hair follicle by normal mode ruby laser pulse. *J. Amer. Acad. Dermatol.* 889–894.

16. Welsh, A.J. and van Gemert, M.V.C. 1995 *Optical–Thermal Response of Laser-Irradiated Tissue.* Plenum Press, ISBN 0306449269.

17. Clement, R.M., Donne, K.D., Thomas, R.A., and Kiernan, M.N. 2000 Thermographic condition monitoring of human skin during laser therapy. *Quality Reliability Maintenance, 3rd International Conference*, St Edmund Hall, University of Oxford, March 30–31, 2000.

18. Andersen, R.R. and Parrish, J.A. 1981 Microvasculature can be selectively damaged using dye lasers. *Lasers Surg. Med.* 1: 263–270.

19. Garden, J.M. and Bakus, W. 1996 Clinical efficacy of the pulsed dye laser in the treatment of vascular lesions. *J. Dermatol. Surg. Oncol.* 19: 321–326.

20. Thomas, R.A., Donne, K.E., Clement, R.M., and Kiernan, M. 2002 Optimised laser application in dermatology using infrared thermography, *Thermosense XXIV, Proceedings of SPIE*, April 1–4, Orlando, USA.

21. Lanigan, S.W. 1996 Port wine stains on the lower limb: Response to pulsed dye laser therapy. *Clin. Exp. Dermatol.* 21: 88–92.

22. Wilson, B.C. and Adam, G. 1983 A Monte Carlo model for the absorption and flux distributions of light in tissue. *Med. Phys. Biol.* 1.

23. Daniel, G. 2002 An investigation of thermal radiation and thermal transport in laser–tissue interaction, PhD thesis, Swansea Institute.

24. Donne, K.E. 1999 Two dimensional computer model of laser tissue interaction. Private communication.

25. Trow, R. 2001 The design and construction of a ruby laser for laser depilation, PhD thesis, Swansea Institute.

26. Thomas, R.A. 1999 *Thermography.* Coxmoor Publishers, Oxford, pp. 79–103.

27. Ring, E.F.J. 1995 History of thermography. In Ammer, K. and Ring, E.F.J., Eds., *The Thermal Image in Medicine and Biology.* Uhlen Verlag, Vienna, pp. 13–20.

49

Thermal Signals and Cutaneous Circulation in Physiological Research and Reconstructive Surgery

David D. Pascoe
Auburn University

Louis de Weerd
*University Hospital of
North Norway*

James B. Mercer
University of Tromsø

Joshua E. Lane
*Mercer University School of
Medicine*

*Emory University School of
Medicine*

Sven Weum
Auburn University

49.1 Overview

In the third edition of the *Biomedical Engineering Handbook* (*Physiology of Thermal Signals*), also republished in this edition, we introduced the reader to skin thermal properties in response to stress, regulation of skin blood flow for heat transfers, modeling equations, and objective thermography [1]. The objective thermography explored the efficiency of heat transport in the hand-reduced blood flow, nerve block and laser Doppler mapping, and sports medicine injury applications. Most of the work in this current publication on thermal signals builds on that foundation of information. However, before we go into further detail on the use of IR thermography, it is important to review some basic principles in thermal physiology.

49.1.1 Skin Thermoregulation Models

The physiological research journal articles reporting skin surface temperatures have almost exclusively obtained these measurements through surface skin probes. This is problematic because the attachment of the probe can alter the microenvironment of the skin, and the probe is only measuring one small location that cannot account for the variance in tissue temperature across the surface area. In an attempt to account for the influence of skin thermoregulation on the thermal homeostasis of the individual, formulas combining the various regions of the body have been created. The challenge in acquiring accurate mean skin temperature measures has been related to the large contoured surface area and the assigned contribution of regional areas to the overall thermal status of the individual. In the literature, 20 measurement sites have been identified and numerous formulas varying in the number of reference sites required by each formula have emerged. Should all sites be given equal representation? While the core environment remains fairly constant, the regional peripheral blood flow and temperatures are variable. To obtain an accurate assessment of mean skin temperature, previous research has focused on four basic formula approaches: (1) unweighted average of the sites recorded; (2) weighted formulas based on regional surface averages as defined within population norms; (3) variable weighting based on individually determined surface areas, often determined by the DuBois linear formula; and (4) weighted formulas that incorporate factors that describe both surface area and the thermoregulatory response to thermal stimuli [2–4]. This fourth approach recognized that while the surface areas of the various regions help to explain the exposed surface available for heat exchange (conduction, convection, and radiation), differences in regional blood flow, temperature, and sweat gland distribution due to evaporative cooling may not be adequately expressed.

49.1.2 Skin Surface Temperature Measurements and Infrared Thermography

In the investigative process, noncontact infrared skin surface thermal maps can provide sensitive measurements (0.05°C) of a region based on a large number of individual reference points (pixels) from which the high, low, and mean temperatures can be derived. This approach utilizing IR thermography can be instrumental in our quest to understand and refine our understanding of skin perfusion, heat transfers, and thermoregulation.

Infrared thermography captures the thermal image of the dynamic heat transfer processes of the skin surface that are critical for the maintenance of our body temperature within a survivable range. As a changing, dynamic process, the thermologist needs to be aware of the factors that influence skin heat transfers, skin blood flow, and sources of heat from the core and external environment. An understanding of thermal responses to various stressors that activate the regulation of skin blood flow can allow the physiologist and clinician to "challenge test" for a better understanding of thermoregulation, assess skin blood perfusion, observe and diagnose vascular pathologies, and evaluate thermal therapies. This chapter will introduce the reader to the emergence of infrared thermography in the practice of plastic surgery and tissue transposition. More specifically, the viability of transposed tissue postsurgery is dependent upon the plastic surgeon's ability to identify the underlying blood vessels and take advantage of the elaborate network of blood vessels to perfuse the transferred tissue.

49.2 Skin Thermal Properties

49.2.1 Radiant Heat and Emissivity

Infrared thermography captures a visual thermal map of the skin. Detectors within the imaging system collect the radiant heat that is emitted from an object. An object's ability to radiate heat is termed emissivity and is compared to a blackbody source that is capable of absorbing and radiating all the electromagnetic heat it encounters. Probably the first research efforts that pointed out the usefulness of infrared emission of human skin as a diagnostic aid in medicine were the series of studies published in 1934–1936 by the American physiologists J. D. Hardy and Carl Muschenheim [5–7]. Their work revealed that the human skin, regardless of its color, is a highly efficient radiator with an emissivity of 0.98. This skin value is close to the emissivity of 1.0 (a perfect blackbody source) and the skin provides the human with a very efficient system for dissipating heat from its surface when blood flow is directed toward the outer layers. The determination of the electromagnetic emissivity of an object is a crucial factor in obtaining accurate temperature measurements. When presenting thermographic data, it is a good practice to reference the emissivity and the blackbody reference temperature.

49.2.2 Perfusion and Heat Transfers

Our skin surface serves as an interactive heat transfer medium between the internal heat produced from our metabolic production within the core and the external thermal conditions of our environment. Changes in skin temperature are primarily modulated by cutaneous perfusion. This perfusion is a function of vascular anatomy and vasoactive control by the autonomic nervous system. Under conditions of hyperthermic stress, skin blood flow can be upregulated to provide a larger surface area for transfers of heat from the body. In contrast, when blood flow is shunted from the skin surface, the cutaneous layer serves as an efficient insulator. Infrared imaging provides a visual map of the skin surface temperature as determined by the perfusion to that region. These temperature measurements are indicative of both spatial and temporal changes to the regional temperature distribution.

However, it should be stressed that an IR image cannot quantify measurements of blood flow to the skin tissue. The infrared image provides a thermal map of the skin that is influenced by blood perfusion to the surface area, but these thermal changes may also be influenced by conductive and/or radiant heat provided from an external thermal stressor.

The interpretation of the dynamic process of skin thermal regulation obtained from thermal imaging requires a basic understanding of physiological mechanisms of skin blood flow and factors that influence heat transfers to the skin. Some researchers and practitioners have combined the use of infrared imagery with methodologies and techniques that provide measurements of blood flow to better understand the complex thermal regulation, functions, and responses of the cutaneous tissue layer. For example, the complementary data obtained from infrared thermography with the more direct measure of blood flow from laser Doppler. The laser Doppler can ascertain the direction of skin blood flow but these measurements are restricted to small surfaces and blood flow which is not quantified but reported as changes in arbitrary Doppler [8]. With this understanding, objective data from IR thermography can add valuable information and complement other methodologies in the scientific inquiry and medical practices. Some plastic surgeons have utilized the complementary methods for pre-, intra-, and postoperative evaluations. A further discussion of infrared imaging, complementary blood flow measurements, and techniques that reveal skin tissue structures, rates, and variability of perfusion can be found in Reference 1.

49.2.3 Skin Blood Flow Perfusion Rates

The ability of the skin to substantially increase blood flow, far in excess of the tissue's metabolic needs, alludes to the tissue's role and potential in heat transfer mechanisms. The nutritive need's of skin tissue has been estimated at 0.2 mL/min per cubic centimeter of skin [9], which is considerably lower than the maximal rate of 24 mL/min per cubic centimeter of skin (estimated from total forearm circulatory measurement during heat stress) [10]. If one were to approximate skin tissue as 8% of the forearm, then skin blood would equate to 250–300 mL/100 mL of skin per minute [11]. Applying this flow rate to an estimated skin surface of 1.8 m² (average individual) suggests that approximately 8 L of blood flow could be diverted to the skin to dissipate heat at rate of 1750 W to the environment [12,13]. This increased blood flow required for heat transfers from active muscle tissue and skin blood flow for thermoregulation is made available through the redistribution of blood flow (splanchnic circulatory beds, renal tissues) and increases in cardiac output [14]. The increased cardiac output has been suggested to account for two thirds of the increased blood flow needs, while redistribution provides the remaining third [12]. Several good reviews are available regarding cutaneous blood flow, cardiovascular function, and thermal stress [14–20].

In summary, the ability of an object to radiate heat is termed "emissivity" and is compared to a perfect blackbody source. The emissivity determination allows thermal imagers to have accurate measurements of sources of radiant heat. The skin is nearly a perfect radiator with an emissivity of 0.98. Skin surface perfusion can be dramatically altered to accommodate thermal conditions that rely on the control of heat transfers from the skin. The importance of the skin as a primary thermoregulatory organ is clearly recognized by its abundance of blood vessels to the skin surface that far exceed the nutritional needs of the tissue. This skin perfusion and accompanying changes in the surface temperature map make infrared thermography an ideal investigative tool.

49.3 Regulation of Skin Blood Flow

49.3.1 Regional Neural Regulation

The acral regions of the body (palms, plantar surface of feet, nose, and ears) are regulated solely by adrenergic sympathetic vasoconstrictor nerves that alter regional skin blood flow and temperature regulation through adjustments to the vasoconstrictor tone [10,21,22]. Within the acral regions, there are an abundance of arteriovenous anastomoses (AVA). The AVAs are thick-walled, low-resistance vessels that direct blood flow from the arterioles to the venules. Sympathetic adrenergic vasoconstriction controls the arterioles and AVA to modulate flow rates to the skin vascular plexus in accordance to prevailing thermal conditions. The opening and closing of the AVAs within the acral areas can substantially alter skin blood flow responses [23]. During vasoconstriction, blood flow is shunted from the subcutaneous region allowing very little heat loss and when the vasoconstriction is relaxed (effectively causing vasodilation) blood flow is increased to the skin vascular plexus allowing heat transfers to dissipate excess heat. The skin sites where these vessels are found are among those where skin blood flow changes are discernible to IR-thermography. While the AVA are most active during heat stress, their thick walls and high velocity flow rates do not support their significant role in heat transfers to adjoining skin tissue [12].

The nonacral regions possess dual sympathetic control regulation of both adrenergic vasoconstrictor and vasodilator nerve activity. This vasodilator response was evidenced in research from the 1930s that demonstrated skin flushing and skin surface temperature changes of sympathectomized limbs and confirmed in the 1950s by Edholm et al. [24,25] and Rodie et al. [26] using nerve blocks. However, the neurotransmitter for active vasodilatation is not yet known. Current investigations postulate cholinergic sudomotor and cotransmitter activation [27–29]. The nonacral regions do not commonly have AVAs.

For a more in-depth discussion of regional sympathetic reflex regulation, see Charkoudian [10] and Johnson and Proppe [13].

49.3.2 Thermal Homeostasis

The regulation of skin blood flow thermoregulation is controlled by the preoptic anterior hypothalamus of the brain based on the fluctuations of internal core and skin temperature sensory information. The thermal stress from the environment can be exacerbated by the influences of radiant heat, high humidity, forced convective flow, and increased amounts of clothing [30]. Internal thermal stress is mostly influenced by the heat production associated with exercise and increased metabolism. Physiologists utilize the "clo" value that factors both physical activity intensity and the amount of clothing, to assess levels of thermal comfort [31]. In the research and clinical settings, a nonexercising slightly dressed individual is in a thermoneutral environment at 20–25°C. Under these conditions, the skin temperature regulation is controlled by a tonically active sympathetic vasoconstrictor system that maintains stable skin and core temperatures, eliciting perceptual sweating or shivering stress responses. This thermoneutral zone provides the basis for the clinical testing standards for room temperatures being set at 18–25°C during infrared thermographic studies. Controlling room test conditions is important when measuring skin temperature responses as changes in ambient temperatures can alter the fraction of flow shared between the musculature and skin [19]. Under the influence of whole-body hyperthermic conditions, removal of the vasomotor vasoconstrictor tone can account for 10–20% of cutaneous vasodilation, while the vasodilator system provides the remaining skin blood flow regulation [10]. Alterations in the threshold (onset of vascular response and sweating) and sensitivity (level of response) in vasodilation blood flow control can be related to an individual's level of heat acclimation [32], exercise training [25], circadian rhythm [33,34], and women's reproductive hormonal status [10]. Recent literature suggests that some observed shifts in the reflex control are the result of female reproductive hormones. Both estrogen and progesterone have been linked to menopausal hot flashes [10].

49.3.3 Challenge Testing

Under thermoneutral testing conditions, the skin temperature remains stable. However, the thermologist and/or clinician may want to provide a stressor or "challenge" test to assess the functioning of the thermal response. Challenge testing can include cold or hot water immersion, convective air flow, and exercise bouts that are designed to alter the skin blood flow. In some functional ergonomic cases, positioning of a body part at a particular angle can create a nerve impingement that can be detected by changes in the thermal temperature and pattern. Under these thermally challenging conditions, the clinical importance of abnormalities of skin blood flow may be more apparent. However, one must also recognize that as heat is being transferred through the various layers of skin, some of the heat is dissipated into the adjoining tissues. The heat decay as the blood traverses the layers of tissue and its dispersion pattern within the circulatory plexus of the skin may disguise the origin of the tissue producing the abnormal thermal response.

In summary, the regulation of blood flow to the skin surface is different for the acral region (sympathetic vasoconstriction) and nonacral regions (sympathetic vasoconstriction and vasodilation). Additionally, the predominance of AVA blood vessels in the acral region provides a structural mechanism for greatly altering blood flow perfusion to the skin. The increased blood flow needs for thermoregulation are made possible by increases to cardiac output and the redistribution of blood flow from the splanchnic circulatory beds and renal tissues without compromising blood pressure. The stability of the skin surface temperatures during thermoneutral conditions and the alterations in blood flow to challenge testing allow the researcher and clinician the opportunity to evaluate the function and regulatory response of the skin to thermal stressors.

49.4 Heat Transfer Modeling of Cutaneous Microcirculation

49.4.1 Vascular Heat Transfers

The modeling of the microcirculation of the cutaneous tissue is developed around the relationships of heat transfers. Models have been created for whole-body thermal responses [35,36] and localized hyperthermia [37,38]. While all heat transfers within the body occur through conduction and convection, the model equation must account for tissue conductivity, tissue density, tissue specific heat, local tissue temperature, metabolic or external derived heat sources, and blood velocity. The equation must also be able to account for vascular architecture and neural regulatory vascular controls which strongly influence heat transfers and transport. The vascular architecture can be complicated by the size of blood vessels and geometric vessel patterns (plexus, countercurrent vessels, AVAs, etc.). The magnitude of the heat transfer between the blood vessels and tissue are dependent on the vessel size. According to Poiseulle's law, the change in radius alters resistance to the fourth power of the change in radius. For example, a twofold increase in radius decreases resistance by 16-fold! Therefore, vessel resistance is exquisitely sensitive to changes in radius. Neural regulation controls the radius of the perfusion vessels and the "perfusion conductivity" depends on the velocity of the local blood flow and tissue–vessel alignment. Thus, large vessels exchange very little energy with the surrounding tissues. In contrast, the small vessels (precapillary arterioles, capillaries, and venules) and the surrounding tissues are close to thermal equilibrium.

49.4.2 Bioheat Equation and Skin Blood Flow Modeling

In 1948, Pennes performed a series of experimental procedures "to evaluate the applicability of heat flow theory to the forearm in basic terms of the local rate of tissue heat production and volume flow of blood" [9]. The model derived from experimental data from this investigation became known as the "Bioheat equation." The importance of this model is that it accounted for the importance of blood as a carrier of heat. Thus, the Bioheat equation calculates volumetric heat that is equated to the proportional volumetric rate of blood perfusion. Many of the current models are modifications developed from this basic premise. The Pennes' model is developed around the assumptions that thermal equilibrium occurs in the capillaries and venous temperatures were equal to local tissue temperatures. Both of these assumptions have been challenged in more recent modeling research. The assumption of thermal equilibrium within capillaries was challenged by the work of Chato [39] and Chen and Holmes in 1980 [40]. Based on this vascular modeling for heat transfer, thermal equilibrium occurred in "thermally significant blood vessels" that are approximately 50–75 mm in diameter and located prior to capillary plexus. These thermally significant blood vessels derive from a tree-like structure of branching vessels that are closely spaced in countercurrent pairs. For a historical perspective of heat transfer bioengineering, see Chato [39], and for a review of heat transfers and microvascular modeling, see Baish [41].

In summary, the capacity and ability of blood to transfer heat through various tissue layers to the skin can be predicted from models. This modeling literature provides a conceptual understanding of the thermal response of skin when altered by disease, injury, or external thermal stressors to skin temperatures (environment or application of cold or hot thermal sources, convective airflow, or exercise). From tissue modeling, we know that tissue is only slightly influenced by the deep tissue blood supply but is strongly influenced by the cutaneous circulation. With the use of infrared thermography, skin temperatures can be accurately quantified and the thermal pattern mapped. However, these temperatures cannot be assumed to represent thermal conditions at the source of the thermal stress. Furthermore, the thermal pattern only provides a visual map of skin surface in which heat is dissipated throughout the skin's multiple microvascular plexuses.

49.5 Vascular Structure of Skin

49.5.1 Work of Manchot, Spalteholz, Salmon, Taylor, and Palmer

One of the earliest studies of value on the vascular anatomy of the skin is that of the medical student Carl Manchot from Hamburg. In 1889, at the age of 23 and studying at the Kaiser-Wilhelm University Medical School in Strassburg, Manchot published his treatise *Die Hautarterien des Menschlichen Körpers*, in the incredible time of 6 months [42]. He gave a detailed description of the deep cutaneous arteries and assigned them to their underlying source vessels. His ink injection studies on cadavers allowed him to chart the cutaneous vascular territories of these source arteries. Manchot did not have the benefit of radiographic contrast studies since Roentgen was not to make his discovery until several years later; nevertheless, the accuracy of his work has mostly stood the test of time. His work was translated in English and published in 1983 under the title *The Cutaneous Arteries of the Human Body* [43].

Another important study was published in 1893 by Werner Spalteholz of Leizig. Based on the gelatin and pigment cadaveric injection studies, he made a distinction between direct cutaneous arteries whose main purpose is to supply the skin and indirect arteries which supply the deeper tissues, especially the muscles [44].

The French anatomist and surgeon Michel Salmon published in 1936 his eminent work on the cutaneous arteries in his book titled *Les Artères de la Peau*. Salmon's work is a reappraisal of the work of Manchot [45]. His detailed radiographic studies of the skin's vasculature using a lead oxide mixture produced excellent images. Based on these images he could divide the cutaneous circulation of the human body in 80 vascular territories, which is approximately twice the number as described by Manchot. Each vascular territory has its own source artery. Salmon noted a difference in density and size of arteries in different regions of the body. He divided regions into hypo- and hypervascular zones.

Taylor and Palmer's radiographic lead oxide injection studies of the blood supply to the skin and underlying tissue of fresh cadavers are a timely rediscovery and expansion of the works of Manchot and Salmon [46]. Their results made it possible to segregate the human body anatomically into three-dimensional vascular territories called angiosomes. These three-dimensional anatomical territories are supplied by a source vessel and its accompanying vein. Each tissue in an angiosome is supplied by branches from the source artery. These composite blocks of skin, bone, muscle, and other soft tissue fit together like the pieces of a jigsaw puzzle. The individual angiosomes varied in size and each angiosome is linked to its neighbor angiosome at every tissue level. These interconnections are mostly by a reduced caliber choke anastomosis but in some cases by simple anastomotic arterial connections without change in the caliber of the vessel. A similar pattern is seen on the venous side with avascular bidirectional or oscillating veins. The watershed zones that separate the angiosomes can be seen on angiograms of the skin as areas with reduced vessel density. The choke vessels are located in these watershed zones.

49.5.2 Blood Supply to Skin

The anatomy of the microcirculation of the skin is well described by Cormack and Lamberty [47]. The human skin consists of two layers. The outer layer or epidermis is a waterproof layer of keratinizing stratified squamous epithelium. The inner layer, or dermis, supports the epidermis and is a layer of connective tissue. This layer contains among others blood vessels, lymphatic vessels, sensory nerves, and receptors and skin appendages like sebaceous glands and hair follicles. The skin is supplied by two vascular plexi, the subdermal plexus and the superficial plexus. The subdermal plexus is located just underneath the dermis and branches from here feed the superficial plexus. The superficial plexus lies at the junction of the dermis and epidermis. The skin relies for its blood supply on the vascular structure of the underlying tissue. The work of Taylor and Palmer, as well as others, has revealed that the skin receives its blood supply from so-called perforators [46,48,49]. Taylor defines a cutaneous perforator as "any vessel that perforates the outer layer of the deep fascia to supply the overlying subcutaneous tissue and skin" [50]. A perforator consists of an artery and its concomitant vein. Perforators arise from a source artery and its concomitant vein and on their course to the skin they may follow the intermuscular septa or pass through a muscle. A perforator that lies in an intermuscular septum is called a septocutaneous perforator. These are most frequently located on the extremities. A perforator that passes through a muscle is called a musculocutaneous perforator. These perforators are mostly found on the trunk. Taylor and Palmer identified an average of 374 major perforators per cadaver [46]. Perforators can be further divided into direct and indirect perforators. This classification was described originally by Spalteholz and used again by Taylor and Palmer [44]. Direct perforators have a straight course to the skin were they connect with the subdermal plexus. Whether they follow the intermuscular septa, or pierce muscles en route, their main destination is the skin. The indirect perforators also arise from a source artery and concomitant vein. Their main purpose is to supply the muscles and after they have perforated the deep fascia, the deeper tissues.

El-Mrakby and Miller studied specifically the vascular anatomy of the lower abdomen [48,49]. They found that direct perforators had a diameter larger than 0.5 mm and kept a constant diameter throughout their straight course to the skin. These large direct perforators feed the subdermal plexus and supply the superficial fat. This is in contrast to the small indirect perforators that contribute to the formation of the deep subcutaneous vascular plexus at the deep fat level. The venous drainage from the skin occurs via a venous plexus that connects with the concomitant veins of the perforators or by superficial veins.

49.6 Applying Infrared Technology

49.6.1 Static versus Dynamic Infrared Thermography

IR thermography may be static in that a single image is taken. This technique involves the observation of the spatial temperature distribution over the area of interest. The interpretation of such an image mainly depends on identifying the distribution of hot and cold spots and asymmetric temperature distributions. One of the assumptions when using this method is that the distribution of body surface temperature is basically symmetrical [51,52].

Dynamic infrared thermography (DIRT) is another technique recently proposed to better understand IR images. Because of the interference from complex vascular patterns, researchers have proposed to monitor the thermal recovery process after exposure of the area of interest to a thermal stress. The dynamic method is able to detect not only spatial but also temporal behavior of skin temperature. By applying a thermal challenge, the subsequent recovery of the skin temperature toward its thermal equilibrium is evaluated. The images can be analyzed with respect to the rate and pattern of recovery. The dynamic method could be classified as a passive method or as an active method. In the active method, an external thermal stress is applied to the area under investigation. In practice, the skin area being examined is subjected to a thermal stress by fan cooling, water immersion, or by applying cold or warm objects to the skin surface. It is, however, important that the subject's skin is prevented from becoming wet during immersion in water. No external thermal stress is needed in the passive method. In the passive method, the temperature reactions of healthy individuals are compared with those of patients when an internal stress is applied to them. A common internal stress can be seen after and during exercise. A special form of DIRT is the perfusion of tissue with warm or cold perfusate. DIRT has been used for the monitoring of rewarming of skin after a cold challenge, after surgical reperfusion, or for monitoring cooling of organs following perfusion of a cold fluid as used occasionally in cardiac surgery or organ transplantation [53–56].

49.6.2 Infrared Imaging for Pandemic Fever Screening

The skin regulates heat transfers from its surface through changes in blood perfusion.

These heat transfers are conducted with the purpose of maintaining the body's thermal homeostasis. In recent years, infrared thermographic pandemic screening has been introduced as a means of detecting individuals with fevers that may be related to infectious diseases. An elevated core temperature of 1–2°C (1.8–3.6°F) is generally regarded as indicating a febrile response, pyrexia, or fever. It should be noted that the skin temperature recorded by the infrared imaging device is capturing a skin surface temperature and can only be considered as an indirect measurement of core temperature. The relationship between the skin and core temperature measurements can be problematic if the infrared devise operator does not operate the screening procedure under standardized conditions. In a recent publication, Ring and colleagues [57] compared the inner canthus eyes of febrile and nonfebrile children eyes and recommended a threshold temperature of 37.5°C to differentiate those with fever. In pandemic fever screening, it should be recognized that not all infectious diseases develop a fever, some diseases have an infectious period that is not concurrent with a fever, and the identification of a threshold temperature would change the sensitivity and specificity of the screening measurement. The fundamental problem with infrared pandemic screening lies with operators and screening locations that do not abide by the published standards. Failure to follow the published standards undermines the efficacy, specificity, and sensitivity of the infrared screening and detection procedures. For a more complete discussion on the International Electrochemical Commission/International Standards Organization standards for "Thermal Images for Human Febrile Temperature Screening," see [58,59], pandemic screening review articles [60,61], or the chapter in this text on pandemic screening [62].

49.7 IR and Sports Medicine

Physiologist and sports medicine practitioners using infrared thermography must adhere to published infrared imaging practice, procedures, and standards for thermal assessments and research. Additionally, they must possess a basic understanding of skin blood flow responses to thermal conditions, be able to identify thermal abnormalities (cold or hot spots, dermatomes), and potentially incorporate challenge testing. Dermatomes are a localized region of skin with innervation via a single nerve from a single nerve root of the spinal cord. Nerve impairments (impingements, cuts, stretch, compression, and impact injury) to a dermatome region may be evidenced by a cooler thermal response to the skin within that specified surface area. Unlike normal thermal maps of the skin, these dermatome nerve impingements produce a thermal pattern that has very discrete borders. In a recent study, Sefton and colleagues [63] performed therapeutic neck and shoulder massage on patients between Cervical 1 and Thoracic 2 vertebrae (dermatomes C3–C5). Significant increases in temperature (60 min posttreatment) were observed in the treated area (anterior upper chest, posterior neck, upper back) and two adjoining areas (right arm and middle of the back; dermatome C6–C8). Physical therapist, occupational therapist, and athletic trainers have used infrared imaging to help in the diagnosis of injury and to provide evidence of the efficacy of various treatment modalities (ice, ultrasound, massage).

49.8 Plastic Surgery

The basis of plastic surgery is to restore form as well as function in patients with, for example, congenital deformities or with tissue defects caused by trauma, tumor surgery, and pressure sores. The treatment of these deformities and injuries relies on techniques for transposition of tissue from one part of the human body to another. The tissue that is transposed is called a flap. Historically, the word *flap* originated from the sixteenth-century Dutch word "flappe," this being anything that hangs broad and loose, fastened only by one side [47]. A flap can consist of, for example, skin, skin and muscle, or skin, muscle, and bone. The term "flap" is now a general term encompassing both pedicled flaps and free flaps. A pedicled flap is an area of tissue, which is detached from its surroundings except from a bridge of tissue. Through this bridge, also called pedicle, blood enters and leaves the flap. The pedicle may also consist of only an artery that supplies the flap and a vein or veins that drain the flap. In a free flap, the flap has an identifiable pedicle of an artery and a vein. After the flap has been detached from its surroundings, the artery and vein are cut at sufficient lengths and the flap is moved from its donor site, that is, the site where the flap is harvested, and transferred to the recipient site, the site to be reconstructed. Here, the blood circulation of the flap has to be reestablished. Under a microscope and using microsurgical techniques, the artery and vein of the flap are connected to the vessels at the recipient site. This procedure is a critical part in free flap surgery as a flap without blood circulation will not survive.

49.8.1 Perforator Flap in Plastic Surgery

In 1989, Koshima and Soeda introduced the perforator flap in reconstructive surgery [64]. A perforator flap can be defined as a flap of skin and subcutaneous tissue, which is supplied by an isolated perforator vessel. Such a perforator consists of an artery and its accompanying vein. Perforators pass from the source vessel to the skin, either through or between the deep tissues. The inclusion of muscle and fascia, previously thought to be necessary to guarantee flap circulation, are no longer required as illustrated in Figure 49.1. As perforator flaps consist only of skin and subcutaneous tissue, they permit excellent "like to like" replacement with minimal donor site morbidity for defects of skin and subcutaneous tissue. Perforator flaps lend themselves to being used as either pedicled or free flaps.

The main advantage of perforator flaps is their low donor site morbidity. The majority of donor sites can be closed directly and as the underlying muscle and its nerve supply are preserved, donor site morbidity is minimal [65]. Studies also suggest faster recovery, less postoperative pain, and shorter hospital stays with the use of perforator flaps compared to the flaps that include a muscle.

The disadvantages of perforator flaps are largely related to the learning curve. Adequate preoperative planning, meticulous surgical techniques and a thorough understanding of the vascular anatomy are crucial for a successful postoperative result. Inadequate perfusion of the flap is a complication that may occur when using this technique, especially by the inexperienced surgeon. Inadequate perfusion of the flap can lead to partial or even to total flap loss. These complications are a devastating experience for a patient as they clearly influence the final postoperative outcome. Besides the psychological effect such a flap loss may have on a patient, it is also an inefficient use of economical and hospital resources as reoperations are often necessary. Great efforts should therefore be made to reduce the risk of postoperative flap complications.

49.8.2 Infrared Thermography in Plastic Surgery

The use of infrared thermography in flap surgery, where the perfusion and reperfusion of the flap, pedicled or free, is an important predictive parameter for the success of the surgery, is limited to a few articles. Theuvenet et al. were probably one of the first to recognize the potential of the use of infrared thermography in flap surgery [66]. In the preoperative planning, they cooled the area where the flap

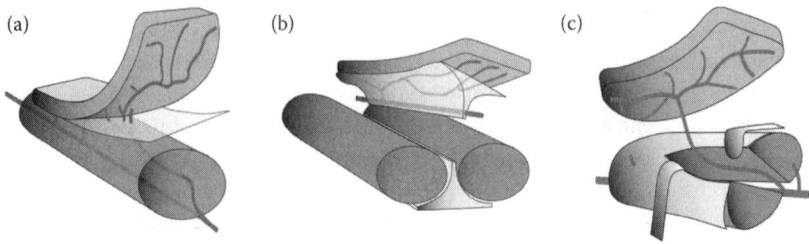

(a)   (b)   (c)

FIGURE 49.1 The evolution from myocutaneous flap (a) to fasciocutaneous flap (b) to perforator flap (c). With the perforator flap, no muscle or fascia is included. In (c), the perforator flap receives its blood supply from a perforator that passes through the muscle and emerges from the source vessel that lies underneath the muscle.

was to be harvested with an ice pack and registered the rewarming of the skin. The locations where hot spots were seen on the infrared images correlated with the locations of perforators as identified during the operation. These flaps were, however, not perforator flaps but musculocutaneous flaps. These musculocutaneous flaps differ from perforator flaps in that a piece of muscle together with a large number of perforators is included in the flap to guarantee flap perfusion. The first to report on the use of infrared thermography in perforator flaps were Itoh and Arai [67]. They illustrated with two clinical cases that a perforator flap could be based on the perforator that was identified by the location of the hot spot on the thermal image during the rewarming of the skin after a cold challenge. Wolff and colleagues used infrared thermography in an experimental study to compare the intraoperative perfusion of different types of flaps [68]. The usefulness of infrared thermography, especially DIRT, has been illustrated in open heart surgery, neurosurgery, and organ transplant surgery [54–56]. We will illustrate in the next section how the use of DIRT can provide the surgeon with valuable information in pedicled and free perforator flap surgery.

49.9 Breast Reconstruction with the Deep Inferior Epigastric Perforator Flap

Breast reconstruction has become an integrated part in the overall treatment of patients diagnosed with breast cancer. The goal of breast reconstruction is to restore a breast mold and to maintain quality of life without affecting the prognosis or detection of recurrence of cancer [69]. Breast reconstruction using tissue from the lower abdomen has become an increasingly popular method after treatment of breast cancer with a mastectomy that is removal of the breast. The lower abdomen is a donor site that remains unmatched in tissue volume, quality, and texture. Patients are specifically pleased with the natural shape, soft consistency, and superior aesthetic results of the reconstructed breast that can be obtained with the use of this donor site [70,71]. An added bonus of an abdominal donor site is for most patients the improved abdominal contour after closure which approximates that of an abdominoplasty or tummy tuck. Although there are several techniques to harvest tissue from the lower abdomen, the technique called the "Deep Inferior Epigastric Perforator" flap or DIEP flap is currently considered the gold standard in breast reconstruction.

The use of the free DIEP flap for breast reconstruction was first described by Allen and Treece in 1994 [72]. The DIEP flap consists of skin and subcutaneous fatty tissue from the lower abdomen. It relies for its blood supply on one of the perforators that arise from the source vessel, the deep inferior epigastric artery and its accompanying vein. After harvest of the DIEP flap on the lower abdomen, the flap is transferred to the thoracic wall. Here, the perforator artery and vein are connected to the internal mammary vessels on the thoracic wall and the blood supply to the flap is reestablished. Finally, a breast is reconstructed. The principle of breast reconstruction with a DIEP flap is illustrated in Figure 49.2.

As with all forms of surgery, breast reconstruction with DIEP flap can be divided into a preoperative phase, an intraoperative phase, and a postoperative phase.

49.9.1 Preoperative Phase

Meticulous planning during the preoperative phase is a prerequisite for successful perforator flap surgery. As the DIEP flap relies for its blood supply on just one perforator, selection of the most suitable perforator to perfuse the flap is crucial for successful surgery. A good perforator can in fact perfuse the whole flap from the lower abdomen.

The perforators of the DIEP flap emerge from the deep inferior epigastric artery and vein, which can be found right underneath the rectus abdominis muscle. While perforators can be located with a handheld Doppler ultrasound probe, studies have shown that this technique is associated with a large number of false-positives [73,74]. The technique is in fact too sensitive and also detects perforators that

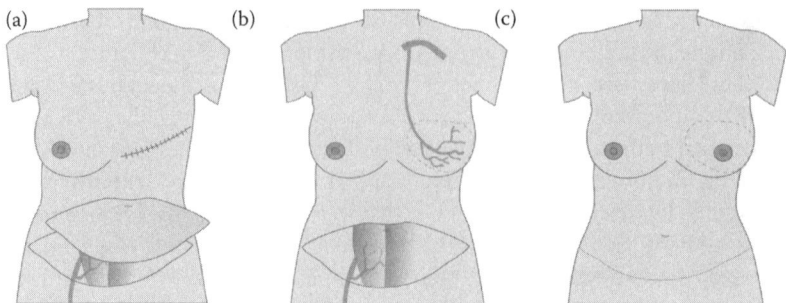

FIGURE 49.2 Breast reconstruction with a DIEP flap. (a) The abdominoplasty flap is harvested from the lower abdomen as a DIEP flap, based on one perforator from the deep inferior epigastric artery and vein. (b) After the flap is transferred to the thoracic wall, its vessels are anastomosed to the internal mammary vessels. (c) A breast is reconstructed and the lower abdomen is closed as an abdominoplasty.

are too small to be used in perforator flap surgery. In 2009, we reported on the value of the use of DIRT in the preoperative planning of the DIEP flap [75]. After the flap had been drawn on the lower abdomen, the locations of arterial Doppler sounds were marked on the skin with a black dot as illustrated in Figure 49.3. All patients were examined in a special examination room with a room temperature of 22–24°C, constant humidity, and air circulation. Typically, the exposed abdomen was subjected to an acclimatization period at room temperature prior to the DIRT examination. A desktop fan was used to deliver the cold challenge by blowing air at room temperature over the abdomen for a period of 2 min. This cold challenge caused visible changes in skin temperature that were well within the physiological range, and had a short recovery period of approximately 5 min. Analysis of the rate and pattern of rewarming of the hot spots allowed a qualitative assessment of all the perforators at the same time. Hot spots that showed a rapid and progressive rewarming could be related to suitable perforators intraoperatively. A rapid rewarming at the hot spot indicates that the perforator is capable of transporting more blood to the skin surface than a hot spot with a low rate of rewarming. A rapid progression of rewarming at the hot spot suggests a better developed vascular network around the hot spot. It appeared that while all first appearing hot spots could be associated with the location of an arterial Doppler sound, not all arterial Doppler sound locations could be related to a hot spot.

The location of the hot spot on the skin could easily be related to the location where the perforator passed through the anterior rectus fascia, although the hot spot as well as the associated Doppler sound were slightly more laterally positioned. The eminent surgeon and anatomist John Hunter (1728–1793)

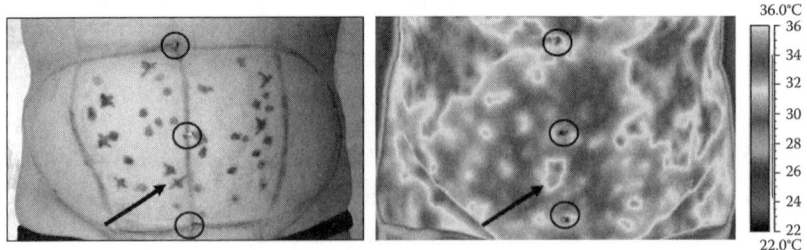

FIGURE 49.3 Left: This photograph of the lower abdomen shows the locations where arterial Doppler sounds were heard and marked with dots. Some of the dots are additionally marked with crosses. The crosses mark arterial Doppler sounds were also associated with hot spots seen in the thermal images shown on the right. The arrows indicate the location where a loud arterial Doppler sound was heard and was associated with a bright hot spot. This perforator could be used to supply a DIEP flap. The circles indicate the positions of small pieces of metal tape used as reference markers.

explained the orientation of vessels as a product of differential growth that had occurred in that area from the stage of fetus to adulthood [76]. Giunta et al. [26] found that the preoperative Doppler location on the skin was located within an average distance of 0.8 cm of that of the exit point of the perforator through the fascia. Interestingly, the selected hot spot on the DIRT images was always associated with an audible Doppler sound and a suitable perforator.

The easiest dissection is reported for those perforators that have a perpendicular penetration pattern through the fascia and a short intramuscular course [73,74,77]. Perforators that are located at the tendineous intersection have these characteristics and are, in addition, larger then average. Interestingly, these perforators were easily identified with DIRT. The short course of the perforator from the source vessel to the skin explains the rapid rewarming of the skin at the hot spot.

In medical infrared thermography, asymmetry on the images has often been associated with pathophysiology [51,78]. The results from our study on the preoperative use of DIRT in the planning of DIEP flaps showed that asymmetry in the distribution and quality of hot spots between both sides on the lower abdomen was more or less a normal finding as can be seen in Figure 49.4. This result is in accordance with other studies related to the preoperative mapping of perforators on the lower abdomen. The use of the modern high-quality IR cameras may be the reason why this nonpathological asymmetry becomes visible now.

Recently, the use of multidetector computed tomography (MDCT) angiography has become increasingly popular for the preoperative planning of perforator flaps, and has become in some hospitals the gold standard [79,80]. The high spatial and temporal resolution achieved with MDCT angiography

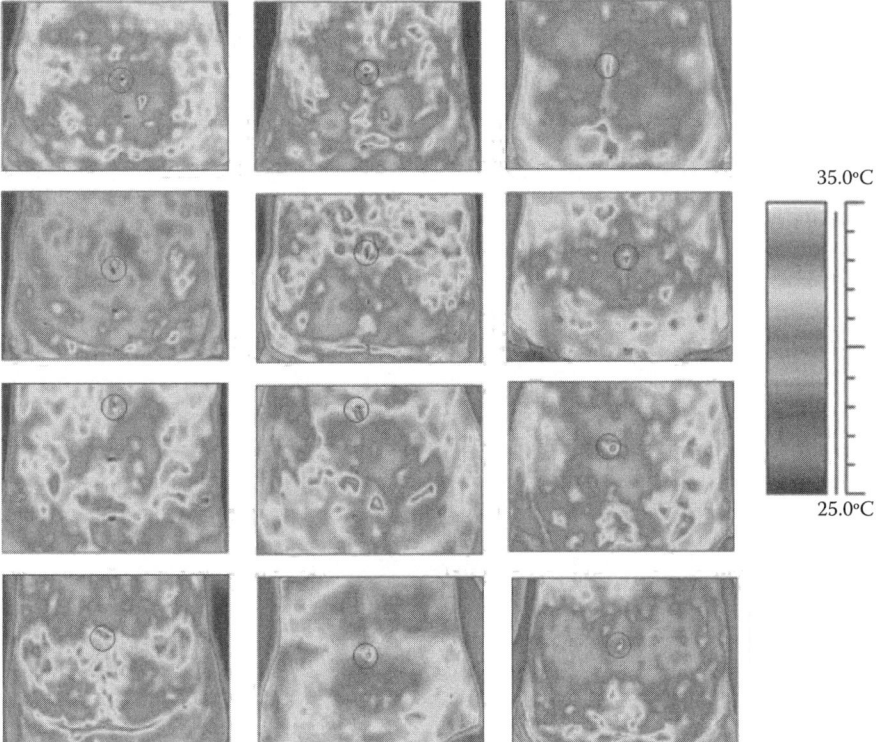

FIGURE 49.4 Preoperative infrared thermal images of the abdominal area of 12 female patients indicating thermal asymmetry. The black circle in each image indicates the position of the navel. The figure illustrates the large variability in the distribution and intensity of hot spots, not only between the left and right side of each individual patient but also between patients.

allows for a precise description of the origin, intramuscular course, and point of fascia penetration of the arterial perforator. MDCT angiography does not provide information on the venous side of the perforator. Such information can be obtained but requires an extra scan. Although DIRT does not show the morphology of the perforators, it identified suitable perforators based on the perforators' physiology.

To adopt MDCT as a routine preoperative imaging modality, the benefit to the patient, for both the reconstructed breast and the abdominal donor site, must outweigh the problems associated with the procedure. These include the risk of intravenous contrast agent, exposure to ionizing radiation, and associated cost. Recent literature cautions against the rising exposure of ionizing radiation to the population due to CT examinations [81,82]. IR thermography has none of these disadvantages.

49.9.2 Intraoperative Phase

During the operation, the DIEP flap is harvested from the lower abdomen (Figure 49.5) and transferred to the thoracic wall where a breast will be reconstructed. On the thoracic wall, the blood circulation to the DIEP flap has to be reestablished. This is a critical part of the whole operation as without blood circulation the flap will not survive. The perforator artery and vein to the DIEP flap are connected to the internal mammary vessels under a microscope and with the use of microsurgical instruments. This connection is called anastomosis. By opening the anastomosis, the flap becomes reperfused. In 2006, we published a study on the intraoperative use of DIRT in free perforator surgery [83]. During the transfer of the DIEP flap from the lower abdomen to the thoracic wall, the flap is a period without blood circulation and as a consequence cools down. After the anastomosis is opened, the flap becomes reperfused and as a consequence rewarms. It showed that the intraoperative use of DIRT allowed to assess perfusion and reperfusion in real time and thus provided the surgeon immediate feedback. The usefulness of DIRT during the period after completion of the anastomosis became readily apparent as partial and total arterial inflow problems were easily detected with analyses of the IR images. Also, venous congestion was easily identified on the IR images. An important advantage of the intraoperative use of DIRT

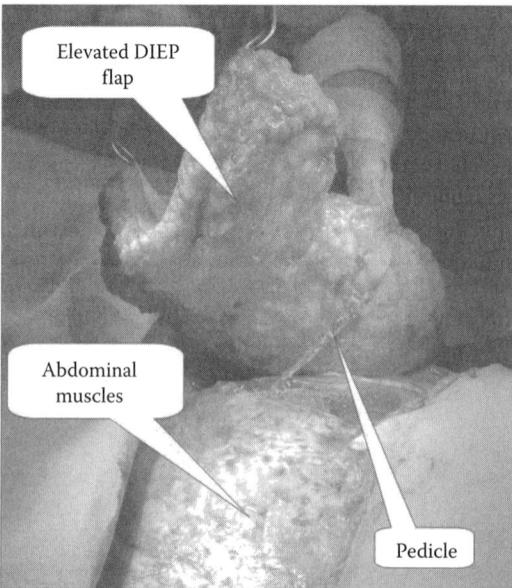

FIGURE 49.5 The skin and subcutaneous tissue of the lower abdomen is elevated as a DIEP flap. The image was taken just prior to transfer of the flap to the thoracic area. The flap receives its blood supply via the pedicle which is the perforator and consists of one artery and one vein. Note no muscle is included.

was that the surgeon could take corrective action when it was most effective, namely during the operation. At the end of the operation, perfusion of the flap could be rapidly and easily evaluated after applying a thermal stress to the skin surface using a cold metal plate and see how the flap rewarms.

49.9.3 Postoperative Phase

During the postoperative phase, the flap is closely monitored for signs of compromised perfusion. Most surgeons rely on clinical observation of skin perfusion using subjective signs such as skin color, capillary refill, skin temperature, and turgor [84]. A typical monitoring protocol includes hourly observations of flaps for the first 24 h and then to extend this to every 4 h for the first three postoperative days. Recognizing the visual cues of a failing flap requires considerable clinical experience. If a flap shows signs of impaired perfusion, whether it is due to an arterial inflow or a venous outflow problem, surgical intervention may be necessary (see Figure 49.6). The success of such secondary microsurgery is inversely related to the time interval between the onset of impaired perfusion and its detection [85,86]. Temperature measurements of skin flaps during the postoperative phase are one of the oldest monitoring methods of free flaps. Measurements of absolute skin surface temperatures of free groin flaps during the postoperative phase was first reported by Baudet et al. in 1976 [87]. Acland promoted the technique of absolute surface temperature monitoring of free flaps and stated that a temperature between 32°C and 30°C was marginal, and a temperature below 30°C was a sign of flap failure [88]. Leonard et al. introduced the concept of differential surface temperature by monitoring

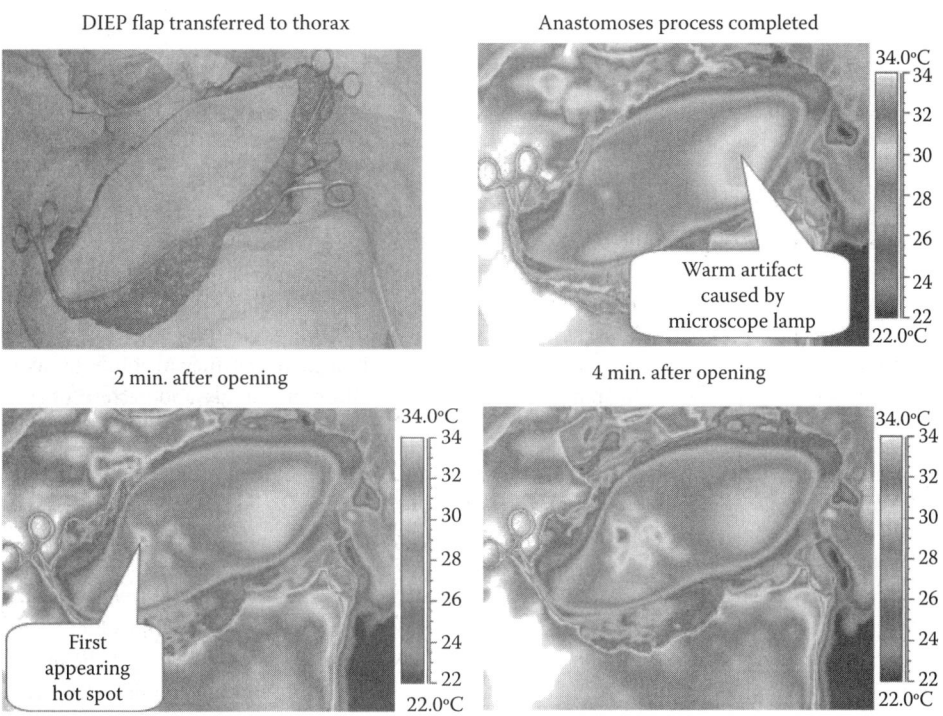

FIGURE 49.6 Digital photograph of a free DIEP flap. The infrared thermal images demonstrate a rewarming of a free DIEP flap after completion of a successful microsurgical anastomosis. The anastomosis was opened in the upper right image. The other images were taken at 2 min intervals after the anastomosis had been opened and the blood flow to the flap was restored. Note the appearance of hot spots that rapidly increase in size and number. A thermal artifact (diffuse warm area) can be seen in the upper left thermal image caused by heating from the microscope lamp. This area cools down after removal of the heat source.

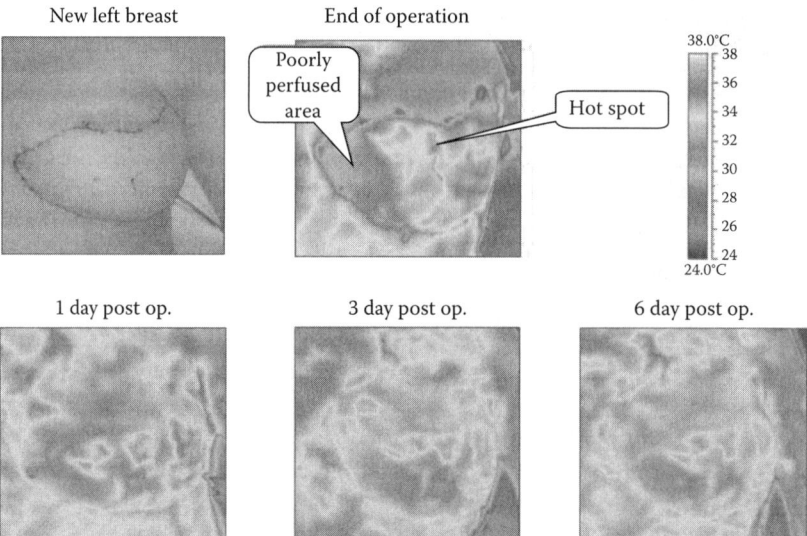

FIGURE 49.7 The photograph on the top left shows a newly reconstructed left breast with a DIEP flap. The infrared thermal images show an improved perfusion over time. Not that part of the newly reconstructed breast is less well perfused at end of operation (indicated by a cooler area) but improves in the days as indicated by the appearance of new hot spots.

the difference between a temperature probe on the flap and a second control temperature probe on adjacent normal skin [89]. Temperature measurements are often included in the protocols of postoperative monitoring of flaps. Recently, Busic et al. criticized the use of temperature measurement in the monitoring of DIEP flaps [90]. We reported on the postoperative use of DIRT on breast reconstruction with a DIEP flap [91]. It appears that the perfusion of DIEP is a dynamic process with a stepwise progression during the first postoperative week. Hot spots are initially seen on the IR images in the area positioned over the location of the entrance point of the perforator in the DIEP flap (Figure 49.7). On subsequent days, the number of hot spots increases, first on the ipsilateral side of the midline and from day three also on the contralateral side. It became clear from this study that the temperature differs from location to location and that the temperature changes over time. Absolute temperature measurements are perhaps less informative then the information on the rate and pattern of rewarming obtained with DIRT.

49.10 Use of Infrared Thermal Imaging to Localize Axial Pedicles in Facial and Nasal Reconstruction

Facial reconstruction is a pivotal component in the treatment of skin cancer as it involves anatomic, functional, and cosmetic challenges. The diagnosis of over one million skin cancers annually exemplifies the increasing prevalence of this condition. The use of Mohs micrographic surgery is the most accurate technique for treatment of all types of skin cancer (melanoma and nonmelanoma) with particular utility on the head and neck. This is due to the high cure rate (exceeding 99%) and superior cosmetic result due to the selective surgical margin that is achieved when performed by fellowship-trained Mohs surgeons.

The Mohs surgical technique yields a surgical defect that must subsequently be repaired. Facial reconstructive techniques encompass a multitude of different options, including primary closure, flaps, grafts, and second intent wound healing. Knowledge of the anatomy, physiology, and flap biomechanics of skin is imperative for successful reconstruction.

There are a multitude of cutaneous flaps in the reconstructive surgeon's armamentarium to repair cutaneous surgical defects. These include primary closures, rotation flaps, advancement flaps, interpolation flaps, allografts, xenografts, and skin grafts, in addition to the numerous variants of each of these. An adequate vascular supply is critical to the success of all of these reconstructive techniques. Reconstruction of the nose specifically mandates a fundamental knowledge of the cutaneous, cartilaginous, and vascular supply for successful reconstruction. A specific reconstruction of larger nasal defects will be utilized to demonstrate the importance of vascular identification and the benefit of adjunctive thermal imaging.

The paramedian forehead flap is an effective surgical technique that can be utilized to reconstruct large surgical defects, primarily of the nasal subunits and/or entire nose [92–94]. This reconstruction relies on a specific arterial supply to maintain patency of the flap. At present, this pedicle flap is identified primarily by the surgeon's knowledge of anatomy and may be confirmed by Doppler ultrasonography.

The use of thermal infrared imaging represents a unique adjunctive technique to allow confirmation of specific arterial sources for cutaneous flaps. Thermal infrared imaging has been shown to provide good sensitivity in the direct imaging of superficial vessels on the face [95]. This fundamental knowledge is applied in the present chapter to a specific artery as it is used in nasal reconstruction.

49.10.1 Anatomy of a Flap

Surgical defects can be repaired with a wide variety of reconstructive techniques. These may include allowing the wound to heal via second intent, primary closure, skin grafts (split thickness and full thickness, allografts, xenografts), and flaps. There are many types of cutaneous flap designs, including transposition, advancement, rotation, and interpolation flaps.

An adequate blood supply is paramount to the survival of a flap. The anatomic vascular characteristics of a flap provide a useful means of classification [96]. Early studies by Manchot and Salmon contributed to the understanding of vascular anatomy, especially in the setting of cutaneous flaps [42,43]. Vascular territories, or angiosomes, are those cutaneous regions that are supplied by a specific vessel or set of vessels.

Proper design of a cutaneous flap must be performed with this angiosome in mind to ensure survival of the flap. In cutaneous flap surgery, arterial supply is characterized as either axial or random pattern [97]. Axial flaps are those that are based on a specific artery, such as the paramedian forehead flap, which is designed around the supratrochlear artery. A random pattern flap is one that is not designed on a specific artery but instead survives on the network of small nonspecified arteries, also known as the subdermal plexus. These vascular territories must be visualized in a three-dimensional view to prevent unintentional transaction of a vessel.

Facial and nasal reconstruction mandates a superior knowledge of anatomy, with particular attention to the vasculature. This allows both the identification of key vessels that are paramount to the survival of a flap in addition to the ability to avoid inadvertent transection of vessels.

The supratrochlear artery traverses the orbital rim between the corrugator and frontalis muscles. It is located above the periosteum as it passes over the medial brow and protected by the corrugator muscle [92–94]. The supratrochlear artery becomes more superficial as it is followed upwards. The artery remains underneath the frontalis muscle until it reaches the mid-forehead, where it then travels through the frontalis muscle and reaches the subdermal position at the superior forehead [93,94]. The supraorbital artery is the dominant artery of the forehead and thus an excellent arterial source for an axial flap [98].

49.10.2 Detection of Vasculature

The surgeon's fundamental knowledge of anatomy is the primary standard for reconstruction. Localization of the supratrochlear artery can be determined by clinical landmarks. This artery is

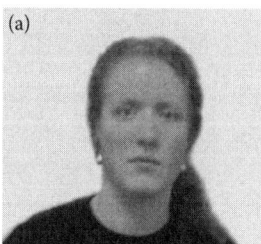 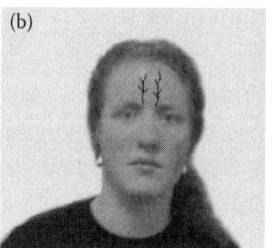 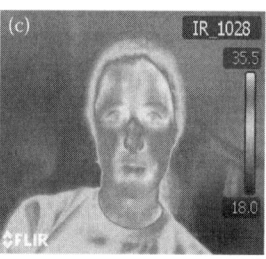

FIGURE 49.8   (a) Digital picture of forehead. (b) The supratrochlear arteries can be localized by clinical land-marks and are typically found originating near the inferior glabellar creases. These near parallel vessels run verti-cally approximately 1.5–2.0 cm from the midline forehead. (c) Infrared image of forehead.

typically found approximately 1.5–2.0 cm from the midline forehead (see Figure 49.8) [98]. Its origin at the lower forehead can be localized by palpation of the supratrochlear foramen and/or visualization of the inferior glabellar crease [98,99].

Continuous wave Doppler ultrasound is commonly used to confirm and track the location of the supratrochlear artery. This is achieved with a handheld vascular probe that allows audible detection of vessels. This is useful provided the target vessel is of sufficient caliber to allow detection. Handheld Doppler ultrasound is not useful in determining vascular characteristics of random-pattern flaps as these vessels are too small.

The use of thermal infrared imaging marks an additional adjunctive tool to localize specific vessels. This technique allows for real-time visualization of the specific artery and/or a vascular plexus, which can be a tremendous aid in the decision-making process of a reconstruction.

Facial segmentation based on thermal signatures of vascular regions has been utilized to demon-strate vascular versus less vascular angiosomes [95]. The work of Buddharaju and Pavlidis with thermal minutia point extraction shows promising results toward increased thermal detection of cutaneous vas-culature [95].

49.10.3 Determinants of Flap Choice

The choice of reconstructive technique is made with consideration of multiple variables. Some of these variables include the location of the surgical defect, the age of the patient, the medical and surgical history of the patient, the type of tumor that was treated, and both functional and cosmetic outcomes from the reconstruction. Additional factors such as the use of tobacco products are significant as nicotine acts as a vasoconstrictor and can decrease arterial flow to a dependent flap [99,100]. The use of surgical delay can be utilized to assist in flaps that are deemed to be risky for a potentially inhibited arterial supply [99,100]. Anatomical differences among various individuals represent another factor that must be considered.

The use of thermal infrared imaging can be used as an adjunctive tool to gauge the vascular health of a cutaneous region. The sensitivity of a camera certainly plays a large part in the amount of information that can be obtained. Imaging for axial versus random pattern flaps has different goals and sensitivi-ties. Imaging for a random pattern flap requires identification of adequate perfusion, while that for an axial flap requires precise localization of a specific vessel. The relatively small caliber vessel in cutaneous flaps makes this more challenging than with the larger vessels due to the decreased thermal signature detected.

49.10.4 Paramedian Forehead Flap

The paramedian forehead flap used today is based on centuries of refinements from surgeons all over the world. In short, this technique classically involves a two-stage transfer of skin from the forehead to

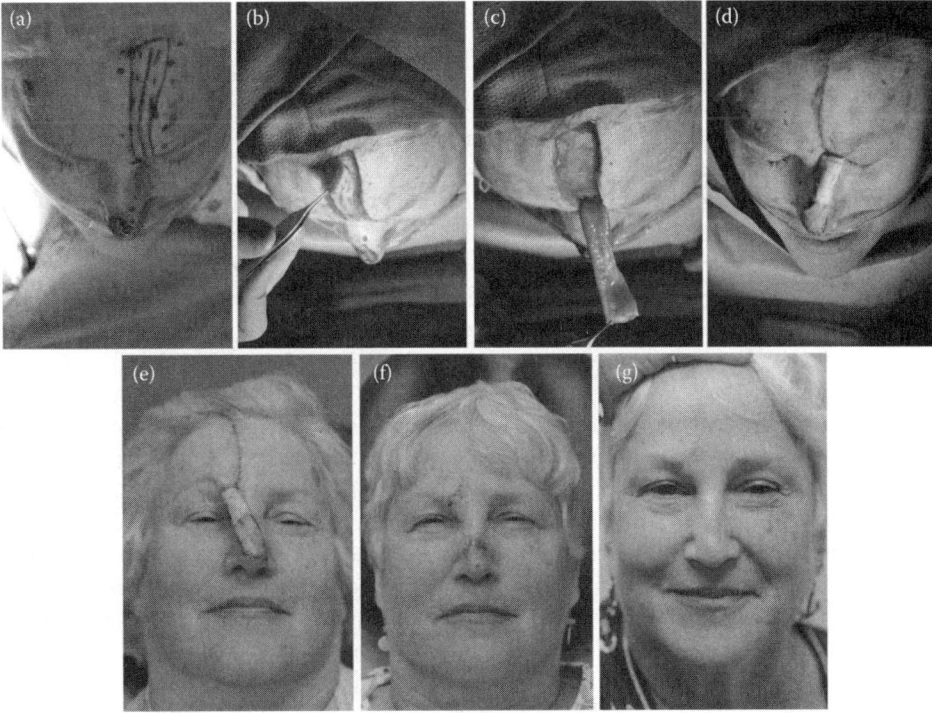

FIGURE 49.9 Paramedian forehead flap reconstruction of a surgical defect following Mohs micrographic surgery for a basal cell carcinoma. The interpolation flap is based on the right supratrochlear artery (a). The flap is elevated superficially at the distal aspect and at the level of the periosteum at the proximal aspect (b, c) to ensure patency of the supratrochlear artery. The flap is subsequently rotated on its proximal base into position to accommodate the surgical defect where it remains for 2–3 weeks (d, e). The second stage of the reconstruction involves taking the flap down (f). The final reconstruction (g) offers a cosmetically acceptable reconstruction.

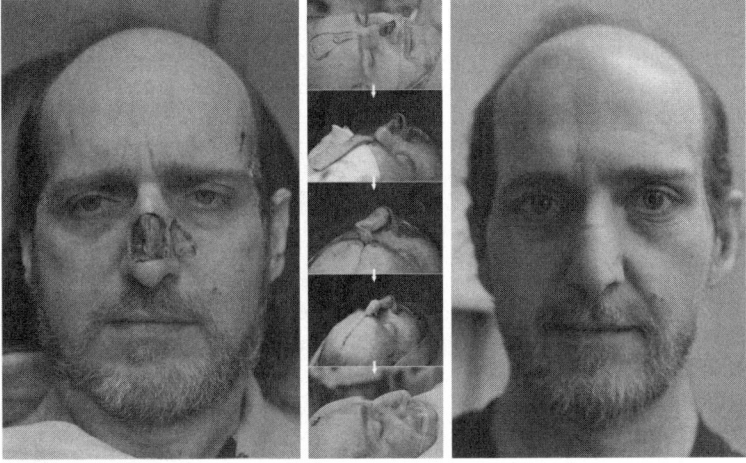

FIGURE 49.10 Paramedian forehead flap reconstruction of a large, infiltrative, morpheaform basal cell carcinoma of the right nasal ala and sidewall treated with Mohs micrographic surgery.

the nose (Figure 49.9). The first English publication of the forehead flap was in 1793; however, this flap is believed to have been used at least since 1440 AD [101,102]. The use of forehead skin to reconstruct the nose is based on its close similarity in both color and texture [92,93]. In addition, the forehead offers a large canvas on which the surgeon can design the flap based on the needed size and thickness.

Multiple optimizations of this flap have been implemented since the initial forehead flap, resulting in a thinner pedicle, less rotation/twisting of the pedicle, and a resultant improved cosmetic outcome [92]. Proper design of the flap with a thinner pedicle requires precise knowledge and localization of the supratrochlear artery. Failure in the identification and/or design of the flap could lead to inadvertent transaction of the artery and subsequent flap necrosis. Basic anatomical landmarks assist in localization of the artery; however, adjunctive techniques for this purpose are always welcome.

Based on the surgical defect and reconstructive requirements, this reconstructive technique may be performed in conjunction with other techniques such as cartilage grafts, nasal mucosal lining flaps and/or grafts, and/or other flaps.

The paramedian forehead flap is well described and thus will only be briefly discussed [103]. As discussed above, proper design of the flap is paramount. Identification of the supratrochlear artery is performed initially based on anatomic landmarks (Figure 49.10) [98,104,105]. This includes multiple different methods such as palpation of foramen and glabellar creases. The use of Doppler ultrasonography is commonly used to localize and/or confirm the course of the supratrochlear artery. Once this axial artery is identified, the flap is designed around the artery based on the necessary dimensions. Incision and elevation of the flap is performed with careful preservation of the supratrochlear artery (Figure 49.4). The flap is incised to the level of the periosteum at the insertion while the level may vary based on surgeon preference at the distal aspect. The interpolation flap is next rotated on its proximal end and placed into position at the surgical defect (Figure 49.3). The flap may be trimmed and tailored for an exact fit and then sutured into position. There are numerous variations on technical aspects of this flap that have been described in detail [92,106]. The donor site on the forehead is repaired as a primary closure, leaving the pedicle intact to maintain an adequate arterial supply to the flap (Figure 49.2d). The flap is typically left in place for 2–3 weeks at which time the flap is divided. This second stage involves removal of the connecting pedicle and fitting the proximal portion of the flap in place (Figure 49.3). There are techniques to perform the paramedian forehead flap in a single stage in addition to three (or more) stages as well.

49.10.5 Utilization of Thermal Imaging as an Adjunctive Tool

The use of thermal infrared imaging offers a safe, real-time visualization of cutaneous vessels. This offers dermatologic, Mohs micrographic, and plastic surgeons an adjunctive tool to assess the vascular characteristics of anatomic regions. The sensitivity of thermal imaging cameras is a critical determinant in this ability to detect the superficial vasculature. This enhanced precision can allow for improvements such as a thinner pedicle to be designed.

Acknowledgments

The schematic diagrams (Figures 49.1 and 49.2) were drawn by Sven Weum, Auburn University, Auburn, Alabama. The images in Figures 49.3 through 49.6 were from patients and volunteers and are courtesy of the Cardiovascular Research Group, Department of Medical Biology, Faculty of Health Sciences, University of Tromsø, Norway and the Department of Hand and Plastic Surgery, University Hospital North Norway, Tromsø, Norway. The infrared thermal images in these examples were taken using an FLIR ThermaCAM®S65-HS uncooled bolometer. The image analysis software used was ThermaCAM researcher ver.2.8(SR2). Examples of IR images (XX) come from the Thermal Lab, Auburn University, Alabama, USA utilizing an FLIR B360. We would like to acknowledge the assistance of Kunal Aswani,

Ryan Ward, and Martha Hart "Ragan" Hart; doctoral students Matt Barberio and David Elmer; and my family for their support and editing (Donna, Corrie, and Annan Pascoe).

References

1. Pascoe D.D., Mercer J.B., DeWeerd L. Physiology of thermal signals. In: *The Biomedical Engineering Handbook; Medical Devices and Systems.* (3rd edition). Joseph D.B. Ed., Boca Raton, FL: CRC Press, Taylor & Francis Group 21.1–21.18, 2006.
2. Nadel E.R., Mitchell J.W., Stowwijk J.A.J. Differential thermal sensitivity in the human skin. *Pflugers Arch.* 340:71–76, 1973.
3. Crawshaw L.I., Nadel E.R., Stolwijk J.A.J., Samford B.A. Effect of local cooling on sweat rate and cold sensation. *Pflugers Arch.* 354:19–27, 1975.
4. Olsen B.W. How many sites are necessary to estimate a mean skin temperature? In: *Thermal Physiology.* Hales J.R.S., Ed., New York: Raven Press, 33–38, 1984.
5. Hardy J.D. The radiation of heat from the human body. III The human skin as a black-body radiator. *J. Clin. Invest.* 13(4): 615–620, 1934.
6. Hardy J.D., Muschenheim C. The radiation of heat from the human body. IV The emission, reflection, and transmission of infra-red radiation by the human skin. *J. Clin. Invest.* 13(5): 817–831, 1934.
7. Hardy J.D., Muschenheim C. Radiation of heat from the human body. V. The transmission of infra-red radiation through skin. *J. Clin. Invest.* 15(1): 1–9, 1936.
8. Ryan T.J., Jolles B., Holti G. *Methods in Microcirculation Studies.* London: H.K. Lewis and Co, Ltd, 1972.
9. Pennes H.H. Analysis of tissue and arterial blood temperatures in resting human forearm. *J. Appl. Physiol.* 1, 93–102, 1948.
10. Charkoudian N. Skin blood flow in adult thermoregulation: How it works, when it does not, and why. *Mayo Clin. Proc.*, 78, 603–612, 2003.
11. Greenfield A.D.M. The circulation through the skin. In: *Handbook of Physiology—Circulation.* Hamilton W.P., Ed., Washington DC: Am. Physiol. Society, Section 3, Vol. II, (Chapter 39), 1325–1351, 1963.
12. Johnson J.M., Brenglemann G.L., Hales J.R.S., Vanhoutte M., Wenger C.B. Regulation of the cutaneous circulation. *Fed. Proc.* 45, 2841–2850, 1986.
13. Johnson J.M., Proppe D.W. Cardiovascular adjustments to heat stress. In: *Handbook of Physiology—Environmental Physiology.* Fregly M.J., Blatteis C.M., Eds., New York/Oxford: Oxford Press, pp. 215–243, 1996.
14. Rowell L.B. Human cardiovascular adjustments to exercise and thermal stress. *Physiol. Rev.* 54, 75–159, 1974.
15. Rowell L.B. Cardiovascular adjustments to thermal stress. In: *Handbook of Physiology—The Cardiovascular System.* Fregly M.J., Blatteis C.M., Eds., Bethesda, MD: Am. Physiol. Society, Section 3, Vol. 5, Part 3, (Chapter 27), 967–1024, 1983.
16. Rowell L.B. *Human Circulation: Regulation during Physiological Stress.* New York: Oxford University Press, 1986.
17. Sawka M.N., Wenger C.B. Physiological responses to acute exercise-heat stress. In: *Human Performance Physiology and Environmental Medicine at Terrestrial Extremes.* KB Pandolf, K.B., Sawka M.N., Gonzales R.R., Eds, Indianapolis, IN: Benchmark Press, pp. 97–151, 1988.
18. Johnson J.M. Circulation to the skin. In: *Textbook of Physiology,* Vol. 2, Patton H.D., Fuchs A.F., Hille B., Scher A.M., Steiner R., Eds, Philadelphia: W.B. Saunders Co., (Chapter 45), 1989.
19. Johnson J.M. Exercise and the cutaneous circulation, *Exercise Sports Sci. Rev.* 20, 59–97, 1992.
20. Charkoudian N. Skin blood flow in adult human thermoregulation: How it works, when it does not, and why. *Mayo Clin. Proc.* 78:603–612, 2003.

21. Gaskell P. Are there sympathetic vasodilator nerves in the vessels of the hands? *J. Physiol.* 131, 647–656, 1956.

22. Fox R.H., Edholm O.G. Nervous control of the cutaneous circulation. *J. Appl. Physiol.* 57, 1688–1695, 1984.

23. Lossius K., Eriksen M., Walloe L. Fluctuations in blood flow to acral skin in humans: Connection with heart rate and blood pressure variability. *J. Physiol.* 460:641–655, 1993.

24. Edholm O.G., Fox R.H., Macpherson R.K. The effect of body heating on the circulation in skin and muscle. *J. Physiol.* 134:612–619, 1956.

25. Edholm O.G., Fox R.H., Macpherson R.K. Vasomotor control of the cutaneous blood vessels in the human forearm. *J. Physiol.* 139:455–465, 1957.

26. Rodie I.C., Shepard J.T., Whelan R.F. Evidence from venous oxygen saturation that the increase in of arm blood flow during body heating is confined to the skin. *J. Physiol.* 134, 444–450, 1956.

27. Kellogg D.L. Jr, Shepard J.T., Whelan R.F. Cutaneous active vasodilation in humans is mediated by cholinergic nerve cotransmission. *Cir. Res.* 77:1222–1228, 1995.

28. Kolka M.A., Stephenson L.A. Cutaneous blood flow and local sweating after systemic atropine administration. *Pflugers Arch.* 410:524–529, 1987.

29. Shastry S., Minson C.T., Wilson S.A., Dietz N.M., Joyner M.J. Effects of atropine and L-NAME on cutaneous blood flow during body heating in humans. *J. Appl. Physiol.* 88:467–462, 2000.

30. Pascoe D.D., Shanley L.A., Smith E.W. Clothing and Exercise I: Biophysics of heat transfer between the individual, clothing, and environment. *Sports Med.* 18(1): 38–54, 1994.

31. Pascoe D.D., Bellinger T.A., McCluskey B.S., Clothing and Exercise II: Influence of clothing during exercise/work in environmental extremes, *Sports Med.* 18(2):94–108, 1994.

32. Roberts M.P., Wenger C.B., Stölwik, Nadel E.R. Skin blood flow and sweating changes following exercise training and heat acclimation *J. Appl. Physiol.* 43, 133–137, 1977.

33. Stephenson L.A., Kolka M.A. Menstrual cycle phase and time of day alter reference signal controlling arm blood flow and sweating *Am. J. Physiol.* 249(2, pt2), R186–R192, 1985.

34. Aoki K., Stephens D.P., Johnson J.M. Diurnal variations in cutaneous vasodilator and vasoconstrictor systems during heat stress. *Am. J. Physiol. Regul. Integr. Comp. Physiol.* 281, R591–R595, 2001.

35. Wissler F.H. Steady State temperature distribution in man. *J. Appl. Physiol.* 16:734–740, 1961.

36. Volpe B.T., Jain R.K. Temperature distribution and thermal responses in humans. I. Stimulation of various modes of whole body hyperthermia in normal subjects. *Med. Physics* 9:506–513, 1982.

37. Chan R.A., Sigelman R.A., Guy A.W. Calculations of therapeutic heat generated by ultrasound in fat-muscle-bone layers. *IEEE Trans. Biomed. Eng.* BME, 21:280–284, 1974.

38. Sekins K.M., Emery A.F., Lehmann J.F., MacDougall J.A. Determination of perfusion field during local hypoerthermia with the adi of finite elements thermal model. *ASME J. Biomech. Eng.* 104:272–279, 1982.

39. Chato J.C. A view of the history of heat transfer in bioengineering. In: *Advances in Heat Transfer*, San Diego/New York/London/Sydney/Boston/Tokyo/Toronto: Academic Press, Vol. 22, pp. 1–19, 1981.

40. Chen M.M., Holmes K.R. Microvascular contributions in tissue heat transfer. In: *Thermal Characteristics of Tumors: Applications in Detection and Treatment.* Jain R.K., Guillino P.M., Eds., Ann N.Y. Acad Sci. 335, 137, 1980.

41. Baish J.W., Microvascular heat transfer, In: *The Biomedical Engineering Handbook.* Bronzino J.D., Ed., Boca Raton, FL: CRC Press/IEEE Press, Vol. II, 98, 1–14, 2000.

42. Manchot C. *Die Hautarterien des Menschlichen Körpers.* Vogel, Leipzig, 1889.

43. Manchot C. *The Cutaneous Arteries of the Human Body.* Springer-Verlag: New York, 1982.

44. Spalteholtz W. Die Vertheilung der Blutgefasse in der Haut. *Arch Anat Entwiecklngs-Gesch (Leipz)* 1:54, 1893.

45. Salmon M. Artères de la peau. Maisson et Cie, Paris, 1936.

46. Taylor G.I., Palmer J.H. The vascular territories (angiosomes) of the body: Experimental study and clinical applications. *Br. J. Plast. Surg.* 40:113–141, 1987.

47. Cormack G.C., Lamberty B.G. The different layers of the integument and functional organization of the microcirculoation. In: *The Arterial Anatomy of Skin Flaps*. Cormack G.C., Lamberty B.G. Eds., New York: Churchill Livingstone, pp. 16–69, 1994.

48. El-Mrakby H.H., Milner R.H. The vascular anatomy of the lower anterior abdominal wall: A micro-dissection study on the deep inferior epigastric vessels and the perforator branches. *Plast. Reconstr. Surg.* 109:539–543, discussion by Taylor GI, 544–547, 2002.

49. El Mrakby H.H., Milner R.H. Bimodal distribution of the blood supply to lower abdominal fat: Histological study of the microcirculation of the lower abdominal wall. *Ann. Plast. Surg.* 50:165–170, 2003.

50. Taylor G.I. The angiosomes of the body and their supply to perforator flaps. *Clin. Plast. Surg.* 30:331–342, 2003.

51. Jiang L.J., Ng E.Y.K., Yeo A.C.B., Wu S., Pan F., Yau W.Y., Chen J.H., Yang Y. A perspective on medical infrared imaging. *J. Med. Eng. Tech.* 29:257–267, 2005.

52. Wilson S.B., Spence V.A. Dynamic thermography imaging method for quantifying dermal perfusion: Potential and limitations. *Med. Biol. Eng. Comput.* 27:496–501, 1989.

53. Miland Å.O., Mercer J.B. Effect of a short period of abstinence from smoking on rewarming patterns of hands following local cooling. *Eur. J. Appl. Phys.* 98:161–168, 2006.

54. Goetz C., Foertsch D., Schoeberger J., Uhl E. Thermography—a valuable tool to test hydrocephalus shunt patency. *Acta Neurochir. (Wien)* 147:1167–1173, 2005.

55. Garbade J., Ulllmann C., Hollenstein M., Barten M.J., Jacob S., Dhein S., Walther T., Gummert J.F., Falk V., Mohr F.W. Modeling of temperature mapping from quantitative dynamic infrared coronary angiography for intraoperative graft patency control. *J. Thor. Card. Surg.* 131:1344–1351, 2006.

56. Gorbach A., Simonton D., Hale A., Swanson S.J., Kirk A.D. Objective real-time, intraoperative assessment of renal perfusion using infrared imaging. *Am. J. Transplant.* 3:988–993, 2003.

57. Ring E.F.J., Jung A., Zuber J., Rukowski P., Kalicki B., Najwa U. Detecting Fever in Polish Children by Infrared Thermography, *QIRT, Proceedings of 9th International Conference on Quantitative Infrared Thermography*, Krakow Poland, Technical University of Ldz. Institute of Electronics, pp. 125–128, 2008.

58. International Standard IEC 80601-2-59, Medical Electrical Equipment-Part 2–59: Particular requirements for basic safety and essential performance of screening thermographs for human febrile temperature screening IEC Geneva (2008) available at www.webstore.ansi.org RecordDetail. aspx? Sku=IEC+8060 1-2-59+Ed.1.0+b%3a2008, 2008.

59. International Organization for Standards ISO/TR 13154:2009, Medical Electrical Equipment-Deployment, implementation, and operational guidelines for identifying febrile humans using a screening thermograph. ISO Geneva, 2009 www.iso.org/iso/iso_catalogue_tc/catalogue_detail. htm?csnumber=51236, 2009.

60. Mercer, J.B., Ring E.F.J. Fever screening and infrared imaging: Concerns and guidelines. *Thermol. Int.* 19, 67–69, 2009.

61. Pascoe D.D., Ring E.F., Mercer, J.B., Snell J., Osborn D., Hedley-Whyte J. International standards for pandemic screening using infrared thermography ISO TC121/SC3-IEC TC/SC62D/JWG 8, Clinical Thermometers, Project Team 1, Thermal Imagers for Human Febrile Temperature Screening. Medical Imaging 2010: Biomedical Applications in Molecular, Structural, and Functional Imaging, Molthen R.C., Weaver J.B., Eds., *Proc. SPIE*, 7626, 76261Z, 2010.

62. Francis J. Ring, EYK Ng, Infrared thermal imaging standards for human fever detection. In: *Medical Infrared Imaging*. Diakides N.A., Bronzino J.D., Eds, Baton Rouge/London/New York: CRC Press.

63. Sefton J.M., Yarar C., Berry J.W., Pascoe D.D. Therapeutic massage of the neck and shoulder produces changes in peripheral blood flow when assessed with dynamic infrared thermography. *J. Alternative Complimentary Med.* 16(7): 1–10, 2010.

64. Koshima I., Soeda S. Inferior epigastric artery skin flaps without rectus abdominis muscle. *Br. J. Plast. Surg.* 42:645–648, 1989.

65. Blondeel P.N. Soft tissue reconstruction with perforator flaps. In: *Tissue Surgery*. Siemionow M.Z., Ed., London: Springer-Verlag, pp. 87–100, 2006.

66. Theuvenet W.J., Koevers G.F., Borghouts M.H. Thermographic assessment of perforating arteries. A preoperative screening method for fasciocutaneous and musculocutaneous flaps. *Scand. J. Plast. Reconstr. Surg.* 20:25–29, 1986.

67. Itoh Y., Arai K. Use of recovery-enhanced thermography to localize cutaneous perforators. *Ann. Plast. Surg.* 34:507–511, 1995.

68. Wolff K.D., Telzrow T., Rudolph K.H. et al. Isotope perfusion and infrared thermography of arterialised, venous flow-through and pedicled venous flaps. *Br. J. Plast. Surg.* 48:61–70, 1995.

69. Cordeiro P.G. Breast reconstruction after surgery for breast cancer. *N. Engl. J. Med.* 359:1590–1601, 2008.

70. Granzow J.W., Levine J.L., Chiu E.S. et al. Breast reconstruction using perforator flaps. *J. Surg. Oncol.* 94:441–454, 2006.

71. Chevray P.M. Update on breast reconstruction using free TRAM, DIEP, and SIEA flaps. *Sem. Plast. Surg.* 18:97–103, 2004.

72. Allen R.J., Treece P. Deep inferior epigastric perforator flap for breast reconstruction. *Ann. Plast. Surg.* 32:32–38, 1994.

73. Blondeel P.N. One hundred free DIEP flap breast reconstructions: A personal experience. *Br. J. Plast. Surg.* 52:104–111, 1998.

74. Giunta R.E., Geisweid A., Feller A.M. The value of preoperative Doppler sonography for planning free perforator flaps. *Plast. Reconstr. Surg.* 105:2381–2386, 2000.

75. de Weerd L., Weum S., Mercer J.B. The value of dynamic infrared thermography (DIRT) in perforator selection and planning of DIEP flaps. *Ann. Plast. Surg.* 63:274–279, 2009.

76. Hunter J. *A Treatise on the Blood, Inflammation and Gunshot Wounds.* John Richardson, London, 1794.

77. Neligan P.C., Blondeel P.N., Morris S.F., Hallock G.G. Perforator flaps: Overview, Classification, and Nomenclature. In: *Perforator Flaps. Anatomy, Technique & Clinical Applications.* Blondeel P.N., Morris S.F., Hallock G.G., Neligan P.C. Eds., St Louis, Missouri: Quality Medical Publishing, pp. 37–52, 2006.

78. Amalu W.C., Hobbins W.B., Head J.F., Elliott R.L. Infrared imaging of the breast: a review. In: *Medical Infrared Imaging.* Diakides N.A., Bronzino J.D. Eds., Boca Raton: CRC Press, Taylor & Francis Group, pp. 9.1–9.19, 2008.

79. Masia J., Clavero J.A., Larrañaga J.R., Alomar X., Pons G., Serret P. Multidetector-row tomography in the planning of abdominal perforator flaps. *J. Plast. Reconstr. Aesthet. Surg.* 59:594–599, 2006.

80. Casey W., Chew R.T., Rebecca A.M., Smith A.A., Collins J., Pockaj A. Advantages of preoperative Computed Tomography in deep inferior epigastric artery perforator flap breast reconstruction. *Plast. Reconstr. Surg.* 123:1148–1155, 2008.

81. Wiest P.W., Locken J.A., Heintz P.H., Mettler Jr F.A. CT scanning: A major source of radiation exposure. *Sem. Ultrasound MRI* 23:402–410, 2002.

82. Brenner D.J., Hall E.J. Computed Tomography: An increasing source of radiation exposure. *N. Engl. J. Med.* 357:2277–2284, 2007.

83. de Weerd L., Mercer J.B., Setså L.B. Intraoperative dynamic infrared thermography and free-flap surgery. *Ann. Plast. Surg.* 57:279–84, 2006.

84. Disa J.J., Cordeiro P.G., Hidalgo D.A. Efficacy of conventional monitoring techniques in free tissue transfer: An 11-year experience in 750 consecutive cases. *Plast. Reconstr. Surg.* 104:97–101, 1999.

85. Jones N.F. Intraoperative and postoperative monitoring of microsurgical free tissue transfers. *Clin. Plast. Surg.* 19:783–797, 1992.

86. Smit J.M., Acosta R., Zeebregts C.J., Liss A.G., Anniko M., Hartman E.H.M. Early reintervention of compromised free flaps improves success rate. *Microsurgery* 27:612–616, 2007.

87. Baudet J., LeMaire J.M., Guimberteau J.C. Ten free groin flaps. *Plast. Reconstr. Surg.* 57:577–595, 1976.
88. Acland R.D. Discussion of "Experience in monitoring the circulation of free flap transfers". *Plast. Reconstr. Surg.* 68:554–555, 1981.
89. Leonard A.G., Brennen M.D., Colville J. The use of continuous temperature monitoring in the postoperative management of microvascular cases. *Br. J. Plast. Surg.* 35:337–342, 1982.
90. Busic V., Das-Gupta R. Temperature monitoring in free flap surgery. *Br. J. Plast. Surg.* 57:588, 2004.
91. de Weerd L., Miland Å.O., Mercer J.B. Perfusion dynamics of free DIEP and SIEA flaps during the first postoperative week monitored with dynamic infrared thermography (DIRT). *Ann. Plast. Surg.* 62:40–47, 2009.
92. Menick F. *Nasal Reconstruction. Art and Practice.* China: Mosby Elsevier, 2009.
93. Menick F.J. Nasal reconstruction: Forehead flap. *Plast. Reconstr. Surg.* 113, 100e–111e, 2004.
94. Moolenburgh S.E., McLennan L., Levendag P.C., Scholtemeijer M., Hofer S.O.P., Mureau M.A.M. Nasal reconstruction after malignant tumor resection: An algorithm for treatment. *Plast. Reconstr. Surg.* 126, 97–105, 2010.
95. Buddharaju P., Pavlidis I. Physiology-based face recognition in the thermal infrared spectrum. In *Medical Infrared Imaging.* Diakides N.A., Bronzino J.D. Eds., New York: CRC Press, pp. 13-1–13-16, 2008.
96. Taylor G.I., Ives A., Dhar S. Vascular territories. In *Plastic Surgery. Vol. 1 General Principles.* Mathes S.J. Ed., Philadelphia, PA: Saunders Elsevier, pp. 317–363, 2006.
97. Mathes S.J., Hansen S.L. Flap classification and applications. In *Plastic Surgery. Vol. General Principles.* Mathes S.J., Ed., Philadelphia, PA: Saunders Elsevier, pp. 365–481, 2006.
98. Vural E., Batay F., Key J.M. Glabellar frown lines as a reliable landmark for the supratrochlear artery. *Otolaryngol. Head Neck Surg.* 123, 543–546, 2000.
99. Stelnicki E.J., Young V.L, Francel T. Randall P. Vilray P. Blair, his surgical descendents, and their roles in plastic surgical development. *Plast. Reconstr. Surg.* 103, 1990, 1999.
100. Riggio E. The hazards of contemporary paramedian forehead flap and neck dissection in smokers. *Plast. Reconstr. Surg.* 112, 346–347, 2003.
101. Antia N.H., Daver B.M. Reconstructive surgery for nasal defects. *Clin. Plast. Surg.* 8, 535, 1981.
102. Reece E.M., Schaverien M., Rohrich R.J. The paramedian forehead flap: A dynamic anatomical vascular study verifying safety and clinical implications. *Plast. Reconstr. Surg.* 121, 1956–1963, 2008.
103. Baker S.R. Interpolated paramedian forehead flaps. In *Local Flaps in Facial Reconstruction.* Baker S.R. Ed., China: Mosby Elsevier, pp. 265–312, 2007.
104. Shumrick K.A., Smith T.L., The anatomic basis for the design of forehead flaps in nasal reconstruction. *Arch. Otolaryngol. Head Neck Surg.* 118, 373–379, 1992.
105. Ugur M.B., Savranlar A., Uzun L, Küçüker H, Cinar F. A reliable surface landmark for localizing supratrochlear artery: Medial canthus. *Otolaryngol. Head Neck Surg.* 138, 162–165, 2008.
106. Angobaldo J., Malcolm M. Refinements in nasal reconstruction: The cross-paramedian forehead flap. *Plast. Reconstr. Surg.* 123, 87–93, 2009.

50

Infrared Imaging Applied to Dentistry

Barton M. Gratt
University of Washington

50.1 The Importance of Temperature

Temperature is very important in all biological systems. Temperature influences the movement of atoms and molecules and their rates of biochemical activity. Active biological life is, in general, restricted to a temperature range of 0–45°C [1]. Cold-blooded organisms are generally restricted to habitats in which the ambient temperature remains between 0°C and 40°C. However, a variety of temperatures well outside of this occurs on earth, and by developing the ability to maintain a constant body temperature, warm-blooded animals; for example, birds, mammals, including humans have gained access to a greater variety of habitats and environments [1].

With the application of common thermometers, elevation in the core temperature of the body became the primary indicator for the diagnosis of fever. Wunderlich introduced fever measurements as a routine procedure in Germany, in 1872. In 1930, Knaus inaugurated a method of basal temperature measurement, achieving full medical acceptance in 1952. Today, it is customary in hospitals throughout the world to take body temperature measurements on all patients [2].

The scientists of the first part of the twentieth century used simple thermometers to study body temperatures. Many of their findings have not been superseded, and are repeatedly confirmed by new investigators using new more advanced thermal measuring devices. In the last part of the twentieth century, a new discipline termed "thermology" emerged as the study of surface body temperature in both health and in disease [2].

50.2 Skin and Skin-Surface Temperature Measurement

The skin is the outer covering of the body and contributes 10% of the body's weight. Over 30% of the body's temperature-receptive elements are located within the skin. Most of the heat produced within the body is dissipated by way of the skin, through radiation, evaporation, and conduction. The range of ambient temperature for thermal comfort is relatively broad (20–25°C). Thermal comfort is dependent upon humidity, wind velocity, clothing, and radiant temperature. Under normal conditions there is a steady flow of heat from the inside of a human body to the outside environment. Skin temperature distribution within specific anatomic regions; for example, the head vs. the foot, are diverse, varying by as much as ±15°C. Heat transport by convection to the skin surface depends on the rate of blood flow through the skin, which is also variable. In the trunk region of the body, blood flow varies by a factor of 7; at the foot, blood flow varies by a factor of 30; while at the fingers, it can vary by a factor of 600 [3].

It appears that measurements of body (core) temperatures and skin (surface) temperature may well be strong physiologic markers indicating health or disease. In addition, skin (surface) temperature values appear to be unique for specific anatomic regions of the body.

50.3 Two Common Types of Body Temperature Measurements

There are two common types of body temperature measurements that are made and utilized as diagnostic indicators.

1. *Measurement of Body Core Temperature.* The normal core temperature of the human body remains within a range of 36.0–37.5°C [1]. The constancy of human core temperature is maintained by a large number of complex regulatory mechanisms [3]. Body core temperatures are easily measured orally (or anally) with contacting temperature devices including: manual or digital thermometers, thermistors, thermocouples, and even layers of liquid temperature-sensitive crystals, and so on [4–6].
2. *Measurement of Body Surface Temperature.* While body core temperature is very easy to measure, the body's skin surface temperature is very difficult to measure. Any device that is required to make contact with the skin cannot measure the body's skin surface temperature reliably. Since skin has a relatively low heat capacity and poor lateral heat conductance, skin temperature is likely to change on contact with a cooler or warmer object [2]. Therefore, an indirect method of obtaining skin surface temperature is required, a common thermometer on the skin, for example, will not work.

Probably the first research efforts that pointed out the diagnostic importance of the infrared emission of human skin and thus initiated the modern era of thermometry were the studies of Hardy in 1934 [7,8]. However, it took 30 years for modern thermometry to be applied in laboratories around the world. To conduct noncontact thermography of the human skin in a clinical setting, an advanced computerized infrared imaging system is required. Consequently, clinical thermography required the advent of microcomputers developed in the late 1960s and early 1970s. These sophisticated electronic systems employed advanced microtechnology, requiring large research and development costs.

Current clinical thermography units use single detector infrared cameras. These work as follows: infrared radiation emitted by the skin surface enters the lens of the camera, passes through a number of rapidly spinning prisms (or mirrors), which reflect the infrared radiation emitted from different parts of the field of view onto the infrared sensor. The sensor converts the reflected infrared radiation into electrical signals. An amplifier receives the electric signals from the sensor and boosts them to electric potential signals of a few volts that can be converted into digital values. These values are then fed into a computer. The computer uses this input, together with the timing information from the rotating mirrors, to reconstruct a digitized thermal image from the temperature values of each small area within the field of observation. These digitized images are easily viewed and can be analyzed using computer software and stored on a computer disk for later reference.

50.4 Diagnostic Applications of Thermography

In 1987, the *International Bibliography of Medical Thermology* was published and included more than 3000 cited publications on the medical use of thermography, including applications for anesthesiology, breast disease, cancer, dermatology, gastrointestinal disorders, gynecology, urology, headache, immunology, musculoskeletal disorders, neurology, neurosurgery, ophthalmology, otolaryngology, pediatrics, pharmacology, physiology, pulmonary disorders, rheumatology, sports medicine, general surgery, plastic and reconstructive surgery, thyroid, cardiovascular and cerebrovascular, vascular problems, and veterinary medicine [9]. In addition, changes in human skin temperature has been reported in conditions involving the orofacial complex, as related to dentistry, such as the temporomandibular joint [10–25], and nerve damage and repair following common oral surgery [25–27]. Thermography has been shown not to be useful in the assessment of periapical granuloma [28]. Reports of dedicated controlled facial skin temperature studies of the orofacial complex are limited, but follow findings consistent with other areas of the body [29,30].

50.5 Normal Infrared Facial Thermography

The pattern of heat dissipation over the skin of the human body is normally symmetrical and this includes the human face. It has been shown that in normal subjects, the difference in skin temperature from side-to-side on the human body is small, about 0.2°C [31]. Heat emission is directly related to cutaneous vascular activity, yielding enhanced heat output on vasodilatation and reduced heat output on vasoconstriction. Infrared thermography of the face has promise, therefore, as a harmless, noninvasive, diagnostic technique that may help to differentiate selected diagnostic problems. The literature reports that during clinical studies of facial skin temperature a significant difference between the absolute facial skin temperatures of men vs. women was observed [32]. Men were found to have higher temperatures over all 25 anatomic areas measured on the face (e.g., the orbit, the upper lip, the lower lip, the chin, the cheek, the TMJ, etc.) than women. The basal metabolic rate for a normal 30-year-old male, 1.7 m tall (5 ft, 7 in.), weighing 64 kg (141 lbs), who has a surface area of approximately 1.6 m^2, is approximately 80 W; therefore, he dissipates about 50 W/m^2 of heat [33]. On the other hand, the basal metabolic rate of a 30-year-old female subject, 1.6 m tall (5 ft, 3 in.), weighing 54 kg (119 lbs), with a surface area of 1.4 m^2, is about 63 W, so that she dissipates about 41 W/m^2 of heat [33,34]. Assuming that there are no other relevant differences between male and female subjects, women's skin is expected to be cooler, since less heat is lost per unit (per area of body surface). Body heat dissipation through the face follows this prediction. In addition to the effect of gender on facial temperature, there are indications that age and ethnicity may also affect facial temperature [32].

When observing patients undergoing facial thermography, there seems to be a direct correlation between vasoactivity and pain, which might be expected since both are neurogenic processes. Differences in facial skin temperature, for example, asymptomatic adult subjects (low temperatures differences) and adult patients with various facial pain syndromes (high-temperature differences) may prove to be a useful criterion for the diagnosis of many conditions [35]. Right- vs. left-side temperature differences (termed: delta T or ΔT) between many specific facial regions in normal subjects were shown to be low (<0.3°C) [40], while similar ΔT values were found to be high (>0.5°C) in a variety of disorders related to dentistry [35].

50.6 Abnormal Facial Conditions Demonstrated with Infrared Facial Thermography

50.6.1 Assessing Temporomandibular Joint (TMJ) Disorders with Infrared Thermography

It has been shown that normal subjects have symmetrical thermal patterns over the TMJ regions of their face. Normal subjects had ΔT values of 0.1°C (±0.1°C) [32,36]. On the other hand, TMJ pain patients were found to have asymmetrical thermal patterns, with increased temperatures over the affected TMJ region, with ΔT values of +0.4°C (±0.2°C) [37]. Specifically, painful TMJ patients with internal derangement and painful TMJ osteoarthritis were both found to have asymmetrical thermal patterns and increased temperatures over the affected TMJ, with mean area TMJ ΔT of +0.4°C (±0.2°C) [22,24]. In other words, the correlation between TMJ pain and hyper perfusion of the region seems to be independent of the etiology of the TMJ disorder (osteoarthritis vs. internal derangement). In addition, a study of mild-to-moderate TMD (temporomandibular joint dysfunction) patients indicated that area ΔT values correlated with the level of the patient's pain symptoms [38]. And a more recent double-blinded clinical study compared active orthodontic patients vs. TMD patients vs. asymptomatic TMJ controls, and showed average ΔT values of +0.2, +0.4, and +0.1°C; for these three groups respectively. This study showed that thermography could distinguish between patients undergoing active orthodontic treatment and patients with TMD [39].

50.6.2 Assessing Inferior Alveolar Nerve (IAN) Deficit with Infrared Thermography

The thermal imaging of the chin has been shown to be an effective method for assessing inferior alveolar nerve deficit [40]. Whereas normal subjects (those without inferior alveolar nerve deficit) show a symmetrical thermal pattern (ΔT of +0.1°C [±0.1°C]); patients with inferior alveolar nerve deficit had elevated temperature in the mental region of their chin (ΔT of +0.5°C [±0.2°C]) on the affected side [41]. The observed vasodilatation seems to be due to blockage of the vascular neuronal vasoconstrictive messages, since the same effect on the thermological pattern could be invoked in normal subjects by temporary blockage of the inferior alveolar nerve, using a 2% lidocaine nerve block injection [42].

50.6.3 Assessing Carotid Occlusal Disease with Infrared Thermography

The thermal imaging of the face, especially around the orbits, has been shown to be an effective method for assessing carotid occlusal disease. Cerebrovascular accident (CVA), also called stroke, is well known as a major cause of death. The most common cause of stroke is atherosclerotic plaques forming emboli, which travel within vascular blood channels, lodging in the brain, obstructing the brain's blood supply, resulting in a cerebral vascular accident (or stroke). The most common origin for emboli is located in the lateral region of the neck where the common carotid artery bifurcates into the internal and the external carotid arteries [43,44]. It has been well documented that intraluminal carotid plaques, which both restrict and reduce blood flow, result in decreased facial skin temperature [43–54]. Thermography has demonstrated the ability to detect a reduction of 30% (or more) of blood flow within the carotid arteries [55]. Thermography shows promise as an inexpensive painless screening test of asymptomatic elderly adults at risk for the possibility of stroke. However, more clinical studies are required before thermography may be accepted for routine application in screening toward preventing stroke [55,56].

50.6.4 Additional Applications of Infrared Thermography

Recent clinical studies assessed the application of thermography on patients with chronic facial pain (orofacial pain of greater than 4 month's duration). Thermography classified patients as being "normal" when selected anatomic ΔT values ranged from 0.0°C to ±0.25°C, and "hot" when ΔT values were >+ 0.35°C, and "cold" when area ΔT values were <–0.35°C. The study population consisted of 164 dental pain patients and 164 matched (control) subjects. This prospective, matched study determined that subjects classified with "hot" thermographs had the clinical diagnosis of (1) sympathetically maintained pain, (2) peripheral nerve-mediated pain, (3) TMJ arthropathy, or (4) acute maxillary sinusitis. Subjects classified with "cold" areas on their thermographs were found to have the clinical diagnosis of (1) peripheral nerve-mediated pain, or (2) sympathetically independent pain. Subjects classified with "normal" thermographs included patients with the clinical diagnosis of (1) cracked tooth syndrome, (2) trigeminal neuralgia, (3) pretrigeminal neuralgia, or (4) psychogenic facial pain. This new system of thermal classification resulted in 92% (301 or 328) agreement in classifying pain patients vs. their matched controls. In brief, ΔT has been shown to be within ±0.4°C in normal subjects, while showing values greater than +0.7°C and less than –0.6°C in abnormal facial pain patients [10], making "ΔT" an important diagnostic parameter in the assessment of orofacial pain [35].

50.6.5 Future Advances in Infrared Imaging

Over the last 20 years there have been additional reports in the dental literature giving promise to new and varied applications of infrared thermography [57–63]. While, infrared thermography is promising, the future holds even greater potential for temperature measurement as a diagnostic tool, the most promising being termed dynamic area telethermometry (DAT) [64,65]. Newly developed DAT promises to become a new more advanced tool providing quantitative information on the thermoregulatory frequencies (TRFs) manifested in the modulation of skin temperature [66]. Whereas the static thermographic studies discussed above demonstrate local vasodilatation or vasoconstriction, DAT can identify the mechanism of thermoregulatory frequencies and thus it is expected, in the future, to significantly improve differential diagnosis [66].

In summary, the science of thermology, including static thermography, and soon to be followed by DAT, appears to have great promise as an important diagnostic tool in the assessment of orofacial health and disease.

Acknowledgment

This chapter is dedicated to Professor Michael Anbar, of Buffalo, New York: A brilliant scientist, my thermal science mentor, and "The Father of Dynamic Area Telethermography."

References

1. Grobklaus, R. and Bergmann, K.E. Physiology and regulation of body temperature. In *Applied Thermology: Thermologic Methods*. J.-M. Engel, U. Fleresch, and G. Stuttgen, Eds., Federal Republic of Germany: VCH, 1985, pp. 11–20.

2. *Applied Thermology: Thermologic Methods*. J.-M. Engel, U. Fleresch, and G. Stuttgen, Eds., Federal Republic of Germany: VCH (1985), pp. 11–20.

3. Kirsch, K.A. Physiology of skin-surface temperature. In *Applied Thermology: Thermologic Methods*. J.-M. Engel, U. Fleresch, and G. Stuttgen, Eds., Federal Republic of Germany: VCH (1985), pp. 1–9.

4. Anbar, M., Gratt, B.M., and Hong, D. Thermology and facial telethermography: Part I. History and technical review. *Dentomaxillofac. Radiol.* (1998), 27: 61–67.

5. Anbar, M. and Gratt, B.M. Role of nitric oxide in the physiopathology of pain. *J. Musc. Skeletal Joint Pain* (1997), 14: 225–254.

6. Rost, A. Comparative measurements with an infrared and contact thermometer for thermal stress reaction. In *Thermological Methods*. J.-M. Engel, U. Flesch, and G. Stuttgen, Eds., Weinheim: VCH Verlag (1985), pp. 169–170.

7. Hardy, J.D. The radiation of heat from the human body: I–IV. *J. Clin. Invest.* (1934), 13: 593–620.

8. Hardy, J.D. The radiation of heat from the human body: I–IV. *J. Clin. Invest.* (1934), 13: 817–883.

9. Abernathy, M. and Abernathy, T.B. International bibliography of thermology. *Thermology* (1987), 2: 1–533.

10. Berry, D.C. and Yemm, R. Variations in skin temperature of the face in normal subjects and in patients with mandibular dysfunction. *Br. J. Oral Maxillofac. Surg.* (1971), 8: 242–247.

11. Berry, D.C. and Yemm, R. A further study of facial skin temperature in patients with mandibular dysfunction. *J. Oral Rehabil.* (1974), 1: 255–264.

12. Kopp, S. and Haraldson, T. Normal variations in skin temperature of the face in normal subjects and in patients with mandibular dysfunction. *Br. J. Oral Maxillofac. Surg.* (1983), 8: 242–247.

13. Johansson, A., Kopp, S., and Haraldson, T. Reproducibility and variation of skin surface temperature over the temporomandibular joint and masseter muscle in normal individuals. *Acta Odontol. Scand.* (1985), 43: 309–313.

14. Tegelberg, A. and Kopp, S. Skin surface temperature over the temporo-mandibular and metacarpophalangeal joints in individuals with rheumatoid arthritis. *Odontol. Klin.*, Box 33070, 400 33 Goteborg, Sweden (1986), Report No. 31, pp. 1–31.

15. Akerman, S. et al. Relationship between clinical, radiologic and thermometric findings of the temporomandibular joint in rheumatoid arthritis. *Odontol. Klin.*, Box 33070, 400 33 Goteborg, Sweden (1987), Report No. 41, pp. 1–30.

16. Finney, J.W., Holt, C.R., and Pearce, K.B. Thermographic diagnosis of TMJ disease and associated neuromuscular disorders. *Special Report: Postgraduate Medicine* (March 1986), pp. 93–95.

17. Weinstein, S.A. Temporomandibular joint pain syndrome—The whiplash of the 1980s. *Thermography and Personal Injury Litigation*, Chapter 7. S.D. Hodge, Jr., Ed., New York, USA: John Wiley & Sons (1987), pp. 157–164.

18. Weinstein, S.A., Gelb, M., and Weinstein, E.L. Thermophysiologic anthropometry of the face in home sapiens. *J. Craniomand. Pract.* (1990), 8: 252–257.

19. Pogrel, M.A., McNeill, C., and Kim, J.M. The assessment of trapezius muscle symptoms of patients with temporomandibular disorders by the use of liquid crystal thermography. *Oral Surg. Oral Med. Oral. Pathol. Oral Radiol. Endod.* (1996), 82: 145–151.

20. Steed, P.A. The utilization of liquid crystal thermography in the evaluation of temporomandibular dysfunction. *J. Craniomand. Pract.* (1991), 9: 120–128.

21. Gratt, B.M., Sickles, E.A., Graff-Radford, S.B., and Solberg, W.K. Electronic thermography in the diagnosis of atypical odontalgia: A pilot study. *Oral Surg. Oral Med. Oral Pathol. Oral Radiol. Endod.* (1989), 68: 472–481.

22. Gratt, B.M. et al. Electronic thermography in the assessment of internal derangement of the TMJ. *J. Orofacial Pain* (1994), 8: 197–206.

23. Gratt, B.M., Sickles, E.A., Ross, J.B., Wexler, C.E., and Gornbein, J.A. Thermographic assessment of craniomandibular disorders: Diagnostic interpretation versus temperature measurement analysis. *J. Orofacial Pain* (1994), 8: 278–288.

24. Gratt, B.M., Sickles, E.A., and Wexler, C.E. Thermographic characterization of osteoarthrosis of the temporomandibular joint. *J. Orofacial Pain* (1994), 7: 345–353.

25. Progrell, M. A., Erbez, G., Taylor, R.C., and Dodson, T.B. Liquid crystal thermography as a diagnostic aid and objective monitor for TMJ dysfunction and myogenic facial pain. *J. Craniomand. Disord. Facial Oral Pain* (1989), 3: 65–70.

26. Dmutpueva, B.C., and Alekceeva, A.H. Applications of thermography in the evaluation of the postoperative patient. *Stomatologiia* (1986), 12: 29–30 (Russian).

27. Cambell, R.L., Shamaskin, R.G., and Harkins, S.W. Assessment of recovery from injury to inferior alveolar and mental nerves. *Oral Surg. Oral Med. Oral Pathol. Oral Radiol. Endod.* (1987), 64: 519–526.

28. Crandall, C.E. and Hill, R.P. Thermography in dentistry: A pilot study. *Oral Surg. Oral Med. Oral Pathol. Oral Radiol. Endod.* (1966), 21: 316–320.

29. Gratt, B.M., Pullinger, A., and Sickles, E.A. Electronic thermography of normal facial structures: A pilot study. *Oral Surg. Oral Med. Oral Pathol. Oral Radiol. Endod.* (1989), 68: 346–351.

30. Weinstein, S.A., Gelb, M., and Weinstein, E.L. Thermophysiologic anthropometry of the face in homo sapiens. *J. Craniomand. Pract.* (1990), 8: 252–257.

31. Uematsu, S. Symmetry of skin temperature comparing one side of the body to the other. *Thermology* (1985), 1: 4–7.

32. Gratt, B.M. and Sickles, E.A. Electronic facial thermography: An analysis of asymptomatic adult subjects. *J. Orofacial Pain* (1995), 9: 222–265.

33. Blaxter, K. Energy exchange by radiation, convection, conduction and evaporation. In *Energy Metabolism in Animals and Man.* New York: Cambridge University Press (1989), pp. 86–99.

34. Blaxter, K. The minimal metabolism. In *Energy Metabolism in Animals and Man.* New York: Cambridge University Press (1989), 120–146.

35. Gratt, B.M, Graff-Radford, S.B., Shetty, V., Solberg, W.K., and Sickles, E.A. A six-year clinical assessment of electronic facial thermography. *Dentomaxillofac. Radiol.* (1996), 25: 247–255.

36. Gratt, B.M., and Sickles, E.A. Thermographic characterization of the asymptomatic TMJ. *J. Orofacial Pain* (1993), 7: 7–14.

37. Gratt, B.M., Sickles, E.M., and Ross, J.B. Thermographic assessment of craniomandibular disorders: Diagnostic interpretation versus temperature measurement analysis. *J. Orofacial Pain* (1994), 8: 278–288.

38. Canavan, D. and Gratt, B.M. Electronic thermography for the assessment of mild and moderate TMJ dysfunction. *Oral Surg. Oral Med. Oral Pathol. Oral Radiol. Endod.* (1995), 79: 778–786.

39. McBeth, S.A., and Gratt, B.M. A cross-sectional thermographic assessment of TMJ problems in orthodontic patients. *Am. J. Orthod. Dentofac. Orthop.* (1996), 109: 481–488.

40. Gratt, B.M., Shetty, V., Saiar, M., and Sickles, E.A. Electronic thermography for the assessment of inferior alveolar nerve deficit. *Oral Surg. Oral Med. Oral Pathol. Oral Radiol. Endod.* (1995), 80: 153–160.

41. Gratt, B.M., Sickles, E.A., and Shetty, V. Thermography for the clinical assessment of inferior alveolar nerve deficit: A pilot study. *J. Orofacial Pain* (1994), 80: 153–160.

42. Shetty, V., Gratt, B.M., and Flack, V. Thermographic assessment of reversible inferior alveolar nerve deficit. *J. Orofacial Pain* (1994), 8: 375–383.

43. Wood, E.H. Thermography in the diagnosis of cerebrovascular disease: Preliminary report. *Radiology* (1964), 83: 540–546.

44. Wood, E.H. Thermography in the diagnosis of cerebrovascular disease. *Radiology* (1965), 85: 207–215.

45. Steinke, W., Kloetzsch, C., and Hennerici, M. Carotid artery disease assessed by color Doppler sonography and angiography. *AJR* (1990), 154: 1061–1067.

46. Hu, H.-H. et al. Color Doppler imaging of orbital arteries for detection of carotid occlusive disease. *Stroke* (1993), 24: 1196–1202.

47. Carroll, B.A., Graif, M., and Orron, D.E. Vascular ultrasound. In *Peripheral Vascular Imaging and Intervention.* D. Kim and D.E. Orron, Eds., St. Louis, MO, Mosby/Year Book (1992), pp. 211–225.

48. Mawdsley, C., Samuel, E., Sumerling, M.D., and Young, G.B. Thermography in occlusive cerebrovascular diseases. *Br. Med. J.* (1968), 3: 521–524.

49. Capistrant, T.D. and Gumnit, R.J. Thermography and extracranial cerebrovascular disease: A new method to predict the stroke-prone individual. *Minn. Med.* (1971), 54: 689–692.

50. Karpman, H.L., Kalb, I.M., and Sheppard, J.J. The use of thermography in a health care system for stroke. *Geriatrics* (1972), 27: 96–105.

51. Soria, E. and Paroski, M.W. Thermography as a predictor of the more involved side in bilateral carotid disease: Case history. *Angiology* (1987), 38: 151–158.

52. Capistrat, T.D. and Gumnit, R.J. Detecting carotid occlusive disease by thermography. *Stroke* (1973), 4: 57–65.

53. Abernathy, M., Brandt, M.M., and Robinson, C. Noninvasive testing of the carotid system. *Am. Fam. Physic.* (1984), 29: 157–164.

54. Dereymaeker, A., Kams-Cauwe, V., and Fobelets, P. Frontal dynamic thermography: Improvement in diagnosis of carotid stenosis. *Eur. Neurol.* (1978), 17: 226–234.

55. Gratt, B.M., Halse, A., and Hollender, L. A pilot study of facial infrared thermal imaging used as a screening test for detecting elderly individuals at risk for stroke. *Thermol. Int.* (2002), 12: 7–15.

56. Friedlander A.H. and Gratt B.M. Panoramic dental radiography and thermography as an aid in detecting patients at risk for stroke. *J. Oral Maxillofac. Surg.* (1994), 52: 1257–1262.

57. Graff-Radford, S.B., Ketalaer, M.-C., Gratt, B.M., and Solberg, W.K. Thermographic assessment of neuropathic facial pain: A pilot study. *J. Orofacial Pain* (1995), 9: 138–146.

58. Pogrel, M.A., Erbez, G., Taylor, R.C., and Dodson, T.B. Liquid crystal thermography as a diagnostic aid and objective monitor for TMJ dysfunction and myogenic facial pain. *J. Craniobandib. Disord. Facial Oral Pain* (1989), 3: 65–70.

59. Pogrel, M.A., Yen, C.K., and Taylor, R.C. Infrared thermography in oral and maxillo-facial surgery. *Oral Surg. Oral Med. Oral Pathol. Oral Radiol. Endod.* (1989), 67: 126–131.

60. Graff-Radford, S.B., Ketlaer, M.C., Gratt, B.M., and Solberg, W.K. Thermographic assessment of neuropathic facial pain. *J. Orofacial Pain* (1995), 9: 138–146.

61. Biagioni, P.A., Longmore, R.B., McGimpsey, J.G., and Lamey, P.J. Infrared thermography: Its role in dental research with particular reference to craniomandibular disorders. *Dentomaxillofac. Radiol.* (1996), 25: 119–124.

62. Biagioni, P.A., McGimpsey, J.G., and Lamey, P.J. Electronic infrared thermography as a dental research technique. *Br. Dent. J.* (1996), 180: 226–230.

63. Benington, I.C., Biagioni, P.A., Crossey, P.J., Hussey, D.L., Sheridan, S., and Lamel, P.J. Temperature changes in bovine mandibular bone during implant site preparation: An assessment using infra-red thermography. *J. Dent.* (1996), 24: 263–267.

64. Anbar, M. Clinical applications of dynamic area telethermography. In *Quantitative Dynamic Telthermography in Medical Diagnosis*. Boca Raton, FL: CRC Press, 1994, pp. 147–180.

65. Anbar, M. Dynamic area telethermography and its clinical applications. *SPIE Proc.* (1995), 2473: 3121–3323.

66. Anbar M., Grenn, M.W., Marino, M.T., Milescu, L., and Zamani, K. Fast dynamic area telethermography (DAT) of the human forearm with a Ga/As quantum well infrared focal plane array camera. *Eur. J. Therol.* (1997), 7: 105–118.

51

Laser Infrared Thermography of Biological Tissues

Alexander Sviridov

Institute for Laser and Information Technologies of Russian Academy of Sciences

Andrey Kondyurin

Institute for Laser and Information Technologies of Russian Academy of Sciences

51.1 Introduction

Laser infrared (IR) thermography of biological tissues is a part of active dynamic thermal (ADT) imaging [1], initially developed for noninvasive remote control of materials [2]. It involves heating of a material by some source of energy at controlled conditions and recording of time-dependent, and nonuniform temperature field on a sample surface by thermal imaging camera. Mathematical analysis of the induced temperature field with adequate modeling allows one to assess the physicochemical processes in the material and its characteristics.

Microwaves, ultrasound devices, xenon lamps, and lasers are commonly used as sources of energy for heating of biological tissues. Laser sources have a number of advantages over alternative heating modalities. A light, emitted by commercial lasers, covers a wide spectral range—from ultraviolet to far IR. It allows one to provide desired penetration depths of a laser beam into tissues ranging from a few microns to about 10 cm. The range of light penetration depths in the tissue may be sufficient to analyze thermally induced processes, to control blood circulation, or for thermal tomography. Modern laser sources become compact and relatively cheap. They are often supplied with a processor-based control of output power, allowing to build a computerized laser system with feedback channels. The spatial profile of a laser beam could be precisely managed by optical elements, such as lenses, axicons, optical fibers, or by fast programmable scanning of a narrow beam on a sample surface. It allows one to generate the required temperature field by spatial and temporal control of laser energy supply into the biological tissue.

Development of systems providing the desired laser heating of a given area of biological tissue with IR radiometric feedback control has a practical significance for medical usages such as laser-induced thermolysis and hyperthermia of malignant tissues [3]. The most important problem to solve is the creation of a programmable temperature field in the given spatial and temporal limits with a laser beam of an appropriate intensity profile. Despite many efforts, of different scientific groups, this problem is not yet solved [4]. In fact, laser intensity distribution should be repeatedly corrected during heating procedure depending on the discrepancy between measured and specified temperature fields. Optimal parameters of the feedback system providing minimal discrepancy may be determined from the modeling of three-dimensional (3D) temperature field induced in the tissue by such laser heating taking into account the accuracy of used devices. To be accurate, such models require information about optical and thermophysical properties of tissues, and their temperature behavior which may be determined by using a similar system with an adequate algorithm for solving the inverse thermal problem.

Programmable laser heating of a local area of the biological tissue with IR thermography of surface temperature field may also be used to control thermal processes, stimulated in the tissue. The first approach involves measurements of volume rate and vector of energy dissipation due to blood flow. The controlled parameters may include dynamics of full temperature field on the tissue surface and laser power, when a chosen local region is heated with a given rate (constant, harmonically, or isothermally). By solving numerically a bio-heat transfer equation with perfusion terms, one could evaluate volume rate and the direction of blood flow in the region of interest. Another potential application of programmable laser heating is a remote calorimetry of the processes such as thermally induced chemical reaction and phase transformation of biological tissue components. Such problems can be important in cases of hyperthermia or in thermoplastics of biological tissues.

In some applications, light-emitting diodes (LED) could also be considered as an excitation source for IR thermography of biological tissues and in many respects they are similar to lasers. Therefore, the term "laser" in the title of this chapter should be considered more generally to include photodiodes, as a heating source. Using LEDs instead of laser systems allow for making an excitation system for IR thermography that is more compact and cheap. However, solving the choice between various excitation sources is determined by specific and technical requirements for a control system.

51.2 Programmable Laser Heating of Biological Tissues

A general scheme of the laser system with IR radiometric feedback control for programmable heating of biological tissues and measurement of optical and thermophysical parameters is presented in Figure 51.1.

The laser output power is controlled by a laser internal processor or a programmable external power supply, an actuator which manages the laser beam shape or beam position on the object surface. According to computer commands, IR camera controls the temperature field of the object surface, the data of IR camera are transmitted to the computer, and digitally processed to provide the control data for the actuators of optical system and laser power.

Let us consider a problem of programmable laser heating of a local region of the biological tissue with IR thermography as feedback control. The typical approach for such a type of problem which is widely used in industrial systems is the so-called three-term control, that is, control of the proportional,

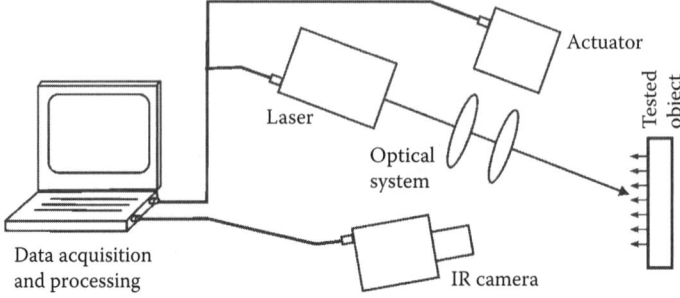

FIGURE 51.1 Block scheme of a laser system with thermovision camera as a feedback control detector.

integral, and derivative values, denoted as *P*, *I*, and *D*, respectively. The weighted sum of these three parameters determines the response of the feedback system to the difference between measured and programmed temperatures at a given point of time. It takes into account the past temperature dynamics, the current temperature, and the rate of temperature change at the current time. Typically, correction of power is performed with some permanent frequency. Depending on the weights of *P*, *I*, and *D* values, one could obtain different temperature time profiles in the region of interest and variations in the laser power, as well. Our goal is to find the optimal set of *P*, *I*, and *D* values to provide a minimal error between measured and programmed temperatures during a whole period of laser operation, also controlling the variations in the laser power. These values are determined by laser beam parameters, as well as thermophysical and optical characteristics of the sample.

To realize this procedure, let us solve a direct heat conduction problem for a laser-heated sample of a biological tissue under the three-term (PID) control operation. It means that the power of laser will be changed with time as follows:

$$P(t) = K_c e(t) + \frac{K_c}{T_i} \int_0^t e(t) \cdot dt - K_c \cdot T_d \frac{de(t)}{dt} + \sigma_P \cdot \text{NRD}, \tag{51.1}$$

where *e(t)* is the difference between measured temperature in the local region (*ValuePoint*) and programmed temperature (*SetPoint*), K_c, K_c/T_i, and $K_c \cdot T_d$ are linearly proportional, integrative and derivative weights, respectively, σ_p is the error of laser power level, a zero-mean normal random distribution (NRD) with a standard deviation of 1. In cylindrical coordinate system, the differential equation to be solved is

$$\frac{\partial T}{\partial t} = \frac{\chi}{r} \frac{\partial}{\partial r}\left(r \frac{\partial T}{\partial r}\right) + \chi \frac{\partial^2 T}{\partial z^2} + f(r,z,t), \tag{51.2}$$

where *z* axis is perpendicular to the sample surface (*z* = 0), *r* is the radial coordinate, *f(r,z,t)* is the heat source function, determined by light absorption. Initial temperature distribution is assumed to be uniform and equal to the room temperature:

$$T(r,z,t = 0) = T_0 \tag{51.3}$$

According to the Newton's law for forced and free convection between the sample and environment, the following conditions were set at the sample boundary:

$$-\chi \frac{\partial T(r,Z,t)}{\partial z}\bigg|_{z=Z} = \beta \cdot T(r,Z,t) - \mu, -\chi \frac{\partial T(R,z,t)}{\partial r}\bigg|_{r=R} = \beta \cdot T(R,z,t) - \mu, \lim_{r \to 0}\left(r\chi \frac{\partial T}{\partial r}\right) = 0, \tag{51.4}$$

where $\beta = h\rho C_p$, $\mu = \beta T_0$, ρ is density, C_p is specific heat, *h* is convective heat transfer coefficient (W mm^{-2} K^{-1}), and *R*, *Z* are radius and thickness of the sample, respectively. The value of *h* was chosen according to the published data [5]. Parameters χ, α, and C_p are assumed to be independent from the temperature, coordinates, and time.

At first approximation, the radiation intensity inside the sample is described by Beer law. Correspondingly, for light beams with Gaussian energy distribution, the function *f(r,z,t)* has been obtained as

$$f(r,z,t) = \left(1 - R_d\right) \frac{\alpha P(t)}{C_p \rho \cdot \pi W_L^2} \exp\left(-2 \cdot \left(\frac{r}{W_L}\right)^2\right) \exp(-\alpha z), \tag{51.5}$$

where α is the total attenuation coefficient (cm^{-1}), W_L is the laser beam radius (mm). ρC_p is the specific heat of a unit volume (J/(cm^3 K)), ρ is the density (g/cm^3), t_{imp} is the laser pulse duration (s), E_0 is the light intensity (W/cm^2), W_L is the laser beam radius (mm), and R_d is the dimensionless diffuse reflectance (for the case of cartilage it was measured earlier with an integrating sphere, $R_d = 0.10$ at $\lambda = 1.56$ μm) [6]. The spatial distribution of the laser radiation power density in an absorbing optically inhomogeneous medium is determined by three optical parameters—absorption, scattering coefficients, and scattering anisotropy. Though, strictly speaking, variations of the intensity are not described by the Beer law, the use of the exponential law with a certain generalized index of exponent α to describe the term heat source in an optically inhomogeneous absorbing medium, such as tissues, seems quite reasonable [7]. We refer to this exponent as the total attenuation coefficient.

The induced temperature field was computed using the finite difference method. An implicit difference scheme was constructed that approximates the heat conduction as Equation 51.2 and boundary conditions (Equation 51.4). In the region of continuous variation of coordinates r from 0 to R and z and from 0 to Z, a uniform grid of $I \times J$ elements with a step of $\Delta r = \Delta z = 0.01$ mm was set. Grid functions $T(r_i, z_j, t_m) = T(i, j, m)$ and $f(r_i, z_j, t_m) = \phi(i, j, m)$ were put into correspondence with functions $T(r, z, t)$ and $f(r, z, t)$. Differential equation (Equation 51.1) and boundary conditions (3) are replaced by the difference in analogs [8]. The laser power at a moment m was calculated according to the PID control:

$$P(m) = K_c\left(e(m) + \frac{1}{T_i} \sum_1^m \frac{e(m-1) + e(m)}{2} \Delta t - T_d \frac{e(m) - e(m-1)}{\Delta t} \right), \qquad (51.6)$$

where $e(m)$ was determined as difference $e(m) = \text{SetPoint}(m) - \text{ValuePoint}(m)$. An error of temperature measurement was taken into account to determine the *ValuePoint*(m): ValuePoint$(m) = \sigma_T \cdot \text{NRD} + u(i_0, j_0, m)$. Here, $u(i_0, j_0, m)$ is the real temperature in the control point (i_0, j_0), σ_T is the error of temperature measurement with thermovision camera ($\sigma_T = 0.05°$C).

The set of optimal PID parameters K_c, T_i, and T_d was found from the solution of the inverse problem, based on minimization of the cumulative square error:

$$\sum_1^M e^2\left(m; K_c, T_i, T_c\right) \to \min_{K_c, T_i, T_c} \qquad (51.7)$$

It was performed with the modified Levenberg–Marquard algorithm [9,10]. The influence of laser beam geometric parameters (W_L), thermophysical characteristics of the tissue (χ, ρC_p), effective attenuation coefficient (α), convective heat transfer coefficient (h) on K_c, T_i, and T_d were studied. A number of calculations for different sets of varied parameters were performed. From Equation 51.5 for $f(r,z,t)$, we assume that the coefficient K_c depends mainly on the combination of the listed parameters, namely:

$$K_c = B_{Kc} \cdot \frac{\rho C_p \pi W_L^2}{\alpha}, \qquad (51.8)$$

where B_{Kc} is phenomenological constant to be determined. A number of calculations of laser heating of the sample with the constant rate at $z = 0$, $r = 0$ substantiated this suggestion if χ, ρC_p, and α are varied in the ranges 0.1–0.2 mm^2/s, 2.5–3.5 J/cm^3/K, and 7.5–15 cm^{-1}, respectively. Calculations have shown that optimal values of T_i are independent of ρC_p and α, as well as the optimal value of T_d is equal to zero for all ρC_p and α. Our analysis also has shown that the variation of h in rather a wide range does not affect the parameters of PID controller. However, B_{Kc} and T_i depend on the heating rate. The data on optimal B_{Kc} and T_i, that is, providing minimal cumulative square error of temperature at laser heating of the local area $z = 0$ and $r = 0$ with constant heating rate are presented in Table 51.1.

TABLE 51.1   Values of B_{Kc} and T_i at Different Heating Rates

Heating Rate (°C/s)	$B_{Kc} \times 10^3$ (s^{-1})	T_i (s)
0.1	2.0	1.46
0.3	3.2	0.84
0.4	4.0	0.69
0.5	4.6	0.58
1.0	5.5	0.52
3.0	9.2	0.31
5.0	12.1	0.26

Similarly, the optimal PID parameters that satisfy condition (Equation 51.7) could be found for any heating scenario of a given local region of the sample. Among them harmonic and isothermal scenarios are more interesting for medical diagnostics and treatment. Significance of PID parameters and its optimization is clearly seen from Figures 51.2 and 51.3, presenting the behavior of temperature and laser power as a function of time with nonoptimal and optimal PID parameters. In the case of nonoptimal PID parameters, the temperature curve has some ripples with amplitudes of ~2°C around the straight line (see Figure 51.2a). On the other hand, the temporal behavior of laser power (Figure 51.2b) looks preferably random. Actually it does not allow the use of power as a measured parameter for control. On the contrary, optimal PID parameters provide stable and smooth behavior both for the temperature and the laser power (see Figure 51.3a,b), making laser thermography a promising tool for control of thermal processes in biological tissues and other materials.

Figure 51.4a demonstrates an experimental realization of programmable laser heating of cartilage by glass Erbium-doped fiber laser illuminating at $\lambda = 1.56$ μm (IRE Polus, Moscow, Russia) with a constant

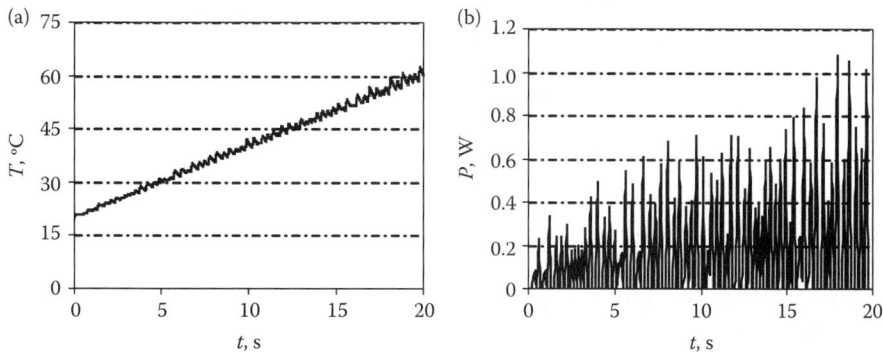

FIGURE 51.2   Temporal behavior of nonoptimal PID parameters: (a) temperature and (b) laser power.

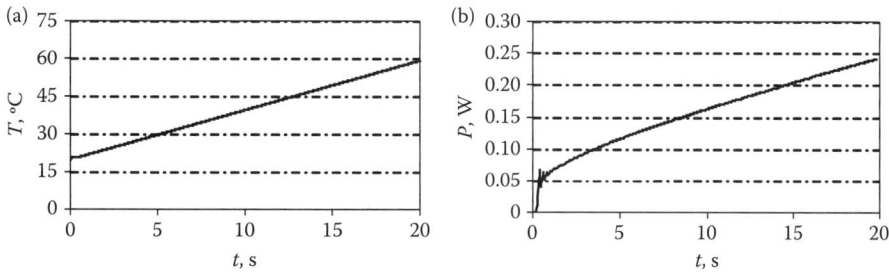

FIGURE 51.3   Temporal behavior of optimal PID parameters: (a) temperature and (b) laser power.

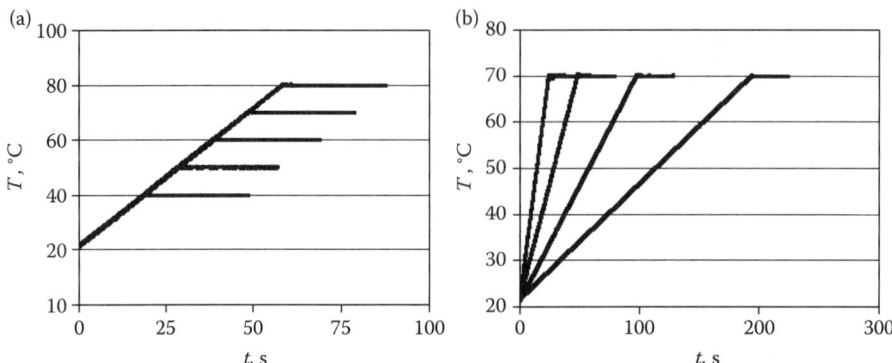

FIGURE 51.4 Examples of experimental realization of programmable laser heating of the cartilage with a given constant rate (1°C/s) up to different temperatures: (a) keeping the rate constant and with different rates up to given temperature (70°C) and (b) keeping the temperature constant.

rate (1°C/s) attaining different temperatures and keeping them at a constant level. Similarly, Figure 51.4b demonstrates regimes of programmable laser heating with different rates attaining 70°C and keeping it at constant level. Temperature control was performed with IR thermograph IRTIS-200 (IRTIS, Moscow, Russia).

51.3 Laser Thermography for Control of Energetic Processes

Successive realization of programmable laser heating with thermal control gave a key for the development of remote calorimetry of energetic processes in open thermodynamic systems. Applying it to biological materials and tissues allows one to implement noninvasive measures of the enthalpy of phase transformation or energetic reactions. The idea is based on the registration of laser power temporal function which may be considered as an analog of heat quantity curve in classical thermal analysis such as differential scanning calorimetry (DSC). Thermophysical processes in biological tissues heated by a laser with constant rate should result in compensation of consumption or release of heat by appropriate correction of laser power. Thus, the nonmonotonic temporal behavior of laser power could become an indicator of energetic processes. The dynamics of temperature field in the full area of sample surface in combination with the power dynamics could be an additional indicator of thermal process. To estimate the sensitivity of laser calorimetry let us consider a programmable laser constant rate heating of the sample with optimal parameters of PID controller at the condition of tentative thermal chemical reaction A → B of first order with given Arrhenius parameters and different enthalpies. In such a statement, the direct problem of temperature field may be solved just by adding the term appropriate energy density on the right side of Equation 51.2 with its subsequent application of the approach described previously:

$$\frac{\partial T}{\partial t} = \frac{\chi}{r}\frac{\partial}{\partial r}\left(r\frac{\partial T}{\partial r}\right) + \chi\frac{\partial^2 T}{\partial z^2} + f(r,z,t) + g(T,r,z,t),\tag{51.9}$$

$$g(r,z,t) = \frac{\Delta_r H}{\rho C_p}\frac{d\xi}{dt}.\tag{51.10}$$

Here, $\Delta_r H$—specific enthalpy of chemical reaction (J/g), ξ—is the factor of substance A conversion in A → B reaction ($\xi = 0$ before reaction, $\xi = 1$ after reaction), and

$$\frac{d\xi}{dt} = k_0 \cdot \exp\left(-\frac{E_a}{RT}\right) \cdot (1 - \xi) \tag{51.11}$$

For numerical computation of the temperature field $u(i,j,m)$ at every node of spatial–temporal grid, it is necessary to express $g(r,z,t)$ by its grid analogs of differential finite increments:

$$\gamma(i,j,m) = \frac{\Delta_r H}{C_p \rho} \frac{\Delta \xi}{\Delta t} = \frac{\Delta_r H}{C_p \rho} \frac{\left(\xi(i,j,m) - \xi(i,j,m-1)\right)}{\Delta t} \tag{51.12}$$

By integrating Equation 51.11 and making a series of algebraic transformations, one could find the following analytical formulas:

$$\gamma(i,j,m) = \frac{\Delta_r H}{C_p \rho \Delta t}\left(-\exp\left[-I\left(u(i,j,m)\right)\right] + \exp\left[-I\left(u(i,j,m-1)\right)\right]\right), \tag{51.13}$$

where

$$I\left(u(i,j,m)\right) = \left(0.5 k_0 \sum_1^m \left(\exp\left(-\frac{E_a}{R \cdot u(i,j,m-1)}\right) + \exp\left(-\frac{E_a}{R \cdot u(i,j,m)}\right)\right)\Delta t\right). \tag{51.14}$$

Notice, as a first result of temperature field calculations, the feedback control system with laser thermography possesses high stability at optimal PID parameters providing constant heating rate by a smooth correction of laser power despite the occurrence of thermal energetic processes. Figure 51.5 demonstrates laser power variations as a function of time at programmable laser heating of a local area of the sample ($r = 0$, $z = 0$) with the Gaussian light beam ($W_L = 4$ mm, $\lambda = 1.56$ μm) under the condition of a tentative endothermic chemical reaction of first order for different enthalpies. The scattering in the power data is due to an intrinsic error of temperature measurement by thermovision camera (0.1°C) and an error of the power control (10 mJ) by laser actuator. One could see bell-shaped curves of laser power which more distinctly manifested as enthalpy increases. As a criterion of minimal enthalpy

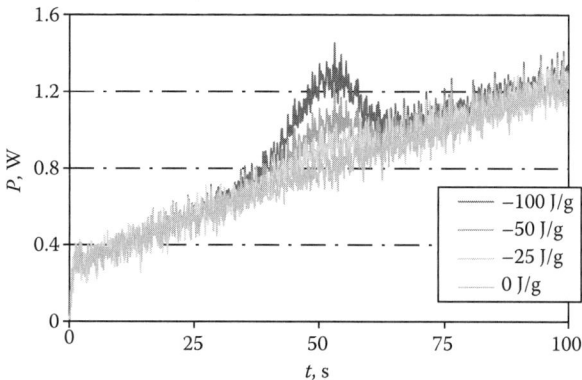

FIGURE 51.5 Temporal behavior of laser power as a function of enthalpy of tentative first-order reaction with Arrhenius-type reaction rate being constant during heating of the local area of the sample with a constant rate 1°C/s. The laser beam has Gaussian intensity distribution $W_L = 4$ mm; $\chi = 0.125$ mm²/s; $\rho C_p = 3.5$ J cm³/°C; $\alpha = 10$ cm⁻¹.

measurement, we have chosen the double standard error excess of the power curve which is caused by correction of energetic processes. In this respect the sensitivity of the presented system to the enthalpy is about 25 J/g. This value is rather large, comparing with a sensitivity of the classical DSC (~1–5 J/g). Note that sensitivity of enthalpy measurement with laser thermography may be substantially improved by increasing the accuracy of temperature measurement and laser power control, as well as by improved data processing. A more sophisticated heating mode and an analysis of laser-induced temperature field can potentially increase sensitivity.

51.4 Laser Thermography for Measurements of Optical and Thermophysical Parameters

Since its emergence in the early 1980s, photothermal radiometry (PTR) has become a very powerful tool for the thermophysical characterization and nondestructive evaluation of broad classes of materials [11–14], including homogeneous materials [15] and layered and/or buried structures [16]. This method combines laser heating and radiometric measurement of the sample surface temperature, making it a natural extension of laser thermography.

PTR is based on the fact that the surface temperature temporal variations, measured by the thermovision camera, are determined by the thermal and optical properties of the material that is being heated locally by the laser. To process experimental thermographic data and to calculate the thermal, and optical parameters, the heat conduction equation should be solved. It includes thermal diffusivity Equation 51.2 with the term heat-source (Equation 51.5), characterizing the rate of temperature increase in the irradiated zone. On the one hand, the term heat-source is defined by the radiation characteristics, that is, the wavelength, exposure power, and duration, and, on the other hand, by optical parameters of the medium, that is, the effective absorption coefficient. Hence, it is the set of optical and thermal parameters that define the temperature response of a biomaterial to laser exposure.

Usually, the effect of optical parameters is eliminated by choosing the appropriate laser wavelength in accordance with the absorption spectrum of basic chromophores of the material. The idea is to provide conditions at which penetration depth is much smaller than laser beam diameter. In this case, the temporal variations of the temperature field are defined only by thermal parameters and the temperature evaluation is reduced by comparing the radiometric signal upon laser heating with the theoretically calculated temperature profiles [15,17].

There exist two basic types of time-dependent methods to measure thermal diffusivity: (1) the transient method and (2) the periodic heat flow method. In the former method, a sample is irradiated with a laser pulse and then the temperature evolution is monitored [18,19]. The thermal diffusivity calculation is based on the integral equation expressing the time dependence of the radiometric image $\Delta M(x,y,t)$ by means of the initial 3D distribution of the temperature induced by short laser pulses. Since the pulse duration is <500 ms, the initial 3D temperature distribution can be represented by the product of two independent components, that is, lateral $T(x,y,t = 0)$ and longitudinal $T(z,t = 0)$. In this case, the radiometric image $\Delta M(x,y,t_2)$ at a point of time t_2 is expressed as a convolution of a specific point spread function $K_r(\Delta t = t_2 - t_1)$ depending on χ and the radiometric image $\Delta M(x,y,t_1)$ recorded earlier. Using the Levenberg–Marquardt algorithm to compare a pair of radiometric images, we determine K_r and calculate the thermal diffusivity χ.

In periodic heat-flow method [20–22] a sample of known thickness is irradiated with a harmonic-modulated laser beam launching a thermal wave and the periodic temperature at the front or the back surface of the sample is monitored at several modulation frequencies f. The frequency-dependent thermal diffusion length ν is given by

$$\nu = \sqrt{\frac{\chi}{\pi f}} \tag{51.15}$$

It is related to the phase shift of the detected temperature wave with respect to the heating source which may be monitored using a lock-in amplifier. The Fourier transform is applied to the measured temperature function, which allows the use of amplitude and phase characteristics instead of temporal characteristics.

Very recently PTR was extended to study the thermal and optical parameters simultaneously. In this work [21], thermal radiometry was applied to characterize both the thermal and optical properties of biomaterials. The dependence of the amplitude and phase on the modulated laser radiation frequency was used to measure the thermal diffusivity $e = (\lambda \rho C_p)^{1/2}$ and the so-called "initial heating coefficient" $g = \mu_{eff}/(\rho C_p)$ where μ_{eff} is the total attenuation coefficient, ρ is the density, and C_p is the specific heat. However, using this method it is impossible to individually and independently determine each of these parameters.

In the paper [23], the noncontact technique to evaluate the thermal and optical properties of biological tissues and materials has been developed. The method is based on a combination of PTR and the solution of the inverse heat conduction problem by the finite difference method. Numerical solution of the heat conduction equation allows rigorous consideration of the heat source distribution over the entire sample volume, which makes it possible to measure the total attenuation coefficient μ_{eff}, characterizing the optical properties of a biomaterial along with the thermal diffusivity χ and specific heat ρC_p.

The calculation of the 3D temperature field induced by IR laser radiation is based on the solution of the classical heat conduction equation, expressed in the cylindrical coordinates, see Equation 51.2.

It has been assumed that the variation of the radiation intensity inside the sample is described by the Beer law; the function $f(r,z,t)$ has been obtained for the light beams with a Gaussian energy distribution (Equation 51.5). The temperature distribution over the sample at the initial time was taken as uniform and equal to the ambient medium temperature T_0. Boundary conditions (Equation 51.4) at the sample surface have been used. The forward heat problem has been solved by the finite-difference method. Similar to Section 51.2, an implicit difference scheme to approximate the heat conduction equation and boundary conditions has been constructed. The determination of the parameters in question ($\chi, \rho C_p, \mu_{eff}$) is reduced to conventional minimization of the squares of deviations of the calculated radiometric temperatures from the experimental:

$$\text{SSE}\left(\chi, \rho C_p, \mu_{eff}\right) = \sum_{l=1}^{L} \sum_{m=1}^{M} \left[u_{exp}\left(r_l, t_m\right) - u_{calc}\left(r_l, t_m; \chi, \rho C_p, \alpha\right) \right]^2, \tag{51.16}$$

where $u_{exp}(r_l, t_m)$ and $u_{calc}(r_l, t_m)$ are respectively, temperatures at the point r_l on the sample surface at the moment t, as measured by the thermovision camera and calculated theoretically.

A temporal series of one-dimensional temperature distributions measured on the back surface of the sample was used in calculations, see Figure 51.6a. We have used Erbium glass laser $\lambda = 1.56 \, \mu m$ with maximal emitting power of 5 W in our experiments. During one laser pulse, the observed temperature increase was up to 6°C. The rate and the shape of the rising temperature front will depend on the distance to the center of the laser beam (Figure 51.6b). The temperature field variations have been recorded as a matrix u_{exp} with size $L \times M$, where L is the number of points with different coordinates r and M is the number of points along the time axis during laser pulse t_{imp}, and some time after the laser is turned off, a substantive cooling of the heated region occurs. The temperature increase at the stage of laser heating depends mostly on the total absorption coefficient α and specific heat ρC_p, while during the cooling phase the temperature is mostly determined by the thermal diffusivity χ. In fact, reliable and accurate measurements of all these parameters proved to be possible, using a few laser pulses and thermovision recordings of the full temperature field induced on the sample surface.

An optimal technique for determining thermal properties should provide both proper accuracy and acceptable speed of calculation. The former depends on both the measurement accuracy of the

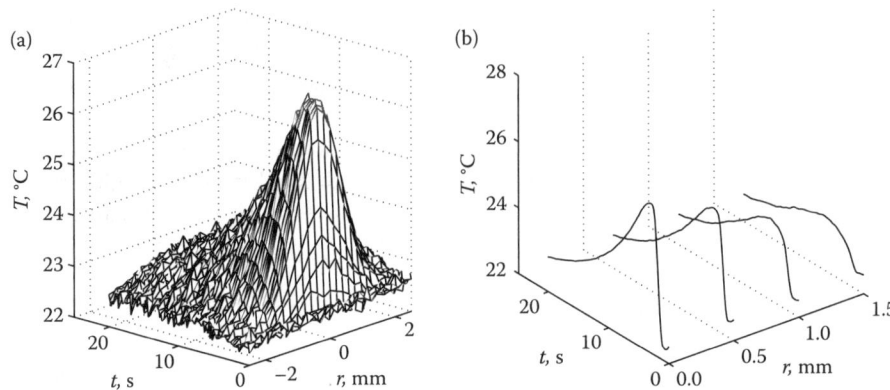

FIGURE 51.6   (a) Variations of the temperature field on the sample surface and (b) examples of temporal profiles of the surface temperature at different distances from the center of the irradiated region.

temperature field and the conditionality of their calculation model [24]. It is necessary to estimate the fraction of the experimental data set that carries the necessary sufficient data for determining all parameters χ, ρC_p, and α with satisfactory accuracy, while keeping the computation time reasonably small. An important stage of testing the technique is also to study the sensitivity of the calculated parameters to the temperature field parameters h and E_0 in the model, which can be a source of certain systematic errors.

The size of the experimental data set is defined by two quantities: L, that is, the number of points of different coordinates r, and M, that is, the number of points along the time axis. To calculate the desired parameters, it is reasonable to use the time dependence of the temperature for points arranged near the center of the irradiated region, since the temperature reaches the maximum exactly in this region (Figure 51.6b). In this case, it is sufficient to use the time dependence of the temperature only for several points from the irradiated region. For these points, the temperature change is several times larger than the temperature measurement error. Quantity L does not affect the calculation time of χ, ρC_p, and α, since the temperature field variations are calculated for the entire sample which is independent of L.

However, the accuracy and computation time of χ, ρC_p, and α depend strongly on the quantity M. The choice of the optimum value of M for calculating the desired parameters consists of three stages [24]:

1. Analysis of the dependences of χ, ρC_p, and α on M;
2. Estimation of the significance of each parameter at various M;
3. Estimation of the accuracy and time for calculating a parameter depending on M.

In addition to the accuracy, quantity M defines the computation time of the desired parameters, which monotonically increases with M. This is because it is necessary to calculate the temperature field variations up to a time point, corresponding to the value of M at each iteration. Thus, computation time of the temperature field variations R_{calc} increases monotonically with M, resulting in an increase of the entire calculation time.

Some arbitrariness in choosing the loss factor h during heat exchange with an ambient medium, which is built into the model for calculating the temperature field variations, is a factor controlling the systematic error of χ, ρC_p, and α measurements. According to the published data, the value of factor h, corresponding to free convection, can differ several times (from 5 to 50 W mm^{-2} K^{-1}) [5]. Therefore, we must determine the sensitivity of the calculated parameters to this parameter. In the paper [23], it has been shown that the dependence of the calculated parameters χ, ρC_p, and α on h can be disregarded if some reasonable value of h, for example, $h = 25$ W mm^{-2} K^{-1} is assumed. It has also been found that optimal M is equal to about 700, providing accuracy of χ, ρC_p, and α measurements in the vicinity of 5%, while $L = 10$.

The error in measurements of the laser radiation intensity E_0 could be the main source of a systematic error in calculating ρC_p, because the quantities E_0 and ρC_p are not independent. In other words, at the same minimum sum of squares error SSE, depending on the value of E_0, one could find the corresponding value of the varied parameter ρC_p. To estimate this factor, it is recommended that the specific heat is to be measured by an independent method such as DSC.

51.5 Tissue-Equivalent Phantoms for Simulation of the Laser-Induced Temperature Fields

Artificial materials, imitating individual physicochemical properties of biological tissues, are more often used to simulate a response caused by various physical interactions. These materials are stable, convenient in applications, allow one to control doses easily and interaction regimes, and simplify the development and tests of the diagnostic medical equipment considerably. Depending on the type of interaction, it is necessary to reproduce various physical properties of biological tissues. At present many phantoms are developed and used to imitate the optical [25–27], acoustic [26–28], electric [29–31], and thermal [29,30,32] properties of biological tissues.

Special interest is of equivalents of biological tissues used to simulate laser-induced heating of tissues. In particular, a moderate heating of biological tissues by laser radiation up to 70–80°C is used for cartilage shaping [33–35], stimulation of regenerative processes, and hyperthermia of malignant tumors. To achieve the therapeutic effect, the temperature field should be reproduced in strictly specified temporal and spatial limits. The spatiotemporal temperature distribution in a biological tissue is determined by the parameters of laser radiation and the absorption, and scattering coefficients specific to heat and thermal diffusivity of the tissue. It is obvious that materials with optical and thermal properties similar to those of biological tissues can be used as their equivalents for simulating laser-induced heating. It is important that all possible thermal and chemical processes would not considerably distort the temperature field and preserve the phase stability.

In the paper [36], the equivalent of biological tissues for simulating temperature fields induced by laser radiation ($\lambda=$) has been developed. The major chromophore, responsible for radiation absorption by biological tissues at wavelength 1.56 µm is water (70–80%). It makes various hydrogels the most convenient basis for obtaining the required tissue equivalent. In the literature different gels were suggested—agar [37], agarose [38], gelatin [39], and polyacrylamide (PAA) hydrogels [29–31]. However, most of these hydrogels easily melt after relatively small heating. Only the PAA hydrogel keeps its elasticity under heating, which makes it possible to synthesize samples of various shapes and to introduce probes and thermocouples into PAA. By synthesizing PAA gels with different monomer concentrations and different degrees of cross-linking, we can obtain a material with thermal and optical properties similar to those of a cartilage tissue.

PAA hydrogels can be easily synthesized by radical copolymerization of acrylamide and N,N'-methylenebisacrylamide in the presence of catalytic amounts of ammonium persulfate and N,N,N',N'-tetramethylethylenediamine [40]. Acrylamide and N,N'-methylenebisacrylamide should be dissolved in distilled water. Then a catalytic amount of $(NH_4)_2S_2O_8$ and N,N,N',N'-tetramethyethylenediamine should be added. At the end of the reaction, the vessel is cooled and hermetically sealed to prevent the evaporation of water.

There are two parameters, which define composition and consequently thermal and optical properties of the PAA hydrogel. The first parameter is the mass content of water in hydrogel. If water is the main absorber of laser radiation, the absorption coefficient of the hydrogel will be proportional to the mass content of water in the hydrogel. The second parameter is the degree of cross-linking, which is equal to the ratio of the initial amounts of N,N'-methylenebisacrylamide and acrylamide and define the value of the scattering coefficient of the hydrogel. PAA hydrogels with water content from 90% to 75% with a degree of cross-linking from 1:9 to 1:24 can be synthesized by the earlier method. On the one hand, the choice of the concentration interval of PAA gels is limited, by the limiting solubility of initial reagents in water, which prevented the preparation of gels with a lower water content, and on the other, by the limiting concentration of initial reagent in water below which gels could not be synthesized.

The thermal analysis of samples performed by the method of DSC shows that the thermal behavior of PAA hydrogels in the temperature range from 25°C to 80°C is stable, and no significant power-consuming processes that could potentially distort the temperature field upon laser heating of the samples, is observed.

51.6 Summary

Feedback control systems combined with a laser as a source of heating, IR radiometer as temperature sensors and PID controller, evaluating and controlling the laser power at a given time could provide programmable heating of the local region of biological tissues with desired temperature variations. Optimal parameters of PID controller could be found by numerically solving a problem of the sample heating under laser radiation. The power of laser is determined by the PID controller to provide minimal integrative error between the current and prescribed temperatures at a given sample area. These errors depend on the optical and thermophysical characteristics of the tissue as well as on the radius of the laser beam. Optimized PID controller provides a smooth and almost linear behavior of the laser power as a function of time when realizing heating of the local sample area with constant rate. Laser power would manifest nonmonotonic behavior if energetic processes are induced in the tissue to compensate its energy consumption/release while the temperature increases linearly. Scattering of laser power data regulated by the PID controller is mainly determined by the errors of temperature measurement by the thermal camera and accuracy of laser power adjustment when performing PID controller commands. Programmable laser heating of tissues could be used to control enthalpies of energetic thermal processes induced in the tissue by the laser.

IR thermography of the temperature field of the tissue surface during postlaser heating allows to express the remote measurement of its total attenuation coefficient, specific heat, and thermal diffusivity simultaneously. The duration of such procedure could be just 10 s while the increment of tissue temperature could be 3–5°C. Since effective thermal diffusivity is strongly related with blood and its volumetric circulation, its measurement may be used for *in vivo* diagnostics of the blood perfusion.

PAA hydrogels may be quite convenient as tissue equivalents to simulate temperature fields induced by the laser radiation in biological tissues as diagnostic and treatment procedures, allowing one to vary the light absorption coefficient by changes in water and organic ratio and light scattering coefficient by changing the concentration of the cross-linking agent. It can also be applied for the calibration of medical devices, based on the interaction of laser light with biological tissues and materials. Laser thermography is proposed to be used as a method to express the characterization of optical and thermophysical properties of such tissue equivalents. Recently, optical and thermophysical equivalents of the cartilage have been developed on the basis of this approach.

References

1. Nowakowski A. (2006). Quantitative dynamic thermal IR-imaging and thermal tomography in medical diagnostic. *Medical Devices and Systems*. Bronzino J. D., Ed. Boca Raton, FL, CRC Press: 22-21-30.
2. Maldague X. P. V. (2001). *Theory and Practice of Infrared Technology for Nondestructive Testing*. New York, J. Wiley & Sons.
3. Zhou J., Chen J. K., Zhang Y. (2010). Simulation of laser-induced thermotherapy using a dual-reciprocity boundary element model with dynamic tissue properties *IEEE Trans. Biomed. Eng.*, 57(2): 238–245.

4. Cheng K.-S., Dewhirst M. W., Stauffer P. F., Das S. (2010). Mathematical formulation and analysis of the nonlinear system reconstruction of the on-line image-guided adaptive control of hyperthermia. *Med. Phys.*, 37(3): 980–994.

5. Orr C. S., Eberhart R. C. (1995). Overview of bioheat transfer. *Optical–Thermal Response of Laser-Irradiated Tissue*. Welch A. J. and van Gemert M. J. C., Ed. New York, Plenum Press, 367–383.

6. Bagratashvili V. N., Bagratashvili N. V., Gapontsev P. V., Makhmutova G. S., Minaev V. P., Omelchenko A. I., Samartsev I. E., Sviridov A. P., Sobol E. N., Tsypina S. I. (1996). Change in the optical properties of hyaline cartilage heated by near-IR laser radiation. *Quantum Electron.*, 31(6): 534–538.

7. Jacques S. L. (1998). Light distributions from point, line and plane sources for photochemical reactions and fluorescence in turbid biological tissues. *Photochem. Photobiol.*, 67(1): 23–32.

8. Samarskii A.A. (1971). *Introduction to the Theory of Differential Schemes*. Moscow, Nauka (in Russian).

9. Marquardt D. W. (1963). An algorithm for least-square estimation of nonlinear parameters. *J. Soc. Indus. Appl. Math.*, 11(2): 431–441.

10. More J. J. (1977). The Levenberg–Marquardt algorithm: Implementation and theory. *Numerical Analysis. Lecture Notes in Mathematics*, Springer. 630: 105–116.

11. Santos R., Miranda L. C. M. (1981). Theory of the photothermal radiometry with solids. *J. Appl. Phys.*, 52(6): 4194–4198.

12. Tom R. D., O'Hara E. P., Benin D. (1982). A generalized model of photothermal radiometry. *J. Appl. Phys.*, 53(8): 5392–5400.

13. Lan T. T., Walther H. G., Goch G., Schmitz B. (1995). Experimental results of photothermal microstructural depth profiling. *J. Appl. Phys.*, 78(6): 4108–4111.

14. Munidasa M., Funak F., Mandelis A. (1998). Application of a generalized methodology for quantitative thermal diffusivity depth profile reconstruction in manufactured inhomogeneous steel-based materials. *J. Appl. Phys.*, 83(7): 3495–3498.

15. Park H. K., Grigoropoulos C. P., Tam A. C. (1995). Optical measurements of thermal-diffusivity of a material. *Int. J. Thermophys.*, 16(4): 973–995.

16. Salazar A., Sanchez-Lavega A., Terron J. M. (1998). Effective thermal diffusivity of layered materials measured by modulated photothermal techniques. *J. Appl. Phys.*, 84(6): 3031–3041.

17. Fujii M., Park S. C., Tomimura T., Zhang X. (1997). A noncontact method for measuring thermal conductivity and thermal diffusivity of anisotropic materials. *Int. J. Thermophys.*, 18(1): 251–267.

18. Milner T. E., Goodman D. M., Tanenbaum B. S., Anvari B., Nelson J. S. (1996). Noncontact determination of thermal diffusivity in biomaterials using infrared imaging radiometry. *J. Biomed. Opt.*, 1(1): 92–97.

19. Telenkov S. A., Youn J. I., Goodman D. M., Welch A. J., Milner T. E. (2001). Non-contact measurement of thermal diffusivity in tissue. *Phys. Med. Biol.*, 46: 551–558.

20. Munidasa M., Mandelis A. (1994). A comparison between conventional photothermal frequency scan and the lock-in rate window method in measuring thermal-diffusivity of solids. *Rev. Sci. Instrum.*, 65(7): 2344–2350.

21. Gijsbertsen A., Bicanic D., Gielen J. L. W., Chirtoc M. (2004). Rapid, non-destructive and non-contact inspection of solids foods by means of photothermal radiometry, thermal effusivity and initial heating coefficient. *Infrared Phys. Technol.*, 45: 93–101.

22. Wang C. H., Mandelis A. (2007). Characterization of hardened cylindrical C1018 steel rods (0.14%–0.2% C, 0.6%–0.9% Mn) using photothermal radiometry. *Rev. Sci. Inst.*, 78(5).

23. Kondyurin A. V., Sviridov A. P., Obrezkova M. V., Lunin V. V. (2010). Noncontact measurement of thermal and optical parameters of biological tissues and materials using IR laser radiometry. *Russ. J. Phys. Chem.*, 83(8): 1405–1413.

24. Draper N. R., Smith H. (1987). *Applied Regression Analysis*. New York, John Wiley & Sons.

25. Gibson A. P., Hebden J. C., Riley J., Everdell N., Schweiger M., Arridge S. R., Delpy D. T. (2005). Linear and nonlinear reconstruction for optical tomography of phantoms with nonscattering regions. *Appl. Opt.*, 44(19): 3925–3936.

26. Spirou G. M., Oraevsky A. A., Vitkin I. A., Whelan W. M. (2005). Optical and acoustic properties at 1064 nm of polyvinyl chloride-plastisol dor use as a tissue phantom in biological optoacoustics. *Phys. Med. Biol.*, 50(14): 141–153.

27. Devi C. U., Sood A. K. (2007). Measurement of visco-elastic properties of breast-tissue mimicking materials using diffusing wave spectroscopy. *J. Biomed. Opt.*, 12(3): 034035-034031–034035-034035.

28. de Korte C. L., Cespedes E. I., van der Steen A. F. W., Norder B., te Nijenhis K. (1997). Elastic and acoustic properties of vessel mimicking material for elasticity imaging. *Ulrtason. Imaging*, 19: 112–126.

29. Bini M., Ignesti A., Millanta L., Olmi R., Rubino N., Vanni R. (1984). The polyacrylamide as a phantom material for electromagnetic hyperthermia studies. *IEEE Trans. Biomed. Eng.*, BME-31(3): 317–322.

30. Andreuccetti D., Bini M., Ignesti A., Olmi R., Rubino N., Vanni R. (1988). Use of polyacrylamide as a tissue-equivalent material in the microwave range. *IEEE Trans. Biomed. Eng.*, 35(4): 275–277.

31. Surowiec A., Shrivastava P., Astrahan M., Petrovich Z. (1992). Utilization of a multilayer polyacrylamide phantom for evaluation of hyperthermia applications. *Int. J. Hyperthermia*, 8(6): 795–807.

32. Arora D., Cooley D., Perry T., Skliar M., Roemer R. B. (2005). Direct thermal dose control of constrained focused ultrasound treatments phantom and *in vivo* evaluation. *Phys. Med. Biol.*, 50(8): 1919–1935.

33. Sobol E. N., Bagratashvili V. N., Sviridov A. P., Omelchenko A. I., Ovchinnikov A. B., Shechter A. B., Helidonis E. (1994). Laser shaping of cartilage. *Proc. SPIE.* 2128: 43–49.

34. Sobol E. N., Bagratashvili V. N., Sviridov A. P., Omelchenko A. I., Shechter A. B., Jones N., Howdle S., Helidonis E. (1996). Cartilage reshaping with holmium laser. *Proc. SPIE.* 2623: 544–547.

35. Wang Z., Pankratov M. M., Perrault D. F., Shapshay S. M. (1995). Laser-assisted cartilage reshaping: *In vitro* and *in vivo* animal studies. *Proc. SPIE.* 2395: 296–302.

36. Kondyurin A. V., Sviridov A. P. (2008). Equivalent of a cartilage tissue for simulations of laser-induced temperature fields. *Quantum* Electron., 38(7): 641–646.

37. Beck G., Akgun N., Ruck A., Stainer R. (1998). Design and characterisation of a tissue phantom system for optical diagnostics. *Lasers Med. Sci.*, 13: 160–171.

38. Saidi I., Jacques S., Tittel F. (1990). Monitoring neonatal bilirubinemia using an optical patch. *Proc. SPIE.* 1201: 569–578.

39. Hielscher A., Liu H., Chance B., Tittel F., Jacques S. (1996). Time-resolved photon emission from layered turbid media. *Appl. Opt.*, 35(4): 719–728.

40. Tanaka T. (1981). Gels. *Sci. Am.*, 244(31): 110–134.

52

Use of Infrared Imaging in Veterinary Medicine

Ram C. Purohit
Auburn University

Tracy A. Turner

David D. Pascoe
Auburn University

52.1 Historical Perspective

In the mid-1960s and early 1970s, several studies were published indicating the value of infrared (IR) thermography in veterinary medicine [1–3]. In the 1965 research study of Delahanty and George [2], the thermographic images required at least 6 min to produce a thermogram, a lengthy period of time during which the veterinarian had to keep the horse still while the scan was completed. This disadvantage was overcome by the development of high-speed scanners using rotating IR prisms which then could produce instantaneous thermograms.

Stromberg [4–6] and Stromberg and Norberg [7] used thermography to diagnose inflammatory changes of the superficial digital flexor tendons in race horses. With thermography, they were able to document and detect early inflammation of the tendon, 1–2 weeks prior to the detection of lameness using clinical examination. They suggested that thermography could be used for early signs of pending lameness and it could be used for preventive measures to rest and treat race horses before severe lameness became obvious on physical examination.

In 1970, the Horse Protection Act was passed by the United States Congress to ban the use of chemical or mechanical means of "soring" horses. It was difficult to enforce this act because of the difficulty in obtaining measurable and recordable proof of violations. In 1975, Nelson and Osheim [8] documented that soring caused by chemical or mechanical means on the horse's digit could be diagnosed as having a definite abnormal characteristic IR emission pattern in the affected areas of the limb. Even though thermography at that time became the technique of choice for the detection of soring, normal thermography patterns in horses were not known. This prompted the USDA to fund research for the uses of thermography in veterinary medicine.

Purohit et al. [9] established a protocol for obtaining normal thermographic patterns of the horses' limbs and other parts of the body. This protocol was regularly used for early detection of acute and chronic inflammatory conditions in horses and other animal species. Studies at Auburn University vet school used an AGA 680 liquid-cooled thermography system that had a black and white and an accessory color display units that allows the operator to assign the array of 10 isotherms to temperature increments from 0.2°C to 10.0°C. Images were captured within seconds rather than the 6 min required for earlier machines. In veterinary studies at Auburn University, the thermographic isotherms were imaged with nine colors and white assigned to each isotherm that varied in temperature between either 0.5°C or 1.0°C.

In a subsequent study, Purohit and McCoy [10] established normal thermal patterns (temperature and gradients) of the horse, with special attention directed toward thoracic and pelvic limbs. Thermograms of various parts of the body were obtained 30 min before and after the exercise for each horse. Thermographic examination was also repeated for each horse on six different days. Thermal patterns and gradients were similar in all horses studied with a high degree of right to left symmetry in IR emission.

At the same time, Turner et al. [11] investigated the influence of the hair coat and hair clipping. This study demonstrated that the clipped leg was always warmer. After exercise, both clipped and unclipped legs had similar increases in temperature. The thermal patterns and gradients were not altered by clipping and/or exercise [10,11]. This indicated that clipping hair in horses with even hair coats was not necessary for thermographic evaluation. However, in some areas where the hair is long hair and not uniform, clipping may be required. Recently, concerns related to hair coat, thermographic imaging, and temperature regulation were investigated in llamas exposed to the hot humid conditions of the southeast [12]. While much of the veterinary research has focused on the thermographic imaging as a diagnostic tool, this study expanded its use into the problems of thermoregulation in various non endemic species.

Current camera technology has improved scanning capabilities that are combined with computer-assisted software programs. This new technology provides the practitioner with numerous options for image analysis, several hundred isotherms capable of capturing temperature differences in the hundredths of a degree Celsius, and better image quality. Miniaturized electronics have reduced the size of the units, allowing some systems to be housed in portable hand-held units. With lower cost of equipment, more thermographic equipment are being utilized in human and animal veterinary medicine and basic physiology studies.

It was obvious from initial studies by several authors that standards needed to be established for obtaining reliable thermograms in different animal species. The variations in core temperature and differences in the thermoregulatory mechanism responses between species emphasizes the importance of individually established norms for thermographic imagery.

A further challenge in veterinary medicine may occur when animal patient care may necessitate outdoor imaging.

52.2 Standards for Reliable Thermograms

Thermography provides an accurate, quantifiable, noncontact, noninvasive measure and map of skin surface temperatures. Skin surface temperatures are variable and change according to blood flow regulation to the skin surface. As such, IR thermography practitioner must be aware of the internal and external influences that alter this dynamic process of skin blood flow and temperature regulation. While imaging equipment can vary widely in price, these differences are often reflective of the wavelength capturing capability of the detectors and adjunct software that can aid in image analysis. The thermographer needs to understand the limitations of their IR system in order to make appropriate interpretations of their data. There have been some published studies that have not adhered to reliable standards and equipment prerequisites, thereby detracting from the acceptance of thermography as a valuable research and clinical technique. In some cases a simple cause–effect relationship was assumed to demonstrate the diagnosis of a disease or syndrome based on thermal responses as captured by thermographic images.

Internal and external factors have a significant effect on the skin surface temperature. Therefore, the use of thermography to evaluate skin surface thermal patterns and gradient requires an understanding of the dynamic changes which occur in blood flow at systemic, peripheral, regional, and local levels [9,10]. Thus, to enhance the diagnostic value of thermography, we recommend the following standards for veterinary medical imaging:

1. The environmental factors which interfere with the quality of thermography should be minimized. The room temperature should be maintained between 21°C and 26°C. Slight variations in some cases may be acceptable, but room temperature should always be cooler than the animal's body temperature and free from air drafts.

2. Thermograms obtained outdoors under conditions of direct air drafts, sunlight, and extreme variations in temperature may provide unreliable thermograms in which thermal patterns are altered. Such observations are meaningless as a diagnostic tool.

3. When an animal is brought into a temperature-controlled room, it should be equilibrated at least 20 min or more, depending on the external temperature from which the animal was transported. Animals transported from extreme hot or cold environments may require up to 60 min of equilibration time. Equilibration time is adequate when the thermal temperatures and patterns are consistently maintained over several minutes.

4. Other factors affecting the quality of thermograms are exercise, sweating, body position and angle, body covering, systemic and topical medications, regional and local blocks, sedatives, tranquilizers, anesthetics, vasoactive drugs, skin lesions such as scars, surgically altered areas, and so on. As stated prior, the hair coat may be an issue with uneven hair length or a thick coat.

5. It is recommended that the IR imaging should be performed using an electronic non contact cooled system. The use of long wave detectors is preferable.

The value of thermography is demonstrated by the sensitivity to changes in heat on the skin surface and its ability to detect temporal and spatial changes in thermal skin responses that corresponds to temporal and spatial changes in blood flow. Therefore, it is important to have well-documented normal thermal patterns and gradients in all species under controlled environments prior to making any claims or detecting pathological conditions.

52.3 Dermatome Patterns of Horses and Other Animal Species

Certain chronic and acute painful conditions associated with peripheral neurovascular and neuromuscular injuries are easy to confuse with spinal injuries associated with cervical, thoracic, and lumbar-sacral areas [13,14]. Similarly, inflammatory conditions such as osteoarthritis, tendonitis, and other associated conditions may also be confused with other neurovascular conditions. Thus, studies have been done over the past 25 years at Auburn University to map cutaneous and differentiate the sensory–sympathetic dermatome patterns of cervical, thoracic, and lumbosacral regions in horses [13,14]. IR thermography was used to map the sensory–sympathetic dermatome in horses. The dorsal or ventral spinal nerve(s) were blocked with 0.5% of mepevacine as a local anesthetic. The sensory–sympathetic spinal nerve block produced two effects. First, blocking the sympathetic portion of the spinal nerve caused increased thermal patterns and produced sweating of the affected areas. Second, the areas of insensitivity produced by the sensory portion of the block were mapped and compared with the thermal patterns. The areas of insensitivity were found to correlate with the sympathetic innervations.

Thermography was used to provide thermal patterns of various dermatome areas from cervical areas to epidural areas in horses. Clinical cases of cervical area nerve compression provided cooler thermal patterns, away from the site of injuries. In cases of acute injuries, associated thermal patterns were warmer than normal cases at the site of the injury. Elucidation of dermatomal (thermatom) patterns provided location for spinal injuries for the diagnosis of back injuries in horses. Similarly, in a case of a dog where the neck injury (subluxation of atlanto-axis) the diagnosis was determined by abnormal thermal patterns and gradients.

52.4 Peripheral Neurovascular Thermography

When there are alterations in skin surface temperature, it may be difficult to distinguish and diagnose between nerve and vascular injuries. The cutaneous circulation is under sympathetic vasomotor control. Peripheral nerve injuries and nerve compression can result in skin surface vascular changes that can be detected thermographically. It is well known that inflammation and nerve irritation may result in vasoconstriction causing cooler thermograms in the afflicted areas. Transection of a nerve and/or nerve damage to the extent that there is a loss of nerve conduction results in a loss in sympathetic tone which causes vasodilation indicated by an increase in the thermogram temperature. Of course, this simple rationale is more complicated with different types of nerve injuries (neuropraxia, axonotomesis, and neurotmesis). Furthermore, lack of characterization of the extent and duration of injuries may make thermographic interpretation difficult.

Studies were done on horses and other animal species to show that if thermographic examination is performed properly under controlled conditions, it can provide an accurate diagnosis of neurovascular injuries. The rationale for a neurovascular clinical diagnosis is provided in the following Horner's Syndrome case.

52.4.1 Horner's Syndrome

In four horses, Horner's Syndrome was also induced by transaction of vagosympathetic trunk on either left or right side of the neck [15]. Facial thermograms of a case of Horner's Syndrome were done 15 min before and after the exercise. Sympathetic may cause the affected side to be warm by 2–3°C more than the nontransected side. This increased temperature after denervation is reflective of an increase in blood flow due to vasodilation in the denervated areas [15,16]. The increased thermal patterns on the affected side were present up to 6–12 weeks. In about 2–4 months, neurotraumatized side blood flow readjusted to the local demand of circulation. Thermography of both non-neuroectomized and neuroectomized sides looked similar and normal [16]. In some cases, this readjustment took place as early as five days and it was difficult to distinguish the affected side. The intravenous injection of 1 mg of epinephrine in a 1000 lb horse caused an increase in thermal patterns on the denervated side, the same as indicating the presence of Horner's Syndrome. Administration of IV acetyl promazine (30 mg/1000 lb horse) showed increased heat (thermal pattern) on the normal non-neuroectomized side, whereas acetylpromazine had no effect on the neurectomized side. Alpha-blocking drug acetylpromazine caused vasodilation and increased blood flow to normal non-neurectomized side, whereas no effect was seen in the affected neurectomized side due to the lack of sympathetic innervation [16–18].

52.4.2 Neurectomies

Thermographic evaluation of the thoracic (front) and pelvic (back) limbs were done before and after performing digital neurectomies in several horses. After posterior digital neurectomy there were significant increases in heat in the areas supplied by the nerves [17]. Within 3–6 weeks, readjustment of local blood flow occurred in the neurectomized areas, and it was difficult to differentiate between the non-neurectomized and the neurectomized areas. At 10 min after administration of 0.06 mg/kg IV injection of acetylpromazine, a 2–3°C increase in heat was noted in normal non-neurectomized areas, whereas the neurectomized areas of the opposite limb were not affected.

52.4.3 Vascular Injuries

Thermography has been efficacious in the diagnosis of vascular diseases. It has been shown that the localized reduction of blood flow occurs in the horse with navicular disease [11]. This effect was more obvious on thermograms obtained after exercise than before exercise. Normally, 15–20 min of exercise will increase skin surface temperature by 2–2.5°C in horses [10,11]. In cases of arterial occlusion, the area distal to the occlusion in the horses' limb shows cooler thermograms. The effects of exercise or administration of alpha-blocking drugs like acetylpromazine causes increased blood flow to peripheral circulation in normal areas with intact vascular and sympathetic responses [17,18]. Thus, obtaining thermograms either after exercise or after administration of alpha-blocking drugs like acetylpromazine provides prognostic value for diagnosis of adequate collateral circulation. Therefore, the use of skin temperature as a measure of skin perfusion merits consideration for peripheral vascular flow, perfusion, despite some physical and physiological limitations, which are inherent in methodology [19].

Furthermore, interference with the peripheral vascular blood flow can result from neurogenic inhibition, vascular occlusion, and occlusion as a result of inflammatory vascular compression. Neurogenic inhibition can be diagnosed through the administration of alpha-blocking drugs which provide an increase in blood flow. Vascular impairment may also be associated with local injuries (inflammation, edema, swelling, etc.) which may provide localized cooler or hotter thermograms. Thus, evaluation using thermography should note the physical state and site of the injury.

52.5 Musculoskeletal Injuries

Thermography has been used in the clinical and subclinical cases of osteoarthritis, tendonitis, navicular disease, and other injuries such as sprains, stress fractures, and shin splints [10,11,20,21]. In some cases thermal abnormalities may be detected 2 weeks prior to the onset of clinical signs of lameness in horses, especially in the case of joint disease [21], tendonitis [10], and navicular problems [11,20].

Osteoarthritis is a severe joint disease in horses. Normally, diagnosis is made by clinical examination and radiographic evaluation. Radiography detects the problem after deterioration of the joint surface has taken place. Clinical evaluation is only done when horses show physical abnormalities in their gait due to pain. An early sign of osteoarthritis is inflammation, which can be detected by thermography prior to it becoming obvious on radiograms [21].

In studies of standard bred race horses, the effected tarsus joint can demonstrate abnormal thermal patterns indicating inflammation in the joint 2–3 weeks prior to radiographic diagnosis [21]. The abnormal thermograms obtained in this study were more distinct after exercise than before exercise. Thus, thermography provided a subclinical diagnosis of osteoarthritis in this study.

Thermography was used to evaluate the efficacy of corticosteroid therapy in amphotericine-B induced arthritis in ponies [22]. The intra-articular injection of 100 mg of methylprednisolone acetate was effective in alleviating the clinical signs of lameness and pain. It is important to note that when compared with clinical signs of nontreated arthritis, it was difficult to differentiate increased thermal patterns between corticosteroid treated vs. non-treated, arthritis-induced joints. However, corticosteroid therapy did not decrease the healing time of intercarpal arthritis, whereas corticosteroid therapy did decrease the time for return to normal thermographic patterns for tibiotarsal joints. In this study, thermography was useful in detecting inflammation in the absence of clinical signs of pain in corticosteroid treated joints and aiding the evaluation of the healing processes in amphotericin B-induced arthritis [22].

The chronic and acute pain associated with neuromuscular conditions can also be diagnosed by this technique. In cases where no definitive diagnosis can be made using physical examination and x-rays, thermography has been efficacious for early diagnosis of soft-tissue injuries [10,23]. The conditions such as subsolar abscesses, laminitis, and other leg lameness can be easily differentiated using thermography [10,11]. We have used thermography for quantitative and qualitative evaluation of anti-inflammatory drugs such as phenylbutazone in the treatment of physical or chemically induced inflammation. The most useful application of thermography in veterinary medicine and surgery has been to aid early detection of an acute and chronic inflammatory process.

52.6 Thermography of the Testes and Scrotum in Mammalian Species

The testicular temperature of most mammalian species must be below body temperature for normal spermatogenesis. The testes of most domestic mammalian species migrates out of the abdomen and are retained in the scrotum, which provides the appropriate thermal environment for normal spermatogenesis [24,25]. The testicular arterial and venous structure is such that arterial coils are enmeshed in the pampiniform plexus of the testicular veins, which provides a counter current heating regulating mechanism by which arterial blood entering the testes is cooled by the venous blood leaving the testes [24,25]. In the ram, the temperature of the blood in the testicular artery decreases by 4°C from the external inguinal ring to the surface of the testes. Thus, to function effectively, the mammalian testes are maintained at a lower temperature.

Purohit et al. [26,27] used thermography to establish normal thermal patterns and gradients of the scrotum in bulls, stallions, bucks, dogs, and llamas. The normal thermal patterns of the scrotum in all species studied is characterized by right to left symmetrical patterns, with a constant decrease in the thermal gradients from the base to the apex. In bulls, bucks, and stallions, a thermal gradient of 4–6°C from the base to apex with concentric hands signifies normal patterns. Inflammation of one testicle increased ipsilateral scrotal temperatures of 2.5–3°C [26,28] If both testes were inflamed, there was an overall increase of 2.5–3°C temperature and a reduction in temperature gradient was noted.

Testicular degeneration could be acute or chronic. In chronic testicular degeneration with fibrosis, there was a loss of temperature gradient, loss of concentric thermal patterns, and some areas were cooler than others with no consistent patterns [26]. Reversibility of degenerative changes depends upon the severity and duration of the trauma. The IR thermal gradients and patterns in dogs [27] and llamas [27,29] are unique to their own species and the patterns are different from that of the bull and buck.

Thermography has also been used in humans, indicating a normal thermal pattern which is characterized by symmetric and constant temperatures between 32.5°C and 34.5°C [30–33]. Increased scrotal IR emissions were associated with intrascrotal tumor, acute and chronic inflammation, and varicoceles [34,35]. Thermography has been efficacious for early diagnosis of acute and/or chronic testicular degeneration in humans and many animal species. The disruption of the normal thermal patterns of the scrotum is directly related to testicular degeneration. The testicular degeneration may cause transient or permanent infertility in the male. It is well established that increases in scrotal temperature above normal causes disruption of spermatogenesis, affects sperm maturation, and contributes toward subfertile or infertile semen quality. Early diagnosis of pending infertility has a significant impact on economy and reproduction in animals.

52.7 Conclusions

The value of thermography can only be realized if it is used properly. All species studied thus far have provided remarkable bilateral symmetrical patterns of IR emission. The high degree of right-to-left symmetry provides a valuable asset in diagnosis of unilateral problems associated with various inflammatory disorders. On the other hand, bilateral problems can be diagnosed due to changes in thermal gradient and/or overall increase or decrease of temperature, away from the normal established thermal patterns in a given area of the body. Various areas of the body on the same side have normal patterns and gradients. This can be used to diagnose a change in gradient patterns. Alteration in normal thermal patterns and gradients indicates a thermal pathology. If thermal abnormalities are evaluated carefully, early diagnosis can be made, even prior to the appearance of clinical signs of joint disease, tendonitis, and various musculoskeletal problems in various animal species. Thermography can be used as a screening device for early detection of an impending problem, allowing veterinarian institute treatment before the problem becomes more serious. During the healing process post surgery, animals may appear physically sound. Thermography can be used as a diagnostic aid in assessing the healing processes. In equine sports medicine, thermography can be used on a regular basis for screening to prevent severe injuries to the horse. Early detection and treatment can prevent financial losses associated with delayed diagnosis and treatment.

The efficacy of noncontact electronic IR thermography has been demonstrated in numerous clinical settings and research studies as a diagnostic tool for veterinary medicine. It has had a strong impact on veterinary medical practice and thermal physiology where accurate skin temperatures need to be assessed under normal conditions, disease pathologies, injuries, and thermal stress. The importance of IR thermography as a research tool cannot be understated for improving the medical care of animals and for the contributions made through animal research models that improve our understanding of human structures and functions.

References

1. Smith W.M. Application of thermography in veterinary medicine. *Ann. NY Acad. Sci.*, 121, 248, 1964.
2. Delahanty D.D. and George J.R. Thermography in equine medicine. *J. Am. Vet. Med. Assoc.*, 147, 235, 1965.
3. Clark J.A. and Cena K. The potential of infrared thermography in veterinary diagnosis. *Vet. Rec.*, 100, 404, 1977.
4. Stromberg B. The normal and diseased flexor tendon in racehorses. *Acta Radiol.* 305(Suppl.), 1, 1971.
5. Stromberg B. Thermography of the superficial flexor tendon in race horses. *Acta Radiol.* 319(Suppl.), 295, 1972.
6. Stromberg B. The use of thermograph in equine orthopedics. *J. Am. Vet. Radiol. Soc.*, 15, 94, 1974.
7. Stromberg B. and Norberg I. Infrared emission and Xe-disappearance rate studies in the horse. *Equine Vet. J.*, 1, 1–94, 1971.
8. Nelson H.A. and Osheim D.L. Soring in Tennessee walking horses: Detection by thermography. *USDA-APHIS, Veterinary Services Laboratories*, Ames, Iowa, pp. 1–14, 1975.
9. Purohit R.C., Bergfeld II W.A. McCaoy M.D., Thompson W.M., and Sharman R.S. Value of clinical thermography in veterinary medicine. *Auburn Vet.*, 33, 140, 1977.
10. Purohit R.C. and McCoy M.D. Thermography in the diagnosis of inflammatory processes in the horse. *Am. J. Vet. Res.*, 41, 1167, 1980.
11. Turner T.A. et al. Thermographic evaluation of podotrochlosis in horses. *Am. J. Vet. Res.*, 44, 535, 1983.
12. Heath A.M., Navarre C.B., Simpkins A.S., Purohit R.C., and Pugh D.G. A comparison of heat tolerance between sheared and non sheared alpacas (*llama pacos*). *Small Ruminant Res.*, 39, 19, 2001.
13. Purohit R.C. and Franco B.D. Infrared thermography for the determination of cervical dermatome patterns in the horse. *Biomed. Thermol.*, 15, 213, 1995.
14. Purohit R.C., Schumacher J., Molloy J.M., Smith, and Pascoe D.D. Elucidation of thoracic and lumbosacral dermatomal patterns in the horse. *Thermol. Int.*, 13, 79, 2003.
15. Purohit R.C., McCoy M.D., and Bergfeld W.A. Thermographic diagnosis of Horner's syndrome in the horse. *Am. J. Vet. Res.*, 41, 1180, 1980.
16. Purohit R.C. The diagnostic value of thermography in equine medicine. *Proc. Am. Assoc. Equine Pract.*, 26, 316–326, 1980.
17. Purohit R.C. and Pascoe D.D. Thermographic evaluation of peripheral neurovascular systems in animal species. *Thermology*, 7, 83, 1997.
18. Purohit R.C., Pascoe D.D., Schumacher J., Williams A., and Humburg J.H. Effects of medication on the normal thermal patterns in horses. *Thermol. Osterr.*, 6, 108, 1996.
19. Purohit R.C. and Pascoe D.D. Peripheral neurovascular thermography in equine medicine. *Thermol. Osterr.*, 5, 161, 1995.

20. Turner T.A., Purohit R.C., and Fessler J.F. Thermography: A review in equine medicine. *Comp. Cont. Education Pract. Vet.*, 8, 854, 1986.

21. Vaden M.F., Purohit R.C., Mcoy, and Vaughan J.T. Thermography: A technique for subclinical diagnosis of osteoarthritis. *Am. J. Vet. Res.*, 41, 1175–1179, 1980.

22. Bowman K.F., Purohit R.C., Ganjan, V.K., Peachman R.D., and Vaughan J.T. Thermographic evaluation of corticosteroids efficacy in amphotericin-B induced arthritis in ponies. *Am. J. Vet. Res.* 44, 51–56, 1983.

23. Purohit R.C. Use of thermography in the diagnosis of lameness. *Auburn Vet.*, 43, 4, 1987.

24. Waites G.M.H. and Setchell B.P. Physiology of testes, epididymis, and scrotum. In *Advances in Reproductive Physiology*. McLaren A., Ed., London: Logos, Vol. 4, pp. 1–21, 1969.

25. Waites G.M.H. Temperature regulation and the testes. In *The Testis*, Johnson A.D., Grones W.R., and Vanderwork N.L., Eds., New York: Academy Press, Inc., Vol. 1, pp. 241–237, 1970.

26. Purohit R.C., Hudson R.S., Riddell M.G., Carson R.L., Wolfe D.F., and Walker D.F. Thermography of bovine scrotum. *Am. J. Vet. Res.*, 46, 2388–2392, 1985.

27. Purohit R.C., Pascoe D.D., Heath A.M. Pugh D.G., Carson R.L., Riddell M.G., and Wolfe D.F. Thermography: Its role in functional evaluation of mammalian testes and scrotum. *Thermol. Int.*, 12, 125–130, 2002.

28. Wolfe D.F., Hudson R.S., Carson R.L., and Purohit, R.C. Effect of unilateral orchiectomy on semen quality in bulls. *J. Am. Vet. Med. Assoc.*, 186, 1291, 1985.

29. Heath A.M., Pugh D.G., Sartin E.A., Navarre B., and Purohit R.C. Evaluation of the safety and efficacy of testicular biopsies in llamas. *Theriogenology*, 58, 1125, 2002.

30. Amiel J.P., Vignalou L., Tricoire J. et al. Thermography of the testicle: Preliminary study. *J. Gynecol. Obstet. Biol. Reprod.*, 5, 917, 1976.

31. Lazarus B.A. and Zorgiotti A.W. Thermo-regulation of the human testes. *Fertil. Steril.*, 26, 757, 1978.

32. Lee J.T. and Gold R.H. Localization of occult testicular tumor with scrotal thermography. *J. Am. Med. Assoc.*, 1976, 236, 1976.

33. Wegner G. and Weissbach Z. Application of palte thermography in the diagnosis of scrotal disease. *MMW*, 120, 61, 1978.

34. Gold R.H., Ehrlich R.M., Samuels B. et al. Scrotal thermography. *Radiology*, 1221, 129, 1979.

35. Coznhaire F., Monteyne R., and Hunnen M. The value of scrotal thermography as compared with selective retrograde venography of the internal spermatic vein for the diagnosis of subclinical varicoceles. *Fertil. Steril.*, 27, 694, 1976.

53

Standard Procedures for Infrared Imaging in Medicine

Kurt Ammer
Ludwig Boltzmann
Research Institute for
Physical Diagnostics

University of Glamorgan

Francis J. Ring
University of Glamorgan

53.1 Introduction

Infrared thermal imaging has been used in medicine since the early 1960s. Working groups within the European Thermographic Association (now European Association of Thermology) produced the first publications on standardization of thermal imaging in 1978 [1] and 1979 [2]. However, Collins and Ring established already in 1974 a quantitative thermal index [3], which was modified in Germany by J.-M. Engel in 1978 [4]. Both indices opened the field of quantitative evaluation of medical thermography.

Further recommendations for standardization appeared in 1983 [5] and 1984, the later related to essential techniques for the use of thermography in clinical drug trials [6]. Engel published a booklet titled *Standardized Thermographic Investigations in Rheumatology and Guideline for Evaluation* in 1984 [7]. The author presented his ideas for standardization of image recording and assessment including some normal values for wrist, knee, and ankle joints. Engel's measurements of knee temperatures were first published in 1978 [4]. Normal temperature values of the lateral elbow, dorsal hands, anterior knee, lateral and medial malleolus, and the first metatarsal joint were published by Collins in 1976 [8].

The American Academy of Thermology published technical guidelines in 1986 including some recommendations for thermographic examinations [9]. However, the American authors concentrated on determining the symmetry of temperature distribution rather than the normal temperature values of particular body regions. Uematsu in 1985 [10] and Goodman in 1986 [11] published the side-to-side variations of surface temperatures of the human body. These symmetry data were confirmed by E.F. Ring for the lower leg in 1986 [12].

In Japan, medical thermal imaging has been an accepted diagnostic procedure since 1981 [13]. Recommendations for the analysis of neuromuscular thermograms were published by Fujimasa et al. in 1986 [14]. Five years later more detailed proposals for the thermal image-based analysis of physiological functions were published in *Biomedical Thermology* [15], the official journal of the Japanese Society of thermology. This chapter was the result of a workshop on clinical thermography criteria.

Recently, the thermography societies in Korea have published a book, which summarizes in 270 pages general standards for imaging recording and interpretation of thermal images in various diseases [16].

As the relationship between skin blood flow and body surface temperature has been obvious from the initial use of thermal imaging in medicine, quantitative assessments were developed at an early stage. Ring developed a thermographical index for the assessment of ischemia in 1980, that was originally used for patients suffering from Raynauds' disease [17]. The European Association of Thermology published a statement in 1988 on the subject of Raynaud's phenomenon [18]. Normal values for recovering after a cold challenge have been published since 1976 [19,20]. A range of temperatures were applied in this thermal challenge test, the technique was reviewed by Ring in 1997 [21].

An overview of recommendations gathered from, the Japanese Society of Biomedical Thermology and the European Association of Thermology was collated and published by Clark and Goff in 1997 [22]. This chapter is based on the practical implications of the foregoing papers taken from the perspective of the modern thermal imaging systems available to medicine.

Finally, a project at the University of Glamorgan, aims to create an atlas of normal thermal images of healthy subjects [23]. This study, started in 2001, has generated a number of questions related to the influence of body positions on accuracy and precision of measurements from thermal images [24,25].

53.2 Definition of Thermal Imaging

Thermal imaging is regarded as a technique for temperature measurements based on the infrared radiation from objects. Unlike images created by x-rays or proton activation through magnetic resonance, thermal imaging is not related to morphology. The technique provides only a map of the distribution of temperatures on the surface of the object imaged.

Whenever infrared thermal imaging is considered as a method for measurement, the technique must meet all criteria of a measurement. The most basic features of measurement are accuracy (in the medical field also named validity) and precision (in medicine reliability). Anbar [26] has listed five other terms related to the precision of infrared-based temperature measurements. When used as an outcome measure, responsiveness, or sensitivity to change is an important characteristic.

53.2.1 Accuracy

Measurements are basic procedures of comparison namely to compare a standardized meter with an object to be measured. Any measurement is prone to error, thus a perfect measurement is impossible. However, the smaller the variation of a particular measurement from the standardized meter, the higher is the accuracy of the measurement or in other words, an accurate measurement is as close as possible to the true value of measurement. In medicine, accuracy is often named validity, mainly caused by the fact, that medical measurements are not often performed by the simple comparison of meter and object. For example, assessments from various features of a human being may be combined to a new construct, resulting in an innovative measurement of health.

53.2.2 Precision

A series of measurements cannot achieve totally identical results. The smaller the variation between single results, the higher is the precision or repeatability (reliability) of the measurement. However, reliability without accuracy is useless. For example, a sports archer who always hits the same peripheral sector of the target, has very high reliability, but no validity, because such an athlete must find the center of the target to be regarded as accurate.

53.2.3 Responsiveness

Both accuracy and precision have an impact on the sensitivity to change of outcome measures. Validity is needed to define correctly the symptom to be measured. Precision will affect the responsiveness also, because a change of the symptom can only be detected if this change is bigger than the variation of repeated measurements.

53.2.4 Sources of Variability of Thermal Images

Table 53.1 shows conditions in thermal imaging that may affect accuracy, precision, and responsiveness.

53.2.5 Object or Subject

As the emittance of infrared radiation is the source of remote temperature measurements, knowledge of the emissivity of the object is essential for the calculation of temperature related to the radiant heat. In nonliving objects emissivity is mainly a function of the texture of the surface.

Seventy years ago, Hardy [27] showed that the human skin acts like an almost perfect black body radiator with an emissivity of 0.98. Studies from Togawa in Japan have demonstrated that the emissivity of the skin is unevenly distributed [28]. In addition, infrared reflection from the environment and substances applied on the skin may also alter the emissivity [29–31]. Water is an efficient filter for infrared rays and can be bound to the superficial corneal layer of the skin during immersion for at least 15 min [32,33] or in the case of severe edema [34]. This can affect the emissivity of the skin.

The hair coat of animal may show a different emissivity than the skin after clipping the hair [35]. Variation in the distribution of the hairy coat will influence the emissivity of the animal's surface [36]. Variation in emissivity will influence the accuracy of temperature measurements.

Homeothermic beings, maintain their deep body (core) temperature through variation of the surface (shell) temperature, and show a circadian rhythm of both the core and shell temperature [37–40]. Repeated temperature registrations not performed at the same time of the day will therefore affect the precision of these measurements.

53.2.6 Camera Systems, Standards, and Calibration

53.2.6.1 The Imaging System

A new generation of infrared cameras has become available for medical imaging. The older systems, normally single element detectors using an optical mechanical scanning process, were mostly cooled by the addition of liquid nitrogen [41–43]. However, adding nitrogen to the system, affects the stability of temperature measurements for a period up to 60 min [44]. Nitrogen-cooled scanners had the effect of limiting the angle at which the camera could be used that restricted operation.

TABLE 53.1 Conditions Affecting Accuracy, Precision, and Responsiveness of Temperature Measures

Condition Affecting	Accuracy	Precision	Responsiveness
Object or subject	X	X	X
Camera systems, standards, and calibration	X	X	X
Patient position and image capture		X	X
Information protocols and resources		X	X
Image analysis	X	X	X
Image exchange	X	X	X
Image presentation	X	X	X

Electronic cooling systems were then introduced, which provided the use of image capturing without restrictions of the angle between the object and the camera. The latest generation of focal plane array cameras can be used without cooling, providing almost maintenance-free technology [45]. However, repeated calibration procedures built inside the camera can affect the stability of temperature measurements [46].

The infrared wavelength, recorded by the camera, will not affect the temperature readings as long as the algorithm of calculation temperature from emitted radiation is correct. However, systems equipped with sensors sensitive in different bands of the infrared spectrum are capable to determine the emissivity of objects [47].

53.2.6.2 Temperature Reference

Earlier reports stipulate the requirement for a separate thermal reference source for calibration checks on the camera [9,48,49]. Many systems now include an internal reference temperature, with manufacturers claiming that external checks are not required. Unless frequent servicing is obtained, it is still advisable to use an external source, if only to check for drift in the temperature sensitivity of the camera. An external reference, which may be purchased or constructed, can be left switched on throughout the day. This allows the operator to make checks on the camera, and in particular provides a check on the hardware and software employed for processing. These constant temperature source checks may be the only satisfactory way of proving the reliability of temperature measurements made from the thermogram [48]. Linearity of temperature measurements which may be questionable in focal plane array equipment, can be checked with two ore more external temperature references. New low-cost reference sources, based on the triple point of particular chemicals, are currently under construction in the United Kingdom [44].

53.2.6.3 Mounting the Imager

A camera stand which provides vertical height adjustment is very important for medical thermography. Photographic tripod stands are inconvenient for frequent adjustment and often result in tilting the camera at an undefined angle to the patient. This is difficult to reproduce, and unless the patient is positioned so that the surface scanned is aligned at 90° to the camera lens, distortion of the image is unavoidable. Undefined angles of the camera view affect the precision of measurements.

In the case of temperature measurements from a curved surface, the angle between the radiating object and the capturing device may be the critical source of false measurements [50–52]. At an angle of view beyond 30° small losses of capturing the full band of radiation start to occur, at an angel of 60° the loss of information becomes critical and is followed by false temperature readings. The determination of the temperature of the same forefoot in different views shows clearly that consideration of the angel of the viewing is a significant task [53]. Unless corrected, thermal images of evenly curved objects lack accuracy of temperature measurements [54].

Studio camera stands are ideal, they provide vertical height adjustment with counterbalance weight compensation. It should be noted that the type of lens used on the camera will affect the working distance and the field of view, a wide-angle lens reduces distance between the camera and the subject in many cases, but may also increase peripheral distortion of the image [55].

53.2.6.4 Camera Initialization

Start up time with modern cameras are claimed to be very short, minutes or seconds. However, the speed with which the image becomes visible is not an indication of image stability. Checks on calibration will usually show that a much longer period from 10 min to several hours with an uncooled system are needed to achieve stable conditions for temperature readings from infrared images [5,46].

53.2.7 Patient Position and Image Capture

Standardized positions of the body for image capture and clearly defined fields of view can reduce systematic errors and increases both accuracy and precision of temperature readings from thermal images recorded in such a manner. In radiography, standardized positions of the body for image capture have been included in the protocol for quality assurance for a long time. Although thermal imaging does not provide much anatomical information compared with other imaging techniques, variation of body positions and the related fields of view affects the precision of temperature readings from thermograms. However, the intra- and inter-rater repeatability of temperature values from the same thermal image was found to be excellent [56].

53.2.7.1 Location for Thermal Imaging

The size of investigation room does not influence the quality of temperature measurements from thermal images, unless the least distance in one direction is not shorter than the distance between the camera and an object of 1.2 m height [57]. Such a condition will result in thermal images out of focus. Other important features of the examination room are thermal insulation and prevention of any direct or reflected infrared radiation sources. Following this proposal will result in an increase of accuracy and precision of measurements.

53.2.7.2 Ambient Temperature Control

This is a primary requirement for most clinical applications of thermal imaging. A range of temperatures from 18 to 25°C should be attainable and held for at least 1 h to better than 1°C. Owing to the nature of human thermoregulation, stability of the room temperature is a critical feature. It has been shown that subjects acclimatized for 40–60 min at a room temperature of 22°C showed differences in surface temperature at various measuring sites of the face after lowering the ambient temperature by 2°C [58]. Whereas the nose cooled on average by 4°C, the forehead and the meatus decreased the surface temperature by only 0.4–0.45%. Similar changes may occur at other acral sites such as tips of fingers or toes, as both regions are highly involved in heat exchange for temperature regulation.

At lower temperatures, the subject is likely to shiver, and over 25°C room temperature will cause sweating, at least in most European countries. Variations may be expected in colder or warmer climates, in the latter case, room temperatures may need to be 1°C to 2°C higher [59].

Additional techniques for cooling particular regions of the body have been developed [60,61]. Immersion of the hands in water at various tempeatures is a common challenge for the assessment of vasospastic disease [21].

Heat generated in the investigation room affects the room temperature. Possible heat sources are not only electronic equipment such as the scanner and its computer, but also human bodies. For this reason the air-conditioning unit should be capable of compensating for the maximum number of patients and staff likely to be in the room at any one time. These effects will be greater in a small room of 2 × 3 m or less.

Air convection is a very effective method of skin cooling and related to the wind speed. Therefore, air-conditioning equipment should be located so that direct draughts are not directed at the patient, and that overall air speed is kept as low as possible. A suspended perforated ceiling with ducts diffusing the air distribution evenly over the room is ideal [62].

A cubicle or cubicles within the temperature-controlled area is essential. These should provide privacy for disrobing and a suitable area for resting through the acclimatization period.

53.2.7.3 Preimaging Equilibration

On arrival at the department, the patient should be informed of the examination procedure, instructed to remove appropriate clothing and jewellery, and asked to sit or rest in the preparation cubicle for a fixed time. The time required to achieve adequate stability in blood pressure and skin temperature is generally considered to be 15 min, with 10 min as a minimum [63–65]. After 30 min cooling, oscillations of the skin temperature can be detected, in different regions of the body with different amplitudes resulting in a temperature asymmetry between left and right sides [64].

Contact of body parts with the environment or with other body parts alters the surface temperature because of the heat transfer by conduction. Therefore, during the preparation the patient must avoid folding or crossing arms and legs, or placing bare feet on a cold surface. If the lower extremities are to be examined, a stool or leg rest should be provided to avoid direct contact with the floor [66]. If these requirements are not met, poor precision of measurements may result.

53.2.7.4 Positions for Imaging

As in anatomical imaging studies, it is preferable to standardize on a series of standard views for each body region. The EAT Locomotor Diseases Group recommendations include a triangular marker system to indicate anterior, posterior, lateral, and angled views [2,67]. However, reproduction of positions for angled views may be difficult, even when aids such as rotating platforms are used [68].

Modern image processing software provides comment boxes that can be used to encode the angle of view which will be stored with the image [69]. It should be noted that the position of the patient for scanning and in preparation must be constant. Standing, sitting, or lying down affect the surface area of the body exposed to the ambient, therefore an image recorded with the patient in a sitting position may not be comparable with one recorded on a separate occasion in a standing position. In addition, blood flow against the influence of gravity contributes to the skin temperature of fingers in various limb positions [70].

53.2.7.5 Field of View

Image size is dependent on the distance between the camera and the patient and the focal length of the infrared camera lens. The lens is generally fixed on most medical systems, so it is a good practice to maintain a constant distance from the patient for each view, in order to acquire a reproducible field of view for the image. If in different thermograms different fields of the same subject are compared, the variable resolution can lead to false temperature readings [71]. However, maintaining the same distance between object and camera, cannot compensate for individual body dimensions, for example, big subjects will have big knees and therefore maintaining the same distance as for a tiny subjects knee is not applicable.

To overcome this problem, the field of view has been defined in the standard protocol at the University of Glamorgan in a twofold way, that is, body position and alignment of anatomical landmarks to the edge of the image [23]. These definitions enabled us to investigate the reproducibility of body views using the distance in pixels between anatomical landmarks and the outline of the infrared images [24–72].

Figure 53.1 gives examples of the views that have been investigated for the reproducibility of body positions. Table 53.2 shows the mean value, standard deviation (SD), and 95% confidence interval (CI) of the variation of body views of the upper and the lower part of the human body. Variations in views of the lower part of the body were bigger than in views of the upper part. The highest degree of variation was found in the view "Both Ankles Anterior," but the smallest variation in the view "Face."

53.2.8 Information Protocols and Resources

Human skin temperature is the product of heat dissipated from the vessels and organs within the body, and the effect of the environmental factors on heat loss or gain. There are a number of further influences that are controllable, such as cosmetics [29], alcohol intake [73–75], and smoking [76–78]. In general terms, the patient attending examination should be advised to avoid all topical applications such as ointments and cosmetics on the day of examination to all the relevant areas of the body [31,47,79,80]. Large meals and above-average intake of tea or coffee should also be excluded, although studies supporting this recommendation are hard to find and the results are not conclusive [81,82].

Patients should be asked to avoid tight-fitting clothing, and to keep physical exertion to a minimum. This particularly applies to methods of physiotherapy such as electrotherapy [83–85], ultrasound [86,87], heat treatment [88–90], cryotherapy [91–94], massage [95–97], and hydrotherapy [31,32,98,99], because thermal effects from such treatment can last for 4–6 h under certain conditions. Heat production by muscular exercise is a well-documented phenomenon [65,100–103].

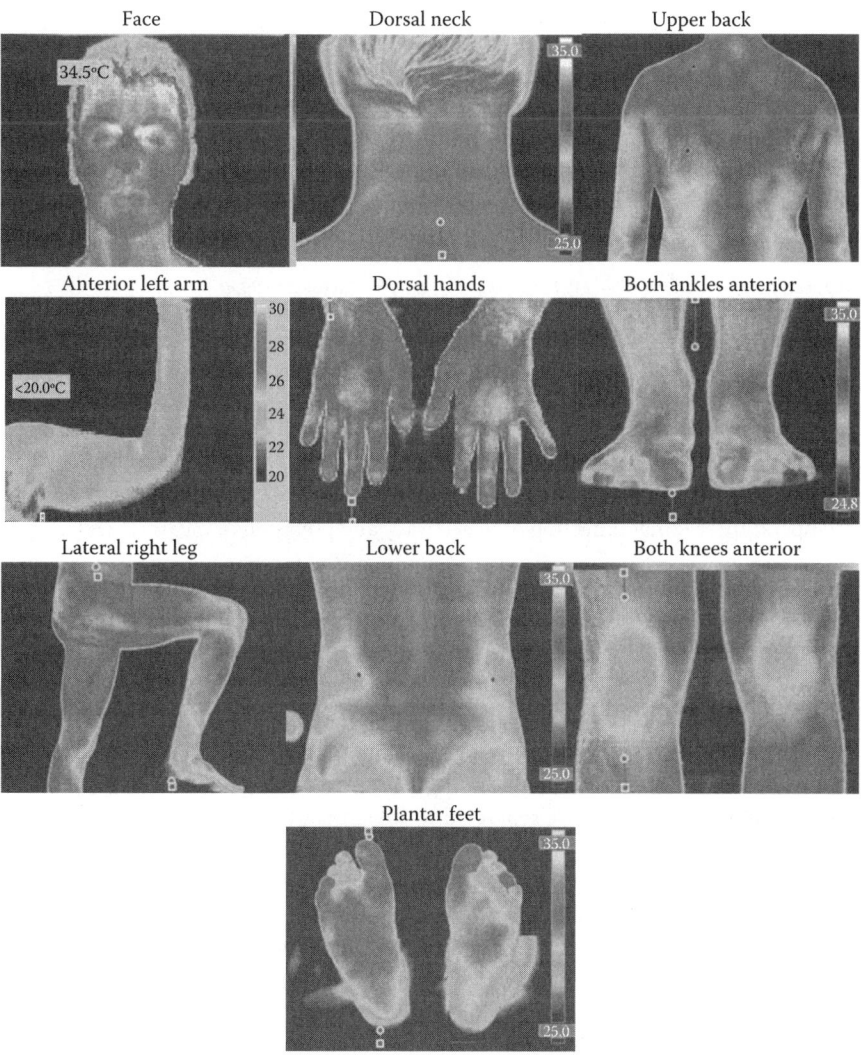

FIGURE 53.1 Body views investigated.

Drug treatment can also affect the skin temperature. This phenomenon was used to evaluate the therapeutic effects of medicaments [6]. Drugs affecting the cardiovascular system must be reported to the thermographer, so that the correct interpretation of thermal images will be given [104–107].

Omitting just one of the aforementioned conditions will result in reduced precision of temperature measurements.

53.2.9 Image Processing

Every image or block of images must carry the indication of temperature range, with color code/temperature scale. The color scale itself should be standardized. Industrial software frequently provides a gray-scale picture and one or more color scales. However, modern image-processing software permits to squeeze the color scale in already-recorded images to increase the image contrast. Such a procedure will affect the temperature readings from thermal images as temperatures outside the compressed

TABLE 53.2 Variation of Positions of All the Investigated Views

View	Upper Edge (Pixel) Mean ± SD (95% CI)	Lower Edge (Pixel) Mean ± SD (95% CI)	Left Side Edge (Pixel) Mean ± SD (95% CI)
Face	0.5 ± 5.3 (−2.2 to 1.9)	4.0 ± 10.9 (−0.03 to 8.2)	
Dorsal neck	−8.4 ± 36.4 (−18.3 to 1.6)	122.6 ± 146.6 (82.6 to 162.6)	
Upper back	4.5 ± 9.9 (0.8 to 8.2)	28.1 ± 22.0 (19.9 to 36.4)	
Anterior left arm	22.4 ± 33.0 (8.7 to 6.0)	15.8 ± 15.4 (9.5 to 22.2)	12.5 ± 16.0 (5.9 to 19.1)
Dorsal hands	41.8 ± 17.8 (35.5 to 48.2)	33.2 ± 22.3 (25.3 to 41.5)	
Both knees anterior	80.7 ± 47.3 (60.7 to 100.7)	84.3 ± 37.0 (68.6 to 99.9)	
Lateral right leg	16.7 ± 21.0 (5.9 to 27.5)	17.2 ± 15.8 (9.0 to 25.3)	
Lower back	17.1 ± 4.2 (8.6 to 25.6)	16.3 ± 4.6 (16.3 to 34.9)	
Both ankles anterior	158.8 ± 12.2 (133.6 to 184.1)	54.9 ± 9.1 (36.1 to 37.8)	
Plantar feet	31.0 ± 24.1 (23.2 to 38.7)	25.7 ± 23.1 (18.3 to 33.1)	

temperature scale will not be included in the statistics of selected regions of interest. This will result in erroneous temperature readings, affecting both accuracy and precision of measurements.

53.2.10 Image Analysis

Almost all systems now use image-processing techniques and provide basic quantitation of the image [108–110]. In some cases, this may be operated from a chip within the camera, or may be carried out through an on-line or off-line computer. For older equipment such as the AGA 680 series several hardware adaptations have been reported to achieve quantitation of the thermograms [111–113].

It has to be emphasized that false color coding of infrared images does not provide means for temperature measurement. If colors are separated by a temperature distance of 1°C, the temperature difference between two points situated in adjacent colors may be between 0.1°C and 1.9°C. It is obvious that false-colored images provide at its best an estimation of temperature, but not a measurement. The same is true for liquid crystal thermograms.

Nowadays, temperature measurements in thermal images are based on the definition of regions of interest (ROI). However, standards for shape, size, and placement of these regions are not available or incomplete. Although a close correlation exists for ROI of different size in the same region [114], the precision of measurement is affected when ROIS of different size and location are used for repeated measurements.

The Glamorgan protocol [23] is the very first attempt to create a complete standard for the definition of regions of interest in thermal images based on anatomical limits. Furthermore, in the view "both knee anterior" the shape with the highest reproducibility was investigated. During one of the Medical Infrared Training Courses at the University of Glamorgan, three newly trained investigators defined on the same thermal image of both anterior knees twice the region of interest in the shape of a box, an ellipsoid or as an hour-glass shape. Similar to the result of a pilot study that compared these shapes for repeatability, the highest reliability was found for temperature readings from the hour-glass shape, followed by readings from ellipsoids and boxes [53]. The repeatability of the regions on the view "Left Anterior Arm," "Both Ankles Anterior," "Dorsal Feet," and "Plantar Feet" were also investigated and resulted in reliability coefficients between 0.7 (right ankle) and 0.93 (forearm). The intraclass correlation coefficients ranged between 0.48 (upper arm) and 0.87 (forearm). Applying the Glamorgan protocol consequently will result in precise temperature measurements from thermal images.

53.2.11 Image Exchange

Most of the modern infrared systems store the recorded thermal images in an own image format, which may not be compatible with formats of thermal images from other manufacturers. However, most of these images can be transformed into established image formats such as TIF, JPEG, GIF, and others. As a thermal image is the pictographic representation of a temperature map, the sole image is not enough unless the related temperature information is not provided. Consequently, temperature measurements from standard computer images derived from thermograms is not possible.

Providing both temperature scale and a scale of gray shades, allows the exchange of thermal images over long distance and between different, but compatible image-processing software [115]. The gray scale must be derived from the original gray shade thermal image. If it has been transformed from a false color image, the resulted black-and-white thermogram may not be representative for the original gray scale gradient as the gray scale of individual colors may deviate from the particular gray shade of the image. This can then result in false temperature readings.

53.2.12 Image Presentation

Image presentation does not influence the result of measurements from thermal images. However, if thermograms are read by eyes, their appearance will affect the credibility of the information in thermal images. This is for instance the case, when thermal images are use as evidence in legal trials [116].

It was stated that for forensic acceptability of thermography standardization and repeatability of the technique are very important features [117]. This supports the necessity of quantitative evaluation of thermal images and standards strictly applied to the technique of infrared imaging will finally result in high accuracy and precision of this method of temperature measurement. At that stage it can be recommended as responsive outcome measure for clinical trials in rheumatology [6,8], angiopathies [107,118], neuromuscular disorders [119], surgery [120], and paediatrics [121].

References

1. Aarts, N.J.M. et al. Thermographic Terminology. *Acta Thermograp.*, 3(Suppl. 2), 1, 1978.
2. Engel, J.M. et al. Thermography in locomotor diseases—Recommended procedure. *Eur. J. Rheum. Inflamm.*, 2, 299, 1979.
3. Collins, A.J. et al. Quantitation of thermography in arthritis using multi-isothermal analysis. *Ann. Rheum. Dis.*, 33, 113, 1974.
4. Engel, J.-M. Quantitative Thermographie des Kniegelenks. *Z. Rheumatol.*, 37, 242, 1978.
5. Ring, E.F.J. Standardisation of thermal imaging in medicine: Physical and environmental factors, in *Thermal Assessment of Breast Health*, Gautherie, M., Albert, E., and Keith, L., Eds., MTP Press Ltd, Lancaster/Boston/The Hague, 1983, p. 29.
6. Ring, E.F.J., Engel, J.M., and Page-Thomas, D.P. Thermologic methods in clinical pharmacology—Skin temperature measurement in drug trials. *Int. J. Clin. Pharm. Ther. Tox.*, 22, 20, 1984.
7. Engel, J.-M. and Saier, U. *Thermographische Standarduntersuchungen in der Rheumatologie und Richtlinien zu deren Befundung.* Luitpold, München, 1984.
8. Collins, A.J. Anti-inflammatory drug assessment by the thermographic index. *Acta Thermograp*, 1, 73, 1976.
9. Pochaczevsky, R. et al. Technical guidelines, 2nd ed. *Thermology*, 2, 108, 1986.
10. Uematsu, S. Symmetry of skin temperatures comparing one side of the body to the other. *Thermology*, 1, 4, 1985.
11. Goodman, P.H. et al. Normal temperature asymmetry of the back and extremities by computer-assisted infrared imaging. *Thermology*, 1, 195, 1986.
12. Bliss, P. et al. Investigation of nerve root irritation by infrared thermography, in *Back Pain—Methods for Clinical Investigation and Assessment*, Hukins, D.W.L. and Mulholland, R.C., Eds., University Press, Manchester, 1986, p. 63.
13. Atsumi, K. High technology applications of medical thermography in Japan. *Thermology*, 1, 79–80, 1985.

14. Fujimasa, I. et al. A new computer image processing system for the analysis of neuromuscular thermograms: A feasibility study. *Thermology*, 1, 221, 1986.

15. Fujimasa, I. A proposal for thermographic imaging diagnostic procedures for temperature related physiologic function analysis. *Biomed. Thermol.*, 11, 269, 1991.

16. Lee, W.-Y. et al. (Eds.) *Practical Manual of Clinical Thermology*, Med Lang, 2004, ISBN 89-954013-04.

17. Ring, E.F.J. A thermographic index for the assessment of ischemia. *Acta Thermograp.*, 5, 35, 1980.

18. Aarts, N.P. et al. Raynaud's phenomenon: Assessment by thermography. *Thermology*, 3, 69, 1988.

19. Acciarri, L., Carnevale, F., and Della Selva, A. Thermography in the hand angiopathy from vibrating tools. *Acta Thermograp.*, 1, 18, 1976.

20. Ring, E.F. and Bacon, P.A. Quantitative thermographic assessment of inositol nicotinate therapy in Raynaud's phenomena. *J. Int. Med. Res.*, 5, 217, 1977.

21. Ring, E.F.J. Cold stress test for the hands, in *The Thermal Image in Medicine and Biology*, Ammer, K. and Ring, E.F.J., Eds., Uhlen-Verlag, Wien, 1995, p. 237.

22. Clark, R.P. and de Calcina-Goff, M. Guidelines for standardisation in medical thermography draft international standard proposals. *Thermol. Österr.*, 7, 47, 1997.

23. Website address, Atlas of Normals, www.medimaging.org.

24. Ammer, K. et al. Rationale for standardised capture and analysis of infrared thermal images, in *Proceedings Part II, EMBEC'02 2. European Medical and Biological Engineering Conference*, Hutten, H. and Krösel, P., Eds. IFMBE, Graz, 2002, p. 1608.

25. Ring, E.F.J. et al. Errors and artefacts in thermal imaging, in *Proceedings Part II, EMBEC'02 2. European Medical and Biological Engineering Conference*, Hutten, H. and Krösel, P., Eds., IFMBE, Graz, 2002, p. 1620.

26. Anbar, M. Recent technological developments in thermology and their impact on clinical applications. *Biomed. Thermol.*, 10, 270, 1990.

27. Hardy, J.D. The radiation of heat from the human body. III. The human skin as a black body radiator. *J. Clin. Invest.*, 13, 615, 1934.

28. Togawa, T. and Saito, H. Non-contact imaging of thermal properties of the skin. *Physiol. Meas.*, 15, 291, 1994.

29. Engel, J.-M. Physical and physiological influence of medical ointments of infrared thermography, in *Recent Advances in Medical Thermology*, Ring, E.F.J. and Phillips, B., Eds., Plenum Press, New York, 1984, p. 177.

30. Hejazi, S. and Anbar, M. Effects of topical skin treatment and of ambient light in infrared thermal images. *Biomed. Thermol.*, 12, 300, 1992.

31. Ammer, K. The influence of antirheumatic creams and ointments on the infrared emission of the skin, in *Abstracts of the 10th International Conference on Thermogrammetry and Thermal Engineering in Budapest 18–20, June 1997*, Benkö, I., Balogh, I., Kovacsics, I., Lovak, I., Eds., MATE, Budapest, 1997, p. 177.

32. Ammer, K. Einfluss von Badezusätzen auf die Wärmeabstrahlung der Haut. *ThermoMed*, 10, 71, 1994.

33. Ammer, K. The influence of bathing on the infrared emission of the skin, in *Abstracts of the 9th International Conference on Thermogrammetry and Thermal Engineering in Budapest 14–16, June 1995*, Benkö, I., Lovak, I., and Kovacsics, I., Eds., MATE, Budapest, 1995, p. 115.

34. Ammer, K. Thermographie in lymphedema, in *Advanced Techniques and Clinical Application in Biomedical Thermologie*, Mabuchi, K., Mizushina, S., and Harrison, B., Eds., Harwood Academic Publishers, Chur/Schweiz, 1994, p. 213.

35. Heath, A.M. et al. A comparison of surface and rectal temperatures between sheared and non-sheared alpacas (*Lama pacos*). *Small Rumin. Res.*, 39, 19, 2001.

36. Purohit, R.C. et al. Thermographic evaluation of animal skin surface temperature with and without haircoat. *Thermol. Int.*, 11, 83, 2001.

37. Damm, F., Döring, G., and Hildebrandt, G. Untersuchungen über den Tagesgang von Hautdurchblutung und Hauttemperatur unter besonderer Berücksichtigung der physikalischen Temperaturregulation. *Z. Physik. Med. Rehabil.*, 15, 1, 1974.

38. Reinberg, A. Circadian changes in the temperature of human beings. *Bibl. Radiol.*, 6, 128, 1975.
39. Schmidt, K.-L., Mäurer, R., and Rusch, D. Zur Wirkung örtlicher Wärme und Kälteanwendungen auf die Hauttemperatur am Kniegelenk. *Z. Rheumatol.*, 38, 213, 1979.
40. Kanamori, T. et al. Circadian rhythm of body temperature. *Biomed. Thermol.*, 11, 292, 1991.
41. Friedrich, K.H. Assessment criteria for infrared thermography systems. *Acta Thermograp.*, 5, 68, 1980.
42. Alderson, J.K.A. and Ring, E.F.J. "Sprite" high resolution thermal imaging system. *Thermology*, 1, 110, 1985.
43. Dibley, D.A.G. Opto-mechanical systems for thermal imaging, in *The Thermal Image in Medicine and Biology*, Ammer, K. and Ring, E.F.J., Eds., Uhlen-Verlag, Wien, 1995, p. 33.
44. Plassmann, P. Advances in image processing for thermology, *Presented at Int. Cong. of Thermology*, Seoul, June 5–6, 2004, p. 3.
45. Kutas, M. Staring focal plane array for medical thermal imaging, in *The Thermal Image in Medicine and Biology*, Ammer, K. and Ring, E.F.J., Eds., Uhlen-Verlag, Wien, 1995, p. 40.
46. Ring, E.F.J., Minchinton, M., and Elvins, D.M. A focal plane array system for clinical infrared imaging. *IEEE/EMBS Proceedings*, Atlanta 1999, p. 1120.
47. Hejazi, S. and Spangler, R.A. A multi-wavelength thermal imaging system, in *Proceedings of the 11th Annual International Conference IEEE Engineering in Medicine and Biology Society*, II, 1989, p. 1153.
48. Ring, E.F.J. Quality control in infrared thermography, in *Recent Advances in Medical Thermology*, Ring, E.F.J. and Phillips, B., Eds., Plenum Press, New York, 1984, p. 185.
49. Clark, R.P. et al. Thermography and pedobarography in the assessment of tissue damage in neuropathicand atherosclerotic feet. *Thermology*, 3, 15, 1988.
50. Clark, J.A. Effects of surface emissivity and viewing angle errors in thermography. *Acta Thermograp.*, 1, 138, 1976.
51. Steketee, J. Physical aspects of infrared thermography, in *Recent Advances in Medical Thermology*, Ring, E.F.J. and Phillips, B., Eds., Plenum Press, New York, 1984, p. 167.
52. Wiecek, B., Jung, A., and Zuber, J. Emissivity-Bottleneck and challenge for thermography. *Thermol. Int.*, 10, 15, 2000.
53. Ammer K. Need for standardisation of measurements, in *Thermal Imaging in Thermography and Lasers in Medicine*, Wiecek, B., Ed., Akademickie Centrum Graficzno-Marketigowe Lodart S.A, Lodz, 2003, p. 13.
54. Anbar, M. Potential artifacts in infrared thermographic measurements. *Thermology*, 3, 273, 1991.
55. Ring, E.F.J. and Dicks, J.M. Spatial resolution of new thermal imaging systems, *Thermol. Int.*, 9, 7, 1999.
56. Melnizky, P., Schartelmüller, T., and Ammer, K. Prüfung der intra-und interindividuellen Verlässlichkeit der Auswertung von Infrarot-Thermogrammen. *Eur. J. Thermol.*, 7, 224, 1997.
57. Ring, E.F.J. and Ammer, K. The technique of thermal imaging in medicine. *Thermol. Int.*, 10, 7, 2000.
58. Khallaf, A. et al. Thermographic study of heat loss from the face. *Thermol. Österr.*, 4, 49, 1994.
59. Ishigaki, T. et al. Forehead–back thermal ratio for the interpretation of infrared imaging of spinal cord lesions and other neurological disorders. *Thermology*, 3, 101, 1989.
60. Schuber, T.R. et al. Directed dynamic cooling, a methodic contribution in telethermography. *Acta Thermograp.*, 1, 94, 1977.
61. Di Carlo, A. Thermography in patients with systemic sclerosis. *Thermol. Österr.*, 4, 18, 1994.
62. Love, T.J. Heat transfer considerations in the design of a thermology clinic. *Thermology*, 1, 88, 1985.
63. Ring, E.F.J. Computerized thermography for osteo-articular diseases. *Acta Thermograp.*, 1, 166, 1976.
64. Roberts, D.L. and Goodman, P.H. Dynamic thermoregulation of back and upper extremity by computer-aided infrared imaging. *Thermology*, 2, 573, 1987.
65. Mabuchi, K. et al. Development of a data processing system for a high-speed thermographic camera and its use in analyses of dynamic thermal phenomena of the living body, in *The Thermal Image in Medicine and Biology*, Ammer, K. and Ring, E.F.J., Eds., Uhlen-Verlag, Wien, 1995, p. 56.

66. Cena, K. Environmental heat loss, in *Recent Advances in Medical Thermology*, Ring, E.F.J. and Phillips, B., Eds., Plenum Press, New York, 1984, p. 81.

67. Engel, J.-M. Kennzeichnung von Thermogrammen, in *Thermologische Messmethodik*, Engel, J.-M., Flesch, U., and Stüttgen, G., Eds., Notamed, Baden–Baden, 1983, p. 176.

68. Park, J.-Y. Current development of medical infrared imaging technology, *Presented at Int. Cong. of Thermology*, Seoul, June 5–6, 2004, p. 9.

69. Plassmann, P. and Ring, E.F.J. An open system for the acquisition and evaluation of medical thermological images. *Eur. J. Thermol.* 7, 216, 1997.

70. Abramson, D.I. et al. Effect of altering limb position on blood flow, O_2 uptake and skin temperature. *J. Appl. Physiol.*, 17, 191, 1962.

71. Schartelmüller, T. and Ammer, K. Räumliche Auflösung von Infrarotkameras. *Thermol. Österr.*, 5, 28, 1995.

72. Ammer, K. Update in standardization and temperature measurement from thermal images, *Presented at Int. Cong. of Thermology*, Seoul, June 5–6, 2004, p. 7.

73. Mannara, G., Salvatori, G.C., and Pizzuti, G.P. Ethyl alcohol induced skin temperature changes evaluated by thermography. Preliminary results. *Boll. Soc. Ital. Biol. Sper.*, 69, 587, 1993.

74. Melnizky, P. and Ammer, K. Einfluss von Alkohol und Rauchen auf die Hauttemperatur des Gesichts, der Hände und der Kniegelenke. *Thermol. Int.*, 10, 191, 2000.

75. Ammer, K., Melnizky, P., and Rathkolb, O. Skin temperature after intake of sparkling wine, still wine or sparkling water. *Thermol. Int.*, 13, 99, 2003.

76. Gershon-Cohen, J., Borden, A.G., and Hermel, M.B. Thermography of extremities after smoking. *Br. J. Radiol.*, 42, 189, 1969.

77. Usuki, K. et al. Effects of nicotine on peripheral cutaneous blood flow and skin temperature. *J. Dermatol. Sci.*, 16, 173, 1998.

78. Di Carlo, A. and Ippolito, F. Early effects of cigarette smoking in hypertensive and normotensive subjects. An ambulatory blood pressure and thermographic study. *Minerva Cardioangiol.*, 51, 387, 2003.

79. Collins, A.J. et al. Some observations on the pharmacology of "deep-heat," a topical rubifacient. *Ann. Rheum. Dis.*, 43, 411, 1984.

80. Ring, E.F. Cooling effects of Deep Freeze Cold gel applied to the skin, with and without rubbing, to the lumbar region of the back. *Thermol. Int.*, 14, 64, 2004.

81. Federspil, G. et al. Study of diet-induced thermogenesis using telethermography in normal and obese subjects. *Recent Prog. Med.*, 80, 455, 1989.

82. Shlygin, G.K. et al. Radiothermometric research of tissues during the initial reflex period of the specific dynamic action of food. *Med. Radiol. (Mosk)*, 36, 10, 1991.

83. Danz, J. and Callies, R. Infrarothermometrie bei differenzierten Methoden der Niederfrequenztherapie. *Z. Physiother.*, 31, 35, 1979.

84. Rusch, F., Neeck, G., and Schmidt, K.L. Über die Hemmung von Erythemen durch Capsaicin. 3. Objektivierung des Capsaicin-Erythems mittels statischer und dynamischer Thermographie, *Z. Phys. Med. Baln. Med. Klim.*, 17, 18, 1988.

85. Mayr, H., Thür, H., and Ammer, K. Electrical stimulation of the stellate ganglia, in *The Thermal Image in Medicine and Biology*, Ammer, K. and Ring, E.F.J., Eds., Uhlen-Verlag, Wien, 1995, p. 206.

86. Danz, J. and Callies R. Thermometrische Untersuchungen bei unterschiedlichen Ultraschallintensitäten. *Z. Physiother.*, 30, 235, 1978.

87. Demmink, J.H., Helders, P.J., Hobaek, H., and Enwemeka, C. The variation of heating depth with therapeutic ultrasound frequency in physiotherapy. *Ultrasound Med. Biol.*, 29, 113–118, 2003.

88. Rathkolb, O. and Ammer, K. Skin temperature of the fingers after different methods of heating using a wax bath. *Thermol Österr.*, 6, 125, 1996.

89. Ammer, K. and Schartelmüller, T. Hauttemperatur nach der Anwendung von Wärmepackungen und nach Infrarot-A-Bestrahlung. *Thermol. Österr.*, 3, 51, 1993.

90. Goodman, P.H., Foote, J.E., and Smith, R.P. Detection of intentionally produced thermal artifacts by repeated thermographic imaging. *Thermology*, 3, 253, 1991.

91. Dachs, E., Schartelmüller, T., and Ammer, K. Temperatur zur Kryotherapie und Veränderungen der Hauttemperatur am Kniegelenk nach Kaltluftbehandlung. *Thermol. Österr.*, 1, 9, 1991.

92. Rathkolb, O. et al. Hauttemperatur der Lendenregion nach Anwendung von Kältepackungen unterschiedlicher Größe und Applikationsdauer. *Thermol. Österr.*, 1, 15, 1991.

93. Ammer, K. Occurrence of hyperthermia after ice massage. *Thermol. Österr.*, 6, 17, 1996.

94. Cholewka, A. et al. Temperature effects of whole body cryotherapy determined by thermography. *Thermol. Int.*, 14, 57, 2004.

95. Danz, J., Callies, R., and Hrdina, A. Einfluss einer abgestuften Vakuumsaugmassage auf die Hauttemperatur. *Z. Physiother.*, 33, 85, 1981.

96. Eisenschenk, A. and Stoboy, H. Thermographische Kontrolle physikalisch-therapeutischer Methoden. *Krankengymnastik*, 37, 294, 1985.

97. Kainz, A. Quantitative Überprüfung der Massagewirkung mit Hilfe der IR-Thermographie. *Thermol. Österr.*, 3, 79, 1993.

98. Rusch, D. and Kisselbach, G. Comparative thermographic assessment of lower leg baths in medicinal mineral waters (Nauheim Springs), in *Recent Advances in Medical Thermology*, Ring, E.F.J. and Phillips, B., Eds., Plenum Press, New York, 1984, p. 535.

99. Ring, E, F.J., Barker, J.R., and Harrison, R.A. Thermal effects of pool therapy on the lower limbs. *Thermology*, 3, 127, 1989.

100. Konermann, H. and Koob, E. Infrarotthermographische Kontrolle der Effektivität krankengymnastischer Behandlungsmaßnahmen. *Krankengymnastik*, 27, 39, 1975.

101. Smith, B.L., Bandler, M.K., and Goodman, P.H. Dominant forearm hyperthermia: A study of fifteen athletes. *Thermology*, 2, 25, 1986.

102. Melnizky, P., Ammer, K., and Schartelmüller, T. Thermographische Überprüfung der Heilgymnastik bei Patienten mit Peroneusparese. *Thermol. Österr.*, 5, 97, 1995.

103. Ammer, K. Low muscular acitivity of the lower leg in patients with a painful ankle. *Thermol. Österr.*, 5, 103, 1995.

104. Ring, E.F., Porto, L.O., and Bacon, P.A. Quantitative thermal imaging to assess inositol nicotinate treatment for Raynaud's syndrome. *J. Int. Med. Res.*, 9, 393, 1981.

105. Lecerof, H. et al. Acute effects of doxazosin and atenolol on smoking-induced peripheral vasoconstriction in hypertensive habitual smokers. *J. Hypertens.*, 8, S29, 1990.

106. Tham, T.C., Silke, B., and Taylor, S.H. Comparison of central and peripheral haemodynamic effects of dilevalol and atenolol in essential hypertension. *J. Hum. Hypertens.*, 4, S77, 1990.

107. Natsuda, H. et al. Nitroglycerin tape for Raynaud's phenomenon of rheumatic disease patients—An evaluation of skin temperature by thermography. *Ryumachi*, 34, 849, 1994.

108. Engel, J.M. Thermotom- ein Softwarepaket für die thermographische Bildanalyse in der Rheumatologie, in *Thermologische Messmethodik*, Engel, J.-M., Flesch, U., and Stüttgen, G., Eds., Notamed, Baden–Baden, 1983, p. 110.

109. Bösiger, P. and Scaroni, F. Mikroprozessor-unterstütztes Thermographie-System zur quantitativewn on-line Analyse von statischen und dynamischen Thermogrammen, in *Thermologische Messmethodik*, Engel, J.-M., Flesch, U., and Stüttgen, G., Eds., Notamed, Baden–Baden, 1983, p. 125.

110. Brandes, P. PIC-Win-Iris Bildverarbeitungssoftware. *Thermol. Österr.*, 4, 33, 1994.

111. Ring, E.F.J. Quantitative thermography in arthritis using the AGA integrator. *Acta thermograp.*, 2, 172, 1977.

112. Parr, G. et al. Microcomputer standardization of the AGA 680 M system, in *Recent Advances in Medical Thermology*, Ring, E.F.J. and Phillips, B., Eds., Plenum Press, New York, 1984, pp. 211–214.

113. Van Hamme, H., De Geest, G., and Cornelis, J. An acquisition and scan conversion unit for the AGA THV680 medical infrared camera. *Thermology*, 3, 205, 1990.

114. Mayr, H. Korrelation durchschnittlicher und maximaler Temperatur am Kniegelenk bei Auswertung unterschiedlicher Messareale. *Thermol. Österr.*, 5, 89, 1995.

115. Plassmann, P. On-line Communication for Thermography in Europe, *Presented at Int. Cong. of Thermology*, Seoul, June 5–6, 2004, p. 50.

116. Ring, E.F.J. Thermal imaging in medico-legal claims. *Thermol. Int.*, 10, 97, 2000.

117. Sella, G.E. Forensic criteria of acceptability of thermography. *Eur. J. Thermol.*, 7, 205, 1997.

118. Hirschl, M. et al. Double-blind, randomised, placebo controlled low level laser therapy study in patients with primary Raynaud's phenomenon. *Vasa*, 31, 91, 2002.

119. Schartelmüller, T., Melnizky, P., and Engelbert, B. Infrarotthermographie zur Evaluierung des Erfolges physikalischer Therapie bei Patienten mit klinischem Verdacht auf Thoracic Outlet Syndrome. *Thermol. Int.*, 9, 20, 1999.

120. Kim, Y.S. and Cho, Y.E. Pre- and postoperative thermographic imaging in lumbar disc herniations, in *The Thermal Image in Medicine and Biology*, Ammer, K. and Ring, E.F.J., Eds., Uhlen-Verlag, Wien, 1995, p. 168.

121. Siniewicz, K. et al. Thermal imaging before and after physial exercises in children with orthostatic disorders of the cardiovascular system. *Thermol. Int.*, 12, 139, 2002.

54

Storage and Retrieval of Medical Infrared Images

Gerald Schaefer
Loughborough University

54.1 Introduction

Advances in camera technologies and reduced equipment costs have led to an increased interest in the application of thermal imaging in the medical fields [7]. Medical infrared images are typically recorded and stored in digital form, and computerized image processing techniques have been used in acquiring and evaluating medical thermal images [13,26] and proved to be important tools for clinical diagnostics. Yet, these tools rely on the digital images to be in a certain format. Unfortunately, manufacturers of medical infrared cameras have their own proprietary image formats with little or no possibility of data interchange between suppliers. There is therefore a need to develop a standardized format for storing and processing thermograms. In the first part of this chapter, we will show that the DICOM (Digital Imaging and Communications in Medicine) medical imaging standard [12] can be adopted for this purpose.

Obviously, the more images are captured the more attention has to be put on necessary resources such as storage space and bandwidth. For example, the images for one person captured according to Reference 14, which suggests 27 standard views, requires, assuming a 12-bit thermal camera with 680×512 resolution, more than 13 megabytes of disk space. The application of compression methods is therefore often a necessary step to reduce these storage requirements. For images, there are two kinds of compression methods: lossless compression which preserves all of the original information and lossy compression which sacrifices some of the visual quality to gain in terms of compression rate. While approaches for lossy compression of medical infrared images have been presented [19,20], clinicians often prefer lossless algorithms to ensure no information is lost. Also, in some countries it is forbidden by law to lossy compress images used for medical diagnosis.

In the second part of the chapter, we evaluate several "standard" lossless image compression algorithms for compressing medical infrared images. Lossless JPEG [10], JPEG-LS [4], JPEG2000 [5], PNG [28], and CALIC [27] are compared on an image set comprising more than 380 thermal images organized into 20 groups according to Reference 14.

Thermograms are typically stored for archival and legal purposes only and are not being retrieved again once a successful diagnosis has been made. In the final part of this chapter, we show how these images of past cases can be used to aid in the diagnosis of new ones. Our approach is based on the concept of content-based image retrieval (CBIR) which has been an active research area in image processing for many years [23]. The principal aim is to retrieve digital images based not on textual annotations but on features derived directly from image data. These features are then stored alongside the image and serve as an index. Retrieval is often performed in a query by example (QBE) fashion where a query image is provided by the user. The retrieval system is then searching through all images in order to find those with the most similar indices which are returned as the candidates most alike to the query.

We consider the application of content-based image retrieval as a generic approach for the analysis and interpretation of medical infrared images. CBIR allows the retrieval of visually similar and hence usually relevant images based on a predefined similarity measure between image features derived directly from the image data. In terms of medical infrared imaging, images that are visually similar to a given sample will also be likely to have medical relevance. These known cases together with their medical reports should then provide a valuable asset for diagnostic purposes.

While the first introduced approach is based on the extraction of image features from the raw (uncompressed) images, we furthermore show that content-based retrieval of medical infrared images can also be performed directly on compressed image data. In particular, we show how retrieval based on wavelet image descriptors allows the retrieval of similar thermograms.

Finally, we also introduce an approach that allows the browsing of whole databases of thermograms, again based on visual features. Utilizing a feature dimensionality reduction method, all thermal images are shown on the computer screen so that images which are close by are also visually similar to provide an alternative method of navigating through these image collections as opposed to standard methods which are restricted to searching by patient name or similar attributes.

The remainder of the chapter is organized as follows. Section 54.2 stresses the need for a standard format for thermograms. Section 54.3 evaluates the performance of several compression algorithms on thermograms, both in terms of compression speed and in terms of compression ratio. Section 54.4 details our methods of applying content-based image retrieval techniques to the domain of thermal medical images and introduces a system of visually navigating collections of thermograms. Section 54.5 concludes the chapter.

54.2 Toward a Standardized Thermogram Format

Various camera suppliers are competing for their share in the market of medical infrared imaging. Unfortunately, each of these also stores the captured images in its own, proprietary file format. This fact makes it hard to impossible to share medical infrared images between users of different systems, despite the urgent need for this facility in the light of increase of telemedicine and other emerging technologies. Thermal imaging packages such as CTHERM [13] allow the capture from various types of cameras and store images in a simple common format; yet this approach is only a step toward a suitable solution.

What is needed is a recognized standard for storage and interchange of thermograms. Clearly this standard needs to be supported by suppliers of both cameras and software packages. Most importantly, such a standard must support the preservation of the original radiometric information. What this also means is that it must support a variety of spatial and radiometric resolutions both of which vary from camera model to camera model. Apart from the storage of the actual image information in digital form, a useful standard format will provide various other properties. Patient identification and the addition of patient information as well as attaching information on the clinicians and treatments should be supported as well as the addition of other information items deemed useful for interpreting the thermogram.

Looking at other medical fields that deal with storage and exchange of digital images, DICOM [12] has emerged as the major standard and is in common use for many imaging modalities such as MRI or CT scans. We therefore want to briefly investigate whether the DICOM standard can be adopted for storing thermograms.

DICOM supports arbitrary image resolutions and various bit depths of data. Saving the radiological information of thermograms accurately will therefore be ensured, though the exact format will need to be specified. Storage of patient and medical information is also provided by default as is the possibility to provide annotations and extra information in the form of tags. This feature can be employed to save information on which part of the anatomy is captured and the storage of region of interest information as suggested in Reference 14 and can hence be used to integrate the efforts of standardization there into a common file format. Furthermore, DICOM supports not only storage of the original image data but also compression thereof which will be investigated in further detail in the next section of this chapter. Overall, DICOM supports the main requirements of a standard for storage and communication of medical thermograms while its application and enforcement will have a major positive impact on the community of users providing them with an effective and efficient way of sharing and interpreting medical infrared images.

54.3 Compression of Thermograms

In this section, we investigate the use of lossless compression algorithms for storing medical infrared images in a more compact manner.

54.3.1 Image Dataset

In order to provide a useful comparison of the performance of compression algorithms, one requires an image set that reflects the diversity of types of thermal images that are typically captured. We have therefore compiled such a data set which follows the standard views introduced in Reference 14. There, 27 standard poses are defined which are designed to capture every view possible necessary for composing an atlas based on infrared imaging. Of these 27 views, we omitted 7 poses which are very similar to some of the other ones due to symmetry reasons (either left/right or anterior/dorsal). Of each of the remaining 20 image groups about 20 images were collected using CTHERM [13]; details regarding each group are given in Table 54.1. With a few exceptions, all images are of size 680×512, and the image bit depth is 7 bits.

54.3.2 Compression Algorithms

We evaluated five popular compression algorithms of which four have also been adapted as international imaging standards. Below, we briefly characterize the algorithms and implementations we used:

- Lossless JPEG—former JPEG committee standard for lossless image compression [10]. The standard describes predictive image compression algorithm with Huffman or arithmetic entropy coder. JPEG is supported by the DICOM standard. The results are reported for the predictor function SV 2, which resulted in the best average compression ratio for the dataset, and Huffman coding.
- JPEG-LS—standard of the JPEG committee for lossless and near-lossless compression of still images [4]. The standard, which is based on the LOCO-I algorithm [25], describes low-complexity predictive image compression algorithm with entropy coding using modified Golomb–Rice family. JPEG-LS is supported by the DICOM standard.
- JPEG2000—a recent JPEG committee standard describing an algorithm based on wavelet transform image decomposition and arithmetic coding [5]. Apart from lossy and lossless compressing and decompressing of whole images, it delivers many interesting features (progressive transmission, region of interest coding, etc.) [1]. JPEG2000 is supported by the DICOM standard.

TABLE 54.1   Image Groups in the Dataset

Abbreviation	Description	Number of Images
ABD	Abdomen, anterior view	19
BAA	Both ankles, anterior view	21
BHD	Both hands, dorsal view	16
BKA	Both knees, anterior view	18
CA	Chest, anterior view	22
DF	Dorsal feet	15
FA	Face	23
LAD	Left arm, dorsal view	15
LB	Lower back, dorsal view	17
LLA	Lower legs, anterior view	20
LLD	Lower legs, dorsal view	19
LRL	Right leg, lateral view	19
ND	Neck, dorsal view	23
PF	Plantar feet	23
TA	Thighs, anterior view	20
TBA	Total body, anterior view	19
TBD	Total body, dorsal view	16
TBR	Total body, right view	17
TD	Thighs, dorsal view	18
UB	Upper body, dorsal view	22
Total		382

- PNG—standard of the WWW Consortium for lossless image compression [28]. PNG is a predictive image compression algorithm using the LZ77 [29] algorithm and Huffman coding. The results are reported for the *sub* predictor function (filter), which resulted in the best average compression ratio for the dataset.
- CALIC—a relatively complex predictive image compression algorithm using arithmetic entropy coder, which because of its usually high compression ratios, is commonly used as a reference for other image compression algorithms [27].

54.3.3 Compression Results

Before detailing the experimental procedure, it should be stressed that, although all evaluated algorithms are lossless, they are only able to preserve the data that is originally presented and which therefore has to be ensured to be radiometrically sound.

Experimental results were obtained on an HP Proliant ML350G3 computer equipped with two Intel Xeon 3.06 GHz (512 kB cache memory) processors, Windows 2003 operating system, and the algorithms were compiled using Intel C++ 8.1 compiler. To minimize effects of the system load and the input–output subsystem, the compressors were run several times. The time of the first run was ignored while the collective time of other runs (executed for at least 1 s, and at least 5 times) was measured and then averaged. The time measured is hence the sum of time spent by the processor in application code and in kernel functions called by the application, as reported by the operating system after application execution.

In Tables 54.2 and 54.3, we show the results obtained by the compression algorithms introduced in Section 54.3.2 for the image dataset described in Section 54.3.1. Results are given in terms of compression speed, expressed in megabytes per second (MB/s), where 1 MB = 2^{20} bytes in Table 54.2 and compression ratio defined as the ratio of the file size of the original image and that of the compressed file, in Table 54.3. The numbers are calculated as an average for all images contained in the group; since not all

TABLE 54.2 Compression Speeds, Given in MB/s

Images	L-JPG	JPEG-LS	JPEG2000	PNG	CALIC
ABD	11.9	17.7	3.8	3.3	4.1
BAA	11.8	18.2	4.0	3.4	4.3
BHD	11.8	17.9	3.8	3.2	4.3
BKA	11.7	14.5	3.5	2.8	3.7
CA	11.6	14.2	3.4	2.6	3.8
DF	11.8	17.6	3.9	3.3	4.2
FA	12.0	20.2	4.1	3.8	4.7
LAD	12.1	22.4	4.3	4.0	5.0
LB	11.6	13.7	3.4	2.6	3.6
LLA	12.2	23.6	4.4	4.3	4.9
LLD	12.0	21.6	4.4	4.0	4.6
LRL	11.9	20.3	4.0	3.8	4.8
ND	11.6	15.3	3.6	2.9	3.8
PF	11.7	17.7	3.9	3.2	4.4
TA	11.8	19.0	4.0	3.7	4.4
TBA	12.4	29.7	4.7	4.9	5.7
TBD	12.5	28.8	4.6	4.9	5.5
TBR	12.5	30.2	4.8	4.8	5.7
TD	12.0	19.6	4.1	3.6	4.5
UB	11.7	14.6	3.5	2.7	3.7
All	11.9	19.6	4.0	3.6	4.5

groups contain the same number of images, the average results for all images may be slightly different from the average of all groups.

Among the tested algorithms the JPEG-LS is clearly the best when we consider the compression speeds listed in Table 54.2. All other algorithms are noticeably slower—from 39% (Lossless JPEG) to 82% (PNG). The speeds of JPEG2000, PNG, and CALIC are similar (CALIC is faster than the remaining two algorithms by 11% and 20%, respectively). Both CALIC and JPEG2000 use an arithmetic entropy coder in contrast to PNG which is based on faster techniques (LZ77 and the Huffman coding). Based on this, we expected PNG to obtain compression speeds close to Lossless JPEG with Huffman coding. Therefore, the low speed of PNG is probably due to the implementation (we used NetPBM). Looking at the results on a group by group basis, the best compression speeds were obtained for groups TBA, TBD, and TBR that is, those groups where the total body is captured. The worst compression speeds were achieved for groups BKA, CA, LB, and UB.

Considering the compression ratios from Table 54.3, we see that the ratios for JPEG-LS and CALIC are higher than those for JPEG2000 which in turn performs better than PNG and Lossless JPEG. While for various continuous tone grayscale images, JPEG2000 has been reported as close to or little worse than JPEG-LS [16], our results indicate that for medical infrared images, JPEG2000 is significantly worse than JPEG-LS which is the best-performing algorithm. CALIC performs slightly worse than JPEG-LS but is also computationally much more complex. Looking at the results for each image group, the highest compression ratios are achieved for the three body groups TBA, TBD, and TBR while images of groups BKA, CA, LB, and UB are least compressible. Correlating this with the compressions speeds from Table 54.2, we see that there is a direct link between efficiency and efficacy.

Overall, it is clear that JPEG-LS is the best-performing algorithm for lossless compression of medical infrared images. Not only does it provide the highest compression ratios, it is also the fastest of the tested methods. Furthermore, JPEG-LS is already included in the DICOM standard and can hence be readily employed.

TABLE 54.3   Compression Ratios

Images	L-JPG	JPEG-LS	JPEG2000	PNG	CALIC
ABD	2.83	3.86	3.48	3.06	3.76
BAA	3.03	4.12	3.73	3.28	4.04
BHD	2.86	3.81	3.41	3.05	3.75
BKA	2.50	3.11	2.85	2.52	3.10
CA	2.41	3.06	2.78	2.55	3.01
DF	3.03	4.04	3.68	3.20	3.99
FA	3.18	4.73	4.23	3.70	4.57
LAD	3.48	5.23	4.68	4.12	4.98
LB	2.36	2.92	2.65	2.41	2.88
LLA	3.75	5.71	5.09	4.27	5.52
LLD	3.64	5.34	4.79	4.06	5.18
LRL	3.24	4.71	4.19	3.66	4.56
ND	2.55	3.33	3.04	2.78	3.28
PF	2.94	3.96	3.59	3.27	3.89
TA	3.14	4.40	3.98	3.44	4.28
TBA	4.21	7.35	6.36	5.42	6.96
TBD	4.20	7.19	6.22	5.36	6.84
TBR	4.26	7.36	6.39	5.64	6.92
TD	3.21	4.49	4.08	3.46	4.36
UB	2.53	3.24	2.95	2.65	3.20
All	3.04	4.21	3.79	3.35	4.11

54.4 Retrieval of Thermograms

While medical infrared images are typically stored for archival purposes, in this section, we demonstrate that a database of images can also be usefully employed for retrieving similar medical cases. For this, we employ concepts initially developed for querying general-purpose image collections.

54.4.1 Content-Based Retrieval

54.4.1.1 Moment Invariant Features

In content-based image retrieval techniques, each image is characterized by a set of features that serve as an index into the database. The features we propose to store as indices for thermal images are invariant combinations of moments of an image. Two-dimensional geometric moments m_{pq} of order $p + q$ of a density distribution function $f(x,y)$ are defined as

$$m_{pq} = \int\limits_{-\infty}^{\infty} \int\limits_{-\infty}^{\infty} x^p y^q f(x, y) \mathrm{d}x \mathrm{d}y \qquad (54.1)$$

In terms of a digital image $g(x,y)$ of size $N \times M$, the calculation of m_{pq} becomes discretized and the integrals are hence replaced by sums leading to

$$m_{pq} = \sum_{y=0}^{M-1} \sum_{x=0}^{N-1} x^p y^q g(x, y) \qquad (54.2)$$

Rather than m_{pq}, often central moments

$$\mu_{pq} = \sum_{y=0}^{M-1}\sum_{x=0}^{N-1}(x - \bar{x})^p(y - \bar{y})^q\,g(x,y) \tag{54.3}$$

with

$$\bar{x} = \frac{m_{10}}{m_{00}} \quad \bar{y} = \frac{m_{01}}{m_{00}}$$

are used, that is, moments with the center of gravity moved to the origin (i.e., $\mu_{10} = \mu_{01} = 0$). Central moments have the advantage of being invariant to translation.

It is well known that a small number of moments can characterize an image fairly well; it is equally known that moments can be used to reconstruct the original image [3]. In order to achieve invariance to common factors and operations such as scale, rotation, and contrast, rather than using the moments themselves, algebraic combinations thereof, known as moment invariants, are used that are independent of these transformations. It is a set of such moment invariants that we use for the retrieval of thermal medical images. In particular, the descriptors we use are based on Hu's original moment invariants given by [3]

$$
\begin{aligned}
M_1 &= 4\mu_{20} + \mu_{02}\\
M_2 &= (\mu_{20} - \mu_{02})^2 + 4\mu_{11}^2\\
M_3 &= (\mu_{30} - 3\mu_{12})^2 + 3(\mu_{21} + \mu_{03})^2\\
M_4 &= (\mu_{30} + \mu_{12})^2 + (\mu_{21} + \mu_{03})^2\\
M_5 &= (\mu_{30} - 3\mu_{12})(\mu_{30} + \mu_{12})[(\mu_{30} + \mu_{12})^2 - 3(\mu_{21} + \mu_{03})^2]\\
&\quad + (3\mu_{21} - \mu_{03})(\mu_{21} + \mu_{03})[3(\mu_{30} + \mu_{12})^2 - (\mu_{21} + \mu_{03})^2]\\
M_6 &= (\mu_{20} - \mu_{02})[(\mu_{30} + \mu_{12})^2 - (\mu_{21} + \mu_{03})^2] + 4\mu_{11}(\mu_{30} + \mu_{12})(\mu_{21} + \mu_{03})\\
M_7 &= (3\mu_{21} - \mu_{03})(\mu_{30} + \mu_{12})[(\mu_{30} + \mu_{12})^2 - 3(\mu_{21} + \mu_{03})^2]\\
&\quad + (\mu_{30} - 3\mu_{12})(\mu_{21} + \mu_{03})[3(\mu_{30} + \mu_{12})^2 - (\mu_{21} + \mu_{03})^2]
\end{aligned}
\tag{54.4}
$$

Combinations of Hu's invariants can be found to achieve invariance not only to translation and rotation but also to scale and contrast [11]

$$
\begin{aligned}
\beta_1 &= \frac{\sqrt{M_2}}{M_1}\\[2mm]
\beta_2 &= \frac{M_3\mu_{00}}{M_1 M_2}\\[2mm]
\beta_3 &= \frac{M_4}{M_3}\\[2mm]
\beta_4 &= \frac{\sqrt{M_5}}{M_4}\\[2mm]
\beta_5 &= \frac{M_6}{M_1 M_4}\\[2mm]
\beta_6 &= \frac{M_7}{M_5}
\end{aligned}
\tag{54.5}
$$

54.4.1.2 Similarity Metric

Each thermal image is characterized by the six moment invariants from Equation 54.5 which form a vector $\Phi = \{\beta_i, i = 1 \ldots 6\}$. It should be noted that in the context of the DICOM standard, these features can be integrated into the thermogram through a set of annotations and can hence be shared by different users.

As similarity metric or distance measure between two thermograms, we use the Mahalanobis norm which takes into account different magnitudes of different components in Φ. The Mahalanobis distance between two invariant vectors $\Phi(I_1)$ and $\Phi(I_2)$ computed from two thermal images I_1 and I_2 is defined as

$$d(I_1, I_2) = \sqrt{(\Phi_1 - \Phi_2)^T C^{-1} (\Phi_1 - \Phi_2)} \tag{54.6}$$

where C is the covariance matrix of the distribution of Φ.

54.4.1.3 Retrieval through Query by Example

One main advantage of using the concept of content-based image retrieval is that it represents a generic approach to the automatic processing of images. Rather than employing specialized techniques which will capture only one type of image or pose (or one kind of disease or defect), image retrieval, when supported by a sufficiently large medical image database, will provide those cases that are most similar to a given one. The QBE method whereby an image is provided to the system and corresponding images from the database are retrieved and returned in order of decreasing similarity, is perfectly suited for this task. Typically, it is sufficient to restrict the attention to the top 20 retrieved images.

The moment invariant descriptors described in Section 54.4.1.1 were used to index an image database of several hundred thermal medical images provided by the University of Glamorgan [8]. An example of an image of an arm was used to perform QBE retrieval on the whole dataset. The result of this query is given in Figure 54.1 which shows those 20 images that were found to be closest to the query (sorted by

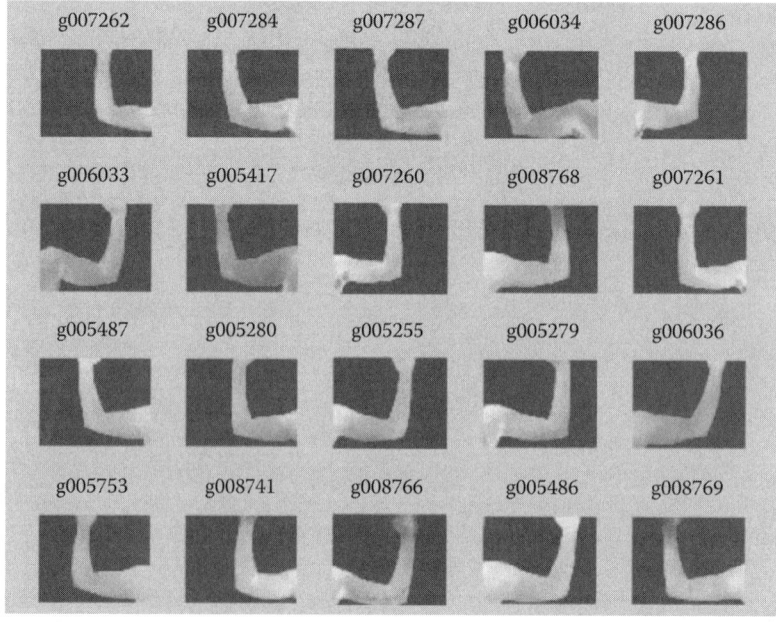

FIGURE 54.1 Example of retrieving thermal images based on a query of an *arm* image. The query image is the one on the top left; the other images are those most similar to the query ordered in decreasing similarity (from left to right, top to bottom).

descending similarity from left to right, top to bottom). As can be seen, all 20 retrieved images are of the same category, that is, arm images. The QBE method can hence be effectively employed to retrieve similar thermograms from an existing medical image repository. If coupled with patient data and related medical records, a powerful information retrieval process supporting clinical diagnosis can be initiated.

54.4.1.4 Comparison with Database of Normals

The QBE paradigm is well suited for checking an existing database of thermal images for similar cases, for example, for cases of the same disease or similar manifestations of a disease. Provided a sufficiently comprehensive database is available, it will hence provide useful results to be used for medical diagnosis. However, in many cases this prerequisite on the database is not realistic. In such instances, an alternative approach based on dissimilarities rather than similarities can be taken. Based on the assumption that a dysfunction will show on the taken thermogram, it can be compared, based on the features and similarity measure described above, to a dataset of healthy subjects captured in the same pose (such a database is described in Reference 14). If the average distance to the healthy subjects is much larger than the intercluster distances within this group of normals, this provides an indication of a certain dysfunction that needs further investigation by the clinician.

Figure 54.2 shows three infrared images of hands. Two of the images depict healthy subjects. However, the third one shows a clear inflammation on one of the fingers and generally cooler hands. Following the strategy laid out above, all hand images in the database were taken and their intercluster distance, that is, the average distance (again, based on the moment invariant features) between any two hand images, calculated. This was then compared with the average distance of the third image to all "healthy" hand thermograms. While the average distance between two images of healthy individuals was 3.53,

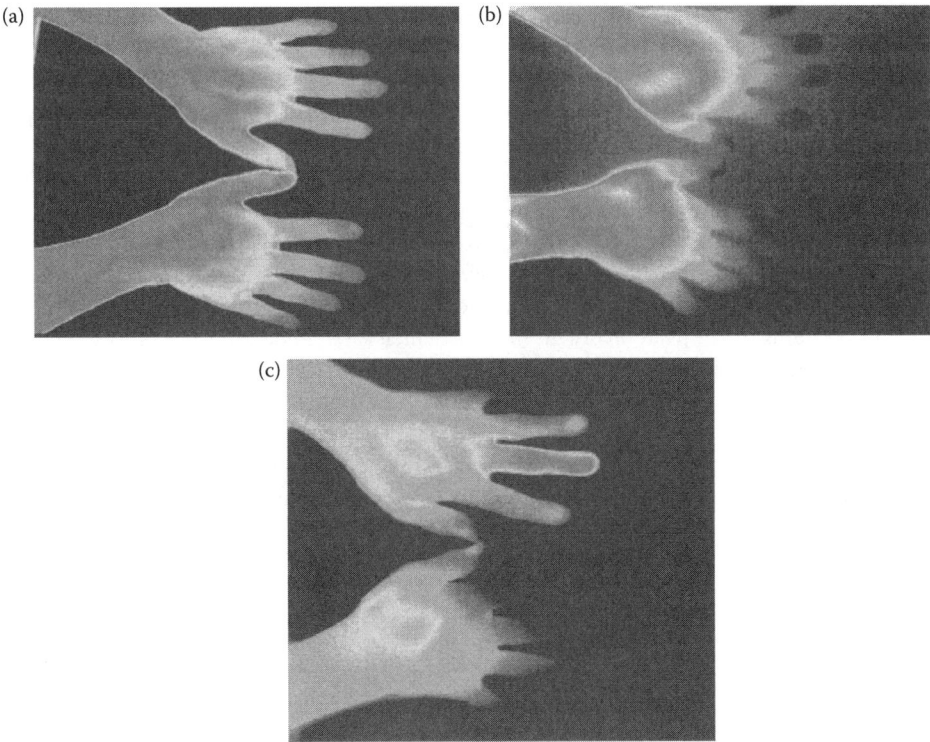

FIGURE 54.2 Thermal hand images of healthy subject (a, b) together with a thermogram showing an inflammation (c).

the distance of the image with the inflammation was 15.78. The difference between the thermogram showing an inflammation and images of healthy subjects is hence calculated as about 4 times the average difference among the images of normals. The presented image indexing techniques can therefore also be employed when no comprehensive database of pathological cases is present. Thermal images falling outside the range of thermograms recorded from healthy subjects can thus be automatically detected and should give a clear indication to the clinician to instigate further investigation.

54.4.2 Compressed-Domain Retrieval

While thermograms are typically stored in uncompressed form, as mentioned earlier in this chapter, image compression techniques can be applied to reduce storage space and resources. For performing content-based retrieval of compressed thermograms, the images would normally need to be uncompressed to allow the calculation of features such as the image moments discussed above, which clearly leads to a computational overhead. Through careful crafting of image descriptors, it is however also possible to perform retrieval directly in the compressed domain of images, for example, for images compressed using a wavelet-based techniques such as JPEG2000 [5].

In wavelet-based compression algorithms, an image is first decomposed using an M-level wavelet transform. The transform of level 1 is obtained in the following way: We start with the original image and apply one-dimensional wavelet low- and highpass filters to the rows of the image. As a result, the image is transformed into low- and high-frequency bands. Then, we apply the transform to rows of bands transforming each band into its respective low- and high-frequency band. The wavelet transform of level 1 produces four bands, each of them of resolution equal to 1/2 of the resolution of the original image. The output band of (double) lowpass filtering is a low-frequency band of level 1 (hence, actually a reduced-size original image), others are high-frequency bands representing fine details oriented at different directions. To obtain a transform of level $N + 1$, we apply the transform of level 1 to the low-frequency band of level N. As a result, we get $3M + 1$ bands of wavelet coefficients in M resolution levels (see Figure 54.3).

In the fast multiresolution image quering method (FMIQ) [6], properties of wavelet coefficients are used directly for the retrieval task. In both variants of the transform, the top-left coefficient represents the average intensity of the image, while the remaining coefficients represent image details of various sizes and orientations (coarsest near the top left corner and finer as we get more distant from there). After decomposition, we threshold the coefficients and only a small number N of wavelet coefficients (we usually choose 100) of largest absolute values (i.e., representing the most important details of image) are used as a "fingerprint of the image." It is also possible to design a special metric that takes into account only these N nonzero wavelet coefficients, thanks to which efficient comparison of fingerprints is possible. Also, depending on the position of a given coefficient, it is weighted using one of six weights (for six ranges of distance from top left corner to coefficient's position). Weights permit adjusting the algorithm to given image types. Images of low resolutions (e.g., 128 × 128), or resized to low resolution, were found sufficient for generating fingerprints.

In Figure 54.4, we show an example of this approach, based on the same image dataset that we have used earlier in this chapter. It can be seen that all 10 retrieved images are similar (i.e., of the same category) to the query image.

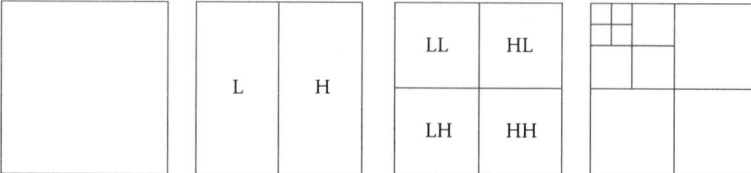

FIGURE 54.3 Wavelet transform (three levels).

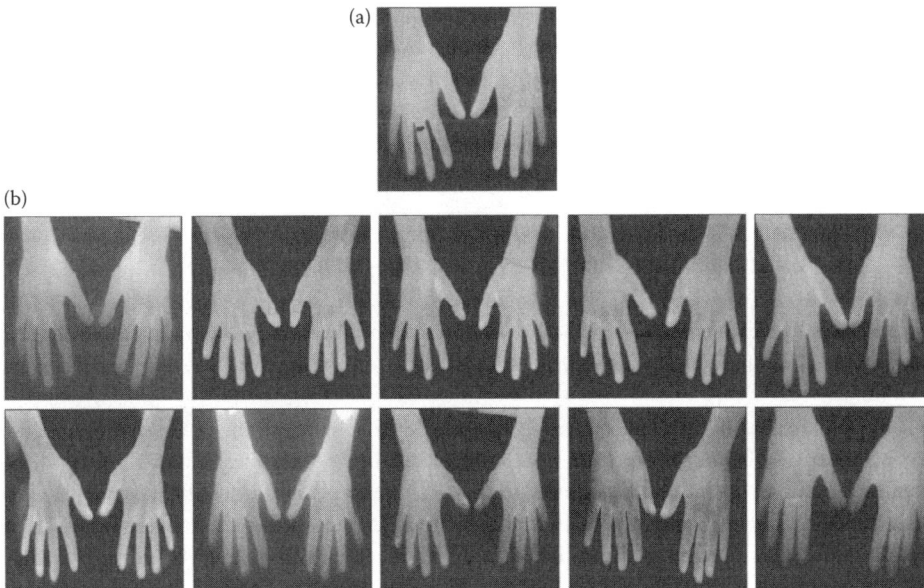

FIGURE 54.4 Example of compressed-domain retrieval showing the top 10 retrieved images based on the query image at the top.

54.4.3 Browsing of Thermal Image Database

When storing thermograms (or other medical images), often little sought is given to the actual organization and management of these image collections. While in typical medical image databases data records are accessed by patient name or other similar attributes, here we present a method that allows access to and navigation through the database based on visual cues. All images in the collection are projected onto a two-dimensional space in such a way that images that are similar to each other are located close to one another in this configuration. The result is then displayed on screen and provides a picture of the complete dataset. That visually similar images are located close to each other (i.e., clustered) is fundamental to this approach as it provides an intuitive and easy-to-understand interface for the user.

54.4.3.1 Features and Similarity Measure

Since the browsing approach taken in this chapter is again based on visual similarity between images, we make use of the features and the similarity metric we introduced and described in Sections 54.4.1.1 and 54.4.1.4, that is, moment invariants and Mahalanobis distance. Doing so allows the same features to be used for both retrieval and browsing without any additional overhead.

54.4.3.2 Multidimensional Scaling

Multidimensional scaling (MDS) [9] expresses the similarities between different objects in a small number of dimensions, allowing for a complex set of interrelationships to be summarized in a single figure. MDS can be used to analyze any kind of distance or similarity/dissimilarity matrix created from a particular dataset.

In this chapter, we follow ideas from Reference 15 and apply MDS for thermal medical image database display and navigation. By applying MDS based on the distances between moment invariant vectors, we produce a way of not only visualizing the retrieved images in terms of decreasing similarities but also according to their common similarities. All images are implanted (based on their similarities) in a two-dimensional Euclidean space where the original distances are preserved as closely as possible.

In detail, first a distance matrix which contains all pairwise distances between the medical images in the databases need to be obtained. As mentioned above, we define as the distance d between two images the Mahalanobis distance between their moment invariant vectors. Euclidean distances $\hat{d}_{i,j}$ are calculated and initially compared using Kruskal's stress formula [9]

$$
\text{Stress} = \frac{\sum_{i,j}(\hat{d}_{i,j} - d_{i,j})}{\sum_{i,j} d_{i,j}^2}
\tag{54.7}
$$

which expresses the difference between the distances d and the Euclidean values $\hat{d}$ between all images. The aim of nonmetric MDS is to assign locations to the input data so that the overall stress is minimal.

Typically, an initial configuration is found through principal component analysis (PCA). While the degree of goodness of fit after this is in general fairly high, it is not optimal. To move toward a better solution, the locations of the points are updated in such a way as to reduce the overall stress. If, for instance, the distance between two specific samples has been overestimated, it will be reduced to correct this deviation. It is clear that this modification will have implications for all other distances calculated. Therefore, the updating of the coordinates and the recalculation of the stress is being performed in an iterative way, where during each iteration the positions are slightly changed until the whole configuration is stable and the algorithm has converged into a minimum where the distances between the projected samples correspond accurately to the original distances. Several termination conditions can be applied such as an acceptable degree of goodness of fit, a predefined maximal number of iterations or a threshold for the overall changes in the configuration. Once the calculation is terminated, the images can then be plotted at the calculated coordinates on the screen.

54.4.3.3 Browsing

Navigation through the image database starts typically with a global display of the entire dataset with images positioned in relation to how similar they are to all others. From here the user has the ability to zoom into certain regions of interest to enlarge for further querying. For each localized visualization occurrence, the images selected in the area have their distance matrix recalculated and MDS reapplied.

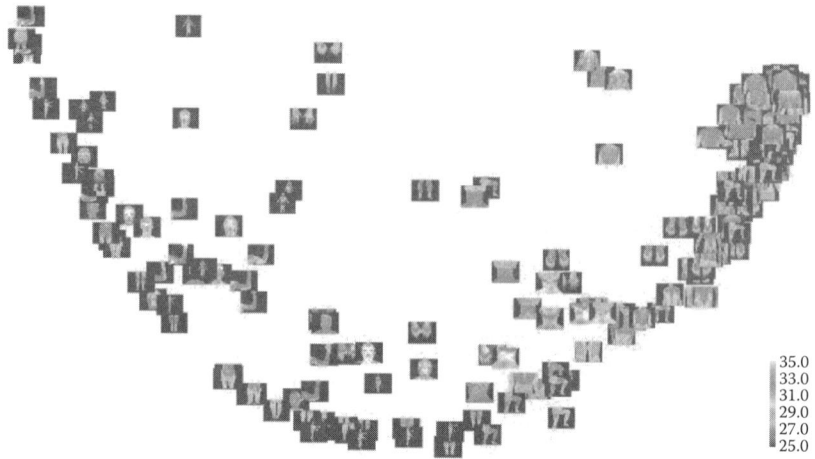

FIGURE 54.5   Global visualization view of complete thermal image database.

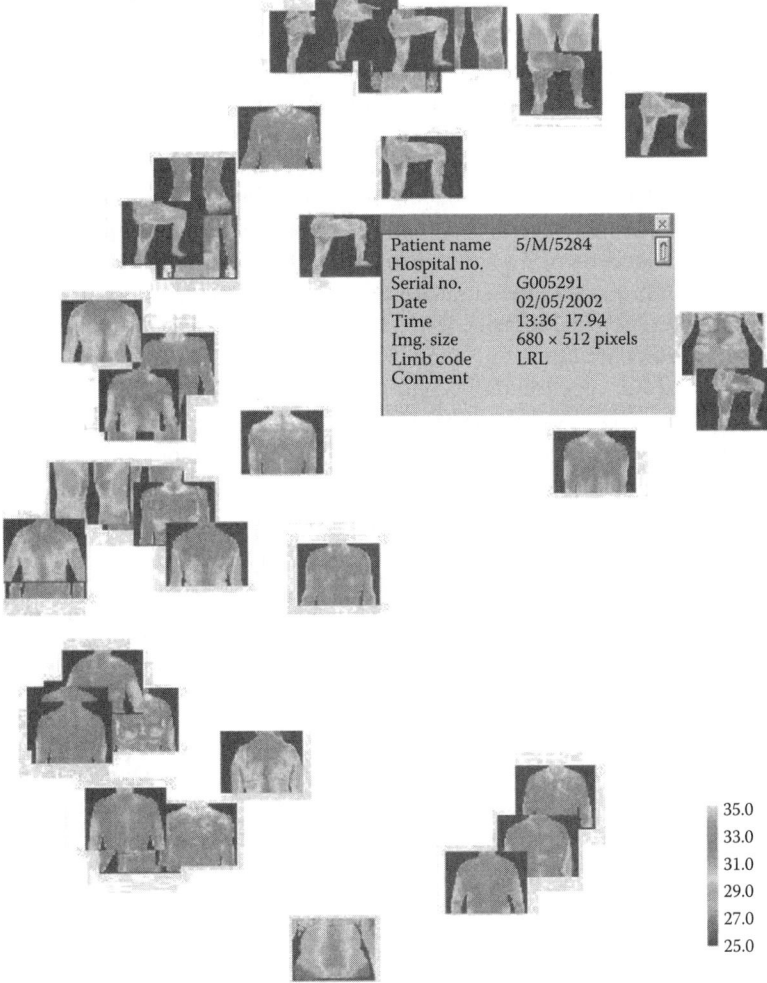

Patient name   5/M/5284
Hospital no.
Serial no.   G005291
Date   02/05/2002
Time   13:36 17.94
Img. size   680 × 512 pixels
Limb code   LRL
Comment

35.0
33.0
31.0
29.0
27.0
25.0

FIGURE 54.6 Zoomed-in area showing leg and upper body images.

The same image database as employed for the retrieval experiments has been used to test our browsing method. The triangular distance matrix between all invariant vectors was obtained using the Mahalanobis distance from Equation 54.6. Based on this distance matrix, multidimensional scaling was applied as explained in Section 54.4.3.2. The resulting global view is shown in Figure 54.5 where all images are projected (although some are occluded by others) onto the visualization plane which is then displayed on screen. It can be see that similar images are indeed placed close to each and that clusters or groups are formed. Typically, the user will then zoom into one of the clusters or areas of interest to narrow down the search as was done to produce Figure 54.6 which displays a zoomed-in area showing mainly *legs* and *upper body* images. MDS is reapplied to the images in the localized area to provide a less cluttered view. Also shown in Figure 54.6 is the possibility to retrieve further information on a certain image which is displayed in a popup window. Clearly, additional medical information such as the patient's medical history, medication, or current diagnosis information can be added to this view which hence provides an intuitive interface.

54.5 Conclusions

In this chapter, we have looked at issues regarding the storage and retrieval of medical infrared images. First, we stressed the need of a standard format for storage and communication of thermograms and suggested the adoption of the DICOM standard for this purpose.

A number of lossless compression algorithms were then evaluated on a large database of thermal medical images. It was shown that, depending on the type of image, compression ratios of up to 1:4 are possible. Furthermore, it was shown that JPEG-LS seems the most suitable algorithm to employ as it provides both the best compression performance and is also the fastest of the tested algorithms. As JPEG-LS is also certified as an international standard and is further integrated into the DICOM standard for the exchange of medical imagery, it could be recommended as a standard for storing and exchanging thermal medical images.

We have also proposed the application of content-based image retrieval to the domain of thermal medical images. Each image can be characterized by a set of moment invariants which are independent to translation, scale, rotation, and contrast. Alternatively, information on wavelet coefficients can be employed which in turn allows for retrieval also directly in the compressed domain. Retrieval is performed by returning those images whose descriptors are most similar to the ones of a given query image. In addition to retrieval, the same features can be used to provide an intuitive interface for browsing a collection of thermograms. Using multidimensional scaling, all images are projected onto a visualization plane so that images that are visually similar are also located close to each other. Experimental results for both techniques have been presented and demonstrated the usefulness of the proposed techniques.

Acknowledgments

This chapter is based on the work published in References 17, 18, 21, 22, 24. The author would like to thank Roman Starosolski (Silesian Technical University), Shao Ying Zhu, and Brian Jones (University of Derby) for their contributions as well as the Medical Computing Research Group at the University of Glamorgan for providing the test image dataset.

References

1. C. Christopoulos, A. Skodras, and T. Ebrahimi. The JPEG2000 still image coding system: An overview. *IEEE Transactions on Consumer Electronics*, 46(4):1103–1127, 2000.
2. Consultative Committee for Space Data Systems. Lossless data compression. *CCSDS Recommendation for Space System Data Standards, CCSDS 121.0-B-1, Blue Book*, 1997.
3. M.K. Hu. Visual pattern recognition by moment invariants. *IRE Transactions on Information Theory*, 8(2):179–187, February 1962.
4. ISO/IEC. Lossless and near-lossless compression of continuous-tone images—Baseline. *ISO/IEC International Standard 14495-1*, 1999.
5. ISO/IEC. JPEG2000 image coding system: Core coding system. *ISO/IEC International Standard 15444-1*, 2002.
6. C.E. Jacobs, A. Finkelstein, and D.H. Salesin. Fast multiresolution image querying. In *SIGGRAPH 95*, pp. 277–286, 1995.
7. B.F. Jones. A reappraisal of infrared thermal image analysis for medicine. *IEEE Transactions on Medical Imaging*, 17(6):1019–1027, 1998.
8. B.F. Jones. EPSRC Grant GR/R50134/01 Report, 2001.
9. J.B. Kruskal and M. Wish. *Multidimensional Scaling*. Beverly Hills, CA: Sage Publications, 1978.
10. G. Langdon, A. Gulati, and E. Seiler. On the JPEG model for lossless image compression. In *2nd Data Compression Conference*, pp. 172–180, 1992.
11. S. Maitra. Moment invariants. *Proceedings of the IEEE*, 67:697–699, 1979.

12. National Electrical Manufacturers Association. Digital Imaging and Communications in Medicine (DICOM). *Standards Publication PS 3.1-2004*, 2004.

13. P. Plassmann and E.F.J. Ring. An open system for the acquisition and evaluation of medical thermological images. *European Journal of Thermology*, 7:216–220, 1997.

14. E.F.J. Ring, K. Ammer, A. Jung, P. Murawski, B. Wiecek, J. Zuber, S. Zwolenik, P. Plassmann, C. Jones, and B.F. Jones. Standardization of infrared imaging. In *26th IEEE International Conference on Engineering in Medicine and Biology*, pp. 1183–1185, 2004.

15. Y. Rubner, L. Guibas, and C. Tomasi. The earth mover's distance, multi-dimensional scaling, and color-based image retrieval. In *Image Understanding Workshop*, pp. 661–668, 1997.

16. D. Santa-Cruz and T. Ebrahimi. A study of JPEG2000 still image coding versus other standards. In *10th European Signal Processing Conference*, pp. 673–676, 2000.

17. G. Schaefer and R. Starosolski. A comparison of two methods for retrieval of medical images in the compressed domain. In *30th IEEE International Conference Engineering in Medicine and Biology*, pp. 402–405, 2008.

18. G. Schaefer, R. Starosolski, and S.Y. Zhu. An evaluation of lossless compression algorithms for medical infrared images. In *27th IEEE International Conference Engineering in Medicine and Biology*, pp. 1125–1128, 2005.

19. G. Schaefer and S.Y. Zhu. Compressing thermal medical images. In *UK Symposium on Medical Infrared Thermography*, 2004. Abstract.

20. G. Schaefer and S.Y. Zhu. Lossy compression of medical infrared images. In *3rd European Medical and Biological Engineering Conference*, 2005.

21. G. Schaefer, S.Y. Zhu, and B. Jones. Retrieving thermal medical images. In *International Conference on Computer Vision and Graphics*, Computational Imaging and Vision. Springer, 2006.

22. G. Schaefer, S.Y. Zhu, and S. Ruszala. Visualisation of medical infrared image databases. In *27th IEEE International Conference Engineering in Medicine and Biology*, pp. 1139–1142, 2005.

23. A.W.M. Smeulders, M. Worring, S. Santini, A. Gupta, and R.C. Jain. Content-based image retrieval at the end of the early years. *IEEE Transactions on Pattern Analysis and Machine Intelligence*, 22(12):1349–1380, 2000.

24. G. Schaefer, J. Huguet, P. Plassmann, S.Y. Zhu, and F. Ring. Adopting the DICOM standard for medical infrared images, *28th IEEE Int. Conference on Engineering in Medicine and Biology*, pp. 236–239, 2006.

25. M.J. Weinberger, G. Seroussi, and G. Sapiro. The LOCO-I lossless image compression algorithm: Principles and standardization into JPEG-LS. *IEEE Transactions on Image Processing*, 9(8):1309–1324, 1996.

26. B. Wiecek, S. Zwolenik, A. Jung, and J. Zuber. Advanced thermal, visual and radiological image processing for clinical diagnostics. In *21st IEEE International Conference on Engineering in Medicine and Biology*, 1999.

27. X. Wu and N. Memon. Context-based adaptive lossless image codec. *IEEE Transactions on Communications*, 45(4):437–444, 1997.

28. WWW Consortium. PNG (Portable Network Graphics) specification. Version 1.0, 1996.

29. J. Ziv and A. Lempel. A universal algorithm for sequential data compression. *IEEE Transactions on Information Theory*, 32(3):337–343, 1977.

55

Ethical Obligations in Infrared Imaging Research and Practice

James Giordano
Potomac Institute for Policy Studies
George Mason University
University of Oxford

Kim Abramson
Institute for BioTechnology Futures

55.1 Introduction

55.1.1 A Perspective on Ethical Issues in the Use of Infrared Technology in Medicine

For the past two decades, technological advancement has led to increased capability and efficacy of functional infrared imaging (fIR). Developments in computerized image acquisition, data processing, and interpretation derived and directly incorporated from formerly classified military applications have increased and solidified the medical utility of fIR. Previous and residual concerns and criticisms of IR as being inadequate to effectively detect thermal signatures that are important to establishing particular differential diagnoses have been assuaged and refuted by the functional sophistication produced through advanced image acquisition and computerized analytic systems. There is recurrent contention surrounding the inapt use of fIR by untrained personnel, and the overuse of IR as an improperly administered or interpreted "diagnostic" test. The aforementioned progress in the technology domains of the field has deepened concerns over the ethical use of fIR, and compels a need for increased stringency in the education, training, and certification of professionally qualified, competent clinicians and technicians to be the sole providers of this technology.

In this chapter, we address the ethical obligations that compel and sustain the use of fIR in medical research and practice. We base this discussion on the premise that medicine is not merely applied science, but rather is a profession that mandates the use of scientific (i.e., theoretical) information in ways that sustain and are resonant to the humanitarian essence of the interaction between clinician and patient (Dell'Oro, 2005). To be sure, there are areas of medicine (e.g., basic science research, epidemiology/public health, etc.) that are not explicitly focused upon the clinical encounter. Yet, their relevance to the clinician–patient relationship, while indirect, implicitly reinforces the scope, tenor, and basis of patient care. This is perhaps most evident in basic sciences' research; while the proximate goal of the basic sciences is the contribution of theoretical knowledge (i.e., "knowledge for knowledge's sake"), this theoretical information contributes to a larger body of epistemic capital that is applied within the context of clinical practice as a fundamental domain of relevant knowledge (Feinstein, 1967). It is in this light that we discuss the imperative to conduct and advance research that is aimed at elucidating the capacities, enhancing the efficacy, and evaluating the outcomes of IR technology as a component of clinical paradigm of detection, discernment, and ultimately diagnosis.

But how this knowledge is utilized is as important as what this knowledge entails, and thus a brief overview of the domains of knowledge that maintain the intellectual virtues important for clinical medicine is provided. For if the information gained from basic sciences' studies of IR is to be the bedrock on which its use in medical practice is to be built, then we must recognize the moral obligations to utilize such knowledge and technical acumen in prudent ways that support the humanitarian dimensions that define medicine as an interpersonal act. This is particularly true when regarding IR technology as a viable method of detection to facilitate diagnosis, as the values in and of diagnosis ultimately establish the subsequent construct(s), content, and the context of care.

Thus, we argue that the use of IR (or any technique or technology) in the medical milieu must be explicitly relevant to and consistent with (if not wholly supportive of) the moral obligations and ethical integrity of clinical encounter between clinical and patient. The clinical encounter is, in essence, a nexus for (1) the multidimensional aspects of medicine as a science, engaging research findings within the context of a complex practice and (2) the enactment of medicine as a humanitarian endeavor, in which the conjoinment of participatory agents who maintain the expectation that the ends, or *telos*, of technically right and morally good care is enabled and provided (Pellegrino, 1983). Therefore, the capacities and limitations of IR must be recognized and explicated, so as to ensure (technically and ethically) appropriate use within the medical fiduciary.

55.1.2 On the Need for Continuing and Progressive Research

Research facilitates the defined *telos* of medicine by affording knowledge that (1) enables the clinician to evaluate the relative value(s), benefits, and risks of particular diagnostic and therapeutic approaches, and ultimately resolve equipoise, and (2) empowers patients to be informed participants in clinical decisions relevant to care, thereby lessening their inherent vulnerability and decreasing the inequalities of knowledge, power, and capacity (Freedman, 1987; Giordano, 2006a). Of course, such research must be methodologically rigorous and ethically sound (Fried, 1974; see Levine, 1986, for review). The relationship of research and practice is reciprocal. Findings from research inform practice, and evaluation of outcomes gained by employing various techniques in practice contributes to a progressive revision and expansion of an evidentiary base of knowledge to instigate and guide further study (Giordano, 2004, 2006a, 2009).

In both cases, the imperative for developing, implementing, and promoting ongoing research to assess and evaluate the capabilities and clinical application(s) of fIR is grounded upon the moral obligation of beneficence (Frankena, 1982). Irrespective of the ethical system that is utilized to guide medical research or care (e.g., employment of *prima facie* principles, casuistic approaches, ethics of care, virtue ethics, etc.), the primacy of patient benefit is critical, if not fundamental to morally sound conduct of clinical research and practice (Giordano, 2007). Pellegrino and Thomasma (1988) have defined beneficence in the clinical encounter as fourfold, encompassing the biomedical (i.e., technical) good, the good as relevant to the choices of the patient, the good for the patient as a (n autonomous) person, and the existential good, in context. Obviously, research is instrumental in determining the technical or practical "good" of a particular technique or technology, such as fIR. But even at this level, application as a meaningful biomedical "good" requires translational studies that evaluate the broader implications of use-in-practice to determine viability in real-world medical settings. In recognizing and achieving the biomedical good the somewhat more passive maxim of non-harm can be concomitantly realized. By understanding the actions, effects and capabilities of fIR, we can also recognize, weigh, and may be able to compensate for (1) inherent limitations of the technology in various applications; (2) potential risks of use or nonuse; and (3) possible burdens incurred to the patient, as well as the medical system.

This knowledge serves to illustrate the potential viability of fIR as a tool within the armamentarium of evaluative techniques that contribute to accurate diagnosis. When coupled to an understanding of the mechanisms of particular pathologies, such knowledge allows the clinician to address whether fIR can, and indeed should, be employed in specific determinative clinical situations. If properly employed, fIR can fortify the informational base necessary toward the resolution of equipoise, and thus allow treatment that is appropriate to the pathologic state, as well as the choices and overall integrity of a particular patient. Ultimately, this process, together with the prudent, practical wisdom of the clinician (i.e., *phronesis*) distinguishes what care *should* be rendered, from what care *can* be rendered (Davis, 1997).

Information fuels this decisional process, and as this volume well illustrates, the technical sophistication of current iterations of fIR enables its utility as a tool in detecting thermal changes that reflect pathologic processes of several disorders (e.g., complex regional pain syndrome, certain vasculopathies, tumorigenesis, etc.). Still, there is equivocal discussion that questions the value and necessity of continuing fIR research. The majority of contention is focused on the incapability of fIR to accurately detect thermal variation with sufficient sensitivity to be relevant to the clinical discernment of particular pathophysiological states. From this assumption would arise the issue that fIR research is impractical, or worse, that time and effort spent pursuing clinical application of fIR are pragmatically, temporally, and economically wasteful and therefore constitute an unethical exploitation of research resources or patient trust and expectation. We do not feel that these criticisms are valid based on the following grounds: first, to reiterate, the wedding of advanced image acquisition systems to state-of-the-art computerized systems using complex statistical data analyses has allowed for increased image clarity and specificity of signal-to-noise discrimination (Kakuta et al., 2002). The technical advancement of current fIR has rendered previous iterations of this technology obsolete (Irvine, 2002). Second, it must be borne in mind that the applied goals of basic (and clinical) research are to address, identify, and develop methods of overcoming problematic issues that affect or impede medical care (Goodman, 2003). But research is not merely a means to these ends; rather it is an end unto itself, being a moral enterprise that must sustain the obligations to patients (as research subjects) and to society as a public good (Giordano, 2006b; Pedroni, 2006). As a public good it should: (1) be effective in achieving goals consistent with stated ends (in this case, of medicine); (2) not be burdensome to individual patient subjects or society (May, 2003); and (3) be relatively self-advancing—that is, maintain a reciprocally translational focus that contributes to the knowledge base that infuses and advances the benefits of patient care (see also Giordano, 2004). Contemporary fIR research satisfies each of these requirements, and thus we argue that contentions against ongoing research in this area are ill informed, improperly directed and hence, unjustified.

But if the knowledge acquired through well-designed and rigorously conducted research studies is to be of any meaningful value, it must be appropriately and effectively used within the clinical encounter. How such knowledge gained from research is to be incorporated within the larger fabric of clinically relevant information is important to both its practical and ethical use, and reflects the intellectual skills necessary to the act of medicine (Pellegrino and Thomasma, 1993; Toulmin, 1975).

55.2 Domains of Knowledge in Clinical Medicine

Arguably, medicine as a science relies on theoretical knowledge that affords understanding of mechanisms of physiological process(es), disease, and diagnostic and therapeutic interventions. Such knowledge is based not only in part on *a priori* understanding of the workings of the world as natural phenomena that are logically consistent, but also on the acquisition of new knowledge that modifies our basic concepts and, as such, provides a somewhat changing epistemological capital of "truth(s)" (Fuller, 2003; Kuhn, 1962). Philosophically, this reflects the essence of science as being self-critical and self-revising as new information is acquired and incorporated into the accepted fund of knowledge

(Nagel, 1961). Theoretical knowledge is gained through research, both as an observational and experimental undertaking; this criticality of epistemic knowledge supports the importance of research to science and medicine, in general, and in the present case, undergirds the importance of progressive research to advance an understanding of the capabilities of fIR.

Given the position that medicine is not just applied science, we believe that its practice involves far more than a theoretical knowledge of physiological systems, pathologies, and the mechanics of particular tests, tools, and interventions. We hold that knowing "what should be done" mandates understanding of "how," "when," and "why" something is done (Giordano, 2006b, 2009). Specifically, knowing whether fIR represents an appropriate detective protocol for a particular clinical case requires understanding not only of the technology (and its capacities and limitations) but also the suspected pathology, the physiological changes it incurs, the viability of fIR to detect such changes, as well as how the technology (of both image acquisition conditions and data analyses) should be employed to meet the particular circumstances. This necessitates experience in differing situations and across time. Experiential knowledge can be gained through an expanding body of research findings, and may be acquired through training and direct activity (Davis, 1997; Giordano, 2006b). The necessity of experiential knowledge in clinical contexts further endorses the need for continued research in mechanisms and applications of fIR, and additionally supports the continued utilization of fIR in practice so as to contribute to a growing database of clinically relevant applications and possibilities. Ultimately, theoretical and experiential knowledge work synergistically when relating current cases to paradigmatic examples (i.e., the casuistic approach), and in this way theory and experience are conjoined to determine if, how and why fIR can and should be utilized as a step in the process of diagnosing particular pathology in a specific patient.

In this situation, contextual knowledge allows the clinician to

1. Utilize technical and experiential knowledge of fIR as a tool in detecting the thermal signatures of certain pathophysiological states.
2. Use this theory and experience to determine whether fIR represents an appropriate evaluative method.
3. Utilize theoretical and experiential understanding to formulate and implement the right conditions for use and interpretation of fIR in a given case.

Taken together, contextual knowledge fuses research to practice (Giordano, 2009), and allows the clinician to avoid a simplistic "one-size-fits-all" approach to assessment of those pathologies for which fIR has been shown to be a valid and effective evaluative tool. Further, fIR provides objective assessment of otherwise subjective diagnostics. Objective measures increase the accuracy of diagnosis and, by extension, the effectiveness of treatment, and are therefore emphasized within most medical disciplines in order to validate subjective information (Johnston et al., 2007; Reinhard et al., 2007; Zhang & Zhou, 2007).

Experiential and contextual knowledge rely on a theoretical foundation, and both require and infuse skill. However, it is important to note that there is an abstract dimension to medicine. Indeed, medicine has been described as both skill and art (i.e., *tekne*) that establishes the distinction between simply applied science and the finesse that empowers its subjective, hermeneutic character (Edelstein, 1967; Owens, 1977; Svenaeus, 2000). The critical intellectual, practical, and moral step in medical practice occurs as description, detection, and differentiation coalesce into the process of diagnosis (Wulff, 1976). It is from this point of determining "what is wrong" with a particular patient that the possibilities for and selection of subsequent treatment can be ascertained (Pellegrino, 1979). Indeed, this is the point at which individual and clinical equipoise are reconciled and resolved on grounds that provide the best choice(s) for ethically good patient care. This process of using theoretical, experiential, and contextual knowledge, together with any and all tools and methods that are nonburdensome, manifest low risk, and which effectively produce reliable data to generate an evidence-based approach, is essential to clinical decision making. *Phronesis*, the intellectual virtue of practical wisdom, is imperative to determine (1) which tools, tests, and approaches best contribute to the diagnostic process; (2) the meaning and relative value(s) of findings; and (3) how these findings facilitate diagnosis (Giordano, 2006a, b, 2007, 2009; see also Davis, 1997). As well, *phronesis* allows the clinician to intuit the nature and power in and of diagnosis as an act of naming the disorder, claiming particular "truths" about the disorder and its care, and framing the patient within a population of those with this disorder and establishing the trajectory of subsequent clinical interaction(s) (Giordano, 2006b, 2007, 2009). The power of this step is exceptional, and as such the inherent responsibilities must be borne by individuals who are capable of integrating multidimensional knowledge, weighing the complex choices arising from diverse circumstances, prudently determining the reasons to guide right action(s), and recognizing and accepting consequences of those actions (Pellegrino, 1979). For fIR to be accurately, effectively, and thus ethically employed, it must be administered and interpreted by individuals who are not simply repeating a task by rote (even if safely, and efficiently), but rather by individuals who exercise practical wisdom in the professional responsibilities of the diagnostic process (i.e., by one who utilizes and embodies *phronesis* by virtue of character—a *phronimos*). By Aristotelian definition, a *phronimos* is concerned not just with knowing the right things, but in using that knowledge in the right ways to achieve the good(s) intrinsic to the practice (Aristotle, 1999; Edelstein, 1967).

55.3 The Contribution of fIR Detection to Diagnostic Value(s)

Assessment, detection, and discernment are not diagnosis; fIR cannot and should not be considered or utilized as a singular method of detection or explicitly diagnostic technique. However, the use of IR evaluation by a competently trained professional, acting prudently to weigh the value of information gained, can serve as an important diagnostic asset. The word diagnosis is derived from the Greek *diagignoskein*, meaning "to distinguish." This distinguishing quality reflects the abilities of the clinician to utilize the aforementioned domains of knowledge to apprehend the features of a disorder as expressed in a particular patient, differentiate these signs and symptoms from other possible disorders, discern the contextual basis of these features and in so doing establish diagnosis, literally as a "... seeing or a knowledge into the problem" (Mainetti, 1992, p. 256). Any and all contributory methods and acts of diagnosis should be oriented toward (1) simplification, (2) ongoing reevaluation and interpretation, (3) synergizing theoretical and contextual understanding and moral intention, and (4) the primacy of the patients' best interest(s) (Sadler, 2004, 2005). Each of these criteria can be met by fIR, for as this volume illustrates, the technical advances that have been made over the past 20 years have allowed fIR to be used to (1) facilitate detection and thus simplify particular diagnoses, (2) afford the ability for (re)evaluation and interpretation of pathological advancement or effects of therapeutic intervention, and (3) incur low/ minimal risk and thus be nonburdensome to the best interest(s) of the patient. In this latter regard, it should be noted that as part of a more expansive diagnostic protocol, fIR may lessen the risks and burdens of medical care through earlier detection of particular pathologies, to prompt better diagnosis and care that ultimately could reduce the extent, duration, as well as negative (personal and financial) impact of subsequent intervention(s). It is clear that this process takes on considerable ethical weight as it provides the basis for prognosis (a knowledge of what could occur), and creates a foundation for the development and implementation of prudent care (Giordano, 2009). Thus, diagnosis also relies at least in part on *phronesis*, as its technical rectitude and moral gravity must be oriented to and consistent with the *telos* of medicine. These telic obligations compel both research to determine those techniques and technologies that enhance diagnoses, as well as the utilization of these approaches in clinical practice (Giordano, 2006b).

55.3.1 Ethical (and Legal) Obligations for Education and Training

If research is to inform practice, and the actions of morally sound practice are reliant on the phronetic integration of distinct types and domains of knowledge, then how can this relationship be fortified to ensure that fIR is aptly utilized? It is notable that the more befouling criticisms of fIR have centered upon its use by poorly trained "technicians" or nonprofessionals, and on unethical claims for financial reimbursement for improper characterization and employment as a "diagnostic" technique. Both of these denunciations reflect inadequacies or improprieties in education and training. Thus, we argue that the technical understanding of fIR technology, use and applications must be provided by stringent programs of didactic pedagogy, practical training, and evaluation that reflect the complexity and advancement of the field, acknowledge the technical and ethical power of this technology in medical diagnosis and care, and uphold a high standard of professionalism. This is not only an ethical question, but a legal one. Improperly or inadequately trained personnel risk negligence resulting in malpractice suits, increasing medical costs, hampering patient trust, and damaging the reputation of the medical provider. Whether personnel simply appear negligent, based on a lack of professionalism, which potentially results in unsuccessful lawsuits, or actually perform an act of malpractice that results in a successful claim against the provider, legal as well as ethical consequences can be dire. We therefore impugn those approaches and programs that claim to "certify" individuals as fIR "technicians" or experts after a course of brief home study, weekend seminar and/or superficial "examination." Such programs are wholly iniquitous, depreciate the field and threaten patient care and the integrity of the medical fiduciary. Rather, we propose that fIR be incorporated into extant training programs of medical imaging, either as an additional curricular focus, or as a specialized program of study. Similarly, we propose that fIR training be provided to licensed medical professionals (i.e., physicians, veterinarians) through continuing education and postgraduate programs that (1) afford thorough information on the technology, conditions and constraints of use, limitations and delimiting factors in clinical application, and (2) mandate practical training and experience in fIR use and methods of data analysis and outcomes evaluation. Progress in technological development should not be ethically undermined by capricious, unprofessional utilization engendered through improper education, training, and certification; and this is sound legal practice, as well, to clearly demonstrate that professional and ethical standards have been instituted.

To be sure, these insurances are demanding, and require revision and ongoing monitoring of research, education, training, and application(s) in practice. Yet, as technology progresses, so too do the responsibilities to utilize and apply such technology in ways that are consistent with an expanding epistemology and are adherent to moral obligations and ethical affirmations for good and nonharm (Jonas, 1973).

55.3.2 The Role of Policy

But while these incentives may affect change on a grass-roots level, meaningful change in the "culture" of medicine (and the economic strata that support it) cannot be fully actualized without "top-down" implementation. This is the role of policy. If positive change is to occur, it must reflect the technological progress in the field, identify and be consonant with the purpose of those individuals who embrace and utilize these developments for identifiably good ends, and enact a process that engages each of the tiers affected (i.e., research, education, training, and application; Light, 2000). The voices of the research, clinical, and patient communities must reflect valuation of fIR as a meaningful clinical tool that requires further study, development, and application, thus necessitating policy that provides enablement and economic support of these endeavors. In this way "bottom-up" values and interests will encourage "top-down" enactment of public policy programs for subsidizing these enterprises. How could this be realistically achieved? First, it is important to recognize that learning must precede change—the vectors for change agency can only be empowered when the potential and possibilities that change incurs are generally appreciated as positive and nonthreatening to some real or perceived status quo. Input from the affected communities, including patients, medical providers and technology developers, is crucial, to identify authentic and perceived risks, fears, and concerns, as well as potential education (for both medical providers and for the general population) and outreach opportunities. By demonstrating the progress in fIR and pragmatically addressing the potential, possibilities, and implications that such progress may afford to healthcare, a pediment to learning can, and hopefully has, been achieved. This is critical for dispelling prior and extant misconceptions, and engendering favorable reappraisal. But "bottom-up" efforts must also reflect a "house cleaning" of sorts, to fortify the field from within, ensuring professionalism that adheres to, and reflects strict ethical standards, as previously described. Without such, any viability of fIR as a technology and technique will be overshadowed by ethical improbity in application, and the value of policy to support further research and clinical use will be abrogated.

The fusion of "bottom-up" and "top-down" change to advance the medical use of fIR requires a multipartite effort of (1) integrating research into formalized education and training, (2) instilling and ensuring high ethical standards for the use of fIR by competent professionals, and (3) instituting public policy to assure ongoing administrative and economic support. The work described by this volume certainly serves both as a cornerstone to such efforts and a catalyst for progress in the ethical use of this technology.

Acknowledgments

This work was supported, in part, by funding from the Institute for BioTechnology Futures (JG and KA), the William H. and Sara Crane Schaefer Endowment (JG), and the Nour Foundation (JG).

References

Aristotle. *The Nicomachean Ethics* (T. Irwin, trans.). Hackett Publishing, Indianapolis, 1999.

Davis FD. Phronesis, reasoning and Pellegrino's philosophy of medicine. *Theoret. Med.*, 1997; 18: 173–198.

Dell'Oro R. Interpreting clinical judgment: Epistemological notes on the praxis of medicine. In: Viafora C. (ed.) *Clinical Bioethics—A Search for Foundations.* Springer, Dordrecht, 2005.

Edelstein L. The professional ethics of the Greek physician. In: Temkin, O. and Temkin, C.L. (eds.) *Ancient Medicine: The Selected Papers of Ludwig Edelstein.* Johns Hopkins Press, Baltimore, MD, 1967.

Feinstein AR. *Clinical Judgment.* Williams & Wilkins, Baltimore, MD, 1967.

Frankena W. Beneficence in an ethics of virtue. In: Shelps, E. (ed.) *Beneficence and Health Care.* D. Reidel, Doredrecht, 1982.

Freedman B. Equipoise and the ethics of clinical research. *N. Engl. J. Med.*, 1987; 317: 141–145.

Fried C. *Medical Experimentation: Personal Integrity and Social Policy.* North-Holland, Amsterdam, 1974.

Fuller S. *Kuhn vs. Popper: The Struggle for the Soul of Science.* Columbia University Press, New York, 2003.

Giordano J. Pain research: Can paradigmatic revision bridge the needs of medicine, scientific philosophy and ethics? *Pain Phys.*, 2004; 7: 459–463.

Giordano J. Good as gold? The randomized control trial—Paradigmatic revision and ethical responsibility in pain research. *Am. J. Pain Manage.*, 2006a; 16: 68–71.

Giordano J. Moral agency in pain medicine: Philosophy, practice and virtue. *Pain Phys.*, 2006b; 9: 71–76.

Giordano J. Pain, the patient and the physician: Philosophy and virtue ethic in pain medicine. In: Schatman M.E. (ed.) *Ethical Issues in Chronic Pain Management.* CRC/Taylor-Francis, Boca Raton, FL, 2007; 1–18.

Giordano J. *Pain, Mind, Meaning and Medicine.* PPM Books, Glen Falls, PA, 2009.

Goodman KW. *Ethics and Evidence-Based Medicine: Fallibility and Responsibility in Clinical Science.* Cambridge University Press, Cambridge, 2003.

Irvine IM. Targeting breast cancer detection with military technology: Applicability of automated target recognition technology to early screening for breast cancer. *Eng. Biol. Med.*, 2002; 21: 36–40.

Johnston DW, Propper C, and Shields MA. Comparing subjective and objective measures of health: Evidence from hypertension for the income/health gradient. Discussion paper. Bonn, Germany: Forschungsinstitut zur Zukunft der Arbeit (Institute for the Study of Labor), 2007.

Jonas H. Technology and responsibility. *Social Res.*, 1973; 40: 31–54.

Kakuta N, Yokoyama S, and Mabuschi K. Human thermal models for evaluating infrared images: Comparing infrared images under various thermal environmental conditions through normalization of skin surface temperature. *Eng. Biol. Med.*, 2002; 21: 63–72.

Kuhn T. *The Structure of Scientific Revolutions.* University of Chicago Press, Chicago, IL, 1962.

Levine RJ. *Ethics and Regulation of Clinical Research*, 2nd ed. Yale University Press, New Haven, CT, 1986.

Light DW. The sociological character of health care. In: Albrecht, G.L., Fitzpatrick, R., and Scrimshaw, S.C. (eds.) *Healthcare Markets, Handbook of Social Studies in Health.* Sage Publications, London, 2000.

Mainetti JA. Embodiment, pathology, diagnosis. In: Pesert J.L. and Gracia D. (eds.) *The Ethics of Diagnosis.* Philosophy and Medicine Series, Vol. 40, Kluwer, Boston, MA, 1992.

May WF. Contending images of the healer in an era of turnstile medicine. In: Walter J.K. and Klein E.P. (eds.) *The Story of Bioethic: From Seminal Works to Contemporary Explorations.* Georgetown University Press, Washington, DC, 2003.

Nagel E. *The Structure of Science: Problems in the Logic of Scientific Explanation.* Harcourt, Brace and World, New York, 1961.

Owens J. Aristotelian ethics, medicine and the changing nature of man. In: Spicker S and Engelhardt HT (eds.) *Philosophical Medical Ethics—Its Nature and Significance*, Vol. 3. D. Reidel, Dordrecht, 1977.

Pedroni J. Going off the gold standard—Pain research beyond the randomized controlled trial. *Am. J. Pain Manage.*, 2006; 16: 61–65.

Pellegrino ED. The anatomy of clinical judgments: Some notes on right reason and right action. In: Engelhardt H.T., Spicker S. and Towers B. (eds.) *Clinical Judgment: A Critical Appraisal.* D. Reidel, Dordrecht, 1979.

Pellegrino ED. The healing relationship: Architectonics of clinical medicine. In: Shelp E (ed.) *The Clinical Encounter: The Moral Fabric of the Patient–Physician Relationship.* Philosophy and Medicine Series, Vol. 4, D. Reidel, Dordrecht, 1983.

Pellegrino ED and Thomasma DC. *For the Patient's Good: The Restoration of Beneficence in Health Care.* Oxford University Press, New York, 1988.

Pellegrino ED and Thomasma DC. *The Virtues in Medical Practice.* Oxford University Press, New York, 1993.

Reinhard MJ, Hinkin CH, Barclay TR, Levine AJ, Mario S., Castellon SA, Longshore D et al. Discrepancies between self-report and objective measures for stimulant drug use in HIV: Cognitive, medication adherence and psychological correlates. *Addictive Behavior*, 1997; *32*(12): 2727–2736.

Sadler JZ. Diagnosis/antidiagnosis. In: Radden J (ed.) *The Philosophy of Psychiatry: A Companion.* Oxford University Press, New York, 2004.

Sadler JZ. *Values and Psychiatric Diagnosis.* Oxford University Press, New York, 2005.

Svenaeus F. *The Hermeneutics of Medicine and the Phenomenology of Health: Steps Toward a Philosophy of Medical Practice*, Kluwer, Dordrecht, 2000.

Toulmin S. Concepts of function and mechanism in medicine and medical science (Hommage a Claude Bernard). In: Engelhardt HT and Spicker S (eds.) *Evaluation and Explanation in the Biomedical Sciences.* Philosophy and Medicine Series, Vol. 1, D. Reidel, Dordrecht, 1975.

Wulff HR. *Rational Diagnosis and Treatment.* Blackwell, Oxford, 1976.

Zhang L and Zhou Z. Objective and subjective measures for sleep disorders. *Neuroscience Bulletin*, 2007; *23*(4).

IV

Medical Informatics

Luis G. Kun
National Defense University

Preface

This new 4th edition of the Medical Informatics section will offer an expanded view of the topic. In addition to the traditional subject matters covered, which have been in several cases updated, new application areas have emerged both at the micro as well as at the macro levels. As shown in Figure IV.1, both areas: molecular and cellular processes (micro) and populations and society (macro) refer to the areas of bioinformatics and public health informatics, respectively. Both have a lot to offer particularly if we want to focus our healthcare delivery systems of the twenty-first century on wellness through disease prevention.

At the bottom of this figure, there are four boxes that represent areas where biomedical engineers, systems engineers, computer scientists, biologists, and others have been doing extensive scientific work. The two boxes in the middle: *Tissues Organs and Systems* and *Individuals (Patients)* represent areas where biomedical engineers have focused their efforts mostly in the past.

Molecular and cellular processes, genetics discovery and populations' (and society) health are areas that have the most to offer if we shift our focus to wellness through prevention. In addition this micro-level segment has a huge impact on the future of personalized medicine. New advancements and discoveries both in sensor as well as on nanotechnology will have an impact as well not only on discovering disease earlier than before but on the way we treat certain conditions. Being able to "attack" diseases while minimizing, for example, secondary effects of drugs and related damages is yet another promising area for advancement. It could be concluded therefore that most of the opportunities for research and development will occur both at the micro and macro levels represented by these two segments.

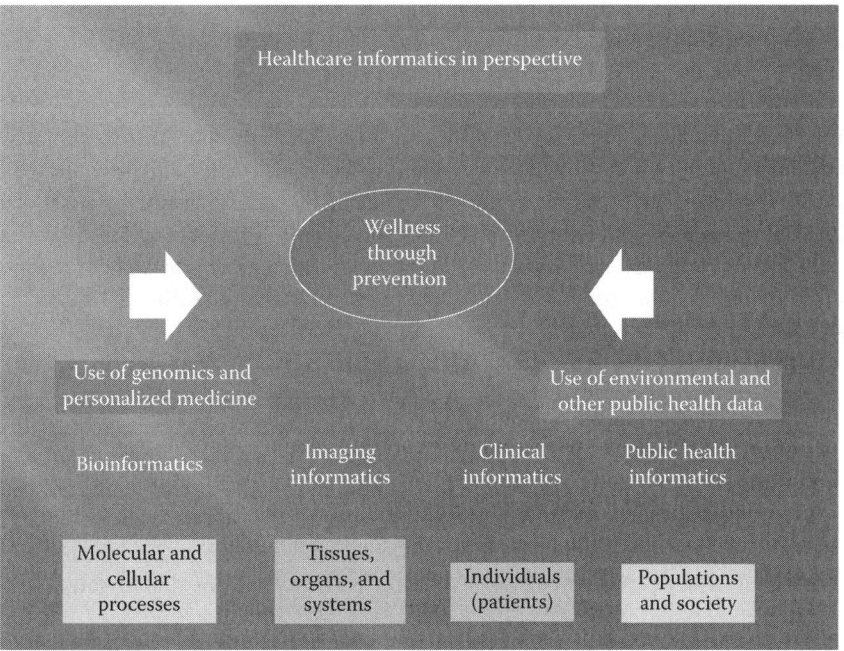

FIGURE IV.1 Healthcare informatics in perspective.

IV.1 Summary of the Medical Informatics Section Covered in the Previous Editions

In the first chapter, Allan Pryor provided us with a tutorial on HIS (hospital information systems). He described not only the evolution of HIS and departmental systems and clinical information systems (CIS) but also their differences. Within the evolution he followed these concepts with the need for the longitudinal patient record and the integration of patient data. This chapter included patient database strategies for HIS, data acquisition, patient admission, and transfer and discharge functions. In addition, patient evaluation and patient management issues were also discussed. From an end-user point of view, a terrific description on the evolution of data-driven and time-driven systems was included, culminating with some critical concepts on HIS requirements for decision support and knowledge base functionality. His conclusions were good indications of his vision.

J. Michael Fitzmaurice followed "Computer-Based Patient Records" (CBPR or CPR). In the introduction, it was explained what CPR is and why it is a necessary tool for supporting clinical decision making and how it is enhanced when it interacts with medial knowledge sources. This was followed by clinical decision support systems (CDSS): knowledge server, knowledge sources, medical logic modules (MLM), and nomenclature. This last issue in particular was one that needed to be well understood. The nomenclature used by physicians and by the CPRs differs among institutions. Applying logic to the wrong concepts can produce misinterpretations. The scientific evidence in this chapter included patient care process, CDSS hurdles, CPR implementation, research databases, telemedicine, hospital, and ambulatory care systems. A table of hospital and ambulatory care computer-based patient records systems concluded this chapter.

On account of the fast convergence of computers, telecommunications, and healthcare applications already in the Third Edition it was impossible to separate these elements (i.e., communications and networks). Both are part of information systems. Soumitra Sengupta provided us in this chapter a tutorial-like presentation that included an introduction and history, impact of clinical data, information types, and platforms. The importance of this section was reflected both in the contents reviewed under current technologies—LANs, WANs, middleware, medical domain middleware, integrated patient database, and medical vocabulary—as well as in the directions and challenges section that included improved bandwidth, telemedicine, and security management. In the conclusions, the clear vision is that networks will become the de facto fourth utility after electricity, water, and heat. Since the publication of the Third Edition, both the Internet and the WWW had taken off in multiple directions, creating a societal vision that is much different than the one most people expected. For example, telemedicine was seen as a tool for rural medicine and for emergency medicine and not for home care for the elderly and for persons suffering from a large number of chronic diseases, both here in the United States and in the rest of the world.

Non-AI decision making was covered by Ron Summers and Ewart R. Carson. This chapter included an introduction that explained the techniques of procedural or declarative knowledge. The topics covered in this section included analytical models and decision theoretic models, including clinical algorithms, and decision trees. The section that followed covered a number of key topics that appear while querying large clinical databases to yield evidence of either diagnostic or treatment or research value; statistical models, database search, regression analysis, statistical pattern analysis, Bayesian analysis, Depster–Shafer theory, syntactic pattern analysis, causal modeling, and artificial neural networks. In the summary, the authors clearly advised the reader to read through this section in conjunction with the expert systems chapters that follow.

The standards section was closely associated with the CPR chapter of this section. Jeffrey S. Blair did a terrific job with his overview of standards related to the emerging healthcare information infrastructure. This chapter gave the reader not only an overview of the major existing and emerging healthcare information standards but an understanding of all (the "then" current) efforts, national and international, to coordinate, harmonize, and accelerate these activities. The introduction summarized how this section was organized. It included identifier standards (patient's, site of care, product, and supply labeling), communications (message format) standards, content, and structure standards. This section was followed by a summary of clinical data representations, guidelines for confidentiality, data, security, and authentication. After that, quality indicators and data sets were described along with international standards. Coordinating and promotion organizations were listed at the end of this chapter, including points of contact that proved to be very beneficial for those who needed to follow up.

Design issues in developing clinical decision support and monitoring systems by John Goethe and Joseph Bronzino provided insight for the development of clinical decision support systems. In their introduction and throughout this chapter, the authors provided a step-by-step tutorial with practical advice and make recommendations on design of the systems to achieve end-user acceptance. After that, a description of a clinical monitoring system, developed and implemented by them for a psychiatric practice, was presented in detail. In their conclusions, the human engineering issue was discussed.

The Third Edition included two new chapters. One was "Introduction to Nursing Informatics" by Kathleen A. McCormick et al. and the other was "Medical Informatics and Biomedical Emergencies: New Training and Simulation Technologies for First Responders," by Joseph M. Rosen et al. Since nurses work side by side with physicians, biomedical engineers, information technologists, and others, the understanding becomes crucial of this profession, and what they do in their daily hospital activities becomes crucial.

Delivering detection, diagnostic, and treatment information to first responders remains a central challenge in disaster management. This is particularly true in biomedical emergencies involving highly infectious agents. Adding inexpensive, established information technologies to existing response system will produce beneficial outcomes. In some instances, however, emerging technologies will be necessary to enable an immediate, continuous response. This chapter identified and described new training, education, and simulation technologies that would help first responders to cope with bioterrorist events.

The Third Edition also had two revisions from the previous edition, made by Ron Summers and Ewart R. Carson and J. Michael Fitzmaurice, respectively.

IV.2 Changes and New Additions to the Fourth Edition

"Genome Informatics" is a new chapter by Konstantinos P. Exarchos, Themis P. Exarchos, and Dimitrios I. Fotiadis provides an overview as well as, in some cases, in-depth information regarding the broad and emerging field of genome informatics. Genome informatics is centered around the development and employment of data analysis algorithms and techniques toward the disentanglement of the inherent genome complexity. They start off with introductory material about evolution and phylogeny, which must always be kept in mind in biology-related studies. Afterwards, they follow by studying genes and their products (i.e., proteins), and moving one step beyond the gene or protein identification and cataloguing, and specifically focus on the interactions among genes/proteins that govern the cellular functioning. This massive interplay among genes and proteins has subsequently spawned a great deal of interest in reference to diseases and their molecular basis. Therefore, the last part of this work is centered around applications of protein interactions in the unraveling of human diseases as well as potential ways to interfere in the diseases' pathway of development and progression, from a genome informatics-oriented point of view.

"Introduction to Informatics and Nursing in the New Healthcare Environment: 2013" by Kathleen A. McCormick, Joyce Sensmeier, Connie Delaney, and Carol J. Bickford is an updated version of their earlier work that was particularly focused on the new environment of health IT and the new agenda and progress of the U.S. Office of the National Coordinator (ONC). Nurses, of course, represent the nursing informatics community at the highest level of the United States Government Policy, Standards, and Meaningful Use committees and workgroups, and as the volume of information system networks has increased in the past five years, so have the volume of nurses prepared to work in these environments. The authors make an excellent summary on how priorities have widened for health information in the form of national and regional health information exchanges, interoperability, transparency, and the widespread goals for the electronic health record (EHR). They also updated the related changes in healthcare policies and standards, demography of the nursing informatics profession, and refreshes the survey data on nursing informatics. Nurses continue to constitute the largest single group of healthcare workers, including experts that serve on national committees and interoperability initiatives focused on standards and terminology development, standards harmonization, and EHR adoption. Nurses are expanding their scopes of practice in hospitals, critical care environments, ambulatory clinics, public health, academic environment, and healthcare and vendor corporations. They focus on the development, implementation, and evaluation of integrated systems that enhance patient care and safety, verify outcomes, assure quality care, and document resource consumption. At the end, an update on the response of the nursing professional associations and organizations in setting the priorities for advanced education for the nursing profession in informatics, and a roadmap for the future through the TIGER Initiative are also provided.

Another new chapter is "eEmergency Healthcare Informatics" by E. Kyriacou, P. Constantinides, A. Panayides, M. S Pattichis, and C. S. Pattichis. The authors look at how advances in communication technologies, IT, and medical technologies facilitate the development of effective systems that can be used in support of emergency healthcare (eEmergency). The objectives of the chapter are to provide an overview of the way that information and communication technologies have been used in order to develop systems for emergency healthcare support, present case studies that have been published in the literature, and describe future trends. This group anticipated that while eEmergency systems can significantly improve the delivery of healthcare during emergency cases, their use in daily practice as well as the monitoring and evaluation of these systems still remains a goal to be achieved. This chapter provides an overview of the main technological components of eEmergency systems. The authors presented the eEmergency systems enabling technologies covering the wireless transmission technologies, mobile computing technologies, biosignals, medical imaging, and video. Later they cover protocols and processes for eEmergency management and response, followed by a review of mobile health eEmergency systems. Their concluding remarks address future challenges.

The new chapter titled "Disaster Response: Roles of Responders and Lessons Learned Since 9/11" by James Geiling, Lindsay Katona, Michael Lauria, and Joseph M. Rosen looks at what happens when disaster strikes a community or nation and many providers and agencies arrive to help. Each of these organizations brings with it a variety of capabilities and resources that may yield different levels of outcome for the victims. A critical challenge, as the authors plan for future disaster response, is how to equalize the playing field so that each response group has sufficient staff, equipment, supplies, technology, and security to provide appropriate care.

This chapter begins by describing the types of emergency responders and categorizing various types of major disasters. A review of the emergency response to recent disasters is offered on a case-study basis, including the Haiti earthquake, Hurricane Katrina, acts of terror such as 9/11, and pandemics and what went right and wrong in each of these, especially with regard to medical informatics.

This portion is followed by a description on how disaster response is supposed to work by reviewing the current national disaster management systems that operate at federal, state, and local levels. This chapter also identifies a series of critical lessons learned from the various successful and failed response efforts during the past decade. Two more areas are covered: (1) modifications to current response systems that will allow medical informatics to improve future response efforts for all types of responders, patients, their contacts, and their families, and (2) a discussion regarding the importance of team, culture, and training. The chapter concludes, with ways to use this information to rethink how we have managed crises like Katrina and Haiti and how we might think differently about fighting future disasters.

"Disaster Response: Potential Improvement with Medical Informatics" by James Geiling, Ron Poropatich, Michael Lauria, Robyn E. Mosher, and Joseph M. Rosen begins by describing two cases from the Haiti earthquake in 2010 and the H1N1 outbreak in 2009, and they describe how both events were worsened by lack of medical technology and informatics. The authors then list the current technologies that exist for disaster management along with a discussion of the gaps in technology that may allow biomedical engineers to create and design innovations to improve future responses to disasters of all types (natural disasters, acts of terror, and pandemics). The medical informatics most applicable in disaster response includes hand-held and portable devices, CIS, and standards and integration architectures. The authors proposed a network-centric architecture as the ideal foundation for emergency response technology, and describe tools that now exist under three subcategories of disaster management informatics: (1) command, control, communications, computers, and intelligence (C4I), (2) medical treatment and evacuation, and (3) managing population health. They also described technology gaps and the critical need for new informatics in five areas: (1) hand-held devices to assist in response and training; (2) increased diagnostics on such devices, including labs for basic tests, examination and pandemic surveillance; (3) mobile healthcare solutions or mHealth; (4) distributed CIS to track populations and affected individuals; and (5) devices and robots to provide remote treatment and telemedicine. This group believes that tools need to be lightweight, easy to carry, and universally understood and reinforce the need for both training and simulation tools, as well as standards and interoperability, so that responders can be fully prepared to use any new technologies and networking for disaster response.

In another new chapter, "Cardiovascular Health Informatics," Carmen C.Y. Poon and Yuan-ting Zhang study cardiovascular disease (CVD) in detail, which according to the World Health Organization has been the leading cause of deaths in most countries and will likely remain the top killer in the near future. CVD claimed the lives of 17.5 million people in 2005, accounting for 30% of all deaths, among which 12.9 million were due to either coronary heart disease or stroke. Some interesting observations are that (1) despite major advances in the treatment of CVD such as coronary artery disease, a large number of victims who appear to be healthy die suddenly of the disease without obvious prior symptoms and (2) nearly two-thirds of people who have a heart attack die before they can reach medical care. This chapter works with the definition of a Cardiovascular Health Informatics and Multimodal E-record (CHIME). This "holistic" e-Record should store relevant health information obtained from all different organ systems. According to the authors, on the spatial scale, information may be found in the order of 10^{-9} m in tRNA and ribosome to the meter range on the human body. On the temporal scale, health information varies from $10 - 6$ s or below for some molecular motions that play a critical role in the transportation of enzymes and chemicals both into and out of cells to 10^9 s for a typical lifetime of a person. Acquiring these multi-scale health information requires a variety of sensing and imaging tools that interacts with the biological system by different modalities, such as optical, magnetic, acoustic, electrical and chemical approaches. The massive, heterogeneous set of information has to be eventually fused together to solve health issues arising from different levels, from personal/individuals to global/ populations.

As always the authors of this section represent industry, academia, and government. Their expertise in many instances is multiple, from developing to actual implementing these technical ideas. I am very grateful for all our discussions and their contributions.

56

Introduction to Medical Informatics

Luis G. Kun
National Defense University

What is medical informatics? In the summer of 2004 I was invited to lecture at Dartmouth. Dr. Rosen, my host, asked me if I could address my interpretation of medical informatics during my lecture. This presentation made me review and reflect on some old and new concepts that have appeared in some cases in the literature. I have observed, for example, that the definition varies greatly depending on the profession of the person who answers this question. A few years earlier, while at the CDC (Centers for Disease Control and Prevention), I had the opportunity to participate in a lecture by Ted Shortliffe, in which he explained a model of medical informatics that appears in his book *Handbook of Medical Informatics.*[*] I also liked portions of the content that appears at the Vanderbilt University[†] website in its program of medical informatics (MI) and finally the work of Musen/Von Bemmel reflected on their *Handbook of Medical Informatics.*[‡]

Healthcare informatics has been defined by these authors, respectively as

- "A field of study concerned with the broad range of issues in the management and use of biomedical information, including medical computing and the study of the nature of medical information itself."[§]
- "The science that studies the use and processing of data, information, and knowledge applied to medicine, healthcare and public health."[¶]

Vanderbilt's MI program uses a *"simplistic definition": Computer applications in medical care* and a *"better definition": Biomedical informatics is an emerging discipline that has been defined as the study, invention, and implementation of structures and algorithms to improve communication, understanding,*

---

[*] Ted Shortliffe, *Handbook of Medical Informatics, Medical Informatics: Computer Applications in Healthcare and Biomedicine (Health Informatics)* Edward H. Shortliffe (Editor), Leslie E. Perreault (Editor), Gio Wiederhold (Editor), Lawrence M. Fagan (Editor), Lawrence M. Fagan (Author).

[†] http://dbmi.mc.vanderbilt.edu/education/

[‡] Von Bemmel J.H., Musen M.A., Eds. *Handbook of Medical Informatics.* AW Houten, Netherlands: Bohn Stafleu Van Loghum; Heidelberg, Germany: Springer-Verlag, 1997.

[§] Shortliffe, E.H., Perreault, L.E., Eds. *Medical Informatics: Computer Applications in Healthcare and Biomedicine.* New York: Springer, 2001.

[¶] Von Bemmel, J.H., Musen, M.A., Eds. *Handbook of Medical Informatics.* AW Houten, Netherlands: Bohn Stafleu Van Loghum; Heidelberg, Germany: Springer-Verlag, 1997.

and management of medical information. The end objective of biomedical informatics is the coalescing of data, knowledge, and the tools necessary to apply that data and knowledge in the decision-making process, at the time and place that a decision needs to be made. The focus on the structures and algorithms necessary to manipulate the information separates biomedical informatics from other medical disciplines where information content is the focus.

The Vanderbilt model shows MI as the intersection of three different domains: biological science, information analysis and presentation (i.e., informatics, computation, statistics) and clinical health services research (i.e., policy, outcomes). The first two at the intersection create bioinformatics, while the second and third create health informatics (through the translation from bench to bedside). Some more definitions: The noun informatics has one meaning; the sciences concerned with gathering and manipulating and storing and retrieving, and classifying recorded information [1]. in.for.mat.ics n. *Chiefly British.* Information science, and bi.o.in.for.mat.ics n. Information technology as applied to the life sciences, especially the technology used for the collection, storage, and retrieval of genomic data [2]. In the *Handbook of Medical Informatics* (Musen/VonBemmel et al.) MI is located at the intersection of information technology (IT) and the different disciplines of medicine and healthcare.

These authors decided not to enter into a fundamental discussion of the possible differences between MI and health informatics, however, several definitions of MI (medical information science, health informatics) were given. Some of these take into account both the scientific and the applied sides of the field. They cited two definitions:

1. Medical information science is the science of using system-analytic tools ... to develop procedures (algorithms) for management, process control, decision making, and scientific analysis of medical knowledge [3].
2. MI comprises the theoretical and practical aspects of information processing and communication, based on knowledge and experience derived from processes in medicine and healthcare [4].

According to Wikipedia: MI is the name given to the application of information technology to healthcare. It is the "understanding, skills, and tools that enable the sharing and use of information to deliver healthcare and promote health" (*British Medical Informatics Society*). MI is often called *healthcare informatics* or *biomedical informatics*, and forms part of the wider domain of *eHealth*. These later-generation terms reflect the substantive contribution of the citizen and nonmedical professions to the generation and usage of healthcare data and related information. Additionally, medical informaticians are active in bioinformatics and other fields not strictly defined as healthcare.

56.1 Convergence of Science and Technology with Medical Informatics

As shown in Figure IV.1, both areas: molecular and cellular processes (micro) and populations and society (macro) refer to the areas of bioinformatics and public health informatics, respectively. Molecular and cellular processes, genetics discovery and populations' (and society) health are areas that have the most to offer if we shift our focus from dealing with disease to wellness through prevention. In addition this micro-level segment has a huge impact on the future of personalized medicine. The convergence of new science with the development of new technologies, new drugs, and new vaccines will change the way we practice medicine.

New advancements and discoveries both in sensor as well as on nanotechnologies will have an impact as well not only on discovering disease earlier than before but on the way we treat certain conditions. Being able to "attack" diseases while minimizing, for example, secondary effects of drugs and related damages is yet another promising area for advancement. It could be concluded then that most of the opportunities for research and development will occur both at the micro and macro levels represented by these two segments.

56.2 Biomedical Informatics: An Evolving Perspective

Some view MI as a basic medical science with a wide variety of potential areas of applications. At the same time, the development and evaluation of new methods and theories are a primary focus of activities in this field. Using the results of experiences, allows, for example, the understanding, structuring, and encoding of knowledge, thus allowing its use in information processing by others, in the same field of specialty (i.e., within the field of clinical informatics) or in other areas (i.e., nursing informatics, dental informatics, and veterinary informatics). In Shortliffe's "biomedical informatics in perspective," his fundamental diagram shows how a clinician or researcher could "move" from basic research to applied research looking at molecular and cellular processes (bioinformatics), tissues and organs (imaging informatics), individual patients (clinical informatics), and populations and society (public health informatics). The important concept is, that a core series of informatics methods, tools and techniques, are the same regardless of the applied research area chosen. This core includes: natural language processing, cognitive science, mathematical modeling and simulation, database theory, statistics, data mining, knowledge management, and intelligent agents. Many of these information technologies were developed in other fields and later applied by the "medical/health" community. In other cases, the reverse has occurred. For example, the skeleton of an expert system developed for a medical diagnosis and treatment application, could be used by others to diagnose and correct problems in a computer system. The basic core mentioned in the previous paragraph, then requires expertise in many different fields that include: biology, biomathematics, medicine, nursing, dentistry, veterinary, computer science—electrical.

Figure 56.1 shows how if we start with the basic sciences and applied fields, we can develop a model that allows, through the use of medical and public health informatics, deal with issues such as national

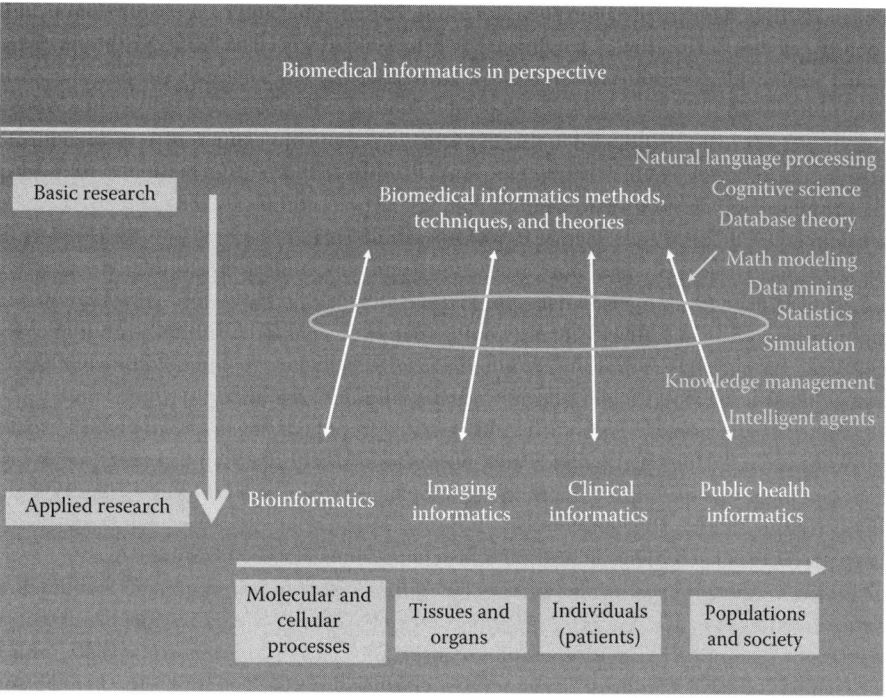

FIGURE 56.1   This figure is a modification of Ted Shortliffe's: "biomedical informatics in perspective." (Adapted from T. Shortliffe: Editorial, *Journal of Biomedical Informatics* 35, 2002, 279–280. Republished with permission of the author.)

and international security and the critical infrastructure protection (CIP) of the public health infrastructure. This figure also shows many of the different professions or areas of expertise involved in the field of MI.

Societal changes have occurred, in particular during the past four decades to information processing. Over the last decade, for those who have observed the Internet and World Wide Web (WWW) evolution, many of these changes come as part of a new resulting culture. The convergence of computers and communications has played a key role in this evolving field of MI. The way physicians, nurses, biomedical engineers, veterinarians, dentists, laboratory technicians, public health specialists, and other healthcare professionals do their "business" regardless if it is clinical, administrative, research and development or academic, requires and demands not only a clear understanding of these terms, but also what their "business process" is all about. For example, around the 1986 timeframe as technical manager for the requirements definition of the nursing point of care system for IBM Federal Systems in Gaithersburg, I had the opportunity to better understand the nursing process of information. Let us assume that a patient falls to the ground as he was having a heart attack. He cut his forehead, his left hand, arm, knee, and twisted his left ankle. When brought into an emergency room in a hospital the medical diagnosis given is myocardial infarction. Yet from a nursing point of view, the patient diagnosis is different. He is assessed and evaluated, classified and care plans are developed for each of the diagnosis (for each of the injuries) according to a list that would include not only the heart attack (and the follow-up ordered by the physician), but the forehead, left hand, left arm, left knee, and left ankle. Following the NANDA (North American Nursing Diagnosis Association) diagnosis there will be a process to be followed for each wound or injury and that would facilitate the patient's discharge. Figure 56.2 depicts biomedical informatics: tools, methods, techniques, and theories applied to individuals interested in the use of medical and public health informatics from a national security perspective. It also shows at the top,

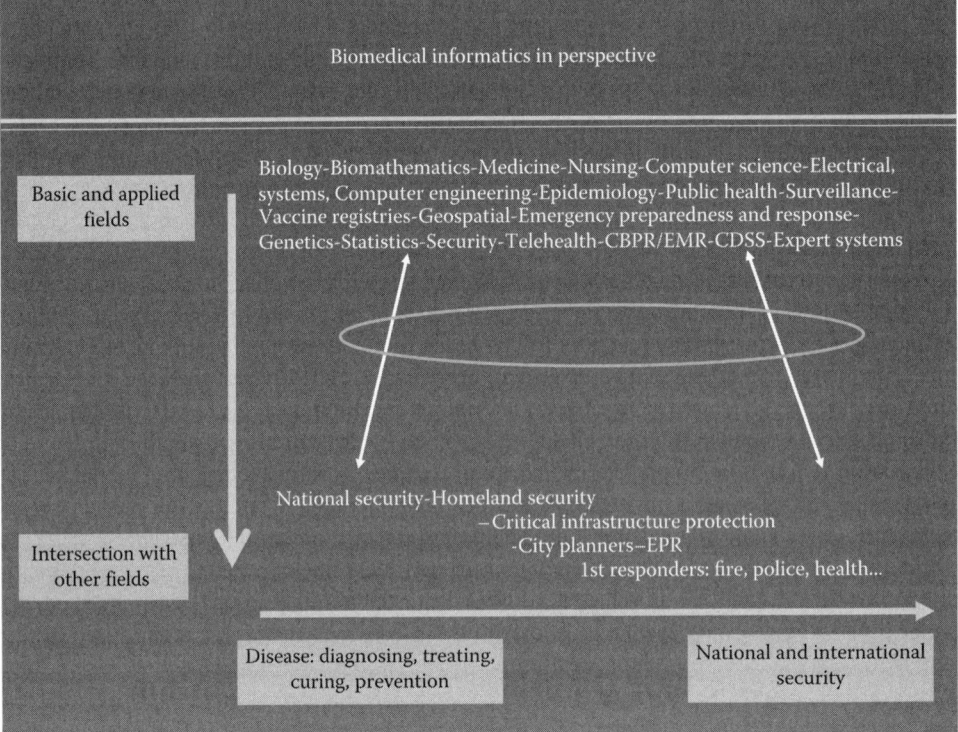

FIGURE 56.2 This is an example of applying the model shown in Figure IV.1, to other disciplines.

some of the different areas of expertise that may be touched by this field. Systems, computer engineering, epidemiology, public health, surveillance, geo-spatial information systems, emergency preparedness and response, genetics, statistics, security, telehealth, computer-based patient records, clinical decision support systems, expert systems, data mining/warehousing, and so on.

Each of the professionals mentioned above, that is, healthcare providers, and so on may have a piece of the patient's health puzzle which may need to be included in their record. In my professional life I have been involved in different activities that included the utilization of different pieces of computer hardware, systems and application software and other devices that acquire, transmit, process, and store information, and in different forms (i.e., signals, voice, images from different modalities: CT, MRI, ultrasound, nuclear, x-ray, scanned/document images, etc.). In my early years at IBM in the late 1970s, the concepts of "patient-centered" information was one of the leading concepts helping us drive toward the implementation of electronic health records (EHR). But in this day and age, we have a significant number of new devices, which were not made for that particular purpose and yet they are being used to collect, transmit, process, or store patient-related information. Biomedical engineers are and will be faced with these new challenges, where patient information may not be flowing from conventional data collection devices. Information now could come from sensing devices, RFID tags and through a myriad of wireless devices and networks. An RFID tag was approved in the 4Q 2004, by the FDA, that could be implanted into a patient. Aside from the issues of privacy and security of that information, the repercussions of such actions can be magnificent. It may improve the life of some or even save lives. Imagine, for example, patients suffering from either Alzheimer's or Parkinson's disease being admitted into an emergency room after an accident and not being able to convey any personal or medical-related information. Having available some basic but critical medical information can identify who the patient is, what medications they may be allergic to, and so on.

Over the past 30 years, the field of MI has grown tremendously both in its complexity and in content. As a result, two types of papers will be written in this handbook.

The first one, represented in some chapters, will be devoted to areas that forma key "core" of computer technologies. These include: hospital information systems (HIS), computer-based patient records (CBPR or CPR), imaging, communications, standards, and other related areas. The second section includes the following topics: artificial intelligence, expert systems, knowledge-based systems neural networks, and robotics. Most of the techniques described in the second section will require the implementation of systems explained in this first section. We could call most of these chapters the information infrastructure required to apply MI techniques to medical data. These topics are crucial because they not only lay the foundation required to treat a patient within the walls of an institution but they also provide the roadmap required to deal with the patient's lifetime record while allowing selected groups of researchers and clinicians to analyze the information and generate outcomes research and practice guidelines information. As an example, a network of associated hospitals in the East Coast (a healthcare provider network) may want to utilize an expert system that was created and maintained at Stanford University. This group of hospitals, HMOs, clinics, physician's offices, and the like would need a "standard" computer-based patient record (CPR) that can be used by the clinicians from any of the physical locations. In addition to access the information, all these institutions require telecommunications and networks that will allow for the electronic "dialogue." The different forms of the data, particularly clinical images, will require devices for displaying purposes, and the information stored in the different HIS, clinical information systems (CIS), and departmental systems needs to be integrated. The multimedia type of record would become the data input for the expert system which could be accessed remotely (or locally) from any of the enterprise's locations. On the application side, the expert system could provide these institutions which techniques that can help in areas such as diagnosis and patient treatment. However, several new trends such as: total quality management (TQM), outcome research, and practice guidelines could be followed. It should be obvious to the reader that to have the ability to compare information obtained in different parts of the world by dissimilar and heterogeneous systems, certain standards need to be followed (or created) so that when analyzing the data, the information obtained will make sense. Many information systems issues described in this introduction will be addressed in this section. The artificial intelligence chapters which follow should be synergistic with these concepts. A good understanding of the issues in this section is required prior to the utilization of the actual expert system. These issues are part of this section of MI, other ones, however, for example, systems integration and process reengineering, will not be addressed here in detail but will be mentioned by the different authors. I encourage the reader to follow up on the referenced material at the end of each chapter, since the citations contain very valuable information.

Several perspectives in information technologies need to be taken into consideration when reading this section. One of them is described very accurately in the book titled *Globalization, Technology and Competition* [5]. The first chapter of this book talks about new services being demanded by end users, which include the integration of computers and telecommunications. From their stages theory point of view, the authors described very appropriately, that "we are currently" nearing the end of the micro era and the beginning of the network era. From an economy point of view, the industrial economy (1960s and 1970s) and the transitional economy (1970s and 1980s) moved into an information economy (1990s and beyond).

In the previous editions I mentioned that: "*Many other questions and answers reflected some of the current technological barriers and users needs. Because of these trends it was essential to include in this Handbook technologies that today may be considered state of the art but when read about 10 years from now will appear to be transitional only. Information technologies are moving into a multimedia environment which will require special techniques for acquiring, displaying, storing, retrieving, and communicating the information. We are in the process of defining some of these mechanisms.*" This is precisely what has occurred. In some instances such as imaging, this handbook contains a full section dedicated to the subject. That section contains the principles, the associated math algorithms, and the physics related to all medical imaging modalities. The intention in this section was to address issues related to imaging as a form of medical information. These concepts include issues related then to acquisition, storage and retrieval, display and communications of document and clinical images, for example, picture archival and communications systems (PACS). From a CPR point of view, clinical and document images will become part of this electronic chart, therefore many of the associated issues will be discussed in this section more extensively. The state of the telecommunications has been described as a revolution; data and voice communications as well as full-motion video have come together as a new dynamic field. Much of what is happening today is a result of technology evolution and need. The connecting thread between evolutionary needs and revolutionary ideas is an integrated perspective of both sides of multiple industries. This topic will also be described in more detail in this section. A Personal (Historical) Perspective on Information Technology in Healthcare: During my first 14 "professional years" I worked with IBM (1978–1992) across the country: Los Angeles, Dallas, Gaithersburg, Dallas, and Houston. As I moved from city to city I noticed that while financial transactions would simply follow me (from place-to-place), that is, with the use of the same credit cards; this was not the case with my medical records. In fact, there wasn't an "electronic" version available. In today's terms my "paper-trail record" was a "cut and paste" document that I had to create and take with me wherever I went. At work, I was engaged since 1983, on the development of concepts of the "All Digital Medical Record" (ADMR), bedside terminals, PACS, Integrated Diagnostics Systems, and other related topics such as Telemedicine. In the 1986 timeframe and while at IBM, Al Potvin (former IEEE-EMBS president) asked me to become part of the IEEE-USA Healthcare Engineering Policy Committee (HCEPC), and I did. I formed and chaired then, the Electronic Medical Record/High-Performance Computers and Communications (EMR/HPCC) working group. Many of these concepts were presented at EMBS [6] and AAMI [7,8] annual meetings, in Biomedical Engineering classes [9,10], and even at National [11–13] and International Conferences/Meetings [14–19]. Nine and ten years ago respectively, we (the HCEPC) had two meetings where the Role of Technology in the Cost of Healthcare were explored [20,21]. At that time, in the early 1990s, and given the rate at which the American Healthcare system was growing, the HCEPC asked me to organize a special Technology Policy session during the 1993 EMBS meeting in San Diego [22]. (After the formal presentations, the participants, who represented the United States, Canada, and Europe had a terrific discussion that lasted well over 3 h from the allotted time for the session.) Costs were the fundamental and center piece of these discussions. The Clinton–Gore administration encouraged the use of IT for healthcare reform and as a consequence we organized a meeting in 1995 [23] to address these needs.

Close to seven years later the book titled: *To Err is Human* [24] changed the focal point from "costs" to "human lives taken by medical errors." Experts estimated that as many as 98,000 people die (in the United States) in any given year from medical errors that occur in hospitals. That's more than those who die from motor vehicle accidents, breast cancer, or AIDS—three causes that receive far more public attention. Indeed, more people die annually from medication errors than from workplace injuries. Add the financial cost to the human tragedy, and medical error easily rose to the top ranks of urgent, widespread public problems. This book broke the silence that has surrounded medical errors and their consequence—but not by pointing fingers at caring healthcare professionals who make honest mistakes. After all, to err is human. Instead, it set forth a national agenda—with state and local implications—for reducing medical errors and improving patient safety through the design of a safer health system. It revealed the often startling statistics of medical error and the disparity between the incidence of error and public perception of it, given many patients' expectations that the medical profession always performs perfectly. A careful examination was made of how the surrounding forces of legislation, regulation, and market activity influenced the quality of care provided by healthcare organizations and then looked at their handling of medical mistakes. (Using a detailed case study, the book reviews the current understanding of why these mistakes happen. A key theme is that legitimate liability concerns discourage reporting of errors—which begs the question, "How can we learn from our mistakes?") Balancing regulatory versus market-based initiatives and public versus private efforts, the Institute of Medicine presented wide-ranging recommendations for improving patient safety, in the areas of leadership, improved data collection and analysis, and development of effective systems at the level of direct patient care. The bottom line was that it asserted that the problem is not bad people in healthcare—it is that good people are working in bad systems that need to be made safer.

A series of efforts, including both private and public sectors, that is, e-Health Initiative [25], occurred which prompted a series of actions, documents, and even proposed legislation in 2003, that is, HR2915 the National Health Information Infrastructure (NHII); and also a National meeting where the requirements for such an infrastructure were agreed upon. A follow-up meeting took place on July 20–23, 2004 here in Washington, DC. *The Secretarial Summit on Health Information Technology launching the National Health Information Infrastructure 2004: Cornerstones for Electronic Healthcare* was well attended by over 1500 people representing the private and public healthcare industry. In challenging both sectors of the healthcare industry, Secretary Tommy G. Thompson stated, "Health information technology can improve quality of care and reduce medical errors, even as it lowers administrative costs. It has the potential to produce savings of 10% of our total annual spending on healthcare, even as it improves care for patients and provides new support for healthcare professionals." A report, titled *The Decade of Health Information Technology: Delivering Consumer-centric and Information-rich Healthcare*, ordered by President George W. Bush in April, was presented on July 21st by David Brailer, the National Coordinator for Health Information Technology, whom the president appointed to the new position in May. The report lays out the broad steps needed to achieve always-current, always-available EHR for Americans. This responds to the call by President Bush to achieve EHRs for most Americans within a decade. The report identifies goals and action areas, as well as a broad sequence needed to achieve the goals, with joint private or public cooperation and leadership. The heads of every agency within DHHS (i.e., AHRQ, NIH,CDC, FDA, CMS, HRSA, etc.) were present and each made a presentation on how the NHII would affect their own area of service (e.g., research and development, education, reimbursement, etc.) For more details about the news coverage on the NHII conference, please link to the following sites:

1. HHS Fact Sheet-HIT Report at-a-glance 7/21/04: http://www.hhs.gov/news/press/2004pres/20040721.html
2. *NY Times* 7/21/04: http://www.nytimes.com/2004/07/21/technology/21record.html

3. Bronz: "2122_s004"—2006/2/24—11:35—page 8—#8 http://www.governmentexecutive.com/dailyfed/0704/072104dk1.htm
4. Center for Health Transformation 7/21/04: http://www.healthtransformation.net/news/chtnews.asp
5. iHealthbeat 7/26/04: http://www.ihealthbeat.org/index.cfm?Action=dspItem&itemid=104473
6. USNews.com 8/2/04: http://www.usnews.com/usnews/tech/articles/040802/2wired.htm

56.3 New Issues of the Information Age

As time passes by, we ("the educated world population") are becoming more accustomed to see how the Internet, for example, is being used to manage the health of the elderly and for homecare purposes. People living in urban, suburban, and rural areas are using telehealth as one of several mechanisms to deal with their personal health. This is one of the many ways that in my opinion healthcare costs have the potential to be reduced [26]. The Balanced Budget Act of 1997 was in fact the first time that the U.S. government decided to measure cost and medical effectiveness through telemedicine, involving elderly patients with diabetes. (A grant of about $28 million was given to Columbia University Medical Center in March 2000 and was renewed in 2004.) In the United States, the constant rising prices of medications, however, are also making the elderly (in particular) look for alternative mechanisms to purchase them, that is, the Internet. The new questions that should be raised are: How can we ensure the quality of those drugs ordered through this mechanism? (i.e., Who is accountable? Who is the producer of such medications? etc.) How many people may be dying (or affected negatively) by those that are self-prescribing medications? Several bills in the U.S. Congress are trying to deal, with some of these issues. The language has the potential to affect prescribing medications during interactive video consultations. The intent of this legislation, to ensure patients have access to safe and appropriate medicine, is a good one; however, it may limit what we will be able to do through this type of technology. Some Internet Rx legislation under consideration includes (bills can be accessed online at http://Thomas.loc.gov)

- S 2464: Internet Pharmacy Consumer Protection Act aka Ryan Haight Act. *Sen. Coleman (MN). Cosponsor: Feinstein.* Requires an in-person medical evaluation in order for a practitioner to dispense a prescription to a patient.
- HR 3880: Internet Pharmacy Consumer Protection Act. *Rep. Davis (VA) Cosponsors: Waxman.* Requires an in-person medical evaluation in order for a practitioner to dispense a prescription to a patient.
- S 2493: Safe Importation of Medical Products and Other Rx Therapies Act of 2004. *Sen. Gregg (NH).Co-sponsors: Smith.* Requires a treating provider to perform a documented patient evaluation (including a patient history and physical examination) of an individual to establish the diagnosis for which a prescription drug is prescribed.
- HR 3870: Prescription Drug Abuse Elimination Act of 2004. *Rep. Norwood (GA). Co-sponsor: Strickland.* Defines treating provider as a healthcare provider who has performed a documented patient evaluation of the individual involved (including a patient history and physical examination) to establish the diagnosis for which a prescription drug involved is prescribed.
- HR 2652: Internet Pharmacy Consumer Protection Act. *Rep. Stupak (MI).* States that a person may not introduce a prescription drug into interstate commerce or deliver the prescription drug for introduction into such commerce pursuant to a sale state requires an in-person medical evaluation in order for a practitioner to dispense a prescription to a patient.

In some cases, the defined requirements or the language used (i.e., in person patient evaluation) may act precisely against the use of that technology (i.e., tele-consultation). It is in the best interest of society, that biomedical engineers, among others get involved in "educating" the law makers regarding the intrinsic value that the technology may bring into the system. Almost a decade later, we still have multiple crises in the US Healthcare System such as the "Meningitis Outbreak" discovered in September 2012 due to the mixing of nonsterile compounds by a pharmaceutical firm in Massachusetts. The importance of protecting the consumer in today's global economy where food as well as medications and vaccines come from everywhere and anywhere is still an unresolved matter and where IT has a great role in either solving and or preventing bigger problems through the use of traceability techniques.

References

1. Word Net 1.7.1 Copyright 2001 by Princeton University. All rights reserved.
2. *The American Heritage*® Dictionary of the English Language, 4th ed. Copyright 2004, 2000 by Houghton Mifflin Company. Published by Houghton Mifflin Company, Boston. All rights reserved.
3. Shortliffe, E.H., The science of biomedical computing. *Med. Inform.* 1984; 9: 185–93.
4. Von Bemmel, J.H., The structure of medical informatics. *Med. Inform.* 1984; 9: 175–80.
5. Bradley, S.P., Hausman, J.A., and Nolan, R.L., *Globalization, Technology, and Competition: The Fusion of Computers and Telecommunications in the 1990s.* 1993.
6. Invited lecturer for the IEEE-EMBS, Dallas/Fort Worth Section. Session Topic—"Paperless Hospital," University of Texas, Arlington, TX; October 1989.
7. Kun, L., Chairman during the *24th Annual AAMI-Association for the Advancement of Medical Instrumentation-Conference*, Session Topic—"The paperless hospital." Presentation: "Trends for the creation of an All Digital Medical Record," St. Louis, Missouri; May 1989.
8. Kun, L., Guest Speaker to the *Association for the Advancement of Medical Instrumentation.* Session: Technology Management in 21st Century Health Care. Topic: "Electronic Community Medical Records." Anaheim, CA; May 1995.
9. Kun, L., Invited lecturer, Trinity College/*The Hartford Graduate Center Biomedical Engineering Seminar Series Fall 1990.* Session Topic—"The Digital Medical Record," Hartford, CT.
10. Kun, L., UTA Biomedical Engineering Dept. Graduate Seminar. Topic— "All Digital Medical Record." Arlington, TX; October 1988.
11. Kun, L., Guest lecturer for the *Emergency Physicians Training Conference.* Session Topic—"All Digital Medical Record at the ER", Infomart, Dallas, TX; June 1990.
12. Kun, L., Guest Speaker to the *1st National Symposium on Coupling Technology to National Need.* Topic: "Impact of the Electronic Medical Record and the High Performance Computing and Communications in Health Care. Albuquerque, New Mexico; August 1993.
13. Kun, L., Distinguished Lecturer and part of a debate panel on the topic: "TheVision of the Future of Health Care Technology and Health Care Reform." Presentation topic: "The Role of the EMR and the HPCC in Controlling the Cost of Health Care." *Sigma-Xi Distinguished Lectureship Program at the University of Connecticut,* April 1994.
14. Kun, L., Applications of Microcomputers in Government, Industry and University. Centro Internacional de Fisica y la Universidad Nacional Quito, Ecuador, Course 4 Topic: *"The All Digital Medical Record. Image, Voice, Signals, Text and Graphics used for Patient Care";* July 1987.
15. Kun, L., Universidad Nacional, Santo Domingo, Dominican Republic. Course 4 Topic: "The All Digital Medical Record. Image, Voice, Signals, Text and Graphics used for Patient Care"; July 1987.
16. Kun, L., *Seminar Manager for the 1 week IBM Europe Institute: "Medical Computing: The Next Decade."* Presentation—"All Digital Medical Record", Garmisch-Partenkirchen, Germany. August 1989.
17. Kun, L., *Seminar Technical Chairman IBM Research/IBM France.* Topic "Medical Imaging Computing: The Next Decade." Presentation—"The Paperless Hospital," Lyon, France; June 1990.
18. Kun, L., Guest speaker and session chairman to the 1994 *2nd International Symposium Biomedical Engineering in the 21st Century.* Topics: "Telemedicine" and "The Computer Based Patient Record."

Center for Biomedical Engineering, College of Medicine, National Taiwan University, Taipei Convention Center, Taipei, Taiwan, R.O.C. September 1994.

19. Kun, L., Invited lecturer to the Director of Health Industry Marketing Asia/Pacific. Session Topic— "The All Digital Medical Record", Tokyo, Japan. Sponsor IBM Japan/Asia Pacific HQ;April 1991.

20. Kun, L., Guest Speaker to the Role of Technology in the Cost of Health Care Conference. Session: "The Role of Information Systems in Controlling Costs." Topic: "The Electronic Medical Record and the High Performance Computing and Communications Controlling Costs of Health Care." Washington, DC; April 1994.

21. Kun, L., Guest speaker to the Role of Technology in the Cost of Health Care: Providing the Solutions Conference. Health Care Technology Policy II Topic: "Transfer & Utilization of Government Technology Assets to the Private Sector in the Fields of Health Care and Information Technologies." Moderator Session: "Use of Information Systems as a Management Tool." Washington, DC; May 1995.

22. Kun, L., Session chairman of a *Special Mini-Symposia on: Engineering Solutions to Healthcare Problems: Policy Issues*, during the *15th Annual International Conference IEEE-EMBS*. Also presenter of the lecture: "Health Care Reform Addressed by Technology Transfer: The Electronic Medical Record & the High Performance Computers & Communications Efforts. San Diego, California; October 1993.

23. Kun, L., Conference Chairman—Health Care Information Infrastructure, Part of *SPIE's 1995 Symposium on Information, Communications and Computer Technology, Applications and Systems.* Philadelphia, Pennsylvania; October 1995.

24. Kohn, L., Corrigan, J.M., and Donaldson, M.S. Editors; Committee on Quality of Health Care in America, Institute of Medicine, To Err is Human: Building a Safer Health System, 2000, Institute of Medicine.

25. Foundation for eHealth Initiative: http://www.ncpdp.org/pdf/eHIOverview.pdf

26. Kun, L., Guest lecture: "Healthcare of the elderly in the 21st century. Can we afford not to use telemedicine?" CIMIC, Rutgers University, NJ; December 12, 1996:http://cimic.rutgers.edu/seminars/kun.html

57

Hospital Information Systems: Their Function and State

T. Allan Pryor
University of Utah

The definition of a hospital information system (HIS) is unfortunately not unique. The literature of both the informatics community and healthcare data processing world is filled with descriptions of many differing computer systems defined as an HIS. In this literature, the systems are sometimes characterized into varying levels of HISs according to the functionally present within the system. With this confusion from the literature, it is necessary to begin this chapter with a definition of an HIS. To begin this definition, I must first describe what it is not. The HIS will incorporate information from several departments within the hospital, but an HIS is not a departmental system. Departmental systems such as a pharmacy or a radiology system are limited in their scope. They are designed to manage only the department that they serve and rarely contain patient data captured from other departments. Their function should be to interface with the HIS and provide portions of the patient medical/administrative record that the HIS uses to manage the global needs of the hospital and patient.

A clinical information system is likewise not an HIS. Again, although the HIS needs clinical information to meet its complete functionality, it is not exclusively restricted to the clinical information supported by the clinical information systems. Examples of clinical information systems are ICU systems, respiratory care systems, nursing systems. Similar to the departmental systems, these clinical systems tend to be one-dimensional with a total focus on one aspect of the clinical needs of the patient. They provide little support for the administrative requirements of the hospital.

If we look at the functional capabilities of both the clinical and departmental systems, we see many common features of the HIS. They all require a database for recording patient information. Both types of systems must be able to support data acquisition and reporting of patient data. Communication of information to other clinical or administrative departments is required. Some form of management support can be found in all the systems. Thus, again looking at the basic functions of the system one cannot differentiate the clinical/departmental systems from the HIS. It is this confusion that makes defining the HIS difficult and explains why the literature is ambiguous in this matter.

The concept of the HIS appears to be, therefore, one of integration and breadth across the patient or hospital information needs. That is, to be called an HIS the system must meet the global needs of those it is to serve. In the context, if we look at the hospital as the customer of the HIS, then the HIS must be able to provide global and departmental information on the state of the hospital. For example, if we consider the capturing of charges within the hospital to be an HIS function, then the system must capture all patient charges no matter which department originated those charges. Likewise, all clinical information about the patient must reside within the database of the HIS and make possible the reporting and management of patient data across all clinical departments and data sources. It is a totality of function that differentiates the HIS from the departmental or restricted clinical system, not the functions provided to a department or clinical support incorporated within the system.

The development of an HIS can take many architectural forms. It can be accomplished through interfacing of a central system to multiple departmental or clinical information systems. A second approach which has been developed is to have, in addition to a set of global applications, departmental or clinical system applications. Because of the limitation of all existing systems, any existing comprehensive HIS will in fact be a combination of interfaces to departmental/clinical systems and the applications/database of the HIS purchased by the hospital.

The remainder of this chapter will describe key features that must be included in today's HIS. The features discussed below are patient databases, patient data acquisition, patient admission/bed control, patient management and evaluation applications, and computer-assisted decision support. This chapter will not discuss the financial/administrative applications of an HIS, since those applications for the purposes of this chapter are seen as applications existing on a financial system that may not be integral application of the HIS.

57.1 Patient Database Strategies for the HIS

The first HISs were considered only as an extension of the financial and administrative systems in place in the hospital. With this simplistic view many early systems developed database strategies that were limited in their growth potential. Their databases mimicked closely the design of the financial systems that presented a structure that was basically a "flat file" with well-defined fields. Although those fields were adequate for capturing the financial information used by administration to track the patient's charges, they were unable to adapt easily to the requirement to capture the clinical information being requested by healthcare providers. Today's HIS database should be designed to support a longitudinal patient record (the entire clinical record of the patient spanning multiple inpatient, outpatient encounters), integration of all clinical and financial data, and support of decision support functions.

The creation of a longitudinal patient record is now a requirement of the HIS. Traditionally the databases of the HISs were encounter-based. That is, they were designed to manage a single patient visit to the hospital to create a financial record of the visit and make available to the care provider data recorded during the visit. Unfortunately, with those systems the care providers were unable to view the progress of the patient across encounters, even to the point that in some HISs critical information such as patient allergies needed to be entered with each new encounter. From the clinical perspective, the management of a patient must at least be considered in the context of a single episode of care. This episode might include one or more visits to the hospital's outpatient clinics, the emergency department, and multiple inpatient stays. The care provider to properly manage the patient, must have access to all the information recorded from those multiple encounters. The need for a longitudinal view dictates that the HIS database structure must both allow for access to the patient's data independent of an encounter and still provide for encounter-based access to adapt to the financial and billing requirements of the hospital.

The need for integration of the patient data is as important as the longitudinal requirement. Traditionally the clinical information tended to be stored in separate departmental files. With this structure it was easy to report from each department, but the creation of reports combining data from different departments proved difficult, if not impossible. In particular in those systems where access to the departmental data was provided only though interfaces with no central database, it was impossible to create an integrated patient evaluation report. Using those systems the care providers would view data from different screens at their terminal and extract with pencil onto paper the results from each department (clinical laboratory, radiology, pharmacy, etc.) the information they needed to properly evaluate the patient. With the integrated clinical database the care provider can view directly on a single screen the information from all departments formatted in ways that facilitate the evaluation of the patient.

Today's HIS is no longer merely a database and communication system but is an assistant in the management of the patient. That is, clinical knowledge bases are an integral part of the HIS. These knowledge bases contain rules and/or statistics with which the system can provide alerts or reminders or implement clinical protocols. The execution of the knowledge is highly dependent on the structure of the clinical database. For example, a rule might be present in the knowledge base to evaluate the use of narcotics by the patient. Depending on the structure of the database, this may require a complex set of rules looking at every possible narcotic available in the hospital's formulary or a single rule that checks the presence of the class narcotics in the patient's medical record. If the search requires multiple rules, it is probably because the medical vocabulary has been coded without any structure. With this lack of structure there needs to be a specific rule to evaluate every possible narcotic code in the hospital's formulary against the patient's computer medication record. With a more structured data model a single rule could suffice. With this model the drug codes have been assigned to include a hierarchical structure where all narcotics would fall into the same hierarchical class. Thus, a single rule specific only to the class "narcotics" is all that is needed to compare against the patient's record.

These enhanced features of the HIS database are necessary if the HIS is going to serve the needs of today's modern hospital. Beyond these inpatient needs, the database of the HIS will become part of an enterprise clinical database that will include not only the clinical information for the inpatient encounters but also the clinical information recorded in the physician's office or the patient's home during outpatient encounters. Subsets of these records will become part of state and national healthcare databases. In selecting, therefore, and HIS, the most critical factor is understanding the structure and functionality of its database.

57.2 Data Acquisition

The acquisition of clinical data is key to the other functions of the HIS. If the HIS is to support an integrated patient record, then its ability to acquire clinical data from a variety of sources directly affect its ability to support the patient evaluation and management functions described below. All HIS systems provide for direct terminal entry of data. Depending on the system this entry may use only the keyboard or other "point and click" devices together with the keyboard.

Interfaces to other systems will be necessary to compute a complete patient record. The physical interface to those systems is straightforward with today's technology. The difficulty comes in understanding the data that are being transmitted between systems. It is easy to communicate and understand ASCII textual information, but coded information from different systems is generally difficult for sharing between systems. This difficulty results because there are no medical standards for either medical vocabulary or the coding systems. Thus, each system may have chosen an entirely different terminology or coding system to describe similar medical concepts. In building the interface, therefore, it may be necessary to build unique translation tables to store the information from one system into the databases of the HIS. This requirement has limited the building of truly integrated patient records.

Acquisition of data from patient monitors used in the hospital can either be directly interfaced to the HIS or captured through an interface to an ICU system. Without these interfaces the acquisition of the monitoring data must be entered manually by the nursing personnel. It should be noted that whenever possible automated acquisition of data is preferable to manual entry. The automated acquisition is more accurate and reliable and less resource intensive. With those HISs which do not have interfaces to patient monitors, the frequency of data entry into the system is much less. The frequency of data acquisition affects the ability of the HIS to implement real-time medical decision logic to monitor the status of the patient. That is, in the ICU where decisions need to be made on a very timely manner, the information on which the decision is based must be entered as the critical event is taking place. If there is no automatic entry of the data, then the critical data needed for decision making may not be present, thus preventing the computer from assisting in the management of the patient.

57.3 Patient Admission, Transfer, and Discharge Functions

The admission application has three primary functions. The first is to capture for the patient's computer record pertinent demographic and financial/insurance information. A second function is to communicate that information to all systems existing on the hospital network. The third is to link the patient to previous encounters to ensure that the patient's longitudinal record is not compromised. This linkage also assists in capturing the demographic and financial data needed for the current encounter, since that information captured during a previous encounter may not be reentered as part of this admission. Unfortunately in many HISs the linkage process is not as accurate as needed. Several reasons explain this inaccuracy. The first is the motivation of the admitting personnel. In some hospitals they perceive their task as a business function responsible only for ensuring that the patient will be properly billed for his or her hospital stay. Therefore, since the admission program always allows them to create a new record and enter the necessary insurance/billing information, their effort to link the patient to his previous record may not be as exhaustive as needed.

Although the admitting program may interact with many financial and insurance files, there normally exists two key patient files that allow the HIS to meet its critical clinical functions. One is a master patient index (MPI) and the second is the longitudinal clinical file. The MPI contains the unique identifier for the patient. The other fields of this file are those necessary for the admitting clerk to identify the patient. During the admitting process the admitting clerk will enter identifying information such as name, sex, birth date, social security number. This information will be used by the program to select potential patient matches in the MPI from which the admitting clerk can link to the current admission. If no matches are detected by the program, the clerk creates a new record in the MPI. It is this process that all too frequently fails. That is, the clerk either enters erroneous data and finds no match or for some reason does not select as a match one of the records displayed. Occasionally the clerk selects the wrong match causing the data from this admission to be posted to the wrong patient. In the earlier HISs where no longitudinal record existed, this problem was not critical, but in today's system, errors in matching can have serious clinical consequences. Many techniques are being implemented to eliminate this problem including probabilistic matching, auditing processes, postadmission consolidation.

The longitudinal record may contain either a complete clinical record of the patient or only those variables that are most critical in subsequent admissions. Among the data that have been determined as most critical are key demographic data, allergies, surgical procedures, discharge diagnoses, and radiology reports. Beyond these key data elements more systems are beginning to store the complete clinical record. In those systems the structure of the records of the longitudinal file contains information regarding the encounter, admitting physician, and any other information that may be necessary to view the record from an encounter view or as a complete clinical history of the patient.

57.4 Patient Evaluation

The second major focus of application development for the HIS is creation of patient evaluation applications. The purpose of these evaluation programs is to provide to the caregiver information about the patient which assists in evaluating the medical status of the patient. Depending on the level of data integration in the HIS, the evaluation applications will be either quite rudimentary or highly complex. In the simplest form these applications are departmentally oriented. With this departmental orientation the caregiver can access through terminals in the hospital departmental reports. Thus, laboratory reports, radiology reports, pharmacy reports, nursing records, and the like can be displayed or printed at the hospital terminals. This form of evaluation functionality is commonly called results review, since it only allows the results of tests from the departments to be displayed with no attempt to integrate the data from those departments into an integrated patient evaluation report.

The more clinical HISs as mentioned above include a central integrated patient database. With those systems patient reports can be much more sophisticated. A simple example of an integrated patient evaluation report is a diabetic flowsheet. In this flowsheet the caregiver can view the time and amount of insulin given, which may have been recorded by the pharmacy or nursing application, the patient's blood glucose level recorded in the clinical laboratory or again by the nursing application. In this form the caregiver has within single report, correlated by the computer, the clinical information necessary to evaluate the patient's diabetic status rather than looking for data on reports from the laboratory system, the pharmacy system, and the nursing application. As the amount and type of data captured by the HIS increases, the system can produce ever-more-useful patient evaluation reports. There exist HISs which provide complete rounds reports to summarize on one to two screens all the patient's clinical record captured by the system. These reports not only shorten the time need by the caregiver to locate the information, but because of the format of the report, can present the data in a more intuitive and clinically useful form.

57.5 Patient Management

Once the caregiver has properly evaluated the state of the patient, the next task is to initiate therapy that ensures an optimal outcome for the patient. The sophistication of the management applications is again a key differentiation of HISs. At the simplest level management applications consist of order-entry applications. The order-entry application is normally executed by a paramedical personnel. That is, the physician writes the order in the patient's chart, and another person reviews from the chart the written order and enters it into the computer. For example, if the order is for a medication, then it will probably be a pharmacist who actually enters the order into the computer. For most of the other orders a nurse or ward clerk is normally assigned this task. The HIS records the order in the patient's computerized medical record and transmits the order to the appropriate department for execution. In those hospitals where the departmental systems are interfaced to the HIS, the electronic transmission of the order to the departmental system is a natural part of the order entry system. In many systems the transmission of the order is merely a printout of the order in the appropriate department.

The goal of most HISs is to have the physician responsible for management of the patient to enter the orders into the computer. The problem for the HISs in achieving this goal has been due to the inefficiency of the current order-entry programs. For these programs to be successful they have to compete favorably with the traditional manner in which the physician writes the order. Unfortunately, most of the current order-entry applications are too cumbersome to be readily accepted by the physician. Generally they have been written to assist the paramedic in entering the order resulting with far too many screens or fields that need to be reviewed by the physician to complete the order. One approach that has been tried with limited success is the use of order sets. The order sets have been designed to allow the physician to easily enter multiple orders from a single screen. The use of order sets has improved the acceptability of the order-entry application to the physician, but several problems remain preventing universal acceptance by the physicians. One problem is that the order set will never be sufficiently complete to contain all orders that the physician would want to order. Therefore, there is some subset of patients' orders that will have to be entered using the general ordering mechanisms of the program. Depending on the frequency of those orders, the acceptability of the program changes. Maintenance issues also arise with order sets, since it may be necessary to formulate order sets for each of the active physicians. Maintaining of the physician-specific order sets soon becomes a major problem for the data processing department. It becomes more problematic if the HIS to increase the frequency of a given order being present on an order set allows the order sets to be not only physician-defined but problem-oriented as well. Here it is necessary to again increase the number of order sets or have the physicians all agree on those orders to be included in an order set for a given problem.

Another problem, which makes use of order entry by the physician difficult, is the lack of integration of the application into the intellectual tasks of the physician. That is, in most of the systems, the physicians are asked to do all the intellectual work in evaluating and managing the care of the patient in a traditional manner and then, as an added task, enter the results of that intellectual effort into the computer. It is at this last step that is perceived by the physician as a clerical task during which the physician rebels. Newer systems are beginning to incorporate more efficiently the ordering task into other applications. These applications assist the physician throughout the entire intellectual effort of patient evaluation and management of the patient. An example of such integration would be the building of evaluation and order sets in the problem list management application. Here, when the care provider looks at the patient problem list he or she accesses problem-specific evaluation and ordering screens built into the application, perhaps shortening the time necessary for the physician to make rounds on the patient.

Beyond simple test ordering, many newer HISs are implementing decision support packages. With these packages the system can incorporate medical knowledge usually as rule sets to assist the care provider in the management of patients. Execution of the rule sets can be carried out in the foreground through direct calls from an executing application or in the background with the storing of clinical data in the patient's computerized medical record. This latter mode is called data-driven execution and provides an extremely powerful method of knowledge execution and alerting. That is, after execution of the rule sets, the HIS will "alert" the care provider of any outstanding information that may be important regarding the status of the patient or suggestions on the management of the patient. Several mechanisms have been implemented to direct the alerts to the care provider. In the simplest form notification is merely a process of storing the alert in the patient's medical record to be reviewed the next time the care provider accesses that patient's record. More sophisticated notification methods have included directed printouts to individuals whose job is to monitor the alerts, electronic messages sent directly to terminals notifying the users that there are alerts which need to be viewed, and interfacing to the paging system of the hospital to direct alert pages to the appropriate personnel.

Execution of the rule sets is sometimes, time-driven. This mode results in sets of rules being executed at a particular point in time. The typical scenario for time-driven execution is to set a time of day for selected rule set execution. At that time each day the system executes the given set of rules for a selected population in the hospital. Time drive has proven to be a particularly useful mechanism of decision support for those applications that require hospital-wide patient monitoring.

The use of decision support has ranged from simple laboratory alerts to complex patient protocols. The responsibility of the HIS is to provide the tools for creation and execution of the knowledge base. The hospitals and their designated "experts" are responsible for the actual logic that is entered into the rule sets. Many studies are appearing in the literature suggesting that the addition of knowledge base execution to the HIS is the next major advancement to be delivered with the HIS. This addition will become a tool to better manage the hospital in the world of managed care.

The inclusion of decision support functionality in the HIS requires that the HIS be designed to support a set of knowledge tools. In general, a knowledge-based system will consist of a knowledge base and an inference engine. The knowledge base will contain the rules, frames, and statistics that are used by the inference applications to substantiate a decision. We have found that in the healthcare area the knowledge base should be sufficiently flexible to support multiple forms of knowledge. That is, no single knowledge representation is sufficiently powerful to provide a method to cover all decisions necessary in the hospital setting. For example, some diagnostic decisions may well be best suited for bayesian methods, whereas other management decisions may follow simple rules. In the context of the HIS, I prefer the term application manager to inference engine. The former is intended to imply that different applications may require different knowledge representations as well as different inferencing strategies to traverse the knowledge base. Thus, when the user selects the application, he or she is selecting a particular inference engine that may be unique to that application. The tasks, therefore, of the application manager are to provide the "look and feel" of the application, control the functional capabilities of the application, and invoke the appropriate inference engine for support of any "artificial intelligence" functionality.

57.6 Conclusion

Today's HIS is no longer the financial/administrative system that first appeared in the hospital. It has extended beyond that role to become an adjunct to the care of the patient. With this extension into clinical care the HIS has not only added new functionality to its design but has enhanced its ability to serve the traditional administrative and financial needs of the hospital as well. The creation of these global applications which go well beyond those of the departmental/clinical systems is now making the HIS the patient-focused system. With this global information the administrators and clinical staff together can accurately access where there are inefficiencies in the operation of the hospital from the delivery of both the administrative and medical care. This knowledge allows changes in the operation of the hospital that will ensure that optimal care continues to be provided to the patient at the least cost to the hospital. These studies and operation changes will continue to grow as the use of an integrated database and implementation of medical knowledge bases become increasingly routine in the functionality of the HIS.

References

1. Pryor T.A., Gardner R.M., Clayton P.D. et al. 1983. The HELP system. *J. Med. Syst.* 7: 213.
2. Pryor T.A., Clayton P.D., Haug P.J. et al. 1987. Design of a knowledge driven HIS. *Proc. 11th SCAMC*, 60.
3. Bakker A.R. 1984. The development of an integrated and co-operative hospital information system. *Med. Inf.* 9: 135.
4. Barnett G.O. 1984. The application of computer-based medical record systems in ambulatory practice. *N. Engl. J. Med.* 310: 1643.
5. Bleich H.L., Beckley R.F., Horowitz G.L. et al. 1985. Clinical computing in a teaching hospital. *N. Engl. J. Med* 312: 756.
6. Whiting-O'Keefe Q.E., Whiting A., and Henke J. 1988. The STOR clinical information system. *MD Comput.* 5: 8.
7. Hendrickson G., Anderson R.K., Clayton P.D. et al. 1992. The integrated academic information system at Columbia-Presbyterian Medical Center. *MD Comput.* 9: 35.
8. Safran C., Slack W.V., and Bleich H.L. 1989. Role of computing in patient care in two hospitals. *MD Comput.* 6: 141.
9. Bleich H.L., Safran C., and Slack W.V. 1989. Departmental and laboratory computing in two hospitals. *MD Comput.* 6: 149.
10. ASTM E1238-91. 1992. *Specifications for Transferring Clinical Observations between Independent Computer Systems*. Philadelphia, American Society for Testing and Materials.
11. Tierney W.M., Miller M.E., and Donald C.J. 1990. The effect on test ordering of informing physicians of the charges for outpatient diagnostic tests. *N. Engl. J. Med.* 322: 1499.
12. Stead W.W. and Hammond W.E. 1983. Functions required to allow TMR to support the information requirements of a hospital. *Proc. 7th SCAMC*, 106.
13. Safran C., Herrmann F., Rind D. et al. 1990. Computer-based support for clinical decision making. *MD Comput.* 7: 319.
14. Tate K.E., Gardner R.M., and Pryor T.A. 1989. Development of a computerized laboratory alerting system. *Comp. Biomed. Res.* 22: 575.
15. Orthner H.F. and Blum B.I. (Eds.). 1989. *Implementing Health Care Information Systems*, Springer-Verlag.
16. Dick R.S. and Steen E.B. (Eds.). 1991. *The Computer-Based Patient Record*, National Academy Press.

58

Computer-Based Patient Records

J. Michael
Fitzmaurice*
*Agency for Healthcare
Research and Quality*

58.1 Electronic Health Records

The objective of this section is to present the electronic health record (EHR) as a powerful tool for organizing patient care data to improve patient care and strengthen communication of patient care data among healthcare providers. The EHR is even more powerful when used in a system that retrieves applicable medical knowledge to support clinical decision making, improving patient safety, and promoting quality improvement. Evidence exists that the use of EHR systems (EHRS) can change both physician behavior and patient outcomes of care. As the speed and cost efficiency of computers rise, the cost of information storage and retrieval falls, and the breadth of ubiquitous networks widens, it is essential that EHRs and

---

* Any opinions expressed in this chapter are those solely of the author and not of the U.S. Department of Health and Human Services or of the Agency for Healthcare Research and Quality.

systems that use them be evaluated for the improvements in and risks to healthcare that they can bring, and for their protection of the confidentiality of individually identifiable patient information.

The primary role of the EHR is to support the delivery of medical care to a particular patient. Serving this purpose, ideally, the EHR brings past and current information about a particular patient to the physician, promotes communication among healthcare givers about that patient's care, and documents the process of care and the reasoning behind the choices that are made. Thus, the data in an EHR should be acquired as part of the normal processes of healthcare delivery by the providers of care and their institutions to improve data accuracy and timeliness of decision support. And these data should be shareable for the benefit of the patient's care, perhaps with the permission or direction of the patient to safeguard confidentiality.

The EHR can also be an instrument for building a clinical data repository that is useful for studying information about which medical treatments are effective in the practice of medicine in the community and for improving population-based healthcare. A clinical data repository may be provider based or patient based; it may be disease specific or geographically specific. Additional applications of EHR data beyond direct patient care can improve population-based care. These applications bring personal and public benefits, but also raise issues that must be addressed by healthcare policy makers.

Since patient information is likely to be located in the medical records of several of the patient's providers, providing high quality of care often requires exchanges of this information among the provider, for example, data about immunizations. The vision of health information technology applications for improving the quality of healthcare contains a role for a nationwide health information network. This network could take many forms but the most likely form is a combination of local or regional networks through which the required exchanges of patient information could take place. Currently, many of these exchanges are still done using faxed messages or phone calls. Sometimes, the patient is just given the information in hard copy to carry to the next provider. The EHR can be an even more powerful tool when it is connected to an electronic network and interoperable with other EHRs. Similar to the use of EHR applications, the use of health information networks also brings issues to be addressed by healthcare policy makers.

Clinical data standards, personal health identification, and communication networks, all critical factors for using EHRs effectively, are addressed separately in other chapters of this book.

58.2 What Is an EHR?

An EHR is a collection of data about a patient's healthcare in electronic form. The EHR, also called an electronic medical record, is part of a system (usually maintained in a hospital, a physician's office, or an Internet or application service provider if it is web based) that encompasses data entry and presentation, storage, and access by the clinical decision maker—usually a physician or a nurse. The data are entered by keyboard, dictation and transcription, voice recognition and interpretation, light pen, touch screen, hand-held computerized notepad, or a wireless hand-held personal digital assistant (perhaps a cell phone) with gesture and character recognition and grouping capabilities. Entry may also be by other means, for example, by direct instrumentation from electronic patient monitors and bedside terminals, nursing stations, bar code readers, radio-frequency identification (RFID), analyses by other linked computer systems such as laboratory autoanalyzers and intensive care unit (ICU) monitors, or another provider's EHRS via a secure network. While the EHR could include patient-entered data, some medical providers may question the validity of such information for making their decisions; others may rely on such data for diagnosis and treatment.

Patient care data collected by an EHRS may be stored centrally or they may be stored in many places (e.g., distributed among the patient's various providers), for retrieval at the request of an authorized user (most likely with the patient's authorization) through a database management system or an electronic health information exchange. The EHR may present data to the physician as text, tables, graphs, sound, images, full-motion video, and signals on an electronic screen, cell phones, pagers, or even paper. The EHR may also point to the location of additional patient data that cannot be easily incorporated into the EHR.

TABLE 58.1   Core Functions of an Electronic Health Record System

- Health information and data
- Results management
- Order entry/management
- Decision support
- Electronic communication and connectivity
- Patient support
- Administrative processes
- Reporting and population health management

Source: Institute of Medicine, Committee on Data Standards for Patient Safety. 2003a. *Key Capabilities of an Electronic Health Record System. Letter Report.* 2003. The National Academies Press, Washington DC.

In too many current clinical settings (hospitals, physicians' offices, and ambulatory care centers), data pertaining to a patient's medical care are recorded and stored in paper medical records. If the paper record is out of its normal location, or accompanying the patient during a procedure or an off-site study, it is not available to the nurse, the attending physician, or the expert consultant. In paper form, data entries are often illegible and are not easily retrieved and read by multiple users one at a time. On the other hand, an electronic form provides legible, clinical information that can be available to all users simultaneously, thus improving timely access to patient care data and communication among care providers. A 2010 survey found that most physicians' offices (82%) were using electronic appointment scheduling, but only 37% of these offices surveyed had completely implemented electronic ordering of tests, imaging, or procedures (Agency for Healthcare Research and Quality, 2010).

Of course, there may be potential harms that are magnified by EHRs, such as when erroneous patient data (say, wrong blood type) are stored or when the clinical decision support information is not kept up-to-date or is faulty (Kaplan, 2009).

Individual hospital departments (e.g., laboratory or pharmacy), often lose the advantages of electronic data when their own computer systems print the computerized results onto paper. The pages are then sent to the patient's hospital floor and assembled into a paper record. The lack of standards for the electronic exchange of these data and the lack of implementation of existing standards, such as using the Logical Observations Identifiers Names and Codes (LOINC) standard for reporting laboratory results or the Digital Imaging and Communications in Medicine (DICOM) standard for exchanging images, hinders the integration of computerized departmental systems. Searching electronic files is often more efficient than searching through paper. The weaknesses of paper medical record systems for supporting patient care and healthcare providers have long been known (Korpman, 1990, 1991).

Many of the functions of an EHR and how it operates within a healthcare information system to satisfy user demands are set out in the Institute of Medicine's (IOM) seminal report "The Computer-Based Patient Record: An Essential Technology for Healthcare" (1991, 1997). In response to a request by the Agency for Healthcare Research and Quality (AHRQ), IOM provided guidance to DHHS in 2003 on a set of "basic functionalities" that an EHR system should possess to promote patient safety (IOM, 2003a), shown in Table 58.1.

This guidance is the basis for a health level seven (HL7, a standards developing organization) standard that specifies the functions of an EHR. This specification is useful for EHR purchasers to specify what functions they want and for vendors of EHRS to describe the functions they offer (HL7, 2004).

58.3 Clinical Decision Support Systems

One of the roles of the EHR is to enable a clinical decision support system (CDSS)—computer software designed to aid clinical decision making—to provide the physician with medical knowledge that is pertinent to the care of the patient. Diagnostic suggestions, testing prompts, therapeutic protocols, practice guidelines, alerts of potential drug–drug and drug–food reactions, evidence-based treatment suggestions, and other decision support services can be obtained through the interaction of the EHR with a CDSS.

58.3.1 Knowledge Server

The existing knowledge about potential diagnoses and treatments, practice guidelines, and complicating factors pertinent to the patient's diagnosis and care is needed at the time treatment decisions are made. The go-between that makes this link is a "knowledge server," which acquires the necessary clinical information for the decision maker from the knowledge server's information sources. The knowledge server can assist the clinical decision maker to put this information, that is, specific data and information about the patient's identification and condition(s) and medical knowledge, into the proper context for treating the patient (Tuttle et al., 1994).

58.3.2 Knowledge Sources

Knowledge sources include a range of options, for example, from internal development and approval by a hospital's staff to external sources outside the hospital, such as the National Guidelines Clearinghouse (see www.guideline.gov) initiated by the AHRQ, the American Medical Association, and the Association of American Health Plans; the Physicians Data Query program at the National Cancer Institute at http://www.nci.nih.gov/cancertopics/pdq; other consensus panel guidelines sponsored by the National Institutes of Health; guidelines developed by medical and other specialty societies and others; and specialized information from private sector knowledge vendors. Additional sources of knowledge include the medical literature, which can be searched for high-quality, comprehensive review articles and for particular subjects using the "PubMed" program to explore the MEDLINE literature database available through the National Library of Medicine at http://www.ncbi. nlm.nih.gov/entrez/query.fcgi?db=PubMed&itool=toolbar. AHRQ-supported evidence-based practice center reports summarizing scientific evidence on specific topics of medical interest are available to support guideline development (see http://www.guideline.gov/search/search.aspx?term=evidence +based+practice+center).

58.3.3 Medical Logic Modules

If medical knowledge needs are anticipated, acquired beforehand, and put into a medical logic module (MLM), software can provide rule-based alerts, reminders, and suggestions for the care provider at the point (time and place) of health service delivery. One format for MLMs is the Arden Syntax, which standardizes the logical statements (ASTM, 1992). For example, an MLM might be interpreted as: "If sex = female, and age is greater than 50 years, and no Pap smear test result appears in the EHR, then recommend a Pap smear test to the patient." If MLMs are to have a positive impact on physician behavior and the patient care process, then physicians using MLMs must agree on the rules in the logical statements or conditions and recommended actions that are based on interactions with patient care data in the EHR. Another format is the guideline interchange format (GLIF), a computer-interpretable language framework for modeling and executing clinical practice guidelines. GLIF uses GELLO, a guideline expression language that is better suited for GLIF's object-oriented data model, is extensible, and allows implementation of expressions that are not supported by the Arden Syntax (Wang, 2004; also see http://www.openclinical.org/gmm_glif.html).

Since MLMs are usually independent, the presence or absence of one MLM does not affect the operation of other MLMs in the system. If done carefully and well, MLMs developed in one healthcare organization can be incorporated in the EHRSs of other healthcare organizations. However, this requires much more than using accepted medical content and logical structure. If the medical concept terminology (the nomenclature and code sets used by physicians and by the EHR) differs among organizations, the knowledge server may misinterpret what is in the EHR, apply logic to the wrong concept, or select the wrong MLM. Further, the physician receiving its message may misinterpret the MLM (Pryor and Hripcsak, 1994). Faulty patient information, say, wrong blood type, can be just as harmful as choosing the wrong guideline.

58.3.4 Nomenclature

For the widespread use of CDSSs, a uniform medical nomenclature, consistent with the scientific literature, is necessary. Medical knowledge is information that has been evaluated by experts and converted into useful medical concepts, options, and rules for decisions. For CDSSs to search through a patient's EHR, identify the medical concepts, retrieve appropriate patient data and information, and provide a link to the relevant knowledge, the CDSS has to recognize the names used in the EHR for the concepts (Cimino, 1993). Providing direction for coupling terms and codes found in patient records to medical knowledge is the goal of the unified medical language system (UMLS) project of the National Library of Medicine (NLM, 2005a). "The UMLS Metathesaurus supplies information that computer programs can use to create standard data, interpret user inquiries, interact with users to refine their questions, and convert the users' terms into the vocabulary used in relevant information sources" (NLM, 2005b). More recently, the National Library of Medicine has developed RxNorm, a specialized vocabulary of terms that doctors can use when ordering drugs. LOINC (developed and maintained by the Regenstrief Institute) is a set of codes for identifying laboratory test results, but as yet there is no reference vocabulary for ordering laboratory tests.

The developers of medical informatics applications need a controlled medical terminology so that their applications will work across various sites of care and medical decision making. The desiderata, or requirements, of a controlled medical terminology as described by Cimino (1998) include: "vocabulary content, concept orientation, concept permanence, nonsemantic concept identifiers, polyhierarchy, formal definitions, rejection of 'not elsewhere classified' terms, multiple granularities, multiple consistent views, context representation, graceful evolution, and recognized redundancy." These remain the most important requirements.

The National Committee on Vital and Health Statistics (NCVHS) is an 18-private-sector-member, federal advisory committee with a 60-year history of advising the Secretary of Health and Human Services (HHS) on issues relating to health data, statistics, privacy, and national health information policy (http://aspe.dhhs.gov/ncvhs/). Recognizing that "[w]ithout national standard vocabularies, precise clinical data collection and accurate interpretation of such data is [sic] difficult to achieve," NCVHS recommended in 2000 that the Secretary of HHS "should provide immediate funding to accelerate the development and promote early adoption of PMRI standards." This recommendation included clinical terminology activities of the National Library of Medicine, the AHRQ, and the Food and Drug Administration to augment, develop, and test clinical vocabularies, and to make them publicly available at low cost (NCVHS, PMRI, 2000, pp. 6, 7–8). The Consolidated Health Informatics work group, a White House, Office of Management and Budget, interagency, eGovernment Initiative dominated by HHS, Department of Veterans Affairs (VA), and Department of Defense (DoD) staff, made similar recommendations over the next 3 years. This encouragement led HHS to negotiate a national license for free use of systematized nomenclature for medicine (SNOMED)–clinical terms (CT), adopt 20 clinical data standards, begin developing drug terminology and structured drug information, map vocabularies to SNOMED–CT, and investigate the standardization of data elements used for reporting patient safety adverse events. This license for free U.S. use was extended for another 5 years in 2007 and funded by the National Library of Medicine.

58.4 Scientific Evidence

58.4.1 Patient Care Processes

Controlled trials have shown the effectiveness of CDSS for modifying physician behavior using preventive care reminders. In an early review of the scientific literature, Johnston et al. (1994) reported that controlled trials of CDSSs have shown significant, favorable effects on care processes from (1) providing preventive care information to physicians and patients (McDonald et al., 1984; Tierney et al., 1987), (2) supporting diagnosis of high-risk patients (Chase et al., 1983), (3) determining the toxic drug dose for obtaining the desired therapeutic levels (White et al., 1987), and (4) aiding active medical care decisions (Tierney et al. 1988). Johnston found that the clinician performance was generally improved when a CDSS was used and, in a small number of cases (3 of 10 trials), significant improvements were made in patient outcomes.

In a randomized, controlled clinical trial, one that randomly assigned some teams of physicians to computer workstations with screens designed to promote cost-effective ordering (e.g., of drugs and laboratory tests), Tierney et al. (1993) reported that patient lengths of stay were 0.89 days shorter and charges generated by the intervention teams were $887 lower, than for the control teams of physicians. These gains were not without an offset. Time and motion studies showed that intervention physician teams spent 5.5 min longer per patient during 10-h observation periods. This study is a rare controlled trial that sheds light on the resource impact and the effectiveness of using a CDSS.

In this setting, physician behavior was changed and resources were reduced by the application of logical algorithms to computer-based patient record information. Nevertheless, a different hospital striving to attain the same results would have to factor in the cost of the equipment, installation, maintenance, and software development plus the need to provide staff training in the use of a CDSS.

Additional evidence, rigorously obtained, shows beneficial effects of the use of EHRs within a CDSS on medical practices. As reported in the response of the Department of HHS to the GAO report, "Health and Human Services' Estimate of Healthcare Cost Savings Resulting from the Use of Information Technology," many studies published in peer-reviewed journals show "substantial improvement in clinical processes" when physicians use EHRs:

> The effects of EHRs include reducing laboratory and radiology test ordering by 9 to 14% (Tierney et al., 1987, 1990; Bates et al., 1999), lowering ancillary test charges by up to 8% (Tierney et al., 1988), reducing hospital admissions, costing an average of $17,000 each, by 2–3% (Jha et al., 2001), and reducing excess medication usage by 11% (Teich et al., 2000; Wang et al., 2003). (GAO, 2005, p. 9)

58.4.2 Incentives

As can be seen from the literature, CDSS can improve quality and, in many cases, can reduce resources needed for treatment. The benefit of this resource reduction, however, most frequently goes to health plans under cost-based reimbursement of providers. The provider of care may need additional incentives to adopt CDSS as part of the regular work process. Otherwise, any added time needed to access and respond to the CDSS prompts and alerts may reduce the provider's personal productivity (see the extra 5.5 min per patient noted above) without offsetting compensation. These additional incentives may be funds for purchase of the hardware and software needed for CDSS, payment for using CDSS, or payment for reporting evidence of improved quality of care or cost reduction. Recognizing this need, Congress provided for incentive payments in the 2009 economic stimulus legislation (P.L. 111-5).

58.4.3 Evaluation

It was recognized early that CDSSs should be evaluated according to how well they enhance performance in the user's environment (Nykanen et al., 1992). If CDSS use is to become widespread and supported, society should judge CDSSs not only on enhanced provider performance but also on whether patient outcomes are improved and system-wide healthcare costs are contained. The evaluation of information systems is extremely difficult because so many changes occur when they are introduced into an existing work flow. Attributing changes in productivity, costs of care, and patient outcomes to the introduction and use of a CDSS or an EHRS is difficult when the work patterns and the culture of the workplace are also changing. Many clinical information system applications have been self-evaluated in their original development site. While impressive findings have been published, the generalizability of those findings needs scientific verification. Nevertheless, federal government support is predicated on this generalizability and on the expected gains from making health information interoperable across EHRS. As noted by Lyman et al. (2010), "[t]he amount of energy and resources that have been devoted to CDS planning efforts in recent years is considerable and impressive."

58.4.4 CDSS Hurdles

In a review of medical diagnostic decision support systems, Miller (1994) examines the development of CDSSs over the past 40 years and identifies several hurdles to be overcome before large-scale, generic CDSSs grow to widespread use. These hurdles include determining (1) how to support medical knowledge base construction and maintenance over time, (2) the amount of reasoning power and detailed representation of medical knowledge required (e.g., how strong a match of medical terms is needed to join medical concepts with appropriate information), (3) how to integrate CDSSs into the clinical environment to reduce the costs of patient data capture, and (4) how to provide flexible user interfaces and environments that adjust to the abilities and desires of the user (e.g., with regard to typing expertise and pointing devices). Although unsolved to date, these hurdles are being strongly attacked in American Recovery and Reinvestment Act–Health Information Technology for Economic and Clinical Health (ARRA–HITECH) activities.

58.4.5 Research Databases

EHRs can have great value for developing research databases, medical knowledge, and quality assurance information that would otherwise require an inordinate amount of manual resources to obtain in their absence. An example of EHR use in research is found in a study undertaken at Latter Day Saints (LDS) Hospital. Using the HELP EHR system to gather data on 2847 surgical patients, this study found that administering antibiotics prophylactically during the 2-h window before surgery (as opposed to earlier or later within a 48-h window) minimized the chance of surgical wound infection. It also reduced the surgical infection rate for this time category to 0.59%, compared to the 1.5% overall infection rate for all the surgical patients under study (Classen et al., 1992).

The same system was used at LDS Hospital to link the clinical information system data (including a measure of nursing acuity) with the financial systems' data. Using clinical data to adjust for the severity of patient illness, Evans et al. (1994) measured the effect of adverse drug events due to hospital drug administration on hospital length of stay and cost. The difference attributable to adverse drug events among similar patients was estimated to be an extra 1.94 patient days and $1939 in costs. Disease registries for specific patient conditions (cancer, diabetes, heart disease, and others) build research databases to develop knowledge about which clinical practices achieve better patient outcomes across many sites of patient care.

58.4.6 Telemedicine

An EHR may hold and exchange radiological and pathological images of the patient taken or scanned in digital form. The advantage is that digital images may be transferred long distances without a reduction in quality of appearance. This allows patients to receive proficient medical advice even when they and their local family practitioners are far from the consulting physicians. It also allows health managers to move such clinical work to take advantage of excess radiology and pathology capacity elsewhere in the system. Further, joint telemedicine consults in real time can also add to the ability of local physicians to become better at diagnosing and treating some conditions (such as those requiring expertise in dermatology) by learning from the long-distance specialist as he or she treats their patients. Nevertheless, while telemedicine has been shown to work in actual practice setting, the scientific literature does not present definitive findings of cost effectiveness or efficacy (Hersh et al., 2001a,b, 2006). Hersh et al. believe that "... the growing use of electronic health records will facilitate systematic data collection that will permit strong observational studies to assess the efficacy of telemedicine" (Hersh et al., 2006).

When personally identifiable healthcare data are electronically transported across state borders for telemedicine uses, the applicability of state laws and policies regarding the confidentiality and privacy of these data is often not obvious to the sender or receiver. This uncertainty raises legal questions for organizations that wish to move these data over national networks for patient management, business, or analytical reasons. When vendors of EHRS plan nationwide distribution of their products, they must consider among other things variation in state laws regarding the validity of electronic information for use in official medical records, the length of time for retention of medical record information, and liability for the consequences of EHR failure. The users of systems that exchange patient information across state borders for treatment must also consider the appropriate state licensing requirements.

58.5 Federal Initiatives for Health Information System Interoperability and Connectivity

For years, the Department of VA (VISTA—Veterans Health Information Systems and Technology Architecture) and the DoD (CHCS-II—Composite Healthcare System) have invested in the development of EHRS to improve care for veterans and active servicemen. The Indian Health Service has adopted and modified the VA's VISTA system for its own EHRS use. HHS has a history of undertaking national terminology development (Humphreys et al., 1998) and medical informatics research (Fitzmaurice et al., 2002). In 2004, however, the federal government began to take the initiative to lay the foundation for improving the coordination of these efforts and promoting the interoperability and connectivity of health information systems across the country.

During the 2004–2005 period, the President placed a greater federal emphasis on using health information technology to improve patient safety and the quality of healthcare. The President in his 2004 State of the Union message said, "By computerizing health records, we can avoid dangerous medical mistakes, reduce costs, and improve care." And on April 26, 2004, "Within ten years, every American must have a personal electronic medical record. That's a good goal for the country to achieve." (Bush, April 26, 2004b). President Obama also adopted this goal.

As recommended by NCVHS (NCVHS, 2001) and others, the President created the Office of the National Coordinator for Health Information Technology (Bush, April 27, 2004a), and on May 6, 2004, the Secretary of HHS (1) appointed David Brailer, MD, PhD, as the first National Coordinator and (2) announced that the medical vocabulary known as SNOMED–CT (a clinical reference language standard created by the College of American Pathologists) could be downloaded for free for use in the United States through HHS' National Library of Medicine (US DHHS, May 6, 2004). By July 21, 2004, the National Coordinator produced a strategic framework to guide the nationwide implementation of health information technology in both the public and private sectors. This plan has four major goals to be pursued in the vision for improved healthcare. They are to build an interoperable national health information system that will

1. Inform clinical practice
2. Interconnect clinicians
3. Personalize care
4. Improve population health (ONC, 2004)

Through its Transforming Healthcare Quality Through Health Information Technology Program, the AHRQ in September 2004 awarded 100 grants ($139 million over 3 years), five state demonstration contracts ($25 million over 5 years), a National Health Information Technology Resource Center contract ($18.4 million over 5 years), and initiated a data standards program ($10 million in 1 year). AHRQ's research program embodies the vision of the federal strategic framework for promoting and invests federal research funds to build a knowledge base of how regional and local information technology networks and applications can improve quality of care and patient safety (AHRQ, 2004).

Recognizing the benefits of EHRS and the exchange of clinical information, the President in his State of the Union message to the American people on February 3, 2005, called for additional investment, saying, "I ask Congress to move forward on … improved information technology to prevent medical error and needless costs …" The federal government has begun to devote resources to support its vision of national networks for the exchange of clinical information to benefit patient care. The vision is one of interoperable clinical applications of health information technology applications over a national set of regional networks and of connectivity to all health providers to these networks.

Health information systems are beginning to rely on intranet networks within the health enterprise to link the information created by disparate applications currently in use (e.g., to link existing (legacy) applications such as laboratory, radiology, and pharmacy information systems), and on private networks to exchange patient information among health providers. These systems use web browsers, object-oriented technology, and document formatting languages, including hypertext markup language (http) and extensible markup language (XML). Indeed, the structure of HL7's Version 3 of its suite of clinical message standards for health institutions' electronic clinical messages employs this technology (HL7, 2001), as does ASTM's proposed Continuity of Care Record standard (ASTM, 2005).

Currently, the health industry does not have acceptable standards for encrypting clinical message exchanges and for electronic signatures that are in widespread use. Although the confidentiality of subjects of personal health information is considered sufficiently protected and the authentication of the sender and receiver is sufficiently assured for those providers who currently exchange clinical information through fax and telephone, pilot tests of electronic prescribing conducted by the Medicare Program should provide additional information on ways to improve protection and authentication for clinical exchanges through electronic networks. These 2006 pilots are mandated by the Medicare Prescription Drug, Improvement, and Modernization Act of 2003 (MMA) (Public Law 108-173, 2003).

58.5.1 President's Information Technology Advisory Committee

The President's Information Technology Advisory Committee (PITAC) is a private sector member committee chartered originally in 1998 to provide the president with independent expert advice on maintaining America's preeminence in advanced information technology. In its 2004 report, *Revolutionizing Healthcare through Information Technology*, PITAC recommended federal leadership in developing a national framework containing four essential elements. These elements are: EHRs, computer-assisted clinical decision support, computerized provider order entry, and "secure, private, interoperable, electronic health information exchange, including both highly specific standards for capturing new data and tools for capturing non-standards-compliant electronic information from legacy systems" (PITAC, 2004, pp. 4–5).

58.5.2 American Recovery and Reinvestment Act–Health Information Technology for Economic and Clinical Health

With the growing support for EHR use in medicine and the need to stimulate the U.S. economy to address recessionary unemployment, Congress passed and President Obama signed (on February 17, 2009) into law the ARRA of 2009 that contained the HITECH provision (P.L. 111-5).

With the enactment of P.L. 111-5 (ARRA, including HITECH) in 2009, and its supporting regulations, the government was charged to provide incentive payments to health providers for demonstrating to the satisfaction of the HHS Secretary the *meaningful use* of *certified* EHRs. Physicians can receive up to $44,000 from the Medicare program or $63,750 from the Medicaid program, spread over 5 years beginning in 2011; hospitals can receive payments from both programs into millions. Under ARRA HITECH, to receive incentive payments, health providers must undertake (1) meaningful use of certified EHR technology, including electronic prescribing; (2) information exchange with EHRs connected to improve quality; and (3) reporting on clinical quality and other measures using EHRs. ARRA also mandated HHS regulations for (1) an initial set of health data standards, (2) implementation specifications, and (3) EHR certification criteria (see http://www.healthit.hhs.gov/portal/server.pt/community/healthit_hhs_gov__home/1204).

58.6 Private Sector Initiatives

The Markle Foundation with support from The Robert Wood Johnson Foundation under its Connecting for Health program and in collaboration with the eHealth Initiative has organized working groups representing the public and private sectors to tackle the barriers to the development of an interconnected health information infrastructure. The Markle Foundation convenes recognized experts and health sector stakeholders to reach consensus on how specific barriers should be tackled and preparing roadmaps for action.

58.6.1 Healthcare Information and Management Systems Society

The Healthcare Information and Management Systems Society (HIMSS) is a membership organization that focuses on providing leadership for the optimal use of healthcare information technology and management systems for better human health. One of its projects, Integrating the Healthcare Enterprise (IHE), is a multiyear initiative that has its goal to create "the framework for passing vital health information seamlessly—from application to application, system to system, and setting to setting—across the entire healthcare enterprise." HIMSS, the Radiological Society of North America (RSNA), and the American College of Cardiology (ACC) work collaboratively with the aim "to improve the way computer systems in healthcare share critical information." At the yearly HIMSS annual conferences, the IHE Connect-a-thon and Interoperability Showcase demonstrates the electronic communication of documents containing patient care information (HIMSS, Integrating the Healthcare Enterprise; see http://www.himss.org/ASP/topics_ihe.asp). Public demonstrations of the applications of health data standards are invaluable for learning what works in the electronic exchange of patient care data and how it works. Essentially, what is learned is how to make health data standards work for specific healthcare applications and how to make them work better.

58.7 Driving Forces for EHRS

58.7.1 Patient Safety

Patient safety is a real concern in the U.S. healthcare system but is not well understood. The publication of the IOM study *To Err Is Human* in 1999 informed the American public that between 44,000 and 98,000 people died of medical errors in hospitals (IOM, 1999). In 2003, Zhan and Miller estimated that complications of often-preventable injuries and complications in hospitals in the United States lead to more than 32,000 deaths, 2.4 million extra days of care, and costs exceeding $9B annually (Zahn and Miller, 2003). Among the conditions studied were accidental puncture and laceration, anesthesia complications, postoperative infections and bedsores, surgical wounds reopening, and obstetric traumas during childbirth. Health information technology is clearly part of the remedy. In a study of

36 hospitals, Barker et al. found that 19% of the doses were in error and that "the percentage of [drug] errors rated potentially harmful was 7%, or more than 40 per day in a typical 300-patient facility." (Barker et al., 2002). Bates et al. (1998) found that the rate of serious medication errors dropped by more than half after a large tertiary teaching hospital implemented a computerized physician order entry system. IOM recommends that "[t]o reduce the number of medical errors, the nation's healthcare system must harness available technologies and build an infrastructure for national health information" (IOM, 2003b).

IOM, which is a foremost advisor to the nation in evaluating scientific evidence and obtaining professional opinion pertaining to patient safety and quality of care, recommends that: "[t]o reduce the number of medical errors, the nation's healthcare system must harness available technologies and build an infrastructure for national health information." More specifically, IOM recommends a seamless national network that requires EHRs, secure platforms for exchange of information among providers and patients, and data standards that would make health information understandable by the information systems of different providers. Further, healthcare organizations must adopt information technology systems that are able to collect and share essential health information on patients and their care (IOM, 2003b).

58.7.1.1 Quality of Care

In *Crossing the Quality Chasm: A New Health System for the 21st Century* (IOM, 2001), IOM noted that a chasm exists between current practice and the best we can do and urged the United States (1) to adopt six attributes of quality care: safe, effective, patient centered, timely, efficient, and equitable, and (2) to use information technology to improve the quality of care.

Quality of care deficiencies are widespread in the United States and one study (McGlynn et al., 2003), based on a random sample of healthcare experiences of adults living in 12 metropolitan areas in the United States over a 2-year period found that study participants received only 54.9% of recommended care. The authors evaluated the health system performance on 439 indicators of quality of care for 30 acute and chronic conditions as well as preventive care, with the participants receiving 53.5%, 56.1%, and 54.9% of the recommended care, respectively, for the three categories. Overall, the proportion of participants receiving the recommended care was 54.9% (McGlynn et al., 2003). In the 12 metropolitan areas studied, Seattle, Washington, received the recommended care 59% of the time (the highest) and Little Rock, Arkansas, received the recommended care 51% of the time (the lowest) (Kerr et al., 2004).

The contribution of EHRS for improving quality of care is to deliver medical knowledge and appropriate patient information to the healthcare decision makers—especially the physician and patient—at the time such information is needed and to aggregate clinical entries to obtain quality measures more efficiently than by combining through paper medical records. Once in place, EHRS can also reduce the cost of obtaining standardized quality measures, compared with manual abstractions of paper medical records, and improve medication ordering and administration (Field et al., 2009; Schedlbauer et al., 2009).

58.7.1.1.1 Rising Healthcare Spending

Healthcare expenditures in the United States totaled $1.8 trillion in 2003 ($6121 per capita) and 15.3% of our gross domestic product. This increase was a 8.4% over 2002 and exceeded the rate of inflation of the consumers price index (2.3%) over threefold (Centers for Medicare and Medicaid Services, 2013; U.S. Department of Commerce, 2013). The concern over rising health spending is a matter of obtaining the value for the dollar spent on healthcare and productive competitiveness. A study by Hussey et al. showed that the United States spends more per capita on healthcare than four other comparable countries: Australia, Canada, New Zealand, and England. However, the United States underperforms on measures such as breast cancer deaths, leukemia deaths, asthma deaths, suicide rates, and cancer screening. The implication is that even though the United States spends more, outcomes are not necessarily better.

58.7.1.1.2 Competition in the U.S. Economy

U.S. firms are concerned that many goods produced in the United States are more expensive than those produced in other parts of the world in part because of the higher costs of healthcare in the United States and the larger portion of healthcare costs they incur as part of their labor costs. Also, if the U.S. healthcare system itself is not as productive as the healthcare systems of other countries, our workers will spend more time obtaining healthcare and recovering from illness, and less time working. As a result, U.S. companies are encouraging health plans to improve the quality of care provided to their employees and to contract with lower-cost providers. The Leapfrog Group and other employer groups are promoting a better health system by encouraging employer purchasers to buy healthcare services from providers using

- Computerized physician order entry to permit computer-generated prompts, alerts, and reminders to inform treatment decisions
- ICU physician staffing—the use of board-certified hospital intensivists, hospital-based physicians that would take over a patient's care in the hospital ICU
- Evidence-based hospital referral—particularly for high-risk surgery and high-risk neonatal intensive care (Birkmeyer et al., 2000)

58.8 Extended Uses of EHR Data

Data produced by such systems have additional value beyond supporting the care of specific patients. For example, subsets of individual patient care data from EHRs can be used for research purposes, quality assurance purposes, developing and assessing patient care treatment paths (planned sequences of medical services to be implemented after the diagnoses and treatment choices have been made), assessments of treatment strategies across a range of choices, and postmarketing surveillance of drugs and medical device technologies in use in the community after their approval by the Food and Drug Administration. When linked with data measuring patient outcomes, EHR data may be used to help model the results achieved by different treatments, sites of care, and organizations of care.

If patient care data were uniformly defined and recorded, accurately linked, and collected into databases pertaining to particular geographical areas, they would be useful for research into the patient outcomes of alternative medical treatments for specific conditions and for developing information to assist consumers, healthcare providers, health plans, payers, public health officials, and others in making choices about treatments, technologies, sites and providers of care, health plans, and community health needs. This is currently an ambitious vision for research considering the presently limited use of EHRs. There are insufficient incentives for validating, storing, and sharing electronic patient record data, plus improvements are needed that push forward the state of the art in measuring the severity of patient illness so that the outcomes of similar patients can be compared. Many healthcare decisions are now based on data of inferior quality or no data at all. The importance of these decisions, however, to the healthcare market is driving higher the demand for uniform, accurate clinical data.

58.9 Federal Programs

Uniform, electronic clinical patient data could be useful to many federal programs that have the responsibility for improving, safeguarding, and financing America's health. For example, AHRQ is charged "to enhance the quality, appropriateness, and effectiveness of health services, and access to such services, through the establishment of a broad base of scientific research and through the promotion of improvements in clinical and health system practices, including the prevention of diseases and other health conditions" (PL 106-129, 1999).

The findings that result from such research should improve patient outcomes of care, quality measurement, and cost and access problems. To examine the influence on patient outcomes of alternative treatments for specific conditions, research needs to account for the simultaneous effects of many patient risk factors, such as diabetes and hypertension. Health insurance claims for payment data do not have sufficient clinical detail for many research, quality assurance, and evaluation purposes. Often, administrative data (such as claims data) must be supplemented with data abstracted from the patients' medical records to be useful. In many cases, the data must be identified and collected prospectively from patients (with their permission) and their providers to ensure availability and uniformity. The use of an EHR could reduce the burden of this data collection, support practice guideline development in the private sector, and support the development, testing, and use of quality improvement measures. Having uniform, computerized patient care data in EHRs would allow disease registries to be developed for many more patient conditions.

Other federal, state, and local health agencies could also benefit from EHR-based data collections. For example, the Food and Drug Administration, which conducts postmarketing monitoring to learn the incidence of unwanted effects of drugs after they are approved, could benefit from analyses of the next 20,000 cases in which a particular pharmaceutical is prescribed, using data collected in an EHR. Greater confidence in postmarket surveillance could speed up the approval of new drug applications. The Centers for Medicare and Medicaid Services (CMS) are providing guidance and information to its Quality Improvement Organizations (QIOs) about local and nationwide medical practice patterns founded on analyses of national and regional clinical data about Medicare beneficiaries. Medicare QIOs could analyze more data from the provider's EHRs in their own states to provide constructive, quality-enhancing feedback providers of care at less expense. As a further example, the Centers for Disease Control and Prevention with access to locally available (and perhaps anonomyzed) EHR data on patient care could more quickly and completely monitor the incidence and prevalence of communicable diseases, and engage in real-time surveillance for monitoring bioterrorism threats. State and local public health departments could allocate resources more quickly to address changing health needs with early recognition of community health problems.

Many of these uses require linked data networks and data repositories that communities and patients trust with their health data, or a filter of data flows that searches for events that would trigger a health alert. A national health information network could provide guidance, governance, and principles for the sharing of electronic patient information. Of paramount importance is the protection of the confidentiality of patient information. This may require an approach that gives patients a choice to opt into such systems of sharing their information to obtain the benefits or to opt out of having the system use their own information.

58.10 Selected Issues

While there are personal and public benefits to be gained from the extended use of EHR data beyond direct patient care, the use of personal medical information for these uses, particularly if it contains personal identification, brings with it some requirements and issues that must be faced. Some of the issues that must be addressed by healthcare policy makers, as well as by private markets, are as follows:

58.10.1 Standards

Standards are needed for the nomenclature, coding, and structure of clinical patient care data; the content of data sets for specific purposes; and the electronic transmission of such data to integrate data efficiently across departmental systems within a hospital and data from the systems of other hospitals and healthcare providers. If benefits are to be realized from rapidly accessing and transmitting patient care data for managing patient care, consulting with experts across long distances, linking physician offices and hospitals, undertaking research, and other applications, data standards are essential (Fitzmaurice, 1994).

The United States has the framework for coordination of U.S. standards developing organizations, development and coordination of the U.S. position on international standards issues, and representation at the technical committee (TC) that develops and approves international health data standards. The Healthcare Informatics Standards Board of the American National Standards Institute coordinates the standards developing organizations that work on such standards in the United States, and produces

TABLE 58.2　HIPAA Administrative Simplification Standards

Transactions and Code Sets (TCS) Rule—October 16, 2002
　Claims attachments—Not released
　TCS revisions—January 2012
Identifiers
　Employer ID—July 30, 2004
　National provider ID—May 23, 2007/2008
　Health plan ID—Expected 2011
　Individual ID—Put on hold by Congress
　Security Rule—April 20, 2005
　Privacy Rule—April 14, 2003

Note:　Small health plans have an additional year before their use of HIPAA standards is mandatory.

special summary reports on administrative and clinical health data standards (ANSI HISB, 1997, 1998). The U.S. Technical Advisory Group of the Organization of International Standards (ISO) TC 215, Health Informatics, develops and represents U.S. positions on international health data standards issues, new work items, and recommends the U.S. vote on international standards ballots. The ISO TC 215, Health Informatics, was formed in 1998 by over 30 countries to provide a forum for international coordination of health informatics standards.

Within the United States, administrative health data standards are mandated in the Health Insurance Portability and Accountability Act (HIPAA) of 1996 (Public Law 104-191). In this law, the Secretary of HHS is directed to adopt standards for nine common health transactions (enrollment, claims, payment, and others) that must be used if those transactions are conducted electronically. Penalties are capped at $100 per violation and a maximum of $25,000 per year for each provision violated. Digital signatures, when adopted by the Secretary, may be deemed to satisfy federal and state statutory requirements for written signatures for HIPAA transactions but there is no industry standard to date. The four categories of HIPAA standards with the dates on which specific standards are mandatory, or the year in which they are expected to be published, are shown in Table 58.2. Published standards are expected to be mandatory about 2 years and 60 days after they are published in the final form.

58.10.2 Security

Confidentiality and privacy of individually identifiable patient care and provider data are the most important issues. For most purposes, the HIPAA Privacy Rule (U.S. Department of Health and Human Services, Office of Civil Rights, 2003) is quite stringent with respect to establishing a privacy floor across all states. It creates a fence around the individually identifiable health information it protects, that is, such information that is in the hands of health plans, clearinghouses, and providers who undertake HIPAA transactions (covered entities). Covered entities may use protected health information only for purposes of treatment, payment, or health operations. Without an individual's authorization, there are only 12 ways for a covered entity to legally disclose or use protected health information. Each of these exceptions has requirements of its own (Table 58.3).

The HIPAA Privacy Rule is an essential cornerstone for building a national health information infrastructure that eases the way for personal health information to be shared. It gives patients new rights and controls nationwide, including the right to see, obtain a copy of, and add amendments to their health information. For uses and disclosures not permitted by the Privacy Rule, HIPAA-covered entities must obtain the individual's authorization. The penalties for violating the Privacy Rule can be expensive and include imprisonment.

System security and integrity become important as more and more information for patient treatment and other uses is exchanged through national networks. This issue relates not only to purposeful

TABLE 58.3 Exceptions to the HIPAA Privacy Rule for Which Individual Authorization Is Not Required for Disclosures and Uses of Protected Health Information

- As required by law
- For public health
- Victims of abuse
- For health oversight activities
- For judicial and administrative proceedings
- For law enforcement
- Disclosures about decedents (coroner, medical examiner)
- To facilitate organ transplantation
- For research
- To avert serious threats to health or safety
- For specialized government functions
- For workers' compensation

violations of privacy but also to the accuracy of medical knowledge for patient benefit. If the system fails to accurately transmit what was sent to a physician—for example, a magnetic resonance imaging (MRI), patient history, a practice guideline, or a clinical research finding—and if a physician's judgment and recommendation is based on a flawed image or other misreported medical knowledge—who bears the legal responsibility for a resulting inappropriate patient outcome due to system failure?

National HIPAA security standards for assuring the confidentiality of electronic protected health information are mandatory as of April 20, 2005. The HIPAA Security Rule addresses the administrative, technical, and physical security procedures that HIPAA-covered entity must use. Some procedure specifications are required; others must be addressed following a risk analysis by the HIPAA-covered entity (Health Insurance Reform, 2003). This rule supports the Privacy Rule in that it establishes what security protections are reasonable to safeguard electronic health information from impermissible uses and disclosures.

Just the financial penalties for violations can be severe. For example, the Health Information Technology for Economic and Clinical Health Act (the HITECH Act), a part of the ARRA of 2009 (Public Law 111-5), increased the potential penalties up to $50,000 for each violation and up to a maximum of $1,500,000 for all violations of an identical HIPAA Privacy or Security Rule requirement, if reasonable diligence was not exercised and the violations are not corrected within 30 days. (CITE) HITECH also extended the scope of the Privacy Rule and provided reporting requirements and penalties for breaches of the security of protected health information.

58.10.3 Data Quality

The quality of stored and exchanged clinical data may be questioned in the absence of organized programs and criteria to assess the reliability, validity, and sufficiency of these data. There should be a natural reluctance to use questionable data for making treatment decisions, undertaking research, and for providing useful information to consumers, medical care organizers, and payers. For proper use and analysis, the user should take special care in judging that the information is of sufficient quality to measure and assess the relevant risk factors influencing patient conditions and outcomes. Providers of care may have reluctance even in relying on data supplied by their own patients without some assurance that it is valid.

58.10.4 Varying State Requirements

Electronically stored records in one state may be considered to be legally the same as paper records, but not in another state. In law, regulation, and practice, many states require pen and ink recording and signatures, apparently ruling out electronic records and signatures. To reduce this inconsistency and uncertainty and to provide national guidance, the Electronic Signatures in Global and National Commerce Act was enacted by the U.S. government effective on October 1, 2000. This law gives electronic signatures the same legality as hand-written ones where all parties agree for transactions that are commercial, consumer, or business in nature (Public Law 106-229, 2000). To add to the variability, state privacy laws that (1) conflict with the HIPAA Privacy Rule and (2) are more stringent override the federal Privacy Rule. Under HITECH, enforcement authority is extended to States' Attorney Generals for the HIPAA Privacy and Security Rules.

Standard unique identifiers for patients, healthcare providers, institutions, and payers are needed to obtain economies and accuracy when linking patient care data at different locations, and patient care data with other relevant data. Under HIPAA, the Secretary of HHS must adopt standards for uniquely identifying providers, health plans, employers, and individuals. Because of national concerns about the confidentiality of personal health information that may be linked using the unique individual health identifier, final implementation of that identifier must await explicit approval by Congress.

Malpractice liability concerns arise as telemedicine and information technology allow physician specialists to give medical advice across state borders electronically to other physicians, other healthcare providers, and patients. Physicians are normally licensed by a state to practice within its own state borders. Does a physician who is active in telemedicine need to obtain a license from each state in which he or she practices medicine from outside the state? If the expert physician outside the patient's state gives bad advice, which state's legal system has jurisdiction for liability considerations?

Benefit–cost analysis methods must be developed and applied to inform investment decision makers about the most productive applications of EHRS. There is a need for a common approach to measure the benefits and the costs for comparing alternative information technology applications. Certainly, this is difficult since so many things change with the introduction of EHRS. As hard as they are to do well, valid business risk and benefit assessments can advance the development and implementation of commercial EHR applications.

Regional health data repositories and information exchange networks for the benefit of patients, providers, employers, hospital groups, consumers, and state health and service delivery programs raise issues about the ownership of patient care data, the use of identifiable patient care data, and the governance of health data repositories. A study by the IOM (1994) examined the power of regional health data repositories for improving public health, supporting better private health decisions, recognizing medically and cost-effective healthcare providers and health plans, and generally providing the information necessary to improve the quality of healthcare delivery in all settings. Since these data may include personally identifiable data and move outside the environment in which they were created, resolving these issues is of paramount importance for the development of regional health networks.

58.10.5 Interoperability

Although EHRs have been emphasized in federal initiatives in the United States since 2004, the passage of HITECH in 2009 set the stage for rewards for the meaningful use of certified EHRs by physicians and hospitals. HITECH provides for incentive payments to eligible health providers who demonstrate their meaningful use of *certified* EHRS to the HHS Secretary's satisfaction. *Such physician providers* receive a 75% increase (the incentive payment) in their fees for services provided to Medicare patients up to a maximum of $44,000 or provided to Medicaid patients up to a maximum of $63,750 over 5 years starting in 2011. Such hospital providers can receive incentive payments into millions. By defining health data standards for health information exchange, EHR certification criteria, and the meaningful use criteria, the federal government aims to provide more certainty to EHR purchasers, more uniformity among EHR vendor products, and, most important, improved healthcare quality, safety, and efficiency.

Throughout the incentive payment period, eligible providers have to report performance measures to the government based on their use of EHRs. Produced jointly by the HHS Office of the National

Coordinator for Health Information Technology (ONC) and the HHS CMS, the performance measures, health data standards needed for providers to exchange clinical information about their common patients, and the EHR certification criteria were published in regulations on a congressionally mandated fast track. Over the 2011–2015 time period, the reporting requirements of providers (demonstrating the performance measures showing meaningful use of certified EHRs) become more numerous and more stringent and involve the exchange of specific health information among health providers and between providers and public health authorities. These exchanges are based on interoperability standards published by ONC.

Finally, under the ARRA HITECH mandates, ONC provides funding for technical assistance to providers through regional extension centers, community demonstration pilot projects, state health information exchanges, evaluation activities, and more.

58.11 Summary

In summary, the benefits of EHRS are becoming better known and accepted. What is unknown are the costs of achieving these benefits in sites other than where the EHRSs were developed and how to successfully overcome institutional obstacles for their implementation. The widespread use of systems that provide clinical decision support depends in good part on the development and use of a common medical terminology or, at least, a reference terminology that contains all the relevant concepts to which different medical terminologies can map. This would enable interoperable electronic health information systems to accurately exchange information about those concepts. Although the HIPAA Privacy Rule gives patients the right to obtain a copy of their health information, research findings are lacking on the benefits of sharing EHR information with the patients themselves, although modeling these potential benefits has been fruitful.

Strong initiatives by the federal government are leading the private and the government sectors to build the infrastructure that is needed to support patient information exchanges by clinical systems for the care of a patient. Indeed, a patient's EHR may not be a real data repository but a set of links to a patient's data that resides in many diverse electronic medical records—a virtual EHR. In addition, the federal government is making substantial investments in regional, often statewide, health information network demonstrations, and in research that studies local health information technology applications. The purpose of these new investments is to learn how these networks can resolve important issues regarding the connectivity of providers to the network, the governance and interoperability of their systems, and how successful they can be for improving patient safety and the quality of care. Many issues must be resolved if the vision of a national health information infrastructure is to be approached in reality. The good news is that there is a national mandate and the leadership to tackle them.

Acknowledgment

The author is a senior science advisor for information technology, Agency for Healthcare Research and Quality in the U.S. Department of Health and Human Services.

References

Agency for Healthcare Research and Quality. 2004. Fact sheet: The Agency for Healthcare Research & Quality Health Information Technology Programs. Accessed on November 30, 2010, at http://healthit.ahrq.gov/portal/server.pt?open=514&objID=5576&mode=2

Agency for Healthcare Research and Quality. 2010. *2010 Preliminary Comparative Results: Medical Office Survey on Patient Safety Culture*. Rockville, MD: Prepared by Westat, Inc., AHRQ Publication No. 11-0015-EF, November 2010; Accessed on November 24, 2010, at http://www.ahrq.gov/qual/mosurvey10/moresults10.pdf

American National Standards Institute, Healthcare Informatics Standards Board. 1997. *HISB Inventory of Health Care Information Standards Pertaining to the Health Insurance Portability and Accountability Act of 1996, P.L. 104-191.* New York.

American National Standards Institute, Healthcare Informatics Standards Board. 1998. *Inventory of Clinical Information Standards.* New York, at http://web.ansi.org/rooms/room_41/public/docs.html

ASTM International. 1992. *E1460-92: Standard Specifications for Defining and Sharing Modular Health Knowledge Bases (Arden Syntax for Medical Logic Modules).* ASTM, Philadelphia, PA.

ASTM International. WK4363 standard specification for the continuity of care record (CCR). 2005. Accessed on November 30, 2010, at http://www.astm.org/SEARCH/sitesearch.html?query=wd4353&cartname=mystore

Barker, K.N., Flynn, E.A., Pepper, G.A., Bates, D.W., and Mikeal, R.L. 2002. Medication errors observed in 36 healthcare facilities. *Arch. Intern. Med.* 162:1897–1903.

Bates, D.W., Kuperman, G.J., Rittenberg, E., Teich, J.M., Fiskio, J., Ma'luf, N., Onderonk, A. et al. 1999. A randomized trial of a computer-based intervention to reduce utilization of redundant laboratory tests. *Am. J. Med.* 106(2):144–150.

Bates, D.W., Leape, L.L., Cullen, D.J., Laird, N., Petersen, L.A., Teich, J.M., Burdick, E. et al. 1998. Effect of computerized physician order entry and a team intervention on prevention of serious medication errors in the JAMA. *J. Am Med. Assoc.* 280: 1311–1316.

Birkmeyer, J. D., Birkmeyer, C.M., Wennberg, D.E., and Young, M. 2000. Leapfrog patient safety standards: The potential benefit of universal adoption. Washington DC: The Leapfrog Group for Patient Safety, Accessed on November 30, 2010, at http://www.leapfroggroup.org/media/file/Leapfrog-Launch-Executive_Summary.pdf

Bush, G.W. 2004a. Incentives for the use of health information technology and establishing the position of the national health information technology coordinator. Executive order (April 27, 2004).

Bush, G.W. 2004b. President unveils tech initiatives for energy. Health Care, Internet. Remarks by the President at American Association of Community Colleges Annual Convention, Minneapolis Convention Center, Minneapolis, Minnesota (April 26, 2004).

Centers for Medicare and Medicaid Services, Office of the Actuary, National Health Statistics Group, Table 1. National Health Expenditures, Centers for Medicare and Medicaid Services, Office of the Actuary, National Health Statistics Group, last accessed on May 4, 2013, and Table 1A. Consumer Price Index for All Urban Consumers (CPI-U), last accessed on May 4, 2013, at http://www.cms.gov/Research-Statistics-Data-and-Systems/Statistics-Trends-and-Reports/NationalHealthExpendData/downloads/tables.pdf.

Chase, C.R., Vacek, P.M., Shinozaki, T., Giard, A.M., and Ashikaga, T. 1983. Medical information management: Improving the transfer of research results to presurgical evaluation. *Med. Care.* 21:410–424.

Cimino, J.J. 1993. Saying what you mean and meaning what you say: Coupling biomedical terminology and knowledge. *Acad. Med.* 68(4):257–260.

Cimino, J.J. 1998. Desiderata for controlled medical vocabularies in the twenty-first century. *Methods Inf. Med.* 37(4–5):394–403.

Classen, D.C., Evans, R.S., Pestotnik, S.L., Horn, S.D., Menlove, R. L., and Burke, J.P. 1992. The timing of prophylactic administration of antibiotics and the risk of surgical wound infection. *New Engl. J. Med.* 326(5):281–285.

Donaldson, M.S. and Lohr, K.N. (eds.) 1994. *Health Data in the Information Age: Use, Disclosure, and Privacy.* National Academy Press, Washington DC.

Evans, R.S., Classen, D.C., Stevens, M.S., Pestotnik, S.L, Gardner, R.M., Lloyd, J.F., and Burke, J.P. 1994. Using a health information system to assess the effects of adverse drug events. *AMIA Proceedings of the 17th Annual Symposium on Computer Applications Medical Care*, McGraw-Hill, Inc., New York, NY, pp. 161–165.

Evans, R.S., Pestotnik, S.L., Classen, D.C., and Burke, J.R. 1993. Development of an automated antibiotic consultant. *M.D. Comput.* 10(1):17–22.

Field, T.S., Rochon, P., Lee, M. et al. 2009. Computerized clinical decision support during medication ordering for long-term-care residents with renal insufficiency. *J. Am. Med. Inform. Assoc.* 16(5):480–485.

Fitzmaurice, J.M. 1994. Health care and the NII. In: Putting the information infrastructure to work: Report of the Information Infrastructure Task Force Committee on Applications and Technology, pp. 41–56. National Institute of Standards and Technology, Gaithersburg, MD.

Fitzmaurice, J.M., Adams, K., and Eisenberg, J.M. 2002. Three decades of research on computer applications in health care. *J. Am. Med. Inform. Assoc.* 9(2):144–160.

General Accounting Office. Health and human services' estimate of health care cost savings resulting from the use of information technology. GAO-05-309R (February 17, 2005), 1–9. Accessed on November 30, 2010, at http://www.gao.gov/new.items/d05309r.pdf

Health Insurance Reform: Security Standards; Final Rule. 2003. Federal Register. Rules and Regulations. 45 CFR Parts 160, 162, and 164.68(34); (February 20, 2003):8334–8381.

Hersh, W.R., Hickam, D.H., and Erlichman, M. 2006. The evidence base of telemedicine: Overview of the supplement. *J. Telemed. Telecare* 12(Suppl. 2):1–2.

Hersh, W.R., Wallace, J.A., Patterson, P.K., Kraemer, D.F., Nichol, W.P., Greenlick, M.R., Krages, K.P., and Helfand, M. 2001b. Telemedicine for the Medicare population: Pediatric, obstetric, and clinician-indirect home interventions. Evidence Report/Technology Assessment No. 24S, Supplement (Prepared by Oregon Health Sciences University, Portland, OR under Contract No. 290-97-0018). AHRQ Publication No. 01-E060. Rockville (MD): Agency for Healthcare Research and Quality. August 2001. Accessed on April 10, 2005, at http://www.ahrq.gov/clinic/tp/telemeduptp.htm

Hersh, W.R., Wallace, J.A., Patterson, P.K., Shapiro, SE, Kraemer, D.F, Eilers, G.M., Chan, B.K.S., Greenlick, M.R., and Helfand, M. 2001a. *Telemedicine for the Medicare Population.* Evidence Report/Technology Assessment No. 24 (Prepared by Oregon Health Sciences University, Portland, OR under Contract No. 290-97-0018). AHRQ Publication No. 01-E012. Rockville (MD): Agency for Healthcare Research and Quality. July 2001a. Accessed on April 10, 2005, at http://www.ahrq.gov/clinic/tp/telemeduptp.htm

HL7 EHR system functional model draft standard for trial use, July, 2004. Dickinson, G., Fischetti, L., and Heard, S. (eds.), Ann Arbor, Michigan: Health Level Seven, Inc., 2004, Accessed on November 30, 2010, at http://www.hl7.org/ehr/downloads/index.asp

HL7 Version 3.0 (Draft), Ann Arbor, Michigan: Health Level Seven. 2001. Accessed on November 30, 2010, at http://www.hl7.org/implement/standards/index.cfm

Humphreys, B.L., Lindberg, D.A., Schoolman, H.M., and Barnett, G.O. 1998. The unified medical language system: An informatics research collaboration. *J. Am. Med. Inform. Assoc.* 5(1):1–11.

Hussey, P.S., Anderson, G.F., Osborn, R., Feek, C., McLaughlin, V., Millar, J., and Epstein, A. 2004. How does the quality of care compare in five countries? *Health Aff.* 23(3):89–99.

Institute of Medicine. 1991. Revised edition, 1997. The computer-based patient record: An essential technology for health care. D.E. Detmer, R.S. Dick, and E.B. Steen (eds.), *Committee on Improving the Patient Record*, National Academy Press, Washington DC.

Institute of Medicine. 1994. *Health Data in the Information Age: Use, Disclosure, and Privacy.* M.S. Donaldson and K.N. Lohr (eds.), National Academy Press, Washington DC.

Institute of Medicine. 1999. *To Err Is Human: Building a Safer Health System.* L.T. Kohn, J. Corrigan, and M.S. Donaldson (eds.), Committee on Quality of Health Care in America. National Academy Press, Washington DC.

Institute of Medicine. 2001. *Crossing the Quality Chasm: A New Health System for the 21st Century.* National Academy Press, Washington DC.

Institute of Medicine, Committee on Data Standards for Patient Safety. 2003a. *Key Capabilities of an Electronic Health Record System. Letter Report.* 2003. The National Academies Press, Washington DC.

Institute of Medicine. 2003b. *Patient Safety: Achieving a New Standard for Care.* P. Aspden, J.M. Corrigan, J. Wolcott, and S.M. Erickson (eds.), Committee on Data Standards for Patient Safety. National Academies Press, Washington DC.

Jha, A.K., Kuperman, G.J., Rittenberg, E., Teich, J.M., and Bates, D.W. 2001. Identifying hospital admissions due to adverse drug events using a computer-based monitor. *Pharmacoepidemiol. Drug Saf.* 10(2):113–119.

Johnston, M.E., Langton, K.B., Haynes, R.B., and Mathieu, A. 1994. Effects of computer-based clinical decision support systems on clinician performance and patient outcome. *Ann. Intern. Med.* 120:135–142.

Kaplan, B. and Harris-Salamone, K.D. 2009. Health IT success and failure: Recommendations from literature and an AMIA workshop *J. Am. Med. Inform. Assoc.* 16:291–299.

Kerr, E.A., McGlynn, E.A., Adams, J., Keesey, J., and Asch, S.M. 2004. Profiling the quality of care in twelve communities: Results from the CQI study. *Health Aff.* 23(3):247–256.

Korpman, R.A. 1990. Patient care automation; the future is now. Part 2. The current paper system—Can it be made to work? *Nurs. Econ.* 8(4):263–267.

Korpman, R.A. 1991. Patient care automation; the future is now. Part 8. Does reality live up to the promise? *Nurs. Econ.* 9(3):175–179.

Lyman, J.A., Cohn, W.F., Bloomrosen, M., and Detmer, D.E. 2010. Clinical decision support: Progress and opportunities. *J. Am. Med. Inform. Assoc.* 17(5):487–492.

Markle Foundation, Connecting for Health, General Resources. 2005. Accessed on December 1, 2010, at http://www.connectingforhealth.org/resources/generalresources.html

McDonald, C.J., Hui, S.J., Smith, D.M., Tierney, W.M., Cohen, S.J., Weinberger, M. et al. 1984. Reminders to physicians from an introspective computer medical record. A two-year randomized trial. *Ann. Intern. Med.* 100:130–138.

McGlynn, E.A., Asch, S.M., Adams, J., Keesey, J., Hicks, J., DeCristofaro, A., and Kerr, E.A. 2003. The quality of health care delivered to adults in the United States. *New Engl. J. Med.* 348(26):2635–2645.

Miller, R.A. 1994. Medical diagnostic decision support systems—Past, present, and future. *J. Am. Med. Inform. Assoc.* 1(1):8–27.

National Committee on Vital and Health Statistics. 2000. Report to the Secretary of the U.S. Department of Health and Human Services on Uniform Data Standards for Patient Medical Record Information. Department of HHS: July 6, 2000. Accessed on December 1, 2010, at http://www.ncvhs.hhs.gov/hipaa000706.pdf.

National Committee on Vital and Health Statistics. 2001. Information for health—A strategy for building the national health information infrastructure: Report and recommendations from the NCVHS. Washington DC: Department of Health and Human Services, November 15, 2001. Accessed on December 1, 2010, at http://www.ncvhs.hhs.gov/nhiilayo.pdf.

National Coordination Office for high performance computing and communication. 1994. *HPCC FY 1995 Implementation Plan.* Executive Office of the President, Washington DC.

National Library of Medicine. 2005a. Unified medical language system, Section 2, Metathesaurus. Accessed on May 7, 2013, at http://www.ncbi.nlm.nih.gov/books/NBK9675/

National Library of Medicine. 2005b. Unified medical language system, Metathesaurus. Accessed on May 7, 2013, at http://www.nlm.nih.gov/pubs/factsheets/umlsmeta.html

Nykanen, P., Chowdhury, S., and Wiegertz, O. 1992. Evaluation of decision support systems in medicine. In: *Yearbook of Medical Informatics.* New York: International Medical Informatics Association, pp. 301–309.

Office of the National Coordinator for Health Information Technology (ONC). 2004. *Strategic Framework: The Decade of Health Information Technology: Delivering Consumer-Centric and Information-Rich Health Care.* July 21, 2004, Washington DC: Department of Health and Human Services. Accessed on December 1, 2010, at http://www.hhs.gov/healthit/frameworkchapters.html.

President's Information Technology Advisory Committee. 2004. Revolutionizing health care through information technology. Arlington, VA: NCO for ITRD National Coordinating Office for Information Technology Research and Development, June 2004.

Pryor, T. Allan and George, H. 1994. Sharing MLMs: An experiment between Columbia-Presbyterian and LDS Hospital. *AMIA Proceedings of the 17th Annual Symposium on Computing Applications Medical Care*, McGraw-Hill, Inc., New York, NY, pp. 399–403.

Public Law 104-191. 1996. The Health Insurance Portability and Accountability Act of 1996, August 21, 1996.

Public Law 105-277. 1998. Department of Transportation and Related Agencies Appropriations Act, October 21, 1998.

Public Law 106-129. 1999. Healthcare Research and Quality Act of 1999, December 6, 1999. Accessed on December 2010, at http://www.ahrq.gov/hrqa99a.htm

Public Law 106-229. 2000. Electronic signatures in Global and National Commerce Act, June 30, 2000. Accessed on December 1, 2010, at http://frwebgate.access.gpo.gov/cgi-bin/getdoc.cgi?dbname=106_cong_public_laws&docid=f:publ229.106.pdf

Public Law 108-173. 2003. Medicare Prescription Drug, Improvement, and Modernization Act of 2003, December 8, 2003. Accessed on December 1, 2010, at http://www.cms.gov/DemoProjectsEvalRpts/downloads/RMBH_Legislation.pdf

Public Law 111-5. 2009. American Recovery and Reinvestment Act, February 17, 2009. TITLE XIII—Health Information Technology Act. Accessed on December 1, 2010, at http://frwebgate.access.gpo.gov/cgi-bin/getdoc.cgi?dbname=111_cong_bills&docid=f:h1enr.pdf

Schedlbauer, A., Prasad, V., Mulvaney, C. et al. 2009. What evidence supports the use of computerized alert and prompts to improve clinicians' prescribing behavior? *J. Am. Med. Inform. Assoc.* 16(5):531–538.

Teich, J.M., Merchia, P.R., Schmiz, J.L., Kuperman, G.J., Spurr, C.D., and Bates, D.W. 2000. Effects of computerized physician order entry on prescribing practices. *Arch. Intern. Med.* 160(18):2741–2747.

Tierney, W.M., McDonald, C.J., Hui, S.J., and Martin, D.K. 1988. Computer predictions of abnormal test results. Effects on outpatient testing. *J. Am. Med. Assoc.* 259(8):1194–1198.

Tierney, W.M., McDonald, C.J., Martin, D.K., and Rogers, M.P. 1987. Computerized display of past test results. Effect on outpatient testing. *Ann. Intern. Med.* 107(4):569–574.

Tierney, W.N. and McDonald, C.M. 1991. Practice databases and their uses in clinical research. *Stat. Med.* 10:541–557.

Tierney, W.M., Miller, M.E., and McDonald, C.J. 1990. The effect on test ordering of informing physicians of the charges for outpatient diagnostic tests. *New Engl. J. Med.* 322(21):1499–1504.

Tierney, W.M., Miller, M.E., Overhage, J.M., and McDonald, C.J. 1993. Physician inpatient order writing on microcomputer workstations. *J. Am. Med. Assoc.* 269(3):379–383.

Tuttle, M.S., Sherertz, D.D., Fagan, L.M., Carlson, R.W., Cole, W.G., Shipma, P.B., and Nelson, S.J. 1994. Toward an interim standard for patient-centered knowledge-access. *AMIA Proceedings of the 17th Annual Symposium on Computer Applications Medical Care*, McGraw-Hill, Inc., New York, NY, pp. 564–568.

U.S. Department of Commerce, Bureau of Economic Analysis; and U.S. Bureau of the Census, last accessed on May 4, 2013, at http://www.bls.gov/cpi/cpid03av.pdf.

U.S. Department of Health and Human Services, Office of Civil Rights. 2003. *Standards for Privacy of Individually Identifiable Health Information; Security Standards for the Protection of Electronic Protected Health Information; General Administrative Requirements Including, Civil Money Penalties: Procedures for Investigations, Imposition of Penalties, and Hearings. Regulation Text (Unofficial Version) (45 CFR Parts 160 and 164);* December 28, 2000 as Amended: May 31, 2002, August 14, 2002, February 20, 2003, and April 17, 2003.

U.S. Department of Health and Human Services Press Release. May 6, 2004. Secretary Thompson, seeking fastest possible results, names first Health Information Technology Coordinator.

U.S. Senate. 1999. Healthcare Research and Quality Act of 1999, Senate Bill. 580. Introduced January 6, 1999, signed into law on December 6, 1999.

Wang, D., Peleg, M., Tu, S.W., Boxwala, A.A., Ogunyemi, O., Zeng, Q., Greenes, R.A., Patel, V.L., and Shortliffe, E.H. 2004. Design and implementation of the GLIF3 guideline execution engine. *Biomed. Inform.* 37(5):305–318.

Wang, S.J., Middleton, B., Prosser, L.A., Bardon, C.G., Spurr, C.D., Carchidi, P.J., Kittler, A.F. et al. 2003. A cost–benefit analysis of electronic medical records in primary care. *Am. J. Med.* 114(5):397–403.

White, R.H., Hong, R., Venook, A.P., Dashbach, M.M., Murray, W., and Mungall, D.R. 1987. Initiation of warfarin therapy: Comparisons of physician dosing with computer-predicted dosing. *J. Gen. Int. Med.* 2:141–148.

Zhan, C. and Miller, M.R. 2003. Excess length of stay, charges, mortality are attributable to medical injuries during hospitalization. *J. Am. Med. Assoc.* 290(14):1868–1874.

59

Overview of Standards Related to the Emerging Healthcare Information Infrastructure

Jeffrey S. Blair
IBM Healthcare Solutions

59.1 Introduction

As the cost of healthcare has become a larger percentage of the gross domestic product of many developed nations, the focus on methods to improve healthcare productivity and quality has increased. To address this need, the concept of a healthcare information infrastructure has emerged. Major elements of this concept include patient-centered care facilitated by computer-based patient record (CPR) systems, continuity of care enabled by the sharing of patient information across information networks, and outcomes measurement aided by greater availability and specificity of healthcare information.

The creation of this healthcare information infrastructure will require the integration of existing and new architectures, products, and services. To make these diverse components work together, healthcare information standards (classifications, guides, practices, terminology) will be required (ASTM, 1994).

This chapter will give you an overview of the major existing and emerging healthcare information standards, and the efforts to coordinate, harmonize, and accelerate these activities. It is organized into the major topic areas of

- Identifier standards
- Communications (message format) standards
- Content and structure standards
- Clinical data representations (codes)
- Confidentiality, data security, and authentication
- Quality indicators and data sets
- International Standards
- Coordinating and promotion organizations
- Summary

59.2 Identifier Standards

There is a universal need for healthcare identifiers to uniquely specify each patient, provider, site of care, and product; however, there is no universal acceptance or satisfaction with these systems.

59.2.1 Patient Identifiers

The social security number (SSN) is widely used as a patient identifier in the United States today. However, critics point out that it is not an ideal identifier. They say that not everyone has an SSN; several individuals may use the same SSN; and the SSN is so widely used for other purposes that it presents an exposure to violations of confidentiality. These criticisms raise issues that are not unique to the SSN. A draft document has been developed by the American Society for Testing and Materials (ASTM) E31.12. Subcommittee to address these issues. It is called the "Guide for the Properties of a Universal Healthcare Identifier" (UHID). It presents a set of requirements outlining the properties of a national system creating a UHIC, includes critiques of the SSN, and creates a sample UHD (ASTM E31.12, 1994). Despite the advantages of a modified/new patient identifier, there is not yet a consensus as to who would bear the cost of adopting a new patient identifier system.

59.2.2 Provider Identifiers

The Healthcare Financing Administration (HCFA) has created a widely used provider identifier known as the Universal Physician Identifier Number (UPIN) (Terell et al., 1991). The UPIN is assigned to physicians who handle Medicare patients, but it does not include nonphysician caregivers. The National Council of Prescription Drug Programs (NCPDP) has developed the standard prescriber identification number (SPIN) to be used by pharmacists in retail settings. A proposal to develop a new national provider identifier number has been set forth by HCFA (1994). If this proposal is accepted, then HCFA would develop a national provider identifier number which would cover all caregivers and sites of care, including Medicare, Medicaid, and private care. This proposal is being reviewed by various state and federal agencies. It has also been sent to the American National Standards, Institute's Healthcare Informatics Standards Planning Panel (ANSI HISPP) Task Force on Provider Identifiers for review.

59.2.3 Site-of-Care Identifiers

Two site-of-care identifier systems are widely used. One is the health industry number (HIN) issued by the Health Industry Business Communications Council (HIBCC). The HIN is an identifier for healthcare facilities, practitioners, and retail pharmacies. HCFA has also defined provider of service identifiers for Medicare usage.

59.2.4 Product and Supply Labeling Identifiers

Three identifiers are widely accepted. The labeler identification code (LIC) identifies the manufacturer or distributor and is issued by HIBCC (1994). The LIC is used both with and without bar codes for products and supplies distributed within a healthcare facility. The universal product code (UPC) is maintained by the Uniform Code Council and is typically used to label products that are sold in retail settings. The national drug code is maintained by the Food and Drug Administration and is required for reimbursement by Medicare, Medicaid, and insurance companies. It is sometimes included within the UPC format.

59.3 Communications (Message Format) Standards

Although the standards in this topic area are still in various stages of development, they are generally more mature than those in most of the other topic areas. They are typically developed by committees within standards organizations and have generally been accepted by users and vendors. The overviews of these standards given below were derived from many sources, but considerable content came from the Computer-based Patient Record Institute's (CPRI) "Position Paper on Computer-based Patient Record Standards" (CPRI, 1994) and the Agency for Healthcare Policy and Research's (AHCPR) "Current Activities of Selected Healthcare Informatics Standards Organizations" (Moshman Associates, 1994).

59.3.1 ASC X12N

This committee is developing message format standards for transactions between payers and providers. It is rapidly being accepted by both users and vendors. It defines the message formats for the following transaction types (Moshman Associates, 1994):

- 834—enrollment
- 270—eligibility request
- 271—eligibility response
- 837—healthcare claim submission
- 835—healthcare claim payment remittance
- 276—claims status request
- 277—claims status response
- 148— report of injury or illness

ASC X12N is also working on the following standards to be published in the near future:

- 257, 258—Interactive eligibility response and request. These transactions are an abbreviated form of the 270/271.
- 274, 275—patient record data response and request. These transactions will be used to request and send patient data (tests, procedures, surgeries, allergies, etc.) between a requesting party and the party maintaining the database.
- 278, 279—healthcare services (utilization review) response and request. These transactions will be used to initiate and respond to a utilization review request.

ASC X12N is recognized as an accredited standards committee (ASC) by the American National Standards Institute (ANSI).

59.3.2 American Society for Testing and Materials

59.3.2.1 Message Format Standards

The following standards were developed within American Society for Testing and Materials (ASTM) Committee E31. This committee has applied for recognition as an ASC by ANSI:

1. ASTM E1238 standard specification for transferring clinical observations between independent systems. E1238 was developed by ASTM Subcommittee E31.11. This standard is being used by most of the largest commercial laboratory vendors in the United States to transmit laboratory results. It has also been adopted by a consortium of 25 French laboratory system vendors. Health level seven (HL7), which is described later in this topic area, has incorporated E1238 as a subset within its laboratory results message format (CPRI, 1994).
2. ASTM E1394 standard specification for transferring information between clinical instruments. E1394 was developed by ASTM Subcommittee E31.14. This standard is being used for communication of information from laboratory instruments to computer systems. This standard has been developed by a consortium consisting of most U.S. manufacturers of clinical laboratory instruments (CPRI, 1994).
3. ASTM 1460 specification for defining and sharing modular health knowledge bases (Arden Syntax). E1460 was developed by ASTM Subcommittee E31.15. The Arden Syntax provides a standard format and syntax for representing medical logic and for writing rules and guidelines that can be automatically executed by computer systems. Medical logic modules produced in one site-of-care system can be sent to a different system within another site of care and then customized to reflect local usage (CPRI, 1994).
4. ASTM E1467 specification for transferring digital neurophysical data between independent computer systems. E1467 was developed by ASTM Subcommittee E31.17. This standard defines codes and structures needed to transmit electrophysiologic signals and results produced by electroencephalograms and electromyograms. The standard is similar in structure to ASTM E1238 and HL7; and it is being adopted by all the EEG systems manufacturers (CPRI, 1994).

59.3.3 Digital Imaging and Communications

This standard is developed by the American College of Radiology—National Electronic Manufacturers' Association (ACR-NEMA). It defines the message formats and communications standards for radiologic images. Digital imaging and communications (DICOM) is supported by most radiology picture archiving and communications systems (PACS) vendors and has been incorporated into the Japanese Image Store and Carry (ISAC) optical disk system as well as Kodak's PhotoCD. ACR-NEMA is applying to be recognized as an accredited organization by ANSI (CPRI, 1994).

59.3.4 Health Level Seven (HL7)

HL7 is used for intra-institution transmission of orders; clinical observations and clinical data, including test results; admission, transfer, and discharge records; and charge and billing information. HL7 is being used in more than 300 U.S. healthcare institutions including most leading university hospitals and has been adopted by Australia and New Zealand as their national standard. HL7 is recognized as an accredited organization by ANSI (Hammond, 1993; CPRI, 1994).

59.3.5 Institute of Electrical and Electronics Engineers, Inc. P1157

59.3.5.1 Medical Data Interchange Standard

Institute of Electrical and Electronics Engineers, Inc. (IEEE) Engineering in Medicine and Biology Society (EMB) is developing the medical data interchange standard (MEDIX) for the exchange of data between hospital computer systems (Harrington, 1993; CPRI, 1994). Based on the International Standards Organization (ISO) standards for all seven layers of the OSI reference model, MEDIX is working on a framework model to guide the development and evolution of a compatible set of standards. This activity is being carried forward as a joint working group under ANSI HISPP's Message Standards Developers Subcommittee (MSDS). IEEE is recognized as an accredited organization by ANSI.

IEEE P1073 Medical Information Bus (MIB): This standard defines the linkages of medical instrumentation (e.g., critical care instruments) to point-of-care information systems (CPRI, 1994).

National Council for Prescription Drug Programs (NCPDP): These standards developed by NCPDP are used for communication of billing and eligibility information between community pharmacies and third-party payers. They have been in use since 1985 and now serve almost 60% of the nation's community pharmacies. NCPDP has applied for recognition as an accredited organization by ANSI (CPRI, 1994).

59.4 Content and Structure Standards

Guidelines and standards for the content and structure of CPR systems are being developed within ASTM Subcommittees E31.12 and E31.19. They have been recognized by other standards organizations (e.g., HL7); however, they have not matured to the point where they are generally accepted or implemented by users and vendors.

A major revision to E1384, now called a standard description for content and structure of the CPR, has been made within Subcommittee E31.19 (ASTM, 1994). This revision includes work from HISPP on data modeling and an expanded framework that includes master tables and data views by user.

Companion standards have been developed within E31.19. They are E1633, A Standard Specification for the Coded Values Used in the Automated Primary Record of Care (ASTM, 1994), and E1239–94, A Standard Guide for Description of Reservation/Registration-A/D/T Systems for Automated Patient Care Information Systems (ASTM, 1994). A draft standard is also being developed for object-oriented models for R-A/D/T functions in CPR systems. Within the E31.12 Subcommittee, domain specific guidelines for nursing, anesthesiology, and emergency room data within the CPR are being developed (Moshman Associates, 1994; Waegemann, 1994).

59.5 Clinical Data Representations (Codes)

Clinical data representations have been widely used to document diagnoses and procedures. There are over 150 known code systems. The codes with the widest acceptance in the United States include

1. International Classification of Diseases (ICD) codes, now in the ninth edition (ICD-9), are maintained by the World Health Organization (WHO) and are accepted worldwide. In the United States, HCFA and the National Center for Health Statistics (NCHS) have supported the development of a clinical modification of the ICD codes (ICD-9-CM). WHO has been developing ICD-10; however, HCFA projects that it will not be available for use within the United States for several years. Payers require the use of ICD-9-CM codes for reimbursement purposes, but they have limited value for clinical and research purposes due to their lack of clinical specificity (Chute, 1991).
2. Current Procedural Terminology (CPT) codes are maintained by the American Medical Association (AMA) and are widely used in the United States for reimbursement and utilization review purposes. The codes are derived from medical specialty nomenclatures and are updated annually (Chute, 1991).
3. The systematized nomenclature of medicine (SNOMED) is maintained by the College of American Pathologists and is widely accepted for describing pathologic test results. It has a multiaxial (11 fields) coding structure that gives it greater clinical specificity than the ICD and CPT codes, and it has considerable value for clinical purposes. SNOMED has been proposed as a candidate to become the standardized vocabulary for CPR systems (Rothwell et al., 1993).

4. Digital imaging and communications (DICOM) is maintained by the American College of Radiology—National Electronic Manufacturers' Association (ACR-NEMA). It sets forth standards for indices of radiologic diagnoses as well as for image storage and communications (Cannavo, 1993).

5. *Diagnostic and Statistical Manual of Mental Disorders* (DSM), now in its fourth edition (*DSM-IV*), is maintained by the American Psychiatric Association. It sets forth a standard set of codes and descriptions for use in diagnoses, prescriptions, research, education, and administration (Chute, 1991).

6. Diagnostic Related Groups (DRGs) are maintained by HCFA. They are derivatives of ICD-9-CM codes and are used to facilitate reimbursement and case-mix analysis. They lack the clinical specificity to be of value in direct patient care or clinical research (Chute, 1991).

7. Unified Medical Language System (UMLS) is maintained by the National Library of Medicine (NLM). It contains a metathesaurus that links clinical terminology, semantics, and formats of the major clinical coding and reference systems. It links medical terms (e.g., ICD, CPT, SNOMED, DSM, CO-STAR, and D-XPLAIN) to the NLM's medical index subject headings (MeSH codes) and to each other (Humphreys, 1991; Cimino et al., 1993).

8. The Canon Group has not developed a clinical data representation, but it is addressing two important problems: clinical data representations typically lack clinical specificity and are incapable of being generalized or extended beyond a specific application. "The Group proposes to focus on the design of a general schema for medical-language representation including the specification of the resources and associated procedures required to map language (including standard terminologies) into representations that make all implicit relations 'visible,' reveal 'hidden attributes,' and generally resolve 'ambiguous references'" (Evans et al., 1994).

59.6 Confidentiality, Data Security, and Authentication

The development of CPR systems and healthcare information networks have created the opportunity to address the need for more definitive confidentiality, data security, and authentication guidelines and standards. The following activities address this need:

1. During 1994, several bills were drafted in Congress to address healthcare privacy and confidentiality. They included the Fair Health Information Practices Act of 1994 (H.R. 4077), the Healthcare Privacy Protection Act (S. 2129), and others. Although these bills were not passed as drafted, their essential content is expected to be included as part of subsequent healthcare reform legislation. They address the need for uniform comprehensive federal rules governing the use and disclosure of identifiable health and information about individuals. They specify the responsibilities of those who collect, use, and maintain health information about patients. They also define the rights of patients and provide a variety of mechanisms that will allow patients to enforce their rights.

2. ASTM Subcommittee E31.12 on CPR is developing Guidelines for Minimal Data Security Measures for the Protection of Computer-based patient Records (Moshman Associates, 1994).

3. ASTM Subcommittee E31.17 on Access, Privacy, and Confidentiality of Medical Records is working on standards to address these issues (Moshman Associates, 1994).

4. ASTM Subcommittee E31.20 is developing standard specifications for authentication of health information (Moshman Associates, 1994).

5. The Committee on Regional Health Data Networks convened by the Institute of Medicine (IOM) has completed a definitive study and published its findings in a book titled *Health Data in the Information Age: Use, Disclosure, and Privacy* (Donaldson and Lohr, 1994).

6. The CPRI's Work Group on Confidentiality, Privacy, and Legislation has completed white papers on "Access to Patient Data" and on "Authentication," and a publication titled "Guidelines for Establishing Information Security: Policies at Organizations using Computer-based Patient Records" (CPRI, 1994).

7. The Office of Technology Assessment has completed a two-year study resulting in a document titled "Protecting Privacy in Computerized Medical Information." It includes a comprehensive review of system/data security issues, privacy information, current laws, technologies used for protection, and models.
8. The U.S. Food and Drug Administration (FDA) has created a task force on Electronic/Identification Signatures to study authentication issues as they relate to the pharmaceutical industry.

59.7 Quality Indicators and Data Sets

The Joint Commission on Accreditation of Healthcare Organizations (JCAHO) has been developing and testing obstetrics, oncology, trauma, and cardiovascular clinical indicators. These indicators are intended to facilitate provider performance measurement. Several vendors are planning to include JCAHO clinical indicators in their performance measurement systems (JCAHO, 1994).

The health employers data and information set (HEDIS) version 2.0 has been developed with the support of the National Committee for Quality Assurance (NCQA). It identifies data to support performance measurement in the areas of quality (e.g., preventive medicine, prenatal care, acute and chronic disease, and mental health), access and patient satisfaction, membership and utilization, and finance. The development of HEDIS has been supported by several large employers and managed care organizations (NCQA, 1993).

59.8 International Standards

The ISO is a worldwide federation of national standards organizations. It has 90 member countries. The purpose of ISO is to promote the development of standardization and related activities in the world. ANSI was one of the founding members of ISO and is representative for the United States (Waegemann, 1994).

ISO has established a communications model for open systems interconnection (OSI). IEEE/MEDIX and HL7 have recognized and built upon the ISO/OSI framework. Further, ANSI HISPP has a stated objective of encouraging compatibility of U.S. healthcare standards with ISO/OSI. The ISO activities related to information technology take place within the Joint Technical Committee (JTC) 1.

The Comite Europeen de Noramalisation (CEN) is a European standards organization with 16 technical committees (TCs). Two TCs are specifically involved in healthcare: TC 251 (Medical Informatics) and TC 224 WG12 (Patient Data Cards) (Waegemann, 1994).

The CEN TC 251 on Medical Informatics includes work groups on: Modeling of Medical Records; Terminology, Coding, Semantics, and Knowledge Bases; Communications and Messages; Imaging and Multimedia; Medical Devices; and Security, Privacy, Quality, and Safety. The CEN TC 251 has established coordination with healthcare standards development in the United States through ANSI/HISPP.

In addition to standards developed by ISO and CEN, there are two other standards of importance. United Nations (U.N.) EDIFACT is a generic messaging-based communications standard with health-specific subsets. It parallels X12 and HL7, which are transaction-based standards. It is widely used in Europe and in several Latin American countries. The READ Classification System (RCS) is a multiaxial medical nomenclature used in the United Kingdom. It is sponsored by the National Health Service and has been integrated into computer-based ambulatory patient record systems in the United Kingdom (CAMS, 1994).

59.9 Standards Coordination and Promotion Organizations

In the United States, two organizations have emerged to assume responsibility for the coordination and promotion of healthcare standards development: the ANSI Healthcare Informatics Standards Planning Panel (HISPP) and the CPRI. The major missions of an ANSI HISPP are

1. To coordinate the work of the standards groups for healthcare data interchange and healthcare informatics (e.g., ACR/NEMA, ASTM, HL7, IEEE/MEDIX) and other relevant standards groups

(e.g., X3, X12) toward achieving the evolution of a unified set of nonredundant, nonconflicting standards.

2. To interact with and provide input to CEN TC 251 (Medical Informatics) in a coordinated fashion and explore avenues of international standards development. The first mission of coordinating standards is performed by the Message Standards Developers Subcommittee (MSDS). The second mission is performed by the International and Regional Standards Subcommittee. HISPP also has four task groups (1) Codes and Vocabulary, (2) Privacy, Security, and Confidentiality, (3) Provider Identification Numbering Systems, and (4) Operations. Its principal membership is composed of representatives of the major healthcare standards development organizations (SDOs), government agencies, vendors, and other interested parties. ANSI HISPP is by definition a planning panel, not an SDO (Hammond, 1994; ANSI HISPP, 1994).

The CPRI's mission is to promote acceptance of the vision set forth in the Institute of Medicine Study report "The Computer-based Patient Record: An Essential Technology for Healthcare." CPRI is a nonprofit organization committed to initiating and coordinating activities to facilitate and promote the routine use of CPR. The CPRI takes initiatives to promote the development of CPR standards, but it is not an SDO itself. CPRI members represent the entire range of stakeholders in the healthcare delivery system. Its major work groups are the: (1) Codes and Structures Work Group; (2) CPR Description Work Group; (3) CPR Systems Evaluation Work Group; (4) Confidentiality, Privacy, and Legislation Work Group; and (5) Professional and Public Education Work Group (CPRI, 1994).

Two work efforts have been initiated to establish models for principal components of the emerging healthcare information infrastructure. The CPR Description Work Group of the CPRI is defining a consensus-based model of the CPR system. A joint working group to create a common data description has been formed by the MSDS Subcommittee of ANSI HISPP and IEEE/MEDIX. The joint working group is an open standards effort to support the development of a common data model that can be shared by developers of healthcare informatics standards (IEEE, 1994).

The CPRI has introduced a proposal defining a public/private effort to accelerate standards development for CPR systems (CPRI, 1994). If funding becomes available, the project will focus on obtaining consensus for a conceptual description of a CPR system; addressing the need for universal patient identifiers; developing standard provider and sites-of-care identifiers; developing confidentiality and security standards; establishing a structure for and developing key vocabulary and code standards; completing health data interchange standards; developing implementation tools; and demonstrating adoptability of standards in actual settings. This project proposes that the CPRI and ANSI HISPP work together to lead, promote, coordinate, and accelerate the work of SDOs to develop healthcare information standards.

The Workgroup on Electronic Data Interchange (WEDI) is a voluntary, public/private task force which was formed in 1991 as a result of the call for healthcare administrative simplification by the director of the Department of Health and Human Services, Dr. Louis Sullivan. They have developed an action plan to promote healthcare EDI which includes: promotion of EDI standards, architectures, confidentiality, identifiers, health cards, legislation, and publicity (WEDI, 1993).

59.10 Summary

This chapter has presented an overview of major existing and emerging healthcare information infrastructure standards and the efforts to coordinate, harmonize, and accelerate these activities. Healthcare informatics is a dynamic area characterized by changing business and clinical processes, functions, and technologies. The effort to create healthcare informatics standards is therefore also dynamic. For the most current information on standards, refer to the "For More Information" section at the end of this chapter.

References

American National Standards Institute's Health Care Informatics Standards Planning Panel, 1994. Charter statement. New York.

American Society for Testing and Materials (ASTM), 1994. *Guide for the Properties of a Universal Health Care Identifier.* ASTM Subcommittee E31.12, Philadelphia.

American Society for Testing and Materials (ASTM), 1994. *Membership Information Packet.* ASTM Committee E31 on computerized systems, Philadelphia.

American Society for Testing and Materials (ASTM), 1994. A standard description for content and structure of the computer-based patient record, E1384–91/1994 revision. ASTM Subcommittee E31.19, Philadelphia.

American Society for Testing and Materials (ASTM), 1994. Standard guide for description of reservation registration-admission, discharge, transfer (R-ADT) systems for automated patient care information systems, E1239–94. ASTM Subcommittee E31.19, Philadelphia.

American Society for Testing and Materials (ASTM), 1994. A standard specification for the coded values used in the automated primary record of care, E1633. ASTM Subcommittee E31.19, Philadelphia.

Cannavo M.J., 1993. The last word regarding DEFF & DICOM. *Healthcare Informatics* 32.

Chute C.G., 1991. *Tutorial 19: Clinical Data Representations.* Symposium on Computer Applications in Medical Care, Washington, DC.

Cimino J.J., Johnson S.B., Peng P. et al., 1993. *From ICD9-CM to MeSH Using the UMLS: A How-to-Guide,* SCAMC, Washington, DC.

Computer Aided Medical Systems Limited (CAMS), 1994. *CAMS News* 4: 1.

Computer-based Patient Record Institute (CPRI), 1994. *CPRI-Mail* 3: 1.

Computer-based Patient Record Institute (CPRI), 1994. Position paper computer-based patient record standards. Chicago.

Computer-based Patient Record Institute (CPRI), 1994. *Proposal to Accelerate Standards Development for Computer-Based Patient Record Systems.* Version 3.0, Chicago.

Donaldson M.S. and Lohr K.N. (Eds.), 1994. *Health Data in the Information Age: Use, Disclosure, and Privacy.* Washington, DC, Institute of Medicine, National Academy Press.

Evans D.A., Cimino J.J., Hersh W.R. et al., 1994. Toward a medical-concept representation language. *J. Am. Med. Inform. Assoc.* 1: 207.

Hammond W.E., 1993. Overview of health care standards and understanding what they all accomplish. *HIMSS Proceedings*, Chicago, American Hospital Association.

Hammond W.E., McDonald C., Beeler G. et al., 1994. *Computer Standards: Their Future within Health Care Reform. HIMSS Proceedings*, Chicago, Health Care Information and Management Systems Society.

Harrington J.J., 1993. *IEEE P1157 MEDIX: A Standard for Open Systems Medical Data Interchange.* New York, Institute of Electrical and Electronic Engineers.

Health Care Financing Administration (HCFA), 1994. Draft issue papers developed by HCFA's national provider identifier/national provider file workgroups. Baltimore.

Health Industry Business Communications Council (HIBCC), 1994. Description of present program standards activity. Phoenix.

Humphreys B., 1991. Tutorial 20: Using and assessing the UMLS knowledge sources. *Symposium on Computer Applications in Medical Care*, Washington, DC.

Institute of Electrical and Electronics Engineers (IEEE), 1994. *Trial-use Standard for Health Care Data Interchange—Information Model Methods: Data Model Framework.* IEEE Standards Department, New York.

Joint Commission on Accreditation of Health Organizations (JCAHO), 1994. *The Joint Commission Journal on Quality Improvement.* Oakbrook Terrace, IL.

Moshman Associates, Inc., 1994. *Current activities of selected health care informatics standards organizations.* Office of Science and Data Development, Agency for Health Care Policy and Research, Bethesda, MD.

National Committee for Quality Assurance, 1993. *Hedis 2.0: Executive Summary.* Washington, DC.

Rothwell D.J., Cote R.A., Cordeau J.P. et al., 1993. *Developing a Standard Data Structure for Medical Language—The SNOMED Proposal.* SCAMC, Washington, DC.

Terell S.A., Dutton B.L., Porter L. et al., 1991. *In Search of the Denominator: Medicare Physicians—How Many are There?* Health Care Financing Administration, Baltimore.

Waegemann C.P., 1994. *Draft—1994 Resource Guide: Organizations Involved in Standards and Development Work for Electronic Health Record Systems.* Medical Records Institute, Newton, Massachusetts.

Workgroup for Electronic Data Interchange (WEDI), 1993. *WEDI report: October 1993.* Convened by the Department of Health and Human Services, Washington, DC.

Further Reading

For copies of standards accredited by ANSI, you can contact the American National Standards Institute, 11 West 42d St., NY, NY 10036 (212), 642–4900. For information on ANSI Health Care Informatics Standards Planning Panel (HISPP), contact Steven Cornish (212) 642–4900.

For copies of individual ASTM standards, you can contact the American Society for Testing and Materials, 1916 Race Street, Philadelphia, PA 19103–1187 (215), 299–5400.

For copies of the "Proposal to Accelerate Standards Development for Computer-based Patient Record Systems," contact the Computer-based Patient Record Institute (CPRI), Margaret Amatayakul, 1000 E. Woodfield Road, Suite 102, Schaumburg, IL 60173 (708) 706–6746.

For information on provider identifier standards and proposals, contact the Health Care Financing Administration (HCFA), Bureau Program Operations, 6325 Security Blvd., Baltimore, MD 21207 (410), 966–5798. For information on ICD-9-CM codes, contact HCFA, Medical Coding, 401 East Highrise Bldg. 6325 Security Blvd., Baltimore, MD 21207 (410), 966–5318.

For information on site-of-care and supplier labeling identifiers, contact the Health Industry Business Communications Council (HIBCC), 5110 N. 40th Street, Suite 250, Phoenix, AZ 85018 (602), 381–1091.

For copies of standards developed by Health Level 7, you can contact HL7, 3300 Washtenaw Avenue, Suite 227, Ann Arbor, MI 48104 (313), 665–0007.

For copies of standards developed by the Institute of Electrical and Electronic Engineers/Engineering in Medicine and Biology Society, in New York City, call (212) 705–7900. For information on IEEE/MEDIX meetings, contact Jack Harrington, Hewlett-Packard, 3000 Minuteman Rd., Andover, MA 01810 (508), 681–3517.

For more information on clinical indicators, contact the Joint Commission on Accreditation of Health Care Organizations (JCAHO), Department of Indicator Measurement, One Renaissance Blvd., Oakbrook Terrace, IL 60181 (708), 916–5600.

For information on pharmaceutical billing transactions, contact the National Council for Prescription Drug Programs (NCPDP), 2401 N. 24th Street, Suite 365, Phoenix, AZ 85016 (602), 957–9105.

For information on HEDIS, contact the National Committee for Quality Assurance (NCQA), Planning and Development, 1350 New York Avenue, Suite 700, Washington, DC 20005 (202), 628–5788.

For copies of ACR/NEMA DICOM standards, contact David Snavely, National Equipment Manufacturers Association (NEMA), 2101 L. Street N.W., Suite 300, Washington, DC 20037 (202), 457–8400.

For information on standards development in the areas of computer-based patient record concept models, confidentiality, data security, authentication, and patient cards, and for information on standards activities in Europe, contact Peter Waegemann, Medical Records Institute (MRI), 567 Walnut, PO Box 289, Newton, MA 02160 (617), 964–3923.

60

Introduction to Informatics and Nursing in the New Healthcare Environment: 2013

Kathleen A.
McCormick*
SAIC-F

Joyce Sensmeier
Healthcare Information and
Management Systems
Society

Connie White
Delaney
University of Minnesota

Carol J. Bickford
American Nurses
Association

* This chapter was written by Kathleen McCormick in her private capacity. No official support or endorsement by SAIC-F or DHHS is intended or should be inferred. The content of this publication does not necessarily reflect the views or policies of the Department of Health and Human Services, nor does mention of trade names, commercial products, or organizations imply endorsement by the U.S. Government.

60.1 Introduction

This chapter updates the information on nursing informatics in this new environment of health information technology (IT) and the new agenda and progress of the U.S. Office of the National Coordinator (ONC). Nurses represent the nursing informatics community at the highest level of United States Government Policy, Standards, and Meaningful Use committees and workgroups. As the volume of information system networks has increased in the past five years, so has the volume of nurses prepared to work in these environments. The priorities have widened for health information in the form of national and regional health information exchanges, interoperability, transparency, and the widespread goals for the electronic health record (EHR).

This chapter updates the changes in healthcare policies and standards, demography of the nursing informatics profession and refreshes the survey data on nursing informatics. Nurses continue to constitute the largest single group of healthcare workers, including experts that serve on national committees and interoperability initiatives focused on standards and terminology development, standards harmonization, and EHR adoption. They are expanding their scopes of practice in hospitals, critical care environments, ambulatory clinics, long-term care and home health, public health, academic environments, and healthcare and vendor corporations. They focus on the development, implementation and evaluation of integrated systems that enhance patient care and safety, verify outcomes, assure quality care, and document resource consumption. This chapter also provides an update on the response of the nursing professional associations and organizations in setting the priorities for advanced education for the nursing profession in informatics, and a roadmap for the future through the TIGER Initiative.

60.2 HITECH, ONC, and Nursing Informatics in National Programs

The Health Information Technology for Economic and Clinical Health (HITECH) Act seeks to improve American healthcare delivery and patient care through an unprecedented investment in health IT. The provisions of the HITECH Act are specifically designed to work together to provide the necessary assistance and technical support to providers, enable coordination and alignment within and among states, establish connectivity to the public health community in case of emergencies and health promotion–disease prevention initiatives, and assure the workforce is properly trained and equipped to be meaningful users of EHRs.

These programs build the foundation for every American to benefit from an EHR, as part of a modernized, interconnected, and vastly improved system of care delivery.

The Office of the National Coordinator for Health Information Technology (ONC) not only coordinates a variety of programs to implement HITECH but also supports the efforts of several related initiatives to facilitate nationwide adoption of health IT (HIT). These initiatives enable ONC to reach diverse stakeholder groups that are imperative to the success of the HITECH Act (HHS, 2010). Five initiatives, which are listed below, serve the needs of a diverse array of stakeholders to foster HIT adoption:

- State Level Health Initiatives—These initiatives are designed to ensure that states and regional efforts can achieve health information exchange (HIE) that are aligned with the national agenda.
- Nationwide Health Information Network (NwHIN)—This program represents a collection of standards, protocols, legal agreements, specifications, and services to enable secure HIEs.
- Federal Health Architecture—This program establishes an e-government line of business initiatives to increase efficiency and effectiveness in all government operations.
- Adoption—This is an initiative that supports two national HIT adoption surveys: one for the physician office and the other for hospitals.

- Clinical Decision Support and the CDS Collaboratory—This is an initiative to provide clinical staff, patients, and other individuals with knowledge and person-specific information, intelligently filtered or presented at appropriate times, to enhance health and healthcare.

Funded by ONC are eight grants programs that specifically support these national initiatives, and which are overseen by informatics nurse, Judy Murphy, ONC Deputy National Coordinator for Programs and Policy:

1. State Health Information Exchange Cooperative Agreement Program: This new grant program supports states or state designated entities (SDEs) in establishing health information exchange (HIE) capability among healthcare providers and hospitals in their jurisdictions.
2. Health Information Technology Extension Program: This program establishes Health Information Technology Regional Extension Centers (RECs) to offer technical assistance, guidance, and information on best practices to support and accelerate healthcare providers' efforts to become meaningful users of EHRs.
3. Strategic Health IT Advanced Research Projects (SHARP) Program: The SHARP grant program funds research focused on achieving breakthrough advances to address well-documented problems that have impeded adoption: (1) Security of Health Information Technology; (2) Patient-Centered Cognitive Support; (3) Healthcare Application and Network Platform Architectures; and (4) Secondary Use of EHR Data.
4. Community College Consortiato Educate Health Information Technology Professionals Program: This new grant program seeks to rapidly create HIT education and training programs at Community Colleges or expand existing programs. Community Colleges funded under this initiative will establish intensive, nondegree training programs that can be completed in six months or less. This is one component of the Health IT Workforce Program.
5. Curriculum Development Centers Program: Curriculum development will be enhanced through another grant program to provide $10 million to institutions of higher education (or consortia thereof) to support HIT curriculum development. This is also a component of the Health IT Workforce Program.
6. Program of Assistance for University-Based Training: To rapidly increase the availability of individuals qualified to serve in specific HIT professional roles requiring university-level training, this grant program has been established to support this training. This is another component of the Health IT Workforce Program.
7. Competency Examination for Individuals Completing Non-Degree Training Program: A grant program has been established to provide $6 million in grants to an institution of higher education (or consortia thereof) to support the development and initial administration of a set of HIT competency examinations. This is yet another component of the Health IT Workforce Program.
8. Beacon Community Program: The Beacon Community Program was established through a grant program for communities to build and strengthen their HIT infrastructure and exchange capabilities. These communities will demonstrate the vision of a future where hospitals, clinicians, and patients are meaningful users of HIT, and together the community achieves measurable improvements in healthcare quality, safety, efficiency, and population health (http://healthit.hhs.gov/portal/server.pt?open=512&objID=1487&parentname=CommunityPage&parentid=2&mode=2&in_hi_userid=10741&cached=true).

60.3 Two National Committees with Nursing Informatics Membership

The American Recovery and Reinvestment Act of 2009 (ARRA) provides that two committees be established related to HIT. The first committee, the Health IT (HIT) Policy Committee makes recommendations to the National Coordinator for Health IT on a policy framework for the develop-ment and adoption of a nationwide health information infrastructure, including standards for the exchange of patient medical information. ARRA provides that the HIT Policy Committee shall at least make recommendations on standards, implementation specifications, and certifications criteria in eight specific areas as previously described above. A coauthor of this chapter (Connie Delaney) sits on this Committee.

Second, the Health IT (HIT) Standards Committee is charged with making recommendations to the National Coordinator on standards, implementation specifications, and certification criteria for the electronic exchange and use of health information. This committee focuses on the same eight areas described above of the Policy Committee and has developed a schedule for the assessment of policy recommendations developed by the Health IT Policy Committee. In developing, harmonizing, and recognizing standards and implementation specifications, this committee provides for the testing of the specifications and standards by the National Institute for Standards and Technology (NIST). Informatics nurses Elizabeth Johnson from Tenet Healthcare Corporation and Tim Cromwell from the Department of Veterans Affairs serve on this Committee.

The ARRA authorizes the Centers for Medicare & Medicaid Services (CMS) to provide reimburse-ment incentives for meaningful use. The Medicare EHR incentive program provides incentive payments to eligible professionals and eligible hospitals for efforts to adopt, implement, or upgrade certified EHR for meaningful use in the first year of their participation in the program and for demonstrating mean-ingful use during each of five subsequent years.

60.4 Definition of "Nursing Informatics"

Health informatics is comprised of multiple discipline-specific information practices; nursing infor-matics is one. Nursing informatics, an applied science, is defined by the American Nurses Association (2008) as a specialty that:

> Integrates nursing science, computer science, and information science to manage and commu-nicate data, information, and knowledge in nursing practice. Nursing informatics facilitates the integration of data, information, knowledge, and wisdom to support patients, nurses, and other providers in their decision-making in all roles, and settings. This support is accomplished through the use of information structures, information processes, and information technology. (p. 65)

60.4.1 Nursing Process

Most nurses have been prepared in their educational programs to use the nursing process as a frame-work to guide thinking and professional practice. Assessment, diagnosis and problem/issue definition, outcomes identification, planning, implementation and evaluation comprise the steps in the nursing process. Employers value the expertise and critical thinking skills of the informatics nurse who uses the nursing process. The nursing process serves as the foundation for the *Informatics Nursing: Scope and Standards of Practice* (ANA, 2008), which provides specific standards of practice and standards of pro-fessional performance statements that assist the informatics nurse in practice. The content can be used when developing position descriptions and performance appraisals, provides a structure for informatics curriculum development for educators, and a supports a research agenda for nursing and interdisciplin-ary research for groups such as bioengineers and nurses.

60.4.2 Demography

Registered nurses comprise the largest professional healthcare group in the United States. Their work environments include traditional hospital, ambulatory clinic, private practice settings, schools, correctional facilities, long-term care, home health, community health, and public health environments. Nurses also provide healthcare services to homeless populations, faith communities, and other disenfranchised, underserved, diverse and uninsured populations. In each setting, the registered nurse serves as the often unrecognized knowledge worker addressing data, information, and knowledge needs of both patients and families, other healthcare providers, and the health system. Record keeping and written and electronic documentation support the necessary communication activities among nurses, other clinicians, the health system, and the patient.

The definition of nursing has evolved over the years. In 2010 the American Nurses Association reaffirmed this contemporary definition that reflects the holistic and health focus of registered nurses in the United States:

> Nursing is the protection, promotion, and optimization of health and abilities, prevention of illness and injury, alleviation of suffering through the diagnosis and treatment of human response, and advocacy in the care of individuals, families, communities, and populations. (ANA, 2010a)

Like other professions, after initial educational preparation and licensure, the registered nurse may continue studies for preparation in a clinical specialty practice, such as, pediatrics, gerontology, cardiology, women's health, and perioperative nursing. Graduate preparation in clinical specialties may lead to designation as an advanced practice registered nurse (APRN) in the role of certified registered nurse anesthetist, certified nurse-midwife, certified nurse practitioner, and clinical nurse specialist. Others may be interested in practice in other areas, such as administration, research, education, case management, or informatics.

In 2012 the nursing profession was ranked as the most trusted profession in the United States by Gallop (Gallop, 2012; ANA, 2010b) for the 13th out of 14 years. Moreover, the landmark Institute of Medicine (IOM) report on "The Future of Nursing: Acute Care" (IOM, 2010) linked the United States's opportunity to transform its healthcare system, and the role nurses can and should play in this transformation. The nursing workforce brings strong assets to the adoption and effective utilization of information systems and other technologies.

Because of the increased national interest in healthcare informatics and implementation of healthcare information systems coupled with the increased numbers of graduate nursing informatics educational programs, the 2008 National Sample Survey of Registered Nurses initial findings report a prevalence of over 9000 informatics nurses from the 3.1 million registered nurses in the United States (HRSA, 2008).

60.5 Nurses: The Largest Group Applying Informatics Competencies and Implementing EHR Systems

In studies since the 1980s, nurses have been identified as the largest users of information systems in healthcare, for example, the hospital and the home. Nurses also constitute the largest single group of healthcare workers, including experts who serve on national committees and interoperability initiatives focused on standards and terminology development, standards harmonization, and EHR adoption. Further, nurses are active in the research, education, implementation, integration and optimization of information systems throughout the healthcare system.

More than three-quarters of informatics nurses are currently developing or implementing nursing/clinical documentation systems according to the 2011 Healthcare Information and Management Systems Society (HIMSS) Nursing Informatics Workforce Survey (HIMSS, 2011a). This survey builds on nursing informatics research that HIMSS released in 2004 and 2007. A total of 660 responses were received to the web-based survey, which was performed to gain a better understanding of the background of informatics nurses, the issues they address on a daily basis, and the tools they use to perform their jobs. The majority of the nurse informaticists who participated in this research continue to work in a hospital setting—48% work at a hospital and another 20% work at the corporate offices of a healthcare system. In comparison to surveys conducted in 2004 and 2007, the 2011 salary data suggest a substantial increase for nurse informaticists as the average salary increased by 17% from 2007 and 42% from 2004. In 2011, electronic medical/health records were reported among the top two highest mentioned applications (following clinical/nursing documentation) that respondents are implementing for the first time since the survey was initiated in 2004.

In addition to identifying the areas with which they were presently developing or implementing solutions, respondents were also asked to identify those areas with which they had overall experience (HIMSS, 2011a). Almost all of the respondents were most likely to report having experience with nursing clinical documentation systems (91%), followed by electronic medical/health records (76%), clinical information systems and CPOE (both at 72%). Respondents were asked to identify the areas that presented the largest barriers to them as a nurse informaticist (they were able to select two barriers). In 2011, almost one-third of respondents mentioned lack of integration/interoperability as one of the top two barriers, followed by lack of financial resources (26%) and lack of administrative support (23%). In 2007, nearly two-thirds of respondents (65%) indicated that availability of financial resources was a top barrier. This was also the top barrier identified in the 2004 survey.

As in previous surveys, the range of nursing titles for respondents to the 2011 survey is varied and mixed. Twenty percent of respondents reported that they have a title of nursing informatics specialist while another 10% reported the title of clinical specialist. Compared to the 2007 survey, the title of nursing informatics specialist is used more often in the 2011 survey, while the use of the clinical specialist title showed a decrease in use. This suggests that the titles specific to informatics are becoming better defined in 2011, moving away from a generic title such as clinical specialist. Seven percent reported the title of consultant and 5% each identified project manager or director of nursing informatics. In 2011, over half of the respondents (56%) reported earning a post-graduate degree.* This represents an increase from the 2007 survey, when 52% of respondents reported this to be the case.

More than half of the nurse informaticists continue to report to the IT department. The reporting structure for nurse informaticists has not changed substantially in the past seven years. The top departments to which respondents identified that they report to are Information Technology (52%), Nursing (32%), and Administration (22%). No other area was reported by more than 6% of respondents. While these items were the top three areas to which nurse informaticists indicated they reported to in the past, there does appear to be a slight shift to Administration and away from Nursing. Based on this survey and compared to the surveys conducted in 2004 and 2007, the healthcare industry is recognizing the value of Nursing Informatics. One metric in particular speaks volumes to the importance of nurse informaticists in the healthcare industry: base salary. Also, the percentage of post graduates (those with master's degree and/or PhDs) increased from 52% in 2007 to 56% in 2011. This represents a statistically significant increase and marks a positive trend that the nurse informaticist profession continues to attract highly qualified and formally educated demographics.

Finally, it is worth noting that the 2011 respondents tended to have less clinical experience than their 2007 and 2004 counterparts, but they have had more experience as nurse informaticists. About two in five nurse informaticists in the 2011 survey have been in this position for 10 years or more, compared to one-third in 2007 and one-quarter in 2004. The increasing maturity of this field is reflected in the substantial increase in salaries, frequency of job promotions and additional staff responsibilities that these respondents have taken on.

60.5.1 Expanding Nursing Informatics Roles

Like the expanding roles of other registered nurses, the role of the informatics nurse reflects significant diversity and expertise. *Nursing Informatics: Scope and Standards of Practice* (ANA, 2008) provides a

---

* Includes master's degree in nursing, master's degree in other field/specialty, PhD in nursing, and PhD in other field/specialty.

listing of functional areas of nursing informatics practice: administration, leadership, and management; analysis; compliance and integrity management; consultation; coordination, facilitation, and integration; development; educational and professional development; research and evaluation. Some of these experts are: analysts, project managers, consultants, educators, researchers, product developers, decision support/outcomes managers, advocate/policy developers, entrepreneurs, chief information officers, and business owners. Most information system vendors have designated a senior executive level nurse, chief nursing officer (CNO), to direct the informatics nurse contingent and patient care software development components of the organization, quite like the CNO in a hospital or multi-facility enterprise. Recent job announcements posted at the HIMSS, AMIA (American Medical Informatics Association), and ANIA (American Nursing Informatics Association) website job banks sought individuals for systems analyst, database administrator, and implementation specialist positions.

Increased organizational appreciation of the value, expertise, and leadership skills of informatics nurse specialists is being reflected by the development of the role and designation of a chief nursing informatics officer (CNIO). The CNIO most often has responsibility for strategic planning and decision-making related to clinical informatics in partnership with the chief medical informatics officer (CMIO). Organizations identify different accountability and reporting mechanisms for the CNIO that fit their operational and structural needs.

60.5.2 What Do Nurses Do That Requires So Much Informatics Background?

The nursing profession is becoming very much the integrator or coordinator of patient care. Within a typical medical surgical unit the majority of nurse's time during a shift is spent predominantly on patient care activities (Hendrich et al., 2008). These activities include assessment and vital sign monitoring (7.2% or 30.9 min). A primary function of nursing is to assess the outcomes of surgery or medication administration, observe for complications and adverse reactions, and evaluate the outcomes of procedures during the day and night following procedures. The delivery of treatments and pain medication results in nurses spending 17.2% or 72 min in medication administration. This includes pills, intramuscular, and intravenous medications and blood. The direct patient care takes 19.2% time or about 81 min which includes such interventions as helping in activities of daily living, changing dressing, and administering procedures. The coordination of care takes 20.6% or 86 min which includes transporting patients for x-ray procedures, laboratory, respiratory, dialysis, and other types of consultations. In addition to procedural coordination, the nurse coordinates and documents the transfers of patients between healthcare environments such as intakes from the emergency room, the intensive care environment, the recovery room, the step-down units, and the transfer to home, long-term care, or rehabilitation environments. The nurse spends 35.3% or 147.5 min documenting all of the above either because the doctor ordered it, or the nursing professional practice, state regulations, hospital quality assurance require it, or because the interaction with the patient demands it. While supporting each of these activities, the nurse is engaged in healthcare education of patients and caregivers. The nursing professional works in a complex system that requires complex systems theory to monitor best practice and adherence to evidence, facilitates decision support and permits documentation of safe, high quality, and effective care.

60.5.3 Strategic Initiatives within Nursing Informatics: The TIGER Initiative

The Technology Informatics Guiding Education Reform (TIGER) initiative has been instrumental in addressing the need for an informatics and technology competent workforce within nursing and the health professions. The TIGER initiative seeks to better prepare practicing nurses, nurse educators, nurse administrators, and nursing students to use technology and informatics to improve the delivery of patient care. The TIGER initiative was formed in 2004 to bring together nursing stakeholders to develop a shared vision, strategies and specific actions for improving nursing practice, education, and the delivery of patient care through the use of HIT. In 2006, the TIGER initiative convened a summit of nursing stakeholders to develop, publish, and commit to carrying out the action steps defined within this plan. The TIGER initiative has published a summary report titled *Evidence and Informatics Transforming Nursing: 3-Year Action Steps toward a 10-Year Vision* (TIGER, 2007).

Before 1990 most nurses did not have training regarding computer use in their nursing or college curriculum unless they returned to school for further education (TIGER, 2007). Therefore, the practicing nurse should be provided with opportunities for learning basic "keyboarding," that is, typing skills and computer basics such as how to use the mouse. This would lessen the anxiety for computer use. Nurses are caring for patients with greater acuity, requiring more documentation and creating higher stress than ever before. Adding the stress of computerization when one is totally unfamiliar with the computer can be a major challenge. Incorporating this challenge into their current work load may seem like an insurmountable task to nurses and could be a large barrier for EHR implementation. Thus, providing educational opportunities as well as designing user-friendly applications for use by the nursing staff can lessen the stress and remove barriers.

Since 2007, hundreds of volunteers have joined the TIGER Initiative to continue the action steps defined at the Summit. Collaborative teams were formed in TIGER Phase Two to accelerate the action plan within nine key topic areas. Each collaborative team researched their subject with the perspective of "What does every practicing nurse need to know about this topic?" The teams identified resources, references, gaps, and areas that need further development, and provided recommendations for industry to accelerate the adoption of IT for nursing. The TIGER Initiative builds upon and recognizes the work of organizations, programs, research, and related initiatives in the academic, practice, and government sector, and references that work within the "references" and "resources" sections of the nine individual collaborative reports. Areas that need further action steps are listed in the "recommendations" section of each collaborative report. The report provides an executive summary of the TIGER activities through 2008, as well as a brief synopsis of each of the findings and recommendations of the nine collaborative teams (TIGER, 2008). The comprehensive report from each of the nine collaborative teams is available on the TIGER website at http://www.thetigerinitiative.org. The nine collaborative teams are: (1) Standards and Interoperability, (2) National Health IT Agenda, (3) Informatics Competencies, (4) Education and Faculty Development, (5) Staff Development, (6) Usability and Clinical Application Design, (7) Virtual Demonstration Center, (8) Leadership Development, and (9) Consumer Empowerment and Personal Health Records.

Phase Three of the TIGER Initiative furthered the application and integration of Phase Two recommendations for the nursing profession, interdisciplinary and allied health groups, and future minority and rural populations. Efforts are underway to create a virtual learning environment to prepare the current practicing workforce, faculty and students for meaningful use goals, as well as future digital participants in the healthcare workforce—with particular focus on minorities, rural populations, and those experiencing the digital divide.

From this grassroots initiative, begun in 2006, with support from over 70 contributing organizations and a grant from the Robert Wood Johnson Foundation, TIGER has emerged, in July 2011, as the TIGER Initiative Foundation, a 501(c) (3) organization operating for charitable, educational, and scientific purposes. TIGER's focus is to engage and prepare the clinical workforce to use technology and informatics to improve the delivery of patient care.

60.6 Informatics Nurses Have a United Voice through the Alliance for Nursing Informatics

The Alliance for Nursing Informatics (ANI) is a growing collaboration of organizations that enables a unified voice for nursing informatics. ANI, sponsored by AMIA and HIMSS, represents more than

TABLE 60.1 Members of the ANI Sponsored by AMIA and HIMSS as of April 2013

ANI Member Organizations
American Medical Informatics Association (AMIA)
American Nursing Informatics Association (ANIA)
American Organization of Nurse Executives (AONE)
Association of periOperative Registered Nurses (AORN)
Association of Women's Health, Obstetric and Neonatal Nurses (AWHONN)
Center for Nursing Classification and Clinical Effectiveness (CNC)
Central Savannah River Area Clinical Informatics Network (CSRA-CIN)
Cerner Nursing Advisory Board
Connecticut Healthcare Informatics Network (CHIN)
CPM Resource Center International Consortium
Croatian Nursing Informatics Association (CroNIA)
Delaware Valley Nursing Computer Network (DVNCN)
Health Informatics of New Jersey (HINJ)
Healthcare Information and Management Systems Society (HIMSS)
Informatics Nurses From Ohio (INFO)
MEDITECH Nurse Informatics program
Midwest Nursing Research Society-NI Research Section (MNRS)
Minnesota Nursing Informatics Group (MINING)
NANDA International
National Association of School Nurses (NASN)
New England Nursing Informatics Consortium (NENIC)
North Carolina State Nurses Association Council on NI (NCNA CONI)
Omaha System
Oncology Nursing Society (ONS)
Puget Sound Nursing Informatics (PSNI)
SNOMED CT Nursing Working Group
South Carolina Informatics Nursing Network (SCINN)
Surgical Information Systems–Clinical Advisory Task Force (SIS)
Taiwan Nursing Informatics Association (TNIA)
Utah Nursing Informatics Network (UNIN)

Note: Also affiliated with the American Nurses Association.

5000 informatics nurses and brings together 30 distinct nursing informatics groups in the United States. Table 60.1 lists the ANI organizations. ANI crosses academia, practice, industry, and nursing specialty boundaries and works in collaboration with more than 3 million nurses in practice today. ANI provides the vehicle for a single, unified voice for nursing informatics that will allow consistent representation and participation in the public healthcare policy process, IT standards development, information systems design, implementation and evaluation, and shared communication and networking opportunities.

ANI member organizations represent multiple nursing informatics stakeholder groups including HIT vendors, terminology developers, user groups and international nursing informatics organizations. Full membership in ANI is extended to organizations that

- Are local, regional, national, or international in scope.
- Are independent organizations or a sub-unit of a multi- or single-disciplinary organization.
- Have open membership structures; membership is open to individuals who are interested in the field of nursing informatics.

- Have a body of knowledge and skills in a defined area relevant to nursing informatics, supported by documentation that might include a core curriculum, publications and research, standards of care/practice, or other documents.

Affiliate membership can be extended to any organization or entity that is not eligible to join as a full member, subject to the approval of the ANI governing directors.

ANI and its members have provided an active voice in helping to shape policy and leverage national IT initiatives. For example, Deborah Aldridge, from the Southern Piedmont Community Care Plan in North Carolina received one of the Beacon Community Awards. She was involved in writing this grant as a representative for the North Carolina State Nurses Association Council on Nursing Informatics (NCNA-CONI, see Table 60.1).

In 2010, ANI was invited to present testimony to the Robert Wood Johnson Foundation Initiative at the IOM. ANI provided a statement on the future of nursing in acute care, focusing on the area of technology (IOM, 2010). ANI's position is that "meaningful use" of HIT, when combined with best practice and evidence-based care delivery, will improve healthcare for all Americans. This is an essential foundation for the future of nursing and informatics nurses must be engaged as leaders in the effective use of IT to impact the quality and efficiency of healthcare services. Thus, nurses must be supported by a healthcare environment that adequately enables their knowledge-based work as

- Leaders in the effective design and use of EHR systems
- Integrators of information
- Full partners in decision making
- Care coordinators across disciplines
- Experts to improve quality, safety, efficiency, and reduce health disparities
- Advocates for engaging patients and families
- Contributors to standardize infrastructure within the EHR
- Researchers for safe patient care
- Educators for preparing the workforce

60.6.1 Ethics and Regulation

Registered nurses have a long tradition of concern about ethics, patient advocacy, safety, and quality of care. Beginning with the first clinical experience, the registered nurse must know the differences and associated practice associated with privacy, confidentiality, and security. Just as for registered nurse colleagues, the *Code of Ethics for Nurses with Interpretive Statements* (ANA, 2001) provides a framework for the informatics nurse. Although primarily focused on support activities for the healthcare environment, the informatics nurse has the obligation to be concerned about issues of privacy, confidentiality, and security surrounding the patient, clinician, and enterprise and the associated data, information, and knowledge.

The federal government's current focus provides numerous ethical and regulatory issues. The current U.S. healthcare environment has yet to resolve the problem of clinical practice and licensure across state lines for individuals working with nurse call centers, telehealth applications, and electronic prescriptions. Another example is related to unequal distribution of resources or the digital divide which is characterized by those without a working personal computer and high-speed Internet at home. Nurses have a strong advocacy role in current initiatives to support consumer health informatics and the development and use of personal health records.

60.6.2 Standards in Vocabularies and Data Sets

Nursing has been developing nomenclatures for over 30 years to address the nursing process components of diagnosis, interventions, and outcomes. Table 60.2 lists the American Nurses Association

TABLE 60.2 American Nurses Association Recognized Nursing Practice Classification Systems

ABC Codes
Clinical Care Classification (CCC) formerly Home Healthcare Classification
International Classification of Nursing Practice (ICNP)
Logical Observation Identifiers Names and Codes (LOINC®)
Nursing Diagnoses, Definitions, and Classification (NANDA)
Nursing Interventions Classification System (NIC)
Nursing Minimum Data Set (NMDS)
Nursing Outcomes Classification (NOC)
Nursing Management Minimum Data Set (NMMDS)
Omaha System
PeriOperative Nursing Data Set (PNDS)
SNOMED CT®
Ozbolt's Patient Care Data Set (PCDS)—retired

recognized classification and nomenclatures developed by the nursing profession. Under the auspices of the International Council of Nurses (ICN) the International Classification of Nursing Practice (ICNP®) was developed as a standardized terminology representing nursing practice and unifying nursing globally. The ICNP is now included in the World Health Organization (WHO) Family of International Classifications (WHO-FIC), as is the International Classification of Diseases (ICD). Further, the International Nursing Minimum Data Set (iNMDS) initiative represents a collaboration of the International Medical Informatics Association-Special Interest Group (SIG) Nursing Informatics (IMIA-NI) and ICN and fosters collaboration to increase nursing's comparative capacity within and across countries (ICN, 2008).

The International Medical Informatics Association (IMIA-NI) SIG Nursing Informatics Working Group developed a Reference Terminology ISO Standard that was approved in 2003. This was accomplished with the international network of nurses who in turn were developing standards for nomenclature and classifications within their respective countries. This group recognized the value of an international effort to compare quality, efficiencies and outcomes of care resulting from nursing care internationally.

60.7 Clinical Information Systems

Healthcare information systems that adequately support nursing practice have not fully advanced over the past decades. Figure 60.1 identifies some of the system components, influencing factors, and relationships that should be considered in describing the complexity of nursing, a profession that relies so heavily on evidence, knowledge, and critical thinking (Androwich et al., 2003). Consequently the requisite detailed analysis and design processes must generate the appropriate and diverse information system components necessary for successful support for nurses and nursing practice.

Nurses have been contributing to the development and harmonization of health data standards through HL7, LOINC, CDISC, SNOMED, and the now retired Healthcare Information Technology Standards Panel (HITSP) committees. Over 130 HITSP specifications were accepted, recognized, and/or adopted by the secretary of the Department of Health and Human Services. These interoperability specifications are being leveraged to advance health information exchange and the widespread adoption of EHRs by 2014.

Wherever health data standards are being developed and applied, nurses are present to consider the input of the professional standards on the work of those committees and working groups. Nurses provide their content expertise throughout the process to ensure that patient care needs are addressed.

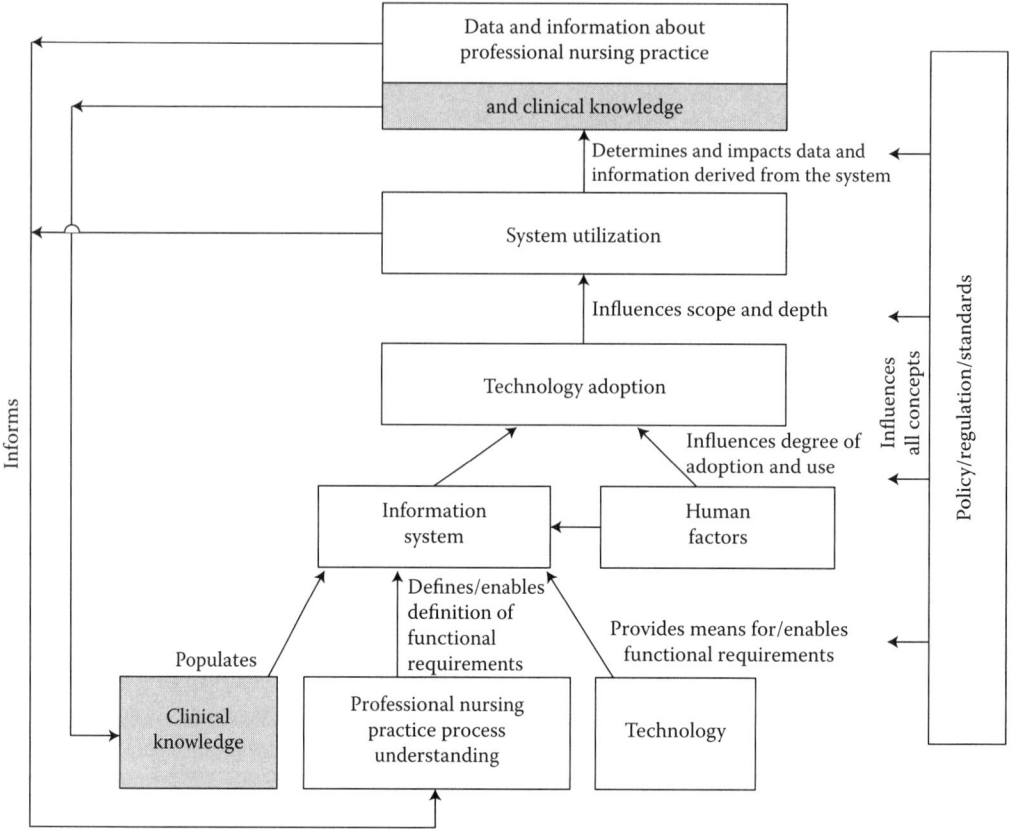

FIGURE 60.1 Organizing framework for clinical information systems: Critical knowledge as the critical factor. (From Androwich IM. et al. 2002. *Clinical Information Systems: A Framework for Reaching the Vision.* Washington, DC: Nursesbooks.org.)

Nurses are at the center of care coordination in almost every healthcare setting. Their data and information must be required in every information system and setting to adequately perform the care coordination from all members of the clinical team.

60.8 Bridging Nursing and Engineering Specialties: The Bioinformatics Partnership of Nurses and Engineers

There are new examples of advanced practice informatics nurses working in partnership with engineering specialties and other interdisciplinary teams in the development of personal health, personalized health, translational research, as well as mobile devices and gaming technology. Because of these new technological advances the need for specialized education for engineers, healthcare professionals, and consumers is paramount.

Relating to personal health, there are services, systems, and host platforms for allowing consumers to centrally store and manage their health information (FNLM, 2009). The basic personal health information that can be entered into a personal health record includes: condition, medications, allergies, immunization profiles, procedures, and laboratory results. Users can opt in or opt out of sharing data with healthcare professionals or other individuals. These records can also be linked to a variety of devices that can monitor conditions from weight to blood pressure to be transmitted to nurses to monitor chronic conditions. Major personal health record systems include the Veteran Administration's MyHealtheVet and Microsoft HealthVault. The primary personal health record system vendors are teamed with large EHR vendors, private pharmacy companies, laboratory chains, healthcare consortia, and large academic medical centers. It is currently not known how many of the major personal health record system vendors employ nursing informatics experts.

Personalized health allows the capture of information so that the diagnosis and treatment can be tailored to an individual's health condition, susceptibility to a condition, and prevention of a condition (Buetow, 2009). The development of personalized science is a paradigm shift in the classic population focused approach to diagnosis and treatment. The shift is toward subclassifying individuals based upon genetic, environmental, and other factors of disease into individualized and tailored treatments for their specific condition. Advances in genomics and microbiology, proteomics, and metabolomics are beginning to identify molecular markers that occur in persons who have a disease, condition, susceptibility to a disease, or a different response to treatment (PricewaterhouseCoopers, 2009). Clinical and populations studies also require massive data collection of biospecimens and biorepositories, as well as biomarker standardized data incorporating the advanced genetic and molecular analyses. Biomedical informatics is also required in personalized medicine. Advances in the new science require the utilization of advanced platforms that support integration, storage on Clouds, and computational analytic skills in biomedical informatics (White House, 2008). Already reshaping this future is the next-generation sequencing, and the collection of open source molecular, tissue, and other biobanking technologies to rapidly identify genetic profiles. Even the clinical trials are changing to adaptive clinical trials that integrate the personal, tissue, and clinical information that informs the patients' individual treatment options (McCormick, 2011).

Integrated databases are a hallmark of consortium science in linking large academic settings to: aggregate data of patients with specific genetic-based diagnostic tests, confirm disease by gender and ethnic groups, and recommend differential treatments. The next quest is the linkage of these personalized data with the patient's individual health records and the EHR (McCormick, 2009). By extending the new personalized health beyond the classic clinical trials, larger populations of patients can be studied, new treatments can be developed, and adverse reporting of treatments can be monitored from diverse populations. This new technology warrants the nursing and engineering scientist to be particularly vigilant to several policy areas, including: technology development, regulations, rules, imaging transmission, interoperability of platforms, common data standards, reimbursement, intellectual property, privacy, and security. New technologies are being invented for both nurses and engineers to become engaged in as the area of personalized health expands.

Translational research bridges the benefits of personal and personalized health to the consumer and the clinicians in hospitals, community healthcare environments, ambulatory care, and the community at large (NCRR, 2010). The technological challenges of translational health offer nursing informatics research and practice challenges. Sixty funded Clinical Translational Research Award sites and their translational research teams engaged in multidisciplinary teams, including nursing. Translational research required the coordination of public and private entities such as academic settings and pharmaceutical companies to transfer the bench finding to bedside application. This shift moved some of the developments for the consumer from the industry to large academic consortia. The integration of longitudinal data to study a health condition also became critical in translational research as the clinical conditions presented themselves over time. Now, the Clinical and Translational Science Awards are administered by the National Center for Advancing Translational Sciences (NCATS) at the National Institutes of Health (NIH) (http://www.ncats.nih.gov, last accessed April 4, 2013).

The Clinical and Translational Science Award (CTSA) Thematic Special Interest Group of Nurse Scientist continues and is led by Dr. Donna Jo McCloskey at the National Institute of Nursing Research (NINR) and Dr. Pamela Mitchell from the School of Nursing at the University of Washington in Seattle. With over 240 members from across the country, the purpose of the CTSA Nurse Scientist Special Interest Group (SIG) is to discuss and implement ways in which clinical and translational nurse scientist investigators can advance nursing contributions to translational research. The group meets on a monthly basis via telecom, coordinates workshops, and meets regionally and nationally during scientific venues (http://www.ctsacentral.org/committee/ctsa-nurse-scientist, last accessed April 4, 2013).

The Clinical and Translational Science Award Thematic Special Interest Group of Nurse Scientist continues and is led by Dr. Donna Jo McCloskey at the National Institute of Nursing Research (NINR) and Dr. Pamela Mitchell from the School of Nursing at the University of Washington in Seattle. With over 240 members from across the country,the purpose of the CTSA Nurse Scientist Special Interest Group (SIG) is to discuss and implement ways in which clinical and translational nurse scientist investigators can be advance nursing contributions to translational research. The group meets monthly via telecom, coordinates workshops, and meets regionally and nationally during scientific venues (http://www.ctsacentral.org/committee/ctsa-nurse-scientist, last accessed April 4, 2013).

The mobile digital technology advances that began over a decade ago have converged on computer power, miniaturization, touch-screen technologies, and high bandwidth for telephones. The new powerful, low-cost platforms are allowing healthcare professionals and consumers to access health information via the smartphones and tablets from almost anywhere. The integration of these devices with entertainment, reminders, monitors, and even avatars, is presenting new opportunities for the development of health applications for almost every major condition. Already these smart phones and tablet computers are changing the ways that nurses can monitor patients with such chronic conditions as congestive heart failure, diabetes, obesity, pain management, and many other chronic symptoms and conditions. The integration of these devices with geographical locators allows consumers to find the nearest healthcare facility, hospital, and 24 h pediatric clinics in addition to finding entertainment places. The application of such technologies to biosurveillance and bioterrorism, and inventory management in healthcare is also expanding.

The need for specialized genetic education for healthcare professionals, engineers, and consumers is being driven by the revolution in science occurring at the bench and the need to quickly transfer this information to those in the field, as well as to consumers who can benefit from the advanced genomic science. Two new National Institutes of Health initiatives have been announced to move the educational endeavors forward. The one educational program is based at the University of Virginia and is funded by the National Human Genome Research Institute (NHGRI, 2009). The other program, the Secretary's Advisory Committee on Genetics, Health and Society has issued a new report to describe the proposals for enhancing *Genetics Education and Training for Healthcare Professionals, Public Health Providers, and Consumers* (NIH, SACGHS, 2010). This report describes the new training and teaching models required, stressing the need for incorporating pedigree maps for family health histories in vendor services, and proposing innovative incentives for reimbursement of healthcare providers who begin to grasp the utilization of genetic information and family histories for patients. All of these new advances have the potential of widening the digital divide for those who are poor, disenfranchised, or culturally diverse.

60.9 Benefits of Using Information Systems in Patient Care

The transformative changes in present-day healthcare throughout the United States include: (1) a focus on population health with services and technologies to support wellness and disease prevention; (2) self-management for those with chronic disease and transitioning resources and services from acute care to community and home; (3) a person-centric focus in care delivery and services for patient empowerment; (4) healthcare system reform using EHRs and other technologies that extend across all levels of services and care settings, including the person's home; and (5) increased resource demands including capacity as well as challenges in the healthcare workforce's skills and preparedness for this new work environment.

The IOM report *To Err Is Human: Building a Safer Health System* (IOM, 1999) served as a wakeup call to the American public by documenting the grave and prevailing deficiency in quality that characterizes healthcare in the United States. This first in a series of reports from the IOMs quality initiative, spoke about the serious needs for improvement and reform. A second report followed, *Crossing the Quality Chasm: A New Health System for the 21st Century* (IOM, 2001), which offered a blueprint for such improvement and urged all organizations, professional groups, policy makers, educators, and healthcare providers to engage in the organic change required to make healthcare safer, effective, timely, efficient, equitable, and patient-centered. This report also called for the essential redesign of health professional education to prepare the numbers and the kinds of providers required to activate and grow a quality-centered healthcare system. A third IOM report titled *Health Professions Education: A Bridge to Quality* (IOM, 2003) offered a strategy for redesigning the education of healthcare professionals to promote and sustain a reformed and responsive healthcare system. Five essential health professional competencies were identified to support and sustain the healthcare system. Health professionals need to be able to (1) provide patient-centered care, (2) work in interdisciplinary teams, (3) employ evidence-based practice, (4) apply quality improvement, and (5) make use of informatics. Fundamentally all of these IOM reports acknowledge the critical role of information. There is a clear synergy among the seismic changes in national and international healthcare environments, huge shifts in nations' health policies, the essential characteristics of the transformative healthcare system, and the areas of essential competencies of healthcare professionals. Informatics is fundamental to enhancing the performance of the other four IOM health professional competencies. The understanding and application of informatics facilitates and augments patient or client-centered care, interdisciplinary teamwork, quality improvement, and the incorporation of evidence into practice. The extensive application of informatics is a critical component of healthcare practice for all professions, and needed to enhance the safety and effectiveness of care.

The concept of using advanced IT to improve treatments and accelerate advances in disease management, is applying the concept of a "rapid learning health system" (IOM, 2010a). In the 2011 IOM book, *Engineering a Learning Healthcare System: A Look at the Future*, the IOM recommends the integration of (1) personalized treatment in diagnosing, planning, and treating patients; (2) tailored care processes in assessing risk, treatment response, and illness; (3) improved use of evidence from research, guidelines, and practice databases; (4) optimized workflow involving peoples' roles, evidence-based protocols, and technology tools such as decision support; (5) and monitored and corrected care delivery processes to determine patient status, clinical outcomes, and trends. These processes together improve the healthcare system, and healthcare delivery.

60.10 The HIMSS Davies Awards of Excellence

A national program that evaluates the impact of IT on the quality and outcomes of care is the Nicholas E. Davies Awards of Excellence sponsored by HIMSS (HIMSS Davies, 2011b). The Davies Award recognizes excellence in the implementation of EHRs in healthcare organizations and primary care practices. Established in 1995 this program has recognized 80 healthcare organizations in the past 17 years. The award categories are: HIMSS Enterprise Davies Award (formerly Organizational) and HIMSS Ambulatory Davies Award, including independent ambulatory practices, HIMSS Community Health Organization Davies Award and HIMSS Public Health Davies Award. Characteristics of Davies winners have been evaluated over time. Key among them is that there were clear objectives and a formal business case. The EHR implementations are each evaluated with regard to their impact on patient care, the planned expenditures, and the anticipated return on investment.

60.10.1 Current Opportunities and Barriers to Creating an Effective Healthcare Information Infrastructure

Informatics nurses have the greatest impact on patient safety, workflow, and user acceptance according to a recent survey of healthcare professionals. A total of 432 responses were received for the HIMSS 2009 Informatics Nurse Impact Survey, sponsored by McKesson (HIMSS, 2009). Making sure that IT does no harm was the concept with the highest rating relative to the area of impact in which informatics nurses have the most success. Eighty-one percent of respondents whose organization was pursuing medical device integration indicated that informatics nurses were involved with this initiative. Survey results also showed that informatics nurses are also highly involved with other emerging technologies including smart devices and remote monitoring.

60.10.2 Opportunities to Create an Effective Healthcare Information Infrastructure

The 24th Annual HIMSS Leadership Survey reflects the opinions of IT professionals in U.S. healthcare provider organizations regarding the use of IT in their organizations (HIMSS, 2013). This study covers a wide array of topics crucial to healthcare IT leaders including IT priorities, issues driving and challenging technology adoption, IT security, as well as IT staffing and budgeting plans. Based on the feedback of 298 healthcare IT professionals, more than one quarter (28%) of the participants in this year's survey indicated that implementation of the systems needed to achieve Meaningful Use as their key IT priority. For the past several years, respondents have identified the lack of adequate financial support as the top barrier to IT implementation. This year, 22% of respondents cited adequate staffing resources as their top challenge, followed by the lack of adequate financial support (15%) and vendors' inability to effectively deliver products or services to respondents' satisfaction (13%). The healthcare CIO respondents of this survey believe that IT can have a positive impact on patient care, either by improving clinical/quality outcomes, reducing medical errors, or helping to standardize care by allowing for the use of evidence-based medicine. Survey results have also recognized the importance of clinical informaticists by identifying the need to increase IT staff to address clinical issues. Among survey respondents, 76% reported that clinicians play some role in the IT process, noting that clinicians are active participants in many aspects of IT use at their organizations, including selecting IT systems for use in their department and acting as project champions.

60.10.3 AACN and NLN Addressing Competencies in Nursing Informatics

In October, 2006 the American Association of Colleges of Nursing (AACN) released a document titled: The Essentials of Doctoral Education for Advanced Nursing Practice, which includes a chapter (Chapter IV) on the necessity of educating in Information Systems/Technology and Patient Care T Technology (AACN, 2006). From 2006 through 2011 AACN has outlined the necessary curriculum content and expected competencies of graduates from baccalaureate (2008), master's (2011), and Doctor of Nursing Practice (2006) programs, as well as the clinical support needed for the full spectrum of academic nursing by approving a series of Essentials documents. (http://www.aacn.nche.edu/education-resources/essential-series).

In May 2008, the National League NLN released the Position Statement *Preparing the Next Generation of Nurses to Practice in a Technology-rich Environment: An Informatics Agenda*, which recommended that faculty develop competence in informatics (NLN, 2008). Recently, NLN have also released an Informatics Education Toolkit. In an effort to assist faculty with this task, the Task Group on Faculty Development Related to Informatics Competencies was formed by the Educational Technology and Information Management Advisory Council to create a web resource with information and links to materials that would assist faculty to develop informatics competence (http://www.nln.org/facultyprograms/facultytoolkits.htm).

The majority of nursing schools have now established innovative training for nursing informatics that focuses on partnerships between academia, the corporate vendor community, and the health systems. For example, the University of Kansas is preparing nursing students to use HIT systems effectively using the Simulated E-Health Delivery System, or SEEDS project. This project teaches students how to coordinate patient care with a fully live Cerner EHR system. In another environment, Johns Hopkins School of Nursing students use a 37-bed simulation laboratory hooked up to an Allscripts Sunrise Clinical Manager System (formerly Eclipsys).

60.11 Summary

Nursing has benefited from teaming with engineers and biomedical engineers in advancing the use of IT in healthcare. This chapter has focused on the ways that nursing works in interdisciplinary teams and can provide information to integrate evidence-based practice, quality improvement, and make use of a broad range of technologies. The nursing profession continues to be supported by national nursing organizational structures and nursing professional organizations to provide policy and curriculum developments to advance the volume and quality of credentials for nurses in informatics. These nurse colleagues also have expert skills in advanced systems implementation, measurement, and evaluation. As we are all challenged with the goals of the United States to provide better healthcare for all, an EHR, and informatics technologies to improve the quality and safety of diverse population, the partnerships previously fostered can be best nurtured by continuous education about our individual disciplines. However, we have continued evidence from HIMSS Leadership Surveys that a major challenge in implementing the technologies are dependent upon having adequate staffing resources who understand the workflow, regulations, standards and organizational behaviors in Healthcare IT. To prepare healthcare professionals, engineers, and computer scientist in Healthcare IT, McCormick and Gugerty have written a textbook that describes Healthcare IT and prepares the engineers and computer scientists to sit for the ONC HIT Pro™ Certifications and the CompTIA® exam (McCormick and Gugerty, 2012).

References

American Association of Colleges of Nursing. (AACN). 2006. *The Essentials of Doctoral Education for Advanced Nursing Practice.* http://www.aacn.nche.edu/publications/position/DNPEssentials.pdf (last accessed April 4, 2013).

American Nurses Association. 2001. *Code of Ethics for Nurses with Interpretive Statements.* Silver Spring, MD: Nursesbooks.org.

American Nurses Association. 2008. *Nursing Informatics: Scope and Standards of Practice.* Silver Spring, MD: Nursesbooks.org.

American Nurses Association. 2010a. *Nursing's Social Policy Statement: The Essence of the Profession.* Silver Spring, MD: Nursesbooks.org.

American Nurses Association. December 3, 2010b. *Public ranks Nurses as Most Trusted Profession: 11th Year in Number One Slot in Gallup Poll.* http://www.nursingworld.org/FunctionalMenuCategories/AboutANA/NationalNursesWeek/MediaKit/NNWFacts.htm (last accessed April 4, 2013).

Androwich, IM et al. 2002. *Clinical Information Systems: A Framework for Reaching the Vision.* Washington, DC: Nursesbooks.org.

Androwich, IM, Bickford, CJ, Button, PS, Hunter, KM, Murphy, J, and Sensmeier, J. 2003. *Clinical Information Systems: A Framework for Reaching the Vision.* Washington, DC: American Nurses Publishing.

Buetow KH. 2009. The Biomedical Informatics GRID (BIG). A platform for 21st century biomedicine. In *Nationwide Health Information Network Advances: Foundation for Interoperable Health Information Exchange Established—Path to Nationwide Production Set.* http://www.hhs.gov/myhealthcare/news/phc_2008_report.pdf (last accessed June 4, 2010).

FNLM. 2009. Personal Health Record. Presentations from the Conference. http://www.fnlm.org/Events_2010_Conference/Events-2010-Conf.html (last accessed April 4, 2013).

Gallop. 2010. Nurses Top Honesty and Ethics List for 11th Year. (December 3, 2010). http://www.gallup.com/poll/1654/honesty-ethics-professions.aspx (last accessed April 4, 2013).

Health and Human Services Health IT Initiatives. 2010. http://healthit.hhs.gov/portal/server.pt?open=512&obj ID=1487&parentname=CommunityPage&parentid=2&mode=2&in_hi_userid=10741&cached=true (last accessed June 1, 2010).

Hendrich, A, Chow, MA, Skierczynski, BA, and Lu, Z. 2008. A 36-Hospital time and motion study: How do medical–surgical nurses spend their time? *The Permanente Journal* 12(3). http://www.ncbi.nlm. nih.gov/pubmed/21331207 (last accessed April 4, 2013).

HIMSS. 2009. HIMSS Informatics Nurse Impact Survey, sponsored by McKesson. http://www.himss.org/ content/files/HIMSS2009InformaticsNurseImpactSurvey.pdf (last accessed June 2, 2010).

HIMSS. 2011a. HIMSS 2011 Nursing Informatics Workforce Survey. http://www.himss.org/content/files/ 2011HIMSSNursingInformaticsWorkforceSurvey.pdf (last accessed March 1, 2011).

HIMSS. 2011b. Davies Awards of Excellence. http://www.himss.org/ASP/topics_FocusDynamic.asp? faid=172 (last accessed April 13, 2012).

HIMSS. 2012. 23rd Annual 2011 HIMSS Leadership Survey. http://www.himss.org/2012 Survey/ (last accessed April 13, 2012).

HIMSS. 2013. 24th Annual HIMSS Leadership Survey. http://himss.files.cms-plus.com/HIMSSorg/ Content/files/leadership_FINAL_REPORT_022813.pdf (last accessed April 10, 2013).

HRSA. 2008. National Sample Survey of Registered Nurses. http://bhpr.hrsa.gov/healthworkforce/ rnsurveys/rnsurveyfinal.pdf (last accessed April 4, 2013).

IOM. 1999. *To Err Is Human.* Washington, DC: National Academy Press.

IOM. 2001. Committee on quality of healthcare in America, Institute of Medicine. *Crossing the Quality Chasm: A New Health System for the 21st Century.* Washington, DC: National Academy Press.

IOM. 2003. *Health Professions Education: A Bridge to Quality.* Washington, DC: National Academy Press.

IOM. 2010. A summary of the October 2009 forum on *The Future of Nursing: Acute Care.* Washington, DC: The National Academies Press.

IOM. 2011. *Engineering a Learning Healthcare System: A Look at the Future.* Washington, DC: The National Academies Press.

McCormick, KA. 2009. *Individualizing Cancer Care with Interoperable Information Systems.* IMIA-NI, Helsinki, Finland, June, 2009.

McCormick, KA. 2011. Future directions. In Saba, VK and McCormick, KA. *Essentials of Nursing Informatics,* 5th ed. New York: McGraw-Hill Medical.

McCormick, KA and Gugerty, B. Healthcare Information Technology Exam Guide for CompTIA® Healthcare IT Technician & HIT Pro™ Certifications. New York: McGraw-Hill, 2012.

National Center for Research Resources. 2010. Translational Science and CTSA. htttp://www.ncrr.nih.gov and http://www.ctsaweb.org (last accessed June 6, 2010).

National Human Genome Research Institute. 2009. *The Genetics/Genomics Competency Center (G2C2) at the University of Virginia.* http://www.genome.gov (last accessed April 4, 2013).

National Institutes of Health. 2010. The Secretary's Advisory Committee on Genetics, Health and Society (SACGHS). *Genetics Education and Training for Healthcare Professionals, Public Health Providers, and Consumers.* http://oba.od.nih.gov/oba/SACGHS/reports/SACGHS_oversight_report.pdf (last accessed April 4, 2013).

National League for Nursing (NLN). 2008. *Next Generation of Nurses to Practice in a Technology-rich Environment: An Informatics Agenda.* http://www.nln.org/facultyprograms/facultyresources/infor-matics.htm (last accessed April 4, 2013).

NCATS. 2012. http://www.ncats.nih.gov (last accessed April 4, 2013).

PricewaterhouseCoopers, LLC. 2009. *The New Science of Personalized Medicine: Targeting the Promise Into Practice.* http://www.pwc.com/us/en/healthcare/publications/personalized-medicine.jhtml (last accessed April 4, 2013).

Science Award Thematic Special Interest Group of Nurse Scientists. http://www.ctsacentral.org/committee/ ctsa-nurse-scientist (last accessed April 4, 2013).

TIGER Initiative. 2007. *The Tiger Initiative: Evidence and Informatics Transforming Nursing: 3-Year Action Steps toward a 10-Year Vision.* http://www.tigersummit.com/Downloads.html (last accessed April 4, 2013).

TIGER Initiative. 2008. *The Tiger Initiative: Collaborating to Integrate Evidence and Informatics into Nursing Practice and Education.* http://www.tigersummit.com/Downloads.html (last accessed April 4, 2013).

White House. 2008. *Priorities for Personalized Medicine.* http://www.whitehouse.gov/files/documents/ostp/PCAST/pcast_report_v2.pdf (last accessed April 4, 2013).

WHO. May 2011. ICN and WHO-FIC. http://www.who.int/classifications/icd/adaptations/icnp/en/ (last accessed April 4, 2013).

61

Non-AI Decision Making

Ron Summers
Loughborough University

Derek G. Cramp
City University

Ewart R. Carson
City University

61.1 Introduction

Non-AI decision making can be defined as those methods and tools used to increase information content in the context of some specific clinical situation without having cause to refer to knowledge embodied in a computer program. Theoretical advances in the 1950s added rigor to this domain when Meehl argued that many clinical decisions could be made by statistical rather than intuitive means [1]. Evidence of this view was supported by Savage [2], whose theory of choice under uncertainty is still the classical and most elegant formulation of subjective Bayesian decision theory, and was very much responsible for reintroducing Bayesian decision analysis to clinical medicine. Ledley and Ludsted [3] provided further evidence that medical reasoning could be made explicit and represented in decision theoretic ways. Decision theory also provided the means for Nash to develop a "Logoscope," which might be considered as the first mechanical diagnostic aid [4].

An information system developed using non-AI decision-making techniques may comprise procedural or declarative knowledge. Procedural knowledge maps the decision-making process into the methods by which the clinical problems are solved or clinical decisions made. Examples of techniques that form a procedural knowledge base are those that are based on algorithmic analytical models, clinical algorithms, or decision trees. Information systems based on declarative knowledge comprise what can essentially be termed a database of facts about different aspects of a clinical problem; the causal relationships between these facts form a rich network from which explicit (say) cause–effect pathways can be determined. Semantic networks and causal probabilistic networks are perhaps the best examples of information systems based on declarative knowledge. There are other types of clinical decision aids, based purely on statistical methods applied to patient data, for example, classification analyses based on logistic regression, relative frequencies of occurrence, pattern-matching algorithms, or neural networks.

The structure of this chapter mirrors to some extent the different methods and techniques of non-AI decision making mentioned earlier. It is important to distinguish between analytical models based on quantitative or qualitative mathematical representations and decision theoretic methods typified by the use of clinical algorithms, decision trees, and set theory. Most of the latter techniques add to an information base by way of procedural knowledge. It is then that advantage can be taken of the many techniques that have statistical decision theoretic principles as their underpinning.

This section begins with a discussion of simple linear regression models and pattern recognition, but then more complex statistical techniques are introduced, for example, the use of Bayesian decision analysis, which leads to the introduction of causal probabilistic networks. The majority of these techniques add information by use of declarative knowledge. Particular applications are used throughout to illustrate the extent to which non-AI decision making is used in clinical practice.

61.2 Analytical Models

In the context of this chapter, the analytical models considered are qualitative and quantitative mathematical models that are used to predict future patient state based on present state and a historical representation of what has passed. Such models could be representations of system behavior that allow test signals to be used so that the response of the system to various disturbances can be studied, thus making predictions of future patient state.

For example, Leaning et al. [5,6] produced a 19-segment quantitative mathematical model of the blood circulation to study the short-term effects of drugs on the cardiovascular system of normal, resting patients. The model represented entities such as compliance, flow, and volume of model segments in what was considered a closed system. In total, the quantitative mathematical model comprised 61 differential equations and 159 algebraic equations. Evaluation of the model revealed that it was fit for its purpose in the sense of heuristic validity, that is, it could be used as a tool for developing explanations for cardiovascular control, particularly in relation to the central nervous system (CNS).

Qualitative models investigate time-dependent behavior by representing patient state trajectory in the form of a set of connected nodes, the links between the nodes reflecting transitional constraints placed on the system [7]. The types of decision making supported by this type of model are assessment and therapy planning. In diagnostic assessment, the precursor nodes and the pathway to the node (decision) of interest define the causal mechanisms of the disease process. Similarly, for therapy planning, the optimal plan can be set by investigation of the utility values associated with each link in the disease–therapy relationship. These utility values refer to a cost function, where cost can be defined as the monetary cost of providing the treatment and cost benefit to the patient in terms of efficiency, efficacy, and effectiveness of alternative treatment options. Both quantitative [8] and qualitative [9] analytical models can be realized in other ways to form the basis of rule-based systems; however, that excludes their analysis in this chapter.

61.3 Decision Theoretic Models

61.3.1 Clinical Algorithms

The clinical algorithm is a procedural device that mimics clinical decision making by structuring the diagnostic or therapeutic decision processes in the form of a classification tree. The root of the tree represents some initial state, and the branches yield the different options available. For the operation of the clinical algorithm, the choice points are assumed to follow branching logic with the decision function being a yes/no (or similar) binary choice. Thus, the clinical algorithm comprises a set of questions that must be collectively exhaustive for the chosen domain and the responses available to the clinician at each branch point must be mutually exclusive. These decision criteria pose rigid constraints on the type of medical problem that can be represented by this method, as the lack of flexibility is appropriate only for a certain set of well-defined clinical domains. Nevertheless, there is rich literature available;

examples include the use of the clinical algorithm for acid–base disorders [10] and diagnosis of mental disorders [11]. A comprehensive guide to clinical algorithms can be found on the website of the American Academy of Family Physicians [12].

61.3.2 Decision Trees

A more rigorous use of classification tree representations than the clinical algorithm can be found in decision tree analysis. Although from a structural perspective, decision trees and clinical algorithms are similar in appearance, for decision tree analysis, the likelihood and cost benefit for each choice are also calculated to provide a quantitative measure for each option available. This allows the use of optimization procedures to gauge the probability of success for the correct diagnosis being made or for a beneficial outcome from therapeutic action being taken. A further difference between the clinical algorithm and decision tree analysis is that the latter has more than one type of decision node (branch point): at decision nodes, the clinician must decide which choice (branch) is appropriate for the given clinical scenario; at chance nodes, the responses available have no clinician control, for example, the response may be due to patient-specific data; and outcome nodes define the chance nodes at the "leaves" of the decision tree. That is, they summarize a set of all possible clinical outcomes for the chosen domain.

The possible outcomes from each chance node must obey the rules of probability and sum to unity; the probability assigned to each branch reflects the frequency of that event occurring in a general patient population. It follows that these probabilities are dynamic, with increasing accuracy, as more evidence becomes available. A utility value can be added to each of the outcome scenarios. These utility measures reflect a trade-off between competing concerns, for example, survivability and quality of life, and may be assigned heuristically.

When the first edition of this chapter was written in 1995, it was noted that although a rich literature describing potential applications existed [13], the number of practical applications described was limited. The situation has changed and there has been an explosion of interest in applying decision analysis to clinical problems. Not only is decision analysis methodology well described [14–17] but there are also numerous articles appearing in mainstream medical journals, particularly *Medical Decision Making*. An important driver for this acceleration of interest has been the desire to contain costs of medical care, while maintaining clinical effectiveness and quality of care. Cost-effectiveness analysis is an extension of decision analysis and compares the outcome of decision options in terms of the monetary cost per unit of effectiveness. Thus, it can be used to set priorities for the allocation of resources and to decide between one or more treatment or intervention options. It is most useful when comparing treatments for the same clinical condition. Cost-effectiveness analysis and its implications are described very well elsewhere [18,19]. One reason for the lack of clinical applications using decision trees is that the underpinning software technologies remain relatively underdeveloped. Babič et al. [20] address this point by comparing decision tree software with other non-AI decision-making methods.

61.3.3 Influence Diagrams

In the 1960s, researchers at Stanford Research Institute (SRI) proposed the use of influence diagrams as representational models when developing computer programs to solve decision problems. However, it was recognized somewhat later by decision analysts at SRI [21] that such diagrams could be used to facilitate communication with domain experts when eliciting information about complex decision problems. Influence diagrams are a powerful mode of graphic representation for decision modeling. They do not replace but complement decision trees and it should be noted that both are different graphical representations of the same mathematical model and operations. Recently, two exciting papers have been published that make the use of influence diagrams accessible to those interested in medical decision making [22,23].

61.4 Statistical Models

61.4.1 Database Search

Interrogation of large clinical databases yields statistical evidence of diagnostic value and in some representations form the basis of rule induction used to build expert systems [24]. These systems will not be discussed here. However, the most direct approach for clinical decision making is to determine the relative frequency of occurrence of an entity, or more likely group of entities, in the database of past cases. This enables a prior probability measure to be estimated [25]. A drawback of this simple, direct approach to problem solving is the apparent tautology of more evidence available leading to fewer matches in the database being found; this runs against common wisdom that more evidence leads to an increase in the probability of a diagnosis being made. Further, the method does not provide a weight for each item of evidence to gauge those that are more significant for patient outcome.

With the completion of the human genome sequence, there has been renewed interest in database search methods for finding data (e.g., single nucleotide polymorphisms—or more simply SNPs) in the many genetic database resources that are distributed throughout the world [26]. Vyas and Summers [27] provide both a summary of the issues surrounding the use of metadata to combine these dispersed data resources and suggest a solution via a semantic web-based knowledge architecture. It is clear that such methods of generating data will have an increasing impact on the advent of molecular medicine.

61.4.2 Regression Analysis

Logistic regression analysis is used to model the relationship between a response variable of interest and a set of explanatory variables. This is achieved by adjusting the regression coefficients, the parameters of the model, until a "best fit" to the data set is achieved. This type of model improves upon the use of relative frequencies, as logistic regression explicitly represents the extent to which elements of evidence are important in the value of the regression coefficients. An example of clinical use can be found in the domain of gastroenterology [28].

61.4.3 Statistical Pattern Analysis

The recognition of patterns in data can be formulated as a statistical problem of classifying the results of clinical findings into mutually exclusive but collectively exhaustive decision regions. In this way, not only can physiologic data be classified but also the pathology that they give rise to and the therapy options available to treat the disease. Titterington [29] describes an application in which patterns in a complex data set are recognized to enhance the care of patients with head injuries. Pattern recognition is also the cornerstone of computerized methods for cardiac rhythm analysis [30]. The methods used to distinguish patterns in data rely on discriminant analysis. In simple terms, this refers to a measure of separability between class populations.

In general, pattern recognition is a two-stage process as shown in Figure 61.1. The pattern vector, P, is an n-dimensional vector derived from the data set used. Let Ω_p be the pattern space, which is the set of all possible values P may assume; then the pattern recognition problem is formulated as finding a way of dividing Ω_p into mutually exclusive and collectively exhaustive regions. For example, in the analysis of the electrocardiogram, the complete waveform may be used to perform classifications of diagnostic value. A complex decision function would probably be required in such cases. Alternatively (and if appropriate), the pattern vector can be simplified to the investigation of subfeatures within a pattern.

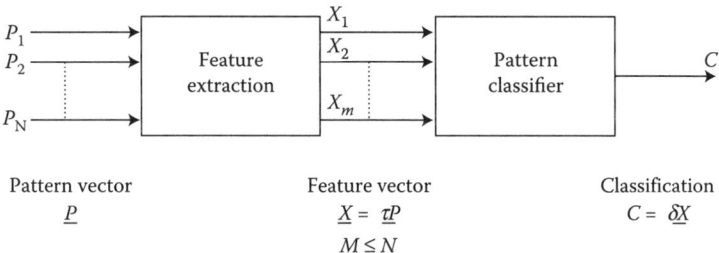

Pattern vector
$\underline{P}$

Feature vector
$\underline{X} = \underline{\tau}\underline{P}$
$M \leq N$

Classification
$C = \underline{\delta}\underline{X}$

FIGURE 61.1 Pattern recognition.

For cardiac arrhythmia analysis, only the *R–R* interval of the electrocardiogram is required, which allows a much simpler decision function to be used. This may be a linear or nonlinear transformation process:

$$X = \tau P$$

where *X* is termed the feature vector and *τ* is the transformation process.

Just as the pattern vector *P* belongs to a pattern space Ω_p, so does the feature vector *X* belong to a feature space Ω_X. As the function of feature extraction is to reduce the dimensionality of the input vector to the classifier, some information is lost. Classification of Ω_X can be achieved using numerous statistical methods, including discriminant functions (linear and polynomial), kernel estimation, *k*-nearest neighbor, cluster analysis, and Bayesian analysis.

61.4.4 Bayesian Analysis

Ever since their reinvestigation by Savage in 1954 [2], Bayesian methods of classification have provided one of the most popular approaches used to assist in clinical decision making. Bayesian classification is an example of a parametric method of estimating class-conditional probability density functions. Clinical knowledge is represented as a set of prior probabilities of diseases to be matched with conditional probabilities of clinical findings in a patient population with each disease. The classification problem becomes one of a choice of decision levels, which minimizes the average rate of misclassification or to minimize the maximum of the conditional average loss function (the so-called minmax criterion) when information about prior probabilities is not available. Formally, the optimal decision rule that minimizes the average rate of misclassification is called the Bayes rule; this serves as the inference mechanism that allows the probabilities of competing diagnoses to be calculated when patient-specific clinical findings become available.

The great advantage of Bayesian classification is that a large clinical database of past cases is not required, thus allowing the time taken to reach a decision to be faster compared with other database search techniques; furthermore, classification errors due to the use of inappropriate clinical inferences are quantifiable. However, a drawback of this approach to clinical decision making is that the disease states are considered as complete and mutually exclusive, whereas in real life, neither assumption may be true.

Nevertheless, Bayesian decision analysis functions as a basis for differential diagnosis and has been used successfully, for example, in the diagnosis of acute abdominal pain [31]. De Dombal first described this system in 1972, but it took another 20 years or so for it to be accepted via a multicenter multinational trial. The approach has been exploited in ILIAD; this is a commercially available [32] computerized diagnostic decision support system with some 850–990 frames in its knowledge base. As it is a Bayesian system, each frame has the prevalence of a disease for its prior probability. There is the possibility however, that the prevalence rates may not have general applicability. This highlights a very real problem, namely, the validity of relating causal pathways in clinical thinking and connecting such pathways to a body of validated (true) evidence. Ideally, such evidence will come from randomized controlled clinical or epidemiological trials. However, such studies may be subject to bias.

To overcome this, Eddy et al. [33] devised the confidence profile method. This is a set of quantitative techniques for interpreting and displaying the results of individual studies (trials), exploring the effects of any biases that might affect the internal validity of the study, adjusting for external validity, and, finally, combining evidence from several sources. This meta-analytical approach can formally incorporate experimental evidence and, in a Bayesian fashion, also the results of previous analytical studies or subjective judgments about specific factors that might arise when interpreting evidence. Influence diagram representations play an important role in linking results in published studies and estimates of probabilities and statements about causality.

Currently, much interest is being generated as to how, what is perceived as the Bayesian action-oriented approach can be used in determining health policy, where the problem is perceived to be a decision problem rather than a statistical problem; see, for instance, Reference 34.

Bayesian analysis continues to be used in a wide range of clinical applications either as a single method or as part of a multimethod approach, for example, for insulin sensitivity [35], for understanding incomplete data sets [36], and has been used extensively for the analysis of clinical trials (e.g., see References 37, 38).

Bayesian decision theory also provides a valuable framework for healthcare technology assessment. Bayesian methods have also become increasingly visible in places where they are being applied to the analysis of economic models [39], being applied particularly to two decision problems commonly encountered in pharmaco-economics and health technology assessment generally, namely, adoption and allocation.

Acceptability curves generated from Bayesian cost-effectiveness analyses can be interpreted as the probability that the new intervention is cost effective at a given level of willingness-to-pay. For Bayesian methods applied to clinical trials with cost as well as efficacy data, see O'Hagan and Stevens [40]. This probabilistic interpretation of study findings provides information that is more relevant and more transparent to decision makers. The Bayesian value of information analysis offers a decision-analytic framework to explore the conceptually separate decisions of whether a new technology should be adopted from the question of whether more research is required to inform this choice in the future [41,42]. Thus, it is a useful analytical framework for decision makers who wish to achieve allocative efficacy.

The Bayesian approach has several advantages over the frequentist approach. First, it allows accumulation and updating of knowledge by using the prior distribution. Second, it yields more flexible inferences and emphasizes predictions rather than hypothesis testing. Third, probabilities involving multiple end-points are relatively simple to estimate. Finally, it provides a solid theoretical framework for decision analyses.

61.4.5 Dempster–Shafer Theory

One way to overcome the problem of mutually exclusive disease states is to use an extension to Bayesian classification put forward by Dempster [43] and Shafer [44]. Here, instead of focusing on a single disorder, the method can deal with combinations of several diseases. The key concept used is that the set of all possible diseases is partitioned into n-tuples of possible disease state combinations.

A simple example will illustrate this concept. Suppose there is a clinical scenario in which four disease states describe the whole hypothesis space. Each new item of evidence will impact on all the possible subsets of the hypothesis space and is represented by a function, the basic probability assignment. This measure is a belief function that must obey the law of probability and sum to unity across the subsets impacted upon. In the example, all possible subsets comprise: one that has all four disease states in it; four, which have three of the four diseases as members; six, which have two diseases as members; and finally, four subsets that have a single disease as a member. Thus, when new evidence becomes available in the form of a clinical finding, only certain hypotheses, represented by individual subsets, may be favored.

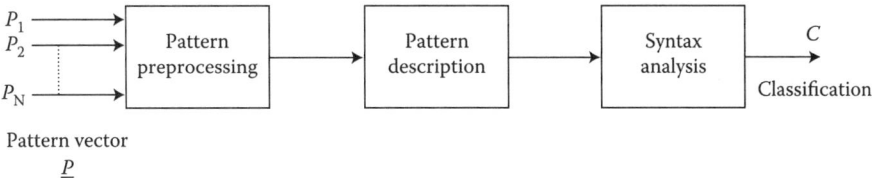

FIGURE 61.2 Syntactic pattern recognition system.

61.4.6 Syntactic Pattern Analysis

As demonstrated earlier, a large class of clinical problem solving using statistical methods involves classification or diagnosis of disease states, selection of optimal therapy regimes, and prediction of patient outcome. However, in some cases, the purpose of modeling is to reconstruct the input signal from the data available. This cannot be done by methods discussed thus far. The syntactic approach to pattern recognition uses a hierarchical decomposition of information and draws upon an analogy to the syntax of language. Each input pattern is described in terms of more simple subpatterns, which themselves are decomposed into simpler subunits, until the most elementary subpatterns, termed the pattern primitives, are reached. The pattern primitives should be selected so that they are easy to recognize with respect to the input signal. Rules that govern the transformation of pattern primitives back (ultimately) to the input signal are termed the grammar.

In this way a string grammar, G, which is easily representable in computer-based applications, can be defined:

$$G = \{V_T, V_N, S, P\}$$

where V_T are the terminal variables (pattern primitives), V_N are the nonterminal variables, S is the start symbol, and P is the set of production rules that specify the transformation between each level of the hierarchy. It is an important assumption that in set theoretic terms, the union of V_T and V_N is the total vocabulary of G, and the intersection of V_T and V_N is the null (empty) set.

A syntactic pattern recognition system therefore comprises three functional subunits (Figure 61.2): a preprocessor—this manipulates the input signal, P, into a form that can be presented to the pattern descriptor, the pattern descriptor that assigns a vocabulary to the signal, and the syntax analyzer that classifies the signal accordingly. This type of system has been used successfully to represent the electrocardiogram [45,46] and the electroencephalogram [47], and for representation of the carotid pulse wave [48].

61.4.7 Causal Modeling

A causal probabilistic network (CPN) is an acyclic multiply-connected graph, which at a qualitative level comprises nodes and arcs [49]. Nodes are the domain objects and may represent, for example, clinical findings, pathophysiologic states, diseases, or therapies. Arcs are the causal relationships between successive nodes and are directed links. In this way, the node and arc structure represents a model of the domain. Quantification is expressed in the model by a conditional probability table being associated with each arc, allowing the state of each node to be represented as a binary value or more frequently as a continuous probability distribution.

In root nodes, the conditional probability table reduces to a probability distribution of all its possible states.

A key concept of CPNs is that computation is reduced to a series of local calculations, using only one node and those that are linked to it in the network. Any node can be instantiated with an observed value; this evidence is then propagated through the CPN via a series of local computations. Thus, CPNs can be used in two ways: to instantiate the leaf nodes of the network with known patterns for given disorders to investigate expected causal pathways; or to instantiate the root nodes or nodes in the graphical hierarchy with, for example, test results to obtain a differential diagnosis. The former method has been used to investigate respiratory pathology [50], and the latter method has been read to obtain pathologic information from electromyography [51].

61.4.8 Artificial Neural Networks

Artificial neural networks (ANNs) mimic their biologic counterparts, although at the present time on a much smaller scale. The fundamental unit in the biological system is the neuron. This is a specialized cell that, when activated, transmits a signal to its connected neighbors. Both activation and transmission involve chemical transmitters, which cross the synaptic gap between neurons. Activation of the neuron takes place only when a certain threshold is reached. This biologic system is modeled in the representation of an ANN. It is possible to identify three basic elements of the neuron model: a set of weighted connecting links that form the input to the neuron (analogous to neurotransmission across the synaptic gap), an adder for summing the input signals, and an activation function that limits the amplitude of the output of the neuron to the range (typically) –1 to +1. This activation function also has a threshold term that can be applied externally and forms one of the parameters of the neuron model. Many books are available that provide a comprehensive introduction to this class of model (e.g., see Reference 52).

ANNs can be applied to two categories of problems: prediction and classification. It is the latter that has caught the imagination of biomedical engineers for its similarity to diagnostic problem solving. For instance, the conventional management of patients with septicemia requires a diagnostic strategy that takes up to 18–24 h before initial identification of the causal microorganism. This can be compared to a method in which an ANN is applied to a large clinical database of past cases; the quest becomes one of seeking an optimal match between present clinical findings and patterns present in the recorded data. In this application, pattern matching is a nontrivial problem as each of the 5000 past cases has 51 data fields. It has been shown that for this problem the ANN method outperforms other statistical methods such as k-nearest neighbor [53].

The use of ANNs in clinical decision making is becoming widespread. A further example of their use in critical care medicine is given by Yamamura et al. [54]. ANNs are used in chronic and acute clinical episodes. An example of the former is their use in cancer survival predictions [55] and an example of the latter is their use in the emergency room to detect early onset of myocardial infarction [56].

61.5 Summary

This chapter has reviewed what are normally considered to be the major categories of approach available to support clinical decision making, which do not rely on what is classically termed artificial intelligence (AI). They have been considered under the headings of analytical, decision theoretic, and statistical models, together with their corresponding subdivisions. It should be noted, however, that the division into non-AI approaches and AI approaches that is adopted in this volume (see the chapter titled "Expert Systems: Methods and Tools") is not totally clear-cut. In essence, the range of approaches can in many ways be regarded as a continuum. There is no unanimity as to where the division should be placed and the separation adopted; here is but one of a number that is feasible. It is therefore desirable that the reader should consider these two chapters together and choose an approach that is relevant to the particular clinical context.

References

1. Meehl R. 1954. *Clinical versus Statistical Prediction*. Minnesota: University of Minnesota Press.
2. Savage L.I. 1954. *The Foundations of Statistics*. New York: John Wiley & Sons.

3. Ledley R.S. and Ludsted L.B. 1959. Reasoning foundations of medical diagnosis. *Science* 130: 9.

4. Nash F.A. 1954. Differential diagnosis: An apparatus to assist the logical faculties. *Lancet* 4: 874.

5. Leaning M.S., Pullen H.E., Carson E.R. et al. 1983. Modelling a complex biological system: The human cardiovascular system: 1. Methodology and model description. *Trans. Inst. Meas. Contr.* 5: 71.

6. Leaning M.S., Pullen H.E., Carson E.R. et al. 1983. Modelling a complex biological system: The human cardiovascular system: 2. Model validation, reduction and development. *Trans. Inst. Meas. Contr.* 5: 87.

7. Kuipers B.J. 1986. Qualitative simulation. *Artif. Intel.* 29: 289.

8. Furukawa T., Tanaka H., and Hara S. 1987. FLUIDEX: A microcomputer-based expert system for fluid therapy consultations. In M.K. Chytil and R. Engelbrecht (Eds.), *Medical Expert Systems.* Wilmslow: Sigma Press, pp. 59–74.

9. Bratko I., Mozetic J., and Lavrac N. 1988. In Michie D. and Bratko I. (Eds.), *Expert Systems: Automatic Knowledge Acquisition.* Reading, MA: Addison-Wesley, pp. 61–83.

10. Bleich H.L. 1972. Computer-based consultations: Electrolyte and acid–base disorders. *Am. J. Med.* 53: 285.

11. McKenzie D.P., McGary P.D., Wallac et al. 1993. Constructing a minimal diagnostic decision tree. *Meth. Inform. Med.* 32: 161.

12. http://www.aafp.org/x19449.xml (accessed February 2005).

13. Pauker S.G. and Kassirer J.P. 1987. Decision analysis. *N. Engl. J. Med.* 316: 250.

14. Weinstein M.C. and Fineberg H.V. 1980. *Clinical Decision Analysis.* London: W.B. Saunders.

15. Watson S.R. and Buede D.M. 1994. *Decision Synthesis.* Cambridge: Cambridge University Press.

16. Sox H.C., Blatt M.A., Higgins M.C., and Marton K.I. 1988. *Medical Decision Making.* Boston: Butterworth Heinemann.

17. Llewelyn H. and Hopkins A. 1993. *Analysing How We Reach Clinical Decisions.* London: Royal College of Physicians.

18. Gold M.R., Siegel J.E., Russell L.B., and Weinstein M.C. (Eds.) 1996. *Cost-Effectiveness in Health and Medicine.* New York: Oxford University Press.

19. Sloan F.A. (Ed.) 1996. *Valuing Health Care.* Cambridge: Cambridge University Press.

20. Babič S.H., Kokol P., Podgorelec V., Zorman M., Šprogar M., and Štiglic M.M. 2000. The art of building decision trees. *J. Med. Syst.* 24: 43–52.

21. Owen D.L. 1984. The use of influence diagrams in structuring complex decision problems. In Howard R.A. and Matheson J.E. (Eds.), *Readings on the Principles and Applications of Decision Analysis*, Vol. 2. Menlo Park, CA: Strategic Decisions Group, pp. 763–772.

22. Owens D.K., Shachter R.D., and Nease R.F. 1997. Representation and analysis of medical decision problems with influence diagrams. *Med. Decis. Mak.* 17: 241.

23. Nease R.F. and Owens D.K. 1997. Use of influence diagrams to structure medical decisions. *Med. Decis. Mak.* 17: 263.

24. Quinlan J.R. 1979. Rules by induction from large collections of examples. In D. Michie (Ed.), *Expert Systems in the Microelectronic Age.* Edinburgh: Edinburgh University Press.

25. Gammerman A. and Thatcher A.R. 1990. Bayesian inference in an expert system without assuming independence. In M.C. Golumbic (Ed.), *Advances in Artificial Intelligence.* New York: Springer-Verlag, pp. 182–218.

26. Goble C.A., Stevens R., and Ng S. 2001. Transparent access to multiple bioinformatics information sources. *IBM Syst. J.* 40: 532–551.

27. Vyas H. and Summers R. 2004. Impact of semantic web on bioinformatics. *Proceedings of the International Symposium of Santa Caterina on Challenges in the Internet and Interdisciplinary Research (SSCCII)*, CD-ROM Proceedings.

28. Spiegelhalter D.J. and Knill-Jones R.P. 1984. Statistical and knowledge-based approaches to clinical decision-support systems with an application in gastroenterology. *J. Roy. Stat. Soc. A* 147: 35.

29. Titterington D.M., Murray G.D., Murray L.S. et al. 1981. Comparison of discriminant techniques applied to a complex set of head injured patients. *J. Roy. Stat. Soc. A* 144: 145.

30. Morganroth J. 1984. Computer recognition of cardiac arrhythmias and statistical approaches to arrhythmia analysis. *Ann. NY Acad. Sci.* 432: 117.

31. De Dombal F.T., Leaper D.J., Staniland J.R. et al. 1972. Computer-aided diagnosis of acute abdominal pain. *Br. Med. J.* 2: 9.

32. Applied Medical Informatics. Salt Lake City, UT.

33. Eddy D.M., Hasselblad V., and Shachter R. 1992. *Meta-Analysis by the Confidence Profile Methods*. London: Academic Press.

34. Lilford R.J. and Braunholz D. 1996. The statistical basis of public policy: A paradigm shift is overdue. *Br. Med. J.* 313: 603.

35. Agbaje O.F., Luzio S.D., Albarrak A.I.S., Lunn D.J., Owens D.R., and Hovorka R. 2003. Bayesian hierarchical approach to estimate insulin sensitivity by minimal model. *Clin. Sci.* 105: 551–560.

36. Crawford S.L., Tennstedt S.L., and McKinlay J.B. 1995. Longitudinal care patterns for disabled elders: A Bayesian analysis of missing data. In Gatsonis C., Hodges J., and Kass R.E. (Eds.), *Case Studies in Bayesian Statistics*, Vol. 2. New York: Springer-Verlag, pp. 293–308.

37. Lewis R.J. and Wears R.L. 1993. An introduction to the Bayesian analysis of clinical trials. *Ann. Emerg. Med.* 22: 1328–1336.

38. Spiegelhalter D.J., Freedman L.S., and Parmar M.K.B. 1994. Bayesian approaches to randomised trials. *J. Roy. Stat. Soc. A* 157: 357–416.

39. Parmigiani G. 2002. *Modeling in Medical Decision Making: A Bayesian Approach*. Chichester: Wiley.

40. O'Hagan A. and Stevens J.W. 2003. Bayesian methods for design and analysis of cost-effectiveness trials in the evaluation of health care technologies. *Stat. Meth. Med. Res.* 11: 469–490.

41. Claxton K. and Posnett J. 1996. An economic approach to clinical trial design and research priority setting. *Health Econ.* 5: 513–524.

42. Claxton K. 1999. The irrelevance of inference: A decision making approach to the stochastic evaluation of health care technologies. *J. Health Econ.* 18: 341–364.

43. Dempster A. 1967. Upper and lower probabilities induced by multi-valued mapping. *Ann. Math. Stat.* 38: 325.

44. Shafer G. 1976. *A Mathematical Theory of Evidence*. Princeton, NJ: Princeton University Press.

45. Belforte G., De Mori R., and Ferraris E. 1979. A contribution to the automatic processing of electrocardiograms using syntactic methods. *IEEE Trans. Biomed. Eng. BME* 26: 125.

46. Birman K.P. 1982. Rule-based learning for more accurate ECG analysis. *IEEE Trans. Pat. Anal. Mach. Intell.* PAMI 4: 369.

47. Ferber G. 1985. Syntactic pattern recognition of intermittant EEG activity. *Meth. Inf. Med.* 24: 79.

48. Stockman G.C. and Kanal L.N. 1983. Problem reduction in representation for the linguistic analysis of waveforms. *IEEE Trans. Pat. Anal. Mach. Intel.* PAMI 5: 287.

49. Andersen S.K., Jensen F.V., and Olesen K.G. 1987. *The HUGIN Core-Preliminary Considerations on Inductive Reasoning: Managing Empirical Information in AI Systems*. Riso, Denmark.

50. Summers R., Andreassen S., Carson E.R. et al. 1993. A causal probabilistic model of the respiratory system. *Proceedings of the IEEE 15th Annual Conference of the Engineering in Medicine and Biology Society*. New York: IEEE, pp. 534–535.

51. Jensen F.V., Andersen S.K., Kjaerulff U. et al. 1987. MUNIN: On the case for probabilities in medical expert systems—A practical exercise. In Fox J., Fieschi M., and Engelbrecht R. (Eds.), *Proceedings of the Ist Conference European Society for AI in Medicine*. Heidelberg: Springer-Verlag, pp. 149–160.

52. Haykin S. 1994. *Neural Networks: A Comprehensive Foundation*. New York: Macmillan.

53. Worthy P.J., Dybowski R., Gransden W.R. et al. 1993. Comparison of learning vector quantisation and nearest neighbour for prediction of microorganisms associated with septicaemia. *Proceedings of the IEEE 15th Annual Conference of the Engineering in Medicine and Biology Society*, New York: IEEE, pp. 273–274.

54. Yamamura S., Takehira R., Kawada K., Nishizawa K., Katayama S., Hirano M., and Momose Y. 2003. Application of artificial neural network modelling to identify severely ill patients whose aminoglycoside concentrations are likely to fall below therapeutic concentrations. *J. Clin. Pharm. Ther.* 28: 425–432.

55. Burke H.B., Goodman P.H., and Rosen D.B. 1997. Artificial neural networks improve the accuracy of cancer survival prediction. *Cancer* 79: 857–862.

56. Baxt W.G., Shofer F.S., Sites F.D., and Hollander J.E. 2002. A neural computational aid to the diagnosis of acute myocardial infarction. *Ann. Emerg. Med.* 39: 366–373.

62

Genome Informatics

Konstantinos
P. Exarchos
University of Ioannina

Themis P. Exarchos
University of Ioannina

Dimitrios I. Fotiadis
University of Ioannina

62.1 Introduction

The aim of this chapter is to provide an overview as well as, in some cases, in-depth information regarding the broad and emerging field of genome informatics. Genome informatics is centered around the development and employment of data analysis algorithms and techniques toward the disentanglement of the inherent genome complexity. We start off with some introductory material about evolution and phylogeny, which must always be kept in mind in biology-related studies. Afterwards, we go on to study genes and their products (i.e., proteins); however, we move one step beyond the gene or protein identification and cataloguing, and specifically focus on the interactions among genes/proteins that govern the cellular functioning. This massive interplay among genes and proteins has subsequently spawned a great deal of interest in reference to diseases and their molecular basis. Therefore, the last part of this chapter is centered around applications of protein interactions in the unraveling of human diseases as well as potential ways to interfere in the pathway of development and progression of diseases, from a genome informatics-oriented point of view.

62.2 Phylogenetics and Evolution

62.2.1 Introduction

Phylogeny and evolution constitute a crucial part of any genome-related analysis. All conclusions derived in the broad field of biology must be coupled with evolutionary background information to gain validity (Dobzhansky and Dobzhansky, 1982; Lewontin, 1997). Evolution refers to the gradual divergence of inherited traits within a population of organisms that lead to the differentiation among species. The process of divergence during a generation is normally quite small; however, the accumulation of changes over time can lead to substantial differentiations in a population. Evolution is based on the passing of the genes from one generation to the next, as well as the interplay among them. Phylogeny on the other hand is the field of biology that studies the evolutionary divergence and relatedness among several groups of organisms, both living (extant) and deceased (extinct).

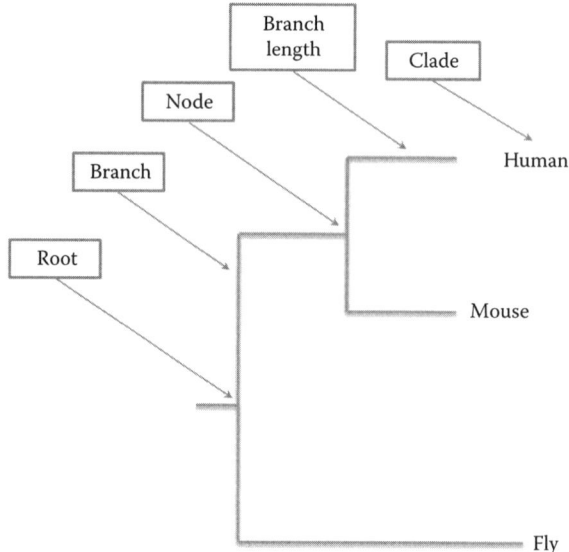

FIGURE 62.1 *Root:* The common ancestor of all taxa. *Branch:* Connector of two nodes that defines the relationships among the taxa in terms of descent and ancestry. *Node:* Represents taxa or taxonomic units. *Branch length:* In scaled trees, the branch length is proportional to the evolutionary divergence, whereas in unscaled trees, the branch length does not have any meaningful correspondence. *Clade:* A group of organisms that includes the most recent common ancestor of all its members and all the descendants of that most recent common ancestor. *Operational taxonomic unit (OTU):* A terminal node. In a phylogenetic tree focused on organisms, it represents an extant taxon. In the case of nucleic acids or proteins, OTUs depict the available sequences.

62.2.2 Nomenclature

In phylogenetic studies, the most common and intuitive way to visually depict evolutionary relationships is the phylogenetic tree. Figure 62.1 presents a simple phylogenetic tree, which is used as a reference to introduce the most frequent terms of phylogenetics.

62.2.3 Tree Building

The initial step toward the formation of a phylogenetic tree is the choice of sequence to study, that is, DNA, RNA, or protein. To define the best way to go, one must bear in mind the question to be answered as well as to take into account a series of nontrivial issues:

- Nucleotide-oriented studies are able to capture potentially significant alterations in the sequence under consideration for both synonymous and nonsynonymous substitutions. On the other hand, amino acid sequence is "opaque" to synonymous substitutions due to the inherent degeneracy of the genetic code. Moreover, by observing and comparing the frequency of occurrence of synonymous and nonsynonymous substitutions, one may infer about positive or negative selection. Positive selection is often indicative of functional differentiation, whereas negative selection tends to maintain the current function, suggesting a critical sequence region (Fay et al., 2001).
- Moreover, the study of protein sequences prevents the phylogenetic analysis of noncoding regions (e.g., introns, 5′ and 3′ untranslated regions), whereas, in such cases, the use of DNA sequences is able to provide adequate conservational information. The same applies more or less with pseudogenes, which by definition do not encode functional proteins (Li et al., 1981; Vanin, 1985).

- Another critical issue has to do with the strength of the phylogenetic signal; more specifically, when dealing with two sequences that have diverged significantly from one another due to multiple mutations, it must be difficult to perform phylogenetic analysis in the four-letter language of DNA. On the other hand, the use of protein sequences is more advisable, since the phylogenetic signal is better represented in the 20-letter language of amino acids. To this end, the persistence of a character is involved, in the sense that a nucleotide changes from one to another in a single step, whereas an amino acid change might be the result of one, two, or even three nucleotide substitutions. Characters that change to another character in one step are called unordered, and characters that need to pass through intermediate states to change are called ordered (Hauser and Presch, 2005; Slowinski, 1993).
- Furthermore, the rate on transitions or transversions must be taken into account when studying a specific organism (Jukes, 1987). For example, transitional substitutions outweigh transversional ones in the case of metazoan, but no significant transition/transversion bias exists for the grasshopper species (Keller et al., 2007). Sometimes, it is also advisable and insightful not only to compare two sequences with one another but also with reference to their ancestor, to unravel mutations otherwise elusive.

The next step in phylogenetic analysis is to perform multiple sequence alignment, a procedure that has been widely reviewed, and is quite definitive of the resulting phylogenetic tree. Basically, sequence alignment involves the application of a program like CLUSTAL W (Larkin et al., 2007), careful manual inspection, and editing of the produced output, which is then fed to a tree-building software.

The resulting alignment is subsequently used to build the tree; tree-building methods can be roughly divided into two principal categories: distance-based and character-based methods. Distance-based methods calculate the pairwise distances between all supplied molecular sequences, using a distance metric, and formulate a tree based on these distances. The most common methods in this category are neighbor-joining (NJ) and unweighted pair group method with arithmetic mean (UPGMA). Character-based methods aim to define ancestral relationships by focusing on specific character substitutions among the sequences. Therefore, character-based methods are far more computationally intensive than distance-based ones. The most important character-based methods for tree-building are maximum parsimony (MP) and maximum likelihood (ML).

Table 62.1 provides a comprehensive list of the state-of-the-art software and web servers for phylogenetic analyses and phylogeny reconstruction.

TABLE 62.1 List of Resources for Phylogenetic Analysis

Resource	Description
Berkeley Phylogenomics Group (Glanville et al., 2007)	A series of tools and methods enabling phylogenetic analyses, provided by the Berkeley Phylogenomics Group
CIPRes (2009)	The Cyberinfrastructure for Phylogenetic Research provides a computational infrastructure for large-scale phylogenetic reconstructions
IBM Genome Annotation Page (2009)	IBM's collection of annotated genomes, along with set of tools for bioinformatics analyses
University of Washington (2009)	Comprehensive list of phylogeny packages
MAVID (Bray and Pachter, 2004)	MAVID performs multiple sequence alignments, constructs phylogenetic trees, and generates graphics
MEGA software (Kumar et al., 2008; Tamura et al., 2007)	MEGA (Molecular Evolutionary Genetics Analysis) is an integrated tool for conducting phylogenetic analyses
MultiPhyl (Keane et al., 2007)	MultiPhyl is a high-throughput implementation of a distributed phylogenetics platform
Phylemon (Tarraga et al., 2007)	A suite of web tools for molecular evolution, phylogenetics, and phylogenomics
Phylogeny.fr (2010)	A set of various components for phylogenetic analyses
TreeView (Page, 2002)	A tool for generating visualizations of phylogenetic trees

62.2.4 Phylogenetics and PPI

Phylogenetic analysis holds a prominent position in the broad and rapidly developing discipline of genome informatics. It is a core part (cornerstone) toward the functional deciphering of proteins solely from the primary sequence; this is based on the assumption that proteins that have evolved in a correlated fashion are likely to be involved in similar functions or act in the same pathway in a complementary manner (Marcotte et al., 1999; Pellegrini et al., 1999). Consequently, phylogenetic analysis is also inherently related to another significant field, that is, the extraction, analysis, and interpretation of gene/protein interaction networks. This is achieved by identifying correlated substitutions or correlated evolution patterns across different sequences.

62.3 Gene/Protein Interaction Networks

In genome informatics, the initial and very important step is to assemble a dataset of genes or proteins that is specific to the problem under consideration. As discussed earlier, the phylogenetic analysis of the input sequences is prone to reveal a great deal of information and provide an added value to the study. However, the mere cataloguing of sequence entities is usually of limited usage, since proteins/genes rarely act in isolation. Therefore, it is of critical significance to identify the interactions that take place among biological entities and thus uncover the molecular basis underlying a biological process. A wide range of methodologies have been proposed to elucidate interactions among biological entities and proteins in particular. These methodologies can be divided into two broad categories: (i) experimental and (ii) computational.

62.3.1 Experimental

In the past few years, a set of high-throughput experimental procedures have revealed a great deal of binary interactions. The most important approaches for experimentally detecting interactions in a genome-wide scale are the yeast two-hybrid system (Y2H), mass spectrometry (MS), and protein microarrays.

62.3.1.1 Yeast Two Hybrid

One of the most common techniques that is being used to study protein–protein interactions is the yeast two-hybrid system (Ito et al., 2001). The basic principle underlying this method is the modular architecture of eukaryotic transcription factors, which are composed of two individually folded units within the same polypeptide chain. This modularity allows for several functions to be performed by a single protein. Two domains are employed, the DNA-binding domain (BD) that recognizes and binds to a specific DNA sequence, and the activation domain (AD) that is capable of activating transcription of the DNA. During the Y2H assay, a protein of interest (X) is fused to the N terminus of the BD to form the "bait" protein and its potential binding partner (Y) is fused to the AD, to create the "prey" protein. If the bait protein interacts with the prey protein, BD and AD are reunited, thus creating a functional transcriptional activator. Consequently, this factor initiates the transcription of a reporter gene, which can be easily detected and measured, indicating the amount of interaction.

62.3.1.2 Mass Spectrometry

Another common technique for identifying potentially novel interactions for a bait protein of interest is mass spectrometry (Aebersold and Mann, 2003; Ewing et al., 2007), which additionally allows for the quantitative evaluation of the detected interactions. A set of bait proteins is carefully selected and introduced into the yeast, where native protein complexes are composed. After the complexes were formed under physiological conditions, the bait was extracted, thus copurifying associated proteins. The resulting proteins are then separated and identified according to their mass. This methodology was initially applied in the yeast genome deciphering a map of invaluable protein interactions, which has also been extrapolated for mammals.

62.3.1.3 Protein Microarrays

Protein microarrays have proven to be an emerging and promising technique for the identification of novel proteins as well as the elicitation of protein interactions (Schweitzer et al., 2003; Walter et al., 2000). Their preparation involves overexpression and high-throughput purification, and turn projection onto a microscopic slide. There are three types of protein microarrays: analytical microarrays, functional microarrays, and reverse phase microarrays. Analytical microarrays are typically employed to study the differential expression during clinical diagnosis. Reverse phase microarrays are used to identify alterations in proteins, which is inherently related to disease abnormalities. The third type of protein microarrays (i.e., functional microarrays) are able to capture biochemical activities of an entire proteome in a single experiment. They are primarily exploited to study a wide range of protein interactions.

62.3.2 Computational

In the literature, several methodologies have been proposed, aiming to extract protein interactions in a more computer-oriented manner. The main approaches are summarized as follows:

- Initial approaches to extract computationally protein–protein interactions in a genome-wide scale have focused on the conservation of adjacent genes (Dandekar et al., 1998; Tamames, 2001). In a similar manner, another group studied the ordering of genes in several microorganisms, deducing pairwise interactions in conserved gene pairs (Overbeek et al., 1999). The so-called gene fusion algorithm (Enright et al., 1999) has proven to be quite beneficial in inferring protein interactions in a genomic scale; basically, if two proteins are located distantly in a single genome or reside in different organisms but have consecutive homologs in a single organism, they are predicted as interacting partners (Marcotte et al., 1999).

- Sequence-based methodologies constitute another significant source of protein–protein interactions. A high percentage of sequence homology is used to extrapolate observed interactions from one organism to another (Matthews et al., 2001). As an added value to this methodology, Wojcik and Schachter (2001) proposed the incorporation of information regarding interacting domains, thus reinforcing the sensitivity and specificity of the inferred interactions. As more and more genomes are being sequenced, protein co-occurrence (i.e., two proteins are either both present or both absent) can be indicative of pairwise interaction. Putative protein interactions can also be extracted by identifying frequently interacting sequence patterns, enriched with geometrical and physicochemical information, indicative of energetically preferred formations (Sprinzak and Margalit, 2001).

- Data mining techniques have revealed a significant amount of protein interactions. To this end, a classifier is trained using sequence-extracted features from known sets of interacting and non-interacting pairs of proteins to recognize potentially novel pairwise interacting partners (Guo et al., 2008).

- One step ahead, the incorporation of full structure information reveals additional information about the three-dimensional structure of the protein, and protein-docking analysis assigns probability of interaction by scoring multiple orientations among multiple protein structures (Aloy et al., 2004; Aloy and Russell, 2002). Such approaches take into account several important properties such as electrostatic forces, potentials, and consequently, energy of interacting docked complexes.

- Furthermore, already constructed valid interaction networks can formulate the basis for extracting previously unknown interactions. Network-related properties stemming from topological

TABLE 62.2 List of Protein–Protein Interaction Repositories

Database Name	Description
HPRD (Prasad et al., 2009)	Human Protein Reference Database (HPRD) is a manually curated database containing interactions among proteins encoded in humans
DIP (Salwinski et al., 2004)	Database of Interacting Proteins (DIP) contains experimentally determined protein interactions curated either manually or computationally
STRING (Jensen et al., 2008)	STRING contains known and predicted interactions from four sources: genomic context, high-throughput experiments, coexpression, and literature
IntAct (Aranda et al., 2010)	IntAct is a free open source repository of interactions from literature data or direct user submissions
BioGRID (Breitkreutz et al., 2008)	The Biological General Repository for Interaction Datasets (BioGRID) contains protein and genetic interactions from major model organism species
MIPS (Mewes et al., 2006)	MIPS is a collection of manually curated high-quality PPI data collected from the scientific literature by expert curators
MINT (Chatr-aryamontri et al., 2007)	MINT focuses on experimentally verified protein–protein interactions mined from the scientific literature by expert curators
I2D (Brown and Jurisica, 2007)	I2D integrates known, experimental, and predicted protein–protein interactions for five model organisms as well as human
BIND (Bader et al., 2001)	BIND stores extensive information about interactions, molecular complexes, and pathways
MiMI (Tarcea et al., 2009)	Michigan Molecular Interactions (MiMI) merges several popular resources of protein–protein interactions
HPID (Han et al., 2004)	The Human Protein Interaction Database (HPID) integrates already available interaction resources but also scores putative interactions
3did (Stein et al., 2008)	The database of 3D Interaction Domains (3did) is a collection of domain–domain interactions in proteins for which high-resolution three-dimensional structures are known
Center for Cancer Systems Biology at Harvard (Han et al., 2004)	This dataset constitutes a proteome-scale map of human binary protein–protein interactions

analysis of the existing proteins can be indicative of new functionally related proteins. The rationale of this approach is that two proteins are likely to interact if they have many mutually interacting neighbors (Goldberg and Roth, 2003).

Besides the great multitude of repositories containing protein–protein interactions, a significant number of software tools and websites have also emerged for network visualization and analysis (Table 62.2). A brief outline of the most common tools is presented in Table 62.3.

However, as each of the aforementioned techniques and methodologies suffers from certain drawbacks, often a careful combination in a complementary manner can be quite fruitful. Moreover, the incorporation of domain knowledge and the enrichment of the network with functional information deposited in other specialized repositories can provide meaningful functional insights about the respective network and at the same time increase the accuracy of mapped interactions by pruning trivial or invalid connections, from a biological point of view. One of the most common and informative mappings in protein interaction networks is the enrichment with gene ontology (Barrell et al., 2009) terms. Gene ontology is a comprehensive and curated repository that aims to assemble and categorize genes and their products, coupled with relevant description and resources.

62.4 Interaction Networks and Diseases

Beyond the identification and cataloguing of existing proteins, it is of utmost importance to unravel interactions that take place among them and subsequently the pathways they participate to carry out certain functionalities. By gaining this knowledge, we are able to gradually and steadily disclose the

TABLE 62.3 List of Resources for Network Visualization and Analysis

Platform Name	Description
	Network Visualization
Cytoscape (Shannon et al., 2003)	Cytoscape is an open source bioinformatics software platform for visualizing molecular interaction networks and integrating these interactions with gene expression profiles and other state data
Osprey (Breitkreutz et al., 2003)	Osprey is a software platform for visualization of complex interaction networks
VisANT (Hu et al., 2009)	VisANT is an integrative visual analysis tool for biological networks and pathways

Application/Server Name	Description
	Network Analysis
ConceptGen (Sartor et al., 2009)	ConceptGen is an enrichment testing and concept mapping tool
NetworkAnalyzer (Assenov et al., 2008) (Cytoscape plugin)	NetworkAnalyzer is a software platform for the analysis and visualization of molecular interaction networks
Pajek (Batagelj and Mrvar, 2002)	Pajek is a software tool for analysis of large-scale networks
Biana (Garcia-Garcia et al., 2010)	Biana is a software framework for compiling biological interactions and analyzing networks
APID (Prieto and De Las Rivas, 2006)	Agile Protein Interaction DataAnalyzer (APID) is an interactive web tool for exploration and analysis of protein–protein interactions

molecular basis of diseases, and possibly to shed some light on their onset, progression, and treatment/confrontation (Ideker and Sharan, 2008). Even though initial approaches to infer protein interactions have been performed in yeast (Ito et al., 2001), substantial effort has been focused on human interactions and pathways (Kann, 2007). To this end, several datasets have been assembled aiming to map the human interactome and their analysis has led to important findings, some of which are summarized as follows:

- Jonsson and Bates (2006) studied the connectivity of a gene interaction network composed of 346 genes that had been implicated with cancers observed in humans. They concluded that cancer proteins, in contrast to noncancer ones, tended to participate in larger and more densely connected clusters. In a similar manner, Wachi et al. (2005) focused on genes that are differentially expressed in lung squamous cancer tissues and assessed their essentiality by means of their connectivity. They showed that differentially elevated genes are much more connected than suppressed ones and also aimed to place this subset of gene interactions within a bigger picture, that is, the context of the living cell.
- The above corollaries were contradicted by Goh et al. (2007) who built a global network of human disorders coupled with their respective disease genes. They found that disease genes mostly localized in the periphery of the network and are nonessential in their majority. On the contrary, hub proteins were encoded by essential genes that play a central role in cellular functions and are therefore expressed in most tissues. The idea was to create a network depicting the complex genetic traits that are indicative of disease susceptibility. Moreover, the resulting network was enriched with gene ontology terms, exhibiting high homogeneity in the localization and functionalities of the genes implicated with a specific disorder.
- Significant efforts have also been devoted to gene association studies, that is, analyses of the interaction among genes involved in a certain disorder to conjecture about novel putative disease-causing genes (Goh et al., 2007). For this purpose, several algorithms have been devised (Lage et al., 2007; Wu et al., 2008, 2009) featuring a broad range of input variables, for example, phenotype and interactions from model organisms, aiming to extrapolate current medical knowledge by identifying which genes are also possibly involved as well as how they participate within the orchestration of the disease interaction map.

- In conceptually similar studies, the authors have not only expanded lists of known state-of-the-art disease genes with inferred potential "culprits," but they have also grouped the genes into subnetworks representing causative disease modules (Calvano et al., 2005; Pujana et al., 2007). The gained results have also been further verified with experimental procedures and case control studies.
- Another significant contribution of gene interaction networks is their utilization/exploitation toward the staging of the diseases or classification of patients according to a risk index. One may superimpose a protein interaction network with gene expression data coupled with clinical profile and discover aggregated lists of genes that may enhance significantly the accuracy in patient stratification studies (Chuang et al., 2007). Furthermore, the incorporation of such information is easily reproducible and extendible and also provides meaningful insights about the underlying molecular mechanisms of the disease.
- This emerging trend has also proven quite beneficial in the analysis of current and experimental drugs and also in the design and development of novel drug agents. More specifically, the drug targets can be systematically analyzed to uncover pathways that are frequently associated with disease onset and progression. Moreover, careful analysis of the interaction network can narrow down the wide range of potential drug targets, leading to enhanced selectivity, and subsequently, reducing possible side effects (Yildirim et al., 2007).

62.5 Closing Remarks

The aim of this chapter is to present a series of intriguing and scientifically active topics centered around the broad field of genome informatics. The core idea is to assemble an interactome map of genes or gene products using a variety of methods and subsequently, exploit it toward the investigation and unraveling of the molecular basis of diseases. Some interesting fields that could benefit from such studies involve identification of novel disease genes, more accurate patient stratification and staging, *in silico* discovery of potential drug targets, and so on. Hence, genome informatics is by all means an open field for scientific research, which also bears immediate impact on the society as a whole.

References

Aebersold, R. and Mann, M. 2003, Mass spectrometry-based proteomics, *Nature*, 422, 198–207.

Aloy, P., Bottcher, B., Ceulemans, H. et al. 2004, Structure-based assembly of protein complexes in yeast, *Science (New York, N.Y.)*, 303, 2026–2029.

Aloy, P. and Russell, R. B. 2002, Interrogating protein interaction networks through structural biology, *Proceedings of the National Academy of Sciences of the United States of America*, 99, 5896–5901.

Aranda, B., Achuthan, P., Alam-Faruque, Y. et al. 2010, The IntAct molecular interaction database in 2010, *Nucleic acids research*, 38, D525–531.

Assenov, Y., Ramirez, F., Schelhorn, S. E. et al. 2008, Computing topological parameters of biological networks, *Bioinformatics (Oxford, England)*, 24, 282–284.

Bader, G. D., Donaldson, I., Wolting, C. et al. 2001, BIND—The Biomolecular Interaction Network Database, *Nucleic Acids Research*, 29, 242–245.

Barrell, D., Dimmer, E., Huntley, R. P. et al. 2009, The GOA database in 2009—An integrated gene ontology annotation resource, *Nucleic Acids Research*, 37, D396–403.

Batagelj, V. and Mrvar, A. 2002, *Pajek—Analysis and Visualization of Large Networks*. Springer, pp. 8–11.

Bray, N. and Pachter, L. 2004, MAVID: Constrained ancestral alignment of multiple sequences, *Genome Res*, 14, 693–699.

Breitkreutz, B. J., Stark, C., Reguly, T. et al. 2008, The BioGRID Interaction Database: 2008 update, *Nucleic Acids Research*, 36, D637–640.

Breitkreutz, B. J., Stark, C., and Tyers, M. 2003, Osprey: A network visualization system, *Genome Biology*, 4, R22.

Brown, K. R. and Jurisica, I. 2007, Unequal evolutionary conservation of human protein interactions in interologous networks, *Genome Biology*, 8, R95.

Calvano, S. E., Xiao, W., Richards, D. R. et al. 2005, A network-based analysis of systemic inflammation in humans, *Nature*, 437, 1032–1037.

Chatr-aryamontri, A., Ceol, A., Palazzi, L. M. et al. 2007, MINT: The Molecular INTeraction database, *Nucleic Acids Research*, 35, D572–574.

Chuang, H. Y., Lee, E., Liu, Y. T. et al. 2007, Network-based classification of breast cancer metastasis, *Molecular Systems Biology*, 3, 140.

Dandekar, T., Snel, B., Huynen, M. et al. 1998, Conservation of gene order: A fingerprint of proteins that physically interact, *Trends in Biochemical Sciences*, 23, 324–328.

Dobzhansky, T. 1951, *Genetics and the Origin of Species*. Columbia University Press, New York.

Enright, A. J., Iliopoulos, I., Kyrpides, N. C. et al. 1999, Protein interaction maps for complete genomes based on gene fusion events, *Nature*, 402, 86–90.

Ewing, R. M., Chu, P., Elisma, F. et al. 2007, Large-scale mapping of human protein-protein interactions by mass spectrometry, *Molecular Systems Biology*, 3, 89.

Fay, J. C., Wyckoff, G. J., and Wu, C. I. 2001, Positive and negative selection on the human genome, *Genetics*, 158, 1227–1234.

Garcia-Garcia, J., Guney, E., Aragues, R. et al. 2010, Biana: A software framework for compiling biological interactions and analyzing networks, *BMC bioinformatics*, 11, 56.

Glanville, J. G., Kirshner, D., Krishnamurthy, N. et al. 2007, Berkeley Phylogenomics Group web servers: Resources for structural phylogenomic analysis, *Nucleic Acids Research*, 35, W27–32.

Goh, K. I., Cusick, M. E., Valle, D. et al. 2007, The human disease network, *Proceedings of the National Academy of Sciences of the United States of America*, 104, 8685–8690.

Goldberg, D. S. and Roth, F. P. 2003, Assessing experimentally derived interactions in a small world, *Proceedings of the National Academy of Sciences of the United States of America*, 100, 4372–4376.

Guo, Y., Yu, L., Wen, Z. et al. 2008, Using support vector machine combined with auto covariance to predict protein-protein interactions from protein sequences, *Nucleic Acids Research*, 36, 3025–3030.

Han, J. D., Bertin, N., Hao, T. et al. 2004, Evidence for dynamically organized modularity in the yeast protein-protein interaction network, *Nature*, 430, 88–93.

Han, K., Park, B., Kim, H. et al. 2004, HPID: The Human Protein Interaction Database, *Bioinformatics (Oxford, England)*, 20, 2466–2470.

Hauser, D. and Presch, W. 2005, The effect of ordered characters on phylogenetic reconstruction, *Cladistics*, 7, 243–265.

http://cbcsrv.watson.ibm.com/Annotations/home.html.

http://evolution.genetics.washington.edu/phylip/software.html.

http://www.phylo.org/.

http://www.phylogeny.fr/.

Hu, Z., Hung, J. H., Wang, Y. et al. 2009, VisANT 3.5: Multi-scale network visualization, analysis and inference based on the gene ontology, *Nucleic acids research*, 37, W115–121.

Ideker, T. and Sharan, R. 2008, Protein networks in disease, *Genome Research*, 18, 644–652.

Ito, T., Chiba, T., Ozawa, R. et al. 2001, A comprehensive two-hybrid analysis to explore the yeast protein interactome, *Proceedings of the National Academy of Sciences of the United States of America*, 98, 4569–4574.

Jensen, L. J., Kuhn, M., Stark, M. et al. 2008, STRING 8—A global view on proteins and their functional interactions in 630 organisms, *Nucleic acids research*.

Jonsson, P. F. and Bates, P. A. 2006, Global topological features of cancer proteins in the human interactome, *Bioinformatics (Oxford, England)*, 22, 2291–2297.

Jukes, T. H. 1987, Transitions, transversions, and the molecular evolutionary clock, *Journal of Molecular Evolution*, 26, 87–98.

Kann, M. G. 2007, Protein interactions and disease: Computational approaches to uncover the etiology of diseases, *Briefings in Bioinformatics*, 8, 333–346.

Keane, T. M., Naughton, T. J., and McInerney, J. O. 2007, MultiPhyl: A high-throughput phylogenomics webserver using distributed computing, *Nucleic Acids Research*, 35, W33–37.

Keller, I., Bensasson, D., and Nichols, R. A. 2007, Transition-transversion bias is not universal: A counter example from grasshopper pseudogenes, *PLoS Genetics*, 3, e22.

Kumar, S., Nei, M., Dudley, J. et al. 2008, MEGA: A biologist-centric software for evolutionary analysis of DNA and protein sequences, *Briefings in Bioinformatics*, 9, 299–306.

Lage, K., Karlberg, E. O., Storling, Z. M. et al. 2007, A human phenome-interactome network of protein complexes implicated in genetic disorders, *Nature Biotechnology*, 25, 309–316.

Larkin, M. A., Blackshields, G., Brown, N. P. et al. 2007, Clustal W. and Clustal X version 2.0, *Bioinformatics (Oxford, England)*, 23, 2947–2948.

Lewontin, R. C. 1997, Dobzhansky's genetics and the origin of species: Is it still relevant?, *Genetics*, 147, 351–355.

Li, W. H., Gojobori, T., and Nei, M. 1981, Pseudogenes as a paradigm of neutral evolution, *Nature*, 292, 237–239.

Marcotte, E. M., Pellegrini, M., Ng, H. L. et al. 1999, Detecting protein function and protein-protein inter-actions from genome sequences, *Science (New York, N.Y.)*, 285, 751–753.

Matthews, L. R., Vaglio, P., Reboul, J. et al. 2001, Identification of potential interaction networks using sequence-based searches for conserved protein-protein interactions or "interologs," *Genome Research*, 11, 2120–2126.

Mewes, H. W., Frishman, D., Mayer, K. F. et al. 2006, MIPS: Analysis and annotation of proteins from whole genomes in 2005, *Nucleic Acids Research*, 34, D169–172.

Overbeek, R., Fonstein, M., D'Souza, M. et al. 1999, The use of gene clusters to infer functional coupling, *Proceedings of the National Academy of Sciences of the United States of America*, 96, 2896–2901.

Page, R. D. 2002, Visualizing phylogenetic trees using TreeView, *Current Protocols in Bioinformatics*, Chapter 6, Unit 6 2.

Pellegrini, M., Marcotte, E. M., Thompson, M. J. et al. 1999, Assigning protein functions by comparative genome analysis: Protein phylogenetic profiles, *Proceedings of the National Academy of Sciences of the United States of America*, 96, 4285–4288.

Prasad, T. S., Kandasamy, K., and Pandey, A. 2009, Human Protein Reference Database and Human Proteinpedia as discovery tools for systems biology, *Methods Mol Biol*, 577, 67–79.

Prieto, C. and De Las Rivas, J. 2006, APID: Agile Protein Interaction DataAnalyzer, *Nucleic acids research*, 34, W298–302.

Pujana, M. A., Han, J. D., Starita, L. M. et al. 2007, Network modeling links breast cancer susceptibility and centrosome dysfunction, *Nature Genetics*, 39, 1338–1349.

Salwinski, L., Miller, C. S., Smith, A. J. et al. 2004, The Database of Interacting Proteins: 2004 update, *Nucleic Acids Research*, 32, D449–451.

Sartor, M. A., Mahavisno, V., Keshamouni, V. G. et al. 2009, ConceptGen: A gene set enrichment and gene set relation mapping tool, *Bioinformatics (Oxford, England)*.

Schweitzer, B., Predki, P., and Snyder, M. 2003, Microarrays to characterize protein interactions on a whole-proteome scale, *Proteomics*, 3, 2190–2199.

Shannon, P., Markiel, A., Ozier, O. et al. 2003, Cytoscape: A software environment for integrated models of biomolecular interaction networks, *Genome Res*, 13, 2498–2504.

Slowinski, J. 1993, Unordered "versus" ordered characters, *Systematic Biology*, 42, 155.

Sprinzak, E. and Margalit, H. 2001, Correlated sequence-signatures as markers of protein-protein interaction, *Journal of Molecular Biology*, 311, 681–692.

Stein, A., Panjkovich, A., and Aloy, P. 2008, 3did Update: Domain-domain and peptide-mediated interactions of known 3D structure, *Nucleic acids research*.

Tamames, J. 2001, Evolution of gene order conservation in prokaryotes, *Genome Biology*, 2, RESEARCH0020.

Tamura, K., Dudley, J., Nei, M. et al. 2007, MEGA4: Molecular Evolutionary Genetics Analysis (MEGA) software version 4.0, *Mol Biol Evol*, 24, 1596–1599.

Tarcea, V. G., Weymouth, T., Ade, A. et al. 2009, Michigan molecular interactions r2: From interacting proteins to pathways, *Nucleic acids research*, 37, D642–646.

Tarraga, J., Medina, I., Arbiza, L. et al. 2007, Phylemon: A suite of web tools for molecular evolution, phylogenetics and phylogenomics, *Nucleic acids research*, 35, W38–42.

Vanin, E. F. 1985, Processed pseudogenes: Characteristics and evolution, *Annual Review of Genetics*, 19, 253–272.

Wachi, S., Yoneda, K., and Wu, R. 2005, Interactome-transcriptome analysis reveals the high centrality of genes differentially expressed in lung cancer tissues, *Bioinformatics (Oxford, England)*, 21, 4205–4208.

Walter, G., Bussow, K., Cahill, D. et al. 2000, Protein arrays for gene expression and molecular interaction screening, *Current Opinion in Microbiology*, 3, 298–302.

Wojcik, J. and Schachter, V. 2001, Protein-protein interaction map inference using interacting domain profile pairs, *Bioinformatics (Oxford, England)*, 17 Suppl 1, S296–305.

Wu, X., Jiang, R., Zhang, M. Q. et al. 2008, Network-based global inference of human disease genes, *Molecular Systems Biology*, 4, 189.

Wu, X., Liu, Q., and Jiang, R. 2009, Align human interactome with phenome to identify causative genes and networks underlying disease families, *Bioinformatics (Oxford, England)*, 25, 98–104.

Yildirim, M. A., Goh, K. I., Cusick, M. E. et al. 2007, Drug-target network, *Nature Biotechnology*, 25, 1119–1126.

63

Cardiovascular Health Informatics

Carmen C.Y. Poon
The Chinese University of Hong Kong

Yuan-ting Zhang
The Chinese University of Hong Kong

Key Laboratory for Health Informatics of Chinese Academy of Science

63.1 Introduction

Cardiovascular disease (CVD) is classified as diseases relating to the heart or blood vessels (arteries and veins) [1]. According to the World Health Organization, CVD has been the leading cause of deaths in most countries and will likely remain the top killer in the near future. CVD claimed the lives of 17.5 million people in 2005, accounting for 30% of all deaths, among which 12.9 million were due to either coronary heart disease or stroke [2]. Despite major advances in the treatment of CVD such as coronary artery disease (CAD), a large number of victims who appear to be healthy die suddenly of the disease without obvious prior symptoms. Nearly two-thirds of the people who have a heart attack die before they can reach medical care. Even when stroke patients managed to get modern, advanced treatment, 60% die or become disabled [3].

The exact number of incidents of sudden cardiac death (SCD) is unknown because internationally accepted classification of death certification does not include a specific category of SCD [4]. SCD is defined as "natural death due to cardiac causes, heralded by abrupt loss of consciousness within 1 hour of the onset of acute symptoms; pre-existing heart disease may have been known to be present, but the time and mode of death are unexpected" [5,6]. The description is clear for many witnessed deaths in the community or in emergency departments; however, for many SCDs that occurred unwitnessed, it is difficult to define for what duration the subject suffered any symptoms prior to death and whether it should be classified as SCD [4]. Therefore, it is presumed that death is sudden if the deceased is known to be in good health 24 h before death for unwitnessed death [4]. The key concept of this definition is the nontraumatic nature of the event and the fact that death is unexpected and instantaneous [6].

Clearly, hospital-oriented care practice that mainly relies on individuals to seek medical consultation when they feel unwell is unable to solve the major issue arising from CVD, particularly SCD. Rather, it is believed that CVD deaths should be prevented through proper treatment and timely lifestyle modification, beginning when subjects still appear to be healthy. It is estimated that preventive approach could reduce CVD deaths by over 90% [7]. Nevertheless, this is only realistic if a system is developed to constantly collect health information from each individual for predicting the risk of developing CVD such that individualized and preemptive treatment can be given ahead of time to prevent sudden cardiac events. Cardiovascular health informatics (CHI), a subdiscipline of health informatics, is therefore an area that deals with the processing, storage, transmission, acquisition, and retrieval (P-STAR) of multiscale and multimodality information at different levels for understanding the pathophysiological mechanisms underlying CVD so as to support making and implementing healthcare decisions to prevent morbidity and mortality resulting from this type of disease [8]. Challenges in the storage and retrieval of information in CHI will be similar to other subdisciplines of health informatics. Therefore, in this chapter, we will highlight the acquisition, transmission, and processing (A-T-P) aspects of the P-STAR of information in CHI.

63.2 Pathology of Cardiovascular Disease and Sudden Cardiac Death

The main pathological process leading to heart attacks and stroke is atherosclerosis, which is characterized by the deposition of atheromatous plaques containing cholesterol and lipids on the innermost layer of the walls of large- and medium-sized arteries [7]. Problems of cardiovascular system usually appear in middle-aged or elderly population, by which time the underlying cause (atherosclerosis) is usually quite advanced and has been developing for some years. Population-based studies in the youth show that the precursors of heart disease begin early in life and progress gradually through adolescence and early adulthood (15–17 years old) [9,10].

The rate of progression of atherosclerosis is accelerated by a number of risk factors: tobacco use, an unhealthy diet and physical inactivity (which collectively cause obesity), elevated blood pressure (hypertension), abnormal blood lipids (dyslipidemia), and elevated blood glucose (diabetes) [2]. Continuous exposure to these risk factors leads to further progression of atherosclerosis, resulting in the development of vulnerable atherosclerotic plaques, narrowing of blood vessels, and obstruction of blood flow to vital organs, such as the heart and the brain [2].

Although atherosclerosis is found to be strongly associated with SCD and the two diseases share many common risk factors, the exact mechanisms leading to SCD are still not well understood. The general accepted paradigm for SCD is it is the result of both a substrate and a trigger for the occurrence of the final dynamic event [11]. In the adult population, two main potential mechanisms leading to SCD are (1) rupture of vulnerable plaque in the coronary artery and (2) the presence of myocardial scarring that can lead to the development of a fatal tachyarrhythmic event even among patients who do not exhibit acute CAD [12]. In younger patients, especially athletes, congenital heart disease, cardiomyopathy, and unexplained left ventricular (LV) hypertrophy are the dominating reasons for SCD [4,6]. Chugh reviewed and summarized the risk factors leading to SCD in patients with CAD, as shown in Figure 63.1 [13].

63.3 Cardiovascular Health Informatics and Multimodal E-Record

Current clinical practice uses severe LV systolic dysfunction, quantified as LV ejection fraction ≤35%, as the only SCD risk stratification and major criterion for primary implantable cardioverter-defibrillator prophylaxis, but the direction of evaluation is undergoing a radical change. Although CVD is the class of diseases that involve the circulatory systems, it is also found closely related to the dysfunction of other organ systems, for example, nervous system, lymphatic/immune system, respiratory system, endocrine system, and excretory system. Apart from depressed LV systolic function and conventional

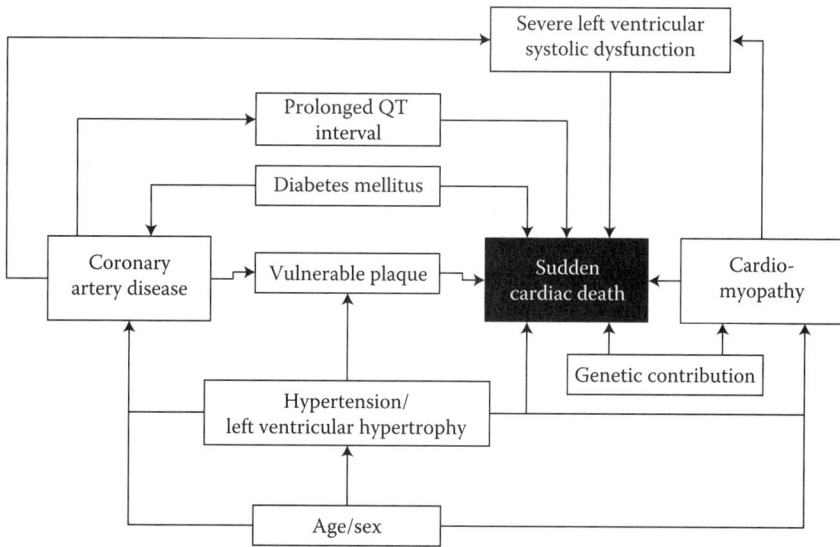

FIGURE 63.1 Risk factors associated with sudden cardiac death in patients with coronary artery disease. (Reproduced from S. S. Chugh, *Nature Reviews Cardiology*, 7, 318–326, 2010.)

risk stratification tools such as age and sex, new markers for plaque vulnerability, specific genetic alterations of the autonomic nervous system, enhanced thrombogenesis, cardiac sarcolemmal and contractile proteins, and familial clustering may better segregate patients with atherosclerotic CAD who are at high risk of SCD from those who may suffer from nonfatal ischemic events [14].

A Cardiovascular Health Informatics and Multimodal E-Record (CHIME) [15] should therefore store relevant health information obtained from all different organ systems. On the spatial scale, information may be found in the order of 10^{-9} m in tRNA and ribosome to the meter range on the human body. On the temporal scale, health information varies from 10^{-6}s or below for some molecular motions that play a critical role in the transportation of enzymes and chemicals both into and out of the cells to 10^{9}s for a typical lifetime of a person. Acquiring these multiscale health information requires a variety of sensing and imaging tools that interact with the biological system by different modalities, such as optical, magnetic, acoustic, electrical, and chemical approaches. The massive, heterogeneous set of information has to be eventually fused together to solve health issues arising at different levels, from personal to global.

63.3.1 Information Acquisition

Figure 63.2 illustrates some potentially useful health information and the corresponding technologies that acquire them for predicting SCD. Three major classes of sensing and imaging tools used for this purpose include (1) quantitative tests for specific genes and biomarkers, (2) multimodal imaging of the vulnerable plaque, and (3) wearable and implantable devices as well as body sensor/area networks (BSN/BAN) that connects them for continuously monitoring the hemodynamics during day-to-day activities.

63.3.1.1 Quantitative Test of Specific Genes and Biomarkers

Studies have demonstrated an independent genetic contribution to SCD. Familial clustering of SCD cases owing to genetic transmission of susceptibility of SCD is observed in a number of studies [13]. Mutations in distinctive genes are found to be associated with the long QT syndrome, which indicates cardiac ion channel dysfunction and increases the risk of SCD. A common variant of chromosome 9p21 is also found to affect the risk of incident CVD [16,17]. Genetic studies of CVD can be carried out by

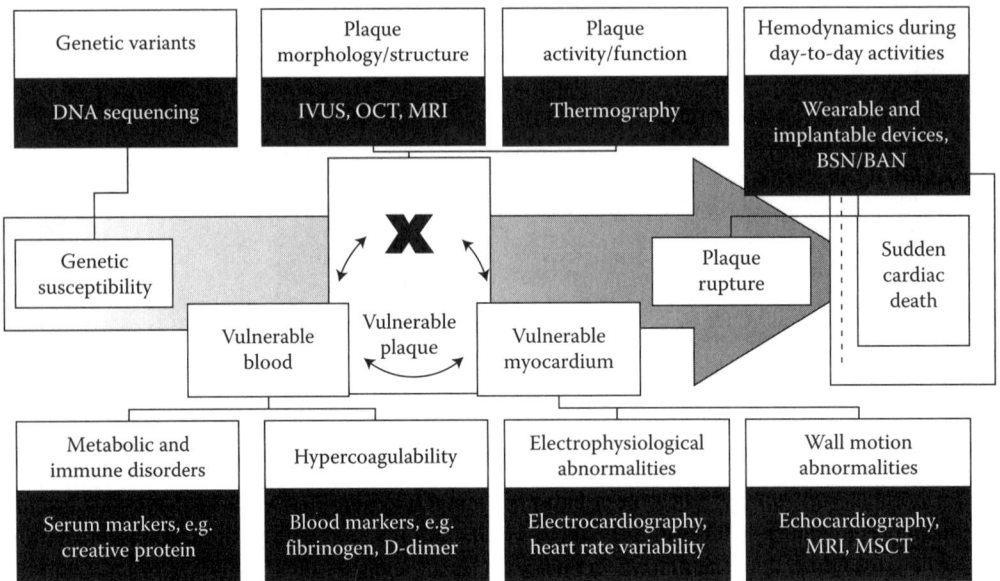

FIGURE 63.2 Multiscale health information and examples of the corresponding acquisition technologies potentially useful for predicting sudden cardiac death. IVUS, intravenous ultrasound imaging; OCT, optical coherence tomography; MRI, magnetic resonance imaging; MSCT, multislice computed tomography; BSN/BAN, body sensor/area network.

examining a candidate gene or identifying regions of common variants in genome-wide association studies [13]. To adopt genetic markers in clinical practice, the functional significance of genetic variants must be better understood.

Biomarker is the biological molecule found in blood, other body fluids, or tissues that is a sign of a normal or abnormal process, or of a condition or disease [18]. Some biomarkers are thought to offer more detailed information of the initiation and progression of CVD [19]. Currently, biomarkers that may reflect a higher risk of CVD include fibrinogen and PAI-1 blood concentrations, homocysteine, asymmetric dimethylarginine, C-reactive protein, and brain natriuretic peptide (also known as B-type) (BNP). A fairly recent emphasis is on the link between low-grade inflammation that hallmarks atherosclerosis and its possible interventions. C-reactive protein (CRP) is an inflammatory marker that may be present in increased levels in the blood in patients at risk for CVD, in particular vulnerable plaque [20]. However, the clinical value of these biomarkers is questionable. Their exact role in predicting disease is the subject of debate, which could not be used as the specific indicators of a specific type and a specific stage of CVD for clinical diagnosis and laboratory research.

Biomarkers are difficult to identify in human serum due to the high abundance of albumin and heterogeneity of plasma lipoproteins and glycoproteins. Common methods of biomarker identification, including gel electrophoresis, chromatography, mass spectrometry, and immunological protein/gene array, have one or more limitations in terms of their sensitivity, resolution, screen time, sample amount, and reproducibility that avoid the identification of the new specific biomarkers to the particular type of CVD [20]. A technical challenge in this aspect is to develop the methods, means, and devices with high sensitivity, high resolution, and high-throughput screening capabilities.

63.3.1.2 Multimodal Imaging of the Vulnerable Plaque

The identification of vulnerable plaque is emerging as a main research topic in risk stratification of CVD [21]. One major difficulty encountered is to provide the ideal criteria for vulnerable plaque. Current

TABLE 63.1 Benefits and Limitations of Different Imaging Techniques in Identifying Vulnerable Plaques

Imaging Modality	Resolution (µm)		Penetration	Calcium	Fibrous Cap	Lipid Core	Thrombus	Inflammation
	Spatial	Axial						
Ultrasound[a]	600	400	9 cm	−	−	−	−	−
MRI	250	3000	NA	+	+	++	+	++
MSCT[b]	400	400	NA	+++	−	+	−	−
SPECT	10,000	NA	NA	−	−	+	+	++
PET	4000	NA	NA	−	−	+	+	++
Coronary angiography	High	UK	Poor	−	−	−	++	−
IVUS[c]	100	100	Total	+++	+	++	+	−
IVUS RF data analysis	40	100	Total	+++	++	++	+	−
Elasto- and palpography	100	225	Total	++	>+	>++	UK	+++
Angioscopy	10	UK	Poor	−	+	++	+++	−
OCT	5	10	1–2 mm	+++	++	+++	++	+
Thermography	500	UK	Poor	−	−	−	−	+++
Spectroscopy	NA	NA	1–2 mm	++	+	++	−	++
Intravascular MRI	100	250	Good	+++	+	++	+	++

Source: Modified from J. G. Kips, P. Segers, and L. M. V. Bortel, *Artery Research*, 2, 21–34, 2008.

Note: NA, not applicable; UK, unknown; MRI, magnetic resonance imaging; MSCT, multislice computer tomography; SPECT, single photon emission computed tomography; PET, positron emission tomography; IVUS, intravenous ultrasound imaging; OCT, optical coherence tomography. +++, sensitivity >90%; ++, sensitivity 80 ~ 90%; +, sensitivity 50 ~ 80%; −, sensitivity <50%.

[a] Ultrasound at 8 MHz.

[b] 64-Slide computer tomography.

[c] IVUS at 40 MHz.

evidences that is largely based on cross-sectional and retrospective studies of culprit plaques suggested in Reference 21 are (1) active inflammation, (2) thin cap with large lipid core, (3) endothelial denudation with superficial platelet aggregation, (4) fissured plaque, and (5) stenosis >90%. As shown in Table 63.1, a number of imaging techniques can provide one or more pieces of the above information [22]; however, none of the current technologies is able to offer a complete picture. Therefore, a multimodal imaging approach is essential for truly reflecting the vulnerability of atherosclerotic plaque. In addition, to identify vulnerable plaques at an early stage, resolution of a number of imaging techniques such as MRI must also be improved.

63.3.1.3 Wearable and Implantable Devices for Continuously Monitoring Hemodynamics during Day-to-Day Activities

While genetic and biological markers as well as structural and functional characteristics of vulnerable plaques or myocardium are snapshots of information essential for evaluating the risk of cardiac death in the long run, wearable and implantable devices are able to supply a continuous stream of health information of the apparently healthy individual during his/her day-to-day activities and fire an alarm or even deliver instantaneous treatment in case of emergency.

At present, an implantable cardioverter-defibrillator is suggested for high-risk patients to prevent SCD due to ventricular fibrillation and ventricular tachycardia. The device is a small battery-powered electrical impulse generator that is programmed to detect cardiac arrhythmia and correct it by delivering a jolt of electricity. Since implanting a device into the body is less acceptable to most subjects who are apparently healthy and are facing low to moderate risk of SCD, the development of wearable devices for long-term continuous monitoring of the health status of an individual becomes an attractive alternative.

Wearable medical devices should entail the following six properties: miniaturized, integrated, networked, digitalized, smart, and standardized (MINDSS) [23]. Miniaturization of devices is achieved by inventing innovative measurement principles to replace traditional technologies that require bulky components. For example, conventional noninvasive blood pressure devices incorporate an occlusive cuff that has to be inflated and deflated for measurement. To miniaturize blood pressure meters into wearable devices, new cuffless principles have been proposed. A major challenge of these cuffless technologies is that they often require an individualized calibration procedure. To calibrate the cuffless technology using simple hand movements that can be carried out even by laymen at home using wearable sensors, a biomodel has been developed [24], that is

$$
\text{PTT} =
\begin{cases}
\dfrac{L\sqrt{\rho b}}{\sqrt{1 + \exp(bP_i)}} & ; h = 0 \\[4ex]
\dfrac{2L}{\sqrt{\rho b g h}} \ln \left| \dfrac{\sqrt{\exp\left[b(P_i - P_h) \right] + \exp(-bP_h)} - \sqrt{\exp(-bP_h)}}{\sqrt{\exp\left[b(P_i - P_h) \right] + 1} - 1} \right| & ; h \neq 0
\end{cases}
, \tag{63.1}
$$

where PTT is pulse transit time found to be correlated with blood pressure, L is the arm length, ρ is the density of blood, g is the acceleration due to gravity, b is a subject-dependent coefficient characterizing the artery properties, h is height difference between the measurement site and heart level, P_i is the blood pressure, and $P_h = \rho \cdot g \cdot h$ is the hydrostatic pressure. For a given set of coefficients $\{L, b\}$, blood pressure can be expressed in terms of PTT while the subject maintains his/her hand at heart level (i.e., $h = 0$ cm):

$$
\text{BP} = \frac{1}{b} \ln \left(\frac{L^2 \rho b}{\text{PTT}^2} - 1 \right) \tag{63.2}
$$

Integration denotes the design of application-specific integrated circuits (ASIC) to reduce the size and power consumption of these wearable devices. Networking devices by BSN/BAN will be further elaborated in the next section. Digitalization implies that new sampling and compression theories are needed for MINDS devices to handle the massive dataset resulting from long-term signal monitoring. Smart devices have to be context aware and resistive to motion artifacts. Last but not least, the development of new standards for these devices is crucial when these devices are designed with different measurement principles as their conventional counterparts. For example, new cuffless blood pressure measurement devices often involve an individualized calibration procedure that is not required in traditional cuff-based blood pressure devices. New protocols should therefore be designed to evaluate cuffless devices [25].

63.3.2 Information Transmission

Seamless transmission of information by standardized protocols is required to build a health information system of multiple levels, from personal to familial, institutional, regional, national, and eventually global. Both healthcare and conventional medical devices used at home and in the hospitals have to be linked up to a server that stores the acquired information by networks such as WiFi, mobile network, LAN, and WAN. Emerging future wireless and network technologies, including new broadband technologies such as WiMAX and other long-term evolution communication systems, will be needed in the next-generation health information systems. For the established networks, security of health information is still a key challenge waiting for a solution.

Among the different networks used for developing the health information system, the emerging BAN/
BSN for connecting biosensors and devices worn on or implanted in an individual is the most underdeveloped. The development of BAN/BSN is critical for many emerging applications in CHI, where
multiple cardiovascular signals and parameters have to be monitored simultaneously. As signals have to
be acquired by on-body or in-body sensors placed on different body parts, setting up a BAN/BSN to connect them helps to optimize the use of resources to satisfy the stringent constraints in these terminals.
For example, health information collected from different sensors can be centralized before being passed
on to external networks for remote analysis, diagnosis, or treatment. In addition, the presence of a BAN
can also enhance the control, scheduling, and programming of the overall system such that it is adaptive to body condition and external environment. For example, some sensors or devices may have to be
reprogrammed from time to time. Since BAN/BSN are extremely limited in power and memory space,
a desirable approach should take into consideration the unique characteristics and resources already
available to develop a lightweight and secured solution for BAN/BSN.

From the user's perspective, unobtrusive connection of wearable and implanted sensors and devices
to form BAN/BSN is highly preferred. Wireless radiofrequency techniques such as Bluetooth, Zigbee,
and ultrawide band (UWB) are some examples that have recently drawn a lot of attention. As for sensor
nodes that are close to each other, they can be connected through "wires." In this respect, a research
group from Georgia Tech [26] proposed the concept of wearable motherboard, where fabric made of
e-textiles is developed into a computer and served as a framework for personalized mobile information
processing [26].

Even more unique, since nodes of BAN are placed in or on the human body, they are inherently
linked by pathways that we named biological channels (biochannels) [27]. Biochannels are commonly
referred to the voltage-gated channels that allow the exchange of selected ions across the otherwise
impermeable cell membrane. In this context, we use biochannels to denote any biological conduit that
is part of the human body and enables the transfer of either exogenous or endogenous information.
Signals transmitted via biochannels can be either processed information or biological data. Some of
the biological data unique to individuals can even potentially be used as an identifier of the owner of
BAN. Thus, a biometrics approach using biochannels could be used to secure wireless communications
in BAN [27].

As illustrated in Figure 63.3, different biosensors of a BSN/BAN for CHI can be collecting health
information that consists of common characteristics unique to an individual, for example, the interpulse intervals from various cardiovascular signals. These intrinsic characteristics can therefore be used
to verify whether two sensors belong to the same individual. The multiple usages of the recorded physiological signals will save resources while adequate security measures are employed.

The method was tested on 99 subjects with 838 segments of simultaneous recordings of electrocardiogram and photoplethysmogram. By using interpulse intervals as the biometric trait, the system achieved
a minimum half total error rate of 2.58%, as shown in Figure 63.4.

The different communication means discussed earlier should be viewed as the complement of each
other. In future, depending on the application, one or more communication means should be used in a
BAN to connect the various sensors and to communicate with the external world, that is, the concept
of hybrid BAN [28].

63.3.3 Information Processing

Statistical tests, including age-adjusted linear regression or logistic regression models, have been most
widely used for predicting risks of cardiovascular incidences or mortality in 5 or 10 years [29–31]. The
Cox's proportional hazards model is formulated as follows:

$$f(x,M) = \beta_1(x_1 - M_1) + \cdots + \beta_p(x_p - M_p), \tag{63.3}$$

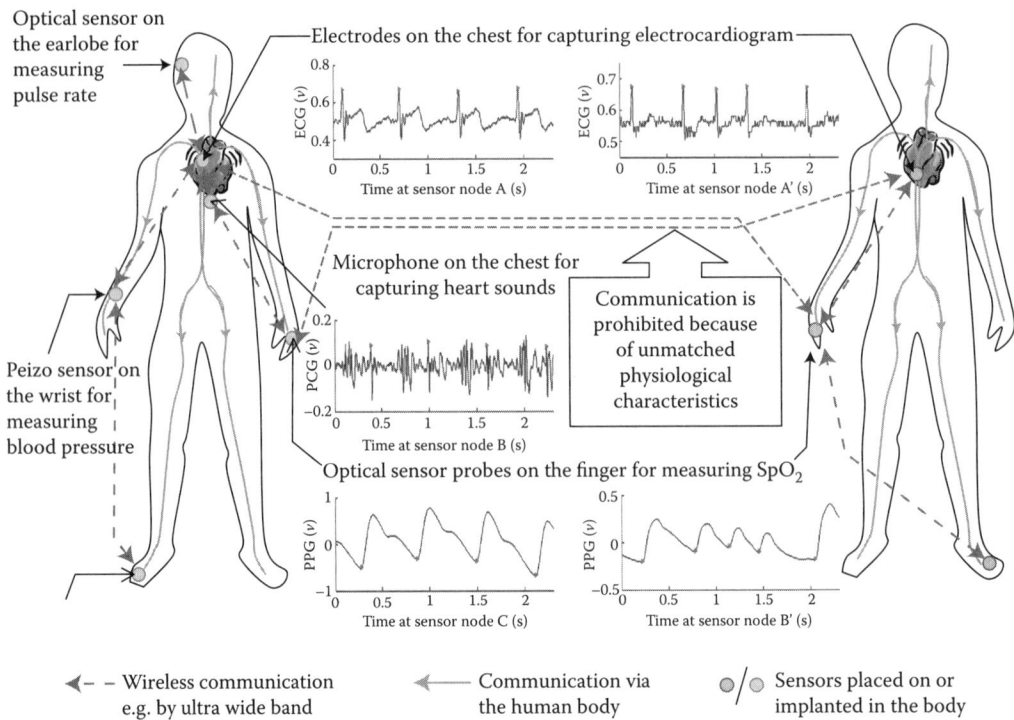

FIGURE 63.3 An illustration of applying the biometrics approach to secure wireless communications between sensors of a body sensor/area network. (From C. C. Y. Poon, Y. T. Zhang, and S. D. Bao, *IEEE Communication Magazine*, 44(4), 73–81, 2006.)

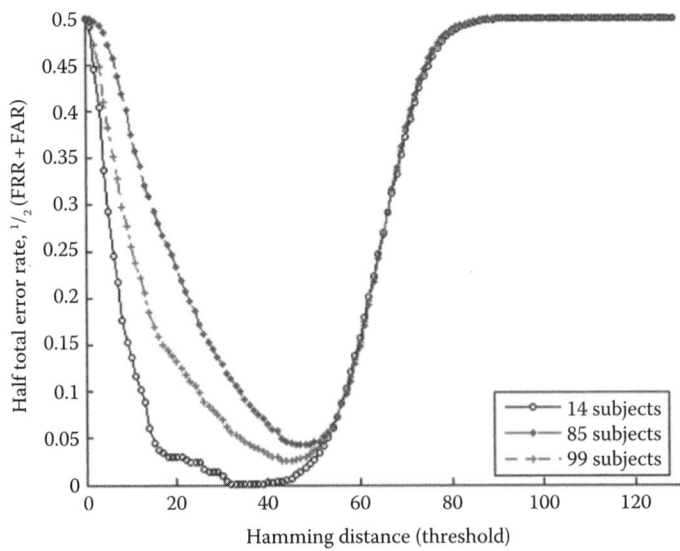

FIGURE 63.4 Performance of the proposed biometrics system using interpulse intervals from electrocardiogram and photoplethysmogram on 99 subjects (from two subject groups with 14 and 85 subjects, respectively). (From C. C. Y. Poon, Y. T. Zhang, and S. D. Bao, *IEEE Communication Magazine*, 44(4), 73–81, 2006. © 2006 IEEE.)

where $\{x_1, \ldots, x_p\}$ are risk factors of CVD or SCD such as age, sex, HDL cholesterol, LDL cholesterol, hypertension, diabetes mellitus, cigarette use, and family history of CVD. A set of coefficients $\{\beta_1, \ldots, \beta_p\}$ is used to weigh each risk factor differently. The area under the receiver operating characteristic curve, which plots sensitivity against false-positive rate at each score, is used as an evaluating parameter of the accuracy of the model.

With the development of new information acquisition methods, researchers have been adding results from new genetic markers and biomarkers together with the list of traditional risk factors to the existing models. The benefits are however not always clear. In a large prospective cohort of White women, genetic variation in chromosome 9p21.3 was found to associate with incidences of CVD but did not improve on the discrimination or classification of predicted risk achieved with traditional risk factors, high-sensitivity C-reactive protein, and family history of premature myocardial infarction [32]. Another study that includes 10 contemporary biomarkers, such as of C-reactive protein, B-type natriuretic peptide, and N-terminal pro-atrial natriuretic peptide, adds only moderately to standard risk factors in predicting the risk of cardiovascular events [19]. However, a study in elderly men with or without prevalent CVD shows that the simultaneous addition of several biomarkers of cardiovascular and renal abnormalities substantially improves the risk stratification for death from cardiovascular causes compared to a model that is based only on established risk factors [33]. One possible reason for the insignificant improvements in incorporating new markers can be because these data are actually reflecting similar information as the traditional risk factors that are acquired by different mortality at different spatial scales.

As the types of health information for CVD or SCD diverge in terms of scale and modality, it is becoming important to develop beyond statistical models for generalizing conclusion from the heterogeneous set of information. Therefore, recent studies on multiscale physiological-based modeling [34] become a very promising area of research to understand the underlying mechanisms of CVD such that health information can be better put together for predicting and preventing CVD and SCD. The idea is to incorporate the concept of personalization in the decision-making procedure, where health information related to an individual acquired up-to-date, including genomic information, personal and family medical history, images of tissue and organs, blood test results, behaviors, and so on, will be used with models of the biological systems and physiological process to support the selection of an optimal and effective healthcare approach for the individual, that is, a tailor-made healthcare decision.

63.4 Conclusion

CVD, particularly SCD, is an unsolved global health issue. Owing to the unexpected nature of cardiac events, health informatics that allows P-STAR of information beyond hospitals is urgently needed for better care for this type of disease. In particular, acquisition, transmission, and processing of cardiovascular health information are three core topics in CHI that require special attention. Emerging technologies in identifying new genetic variants and biomarkers, wearable devices, body area/sensor networks, and individualized physiological-based modeling are anticipated to play important roles in the management of CVD and SCD in the future.

Acknowledgments

The authors would like to thank Ms Jie Meng and Ms Wenbo Gu for their help in organizing related literatures. This work was supported in part by the Hong Kong Innovation and Technology Fund (ITF), the 973 Project Fund (2010CB732606), and the Guangdong Innovation Team Fund in China. The authors are grateful to Standard Telecommunication Ltd., Jetfly Technology Ltd., Golden Meditech Company Ltd., Bird International Ltd., Bright Steps Corporation, and PCCW for their support to the ITF projects.

References

1. A. Maton, *Human Biology and Health*. Englewood Cliffs, New Jersey: Prentice Hall. ISBN 0-13-981176-1. 1993.
2. World Health Organization, *Prevention of Cardiovascular Disease: Guidelines for Assessment and Management of Cardiovascular Risk*, 2007
3. World Health Organization, *Avoiding Heart Attacks and Strokes: Don't Be a Victim—Protect Yourself*, 2005.
4. P. J. Gallagher, The pathological investigation of sudden cardiac death, *Current Diagnostic Pathology*, 13, 366–374, 2007.
5. R. J. Myerburg and A. Castellanos, Cardiac arrest and sudden cardiac death. In: Braunwald E, ed. *Heart Disease: A Textbook of Cardiovascular Medicine*. New York, NY: WB Saunders Publishing Co., 1997, pp. 742–779.
6. S. G. Priori, E. Aliot, C. Blomstrom-Lundqvist, L. Bossaert, G. Breithardt et al., Task force on sudden cardiac death of the European Society of Cardiology, *European Heart Journal*, 22, 1374–1450, 2001.
7. O. S. Randall and D. S. Romaine, *The Encyclopedia of the Heart and Heart Disease*, New York, NY: Facts on File, ISBN 081606637X, 2005.
8. Y. T. Zhang and C. C. Y. Poon, Editorial note on bio, medical, and health informatics, *IEEE Transactions on Information Technology in Biomedicine*, 14(3), 543–545, 2010.
9. A. W. Zieske, G. T. Malcom, and J. P. Strong, Natural history and risk factors of atherosclerosis in children and youth: The PDAY study, *Pediatric Pathology & Molecular Medicine*, 21(2), 213–237, 2002.
10. H. C. McGill, Jr, C. A. McMahan, and S. S. Gidding, Preventing heart disease in the 21st century: Implications of the pathobiological determinants of atherosclerosis in youth (PDAY) study, *Circulation*, 117, 1216–1227, 2008.
11. D. P. Zipers and H. J. Wellens, Sudden cardiac death, *Circulation*, 98, 2334–2351, 1998.
12. A. J. Moss and I. Goldenberg, Prevention of sudden cardiac death: Need for a plaque stabilizer, *American Heart Journal*, 159(1), 15–16, 2010.
13. S. S. Chugh, Early identification of risk factors for sudden cardiac death, *Nature Reviews Cardiology*, 7, 318–326, 2010.
14. N. El-Sherif, A. Khan, J. Savarese, and G. Turitto, Pathophysiology, risk stratification, and management of sudden cardiac death in coronary artery disease, *Cardiology Journal*, 17(1), 4–10, 2010.
15. Y. T. Zhang, C. C. Y. Poon, and E. Macpherson, Editorial note on health informatics, *IEEE Transactions on Information Technology in Biomedicine*, 13(3), 281–283, 2009.
16. A. Helgadottir, G. Thorleifsson, A. Manolescu, S. Gretarsdottir, T. Blondal et al., A common variant on chromosome 9p21 affects the risk of myocardial infarction, *Science*, 316, 1491–1493, 2007.
17. R. McPherson, A. Pertsemlidis, N. Kavaslar, A. Stewart, R. Roberts et al., A common allele on chromosome 9 associated with coronary heart disease, *Science*, 316, 1488–1491, 2007.
18. U.S. National Institutes of Health, *NCI Dictionary of Cancer Terms*.
19. T. J. Wang, P. Gona, M. G. Larson, G. H. Tofler, D. Levy et al. Multiple biomarkers for the prediction of first major cardiovascular events and death, *New England Journal of Medicine*, 355, 2631–2639, 2006.
20. T. J. Wang, M. G. Larson, D. Levy, E. J. Benjamin, E. P. Leip, T. Omland, P. A. Wolf, and R. S. Vasan, Plasma natriuretic peptide levels and the risk of cardiovascular events and death, *New England Journal of Medicine*, 350(7), 655–663, 2004.
21. M. Naghavi, P. Libby, E. Falk, S. W. Casscells, S. Litovsky et al., From vulnerable plaque to vulnerable patient: A call for new definitions and risk assessment strategies: Part I, *Circulation*, 108, 1664–1672, 2003.
22. J. G. Kips, P. Segers, and L. M. V. Bortel, Identifying the vulnerable plaque: A review of invasive and non-invasive imaging modalities, *Artery Research*, 2, 21–34, 2008.

23. Y. T. Zhang, Y. S. Yan, and C. C. Y. Poon, Some perspectives on affordable healthcare systems in China, in *Proc. 29th Ann. Int. Conf. IEEE Eng. Med. Biol. Soc.*, France: 6154, 2007.

24. C. C. Y. Poon, Y. T. Zhang, and Y. B. Liu, Modeling of pulse transit time under the effects of hydrostatic pressure for cuffless blood pressure measurements, in *Proc 3rd IEEE-EMBS Int. Summer School Sym. Medical Devices Biosensors*, Cambridge, MA, USA, September 4–6, 2006, pp. 65–68.

25. I. R. F. Yan, C. C. Y. Poon, and Y. T. Zhang, Evaluation scale to assess the accuracy of cuff-less blood pressure measuring devices, *Blood Pressure Monitoring*, 14(6): 257–267, 2009.

26. S. Park and S. Jayaraman, Enhancing the quality of life through wearable technology, *IEEE Engineering in Medicine and Biology Magazine*, 22(3), 41–48, 2003.

27. C. C. Y. Poon, Y. T. Zhang, and S. D. Bao, A novel biometrics method to secure wireless body area sensor networks for telemedicine and m-Health, *IEEE Communication Magazine*, 44(4), 73–81, 2006.

28. C. H. Chan, C. C. Y. Poon, R. C. S. Wong, and Y. T. Zhang, A hybrid body sensor network for continuous and long-term measurement of arterial blood pressure, in *Proc 4th IEEE-EMBS Int. Summer School Sym. Medical Devices Biosensors*, Cambridge, UK, August 19–22, 2007, pp. 121–123.

29. P. W. F. Wilson, R. B. D'Agostino, D. Levy, A. M. Belanger, H. Silbershatz, and W. B. Kannel, Prediction of coronary heart disease using risk factor categories, *Circulation*, 97, 1837–1847, 1998.

30. A. Menotti, M. Lanti, P. E. Puddu, and D. Kromhout, Coronary heart disease incidence in northern and southern European populations: A reanalysis of the seven countries study for a European coronary risk chart, *Heart*, 84, 238–244, 2000.

31. Y. F. Wu, X. Q. Liu, X. Li, Y. Li, L. C. Zhao et al., Estimation of 10-year risk of fatal and nonfatal ischemic cardiovascular diseases in Chinese adults, *Circulation*, 114, 2217–2225, 2006.

32. N. P. Paynter, D. I. Chasman, J. E. Buring, D. Shiffman, N. R. Cook, and P. M. Ridker, Cardiovascular disease risk prediction with and without knowledge of genetic variation at chromosome 9p21.3, *Annals of Internal Medicine*, 150(2), 65–72, 2009.

33. B. Zethelius, L. Berglund, J. Sundström, E. Ingelsson, S. Basu, A. Larsson, P. Venge, and J. Ärnlöv, *New England Journal of Medicine*, 358, 2107–2116, 2008.

34. P. Hunter, P. Robbins, and D. Noble, The IUPS human hysiome project, *European Journal of Physiology*, 445, 1–9, 2002.

64

eEmergency Healthcare Informatics

E. Kyriacou
Frederick University

P. Constantinides
University of Warwick

A. Panayides
Imperial College

M.S. Pattichis
University of New Mexico

C.S. Pattichis
University of Cyprus

64.1 Introduction

The emerging development of emergency healthcare systems and services (eEmergency) in the last decade was made possible due to the recent advances in wireless and network technologies, linked with recent advances in nanotechnologies, compact biosensors, wearable devices and clothing, and pervasive and ubiquitous computing systems. These advances have a powerful impact in the provision of mHealth (mobile health), and eHealth services at large, and reshape the workflow and practices in the delivery of healthcare services [1,2]. The objective of this chapter is to provide a review of the status and challenges of eEmergency systems, covering both eEmergency management and response processes, and mobile health eEmergency systems.

One consistent challenge for emergency management and response is communication and information management [3–5]. Effective response requires a moment-to-moment situational analysis and real-time information to assess needs and available resources that can change suddenly and unexpectedly [5]. Accurate information from the field about the incident impacts the utilization and preparedness of resources such as emergency units, hospitals, and intensive care units. Similarly, information on available and accessible hospital, emergency units, and ambulance resources alters the management and disposition of victims at the scene [4].

The timely and effective way of handling emergency cases can prove essential for patient's recovery or even for patient's survival. Especially in cases of serious injuries of the head, the spinal cord, and internal organs, the way of transporting and generally the way of providing care are crucial for the future of the patient. Furthermore, during cardiac disease cases, much can be done today to stop a heart attack or resuscitate a victim of sudden cardiac death (SCD). Time is the enemy in the acute treatment of a heart attack or SCD. The first 60 min (the golden hour) are the most critical regarding the long-term patient outcome. Therefore, the ability to remotely monitor the patient and guide the paramedical staff in their management of the patient can be crucial. eEmergency becomes important in facilitating access to effective and specialist-directed care. Some benefits of prehospital transmitted ECG, for example, as documented by Giovas et al. [6], are the following: reduction of hospital delays, better triage, continuous monitoring, ECG data accessible for comparison, computer-aided analysis and decision making, and prehospital therapy in eligible subjects with acute myocardial infarction (AMI).

This chapter provides an overview of the main technological components of eEmergency systems. The chapter is organized as follows. Section 64.2 presents the eEmergency system enabling technologies covering the wireless transmission technologies, mobile computing technologies, biosignals, medical imaging, and video. In Section 64.3, protocols and processes for eEmergency management and response are covered. This is followed by a review of mobile health eEmergency systems in Section 64.4. Section 64.5 presents the concluding remarks and future challenges.

64.2 Enabling Technologies

64.2.1 Wireless Communication Networks and Standards

Mobile telemedicine systems are based on different types of wireless technologies depending on the target application. In general, systems are based on the following wireless technologies: well-established second-generation (2G), 2.5G and 3G, and recently 3.5G of mobile telecommunication systems, wireless local area networks (WLANs), mobile ad hoc networks (MANETs), wireless sensor networks (WSNs), and satellite links. Home/personal/body area networks also drive growth in mobile telemedicine systems. Long-term evolution (LTE) (toward 4G) and WiMax technologies are expected to significantly advance available wireless data rates.

Starting from voice call GSM (2G) in the early 1990s, the evolution of mobile telecommunication systems facilitates a continuous increase in available data rates as well as "always on" model (compared to original circuit-switch mode of GSM). iDEN (64 kbps), GPRS (171 kbps), and EDGE (384 kbps) are considered as 2.5G technologies, while 3G (W-CDMA, CDMA2000, TD-CDMA) enable a theoretical 14.4 Mbps. Nowadays, 3.5G (HSPA and HSPA+) extend the available data rates above 20 Mbps (56 Mbps in theory). LTE (4G) utilizing multiple in multiple out (MIMO) technologies target 100 Mbps in the downlink and 50 Mbps in the uplink. Coverage typically extends over 90% and 80% of a country region for GSM (2G) and 3G beyond systems, respectively. WLANs transmit and receive data over the air offering data speeds of up to 54 Mbps. However, WLAN coverage is limited up to a distance of about 100 m per cell (access point). Home/personal/body area networks allow connectivity of devices in the vicinity of tens of meters utilizing Bluetooth, RF, ZigBee, and Ultra-wideband technologies. WiMax, on the other hand, can provide broadband wireless access of 45 Mbps up to 50 km for fixed stations and 5–15 km for mobile stations. In this fashion, it can be used for wireless "metropolitan area networks" (WMANs). MANETs and WSNs do not require infrastructure acting as a gateway to a wired backbone network; instead, they interact on the move with geographically adjacent mobile nodes parting their network over the wireless medium. With satellite links, a variety of data transfer rates from 2.4 kbps up to 2×64 kbps and beyond can be supported. They provide worldwide coverage enabling the use over the sea or in areas with no other infrastructure. For more details regarding the aforementioned technologies, we refer to Reference 2.

64.2.2 Mobile Computing Platforms

The introduction of portable devices such as PDAs, smart phones, small-sized laptops, and pen-tablet PCs enables eEmergency system application developers to create more efficient systems with respect to computing power and functionality, which consume less power, and are more compact and smaller.

Such systems have already appeared in the last decade, and will certainly continue to appear in the coming years.

In a recent study, where mobile and fixed computer use by doctors and nurses on hospital wards was investigated, it was found that the choice of the device was related to clinical role, nature of the clinical task, and degree of mobility required [7]. Nurses' work and clinical tasks performed by doctors during ward rounds require highly mobile computer devices, and they showed a strong preference for generic computers on wheels (including laptops) over all other devices. Tablet PCs were selected by doctors for only a small proportion of clinical tasks. It should be noted that even when using mobile devices, clinicians completed a very low proportion of observed tasks at the bedside [7].

A systematic review of PDA usage surveys by healthcare providers was carried out by Garritty and coworkers [8]. It was documented that younger physicians and residents and those working in large and hospital-based practices are more likely to use a PDA. Moreover, it appeared that professional PDA use in healthcare settings involved more administrative and organizational tasks than those related to patient care. They concluded that physicians are likely accustomed to using a PDA; however, there is still a need to evaluate the effectiveness and efficiency of PDA-based applications [8].

Another exhaustive review of the existing literature research on the use of PDAs (from 1996 to 2008) among personnel and students in healthcare was carried out by Lindquist et al. [9]. This overview of the use of PDAs revealed a positive attitude toward the PDA, which was regarded as a feasible and convenient tool. The possibility of immediate access to medical information has the potential to improve patient care. However, there is a need for further intervention studies, randomized controlled trials, action research, and studies with various healthcare groups to identify its appropriate functions and software applications [9].

64.2.3 Biosignals

The biosignals usually collected in an eEmergency system include the following: ECG up to 12 leads, depending on the monitor used, oxygen saturation (SpO_2), capnography (CpO_2), heart rate (HR), noninvasive blood pressure (NIBP), invasive blood pressure (IP), temperature (Temp), respiration (Resp), and their corresponding trends and alarms based on preset settings. ECG signals are sampled at a rate of 200 samples/s at 12 bits/sample (at least) (depending on the monitor used), thus resulting in a generation of at least 2400 bits/s per ECG channel. SpO_2 and CpO_2 waveforms are sampled at a rate of 100 samples/s by 10 bit/sample, thus resulting in a generation of 1000 bits/s for one channel. Trends for SpO_2, HR, NIBP, BP, Temp, Resp, and monitor data are updated with a refresh rate of one per second, thus adding a small fraction of data to be transmitted approximately up to 200 bits/s.

The collection of biosignals [10–13], such as ECG, until now was performed using expensive devices that could only be handled and supported by medical personnel. More recently, the collection of biosignals, such as ECG, can be performed by very small devices. These are not always devices on their own but they might connect to a smart phone, PDA, laptop, or PC to display or send the signals, and usually have Bluetooth or GPRS connectivity to wirelessly transfer the signals. They might be wearable, have the shape and weight of a necklace, and so on. These devices will enable the use of wireless telemedicine systems almost anywhere and at less cost. Such devices can be used for home care purposes much easily than the standard medical devices.

Biosignal compression is very desirable for eEmergency applications or long-term recordings. Efficient compression algorithms achieve a reduction of the number of bits required to describe a biosignal that could facilitate data transmission. However, this must be done with great care without affecting the diagnostic loss of information. According to Hadjileontiadis [14], although new emerging data compression techniques with very promising results are seen in the recent years, some problems have not been entirely addressed. In particular, the lack of the following items are still under consideration: (i) widely adopted compression quality assurance criteria and standards, (ii) widely available benchmark biosignal databases, and (iii) interoperability of data acquisition and processing equipment, and exchange of compressed data between databases from different research groups and/or manufacturers because of their incompatibility.

The SCP-ECG (ISO/IEEE 11073), HL7 aECG, and DICOM-ECG are three widely used open standards facilitating the exchange of ECG signals. These three open standards are supported by the ECG toolkit, recently published by van Ettinger and coworkers [15]. In this paper, it is documented that SCP-ECG gives the smallest size of the file, requiring the smallest bandwidth; however, it is complex to implement; HL7 aECG supports XML textfiles (and it can be easily compressed by gzip, or any other compression utility), and is the preferred standard for exchanging and comparing ECGs required by the FDA for drug trials; DICOM allows integration of ECGs with other imaging modalities; however, very few DICOM viewers support the proper ECG display. Moreover, the need still exists to develop eHealth systems integrating the ISO/IEEE11073 SCP-ECG standard, and the EN13606 Electronic Healthcare Record (EHR) standard, thus facilitating an end-to-end standard-based solution, as it has recently been demonstrated in Reference 16.

64.2.4 Transmission of Digital Images

The use of digital images in medicine has benefited from the formation of the Digital Imaging and Communications in Medicine (DICOM) committee [17]. The committee was formed in 1983 by the American College of Radiology (ACR) and the National Equipment Manufacturers Association (NEMA). For still images, DICOM has adopted various JPEG variants such as lossless JPEG (JPEG-LS) [18] and JPEG 2000 [19].

We first consider lossless image compression methods that provide for exact reconstruction of the input images. Lossless image compression eliminates the need for diagnostic validation of compression artifacts [20,21]. Unfortunately, lossless methods provide limited compression ratios, usually ranging between 2 and 3.7 [22]. Lossy image compression methods can provide much better compression ratios. However, the use of lossy image compression requires a careful evaluation of the effect of compression artifacts on diagnostic performance [23]. While not directly relevant to diagnostic performance, lossy image compression of general images attempts to be perceptually lossless. Here, a compressed image is termed *perceptually lossless* if an (average) human observer cannot differentiate it from its uncompressed version. In general, optimal performance requires the study of the impact of lossy compression for different clinical scenarios.

A general lossy compression approach that can be directly applied to medical images is to use diagnostic regions of interest (ROIs). Here, the parts of an image that are of diagnostic interest will see little or no compression. On the other hand, the parts that are not of diagnostic interest can be compressed significantly. For example, if the ROI covers about 20% of the entire image, average compression ratios of about 15:1 have been reported using JPEG-LS, while an average compression ratio of only 2.58 was achieved when using the entire image as the ROI [24].

Similar to perceptually lossless compression for general images, another approach is to use lossy compression that does not allow clinicians to differentiate between the compressed image from the uncompressed. Clearly, if the uncompressed image cannot be identified, then the (clinical) visual inspection of the compressed images should not impact the diagnosis [24]. This technique leads to near lossless techniques where the uncompressed image differs from the original in only a small number of levels (±1, ±2 out of a possible 4096 levels). For comparison, JPEG-LS in lossless mode provides for an average compression ratio of 2.58 that improves to 3.83 in the near-lossless mode (±1 levels) [24]. In addition, for a ROI that covers 20% of the image region, the average compression ratio improves from 15.1 to 22.0 [24].

64.2.5 Transmission of Digital Video

The DICOM committee has adopted two MPEG-2 standards for digital video [25]. While adoption of these standards is inadequate for eEmergency applications, they do provide an important reference framework for frame sizes and frame rates for future applications. We will begin with the DICOM standards and conclude this section with specific recommendations for emerging and future applications.

We have the following DICOM standards [25]:

- MPEG2 MP@ML supports conversion from: (i) 525-line NTSC at a maximum size of 480×720 pixels at 29.97 frames per second (fps), and (ii) 625-line PAL at a maximum size of 576×720 pixels at 25 fps.
- MPEG2 MP@HL supports high definition TV (HDTV) formats with sizes of 720×1280 and 1080×1920 and frame rates from 25 to 60 fps.

The DICOM standard does not provide any guidelines for image and video compression. Furthermore, another limitation is the MPEG-2 requirement for constant delay method for frame synchronization [26,27]. The constant delay requirement is not supported by ATM networks, making it difficult to deliver real-time MPEG-2 video over ATM [27]. On the other hand, the transmission of offline video is still possible.

We distinguish among the requirements for real-time video transmission, offline video transmission, medical video and audio for diagnostic applications, and nondiagnostic video and audio. Real-time video transmission for diagnostic applications is clearly the most demanding. Offline video transmission is essentially limited by the requirement to provide patient–doctor interaction. Real-time diagnostic audio applications may include the transmission of stethoscope audio, or the transmission of the audio stream that accompanies the diagnostic video. Good-quality diagnostic audio at 38–128 kbps using Dolby AC-2 has been achieved, while MPEG-1 Layer 2 audio (32–256 kbps) or Dolby AC-3 (96–768 kbps) may also be used [27]. For nondiagnostic applications in video teleconferencing, H.261 (64 kbps–1.92 Mbps) and H.263 (15–64 kbps) may be acceptable [27]. A typical application will require a diagnostic audio and video bitstream, in addition to a standard teleconferencing bitstream. Digital video modalities include real-time patient video and ultrasound video.

Owing to the high bandwidth requirements and the frame synchronization problem, successful methods for real-time diagnostic video transmission will most likely require the adoption of the MPEG-4 part 10 standard (or H.264/AVC standard). The frame synchronization problem is alleviated since MPEG-4 part 2 via the use of timestamps on each frame [28,29]. A possible method for achieving acceptable video compression for diagnostic purposes may be possible through the use of object-based encoding and decoding. In object-based encoding and decoding, different bitrates are allocated to different parts of the digital video, according to the level of diagnostic importance. The advantage of this approach is that it can significantly reduce the required bandwidth while maintaining high-quality video images of the regions of diagnostic interest. As an example, in the transmission of patient video, the transmission of the face and injured parts are of far more diagnostic importance than the background. For stroke risk assessment, the most important diagnostic regions include the atherosclerotic plaque and the arterial walls [30]. A disadvantage of object-based coding is that it is not always clear which part of the video is of diagnostic importance. This obstacle can be overcome by letting the users interactively select the ROIs.

For eEmergency applications, the DICOM standard is clearly insufficient. Real-time video conferencing requires the adoption of H.264/AVC technologies and diagnostically relevant metrics. Wireless video transmission also requires that we provide bandwidth requirements for specific clinical scenarios and evidence of error-resilient behavior.

64.3 Protocols and Processes for eEmergency Management and Response

64.3.1 Importance of Emergency Management and Response

Research on medical informatics has examined in depth the role of accurate and real-time information on effective emergency management and response [31–34]. In particular, research in this area in combination with research in computer science has led to the development of the so-called smart devices, third-generation wireless connectivity, and positioning technologies, all of which have application in emergency management and response because they are location-aware, that is, they combine timely, clinical information with accurate geographic information. For example, geo-position tracking and smart devices have been tested on soldiers and medics in the military battlefield [35]. Ambulances have been linked via wireless communication devices to the Internet to transmit and relay clinical data to emergency departments while in transit [36]. In addition, recent advances in triage tagging technology have focused on the use of mobile wireless data acquisition to individually identify and track victims of disasters by assigning a unique identifier to each individual and linking that identifier with triage status [37,38]. For example, the patient barcode registration system developed in the Netherlands has linked patient identification and registration data with out-of-hospital and in-hospital medical data. By scanning patient wristbands at various locations (emergency site, ambulance unit arrival, hospital location), the system can passively track and provide the approximate locations of patients [39,40].

These technologies are being evaluated to improve and enhance patient care and tracking; foster greater provider safety; enhance incident management at the scene and coordination of emergency medical services and hospital resources; and greatly enhance informatics support at the scene and at receiving emergency departments and hospitals.

64.3.2 Challenge of Coordination: Role of Standardized Priority Dispatch Protocols

Despite these advances, however, many of the logistical problems faced in emergencies are not caused by shortages of medical and technological resources, but rather from failures to coordinate their distribution [41], with significant possibilities for error and destruction, as occurred at New York's World Trade Center command post on September 11, 2001 [42,43].

To address the challenge of coordination, emergency dispatch centers around the world are increasingly using some form of priority dispatch protocol when handling emergency calls. The key objective behind these protocols is to ensure that the right response is sent to the right incident at the right time in the right way and to carry out the right procedures until professional help arrives [44].

Over the last 30 years or so, organizations such as the European Emergency Number Association (http://www.eena.org) and the National Academies for Emergency Dispatch in North America (http://www.emergencydispatch.org) have established standards for the development of priority dispatch protocols with which to help the coordination of medical and technological resources toward the effective management and response to emergency incidents. The most popular system of priority dispatch protocols is the medical priority dispatch system (MPDS), developed by the National Academies for Emergency Dispatch in collaboration with the National Association of Emergency Management Physicians, the American Society for Testing and Materials, the American College of Emergency Physicians, the U.S. Department of Transportation, the National Institutes of Health, and the American Medical Association. The original set of protocols contained 29 sets of two 8-inch-by-5-inch cards. Each caller complaint was listed in alphabetical order, as they are today, and reflected either a symptom (e.g., abdominal pain, burns, cardiac/respiratory arrest) or an incident (e.g., electrocution, drowning, or traffic injury accident). The core card contained three color-coded areas: key questions, prearrival instructions, and dispatch priorities. The MPDS has since gone through 18 revisions to reflect advances in medicine, such as the addition of chest compressions prior to any other form of cardiopulmonary resuscitation (CPR), and it shares the stage with protocol designed for police and fire dispatch centers. The MPDS now contains 34 chief complaint protocols, case entry and exit information, call termination scripts, and additional verbatim instruction protocols for ambulance and emergency dispatch, cardiopulmonary resuscitation, childbirth assistance, tracheostomy airway and breathing, and the Heimlich maneuver. The MPDS is now used by more than 3000 emergency dispatch centers and in 23 countries worldwide, including Great Britain, Ireland, Germany, Italy, Azerbaijan, New Zealand, and Australia.

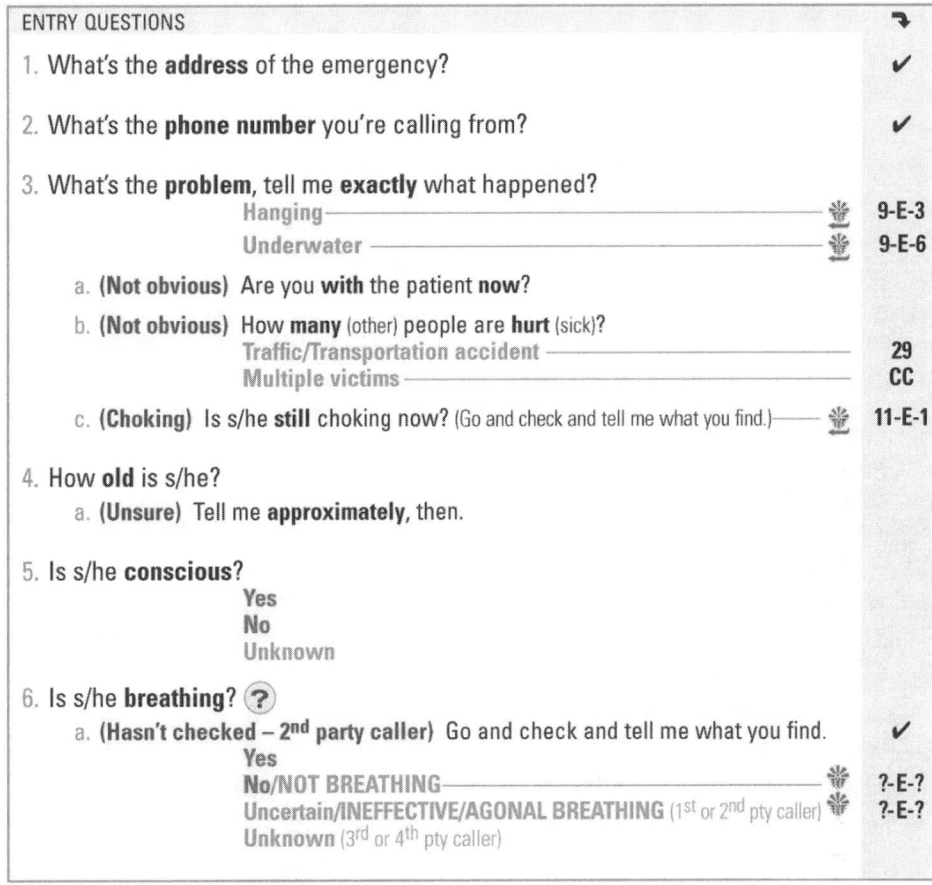

For use under MPDS® licence agreement only. © 2005 Priority Dispatch Corp. All rights reserved.

FIGURE 64.1 Case entry protocol for priority medical dispatch.

Priority Dispatch Corporation is licensed to design and publish the MPDS and associated support products (http://www.prioritydispatch.net). Figure 64.1 provides an illustration of the set of case entry questions employed in MPDS leading to an identification of a convulsion/fitting incident (Figure 64.2), and to a set of prearrival instructions (Figure 64.3).

As evident from the table in Figure 64.1, the process starts with the dispatcher asking a set of so-called Entry Questions to establish the exact location of the incident, the phone number of the caller, the exact type of problem, age of the victim, and whether they are conscious and breathing. These questions are then followed by more specific questions according to the answers received, through which the dispatcher identifies the type of "Chief Complaint"—in this case, a "convulsions/fitting" incident (see Figure 64.2). Depending on the answers to such questions as "does s/he have a history of heart problems" and "is s/he an epileptic or ever had a fit before," the dispatcher assigns a severity score to the call according to different "determinant descriptors," which allow him/her to categorize the call into one of four priority dispatch levels from A to D. Level A would indicate that the victim is in a stable, nonemergency condition, thus, not requiring immediate assistance, especially if units are required for other incidents. Level B would indicate a response, but still not immediate, whereas levels C and D would indicate the need for immediate responses with an advanced life support ambulance (see Figure 64.2). After having triaged the call and dispatched an ambulance, the dispatcher would continue to give instructions to the caller until the ambulance arrived at the scene of the incident. Depending on answers to such questions

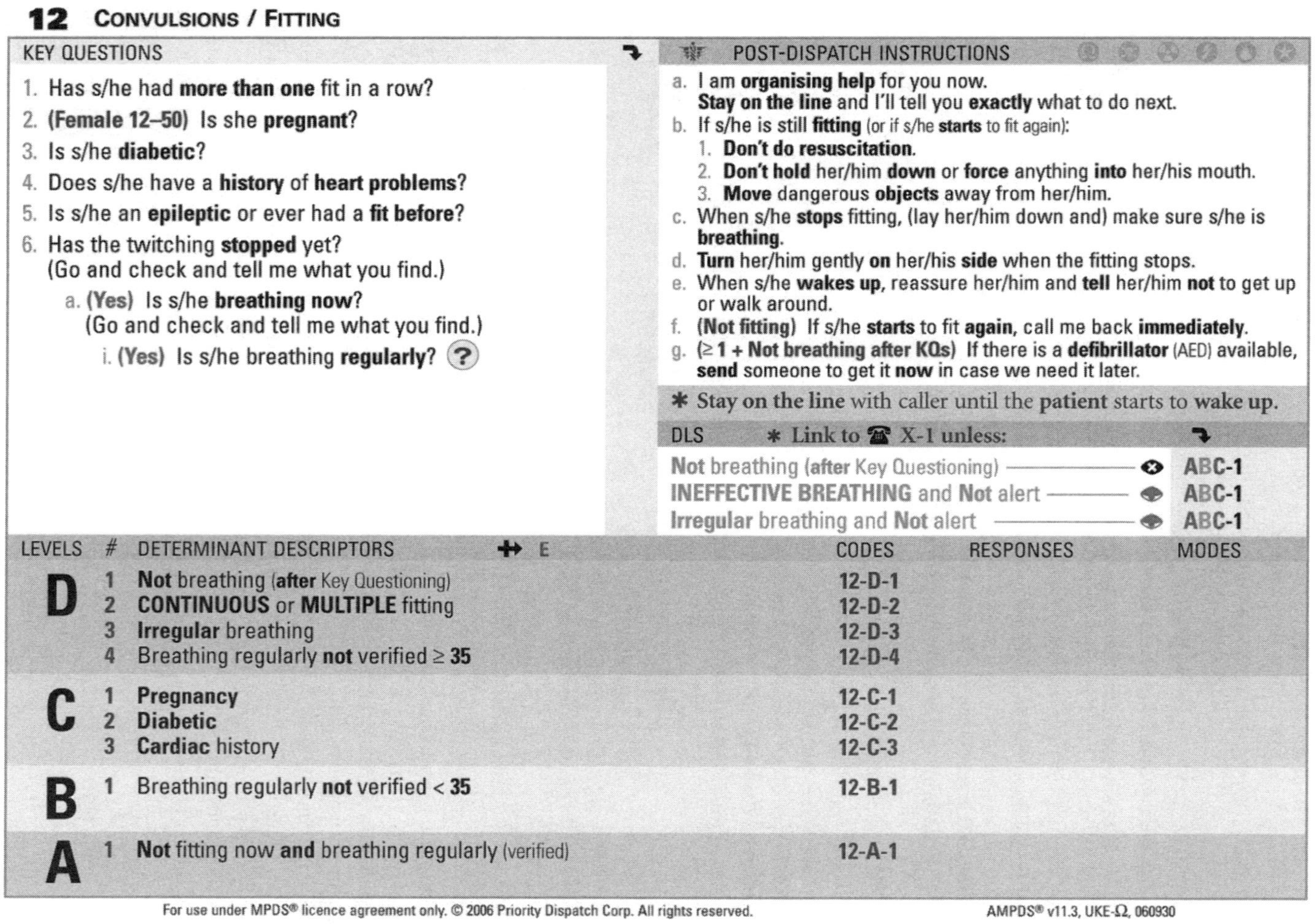

12 CONVULSIONS / FITTING

KEY QUESTIONS

1. Has s/he had **more than one** fit in a row?
2. **(Female 12–50)** Is she **pregnant**?
3. Is s/he **diabetic**?
4. Does s/he have a **history** of **heart problems**?
5. Is s/he an **epileptic** or ever had a **fit before**?
6. Has the twitching **stopped** yet?
   (Go and check and tell me what you find.)
   a. **(Yes)** Is s/he **breathing now**?
      (Go and check and tell me what you find.)
      i. **(Yes)** Is s/he breathing **regularly**? ?

POST-DISPATCH INSTRUCTIONS

a. I am **organising help** for you now.
   Stay on the line and I'll tell you **exactly** what to do next.
b. If s/he is still **fitting** (or if s/he **starts** to fit again):
   1. **Don't do resuscitation.**
   2. **Don't hold** her/him **down** or **force** anything **into** her/his mouth.
   3. **Move** dangerous **objects** away from her/him.
c. When s/he **stops** fitting, (lay her/him down and) make sure s/he is **breathing**.
d. **Turn** her/him gently **on** her/his **side** when the fitting stops.
e. When s/he **wakes up**, reassure her/him and **tell** her/him **not** to get up or walk around.
f. **(Not fitting)** If s/he **starts** to fit **again**, call me back **immediately**.
g. **(≥ 1 + Not breathing after KQs)** If there is a **defibrillator** (AED) available, **send** someone to get it **now** in case we need it later.

*** Stay on the line** with caller until the **patient** starts to **wake up**.

DLS *** Link to ☎ X-1 unless:**

Not breathing (**after** Key Questioning) —— ABC-1
INEFFECTIVE BREATHING and **Not** alert —— ABC-1
Irregular breathing and **Not** alert —— ABC-1

LEVELS	#	DETERMINANT DESCRIPTORS	CODES	RESPONSES	MODES
D	1	**Not** breathing (**after** Key Questioning)	12-D-1		
	2	**CONTINUOUS** or **MULTIPLE** fitting	12-D-2		
	3	**Irregular** breathing	12-D-3		
	4	Breathing regularly **not** verified ≥ **35**	12-D-4		
C	1	**Pregnancy**	12-C-1		
	2	**Diabetic**	12-C-2		
	3	**Cardiac** history	12-C-3		
B	1	Breathing regularly **not** verified < **35**	12-B-1		
A	1	**Not** fitting now **and** breathing regularly (verified)	12-A-1		

AMPDS® v11.3, UKE-Ω, 060930

FIGURE 64.2 Chief complaint protocol for convulsions/fitting.

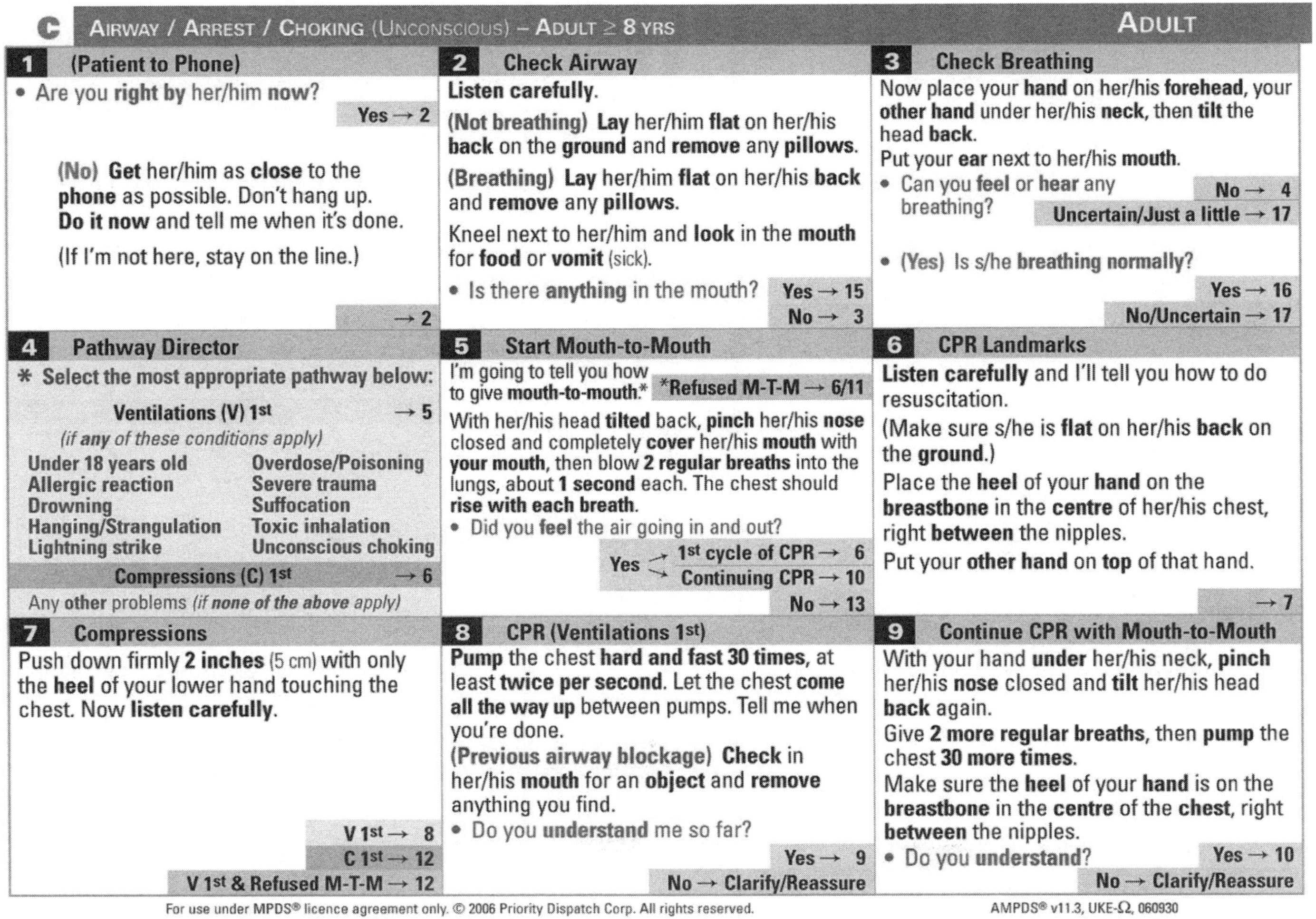

C AIRWAY / ARREST / CHOKING (UNCONSCIOUS) – ADULT ≥ 8 YRS | **ADULT**

1 (Patient to Phone)

- Are you right by her/him now?
  Yes → 2

(No) Get her/him as close to the phone as possible. Don't hang up. Do it now and tell me when it's done.

(If I'm not here, stay on the line.)
→ 2

2 Check Airway

Listen carefully.

(Not breathing) Lay her/him flat on her/his back on the ground and remove any pillows.

(Breathing) Lay her/him flat on her/his back and remove any pillows.

Kneel next to her/him and look in the mouth for food or vomit (sick).

- Is there anything in the mouth?
  Yes → 15
  No → 3

3 Check Breathing

Now place your hand on her/his forehead, your other hand under her/his neck, then tilt the head back.

Put your ear next to her/his mouth.

- Can you feel or hear any breathing?   No → 4   Uncertain/Just a little → 17
- (Yes) Is s/he breathing normally?
  Yes → 16
  No/Uncertain → 17

4 Pathway Director

* Select the most appropriate pathway below:

Ventilations (V) 1st → 5
(if any of these conditions apply)

Under 18 years old	Overdose/Poisoning
Allergic reaction	Severe trauma
Drowning	Suffocation
Hanging/Strangulation	Toxic inhalation
Lightning strike	Unconscious choking

Compressions (C) 1st → 6

Any other problems *(if none of the above apply)*

5 Start Mouth-to-Mouth

I'm going to tell you how to give mouth-to-mouth.*   *Refused M-T-M → 6/11

With her/his head tilted back, pinch her/his nose closed and completely cover her/his mouth with your mouth, then blow 2 regular breaths into the lungs, about 1 second each. The chest should rise with each breath.

- Did you feel the air going in and out?
  Yes → 1st cycle of CPR → 6
       → Continuing CPR → 10
  No → 13

6 CPR Landmarks

Listen carefully and I'll tell you how to do resuscitation.

(Make sure s/he is flat on her/his back on the ground.)

Place the heel of your hand on the breastbone in the centre of her/his chest, right between the nipples.

Put your other hand on top of that hand.
→ 7

7 Compressions

Push down firmly 2 inches (5 cm) with only the heel of your lower hand touching the chest. Now listen carefully.

V 1st → 8
C 1st → 12
V 1st & Refused M-T-M → 12

8 CPR (Ventilations 1st)

Pump the chest hard and fast 30 times, at least twice per second. Let the chest come all the way up between pumps. Tell me when you're done.

(Previous airway blockage) Check in her/his mouth for an object and remove anything you find.

- Do you understand me so far?
  Yes → 9
  No → Clarify/Reassure

9 Continue CPR with Mouth-to-Mouth

With your hand under her/his neck, pinch her/his nose closed and tilt her/his head back again.

Give 2 more regular breaths, then pump the chest 30 more times.

Make sure the heel of your hand is on the breastbone in the centre of the chest, right between the nipples.

- Do you understand?
  Yes → 10
  No → Clarify/Reassure

AMPDS® v11.3, UKE-Ω, 060930

FIGURE 64.3 Ambulance prearrival instruction protocol.

as "is s/he breathing?" the dispatcher would give instructions to check the airway, to check breathing, and to administer cardiopulmonary resuscitation (see Figure 64.3, steps 1–9).

64.3.3 Computer-Aided Medical Dispatch Systems

Since the early 1990s, there has been a consistent effort to implement the MPDS and similar priority dispatch protocols through computer-based systems in an effort to automate processes and further minimize human error rates [45]. We have carried out a literature review of empirical case studies illustrating the advantages and disadvantages of computer-aided dispatch systems using priority dispatch protocols.

The search was initially carried out in the database *Science Direct* using the term "Computer-aided Medical Dispatch Systems" across "All fields." We limited our search to the years 2000–2010 to focus on computer and telecommunication developments of the last decade. The search resulted in 169 articles. Many of these articles were found in subject areas not related to emergency care so the results were filtered according to the following subjects: "Computer Science" + "Decision Sciences" + "Medicine and Dentistry" + "Nursing and Health Professions." This search resulted in 84 articles. Then, we further filtered our results down to 38 articles, by keeping only articles from journal titles directly related to emergency care, including *Resuscitation* (13), *Prehospital Emergency Care* (9), *Air Medical Journal* (4), *Annals of Emergency Medicine* (4), *International Journal of Medical Informatics* (4), *American Journal of Preventive Medicine* (1), *Disaster Management & Response* (1), *Journal of the American Medical Informatics Association* (1), and *The Journal of Emergency Medicine* (1). To triangulate our filtered results, we carried out a further search in the databases *PubMed* and the *Cumulative Index to Nursing & Allied Health Literature* (via EBSCOhost), using the same term "Computer-aided Medical Dispatch Systems" and came up with five more articles. From these combined results, we excluded review and editorial articles that did not report on empirical research findings on the direct or indirect impact of computer-aided medical dispatch systems on the outcome of emergency care provided by emergency teams, including the success rate of dispatchers' decisions on the severity of emergency calls. Table 64.1 lists the 10 most representative articles found in our literature review.

The key findings reported in these empirical case studies show that, despite the evident advantages of computer-aided dispatch systems utilizing priority dispatch protocols, effective emergency management and response cannot be minimized in ritualistic behavior through "blind" protocol-following [56,57]. Protocols should be used as standardized, guidance tools, but emergency professionals should not rely on them to complete their tasks. This is because it is impossible to create workflow scenarios that will adequately handle every type of call a dispatcher will take. Further, the criteria in these workflow guides are not based on a strict yes or no answer and the questions are listed so that dispatchers can easily guide a caller into follow-up questions, but not necessarily to make a final diagnosis. More importantly, the effective management of emergency incidents is very much dependent on team characteristics such as, how long have emergency team members spent on the same team, whether team members share the same levels of knowledge and expertise in dealing with different incidents, whether team members trust one another to complete a task successfully, and whether a task is an easy routine or involves a more complex scenario such as a mass accident [58,59].

64.4 mHealth eEmergency Systems

Technological applications for emergency healthcare support appeared in the literature more than a 100 years ago [60] where Einthoven demonstrated a telemedicine application by connecting his lab with the University Hospital in Holland at a distance of 1.5 km. Since then, many studies have been presented. Recent advances in mobile communications have also impacted mHealth eEmergency systems. In this section, we present a literature review for studies published in journals related to mobile systems for emergency healthcare support (eEmergency, mHealth systems) that appeared since 2000.

TABLE 64.1 Empirical Case Studies on the Impact of Computer-Aided Dispatch Systems in Emergency Management and Response

Author/Year	Country of Study	Key Objective	Key Findings
1. Garza et al. 2003 [46]	USA	Analyze the accuracy of dispatchers in predicting cardiac arrest through computer-aided dispatch protocols and assess the effect of the caller party on dispatcher accuracy.	A higher level of medical training may improve dispatch accuracy for predicting cardiac arrest. The type of calling party influenced the dispatcher-assigned condition.
2. Dale et al. 2003 [47]	UK	Investigate the potential impact for ambulance services of telephone assessment and computer-aided triage for nonserious emergency calls as classified by ambulance service call takers.	Telephone assessment and computer-aided triage can identify nonserious calls, which could have a significant impact on emergency ambulance dispatch rates. Nurses were more likely than paramedics to assess calls as requiring an alternative response to emergency ambulance dispatch, but the extent to which this relates to aspects of training and professional perspective is unclear.
3. Michael and Sporer 2005 [48]	USA	Evaluate a group of computer-aided dispatch protocols defined as requiring advanced life support (ALS) intervention.	There was variation in clinical practice toward ALS intervention due to the more precautionary approach to care found in this computer-aided dispatch system.
4. Deakin et al. 2006 [49]	UK	Examine patients with acute coronary syndrome (ACS) to identify whether a computer-aided dispatch system enabled dispatchers to allocate an appropriate emergency response.	The system was found not to be an appropriate tool designed for clinical diagnosis, and its extension into this field does not enable accurate identification of patients with ACS. However, the system can be used to guide the appropriate level of clinical response to different emergency incidents.
5. Flynn et al. 2006 [50]	Australia	Undertake a sensitivity/specificity analysis to determine the ability of a computer-aided dispatch system to detect cardiac arrest.	The system correctly identified 76.7% of cardiac arrest cases, but the number of false negatives suggests that there is room for improvement to maximize chances for survival in out-of-hospital cardiac arrest.
6. Reilly 2006 [51]	USA	Assess the relationship between dispatches of a cardiac nature through a computer-aided dispatch system, and the actual clinical diagnosis as determined by an emergency department physician.	The system may over-triage emergency medical responses to cardiac emergencies. This can result in the only advanced life support unit in the community being unavailable in certain situations. Future studies should be conducted to determine what level of over-triage is appropriate when using such systems.
7. Feldman et al. 2006 [52]	Canada	To determine the relationship between a computer-aided dispatch system and an out-of-hospital patient acuity scale.	The system exhibits at least moderate sensitivity and specificity for detecting high acuity of illness or injury. This performance analysis may be used to identify target protocols for future improvements
8. Clawson et al. 2007 [53]	UK	Establish the accuracy of the emergency medical dispatcher's decisions to override the automated computer-aided dispatch system's triage recommendations based on at-scene paramedic-applied transport acuity determinations and cardiac arrest findings.	Automated, protocol-based call taking is more accurate and consistent than the subjective, anecdotal, or experience-based determinations made by individual emergency medical dispatchers.

TABLE 64.1 (continued)   Empirical Case Studies on the Impact of Computer-Aided Dispatch Systems in Emergency Management and Response

Author/Year	Country of Study	Key Objective	Key Findings
9. Buck et al. 2009 [54]	USA	Assess the diagnostic accuracy of the current national protocol guiding dispatcher questioning of emergency callers to identify stroke.	Dispatcher recognition of stroke calls using a computer-aided dispatch system algorithm is suboptimal, with failure to identify more than half of stroke patients as likely stroke. Revisions to the current national dispatcher structured interview and symptom identification algorithm for stroke may facilitate more accurate recognition of stroke by emergency medical dispatchers.
10. Johnson and Sporer (forthcoming) [55]	USA	Evaluate the number of emergency dispatches per cardiac arrest in cardiac arrest and noncardiac arrest determinants found in a computer-aided dispatch system.	The system was designed to detect cardiac arrest with high sensitivity, leading to a significant degree of mistriage. The number of dispatches for each cardiac arrest may be a useful way to quantify the degree of mistriage and optimize emergency dispatch.

64.4.1 Overview

The MEDLINE and IEEE Explore databases were searched with the following keywords: wireless telemedicine emergency, wireless telemedicine ambulance, wireless telemedicine disaster, wireless ambulance, wireless disaster, and wireless emergency. The number of journal papers found to be published under these categories is around 220. Out of these, a total of 40 applications were selected and are briefly summarized in Tables 64.2 through 64.4. We tried to select systems that cover the whole spectrum of medical informatics applications for emergency cases that have been published in the last decade.

These papers are grouped under the following eEmergency areas as ambulance systems (see Table 64.2), rural health center systems and in-hospital systems (see Table 64.3), and civilian systems (see Table 64.4). The headings in these tables are coded as follows: ECG; other biosignals for biosignals such as SpO_2, CO_2, heart rate, blood pressure, temperature, respiration, and others; images for SCN: incident/patient scenery, x-ray, CT: computed tomography imaging, and MRI: magnetic resonance imaging; video for SCN: incident/patient scenery, US: ultrasound; and communication link for WT: GSM/GPRS/3G, SAT: satellite, WLAN: wireless LAN, BLUET: Bluetooth, and SENSN: sensor networks.

As illustrated in Table 64.2, most of the mHealth eEmergency systems fall under the category of ambulance systems. These systems exploit the wireless telephone connectivity GSM/GPRS/3G. Almost all of the systems supported ECG transmission, and other biosignals, whereas a few recent studies supported the ultrasound video transmission. Systems tabulated in Table 64.3 for eEmergency systems in rural health centers and in-hospital cover mainly the transmission of medical images, including x-ray, CT, and MRI, as well as two applications that supported the ultrasound video transmission.

Civilian eEmergency systems cover mainly the transmission of ECG in emergency cases (see Table 64.4). The system introduced by Virgin Atlantic Airways in 2006 [95] supports the monitoring of a passenger's blood pressure, pulse rate, temperature, ECG, blood oxygen, and carbon dioxide levels in emergency cases in the aircraft via the satellite communications link. Etihad Airlines has recently also announced the installation of an eEmergency system for monitoring the condition of passengers who display signs of illness that might require immediate medical attention [96].

TABLE 64.2 Selected mHealth eEmergency Ambulance Systems

Application Area	Author	Year	ECG	Other Biosignals	Images	Video	Communication Link	Comments
Ambulance systems	Karlsten and Sjoqvist [61]	00	√	√			WT	Triage support
	Yan Xiao et al. [62]	00	√	√		SCN	WT	Ambulance neurological examination support
	Anantharaman and Swee Han [63]	01	√	√			WT	Prehospital support
	Rodrvguez et al. [64]	01	√	√			WT	Cardiac arrest treatment
	Istepanian et al. [65,66]	01	√	√	SCN		WT	Transmission of ECG data and still images for emergency use. Compression of ECG using a wavelet compression method
	Pavlopoulos et al. [36]	01	√	√			WT	Portable teleconsultation medical device
	Chiarugi et al. [67]	03 05	√				WT	Transmission of 12-lead ECG to support ambulance and rural health centers emergencies (HygeiaNet)
	Garrett et al. [68]	03				US	WT	Echocardiogram transmission in cardiac emergency from an ambulance in transit to a tertiary care facility
	Kyriacou et al. [69]	03	√	√	SCN		WT	Wireless transmission of biosignals and images from a moving ambulance vehicle to a central hospital
	Chu and Ganz [70]	04	√		SCN	SCN	WT	Trauma care through transmission of patient's video, medical images and ECG
	Clarke [71]	04	√				WT	Wireless connection to sensors and transmission of data from an ambulance
	Clemmensen et al. [72]	05	√				WT	Transmission of ECG signals directly to a cardiologist's PDA to improve time to reperfusion
	Campbell et al. [73]	05	√				WT	Wireless transmission of ECG from the emergency scenery to the department and then through a wireless LAN to the on-call cardiologist who is carrying a PDA
	Giovas et al. [6]	06	√				WT	Wireless transmission of 12-lead ECG from a moving ambulance vehicle to a central hospital
	Sillesen et al. [74]	06	√				WT	Transmission of ECG signals to a cardiologist's PDA to improve time for PCI treatment
	Kontaxakis et al. [75]	06				US	WT	Tele-echography system and 3D-ultrasound
	Garawi et al. [76]	06				US	WT	Tele-operated robotic system for mobile tele-echography (OTELO-Project)
	Tsapatsoulis et al. [77]	07				US	WT	Low-bitrate ultrasound video coding based on the region of interest
	Doukas and Maglogiannis [78]	08				√	WT	Adaptive transmission of medical video and images using scalable video coding and context aware scheme based on the case needs
	Panayides et al. [79]	08				US	WT	Efficient H.264 coding of medical ultrasound video over wireless channels

Note: SCN, incident/patient scenery; US, ultrasound; WT, GSM/GPRS/3G.

TABLE 64.3 Selected mHealth eEmergency Rural Health Center Systems and In-Hospital Systems

Application Area	Author	Year	ECG	Other Biosignals	Images	Video	Communication. Link	Comments
					Data Transmitted			
Rural health center	Strode et al. [80]	03				US	SAT	Examination of trauma using focused abdominal sonography (military)
	Chiarugi et al. [67], Kouroubali [81]	03 05	√				WT	Transmission of 12-lead ECG to support ambulance and rural health centers emergencies (HygeiaNet)
	Kyriacou et al. [82]	03	√	√	SCN		WT	Wireless transmission of biosignals and images from a moving ambulance vehicle to a central hospital
	Garawi et al. [76], Vieyres et al. [83], Canero et al. [84]	06				US	WT SAT	Tele-operated robotic system for mobile tele-echography (OTELO-Project)
	Reponen et al. [85]	00			CT		WT	Transmission of CT scans using GSM and PDAs. Images transmitted to a neuroradiologist for a preliminary consultation
	Oguchi et al. [86],	01			CT		WT	Use of a personal handyphone system to transmit CT images using a web-based application
	Voskarides et al. [87], Hadjinikolaou et al. [88]	03			X-ray		WT	Transmission of x-ray images in emergency orthopedics
In-hospital systems	Hall et al. [89]	03					WT WLAN	Wireless access to electronic patient record
	Pagani et al. [90]	03			CT		WLAN	Web-based transmission of cranial CT images
	Lorincz et al. [91]	04	√				SENSN	Sensor networks for emergency response. System tested using two vital signs monitors
	Campbell et al. [73]	05	√				WLAN	Wireless transmission of ECG from the emergency scenery to the department and then through a wireless LAN to the on-call cardiologist who is carrying a PDA
	Kim et al. [92]	05			CT MRI		WLAN	Transmission of CT and MRI images through a PDA and wireless high-bandwidth net to neurosurgeons
	Kim et al. [93]	09				√	WLAN	Transmission of video and audio to consult on the treatment of acute stroke patients

Note: CT, computed tomography; MRI, magnetic resonance imaging; SCN, incident/patient scenery; US, ultrasound; WT, GSM/GPRS/3G; SAT, satellite; WLAN, wireless LAN.

TABLE 64.4   Selected mHealth eEmergency Civilian Systems

Application Area	Author	Year	ECG	Other Biosignals	Images	Video	Communication Link	Comments
Civilian systems	Salvador et al. [94]	05	√				WT	Transmission of ECG and other parameters to support patients with chronic heart diseases during an emergency case
	Virgin Atlantic Airways [95]	06	√	√	SCN		SAT	The Tempus 2000 device will be used for monitoring a passenger's blood pressure, pulse rate, temperature, ECG, blood oxygen, and carbon dioxide levels in emergency cases in the aircraft
	Etihad Airways [96]	10	√	√	SCN		SAT	Tempus IC will be installed on long-haul aircraft flights for monitoring the condition of passengers who display signs of illness that might require immediate medical attention
	Maki et al. [97]	04	√				SENSN	Wireless monitoring of sensors on persons that need continuous monitoring; when an emergency occurs the specialized personnel listens a sound alarm or a notification through mobile phone
	Palmer et al. [98]	05		√			WLAN	Wireless blood pulse oximeter system for mass casualty events designed to operate in WiFi hotspots. The system is capable of tracking hundreds of patients. Suitable for disaster monitoring
	Lenert et al. [99]	05	√				WLAN	Medical care during mass casualty events, transmission of signals, and alerts monitor
	Nakamura et al. [100]	03					WLAN	Wireless emergency telemedicine LAN with over 30 km distance coverage, used in the Japan Alps for monitoring mountain climbers in emergency cases
	Lee et al. [101]	07	√	√			WT	Patient continuous monitoring/alert in case of emergency. Signals are transmitted through GSM and acquisition to device is through Bluetooth
	Chin-Teng et al. [102]	10	√				BLUTH	A wearable system to detect atrial fibrillation using expert systems

Note: SCN, incident/patient scenery; WT, GSM/GPRS/3G; SAT, satellite; WLAN, wireless LAN; BLUTH, bluetooth; SENSN, sensor networks.

64.4.2 Case Studies

Two case studies were selected and presented here to show examples of the evolution of medical informatics used for emergency healthcare support.

Case Study 1: Emergency Telemedicine: The Ambulance and Emergency-112 Projects

The availability of prompt and expert medical care can meaningfully improve healthcare services at understaffed rural or remote areas. The provision of effective emergency telemedicine and home monitoring solutions are the major fields of interest of Ambulance HC1001 and Emergency-112 HC4027 projects that were partially funded by the European Commission/DGXIII Telematics Application Programme.

The aim of the Ambulance [36] project was the development of a portable emergency telemedicine device that supports real-time transmission of critical biosignals as well as still images of the patient using initially the GSM link, and then the GPRS, and 3G links. This device can be used by paramedics or nonspecialized personnel that handle emergency cases, to get directions from expert physicians. The system comprises of two different modules: (i) the mobile unit, which is located in an ambulance vehicle near the patient, and (ii) the consultation unit, which is located at the hospital site and can be used by the experts to give directions. The system allows telediagnosis, long distance support, and teleconsultation of mobile healthcare providers by experts located at an emergency coordination center or a specialized hospital.

Emergency-112 [103,104], which was the extension of the Ambulance project, aimed for the development of an integrated portable medical device for emergency telemedicine. The system enables the transmission of critical biosignals (ECG, BP, HR, SpO_2, temperature) and still images of the patient, from the emergency site to an emergency call center, thus enabling physicians to direct prehospital care in a more efficient way, improving patients outcome and reducing mortality. The system was designed to operate over several communication links such as satellite, GSM/GPRS/3G/HSPA, POTS, ADSL, and ISDN. In Emergency-112, emphasis was given on maximizing the system's future potential application, through the utilization of several communication links (both fixed and wireless), as well as through the increase of the overall system's usability, focusing on advanced user interface and ergonomics. The system comprises of two different modules: (i) the patient unit, which is the unit located near the patient and which can operate automatically over several communication means and has several operating features (depending on the case used), and (ii) the physician's unit, which is the unit located near the expert doctor and which can operate over several communication links (depending on the place where the expert doctor is located). A snapshot from the transmitted biosignals between the two units can be seen in Figure 64.4. This system was further expanded through an Interreg III Archimed project called "Intermed." The current version of the portable unit of the system titled "Abaris" is shown in Figure 64.5. According to Greek mythology, "Abaris" was an ancient magician who had the gift to travel from place to place on his arrow and cure people. The new system consists of a "Welch Allyn" monitor that is connected to a netbook that has the software and the control of the unit. The communication link is achieved via a "Vodafone" 3G modem.

The final system was used in emergency healthcare provision via different scenario: in ambulance vehicle, in rural health centers, in navigating ships, and others.

Case Study 2: Wireless Ultrasound Video Transmission Using H.264/AVC for Emergency Telemedicine

The second system presented facilitates the wireless transmission of ultrasound video for emergency healthcare support. In this case, we present a diagnostically driven system for the transmission of wireless ultrasound video of the carotid artery using H.264/AVC [105].

Unique requirements associated with the transmission of medical video over bitrate-limited error-prone wireless channels dictate that careful planning should precede the actual development of such systems. Source encoding should match the available bitrate, while adaptation to varying network's conditions when streaming in real time may prove particularly efficient. Yet, delay, jitter, and packet losses introduced by wireless channels may make the transmitted data clinically unacceptable. Hence,

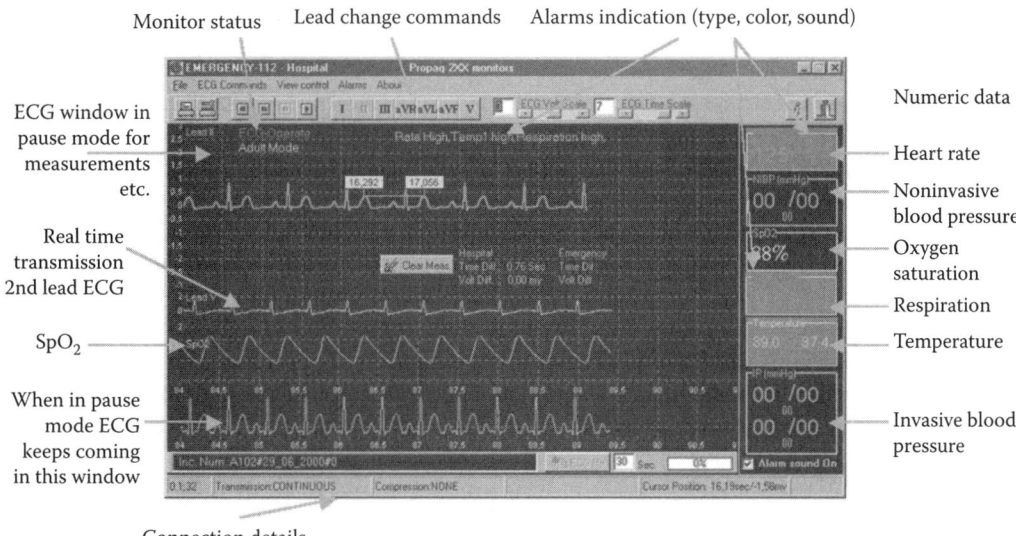

Monitor status   Lead change commands   Alarms indication (type, color, sound)

ECG window in pause mode for measurements etc.

Real time transmission 2nd lead ECG

SpO₂

When in pause mode ECG keeps coming in this window

Connection details

Numeric data

Heart rate

Noninvasive blood pressure

Oxygen saturation

Respiration

Temperature

Invasive blood pressure

FIGURE 64.4 eEmergency system biosignal transmission from the mobile unit (from the location of the incident or from the ambulance) to the base unit (that is installed usually in the hospital).

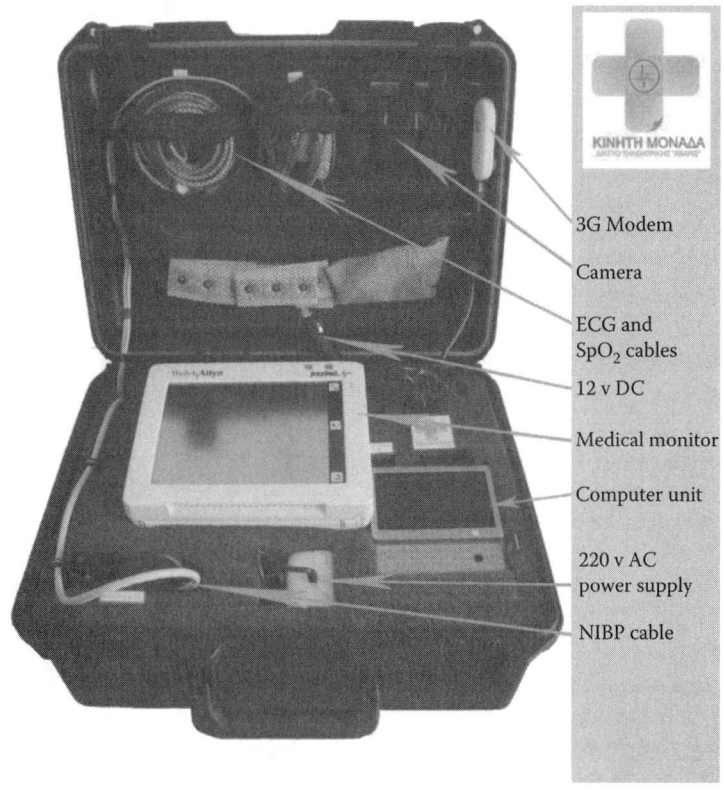

3G Modem

Camera

ECG and SpO₂ cables

12 v DC

Medical monitor

Computer unit

220 v AC power supply

NIBP cable

FIGURE 64.5 The mobile unit of the "Abaris" eEmergency ambulance system.

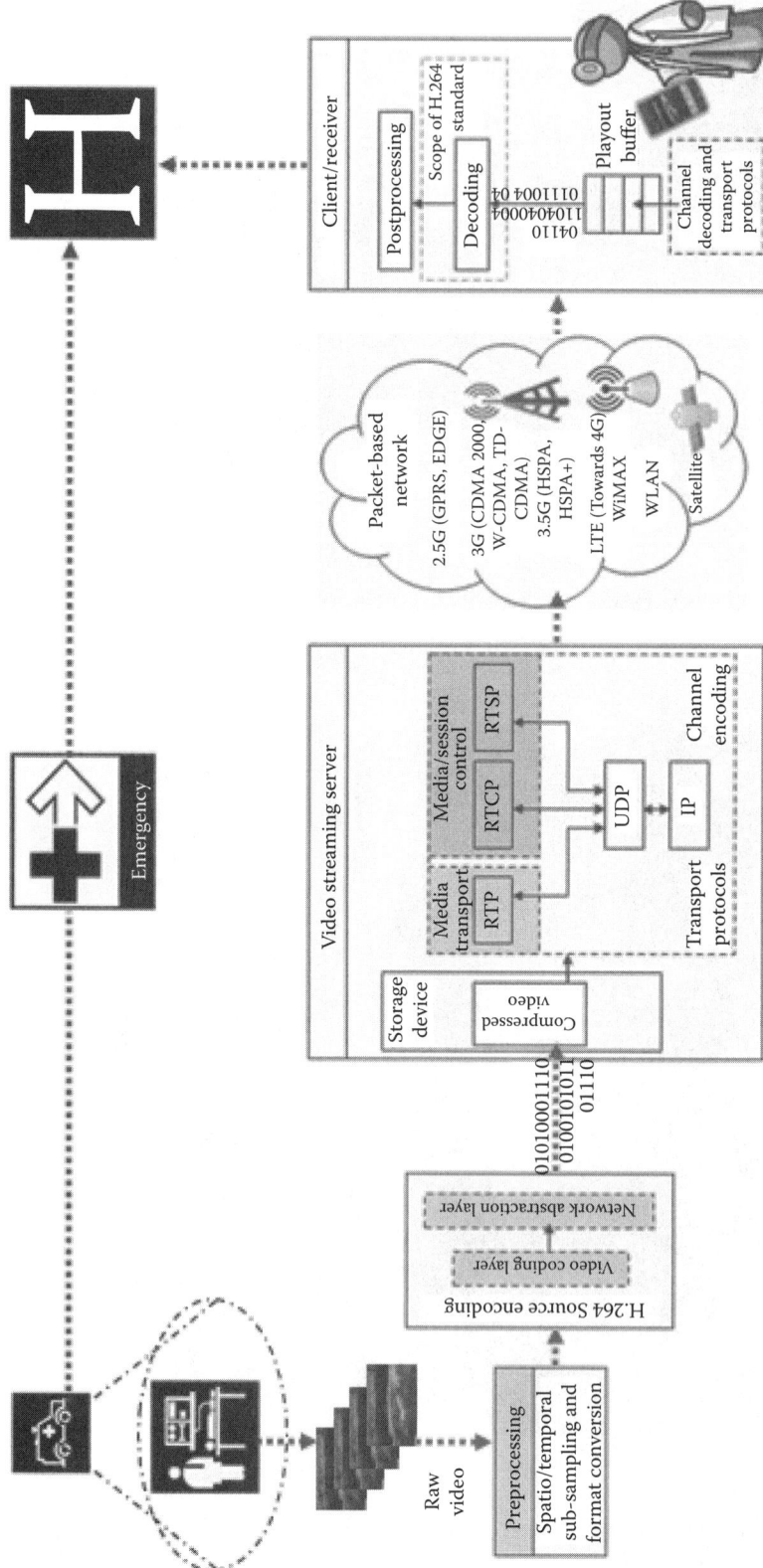

FIGURE 64.6 Wireless ultrasound video transmission using H.264/AVC for emergency telemedicine. A portable ultrasound device residing in the ambulance is used to capture the ultrasound video. Following preprocessing (resolution, frame rate, format conversion), the ultrasound video is fed to the H.264/AVC encoder for source encoding. Video coding layer (VCL) tackles compression (to match the available data rate) and error resilience (to shield against errors introduced by error-prone wireless channels), while the network abstraction layer (NAL) adapts VCL content to the appropriate wireless transmission medium format. Typically, H.264/AVC to RTP/UDP/IP is performed. At the receiver's end (remote medical expert and/or hospital premises), the reverse procedure is followed, including decoding, postprocessing, and error recovery. Assistance with the diagnosis and preparations for the patient's admission to the hospital are performed.

error-resilient techniques must be included in the design considerations, while diagnostic validation of the decoded video will verify the clinical performance. The presented case study tries to address aforementioned implications. Figure 64.6 depicts the system's architecture and all the involved steps.

In this study, quantization levels are spatially varying as a function of the diagnostic significance of each video region. Diagnostic ROIs include atherosclerotic plaque boundaries, arterial walls, and ECG signal (when available) (see Figure 64.7), and are derived using segmentation algorithms [106]. H.264/ AVC Flexible Macroblock Ordering (FMO) type 2 is used to encode diagnostic ROIs as independently transmitted and decoded slices, while redundant slices (RS) utilization increases the error resilience

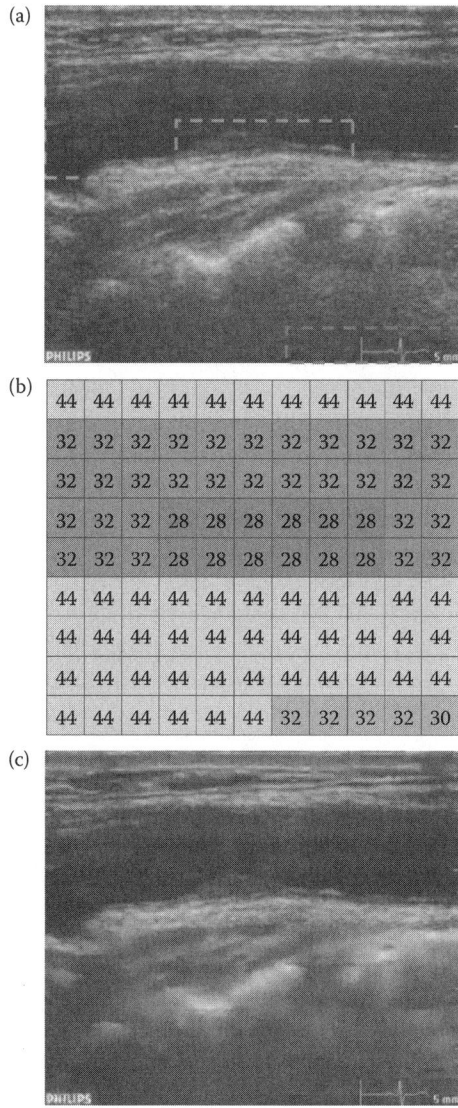

FIGURE 64.7 Variable quality region of interest encoding: (a) ROI boundaries are derived using segmentation algorithms. (b) A quantization parameter allocation map (QPAmap) is used to track spatially varying quantization levels. (c) The corresponding compressed video. Here, with QPs 44/32/28 (28: atherosclerotic plaque ROI, 32: arterial walls and ECG signal ROIs, 44: background and other components (necessary for plaque detection)).

capacity of the transmitted bitstream. In this manner, a diagnostically robust system for transmission over 3G wireless networks is achieved. A new clinical rating system that provides for assessing independent parts of the video that contribute to the overall diagnosis is used (see Tables 64.5 and 64.6). Both subjective (clinical ratings) and objective video quality assessment (VQA) show that the proposed system preserves diagnostic quality at high error rates while achieving significant bandwidth demand reductions.

In Figure 64.8 and Tables 64.5 and 64.6, we demonstrate a portion of the objective and subjective video quality assessment findings of the presented case study. Figure 64.8a depicts the bitrate savings attained by the proposed method (FMO ROI and FMO ROI RS), which allocates quantization parameters as a function of the diagnostic significance of the video, compared to the conventional encoding (FMO). Given that the clinically important factors are encoded in high quality, hence not compromising diagnostic quality, the bitrate savings for the particular video are depicted.

TABLE 64.5　Clinical Evaluation, CIF Resolution Video, 25 fps, No ECG Lead

FMO[a]	QP[b]	36/36/**36**	32/32/**32**	28/28/**28**	24/24/**24**
	Bitrate (kbps)	121	247	523	976
Plaque boundary		5	5	5	5
Artery stenosis		4	4	5	5
Plaque type		4	4	5	4
FMO ROI	QP	48/40/**36**	44/36/**32**	44/32/**28**	40/28/**24**
	Bitrate (kbps)	61	111	217	431
Plaque boundary		5	5	5	5
Artery stenosis		4	4	5	5
Plaque type		4	4	5	5
FMO ROI RS	QP	48/40/**36**	44/36/**32**	44/32/**28**	40/28/**24**
	Bitrate (kbps)	53	107	230	471
Plaque boundary		5	5	5	5
Artery stenosis		4	4	5	5
Plaque type		4	4	5	5

Note:　1: Lowest quality; 5: highest quality.

[a] We use FMO, FMO ROI, and FMO ROI RS for constant QP FMO encoding, variable QP FMO encoding, and variable QP FMO with RS, respectively.

[b] Quantization parameters (QPs) are given in the order of background/ wall and ECG ROIs/plaque ROI (in bold).

TABLE 64.6　Clinical Evaluation, CIF Resolution Video, 25 fps, No ECG Lead Plaque ROI QP 28

	FMO[a]	FMO ROI	FMO ROI RS
QP[b]	28/28/**28**	44/32/**28**	44/32/**28**
Bitrate (kbps)	**523**	**217**	**230**
Loss rates (%)	**5/8/15**	**5/8/15**	**5/8/15**
Plaque boundary	4/4/3	4/4/3	4/4/4
Artery stenosis	4/4/3	4/4/3	4/4/4
Plaque type	4/3/3	4/3/3	4/4/4

Note:　1: Lowest quality; 5: highest quality.

[a] We use FMO, FMO ROI, and FMO ROI RS for constant QP FMO encoding, variable QP FMO encoding, and variable QP FMO with RS, respectively.

[b] Quantization parameters (QPs) are given in the order of background/wall and ECG ROIs/plaque ROI (in bold).

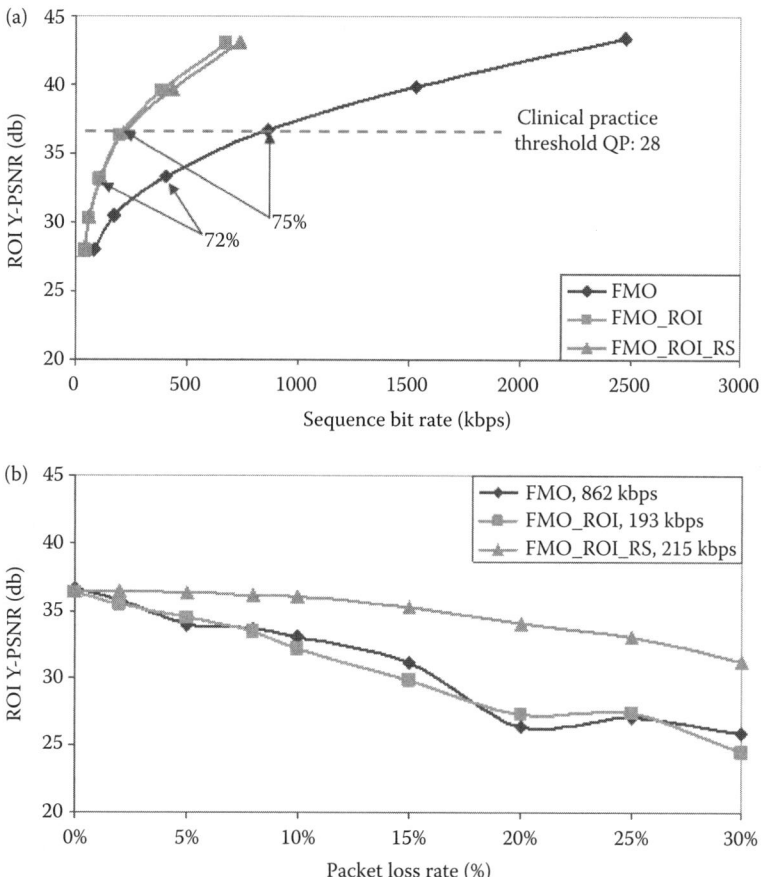

FIGURE 64.8 Rate-distortion and packet loss evaluation for carotid ultrasound video transmission. (a) Variable QP FMO (FMO ROI and FMO ROI RS) and constant QP FMO achieve similar PSNR ratings as expected (since atherosclerotic plaque region is encoded with equal QP for all cases). The key point is the significantly reduced bitrate without compromising clinical quality. Indicatively, for this particular video, FMO ROI RS requires 72% and 75% less bitrate than conventional FMO for QPs of 32 and 28, respectively. (CIF resolution (352 × 288) in macroblocks (MB): 396. ROI dimensions in MB: plaque ROI (33), wall ROI (121), ECG ROI (20) (see Figure 64.7)). (b) Noisy channels quality assessment: PSNR versus loss rate curve for diagnostic ROI (atherosclerotic plaque) with QP 28. FMO ROI RS achieves graceful degradation of video quality in the presence of severe loss rates. The medical expert is able to provide diagnosis at PLR of 15%. FMO ROI and FMO attain similar ratings, the former requiring significantly less bandwidth than the latter as illustrated in (a).

Clinical evaluation performed by a medical expert shown in Table 64.5 on the whole video, at its original dimensions, verified diagnostic quality. Interestingly, for ROI QP of 28, the medical expert could identify almost as much information in the compressed video as in the original. Thus, a selection of ROI QPs of 28 and lower were found to qualify for clinical practice. Figure 64.8b demonstrates the error resilience of the scheme incorporating RS (FMO ROI RS) over severe packet loss rates (PLR), likely to occur when transmitting over error-prone wireless channels. As deducted by the clinical evaluation in Table 64.6, the medical expert is able to provide a confident diagnosis even at 15% PLR (achieving a diagnostically acceptable rating of 4) or PSNR ratings above 35 db. In Figure 64.7, CIF resolution video at 25 fps with ECG lead is depicted, while Tables 64.5 and 64.6 record the clinical ratings on a CIF video with no ECG lead. Reported results are video specific. However, similar trends were observed for all investigated videos.

64.5 Concluding Remarks and Future Challenges

This chapter reviews information technology protocols and processes for emergency management, response, and support of eEmergency systems. The importance and benefits for using these technologies in emergency care are clearly demonstrated, as well as the need for their wider deployment.

The development and continuous improvement of computer-aided priority dispatch protocols supporting the automated implementation of these protocols in practice has greatly improved emergency management and response. However, further research is needed to address emerging organizational and technological challenges. First, emergency centers need to consider enforcing a number of adaptive learning processes to address organizational challenges. Organizational challenges include the diversity in the knowledge and experience of different emergency team members, issues of trust, and task complexity. These could include cross-training and/or role-rotation systems between ambulance crew members and dispatchers, weekly presentations, and postbriefings of different emergency incidents by and for team members, as well as more specialized training to help team members identify the level of complexity of each task. These learning processes could help minimize knowledge diversity levels and establish better trust between team members, as well as set some guidelines for dealing with task complexity. Second, in relation to technological challenges related to computing and networking for facilitating the instant availability and access to emergency-related information, emergency centers in collaboration with technology services providers and policy organizations could establish a number of standards and policies. These could include mechanisms for tuning in various satellite systems for geolocation of ambulances in real time, as well as communicating with other emergency-related systems, such as fire and police dispatching systems so as to better coordinate efforts.

Emerging eEmergency telemedicine systems can support the transmission of 2-D/3-D ultrasound and patient video (optical). Wireless medical video transmission has benefited from bitrate availability and extended coverage offered by 3G or current 4G mobile networks. However, the development of reliable eEmergency systems requires efficient encoding that matches achievable data rates and the use of error-resilient methods for dealing with error-prone transmissions. Furthermore, the overall systems also need extensive clinical validation using diagnostically relevant VQA metrics. On the other hand, forthcoming 4G systems targeting theoretical data rates of up to 100 Mb/s may reduce the needs for efficient video encoding.

A large-scale study by the telemedicine program at the State University of New York at Buffalo, School of Medicine, and the Erie County Medical Center (UB/ECMC) [107] has documented the success, experience, and benefits of clinical services in emergency telemedicine. It was shown that the use of emergency telemedicine services could result in an approximately 15% decrease in ambulance transports when it is added to the prehospital care provider's services, with emphasis given on younger subjects [108]. The publication of additional studies with encouraging findings, similar to this one, can facilitate the wider deployment of eEmergency systems.

Research in the aforementioned areas has so far examined either the technological or the organizational challenges associated with emergency management and response, but not both together. We argue that there is a need for a more holistic approach to understanding emergency management and response, which would require interdisciplinary research from disciplines such as computer science, medical informatics, and healthcare management.

To conclude, eEmergency systems can significantly impact the delivery of healthcare. However, their use in daily practice as well as the monitoring and evaluation of these systems still remains a goal to be achieved. Ultimately, the use of eEmergency systems should provide a better service to the citizen.

References

1. R.H. Istepanian, S. Laxminarayan, and C.S. Pattichis, Eds., *M-Health: Emerging Mobile Health Systems*, New York: Springer, 2006.

2. E. Kyriacou, M.S. Pattichis, C.S. Pattichis, A. Panayides, A. Pitsillides, m-Health e-emergency systems: Current status and future directions, *IEEE Antennas and Propagation Magazine*, 49(1), 216–231, 2007.

3. Office of U.S. Foreign Disaster Assistance. *Disaster History: Significant Data on Major Disasters Worldwide, 1900–Present.* Washington, DC: Agency for International Development, 1995.

4. T.C. Chan, J. Killeen, W. Griswold, and L. Lenert, Information technology and emergency medical care during disasters, *Academic Emergency Medicine*, 11(11), 1229–1236, 2004

5. Auf der Heide E. *Disaster Response: Principles of Preparation and Coordination*, ed 1. St. Louis, MO: Mosby, 1989. Free online edition: Center for Excellence in Disaster Management and Humanitarian Assistance, updated 2002.

6. P. Giovas, D. Thomakos, O. Papazachou, and D. Papadoyannis, Medical aspects of prehospital cardiac telecare, in *M-Health: Emerging Mobile Health Systems*, R.H. Istepanian, S. Laxminarayan, C.S. Pattichis, Eds., New York: Springer, 2006, pp. 389–400.

7. P. Andersen, A.M. Lindgaard, M. Prgomet, N. Creswick, and J.L. Westbrook, Mobile and fixed computer use by doctors and nurses on hospital wards: Multi-method study on the relationships between clinician role, clinical task, and device choice, *Journal of Medical Internet Research*, 11(3), e32, August 4, 2009.

8. C. Garritty, and K. El Emam, Who's Using PDAs? Estimates of PDA Use by health care providers: A systematic review of surveys, *Journal of Medical Internet Research*, 8(2), e7, April–June 2006. Published online May 12, 2006. doi: 10.2196/jmir.8.2.e7.

9. A.M. Lindquist, P.E. Johansson, G.I. Petersson, B.I. Saveman, and G.C. Nilsson, The use of the personal digital assistant (PDA) among personnel and students in health care: A review, *Journal of Medical Internet Research*, 10(4), e31, October 28, 2008.

10. F. Axisa, C. Gehin, G. Delhomme, C. Collet, O. Robin, and A. Dittmar, Wrist ambulatory monitoring system and smart glove for real time emotional, sensorial and physiological analysis, in *Proceedings of the 26th Annual International Conference of the IEEE EMBS*, San Francisco, CA, pp. 2161–2164, 2004.

11. M. Bolaños, H. Nazeran, I. Gonzalez, R. Parra, and C. Martinez, C., A PDA-based electrocardiogram/blood pressure telemonitor for telemedicine, in *Proceedings of the 26th Annual International Conference of the IEEE EMBS*, San Francisco, CA, pp. 2169–2172, 2004.

12. Wealthy Project: Wearable Health Care System, IST 2001-3778, Commission of the European Communities; http://www.wealthyist.com.

13. E. Jovanov, and D. Raskovic, Wireless intelligent sensors, in *M-Health: Emerging Mobile Health Systems*, R.H. Istepanian, S. Laxminarayan, C.S. Pattichis, Eds., New York: Springer, 2006, pp. 33–49.

14. L.J. Hadjileontiadis, Biosignals and compression standards, in *M-Health: Emerging Mobile Health Systems*, R.H. Istepanian, S. Laxminarayan, C.S. Pattichis, Eds., New York: Springer, 2006, pp. 277–292.

15. M.J.B. Van Ettinger, J.A. Lipton, M.C.J. de Wijs, Nvan der Putten, and S.P. Nelwan, An open source ECG toolkit with DICOM, *Computers in Cardiology*, 35, 441–444, 2008. Online: http://www.open-ecg-project.org, August 2010.

16. I. Martínez, J. Escayola, J. Trigo, P. Muñoz, J. García, M. Martínez-Espronceda, and L. Serrano, Implementation guidelines for an end-to-end standard-based platform for personal health, in *Fourth International Multi-Conference on Computing in the Global Information Technology, 2009*, ICCGI, pp. 123–131, 2009.

17 National Electrical Manufacturers Association (NEMA), *Digital Imaging and Communications in Medicine (DICOM) Publication PS 3*, Rosslyn, Virginia, 1996.

18. ISO/IEC 14995-1 Final Draft International Standard (FDIS), Information Technology—Lossless and Near-Lossless Coding of Continuous-Tone Still Images: Baseline, JPEG-LS Standard, Part 1, March 1999.

19. M. Boliek, C. Christopoulos, and E. Majani, Eds., JPEG2000 Part I Final Draft International Standard, ISO/IEC FDISI5444-1, ISO/IEC JTC1/SC29/WGINI855, August 18, 2000.

20. S. Wong, L. Zaremba, D. Gooden, and H.K. Huang, Radiologic image compression—A review, *Proceedings of the IEEE*, 83(2), 194–219, 1995.

21. P.W. Jones, and M. Rabbani, JPEG compression in medical imaging, Chapter 5, in *Handbook of Medical Imaging: Vol. 3 Display and PACS*, Y. Kim and S.C. Horii, Eds., Bellingham, Washington: SPIE Press, 2000, pp. 221–275.

22. J. Kivijarvi et al., A comparison of lossless compression methods for medical images, *Computerized Medical Imaging and Graphics*, 22, 323–339, 1998.

23. H. MacMahon et al., Data compression: Effect on diagnostic accuracy in digital chest radiography, *Radiology*, 178, 175–179, 1991.

24. S.S. Young, B.R. Whiting, and D.H. Foos, Statistically lossless image compression for CR and DR, *Proceedings of the SPIE Medical Imaging*, 3658, 406–419, 1999.

25. Digital Imaging and Communications in Medicine (DICOM), Part 5: Data Structures and Encoding [Online]. Available: ftp://medical.nema.org/medical/dicom/2009/09_05pu3.pdf, August 2010.

26. MPEG-2 CD, Committee Draft, ISO/IEC 13818 JTC1/SC29/WG11, ISO, March 25, 1994.

27. C. Lau, J.E. Cabral, Jr., D.R. Haynor, and Y. Kim, Telemedicine, Chapter 7, in *Handbook of Medical Imaging: Vol. 3 Display and PACS*, Y. Kim and S.C. Horii, Eds., Bellingham, Washington: SPIE Press, 2000, pp. 305–331.

28. ISO/IEC JTC1/SC29/WG11, MPEG-4 Overview, N2323, July, 1998.

29. MPEG-4 Video Group, Coding of Audio-Visual Objects: Video, ISO/IEC JTC1/SC29/WG11 N2202, March 1998.

30. A. Panayides, M.S. Pattichis, and C.S. Pattichis, Wireless ultrasound video transmission for stroke risk assessment: Quality metrics and system design, in *International Workshop on Video Processing and Quality Metrics for Consumer Electronics*, (VPQM 2010), Scottsdale, Arizona, January 2010.

31. J.M. Teich, M.M. Wagner, C.F. MacKenzie, and K.O. Schafer, The informatics response in disaster, terrorism, and war, *Journal of the American Medical Informatics Association*, 9, 97–104, 2002.

32. V. Garshnek, and F.M. Jr Burkle, Applications of telemedicine and telecommunications to disaster medicine: Historical and future perspectives, *Journal of the American Medical Informatics Association*, 6, 26–37, 1999.

33. V. Garshnek, and F.M. Jr Burkle, Telecommunications systems in support of disaster medicine: Applications of basic information pathways, *Annals of Emergency Medicine*, 34, 213–218, 1999.

34. D. Bravata et al., *Bioterrorism Preparedness and Response: Use of Information Technologies and Decision Support Systems*. Evidence report/technology assessment no. 59. AHRQ publication no. 02–E028. Rockville, MD: Agency for Healthcare Research and Quality, June 2002.

35. R.M. Satava, and S.B. Jones, Military applications of telemedicine and advanced medical technologies, *Army Medical Department Journal*, 16–21, November–December 1997, (OCLC) 32785416, ISSN 1524-0436.

36. S. Pavlopoulos, E. Kyriacou, A. Berler, S. Dembeyiotis, and D. Koutsouris. A novel emergency telemedicine system based on wireless communication technology—AMBULANCE, *IEEE Transactions on Information Technology in Biomedicine–Special Issue on Emerging Health Telematics Applications in Europe*, 2(4), 261–267, 1998.

37. Achieving better patient care through supply management technology. *Urgent Matters Online Newsletter*, 1(1), December 2003.

38. J. Berman, Exclusive: Center to test RFIDs to track patients, equipment. *Health IT World News*, June 29, 2004.

39. J.H. Bouman, R.J. Schouwerwou, K.J. VanderEijk, A.J. Van Leusden, and T.J.F. Savelkoul, Computerization of patient tracking and tracing during mass casualty incidents, *European Journal of Emergency Medicine*, 7, 211–216, 2000.

40. G.J. Noordergraaf et al., Development of computer-assisted patient control for use in the hospital setting during mass casualty incidents, *American Journal of Emergency Medicine*, 14, 257–261, 1996.

41. E. Aufderheide, Disaster planning, part II: Disaster problems, issues, and challenges identified in the research literature, *Emergency Medicine Clinics of North America*, 14, 453–480, 1996.
42. Improving NYPD Emergency Preparedness and Response. Post-9/11 Report of the NYPD. New York: McKinsey & Company, August 2002.
43. Post-9/11 Report of the Fire Department of New York (FDNY). McKinsey & Company, August 2002.
44. B.S. Zachariah and P.E. Pepe, The development of emergency medical dispatch in the USA: A historical perspective, *European Journal of Emergency Medicine*, 2(3), 109–112, 1995.
45. B.S. Zachariah, P.E. Pepe, and P.A. Curka, How to monitor the effectiveness of an emergency medical dispatch system: The Houston model. *European Journal of Emergency Medicine*, 2(3), 123–127, 1995.
46. A.G. Garza et al., The accuracy of predicting cardiac arrest by emergency medical services dispatchers: The calling party effect, *Academy Emergency Medicine*, 10(9), 955–960, 2003.
47. J. Dale et al., Computer assisted assessment and advice for "non-serious" 999 ambulance service callers: The potential impact on ambulance dispatch, *Emergency Medicine Journal*, 20(2), 178–183, 2003.
48. G.E. Michael, and K. Sporer, Validation of low-acuity emergency medical services dispatch codes, *Prehospital Emergency Care*, 9(4), 429–433, 2005.
49. C.D. Deakin et al., Does telephone triage of emergency (999) calls using advanced medical priority dispatch (AMPDS) with Department of Health (DH) call prioritisation effectively identify patients with an acute coronary syndrome? An audit of 42 657 emergency calls to Hampshire Ambulance Service NHS Trust, *Emergency Medicine Journal*, 23, 232–235, 2006.
50. J. Flynn et al., Sensitivity and specificity of the medical priority dispatch system in detecting cardiac arrest emergency calls in Melbourne, *Prehospital and Disaster Medicine*, 21(2), 72–76, 2006.
51. L.J. Reilly, Accuracy of a priority medical dispatch system in dispatching cardiac emergencies in a suburban community, *Prehospital and Disaster Medicine*, 21(2), 77–81, 2006.
52. Feldman et al., Comparison of the medical priority dispatch system to an out-of-hospital patient acuity score, *Academy Emergency Medicine*, 13(9), 954–960, 2006.
53. J. Clawson et al., Accuracy of emergency medical dispatchers' subjective ability to identify when higher dispatch levels are warranted over a medical priority dispatch system automated protocol's recommended coding based on paramedic outcome data, *Emergency Medicine Journal*, 24, 560–563, 2007.
54. B. Buck et al., Dispatcher recognition of stroke using the national academy medical priority dispatch system, *Stroke*, 40, 2027–2030, 2009.
55. N. Johnson, and K. Sporer, How many emergency dispatches occurred per cardiac arrest. *Resuscitation*, 8(11), 1499–1504, 2010.
56. T.E. Drabek and D.A. McEntire, Emergent phenomena and the sociology of disaster: Lessons, trends and opportunities from the research literature, *Disaster Prevention and Management*, 12(2), 97–112, 2003.
57. K.J. Tierney, M.K. Lindell, and R.W. Perry, *Facing the Unexpected: Disaster Preparedness and Response in the United States*. Joseph Henry Press, Washington DC, 2001.
58. A. Majchrzak, S.L. Jarvenpaa, and A.B. Hollingshead, Coordinating expertise among emergent groups responding to disasters, *Organization Science*, 18(1), 147–161, 2007.
59. P. Constantinides, A. Kouroubali, and M. Barrett, Transacting expertise in emergency management and response, in *Proceedings of the International Conference of Information Systems*, Paris, France, December 8–10, 2008.
60. W. Einthoven, Le telecardiogramme, *Archives Internationales Physiologie*, IV, 132–164, 1906.
61. R. Karlsten and B.A. Sjoqvist, Telemedicine and decision support in emergency ambulances in Uppsala, *Journal of Telemedicine and Telecare*, 6(1), 1–7, 2000.
62. Yan Xiao, D. Gagliano, M. LaMonte, P.Hu, W. Gaasch, and R. Gunawadane. Design and evaluation of a real-time mobile telemedicine system for ambulance transport, *Journal of High Speed Networks*, 9(1), 47–56, 2000.

63. V. Anantharaman and L. Swee Han, Hospital and emergency ambulance link: Using IT to enhance emergency pre-hospital care, *International Journal of Medical Informatics*, 61(2–3), 147–161, 2001.

64. A. Rodrvguez, J.L. Villalar, M.T. Arredondo, M.F. Cabrera, and F. Del Pozo, Transmission trials with a support system for the treatment of cardiac arrest outside hospital, *Journal of Telemedicine and Telecare*, 7(Suppl 1), 60–62, 2001.

65. R.S. Istepanian, L.J. Hadjileontiadis, and S.M. Panas, ECG data compression using wavelets and higher order statistics methods, *IEEE Transactions on Information Technology in Biomedicine*, 5(2), 108–115, 2001.

66. R.S Istepanian, E. Kyriacou, S. Pavlopoulos, and D. Koutsouris, Effect of wavelet compression on data transmission in a multipurpose wireless telemedicine system, *Journal of Telemedicine and Telecare*, 7(Suppl 1), 14–16, 2001.

67. F. Chiarugi et al., Continuous ECG monitoring in the management of pre-hospital health emergencies, *Computers in Cardiology*, 205–208, September 2003.

68. P.D. Garrett et al., Feasibility of real-time echocardiographic evaluation during patient transport, *Journal of American Society of Echocardiography*, 16(3), 197–201, 2003.

69. E. Kyriacou et al., Multi-purpose healthcare telemedicine systems with mobile communication link support, *BioMedical Engineering OnLine*, http://www.biomedical-engineering-online.com, 2(7), 2003.

70. Y. Chu and A. Ganz, A mobile teletrauma system using 3G networks, *IEEE Transactions on Information Technology in Biomedicine*, 8(4), 456–462, 2004.

71. M. Clarke, A reference architecture for telemonitoring, *Studies in Health Technology and Informatics*, 103, 381–384, 2004.

72. P. Clemmensen et al., Diversion of ST-elevation myocardial infarction patients for primary angioplasty based on wireless prehospital 12-lead electrocardiographic transmission directly to the cardiologist's handheld computer: A progress report, *Journal of Electrocardiology*, 38(4), 194–198, 2005.

73. P.T. Campbell et al., Prehospital triage of acute myocardial infarction: Wireless transmission of electrocardiograms to the on-call cardiologist via a handheld computer, *Journal of Electrocardiology*, 38(4), 300–309, 2005.

74. M. Sillesen et al., Telemedicine in the transmission of prehospitalisation ECGs of patients with suspected acute myocardial infarction, *Ugeskr Laeger*, 168(11), 1133–1136, 2006.

75. G. Kontaxakis, G. Sakas, and S. Walter, Mobile tele-echography systems—TELEINVIVO: A case study, in *M-Health: Emerging Mobile Health Systems*, R.H. Istepanian, S. Laxminarayan, C.S. Pattichis, Eds., New York: Springer, 2006, pp. 445–460.

76. S. Garawi, R.S.H. Istepanian, and M.A. Abu-Rgheff, 3G wireless communications for mobile robotic tele-ultrasonography systems, *IEEE Communications Magazine*, 44(4), 91–96, 2006.

77. N. Tsapatsoulis, C. Loizou, and C. Pattichis, Region of interest video coding for low bit-rate transmission of carotid ultrasound videos over 3G wireless networks, in *Proceedings of IEEE EMBC'07*, Lyon, France, August 23–26, 2007.

78. C. Doukas and I. Maglogiannis, Adaptive transmission of medical image and video using scalable coding and context-aware wireless medical networks, *EURASIP JWCN*, vol. 2008, Article ID 428397, 2008.

79. A. Panayides, M.S. Pattichis, and C.S. Pattichis, Wireless medical ultrasound video transmission through noisy channels, in *Proceedings of IEEE EMBC'08*, Vancouver, Canada, August 28–30, 2008.

80. C.A. Strode et al., Wireless and satellite transmission of prehospital focused abdominal sonography for trauma, *Prehospital Emergency Care*, 7(3), 375–379, 2003.

81. A. Kouroubali, D. Vourvahakis, and M. Tsiknakis, Innovative practices in the emergency medical services in Crete, in *Proceedings of the 10th International Symposium on Health Information Management Research—iSHIMR 2005*. P.D. Bamidis et al., Eds., pp. 166–175, 2005.

82. E. Kyriacou, S. Pavlopoulos, D. Koutsouris, A. Andreou, C. Pattichis, and C. Schizas. Multipurpose health care telemedicine system, in *Proceedings of the 23rd Annual International Conference of the IEEE/EMBS*, Istanbul, Turkey, 2001.

83. P. Vieyres et al., A tele-operated robotic system for mobile tele-echography: The OTELO project, in *M-Health: Emerging Mobile Health Systems*, R.H. Istepanian, S. Laxminarayan, C.S. Pattichis, Eds., New York: Springer, 2006, pp. 461–473.

84. C. Canero et al., Mobile tele-echography: User interface design, *IEEE Transactions on Information Technology in Biomedicine*, 9(1), 44–49, 2005.

85. J. Reponen, E. Ilkko, L. Jyrkinen, O. Tervonen, J. Niinimδki, V. Karhula, and A. Koivula, Initial experience with a wireless personal digital assistant as a teleradiology terminal for reporting emergency computerized tomography scans, *Journal of Telemedicine and Telecare*, 6(1), 45–49, 2000.

86. K. Oguchi et al., Preliminary experience of wireless teleradiology system using Personal Handyphone System, *Nippon Igaku Hoshasen Gakkai Zasshi*, 61(12), 686–687, 2001.

87. S.Ch, Voskarides, C.S. Pattichis, R. Istepanian, C. Michaelides, and C.N. Schizas, Practical evaluation of GPRS use in a telemedicine system in Cyprus, in *CD-ROM Proceedings of the 4th International IEEE EMBS Special Topic Conference on Information Technology Applications in Biomedicine*, Birmingham, UK, 4 pages, 2003.

88. M.G. Hadjinicolaou, R. Nilavalan, T. Itagaki, S.Ch. Voskarides, C.S. Pattichis, and A.N. Schizas, Emergency tele-orthopaedics m-health system for wireless communication links, *IET Communications*, 3, 1284–1296, 2009.

89. E.S. Hall, D.K. Vawdrey, C.D. Knutson, and J.K. Archibald, Enabling remote access to personal electronic medical records, *IEEE Engineering in Medicine and Biology Magazine*, 22(3), 133–139, 2003.

90. L. Pagani et al., A portable diagnostic workstation based on a Webpad: Implementation and evaluation, *Journal of Telemedicine and Telecare*, 9(4), 225–229, 2003.

91. K. Lorincz et al., Sensor networks for emergency response: Challenges and opportunities, *IEEE Pervasive Computing*, 3(4), 6–23, 2004.

92. D.K. Kim, S.K. Yoo, and S.H. Kim, Instant wireless transmission of radiological images using a personal digital assistant phone for emergency teleconsultation, *Journal of Telemedicine and Telecare*, 11(2), S58–S61, 2005.

93. D.K. Kim et al., A mobile telemedicine system for remote consultation in cases of acute stroke, *Journal of Telemedicine and Telecare*, 15 102–107, 2009.

94. C.H. Salvador et al., Airmed-cardio: A GSM and Internet services-based system for out-of-hospital follow-up of cardiac patients, *IEEE Transactions on Information Technology in Biomedicine*, 9(1), 73–85, 2005.

95. Virgin to upgrade telemedicine across fleet, *E-Health Insider*, available at: http://www.e-health-insider.com/news/item.cfm?ID=1925, Announced: June 6, 2006.

96. Etihad to install onboard health monitor system on long-haul fleet, http://www.airlinesanddestinations.com/airlines/etihad-to-install-onboard-health-monitor-system-on-long-haul-fleet/, July 30, 2010.

97. H. Maki et al., A welfare facility resident care support system, *Biomedical Sciences Instrumentation*, 40, 480–483, 2004.

98. D.A. Palmer, R. Rao, and L.A. Lenert, An 802.11 wireless blood pulse-oximetry system for medical response to disasters, in *Proceedings of the AMIA Annual Symposium*, pp. 1072, 2005.

99. L.A. Lenert, D.A. Palmer, T.C. Chan, and R. Rao, An intelligent 802.11 triage tag for medical response to disasters, in *Proceedings of AMIA Annual Symposium*, pp. 440–444, 2005.

100. M. Nakamura, Y. Yang, S. Kubota, H. Shimizu, Y. Miura, K. Wasaki, Y. Shidama, and M. Takizawa, Network system for alpine ambulance using long distance wireless LAN and CATV LAN, *Igaku Butsuri*, 23(1) 30–39, 2003.

101. R.G. Lee et al., A mobile care system with alert mechanism, *IEEE Transactions on Information Technology in Biomedicine*, 11(5), 507–517, 2007.

102. L. Ching-Teng et al. An intelligent telecardiology system using a wearable and wireless ECG to detect atrial fibrillation, *IEEE Transactions on Information Technology in Biomedicine*, 14(3), 726–733, May 2010.

103. C. Antoniades, A. Kouppis, S. Pavlopoulos, E. Kyriakou, A. Kyprianou, A.S. Andreou, C. Pattichis, and C. Schizas, A novel telemedicine system for the handling of emergency cases, in *Proceedings of the 5th World Conference on Injury Prevention and Control*, World Health Organisation (WHO), New Delhi, India, 2000.

104. E. Kyriacou, S. Pavlopoulos, A. Bourka, A. Berler, and D. Koutsouris, Telemedicine in emergency care, in *Proceedings of the VI International Conference on Medical Physics, Patras 99*, Patra, Greece, pp. 293–298, September 1999.

105. A. Panayides, M.S. Pattichis, C.S. Pattichis, C.P. Loizou, M. Pantziaris, and A. Pitsillides, Robust and efficient ultrasound video coding in noisy channels using H.264, in *Proceedings of IEEE EMBC'09*, Minnesota, USA, September 2–6, 2009.

106. C.P. Loizou, C.S. Pattichis, M. Pantziaris, and A. Nicolaides, An integrated system for the segmentation of atherosclerotic carotid plaque, *IEEE Transaction on Information Technology in Biomedicine*, 11(5), 661–667, 2007.

107. D.G. Ellis and J. Mayrose, The success of emergency telemedicine at the State University of New York at Buffalo, *Telemedicine Journal and e-Health*, 9(1), 73–79, 2003.

108. P.A. Haskins, D.G. Ellis, and J. Mayrose, Predicted utilization of emergency medical services telemedicine in decreasing ambulance transports, *Prehospital Emergency Care*, 6(4), 445–448, 2002.

65

Disaster Response: Roles of Responders and Lessons Learned since 9/11

James Geiling*
Geisel School of Medicine at Dartmouth
Veterans Affairs Medical Center, White River Junction, Vermont

Lindsay Katona
University of New England College of Osteopathic Medicine

Michael Lauria†
Dartmouth-Hitchcock Medical Center

Joseph M. Rosen
Geisel School of Medicine at Dartmouth
Veterans Affairs Medical Center, White River Junction, Vermont

65.1 Introduction: Setting the Stage

On March 11, 2011, a 9.03 Mw earthquake originating 70 km off the Japanese coast resulted in the multi-disaster Great East Japan Earthquake. In its wake, not only did the region suffer the consequences of the earthquake itself, but it also led to severe flooding from powerful tsunami waves of over 40 meters in height. Both the earthquake and tsunamis damaged the Fukushima Daiichi Nuclear Power Plant complex, resulting eventually in three reactors suffering meltdowns with radioactive material release. This overwhelming, multi-dimensional disaster caused approximately 16,000 deaths, 6000 injuries, and 3000 missing persons, at a cost of $235 billion (U.S. dollars), the costliest disaster on record.

In October 2012, Hurricane Sandy came out of the Caribbean and skirted the East Coast of the United States, affecting 24 states. It was the largest Atlantic hurricane on record and resulted in 72 direct deaths and approximately $75 billion (U.S.) in damage; it was the deadliest hurricane to hit the U.S. mainland since Hurricane Katrina in 2005. In New Jersey, three towns were destroyed with many beachfront communities severely damaged, with total damage estimates at approximately $30 billion (U.S.). In New York, the Stock Exchange closed for two consecutive days, the first such weather closure since 1888. Large sections of Lower New York City were flooded, destroying or damaging buildings; disrupting businesses and the subway train system, which had to close seven subway tunnels. On Long Island, approximately 100,000

---

* The views expressed in this chapter are those of the author and do not necessarily reflect the official policy of the U.S. Government or the Department of Veterans Affairs.

† The views expressed in this chapter are those of the author and do not necessarily reflect the official policy of the U.S. Government, the U.S. Department of Defense, or the U.S. Air Force.

homes were destroyed or damaged. Several city hospitals also closed, requiring relocation of their patients and staff.

On January 12, 2010 at 4:53 in the afternoon, a 7.0 earthquake rocked Haiti, flattening buildings and sending citizens into the streets for refuge. Shortly thereafter, search and rescue teams from around the world began to deploy to help find the many victims trapped inside the debris and to treat the wounded survivors who were in makeshift camps all around the city. Many thousands of emergency responders and medical personnel also arrived to support various other rescue efforts and overwhelming medical needs.

On September 11, 2001, the United States was struck with the worst terrorist attack in the nation's history. With the collapse of the twin towers in New York City and the attack on the Pentagon came massive devastation. In spite of the dangers of explosion and building collapse or the threat of additional attacks, first responders flocked to each scene to fight the fires, provide first aid and support, and conduct search and rescue operations.

This section compares the Haiti earthquake and September 11 disaster, for which the authors, James Geiling and Joseph Rosen, were involved in medical response missions (James Geiling with both events; Joseph Rosen with Haiti). These two disasters were caused by very different mechanisms, but adjusting for the massive number of victims in the Haiti earthquake, they resulted in similar outcomes. Both disasters required massive external response, coordinated delivery of care, and a rapid mobilization of resources. (In 9/11, hospitals sadly mobilized for many injured who did not come—but they did mobilize.) Given the similar outcomes, one might ask the following question: In the almost 10 years between these two similar disasters, have emergency management programs evolved and have the organizations responsible for supporting our responders kept pace with the rapidly changing technologies available for training, educating, and equipping them?

This chapter explores these questions. We outline how emergency responders' roles, their handling of disasters, and relevant technology may vary based on the type of disaster, and we describe response doctrines of either treatment in place or evacuation (for sudden-impact events) versus isolation and quarantine (for biological events). Later in the chapter, we outline the current systems of emergency management in the United States; we describe what challenges exist in our approach, and we identify a series of lessons learned in the decade since 9/11. To close this second section, we describe the key elements of a good response, including "team, culture, and training." To better prepare for, respond to, and learn from large-scale disasters, we must make fundamental changes to our team culture, improve the way we train, and incorporate technology-enabled communication solutions that coordinate the response of numerous organizations.

This chapter's discussion serves as an introduction to the follow-on Chapter 66 where we explain how new communication, treatment, training, and simulation technologies can better prepare emergency responders to cope with a full spectrum of both natural and human-made disasters.

65.1.1 Types of Responders

Emergency and medical personnel who respond to and support disasters assume a variety of roles, depending on their training and skills, and the setting. For this chapter, we define *first responder* as one category of *emergency responder*—those who are immediately activated in the wake of a disaster. Conventionally, the term refers to firefighters, police, emergency medical technicians (EMTs) and paramedics: the people who are first on the scene to rescue and aid victims of sudden-impact events, such as earthquakes, hurricanes, accidents, fires, and so on. These first responders treat and transport the victim to the hospital for ongoing treatment by *first receivers*, e.g., hospital-based nurses, doctors, and other healthcare professionals.

The doctors and nurses who went to support relief efforts in Haiti may be referred to as *disaster responders* who provided support as field-based rather than hospital-based providers. In this setting, these providers have a combination of skills—primarily hospital-based care, but in an austere environment. These providers still differ from the classic *first responders* who, in this setting, act primarily in an effort to search, rescue, and render care.

A pandemic disaster is somewhat unique since it involves a time delay—an incubation period, in which many patients may spread illness before they know they are infected or seek help. In a pandemic, the first responders who care for the patient are often family members, local healthcare providers, and public health practitioners. In a pandemic, the public health officials and local doctors may also serve as responders. We would not call them emergency responders, per se, because that is not their normal discipline.

This chapter is written for all these types of medical personnel who respond to disasters; these people may or may not be first responders, depending on the event, and they may or may not be disaster or emergency responders.

65.1.2 Types of Disasters

Disasters take many forms and have a variety of characteristics (see Tables 65.1 and 65.2).

This chapter classifies disasters and responses into three broad categories:

1. *Sudden-impact disasters* (hurricanes, earthquakes, cyclones, tsunamis, and also transportation accidents, environmental accidents, etc.)
2. *Terrorist attacks*, including chemical, radiological, explosive, cyber terrorism, and other events designed by humans to cause harm
3. *Biological catastrophes* (noncontagious vs. contagious), such as pandemics or severe lab accidents that may occur naturally, accidentally, or intentionally

Disaster management has four phases—mitigation, preparation, response, and recovery. *Consequence management* focuses on the recovery and reconstitution mission. This chapter deals mostly with preparation and response capabilities.

Just as disasters take many forms, the response can take different forms. Note that there is some overlap in the categories above (e.g., a pandemic is both a biological disaster and can also be an act of terror if caused by humans). Also important to note is that some disaster events could be either human-made or from natural causes, for example, a fire or oil spill might result from an earthquake, but might also

TABLE 65.1 Types of Disasters

External	Internal
Natural	Power failure
Earthquake	Flood
Tornado	Water loss
Hurricane	Chemical or radiation accident/fumes
Flood	Fire/explosion
Storm	Loss of medical gases
Fire	Violence/bomb threat or explosion
Human-made	Inability of staff to reach hospital
Terrorism	Elevator emergencies
Transportation	
Chemical/radiation accident	
Mass gathering-hysteria/unrest	

Source: Adapted from Rosen, J.M. et al. 2003. In *Integration of Health Telematics into Medical Practice*, 95–114. Amsterdam: IOS Press.

TABLE 65.2   Characteristics of Disasters

Origin
1. Natural (geophysical or weather-related)
2. Human-made

Location
1. Single site (single or multiple occurrence)
2. Multiple sites (single or multiple occurrence)

Predictability
1. Fairly predictable
2. Unpredictable

Onset
1. Gradual
2. Sudden

Duration
1. Brief
2. Extended

Frequency
1. Common
2. Rare

Determinants of magnitude
1. Size of involved area
2. Extent of damage to people/
   property damage
3. Extent to which community
   resources are overwhelmed

Source: Adapted from Rosen, J.M. et al. 2003. In *Integration of Health Telematics into Medical Practice*, 95–114. Amsterdam: IOS Press.

occur from human error or mistakes. Even human-made incidents break down into two subcategories: intentional malice versus human mistakes or stupidity.

Each type of disaster can be further categorized by magnitude and duration. For example, an earthquake is large (in magnitude) and short (in duration); a pandemic is "large and long." Some events become a megadisaster, that is, a disaster that completely overwhelms the existing emergency management infrastructure and capacity to respond, so that outside leadership and other capabilities are called in to provide support.

In theory, no matter whether a disaster's cause is natural or due to humans, the response structure should be the same, as should the information management. For example, in a nuclear accident like Chernobyl, responders would decontaminate and triage the victims, keep statistics on victims, and so on, in the same way, regardless of whether the cause of the leak had been human error or an earthquake.

How much the medical response is independent of causes depends on where the disaster occurs and what that country's laws specify. Human-made terrorist events are crimes, whereas human accidents and natural disasters are not. This can add a different perspective to the response effort. In the United States, under U.S. Department of Human Services (DHS), if an incident is human-made/accidental/natural, the Federal Emergency Management Agency (FEMA) oversees the response, and if it a terrorist incident, it is managed by the Department of Justice and the Federal Bureau of Investigation. Additionally, if the event occurs overseas, as in the Kenya Embassy bombing, the U.S. State Department takes the lead. Law enforcement officials view the world differently than medical responders: medical personnel want to rescue and then recover, but police may see this as interference in the investigation—because all material, including patients, are evidence.

65.1.2.1 Sudden-Impact Disasters

The 2010 earthquake in Haiti and 2005 hurricane in the U.S. Gulf Coast were natural sudden-impact events that became megadisasters. With each year, additional disasters appear, such as the Great East Japan Earthquake in 2011 and Hurricane Sandy in 2012. While the impacts of these two recent mega-disasters continue to unfold, both the Haiti Earthquake and Hurricane Katrina offer useful case studies on these types of events. Effective response to megadisasters requires the rapid augmentation of local resources with remote surge capacity that integrates the country's own response system seamlessly with local capability.

65.1.2.1.1 Case Study: Haiti Earthquake, 2010

The earthquake that struck Haiti in January 2010 caused approximately 230,000 deaths, an estimated 300,000 serious injuries, and abruptly made over one million people homeless. Much of the country's modest infrastructure was destroyed. Critical transportation assets such as docks, bridges, highways, and airport facilities were rendered unusable. Further, Haiti's centers of commerce and healthcare were leveled. Gone were the Presidential Palace, the National Assembly building, and the Ministry of Health with all of its records.

On the medical front, the earthquake resulted in an overwhelming number of traumatic injuries, many of which required amputations, and treatment of widespread illness. These problems were magnified given the challenges that Haiti already faced in its public health and patient care systems prior to the megadisaster [15]. Also, Haiti's medical education and training system immediately ceased; for example, the nursing school at University Hospital in Port-au-Prince was flattened with many students and instructors trapped or killed inside.

Governmental agencies, the U.S. military, and nongovernmental organizations (NGOs) poured into the country in an initially haphazard and uncoordinated fashion to provide rescue efforts, and then to support the long-term recovery. Medical teams, with little coordination, worked to find ways to provide surgical care and support.

Hospital-based providers from modern, Western settings were often challenged by the austere conditions of the Haiti disaster. Technological solutions common in their home environments no longer worked, or the infrastructure to support such technology did not exist. First responders had to bring their own food, water, housing, and security. Even when they brought their own communications equipment, teams or agencies from different countries often could not easily communicate. Cell service was intermittently available, but there was little Internet access unless groups brought their own capability. Even the resource-and technology-rich military was limited: the U.S. Army 82nd Airborne and the U.S. Navy hospital ship *Comfort*, who both responded, could not communicate. This situation complicated patient movement priority under the care of NGOs, many of whom actually had functioning landlines (Jim Geiling, personal observation). Military communications systems clearly set a standard for deployable capability, but these networks are often not available to the wide range of responders at an international disaster site. Without a common communications standard, responders are left to a patchwork system of connectivity.

Many emergency responders brought their own medical supplies to Haiti, but logistical support was spotty and disjointed. Basic systems, such as electricity to run equipment (including that for potable water), oxygen, laboratory support, and x-rays were dependent on fuel-intensive generators. Medically, normal processes and procedures were often abandoned, and innovation was critical. Medical personnel who had either practiced in these conditions previously or had trained before Western medicine became so dependent on technology, were sought for their advice and support. As we later describe in the section on new technologies for disaster response, it is important that technologies used in disaster response can be self-sustaining or deployable as a fully integrated package, when possible.

The most important point about technology during disaster relief efforts is that responders need to bring their own. Often, military medical teams can provide the highest standard of care because they deploy with a preset package of trained personnel, equipment, supplies, communications gear, and security. Independent groups, NGOs, and others that rely on other disaster responders or an intact host-nation for support cannot duplicate the military's model, especially for sustained periods, and hence the care standards and capabilities may at times be different. *A question in desperate need of technological solutions, support, and innovation is: how can we standardize and equalize the resources so that all response groups have sufficient staff, equipment, supplies, technology, and security that they will need to coordinate assets and provide optimal care (communications, logistics distribution, and personnel allocation)?* Given that the military has enormous assets that other organizations may lack, how can we create cost-efficient technologies to help all response agencies, including NGOs, to network and collaborate with the military and academic responders for an effective response to any disaster? The larger goal should be to set a common international standard for collaboration, based on very basic protocols, so that people can communicate and provide effective response, no matter what they bring. Unfortunately, Haiti is not the first event to demonstrate that need.

65.1.2.1.2 Case Study: Katrina, 2005

On August 26, 2005, the Miami Hurricane Simulation Center predicted a landfall of a category 4 or 5 hurricane in and around New Orleans. Despite this early warning, U.S. Federal officials did not initiate the emergency response system to evacuate the city in advance. On August 29, a category 4/5 storm reached New Orleans and the surrounding areas, causing multiple broken levees and widespread flooding throughout the city. This resulted in multiple infrastructure failures and many drowning deaths. First responders from the city were either occupied with their own individual issues or under-resourced in an uncoordinated fashion; many even failed to respond because of being personally overwhelmed with the magnitude of the event and its impact on their personal and family well-being. Further, many critically ill patients in hospitals throughout the city died as a result of failure of evacuation, which could have happened on August 27 or 28 ahead of the storm. Figure 65.1 illustrates how the National Response Plan was delayed and how it should ideally have worked during Katrina.

The Katrina response demonstrated how the United States is particularly vulnerable with regard to emergency response capability. By the time the event began, it was impossible to move assets into the stricken region with any chance at containment or evacuation until the hurricane passed. A lack of training among local authorities, and a lack of timely decisions and response thereby made the disaster response itself a failure. As U.S. President George Bush acknowledged at the time, "the system, at every level of government, was not well-coordinated, and was overwhelmed in the first few days" [32]. The failures of Katrina were analyzed by the U.S. government [31] as an attempt to learn and improve future disaster response.

65.1.2.2 Terrorism

Terrorist events can occur anywhere in the world, at any time, and encompass chemical, biological, radiological, nuclear, and explosive (CBRNE) attacks; as well as attacks involving transportation vehicles (e.g., 9/11), or a bomb on an airplane, or aircraft being shot down from the ground via handheld devices like Stinger missiles. Airplanes can also spread biological agents, as shown during 2003 SARS and 2009/2010 H1N1. Starting in the early incubation phase of H1N1, airplanes could connect the globe within hours and spread the virus. The worst terrorist attack on U.S. soil in this century was the 9/11 attacks, with over 2981 fatalities (more than 2600 people died at the World Trade Center; 125 died at the Pentagon; 256 died on the four planes). The death toll surpassed that at Pearl Harbor in December 1941 [30]. Owing to heightened post-9/11 airline security, a repeat terrorist attack using an airplane as a weapon is less likely. However, terrorist events have occurred worldwide in the decade following 9/11, including Russia's 2004 Beslan school siege (365 fatalities), Madrid's 2004 bombing (191 deaths), London's 2005 bombings (56 deaths), Sadr City, Iraq's 2006 bombings (215 deaths), Mumbai, India's 2006 train bombing (209 deaths), and Qahtaniya, Iraq's 2007 bombings (796 deaths) [6]. These were all

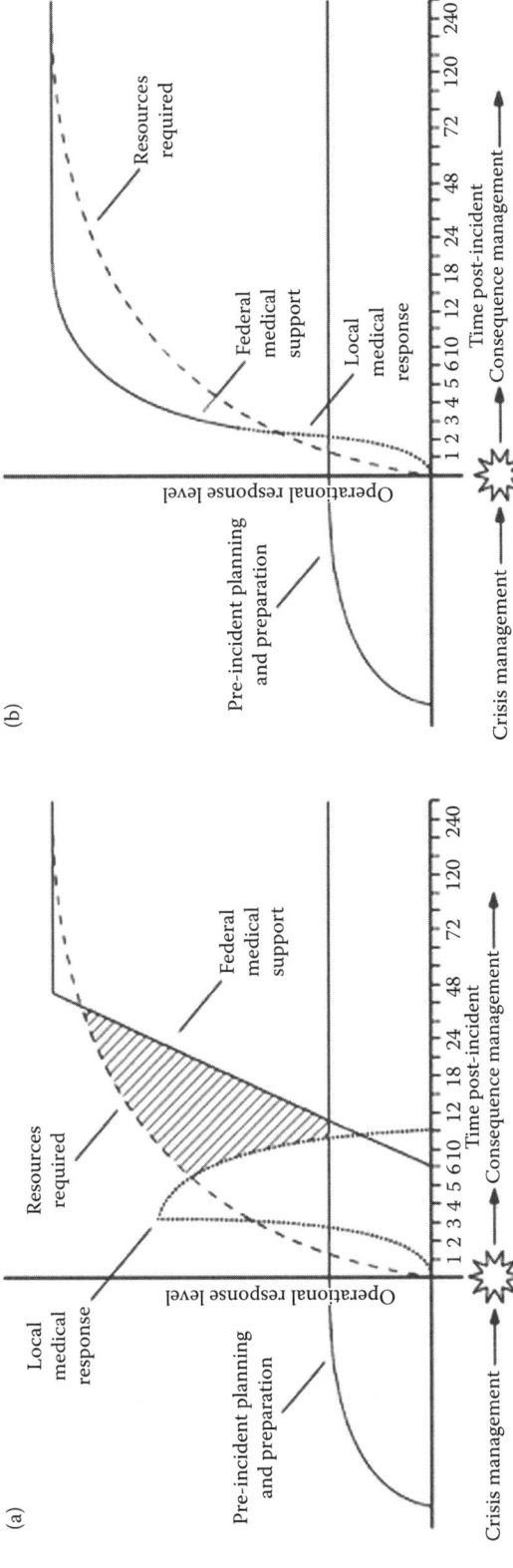

FIGURE 65.1 What happened when the U.S. National Response Plan was delayed in Hurricane Katrina in 2005 by lack of resources for evacuation and care of patients on 8/29/2005, (b) how the U.S. National Response Plan should have worked ahead of storm. (Rosen, J.M., Grigg, E.B., McKnight, M.F. et al. Transforming medicine for biodefense and healthcare delivery: Developing a dual-use doctrine that utilizes information superiority and network-based organization. *IEEE Engineering in Medicine and Biology* 23:89–101. © 2004 IEEE.)

examples of small and short events, with less than 1000 casualties and duration from a few minutes to 24 hours. These are the types of events that classically impact first responders—sudden and overwhelming, with often constrained communications.

A failed car-bombing attempt in Times Square, New York City in May 2010 [18] demonstrated the continued threat of terrorism in the United States. Despite our heightened post-9/11 security in government buildings and airlines, U.S. intelligence and law enforcement agencies cannot be everywhere and see everything. Robust search and seizure capabilities will inevitably be restrained in a society that balances security with civil rights and individual freedom.

65.1.2.3 Biologic Pandemics

Biological events played a major role in destabilizing great empires, past and recent. For example, between 250 and 650 AD, the Roman Empire "was assaulted by successive waves of pandemics that reduced the population by at least one-quarter ..." [5]. In pandemics from Europe's Black Plague to the 1918 flu pandemic, cultures experienced lost economic productivity, a declining agricultural and tax base, and severe shortages in military power. Germs, even more than military enemies, decimated great civilizations—the Germans and Austrians may have lost World War 1 because of flu-related manpower losses [23]—and can have profound economic impact worldwide [1].

In contrast to past naturally occurring pandemics, modern pandemics can also stem from human accident or intent. Accidents may occur during research or industrial operations, while scientists are making vaccines or biological agents, and strains may become mixed. Pandemics could also be masterminded by terrorists who want to cause extreme harm [12]. Pandemics are a serious challenge for emergency responders because they spread, and may cause enormous damage to people and social infrastructures. Pandemics will travel as quickly as people do in our modern world. Pandemics spread via individuals, often in the home or the workplace, as victims often unwittingly pass the disease to others. When patients eventually realize they are ill, they often go directly to the hospital or clinic for care, bypassing fire, police, and EMTs. During the incubation period, victims may infect others, especially those particularly susceptible because of comorbidities (immunocompromised people, pregnant women). Although most pandemic agents affect the very young and the very old—"U curve" (where, if we plot the number of incidents by age, the plot looks like a "U" with peaks at both young and old ages)—in rare instances like the 1918 flu, and the 2009/2010 H1N1 flu, the distribution of those infected follows a "W curve" (where, if we plot the number of incidents by age, the plot looks like a "W" with peaks at young, middle, and old ages [29]), the "W" including previously healthy individuals aged in their twenties and thirties either as a result of absolute immunological naïveté or exaggerated immunological response to the contagion, the so-called cytokine storm.

Because biological agents are silent, unpredictable, and have an asymptomatic incubation time, they are especially effective for terrorist attacks [27]. Five characteristics make terrorists prefer biological weapons to nuclear, chemical, or even radiological weapons: (a) Biological agents are easily concealed in small containers that can carry enough pathogen to infect entire communities. Alternatively, the container can be a human vector (Luis Kun, personal communication). (b) Incubation periods enable terrorists to silently disperse and transmit bio-agents into target populations in a manner that may be indistinguishable from naturally occurring phenomena (e.g., H1N1 has an asymptomatic incubation period when a patient is contagious for a day prior to onset of symptoms). (c) Biological attacks can incapacitate the very public health personnel needed to detect, contain, treat, and respond to the disaster.* (d) The longer a biological attack remains undetected, the more difficult it becomes to prevent its proliferation. Unlike a static strike with conventional weapons, the damage caused by a bioterrorist

---

* In one set of war games (in 1990 in California), a scenario of planned bioterror was modeled, in which two biological agents were deployed—the first agent, which was treatable, was transmitted to the public to attract the public health service key personnel; then, the second agent was deployed to cause untreatable casualties within the critical group of responders.

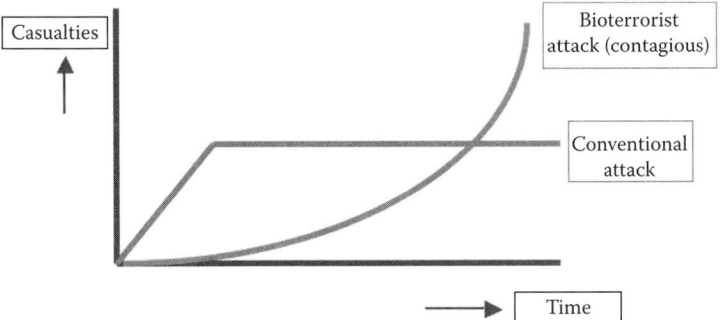

FIGURE 65.2 Conventional and bioterror attacks. (Courtesy of Joseph M. Rosen, MD. With permission.)

attack with a contagious agent can grow geometrically (see Figure 65.2). This is mostly from airborne transmission, which is why smallpox, pneumonic plague, and hemorrhagic fever viruses may be so effective, as airborne-size particles can be transmitted from person to person [10]. (e) Finally, caring for illness is more costly to society than weapons causing immediate deaths. That is one reason why conventional enemies often desire to wound rather than kill enemy soldiers, as it ties up medical, logistics, transportation, and other costly assets.

U.S. government simulations have revealed that existing local, state, and federal resources are not capable of easily responding to, and containing, events of biological warfare. Resources often cannot be allocated and distributed efficiently [24]. Emergency response systems must quickly detect and contain such an event and treat patients rapidly. We need a new paradigm for responding to a pandemic. This will require new roles for emergency responders to deliver critical supplies to the home, along with technology like Remote Platforms [4] that can be placed in each home so families can receive critical medical advice to better care for sick individuals without requiring transport to a clinic or hospital environment. It will also require technologies to enable early detection of the virus and keep people at home before it spreads. Emergency or public health responders could be involved in these new, preventive efforts for detection, treatment at home, and limiting the spread of disease.

If we cannot reliably predict pandemics, we can be proactive in trying to stockpile vaccines and antivirals for viruses such as H1N1 or H5N1. Technology plays a role because we need to discover ways to manufacture such vaccines quickly and efficiently and in large doses [1]. In 2010, the H1N1 vaccine was given to many patients too late to be effective—not months ahead of flu season, in the summer, but well after the flu had begun.

International, federal, state, and local officials must respond to future attacks of CBRNE agents with planning, practice, simulation, and the best technology solutions available in both the military and civilian domains.

65.2 Current Response Systems and Potential Improvements to Disaster Response Paradigms: Lessons Learned since 9/11

All major disasters are global because all nations are connected in the modern world via robust transportation systems that can facilitate dissemination. The 2003 SARS pandemic spread from Asia to Canada rapidly because of the speed of people traveling internationally. The volcano eruption in Iceland in April 2010 disrupted air travel from Africa through Europe and into the United States and back. The U.S. Gulf of Mexico oil spill in 2010 impacted countries worldwide because food supplies from the Gulf were shipped internationally. This disaster had as-yet-unknown, long-term environmental effects. And in many disasters, owing to media coverage and the Internet, the whole world is aware. People around the world watched and many cried as events unfolded on the day of the U.S. 9/11 disasters; in the 2010 Haiti earthquake, 2011

Japan disasters, 2012 U.S. Hurricane Sandy, and other ongoing disasters, we continue to observe, read, and weep for those victims from countries far away.

It is beyond the scope of this chapter to describe current emergency response systems worldwide but it is an international goal to have such agencies continue to build networks of technology and cooperation in disaster response. In this section, we describe disaster response systems in the United States as an example. While the specifics are U.S.-centric, the concepts of distributed command and control are universal.

65.2.1 Current Disaster Response Systems

Although the U.S. government recognizes the potential threats of natural disasters, terrorism, and pandemics, the current federal emergency response system cannot adequately respond to a large-scale catastrophe. Americans often assume that in a severe disaster, the government (authority) will respond quickly. This may not be true in a huge disaster, or when local or national response systems fail, as was the case with Katrina and the 2010 Gulf oil spill.

Present disaster response systems are based on a vertical, often rigid, hierarchy. In the future, we need a dynamic, adaptive, agile response system from first responder all the way to command and control. This section briefly describes the nation's disaster response efforts under the National Response Framework (NRF) [22] and its medical arm, the National Disaster Medical System (NDMS) [20], including their interactions, limitations, and proposed improvements.

The current disaster response systems stem from a failed response to Alaska's 1964 9.2 earthquake. The Disaster Relief Act of 1974 attempted to coordinate federal response efforts, including the creation of FEMA in 1979, though its focus at the time was to respond to Cold War needs. The mission of FEMA is to "support our citizens and first responders to ensure that as a nation we work together to build, sustain, and improve our capacity to prepare for, protect against, respond to, recover from, and mitigate all hazards" [2]. The current basis for a federal disaster response in the United States is PL 93-288 (later amended in PL 100-707), the Robert T. Stafford Disaster Relief and Emergency Assistance Act (most commonly known as the "Stafford Act") [28]; in summary, all disasters are local and state events unless the governor specifically asks for federal support, which is granted by the President's declaration of a disaster.

65.2.1.1 Local and State Disaster Response Systems

Emergency response systems typically begin at the local level; later, state or federal resources may be called in, depending on the escalation and duration of the event and number of casualties. And while the federal government, through FEMA, may provide substantial financial support in the aftermath of large-scale disasters, state and local governments will still conduct most of the hands-on disaster recovery efforts [7].

The local and state response capability includes a variety of organizations, including many funded by the federal government. Typically, the local response includes fire, police, and EMS along with public health officials in a medical event. Local Emergency Planning Committees are multiagency groups that provide additional assets to the response. Substate regions may develop All-Hazards Health Regions as done in New Hampshire with their own Neighborhood Health Clinics for minor, primary care, and Points of Distributions under the recently developed Modular Emergency Management System program (MEMS) [8]. Federal assets that work in the community include the Surgeon General's Medical Reserve Corps Teams and FEMA's Community Emergency Response Teams or Metropolitan Medical Response Systems. Some communities have U.S. Department of Defense (DOD) bases, hospitals, or Veterans Affairs (VA) hospitals that can be used locally in a disaster. States may have their own State Emergency Management Agencies that oversee Hazardous Materials (HAZMAT) teams, along with their state National Guards, including the newly created Weapons of Mass Destruction Civil Support Teams. States may also reach across borders to other states, without asking for federal support, by invoking the Emergency Management Assistance Compact.

65.2.1.2 Federal Disaster Response Systems

When local and state resources and processes have been exhausted, a state governor may request federal assets. Disaster support from the national level has changed over the past few years from the Federal Response Plan prior to 9/11 to the National Response Plan to its current NRF [9] (see Figure 65.3). "National" is intentional as it describes the full response effort, not just federal assets.

65.2.1.2.1 National Response Framework

The National Response Framework (NRF) [22] is designed to be all-hazards and broad in scope, from the smallest incident to the largest catastrophe. It is designed to be scalable, flexible, and adaptable; always be in effect; and to articulate clear roles and responsibilities among local, state, and federal officials [35]. Importantly, the NRF is multidimensional. While we tend to think of only its medical response efforts, it entails 15 essential support functions (ESFs) covering everything from transportation (ESF 1) to external affairs (ESF 15). Each ESF has a coordinating federal agency in charge. National medical support falls under ESF 8, Public Health and Medical Services coordinated by the U.S. Department of Health and Human Services (DHHS) and its NDMS.

65.2.1.2.2 National Disaster Medical System

According to FEMA, "The overall purpose of the NDMS is to establish a single, integrated national medical response capability for assisting state and local authorities in dealing with the medical impacts of major peacetime disasters. National Disaster Medical System (NDMS), under (NSF) Emergency Support Function #8—Public Health and Medical Services, supports Federal agencies in the management and coordination of the Federal medical response to major emergencies and federally declared disasters" [22]. Currently, NDMS operates under DHHS' Assistant Secretary for Preparedness and Response, and collaborates with the Department of Defense, the Department of Veterans Affairs, and FEMA in providing disaster medical support. NDMS' medical assets have been categorized into several groups of teams [20]:

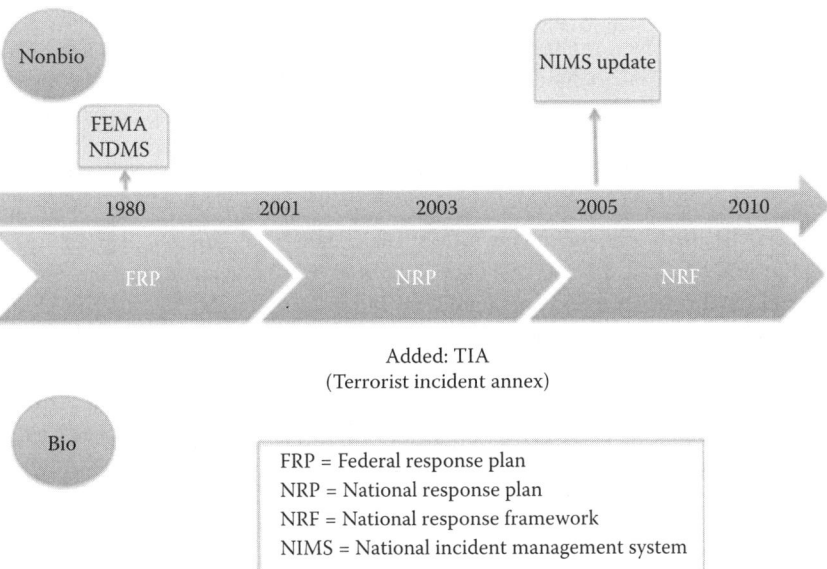

FRP = Federal response plan
NRP = National response plan
NRF = National response framework
NIMS = National incident management system

FIGURE 65.3 Development of Current National Response Framework. (Courtesy of Joseph M. Rosen, MD. With permission.)

- Disaster Medical Assistance Team—provides medical care during a disaster or other incident.
- National Medical Response Team—provides mass decontamination and medical care to victims of a release of weapons of mass destruction, or a large-scale release of hazardous material.
- Disaster Mortuary Operational Response Team—provides victim identification and mortuary services during a disaster or other incident.
- National Veterinary Response Team—provides assistance in assessing the need for veterinary services following major disasters or emergencies.
- Federal Coordinating Centers—recruit hospitals and maintain local non-Federal hospital participation in the NDMS and coordinate exercise development and emergency plans.
- National Pharmacy Response Teams—assist in chemoprophylaxis or the vaccination of a large number of Americans in response to an emergency such as a disease outbreak.
- International Medical Surgical Response Team (IMSuRT)—IMSuRT is widely recognized as a specialized team, trained and equipped to establish a fully capable field surgical facility anywhere in the world.
- National Nurse Response Team (NNRT)—The NNRT will comprise 10 regionally based teams of 200 registered nurses who could be called upon, for example, to assist in the vaccination of hundreds of thousands or millions of Americans, if needed.

65.2.1.2.3 Incident Command System and National Incident Management System

The original *command and control system* that coordinated multiple agencies from many organizations in disaster response was the incident command system (ICS) [11]. The use of ICS began in 1970 following a large number of fires in southern California, which in 13 days, destroyed 600,000 acres, 772 structures, and caused 16 deaths. The 13 largest fires crossed federal, county, and city jurisdictions simultaneously. Following this disaster, the U.S. Department of Agriculture's Forest Service reviewed and analyzed the efforts of the responding federal, state, county, and city organizations. This 1971 project identified six major problem areas that impeded an efficient response effort: lack of a common organization; poor on-scene and interagency communications; inadequate joint planning; lack of valid and timely intelligence; inadequate resource management; and limited prediction capability [17, pp. 135–136]. The basic philosophical foundation of the ICS, ideally, includes autonomy of the agencies, management by objectives, unit integrity, and functional clarity [17, p. 138]. In addition, ICS requires an effective span-of-control, modularity to the organization, common terminology, integrated communications, and comprehensive resource management [17, pp. 139–141].

ICS has become an integral component of the U.S. National Incident Management System (NIMS) [21]. Also developed in California is a hospital incident command system (HICS), which is becoming a part of most U.S. hospitals' disaster response organization. The unified structure of incident management requires all federal agencies to use NIMS in their incident management, prevention, response, and recovery activities. Additionally, all state, tribal, and local organizations using federal funding for training and support must also be compliant with NIMS. The system is built upon the principles of flexibility and standardization. While ICS is its most functional and well-known component, it also includes a multiagency coordination system and public information systems.

The principles of distributed command and control could apply in any worldwide disaster and its medical response. Leaders should supervise three to seven sections, ideally five, and have a distribution of areas to supervise, including planning, operations, finance/administration, and logistics sections. ICS is a model that meets those requirements, and can be expanded or contracted as needed. ICS comes from basic military command and control that is used worldwide.

65.2.2 Gaps and Potential Improvements in Current Systems

In the current response framework, first responders often respond as local teams. State and federal resources then become available only after the declaration of a state of emergency—a process that can take hours, if not days. By the time a disaster is detected, its scale fully understood, and federal resources arrive, it may be too late: an event may escalate beyond the incident area, or become exponentially greater (see Figure 65.1a). Though "federal personnel [might] deal with the horrendous aftermath, [they] would typically not be involved in the direct response" [26]. Ideally, medical response assets would be prepositioned and/or preauthorized to rapidly surge to meet demand in concert with local assets (see Figure 65.1b), thereby avoiding the response gap in normal response scenarios.

An additional challenge may be the potential use of decoy or multiple targets by terrorists, leaving federal resources playing "whack-a-mole" in trying to deliver resources to overwhelmed local and state groups in multiple targets and locations. The system needs to evolve to foster improved coordination between federal authorities and first responders at the state and local levels; to revamp our response systems and training programs; and to enhance all of the above with new technology.

65.2.3 Specific Examples of Gaps in Current Systems

65.2.3.1 Sudden-Impact Natural or Human-Made Disasters

NDMS was originally set up for an event like an earthquake, and thus an evacuation of up to 100,000 casualties. In the case of a hurricane, with forewarning, NDMS was ideally suited to save thousands of lives during Katrina, had it been activated in time [14]. This was not a failure of the NDMS, which was ideally designed for this type of evacuation; rather, it was a failure of leadership, which did not have the foresight to request or move NDMS assets ahead of the storm. Although significant improvements have occurred since Hurricane Katrina, a multi-dimensional disaster such as the Great East Japan Earthquake with both earthquake, tsunami and flood damage, coupled with radiation exposure would test even the best of plans. Even in 2012, although Hurricane Sandy mirrored in some ways the types of damages seen with Katrina, the sheer magnitude and scope of the storm affecting the most populous region in the United States identified further gaps in preparedness and response.

65.2.3.2 Terror Attacks

The September 11 Commission report illuminated failures to coordinate U.S. intelligence among agencies [4]. As a result of this incident, the National Counter-Terrorism Center (NCTC) was established in 2005 [19]. Its role was to integrate key information across all 16 agencies that deal with counter-terrorism. In response to persistent stove-piped intelligence gathering, the Director of National Intelligence (DNI) was established; however, both the DNI and NCTC have not filled the gap that was pointed out by the 9/11 report. The 2009 "Christmas Day Bomber" is an example of a failure to integrate multiple agencies. The first responders should be able to report suspicious events, through their appropriate chain of command, to the NCTC, which would then assign staff to investigate how individual observations fit into a broader upcoming surprise event. Unfortunately, this has not happened and remains to be addressed.

65.2.3.3 Biological Disasters

A continuous, integrated response is particularly needed in biological disaster scenarios. Casualties should be treated onsite or screened before evacuation to remote medical facilities; otherwise, centralized, tertiary care hospitals without appropriate infection-control measures in place, and lacking proper utilization of HICS, will become overwhelmed and may become a place where infections can propagate. If providers fall ill, we will lose a node in the public health network. Adequate staging of personnel, equipment, and supplies is necessary to prevent such secondary effects of a primary disaster. Isolation and quarantine would need to be utilized for a contagious agent.

A terrorist attack of national scope will inevitably initiate "a multi-agency operation requiring sophisticated (and sometimes chaotic) communications and coordination" [25]. A primary objective for first responders and federal agencies is to enhance interoperability across functional and geographic jurisdictions, including improving communications networks and enhancing incident command and control (C^2). Chief among them is the adoption of new doctrines for evacuation, isolation in place, hospitalization, and treatment.

65.2.4 Lessons Learned in Disaster Response during the Decade since 9/11: Setting the Stage for Systematic Improvement

In the aftermath of Hurricane Katrina and other recent disasters (see Table 65.3), emergency responders and government officials at local, state, and federal levels have collaborated to refine and improve our response systems. For example, DOD created U.S. Northern Command (Northcom) [34], which coordinates all continental United States (CONUS) DOD assets integrated into the federal response and, as needed or tasked, plays a leading role in coordination capabilities among relevant federal, state, and local agencies. The real question is what lessons learned from Haiti, Japan, and other recent incidents will provide guidance for future international disasters, and who will be in charge of these megadisasters? Additionally, how can these various entities coordinate a robust, integrated response effort?

Recent U.S. legislative and organizational changes have resulted in the appropriation of resources and people (e.g., the new Department of Homeland Security), but the response effort remains disjointed. The paradigm of training and integrating these multiagencies and groups needs to adapt to the increasing complexity of disaster response. In some ways, human-made terrorist groups are succeeding in scrambling our response construct. Our response ethos, training techniques, and use of technology all need to adjust to overcome the organizational turf battles that impair a coordinated response. If not, our adversaries, natural or human-made, will find this "white space" and exploit our deficiencies.

To improve response, clearly, we need a way to equalize and link the resources for various emergency responders, both military and civilian, as mentioned in Section 65.1. We also suggest a fundamental change in how we describe personnel responding to an incident: we might reclassify them as (a) untrained first responders and (b) professional responders—both of which play complementary

TABLE 65.3 Natural Disasters in the Decade since 9/11

Year	Name	Death Toll (apx)	Source of Data
2003	SARS pandemic, Canada, Asia	813	http://www.phac-aspc.gc.ca/publicat/sars-sras/naylor/1-eng.php
2004	Tsunami, Indian Ocean	230,000	http://en.wikipedia.org/wiki/List_of_natural_disasters
2005	Kashmir earthquake, Pakistan	79,000	http://www.msnbc.msn.com/id/9626146/ns/world_newssouth_and_central_asia/
2005	Hurricane Katrina, United States	1836	http://www.hurricanekatrinarelief.com/faqs.html#What%20is%20the%20death%20toll%20of%20Hurricane%20Katrina
2008	Cyclone, Myanmar	138,000	http://en.wikipedia.org/wiki/List_of_natural_disasters
2009	H1N1 pandemic, Mexico and worldwide (*)	284,000	http://www.cidrap.umn.edu/cidrap/content/influenza/panflu/news/jun2712deaths.html
2010	Earthquake, Haiti	316,000	http://earthquake.usgs.gov/earthquakes/eqarchives/year/2010/2010_deaths.php
2011	Japan earthquake-tsunami	19,850	http://reliefweb.int/report/world/annual-disaster-statistical-review-2011-numbers-and-trends http://reliefweb.int/sites/reliefweb.int/files/resources/2012.07.05.ADSR_2011.pdf
2012	Hurricane Sandy, United States	133	http://www.guardian.co.uk/news/datablog/2012/oct/31/hurricane-sandy-death-toll
Annually	Seasonal influenza	250,000–500,000	http://www.who.int/mediacentre/factsheets/fs211/en/

roles. In recent responses, the people who were not medical providers but acted to help people could make a big difference. After one helicopter crash, a U.S. soldier observed that "it was a good thing some of these guys who responded remembered the info in their buddy aid class" (Michael Lauria, personal communication). The U.S. military trains everybody in first aid for a reason, and that system works pretty well: When a medic cannot get to a person, an infantryman can help apply a tourniquet. If we extended this training to civilians, we would have a corps of volunteers who might assist clinical responders in a disaster, especially a pandemic that might require quarantine care at home in the community. We could structure the response like an image of a pyramid, whose base would be citizens, people at the scene with basic knowledge who can make an immediate difference. This worked very well in the German case study, described below.

For combat casualty care, the present paradigm is "the right care, at the right time, in the right place, by the right person" (John Holcomb, personal communication). In a similar analogy, the first responder during a civilian disaster has the same requirements: (1) the team and its culture, (2) the training of the team, and (3) the technologies utilized by the team. The first two are discussed here; the third is covered in Chapter 66.

65.2.4.1 Team Culture

We believe that the culture of the team greatly influences the success of the response to the event. Different cultures can have the view that (a) the whole population must help in emergency response—everyone is responsible or (b) citizens should wait for government to come rescue them. There are two excellent examples of an all-population response—from Germany and Vietnam, respectively.

65.2.4.1.1 Germany

On October 3, 1998, in Eschede, Germany, there was an intercity express (ICE) train accident, in which 287 passengers had been traveling around 200 km/h [16]. The front wheel cracked, and the train derailed 1 km before an underpass and slammed into the underpass. The Germans have a culture of involving all members of society in their response system. They also had been preparing for several years for a train catastrophe in which a train could derail within a tunnel in the Alps. They had done multiple training exercises, and had set up specific requirements, such as integrating command centers within 15 minutes following the disaster. The command centers, along with the individual in charge, were responsible for controlling all resources and bringing them to bear during a train (or other) disaster. Within 6 minutes, the first emergency responders arrived at the site of the disaster. Over 2000 responders were mobilized, and 40 airborne transport vehicles were brought in for evacuation. Two local hospitals and 20 distant hospitals were placed under the command of the individual in charge, who happened to be a physician. Traffic was diverted to create capacity for the victims. Eighty-seven victims were evacuated to these 22 facilities within a 100-mile radius. There was one additional victim who had to be cut out of a high-speed car, which took an additional 2 hours. The response to this German event demonstrated an unprecedented level of team coordination, training, and use of technology. In particular, handheld devices were introduced that enabled victims to be identified and triaged.

65.2.4.1.2 Vietnam

Vietnam's response to SARS in 2003 was well coordinated and orchestrated by the government, despite limited resources in comparison to other countries that were also hit. Having distributed the "Ten Measures for Prevention against SARS" in December 2002 (approximately 2 months before the first case presented), the general population was well prepared for a potential disaster. This document included a set of requirements for the general population to follow to keep the pandemic under control. These guidelines were followed because there exists a culture in Vietnam to listen to the government and to work as a community in response to threats. Initially, SARS presented at the French Hospital in Hanoi, but patients were also directed to the Tropical Medicine Institute at Bach Mai Hospital. The response was coordinated by the Vietnamese government's Vice Premier, who had control of all resources that would need to be mobilized for this effort. The initial intention to alert the population and government about SARS was made by the Italian Dr. Carlo Urbani at the World Health Organization (WHO), which immediately enabled the Vietnamese government and Ministry of Health to respond quickly and effectively.

Vietnam's response to SARS can be compared to Toronto's less effective response to SARS, where many more people were infected and killed due to a less coordinated and inefficient response effort. While the Vietnamese government issued a preparatory "Ten Measures" document 2 months before the outbreak occurred, Canada only issued instructions once the outbreak was already in full swing. In Vietnam, SARS patients were directed to two major hospitals (the French Hospital and Bach Mai Hospital), while in Canada patients stayed where they presented, which became a logistical nightmare for providers. After the WHO put a 2-month quarantine in place in both countries, Vietnam responded by deciding to keep the quarantine in place beyond the 2-month timeframe, while Toronto let their quarantine end, which resulted in another wave of SARS cases. Toronto used high-technology methods of isolation and venting in the hospital rooms of infected patients, whereas Hanoi used a simple, low-technology approach of opening the windows of hospital rooms, and lettings the virus dilute into the outdoors harmlessly. While Toronto relied on voluntary isolation of people who had been exposed, Hanoi used a mandatory compulsory system with guards to ensure that exposed people did not spread the virus. Overall, Hanoi was more aggressive in their response, capitalizing on a culture that submitted more easily to the government, and worked closely together to gain control of the pandemic. In Toronto, the virus remained out of control for a longer period of time, resulting in many more overall deaths. Toronto suffered 375 cases and 44 deaths, while Hanoi only suffered 63 cases and six deaths [10].

In Germany and Vietnam, team culture, training, and technology all played a major role. Although this chapter and Chapter 66 seek new ways to address these challenges, including the use of high technology, it is interesting to note that sometimes an effective response can involve the less costly, low-technology, yet still coordinated response efforts. For example, instead of using high technology, the Vietnamese used "low technology" (opening windows) and centralized authority to mount an overwhelming response to the threat of SARS to both the population and the economy.

65.2.4.2 Team Training

In the German example, success came from having the right team culture, training, and technology. In the United States, despite the efforts to improve response agencies and communication, first responder training often falls to a diverse collection of agencies possessing disparate sources of authority, funding, and information. The U.S. Department of Energy, for example, oversees training for nuclear and radiological attacks. The DHHS, with the Centers for Disease Control as a principal agency, oversees bioterrorism programs. The Departments of Justice and Homeland Security each provide a broad spectrum of grants and training programs for fire, law enforcement, and emergency medical personnel. And finally, the Department of Defense has its own combined and service-specific training for its medical personnel. The result is an unwieldy and extraordinarily complex bureaucratic web. If we could find one of the existing organizations to take the lead, standardize the training program, and implement it, that would be key.

Significant challenges also exist at the state and local level. Most training occurs under the auspices of local departments, sometimes supported by federal, state, or regional academies, and the level of preparedness often varies across jurisdictions and agencies. The result is a patchwork quilt that covers some areas, but leaves others woefully bare.

Between an earthquake and a pandemic, 80% of first responder training is the same; 20% is different. The event may be large-scale, short-duration, like an earthquake, or medium- or large-scale but long-duration, like a pandemic. The doctrine may include evacuation for some events versus quarantine for others. After 72 hours, Disaster Medical Assistance Team (DMAT) supplies start to run out. If up to

20% of the population could respond quickly, and had the aptitude and training to do so, we might have a better chance to "overwhelm the disaster" (with a 3:1 ratio of responders to victims) and shorten its duration. But we also need longer-term plans for large-and-long events.

Training people to respond to both military and civilian incidents should also involve a long hard look at public education. The American Heart Association (AHA)–standardized CPR training presents a single curriculum on a national scale to teach people how to provide on-the-spot resuscitation efforts. The widespread use by bystanders in Seattle has resulted in a 30% victim survival rate, compared to 1–2% in New York City, where it is implemented less often [3]. It is important to not only redefine the general population as "first responders" but also to consider public education as an important part of disaster response in our country.

Finally, the construct of training needs to change. For example, the single technology that best bridges education and delivery of care is simulation. In the disaster relief arena, responders could simulate various emergency and relief scenarios to better prepare for an eventual disaster. Simulation provides a number of advantages, including

- Accelerating development of expertise, self-confidence, and motivation
- Providing for experiential learning that is readily and predictably available
- Connecting knowledge with action
- Providing opportunities for frequent practice and feedback
- Fostering teamwork
- Providing a means for rational assessment of skills

Trainees can also benefit from simulators based on a variety of technologies, including computers, broadband networks, and multimedia (still and moving graphics, still photos and video, audio, text). Simulators can be stand-alone (single-user) or deployed in a multiuser online virtual world (e.g., Second Life® or its open-source derivatives). And finally, the simulators can be partial-task, dealing with one aspect of a patient encounter, or they can be comprehensive, addressing knowledge, skills, and attitudes associated with a given patient-care situation. In short, medical training needs to evolve from "death by Powerpoint" to live, interactive learning in a no-threat environment, conducive to the adult learner, while employing the tools today's young learners have come to expect. One example is Dartmouth's Interactive Media Laboratory Virtual Clinic [13].

Training, like medical care and medical response, needs to move toward a model that is needs-based, cross-platform, and cross-cultural. We believe that in the future, training and improved performance can be combined. Just-in-time training can be incorporated in new technologies to train first responders to meet the challenges of new and unique events. We call this a "performance machine," which can take various forms—from simple, handheld devices, to computers, to virtual environments. Chapter 66 gives more details on these concepts.

65.3 Conclusions

As the threat of global terrorism grows, so does the need for a corps of fire, police, and EMTs trained to take the initiative in chaotic, dynamic events. The ideal first responder must be well rounded; an expert in his or her field; prepared for an eventuality; and capable, when necessary, of working alone. These characteristics may be innate, but can also be learned. Enabling local decision making is a necessary first step in creating a technology-based crisis response paradigm in which other disaster information flows horizontally among all components of the Homeland Security architecture.

In the future, we will use the "three Ts"—*team culture, training,* and *technology*—to expand the category of first responder to include family members, volunteers, and public and private health personnel. In an event that is distributed and involves one-third of the population, such as a pandemic, or an unforeseen nuclear or environmental catastrophe, we will need everyone who is alive, able-bodied, and

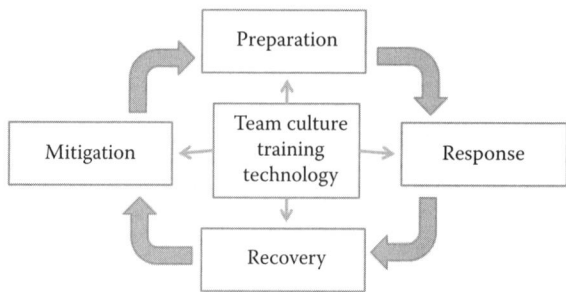

FIGURE 65.4 Integration of team culture, training, and technology into disaster phases. (Courtesy of Joseph M. Rosen, MD. With permission.)

available to join the emergency response—including civilians and nonclinicians who have been trained in basic first aid (see Figure 65.4).

Team culture: Response culture may come into play. In the German model, they overwhelmed the disaster with responders, for a swift and successful response. Other responses failed because we let the disaster overwhelm the responders. In the United States, traditionally the culture was to assume that someone in uniform would lead the rescue and citizens might passively wait for help. However, there were recent exceptions in which heroic civilians "swam upstream" to help victims at the event, such as in the Boston Marathon bombing in April 2013.

Training: We can not only improve the first responder system but we must also change the system to network-based, and change the process to mission command and control versus hierarchical. The military calls this "mission orders," which means to give responders a specific mission or task and let them find the most effective means given the information at hand, on scene. In this way, each small team has a role to play and can pursue this in their designated area, with independence, but connected to the overall response. The training then also needs to include senior leaders and command structures as well as individual providers and middle-level managers to exercise this distributive response effort.

Technology: Ultimately, there will be a convergence of technologies, and of all the disasters, and with the roles of the first responders in each type of disaster. There will be a time shift of the response to the left—that is, first responders will be proactive earlier in the onset of the disaster. They will triage and treat in the prehospital environment before the victim needs to go the hospital. They will contain the spread of disease and prevent both disease and needed response from reaching epic proportions. This will apply to hurricanes and pandemics.

In conclusion, this chapter has described how team culture and training may improve paradigms for responding to various types of disasters. The impact of the third and perhaps most important "T"—technology—on improving disaster response is covered in Chapter 66. The integration of these improvements will then cross all disaster phases, leading to a more effective response effort (Figure 65.4).

Acknowledgments

The authors wish to thank Matthew McKnight for many thoughtful comments and editing to improve this chapter, and Robyn Mosher for extensive editorial assistance.

References

1. 2005 Congressional Report on Pandemic Economic Consequences. Available at: http://www.cbo.gov/sites/default/files/cbofiles/ftpdocs/69xx/doc6946/12-08-birdflu.pdf. Accessed 4/23/13.
2. About FEMA. Available at: http://www.fema.gov/about-fema. Accessed 4/23/13.

3. American Heart Association. Cardiopulmonary Resuscitation (CPR) Statistics. Available at: http://www.heart.org/HEARTORG/CPRAndECC/WhatisCPR/CPRFactsandStats/CPR-Facts-and-Stats_UCM_302910_SubHomePage.jsp. Accessed 4/23/13.
4. Bosch Healthcare—Telehealth. Available at: http://www.bosch-telehealth.com/en/us/products/health_buddy/health_buddy.html. Accessed 4/23/13.
5. Cantor, N.F. 2001. *In the Wake of the Plague: The Black Death and the World It Made.* New York, NY: Free Press.
6. Death Tolls in Terror Attacks. Available at: http://en.wikipedia.org/wiki/List_of_battles_and_other_violent_events_by_death_toll#Terrorist_attacks. Accessed 4/23/13.
7. GAO Report: Disaster Recovery: Past Experiences Offer Insights for Recovering from Hurricanes Ike and Gustav and Other Recent Natural Disasters. September 2008. Available at: http://www.gao.gov/products/GAO-08-1120. Accessed 4/23/13.
8. Gougelet, R. Modular Emergency Medical Systems (MEMS) for All Types of Catastrophic Emergencies: A Guide for Community Preparedness. Available at: http://geiselmed.dartmouth.edu/necep/pdf/mems.pdf. Accessed 4/23/13.
9. Gougelet, R.M. and Geiling, J. 2012. The National Response Framework – How will the nation support a local disaster? In *The Oxford American Handbook of Disaster Medicine* (Eds. R. A. Partridge, L. Proano, D. Marcozzi, A. G. Garza, I. Nemeth, K. Brinsfield, E. S. Weinstein), New York: Oxford University Press.
10. Grigg, E., Rosen, J., and Koop, C.E. 2006. The biological disaster challenge. Why we are least prepared for the most devastating threat and what we need to do about it. *Journal of Emergency Management* 4(1): 23–35.
11. Incident Command System (ICS) under National Incident Management System (NIMS). Available at: http://www.fema.gov/incident-command-system. Accessed 4/23/13.
12. Intentional Terror Acts. http://www.cbsnews.com/stories/2007/07/02/terror/main3004644.shtml. Accessed 4/23/13.
13. Interactive Media Laboratory, Dartmouth Medical School. Primary Care of the HIV/AIDS Patient: A Virtual Clinic. Available at: http://iml.dartmouth.edu/education/cme/HIV_Primary_Care/index.html. Accessed 4/23/13.
14. Katrina GAO Report. Hurricane Katrina: Providing Oversight of the Nation's Preparedness, Response, and Recovery Activities. GAO-05-1053T. Available at: http://www.gao.gov/new.items/d051053t.pdf. Accessed 4/23/13.
15. Kidder, T. 2003. *Mountains beyond Mountains.* New York: Random House. (Biography of Paul Farmer, MD, founder of Partners in Health in Haiti).
16. Langley, D., Lockhardt, S.M., Lockhardt, J.M., Rosen, J.M., and McKnight, M.F. 2004. *ICE 884: Response to Disaster.* Durham, NH: Team Hill Studios.
17. Lewis, C.P. and Aghababian, R.V. 1996. Disaster planning, Part I; Overview of hospital and emergency department planning for internal and external disasters. *Emergency Medicine Clinics of North America* 14(2):135–6.
18. May 2010 NYC Bomb Threat. Described in: http://www.nytimes.com/2010/05/02/nyregion/02timessquare.html. Accessed 4/23/13.
19. National Counter-Terrorism Center (NCTC). Available at: http://www.nctc.gov/. Accessed 4/23/13.
20. National Disaster Medical System. Available at: http://www.phe.gov/Preparedness/responders/ndms/Pages/default.aspx. Accessed 4/23/13.
21. National Incident Management System (NIMS). Available at: http://www.fema.gov/national-preparedness/national-incident-management-system. Accessed 4/23/13.
22. National Response Framework (NRF) News Release. Available at: http://www.fema.gov/pdf/emergency/nrf/whatsnew.pdf Release Date: January 22, 2008 (Release Number: FNF-08-008). Also: NRF Info with definition of National Disaster Medical System (NDMS). Available at: http://www.fema.gov/pdf/emergency/nrf/nrf-glossary.pdf. Accessed 4/23/13.

23. Price-Smith, A. 2009. *Contagion and Chaos*. Cambridge, MA: MIT Press.

24. Report to the President on US Preparations for 2009-H1N1 Influenza. Available at: http://www. whitehouse.gov/assets/documents/PCAST_H1N1_Report.pdf. Accessed 4/23/13.

25. Rosen, J.M., Grigg, E., McGrath, S., Lillibridge, S., and Koop, C.E. 2003. Cybercare NDMS: An improved strategy for biodefense using information technologies. In *Integration of Health Telematics into Medical Practice*, eds. M. Nerlich and U. Schaechinger, 95–114. Amsterdam: IOS Press.

26. Rosen, J.M., Grigg, E.B., McKnight, M.F. et al. 2004. Transforming medicine for biodefense and healthcare delivery: Developing a dual-use doctrine that utilizes information superiority and network-based organization. *IEEE Engineering in Medicine and Biology* 23 (1):89–101.

27. Rosen, J.M., Koop, C.E., and Grigg, E.B. 2002. Cybercare: A system for confronting bioterrorism. *The Bridge* 32:34–50.

28. Stafford Act. Available at: http://www.fema.gov/robert-t-stafford-disaster-relief-and-emergency-assistance-act-public-law-93-288-amended. Accessed 4/23/13.

29. Taubenberger, J.K. and Morens, D.M. 2006. 1918 Influenza: The mother of all pandemics. *Emerging Infections Diseases* (12):1. Figure 2. "U-" and "W-" shaped combined influenza and pneumonia mortality. Available at: http://wwwnc.cdc.gov/eid/article/12/1/05-0979_article.htm. Accessed 4/23/13.

30. The 9/11 Commission Report, Executive Summary. Available at: http://www.c-span.org/pdf/911finalreportexecsum.pdf. Accessed 4/26/13. Full report: National Commission on Terrorist Attacks upon the United States, Washington, DC, July 22, 2004.

31. The Federal Response to Hurricane Katrina: Lessons Learned. February 2006 Publication from the US President Bush and the White House. Available at: http://www.au.af.mil/au/awc/awcgate/whitehouse/katrina/katrina-lessons-learned.pdf. Accessed 4/26/13.

32. The White House, President Discusses Hurricane Relief in Address to the Nation, News Release, September 15, 2005. Available at: http://georgewbush-whitehouse.archives.gov/news/releases/2005/09/20050915-8.html. Accessed 4/26/13.

33. United States Northern Command (Northcom). Available at: http://www.northcom.mil/about/index.html. Accessed 4/26/13.

34. What's New in the National Response Framework. January 22, 2008. Available at: www.fema.gov/pdf/emergency/nrf/whatsnew.pdf. Accessed 4/26/13.

66

Disaster Response: Potential Improvement with Medical Informatics

James Geiling*
Geisel School of Medicine at Dartmouth

Veterans Affairs Medical Center, White River Junction, Vermont

Ron Poropatich
University of Pittsburgh

Michael Lauria†
Dartmouth-Hitchcock Medical Center

Robyn E. Mosher
Dartmouth College

Joseph M. Rosen
Geisel School of Medicine at Dartmouth

Veterans Affairs Medical Center, White River Junction, Vermont

66.1 Introduction

66.1.1 Background

Significant disasters occur with some regularity, including the Great East Japan Earthquake-tsunami-nuclear disaster in 2011; Hurricane Sandy in the United States and Caribbean in 2012; and most recently, with smaller scale, the Boston Marathon bombing in 2013. While these disasters and their medical responses continue to be studied, this chapter analyzes two other recent disasters, the Haiti earthquake in 2010 and the H1N1 outbreak in 2009, in which an efficient medical response was hampered by a lack of medical informatics that would have supported the responders at many levels. One example in Haiti was that cell phone communications, which would normally connect responders to each other and to critical information, were unreliable, as were electric power and sanitation (James Geiling, personal observation). There was also partial to complete destruction of any existing technology. When many responders arrived at one time at this chaotic disaster scene, they had disparate and often incompatible equipment, technologies, resources, networks, and even languages. By examining the response to Haiti

---

* The views expressed in this chapter are those of the author and do not necessarily reflect the official policy of the U.S. Government or the Department of Veterans Affairs.
† The views expressed in this chapter are those of the author and do not necessarily reflect the official policy of the U.S. Government, the U.S. Department of Defense, or the U.S. Air Force.

and other recent disasters, we hope to improve future response capacity by using medical informatics, technology, and networking that will function even in the presence of chaos.

Chapter 65 describes how disaster response systems are designed to work, and in what ways they have sometimes failed in recent disasters. That chapter classifies the types of personnel who respond to disasters, and also classifies the various types of disasters, including natural disasters, terrorist events, and pandemics—giving case studies of several disaster and response scenarios.

This chapter builds on the earlier chapter, using cases to illustrate how medical informatics may facilitate disaster response. In the ideal disaster response, diverse responders would use the latest military-grade technology (particularly hand-held and mobile devices) and employ a standardized network-centric infrastructure that would allow all agencies (military and others) to communicate and provide needed medical relief. We support the goal of establishing an international network architecture for disaster response: specifically, a broadband network that could seamlessly integrate voice, data, image, video, and multimedia content, and support interagency and cross-jurisdictional communications. While such a network remains a long-term deliverable, we can focus on the current technologies that exist for disaster management and what informatics gaps might be filled in the near term. The specific gaps and needs, listed below, are described in more detail in Section 66.3.

- *Hand-held devices* for technologies to assist in response, and devices to train on
- *Increased diagnostics* on these devices—laboratories for basic tests, examination, and pandemic surveillance
- *Mobile healthcare solutions or mHealth*, which refers to the use of emerging mobile devices and network technologies for healthcare systems to form a virtual "hospital without walls" for disasters
- *Distributed clinical information systems* to track populations and affected individuals
- *Telemedicine* and remote treatment—on remote devices (robots)—when needed (unsafe or contaminated sites, etc.)

By discussing the gaps in technologies for disaster responders, we hope to foster the creation and design of products to improve future responses to disasters of all types (natural disasters, acts of terror, and pandemics). Along with the technology itself, there is a need for developing trainers and simulators to help responders gain expertise with the technology.

66.1.2 Haiti, 2010: A View from Downtown Port-au-Prince*

The earthquake that struck Haiti in January 2010 was a complex, sudden-impact event with long-term consequences that are still being realized. Unfortunately, the decayed socioeconomic state of Haiti before the earthquake, combined with the magnitude of the earthquake and the limitations of the relief effort, all hindered the response capability. Although many groups and agencies labored to provide effective medical support, the efforts were often uncoordinated, and technology did not work properly for communication or provision of medical care—resulting in delays in care or even unnecessary patient deaths.

Haiti was an especially complex humanitarian assistance operation, with support coming from military and civilian groups around the world. The Haitian government itself was decimated, thereby causing severe deficiencies in overarching control of the event. Because of its proximity and significant cultural relationship with Haiti, the U.S. military took the lead in organizing airport security operations. The United Nations (UN) oversaw search and rescue efforts, but in reality, many teams arrived and then operated independently of the UN. Once additional medical resources and nongovernmental organizations (NGOs) arrived, the response situation became more complex. For example, at the

---

* The Haiti scenario is based on the experiences of author James Geiling, MD, who led a response team there in early 2010. Dr. Rosen and Dr. Geiling led a medical team that returned to Haiti in 2011, one year following the earthquake, to conduct plastic and reconstructive surgery.

University Hospital in downtown Port-au-Prince, on January 29, 2010, there were U.S. military forces that provided security, along with the Haitian hospital staff (who were mostly not available due to their own personal or family emergencies), and 23 NGOs to provide or support direct care.

What was unique about Haiti is that it was more like a war zone than a typical disaster. Almost all aspects of critical infrastructure (security, housing, water, food, and sanitation) were destroyed, requiring the military to restore infrastructure and replace missing key platforms, such as hospitals, using a military hospital ship. This type of coordination at present only truly exists within a military operation, but making it available for civilian disaster response is a present and future priority. Sharing technology via medical informatics may help level the playing field between the resource-rich military and other relief agencies with limited resources.

The provision of care in Haiti was difficult because of both the magnitude of the event and the complexity of the response effort. Table 66.1 highlights some of the observed areas and problems in downtown Port-au-Prince that need innovative solutions.

66.1.3 H1N1: A Close Call*

The 2009 H1N1 outbreak was first detected in Veracruz, Mexico in March 2009, and the first U.S. cases were presented in San Diego on April 1 and 2, 2009. At this point, the particular H1N1 strain was identified as a new virus—a combination of swine, avian, and human strains that had not been seen before. Initially, this H1N1 strain had the potential to be as deadly as the 1918 pandemic due to its genetic similarity. Its characteristics made it a potential global threat if its virulence evolved from less than 0.01% initially to 0.1% or even 1%. Ultimately, H1N1, like most pandemic flu strains, infected one-third of the U.S. population of 313 million [25], or about 100 million people. A virulence of 1% would thus have resulted in 1 million deaths.† Fortunately, this did not happen. However, there was no guarantee in April of 2009, when the initial cases presented, that the strain would not evolve to become more virulent. Surveillance and detection technologies, discussed later in this chapter, could have been very important to mitigate the outcome of a more virulent H1N1. These technologies enable detection, identification, and treatment of the virus, along with tracking the members of the population who have been exposed, infected, treated, and/or isolated.

In the case of H1N1, the vaccine was not ready in time for the second wave—while it should have been given in the summer of 2009, it was only ready in the fall of 2009, and an insufficient quantity was initially produced [24], which led to rationing for those at greatest risk and long wait lines. Ironically, in spring 2010, as the pandemic ebbed, about 71 million doses—out of 229 million doses originally bought by the United States—had to be discarded [4]. Technological innovations are needed to speed the development of vaccines and antivirals for new or rapidly evolving virus strains—the quicker and more efficient the process can be made, the better we can provide almost on-demand delivery, so that neither too little nor too much vaccine is produced.

Pandemics differ from other types of disasters, in that the victims should ideally be isolated, not evacuated. If victims were evacuated, then the disease might spread outside of its present domain, ultimately resulting in a huge increase in the population exposed to the pandemic. Pandemics require social distancing—isolation, restricted movement, personal separation, and in some extreme cases, even quarantine to prevent the potentially rapid spread of disease. Technology and training exercises are important to allow a response system that is usually involved in direct care to be mobilized to provide remote care to support such quarantine.

---

* The H1N1 flu scenario was written by author Joseph Rosen, MD, who was involved with planning and prevention of that event as well as working on pandemic response and prevention back in the severe acute respiratory syndrome (SARS) episode of 2003.
† *Note:* 1% equaling 1 million would mean that 100% is 100 million—if 100 million was 1/3 of the population, this would imply population is ~300 million in the United States—this matches the latest U.S. Census data from 2009 of 307 million.

TABLE 66.1 Technological Challenges to Providing Care during a Disaster (Haiti, 2010)

Technology	Challenges and Needs for Improved Design
Command and control	While hospital leadership was present, the lack of local staff and the overwhelming numbers of NGOs present impaired on-scene healthcare coordination. Each NGO has its own infrastructure and two primary constituents to support. The NGO is there to serve the needy on the ground, but also must market their efforts to donors at home. For example, on the ground, there may be a need to provide primary care medicine, but if a major donor has given surgical supplies, the NGO may focus some of its efforts on surgery. Only AT&T™-capable U.S. phones worked; Verizon™ and other vendors did not.
Communications and computers	U.S. Department of Defense (DOD) communications were limited by service and location—for example, there was no direct communication between the U.S. medical forces at the hospital, the medical regulator at the helicopter landing zone, or the U.S. Comfort hospital ship. Handwritten notes were the only means of communication between the hospital and the ship. No wide area network (WAN) or consistent Internet access existed. Cellular broadband was slow and overwhelmed.
Intelligence	No technology or processes existed to convey information from the situation in the city to the medical planners at the hospital. There was no organized medical control system to designate patients within the various healthcare entities. For example, one evening, representatives came from the Israeli Medical Hospital looking for orthopedic patients because they had excess capacity.
Patient care—Diagnostics	Initially, no diagnostic capability existed. Many patients had indigenous tuberculosis (TB) and human immunodeficiency virus (HIV) infections, yet responding doctors had to diagnose them by their appearance and how their lungs sounded. The first laboratory test available was HIV, followed shortly by complete blood count (CBC) and basic metabolic panel. Limited transfusion capability came later. Radiology capability required generator power. Only one antiquated, nondigital machine was available, which had plain film using chemicals, and it took providers 4 hours to get the patient to x-ray and back with the film. This created havoc, given that so many earthquake victims had multiple broken bones: it was an "orthopedic disaster." Monitoring capability was primarily by physical signs except in the operating room—blood pressure cuffs and pulse oximeters were useful, but in the chaos, both were later stolen.
Patient care—Logistics	Supplies came in poorly labeled boxes and required significant time and people resources to "sort." Oxygen was severely in short supply, and often, large H tanks came without necessary regulators.
Patient care—Preventive medicine and infectious disease control	HIV and tuberculosis are very prevalent in Haiti. Management of those patients should have employed necessary laboratory and personal protective equipment (e.g., N95 masks) for providers—none of which was available except for the basic blood HIV test. Their condition and treatment were based upon clinical findings.
Patient care—Therapeutics and triage	Record keeping and patient tracking were either nonexistent or consisted of "Sharpie" notes on bandages. Nurses developed their own system on plain paper. Initially, no provider-directed care occurred in the overnight shift due to limited resources and security concerns. IV drips, pain medications, antibiotics, and so on all needed innovative means of administration to ensure that patients received their needed medications. Collating patients to triage for evacuation required the "triage officer" to physically walk around the hospital grounds to see each tent to help determine who would go—eventual evacuation was dependent on U.S. DOD ambulances' availability and capability, and was also limited by the communication challenges already noted. Little patient movement occurred between NGO facilities because of limited situational awareness on their capabilities.

In summary, H1N1 in 2009/2010 did not develop the virulence to reproduce the catastrophe of 1918. However, it is possible and likely that we will, in the future, face a new virus with increased virulence, which will call for a restructuring of our National Response Framework (NRF) to respond effectively. This will necessitate a network-centric approach to optimize the response, using all the resources within the United States directed remotely to the affected areas. This will take appropriate technology, training, and encouraging a multidisciplinary, global-networked culture where everyone is part of the response.

66.2 Emergency Management Infrastructure: Network-Centric

Most medical response systems are based on specialized, proprietary networks, and organizations run by different public safety agencies in different geographic locales. Emergency responders will need to transition, over time, to a distributed network that would ideally be built and supported in concert with as many agencies as possible, worldwide. Individual response groups will communicate most effectively in disasters if they are willing to collaborate in using communications and technology that individual agencies do not exclusively own and control [7]. The network may be flexible to support local needs, but such flexibility needs to exist under a larger interoperable network.

We support the idea of a government-mandated and ultimately global network-centric infrastructure for disaster management—one that merges key concepts from (1) the current systems used in the U.S. military for network-centric warfare, which can be adapted to emergency response [22] and medicine [9] and (2) civilian networks including the Internet and social networking. During a disaster, there should be technology and systems for command and control (C2), communications, computers, intelligence, and medical treatment, which would employ this network to deliver timely information wherever it is needed, to enable rapid and quality decision making for medical responders, as well as the general public and accident victims. The network-based system would have centralized C2 such as the military systems, but would support independent decision making for responders when needed. It would have redundancy and could be distributed to provide backup for localized damage. The system should incorporate methods to avoid "information overload" by filtering out peripheral or extraneous information, and to check what sources of information are reliable [22].

The vision would be to link all agencies into a network of networks. Hatfield and colleagues refer to a *next generation network* (NGN) for public safety and define this as *broadband, Internet protocol (IP)-based and capable of handling voice, data, image, video, and multi-media content* [7]. Such a network must be reliable, secure, open, modular, extensible, redundant, and based on commercial or broadly supported standards [7]. The network must have backward compatibility with existing narrowband systems and must have governance standards [7]. It will likely take a national or international government mandate to deploy a network-centric disaster management system—just as it took a mandate to build the U.S. interstate highway network in the last century: a massive undertaking, but one that drastically and forever improved the U.S. transportation system for the better [9].

66.2.1 Infrastructure: Eventually Global and Network-Centric But Now, What?

In the absence of a standard network infrastructure or a master plan, we have only various devices and small networks that may not interoperate well. Using a simplistic analogy, this is like having 100 people meet in an airport, each speaking one unique language, with no one able to communicate at all, even though all are highly intelligent and will eventually get on the same plane headed for the same destination. Additionally, each one also answers to a parent supervisor or organization back home, thereby impeding a coordinated effort on scene. Given that we do not yet have a global, network-centric emergency response network, which may take some time to develop, any new technologies should, at the very least, be backward compatible, standardized, and as interoperable as possible.

66.3 Medical Informatics Technologies for Disaster Response

Medical informatics during a disaster can be as simple as reporting a patient's condition to physicians while en route to the hospital, or as complex as managing triage in a mass-casualty, multiple-incident terrorist attack. In both instances, emergency responders collect, categorize, and communicate casualty information to other disaster management workers. In the latter scenario, the scope of the events is more complex, and their nature is more sensitive, requiring careful management of patients and resources alike. Both instances use information technology (IT) to significantly improve the access to available information. Regardless of the cause, the disaster response and consequence management is essentially the same. From a technology standpoint, the information management (IM) and the informatics are identical.

Technology's prevalence in everyday life, from laptops to smart phones, makes it easier to incorporate into the medical arena and specifically into medical response to disasters. As the above case studies demonstrate, there is a critical need for both a standard network infrastructure and more simple, portable, and mobile technology that will support optimal disaster response—such as cell phones that are ubiquitous worldwide. The section below describes various technologies and needs for further development.

66.3.1 Command, Control, Communications, Computers, and Intelligence

Technologies that support optimal command, control, communications, computers, and intelligence (C4I) during a disaster allow responders and controllers to make faster and better decisions, which in turn allows for immediate response where and when it is needed.

66.3.1.1 Command and Control

C2 should be distributed (see Figure 66.1) with both a central command in a central location and multiple distributed local sites (in the United States, the central command would be in Washington DC and the local sites might be emergency operation centers, which are located in various government sites and even in corporations). There should also be virtual operation centers in all locations where people can

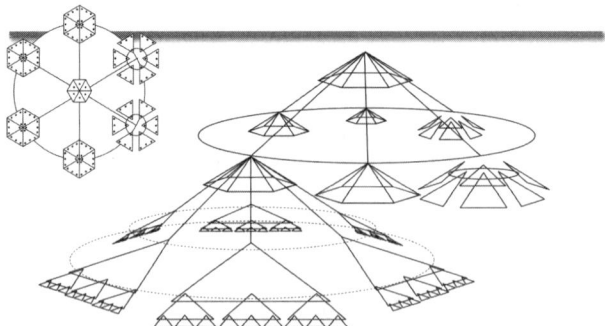

FIGURE 66.1 Model of distributed command and control (C2) disaster response using network-centric architecture. The diagram on the left shows central command connected to multiple distributed command centers—but the distributed command centers could take over control anywhere in the network. If the central command fails, or the local command at the site of a disaster began to fail, any part of the command structure in a network is designed to support other sites in the command structure. The diagrams on the right side show more of a three-dimensional view of how the network fits together. (Rosen, J.M., Grigg, E., Lanier, J. et al. Cybercare: The Future of Command and Control for Disaster Response. *IEEE Engineering in Medicine and Biology* 21(5): 56–68 © 2002 IEEE. Rosen, J.M., Grigg, E.B., McKnight, M.F. et al. Transforming Medicine for Biodefense and Healthcare Delivery. *IEEE Engineering in Medicine and Biology Magazine* 23(1):89–101. © 2004 IEEE.)

visualize any part of the disaster space, so that remote C2 outside the disaster zone can be brought into play to manage resources within the disaster. Having such distributed virtual C2 would avoid problems such as those that occurred in 9/11, in which the C2 center was within the zone of injury, and thus was crippled. Engineers could also expand the virtual command centers to be used as simulation tools for responders.

There must be interplay between the central C2 and responders in the field, such that local commanders can make independent decisions given mission or strategic orders from central command; senior leaders, with their increased connectivity and virtual presence, must avoid micromanagement of local commanders.

66.3.1.2 Communications and Computers

Communications are used during a disaster to reach out, ask for help, get advice, and let the next echelon know what is coming. "During a crisis event, bringing the right information, at the right time, to the right person, can significantly impact the quality of decision making for medical responders as well as the general public" [26].

In the United States, the ability to integrate multiple communication systems within a common framework during a disaster is currently available only through military C4I assets. No disaster exercise or real event has had "excellent communications and coordination" as one of its after-action comments. Communications during a disaster remain disjointed due to fragmented C2 with each response entity reporting through its channels, on its communication devices. In Haiti, despite having high-tech equipment, at one point, handwritten messages were physically carried from the hospital to its support ship as the only means of direct communication (James Geiling, personal observation).

Ultimately, it would be best to have *interagency and cross-jurisdictional* communications that are jointly developed by disparate responders [7] and worldwide governmental cooperation to the extent possible.

Historically, the most effective communication medium in disasters has been low-bandwidth voice communication over a phone or similar device, either hard wired (i.e., POTS—plain old telephone system) or wireless. Video links, at the risk of more bandwidth requirements, may enhance this capability through movement or body-language visualization, but often for strictly C2, POTS suffices. Video clearly enhances clinical capabilities, including the ability to interview patients, and partially examine them, remotely.

A simple technology that is greatly useful in emergency response is Apple™'s iPhone™/iPad™ technology; Google™, Microsoft™ and other companies also have similar technologies. Responders can use iPhones to facilitate all points of care—C2, diagnostics, determining the location of personnel and supplies, and evaluating and treating injuries. The iPad can have four screens up at once in which the user can simultaneously look at four different functions to store and download information. During events such as the earthquake in Haiti, there is the potential that broadcasts, social networks, wireless devices, and the convergence of emerging technologies (e.g., mobile phones, iPads, blackberries, Internet, etc.) might advise citizens that the water or food in their neighborhood is contaminated, and what alternative places they might go to, and so on.

Cell phones play a strong role in mHealth. The mHealth Alliance was chartered in 2009 to accelerate mHealth and to deliver quality healthcare via wireless networks in the developing world, in partnership with the UN Central Emergency Response Fund, IEEE, Palm, Telecoms Sans Frontieres, Vodaphone, and other partners [14].

The military and civilian domains often exchange and codevelop technology. In the past, new technology was often initially developed by the military and was later adapted for civilian use. Recently, the military has taken commercial, off-the-shelf ("COTS") technology, everything from cell phones to robots, and "ruggedized" it for military use. Among the most sought-after technology from factors cited by U.S. Army, USMC, and U.S. Air Force medic first responders participating

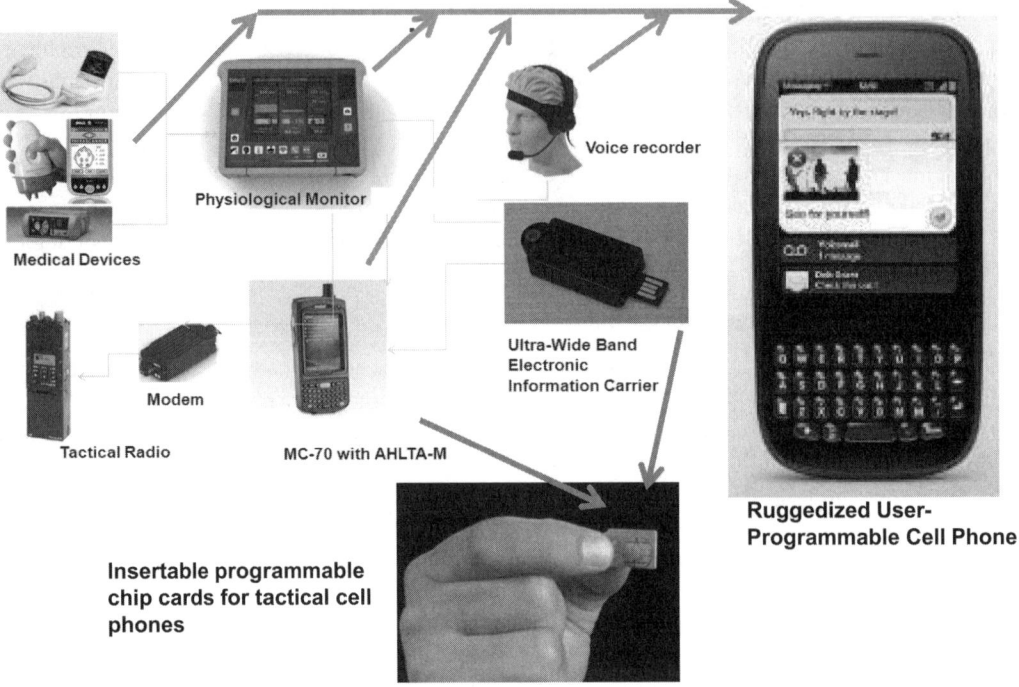

Medical Devices

Physiological Monitor

Voice recorder

Ultra-Wide Band Electronic Information Carrier

Tactical Radio

Modem

MC-70 with AHLTA-M

Insertable programmable chip cards for tactical cell phones

Ruggedized User-Programmable Cell Phone

FIGURE 66.2 Combat casualty care informatics and telemedicine—first responder medic. Notional schema for integrating multiple image and audio devices into a medical monitor that can communicate with a "ruggedized" cell phone to transmit medical data to a higher echelon or off-site medical facility. (Courtesy of Ronald K. Poropatich, MD. With permission.)

in the U.S. Joint Forces Command (USJFCOM), Joint Medical Distance Support and Evacuation (JMDSE), Joint Capabilities Technology Demonstration (JCTD) is a ruggedized, user-programmable cell phone that can address a wide range of technological and communications integration issues with civilian and military networks within the Joint Combat Casualty Care System (JCCCS) component of the JMDSE JCTD. Most of the technical telemedicine and medical information capture and transmission capabilities being integrated for the JCTD could be combined into such a ruggedized, cell-phone type of device. This would combine the best features of various devices, as conceptualized in Figure 66.2.

Commercial satellite phones are an important technology to help provide both communications and C2 in humanitarian assistance for disaster relief. One program is the International Maritime Satellite (Inmarsat)/Broadband Global Area Network (BGAN), which uses 11 satellites to provide worldwide coverage that, with new technology from Boeing, will soon extend to 50 megabits/s [8].

mHealth's role in humanitarian assistance and disaster relief situations extends to the fairly extensive *open-source software applications* that are being used in various public health situations currently; below is a list of some open sources for consideration:

- *Open data kit (ODK)*—Developed by University of Washington engineering students, this application provides a complete end-to-end suite of tools for data collection and device management, and leverages Google's free and robust web services (currently, only working on Android™ phones). The phones require a subscriber identity module (SIM) and portable memory card with an active data plan.

- *FrontlineSMS* is an open-source Java software that transforms any computer and a globalization management system (GMS) mobile device into a bulk short message service (SMS)* messaging center (hub to many mobile devices). Its uses are in alerting, surveys, voting-based competitions, and entry-level data collection on a large scale; the alerting and data collection features would have medical applications.
- *EpiSurveyor*—Developed by DataDyne™, this is a freely hosted web application with a mobile-phone-based component for data collection to empower global health and international development initiatives. The World Health Organization (WHO) uses this application in 13 African countries.
- *GATHERdata*—With funding from many sources, and code publicly released in 2009, applications range from rural health centers doing routine data collection to community health workers surveying at the field level.
- *eMOCHA*—Developed by Johns Hopkins University, this application was designed to assist health programs in developing countries to improve provider communication and education as well as patient care. It uses the ODK Collect application, and transforms smart phones into global positioning system (GPS)-linked clinical gathering tools, interactive training devices, and medical consultation systems.

66.3.1.3 Intelligence: Situational Awareness, Actionable Intelligence, and Patient Tracking

66.3.1.3.1 *Situational Awareness*

Situational awareness can be defined as a comprehensive understanding of the current operational environment, information sources, and impact of actions. One poignant example demonstrates how a failure of situational awareness during a disaster led to loss of life. In the South Tower of the World Trade Center on 9/11, people trapped on high floors above the jet impact were not told of a possible escape route that existed: for a limited time following the impact, one of three exit stairways was still open, which they could have used to go down past the impact area, all the way to ground level and safety. Despite one worker who was trapped on a high floor speaking by cell phone to his wife, who was simultaneously watching TV for information and also talking to a 9/11 dispatcher, no one delivered the right information at the right time to tell the man and his colleagues how to safely descend. He and others died—more from loss of information, in this case, than from the primary disaster [16].

To meet the challenges of exerting C2 and building situational awareness in a complex, chaotic, and dangerous environment, civilian emergency responders can build on existing military models, which employ the latest technology and a network-centric model [22]. Typically, military medical units deploy with a package of technological assets, including communications, logistics, and security support. They also normally have a robust intelligence network that gives them real-time information on the extent of a disaster, its geospatial dimensions, and its infrastructure and human impact. However, both the military and especially nonmilitary groups such as NGOs often go into harm's way with little situational awareness of events on the ground. Open-source data and information that might be useful exists, but attaining that information in a useful format can be challenging. One technology that has become operational is the integration of information from e-mails, tweets (from Twitter™), geo-tagged photos, and other similar information—the so-called "crisis mapping." Currently, some require active submission, such as the USHAHIDI-HAITI project from Tufts University, which has an online crisis map of Haiti that, according to its website, *represents the most comprehensive and up-to-date crisis map available to the humanitarian community. The information here is mapped in*

---

* SMS is the "text communication service component of phone, web or mobile communication systems, using standardized communications protocols that allow the exchange of short text messages between fixed line or mobile phone devices" (definition by http://en.wikipedia.org/wiki/SMS).

near real time and gathered from reports coming from inside Haiti via: SMS, Web, Email, Radio, Phone, Twitter, Facebook™, Television, List-serves, Live streams, Situation Reports [29]. Other crisis mapping tools will eventually combine open-source information automatically. This technology would be most applicable if it could be carried in the hands of first responders. If it was web based and if Internet access was available, this real-time situational awareness tool could be extremely useful to those on the scene.

While social networking could be used to communicate in a disaster, we need to avoid information overload—and sort out "what info is pertinent, what is peripheral, what is extraneous" as well as determining what sources of information are reliable [22].

For biological disasters, cell phones are being developed "with a tiny silicon chip that works a bit like a nose" [13] to detect airborne toxins—upon detection, the intelligent chip would notify emergency responders via their cell phones that an infectious pathogen was present. The success of the device would depend upon many users carrying such cell phones. In that case, in the event of an accidental gas leak or terrorist release of a biological weapon, the tiny sensors could map the location and size of the biohazard. *"Cell phones are everywhere people are,"* said Michael Sailor, professor of chemistry and biochemistry at the University of California, San Diego who heads the research effort. *"This technology could map a chemical accident as it unfolds"* [13].

66.3.1.3.2 Actionable Intelligence

In a disaster-recovery effort, actionable intelligence is a key concept—involving technologies that can track a population of people, use sensors to do diagnostics, and determine which people need treatments. On a large design scale, responders could benefit if engineers could design simpler versions of military technologies such as unmanned aerial vehicles (UAVs) for actionable intelligence. These vehicles provide the military with a lot of information: live video feed plus the ability to see in the dark using infrared cameras, which allows personnel to learn about a scene from a bird's-eye view. On a simpler scale, being able to have situational awareness and actionable intelligence delivered by a cell phone to responders would meet many needs.

66.3.1.3.3 Patient Tracking

There are new technologies now available to track populations that have sustained injuries from disasters, part of a suite of new technologies in IT/IM developed by agencies such as the U.S. Department of Defense (DoD), Health Affairs. In particular, medical situational awareness in theatre (MSAT) is an example of a technology that enables the DoD to keep a constant situational awareness of the health of a population of deployed personnel [15]. The MSAT is an actionable intelligence system to track casualties and the dead, and would operate under a network-centric C2 system to allow coordination of the multiple NGOs and other resources. The MSAT, or a civilian-designed version of it, could be used in general disaster response to identify, triage, and track the care and treatment of individuals. It could also be used to help predict the impact of loss of important individuals in the continued sustainment of critical infrastructures.

A commercial patient-tracking system, Raytheon™ Company's emergency patient-tracking system (EPTS), employs wristbands with bar-coded patient medical information and mobile technology that allows responders to automatically collect and communicate patient information—through the stages of triage, transportation, treatment, and discharge. Each patient's status is continually updated in a web-enabled, secure central database that ensures patient privacy, yet provides a regulatory/reporting audit trail. EPTS "has allowed real-time communication between first responders, emergency management, and hospital officials, allowing authorities to balance resources, minimize hospital overcrowding, and increase survival rates," according to the manufacturer [18].

FalconView™ is a mapping application, based on Microsoft Windows® that shows map types with various overlays, especially related to aviation, but which might potentially be adapted for disaster management, especially now that it has become available in an open-source version [5].

The iPhone/iPad applications (and similar systems by other vendors) are important tools because they incorporate a program on a smart phone system that many people are familiar with, and use an already existing technological infrastructure. If responders could have an easily portable phone-based tool to track patients from the field to treatment and beyond, that would be "awesome"; in the words of one responder: "I can only imagine how effective it could be if I could talk into an iPhone, have it record a patient chart, save/transcribe that information, including patient photos taken with the phone, and then be able to send the data and files to the patient's hospital or other providers" (Mike Lauria, personal observation). As mentioned above, this could work, but all responders would need to be "on the same page" with technology and networking.

There are a number of practical issues to keep in mind for the tracking technologies. The tracking devices themselves (transmitters) must be lightweight and easily carried by responders; very durable (resistant to dirt, sand, water, and impacts); easy to employ; and unconditionally reliable. Disaster responders currently just use the waterproof paper patient tags—a simple innovation would entail having the same information be transferred from these to an electronic barcode format on the tag, which needs to be operator- and responder-friendly.

66.3.1.3.4 Summary (Situational Awareness, Actionable Intelligence, and Patient Tracking)

To optimize triage and treatment in any conventional disaster, we must systematically collect, disseminate, and store information about the casualties. For emergency responders to successfully manage consequences, we must understand the nature and location of the incident, the current condition of the victims, and the likely cause. Providing such information in a complex event may require a brute-force scaling of current health information systems, together with significant increases in telecommunications bandwidth. Depending on the scenario, especially if communication nodes have been destroyed or overwhelmed, engineers and/or responders will need to establish a disaster network, or an expanded regional Wi-Fi capability, to help facilitate information flow. The existing care systems must be enhanced, rather than simply being augmented. Making this scenario work will require significant investments in public health, combined with leadership, strategy, and funding to increase technology to facilitate disaster recovery [9].

66.3.2 Medical Treatment and Evacuation

66.3.2.1 Point-of-Care Technologies

Point-of-care testing refers to diagnostic testing done at or near the site of patient care [10]. In a disaster, when patients cannot be moved or even hospitals may not be functioning, simple point-of-care test systems such as test strips can help detect drugs or pathogens. Eventually, these may not require specimens but may employ noninvasive detectors that are biometrically linked to the patient in a database. If smart cell phones could transmit the results of such tests to a central network or a database, it could facilitate patient diagnosis and care, and could potentially expedite public health epidemiology (tracking and follow-up), as in a pandemic.

66.3.2.2 Smart Treatment Technologies

66.3.2.2.1 Recovery of Wounded Using Unpeopled, High-Technology Approaches

Currently, wounded disaster victims sometimes require the rescuer to put himself or herself into harm's way to provide care or extract the victim. Technologies may soon exist to provide accident victims with personal monitoring equipment or other equipment that tells the central control about their location and physiological status. In a future scenario, an automated "rescue robot" would go to the injured or ill victim and bring him or her to a predetermined safe, casualty collection point. The robot could then place the victim into a treatment vehicle or "pod" where the patient could be imaged, and have a medical robot do their wound and hemorrhage control and apply their dressings. The patient could be connected to a Life Support for Trauma and Transport (LSTAT™) system by Integrated Medical Systems™, a portable "suitcase"-sized device that contains the capabilities of an intensive care room (ICU) condensed on a 6-inch platform that underlies a standard rescue stretcher, that can travel with a sick patient in transport [12,28]. Finally, an unmanned helicopter could evacuate the victim, if needed, for transport to a care facility. No humans would have to be endangered or even present, except remotely, during the rescue.

The above model sounds futuristic, but may be implemented by the U.S. military within 15 years, and could be available to civilians soon thereafter. Some technologies such as this are being developed by the Defense Advanced Research Projects Agency (DARPA) [3] and the Telemedicine and Advanced Technology Research Center (TATRC) [23]. The existing models can follow that of the U.S. Air Force's Critical Care Air Transport Teams (CCATTs)—a system designed not simply to transport critically ill soldiers from war zones, but to continue the critical care treatment process from the point of injury or illness to the highest capability facility [2].

66.3.2.2.2 Technology for Trauma Victims

The TATRC [23] is an office of the headquarters of the U.S. Army Medical Research and Materiel Command (USAMRMC) that supplements DoD medical research programs with a focus on health informatics, telemedicine/mHealth, medical training systems, and computational biology.

The Combat Application Tourniquet "Emergency Medical Tourniquet" bandage [1] is one simple example of a product that has been adapted from military use for civilian emergency responders. It is lightweight and easy to deploy and store, and adheres during patient transport.

66.3.2.3 Diagnostic Capabilities

66.3.2.3.1 Laboratory and Radiology Services

In a disaster during which hospitals may lack power or may have older (analog) radiology equipment, or alternately, in disasters that happen in remote regions, there is a critical need to have portable imaging systems. X-ray is critical in disasters such as the earthquake in Haiti where patients have multiple fractured bones from earthquake trauma. Ultrasound images can be transported from remote regions via telemedicine [17]. Ideally, clinicians would conduct imaging on portable radiology machines, and, as with laboratory results, cell phones could securely transport results back to a central database.

66.3.2.3.2 Virus Detection and Vaccinations

A key diagnostic technology that could be employed in a pandemic is a hand-held device that can rapidly detect that someone is infected with the novel virus or other agent in real time. Another technology could be used to identify the strain of the virus to confirm that it is a new or more lethal genomic strain. Finally, the infected individual would have to be treated with appropriate countermeasures (not only antivirals but also quarantine if appropriate, hand washing, elbow rubs, etc.). Antivirals might also be used to mitigate the effect of the virus and vaccines could also be a potential option. However, vaccines need to be ready in time to be given to the population to prevent transmission of the virus. There are new methodologies to prepare an influenza vaccine faster, by growing the vaccine in tobacco or on cell culture, rather than in eggs. There are also technologies being developed to more rapidly test the efficacy of the vaccines. To be optimally efficient, we would simultaneously develop improved methods to detect, identify, and treat a virus immediately, as opposed to waiting for the development of a vaccine.

66.3.2.4 Telehealth, Remote Medicine, and the Hospital without Walls

Using telemedicine and telehealth, clinicians can diagnose the ill during a disaster even if they are located far away. Telemedicine helps make disaster response "all-hazards" to encompass pandemics and biological events, including hybrid events, such as a hurricane or cyclone that creates an environment for cholera or airborne-transmissible diseases. Disaster recovery teams could use the same telemedicine systems now used in remote areas of the world, or on ships and airplanes, to remotely consult with medical experts [9,17]. Providing care to pandemic victims who are quarantined is possible through the implementation of telemedicine, teleconsultation, telemonitoring, and telerobotics over a network-based healthcare system [9]. Telemonitoring currently allows clinicians to remotely monitor patients who have known medical conditions, who wear (or have implanted) sensors, and who may have other equipment at home to conduct laboratory tests and transmit results to clinicians [9]. This technology could be expanded for disaster relief efforts to help coordinate the various responders, including families who provide direct care to victims, first responders, healthcare providers, both prehospital and in-hospital, and experts who provide care from a distance.

A pilot project in Vietnam is testing a Short Message Service (SMS) surveillance system that leverages existing mobile phone technology to aggregate disease data for analysis, distribution, and real time response. Vietnamese healthcare workers at community health clinic stations were trained to directly report disease information (on diarrhea and influenza for the purposes of the pilot) to a central data repository using their mobile phones and an intuitive, user-friendly platform (Joseph Rosen and Lindsay Katona, personal observations, Hanoi, Vietnam trips, 2010–2013).

Technologies for mobile health are crucially relevant in emergency response, especially in achieving the goal of making prehospital care and hospital care as seamless as possible. The term "hospital without walls" is a useful term. Perhaps the most important aspect of this is to develop a system in which we treat everyone as soon as we can, by whomever is adequately or best trained, or closest to the biomedical casualty. Telemedicine will complement hospital care in disasters as it does in daily medical care. Hospitals represent a collaboration and convergence of medical informatics technologies into a central, physical "brick and mortar" location. Hospital care is important for critically ill patients because of the intensity of support they require, whereas remote care for less acutely ill patients is more functional. The technologies to support both settings fall into those domains already discussed, namely, C4I, diagnostics, medical treatment, evacuation, and epidemiological evaluation and analysis.

66.3.3 Population Health and Patient Data Collection

In large-scale, long-duration events, diagnostic information will need to be supplemented with geo-spatial information regarding the location of victims and multiple incident sites, together with the positions of both materiel and medical personnel. Ideally, a dynamic, integrated health information system would combine GPS and geographical information system (GIS) technologies to provide first responders and incident commanders alike with a seamless data source. MSAT is an example of this. Likewise, logistical and environmental data would prove invaluable in tracking not only casualties but also the potential spread of a biological, chemical, or radiological plume beyond the initial incident zone.

The Haiti IT (HIT) Rescue project is "a collaboration of multiple agencies, volunteers and corporations that are conducting a trial of multiple electronic patient tracking and medical record systems" at the Fond Parisien Treatment center in Haiti. This is a modified iPhone-based application that has registered over 600 patients, reunited 15 children with their families using a tracking feature, and identified and tracked 20 amputee victims [6]. This project was piloted at the request of the UN Technology Cluster, by a team from the Operational Medicine Institute (OMI). The OMI-driven Comprehensive Amputee Identification and Rehabilitation (CAIR) Consortium is also using this system to coordinate care and track data for amputees.

In summary, patient data should be tracked and studied to determine the disaster's dimensions, movement or progression, and pace of evolution, in the case of a pandemic. The goal is to better understand the changes, in real time, to effect treatment changes and social distancing requirements.

66.3.4 Training and Simulation

Technologies play a central role in training and simulation. Both Fortune 500 companies and the U.S. DoD use computer-based training. Trainees can develop advanced skills through interactive videoconferencing and simulations, which reduce the time necessary for hands-on training, yet improve trainees' knowledge for subsequent field drills. By using standardized, computer-based curricula for training disaster responders, small training cadres from the federal government could supplement local and regional programs whenever necessary.

66.3.4.1 Training

In Chapter 65, we explored team culture and training opportunities to enhance disaster response efforts. Emergency personnel, to provide an effective response, must maintain proficiency. It is important to provide ongoing training and to offer responders performance machines [19] to augment their skills and cognitive performance (on the way to the event or during the event). In the past, training had to be done in a central facility, but now, high-level training can be done in a distributed remote manner. This should help overcome a high variability in training regimes. Any first-responder training program must provide a core set of skills that could be used by all diverse care providers (doctors, nurses, firefighters, EMTs, military, police, and others) who might respond to a disaster. Additionally, the training must be of sufficient scope and breadth or available "just in time" for these providers to expand their care into domains where they do not normally operate, such as working in hospitals or providing home-based care. Each profession brings its own knowledge to an incident site and agreed frameworks for cooperation will facilitate communication as well as C2.

66.3.4.2 Simulation

Just as war games are invaluable in military planning and training ("train as you fight, fight as you train") [29], simulated crisis scenarios will likely prove instrumental in teaching first responders, as well as managers and senior leaders, to cope with a broad spectrum of disaster situations. The simulations should not be designed to make the first responders and leadership comfortable, but rather they should be designed to maximize improvement in their readiness for both disasters and megadisasters to essentially face the stress, shock, and uncertainty that comes with any disaster. In addition to providing cost-effective technologies for regular drills, virtual reality (VR)* and augmented reality (AR)† trainers, now widely used in the U.S. military,‡ would enable personnel from various professional and jurisdictional backgrounds to simulate different operational roles. Frontline firefighters or police officers might play incident commanders, and state and federal decision makers could simulate first-responder duties; all this would help individuals to cross-train and understand other team members' functions.

Finally, these same technologies may also improve the use of medical informatics in crisis situations. The very hardware and software used for simulation or instruction purposes could carry real-time information regarding the condition, location, and status of victims in a multiple-casualty event. Combined with GPS and GIS technology, VR programs might link physicians in remote hospitals with first responders at the incident site—a particularly valuable interface in biological weapon attacks, or other scenarios that involve chemical, biological, radiological, nuclear, and high-yield explosives (CBRNE) and that require swift treatment and effective containment [20]. But providers must possess sufficient and appropriate training to operate in a communication-deprived setting, and understand the basic tasks necessary for the given disaster situation.

---

* Virtual reality refers to computer-simulated environments that depict real-life or imagined situations, using visual information displayed to the user on a screen or stereoscopic (hand or head mounted) displays, and which may include sound, or touch/force feedback information.

† Augmented reality "is a term for a live direct or indirect view of a physical real-world environment whose elements are augmented by virtual computer-generated imagery" (http://en.wikipedia.org/wiki/Augmented_reality); for example, a cell phone view of a mountain in front of a hiker, with GPS information overlaid on top of it to guide the viewer.

‡ For example, at Fort Drum and the Uniformed Services University of the Health Sciences (USUHS)—Joseph Rosen, personal communication.

66.3.5 Interoperability

To effectively design, integrate, and employ medical technology for disaster response will require biomedical engineers to resolve both hardware and software issues to establish interoperability and coordination across a broad spectrum of probable disaster situations. Wetware (humans), hardware (machines), and software (programs) are all important elements to integrate. In the past, they were not successfully integrated, due to barriers that included poor graphical user interfaces and systems that were not intuitive to the user. Newer platforms have made significant progress in overcoming such barriers (e.g., iPhone). To establish a network-centric disaster response domain, emergency personnel must first know how to use the systems in question and must be able to develop doctrines that codify best practices. Training and simulation will play a critical role in bringing new systems online. But the best is the notion of a merger or convergence, in which training and performance will become one thing: you are trained as you perform.

66.4 Conclusions

Disasters occur globally without respect for any group or nation. Engineers, in collaboration with emergency response personnel worldwide, continue to make progress in developing technologies and products to help response efforts. But with each new event, we identify recurring opportunities to improve those capabilities. Clearly, the organization of most emergency response systems remains regimented and linear, rather than distributive and network-centric. A computerized, network-centric, government or centrally controlled emergency management system is the ideal model, but to implement this may require a paradigm shift that could take years—years that policy makers and the public may not have. In the meantime, if we can design and deploy standardized, easy-to-use, mobile technology and information management, we will improve the efficiency and outcome of the response to any kind of disaster, anywhere in the world.

The ultimate goal for civilian disaster response is that small teams can perform complex tasks without a centralized command guiding their every move—as seen in the system of MSAT in a disaster or pandemic, combined with public health systems for pandemic or biological surveillance. For medical treatment, we need to employ the model of a hospital without walls—in which we treat everyone as soon as possible, by whomever is adequately or best trained, or closest to the biomedical casualty. New training and simulation systems (as described in Chapter 65, and in Reference 21) will help responders to effectively use new tools, ranging from the simplest hand-held devices through remote robotics and telemedicine. The technologies converge with a network-centric infrastructure to provide the real-time epidemiology of the storm/earthquake/hurricane/pandemic.

Any technologies for medical response need to be lightweight, easy to carry, and universally understood. Phone-based applications (iPhone or others) are a great platform, especially if we solve the challenge of how to develop a larger network that can integrate these systems in the field with other care providers and facilities. Tracking technologies for patients are universally used and recognized, and if they could run on phones connected to a central, secure database, it would greatly help responders. For communications, civilian responders might look to the U.S. military, all of whose services employ very similar communication systems; can our civilian communication modalities also be made uniform? This applies to radios, scanners, computers, and other communication devices. Finally, we will need training and technologies for educating lay people (as well as responders) and changing the team culture: in large disasters, everyone needs to be a responder. A question remaining to be seen over time is whether the emergency response community can adapt quickly to new technologies, and what can we do to facilitate their adoption over older, proven techniques [12].

Each unique disaster has its own epidemiology of casualties. However, a coordinated response effort can overcome the chaos of the moment and mitigate the effect of the tragedy. This response capability requires preparation, training, and coordination to reduce deaths, sickness, terror, and economic damage. A more rapid and coordinated response action, enhanced by medical informatics and technological innovations, lessens the harm and leads to recovery more rapidly.

Acknowledgments

The authors wish to thank Lindsay Katona and Matthew McKnight for concept development and assistance in editing this manuscript.

References

1. Combat Application Tourniquet by Composite Resources. Available at: http://combattourniquet. com. Accessed 4/24/13.
2. Critical Care Air Transport Teams (CCATT) at San Antonio Military Medical Center. Available at: http://www.whasc.af.mil/departments(clinics)/cirticalcareairtransportteam.asp. Accessed 4/24/13.
3. Defense Advanced Research Projects Agency (DARPA) website. Available at: http://www.darpa. mil/. Accessed 9/19/10.
4. Drummond, K. 2010. Once scarce, H1N1 vaccines now getting dumped. AOL News, Health, April 1, 2010. Available at: http://www.aolnews.com/2010/04/01/once-hard-to-get-h1n1-vaccines-now-getting-dumped/. Accessed 4/24/13.
5. FalconView Mapping Application. Available at: http://www.falconview.org/trac/FalconView. Accessed 4/24/13.
6. Haiti IT Rescue Project. Operational Medicine Institute. Available at: http://www.opmedinstitute. org/. Accessed 4/24/13.
7. Hatfield, D. N. and Weiser, P. J. 2007. Toward a next generation network for public safety communications. Silicon Flatirons Telecommunications Program, University of Colorado School of Law, May 17, 2007.
8. Inmarsat, the mobile satellite company, broadband network. Available at: http://www.inmarsat. com/index.htm. Accessed 4/24/13.
9. Koop, C.E., Mosher, R., Kun, L. et al. 2008. Future delivery of health care: Cybercare. *IEEE Eng Med Biol* 27: 29–38.
10. Kost, G.J. 2002. Goals, guidelines and principles for point-of-care testing. In: *Principles & Practice of Point-of-Care Testing*. Kost G.J, Ed. Hagerstown, MD: Lippincott Williams & Wilkins. pp. 3–12. ISBN 0-7817-3156-9.
11. Life Support for Trauma and Transport (LSTAT) by Integrated Medical Systems. Available at: http:// www.lstat.com/. Accessed 4/25/13.
12. McGrath, D. and McGrath, S.P. 2005. Simulation and network-centric emergency response. *Paper presented at the Interservice/Industry Training, Simulation, and Education Conference (I/ITSEC)*, 2005, Orlando, FL.
13. Science Daily. Tiny Sensors Tucked into Cell Phones Could Map Airborne Toxins in Real Time. May 14, 2010. Article about Michael Sailor research team at University of California, San Diego. Available at: http://www.sciencedaily.com/releases/2010/05/100513093739.htm. Accessed 4/25/13.
14. mHealth Alliance. Available at: http://www.unfoundation.org/what-we-do/partners/organizations/ mhealth-alliance.html. Accessed 4/25/13.
15. Military Health System, US Department of Defense, Defense Health Information Management System: Medical Situational Awareness in Theater (MSAT). Available at: http://dhims.health.mil/ products/theater/msat.aspx. Accessed 4/25/13.
16. Pauls, J., Groner, N., Gwynne, S. et al. 2009. Informed emergency responses through improved situation awareness. National Research Council of Canada. July 13, 2009 [NRCC-51388] Available at: http://nparc.cisti-icist.nrc-cnrc.gc.canpsi/ by searching on author and title. Accessed 4/25/13. A

version of this document is also published in the *Proceedings of the 4th International Symposium on Human Behaviour in Fire* (Robinson College, Cambridge, UK, July 13, 2009), pp. 531–42.

17. Popov, V., Popov, D., Kacar, I., and Harris, R.D. 2007. The feasibility of real-time transmission of sonographic images from a remote location over low-bandwidth Internet links: A pilot study. *AJR Am J Roentgenol* 188(3):W219–22.

18. Raytheon Emergency Patient Tracking System. Available at: http://www.raytheon.com/capabilities/products/epts/. Accessed 4/25/13.

19. Rosen, J.M., Laub, Jr. D.R., Pieper, S.D., Mecinski, A.M., Soltanian, H., McKenna, M.A., Chen, D., Delp, S.L., Loan, J.P., Basdogan, C. Virtual reality and medicine: from training systems to performance machines. *Proceedings of the IEEE 1996 Virtual Reality Annual International Symposium*, March 30–April 3, 1996, Santa Clara, CA.

20. Rosen, J.M., Grigg, E.B., McKnight, M.F. et al. 2004. Transforming medicine for biodefense and healthcare delivery. *IEEE Eng Med Biol* 23(1): 89–101.

21. Rosen, J.M., Long, S.A., McGrath, D.M., and Greer, S.E. 2009. Simulation in plastic surgery training and education: The path forward. *Plast Reconstr Surg* 123(2): 729–38; discussion 739–40. Review.

22. Stanovich, M. 2005. "Network-centric" emergency response: The challenges of training for a new command and control paradigm. Publication of the Emergency Readiness and Response Research Center, Institute for Security Technology Studies, Dartmouth College, Hanover, NH.

23. Telemedicine and Advanced Technology Research Center (TATRC) website. Available at: http://www.tatrc.org/. Accessed 4/25/13.

24. United Press International (UPI). 2009. Health News, November 6, 2009. Double H1N1 vaccine, but still not enough. Available at: http://www.upi.com/Health_News/2009/11/06/Double-H1N1-vaccine-but-still-not-enough/UPI-96621257547831/. Accessed 4/25/13.

25. United States Census Bureau. 2012. US Population Estimates, National Totals: Vintage 2012. Available at: http://www.census.gov/popest/data/national/totals/2012/index.html. Accessed 4/25/13.

26. University of California at Irvine (UCI), Center for Emergency Response Technologies (CERT). Available at http://cert.ics.uci.edu/. Accessed 4/25/13.

27. USHAHIDI crisis mapping project. Available at : http://findingwhatworks.org/2012/05/08/ushahidi-collaborative-crisis-mapping/. Accessed 4/25/13.

28. Velmahos, G.C., Demetriades, D., Ghilardi, M., Rhee, P., Petrone, P., and Chan, L.S. 2004. Life support for trauma and transport (LSTAT): A mobile ICU for safe in-hospital transport of critically injured patients. *J Am Coll Surg* 199: 62–8.

29. Wodka-Gallien, P. 2001. Train as you fight, fight as you train. *J Electron Def* 24(6): 63. Available at: http://connection.ebscohost.com/c/articles/4824472/train-as-you-fight-fight-as-you-train. Accessed 4/25/13.

Index

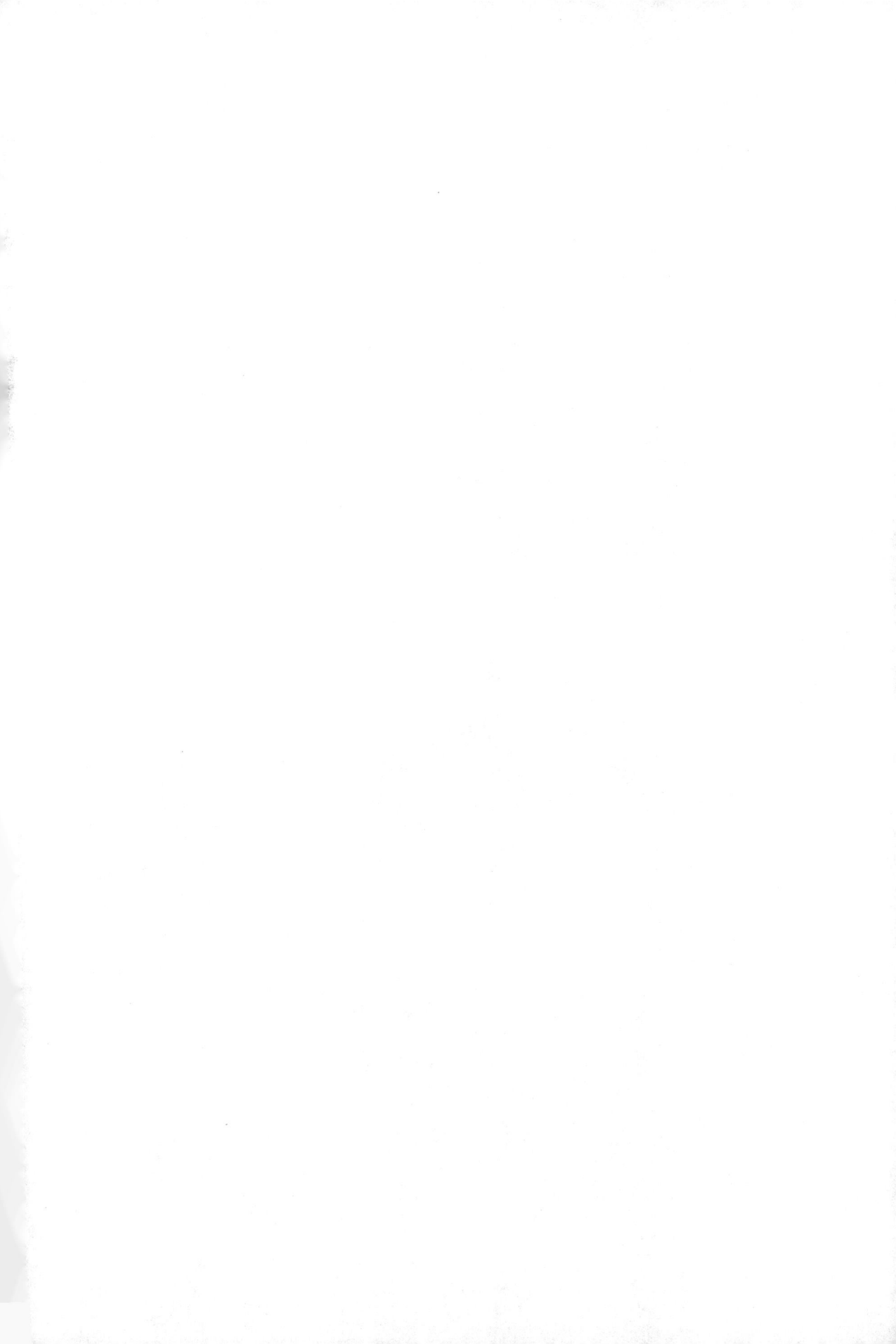